FDA Pregnancy Safety Categories

Category A: Adequate studies indicate no risk to the fetus in the first trimester of pregnancy, and there is no evidence of risk in later trimesters.

Category B: Animal reproduction studies have not demonstrated a risk to the fetus, but there are no well-controlled studies in pregnant women.

Category C: Animal reproduction studies have reported an adverse effect on the fetus, but there are no adequate studies in humans; the benefits of the drug in pregnant women may be acceptable despite its potential risks.

or

There are no animal reproduction studies and no adequate studies in humans.

Category D: There is evidence of human fetal risk, but the potential benefits from the use of the drug in pregnant women may be acceptable despite its potential risks—if safer drugs are not available or are ineffective.

Category X: Studies in animals or humans demonstrate fetal abnormalities, or adverse reaction reports indicate evidence of fetal risk. The risk of use in a pregnant woman clearly outweighs any possible benefit. These drugs should not be used in pregnant women.

Mosby's
Pharmacology in Nursing

Revised and Updated
21st Edition

Leda M. McKenry, PhD, CRN, FNP, FAAN
Associate Professor and Director of Academic Outreach,
School of Nursing,
University of Massachusetts,
Amherst, Massachusetts

Evelyn Salerno, RPh, BS, PharmD, FASCP
Courtesy Professor,
School of Nursing,
Florida International University;
Clinical Assistant Professor,
Nova-Southeastern College of Pharmacy,
Miami, Florida

with 212 illustrations

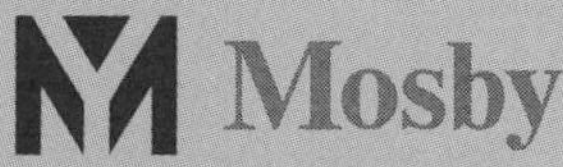

An Affilate of Elsevier Science
St. Louis London Philadelphia Sydney Toronto

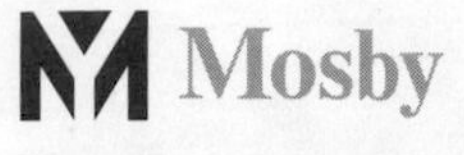

An Affiliate of Elsevier Science

11830 Westline Industrial Drive
St. Louis, Missouri 63146

MOSBY'S PHARMACOLOGY IN NURSING ISBN 0-323-01822-X

NOTICE

Pharmacology is an ever-changing field. Standard safety precautions must be followed, but as new research and clinical experience broaden our knowledge, changes in treatment and drug therapy may become necessary or appropriate. Readers are advised to check the most current product information provided by the manufacturer of each drug to be administered to verify the recommended dose, the method and duration of administration, and contraindications. It is the responsibility of the licensed prescriber, relying on experience and knowledge of the patient, to determine dosages and the best treatment for each individual patient. Neither the publisher nor the author assumes any liability for any injury and/or damage to persons or property arising from this publication.

The Publisher

REVISED AND UPDATED TWENTY-FIRST EDITION

Previous editions copyrighted 2001, 1998, 1995, 1992, 1989, 1986, 1982, 1979, 1976, 1973, 1969, 1966, 1963, 1960, 1955, 1951, 1948, 1945, 1942, 1940, 1936

Vice President, Publishing Director: Sally Schrefer
Executive Editor: Robin Carter
Managing Editor: Lee Henderson
Senior Developmental Editor: Kristin Geen
Publishing Services Manager: Deborah L. Vogel
Senior Project Manager: Jodi M. Willard
Design Manager: Bill Drone

CL/QKT

Printed in the United States of America

Last digit is the print number: 9 8 7 6 5 4 3 2 1

Reviewers

Laura H. Clayton, MSN, RN, FNP
Assistant Professor of Nursing Education,
Shepherd College,
Shepherdstown, West Virginia

Cathy E. Flaser, MSN, RN, CS, FNP
Assistant Professor of Nursing,
Jewish Hospital College of Nursing and Allied Health,
Washington University Medical Center,
St. Louis, Missouri

Elizabeth Green, BScN, MEd, RN
Professor of Nursing,
St. Clair College Thames,
Chatham, Ontario

Natasha Leskovsek, MBA, JD, RN
Nurse Attorney,
Fox, Bennett, & Turner,
Washington, D.C.

Karen S. March, MSN, RN, CS, CCRN
Assistant Professor of Nursing,
University of Pittsburgh at Bradford,
Bradford, Pennsylvania

Tippie Pollard, MSN, EdD, RN
Professor of Nursing and Chair of Undergraduate Studies in Nursing,
Carson-Newman College,
Jefferson City, Tennessee

Susan Klasson Zareksi, MN, RNC, CNS
Professor of Nursing,
El Camino College,
Torrance, California

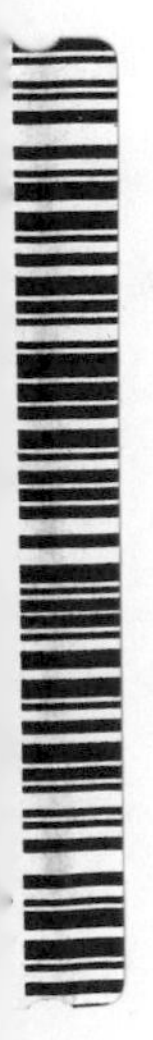

PREFACE

Mosby's Pharmacology in Nursing—now in its twenty-first edition for the twenty-first century—is a classic text with a long and distinguished tradition of providing nurses with a sound basis for the clinical application of pharmacology. It remains one of the most comprehensive and current pharmacology texts available for nurses. Through twenty-one editions, it has enjoyed tremendous success as a textbook for students who, when confronted with the rigorous content of their pharmacology course work, find our organization and presentation both accessible and conducive to learning.

The focus of *Mosby's Pharmacology in Nursing* is on a sound understanding of the pharmacologic properties of major drug classes and individual drugs, with special emphasis on clinical application of drug therapy through the nursing process.

Nursing students undertaking the study of pharmacology today face a growing challenge: how to master a body of knowledge that is growing at the speed of the digital age while also studying in an increasingly compressed time frame. *Mosby's Pharmacology in Nursing* equips students to meet that challenge by covering each major drug and drug class in concise, easy-to-locate passages of text, which we call **drug monographs.** It also provides **specific applications of the nursing process** to each major drug and drug class. As an additional tool to help students grasp the action of drug classes, *Mosby's Pharmacology in Nursing* identifies **key drugs** throughout; these are noted with a special key icon ( ) and the use of color. Mastering the content of the key drugs helps students better grasp the pharmacologic properties of all drugs in the same class.

Mosby's Pharmacology in Nursing has additional appeal as **a pharmacology reference** because of its thorough coverage of the very latest drug classes and individual drugs and its emphasis on clinical nursing management. This makes the book useful both as a primary textbook and as a clinical reference for nursing practice.

The revised and updated twenty-first edition provides thorough coverage of more than 1100 drugs, including **approximately 130 new drugs** approved by the FDA since the last edition. Content has been carefully updated throughout, with **increased emphasis on pharmacology in the community.**

ORGANIZATION

Macrostructure

The book is divided into two major parts. Part One: Basic Concepts includes four units: Unit 1, Principles of Pharmacology; Unit 2, The Nursing Process and Pharmacology; Unit 3, Biopsychosocial Aspects of Pharmacology; and Unit 4, Current Issues in Pharmacology. Unit 4 includes chapters that cover over-the-counter medications (Chapter 11) and **complementary and alternative pharmacology** (Chapter 12). The subject of complementary and alternative pharmacology has grown tremendously in importance since the publication of the previous edition. To complement this important chapter, we have included **17 Complementary and Alternative Therapies boxes** throughout the book; these boxes highlight the most common herbal therapies in use today.

Part Two: Clinical Concepts consists of broad pharmacologic units and makes up the largest portion of this text. In general, the 16 units in Part Two begin with a chapter that reviews the body system and then proceed with chapters on the major drug categories used for that system.

Chapter Organization

Each chapter of *Mosby's Pharmacology in Nursing* begins with a **Chapter Focus,** followed by **Learning Objectives** and lists of **Key Terms** (boldfaced in the text) and **Key Drugs** to help students focus on important material in the chapter. Summary tables and boxes are included throughout to supplement, reinforce, and help the student make comparisons among similar drugs.

The drug chapters that make up the bulk of *Mosby's Pharmacology in Nursing* begin with a discussion of a drug group. Individual drugs are then discussed by generic name, followed by a **pronunciation guide** and **U.S. and Canadian trade names.** (Canadian trade names are highlighted with a maple leaf icon, .) If the generic name is a key drug, it is highlighted with the use of color and a key icon and receives special, in-depth coverage. The drug monograph continues in a step-by-step, clinically oriented format that includes mechanism of action, indications, pharmacokinetics, side effects/adverse reactions, significant drug interactions (when appropriate), and dosage and administration; it concludes with a Nursing Management section.

The Nursing Management section uses the following nursing process format:

- Assessment
- Nursing diagnosis
- Implementation (with subheads for monitoring, intervention, and education, when appropriate)
- Evaluation

When the nurse must be aware of significant potential drug interactions, the assessment portion of the nursing management section includes a two-column **drug interactions overview** that consists of Drug/Possible Effect and Management columns. The use of bold type and color in this material highlights the most serious interactions.

The text of each chapter concludes with a **summary** that provides students with a succinct review of the chapter. Following the summary, **Critical Thinking Questions** present "real-life" scenarios to help the student apply the chapter material. (Answer guidelines for these questions are now available on the book's MERLIN website, as well as in the *Instructor's Electronic Resource* CD-ROM, which is available free to programs adopting classroom quantities of the book.) **Collaborative Learning Activities**—new to the twentieth edition and expanded in the twenty-first edition—are now posted on the MERLIN website. These activities encourage students to work in groups to apply their knowledge to specific situations. A **bibliography** wraps up each chapter.

ALSO NEW TO THIS EDITION

New to the twenty-first edition is an expanded focus on **women's health issues** in Chapter 52, which is now entitled "Drugs Affecting Women's Health and the Female Reproductive System."

The twenty-first edition also features a unique series of 12 resource boxes called **TechnologyLink**, which are updated for the revised and updated twenty-first edition. These boxes provide lists of video, audio, and Web resources that can serve as a springboard to student research in the constantly shifting science of pharmacology. (As you use these TechnologyLink boxes, you'll want to keep in mind that change is in the nature of Web addresses; if you find that a specific website has moved, type in the *general* web address of the parent organization to search for the specific document.)

This edition also includes twice as many pediatrics boxes as in the previous edition, and these boxes are now called **Special Considerations for Children.** Likewise, the geriatrics and culture boxes have been retitled **Special Considerations for Older Adults** and **Cultural Considerations,** respectively, and the home health boxes have been retitled **Community and Home Health Considerations.**

Because **evidence-based practice** is as important in pharmacology as in any other aspect of nursing—and perhaps more important—the **Nursing Research boxes** in *Mosby's Pharmacology in Nursing* have been carefully reviewed (and in some cases replaced) to ensure that they reflect the latest research. These boxes have also been redesigned for improved reader access and, as with all special boxes in the twenty-first edition, are distinguished by **eye-catching icons** that help to differentiate each type of box.

Also new to this edition is an **improved graphic design** that better distinguishes where one Nursing Management section ends and the next drug monograph begins.

At the end of the book, the student will find an updated appendix (Appendix F) that lists the **100 most commonly prescribed brand-name drugs.** Together with the Key Drugs lists, this appendix will help time-pressed students focus more efficiently on the most important and most commonly used drugs.

Additional time-saving tools are the book's **thoroughly reengineered indexes**—a Comprehensive Index and a Disorders Index. The Comprehensive Index includes entries for every single generic and trade name in the book, with page numbers for drug monographs highlighted in bold type. The Disorders Index is a convenient tool for programs in which pharmacology is integrated throughout the curriculum.

ADDITIONAL FEATURES

Grasping the underlying principles of pharmacology and mastering the body of knowledge encompassing contemporary drug therapy is a significant challenge. To help students meet this challenge, *Mosby's Pharmacology in Nursing* includes a number of additional features:

- **Pregnancy Safety boxes**
- **Case Studies**
- **Nursing Care Plans**
- **Management of Drug Overdose boxes**

ALSO NEW TO THE REVISED REPRINT

This revised and updated twenty-first edition now functions as an interactive textbook, with distinctive in-text icons that send students online for a variety of resources and activities, including:

- More than 40 **web-based Case Studies**
- 10 interactive, **web-based Concept Maps**
- Links to *Mosby's Drug Consult* for detailed information on more than 30 new drugs

Herbal Interactions are now included throughout and are highlighted with a special icon. Nursing diagnoses are updated throughout to reflect the **2001-2002 NANDA list** of approved nursing diagnoses. The **top 100 drugs by prescription** are now highlighted in the text with a special icon to help focus study time on the drugs seen most often in clinical practice. A new appendix entitled **Drug Therapy in End-of-Life Care** (Appendix I) has been added.

ANCILLARIES

Mosby's Pharmacology in Nursing, twenty-first edition, is not just a textbook but the core of a state-of-the art learning system.

For students, we have created a printed **Student Learning Guide.** This guide now includes additional multiple-choice questions and a variety of student-friendly activities.

For both students and instructors, we offer three electronic resources: a MERLIN website, *Mosby's Drug Consult,* and the Mosby/Saunders ePharmacology Update. The **MERLIN website** (mosby.com/MERLIN/McKenry/) includes a continually updated library of WebLinks, Content Updates, interactive Case Studies and Concept Maps, and more. ***Mosby's Drug Consult***—an authoritative Internet drug reference—is available free for 6 months to everyone who purchases the twenty-first edition. The **ePharmacology Update,** written by Evelyn Salerno, PharmD, is an e-mail newsletter delivered twice each semester to keep students and instructors up-to-date on the latest new drugs, warnings and precautions, questions and answers, and much more.

For instructors, we provide an *Instructor's Electronic Resource* CD-ROM, along with two additional electronic ancillaries: the *Electronic Image Collection for Pharmacology,* and the web-based *Nursing Pharmacology PowerPoint Presentations.*

The **Instructor's Electronic Resource** is a three-part, CD-ROM–based ancillary consisting of a *LectureView* PowerPoint presentation, an electronic *Instructor's Manual* (word processing files for Windows and Macintosh), and a *Test Bank* (word processing files for Windows and Macintosh). The *LectureView* consists of approximately 150 PowerPoint word slides and 75 PowerPoint image slides selected from the textbook. The *Instructor's Manual* consists of chapter teaching strategies for each chapter, strategies for teaching pharmacology in an integrated curriculum, answer guidelines for all Critical Thinking Questions in the textbook, and five home medication administration sheets. The *Test Bank* consists of 750 new and thoroughly revised NCLEX-style questions, an increased percentage of them emphasizing higher-level thinking. Carefully prepared to reflect the most important points from the text, the questions are now coded for cognitive type, nursing process step, and NCLEX client needs category.

The **Electronic Image Collection for Pharmacology** is a versatile, CD-ROM–based ancillary containing 150 images suitable for incorporation into lectures.

The newly revised **Nursing Pharmacology PowerPoint Presentations,** written by Robert S. Aucker, PharmD, are organized by body system into 18 presentations covering the principles of pharmacology and key drug information. The presentations can be used without modification or customized to suit specific classroom needs.

We believe this package of ancillary materials will provide both students and instructors with the best teaching/learning tools to make the most effective use of their time both inside and outside the classroom. The ancillary package is also geared to encourage student involvement and to facilitate the comprehension of key content related to pharmacology for nurses.

ACKNOWLEDGMENTS

We would like to thank the many people who have contributed to the development of the revised and updated twenty-first edition. Students, classroom instructors, and reviewers have provided suggestions and constructive comments that were most helpful in guiding us through this revision.

In addition, the entire editorial staff and associates at Mosby were outstanding in their professional support of this project. We are grateful to Executive Editor Robin Carter and Publishing Services Manager Debbie Vogel. Thanks also to Design Manager Bill Drone for his beautiful cover design and for his deft refinements to the book's typography. Special thanks to Senior Developmental Editor Kristin Geen, who contributed creative ideas and essential support during the crucial, formative stages of this revision. Thanks, too, to Managing Editor Lee Henderson for his ideas and assistance during the production stage. We would also like to give special mention to Senior Project Manager Jodi Willard for her exceptional work on this edition. Special thanks to Susan J.T. Henderson, R.N., M.A., and Gail M. Marchigiano, R.N., M.S.N., A.N.P.-C, of Saint Joseph's College of Maine; their web-based case studies bring a new dimension of teaching and learning to the revised and updated twenty-first edition.

Finally, we would like to thank our families, friends, and colleagues for their patience and encouragement. Without your support, this edition would not have been possible.

Leda M. McKenry
Evelyn Salerno

PUBLISHER'S HISTORICAL PERSPECTIVE

Mosby's Pharmacology in Nursing has a tradition of providing the nursing student, educator, and practicing nurse with thorough and up-to-date coverage of pharmacology and nursing management.

Through twenty editions, this book has sold well over 2,000,000 copies, making it the most widely used and successful nursing pharmacology textbook ever published.

Currently in its twenty-first edition, *Mosby's Pharmacology in Nursing* has its roots in *A Textbook of Materia Medica for Nurses* by A. L. Muirhead, which was published in 1919. In 1936, Hugh Alister McGuigan became the primary author, at which time the book was renamed *Materia Medica and Pharmacology.* In 1940, Elsie E. Krug joined McGuigan as co-author—a role she was to hold until 1948, when she became the primary author. After 10 successful editions, the book was renamed *Pharmacology in Nursing* in 1955.

In recognition of the book's long history, the chapter opener pages in each unit of this edition display a graceful photograph by Jim Leick of historical medicinal items from the private collection of Evelyn Salerno. We are grateful for her generosity in allowing us to include some of her personal treasures in this twenty-first edition.

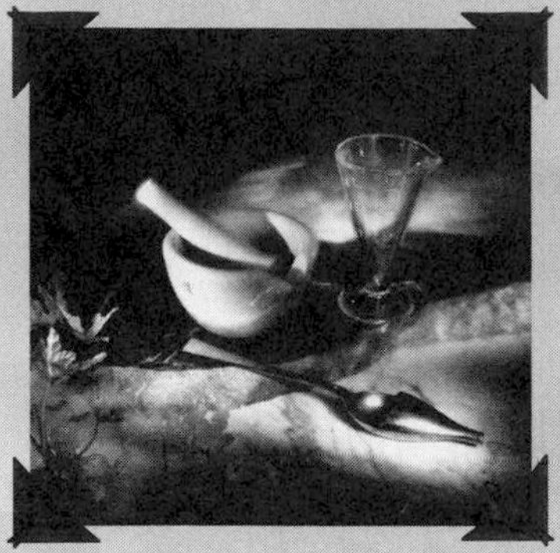

UNIT 1 Principles of Pharmacology

A mortar and pestle, measuring graduate, and dosing spoon are a few early examples of equipment used at the turn of the century for the preparation and administration of medicines. The earthenware mortar and pestle was used to reduce solids into the powdered substances used in medicines. The glass measuring graduate, with teaspoon and tablespoon graduations, was used to measure liquid medications before administration. The medical spoon is a special half-covered spoon that was used to prevent spilling. It was ideal for babies and others who were difficult to medicate.

UNIT 2 The Nursing Process and Pharmacology

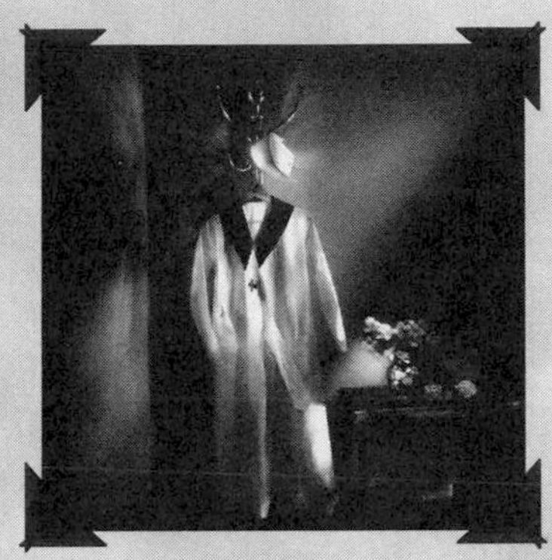

Nursing is an art; and if it is to be made an art,
it requires as exclusive a devotion, as hard a preparation,
as any painter's or sculptor's work;
for what is the having to do with dead canvas or cold marble,
compared with having to do with the living body—
the temple of God's spirit?
It is one of the Fine Arts;
I had almost said,
the finest of the Fine Arts.
—Florence Nightingale

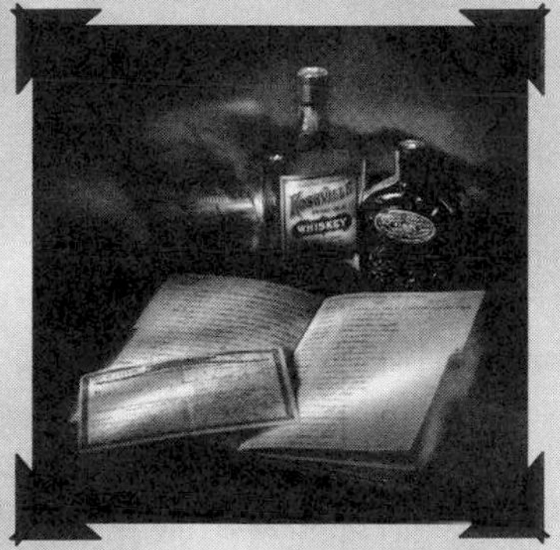

UNIT 3 Biopsychosocial Aspects of Pharmacology

The National Prohibition Act (1919-1933) restricted the sale of beverage alcohol but permitted the legal distribution of alcohol by prescription for the treatment of a known ailment. Physicians and pharmacists had to have a federal permit to prescribe or dispense medicinal spirits or whiskey. The whiskey bottles dispensed had a warning on the label: "For Medicinal Purposes Only." Physicians were required to write their alcohol orders on a U.S. Internal Revenue form and also had to record each prescription in a government-issued Physician's Record book. The entries for pints of whiskey in the record book shown here indicate that alcohol was prescribed for ailments such as slight colds, acute gastritis, bronchitis, and pneumonia. Pharmacologically, alcohol has little if any effect on these conditions, and in fact it is reported to cause gastritis.

UNIT 4 Current Issues in Pharmacology

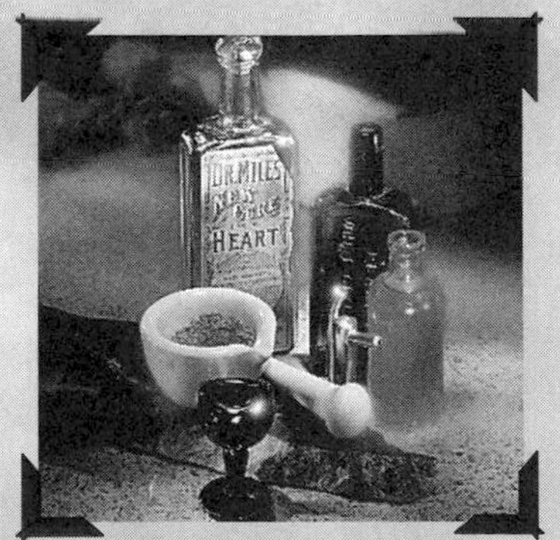

Before the twentieth century, diseases and illnesses were treated primarily with home remedies, vegetable concoctions, or narcotic-laced nostrums. At that time, trained health care professionals were few, and drug legislation was limited. Today, public interest in self-care management is at an all-time high. Thus the nurse should be knowledgeable about the major categories of over-the-counter drugs and the complementary and alternative therapies available for self-treatment.

UNIT 5 Drugs Affecting the Central Nervous System

The old medications featured here include the Pain-Expeller, a preparation containing 49% alcohol that was promoted as a liniment and inhaler. The Tongaline tablet container states that it is "a thorough eliminative for the various forms of Rheumatism and Neuralgia, and also La Grippe, Nervous Headache, Gout and Sciatica or wherever the salicylates are indicated." The ingredients are not listed. Bromo-Lithia Effervescent consisted of acetanilide combined with caffeine citrate, lithium bitartrate, and sodium bromide in a pure fruit acid. The indications for Bromo-Lithia were headache, biliousness, and rheumatism, whereas the Bromo Caffeine for Brain Workers contained effervescent hydrobromate of caffeine and according to the label was a "remedy for relief of the nervous headache resulting from overtaxed mental energy or excitement, acute attacks of indigestion, the depression following alcoholic excesses, the supra-sensitiveness of chloral, morphia, and opium habituates and with ladies, the headache and backache of neurasthenia, hysteria, dysmenorrhea and kindred disorders." Several of the drugs in these preparations are still in use today, such as lithium for the treatment of mania and caffeine with aspirin. Bromides and acetanilide have been replaced with safer products.

UNIT 6 Drugs Affecting the Autonomic Nervous System

The Microbeater was an early version of a nasal inhaler; the client inserted one metal arm in the mouth and the second curved arm in the nose and blew. This product was promoted as a cure for headache, neuralgia, colds, coughs, and catarrh. This device was probably a precursor to the inhalers in use today.

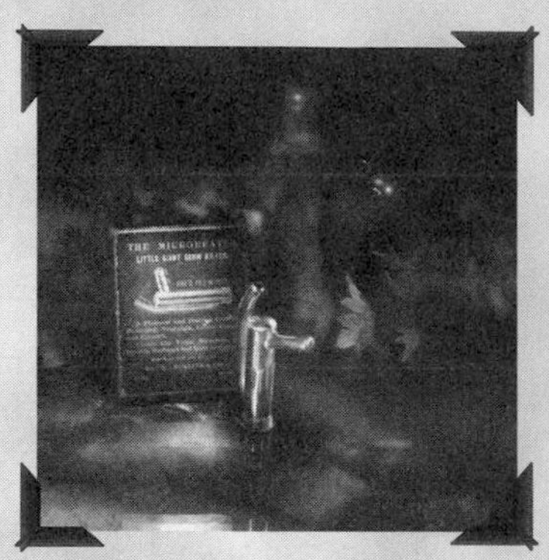

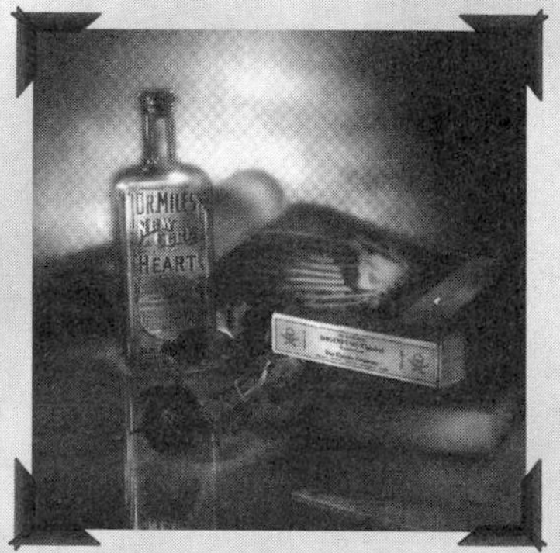

UNIT 7 Drugs Affecting the Cardiovascular System

The preparations on display are illustrative of the medicines used in the late 1800s to early 1900s for the treatment of heart disease. In 1885 Dr. Franklin Miles began to market his remedies, such as Dr. Miles New Cure for the Heart (and stomach, lungs, kidneys, and so on). The laws of the day did not require makers of patent medicines to list their ingredients, but the testimonials used in their advertising implied that the ingredients were digitalis and cactus. However, laboratory analysis revealed this cure to contain only a small amount of iron, phosphate, glycerin, and alcohol colored with caramel; no digitalis was found. This bottle dates between 1888 and 1920, when the name of the product changed to Heart Treatment. It was taken off the market in 1938. Diginfuse contains tablets of *Digitalis purpurea* leaves. The two active cardiac glycosides isolated from digitalis leaves are digoxin and digitoxin. These glycosides are more stable and reliable and have replaced the types of early products shown here.

UNIT 8 Drugs Affecting the Blood

This photograph shows two types of Civil War–era bleeding devices and Pinkham's Liver Pills. The center device is a venesection knife, and the bottom instrument is a combination tenaculum and lancet. Such devices were used to "bleed" patients to remove "excesses" from the blood. Overzealous physicians may have hastened their patients' death with this practice. It has been reported that George Washington had 9 pints of blood removed in 24 hours for the treatment of an infected throat. He died as a result of this "throat infection."

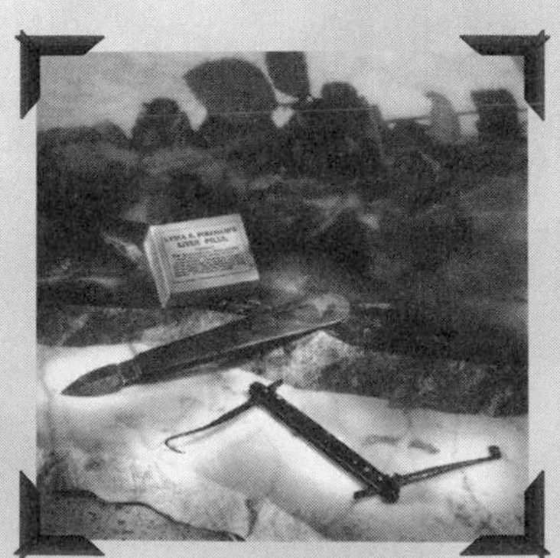

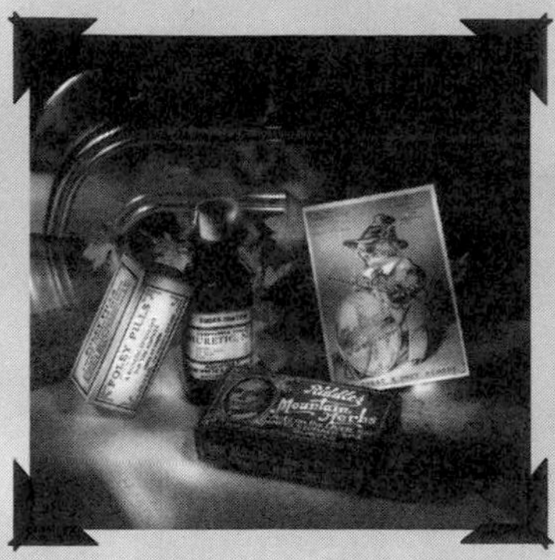

UNIT 9 Drugs Affecting the Urinary System

This photo shows an advertising card and a variety of turn-of-the-century medications used to treat kidney disease. The Mountain Herbs product lists approximately 30 disease states, as well as a number of testimonials. All three products contain herbs or plant ingredients, with the diuretic product also containing digitalis. This is an interesting assortment of early kidney medications.

UNIT 10 Drugs Affecting the Respiratory System

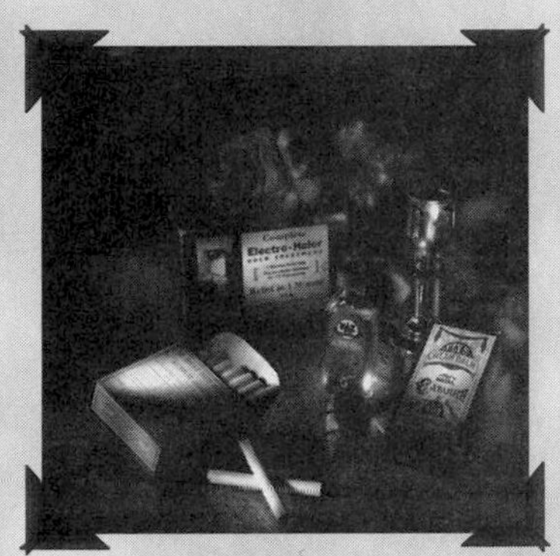

The equipment and products pictured here were used to treat respiratory illnesses. For example, Dr. Guild's Green Mountain Asthmatic Cigarettes were used to relieve attacks and paroxysms of asthma. Ingredients included stramonium and belladonna with directions to "put tube end into mouth and light closed end, same as ordinary cigarettes, but the smoke should be inhaled deeply.... An adult should not exceed 6 cigarettes or a child 3 cigarettes per 24 hours." The Electro-Halor Cold Treatment was said to provide relief in 1 minute from head colds, lung colds, coughs, and hay fever. Shown next to it are the contents of the box: the Kaz inhalant and the electrical cup for inhalation. Ely's Cream Balm was for nasal catarrh or cold in the head. A government analysis of this preparation stated that it contained mainly liquid petrolatum (mineral oil) with small amounts of thymol and menthol. The chemist reported that a 69-cent bottle of Ely's contained approximately a half-cent's worth of liquid petrolatum.

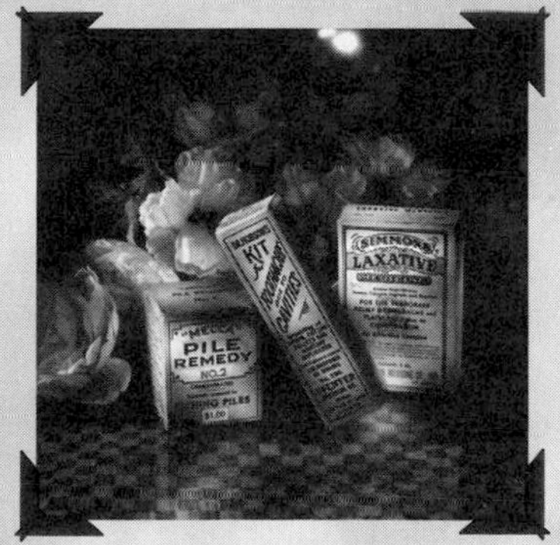

UNIT 11 Drugs Affecting the Gastrointestinal System

The three drug packages pictured include Mecca Pile Remedy No. 2 "for blind bleeding and protruding piles...." It contained carbolic acid. Dr. Hobson's Kit for Toothache Due to Cavities contained a bottle, cotton pellets, and tweezers. The liquid in the bottle contained chloroform, creosote, oil of cloves, oil of camphor, and phenol. Simmons Laxative Medicine was used for the temporary relief of headache and flatulence due to constipation. This powder contained senna, cascara sagrada, and gentian. Carbolic acid or phenol was used in the Mecca package as an antiseptic for hemorrhoids, but today both the safety and the efficacy of this use are questionable. Phenol has been approved by the FDA for the relief of teething in infants 4 months of age and older. Currently, the FDA states there to be no effective over-the-counter product that can be placed in the tooth cavity to relieve toothache.

UNIT 12 Drugs Affecting the Visual and Auditory Systems

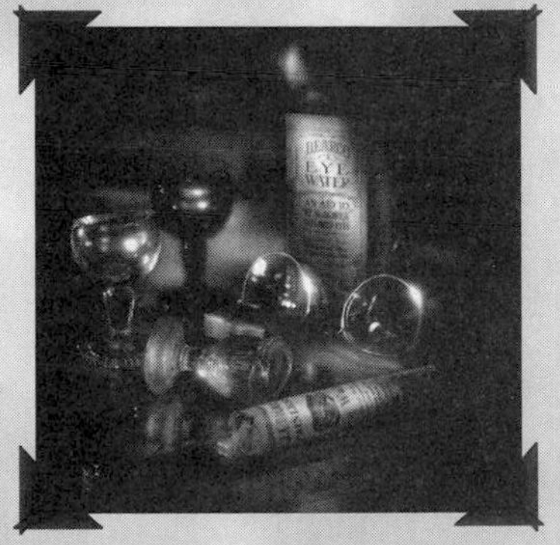

The two large eye cups shown in this photo have patent dates of 1917, and the Dearco Eye Water is advertised as "excellent for automobiles and others subjected to dust and winds" (1928). Dr. Dickey's Painless Eye Water has a copyright date of 1908. According to *Nostrums and Quackery* (1912), Dr. Pettit's Eye Salve contained morphine—an unusual ingredient for an eye preparation. Many of these products were astringents or eye washes.

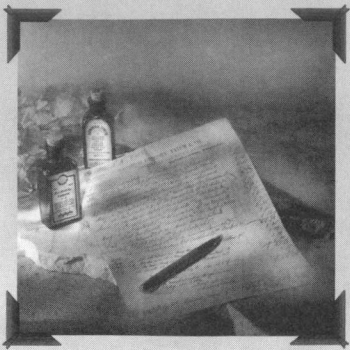

UNIT 13 Drugs Affecting the Endocrine System

This photograph shows two turn-of-the-century glandular products, an original druggist's bill dated 1863, and an instrument. The bottles contained suprarenal gland, with the Pluriglandular Compound also containing thyroid and ovarian residue. The druggist's bill was from Tallahassee, Florida, and it lists items purchased by General R.K. Call from 1861 to 1862. (An R.K. Call was governor of territorial Florida in 1836 and 1841.)

UNIT 14 Drugs Affecting the Reproductive System

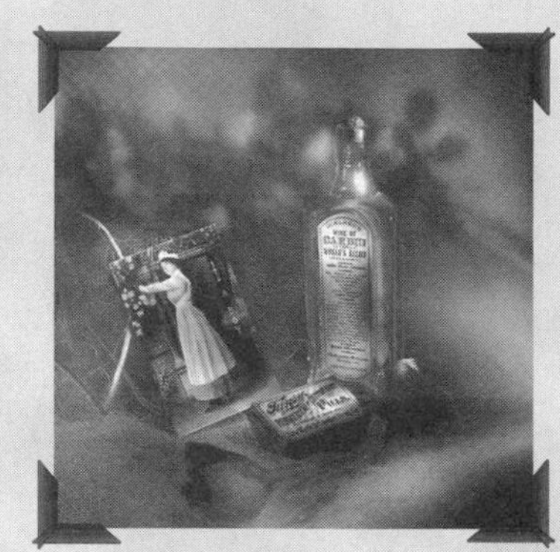

The "It's a Boy" postcard is an early example of an announcement of the birth of a baby boy, and McElree's Wine of Cardui or Woman's Relief was promoted as a remedy for the treatment of female diseases. The label indications include its use for "suppressed or delayed menses, painful menstruation, profuse or too frequent flow of menses, whites, falling of the womb, change of life and as a general restorative for delicate women." The label states it contains 20% alcohol. The tin contains Tansy Pennyroyal and Cotton Root Pills, a Reliable, Female Regulating Pills. Dated 1896, the insert states, "It is best, in beginning the use of these pills, that the bowels should be thoroughly opened by some good cathartic....It is also well, while using these pills, to make use of a warm foot bath every night, which may be made further efficient by the addition of a small quantity of mustard, salt or salsoda...."

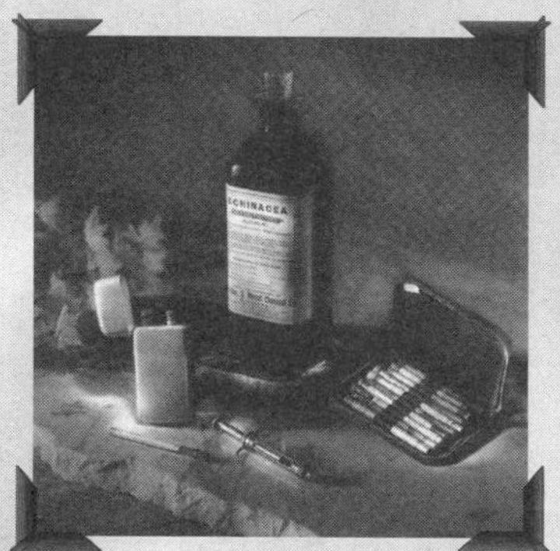

UNIT 15 Drugs Used in Neoplastic Diseases

The photograph shows a turn-of-the-century bottle of Echinacea, a substance used to treat cancer, blood poisoning, syphilis, rabies, reptile bites, and many other disease states. The two small doctor kits contain vials of hypodermic tablets (e.g., strychnine, morphine, atropine). The kit on the left also contained a syringe (pictured in front) and needles. Note that the syringe barrel is similar to the injector unit commonly used today. These items date from the nineteenth century to the early twentieth century.

UNIT 16 Drugs Used in Infectious Diseases and Inflammation

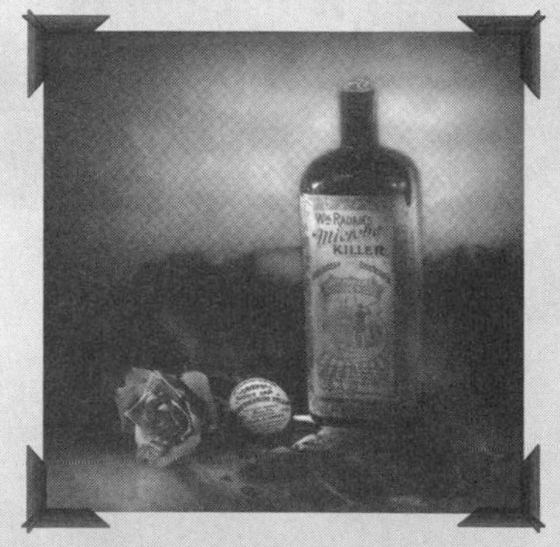

William Radam, a gardener, made a concoction of muriatic acid, sulfurous acid, red wine, and water and sold it as a cure for cancer, consumption, diabetes, diphtheria, yellow fever, paralysis, and men's diseases. The government charged the company with quackery and then seized and destroyed cases of this product. On analysis, this product contained 99.381% water. Note the embossment on the label and the back of the bottle that pictures a man clubbing a skeleton. The trademark is registered 1887 and 1893 on the label. The Dref's Gout and Rheumatism Pill tin is dated 1916 and has explicit instructions: "One pill at night when required. Cannot be given to children." The ingredients of this pill are unknown.

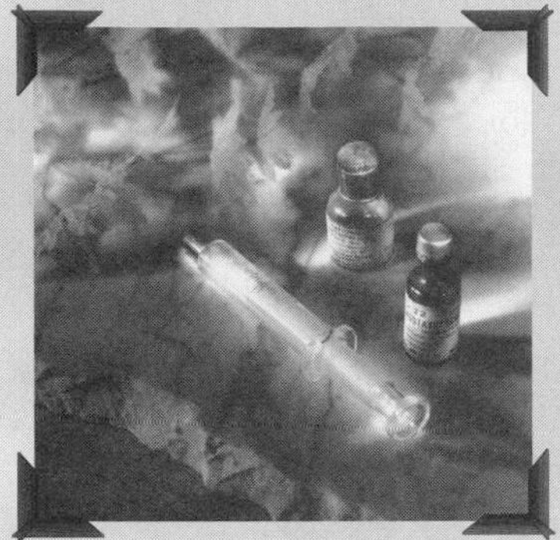

UNIT 17 Drugs Affecting the Immunologic System

A glass syringe lies next to two early injectable vials. The Hemostatic (Hemoplastin) labeled vial has a U.S. License No. 1 on the label, and the second vial is Erysipelas Vaccine, a bacterial vaccine made from *Streptococcus*.

UNIT 18 Drugs Affecting the Integumentary System

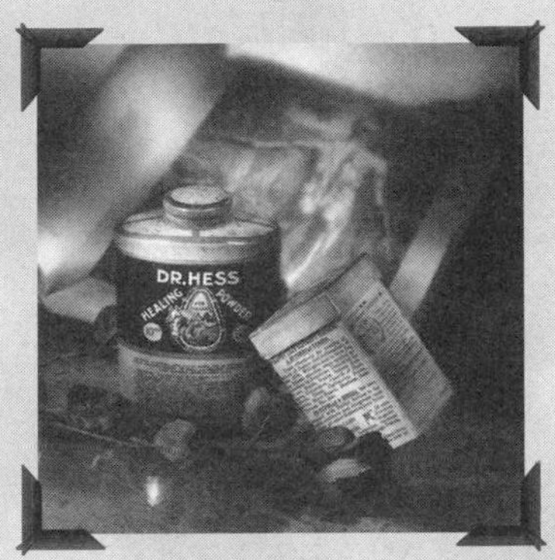

Dr. Hess Healing Powder is a good example of a product for multiple uses, a patent medicine "good for man and beast." The front of this tin lists all of the human reasons for using the product, and the back lists a variety of animal conditions. Mail order medicines were common on the frontier, and products that could serve everyone in the household were preferred. The second item is Velvet Leaf Ointment Compound, a substance promoted for treating all diseases of the rectum (piles, hemorrhoids, tumors, fissures, and rectal ulcers), blood poisoning, rattlesnake bite, eczema, abscesses, lumps and tumors, cuts, burns, scalds, head congestion, deafness, sore throat, and other conditions. This product has the 1906 Food and Drugs Act Guarantee. The legislation and marketing of drug products has changed in the twentieth century. Although similar drugs may still be commonly used in humans and animals, veterinary medicine has in general developed as a separate specialty.

UNIT 19 Intravenous and Nutritional Therapy

An invalid or sick feeder is shown with Stearns' Tonic and Iron, Quinine and Strychnine No. 2 tablets. The latter product was used as a hematinic and bitter tonic. Strychnine was used in tonics because of its bitter taste, which was believed to stimulate gastric secretion and appetite. Stearns' Tonic came in a triangular bottle and contained beef and cod liver peptones, calcium, iron, and ammonium citrate. It was promoted as the ideal tonic for older adults, for weak, pale, and delicate children, and for convalescents.

UNIT 20 Miscellaneous Agents

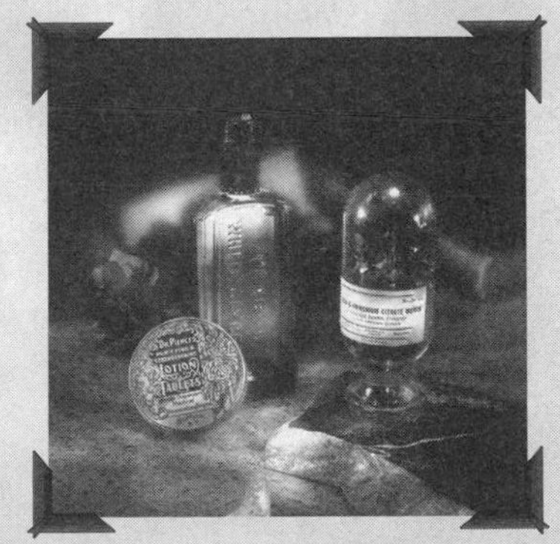

The items in this photograph include Dr. Pierces Lotion Tablets, a cobalt bottle of Pearl's White Glycerine, and a pharmacy display bottle. Dr. Pierces tablets were crushed and dissolved in hot water to make an antiseptic lotion. The Iron & Ammonium Citrate Merck pharmacy bottle is an inverted show bottle that was used to display chemicals. At the turn of the century, many pharmacists displayed these bottles in their prescription areas.

CONTENTS

1 ORIENTATION TO PHARMACOLOGY

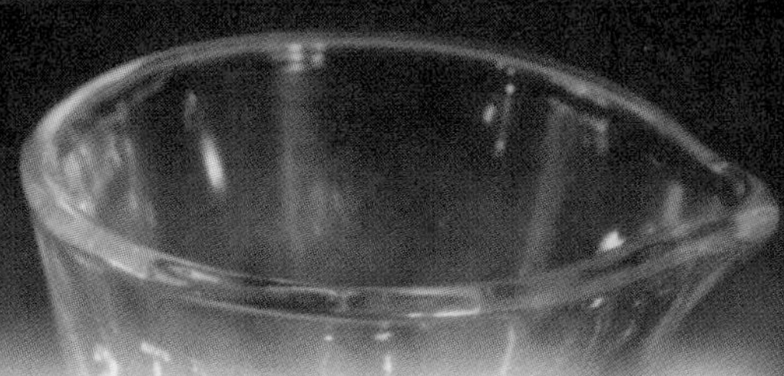

Chapter Focus

In order to administer medications safely and teach clients and caregivers how to manage a therapeutic drug regimen effectively, nurses need to understand and apply the principles of pharmacology. This chapter will focus on the historical development of pharmacology as a science for the improvement of health, the terminology associated with it, and the scope of nursing practice related to it.

Learning Objectives

1. Define key terms used in pharmacology.
2. Cite significant historical events in the development of pharmacology.
3. Describe the difference between chemical, generic, and trade names of drug products.
4. Name four main sources of drug and biologic products.
5. Differentiate between alkaloid, glycoside, gum, resin, and oil.
6. Identify authoritative sources for drug information.
7. Identify the scope of nursing responsibilities related to pharmacology.
8. Correlate the steps of the nursing process with the study of pharmacology.

Key Terms

chemical name, p. 3
collaborative problems, p. 8
dosage, p. 8
drug, p. 3
generic (nonproprietary) name, p. 3
indications, p. 8
mechanism of action, p. 8
nonprescription or over-the-counter (OTC) drug, p. 4
pharmacokinetics, p. 8
pharmacopeia, p. 2
pregnancy safety, p. 8
prescription drug or legend drug, p. 4
side effects/adverse reactions, p. 8
trade, brand, or proprietary name, p. 3

Pharmacology is a science that studies the effects of drugs within a living system. It deals with all legal and illegal drugs used in society today, including street, prescription, and nonprescription or over-the-counter medications. The pharmacologic agents available today have controlled, prevented, cured and, in a few instances, eradicated disease. The result has been an improved quality of life and, perhaps, an extension of the life span.

However, medications can also potentially harm the client, which is reflected by the fact that the term *pharmaceutical* is actually derived from the Greek word for poison (Siler et al., 1982). Therefore the nurse should have a thorough understanding of any medication *before* giving it to a client. The nurse must know the usual dosage, route of administration, indication(s), significant side effects and adverse reactions, major drug interactions, contraindications, and the appropriate nursing assessment, planning, implementation, and evaluation techniques necessary to administer the drug safely.

A number of terms are fundamental to the knowledge base of nurses. Lists of key terms that are essential for nurses to understand are found at the beginning of this chapter and future chapters along with the pages on which the definitions may be found.

HISTORICAL TRENDS

Since the beginning of time people have searched for substances to treat illness and cure disease. The oldest known prescriptions were found on a clay tablet written by a Sumerian physician in approximately 3000 BC, or about 5000 years ago.

Primitive people through the Egyptian period believed that evil spirits living in the body caused disease. Asclepios, who lived between 600 and 700 BC, was considered the principal Greek god of healing. He combined religion and healing in a temple setting, and his large family represented health or medical ideology. For example, his wife Epione soothed pain; daughter Hygeia, the goddess of health, represented the prevention of disease; and Panacea, another daughter, represented treatment. His large temple settings were used to treat both the rich and poor to cure their illnesses.

Hippocrates (fifth century BC) advanced the idea that disease resulted from natural causes and could be understood only through a study of natural laws. He believed the body to have recuperative powers and saw the role of the health care provider as assisting the recuperative process. Called the Father of Medicine, Hippocrates influenced the principles that control the practice of medicine today.

The fall of the Roman Empire marked the beginning of the medieval period (400 to 1580 AD). Germanic barbarians overran Western Europe, which reverted to a medicine of folklore and tradition similar to that of the Greeks before Hippocrates. At the same time, Christian religious orders built monasteries that became sites for all learning, including pharmacy and medicine. They aided the sick and needy with food, rest, and medicinals from their monastery gardens. The Arabs' interest in medicine, pharmacy, and chemistry was reflected in the hospitals and schools they built, the many new drugs they contributed, and their formulation of the first set of drug standards.

In 1240 AD Emperor Frederick II declared pharmacy to be separate from medicine, but pharmacy was not truly established separately until the sixteenth century, when Valerius Cordus wrote the first pharmacopeia as an authoritative standard. A **pharmacopeia** is the total of all authorized drugs available within a country; it contains descriptions, recipes, strengths, standards of purity, and dosage forms for the drugs.

Paracelsus (1493-1541), professor of physics and surgery at Basel, denounced "humoral pathology" and substituted the idea that diseases were actual entities to be combated with specific remedies. He improved pharmacy and therapeutics for succeeding centuries, introducing new remedies and reducing the overdosing so prevalent in that period.

Great progress was made in pharmacy and chemistry during the seventeenth and eighteenth centuries. The first London pharmacopeia appeared in 1618, and many preparations introduced then are still in use today, including opium tincture, coca, and ipecac. The first important national pharmacopeia was the French *Codex* (1818); this was followed by the *United States Pharmacopeia* in 1820, Great Britain in 1864, and Germany in 1872. See Table 1-1 for a summary of major drug discoveries.

The study of accurate dosages in the nineteenth century led to the establishment of large-scale manufacturing plants for the production of drugs. Drug dosages and knowledge of their expected action became more precise. Rational medicine had begun to replace empiricism. In the twenty-first century, change will continue to reform the health care systems in the United States and Canada. The emphasis on providing quality health care in a more cost-effective manner is leading to a redefinition of professional roles and decision-making responsibilities among health care professionals (Blumengold, 1995; van de Ven, 1996). More clients and health care providers are using complementary and alternative therapies for health promotion and the treatment of illness and injury. An integrated health care delivery team is evolving; this team centers on client-focused care that at a minimum includes assessment, planning, monitoring, client counseling, accountability for therapeutic outcomes, and client advocacy. A health promotion focus and managed care approaches are changing the content of professional education. Drug therapy is the mainstay in the application of restorative and rehabilitative care, and therefore the nurse needs to have a solid foundation in pharmacology.

As a result of the current and projected trends, the health care consumer will be asking for more information; one of the persons most often questioned is the nurse. Nurses in all practice roles and settings need to understand the therapeutic uses of and potential for injury with prescription, over-the-counter, herbal/complementary, and illicit drugs. Nursing roles—which include administering medications in

TABLE 1-1 Summary of Major Drug Discoveries

Drug	Time Period	Comments
opium tincture, coca (cocaine), and ipecac	17th century	Important drugs; still used today
digitalis	1785	Cardiac medication; source of cardiac glycosides (digoxin, digitoxin)
smallpox vaccine	1796	Important vaccine in its time; smallpox has now been eradicated worldwide
morphine	1815	Most important analgesic derived from opium; used to treat severe pain
quinine, atropine, and codeine	19th century	Still available for use today
ether and chloroform	1840s	First general anesthetics; rare or obsolete today
insulin	1922	Most important discovery for treatment of diabetes mellitus
penicillin	mid-1940s	Revolutionized treatment of microbial infections; precursor of many other antibiotics
cortisone	1949	Important hormone from adrenal gland cortex; also synthetically prepared
polio vaccines	1955, 1961	Discovery of inactivated and live oral poliovirus vaccines very significant in eliminating polio epidemics
oral contraceptives	late 1950s	Chemicals similar to natural estrogen or progesterone hormones; have been used by millions of women worldwide
antivirals	mid-1970s	Useful for the prophylaxis and treatment of viral diseases
zidovudine (AZT)	1987	First antiretroviral agent
HIV protease inhibitors	1996	Potent class of antiretroviral agents; dramatically reduces mortality when used in combination with other drugs

health care agencies, community, and home care settings; teaching clients safe and effective self-administration of medications; and detecting drug-related problems—require thorough preparation with comprehensive and current knowledge (Naegle, 1994). Nurses will assume greater responsibility for professional judgment in the administration and supervision of drug therapy and, in advanced roles, prescriptive authority (Cheek, 1997). Therefore nurses must know about and use drug information to better care for their clients. This nursing activity is made more complex by the knowledge that a single drug may bear many names.

NAMES OF DRUGS

A **drug** is any substance used in the diagnosis, cure, treatment, or prevention of a disease or condition. A drug collects three different types of names as it passes through the investigational stages before being approved and marketed. The first is the chemical name, the second is the generic or nonproprietary name, and the third is the trade, brand, or proprietary name.

The **chemical name** is a precise description of the chemical composition and molecular structure of the drug. This name is particularly meaningful to the chemist. For example, the chemical name of a popular analgesic is N-(4-hydroxyphenyl) acetamide. Its generic name is acetaminophen, and it is also sold under a number of brand or trade names—Tylenol, Tempra, and Panadol, among others.

The manufacturer, with the approval of the United States Adopted Name Council (USAN), often assigns the **generic** or **nonproprietary name.** Because the generic name is simpler than the chemical name, it is the official name listed in official compendiums, such as the *United States Pharmacopeia (USP).* When drug companies market a particular drug product, they often select and copyright a **trade, brand,** or **proprietary name** for their drug. This copyright restricts the use of the name to only the individual drug company. Because numerous brand names may exist for the same ingredient, such as for acetaminophen, prescribers are encouraged to use the generic name. The use of generic names is also widely advocated to avoid confusion between similar-sounding trade names. The brand, trade, or proprietary name of drugs discussed in this text will be enclosed in parentheses following the generic name.

With some exceptions, the majority of generic drug products sold are considered therapeutically equivalent to the trade name product. Most states allow pharmacists to substitute generic drugs when filling a prescription unless the prescriber has indicated that the trade name form of the drug is essential. Generic products are often much less expensive than trade name drugs.

Extensive advertising is usually necessary to encourage health care provider prescribing and to promote sales of the trade name drug. Pharmaceutical manufacturers are now extensively advertising prescription drugs directly to consumers, with the expense of this advertising borne mainly by the consumer. However, much of the research in new drugs is performed in laboratories of reputable drug firms. To realize a legitimate return for the cost of research, drug companies need to patent their products and have exclusive rights to their manufacture and sale for a specified time period.

A drug may be considered a **prescription drug** or a **legend drug**, which means it requires a legal prescription in order to be dispensed; or it may be a **nonprescription** or **over-the-counter (OTC) drug**, a drug that may be purchased without a prescription. Some prescription drugs may be purchased in lower doses that are considered relatively safe for sale over-the-counter. Such a drug is ibuprofen, which is sold as an OTC drug in its 200-mg strength (Advil or Motrin IB) but requires a prescription for the 300-, 400-, 600-, or 800-mg tablet.

SOURCES OF DRUGS

Drugs and biologic products are identified or derived from four main sources: (1) plants, from which drugs such as digitalis, vincristine, and colchicine are obtained; (2) animals and humans, from which drugs such as epinephrine, insulin, and adrenocorticotropic hormone are obtained; (3) minerals or mineral products, such as iron, iodine, and zinc; and (4) synthetic or chemical substances made in the laboratory. The drugs made of chemical substances are pure drugs, and some of them are simple substances, such as sodium bicarbonate and magnesium hydroxide. Others are products of complex synthesis, such as the sulfonamides and the adrenocorticosteroids.

The leaves, roots, seeds, and other parts of plants may be dried or otherwise processed for use as a medicine and, as such, are known as crude drugs. The chemical substances they contain produce their therapeutic effect. When the pharmacologically active constituents are separated from the crude preparation, the resulting substances are more potent and usually produce effects more reliably than does the crude drug. Some of the types of pharmacologically active compounds found in plants, grouped according to their physical and chemical properties, are alkaloids, glycosides, gums, and oils:

1. *Alkaloids* are organic compounds that are alkaline in nature and are chemically combined with acids in the laboratory to form water-soluble salts such as morphine sulfate and atropine sulfate. Synthetic alkaloids formulated in the laboratory have activity similar to that of plant alkaloids.
2. *Glycosides* are active plant substances that, on hydrolysis, yield a sugar plus one or more additional active substances. The sugar is believed to increase the solubility, absorption, permeability, and cellular distribution of the glycoside. An important cardiac glycoside used in medicine is digoxin.
3. *Gums* are plant exudates. Some of them swell and form gelatinous masses when water is added. Others remain unchanged in the gastrointestinal tract, where they act as hydrophilic (water-attracting) colloids; they absorb water, form watery bulk, and exert a laxative effect. Agar and psyllium seeds are examples of natural laxative gums, whereas methylcellulose and sodium carboxymethylcellulose are synthetic colloids.
4. *Oils* are highly viscous liquids and are generally of two types: volatile or fixed. A volatile oil imparts an aroma to a plant; because of their pleasant odor and taste, these oils were often used as flavoring agents. Peppermint and clove oil are examples of volatile oils occasionally used in medicine. Fixed oils are generally greasy and, unlike volatile oils, do not evaporate easily. Olive oil is a fixed oil used in cooking, whereas castor oil is an example of a fixed oil used in medicine.

DRUG CLASSIFICATION

Drug classification can be approached from two perspectives: clinical indication or body system. This book uses both approaches where appropriate. Examples of drugs classified by clinical indication include the following:

Chapter 38: Mucokinetic and Bronchodilator Drugs
Chapter 60: Antifungal and Antiviral Drugs

An example of drugs classified by body system is the following:

Unit Five: Drugs Affecting the Central Nervous System

These drug groupings can assist the nurse in understanding and learning about the individual agents available for drug therapy. Pharmacology becomes easier when one understands the common characteristics of each drug classification and when a *key* or *prototype* drug within each group is studied thoroughly. When a new drug becomes available, the nurse will then be able to associate it with its drug classification and make inferences about many of its basic qualities before reading about its specific properties. Learning which of the qualities of a new drug are different from those of the prototype drug and its dosage is extremely helpful.

The basic information to be learned about each major drug includes its generic name and original trade name, the category to which it belongs, its clinical uses, mechanism of action, side effects/adverse reactions, contraindications, precautions, significant drug interactions, and other specifics associated with the nurse's role in the administration of, evaluation of, and client teaching about that drug. "Looking it up" should become second nature to both nursing students and practicing nurses. *Nurses are professionally, morally, legally, and personally responsible for every dose of medication they administer.*

The release of new drugs, as well as new information on old drugs, is an ongoing event. News releases and numerous articles, journals and books are written in an attempt to keep up with the new discoveries. It is unrealistic to believe that one can know everything about all medications on the market; therefore the practitioner must know how and where to obtain general and detailed drug information. Many excellent drug references are available, each with its own focus and/or emphasis. Because no single reference is a complete source of drug data to meet the varied and specialized needs of clinical practice today, the nurse should be familiar with the primary drug reference sources available. Drug information resources are listed in Table 1-2.

TABLE 1-2 Drug Information Resources

Reference	Comments
American Hospital Formulary Service (AHFS) Drug Information (Bethesda, MD: American Society of Hospital Pharmacists, Inc.)	Objective overview in monograph form Comprehensive source of comparative, unbiased drug information on nearly every available drug in United States Issues supplements; updated annually Widely used drug information source for all health care professionals
United States Pharmacopeia Dispensing Information (USP DI) (Rockville, MD: U.S. Pharmacopeial Convention)	Available in several volumes; Volume I is for health care professionals, and Volume II offers advice for clients in lay language Consists of extensive drug monographs with practical information Highlights clinically significant information to reduce drug risks Issues monthly updates; updated annually Highly recommended drug reference for all health care professionals
Physicians' Desk Reference (PDR) (Oradell, NJ: Medical Economics)	Widely used source for health care professionals Pharmaceutical industry finances the book Drug information same as drug package insert Lacks comparative information on safety and efficacy Lacks nursing information Contains drug product identification section and manufacturers' addresses and phone numbers
Mosby's GenRx (St. Louis, MO: Mosby)	Comprehensive drug information Contains drug product identification charts Includes product ratings (equivalent/not equivalent classifications) from FDA Has drug costs comparisons Published annually
Drug Facts and Comparisons (St Louis, MO: Facts and Comparisons, Inc.)	Loose leaf edition updated monthly Comprehensive drug information arranged to facilitate comparisons and evaluations Contains package sizes and strengths plus cost index information Contains manufacturers' addresses and phone numbers Contains section for orphan drugs, diagnostic aids, radiopaque agents, antidotes, and drugs in development Widely used reference source, especially for pharmacists
The Medical Letter (New Rochelle, NY: The Medical Letter, Inc.)	Biweekly newsletter with evaluation of the efficacy, safety, rationale, and price comparison of current medications Objective summaries Valuable newsletter, highly recommended
Handbook of Nonprescription Drugs (Washington, DC: American Pharmaceutical Association)	Comprehensive OTC drug information Reviews physiology, the primary minor illnesses, and the drugs used in treatment Has tables with specific OTC drug information
Compendium of Pharmaceuticals and Specialties (CPS) (Ottawa, Ontario, Canada: Canadian Pharmaceutical Association)	Widely used reference source in Canada for all health care professionals Published annually Contains manufacturers' addresses and phone numbers
Various drug handbooks for nurses	Gives brief overviews of drugs in outline format Helpful as a quick refresher on the unit to remind nurse of important points once nurse has had a course in pharmacology Drug information is formatted according to the nursing process; gives nursing considerations
Computerized pharmacology databases	Available in some health agencies Allow drug information to be printed so clients have it for personal use Some systems allow individualization of information for clients

Any nursing process is only as effective as the knowledge base and the analytic thought that go into it. Logic and judgment improve as the nurse's information base is perfected, partly as experience is tested against knowledge. Nowhere is ongoing self-learning more essential than in nursing pharmacotherapeutics. The "need to know" escalates, for example, when a nurse who is responsible for administering medications is confronted with an order for an unfamiliar drug or with an unexpected client symptom not usually associated with the diagnosis.

Drug information centers are located throughout Canada and the United States to disseminate information about the clinical uses of drugs and related equipment. These centers are often located within large medical center settings. Both general and specific information can be obtained, with advice based on scientific literature. Many difficult pharmacologic questions related to client care can be dealt with quickly by contacting the nearest drug information center. In addition, drug manufacturers, package inserts, and pharmacists are usually available to provide similar information.

Health care agencies commonly furnish similar sources of information. The area or unit in which a nurse works often has a card file of package inserts; ideally, a nursing library shelf within the clinical setting contains pharmacology information and other material of interest. Any nurse can initiate the development of such material and request funds or supplies. The agency's nursing staff development department is responsible for promoting ongoing and updated learning and can facilitate audiovisual aids, references, or a seminar program. Building a personal library and keeping it current are also important professional activities.

With the proliferation of medical sites on the Internet, many search engines and directories are available to provide both general and specialized drug information for health care professionals and clients. It has been estimated that more than 10,000 medical sites are available on the Internet (Hutchinson, 1997). Many professional journals (nursing, pharmacy, medical) also provide current drug information, and a number of them are also available on the Internet. The student is urged to select the Internet site carefully when seeking drug information, because erroneous information may also be posted. There is no screening tool for Internet information, and thus the best approach is to be knowledgeable about the reputation of the provider of the information, for example, drug information from drug information centers; pharmacy, medical, or nursing school posted information; professional journals; and the American Cancer Society, the Food and Drug Administration (FDA), the National Institutes of Health, and numerous other organizations.

No one text is a complete source of all the pharmacology information necessary for nursing practice. The nurse must gather reliable information from various sources to meet clinical needs.

THE SCOPE OF NURSING MANAGEMENT OF DRUG THERAPY

Drugs can either help or harm. Nurses, physicians, and clinical pharmacists are held legally responsible for safe and therapeutically effective drug administration. Specifically, nurses are liable for their actions and omissions and for the duties they delegate to others, including medication technicians, pharmacy technicians, practical nurses, and even physicians. They are personally responsible—legally, morally, and ethically—for every drug they administer or have administered, no matter who actually prescribed it. Indeed, all members of a health care team may be held liable for a single injury to a client. The increase in litigation against nurses and physicians indicates that society tolerates only a minimal margin of error in relation to human injury and life. Claims have been brought against health care professionals for drug errors that caused loss of life and permanent injury. When these claims are supported with evidence that the conduct of one or more health care professionals helped to bring about the loss or injury, those parties may be held liable. The law, a legal and social norm, requires health care professionals to be safe and competent practitioners and permits compensation to those harmed or injured.

However, the law is also a protective force for the knowledgeable, competent, and responsible nurse. Nurses who are determined to safeguard clients from drug-induced harm will, for example:

- Keep their knowledge base current
- Refer to authoritative sources in professional literature and to physicians, pharmacists, and other colleagues
- Use correct techniques and precautions
- Observe and chart drug effects explicitly
- Question a drug order that is unclear or that appears to contain an error
- Refuse to administer or refuse to allow others to order or administer a drug if there is reason to believe it will be harmful

The law, in turn, protects such nurses from unfair litigation. Chapter 2 discusses in greater detail the legal role of the nurse related to drug therapy.

Much remains to be learned about the actual mode of action of many commonly prescribed drugs, as well as the effects from prolonged use. Furthermore, there is increasing concern about drug-induced disease. Fortunately, drug therapy is temporary for most conditions or for illness prevention. Some diseases require lifelong use of drugs to sustain life (such as insulin for type 1 diabetes mellitus) or prolonged use to maintain relatively normal physiologic or psychologic functioning (such as phenytoin [Dilantin] for seizure disorders).

Nurses are entrusted with potent and habit-forming drugs, and they must not abuse or misuse this trust. Drugs are comforting and lifesaving when used respectfully and intelligently, but they can lead to tragedy when used unwisely or with undue dependence. The nurse who combines diligent and intelligent observation with moral integrity and factual knowledge is a safe and competent practitioner and a credit to the nursing profession.

In addition, the nurse must establish with the client a "therapeutic alliance," a respectful and trusting relationship to facilitate the highest attainable level of self-care. The client is the most important participant in the team effort for safe and effective drug administration. Clients are not expected to be submissive, acquiescent, and unquestioning followers of the health team's instructions; they must be motivated to assume responsibility for their own care. Nurses must recognize that the willingness to participate is ultimately the client's. All the nurse's knowledge, skill, and ability are brought to bear on the establishment of a therapeutic alliance to facilitate the most appropriate level of self-care related to medications.

Paying close attention to all drugs the nurse administers helps the nurse learn to identify them, tailor their application, and spot errors before they occur. Expertise is built in just this fashion. Learning the names of drugs, their formulations, and their pharmacologic actions is best accomplished in small increments and in a systematic way by making associations with information about a known drug in a classification, its close analogues, and clients for whom the nurse has provided care. The learning value of the analysis and synthesis of data in actual practice far outweighs that of memorizing long lists of unrelated drugs and their properties.

Nurses in emergency departments and in community health practices are often challenged to identify medications from a client's personal unlabeled pillboxes or containers. Often many varieties of drugs and pieces of tablets are mixed together. Clients are often unable to assist in identifying their drugs, having never been properly educated by health care providers. The *Physician's Desk Reference (PDR)*, the *USP DI*, and *Mosby's GenRx* provide actual photographs of drugs to assist the health care professional in identifying an unknown tablet or capsule. In addition, manufacturers often place an identification code consisting of letters or numbers on their solid oral dosage forms. Although these markings may not be meaningful to the practicing nurse, pharmacists and local drug information centers can use them to assist in the identification of generic and trade products. Difficult identification problems may be referred to the FDA Drug Listing Branch or the FDA Division of Poison Control, both of which are located in Rockville, Maryland.

Pharmacology applies knowledge from many different disciplines, including anatomy and physiology, pathology, microbiology, organic chemistry and biochemistry, mathematics, anthropology, psychology, and sociology. Thus clinical drug therapy can be considered an applied science. The thousands of drugs available would present a formidable study if they had to be approached as individual agents. Fortunately, drugs can be systematically classified into a reasonable number of drug groups on the basis of chemical, pharmacologic, or therapeutic relatedness.

Understanding the characteristic effects of a particular class of drugs at the cellular, tissue, organ, and functional system levels permits the student or practitioner to extrapolate information to a wide variety of drugs. A typical representative drug can be selected and studied and its specific characteristics compared with those of others in the same class. In this way the individual gradually builds a knowledge base.

Lists of drugs, dosages, and their indications should not be regarded as dogma. Laboratory research and new scientific methods of evaluation are constantly generating new information. Sometimes there are reports that a drug, even an old and trusted one, is suspected of causing mutations, birth defects, cancer, or less serious secondary effects. Not only nursing students but also practicing nurses are challenged by the proliferation of drugs; most of the drugs on the market today were developed recently. Change is the only constant in pharmacology.

Pharmacology books must be kept up-to-date in the nurse's library. In addition, official current literature on drugs must be followed carefully, because new drugs only slowly make their way into more permanent literature. For the nurse working in a hospital or home health service, physicians, instructors, in-service educators, and pharmacists are on hand to help. In a more isolated practice, greater personal effort is required to maintain currency. In any case, nurses must pay close attention to the drug therapy of their clients.

Learning is an active process. Therefore clinical experience with drugs is invaluable, because it enables the student to do the following:

- Note which drugs are most commonly used to treat certain diseases or specific signs and symptoms
- Note the dosage of and the frequency with which drugs are administered
- Observe which drugs are most effective in relieving particular signs and symptoms
- Witness individual differences in clients' reactions to a specific drug
- Relate knowledge obtained from authoritative sources to real-life situations

Regardless of what is to be learned, reasoning and the ability to analyze and synthesize information are prerequisites to understanding. These cognitive skills, along with perceptual skills, permit a student to see meaningful relationships, make comparisons, and determine significance, all of which are essential for sound decision making in nursing.

THE NURSING PROCESS AND DRUG ADMINISTRATION

The *nursing process* is a systematic method for identifying actual or potential health care problems or impediments to the activities of daily living. It points the way to rational nursing actions and the objective evaluation of care.

The direction of the nursing process is fairly universal in the field, although its structure may vary from the widely used pattern of four phases or steps: (1) assessment of data (which may culminate in a nursing diagnosis), (2) planning, (3) implementation, and (4) evaluation.

To apply the nursing process to drug therapy, nurses *assess* the medication needs of their clients partly in terms of how these needs are matched by the prescriber's orders; to do this they consider the indications of the drug, the client's preexisting heath conditions, and any medications the client is currently taking. The result of this assessment is the *nursing diagnosis*. Nurses make *plans*, which include goals that directly relate to the client's nursing diagnoses and specific outcome criteria. The stage is then set for *implementation* of the goals using specific, rationale-based nursing actions. Implementation may include the following: *monitoring* the client for therapeutic and nontherapeutic effects of the drug and ability to manage the therapeutic regimen; *intervention* related to preparing and administering a medication as ordered or to withholding a dose and obtaining a change in the medication order; and *client education* for the safe and accurate self-administration of the drug. The final step is the *evaluation* of the nursing care provided based on the level of achievement of the outcome criteria for which the client and nurse have planned. Each time nursing care is evaluated, the knowledge bases of the nurses increase and become more valuable. The nursing process is discussed in more detail in Unit 2, The Nursing Process and Pharmacology.

GOALS OF THIS TEXT

This text orients the reader to nursing pharmacology and therapeutics by presenting a firm theoretic foundation and a practical approach to drug therapy that is applicable in many settings—the home, the clinic, the extended care facility, the office, the classroom, and the hospital.

Part I provides general principles, theories, and facts about drugs and their administration. Practical information about the integration of the nursing process with pharmacology is presented, and general principles of action are given to facilitate a student nurse's learning in both academic and clinical environments. The rest of the book presents specific drug information about clinical applications and nursing management of the care of clients receiving specific medications. Thus this book can be used both as a text and as a reference.

To find information about a particular drug in this book, do the following:

1. Look it up in the index.
2. When you find the information about the drug, refer back to the beginning of the chapter or unit and read the material that precedes the specific discussion.

Reading only the pages listed in the index will illuminate only the specifics of the drug, which will be out of context and without the necessary fundamental information about that class of drugs. Reading the background information offers an overall view and places the drug information into an understandable framework.

One of the more effective ways to study pharmacology is to understand the pharmacologic characteristics of a classification of drugs: its major uses; mechanisms of action; absorption, distribution, metabolism, and excretion; onset and duration of action; and adverse reactions. Throughout the book, key drugs are highlighted with the symbol ✔. These drugs can be studied as representatives of the drug classification under discussion. Other drugs within the classification can then be identified by the manner in which they differ from the prototype. This approach will enhance learning rather than the rote memorization of a multiplicity of facts about each and every drug.

The specific drug information in the text summarizes what is needed to administer drugs safely and competently. Each discussion is titled with some of the common names by which the particular drug is known. The trade names of drugs that are available in Canada but not in the United States are followed by a Maple leaf symbol (🍁).

In the sections that present specific drug information, the **mechanism of action** section explains how the drug acts at the biochemical or cellular level to produce its therapeutic effects. The officially approved therapeutic purposes of the drug or the conditions for which it is used are detailed as **indications.** The **pharmacokinetics** section specifies how the drug is absorbed, distributed, associated with tissue, biotransformed or metabolized, and excreted. The section titled **side effects/adverse reactions** details most of the common secondary effects that may be experienced when the drug is administered. The **dosage** section presents the currently approved regimen governing the size, frequency, and number of doses of a therapeutic agent. It must be noted that not all drugs have been tested for safety and efficacy in administration to older adults, pregnant women, women who are breastfeeding, or children. The routes and special techniques for drug preparation are also listed here in each monograph. **Pregnancy Safety** boxes list the FDA pregnancy safety category associated with various drugs, which indicates the documented problems with the use of a drug during pregnancy.

The nursing management sections describe distinctive nursing measures:

Assessment involves gathering data about an individual's experience with medications and allergies, identifying preexisting medical conditions that might influence the choice of dosage of drug and/or concurrent drugs that might cause significant interactions, determining the potential outcome and suggested management of such interactions, and performing baseline observations that are essential for measuring changes in the client's health status during the medication regimen or for determining whether administration of the drug is appropriate.

Nursing diagnosis involves identifying selected nursing diagnoses that nurses, by virtue of their education and experience, are able and licensed to treat, as well as **collaborative problems,** which are physiologic complications that nurses monitor to detect their onset or changes in status (Carpenito, 2000).

Planning is an important step in the nursing process. However, to prevent redundancies within each drug monograph, modifications to administration of the drug are found in the intervention section, and outcome criteria are discussed in the evaluation section.

Implementation incorporates the nursing activities of monitoring, intervention, and education, which need to be planned in order to administer a specific drug safely and accurately:

Monitoring: significant observations relative to the client's health status, including diagnostic and laboratory tests that ensure a safe and effective drug regimen

Intervention: special handling, timing of doses, and other significant aspects of the actual administration of a drug

Education: client teaching to enable the client and/or caregiver to effectively manage the therapeutic medication regimen at home

Evaluation provides the planned outcome criteria or nursing outcomes for reviewing care of the client in regard to safe and effective drug therapy.

Safe, therapeutically effective drug administration is a major responsibility of nurses. It depends on sound, current knowledge of medications and careful monitoring of their effects on clients. With increasingly shorter lengths of stay by clients in acute and subacute care settings, nurses have an increasing responsibility to ensure that clients and caregivers can effectively manage the medication regimen at home. Ongoing laboratory and clinical research modifies and enlarges available drug information, necessitating a continual effort to keep one's knowledge up-to-date. The modes of action of many commonly prescribed drugs, the effects of their prolonged use, and the possibility of drug induced disease are yet to be completely understood. There are many sources of current drug information, but even the most diligent student of these sources requires clinical experience to develop competence in drug administration. Few areas of nursing demand more intellectual curiosity, integrity, factual knowledge, and motivation to use reference sources.

SUMMARY

Pharmacology, the study of drug effects within a living system, has always been linked to our concept of health and illness and therefore has held importance for humanity through the ages.

Each drug is identified by three names: the chemical name; the generic (nonproprietary) name, generally a simplification of the chemical name; and the trade, brand, or proprietary name under which the pharmaceutical company markets the drug. Because generic drugs are less expensive than trade name drugs, most states allow pharmacists to substitute them for trade name drugs within limitations.

Plants, animals and humans, minerals, and chemical substances are the four sources of drugs. The pharmacologically active compounds derived from plants are alkaloids, glycosides, gums, resins, and oils.

Drugs are classified either by clinical indication or by body system. Drug classifications facilitate the nurse's understanding of pharmacology by allowing the conceptualization of the common characteristics of each grouping and prototype drug and the association of new drugs with a particular classification.

Pharmacology is a field of ever-increasing importance for nursing. Because nurses are held by law to be responsible for the drugs they administer, they should maintain a current knowledge base and be competent in the assessment, planning, implementation, and evaluation of the client's nursing care. The goal of this text is to assist the learner in achieving that knowledge and competence within pharmacology.

Critical Thinking Questions

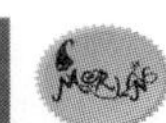

1. Why is the study of pharmacology important for nurses? Think of three clinical examples that would indicate its importance to the care of clients.
2. Review the structure of one of the later chapters that discusses a classification of drugs. Consider how you might go about studying for an examination on that chapter.
3. A nurse in the process of administering medications is confronted with a prescriber's order for a drug with which he or she is not familiar. What sources of drug information could he or she use?

Collaborative Learning Activities

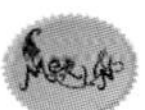

For Collaborative Learning Activities, go to mosby.com/MERLIN/McKenry/.

BIBLIOGRAPHY

Alcock, D., Jacobson, M.J., & Sayre, C. (1997). Competencies related to medication administration and monitoring. *Canadian Journal of Nursing Administration, 10*(3), 54-73.

Anderson, K.L., Anderson, L.E., & Glanze, W.D. (Eds.). (1998). *Mosby's medical, nursing, and allied health dictionary* (5th ed.). St. Louis: Mosby.

Atkinson, L.D. & Murray, M.E. (1995). *Clinical guide to care planning: Data to diagnosis.* New York: McGraw-Hill.

Blumengold, J.G. (1995). Strategic and financial considerations for integrated health care delivery. *Medical Interface, 8*(5), 77-79, 83, 85.

Carpenito, L.J. (1995). *Nursing care plans and documentation: Nursing diagnoses and collaborative problems* (2nd ed.). Philadelphia: J.B. Lippincott.

Carpenito, L.J. (2000). *Nursing diagnosis: Applications to clinical practice* (8th ed.). Philadelphia: J.B. Lippincott.

Cheek, J. (1997). Nurses and the administration of medications: Broadening the focus. *Clinical Nursing Research, 6*(3), 253-274.

Drug Facts and Comparisons. (2000). St. Louis: Facts and Comparisons.

Hutchinson, D. (1997). *A pocket guide to the medical Internet.* Sacramento, CA: New Wind Publishing.

Leake, C.D. (1975). *An historical account of pharmacology to the twentieth century.* Springfield, IL: Charles C. Thomas.

Lyons, A.S., & Petrucelli, R.J. II. (1978). *Medicine: An illustrated history.* New York: Harry N. Abrams.

Mosby's GenRx (9th ed.). (1999). St. Louis: Mosby.

Naegle, M.A. (1994). Prescription drugs and nursing education: Knowledge gaps and implications for role performance. *Journal of Law, Medicine & Ethics,* 22(3), 257-261.

O'Donnell, J. (1994). Drug therapy: 20 ways your role will change. *Nursing,* 24(3), 46-48.

Roger, F.B. (1972). *A syllabus of medical history.* Boston: Little, Brown.

Siler, W.A. et al. (1982). *Death by prescription.* Tallahassee, FL: Rose Publishing.

United States Pharmacopeia Dispensing Information (USP DI): Drug information for the health care professional (19th ed.). (1999). Rockville, MD: United States Pharmacopeial Convention.

van de Ven, W.P. (1996). Market-oriented health care reforms: Trends and future options. *Social Science & Medicine,* 43(5), 655-666.

2 Legal and Ethical Aspects of Medication Administration

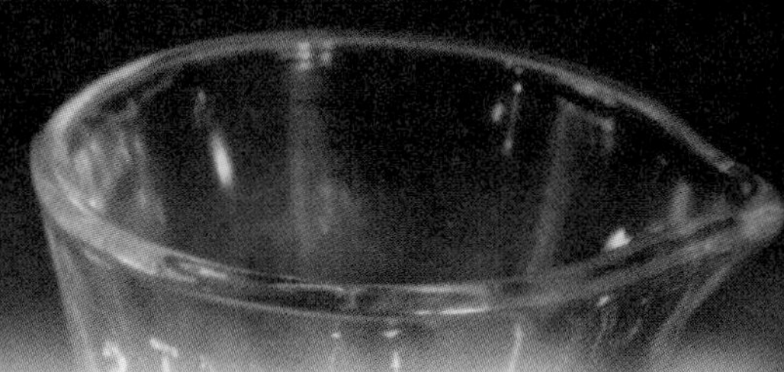

Chapter Focus

As the professional role has grown in nursing, nurses have become more autonomous in their practice. With this autonomy has come a growing legal accountability, and nurses need to consider this responsibility as they practice. However, even the law and the technologic advances in health care are not sufficient to cope with many of the ethical dilemmas faced by nurses. This chapter will discuss the legal foundations and ethical considerations for the use of drugs.

Learning Objectives

1. Identify the process used in the development and evaluation of a new drug before marketing.
2. Differentiate between over-the-counter and prescription drugs.
3. Describe the procedure for evaluating over-the-counter drugs and prescription drugs for safety and effectiveness.
4. Identify legislative or authoritative source(s) for drug standards.
5. Describe the difference between permissive and mandatory drug substitution in the United States.
6. Describe the Food and Drug Administration's pregnancy categories for drugs.
7. Discuss the nurse's role in drug research.
8. Discuss the changing nursing roles related to drug administration.
9. Discuss the ethical issues involved in the administration of medications.

Key Terms

assay, p. 19
beneficence, p. 29
bioassay, p. 19
controlled substances, p. 14
Controlled Substances Act, p. 14
Five Rights of Medication Administration, p. 28
informed consent, p. 22
International Narcotics Control Board, p. 20
malpractice, p. 28
nonmalfeasance, p. 29
Nuremberg Code, p. 22
orphan drug, p. 12
product liability, p. 14
Pure Food and Drug Act, p. 12
therapeutic index, p. 20

Many remedies of the past lacked the information taken for granted today, such as the strength of the substance in a preparation or even the ingredients themselves. This type of medical practice, although not always ineffective, extended well into the nineteenth century. Not until the twentieth century were standards for drug identification, drug preparation, and proof of drug effectiveness and safety required.

UNITED STATES DRUG LEGISLATION

Before 1906 patent medicines and remedies were sold by medicine men in traveling wagon shows, in drugstores, by mail order, and by doctors, real or self-titled. Such products were not required to have a list of ingredients on the label, so many contained potent and dangerous drugs such as opium, morphine, heroin, chloral hydrate, and alcohol. Many persons (especially infants) were reportedly injured, became addicted, or died as a result of ingesting the ingredients contained in these preparations.

In 1906 the first U.S. law, the federal **Pure Food and Drug Act,** was passed to protect the public from adulterated or mislabeled drugs. The law required a drug company to declare on the package label the presence of any of 11 drugs identified as being dangerous and perhaps addictive (some of which were in the list just mentioned). However, this first law had loopholes that were used by the patent medicine dealers for their own gain. For example:

1. False and misleading claims about the curative value of the product were not allowed *on the package,* which was described as a bottle, label, or wrapper that encircled the bottle. Claims made in advertisements, newspapers, or drug almanacs; by word of mouth; or on signs in store windows were not covered under the law. Unscrupulous nostrum dealers took full advantage of this oversight.
2. Serial numbers were required for products containing any of the 11 dangerous drugs, and each label was to bear the words "Guaranteed under the Food and Drug Act." This meant that the dealer had registered the product and was legally responsible for it if it was improperly sold. However, many patent medicine dealers implied that this label was the government's seal of approval. In response to this abuse, this clause was abolished in 1919.
3. Only drugs sold in interstate commerce (made in one state and sold to persons living in other states) were covered. Drugs made and sold within the same state did not fall under the jurisdiction of this law.

The Pure Food and Drug Act of 1906 designated the *United States Pharmacopeia* and the *National Formulary* as official standards and empowered the federal government to enforce them. Drugs were required to comply with the standards of strength and purity professed for them, and labels had to indicate the type and amount of morphine or other narcotic ingredients present. In 1912 Congress passed the Sherley Amendment, prohibiting the use of fraudulent therapeutic claims.

A further update of the drug legislation occurred in 1938 with the passage of the federal Food, Drug, and Cosmetic Act. More than 100 deaths occurred in 1937 as a result of ingestion of a diethylene glycol solution of sulfanilamide. This preparation had been marketed as an "elixir of sulfanilamide" without investigation of its toxicity. Under the 1906 law the only charge that could be made against the drug company was mislabeling, since it was labeled an "elixir" and the drug failed to meet the definition of an elixir as an alcoholic solution. The 1938 act prevented new drugs from being marketed before being properly tested for safety.

The Durham-Humphrey Amendment of 1952 further changed the 1938 drug act by specifying how legend, or prescription, drugs and refills could be ordered and dispensed (Box 2-1). This amendment also recognized a second class of drugs, over-the-counter drugs (OTCs), for which prescriptions are not required.

In 1958 a U.S. Senate investigation into the drug industry was begun when it became known that drug companies were making huge profits and that some drug promotion was false or misleading. This investigation received little support until given impetus by the thalidomide tragedy, although for the United States it was more a might-have-been catastrophe than a real one. Thalidomide, a hypnotic marketed in Europe, was found to be responsible for severe deformities in infants whose mothers had taken the drug during the early stages of pregnancy. These events led to passage of the Kefauver-Harris Amendment in 1962. (Thalidomide is currently available in the United States for the treatment and maintenance therapy of erythema nodosum leprosum [leprosy]. It is also available as an **orphan drug**—a drug developed under special funding through the Orphan Drug Act [see Orphan Drug Act, p. 13]—for use in bone marrow transplantation, acquired immunodeficiency syndrome (AIDS) and several other conditions.)

BOX 2-1
Prescription (Legend) Drugs

Legend drugs must bear the legend "Caution: Federal law prohibits dispensing without prescription." These include all drugs given by injection as well as the following:

1. Hypnotic, narcotic, or habit-forming drugs or derivatives thereof as specified in the law
2. Drugs that because of their toxicity or method of use are not safe unless administered under the supervision of a licensed practitioner (physician, dentist, or nurse practitioner)
3. New drugs that are limited to investigational use or new drugs that are not considered safe for indiscriminate use by the public

The Kefauver-Harris Amendment required proof of both the safety and efficacy of a new drug before it could be approved for use. This meant that all drugs introduced under the safety-only criteria in effect from 1938 to 1962 had to be evaluated. To do this the Food and Drug Administration (FDA) signed a contract in 1966 with the National Academy of Sciences and the National Research Council (NAS/NRC) to study all supporting data for all therapeutic claims. This program of study was called the Drug Efficacy Study Implementation (DESI).

Thousands of drugs and therapeutic claims have been evaluated and many ineffective drugs have been withdrawn from the market. For example, guaifenesin (Robitussin) is the only expectorant classified as effective; others, such as terpin hydrate and ammonium chloride, are not approved for sale as expectorants but may be available on the market for other approved uses. Those rated as "possibly effective" or "probably effective" are being withdrawn or reformulated; a drug may remain on the market while claims are being modified and scientific data collected to substantiate the claims. However, an approved drug can be prescribed for a disorder for which the drug has not been FDA approved. Informed consent for this non-research application is generally not required. Box 2-2 provides a summary of important legislation.

BOX 2-2

Important Drug Legislation (United States)

Food, Drug, and Cosmetic Act of 1938
Mandated that drug manufacturers must test all drugs for harmful effects and that drug labels must be accurate and complete

Wheeler-Lea Act of 1938
Defined criteria for nonfraudulent advertising

Durkham-Humphrey Amendment of 1952
Distinguished more clearly between drugs that can be sold with or without a prescription and those that cannot be refilled

Drug Amendment of 1962 (Kefauver-Harris Act)
Tightened controls over drug safety and statements about adverse reactions and contraindications, drug testing methods, and drug effectiveness criteria

Controlled Substances Act of 1970 (Comprehensive Drug Abuse Prevention and Control Act of 1970)
Categorized controlled substances on the basis of their relative potential for abuse

Drug Regulation Reform Act of 1978
Shortened the drug investigation process to release drugs sooner to the public

Over-the-Counter Drug Review

Of the estimated 400,000 drug products marketed in the United States, more than 300,000 are OTC drugs (Covington, 1996). These 300,000 individual drug products contain approximately 700 to 1000 active ingredients. In 1972 the FDA assembled an advisory review panel to perform an ingredient review, asking primarily the following questions: Are the ingredients safe and effective for consumers to self-medicate, and are the labeling, indications, dosage instructions, and warnings sufficient? If they were found lacking, appropriate recommendations had to be developed.

This study, completed in 1983, found that approximately one third of the ingredients reviewed were safe and effective for the labeled indications. Ingredients found particularly or potentially dangerous were either transferred to prescription status only (e.g., hexachlorophene, an antibacterial topical with a potential for inducing neurologic toxicities) or removed entirely from the market (e.g., camphorated oil or camphor liniment). (See Chapter 11 for a discussion of OTC medications.)

Prescription Drugs Switched to Over-the-Counter Drug Status

In the United States, the OTC review panels are primarily responsible for switching a number of prescription drugs to nonprescription or OTC status. These drug products are considered to be safe for self-treatment by consumers without professional guidance. Cimetidine (Tagamet HB), famotidine (Pepcid AC), diphenhydramine (Benadryl), and topical hydrocortisone are examples of products switched from prescription to OTC status. However, drugs such as cimetidine, famotidine, and topical hydrocortisone still require a prescription in Canada.

Orphan Drug Act

In 1983 the Orphan Drug Act authorized the FDA to provide pharmaceutical researchers with grants to encourage drug research for the treatment of rare chronic diseases. Because this type of research is typically unprofitable, it was limited before the passage of this Act. Among the disorders that benefit from this research are cystic fibrosis, von Willebrand's disease, leprosy (Hansen's disease), AIDS, and rare cancers. Nearly 500 drugs have been discovered under this Act (*Drug Facts and Comparisons*, 2000).

Control of Opioids (Narcotics) and Other Dangerous Drugs

Narcotic and Substance Abuse Laws. The Harrison Narcotic Act (1914) was the first federal law aimed at curbing drug addiction or dependence. This law not only established the word "narcotic" as a legal term but also regulated the importation, manufacture, sale, and use of opium and cocaine and all of their compounds and derivatives. Marijuana and its derivatives were also included in this Act, as were many synthetic analgesic drugs that proved to produce or sustain either physical or psychologic dependence.

This Act and other substance abuse amendments now have only historical import; they have been superseded by the Comprehensive Drug Abuse Prevention and Control Act of 1970,* which is also called the **Controlled Substances Act (CSA)** and became effective May 1, 1971. This law was designed to provide increased research into, as well as prevent, substance abuse and dependence and to provide for the treatment and rehabilitation of drug abusers and drug dependent persons. It also was to improve the administration and regulation of the manufacturing, distribution, and dispensing of **controlled substances** (drugs covered by this act, which are classified according to their use and abuse potential) by legitimate handlers of these drugs to help reduce their widespread dispersion into illicit markets.

The CSA classifies controlled substances solely according to their potential for use and abuse. Drugs are classified into numbered levels, or schedules, from Schedule I to Schedule V (Table 2-1). Drugs with the highest abuse potential are placed in Schedule I; those with the lowest potential for abuse are in Schedule V. These classifications are flexible because drugs may occasionally be added or changed from one schedule to another without new legislation. It might be anticipated, for example, that marijuana would be changed to another schedule if and when it is accepted for use in treating the nausea associated with cancer chemotherapy or for treatment of glaucoma. Certain drugs with a potential for dependence, such as ethanol and certain analgesics, are not listed as controlled substances. Anyone handling controlled substances must follow the more inclusive or stringent requirements of federal and state laws.

In July 1973 the Drug Enforcement Administration (DEA), in the Department of Justice, became the sole legal drug enforcement agency in the United States.

Possession of Controlled Substances. It is unlawful for any person to possess a controlled substance unless it has been obtained by a valid prescription or order or unless its possession is pursuant to actions in the course of professional practice. It is a federal offense to transfer a drug listed in Schedule II, III, or IV to any person other than the individual for whom the drug was ordered.

Drug suppliers and hospitals—as well as physicians, pharmacists, and nurses—are individually and collectively responsible for accounting for the inventory and management of the flow and distribution of controlled substances. Institutional control of the flow of controlled substances is maintained by carefully recorded checks of the balance on hand, supplies added, and doses administered. All doses of controlled substances should be kept in double-locked cabinets or other secure areas, with the keys in the custody of a designated nurse. The nurse who carries the keys to the "narcotics box" is responsible for stock supplies of controlled substances. This person is required to perform actual counts of the doses of each controlled substance in the unit's stock at the beginning and end of each shift or workday. Many health care agencies use computerized systems for the dispensing of controlled substances; these systems tabulate the counts, thus eliminating the physical counting of these substances at the beginning and end of the shift. Complete documentation and high accountability are demanded of the nurses who do this counting and of all those who handle controlled substances during the work period. Each dose is accounted for as it is administered, discarded, wasted, or withheld. Although these protocols may seem to entail a needless waste of time, they are necessary to safeguard the control of drug flow.

*Current regulations can be obtained from the nearest Regional Director, Drug Enforcement Administration, or from the Drug Enforcement Administration, Department of Justice, Washington, DC 20004.

Additional Regulatory Bodies or Services

Food and Drug Administration. The FDA is charged with enforcement of the federal Food, Drug, and Cosmetic Act. The seizure of offending (improperly manufactured or packaged) goods and the criminal prosecution of responsible persons or firms in federal courts are among the methods used to enforce the Act. At regular intervals, pharmaceutical firms must report to the FDA all adverse effects associated with their new drugs.

The FDA also has an adverse-reaction reporting program. Although there may be large, well-designed clinical trials before the FDA approves a drug, not every problem with a drug may be evident before it is marketed. Adverse events may occur once a product is on the open market and widely used—often by clients who have multiple health problems and are taking many other drugs. All health care professionals, including nurses, are encouraged to report an unusual occurrence or an unusually high number of occurrences associated with a drug, its formulation, its packaging, and so forth. Communication may be made directly to the FDA by telephone or by completing a MedWatch form. A response from the FDA will follow. The purpose of this program is to detect reactions that have not been revealed by previous clinical or pharmaceutical studies. Such reports may lead to changes in the drug package insert, and in some instances the drug may be withdrawn from the market.

Public Health Service. The Public Health Service is part of the Department of Health and Human Services. One of the many functions of this agency is the regulation of biologic products. This refers to viral preparations, serums, antitoxins, or analogous products that are used for the prevention, treatment, or cure of diseases. The Public Health Service exercises control over these products by inspecting and licensing the establishments that manufacture them and also by examining and licensing the products themselves.

Product Liability. In a majority of the states the rule of strict manufacturer's liability has been adopted. This doctrine holds manufacturers liable for injuries caused by defects in their products, drugs, or devices. **Product liability**

TABLE 2-1 Schedule of Controlled Substances

Schedule	Characteristics	Dispensing Restrictions	Examples
I	High abuse potential No accepted medical use—for research, analysis, or instruction only May lead to severe dependence	Approved protocol necessary	Heroin, marijuana (cannabis), tetrahydrocannabinols, LSD, mescaline, peyote, psilocybin, methaqualone
II	High abuse potential Accepted medical uses May lead to severe physical and/or psychologic dependence	Written prescription necessary (signed by the practitioner)—emergency verbal prescriptions must be confirmed in writing within 72 hours No prescription refills allowed Container must have warning label*	Opium, morphine, hydromorphone, meperidine, codeine, oxycodone, methadone, secobarbital, pentobarbital, dextroamphetamine, methylphenidate, cocaine, and others
III	Less abuse potential than Schedules I and II Accepted medical uses May lead to moderate/low physical dependence or high psychologic dependence	Written or oral prescription required Prescription expires in 6 months No more than 5 prescription refills allowed within a 6-month period Container must have warning label*	Preparations containing limited opioid quantities or combined with one or more active ingredients that are noncontrolled substances: acetaminophen with codeine, aspirin with codeine, and others Also paregoric, nandrolone, stanozolol, testosterone, and others.
IV	Lower abuse potential than Schedule III Accepted medical uses May lead to limited physical or psychologic dependence	Written or oral prescription required Prescription expires in 6 months with no more than 5 prescription refills allowed Container must have warning label*	Phenobarbital, chloral hydrate, meprobamate, chlordiazepoxide, diazepam, oxazepam, clorazepate, flurazepam, lorazepam, propoxyphene, pentazocine, mazindol, alprazolam, and others
V	Lower abuse potential than Schedule IV Accepted medical uses May lead to limited physical or psychologic dependence	May require written prescription or may be sold without prescription (check state law)	Medications (generally for relief of coughs or diarrhea) that contain limited quantities of certain opioid controlled substances: terpin hydrate with codeine, and others

Information from *Mosby's GenRx.* (1999). St. Louis: Mosby.
*The warning label states the following: "Caution: Federal law prohibits the transfer of this drug to any person other than the client for whom it was prescribed."

exists if (1) a product is defective or not fit for its reasonably foreseeable uses, (2) the defect arose before the product left the control of the manufacturer, and (3) the defect caused some person harm. If these three criteria are met, the manufacturer must pay monetary damages for harm unless the liability can be shifted to some other party. Anyone harmed by a defective product has the right to sue the manufacturer for compensation.

Manufacturers are legally responsible for knowing the effects of their products. If an unknown risk could have been discovered through a reasonable amount of research, the manufacturer is held liable for any resulting harm. Because nurses are accountable, they need to stay alert to defects in the drugs they administer. Despite manufacturers' quality assurance programs, drug products are susceptible to errors in the manufacturing, packaging, and delivery processes. Although the detection of chemical defects is usually outside the nurse's province, the detection of observable physical defects is not. Nurses should learn to be keenly aware of the physical characteristics of the drugs they administer and make comparisons before administering them. For example, unusual discolorations, precipitates, other inconsistencies, or foreign bodies in parenteral fluids should be considered suspect. Such observations warrant withholding the drug and contacting the pharmacy department or other authoritative source. Recall of defective drugs is necessary to prevent client harm.

Occasionally, human error can be expected to cause the wrong medication to be dispensed from the pharmacy. Again, the nurse is responsible for every medication administered. In this case both the nurse who administers the wrong drug and the pharmacist who labeled it may be held liable for any resulting client harm. This liability has been sustained in the courts on several occasions. Helpful color photographs of many drug formulations can be found in the *Physician's Desk Reference, Mosby's GenRx,* and the *United States Pharmacopeia Dispensing Information: Drug Information for the Health Care Professional (USP DI).* The pharmacist can be contacted for assistance in the verification of any questionable medication.

Drug Substitution

Although the prescriber retains the prerogative to require the dispensing of a particular brand of drug, nearly every state has a drug substitution law that either permits or mandates substitution on the part of the pharmacist. In permissive states the prescriber must give express permission for substitution by either signing a special section on the prescription form or by checking the correct phrase on the prescription. If substitution is not wanted, the prescriber may note this by indicating "dispense as written," "brand necessary," or "medically necessary."

In states with a mandatory law, the pharmacist is required to dispense approved, less expensive, generic drugs to the client. Several exceptions apply in such situations; for example, the client's consent may be required before substitution, or the prescriber may mark the individual prescription with a term that prohibits substitution, such as "medically necessary."

CANADIAN DRUG LEGISLATION

In Canada the Health Protection Branch (HPB) of the Department of National Health and Welfare is responsible for the administration and enforcement of the Food and Drugs Act as well as the Proprietary or Patent Medicine Act and the Narcotic Control Act. These Acts are designed to protect the consumer from health hazards and fraud or deception in the sale and use of foods, drugs, cosmetics, and medical devices. Canadian drug legislation began in 1875 when the Parliament of Canada passed an act to prevent the sale of adulterated food, drink, and drugs. Since that time foods and drugs have been controlled on a national basis.

Canadian Food and Drugs Act. In 1953 the present Canadian Food and Drugs Act was passed by the Senate and House of Commons of Canada, and since that time the law has been amended often. The Act stipulates that no food, drug, cosmetic, or device is to be advertised or sold to the general public as a treatment, preventive, or cure for certain diseases listed in Schedule A of the Act. Among the diseases included in the list are alcoholism, arteriosclerosis, and cancer. When it is necessary to provide adequate directions for the safe use of a drug to treat or prevent diseases mentioned in Schedule A, that disease or disorder may be mentioned on the labels and inserts accompanying the drug. In addition, the Act prohibits the sale of drugs that are contaminated, adulterated, or unsafe for use and those whose labels are false, misleading, or deceptive. According to the Act, drugs must comply with prescribed standards as stated in the recognized pharmacopoeias and formularies listed in Schedule B of the Act, or with the professed standards under which the drug is sold. Recognized pharmacopoeias and formularies include the following:

- *Pharmacopoeia Internationalis*
- *British Pharmacopeia*
- *United States Pharmacopeia*
- *Pharmacopée Française*
- *Canadian Formulary*
- *British Pharmaceutical Codex*

The legend "Canadian standard drug" or the abbreviation CSD must appear on the inner and outer labels of a drug to signify that it meets the standards prescribed for it.

The sale of certain drugs is prohibited unless the premises where the drug was manufactured and the process and conditions of manufacture have been approved by the Minister of National Health and Welfare. These drugs are listed in Schedules C and D and include injectable liver extracts, all insulin preparations, anterior pituitary extracts, radioactive isotopes, antibiotics for parenteral use, serums and drugs other than antibiotics prepared from microorganisms or viruses, and live vaccines. The distribution of samples of drugs is also prohibited, with the exception of distribution to duly licensed individuals such as physicians, dentists, or pharmacists. Schedule F of the Act contains a list of drugs that can be sold and refilled only on prescription. Refills

BOX 2-3

Canadian Prescription and Restricted Drugs

Prescription Drugs

Schedule F

May be used only after professional consultation
Includes more than 200 drugs
Identified by Pr on the label

Schedule G

Also called "controlled drugs"
Affect the central nervous system (stimulants, sedatives)
Identified by ◈ on the label

Restricted Drugs

Schedule H

Available only to institutions for research
Present dangerous physiologic and psychologic side effects and have no recognized medical use

may be permitted at specified intervals but cannot exceed 6 months. The drugs listed in Schedule F include antibiotics, hormones, and tranquilizers. They must always be properly and clearly labeled and include directions for use. Labels on containers of Schedule F drugs must be marked with the symbol Pr (prescription required). These drugs cannot be advertised to the general public other than giving the name, price, and quantity of the drug. Box 2-3 contains a summary of Canadian prescription (Schedules F and G) and restricted (Schedule H) drugs.

Controlled drugs for Canada are those listed in Schedule G of the Act and include amphetamines, barbituric acid and its derivatives (barbiturates), and phenmetrazine. Controlled drugs must be marked with the symbol ◈ in a clear and conspicuous color and size on the upper left quarter of the label. The proper name of the drug must appear on the labels either before or after the proprietary or trade name. Controlled drugs can be dispensed only by prescription.

When a controlled drug is dispensed by prescription, the labels must carry the following:

1. Name and address of the pharmacy or pharmacist
2. Date and number of the prescription
3. Name of the person for whom the controlled drug is dispensed
4. Name of the practitioner
5. Directions for use
6. Any other information that the prescription requires be shown on the label

Prescriptions for controlled drugs cannot be refilled unless the practitioner so directed in writing at the time the prescription was issued and also specified the number of refills and the dates for or intervals between refilling. All information on the labels must be clearly and prominently displayed and readily discernible. Controlled drugs cannot be advertised to the general public.

Designated drugs are the following controlled drugs: (1) amphetamines, (2) methamphetamines, (3) phenmetrazine, and (4) phendimetrazine. Physicians may prescribe a designated drug for the following conditions: (1) narcolepsy, (2) hyperkinetic disorders in children, (3) mental retardation (minimal brain dysfunction), (4) epilepsy, (5) parkinsonism, and (6) hypotensive states associated with anesthesia. Permission can be obtained to prescribe amphetamines for clients with diagnoses other than those listed.

Restricted drugs are those listed in Schedule H of the Act and include the hallucinogenic drugs lysergic acid diethylamide (LSD), diethyltryptamine (DET), dimethyltryptamine (DMT), and dimethoxyamphetamine (STP, DOM). The sale of these drugs is prohibited. These drugs may be obtained for research by a qualified investigator if authorized by the Minister of National Health and Welfare. Precautions must be taken to ensure against the loss or theft of a restricted drug.

The following list includes some of the additional requirements found in the Canadian Food and Drugs Act:

1. Labels of drugs must show the following:
   a. Proper name of the drug immediately preceding or following the proprietary or brand name.
   b. Name and address of the manufacturer or distributor.
   c. Lot number of the drug.
   d. Adequate directions for use.
   e. Quantitative list of medicinal ingredients and their proper or common names.
   f. Net amount of drug.
   g. Common or proper name and proportion of any preservatives used in parenteral drugs.
   h. Expiration date if the drug does not maintain its potency, purity, and physical characteristics for at least 3 years from the date of manufacture.
   i. Recommended single and daily adult dose; if the drug is for children, the label must state "Children: As directed by physician" or:

Age (in years)	Proportion of Adult Dose
10-14	One-half
5-9	One-fourth
2-4	One-sixth
Under 2	As directed by physician

   j. A warning that the drug be kept out of the reach of children and any precautions to be taken (e.g., "Caution: May be injurious if taken in large doses for a long time. Do not exceed the recommended dose without consulting a physician.") This warning is to be preceded by a symbol—octagonal in shape, red in color, and on a white background.
   k. Contraindications and side effects of nonprescription drugs.
   l. On and after July 1, 1974, the drug identification number assigned to the drug, preceded by the words "Drug Identification Number" or the abbreviation "D.I.N." is to be shown on the main labels of a drug sold in dosage form (i.e., one ready for use by the consumer).
2. Other specific regulations are the following:
   a. Manufacturers must be able to demonstrate that a drug in oral dosage form represented as releasing the drug at certain time intervals actually is released and available as represented.
   b. Oral tablets must disintegrate within 45 minutes. Enteric-coated tablets must not disintegrate for 60 minutes when exposed to gastric juice but must disintegrate within an additional 60 minutes when exposed to intestinal juices.
   c. Drugs containing boric acid or sodium borate as a medicinal ingredient must carry a statement that the drug should not be administered to infants or children under 3 years of age.
   d. Safety factors such as sterility and the absence of pyrogens must be ensured in parenteral drugs.

These regulations allow the government to withdraw from the market any drugs found to be unduly toxic. New drugs introduced to the market must have demonstrated effectiveness and safety in human clinical studies to the satisfaction of the manufacturer and the government.*

Canadian Narcotic Control Act. The regulations of the Canadian Narcotic Control Act govern the possession, sale, manufacture, production, and distribution of narcotics. The Canadian Narcotic Control Act was passed in 1961 and revoked the Canadian Opium and Narcotic Act of 1952. The 1961 Act has been amended a number of times.

Only authorized persons can be in possession of a narcotic. Authorized persons include a licensed dealer, pharmacist, practitioner, person in charge of a hospital, or a person acting as an agent for a practitioner. A licensed dealer is one who has been given permission to manufacture, produce, import, export, or distribute a narcotic. Practitioners include persons registered under the laws of a province to practice the profession of medicine, dentistry, or veterinary medicine. However, persons other than these may be licensed by the Minister of National Health and Welfare to cultivate and produce opium poppy or marijuana or to purchase and possess a narcotic for scientific purposes. Members of the Royal Canadian Mounted Police and members of technical or scientific departments of the government of Canada or of a province or university may possess narcotics in connection with their employment. A person who is undergoing treatment by a medical practitioner and requires a narcotic may possess a narcotic obtained on prescription. This person may not knowingly obtain a narcotic from any other medical practitioner without notifying that practitioner that he or she is already undergoing treatment and obtaining a narcotic on prescription.

All persons authorized to be in possession of narcotics must keep a record of the name and quantity of all narcotics received, from whom the narcotics were obtained, and to whom the narcotics were supplied (including quantity, form, and dates of all transactions). In addition, they must ensure the safekeeping of all narcotics, keep full and complete records on all narcotics for at least 2 years, and report any loss or theft within 10 days of discovery.

The schedule of the Act lists those drugs—as well as their preparations, derivatives, alkaloids, and salts—that are subject to the Canadian Narcotic Control Act. Included in the schedule are opium, coca, and marijuana. Before a pharmacist may legally dispense a drug included in the schedule or a medication containing such a drug, he or she must receive a prescription from a physician. A signed and dated prescription issued by a duly authorized physician is essential in the case of any narcotic medication prescribed as such or any preparation containing a narcotic in a form intended for parenteral administration. Medications containing a narcotic and two or more nonnarcotic ingredients may be dispensed by a pharmacist on the strength of a verbal prescription received from a physician who is known to the pharmacist or whose identity is established. Prescriptions of any narcotic drug may not be refilled.

There is one exception to the prescription requirement. Certain compounds with a small codeine content may be sold to the public by a pharmacist without a prescription. In such instances the narcotic content cannot exceed 8 mg per tablet or 20 mg/28 mL. In products of this type, codeine must be in combination with two or more nonnarcotic substances and in recognized therapeutic doses. In addition, the labels for items of this nature are required to show the true formula of the medicinal ingredients and contain a caution to the following effect: "This preparation contains codeine and should not be administered to children except on the advice of a physician." These preparations cannot be advertised or displayed in a pharmacy. It is also unlawful to publish any narcotic advertisement for the general public.

Labels of containers of narcotics must legibly and conspicuously bear the proprietary and proper or common names of the narcotic, the names of the manufacturer and distributor, the symbol "N" in the upper left-hand quarter, and the net contents of the container and of each tablet, capsule, or ampule.

Although the administration of the Canadian Narcotic Control Act is legally the responsibility of the Department of National Health and Welfare, enforcement of the law has been made largely the responsibility of the Royal Canadian Mounted Police. Prosecution of offenses under the Act is handled through the Department of National Health and Welfare by legal agents specially appointed by the Department of Justice.

The Narcotic Control Act defines a narcotic addict as "a person who through the use of narcotics has developed a desire or need to continue to take a narcotic, or has developed a psychological or physical dependence upon the effect of a narcotic." A person brought into court for a narcotic offense may be placed in custody by the court for observation and examination. If the person is convicted of the offense and found to be a narcotic addict, the court can sentence him or her to custody for treatment for an indefinite period.

Amendments to this Act place special restrictions on methadone. No practitioner can administer, prescribe, give, sell, or furnish methadone to any person unless the practitioner has been issued an authorization by the Minister of National Health and Welfare.

Application to Nursing. A nurse may be in violation of the Canadian Narcotic Control Act if he or she is guilty of illegal possession of narcotics. Ignorance of the content of a drug in the nurse's possession is not considered a justifiable excuse. Proof of possession is sufficient to constitute an offense. Legal possession of narcotics by a nurse is limited to times when a drug is administered to a client on the order of a physician, when the nurse is acting as the official custodian of narcotics in a department of a hospital or clinic, or when the nurse is a client for whom a physician has prescribed narcotics. A nurse engaged in illegal distribution or transportation of narcotic drugs may be held liable, and heavy

*For more specific information, see *Health Protection and Drug Laws* from Supply and Services Canada, Canadian Government Publishing Centre, Ottawa, Canada, KIA 059.

penalties are imposed for violation of the Canadian Narcotic Control Act.

Apart from the general rules for prescription drugs, certain rules for controlled drugs apply in most health agencies:

1. A prn order (an "as required for pain" order) for narcotics must be rewritten every 7 days in Canada.
2. A standing order (i.e., drug dose administered by the nurse for the physician without obtaining a signed order) is not permitted for narcotic drugs.
3. In an emergency situation a verbal order is permitted if the nurse documents the nature of the emergency in the chart and validates the order within 24 hours.
4. When a narcotic drug is administered to a client, the nurse must record the date, time of administration, client's name, and physician's name, and he or she must sign the entry.
5. When a client refuses a dose of narcotic, it should be placed in the sewage system in the presence of a witness. If a dose of the drug is contaminated or wasted, the nurse should make an entry in the records book explaining how the dose was disposed of, and a witness should sign the entry.
6. All controlled substances stored on nursing units must be kept in locked cabinets so that only authorized personnel have access to them.

STANDARDIZATION OF DRUGS

Drugs may vary considerably in strength and activity. Drugs obtained from plants (e.g., opium and digitalis) may fluctuate in strength from plant to plant depending on where the plants are grown, the age at which they are harvested, and how they are preserved. Because accurate dosage and reliability of a drug's effect depend on uniformity of strength and purity, standardization is necessary.

The technique, either chemical or biologic, by which the strength and purity of a drug are measured is known as **assay.** Chemical assay is a chemical analysis to determine the types and amounts of ingredients present. For example, opium is known to contain certain alkaloids, and these may vary greatly in different preparations. The United States official standard demands that opium contain not less than 9.5% and not more than 10.5% of anhydrous morphine. Opium of a higher morphine content may be reduced to the official standard by admixture with opium of a lower percentage or with certain other pharmacologically inactive diluents such as sucrose, lactose, glycyrrhiza, or magnesium carbonate.

With some drugs, either the active ingredients are not known or there are no available methods of analyzing and standardizing them. These drugs may be standardized by biologic methods in a process called bioassay. **Bioassay** is performed by determining the amount of a preparation required to produce a defined effect on a suitable laboratory animal under certain standard conditions. For example, the potency of a certain sample of insulin is measured by its ability to lower the blood sugar of rabbits.

Drug Standards in the United States. Since 1980 the only official book of drug standards in the United States has been the *USP.* Any drug included in this book has met high standards of quality, purity, and strength. Drugs meeting these criteria can be identified by the letters "USP" following the official name. The *National Formulary (NF),* was established in 1888 by the American Pharmaceutical Association, and through the years it has been the project of pharmacists. When the first Food and Drug Act was passed in 1906, both of these privately issued compendia—the *USP* (revised primarily by physicians) and the *National Formulary*—were established as the official standards by the United States government. Since 1980 the only official book of drug substances and dosage forms in the United States has been the *USP* (Cowen & Helfand, 1990).

Although numerous additional reference books and guides are available on the market, two very valuable resources for drug information in a clinical setting are the *USP DI* and the *American Hospital Formulary Service (AHFS) Drug Information.* The *USP DI* contains information for both the health care provider and the client. Drug information resources are reviewed in Chapter 1.

Drug Standards in Great Britain and Canada. The *British Pharmacopoeia (BP)* is similar to the *USP* in scope and purpose. Drugs listed in the *British Pharmacopoeia* are considered official and subject to legal control in the United Kingdom and in those parts of the British Commonwealth in which the *British Pharmacopoeia* has statutory force. The *USP* is used a great deal in Canada, and some preparations used in Canada conform to the *USP* instead of the *British Pharmacopoeia* because many of the drugs used in Canada are manufactured in the United States.

The *British Pharmaceutical Codex* is published by the Pharmaceutical Society of Great Britain. In general, it resembles the *National Formulary.* The Canadian formulary contains formulas for preparations used extensively in Canada. It also contains standards for new drugs prescribed in Canada but not included in the *British Pharmacopoeia.* The publication has been given official status by the Canadian Food and Drugs Act.

The *Physician's Formulary* contains formulas for preparations that are representative of the needs of medical practice in Canada. It is published by the Canadian Medical Association.

INTERNATIONAL DRUG CONTROL

International control of drugs legally began in 1912 when the first "Opium Conference" was held in The Hague, Netherlands. International treaties were drawn up legally obligating governments to (1) limit to medical and scientific needs the manufacturing of and trade in medicinal opium, (2) control the production and distribution of raw opium, and (3) establish a system of governmental licensing to control the manufacture of and trade in drugs covered by the convention.

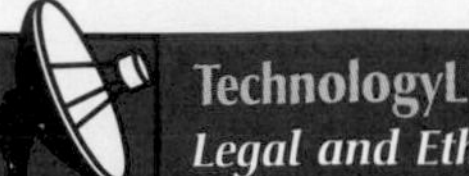

TechnologyLink
Legal and Ethical Aspects of Medication Administration

Video Resources

Mosby's Legal and Ethical Issues in Nursing Video Series, ISBN 0-8151-6010-0

Mosby, Inc., 11830 Westline Industrial Drive, St. Louis, MO 63146; (800) 426-4545; www.mosby.com.

Ethical Dilemmas and Decision Making, ISBN 0-8151-6067-4

Intro to Legal Issues and Terminology, ISBN 0-8151-6069-0

Legal Aspects of Nursing Documentation, ISBN 0-8151-6068-2

Patient Self-Determination, ISBN 0-8151-6071-2

The Nurse's Right as an Employee, ISBN 0-8151-6072-0

Minimizing Legal Liability, ISBN 0-8151-6070-4

Web Resources

American Nurses Association (www.ana.org)

This site contains the ANA Code for Nursing, which includes guidelines for self-determination of clients, social and economic status of clients, and patient rights.

Nursing Ethics Resources (www.nursingethics.ca/)

This site is a good source of general nursing ethics resources, such as codes of ethics, nursing ethics in the news, books and articles on nursing ethics, and links to other biomedical and health care ethics websites.

Nursing Ethics Network (NEN) (www.nursingethicsnetwork.org)

The Nursing Ethics Network is a nonprofit organization of professional nurses committed to the advancement of nursing ethics in clinical practice through research, education, and consultation.

Nursing Ethics Network (NEN) (www.bc.edu/bc__org/avp/son/ethics/nen.html)

The Nursing Ethics Network is an organization of professional nurses dedicated to advancing nursing ethics in clinical settings. It is supported by the Boston College of Nursing.

National Council of State Boards of Nursing (www.ncsbn.org/)

This site contains a variety of nursing resources and documents. This organization is also the developer of the NCLEX examinations.

Truman State University Indexes & Abstracts—Health Nursing, Medicine (www2.truman.edu/pickler/web2000/resources/abstracts/health.html/)

This site has a large bibliography on bioethics, a health information database (free to the public), and other abstracts and databases for nurses and allied health professionals.

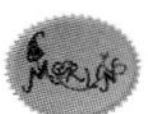

For additional WebLinks, a free subscription to the "Mosby/Saunders ePharmacology Update" newsletter, and more, go to mosby.com/MERLIN/McKenry/.

In 1961 government representatives formulated the "Single Convention on Narcotic Drugs," which became effective in 1964. This act consolidated all existing treaties into one document for the control of all narcotic substances by doing the following:

1. Outlawing their production, manufacture, trade, and use for nonmedicinal purposes
2. Limiting the possession of all narcotic substances to authorized persons for medical and scientific purposes
3. Providing for international control of all opium transactions by the national monopolies (countries designated to produce opium, such as Turkey) and authorizing production only by licensed farmers in areas and on plots designated by these monopolies
4. Requiring import certificates and export authorizations

An **International Narcotics Control Board** was established to enforce this law. This Board is an international organization of governmental representatives established to enforce the "Single Convention on Narcotic Drugs." Enforcement is an immense task, and it is impossible to prevent illicit trafficking in drugs. For example, during a 1-year period it was estimated that 1200 tons of opium were circulated in the illicit market when only 800 tons were considered sufficient to meet world medical needs. Laws need to be frequently updated and strictly enforced, but the unfortunate fact is that financial support for regulation and enforcement is sometimes not equal to the task.

INVESTIGATIONAL DRUGS

The multibillion dollar pharmaceutical industry is constantly screening substances that have the potential to be marketed as new drugs. It may take years and huge amounts of capital for a prospective drug to progress through the following FDA-required testing sequence:

A. Animal studies, to ascertain the following:
   1. Toxicity
      a. Acute toxicity as represented by the LD_{50} (the median lethal dose—the dose that is lethal to 50% of the laboratory animals tested)
      b. Subacute toxicity
      c. Chronic toxicity
   2. **Therapeutic index**—a quantitative measure of the relative safety of a drug; the ratio of the median lethal dose to the median effective dose (the dose that has a therapeutic effect in 50% of the animals tested)
   3. Modes of absorption, distribution, metabolism (biotransformation), and excretion

B. Human studies
   1. Phase I—initial pharmacologic evaluation
   2. Phase II—limited controlled evaluation
   3. Phase III—extended clinical evaluation

A noteworthy lack of correlation exists between levels of toxicity in animals and adverse effects in humans. In addition, many symptoms of adverse effects in humans simply cannot be determined in animals. A partial list of common human symptoms that are not measurably distinguishable in animals includes dizziness, nausea, drowsiness, nervousness, indigestion, headache, and weakness.

FDA Approval Process. The FDA approval process and specifications are as follows:

1. *Investigational New Drug (IND).* An IND application must be completed and submitted to the FDA if a pharmaceutical company or individual wants to investigate either a new drug substance or an old drug for a new indication or at a different, unapproved dosage in humans. The IND will include evidence of drug safety by providing animal or clinical information, proof of the investigator's qualifications to perform this research, and evidence of the drug product's proven quality and strength. The investigation covered under the IND is divided into three phases:
   - *Phase I:* initial pharmacologic evaluation. A small number of normal individuals (usually volunteers) take the drug so that the investigators can determine the pharmacokinetics of the agent (absorption, distribution, metabolism, routes of elimination or excretion). Blood tests, urine analysis, vital signs, and specific monitoring tests are performed during this phase.
   - *Phase II:* limited controlled evaluation. The drug is now administered at gradually increasing dosages to selected individuals with the targeted disease. For example, if the product is believed to have antihypertensive properties, individuals with documented hypertension are chosen for this phase. During this phase the individual is closely monitored for drug effectiveness and side effects. If no serious side or adverse effects occur, the study progresses to phase III.
   - *Phase III:* extended clinical evaluation. The drug is now ready for testing in various centers in the United States in larger numbers of individuals. Standards (protocols) have been developed and are to be followed at all investigative sites. The three objectives for this phase are: (1) determination of clinical effectiveness, (2) determination of drug safety, and (3) establishment of tolerated dosage or dosage range.

   Several other factors are involved with this program. First, the investigator reports to the FDA after completion of each phase and needs its approval before progressing to the following phases. Second, a double-blind study may be instituted, usually in phase II or phase III. A double-blind study involves the administration of the research drug or a placebo (such as lactose) and/or a marketed drug with the same pharmacologic effects as the drug being studied. All of the products are formulated to look the same and are then packaged, usually by code numbers. In general, no one involved with the study knows if the client is taking the study drug (the active drug) or the placebo. This eliminates bias and allows the evaluation to be performed accurately—on the basis of therapeutic response.
2. *New Drug Application (NDA).* After completing phase II of the IND, and assuming the data collected indicate that the new drug is very promising, investigators submit all data to the FDA. After careful review of the information, the FDA may approve or reject the NDA. If the NDA is approved, the drug product can be marketed for the selected indication in the dosing schedules as studied. If the NDA is rejected, the FDA may require additional studies or information before reconsideration.
3. *Abbreviated New Drug Application (ANDA) (for generic drug approval).* Generic formulations of currently marketed medications are not usually required to repeat all of the previous steps before marketing. A company is required to prove that its product can produce the same therapeutic effects as the already marketed drug. Although nearly all generic drugs require the ANDA, the FDA may require different methods to prove generic equivalency, depending on the drug. For example, chlordiazepoxide (Librium) and amitriptyline (Elavil) require in vivo studies; the generic drug must be given to humans, and data from blood and urine studies should be equivalent to data obtained when the name brand product is given, according to statistical analysis. Other drug products, such as chlorpheniramine (Chlor-Trimeton) and dexamethasone (Decadron) need only prove that the manufacturing process is in compliance with Good Manufacturing Practice guidelines and that their quality control standards are equivalent. Thus the FDA establishes criteria according to the drug product, the possibility of bioequivalency problems, or the lack of such problems. Drugs marketed before 1938, such as chloral hydrate and phenobarbital, do not require an approved ANDA before marketing.

The nurse should be aware of several of the limitations of the testing and marketing process. The number of persons studied and the time allotted for the study are limited. In addition, certain types of individuals are excluded from the study, such as children, pregnant women, persons with multiple disease states, persons on multiple medications, and the older adults. A drug is marketed if it is considered safe and effective during the time of study, with the previously mentioned limitations.

Once marketed, the drug is used in much greater numbers of clients and probably for longer periods; thus it is inevitable that the drug will be reported to produce additional

BOX 2-4

FDA Classifications for Newly Approved Drugs*

To assist the professional in immediately classifying new drug entities, the FDA has developed the following method of drug classification. A number and a letter are assigned to each new drug at the IND phase or at the NDA review by the FDA. The manufacturer has a right to contest this classification and have it changed before the final classification is established.

Numerical Classification

1—A new molecular drug
2—A new salt of a marketed drug
3—A new formulation or dosage form not previously marketed
4—A new combination not previously marketed
5—A drug that is already on the market; a generic duplication
6—A product already marketed by the same company (This designation is used for new indications for a marketed drug.)

Letter Classification

A—Drug offers an important therapeutic gain.
B—Medication offers a modest therapeutic gain over drugs already on the market.
C—Drug offers little or no therapeutic gain over other marketed drugs.
M—Drug is marketed in a foreign country.
R—Drug has individual unique conditions for approval that are outlined in NDA approval letter.
T—Drug has toxicity problem (such as carcinogenicity in animals).
U—Drug is apt to be used for treatment of children.
D—Drug has less safety or is less effective as compared with marketed drugs but has a compensating virtue (such as being available for persons who have not responded to or are unable to tolerate the alternative available drugs on the market).
P—The important feature of the product is the container or package, not the drug.

New FDA Classification System

In January 1992 the FDA added a new drug classification system that replaces the A, B, and C ratings. Drugs are now rated P for priority—a new therapeutic advance—or S for standard—a drug that is similar to drugs already on the market. This rating is issued by the FDA when a New Drug Application is received. Drugs approved in 1991 or before will have the A, B, or C rating.

*This classification is available by request from the Freedom of Information Staff at the Bureau of Drugs (Food and Drug Administration, 5600 Fishers Lane, Rockville, MD 20857).

effects (possibly therapeutic but often adverse) that were not noted during the trial studies. Therefore a phase IV, or postmarketing surveillance period, has been advocated to monitor and tabulate information about new drugs and disseminate it to health care professionals and consumers. This is a more difficult phase to supervise because it depends on the voluntary reports of persons in the medical field. The importance of this phase should not be underestimated—it affects many more people than the previous three phases combined. Classifications for newly approved drugs are listed in Box 2-4.

In 1993 the FDA initiated MedWatch, a voluntary program to enhance the reporting by health care professionals of adverse effects they suspect to be related to medications and medical devices. The nurse need not verify the cause of an adverse effect but does need to inform the agency of medication- or medical device–related events that are suspected to have resulted in death or the risk of death, hospitalization, persistent or permanent disability, birth defects, or the need for medical intervention to prevent permanent impairment. The FDA requests that nurses provide information about products even if clients are not involved (e.g., contaminated products or product labeling that might be confusing). Nurse and client confidentiality are maintained in the reporting. The paperwork is a one-page form that can be obtained from the hospital's risk manager or copied from any of the drug reference books previously discussed (Figure 2-1). The American Nurses Association was involved in the development of MedWatch and supports the program for providing another way in which nurses can advocate for client safety.

Informed Consent. All participants in experimental drug studies should be true volunteers and not subjected to any coercion. **Informed consent** must be obtained from all participants. This is the written consent to an experimental procedure by an individual after he or she has been given a careful explanation of the purpose of the study, the procedure to be used, the expected effects, and the risks involved. New drug studies in children require special consideration. In 1983 new rules were created that stipulate the requirement of both children's and parents' consent for research that involves children for studies funded by the Department of Health and Human Services. In addition, researchers must follow more rigorous guidelines to protect a child's rights. The rights of human participants in medical research have come to be protected under the umbrella of the **Nuremberg Code.** This code was developed under the aegis of American physicians as a result of the post–World

MEDWATCH FORM

Form Approved: OMB No. 0910-0291 Expires: 1/31/99
See OMB statement on reverse

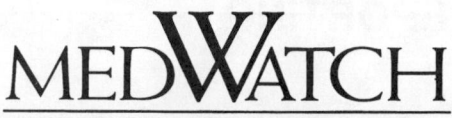

For VOLUNTARY reporting by health professionals of adverse events and product problems

Page ___ of ___

FDA Use Only (AHFS)

Triage unit sequence #

A. Patient information

1. Patient identifier — In confidence
2. Age at time of event: or Date of birth:
3. Sex ☐ female ☐ male
4. Weight ___ lbs or ___ kgs

B. Adverse event or product problem

1. ☐ Adverse event and/or ☐ Product problem (e.g., defects/malfunctions)
2. Outcomes attributed to adverse event (check all that apply)
   - ☐ death ______ (mo/day/yr)
   - ☐ life-threatening
   - ☐ hospitalization – initial or prolonged
   - ☐ disability
   - ☐ congenital anomaly
   - ☐ required intervention to prevent permanent impairment/damage
   - ☐ other: ______
3. Date of event (mo/day/yr)
4. Date of this report (mo/day/yr)
5. Describe event or problem
6. Relevant tests/laboratory data, including dates
7. Other relevant history, including preexisting medical conditions (e.g., allergies, race, pregnancy, smoking and alcohol use, hepatic/renal dysfunction, etc.)

C. Suspect medication(s)

1. Name (give labeled strength & mfr/labeler, if known) #1 #2
2. Dose, frequency & route used #1 #2
3. Therapy dates (if unknown, give duration) from/to (or best estimate) #1 #2
4. Diagnosis for use (indication) #1 #2
5. Event abated after use stopped or dose reduced
   - #1 ☐ yes ☐ no ☐ doesn't apply
   - #2 ☐ yes ☐ no ☐ doesn't apply
6. Lot # (if known) #1 #2
7. Exp. date (if known) #1 #2
8. Event reappeared after reintroduction
   - #1 ☐ yes ☐ no ☐ doesn't apply
   - #2 ☐ yes ☐ no ☐ doesn't apply
9. NDC # (for product problems only) – –
10. Concomitant medical products and therapy dates (exclude treatment of event)

D. Suspect medical device

1. Brand name
2. Type of device
3. Manufacturer name & address
4. Operator of device
   - ☐ health professional
   - ☐ lay user/patient
   - ☐ other: ______
5. Expiration date (mo/day/yr)
6. model # ______ catalog # ______ serial # ______ lot # ______ other #
7. If implanted, give date (mo/day/yr)
8. If explanted, give date (mo/day/yr)
9. Device available for evaluation? (Do not send to FDA) ☐ yes ☐ no ☐ returned to manufacturer on ______ (mo/day/yr)
10. Concomitant medical products and therapy dates (exclude treatment of event)

E. Reporter (see confidentiality section on back)

1. Name, address & phone #
2. Health professional? ☐ yes ☐ no
3. Occupation
4. Also reported to
   - ☐ manufacturer
   - ☐ user facility
   - ☐ distributor
5. If you do NOT want your identity disclosed to the manufacturer, place an " X " in this box. ☐

FDA

Mail to: MEDWATCH 5600 Fishers Lane Rockville, MD 20852-9787 *or* FAX to: 1-800-FDA-0178

FDA Form 3500 (6/93)

Submission of a report does not constitute an admission that medical personnel or the product caused or contributed to the event.

Figure 2-1 MedWatch form and advice about voluntary reporting. (From MedWatch: The FDA Medical Products Reporting Program. Rockville, MD: Department of Health and Human Services, Public Health Service, Food and Drug Administration.)

Continued

ADVICE ABOUT VOLUNTARY REPORTING

Report experiences with:
- medications (drugs or biologics)
- medical devices (including in-vitro diagnostics)
- special nutritional products (dietary supplements, medical foods, infant formulas)
- other products regulated by FDA

Report SERIOUS adverse events. An event is serious when the patient outcome is:
- death
- life-threatening (real risk of dying)
- hospitalization (initial or prolonged)
- disability (significant, persistent or permanent)
- congenital anomaly
- required intervention to prevent permanent impairment or damage

Report even if:
- you're not certain the product caused the event
- you don't have all the details

Report product problems – quality, performance or safety concerns such as:
- suspected contamination
- questionable stability
- defective components
- poor packaging or labeling

How to report:
- just fill in the sections that apply to your report
- use section C for all products except medical devices
- attach additional blank pages if needed
- use a separate form for each patient
- report either to FDA or the manufacturer (or both)

Important numbers:
- 1-800-FDA-0178 to FAX report
- 1-800-FDA-7737 to report by modem
- 1-800-FDA-1088 for more information or to report quality problems
- 1-800-822-7967 for a VAERS form for vaccines

If your report involves a serious adverse event with a device and it occurred in a facility outside a doctor's office, that facility may be legally required to report to FDA and/or the manufacturer. Please notify the person in that facility who would handle such reporting.

Confidentiality: The patient's identity is held in strict confidence by FDA and protected to the fullest extent of the law. The reporter's identity may be shared with the manufacturer unless requested otherwise. However, FDA will not disclose the reporter's identity in response to a request from the public, pursuant to the Freedom of Information Act.

Figure 2-1, cont'd MedWatch form and advice about voluntary reporting. (From MedWatch: The FDA Medical Products Reporting Program. Rockville, MD: Department of Health and Human Services, Public Health Service, Food and Drug Administration.)

War II Nuremberg trials of Nazi physicians who had conducted experiments on political prisoners without their consent. In essence, the Code states the following:

1. Truly voluntary consent of the human subject is critical.
2. The experiment must be proved to be valid or made possible only through the use of human subjects.
3. The results and risks are justified by the study.
4. Unnecessary suffering, death, or disability will be avoided.
5. The experiment will be conducted in a careful and professional manner by scientifically qualified persons.
6. The subject or the investigator may terminate the experiment at any point that it is felt unendurable or impossible.

Additionally, any experimental drug trials using humans, if supported by the Department of Health and Human Services, must also meet federal guidelines for the protection of participants. Institutions supporting such investigational research have review boards that evaluate aspects of the research as it affects human subjects and that formally approve or disapprove research proposals accordingly.

Pregnancy Safety Categories. Before any drug is used during pregnancy, the expected benefits should be considered against the possible risks to the fetus. The FDA has established a scale to indicate drugs that may have documented problems in animals and/or humans during pregnancy, but for many drugs this information is unknown. The prescriber, nurse, and client should carefully review any precautionary information before using the drug product. The categories are as follows (*Drug Facts and Comparisons*, 2000):

Category A: Adequate studies indicate no risk to the fetus in the first trimester of pregnancy, and there is no evidence of risk in later trimesters.

Category B: Animal reproduction studies have not demonstrated a risk to the fetus, but there are no well-controlled studies in pregnant women.

Category C: Animal reproduction studies have reported an adverse effect on the fetus, but there are no adequate studies in humans; the benefits of the drugs in pregnant women may be acceptable despite its potential risks.

or

There are no animal reproduction studies and no adequate studies in humans.

Category D: There is evidence of human fetal risk, but the potential benefits from the use of the drug in pregnant women may be acceptable despite its potential risks—if safer drugs are not available or ineffective.

Category X: Studies in animals or humans demonstrate fetal abnormalities, or adverse reaction reports indicate evidence of fetal risk. The risk of use in a pregnant woman clearly outweighs any possible benefit. These drugs should not be used in pregnant women.

NURSES AND DRUG RESEARCH

Nurses involved in research projects involving human subjects must be knowledgeable about the precepts of the Nuremberg Code and must protect clients by being ever alert to the possibility of subtle errors in protocol or oversights in adherence to the tenets of the Code. The most important elements of the Code relate to a client's right to informed consent and to participation that is fully voluntary and without coercion.

Informed consent must be obtained in writing. This particular consent is heir to the flaws of other client consents: the information conveyed may be incomplete or not delivered in nonmedical language or perhaps presented at a time when the client is sleepy or sedated and not fully cognizant of the ramifications of what is being signed. It is the nurse's obligation to ensure that this does not happen and that it is the researcher or the physician, not the nurse, who gives a full explanation and answers pertinent questions.

Expanding roles in nursing often include nurses on a team that is researching experimental drug development. Indeed, more nurses than ever before are conducting research of their own using human subjects; much of this research is clinical even if not directly related to investigational drugs. Because of a healthy professional commitment to client well-being, nurses may find themselves caught in an ethical conflict. They likely may feel ambivalent about a client's right to know (vis-a-vis the Patient's Bill of Rights) and yet be uncomfortably aware that too much information may unduly influence a person's behavior or condition in some way and thereby adversely influence the variable under study. This area of ethics awaits further study.

Nurses involved in clinical drug studies should be fully informed about the study and the drug under investigation. All information available to the prescriber, researcher, or pharmacist should also be available to the nurse. Ethical and legal responsibilities mandate that a nurse's actions be based on adequate knowledge and skill and that clients be protected from foreseeable harm. This necessitates that the nurse know the recommended dosage range and route of administration, the desired therapeutic effect, and the undesired and toxic effects of the drug being investigated. Throughout the entire investigation the nurse must strictly adhere to the protocols of the study. Recordings of all observations should be as precise as possible because they will have a direct influence on the outcome of the study.

NURSING LEGISLATION

Nursing practice is regulated not only by the previous drug standards and legislation but also by individual state nurse practice acts; joint policy statements among the state nursing associations, medical associations, and hospital associations; and institutional and agency policies. Institutions and agencies may set policies that interpret more specifically those actions allowable under state nursing practice acts, but they may not modify, expand, or restrict the intent of such acts. Personal and professional ethical standards further govern actual nursing decisions and judgments in practice.

The nurse practice acts of individual states define conditions under which nurses may be licensed to practice professionally. One of the functions of these acts is to protect the public from unskilled, undereducated, or unlicensed nurses and to delineate clearly the scope of nursing as a health care profession. Another function is to protect nurses by clearly defining their responsibilities and freedoms. Every state nurse practice act includes laws and regulations on reciprocity and suspension or revocation of nurse licenses.

Changing Nursing Roles. Clearly the traditional roles of the nurse are changing and expanding along with newer techniques and approaches to drug therapy. These expanding roles often find the nurse in activities beyond traditionally accepted nursing practices, which challenge the judgment and accountability of the nurse legally. Two such areas are prescription writing and certain modes of drug administration.

In the past, prescribing medications was a purely medical function as determined by state law, and medication administration was usually delegated to nurses and occasionally to licensed pharmacists and other trained personnel. In reality, astute nurses have been indirectly prescribing for many years, using diplomatic ploys with physicians to attend to changing client needs: "Will you write an order for Dulcolax for Mrs. Rommel? She hasn't had a bowel movement for 3 days." Today certain expanding roles in nursing, along with increased education and expertise (e.g., certification as a nurse practitioner by the American Nurses Credentialing Center and other organizations), have led states to legitimize the prescribing function of nurse practitioners.

Two reports have helped to define this prescribing role, one from the American Medical Association in 1970 and the other from the Department of Health, Education, and Welfare in 1971. Both clearly state that the prescribing of medications "may be the practice of medicine when carried out by a physician and the practice of nursing when carried out by the nurse." As a result of this change, all states have amended their nurse practice acts. These amendments have predominantly given authorization to the nurse practitioner to write prescriptions according to established protocols or under physician supervision or collaboration. As of September 1998, nurse practitioners in all 50 states and the District of Columbia have legislative authority to prescribe (Pearson, 2000). However, within these states there is a wide disparity, with some states having almost no prescription barriers to nurse practitioner practice and others having barriers that are still significant (Box 2-5).

Many states and institutions have developed protocols for designating the types of clients to be treated by nurse practitioners. They have also developed formularies to aid in their selection of prescribed drugs and to provide reviews of their prescribing activities, usually by periodic chart audits. One evaluative study of 1000 nurse practitioner–generated prescriptions demonstrated high levels of accuracy, accountability, and legibility. Of these prescriptions, 25% were for relief of discomfort, 25% were for contraceptive purposes (one fourth of these were for diaphragms), 40% were for antibiotics, 6% were for the treatment of chronic stabilized disorders, and a small number were written in consultation with a physician for controlled substances. Nonprescription preparations such as antacids, aspirin, and vitamin supplements were also recommended by nurse practitioners. Of the drugs ordered, 99% were consistent with the related protocol. There was no evidence of any complications arising from the medication prescribed, and all were deemed appropriate in terms of safety and therapeutic usefulness. It is of interest to note that the ratio of drug prescriptions to clients was lower among the nurse practitioners than among the physicians (Nichols, 1992).

The Socioeconomic Monitoring System of the American Medical Association has ascertained that physicians who employ nurse practitioners or physician assistants are able to charge less for visits and to manage approximately 20% more client visits per week than those who do not. Physicians who employ nurse practitioners report being generally pleased. Physicians who were polled stated that they fully expected more nurse practitioners to be part of the health care delivery system in the future and that this would be for the better. The plethora of studies attesting to the nurse practitioner's functional effectiveness, safety, and acceptance by the client may offer one solution to the high costs, long waits, and depersonalization in health care today.

For a very long period in health care history, drug administration was a function of physicians only. In fact, nurses were kept ignorant of the medications the client might be receiving. Gradually, medication administration has become an interdependent function. Now nurses find themselves assuming increasing responsibility for suggesting and selecting drugs and their dosages and regulation. For example, in the specialty units of some acute care hospitals nurses assume responsibility for titrating the infusion rates and dosages of potent antihypertensive medications against blood pressure parameters. They often are responsible for titrating intravenous (IV) fluids to replace gastrointestinal drainage milliliter for milliliter. In the past, nurses were authorized to administer large-volume, continuous IV infusions. Nurses now also administer medications by small-volume, intermittent IV infusion (by "piggyback," "rider," or "add-a-line"). Many hospitals, particularly in specialized care units, authorize nurses to give very small-volume, undiluted medications either directly into a vein by IV "push" or into IV tubing.

In general, changing roles and functions and the laws that govern them are not enacted simultaneously. Usually a time lag exists between the adoption of a new function and official approval. Thus nurses who fill drug reservoirs for epidural administration of analgesia and inject some medications intravenously are breaking new legal ground. Such procedures are potentially more risky than other medication procedures, and nurses who perform them are probably placing themselves in a tenuous legal position unless (1) they are qualified by virtue of adequate training, education, and experience; and (2) there exists written sanction. Health agency policy provides solid grounding for the nurse to follow in the interpretation of role responsibilities (*Treinis v. Deepdale General Hosp.*—570 N.Y.S. 2d 185, 1991). Policies should be drawn up jointly by the administration of the health care agency

BOX 2-5

Prescriptive Authority for Nurse Practitioners within the United States

States with Independent Nurse Practitioner Prescribing Authority*

Including controlled substances:

Alaska	Maine	Utah†
Arizona	Montana	Washington
District of Columbia	New Hampshire	Wisconsin
	New Mexico	Wyoming
Iowa	Oregon	

States with Dependent Nurse Practitioner Prescribing Authority

Including controlled substances:

Arkansas	Louisiana	Ohio
California	Maryland	Oklahoma
Colorado	Massachusetts	Pennsylvania
Connecticut	Michigan	Rhode Island
Delaware	Minnesota	South Carolina†
Georgia‡	Nebraska	South Dakota
Hawaii	Nevada	Tennessee
Idaho	New Jersey	Vermont
Illinois	New York	Virginia
Indiana	North Carolina	West Virginia
Kansas	North Dakota	

Excluding controlled substances:

Alabama	Kentucky	Missouri
Florida	Mississippi	Texas

Modified from Pearson, L.J. (2002). Annual legislative update: How each state stands on legislative issues affecting advanced nursing practice. *Nurse Practitioner* 27(1), 10-52, Springhouse Corporation, www.springnet.com.

*Independent prescribing means that prescribing is defined by the State Board of Nursing of a state as an activity within the actual practice of a nurse practitioner. It is not statutorily defined as a delegated medical act and so does not require physician collaboration or supervision.

†Schedule IV and/or V controlled substances only.

‡State does not have written prescribing or dispensing authority; falls under delegated medical authority.

and nursing representatives. These policy statements should carefully delineate the roles of nurses, nurse practitioners, and physicians and should present guidelines for these procedures. These statements should also include a list of drugs and routes to be used only by physicians and a list of criteria for permitting nurses to give medications by an IV route or other system. Currently a trend exists in which pharmacy department personnel to draw up and prepare admixtures in large-volume IV solutions before delivering the medication to the nursing area. This procedure is performed under controlled conditions in agency pharmacies, with the goal of reducing IV solution contamination.

At the implementation stage, three conditions should be met before a nurse may legally begin to administer a medication by any mode:

1. The medication order must be valid.
2. The physician/prescriber and the nurse must be licensed. The nonphysician prescriber must be prescribing within the regulations of the state.
3. The nurse must know the purpose, actions, effects, and major side effects and toxic effects of the drug, as well as the teaching required to enable the client or caregiver to self-administer the drug safely and accurately.

A valid order is one that leaves no room for doubt regarding the medication prescribed, its dosage and route, the dosing interval, and the prescriber's name/signature. Moreover, the drug must also be deemed appropriate for that specific client. Because nurses are legally, morally, and ethically responsible for their actions, they must assess the medication order for its preciseness, accuracy, and appropriateness.

The medication order must be written and worded in a way that is correct, complete, legible, and clearly understandable. If it is not, clarification must be sought from the prescriber. Creating a healthy, open, questioning atmosphere in the prescriber-nurse relationship avoids the very real hazard lurking behind "guessing," "assuming," and "not wanting to bother the doctor."

Although not every medication given in error results in actual client harm, the potential always exists. It is wise to avoid such incidents by clarifying the prescribing situation in the ways discussed in the following sections.

Verbal Order. A prescriber's order may be given verbally (often at a client's bedside): "Just give her a little antacid." It is then appropriate to remind the prescriber that nurses cannot give medication unless the order is in writing. If the order is not written at that time, it is often forgotten. If the medication has already been given and it has not been "signed for" by the prescriber, it is illegal until the order is written and signed. Managing this before the prescriber leaves the area is often not possible.

Telephone Order. An order given over the telephone can easily be miscommunicated, misinterpreted, or not clearly heard, and such an order often remains unsigned by the prescriber for too long. Nursing students should not follow or transcribe any unsigned telephone or verbal orders except in emergencies. Many institutions have a specific policy that limits the acceptance of verbal or telephone orders to emergency situations only. In any event, the prescriber should sign all orders as soon as possible.

Incomplete Order. Orders that are not complete in medication name, dosage, route, time, or signature must be clarified with the prescriber and completed before administration. Orders for medications to be given by the IV route are the ones most often found incomplete; often the rate of infusion is missing from the order.

Incorrect or Inappropriate Order. The order may be judged by the nurse to be incorrect or inappropriate for the client. An example of this would be a dose too high for a client of low body weight or impaired renal function as evidenced by low creatinine clearance or a medication that is noted to have secondary effects of tachycardia or dysrhythmias and is ordered for a client with a recent myocardial infarction. Such a situation may be quite intimidating to the nurse, who is now in the position of challenging the judgment of the prescriber at the risk of incurring embarrassment, a job threat, or both. Of course, such intimidation is not justifiable. It is the nurse's or nursing student's absolute right and responsibility to question any proposed action that is potentially harmful to a client. Medications are written by the prescriber at a given time in the treatment of the client. However, the condition of the client may change, and thus the nurse must exercise critical judgment regarding the appropriateness of each dose for that client before administering it.

Prescribers and some nurses (and many consumers) often are under the mistaken impression that nurses who merely act by following a prescriber's order are absolved from any untoward results of that act. Actually, *no one can relieve a nurse of responsibility for his or her actions*; for a nurse to carry out an order that he or she knows to be incorrect constitutes negligence. Changing an order by modifying any part of it without consultation with the prescriber is similarly illegal.

If an order is believed to be in error, some suggested actions are as follows:

1. Validate the order by consulting an authoritative reference source, such as the *USP DI* or *AHFS Drug Information*.
2. If the order is apparently incorrect, objectively report the conflicting facts and discuss it with the prescriber in a factual, nonblaming manner.
3. If the prescriber still wants the medication given as ordered after the nurse's objections have been raised, can the nurse give the medication if the prescriber takes full responsibility? Again, *no one* can release nurses from full responsibility for every medication they give just because they are acting under a prescriber's order. To do so is to court a lawsuit for negligence. This fact must be made clear to the prescriber as the rationale for the nurse's refusal to medicate.

If the prescriber chooses to administer the medication personally after the nurse refuses to do so in the belief that it could be potentially harmful to the client, the nurse should see that the facts of the situation are made known to the immediate supervisors, and consultation should be sought if necessary. Every health care agency should have in place a mechanism for such reporting (*Campbell v. Pitt County Mem. Hosp.*—352 S.E. 2d 902-N.C., 1991). If the drug is given, the medication record should reflect that it was the prescriber who gave it.

Invalid Order. Orders signed by medical students, physician assistants and, in some states, nurse practitioners are not legally accepted as having been signed by a duly licensed physician (this is the wording of many nursing practice acts) and should not be until a physician actually signs it (unless the law is changed). Nurses should be aware of the policy of their health agency and state regulation. The validity of orders written and signed by an unlicensed intern or resident may be equivocal depending on local law or policy.

Order for Unfamiliar Drug. Orders for a medication that is unfamiliar to the administering nurse must stimulate a nearly reflex reaction to "look it up" or to "ask the pharmacist." Administering an unfamiliar drug while remaining in ignorance of its actions, its intended effects and side effects, and its adverse reactions (at the very minimum) is considered nursing negligence if it results in harm to the client. In one instance a nurse was found liable when a 3-month-old infant died after being given an injectable form of digoxin instead of the pediatric elixir. In another instance hospital staff members were found negligent when prolonged infiltration of a dopamine infusion went unobserved, causing permanent injury (*Macon-Bibb Hosp. Authority v. Ross*—335 S.E. 2nd 633-GA) (Box 2-6).

Safeguards. Astute nurses are alert not only to the set limits of functioning but also to the quality of functioning within those limits. Although lawsuits can be initiated when a nurse exceeds the limits of accepted practice, few have actually been instituted. However, more lawsuits can be anticipated in the near future as the public becomes more aware of the liability of nurses. Most lawsuits are brought by clients or families who feel they have been subjected to a behavior or procedure that was not of the quality reasonably expected of someone with a nurse's professional education and experience and under the particular circumstances. This is identified legally as **malpractice**. The nurse can take precautions against malpractice resulting from errors of medication administration by observing the **Five Rights of Medication Administration**:

1. The *right medication* (the one that was prescribed and one that is not contraindicated)
2. The *right client* (not someone else's medication by mistake, or someone in the next bed)
3. The *right dose* as prescribed and appropriate (this may involve simple mathematical computations)
4. The *right route, form of the drug, and administration technique* as prescribed
5. The *right time* for the dose (usually within half an hour

BOX 2-6

Legal Aspects of the Nursing Role

How often do nurses encounter an infiltrating IV in the routine care of clients? The assessment and action taken by the nurse can be significant for the client, as in the case of *Macon-Bibb Hosp. Authority v. Ross* (335 S.E. 2d 633-GA).

Ms. Ross was brought to the emergency department with dyspnea, bradycardia, and a blood pressure of 250/150 mm Hg. She went into respiratory arrest at 2:55 PM; she was intubated with an endotracheal tube, and nitroprusside was administered intravenously to decrease her blood pressure. Because of the rapid drop in blood pressure, an IV administration of dopamine was started at 3:28 PM in her right wrist to increase her blood pressure. When her blood pressure stabilized, she was transferred to the cardiac care unit at 4:30 PM. At midnight, a nurse noted that the IV site had a "bruise bluish in color." The next notation was at 11:00 AM the following day, in which it was recorded that the client's right arm was swollen and painful with a large blistered area around the IV site. The same notation was made at 4:00 PM. It was not until 6:50 PM that a note indicated that a physician was informed of the infiltration. As a result of the extravasation of dopamine, the client's lower right arm was permanently scarred. On a jury verdict, the court entered judgment for the client.

The hospital appealed, but the court of appeals affirmed the judgment of the lower court. It was noted that although an infiltration may result from an improper technique, it may also be due to the size of the needle, the status of the client's veins, or a particular intolerance to an IV. According to the expert nurse's testimony and supported by suitable references, dopamine should be infused into a "large vein," such as in the antecubital fossa, to minimize the risk of extravasation. In addition, dopamine should be monitored continuously for free flow. If extravasation of dopamine occurs, the recommended treatment of the site is infiltration with a saline solution of phentolamine (Regitine) within 12 hours.

The nurses were criticized for not being sufficiently knowledgeable regarding dopamine, which resulted in their failure to notify a physician of the client's impaired tissue integrity.

Critical Thinking Questions

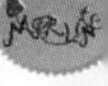

- How could the emergency department nurse caring for Ms. Ross have prevented this incident?
- What action should have been taken by Ms. Ross's admitting nurse in the intensive care unit to prevent this incident?
- What action should have been taken by the nurse who noted that the IV site had a "bruise bluish in color"?
- In what way could this hospital prevent a similar occurrence in the future?

of the time indicated and at beneficial intervals as ordered)

The following are examples of nursing actions that support and facilitate meeting these five rights:

- Refusing to allow administration of a drug against good nursing judgment
- Preparing medications in a quiet, undisturbed environment conducive to thoughtfulness and accuracy
- Comparing the information on the medication Kardex or computer printout sheet with the prescriber's order and medication chart to prevent administering the wrong dose, double-dosing, or making similar errors
- Looking up information about all new or unfamiliar drugs before administering them
- Reading medication labels three times: when taking the drug container from its storage place, when preparing the dose, and when returning the drug container to its storage place
- Carefully calculating the dose as necessary, especially when working with decimals
- Administering only drug doses that were self-prepared
- Positively identifying the client by comparing the arm band with the name on the medication administration record
- Listening intently to clients when they question the administration of a particular drug, state a possible allergy, or question the drug's color, size, or dose; clients often give nurses crucial data in this manner
- Recording the administration of each dose as soon as possible
- Observing carefully for side effects and adverse effects, reporting them, and documenting the actions taken

For the nurse's part, *accountability* is a term that has gained increasing importance, particularly as related to pharmacotherapeutics. Nurses are no longer considered to be merely "physicians' handmaidens" or to be accorded "umbrella protection from litigation" by the prescriber and the health care agency. Nurses are increasingly expected to take the responsibility for and be answerable for the service they provide or make available.

In summary, the basic guidelines to litigation-free, professional nursing practice and to medication administration in particular include the following:

1. Knowing the limitations of nursing practice in the community by being aware of and abiding by agency policies, joint medical and nursing practice statements, nursing practice acts, and state and federal laws.
2. Knowing the limitations of one's own skills, expertise, knowledge, and experience and never exceeding them.
3. Informing involved personnel of and documenting thoroughly and carefully all happenings related to client care, especially those with potential legal implications.
4. Maintaining a professional, caring, and collaborative relationship with clients and their families. Aside from this approach being proper, it can act to dissolve the potential dissatisfaction of clients with health care, the institution, or its policies.

ETHICAL CONSIDERATIONS

Value conflicts for nurses occur as a result of the changing legislation governing many of their activities in relation to medication administration , the increasing role of nurses in clinical research in pharmacotherapeutics, and day-to-day practice in which nurse, client, and prescriber may have differing opinions as to what measures to take in a specific situation.

Probably the most powerful fundamental force at work in the actual implementation of right and proper nursing practice is the nurse's own concept of ethical and moral correctness and responsibility. The American Nurses Association (1985), the Canadian Nurses Association (1980), and the International Council of Nurses (1973) (Ellis & Hartley, 1995) have adopted similar codes of ethics for nurses, which can serve as guides to standards of conduct, relationships, and practice. The nurse's responsibilities to clients as defined by these codes of ethics are to promote health, prevent illness, restore health, and alleviate suffering. The core of any such professional code is that its precepts spring from the reality that the client is a person with rights and dignity not to be subsumed under the needs or rights of any other person or the machinations of a health care agency or society at large. Thus nurses are obligated to respect the wishes of clients and to treat them with dignity. For example, a client has every right to know the necessary information about a drug he or she is receiving and to refuse to take a drug after having been given an explanation, no matter what the consequences. A client's right to respect from the nurse is independent of nationality, race, creed, color, age, sex, politics, or physical or social status.

When ethical dilemmas occur, nurses may experience conflicting loyalties to their profession, colleagues, clients, agencies, and society. Nursing ethics, which provide guidance for nursing action, are based on the principles of **nonmalfeasance** (the duty to do no harm), **beneficence** (the duty to do good), client autonomy, truthfulness, justice, fidelity (faithfulness to one's obligations), and integrity (being true to one's word). These issues are essential to the bond of trust in the nurse-client relationship and demonstrate the caring perspective that is at the heart of nursing practice. The tenets of the codes of practice for nurses assure the client that the nurse will act in the client's best interest.

This obligation of the nurse to the client includes respecting the client's values, whether or not the nurse agrees with the client's decision in relation to his or her health care. For example, some clients might value remaining mentally alert and in control of their experiences over taking medications that would offer pain relief but could also alter their thought processes. The responsibility of the nurse is to assist the client in the decision-making process by ensuring that the client is informed of the risks and benefits of the therapy and can make a knowledgeable decision.

NURSING PRACTICE

Early in a nursing career, the study of legal issues related to the administration of medications can seem a somewhat less than fascinating exercise. However, as the nurse builds practical experience, this study proves its worth time and time again. Laws, acts, codes, and regulations shaping pharmacologic practice provide the boundaries for safe practice. Experience proves that knowing the accepted scope of nursing practice of one's nation, state, locale, and institutional community provides security and support for the nurse who aspires to provide harm-free care. Legal statutes only guide; nurses must translate these guides into action. Often what provides the best guidance within legal constraints is the judgment of the individual nurse on the basis of his or her own code of ethics, professionalism, and sense of accountability. A fundamental precept is that what is best for the client usually turns out to be best for the nurse.

There are few hard and fast rules in nursing practice. Many specific questions about legalities in drug administration must be answered, and the answer is often "It depends. . . ." This should not immobilize nurses and prevent them from acting in healthy, assertive ways. If they function within the accepted boundaries of practice, continue to stretch for new knowledge, and act accountably for the benefit of their clients, little exists that can harm their clients, themselves, their professional reputations, or their jobs. The sureness that comes with experience flourishes as these skills are exercised. Exercising these skills often demands standing up for what is right in client care despite pressures generated by time constraints or by others who want them to "just get on with it." Being human, nurses will occasionally fail to use the best judgment or to be perfect. This is reasonable, but it is also reasonable for nurses to aspire to structure their practice in ways that make it difficult to fail.

The neophyte nurse may be somewhat shaken by the wealth of background information necessary to safe practice. The more experienced nurse will probably grapple with the temptation to become complacent and to make dangerous assumptions about the limits of his or her practice. Both have an equal need to continue to read and question in order to improve the quality of their decisions, whether the issues stem from legal, ethical, or moral considerations.

Although sophisticated and well regulated in theory, the art of drug development, evaluation, and prescribing may sometimes be inadequate in practice. Because all chemical substances create side effects, adverse reactions, and interactions and because many have been identified as having questionable efficacy, it becomes increasingly compelling to avoid medicating when feasible and to substitute rational nursing measures. For example, if instituted effectively and early in the pain cycle, nursing interventions to promote comfort can often substantially reduce pain so that "as necessary" medications become less necessary.

SUMMARY

Although substances to treat illness and cure disease have always existed, it was not until the twentieth century that the need to standardize and regulate such substances became apparent. In the United States the Pure Food and Drug Act of 1906 was the first to limit false and misleading claims for drugs, but only those involved in interstate commerce. *USP* and the *National Formulary* were established as official standards for drugs. Further legislation in 1938 required the testing of drugs for safety, and in 1952 the requirements for distinction between legend drugs and OTCs were established. Since that time both types of preparations have proliferated and there has been constant review to ensure their safety and efficacy.

The Harrison Narcotic Act of 1914 was the first law passed by any nation to regulate opium and other substances producing drug dependence. Currently such drugs are governed by the Controlled Substances Act which, in addition to other regulation, classifies controlled substances into their compared use and abuse potential. This law influences the daily routine of many nurses; a controlled substances count is performed at the beginning and end of every shift in settings where supplies of these drugs are maintained. Other protection in effect for consumers includes the reporting of drug reactions by clinicians to the FDA, the regulation of biologic products by the Public Health Service, and the legislation of product liability by many states.

Similar legislation exists in Canada for the protection of its citizens. Although often amended, the Canadian Food and Drugs Act of 1953 stipulates the standards for drugs through a variety of pharmacopoeias and formularies, prohibits the sale of unsafe drugs and those with misleading labels, and in general regulates biologic, legend, controlled, and designated drugs. The Canadian Narcotic Control Act of 1961 governs the possession, sale, manufacture, production, and distribution of narcotics. By this Act a nurse can be in legal possession of a narcotic only when administering a drug on the order of a physician, acting as the official custodian of narcotics in a hospital or clinic, or being a client for whom a physician has prescribed a drug.

Because drugs vary in strength and activity, standardization is necessary to ensure uniformity of strength and purity by either chemical or biologic assay. The only official book of drug standards in the United States is the *USP,* whereas Canada uses the *USP,* the *Canadian Formulary,* and the *British Pharmacopoeia.*

The progress of any drug from concept to acceptance in general practice is lengthy and costly. The FDA approval process ensures that each drug progresses sequentially after being classified as an Investigational New Drug, with an initial pharmacologic evaluation, a limited controlled evaluation, and an extended clinical evaluation. If the drug is promising, an NDA is submitted to the FDA for approval. If the NDA is approved, a postmarketing surveillance period follows. All participants in the experimental studies of this process should have given informed consent. Because nurses have increasing contact with clinical drug studies, they need to understand the precepts of the Nuremberg Code and be alert to the protection of clients' rights.

Nurses in their practice are regulated not only by the legislation previously discussed but also by the nurse practice acts of the individual state in which they practice. These statutes define the scope of nursing practice as a health care profession within that state. As the roles of nurses change and expand in drug therapy, all states are allowing nurse practitioners to prescribe within limitations. Even for nurses without a practitioner qualification, medication administration has become more of an interdependent function. Three conditions are essential for the administration of any drug by a nurse: (1) the medication order must be valid; (2) the physician/prescriber and the nurse must be licensed; and (3) the nurse must be knowledgeable about the drug. In addition, nurses can safeguard themselves from errors of medication administration by observing the Five Rights of Medication Administration. With increasing accountability for their role in pharmacotherapeutics, nurses should be aware of guides to litigation-free, professional nursing practice.

Critical Thinking Questions

1. A nurse is working with a client with advanced cancer for whom the physician orders chemotherapy. The client has reservations about starting the chemotherapy regimen and asks numerous questions about the benefits and risks associated with it. The nurse has been told that the client's condition is terminal and knows that the chemotherapy may alter the client's comfort with severe nausea and vomiting. Although the nurse realizes that the physician recommends the chemotherapy, she feels a conflict with her role as client advocate. What action should the nurse take?
2. A nurse is preparing to administer medications to a client in a home setting when she notices that the container for one of the medications, instead of having a drug name, bears a number as an experimental drug with instructions to be given "one tablet three times a day." What action should the nurse take?

Collaborative Learning Activities

For Collaborative Learning Activities, go to mosby.com/MERLIN/McKenry/.

BIBLIOGRAPHY

American Nurses Association. (1985). *Code for nurses with interpretive statements.* Kansas City, MO: Author.

Anderson, KN, Anderson, L.E., & Glanze, W.D. (Eds.). (1998). *Mosby's medical, nursing, & allied health dictionary* (5th ed.). St. Louis: Mosby.

Benjamin M. & Curtis J. (1992). *Ethics in nursing* (3rd ed.). New York: Oxford University Press.

Blake J.B. (Ed.). (1968). *Safeguarding the public: Historical aspects of medicinal drug control.* Baltimore: The Johns Hopkins University Press.

Canadian Nurses Association. (1980). *CAN code of ethics: An ethical basis for nursing in Canada.* Ottawa: Author.

Couig, M.P. & Merkatz, R.B. (1993). MedWatch: The new medical products reporting program. *American Journal of Nursing, 93*(8), 66.

Covington, T.R. (Ed.). (1996). *Handbook of nonprescription drugs* (10th ed.). Washington, DC: American Pharmaceutical Association.

Cowen, D.L. & Helfand, W.H. (1990). *Pharmacy: An illustrated history.* New York: Harry N. Abrams.

Dippel, J.V.H. (1993). Legally speaking: Reporting to the FDA. *RN, 56*(12), 61-62.

Drug Enforcement Administration. (1990). *Pharmacist's manual: An informational outline of the Controlled Substance Act of 1970.* Washington, D.C.: Department of Justice.

Drug Facts and Comparisons. (2000). St. Louis: Facts and Comparisons.

Ellis, J.R. & Hartley, C.L. (1995). *Nursing in today's world: Challenges, issues, and trends.* Philadelphia: J.B. Lippincott.

Farley, D. (1987/1988). Getting outside advice for the "close calls" . . . advise FDA about the safety and effectiveness of drugs and biological products. *FDA Consumer, 21*(10), 14.

Farley, D. (1987/1988). How FDA approves new drugs. *FDA Consumer, 21*(10), 6.

Gift, A.G. (1993). Informed consent and vulnerable subjects. *Clinical Nurse Specialist, 7*(4), 183.

Johnson, J.M. (1986). Clinical trials: New responsibilities and roles for nurses. *Nursing Outlook, 34*(3), 149.

Kallet, A. & Schlink, F.J. (1933). *100,000 guinea pigs: Dangers in everyday foods, drugs, and cosmetics.* New York: The Vanguard Press.

Kessler, D.A. (1993). Introducing MedWatch: A new approach to reporting medication and devise adverse effects and product problems. *Journal of the American Medical Association, 269*(21), 2765-2768.

Mahoney, D.F. (1994). Appropriateness of geriatric prescribing decisions made by nurse practitioners and physicians. *Image, 26*(1), 41-45.

Modell, W. & Lansing, A. (1967). *Drugs.* New York: Life Science Library, Time.

New FDA classification system. (1992). *American Pharmacist, NS32*(4), 11.

Nichols, L.M. (1992). Estimating the cost of underusing advanced practice nurses. *Nursing Economics, 10*(5), 343.

Pearson, L.J. (2000). Annual legislative update: How each state stands on legislative issues affecting advanced nursing practice. *Nurse Practitioner, 25*(1), 16-21.

Shapiro, R.S. (1994). Legal bases for the control of analgesic drugs. *Journal of Pain & Symptom Management, 9*(3), 153-159.

Tabak, N. (1995). Decision making in consenting to experimental cancer therapy. *Cancer Nursing, 18*(2), 89-96.

United States Pharmacopeia Dispensing Information (USP DI): Drug information for the health care professional. (1999). (19th ed.). Rockville, MD: United States Pharmacopeial Convention.

Young, J.H. (1961). *The toadstool millionaires: A social history of patent medicines in America before federal regulation.* Princeton, NJ: Princeton University Press.

3 Principles of Drug Action

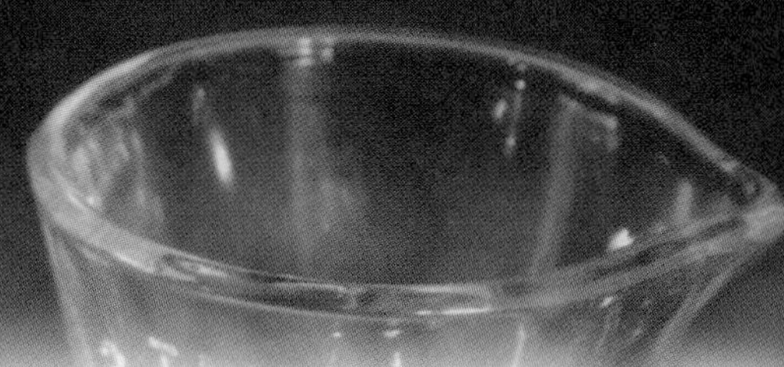

Chapter Focus

The number of drugs used therapeutically is increasing tremendously, and because of this the nurse's responsibilities concerning these agents have also expanded. To approach the level of knowledge needed to meet these increased responsibilities, all health care professionals must develop a fundamental theoretical framework within which to study and apply an understanding of drug therapy. This chapter presents theories of drug action, physiologic processes mediating drug action, variables affecting drug action, and unusual and adverse reactions to drug therapy. The nurse can transfer this knowledge to the care of the unique problems of individual clients.

Learning Objectives

1. Discuss the three general properties of drugs.
2. Describe the three phases of drug activity: pharmaceutical, pharmacokinetic, and pharmacodynamic.
3. Cite examples of drug properties that influence pharmacokinetics.
4. Describe the physiochemical processes mediating drug action.
5. Discuss the client variables that influence the rate and extent of absorption, distribution, metabolism, and elimination.
6. Explain current theories of drug action: drug-receptor interaction, drug-enzyme interaction, and nonspecific drug interaction.
7. Discuss conditions that can alter the body's response to drugs.
8. Use nursing assessments that can identify unusual and adverse reactions to drug therapy.
9. Implement nursing management of drug therapy related to client variables that alter drug responses.

Key Terms

absorption, p. 35
bioavailability, p. 45
biotransformation, p. 41
dissolution, p. 33
distribution, p. 39
excretion, p. 42
half-life, p. 45
iatrogenic, p. 48
loading or priming dose, p. 36
maintenance dose, p. 36
pharmaceutics, p. 33
pharmacodynamics, p. 43
pharmacokinetics, p. 34
receptor, p. 43
therapeutic index, p. 45

Nurses have traditionally administered drugs to clients. In many health care delivery settings today, the nurse's responsibility has shifted to client education for the safe and effective administration of drugs, as well as the observation, interpretation, and documentation of the client's response to drug therapy. The nurse may also be responsible for ensuring the safe administration of drugs by delegation of that task to a variety of specially educated health workers. Because the moral, ethical, and legal responsibilities remain the nurse's, an understanding of the principles of drug action—pharmacokinetics and pharmacodynamics—is essential.

GENERAL PROPERTIES OF DRUGS

As stated earlier, a drug is a chemical that interacts with a living organism to produce a biologic response. This text deals with drugs administered in doses that obtain therapeutic, prophylactic, or diagnostic effects. These effects are achieved through a biochemical and/or physiologic interaction between the drug and a functionally important tissue component (usually a receptor) in the body. It is important to recognize the following general properties of drugs:

1. *Drugs do not confer any new functions on a tissue or organ in the body; they only modify existing functions.* Therefore the effects of drugs can be recognized only by alterations of a known physiologic function or process, such as replacing, interrupting, or potentiating a physiologic process in specialized tissues. For example, drugs used to treat anemia can replace iron to restore the adequate production of red blood cells. On the other hand, atropine reduces the rate of salivation in preoperative clients, which is essentially an abnormal state but a necessary one to decrease the surgical risk of aspiration. The administration of a cathartic can potentiate the rate of evacuation of the large intestine.
2. *In general, drugs exert multiple actions rather than a single effect.* Consequently, drugs may produce undesirable responses to varying degrees because of their potential to modify more than one function of the body. These unwanted effects may be avoided somewhat by administering more specific or more selective drugs. For example, metaproterenol (Alupent) is a selective beta$_2$-adrenergic agent used to produce bronchodilation, and a common side effect is beta$_2$-mediated muscle tremors.
3. *Drug action results from a physicochemical interaction between the drug and a functionally important molecule in the body.* Some drugs act by combining with a small molecule (e.g., antacids neutralize gastric acid) or by altering cell membrane activity (e.g., local anesthetics). However, the major mechanism by which drugs interact is by combining with macromolecular components of tissues, such as receptors.

MECHANISMS OF DRUG ACTION

To produce its optimal effect, a drug must reach the appropriate concentrations at its site of action. This means that the molecules of the chemical compound must proceed from the point of entry into the body to the tissues with which they react. In addition, the magnitude of the response depends on the dose and the frequency of doses of the drug in the body. Therefore the concentration of the drug at its site of action is influenced by various processes that may be divided into three phases of drug activity: pharmaceutical, pharmacokinetic, and pharmacodynamic. The sequential order of these phases is depicted in Figure 3-1.

Pharmaceutical Phase

Pharmaceutics is the study of the ways in which various drug forms influence pharmacokinetic and pharmacodynamic activities. A drug may appear in solid form (tablet, capsule, or powder) or in liquid form (solution or suspension).

Disintegration of solid dosage forms must occur before absorption can occur. The process by which a drug goes into solution and becomes available for absorption is known as **dissolution.** The dosage form of the drug is important—the more rapid the rate of dissolution, the more readily the compound crosses the cell membrane to achieve absorption. Obviously, oral drugs in liquid form are more rapidly avail-

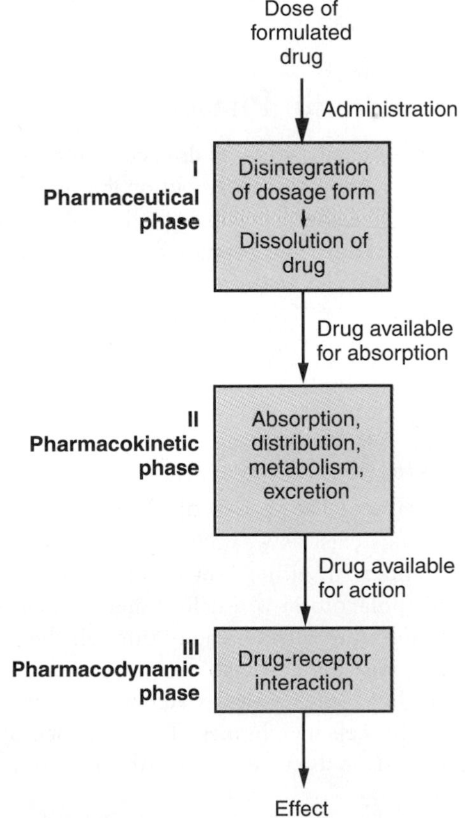

Figure 3-1 Phases of drug activity.

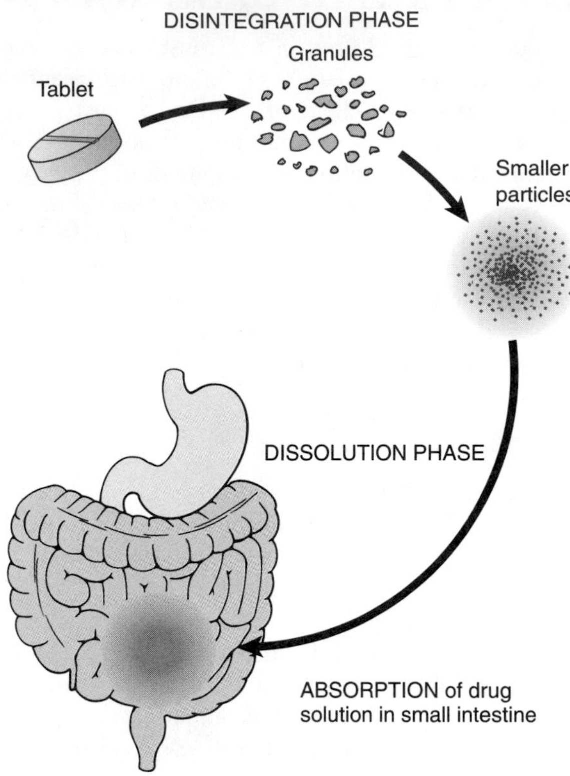

Figure 3-2 Pharmaceutical phase.

able for gastrointestinal absorption than those in solid form (Figure 3-2 and Box 3-1).

Pharmacokinetic Phase

Pharmacokinetics is the study of drug concentrations during the processes of absorption, distribution, biotransformation, and excretion. The concentration of a drug at the site of its action is influenced by four primary factors: the rate and extent to which a drug is (1) absorbed into body fluids, (2) distributed to sites of action or storage areas, (3) biotransformed or metabolized to breakdown or active metabolites, and (4) excreted from the body by various routes (Figure 3-3).

Properties That Influence Pharmacokinetic Activity

Physiochemical Properties of Drugs

In general, drugs exist as weak acids or weak bases and in body fluids appear in either ionized or nonionized forms. The ionized (polar) form is usually water soluble (lipid insoluble) and does not diffuse readily through the cell membranes of the body. By contrast, the nonionized (nonpolar) form is more lipid soluble (less water soluble) and is more apt to cross the cell membranes. The influence of pH on these compounds is discussed under Absorption, p. 35.

Physiochemical Properties of Cell Membranes

The extent to which a drug attains pharmacokinetic activity (absorption, distribution, biotransformation, and excretion)

BOX 3-1

Absorption of Dosage Forms

Dosage form	Rate
Liquids, Elixirs, Syrups	Fastest
Suspension solutions	↓
Powders	
Capsules	
Tablets	
Coated tablets	↓
Enteric-coated tablets	Slowest

depends on the rate at which it crosses the cell membrane. The cell membrane consists of a bimolecular layer of lipids. Protein molecules are irregularly dispersed throughout this lipid bilayer and may act as carriers, enzymes, receptors, or antigenic sites. Drugs that are lipid (fat) soluble pass easily through the lipid membrane, whereas ionized or water-soluble drugs have difficulty crossing cell membranes. The membrane, which appears to contain pores, permits the passage of small water-soluble substances such as urea, alcohol, electrolytes, and water.

Drug molecules, when free to move to sites of action, are transported from one body compartment to another by way of the plasma. However, free movement can be somewhat limited because these various sites are enclosed by membranes. Barriers to drug transport may consist of a single layer of cells (e.g., the villus in intestinal epithelium) or several layers of cells (e.g., the skin). A drug must penetrate these cell membranes in order to gain access to the interior of a cell or body compartment. All of the physiologic processes mediating drug action—absorption, distribution, metabolism, and excretion—are predicated on two physiochemical properties: passive transport and active transport.

Passive Transport. Passive transport, or diffusion, of drugs occurs when the membrane is not required to generate energy to carry out the process. This mechanism involves the random movement of a substance from a region of higher concentration to a region of lower concentration until equilibrium is established at the membrane. The vast majority of drugs are transported via this mechanism. This transport mechanism also forms the basis for many extended-release tablets and rectal formulations (Sjoqvist, Borga, Dahl, & Orme, 1997).

Active or Carrier Transport. Active or carrier transport is usually more rapid than passive diffusion. This mechanism involves the movement of drug molecules against the concentration gradient (from areas of low concentration to areas of high concentration) or, in the case of ions, against the electrochemical potential gradient (such as occurs with the "sodium pump"). An energy source is therefore required. Active or carrier transport is necessary for the transport of moderate-sized ions and water-soluble molecules such as amino acids, glucose and a few drugs (e.g., methyldopa [Aldomet] and levodopa [L-Dopa]). These drugs are transported by carriers that form complexes with

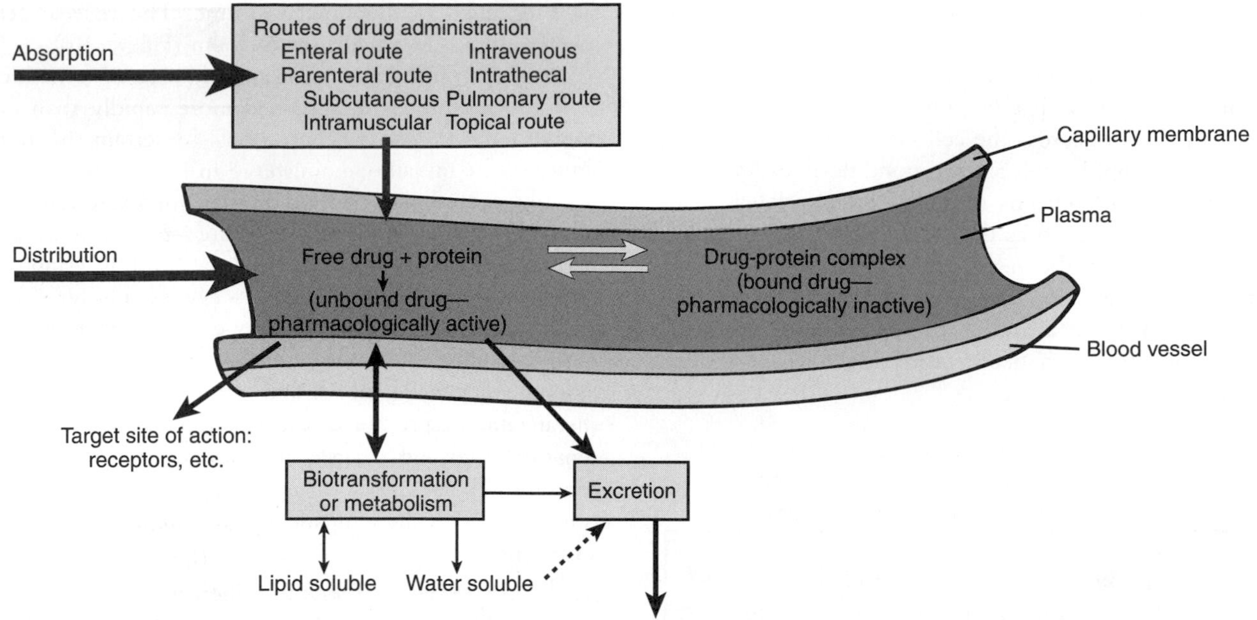

Figure 3-3 Schema of pharmacokinetic phase of drug action. Note that only free drug is capable of movement for absorption, distribution to the target site of action, biotransformation, and excretion. The drug-protein complex represents bound drugs; because the molecule is large, it is trapped in the blood vessel and serves as a storage site for the drug.

drug molecules on the membrane surface, carry them through the membrane, and dissociate from them.

Pharmacokinetic Activities

Absorption

Absorption is a process involving the movement of drug molecules from the site of entry into the body to the circulating fluids. Absorption begins at the site of administration and is essential to the three subsequent processes of distribution, metabolism, and excretion. The rate of drug absorption is significant because it determines when a drug becomes pharmacologically available to exert its action. Of importance is that both the duration and the intensity of drug action are greatly influenced by the rate of this process. The type of response depends on the selection of the *route* of administration, the *dose* of the drug, and the *dosage form* (tablet, capsule, or liquid) of the agent administered.

Variables That Affect Drug Absorption. The rate at and extent to which a drug is absorbed are influenced by the following:

Nature of the Absorbing Surface (Cell Membrane) Through Which the Drug Must Traverse. Transport of a drug molecule is faster through a single layer of cells (intestinal epithelium) than through several layers of cells (skin). The size of the surface area of the absorbing site also is an important determinant of drug absorption. In general, the more extensive the absorbing surface, the greater the drug absorption and the more rapid its effects. Anesthetics are absorbed immediately from the pulmonary epithelium because of the vast surface area. Absorption from the small intestine, which offers a massive absorbing area, is more rapid than from a smaller absorbing surface such as the stomach.

Blood Flow to the Site of Administration. Circulation to the site of administration is a significant factor in the absorption of drugs. A rich blood supply (sublingual route) enhances absorption, whereas a poor vascular site (subcutaneous route) delays it. An individual in shock, for example, may not respond to intramuscularly administered drugs because of poor peripheral circulation. On the other hand, drugs injected intravenously are placed directly into the circulatory system and are totally available. Intravenous administration is desirable when speedy drug effects are necessary, but this mode of administration carries the potential danger of temporarily toxic responses in vital organs such as the heart or brain. To prevent such deleterious effects, most drugs must be injected slowly. In addition, the decreased peripheral blood flow in clients with congestive heart failure or circulatory shock may cause a significant reduction in the rate of transport of injected drugs to target tissues, thereby considerably altering their efficacy.

Solubility of the Drug. To be absorbed, a drug must be in solution; the more soluble the drug, the more rapidly it is absorbed. Because cell membranes contain a fatty acid layer, lipid solubility is a valuable attribute of drugs to be absorbed from certain areas, such as the alimentary tract and the placental barrier. Chemicals and minerals that form insoluble precipitates in the gastrointestinal tract (e.g., barium salts) or drugs that are not soluble in water or lipids cannot be absorbed. Parenterally administered drugs prepared in oily vehicles, such as estradiol, are absorbed more slowly than drugs dissolved in water or isotonic sodium chloride; this allows for weekly injections to maintain the drug in a steady state in the body.

pH. When in solution, drugs are a mixture of ionized and nonionized forms. The nonionized drug is lipid soluble and readily diffuses across the cell membrane, whereas the ionized drug is lipid insoluble and nondiffusible. An acidic drug (e.g., aspirin) remains relatively undissociated in an acidic environment such as the stomach and therefore can readily diffuse across the membranes into the circulation. In contrast, a basic drug tends to ionize in the same acidic environment and is not absorbed through the gastric membrane. Absorption is enhanced in the less acidic or more basic sites, such as the small intestine. The reverse occurs when a drug is in an alkaline medium (Figure 3-4).

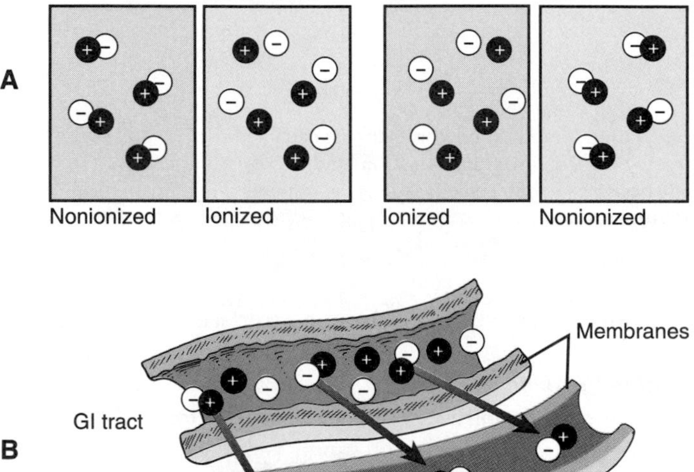

Figure 3-4 Effect of pH on drug ionization and transport. **A,** Effects of pH on drug molecules. **B,** Effects of pH on the transport of drug molecules through membranes.

Drug Concentration. Drugs administered in high concentrations tend to be absorbed more rapidly than drugs administered in low concentrations. In certain situations a drug may be initially administered in large doses that temporarily exceed the body's capacity for excretion of the drug. In this way active drug levels are rapidly reached at the receptor site. Once an active drug level is established, smaller daily doses of the drug can be administered to replace only the amount of the drug excreted since the previous dose. The initial, temporary large doses of the drug are **loading,** or **priming doses** and are used to obtain a rapid therapeutic drug response; the smaller daily doses are **maintenance doses** and are used to maintain a therapeutic drug response (Figure 3-5). Such manipulation of drug doses is often used with digitalis and steroid preparations in acute situations.

Dosage Form. Drug concentrations can be manipulated by pharmaceutical processing. It is possible to combine an active drug with a resin or other substance from which it is slowly released or to prepare a drug in a vehicle that offers relative resistance to the digestive action of stomach contents (enteric coating). Enteric coatings on drugs are used to (1) prevent decomposition of chemically sensitive drugs by gastric secretions (penicillin G and erythromycin are unstable in an acidic pH), (2) prevent dilution of the drug before it reaches the intestine, (3) prevent nausea and vomiting induced by the drug's effect in the stomach, and (4) provide delayed action of the drug.

Routes of Drug Administration. The mode of drug administration affects both the rate at which onset of action occurs and the magnitude of the therapeutic response that results. Therefore the choice of route of administration is crucial in determining the suitability of a drug for an individual client. For example, a client who is vomiting will have little or no appreciable gastrointestinal absorption of a drug when it is administered orally. In such a case rectal or par-

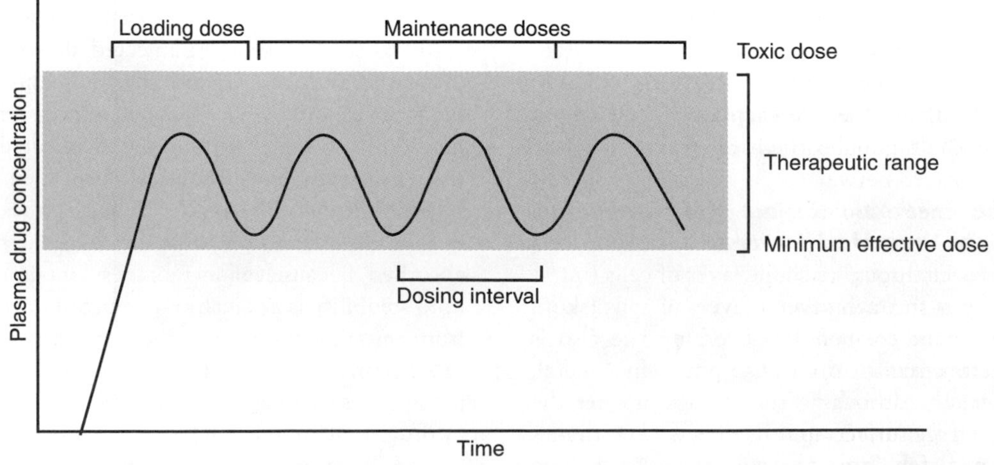

Figure 3-5 A loading dose is administered to reach a therapeutic response level rapidly. Maintenance doses are administered at prescribed intervals to maintain a therapeutic drug response.

enteral administration would be more beneficial in obtaining a therapeutic drug response.

Drugs are given for either local or systemic effects. The local effect of a drug usually occurs at the immediate site of application, in which case absorption is a disadvantage. When a drug is given for a systemic effect, absorption is an essential first step before the agent appears in the circulation and is distributed to a location distant from the site of administration.

A drug may enter the circulation either by being injected directly (intravenously) or by being absorbed from depots in which it has been placed. The routes of drug administration can be classified into the following categories: (1) enteral (administered along any portion of the gastrointestinal tract); (2) parenteral (administered subcutaneously, intramuscularly, intravenously, or intrathecally); (3) pulmonary; and (4) topical (see Figure 3-3).

Enteral Route. In general, oral or enteral ingestion is the most commonly used method of drug administration. It is also the safest (because the drug may be retrieved), most convenient, and most economical route of administration. However, the frequent changes of the gastrointestinal environment produced by food, emotion, and physical activity may make it the most unreliable and slowest of the commonly used routes. Drugs are absorbed from several sites along the gastrointestinal tract.

Oral Absorption. The oral cavity is lined with mucous membranes that consist of epithelial cells; these cells secrete saliva to begin food digestion. Although the oral cavity possesses a thin lining, a rich blood supply, and a slightly acidic pH, little absorption occurs in the mouth. However, despite its small surface area, the oral mucosa is capable of absorbing certain drugs as long as they dissolve rapidly in the salivary secretions. The oral mucosa absorbs drugs given by the sublingual and buccal routes. In sublingual administration the drug is placed under the tongue to permit tablet dissolution in salivary secretions. Nitroglycerin is administered in this manner, and the client is advised to refrain as long as possible from swallowing the saliva containing the dissolved drug. Because nitroglycerin is nonionic with high lipid solubility, the drug readily diffuses through the lipid mucosal membranes. After absorption it enters the systemic circulation without preliminary passage through the liver. Absorption is therefore rapid, and the effects of the drug may become apparent within 2 minutes. In buccal administration the drug (tablet) is placed between the gum and the mucous membrane of the cheek. Some hormones and enzyme preparations are administered by this route and are rapidly absorbed. Both the sublingual and the buccal routes avoid drug destruction by gastrointestinal fluids by bypassing the stomach; they also avoid the first-pass effect of the liver by bypassing the portal circulation.

Gastric Absorption. Although the stomach has a rich blood supply and a large surface area, both of which provide an excellent potential for drug absorption, it is not an important absorption site. The length of time a substance remains in the stomach is a significant variable in determining the extent of gastric absorption. This is governed by gastric motility and the pH of the drug.

In the stomach the pH is low (approximately 1.4), and drugs such as the barbiturates, which are slightly acidic, tend to remain nonionized and thus are readily absorbed into the circulation. Morphine and quinine are slightly basic; they ionize in the stomach and thus are poorly absorbed. A large majority of drugs are weak bases and are absorbed upon entering the small intestine because of the alkaline pH of that environment.

In general, slowing the gastric emptying rate decreases drug absorption, whereas increasing the gastric emptying rate increases drug absorption. Therefore many drugs are administered on an empty stomach with sufficient water (8 ounces) to ensure dissolution, rapid passage into the small intestine, and drug absorption in the larger surface area. Drugs that cause gastric irritation are usually given with food. After the administration of a solid, the client should be encouraged to sit upright for at least 30 minutes to hasten gastric emptying time (time required for the drug to reach the small intestine) and to reduce the potential for tablets or capsules to lodge in the esophageal area. Prolonging gastric emptying time increases the risk of destruction of unstable drugs (e.g., acetaminophen [Tylenol]) by gastric juices.

Absorption in the Small Intestine. The small intestine with its many villi has a larger absorption area than the stomach and is highly vascularized. Drugs that are poorly soluble in the stomach pass into this region and are absorbed primarily in the upper part of the small intestine. The pH of the intestinal fluid is alkaline (7 to 8), which strongly influences the rate of absorption of the nonionized basic drugs. Increased intestinal motility caused, for example, by diarrhea or cathartics may decrease exposure to the intestinal membrane and thereby diminish absorption. Prolonged exposure allows more time for absorption.

Rectal Absorption. Although the surface area of the rectum is not very large, drug absorption can occur because of extensive vascularity. Drugs administered rectally are not immediately subjected to hepatic alteration because the blood that perfuses this region initially bypasses the liver. Disadvantages to rectal drug administration include erratic absorption because of rectal contents, local drug irritation with some medications, and uncertainty of drug retention.

Parenteral Route. The parenteral route refers to the administration of drugs by injection.

Subcutaneous Route. A subcutaneous (SC) injection is given beneath the skin into the connective tissue or fat immediately underlying the dermis. This site is used only for drugs that are not irritating to the tissue; otherwise severe pain, necrosis, and sloughing of tissue may occur. The rate of absorption is slow and can provide a sustained effect.

Intramuscular Route. With intramuscular (IM) administration, a drug is injected into skeletal muscle. Absorption occurs more rapidly than with SC injection because of greater tissue blood flow.

Intravenous Route. The intravenous (IV) route produces an immediate pharmacologic response because the desired concentration of drug is injected directly into the bloodstream, thereby circumventing the absorption process. IV drugs should be administered slowly to prevent adverse reactions.

Intrathecal Route. Many compounds cannot enter the cerebrospinal fluid or are absorbed in this region very slowly because of the protective properties of the blood-brain barrier. With intrathecal administration, the drug is injected directly into the spinal subarachnoid space, thereby bypassing this blood-brain barrier. This route may be used when rapid effects are desired, such as in spinal anesthesia or in the treatment of acute infection of the central nervous system (CNS).

Epidural Route. With epidural administration, a drug is injected via a small catheter into the epidural space of the spinal column—the space outside of the dura mater. This route is increasingly being used with opioids for pain management.

Other Parenteral Routes. Drugs may be injected into other cavities of the body. Intraarticular administration delivers the medication into the synovial cavity of a joint, usually to relieve pain, reduce inflammation, and maintain joint mobility. Intraosseous administration delivers drugs or blood into the bone marrow when IV access is difficult. Intraperitoneal and intrapleural administration of antineoplastic agents allows these drugs to be delivered directly to tumor sites.

Pulmonary Route. To ensure that the normal gas exchange of oxygen and carbon dioxide is continuous in the lungs, drugs must be in the form of gases or fine mists (aerosols) when administered by inhalation. The lungs provide a large surface area for absorption, and the rich capillary network adjacent to the alveolar membrane tends to promote ready entry of medication into the bloodstream. Drugs such as bronchodilators, mucolytics, and antibiotics are administered by various inhalation devices (oral inhalers, nebulizers) that propel the agents into the alveolar sacs and produce primarily local effects and, at times, unwanted systemic effects. In addition, epinephrine may be administered into the intratracheal tube to restore cardiac rhythm in cardiac arrest.

Topical Route. In general, drugs applied topically to the skin and mucous membranes of various structures in the body are absorbed rapidly (see the Nursing Research box below).

Skin. Drugs applied to the skin are used to produce a local or systemic effect through ointments or transdermal patches. Only lipid-soluble compounds are absorbed through the skin, which acts as a lipid barrier. To provide a consistent rate of absorption, only intact skin surfaces are used for the application of most topical agents. Adverse reactions might occur from the systemic absorption of certain topical agents through broken or excoriated skin. Massaging the skin enhances drug absorption because capillaries become dilated and local blood flow is increased as a result of the warmth created by the friction of rubbing.

Transdermal. Transdermal drugs usually consist of a disk or patch that contains a day's to a week's supply of medica-

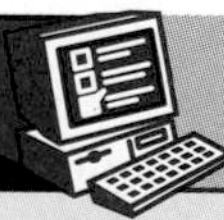

Nursing Research

Perspectives on New Approaches to Drug Delivery

Recent developments in both applied dermal physiology and pharmaceutical technology are expanding the more nontraditional routes of drug administration; this will have an effect on nursing practice. Among these approaches, transdermal and transmucosal applications appear particularly promising because of the accessibility, noninvasiveness, compliance, safety, and efficacy associated with the techniques.

Under normal clinical conditions, the transdermal patch delivers the drug at a rate below the absorbing capacity of the skin. Uptake of the drug by local blood flow then lowers the concentration of the drug in the skin, which maintains the concentration gradient between the transdermal reservoir and the skin. Fentanyl, the prototypical opioid for transdermal applications, is available for general clinical use in the pain management of clients with cancer.

Newly developed for transmucosal administration is a fentanyl lozenge that allows for the comfortable premedication, anxiolysis, and sedation of both children and adults within 20 to 40 minutes. The drug was readily accepted in a candy matrix, provided a rapid onset of action, and provided a high rate of "good to excellent" induction conditions, but dose-related respiratory depression, facial pruritus, nausea, and vomiting also occurred.

The potent synthetic opioid sufentanil and the tranquilizer midazolam have established therapeutic efficacy with intranasal instillation. Despite some limitations, practitioners have developed great skill at administering carefully titrated amounts of premedicant drugs to children and adults.

Nontraditional approaches to the administration of medications are currently under extensive investigation. As these technologies become refined, the ability to achieve and control therapeutic concentrations of drugs within the body will be realized.

Critical Thinking Questions

- What might occur if a client wearing a transdermal patch experiences very low cutaneous blood flow from, for example, hypothermia or low cardiac output?
- What might be of ethical concern with fentanyl lozenges?

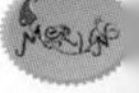

tion. After being applied to the skin, the medication is absorbed at a steady rate. Examples of drugs that are applied transdermally are nitroglycerin (Nitrodisc) and scopolamine (Transderm-Scop).

Eyes. The administration of drugs in the eye produces a local effect on the conjunctiva or anterior chamber. Movement of the eyeball promotes distribution of the drug over the surface of the eye.

Ears. The administration of drops into the auditory canal may be chosen to treat local infection, inflammatory conditions, or wax in the external ear.

Nasal Mucosa. Drugs may be instilled in droplet form or in a prepackaged specific-dose swab intended for direct intranasal application. This mode of administration can be used for systemic absorption or to facilitate shrinkage of the mucosa to enhance breathing or to enable insertion of a nasotracheal tube.

Distribution

Once absorbed, a drug is immediately distributed throughout the body by blood circulation. **Distribution** is defined as the transport of a drug in body fluids from the bloodstream to various tissues of the body and ultimately to its site of action (see Figure 3-3). The rate at which a drug enters the different areas of the body depends on the permeability of capillaries to the molecules of the drug. As already discussed, lipid-soluble drugs can readily cross capillary membranes to enter most tissues and fluid compartments, whereas lipid-insoluble drugs require more time to arrive at their point of action. Cardiac functions also affect the rate and extent of drug distribution; specifically, cardiac output (the amount of blood pumped by the heart each minute) and regional blood flow (the amount of blood supplied to a specific organ or tissue) determine how much time is required. Most of the drug is first distributed to organs that have a rich blood supply, such as the heart, liver, kidney, and brain. Afterward, the drug enters organs with a poor blood supply, such as muscles and fat.

Drug Reservoirs. Storage reservoirs allow a drug to accumulate by binding to specific tissues in the body. This sustains the pharmacologic effect of a drug at its point of action. Storage reservoirs in the body involve two general types of drug pooling: plasma protein binding and tissue binding.

Plasma Protein Binding. On entry into the circulatory system, drugs may become attached to proteins, mainly albumin contained in the blood. As a free drug enters the plasma, it binds to the protein to form a drug-protein complex. This combination can also be reversed:

Free drug + Protein = Drug-protein complex

This formula indicates that equilibrium is established between the amount of free drug and the amount of drug that is bound to protein (drug-protein complex). Protein binding decreases the concentration of free drug in the circulation, thereby limiting the amount that travels to the site of action. Because the drug-albumin molecule is too large to diffuse through the membrane of the blood vessel, the bound molecule is trapped in the bloodstream and is pharmacologically inactive. It thus becomes a circulating drug reservoir or storage depot (see Figure 3-3).

The equilibrium process is dynamic. As free drug is eliminated from the body, the drug-protein complex begins to dissociate so that more free drug is released to replace what is lost. Temporary storage of drug molecules in the drug-protein complex allows the drug to be available for a longer period of time. For example, a sulfonamide is highly bound to protein; because free drug molecules are released slowly from the bound form, the antiinfective action of the antibiotic is long lasting.

Degree of Drug Binding. Plasma protein binding is expressed as a percentage, which represents the percent of total drug that is bound. Among the *highly protein-bound* drugs are warfarin (Coumadin), which is 99% protein bound, and diazepam (Valium), which is 98% protein bound. Accordingly, a ratio exists between free and bound drug. In the case of propranolol (Inderal), 99% is bound to plasma proteins at any given time; only 1% of free drug is available for therapeutic use, eventual biotransformation, and excretion. If more than 1% of the drug is free to act within this same period, toxicity may occur. The *United States Pharmacopeia Dispensing Information (USP DI)* (1999) defines protein binding in general terms with ranges as follows:

- Very high: >90%
- High: 65% to 90%
- Moderate: 35% to 64%
- Low: 10% to 34%
- Very low: <10%

Competition for Binding Sites. Because albumin and other plasma proteins provide a number of binding sites, two drugs can compete with one another for the same site and displace each other. This competition may have dangerous consequences if particular combinations of drugs are administered. For example, serious problems can arise when a client who is satisfactorily stabilized on maintenance doses of warfarin, an anticoagulant, is simultaneously given aspirin, an analgesic. The aspirin may displace some of the protein-bound warfarin, thereby increasing the level of free drug. Although this would seem to increase the drug effect and produce a toxicity that causes severe hemorrhage, the body is an open system capable of eliminating the unbound drug (Katzung, 1998). When the amount of unbound drug increases, the rate of elimination increases if drug clearance (the removal of a substance from the blood via the kidneys) remains unchanged. After four half-lives the unbound concentration returns to its previous steady state if clearance is unchanged. According to Katzung (1998), "When drug interactions associated with protein binding displacement and clinically important effects have been studied, it has been found that the displacing drug is also an inhibitor of clearance, and it is the change in *clearance* of the unbound drug that is the relevant mechanism explaining the interaction." However, Benet, Kroetz, and Sheiner (1996) state that "for narrow therapeutic index drugs, a transient change in unbound concentrations occurring immediately following the dose of a displacing drug could be of concern." Therefore the nurse must be alert to the potential dangers of possible drug interactions when multiple agents are prescribed concurrently.

The more common problem of the competition of drugs for plasma protein is the tendency to misinterpret the results of determinations of serum levels of drugs, because most determinations do not distinguish free from protein-bound drugs.

Hypoalbuminemia. Hypoalbuminemia is characterized by low levels of albumin in the blood. This condition may be caused by malnutrition, hepatic damage (e.g., cirrhosis of the liver), or some type of body cavity drainage. Furthermore, failure of the liver to synthesize enough of the plasma proteins needed to bind drugs means that more free drug is available for distribution to tissue sites. When a client with low plasma protein is given the normal dosage of a drug that normally has plasma protein binding (plasma albumin for acidic drugs and alpha$_1$-acid glycoprotein for basic drugs), more of the free form of drug is allowed into the circulation, resulting in possible overdosage and toxicity. The drug dosage should be adjusted (reduced) until a normal level of plasma protein is reported.

Tissue Binding

Fat. Lipid-soluble drugs have a high affinity for adipose tissue, and this is where these drugs are stored. The relatively low blood flow in fat tissue makes it a stable reservoir for drugs. For example, a lipid-soluble drug such as thiopental (Pentothal) may stay in low concentrations in body fat for as long as 3 hours after administration. Administering this drug again before all of it has been excreted can produce a cumulative effect, because an additional amount of the agent will be stored in the fat tissue.

Bone. Some drugs have an unusual affinity for bone; for example, tetracycline, an antibiotic, accumulates in bone after being absorbed onto the bone-crystal surface. Tetracycline can interfere with bone growth when it accumulates in the skeletal tissues of the fetus (by crossing the placenta from the mother) or young children. Tooth discoloration results when this drug is distributed to unerupted teeth in a fetus or young child. Brownish pigmentation of permanent teeth also may result if this drug is given during the prenatal period or early childhood. Box 3-2 lists specific actions of drugs in fetal tissues.

BOX 3-2

Actions of Drugs in Fetal Tissues

Two major types of drug effects occur in the fetus. When given during the first trimester of pregnancy, some drugs induce the aberrant development of organs and systems during the formation of these structures. This type of drug is known as a teratogenic drug, which is defined as an agent that causes physical defects in a developing embryo. Many drugs that cause anomalies are known to cross the placenta and exhibit teratogenicity.

The second type of drug affects the second half of pregnancy as well as delivery, causing respiratory depression in the newborn because of the underdeveloped capacity of the infant to biotransform the drug and excrete it.

The rate of maternal blood flow to the placenta limits the availability of the drug to the fetus. Because the passage of drugs is delayed, drugs take action in the mother more rapidly than in the fetus. This fact explains why an alert infant can be delivered to an anesthetized mother, provided that delivery occurs within 10 to 15 minutes of the time the drug is administered to the mother. Long-term administration of drugs to the mother, however, may produce adverse reactions with the fetus. For example, infants born to mothers dependent on narcotics or cocaine manifest withdrawal symptoms after delivery and removal from the flow of the products through the mother.

Unfortunately, the teratogenic effects of many drugs have not been adequately studied. In addition, a potentially dangerous drug may be administered to a woman who is not aware of her pregnancy. Sexually active women of childbearing years who are not using contraception should be considered at risk. It should be assumed that any drug is able to pass the placental barrier, and the nurse must advise pregnant women not to take any drug without consulting her prescriber or nurse-midwife. Drugs should be administered during pregnancy only when the advantages greatly outweigh the potential risks to the fetus.

Barriers to Drug Distribution. Specialized structures made up of biologic membranes can serve as barriers to the passage of drugs at certain sites in the body. These include the blood-brain barrier and the placental barrier.

Blood-Brain Barrier. The blood-brain barrier is a special anatomic arrangement that allows the distribution of only lipid-soluble drugs (e.g., general anesthetics, barbiturates) into the brain and cerebrospinal fluid. The blood-brain barrier consists of a row of capillary endothelial cells covered by a fatty sheath of glial cells joined by continuous tight intercellular junctions. Consequently, compounds that are strongly ionized and poorly soluble in fat cannot enter the brain. Antibiotics that are limited in their ability to cross the blood-brain barrier cannot be used to treat infections of the CNS. If the drug is instilled intrathecally, however, it bypasses the blood-brain barrier and directly treats the bacterial infection.

Placental Barrier. The membrane layers that separate the blood vessels of the mother and the fetus constitute the placental barrier. Tissue enzymes in the placenta can metabolize certain agents (e.g., catecholamines) by inactivating them as they travel from the maternal circulation to the embryo. Despite the thickness of the placenta, it does not afford complete protection to the fetus. Unlike the relative impermeability of the blood-brain barrier, the nonselective passage of drugs across the placenta to the fetus is a well-established fact. Although lipid-soluble substances preferentially diffuse across the placenta, the barrier is also permeable to a great number of lipid-insoluble drugs. Consequently, many agents intended to produce a therapeutic response in the mother may also cross the placental barrier and exert harmful effects on the developing embryo. Among the drugs easily transported across the placenta are steroids, narcotics, anesthetics, and some antibiotics.

Metabolism or Biotransformation

Drug metabolism, or **biotransformation,** is the process of chemically inactivating a drug by converting it into a more water-soluble compound or metabolite that can then be excreted from the body (see Figure 3-3). The liver is the primary site of drug metabolism, but other tissues may be involved in the process, such as the plasma, kidneys, lungs, and intestinal mucosa.

Hepatic Biotransformation. The vast majority of drugs are metabolized in the liver by the hepatic microsomal enzyme system. A key element of the hepatic microsomal enzyme system is the cytochrome P-450 system. The microsomal enzymes (and subvariants) usually affect the biotransformation of lipid-soluble, nonionized drugs. To increase ionization or water solubility, they undergo one or both of two general types of chemical reactions. One type of transformation consists of the chemical reactions of oxidation, hydrolysis, or reduction to increase the water solubility of drug molecules. The second type of transformation, conjugation, involves the union of the polar group of a drug with another substance in the body—glucuronide, glycine, methyl, or other alkyl groups. The conjugated molecule also becomes more ionized, or more water soluble, and therefore the result is an acceleration in renal excretion. In general, these responses convert an active drug to an inactive substance (a decrease or loss of pharmacologic activity) and to a substance that is more easily excreted in the urine.

Secondly, many drugs can affect the hepatic enzymes by either increasing or decreasing their activity. The metabolism of some drugs can be enhanced by induction, or increasing hepatic enzymes, so that drug effectiveness is decreased. By inhibiting hepatic enzymes, such as the cytochrome P-450 system, drug metabolism is decreased and the potential for drug interactions and toxicity is possibly increased. Cimetidine (Tagamet) inhibits the P-450 system, which then can diminish the metabolism of warfarin (Coumadin), phenytoin (Dilantin), and many other drugs and lead to toxic reactions.

A third example of hepatic metabolism is the chemical or enzymatic alterations needed to activate a pro-drug. A pro-drug is an inactive substance that must be converted to an active substance in the liver so that the metabolic product can subsequently exhibit the desired pharmacologic response (DiPiro et al., 1997). Some examples of pro-drugs include losartan (Cozaar), benazepril (Lotensin), and sulindac (Clinoril).

The fourth example of hepatic metabolism is the conversion of an active drug to other active metabolites with similar therapeutic effects. Examples include the partial conversion of codeine to morphine, which increases the analgesic effect of codeine. Another is the conversion of the antidepressant amitriptyline (Elavil) to the active metabolite nortriptyline, which was later marketed individually as Aventyl and Pamelor.

In summary, drug metabolism may result in (1) inactivation of the drug; (2) alteration of the drug molecule to increase renal excretion of the drug; (3) induction (increasing) or inhibition of the liver metabolizing enzyme (P-450), which may affect the metabolism of other medications administered (e.g., decreasing drug effectiveness or increasing the potential for drug toxicity); (4) activation of a pro-drug to an active substance; or (5) conversion of an active drug to active metabolite(s) with similar effects. Significant drug interactions are discussed in the individual drug monographs throughout this text.

Other Considerations. Individuals vary considerably in the rates at which they metabolize drugs. The microsomal enzyme system can be depressed by conditions that affect hepatic function, such as starvation and obstructive jaundice. Individuals with liver disease, severe cardiovascular dysfunction, or renal problems may be expected to have prolonged or decreased drug metabolism. Infants with immature metabolizing enzyme systems and older adults with degenerative enzyme function are the major groups that experience depressed biotransformation.

Genetically determined differences also affect metabolism. Some drugs (e.g., procainamide [Pronestyl], hydralazine [Apresoline], and isoniazid [INH]) are metabolized by the acetyltransferase system. This system divides the population into "rapid acetylators" and "slow acetylators." The rapid acetylators metabolize a greater proportion of a drug dose than do the slow acetylators. The rapid (extensive) acetylators may develop reactions caused by the metabolic products of a drug, whereas the slow (poor) acetylators may appear more sensitive to a drug by experiencing severe toxic effects. For example, an individual who is a slow acetylator and is receiving hydralazine (Apresoline) is apt to develop a lupus-like syndrome—a serious adverse reaction. An individual who is a rapid acetylator of the same drug might require higher doses of hydralazine to control hypertension.

If drug metabolism is delayed, cumulative drug effects may be expected and may be manifested as excessive or prolonged responses to ordinary doses of drugs. If drug metabolism is stimulated, a state of apparent drug tolerance is produced. A number of substances cause increased activity by hepatic microsomal enzymes, including CNS depressants, xanthines, pesticides, food preservatives, and dyes. Repeated administration of some drugs may stimulate the formation of new microsomal enzymes. This is the case with some hypnotic drugs (e.g., barbiturates, whose effect diminishes with prolonged administration).

Hepatic First-Pass Effect. Orally administered drugs absorbed from the gastrointestinal tract normally travel first to the venous portal system and the liver before entering the general circulation. Some drugs are first taken up by the hepatic microsomal enzyme system, and a significant amount of the drug is metabolized before ever reaching the systemic circulation. Consequently, only a small fraction of the dose is available for distribution to produce a pharmacologic effect. With such medications, the oral drug dose is calculated to compensate for this effect. For example, propranolol (Inderal) has a very significant hepatic first-pass effect; the oral dose may range from 10 mg to 80 mg, whereas the parenteral usual dose is usually 1 mg to 3 mg to achieve the same therapeutic effect. The hepatic first-pass effect helps to explain why an IV dose of some drugs is so much smaller than an equally potent oral dose.

Some drugs may have a hepatic first-pass effect that totally eliminates pharmacologic activity. These medications, such as lidocaine, require a different route of drug administration (e.g., parenteral) to enter the general circulation, thereby preventing the significant biotransformation as a result of first pass through the liver.

Excretion

A drug continues to act in the body until it is biotransformed or excreted. Drug molecules (intact, changed, or inactivated) must ultimately be removed from their sites of action by physiologic channels involving mechanisms of excretion. **Excretion** is a process by which drugs and pharmacologically active or inactive metabolites are eliminated from the body, primarily through the kidneys.

Kidneys. Drug excretion via the kidneys is the most important route for elimination. Some drugs are excreted unchanged in the urine, whereas other drugs are so extensively metabolized that only a small fraction of the original chemical substance is excreted intact.

Excretion is accomplished through passive glomerular filtration, active tubular secretion, and partial reabsorption (Figure 3-6). The availability of a drug for glomerular filtration depends on its concentration in unbound form in plasma. Free, unbound drugs and water-soluble metabolites are filtered by the glomeruli, whereas protein-bound substances do not pass into the tubular filtrate through the glomeruli. After filtration, lipid-soluble compounds are not excreted but instead are reabsorbed by the tubular nephron and reenter the systemic circulation. The water-soluble compounds fail to be reabsorbed and therefore are eliminated from the body.

Urinary pH varies between 4.6 and 8.2 and affects the amount of drug reabsorbed in the renal tubule by passive diffusion. By altering the pH of urine, increased elimination of certain drugs can be facilitated, thus preventing prolonged action or overdosage of a toxic compound. Weak acids are excreted more readily in alkaline urine and more slowly in acidic urine; the reverse is true for weak bases. Alkalinizing the urine can result in increased urinary drug excretion in cases of poisoning by weak organic acids such as aspirin or phenobarbital. Raising the pH of the urine causes weak acids to become ionized, and subsequently these agents are excreted. Urine may be alkalinized by administering sodium bicarbonate or tromethamine (Tham). In contrast, high doses of vitamin C or ammonium chloride acidify the urine and promote the excretion of alkaline drugs.

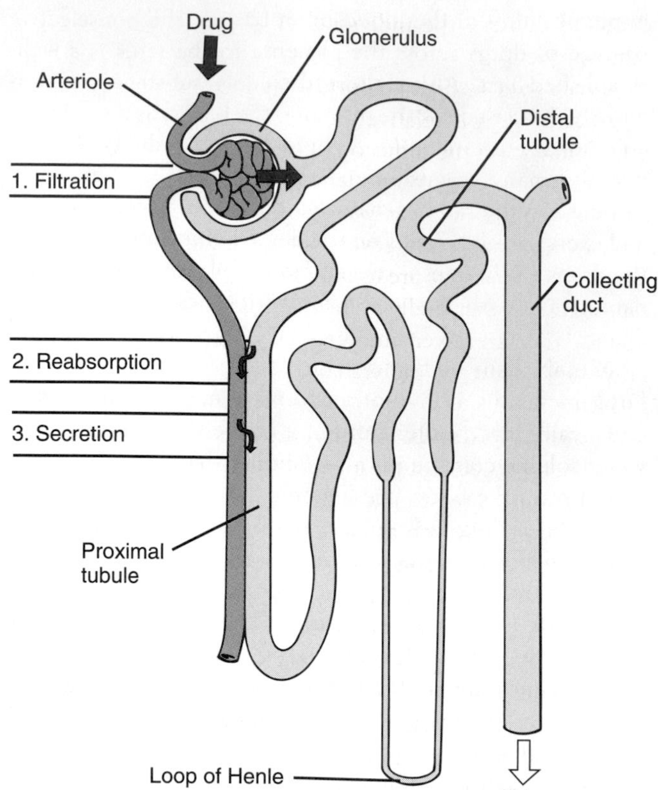

Figure 3-6 The drug excretion process.

Another technique to alter the rate of excretion of a drug is to produce a competitively blocking effect. For example, probenecid may be used to block the renal excretion of penicillin. This prolongs the effect of the antibiotic by maintaining a higher therapeutic plasma level.

Additional Excretion Sites

Gastrointestinal Tract. Some drugs may be excreted by biliary excretion. After metabolism by the liver, the metabolite is secreted into the bile, passed into the duodenum, and eliminated with feces.

Other drugs such as fat-soluble agents may be reabsorbed by the bloodstream from the intestine and returned to the liver. This is the enterohepatic cycle. These compounds are later excreted by the kidney.

Lungs. Gases and volatile liquids (general anesthetics) are administered and excreted via the pulmonary route, generally in intact form. On inspiration, these agents enter the bloodstream and, after crossing the alveolar membrane, are distributed by the general circulation. The rate of gas loss depends on the rate of respiration. Therefore exercise or deep breathing, which causes a rise in cardiac output and a subsequent increase in pulmonary blood flow, promotes excretion. In contrast, decreased cardiac output, such as that which occurs in shock, prolongs the period of drug elimination. Other volatile substances such as ethyl alcohol and paraldehyde are highly soluble in blood and are excreted in limited amounts by the lungs. These substances are easily detected because the individual exhales the gases into the atmosphere.

Sweat and Salivary Glands. Drug excretion through sweat and saliva is relatively unimportant because this process depends on the diffusion of lipid-soluble drugs through the epithelial cells of the glands. The elimination of drugs and metabolites in sweat may be responsible for side effects such as dermatitis and several other skin reactions. Drugs excreted in the saliva are usually swallowed and undergo the same fate as other orally administered agents. Certain compounds that are given intravenously may be excreted into saliva and cause the individual to complain of the "taste of the drug."

Mammary Glands. Many drugs or their metabolites cross the epithelium of the mammary glands and are excreted in breast milk. Breast milk is acidic (pH 6.5), and therefore basic compounds such as narcotics (e.g., morphine and codeine) achieve high concentrations in this fluid. A major concern arises over the transfer of drugs from mothers to their breastfed babies, which can result in a cumulative drug effect because of the infant's undeveloped metabolizing system. The nursing mother should be warned against taking any medications without approval of her health care provider.

Hemodialysis. Drugs may also be eliminated through the use of extracorporeal dialysis, which was originally designed to substitute for renal function in cases of severe but temporary renal shutdown. Overdosage of drugs may lead to just such a situation. By an artificial process resembling glomerular filtration, dialysis can rapidly reduce high plasma levels of a drug. As a general rule, substances that are completely or almost completely excreted by the normal kidney can be removed by hemodialysis. Such substances include some CNS stimulants and depressants, some nonnarcotic analgesics, and metals.

Pharmacodynamic Phase

Pharmacodynamics is the study of the mechanism of drug action on living tissue, or the response of tissues to specific chemical agents at various sites in the body. Whereas *pharmacokinetics* refers to the way the body processes or handles the drug, *pharmacodynamics* refers to the *effect* the drug has on the body (Katzung, 1998). The effects of drugs can be recognized only by alterations of a known physiologic function; drugs modify physiologic activity but do not confer any new function on a tissue or organ in the body. They may increase, decrease, or replace enzymes, hormones, or body metabolic functions. Some drugs inhibit or destroy foreign organisms or malignant cells in the body, whereas other drug substances protect cells from foreign agents. The goal of drug therapy is to attain a therapeutic effect in an individual. In this context, some drugs are used to treat symptoms and cure disease, and others are used to diagnose or prevent disease.

The means by which drugs produce an alteration in function at their sites of action is known as the mechanism of action. The mechanism of action of most compounds is believed to involve a chemical interaction between the drug and a functionally important component of the living system. Most drugs produce their effects in one of the following ways: a drug-receptor interaction, a drug-enzyme interaction, or a nonspecific drug interaction.

Drug-Receptor Interaction. Structural specificity is an essential premise of the receptor theory of drug action. This theory hypothesizes that drugs are selectively active substances with a high affinity for a specific chemical group or a particular constituent of a cell. In essence the drug-receptor interaction theory states that a certain portion (active site) of the drug molecule selectively combines or interacts with some molecular structure (a reactive site on the cell surface or within the cell) to produce a biologic effect. The **receptor** is the reactive cellular site with which a drug interacts to produce a pharmacologic response. The relationship of a drug to its receptor has often been likened to that of the fit of a key in a lock. The drug represents the key that fits into the lock, or receptor. Thus some sort of reciprocal or complementary relationship exists between a certain portion of the drug molecule and the receptor site of the cell.

It has been postulated that the drug molecule with the best fit to the receptor will produce the greatest response from the cell. It has also been suggested that some force must attract a receptor and hold it in combination with a specific drug long enough to produce a pharmacologic response. Following absorption, a drug gains access to the receptor after it leaves the bloodstream and is distributed to tissues that contain receptor sites. Box 3-3 lists terms that are essential to understanding drug-receptor interaction.

Drug-Enzyme Interaction. The second method by which a drug may produce an effect is the interaction between the drug and a cellular enzyme. Enzymes are indispensable biologic catalysts that control all biochemical reactions of the cell. Drugs can inhibit the action of a specific enzyme and alter a physiologic response. For example neostigmine (Prostigmin) is an agent used to manage the muscle weakness caused by myasthenia gravis, a degenerative neurologic disease. Neostigmine acts chemically by combining with the enzyme acetylcholinesterase to prevent it from inactivating the neurotransmitter acetylcholine at the neuromuscular junction.

Drugs that combine with enzymes are thought to do so by virtue of their structural resemblance to an enzyme's substrate molecule (the substance acted on by an enzyme). A drug may resemble an enzyme's substrate so closely that the enzyme combines with the drug instead of with the normal substrate. Drugs resembling enzyme substrates are termed "antimetabolites" and can either block normal enzymatic action or result in the production of other substances with unique biochemical properties. The antimetabolites, then, become the receptors for the enzyme. However, although enzymes may be receptors, not all receptors are enzymes. An example of an antimetabolite is the anticancer drug methotrexate, which inhibits the enzyme that allows the reduction of folic acid for DNA, RNA, and protein synthesis.

Nonspecific Drug Interaction. Some drugs demonstrate no structural specificity and presumably act by producing more general effects on cell membranes and cellular

BOX 3-3

Drug-Receptor Interaction Terms

affinity The propensity of a drug to bind or attach itself to a given receptor site.

agonist A drug that combines with receptors and initiates a sequence of biochemical and physiologic changes; possesses both affinity and efficacy.

antagonist An agent designed to inhibit or counteract the effects produced by other drugs or the undesired effects caused by cellular components during illness.

competitive antagonist An agent with an affinity for the same receptor site as an agonist; competition with the agonist for the site inhibits the action of the agonist; increasing the concentration of the agonist tends to overcome the inhibition. Competitive inhibition responses are usually reversible.

efficacy (intrinsic activity) The ability of a drug to initiate biologic activity as a result of binding to a given receptor.

noncompetitive antagonist An agent that combines with different parts of the receptor mechanism and inactivates the receptor so that the agonist cannot be effective regardless of its concentration. Noncompetitive antagonist effects are considered to be irreversible or nearly irreversible.

partial agonist An agent that has affinity and some efficacy but may antagonize the action of other drugs that have greater efficacy. Not infrequently, antagonists share some structural similarities with their agonists.

BOX 3-4

Plasma Level Profile Terms

duration of action The period from onset of drug action to the time when a response is no longer perceptible.

minimal effective concentration The lowest plasma concentration that produces the desired drug effect.

onset of action (latent period) The interval between the time a drug is administered and the first sign of its effect.

peak plasma level The highest plasma concentration attained from a dose.

termination of action The point at which a drug effect is no longer seen.

therapeutic range The range of plasma concentrations that produce the desired drug effect without toxicity (the range between minimal effective concentration and toxic level).

toxic level The plasma concentration at which a drug produces serious adverse reactions.

processes. These drugs may penetrate into cells or accumulate in cellular membranes, where they interfere, by physical or chemical means, with some cell function or some fundamental metabolic processes.

Cell membranes are complex lipoprotein structures that regulate the flow of ions and metabolites in a highly selective manner, thereby maintaining an electrochemical gradient between the interior and exterior surfaces of the cell. Structurally nonspecific drugs are exemplified by the general anesthetics, which are lipid-soluble compounds that have unrelated chemical structures but similar properties. It is believed that the general anesthetics alter the properties of lipids in the cell membranes of nerves rather than act on specific receptors.

Other structurally nonspecific drugs may act by biophysical means that do not affect cellular or enzymatic functions. Drugs acting as a result of their obvious physical properties include the ointments and emollients. Hydrophilic indigestible substances exert a cathartic effect because of their physical action on the bowel. Examples of true chemical reactions that produce biologic effects are the interaction of a molecule such as lead with an antidotal drug and the neutralization by antacid drugs of the hydrochloric acid present in gastric juice. Neither is considered a receptor interaction because no macromolecular tissue elements are involved. Detergents, alcohol, hydrogen peroxide, and phenol derivatives such as Lysol are also structurally nonspecific and act by irreversibly destroying the functional integrity of the living cell.

Drug-Response Relationship

After administration, each drug has its own characteristic pharmacokinetics, which can be analyzed by performing a plasma level profile. In many instances nurses are required to monitor serum drug levels to help the prescriber determine the dose, scheduling, and route of administration for an individual client. These data provide information concerning the degree of therapeutic effectiveness as well as toxic levels or levels below the therapeutic range so that potential adverse reactions can be predicted and serious clinical problems can be prevented.

Plasma Level Profile of a Drug. The plasma or serum level profile graphically demonstrates the relationship between the plasma drug concentration and the level of therapeutic effectiveness over time. After one dose is administered, the time course of the amount of drug in the body depends on the rates of absorption, distribution, metabolism, and elimination. For example, the drug in Figure 3-7 has an onset of action of approximately 2 hours, a peak level at 5 hours, and a 10-hour duration of action or effect. By monitoring the plasma level of a compound, the efficacy and safety of drug therapy can be more closely controlled. Box 3-4 lists important terms used in plasma level profiles and explains their interrelationships.

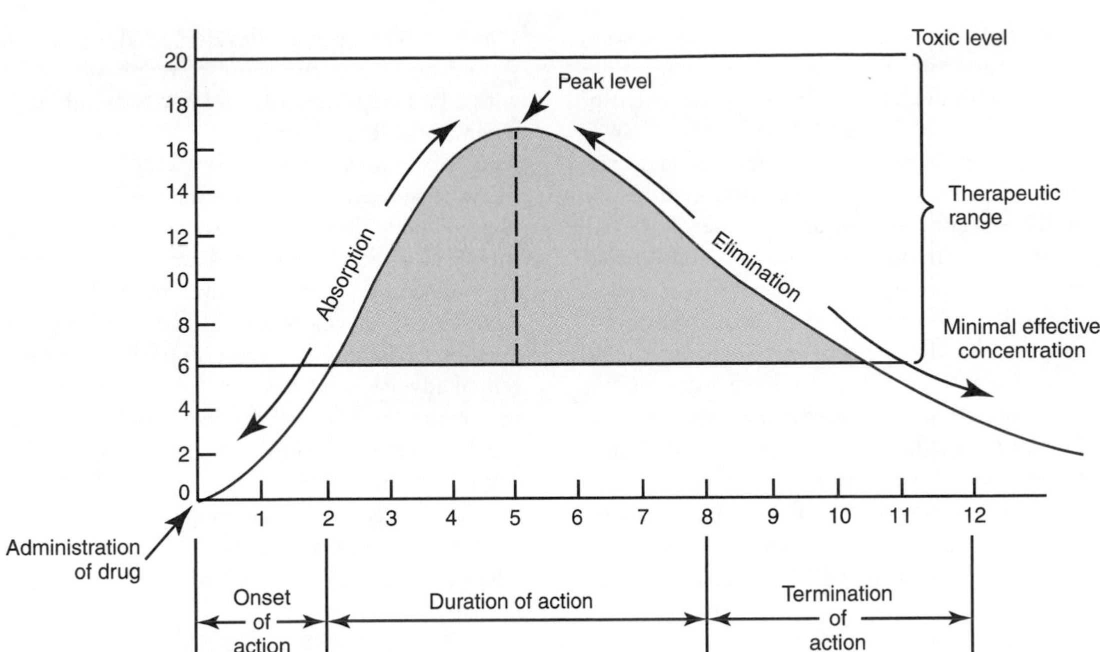

Figure 3-7 Plasma level profile of a drug.

Biologic Half-Life. The rate of biotransformation and excretion of a drug determines its biologic **half-life** (t½), the time required to reduce by one half the amount of unchanged drug in the body at the time equilibrium is established. The duration of a dose can be demonstrated by the biologic half-life, which differs for each drug. A drug with a short t½, such as 2 or 3 hours, needs to be administered more often than one with a long t½, such as 12 hours.

The half-life does not change with the size of the drug dose; it always takes the same amount of time to eliminate one half of the drug present in the body. If, for example, 10,000 units of a drug are administered and that drug has a half-life of 4 hours, then 5000 units of the drug will be excreted in 4 hours. In the next 4 hours, 2500 units will be excreted, with 1250 units more being excreted in the third 4-hour period. Drug elimination may be prolonged and drug half-life lengthened in individuals with hepatic dysfunction or renal disorders; this usually necessitates reduction of the drug dose.

Therapeutic Index. The **therapeutic index** (TI) provides a quantitative measure of the relative safety of a drug. It represents a ratio between two factors: (1) lethal dose (LD_{50}), the drug dose that is lethal in 50% of laboratory animals tested; and (2) effective dose (ED_{50}), the dose required to produce a therapeutic effect in 50% of a similar population. The therapeutic index is calculated as follows:

$$TI = \frac{LD_{50}}{ED_{50}}$$

The closer the ratio is to 1, the greater the danger involved in administering that drug to human beings. In humans the dose that promotes a side effect or the first sign of a toxic response is obviously of greater importance than the therapeutic index of the drug, because the prescriber's major concern is avoiding even an isolated fatality caused by drug toxicity.

Drug Bioavailability. Bioavailability refers to the percentage of active drug substances absorbed and available to reach the target tissues following drug administration. Drugs are considered to be biologically equivalent if they attain similar concentrations in blood and tissues at similar times; they are therapeutically equivalent if they provide equal therapeutic effectiveness in clinical trials. Of importance is the similarity of the absorption and therapeutic performances of drugs, which can be altered markedly by the ingredients and method of drug manufacture. Different brands of the same drug can vary, and even different lots from a single manufacturer may show different levels of effectiveness. Thus the Food and Drug Administration is paying more attention to drug preparation and trying to ensure that the bioavailability of a drug conforms to uniform standards. Both the proportion of active drug and the percentage of its absorption are essential in attaining therapeutic equivalence among all chemically similar drugs.

SIDE EFFECTS/ADVERSE REACTIONS

In addition to producing therapeutic effects, drugs have the potential of causing undesirable responses, such as side effects or adverse reactions. Side effects are usually a predictable and, in many instances, an unavoidable secondary effect produced by the drug at the usual therapeutic drug doses. For example, an opioid analgesic often causes the side effects of drowsiness and constipation. These effects occur at the usual prescribed dose, with drowsiness occurring soon after drug administration and constipation often being a delayed side effect that occurs later in therapy. The intensity of the side effects is often dose dependent.

The most commonly reported side effects are anorexia, nausea, vomiting, dizziness, drowsiness, dry mouth, abdominal gas or distress, constipation, and diarrhea. For some side effects, health care providers can provide nonpharmacologic advice, such as advising the individual to use caution when getting up suddenly from a lying or sitting position to reduce the potential for dizziness or hypotension, to use sugarless gum or candy or ice chips to relieve a dry mouth, or to not drive or use dangerous machinery until the individual's response to the medication can be assessed. Persistent or troublesome side effects may require pharmacologic interventions such as laxatives, antiemetics, and antidiarrheals for constipation, vomiting, and diarrhea, respectively. In general, the side effects are manageable, and in some instances tolerance may develop to the side effect. Clients should be taught the most common side effects reported with a particular medication, how to avoid or self-manage it when possible, and when to report especially persistent effects to the prescriber.

Adverse reactions are unintended, undesirable, and often unpredictable drug effects. Every medication has a potential for causing harm. Sometimes adverse reactions are immediately apparent, whereas at other times they may take weeks or months to develop. Because only up to several thousand persons are exposed to each drug before release, not all potential adverse reactions may be detected before the drug is marketed. Therefore the nurse should be alert to any unusual individual responses to drugs, especially with newly released medications.

Adverse reactions can range from mild to fatal. With increasing numbers of drugs being used, the incidence of adverse reactions has increased and is presently a sig-

TABLE 3-1 Factors That Modify Cell Conditions and Drug Activity

Factor	Nursing Considerations
Age	
Infants—immature body systems	Modify dosages.
Children—dosage adjustment usually necessary	Children have a different physiologic profile and body mass distribution. Thus the dose per kilogram is individualized and can be more or less than in an adult.
Older adults—depressed hepatic and renal systems	Older adults may also have concomitant physical conditions that alter drug effects; an altered excretion mechanism may also necessitate less drug or different scheduling of medication. Older adults are also at risk for drug interactions resulting from the use of multiple drugs.
Body Mass	
The greater the volume of distribution of the drug in body mass, the lower the concentration of the drug in the body compartments Calculation: average adult dose is based on a drug quantity that will produce a particular effect in 50% of population between the ages of 18 and 65 and approximately 150 pounds (70 kg) in weight	Adjust dosage in proportion to body mass. For children, dosage often is determined on the basis of an amount of drug per kilogram of body weight or body surface area.
Sex	
Women—smaller than men; definite differences during pregnancy and in relative proportions of fat and water; drugs vary by water or fat solubility	Allow for size differential and whether a drug is water or lipid soluble. Avoid drugs during pregnancy unless an absolute necessity exists.
Environmental Milieu	
Mood and behavior modified by (1) drug itself, (2) personality of the user, (3) environment of the user, and (4) interaction of these three factors Other factors: sensory—deprivation or overload; physical environment—cold vs. heat; oxygen deprivation (altitude)	Be aware of the physical situation of the client with regard to heat and cold, interactions with other individuals, drug effects, and the way the client generally reacts to situations.

nificant problem in clinical practice (Nies & Spielberg, 1996).

Predictable Adverse Reactions

Factors such as age, body mass, sex, environment, time of administration, pathologic state, genetics, and psychologic characteristics can alter an individual's response to drug therapy. Deviant drug reactions are often traced to the predictable influence of such variables. The nurse must be cognizant of characteristics that modify cell conditions and, therefore, the activity of a drug (Table 3-1).

Age. Young children and older adults are usually highly responsive to medications. Infants often have immature hepatic and renal systems and, therefore, incomplete metabolic and excretory mechanisms. Older adults may demonstrate different responses to drug therapy because of a decline in hepatic and renal function, which is often accompanied by a concurrent disease process.

Body Mass. The relationship between body mass and amount of drug administered influences the distribution and concentration of a drug. To maintain a desired drug concentration in individuals of various sizes, the drug dosage must be adjusted in proportion to body mass. For any given drug dose, the greater the volume of distribution, the lower the concentration of drug reached in various body compartments. Because the volume of interstitial and intracellular water is related to body mass, weight has a marked influence on the quantitative effects produced by drugs. The average adult drug dosage is calculated on the basis of the drug quantity that produces a particular effect in 50% of persons who are between the ages of 18 and 65 and weigh approximately 150 pounds (70 kg). With children and very lean or very obese individuals, drug dosage is commonly deter-

TABLE 3-1 Factors That Modify Cell Conditions and Drug Activity—cont'd

Factor	Nursing Considerations
Time of Administration	
Food—presence or absence	Give irritating drugs when food is in the client's stomach. The presence of food in the stomach may delay the absorption of oral drugs. Follow manufacturer's recommendations.
Biologic rhythms—sleep-wake cycle, drug-metabolizing enzyme rhythms, corticosteroid secretion rhythm, blood pressure rhythms, circadian (24-hour) cycle in absorption and urinary excretion; also rhythm of drug receptor susceptibility	Make every effort to understand the client's normal and abnormal rhythms, and seek possible relationships between the client's biologic rhythms and reactions to drug therapy.
Insufficient fluid intake with solid dosage forms	Administer drugs at the same time each day with a full glass of water.
	Altered body cycles (shift workers) may result in an altered response to a drug.
Pathologic State	
Presence and severity of pathologic state—pain intensifies the need for opioids; anxiety may produce resistance to large doses of tranquilizing drugs; the presence of circulatory, hepatic, and/or renal dysfunctions interferes with physiologic processes of drug action	Take into account any pain, disease, or altered metabolic state of the client and adjust dosage accordingly.
Genetic Factors	
Genetically determined abnormal susceptibility to a chemical, or "idiosyncratic response"	Be aware that any client may show an idiosyncratic response. Always monitor closely for abnormal susceptibility, especially when beginning therapy. Be aware of common drug idiosyncrasies.
Psychologic Factors	
Symbolic investment in drugs and faith in their efficacy Placebo effect Hostility toward or mistrust of medicine or health personnel	Be aware of the attitude and impression the nurse creates at the time of drug administration, and use them to enhance the effects of the drug.

mined on the basis of amount of drug per kilogram of body weight or body surface area.

Sex. Differences in drug effects related to sex result in part from the size differences between men and women. Women are usually smaller than men, which may lead to higher drug concentrations in women if the drug dosage is prescribed indifferently. Demonstrable differences also exist in relative proportions of fat and water in the bodies of men and women, and some drugs may be more soluble in one or the other. Because drugs taken by a pregnant woman might affect the fetus as a result of placental transfer, the use of drugs is best avoided during pregnancy unless an absolute necessity exists.

Environmental Milieu. Drugs affecting mood and behavior are particularly susceptible to the influence of environment. With such drugs one must consider the effects of (1) the drug itself, (2) the personality of the user, (3) the environment of the user, and (4) the interaction of these three components. Sensory deprivation and sensory overload may also affect responses to drugs. The physical environment can modify drug effects. For example, temperature affects drug activity, with heat relaxing the peripheral vessels and thus intensifying the actions of vasodilators; cold has the opposite effect. The relative oxygen deprivation at high altitudes may increase sensitivity to some drugs.

Time of Administration. It is well known that drugs are absorbed more rapidly if the gastrointestinal tract is free of food and that irritating drugs are more readily tolerated if there is food in the stomach. Research has indicated that the time of drug administration in relation to human biologic rhythms can significantly affect the response to certain medications. It seems quite plausible that in humans the sleep-wake rhythm, drug–metabolizing enzyme rhythms, and circadian (24-hour) variations contribute to the effective, ineffective, adverse, or toxic response to particular drugs. For example, cyclophosphamide (Cytoxan), an antineoplastic agent, should be administered in the morning to reduce the risk of hemorrhagic cystitis (blood in the urine) (*United States Pharmacopeia Dispensing Information*, 1999). Chronopharmacology (pharmacology concerned with the effects of drugs relative to body rhythms) and chronotoxicology (the study of poisons and their effects relative to body rhythms) are new areas that health care professionals are monitoring with great interest.

Pathologic State. The presence of a pathologic condition and the severity of symptoms may call for careful consideration of the type of drug administered and for an adjustment in dosage. For example, the presence of severe pain tends to increase a client's requirement for an analgesic, and an extremely anxious individual can prove resistant to very large doses of tranquilizing and sedating drugs. Aspirin administered to a client with a fever will produce a decrease in temperature, whereas a client taking the drug for its analgesic effects will show no temperature change at all. In addition, it bears repeating that the presence of circulatory, hepatic, or renal dysfunctions will interfere with the physiologic processes of drug action.

Genetic Factors. Genetic differences may affect an individual's response to a number of drugs. Such differences may arise from genetically conditioned deficiencies in drug metabolism or in receptor sensitivity. These pharmacogenetic abnormalities often manifest themselves as "idiosyncrasies" and may be mistakenly diagnosed as drug allergies. For example, some individuals may lack pseudocholinesterase activity in their plasma. If they receive an injection of succinylcholine (Anectine), which is normally hydrolyzed by plasma cholinesterase, they may become paralyzed and remain that way for a long time. Malignant hyperpyrexia with general anesthesia is another example of a genetically based difference (Edwards, 1997). The field of pharmacogenetics is of great interest because it may provide a rational explanation for many so-called drug idiosyncrasies.

Psychologic Factors. A client's symbolic investment in drugs and faith in their effects strongly influence and usually potentiate drug effects. The placebo effect is an outstanding example of how strong motivation can influence the emergence of desired drug effects, whereas hostility and mistrust of medicine and health personnel can diminish drug effects. It is important for nurses to realize that their attitudes and the impressions created at the time of drug administration may influence the therapeutic result.

Iatrogenic Responses

An **iatrogenic** condition is any adverse mental or physical condition induced in a client by a prescribed treatment or diagnostic procedure. Because these often involve prescribed medications, this term has also been used to define a disease caused by a prescriber (e.g., the use of phenothiazines in psychotic persons, which results in drug-induced Parkinson's disease). Other drug-induced diseases may include blood dyscrasias, hepatotoxicity, nephrotoxicity, and teratogenicity. With careful prescribing and monitoring, iatrogenic conditions are usually avoidable. With careful evaluation of a client's response to a drug, the nurse may be able to avoid or limit an iatrogenic disease.

Unpredictable Adverse Reactions

Adverse drug reactions are one way of characterizing unpredictable and sometimes inexplicable drug responses that have not been clearly and distinctly defined. The most common and best-defined adverse drug reactions are described in the following sections.

Allergic Drug Reactions

A drug allergy is an altered state of reaction to a drug that results from previous sensitizing exposure and the development of an immunologic mechanism. Substances foreign to the body act as antigens to stimulate the production of antibodies or immunoglobulins (IgE, IgG, IgM). When a previously sensitized individual is again exposed to the foreign substance, the antigen reacts with the antibodies to release substances such as histamine, which then provoke allergic symptoms. *Hypersensitivity, drug allergy,* and *chemical allergy* are all terms used to describe an allergic drug reaction (Klaassen, 1996). There are four different types of allergic drug reactions: Type 1, type 2, type 3, and type 4.

Type I (anaphylactic reaction) is an immediate reaction that occurs in a previously sensitized person within minutes of exposure to the chemical. This reaction is mediated by IgE antibodies located on the surface of mast cells and basophils. An immediate, severe reaction results and may be fatal if not recognized and treated quickly. The most dramatic form of anaphylaxis is sudden and severe bronchospasm, vasospasm, severe hypotension, and rapid death. Signs and symptoms are largely caused by the contraction of smooth muscles and may begin with irritability, extreme weakness, nausea, and vomiting and may proceed to dyspnea, cyanosis, convulsions, and cardiac arrest. Drugs associated with this type of reaction include penicillins and cephalosporins. Antihistamines, epinephrine, and bronchodilators are indispensable in the treatment of anaphylactic shock.

Type II (cytotoxic reaction) involves a drug and IgG or IgM; it has sometimes been called an autoimmune response. This reaction manifests as hemolytic anemia (methyldopa [Aldomet] or penicillin induced), thrombocytopenia (quinidine [Quinaglute] induced), or lupus erythematosus (procainamide [Pronestyl] induced). Removal of the medication usually results in improvement, but it may take several months for the reaction to subside.

Type III (or Arthus reaction, an immune complex reaction) is sometimes called "serum sickness." With this reaction the drug forms a complex with IgG antibodies in the blood vessel, resulting in angioedema, arthralgia, fever, swollen lymph nodes (lymphadenopathy), and splenomegaly approximately 1 to 3 weeks after drug exposure. Penicillins, sulfonamides, and phenytoin (Dilantin) can cause this type of delayed reaction.

Type IV is a cell-mediated or delayed hypersensitivity reaction. For example, direct skin contact between the drug and sensitized cells results in an inflammatory reaction, such as contact dermatitis from poison ivy. This type of reaction involves sensitized T lymphocytes and macrophages (Klaassen, 1996).

Drug-Induced Reactions

An individual who has had a mild allergic response to a particular drug should avoid reexposure to that drug and, optimally, should have skin tests performed to more definitively diagnose the response. Mild allergic reactions may be characterized by the development of a rash, angioedema, rhinitis, fever, asthma, and pruritus. Reinstitution of therapy with the same drug in a client who manifests allergic reactions is always dangerous because an anaphylactic reaction may occur. Important drug-induced reactions are discussed in the following paragraphs.

Tolerance refers to a decreased physiologic response that occurs after repeated administration of a drug or a chemically related substance. This type of reaction necessitates an increase in dosage to maintain a given therapeutic effect. A cross tolerance to pharmacologically similar drugs may also develop, and drugs that act at the same receptor sites may also need their dosage increased to maintain an effect.

Although the actual mechanism of tolerance is unknown, multiple mechanisms have been proposed, such as an increase in hepatic drug metabolizing enzymes and pharmacodynamic tolerance. Pharmacodynamic tolerance refers to chronic or long-term drug use in an individual who requires larger drug doses to achieve the same effect as before. Drugs well known for their propensity to produce tolerance are tobacco, opium alkaloids, nitrates, and ethyl alcohol. The exact reason for this is unknown, but it is believed that receptor or cellular adaptation may occur (Nies & Spielberg, 1996).

Tachyphylaxis refers to a quickly developing tolerance that occurs after repeated administration of a drug. It is rapid in onset, and the client's initial response to the drug cannot be reproduced, even with larger doses of the drug. Nitroglycerin transdermal is an example of a drug that requires an intermittent dosing schedule (12 hours on, 12 hours off) to maintain its effect.

A *cumulative effect* occurs when the body cannot metabolize one dose of a drug before another dose is administered. When drugs are excreted more slowly than they are absorbed, each new dose adds more to the total quantity in the blood and organs than is lost in the same amount of time by excretion. Unless drug administration is adjusted, high concentrations can be reached, producing toxic effects. Cumulative toxicity can occur rapidly, as dramatically illustrated in ethyl alcohol intoxication, or it can occur insidiously, as is the case in poisoning with heavy metals such as lead. Lead is stored in many body tissues and deposited in bones, thus having prolonged effects on the body while accumulation continues.

Idiosyncrasy is any abnormal or peculiar response to a drug, which may manifest itself by (1) overresponse or abnormal susceptibility to a drug; (2) underresponse, which demonstrates abnormal tolerance; (3) a qualitatively different effect from the one expected, such as excitation after the administration of a sedative; or (4) unpredictable and unexplainable symptoms. Idiosyncratic reactions are generally thought to result from genetic enzymatic deficiencies that lead to an abnormal mechanism of drug metabolism. This term has been used rather vaguely to describe drug reactions that are qualitatively different from the usual effects obtained in the majority of patients and that cannot be attributed to drug allergy.

Drug dependence is the term preferred over the previous terminology of "habituation" and "addiction." The World Health Organization has suggested the use of the term *dependence* in conjunction with the drug being described (e.g., barbiturate dependence or opiate dependence). Dependence can be physical or psychologic. Physical dependence refers to a state of physiologic drug adaptation that manifests itself by intense physical disturbance when the drug is withdrawn. Psychologic dependence is a state of emotional reliance on a drug to maintain an effect. Its manifestations may range from a mild desire for a drug to craving to compulsive use of the drug. Drug dependence is explored in greater detail in Chapter 9.

Drug interaction occurs when the effects of one drug are modified by the prior or concurrent administration of another drug, thereby increasing or decreasing the pharmacologic action of each. Drug interactions may be either beneficial (e.g., probenecid [Benemid] prolongs the action of penicillins) or detrimental (e.g., aspirin increases the action of anticoagulants, causing hemorrhage).

Drug antagonism occurs when the combination effect of two drugs is less than the sum of the drugs acting separately.

Summation (addition or additive effect) occurs when the combined effect of two drugs produces a result that equals the sum of the individual effects of each agent. The mathematical equivalent is $1 + 1 = 2$. For example, codeine and aspirin both act as analgesics and when given together they provide an additive or greater pain relief than when either one is used alone. This combination allows the administration of a lower dose of each drug, with a resultant decrease in adverse reactions.

Synergism describes a drug interaction in which the combined effect of drugs is greater than the sum of each individual agent acting independently. Mathematically the response can be written as $1 + 1 = 3$ or more. Synergism can be exemplified by the use of a combination of drugs in treating hypertension. Each of the drugs lowers blood pressure but in a different way; the combined effect produces a greater decrease in hypertension than if either drug is given alone.

Potentiation refers to the concurrent administration of two drugs in which one drug increases the effect of the other drug.

NURSING MANAGEMENT OF DRUG THERAPY

The nurse's responsibilities in the administration of drugs require more than the memorization of specific drugs, their actions, and their dosages. Effective implementation depends on a sound comprehension of the theories of drug action, constituting clinical judgment that the nurse can apply to the individual client, each with a specific diagnosis and definable individual needs. Such a background necessitates the understanding of theories of drug action, physiologic processes mediating drug action, variables affecting drug action, and unusual and adverse reactions to drug therapy.

The application of critical thinking in the nursing management of a client's therapeutic regimen is essential. A prescriber's order for a specific medication for an individual client is written at a particular time when such a pharmacologic intervention is determined to be appropriate. However, circumstances change and a client may have a different response to a medication than was intended. The nurse must assess whether each dose is appropriate for that client each time it is to be administered. An analogy would be that the prescriber's order exists in time and space much like a pedestrian sign flashing "walk" or "don't walk" regardless of what is occurring in the environment. What is important is whether it is safe to cross the street at a given time—that the traffic has really stopped—regardless of what the sign indicates. In the same way, the nurse monitors for the therapeutic and nontherapeutic effects of the client's medications on an ongoing basis with each and every dose to ensure safe administration of the drug therapy.

On entry into the body, a drug initiates a series of physiologic events before it reaches its site of action. The extent of drug absorption depends on the form of the drug. Assessment of the client's ability to tolerate a particular form or route is essential (e.g., testing the client's ability to swallow before an oral medication is administered). Tablets or capsules must first disintegrate and then be dissolved before absorption through the intestinal membrane can occur. However, the nurse should never crush an enteric-coated tablet, because the coating protects the tablet from destruction by the acid pH of the stomach. A drug is produced in this form so it can disintegrate and dissolve in the alkaline pH of the intestine and maintain its effectiveness. Drugs that irritate the gastric mucosa are also coated.

The time of administration is another important concern of the nurse. Drugs that require multiple daily doses and steady-state serum levels need to be evenly spaced throughout a 24-hour period. Drugs with more infrequent dosing need to be taken at the same time each day. To obtain the maximal pharmacokinetic benefit, oral drugs should be given with a glass of water (8 ounces) ½ hour to 1 hour before meals. It is important to remember that the presence of food, which delays stomach emptying, tends to diminish the therapeutic effect of the drug. Occasionally, an agent must be administered with meals to prevent gastrointestinal irritation. The nurse should anticipate a rapid response when a drug is administered intravenously, because the full dose is placed directly into the bloodstream, thus bypassing the need for absorption.

Individuals with hepatic dysfunction are susceptible to drug overdosage, especially if the drug is highly bound to plasma proteins. In addition, the nurse should be alert to the client's response to a drug if there is renal dysfunction. Because most agents are excreted by the kidneys, the client should be observed for a cumulative effect that may result from the continued administration of the drug. Usually drug dosage is adjusted in individuals with hepatic or renal disorders so that adverse reactions are prevented.

In instances in which the nurse is required to monitor serum drug levels, careful observations of the client's response to the drug provide information that aids the prescriber in determining the dosage of a drug, the frequency of administration, and the route of administration. The data are essential for promoting the optimal therapeutic benefit to the client and at the same time preventing potential adverse reactions.

Finally, the nurse should advise a pregnant woman about the danger of taking medications and, to prevent teratogenic effects, should instruct her to check with her prescriber or licensed nurse midwife before taking any drug. If a medication is required, the lowest possible dose of the prescribed drug should be administered.

Unit 2, The Nursing Process and Pharmacology, provides the principles upon which the nursing judgment necessary for the safe and accurate administration of medications can be developed.

SUMMARY

Drugs are chemicals that interact with a living organism to produce biologic responses. They produce these responses according to certain theories of drug action, physiologic processes mediating drug action, variables affecting drug action, and unusual and adverse reactions to drug therapy. Drugs modify only existing functions and exert multiple actions rather than a single effect. These actions result from a physiochemical interaction between the drug and a functionally important molecule in the body.

To produce the desired effect, a drug must have an appropriate concentration at its site of action. This concentration is influenced by a number of processes that can be divided into three phases: pharmaceutical, pharmacokinetic, and pharmacodynamic. The pharmaceutical phase focuses on the form of the drug, solid or liquid, and its dissolution to achieve absorption. The pharmacokinetic phase is concerned with the concentration of the drug during the processes of absorption, distribution, biotransformation, and excretion. Absorption involves the movement of drug molecules from the site of entry into the body to the circulating fluids. Several factors influence absorption: the nature of the absorbing surface through which the drug must pass, blood flow to the site of administration, solubility of the drug, pH, drug concentration, and dosage form. Drugs may be given for their local or systemic effect. The routes of drug administration are classified as enteral, parenteral, pulmonary, and topical. Distribution is the transport of a drug in body fluids to various tissues of the body and ultimately to the site of action. It is influenced by the body's storage reservoirs for drugs—plasma protein binding and tissue binding—as well as by barriers to drug distribution, such as the blood-brain barrier and the placental barrier. In biotransformation the liver, the primary site for drug metabolism, inactivates the drug by converting it to a metabolite that can be excreted from the body. Excretion, elimination of pharmacologically active or inactive metabolites from the body, occurs primarily through the kidneys, with some elimination through the intestine, lungs, mammary glands, and sweat and salivary glands.

The pharmacodynamic phase is concerned with the response of tissues to specific chemical agents at various sites in the body. The mechanism for action between the drug and a functionally important component of the living system may be a drug-receptor interaction, a drug-enzyme interaction, or a nonspecific drug interaction. Because each drug has its own characteristic pharmacokinetic activity, it may be necessary to monitor a client by obtaining a plasma level of a drug. The biologic half-life and the therapeutic index of a drug also provide information to assist the prescriber in determining the dose, scheduling, and route of administration for an individual client.

No drug is totally safe; it can sometimes react in the body to produce unpredictable and harmful effects. However, some identifiable factors do alter the response to drug therapy: age, body mass, sex, environmental milieu, time of administration, pathologic states, genetic factors, and psychologic factors. The adverse reactions caused unintentionally by treatment are known as iatrogenic disease. With drug therapy, iatrogenic diseases may be manifested in five major ways: blood dyscrasias, hepatic toxicity, renal damage, teratogenic effects, and dermatologic effects. Other, somewhat unpredictable adverse reactions may be evidenced as drug allergy, tolerance, tachyphylaxis, cumulation, idiosyncrasy, drug dependence, drug interaction, drug antagonism, summation, synergism, potentiation, or immediate reactions such as anaphylaxis.

It is important that the nurse understand the principles involved in drug action and their influence on nursing practice in order to administer each medication with the greatest safety and efficacy.

Critical Thinking Questions

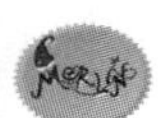

1. If you were administering a medication with a long half-life, what types of clients would be more at risk for cumulative effects?
2. Both diazepam (Valium), an anxiolytic drug, and warfarin (Coumadin), an oral anticoagulant, are highly protein-bound medications. If you were administering both of these medications to the same client, what assessments of the client would be particularly important?
3. How can a drug that has CNS activity but cannot cross the blood-brain barrier be administered for effectiveness?

Collaborative Learning Activities

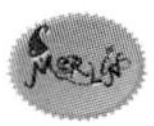

For Collaborative Learning Activities, go to mosby.com/MERLIN/McKenry/.

CASE STUDY

For a Case Study that will help ensure mastery of this chapter content, go to mosby.com/MERLIN/McKenry/.

BIBLIOGRAPHY

Benet, L.Z., Kroetz, D.L., & Sheiner, L.B. (1996). Pharmacokinetics: The dynamics of drug absorption, distribution, and elimination. In J.G. Hardman & L.E. Limbird (Eds.), *Goodman & Gilman's The pharmacological basis of therapeutics* (9th ed.). New York: McGraw-Hill.

Daly, S. (Ed.) (1993). *Giving drugs by advanced techniques.* Springhouse, PA: Springhouse.

DiPiro, J.T., Talbert, R.L., Yee, G.C., Matzke, G.R., Wells, B.G., & Posey, L.M. (Eds.). (1997). *Pharmacotherapy: A pathophysiological approach* (4th ed.). Stamford, CT: Appleton & Lange.

Edwards, I.R. (1997). Pharmacological basis of adverse drug reactions. In T.M. Speight & N.H.G. Holford (Eds.), *Avery's Drug Treatment* (4th ed.). Auckland, New Zealand: Adis International.

Hardman, J.G., & Limbird, L.E. (Eds.). (1998). *Goodman & Gilman's The pharmacological basis of therapeutics* (10th ed.). New York: McGraw-Hill.

Katzung, B.G. (1998). *Basic & clinical pharmacology* (7th ed.). Stamford, CT: Appleton & Lange.

Klaassen, C.D. (1996). Principles of toxicology and treatment of poisoning. In J.G. Hardman & L.E. Limbird (Eds.), *Goodman & Gilman's The pharmacological basis of therapeutics* (9th ed.). New York: McGraw-Hill.

Mallet, L. (1992). Counseling in special populations: The elderly patient. *American Pharmacist NS, 32*(10), 71.

Miller, S.W., & Strom, J.G., Jr. (1990). Drug-product selection: Implications for the geriatric patient. *Consultant Pharmacist 5*(1), 30.

Nies, A.S., & Spielberg, S.P. (1996). Principles of therapeutics. In J.G. Hardman & L.E. Limbird (Eds.), *Goodman & Gilman's The pharmacological basis of therapeutics* (9th ed.). New York: McGraw-Hill.

Sjoqvist, F., Borga, O., Dahl, M.L., & Orme, M.L.E. (1997). Fundamentals of clinical pharmacology. In T.M. Speight & N.H.G. Holford (Eds.), *Avery's drug treatment* (4th ed.). Auckland, New Zealand: Adis International.

United States Pharmacopeia Dispensing Information (USP DI): Drug information for the health care professional (19th ed.). (1999). Rockville, MD: United States Pharmacopeial Convention.

Young, L.Y. & Koda-Kimble, M.A. (Eds.). (1995). *Applied therapeutics: The clinical use of drugs* (6th ed.). Vancouver, WA: Applied Therapeutics.-

4 Assessment, Nursing Diagnosis, and Planning

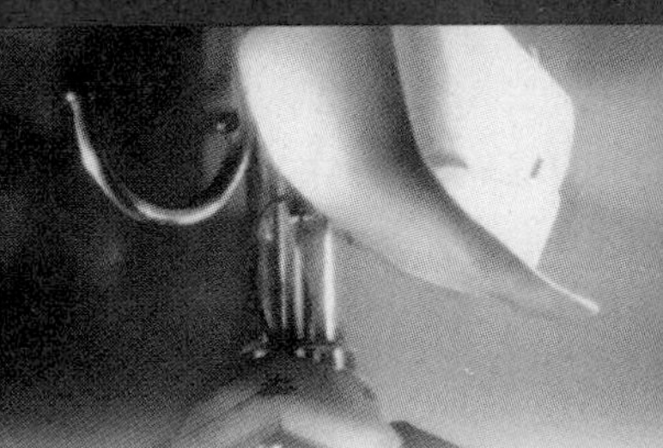

Chapter Focus

Whether contact with clients occurs in the home, ambulatory care setting, extended care facility, or hospital, the nurse uses the nursing process to work with clients in relation to drug therapy. When its five components—assessment, nursing diagnosis, planning, implementation, and evaluation—are applied to drug therapy, the nurse develops a systematic and organized approach to handling the wealth of data about clients and their drugs. This chapter discusses the first three components of the nursing process: assessment, nursing diagnosis, and planning.

Learning Objectives

1. Obtain an accurate and thorough drug history from a client.
2. Articulate the components and types of drug orders essential for safe, effective drug administration.
3. Assess contraindications to the administration of a drug and take appropriate action.
4. Identify the variables influencing drug interactions, as well as common drug interactions and incompatibilities.
5. Describe the components and purpose of the nursing diagnosis.
6. Identify the most common nursing diagnoses for any client receiving medication.
7. Discuss the three domains of nursing interventions.
8. Explain the importance of setting nursing or other outcome criteria for nursing care related to drug therapy.
9. Apply the nursing process steps of assessment and planning as they relate to drug therapy of a client.

Key Terms

analysis, p. 65
collaborative domain, p. 68
collaborative problems, p. 65
contraindications, p. 60
dependent domain, p. 68
drug history, p. 54
incompatibilities, p. 64
independent domain, p. 68
nursing diagnosis, p. 65
nursing outcomes, p. 69
nursing process, p. 54
outcome criteria, p. 69
prn order, p. 58
protocol, p. 58
routine order, p. 58
single order, p. 58
stat order, p. 58

When applied to drug therapy, the **nursing process** provides the nurse with a systematic observational and problem-solving technique to collaborate with the client on appropriate medication-related interventions and to evaluate the effectiveness of these interventions. It provides direction for rational nursing actions to prevent and manage problems related to drug therapies. Its process and phases are analogous to scientific and problem-solving methods. Although other variations exist, the nursing process is described in this text as four phases: (1) assessment, which culminates in nursing diagnoses and collaborative problems; (2) planning; (3) implementation; and (4) evaluation. Figure 4-1 diagrams these phases or steps, which are discussed in this chapter and in Chapter 5. It should be kept in mind that the steps of the nursing process have an ongoing, cyclic nature—no step should be considered complete or static.

ASSESSMENT

The assessment phase of the nursing process is both the first phase and a continuous processing of client-related data. During assessment of data, all the facts relating to clients and their drug therapy, relationships with others, health history, and environment are collected and organized so the nurse can begin to make inferences about the client's drug therapy. The data that are collected and analyzed form the basis for the development of nursing diagnoses and/or collaborative problems.

The client's status and the assessment data derived from these indicated sources will constantly change. As a result, the nursing diagnostic statements also will change. In collaboration with the prescriber, these changes may result in revision of the treatment plan, such as drug deletions, additions, or dosage changes.

Nurses must have a sound base of knowledge about a client's health issues and the drugs being administered, as well as the skill to use references to answer questions that arise. The ability to ask questions and seek answers about the data collected will form a solid foundation for the planning, implementation, and evaluation phases of the nursing process.

Drug History Guidelines

Obtaining a **drug history,** the process of gathering information that is relevant to the management of a client's medication regimen, is essential for planning nursing interventions and client education. Obtaining a comprehensive drug history requires a combination of nursing knowledge, interviewing skills, and a review of specific drug reference resources whenever necessary. A drug history should explore the client's use of prescription medications, use of over-the-counter (OTC) medications, self-treatment with herbal or home remedies, general and specific health history and, when possible, specific cultural factors that influence individual drug therapies. Particular attention should be given to other substances the client may be taking but may not consider medications, such as home remedies and OTC medications. Stoehr, Ganguli, Seaberg, Echement, and Belle (1997) determined that 87% of their study participants took one OTC drug and that 5.7% took more than five. The client's readiness and ability to provide information should be assessed. The purpose of a drug history should be explained so the client understands why some

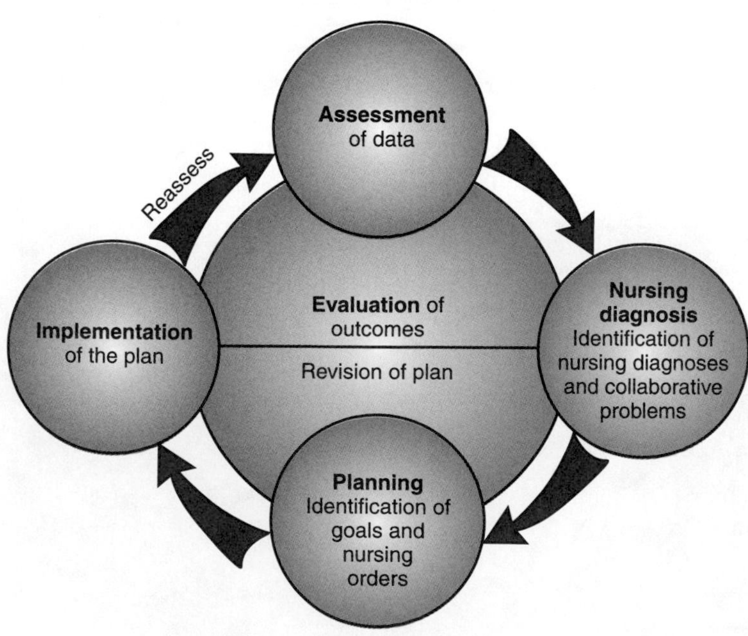

Figure 4-1 The nursing process.

questions may sound personal. Figure 4-2 shows a sample drug history form.

A thorough drug history can provide extremely useful information for the entire health care team. For example, it can do the following:

1. Explain a mysterious new symptom reported in the client
2. Provide clues about unreported chronic disorders
3. Reveal learning needs or concerns regarding the client's effective management of a therapeutic regimen
4. Provide information crucial to prevent drug interactions, allergies, or side effects/adverse reactions
5. Help interpret laboratory tests reliably
6. Identify the risk for drug-drug and drug-food interactions

When obtaining a drug history, it is important to communicate at the level of understanding appropriate for the client. Medical terms may be confusing to the nonmedically trained person; therefore the nurse should be familiar with local observances and, when applicable, ethnic or cultural terms for specific diseases, illnesses, symptoms, and other information. The client's own words should be used if appropriate. Rapport must be established if the transfer of relevant information is to be made freely.

Open-ended questioning is preferred to direct "yes" or "no" questions during the interview. For example, in obtain-

DRUG HISTORY

Client's name__________ Sex ______ Age ____ Date of interview __________

Occupation __________ Physician(s) or other health care provider(s) __________

Diagnosis and past medical history (if relevant):

Current prescribed medications; include name, strength, daily dosage, indication, and therapeutic/nontherapeutic responses (note client's knowledge about medications and the need for teaching):

Prescription medications taken during the previous 3 months:

Allergies/drug reactions (food and/or drugs; describe reaction, approximate date, and action taken or outcome):

Close family members with drug allergies (relationship, drug, and reaction):

Over-the-counter medications and herbal preparations:
List medications, dose, frequency, and when last dose was taken for the following:

Constipation (laxatives):
Diarrhea (antidiarrheals):
Gastric upset/heartburn (antacids):
Aches and pains, headache (analgesics):
Cold medication (antihistamine, decongestants):
Cough medicine (syrups/other forms):
Drugs for sleep:
Drugs to stay awake:
Drugs for menstrual conditions in premenopausal women:
Drugs for control of menopausal symptoms:
Drugs for nerves:
Drugs for fluid retention:
Do you take any other over-the-counter medications, herbal remedies, or health food products? Obtain a complete listing and daily consumption.
Do you use any salt substitutes (obtain brand name; Morton Lite Salt, CoSalt, etc.)
Do you use any food supplements? Name and quantity per day:
Do you take vitamins/minerals/iron? Note type, strength, and amount per day:

Frequency of meals? Special diet, prescribed or self-imposed:

Caffeine intake: (type & amount) Type /daily consumption of alcohol: Smoking (type and amount):

Nurse __________

Figure 4-2 Sample drug history form.

ing information about a client's use of analgesics, a "yes" or "no" question would be "Do you take analgesics? If 'yes,' name them." If the person is unsure of the meaning of the term *analgesic*, a "no" answer might be the natural response. The more descriptive information the nurse is seeking may be elicited if the question is reworded to ask "What do you take when you have pain, such as a headache, backache, muscle sprain, or other type of ache or pain?" Reminders must often accompany questions concerning OTC drugs; commonly used product names or currently advertised brands may be suggested to jog the memory of the client. For example, aspirin is an ingredient in hundreds of OTC preparations; therefore simply asking the client if he or she consumes aspirin may limit the answer to only products labeled as aspirin. Suggesting trade name products, such as Anacin, Bufferin, or Alka-Seltzer, increases the possibility of obtaining a more thorough drug history.

If the interview is performed in the client's living quarters, the nurse should ask to see the medications. In an ambulatory care setting, the client should be asked to bring all of his or her medications into the office for review. Many individuals, especially older adults, forget to report all the medications they have on hand for self-medicating purposes. The storage place for medications should be noted; this information may be important if a potentially hazardous site is used. Storage in a bathroom cabinet or over a kitchen sink or stove may adversely affect many medications. Areas of heat and moisture are not recommended as proper storage areas for most drugs. Unless they are to be refrigerated, almost all medications are to be stored below 40° C (104° F), preferably between 15° and 30° C (59° and 86° F), and are to be protected from freezing.

Evaluating the client's knowledge about the proper disposal of drugs (via the sink or toilet), ability to read the print and the language and understand the terms and instructions on the medication labels, and ability to locate expiration dates is part of assessing the individual's ability to store and consume medications safely. Studies have indicated that many persons (from one third to one half of various older adult populations) cannot read or do not understand drug package labels. This high incidence clearly indicates an area of concern that requires nursing assessment.

Information should also be obtained regarding the client's general lifestyle, dietary patterns, consumption of alcohol, use of caffeine-containing products, and smoking habits. All of these factors may affect or modify a typical drug response. (See Drug Interactions, p. 61, for further information.)

Client and Environmental Data

Client and environmental data are collected from the clients, their friends, or their relatives through subjective and objective observations. In addition to observing clients and their environment, other sources of data are the interactions of clients with others and notes from the history and physical examination sections of the clinical record. At the initial interview the health care provider notes a client's past health history and performs a physical examination to assess the client's current health status. The resulting prioritized problem list helps to direct the therapeutic approach of the health care team. The client's history and physical examination should be reviewed by the nurse for relevant data in assessing the appropriateness of the planned drug therapy. If drug dosages and routes of administration are not carefully selected, alterations in the various systems may result in either an increased or exaggerated drug effect or a decrease in drug response. Table 4-1 lists the major client and environmental data to be obtained before initiating drug therapy.

Current Client Drug Data

Drug data include information derived from a prescriber's orders or prescription and that gained from assessing the effects of the drugs on the client on the basis of observation, examination (including vital signs), and laboratory reports. The characteristics of the drugs administered and the way the prescriber orders them to be administered have an impact on the client's nursing care.

Drug Orders and Prescriptions

"Medicating" a client begins when the medication is suggested and authorized by a legally sanctioned prescriber, usually a licensed physician or dentist. In many states nurse practitioners, pharmacists, or physician assistants are given this function legally within specified limitations. Practicing nurses should be aware of and follow the limitations outlined in the state nurse practice act for the state in which they practice.

The prescriber's orders are meant for the individual who dispenses the medication. There are two different formats: the prescription blank and the order sheet. The prescription blank is given to clients in an ambulatory care setting or on discharge from the health care agency and is to be filled by a community pharmacist; it may look similar the one shown in Figure 4-3. For clients in an institutional setting, the order is written on an order sheet found in the client's chart (Figure 4-4). It is filled by the pharmacy within the institution or contracted for by the institution and sent to the medication area on the client's unit for access by the client's medication nurse. Many health care settings have computerized the process of ordering medications for clients, but the principles remain the same, with the computer printouts often resembling the former noncomputerized hospital stationery for medication administration.

The prescriber's order has seven elements that should be present and identifiable. These elements and the associated "Five Rights" of medication administration are included in Box 4-1. All parts of the order should be legible and clearly expressed. If there is any doubt, the *prescriber must be contacted* to validate or clarify. Obviously, to administer a drug under questionable instructions is to risk harm to the client in an area with a high potential for error (see Chapter 5) (*Adverse drug reaction*, 1997).

TABLE 4-1 Client and Environmental Data for Drug Therapy

Factor	Questions for Evaluation	Rationale
Medical diagnosis	Are the drugs ordered clinically indicated and corroborated by the best judgments according to authoritative literature?	The client must be protected from wrongful harm; the administering nurse may be held legally accountable.
Age	Has the client's age been considered? Have drug reactions occurred in the past?	Very young children and older adults are subject to a wide range and great intensity of side effects and adverse reactions because of reduced functioning of body systems that absorb, transport, affect the metabolism of, and excrete drugs (see also Chapters 7 and 8).
Body mass	Was the dosage assessed in relation to total body weight, body surface area (weight-to-height ratio), and lean body mass?	For prescribing purposes, a person up to 12 years old is usually considered a child and is given a pediatric dosage. The dosage is based on the different physiologic and pharmacokinetic factors in the neonate, infant, or older child. The average weight of a 12-year-old child is approximately 90 pounds; an "average" adult weighs 150 pounds. An adult at or near the weight of 90 pounds who receives the "average adult dosage" may exhibit signs of overdose.
Inherited factors	Have genetic differences (pharmacogenetic variations) in enzyme production or destruction—which may cause apparent therapeutic failure or secondary effects when a drug is metabolized too rapidly, too slowly, or incompletely—been considered?	Many aberrant reactions (termed *idiosyncrasy*) are often acutely caused by genetic abnormalities. An example is the lack of the enzyme glucose-6-phosphate dehydrogenase, which occurs in a small percentage of people of Mediterranean descent (Italians, Greeks, Arabs, and Sephardic Jews), in approximately 10% of African-American males, and less often in African-American females. If these susceptible people ingest fava beans and medications such as aspirin, antimalarials, and sulfonamides, they may experience hemolytic anemia. In addition, hypersensitivity (allergy) to specific medications often correlates with a tendency toward common allergies to certain foods, grasses, trees, molds, or animal dander.
Coexisting conditions	Are there disorders that affect any of the major body systems—especially those of the gastrointestinal tract or the circulatory, hepatic, or renal system—that will interfere with the normal digestion, absorption, transport, metabolism, degradation, and detoxification or excretion of the drugs prescribed?	Impaired capacity for biotransformation may alter drug action and increase the possibility of toxic effects or therapeutic failure. Pregnancy or breastfeeding precludes the administration of all but essential medications (see Chapter 7).
Management of therapeutic regimen	Is there a past history or other factors to indicate that the client, if self-medicating, will not follow medication instructions? (See Chapter 6 for a full discussion of client management of the therapeutic regimen.)	Attitudes and behavior conducive to positive health behaviors depend on psychosocial, cultural, economic, cognitive, and physical factors—how the client views and values health and illness; how the client understands or accepts illness; what he or she knows about the drug in question; how he or she relates to the health care surroundings, system, and practitioners; how the client assigns control and decision making; whether the client communicates and thinks logically; how he or she has been educated; and whether he or she has manipulative skills, among others. Studies show that having faith in a therapy has a decidedly favorable effect on its outcome. A subtle approach is needed to evaluate these parameters.

DEA # ____________

KEVIN NATHANSON, M.D.
EMILY KATE ZIMMERMAN, A.N.P.-C
OAK HILLS HEALTH CENTER
2901 OAK HILLS DRIVE
REDLANDS, CA 92373

Name ____________

ADDRESS ____________ DATE ____________

℞

☐ Label

Refill ______ times PRN NR

To ensure brand name dispensing, prescriber must write 'Dispense As Written' on the prescription.

Figure 4-3 Example of a prescription pad order form.

Safe nursing practice requires following approved procedures in the particular work environment and administering only drugs that are ordered in writing. Nursing students should be aware of special limitations imposed on their actions by the educational and/or clinical institution. In particular, they should be advised to follow only written orders. However, a verbal or telephoned order from a prescriber, often in response to the nurse's telephoned request, is sometimes unavoidable. When this occurs it is best for the nurse, not a student, to copy the order as it is being given, then verify it by repeating it back to the prescriber. Verbal or telephoned orders should be rare and involve circumstances of some urgency rather than convenience. Such orders must be clearly communicated and noted on the client's chart by the nurse. The prescriber must countersign the order, usually within 24 hours in most institutions, in order for it *to be legal*. Allowing the order to remain unsigned is careless and negligent because it violates both the law and institutional policy. This allows a precarious period of nursing vulnerability to malpractice charges (see Chapter 2).

Types of Drug Orders

It is probably obvious by now that although clients in the community are free to medicate themselves with any accessible medication, usually neither the client nor the nurse may legally administer any medication without a written order once an individual is admitted to a clinical institution. The content of the prescriber's orders dictates the conditions under which the ordered drug may be administered. Several types of orders are described in the following sections.

BOX 4-1

Elements Essential For Medication Administration

Five Rights	Elements of Prescriber's Order
Right client	1. Client's name
	2. Date order written
Right drug	3. Medication name
Right dose	4. Dosage
Right route	5. Route
Right time	6. Frequency
	7. Prescriber signature

In addition, the medication should be correctly documented before its administration is considered to be complete. Documentation may be the sixth "right" essential for medication administration.

Routine Order. The most common type of order is the **routine order,** in which the drug is to be regularly administered as ordered until a formal discontinuation order is written or until a specified termination date is reached. Automatic termination or "automatic stops" may be explicit in agency policy. Automatic stop policies may be mandated for institutional accreditation or licensure requirements, or they may be applied variously by institutions. Such policies act as a stimulus to the prescriber to reevaluate the client's continued need for drugs that require especially close attention.

prn Order. A **prn order** is an order for drugs to be administered according to client need. Within the other criteria specified by the order, the decision of when to medicate is left to the nurse's judgment. This type of order has implications for nursing autonomy similar to protocol orders.

Medications to reduce the perception of pain make up the bulk of prn orders. Keen nursing assessments of pain are required to carry out these prn orders appropriately. (See Chapter 14 for specifics for the evaluation of pain.) It is sufficient to note that pain is a very complex phenomenon that is influenced by factors of subjectivity, emotions, and age, among others. The most dependable guide is that the pain is what and when the client says it is; assumptions by the nurse are not as reliable. Research has demonstrated that clients are often undermedicated for pain (Jacox, Ferrell, Heidich, Hester, & Miaskowski, 1992). Children in particular are often left to suffer, undermedicated for pain, under the assumption that their pain is less severe than it seems.

Single Order. A **single order** is an order for a drug to be administered only once at the time indicated. An example is an order for a preoperative medication.

Stat Order. A **stat order** is an order for a drug to be administered as a single dose immediately.

Protocol. A **protocol** is a set of criteria that serves as a directive under which medication may be given. Protocols may typically be one of two types: standing orders or flow diagram protocols. Standing orders are officially accepted sets of orders (not only for medications) that are to be ap-

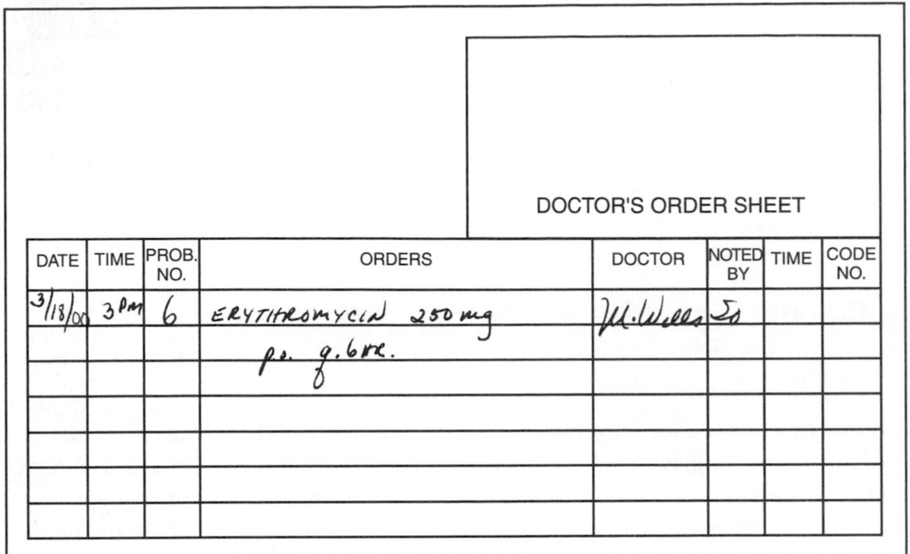

DOCTOR'S ORDER SHEET

DATE	TIME	PROB. NO.	ORDERS	DOCTOR	NOTED BY	TIME	CODE NO.
3/18/00	3 PM	6	ERYTHROMYCIN 250 mg	M. Wells	Sd		
			p.o. q.6hr.				

Figure 4-4 Example of an order sheet.

plied routinely by nurses in caring for clients with certain conditions or under certain circumstances (e.g., as part of admission orders in some critical care units). Flow diagram protocols are criteria that give nurses guidelines for the administration of certain treatments and medications on the basis of client variables. Of all the types of orders, protocols provide the widest scope for the application of nursing judgment and decision making. Criteria and direction may be either very specific, for those with limited expertise or responsibility, or less specific and allow for greater latitude, self-reliance, and sophistication in decision making.

Assessment of Medication Orders

Client. Every possible effort should be made to ensure that the client receives the intended medication in the manner planned by the prescriber. Toward this end, clients with similar names should be widely separated in the health care setting, and all their paperwork must be clearly distinguishable. An identifying wristband must be kept on every client in an institutional setting and compared with the identifying information that accompanies each dose of medication.

Date. The date that a medication order was written must be checked against other information for accuracy or for confirmation of when the last dose is to be given.

Medication. The name of the medication may be written in either generic or trade form. Clients should be familiar with the names of their medications. They should be told the names of their drugs when the drugs are administered. Doing so begins the educational process so that clients may effectively manage their medication regimen at home. It is dangerous for clients not to know their medications. Exact names and dosages are crucial drug information for clients to provide to health care providers if, for example, multiple providers are used or emergency treatment is needed.

Dosage and Frequency. Drug dosages should be given as prescribed in the medication order unless nursing judgment detects, for example, that the ordered amount falls outside the range of usual limits or that there are intervening individual client factors that would affect the appropriateness of the dosage, frequency, or route of administration of the drug. In such a case the drug is not administered; this omission is documented, and the prescriber is consulted as soon as possible.

During the development of a drug, the manufacturer makes determinations regarding the optimal range of dosage, frequency, and effective route of administration for most people. These determinations are based on the known pharmacokinetics and pharmacodynamics of the drug. For example, a drug that routinely undergoes a slow biotransformation may remain in the body system longer and produce more prolonged effects than another drug. This type of drug may therefore be given effectively on a once-a-day basis; a drug that is excreted rapidly may need to be given every 4 hours around-the-clock if effective serum levels are to be maintained. Nursing judgments must be made in order to align an individual client's medication schedule with agency policy at appropriate intervals or to keep to a single schedule to meet a specific drug requirement (e.g., before or after meals) or a special need of the client. Reasons to individualize administration time include client convenience and the avoidance of disturbing the client's rest, sleep, meals, visiting hours, activities, or treatments. The rationale for other modifications in the therapeutic regimen should be discussed with the prescriber.

Route. Every medication order should include a specified route for administration. Making assumptions in this area is negligent. The choice of the actual *site* of administration of injectables is a nursing or nurse-client decision. For example, SC, IM, and IV sites to avoid include any areas of obvious injury, disease, or lesions, even if minor; any areas that are noticeably erythematous (reddened), vesicular (blistered), open and weeping or pustular, ecchymotic (bruised),

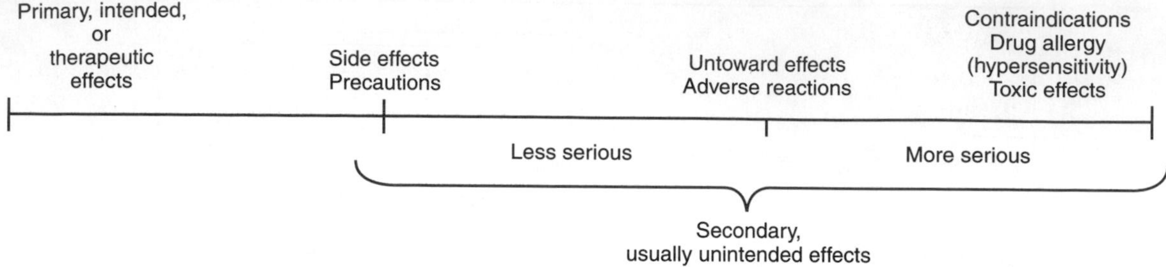

Figure 4-5 Terms indicating relative severity of medication effects—a continuum.

or scarred; and areas previously overused for injection. Such areas may have impaired circulation or may be adversely affected by the injection itself or by the material injected. Injection sites are rotated to avoid tissue damage from injections. (Details may be found in Chapter 5.)

The ordered route of administration should be assessed routinely for efficacy, feasibility, or practicality. For example, the oral route would naturally be precluded for a client who is nauseated or vomiting. Prior consultation with the prescriber must be made before administering a drug by a different route, because dosage or other factors may need to be readjusted if bioavailability is affected by such changes.

Evaluation of Primary and Secondary Effects

The ultimate effects of drugs on the body can be divided into two types. The main purpose of administering a medication is for its primary or therapeutic effect. All other consequences can be considered secondary effects, which are largely unintended and often nontherapeutic. Figure 4-5 illustrates the association among common terms that are used to describe the relative severity of secondary effects.

Drugs are developed and formulated to promote special effects, and the appearance of secondary effects demonstrates a continuing challenge to drug manufacturers. The crux of this problem is that most drugs are not selective enough to target only one body system, organ, tissue, or cell. When the drug is circulated or distributed to other areas, reactions may range in severity from merely inconvenient or annoying to very serious. Under certain circumstances a side effect may actually be the sought-after primary effect or may be exploited by the prescriber as a therapeutic effect along with the primary effects. For example, diphenhydramine (Benadryl) is an antihistamine that produces a high incidence of drowsiness or sedation-type side effects. If this antihistamine is prescribed for an irritable child afflicted with an itching, poison ivy rash, the effect of sedation becomes a desired secondary effect. In fact, diphenhydramine is a common ingredient in OTC medications for sleep. However, sedation is undesired for a person who handles dangerous machinery or drives a commercial vehicle for a living. In such instances, the prescriber should probably select an antihistamine that does not have a significant sedative side effect.

Primary and secondary effects are often dose related—directly related to increases in dosage—or they may be related to the duration of that specific therapy.

In the assessment phase of the nursing process, it is essential to discover any **contraindications**—conditions that would preclude the administration of a drug. A contraindication to the administration of a drug has the potential to be more harmful than do side effects and adverse reactions, which may be discerned only in the evaluation phase (see Chapter 5)—after the administration of the drug. It is essential that the medicating process be assessed with regard to each medication's clinical indications and potential efficacy and any contraindications, especially any allergy or pathologic condition that would preclude its administration. Box 4-2 summarizes the medications often implicated in allergic reactions.

The client's allergy history, even if unrelated to the medication, must be explored to rule out and prevent any possible allergic reaction. The occurrence of drug allergy reactions is extremely individualized, unpredictable except for history, and not usually closely dose related. The reaction may result in a very serious and life-threatening situation; consequently the drug must not be given. Reactions may vary from mild rash to severe exfoliative dermatitis and from asthma to anaphylactic shock. They may include urticaria, angioneurotic edema, and drug fever.

An allergic drug response is caused by a specific reaction between a drug and the immune system. Most drugs are organic molecules with molecular weights of less than 1000 daltons. (A dalton is an arbitrary unit of mass equivalent to 1.657×10^{-24} g.) Such small molecules act as haptens, in which they take on the ability to act as allergens as they are bound to carrier proteins. An immune response is stimulated and an allergic response is provoked only when the drug or its metabolite combines with tissue or plasma proteins to form the drug-protein complex—the complete allergen. At initial exposure to the drug, sensitive persons may exhibit a latent period of 10 to 20 days before the allergic reaction occurs. Reactions upon reexposure to the drug may occur sooner, even immediately.

It is essential to place alerting stickers or notations regarding the client's allergic history in the clinical record, computerized information system, Kardex, or other places according to agency policy. These locations need to be

BOX 4-2

Medications Commonly Implicated in Allergic Reactions

Antibiotics: penicillin (the most common cause of drug-induced anaphylaxis), cephalosporins, tetracyclines, streptomycin, erythromycin, neomycin, nitrofurantoin, and sulfa drugs (very common)

Other drugs: aspirin, hydantoins, acetaminophen, tolbutamide, gold salts, phenothiazines, histamines, iodides, iron dextran, methylergonovine, quinidine, aminosalicylic acid, tranquilizers, anesthetics such as benzocaine (particularly troublesome because they are often used for topical application to irritated or delicate mucous membranes), tetracaine, procaine, lidocaine, and cocaine

Diagnostic agents such as iodinated contrast media (e.g., dye for intravenous pyelogram [IVP]), iopanoic acid (Telepaque), dehydrocholic acid (Decholin), Congo red dye

Biologicals such as antitoxins, vaccines, gamma globulin, insulin, adrenocorticotropic hormone (ACTH), enzymes, and their preservatives such as thimerosal and parabens

checked before any medications are given. Records may denote "no known allergy" (NKA), but this notation usually refers to drugs. Because a correlation often exists between one allergic response and the development of another, the client's description of any past allergic manifestations—to drugs, inhalants, foods (typically eggs, orange juice, chocolate, shellfish, or strawberries), or whatever—must be clarified and evaluated. Often the client erroneously defines an unexpected response as an allergic one. For example, the nausea that occurs following a meperidine (Demerol) injection may be labeled an allergic reaction by the client, when in actuality it is likely to be only a normal, if exaggerated, side effect. Correcting such misinformation with the client and in the records may be important because it makes that drug available for therapy when necessary. Before any questionable medications are administered, nurses should specifically inquire about previous experiences with these agents and, if necessary for a client who has many allergies, discuss with the prescriber the need for a test dose. Special methods for those who must take a medication to which they are allergic (e.g., aspirin, local anesthetics, or contrast media in diagnostic agents) include pretreatment medications in the form of antihistamines, prednisone, and ephedrine or cautiously increasing dosages of the allergy-provoking drug under supervision. Clients may also have allergies to the additives found in foods and drug products (Box 4-3).

Other contraindications to drug therapy must be assessed before administration. Clients may have medical problems that contraindicate a given drug or, if the drug is deemed necessary, that require careful consideration of the risk-benefit ratio and careful monitoring of the client. For example, opioid analgesics are contraindicated in clients with acute respiratory depression, because the respiratory depressive effects of the drug would exacerbate the condition. Most drugs, including opioid analgesics, would be administered with caution and probably with dosage modifications to clients with hepatic or renal function impairment because these drugs are metabolized in the liver and excreted by the kidneys. It is essential to assess for and plan the pharmacologic therapeutic regimen to minimize the adverse effects and provide for client safety.

BOX 4-3

Allergic Reactions to Food Additives

Allergic reactions have been reported after the ingestion of food additives such as monosodium glutamate (MSG), tartrazine, and sulfites. Tartrazine and sulfites are also used as additives, preservatives, and antioxidants in various medications. The most serious adverse reaction has occurred most often in clients who are asthmatic and has resulted in some reported deaths. Current lists of foods and drug products containing tartrazine and sulfites should be reviewed in assessing reported allergic reactions.

Drug Interactions

The complexity of modern pharmacotherapy is nowhere more obvious than in the ever-growing list of drugs that either interact nontherapeutically with one another, with foods, and with fluids or distort laboratory test results. That these chemical substances interact with or potentiate one another is not surprising. This fact should always be kept in mind when medications appear either ineffective or harmful or when the accuracy of laboratory tests is crucial.

Variables influencing drug interaction include (1) intestinal absorption, (2) competition for plasma binding, (3) drug metabolism or biotransformation, (4) action at the receptor site, (5) renal excretion, and (6) alteration of electrolyte balance. The following are examples of effects that interact nontherapeutically with other drugs, food, juices, and other liquids and distort many laboratory test results:

1. *Intestinal absorption.* Foods or antacids that contain calcium, magnesium, or aluminum (e.g., antacids or dairy products) may form a complex with or bind tetracycline, resulting in reduced absorption of the antibiotic.
2. *Competition for plasma protein binding.* Tolbutamide (Orinase), an oral antihyperglycemic agent, can be displaced from its binding on plasma proteins by sulfonamides, resulting in severe hypoglycemia. Many drugs are weak acids that are bound largely to plasma proteins. These weak acids may compete for binding sites on plasma proteins, thus increasing the free, active drug, which may have potent effects.

3. *Drug metabolism or biotransformation.* The monoamine oxidase inhibitors prevent the biotransformation of tyramine, which is present in aged cheese, liver, overripe fruit, and preserved meat (sausage, bologna, pepperoni, salami) and may provoke a hypertensive crisis (a rapid and severe increase in blood pressure). Grapefruit juice inhibits the metabolism of carbamazepine (Tegretol) and other drugs in the gastrointestinal tract, which allows more of the drug to be absorbed. Higher carbamazepine levels can cause nausea, dizziness, tremor, and confusion (Garg, Kumar, Bhargava, & Prabhakar, 1998).
4. *Action at the receptor site.* Numerous examples exist of one drug intensifying or antagonizing the action of another drug at the receptor site. For example, the antihistaminics decrease many effects of histamine, whereas cocaine increases the actions of epinephrine.
5. *Renal excretion.* Probenecid (Benemid) inhibits the renal clearance of penicillin because it inhibits the active renal tubular secretion of many weak organic acids, of which penicillin is one.
6. *Alteration of electrolyte balance.* The thiazide diuretics may cause hypokalemia, which predisposes to digitalis toxicity, because there is increased renal secretion of potassium with their use.

In addition to these drug interactions, the nurse should also consider drugs that have a pharmacodynamic interaction. Pharmacodynamic interactions are caused by the concurrent administration of two drugs that have the opposite effect or similar effects. The interactions of drugs having similar effects (e.g., alcohol and sedatives, or drugs having hypotensive effects) may be easier to identify than the interactions of drugs having opposite effects. An example of such an interaction is a client with asthma who is being treated with a beta-adrenergic drug such as albuterol (Proventil, Ventolin) for its bronchodilating effects while also being given a beta-adrenergic blocking drug, which has bronchoconstricting properties, as an antihypertensive agent.

Not all drug interactions are dangerous; some are relatively insignificant or even beneficial. In the hospital setting, tables listing known harmful drug interactions should be posted in the medication area as a reference for nurses. Most nurses practicing in the home setting carry drug handbooks that list significant drug interactions.

Drug-Drug Interactions

Some drugs commonly involved in clinically significant drug-drug interactions include antacids, warfarin (Coumadin), aspirin, tricyclic antidepressants (monoamine oxidase [MAO] inhibitors), aminoglycosides, amphetamines, corticosteroids, digitalis glycosides, diuretics, cimetidine (Tagamet), sulfonamides, alcohol, phenytoin (Dilantin), quinidine (Quinaglute), antihypertensives, beta blockers, and theophylline (Elixophyllin). Before any such medication is given, an appropriate source should be consulted to assess the drug, its mechanism, and any other medications given concurrently to determine the probability of interactions. This text provides this information in the context of specific drug monographs.

Other Drug Interactions

Drug-Induced Malabsorption of Foods and Nutrients. Drugs that change gastric or intestinal motility can alter the digestion or absorption of other drugs and nutrients. Important drugs that affect these changes are gastrointestinal prokinetic drugs such as cisapride (Propulsid), metoclopramide (Reglan), and stimulant cathartics, which increase bowel motility; at the other extreme are anticholinergics and narcotics, which inhibit bowel motility. Cholestyramine (Questran) and colestipol (Colestid), drugs indicated for hypercholesteremia, adsorb and combine with bile acids to form an insoluble complex that is excreted through the feces; this loss of bile acids lowers blood cholesterol levels. However, these drugs also adsorb other medications, as well as the fat-soluble vitamins A, D, E, and K; these substances are then excreted from rather than absorbed into the body. Some oral contraceptives impair the absorption of folic acid in undernourished clients.

Food-Induced Malabsorption of Drugs. Fatty foods and foods low in fiber delay stomach emptying by up to 2 hours, which may result in delayed and/or reduced drug absorption. Other medications, such as griseofulvin (Grisactin), exhibit enhanced bioavailability (absorption) following a high-fat meal. Many tetracyclines can form insoluble complexes in the gastrointestinal tract if given at the same time as foods or drugs containing ions of calcium, aluminum, magnesium, or iron. Thus administering tetracycline medication along with milk-based tube feedings, dairy products, or common antacids should be avoided. Ascorbic acid from citrus fruits or juices enhances the absorption of iron, but carbonated soft drinks or acid juices (fruit or vegetable) can cause drugs to dissolve more quickly in the stomach than in the intestine or can neutralize them, thereby changing the intended rate or completeness of absorption (Lowenthal & Parnetti, 1996). Grapefruit juice interacts with most calcium channel blockers, lovastatin (Mevacor), and triazolam (Halcion), among other drugs.

Milk, coffee, eggs, tea, whole-grain breads and cereals, dietary fiber, and foods containing bicarbonates, carbonates, phosphates, or oxalates may reduce iron absorption if given concurrently. Iron products should be ingested no sooner than 1 hour before or 2 hours after the mentioned food substances are given.

Alteration of Enzymes. Enzyme alterations, either induction or inhibition, may affect the metabolism of a food or drug. An increased synthesis of cytochrome P-450 by a drug, such as the anticonvulsant carbamazepine (Tegretol), induces the biotransformation of other drugs and its own metabolism. In the case of carbamazepine it is metabolized to its reactive form so that increased induction is associated with increased toxicity. With certain other drugs, such as barbiturates, increased induction decreases the availability of the parent drug and other drugs as they are metabolized to inactive substances. In the example of barbiturates, this activity contributes to the development of drug tolerance.

The natural extract of black licorice is chemically similar to that of steroids; therefore if taken in excess, licorice can cause hypokalemia, sodium and water retention with resultant hypertension, and alkalosis. The ingestion of large amounts of black licorice is contraindicated for clients who are concurrently taking potassium-losing diuretics or for those who have cardiovascular disease.

Similarly, the consumption of large amounts of foods high in vitamin K (such as liver and green leafy vegetables) may reduce or antagonize the effectiveness of oral anticoagulants. Difficulty in maintaining the desired anticoagulant response with the appropriately prescribed dosages indicates the need for an assessment of food and drug consumption.

MAO inhibitors (tricyclic antidepressants) act by inhibiting the breakdown of norepinephrine, a vasopressor substance. The excess norepinephrine is stored in the neurons. Ingesting certain tyramine-containing foods (aged cheeses, beef and chicken liver, pickled herring, broad beans, canned figs, bananas, avocados, soy sauce, active yeast preparations, beer, sherry in large quantities, Chianti wine, chocolate, anchovies, caffeine, mushrooms, raisins, sausages, dried fish, tuna fish, cola drinks, and many fermented foods) may elevate the quantity of norepinephrine to toxic levels and precipitate a hypertensive crisis. OTC cold remedies containing ephedrine, phenylephrine, and phenylpropanolamine, as well as amphetamines in general can act similarly, releasing stored quantities of norepinephrine. The net effect may be a headache, a sudden climb in blood pressure to dangerous levels, cardiac dysrhythmias, or intracranial bleeding.

Alcohol Consumption. It is important to elicit information about patterns of alcohol consumption when obtaining a history (Bird, 1997). Of the more than 100 most commonly prescribed drugs, more than half contain at least one ingredient known to interact adversely with imbibed alcohol. An interaction is probable if the drug is known to affect the central nervous system (CNS) or is metabolized by the liver. The effects are dose related, and whether quantities of alcohol are used habitually, chronically, or only occasionally often makes a distinct difference in the direction of interactive effects. Patterns of alcohol consumption are likely to affect the client's concurrence with drug treatment and follow through. Alcohol consumption should be limited or completely avoided if a client is taking narcotics, tranquilizers, sedatives, and other CNS depressant–type drugs, which may cause additive or synergistic respiratory and CNS depression.

The fact that many elixirs and tinctures are liquid formulations of drugs dissolved in alcohol is significant, especially in the assessment of pharmacotherapy for children, who are more at risk for the hypoglycemic effects of alcohol. Preparations with ethanol content must be reassessed and cannot be assumed to have the same rates and degrees of absorption as the same drugs in aqueous solution, because bioavailability may be altered.

Cigarette Smoking. The main pharmacokinetic effect of heavy cigarette smoking is the lowering of drug plasma levels by the induction of microsomal enzyme systems responsible for increased drug metabolism or excretion. The rate of theophylline (Theo-Dur) breakdown is increased, necessitating an increase of 1.5 times to twice the average dose. The usual doses of other drugs have diminished effectiveness in the heavy cigarette smoker, such as with the antidepressant imipramine (Tofranil); analgesics such as pentazocine (Talwin) and propoxyphene (Darvon); vitamins C, B_{12}, and B_6; and the influenza vaccine. The absorption rate of insulin by the SC route is twice as slow as usual. Smoking also interacts with furosemide (Lasix) and propranolol (Inderal). Drowsiness and depression of the CNS are less common with diazepam (Valium), and drowsiness is reduced with chlorpromazine (Thorazine). The risk of heart attack, stroke, and other circulatory disorders increases when smoking is combined with the use of estrogens.

Laboratory test results may also be somewhat outside the range of normal, depending on inhalation practices and the duration of smoking history. The white cell count is increased (in the absence of clinical infection); hemoglobin concentration, hematocrit, and red blood cell size are increased; and clotting time is reduced. Some investigators of cigarette smoking have found an abnormal increase in cholesterol, and others have found carcinoembryonic antigen levels as high as for persons with colon cancer, yet without other evidence of it. Therefore smokers sometimes can be expected to exhibit more numerous drug therapy "failures" or adverse effects, or they may even have fewer or different reactions to drugs than do nonsmoking clients. Certain laboratory test results must be interpreted in light of the client's history of smoking.

Caffeine Consumption. Caffeinated beverages present a medical problem in that many people consume enough caffeine to produce substantial effects on a number of organ systems. Caffeine stimulates the CNS and cardiac muscle, and it acts on the kidney to produce diuresis. Individuals ingesting caffeine or caffeinated beverages usually experience less drowsiness and fatigue and more rapid and clearer flow of thought. As the dose is increased, however, signs of progressive CNS stimulation occur, including nervousness, anxiety, restlessness, insomnia, and tremors. Caffeine produces tachycardia and, in higher doses, dysrhythmias. Increases in blood pressure with caffeine ingestion are the result of an increase in systemic vascular resistance. Caffeine causes the secretion of both pepsin and gastric acid from the parietal cells of the stomach. The cardiac-stimulating effects of caffeine may inhibit the therapeutic effect of beta-adrenergic blockers. Excessive CNS stimulation may occur with the concurrent use of caffeine and other CNS stimulants, progressing from nervousness to possibly convulsions or cardiac dysrhythmias. Caffeine inhibits the absorption of calcium and promotes the excretion of lithium and other drugs. Caffeine may also produce severe hypertension when combined with MAO inhibitors.

Food-Initiated Alteration of Drug Excretion. Because pH influences the ionization of weak acids and bases, changes in the pH of urine caused by food (making the urine overly acidic or alkaline) can have a significant effect on the excretion rates of some drugs. A drug in a nonionized state will diffuse more easily from the urine back into the blood, thereby prolonging drug action. For this reason, the action of acidic drugs is prolonged when urine is acidic. Although it is quite difficult to override the ability of the kidney's to regulate urine pH, an alkaline-ash or acid-ash diet, whether or not it is intentional, can drive urinary pH above 8 or below 5 and create a medium for potential drug reactions. The continued use of many antacid tablets each day in concert with quinidine administration has been seen to create quinidine intoxication by shifting urinary pH toward the alkaline levels and causing a dysrhythmia serious enough to require hospitalization.

Drug Incompatibilities

Interactions that occur when drugs are mixed before administration, as in a single syringe or in IV fluids, are termed drug **incompatibilities.** Drugs that are physically incompatible may produce unwanted changes through processes such as liquefaction, deliquescence, or precipitation. Chemical incompatibilities may result when ingredients interact to form new compounds or are neutralized (see the Nursing Research box below). Separate administration routes should be sought if drug incompatibilities are anticipated.

Some drugs are highly incompatible in solution with many other drugs. Because solution incompatibilities are often time dependent, fewer difficulties may be associated with mixing drugs in one syringe than with IV solutions; both drugs should be administered as soon after mixing as possible. Drugs that are noted for being incompatible with many other drugs in a syringe include chlordiazepoxide (Librium), diazepam (Valium), pentobarbital (Nembutal), phenobarbital (Luminal), phenytoin (Dilantin), secobarbital (Seconal), and sodium bicarbonate; these drugs should be administered alone.

Many drugs have explicit manufacturer's instructions for preparation (dilution and method of adding to select parenteral solutions); these instructions should be followed closely. A check for drug compatibility is indicated before two or more drugs are added to the same IV solution. Standard IV parenteral drug charts and guides are available for reference use. Most hospital pharmacies provide an IV preparation service that screens for incompatibilities before preparation and delivery to the nursing area or the client's home.

With the increase in the number of potent drugs and the variety of combinations, use of the pharmacist's expertise in a controlled environment is probably a wise policy. If the

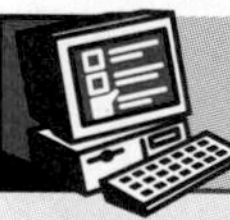

Nursing Research
Incompatible Drug Infusions Via Multilumen Catheters

Citation: Collins, J.L. & Lutz, R.J. (1991). In vitro study of simultaneous infusion of incompatible drugs in multilumen catheters. *Heart Lung, 20*(3), 271.

Abstract: Nurses have long been alert to the occurrence of incompatibilities when mixing multiple medications in the same syringe. With the increased use of multilumen catheters to maintain long-term, reliable central venous access for frequent administration of multiple drugs and hyperalimentation solutions, as well as for blood sampling and transfusions, consideration needs to be given to the possibility of such incompatibilities occurring in vivo.

Collins and Lutz used an in vitro model venous flow system to examine the physicochemical phenomena that occur when two incompatible drugs (phenytoin and total parenteral nutrition) are simultaneously administered through multilumen catheters. In this system, flow conditions and drug infusions mimicked in vivo clinical situations to evaluate two central venous catheter types: a double-lumen catheter and a triple-lumen catheter. Video recordings were made of drug interactions, and assays of phenytoin concentration were performed on samples of the circulating fluid. White clouds of phenytoin precipitation were observed near the tip of the double-lumen catheter but not the triple-lumen catheter. Infusion through the double-lumen catheter resulted in an average loss of phenytoin of 6%, the precipitate of which, on microscopic examination, appeared as spindle-shaped crystals 25 to 50 μm in length and 5 to 10 μm wide. In some instances, millimeter-sized fragments of phenytoin were seen to dislodge from the tip of the double-lumen catheter. The adjacent orifices at the tip of the double-lumen catheter appeared to permit interaction of the two effusing streams of incompatible drugs, whereas the staggered orifices of the triple-lumen catheter minimized this interaction. Although the clinical significance of in vivo precipitate incompatibility has yet to be determined, theoretically possible complications would include reduced bioavailability of the drug, thrombophlebitis from particulate matter, pulmonary emboli from larger precipitate fragments, and occlusion of the catheter.

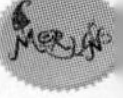

Critical Thinking Questions

- In what way do you think this research could affect the use of central venous catheters with clients on multidrug regimens?
- If you were administering precipitate-incompatible drugs to a client with a double-lumen central venous catheter, how would you modify your nursing care?

nurse is required to prepare IV solutions on the nursing unit, adequate references, including a list of incompatibilities, should be posted in the area where this duty is performed. Open and regular communication with the pharmacy department is necessary for obtaining new or additional information and assistance whenever necessary.

ANALYSIS OF DATA

When data from the nursing assessment have been collected, the next phase is **analysis**—the critical evaluation of information to determine its meaning and importance. It is the process of interpreting data based on sound pharmacologic and nursing principles. As with all phases of the nursing process, analysis is continuous.

The nurse may follow several steps to facilitate analysis. Initially, data are organized into categories. These data include the client's history of preexisting health conditions and present health status, concurrent medication regimen, understanding of the drug and the condition for which the drug is prescribed, and ability to manage a therapeutic regimen. Categorization of information is accomplished with a planned systematic assessment, and gaps in data are noted. Once identified, this missing information can be obtained to complete the assessment. Accepted standards and norms are then applied to determine discrepancies between what is and what should or could be, and conclusions are drawn regarding what actual problems may be present and those for which the client may be at high risk (Crow, Chase, & Lamond, 1995). The culmination of analysis is the diagnostic statement, which includes nursing diagnoses and collaborative problems toward which nursing care may be directed.

NURSING DIAGNOSES/ COLLABORATIVE PROBLEMS

The North American Nursing Diagnosis Association (NANDA) defines a **nursing diagnosis** as a clinical judgment about individual, family, or community responses to actual or potential health problems/life processes. A nursing diagnosis provides the basis for the selection of nursing interventions to achieve outcomes for which the nurse is accountable (North American Nursing Diagnosis Association, 1997). NANDA is the formal organization sanctioned by the American Nurses Association (ANA) to govern the development of a classification system for nursing diagnoses. Proposed nursing diagnoses are submitted to NANDA for official acceptance.

Until 1992 the phrase "potential for" was used if the client was at risk of developing a particular nursing diagnosis. Since then, "high risk for" or "risk for" has been the appropriate terminology and is defined by NANDA (1997) to indicate "a clinical judgment that an individual, family, or community is more vulnerable to develop the problem than others in the same or similar situation." In the current health care climate the cost of health care may limit nurse-client interaction, and thus the use of "high risk for" nursing diagnoses assist nurses to identify the most vulnerable clients, families, and community populations.

Collaborative problems are "certain physiologic complications that nurses monitor to detect onset or changes of status. Nurses manage collaborative problems utilizing physician-prescribed and nursing-prescribed interventions to minimize the complications of the events" (Carpenito, 2000). With nursing diagnoses, assessment involves detecting signs and symptoms of actual problems and risk factors for high-risk nursing diagnoses, whereas the assessment for collaborative problems focuses on determining the status of the collaborative problem, that is, that certain conditions are present that increase the client's vulnerability to the complication, or that the client has experienced the complication. The nurse's responsibility is to monitor the client's physiologic status, perform specific activities to manage and minimize the severity of the situation, and consult with a health care provider to obtain orders for appropriate interventions. Collaborative problems can be written as "Potential complication: (specify)." An example of a collaborative problem with the administration of a nonsteroidal antiinflammatory analgesic would be "Potential complication (PC): gastrointestinal bleeding," or with methotrexate, an antineoplastic agent, "PC: hepatotoxicity."

The nurse makes independent decisions for both nursing diagnoses and collaborative problems. The difference is that in nursing diagnoses, nursing prescribes the definitive treatment, whereas with collaborative problems both nursing and medicine prescribe for the definitive treatment to achieve the desired outcomes for client care.

The nursing profession is working actively toward a classification for nursing practice. Standardization of terminology facilitates communication among practitioners. An aim is to classify groups of nursing diagnoses so that patterns will emerge, leading to categories of diagnoses. NANDA has endorsed a classification of nursing diagnoses by human response patterns with approved terminology (McCourt & Carroll-Johnson, 1992). Diagnostic statements used in this book are drawn from the list of NANDA-approved nursing diagnoses whenever possible. The NANDA list and other widely circulated lists are not considered complete; nurses are encouraged to test nursing diagnoses and develop new ones.

Several examples of nursing diagnoses follow. There are countless ways to convey the same thoughts, all equally correct; variations arise from differences among individuals constructing the diagnoses and from the wording chosen. All nursing diagnoses include two main components: a description of altered health status and an inferred reason for it (etiology or risk factors). If the nursing diagnosis is an actual one rather than one for which the client is at risk, the symptoms by which the client demonstrates the problem are included in the statement for completeness. The following list presents some sample nursing diagnoses:

- Risk for impaired urinary elimination: urinary retention related to history of benign prostatic hypertrophy and concurrent anticholinergic therapy

- Risk for constipation related to morphine sulfate administration
- Excess fluid volume: edema related to steroid therapy evidenced by 2+ pitting edema of ankles and weight gain of 4 pounds over 3 days
- Ineffective therapeutic regimen management: failure to refill prescriptions related to inadequate financial resources to buy drugs as evidenced by client's statement "I wish I could afford my heart pills"

Box 4-4 contains the current list of NANDA-approved nursing diagnoses; the ones that more commonly result from drug therapy are noted by asterisks. However, the nurse should consider the full range of nursing diagnoses during assessment.

For each medication there is a combination of nursing diagnoses and collaborative problems that should be anticipated or for which the client needs to be assessed. In addition to quite specific ones that may be particular to the individual client, assessment for the following eight specific nursing diagnoses/collaborative problems are basic to the management of every client's drug regimen:

1. *Client issues related to the client's preexisting health status.* These may be stated as "Potential complication (PC): (specify the physiologic complication related to the client's preexisting medical conditions, age, and childbearing status)," such as "PC: acute respiratory depression related to client's preexisting chronic obstructive pulmonary disease and the administration of morphine." On the other hand, a number of nursing diagnoses might also relate to the client's preexisting health status and the administration of morphine, such as "Risk for constipation related to the client's age (76 years), low fiber intake, and the administration of morphine" or "Risk for urinary retention related to client's history of benign prostatic hypertrophy and the administration of morphine."
2. *Client issues related to concurrent drug therapy.* "PC: (specify the physiologic complication related to concurrent drug therapy)," such as "PC: digoxin toxicity related to the concurrent administration of digoxin and diuretic therapy." An appropriate nursing diagnosis related to concurrent drug therapy might be "Risk for injury related to postural hypotension secondary to the concurrent administration of propranolol (Inderal) and diuretic therapy."
3. *Client issues related to the ineffectiveness of the drug.* "PC: (specify the physiologic complication of the client's underlying condition related to the ineffectiveness of the drug)," such as "PC: sepsis related to the ineffectiveness of antibiotic therapy." A nursing diagnosis related to the ineffectiveness of therapy might be "Chronic pain related to ineffective pain management program." The assessment of the effectiveness of the client's drug regimen is essential. If the outcome criteria for the client's drug therapy are not met, the drug is considered to be ineffective and the prescriber will need to alter the client's medications.
4. *Client issues related to the side effects/adverse reactions.* "PC: (specify the physiologic complication related to the side effects/adverse reactions of the administered drug)," such as "PC: thrombocytopenia related to heparin therapy" or "PC: GI bleeding related to aspirin therapy." An appropriate nursing diagnosis related to drug side effects might be "Disturbed sleep pattern related to caffeine ingestion." Carpenito (2000) has described "PC: medication therapy adverse effects" as well as specific potential complications for anticoagulant, antianxiety, adrenocorticosteroid, antineoplastic, anticonvulsant, antidepressant, antiarrhythmic, antipsychotic, antihypertensive, beta-adrenergic blocker, calcium channel blocker, and angiotensin-converting enzyme therapy.
5. *Risk for poisoning: drug toxicity,* which is the accentuated risk of accidental exposure to or ingestion of drugs or dangerous products in doses sufficient to cause poisoning. Older adults are particularly prone to this nursing diagnosis because of reduced vision, forgetfulness, polypharmacy, and the effects of drugs in the aging body.
6. *Deficient knowledge related to initiation of or change in the medication regimen.* Although deficient knowledge, the state in which an individual or group experiences a deficiency in cognitive knowledge or psychomotor skills concerning the condition or treatment plan, is listed as a nursing diagnosis, it does not represent a human response, alteration, or pattern of dysfunction (Jenny, 1987). However, each client must be assessed for the level of knowledge related to his or her health condition and medication regimen. Client education is necessary if the client requests information or expresses inadequate knowledge of his or her health condition or medications to self-administer the prescribed drugs accurately and safely.
7. *Noncompliance,* the state in which an individual or group desires to comply but is prevented from doing so by factors that deter adherence to health-related advice given by health care professionals, is another nursing diagnosis that should be considered in the client's assessment. Indicators that noncompliance may be an issue are that the client does not participate in therapy, the client's symptoms persist, the disease progresses, and drug therapy outcome criteria are not met. The nursing diagnosis "noncompliance" is not used to describe a client who has made an informed autonomous decision not to comply (Cassells & Redman, 1989).
8. *Ineffective therapeutic regimen management related to (specify)* is a pattern in which the individual experiences or is at high risk to experience difficulty integrating into daily living a program for the treatment of illness and its sequelae to meet specific health goals (NANDA, 1997). Factors that contribute to ineffective management may be a lack of trust in health care providers or insufficient confidence, knowledge, or resources.

BOX 4-4

Nursing Diagnoses Approved by the North American Nursing Diagnosis Association (2001-2002)

*Activity intolerance
*Activity intolerance, risk for
Adjustment, impaired
Airway clearance, ineffective
Allergy, latex response
Allergy, latex response, risk for
*Anxiety
Anxiety, death
*Aspiration, risk for
Attachment, impaired parent/infant/child, risk for
Autonomic dysreflexia
Autonomic dysreflexia, risk for
Body image, disturbed
Body temperature, imbalanced, risk for
Bowel incontinence
*Breastfeeding, effective
Breastfeeding, ineffective
Breastfeeding, interrupted
*Breathing pattern, ineffective
Cardiac output, decreased
Caregiver role strain
Caregiver role strain, risk for
Comfort, impaired
Communication, impaired verbal
Conflict, decisional
Conflict, parental role
Confusion, acute
Confusion, chronic
*Constipation
Constipation, perceived
Constipation, risk for
Coping, defensive
Coping, family, compromised
Coping, family, disabled
Coping, family, readiness for enhanced
*Coping, ineffective
Coping, ineffective, community
Coping, readiness for enhanced community
Denial, ineffective
Dentition, impaired
Development, risk for delayed
*Diarrhea
Disuse syndrome, risk for
Diversional activity, deficient
Energy field, disturbed
Environmental interpretation syndrome, impaired
Failure to thrive, adult
*Falls, risk for
Family processes, dysfunctional: alcoholism
Family processes, interrupted
*Fatigue
Fear
Fluid volume, deficient
*Fluid volume, deficient, risk for
*Fluid volume, excess
Fluid volume, imbalanced, risk for
*Gas exchange, impaired
Grieving
Grieving, anticipatory
Grieving, dysfunctional
Growth and development, delayed
Growth, disproportionate, risk for
*Health maintenance, ineffective
*Health-seeking behaviors (specify)
*Home maintenance, impaired
Hopelessness
Hyperthermia
Hypothermia
Identity, disturbed personal
Incontinence, functional urinary
Incontinence, reflex urinary
Incontinence, stress urinary
Incontinence, total urinary
Incontinence, urge urinary
Incontinence, urge urinary, risk for
Infant behavior, disorganized
Infant behavior, disorganized, risk for
Infant behavior, readiness for enhanced organized
Infant feeding pattern, ineffective
*Infection, risk for
*Injury, risk for (specify)
Injury, risk for perioperative-positioning
*Intracranial, decreased adaptive capacity
Knowledge, deficient (specify)
Loneliness, risk for
Memory, impaired
Mobility, impaired bed
Mobility, impaired physical
Mobility, impaired wheelchair
Nausea
Neglect, unilateral
*Noncompliance (specify)
*Nutrition, imbalanced: less than body requirements
Nutrition, imbalanced: more than body requirements
Nutrition, imbalanced: more than body requirements, risk for
*Oral mucous membrane, impaired
Pain, acute
Pain, chronic
Parenting, impaired
Parenting, impaired, risk for
Peripheral neurovascular dysfunction, risk for
*Poisoning, risk for
Post-trauma syndrome
Post-trauma syndrome, risk for
Powerlessness
Powerlessness, risk for
*Protection, ineffective
Rape-trauma syndrome
Rape-trauma syndrome: compound reaction
Rape-trauma syndrome: silent reaction
Relocation stress syndrome
Relocation stress syndrome, risk for
Role performance, ineffective
Self-care deficit: bathing/hygiene
Self-care deficit: dressing/grooming
Self-care deficit: feeding
Self-care deficit: toileting
Self-esteem, chronic low
Self-esteem, situational low
Self-esteem, situational low, risk for
Self-mutilation
Self-mutilation, risk for
*Sensory perception, disturbed (specify) (visual, auditory, kinesthetic, gustatory, tactile, olfactory)
*Sexual dysfunction
*Sexual patterns, ineffective
*Skin integrity, impaired
*Skin integrity, impaired, risk for
Sleep deprivation
*Sleep pattern, disturbed
Social interaction, impaired

Modified from North American Nursing Diagnosis Association (2002). *Nursing diagnoses: Definitions and classification* 2001-2002. Philadelphia: Author.
*Nursing diagnoses commonly seen with drug therapy.

Continued

BOX 4-4

Nursing Diagnoses Approved by the North American Nursing Diagnosis Association (2001-2002)—cont'd

Social isolation
Sorrow, chronic
Spiritual distress (distress of the human spirit)
Spiritual distress, risk for
Spiritual well-being, readiness for enhanced
Suffocation, risk for
Suicide, risk for
Surgical recovery, delayed
*Swallowing, impaired
Therapeutic regimen management, effective
*Therapeutic regimen management, ineffective
Therapeutic regimen management, community, ineffective
Therapeutic regimen management, family, ineffective
Thermoregulation, ineffective
*Thought processes, disturbed
Tissue integrity, impaired
*Tissue perfusion, impaired (specify) (renal, cerebral, cardiopulmonary, gastrointestinal, peripheral)
Transfer ability, impaired
Trauma, risk for
Urinary elimination, impaired
*Urinary retention
Ventilation, impaired spontaneous
Ventilatory weaning response, dysfunctional (DVWR)
Violence, risk for: directed at others
Violence, risk for: self-directed
Walking, impaired
Wandering

Modified from North American Nursing Diagnosis Association (2001). *Nursing diagnoses: Definitions and classification 2001-2002*. Philadelphia: Author.
*Nursing diagnoses commonly seen with drug therapy.

In the interests of producing a text that is still manageable in size, these eight client issues will not be listed with every drug when client assessment is discussed. However, the reader should keep all of these issues in mind, because they are considered to be universal and are relevant to every medication.

Nursing diagnoses and collaborative problems form the basis for the design of subsequent phases of the nursing process—planning, implementation, and evaluation. The nursing diagnostic statement differentiates among actual problems, possible problems, and those that the client is at risk for developing. Table 4-2 defines these three types of problems and the corresponding focus of nursing interventions for each.

Nature of Nursing Actions

Nursing interventions may be categorized into three domains: dependent (or delegated), collaborative, and independent. Medicine both diagnoses and treats pathologic or cellular responses, whereas nursing both diagnoses and treats the human response. Activities that legally require a physician directive, or in some states a nurse practitioner or physician assistant, are considered to be within the **dependent domain** of nursing interventions; these activities constitute a significant portion of nursing practice related to pharmacology. A significant number of interventions within the **collaborative domain** involve interdependent activity between nurses and other health care providers. Client conditions require different ratios of medical (or other health care provider) input and nursing input (Figure 4-6). Neither nurses nor other health care providers possess exclusive responsibility for the diagnosis and treatment of collaborative problems. Each group maintains its own responsibility throughout its involvement with the client. The **independent domain** involves the diagnosis and treatment of problems that are primarily nursing in nature. The nurse identifies these problems and assumes primary responsibility for ordering the necessary interventions.

Utility of Nursing Diagnoses

By describing human responses, a nursing diagnosis distinguishes nursing from other health care disciplines. Nursing diagnoses are most useful in the independent domain. A nursing diagnosis is a clear, concise description of a problem that is uniquely addressed by nurses; the use of nursing diagnoses provides a focus for goals and interventions. The development of nursing diagnoses has added much to the refinement and description of nursing care by providing structure, focus, and language for clear communication.

Because of the continuing development of nursing diagnoses, their implementation is hampered by divergent views, conceptual controversies, and confusing terminology. The nursing profession's health-related, client-strength emphases are not easily addressed by currently accepted nursing diagnoses, and it may be unrealistic to expect nursing diagnoses to describe all of nursing practice. Much of the nurse's role in pharmacotherapeutics encompasses the dependent and collaborative domains; these areas are not thoroughly addressed by nursing diagnoses but are more appropriately addressed by the identification of collaborative problems as potential complications. Throughout this text the use of nursing diagnosis is encouraged but not forced on situations in which it is inappropriate. As the evolution of nursing diagnoses continues, their application to pharmacotherapeutics will become increasingly appropriate and useful.

TABLE 4-2 Nursing Diagnoses and Related Interventions

Type	Definition	Focus of Nursing Interventions
Actual (is present)	Validated major signs and symptoms	To reduce or eliminate signs and symptoms or promote positive diagnoses
Risk (may happen)	Presence of risk factors	To prevent onset
Readiness (may be present)	Suspected to be present	To obtain additional data to rule out or confirm diagnosis

Modified from North American Nursing Diagnosis Association. (2001). *Nursing diagnoses: Definitions and classification 2001-2002.* Philadelphia: Author.

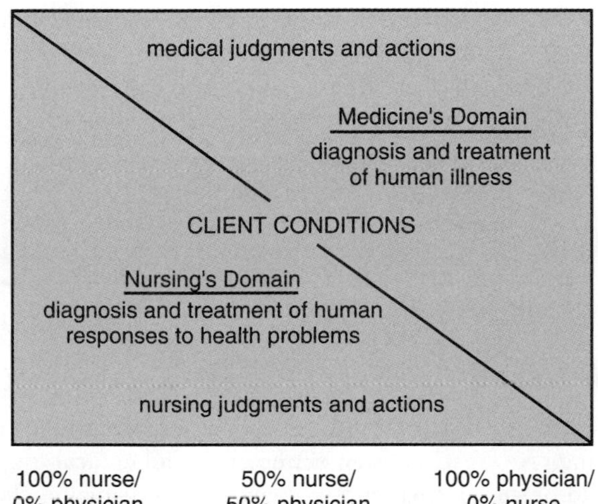

Figure 4-6 Nursing and medical responsibilities. (From McLane, A.M. (Ed.). (1987). *Classification of nursing diagnoses: Proceedings of the seventh conference.* St. Louis: Mosby.)

PLANNING FOR DRUG THERAPY

The planning phase of the nursing process has two parts: setting goals and creating specific plans for interventions that will implement those goals. Goals are usually stated as **nursing outcomes** (nursing-sensitive client outcomes to evaluate nursing interventions) or other **outcome criteria** (statements of observable or measurable results that should occur as the result of nursing and other health service activities). Goals for the effective management of the client's pharmacotherapeutic regimen include nursing outcomes and other outcome criteria because of the dependent, collaborative, and independent nature of the nursing activities involved. The planning to meet the pharmacotherapeutic nursing needs of clients should be characterized by an orientation to (1) the client, (2) resources in the environment, and (3) the future. The desired outcomes are to be established in collaboration with the client and others on the health care team, and in turn they should be characterized by a balance between the real and the ideal.

Outcome criteria associated with the medication needs of clients may be stated in many ways to encompass these three orientations. They must actually be stated (e.g., in the nursing care plan or protocol of care) to provide communication with the rest of the staff and to give clear direction for the subsequent implementation and evaluation phases. Without such statements, the implementation and evaluation of the client's care will be based on vague events and partially remembered and incomplete actions. When written as part of the goals for the resolution of nursing diagnoses in the nursing care plan, the outcome criteria are known as nursing outcomes. Nursing outcomes usually focus on enhancing the client's compliance behavior and resolving any knowledge deficits the client might have about his or her medication. Other outcome criteria are more the result of collaboration between the nurse and the prescriber. The nursing role focuses on monitoring for the "onset or any change in the client's status of physiological complications and responding to any such changes with prescriber- and nurse-prescribed nursing interventions" (Carpenito, 2000). Such therapeutic outcomes might relate to the normalization of the white blood cell count, maintenance of adequate control of blood glucose, control of hypertension, or elimination of fever.

Nursing outcomes or other outcome criteria are objectives to be met sometime in the future. Therefore the use of the words "will be" in the outcome statement is appropriate. An approximation of time limits for accomplishing the outcome should be included in the statement to provide a way of measuring progress toward the outcome, whether short term, intermediate, or long term (e.g., "by date of discharge," "in 3 days," "three weeks after surgery"). The time limit should be the best estimate, not an edict carved in stone. The outcome indicator or criterion should be client oriented in that it *should describe what the client's condition or behavior will be at the outcome of nursing care,* not what the nurse intends to do for the client. For example, an outcome is best stated as "Client will demonstrate the safe and accurate self-administration of insulin in 3 days," rather than "To promote understanding of the drug regimen by the time of discharge from the hospital." If the goal describes only what nurses do, nurses could work diligently to promote a client's understanding of a drug regimen, with success being measured only in terms of what procedures were performed; however, the client may never have actually learned, which is the in-

Nursing Care Plan
Selected Nursing Diagnoses Related to Client-Oriented Outcome Criteria

Nursing Diagnosis	Goals/Expected Outcomes	Nursing Interventions
Deficient knowledge related to new drug regimen of digoxin, furosemide, and potassium chloride	Before discharge, Ms. Strauss will do the following: State the action of each drug and how it relates to her cardiac status. Identify at least three untoward reactions that should be reported to her health care provider. Weigh herself accurately and report results to nurse daily. Demonstrate the ability to take her own pulse accurately.	1. Discuss with Ms. Strauss the action of each drug and how it relates to her cardiac status. 2. Instruct her about the possible side effects/adverse reactions of each drug. 3. Instruct her to report to her health care provider symptoms such as palpitations, a resting pulse rate of <60 or >100, a sudden change in weight, anorexia, nausea, or lethargy. 4. Discuss the importance of weighing daily and reporting a weight gain of 2 pounds or more. 5. Instruct in pulse taking, using daily practice. 6. Include her significant other/caretaker in the teaching, if possible. 7. Provide her with written instructions concerning all of her care as a guide for her use at home.

tent of the goal. The sample nursing care plan above illustrates client-oriented outcome criteria.

The nurse can prevent the blurring of the distinction between outcomes and interventions—two entirely different phases of the nursing process—by stating nursing or other outcome criteria in terms of behavioral objectives for the client. If criteria are stated in words that depict nursing interventions or actions, such as "prevent," "provide," "promote," or "maintain," the evaluation of care becomes more an appraisal of what the nurse did than of the client's condition.

Finally, nursing outcomes and outcome criteria related to each nursing diagnosis or potential complication identified earlier may be ranked in priority to meet the client's needs.

The rest of the planning phase lays the groundwork for carrying out specific actions in the implementation phase. Such plans for nursing actions should be supportable by research for best practice.

Development of a positive, accountable attitude by setting goals with expected outcomes and planning for each nursing action strengthens what nurses do for clients and why. The completed abbreviated nursing care plan, as a blueprint for action, can be entered in writing in the Kardex, in the computerized nursing information system, or on the client's chart and makes up the plan for nursing management of the client's nursing care. The nursing outcomes and other outcome criteria related to drug therapy may also be incorporated into interdisciplinary protocols for care, such as critical paths or protocols for client care. Outcome criteria and specific planning provide documentation for peers and preclude legal challenge while first and foremost guiding the selection of appropriate caring actions.

SUMMARY

Although its structure and terminology may change, the nursing process remains an extremely useful clinical tool. It should be approached as a framework for organizing client care in creative and satisfying ways.

Professional nurses enhance their decision-making skills by critically reviewing their clients' medication plans and maintaining a strong knowledge base about medications and their indications, mechanisms, pharmacokinetics, and dosages.

The quality of nursing assessment relies on the nurse's ability to observe significant cues, to make sound inferences, and to recognize the client's individuality and establish rapport. Thus a nurse can develop a valid diagnosis, establish realistic goals with the client, and shape an effective nursing plan.

Medication administration is a highly visible, legal function of nurses. Because it depends heavily on the structure and content of a prescriber's orders, conscientious assessment of the drug order becomes a very healthy habit. Professional accountability for all disciplines demands open collaboration on questions about clients' medication orders and plans. Underlying the routine of assessing medication therapy is the major goal of preventing harm. Assessment should emphasize protecting the client from receiving drugs that will complicate a preexisting health condition; will interact, be incompatible, or evoke an allergic response; will not be degraded or excreted adequately; or will be transferred to a fetus or nursing infant. Creative nursing consists of finding ways to reschedule or space intervals between doses of interactive drugs. If there is any question about pregnancy or breastfeeding, drug administration should be suspended and the prescriber contacted for consultation. Allergic reactions, if anticipated, are usually grounds for a prescriber's decision to change drugs. However, it is often the nurse who notes the offending allergenic substance via a client's history and other data. Again, effective nursing assessment can improve compliance, enhance therapeutic outcomes, and avoid negative secondary effects.

The nursing assessment culminates in the identification of nursing diagnoses (actual, at risk, wellness, or possible) and collaborative problems as potential complications. Although any number of issues are possible within nursing pharmacotherapeutics, eight issues must be considered with every medication to be administered:

1. Client issues related to the client's preexisting medical conditions, age, and childbearing status
2. Client issues related to concurrent drug therapy
3. Client issues related to the physiologic complication of the client's underlying condition related to the ineffectiveness of the drug
4. Client issues related to the physiologic complication related to the side effects/adverse reactions of the administered drug
5. Risk for poisoning: drug toxicity
6. Deficient knowledge related to initiation of or change in the medication regimen
7. Noncompliance (specify)
8. Ineffective therapeutic regimen management (individual or family)

Interventions by the nurse to address identified problems may involve collaborative interventions with physicians and other health care providers or interventions that are solely the domain of nurses. Problems falling within the independent nursing domain are best described by the nursing diagnosis, which is a concise statement of a problem that is uniquely addressed by nurses. The potential complications of the pharmacotherapeutic regimen are generally seen as collaborative problems.

After the identification of problems and the formulation of nursing diagnoses and collaborative problems, goals in the form of nursing outcomes and other outcome criteria are established. A specific plan is developed to direct nursing care toward meeting all of the outcomes. The development of goals and clear planning form the basis for implementing and evaluating nursing care.

Critical Thinking Questions

1. What might be the possible consequences to the client if a client's medication history and medication-taking behaviors are not obtained or are inadequate?
2. What nursing actions could be taken to minimize the different types of drug interactions discussed in this text?
3. Using information from the drug history of a client, discuss the potential for each of the eight problems within the nursing diagnoses that could be applied to the medications possibly prescribed for that client.

Collaborative Learning Activities

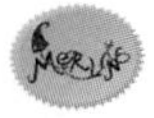

For Collaborative Learning Activites, go to mosby.com/MERLIN/McKenry/.

BIBLIOGRAPHY

Adverse drug reaction: nurse neglect not to clarify orders and to give patient's at-home medications. (1997). *Legal Eagle Eye Newsletter for the Nursing Profession, 5*(12), 2.

American Hospital Formulary Service. (1998). *AHFS drug information '98*. Bethesda, MD: American Society of Hospital Pharmacists.

Anderson, K.N., Anderson, L.E., & Glanze, W.D. (1998). *Mosby's medical, nursing, & allied health dictionary.* (5th ed.). St. Louis: Mosby.

Bird, R. (1997). The use of prescribed medication by problem drinkers: "painting over the rust?" *Journal of Substance Misuse of Nursing, Health & Social Care, 2*(3), 167-176.

Carpenito, L.J. (2000). *Nursing diagnosis: Application to nursing practice.* (8th ed.). Philadelphia: J.B. Lippincott.

Cassells, J.M. & Redman, B.K (1989). Preparing students to be moral agents in clinical nursing practice. *Nursing Clinics of North America, 24*(2), 463-473.

Collins, J.L. & Lutz, R.J. (1991). In vitro study of simultaneous infusion of incompatible drugs in multilumen catheters. *Heart Lung, 20*(3), 271.

Craig, C. (1995). Teaching food drug interactions. *Journal of Psychosocial Nursing, 33*(2), 44-46.

Crow, R.A., Chase, J., & Lamond, D. (1995). The cognitive component of nursing assessment: An analysis. *Journal of Advanced Nursing, 22*(2):206-212.

Garg, S.K., Kumar, N., Bhargava, V.K., & Prabhakar, S.K. (1998). Effect of grapefruit juice on carbamazepine bioavailability in patients with epilepsy. *Clinical Pharmacology & Therapeutics, 64*(3), 286-288.

Hardman, J.G. & Limbird, L.E. (Eds.) (1996). *Goodman & Gilman's The pharmacological basis of therapeutics.* (9th ed.). New York: Macmillan.

Iowa Outcomes Project. (1997). *Nursing outcomes classification (NOC).* St. Louis: Mosby.

Jacox, A., Ferrell, B., Heidich, G., Hester, N., & Miaskowski, C. (1992). A guideline for the nation: Managing acute pain. *American Journal of Nursing, 92*(5), 49-55.

Jenny, J. (1987). Knowledge deficit: Not a nursing diagnosis. *Image, 19*(4), 184-185.

Lowenthal, D.T., & Parnetti, L. (1996). Drug-food interaction: real, problematic, and potentially harmful. *Consultant, 36*(10), 2149-2152.

McCourt, A., & Carroll-Johnson, R.M. (Eds.). (1992). *Classification of nursing diagnosis: Proceedings of the ninth NANDA national conference.* Philadelphia: J.B. Lippincott.

McFarland, G.K. & McFarland, E.A. (1997). *Nursing diagnosis & intervention: Planning for patient care.* (3rd ed.). St. Louis: Mosby.

McPherson, M.L. (1996). Taking an accurate medication history. *Home Health Care Practice, 5*(4), 35-40.

North American Nursing Diagnosis Association. (1997). *Nursing diagnoses: Definitions and classification 1997-1998.* Philadelphia: Author.

North American Nursing Diagnosis Association. (2001). *Nursing diagnoses: Definitions and classification 2001-2002.* Philadelphia: Author.

Stoehr, G. P., Ganguli, M., Seaberg, E.C., Echement, D.A., & Belle, S. (1997). Over-the-counter medication use in an older rural community: the MoVIES Project. *Journal of the American Geriatrics Society, 45*(2), 158-165.

United States Pharmacopeia Dispensing Information (USP DI): Drug information for the health care professional (19th ed.). (1999). Rockville, MD: United States Pharmacopeial Convention.

5 Implementation and Evaluation

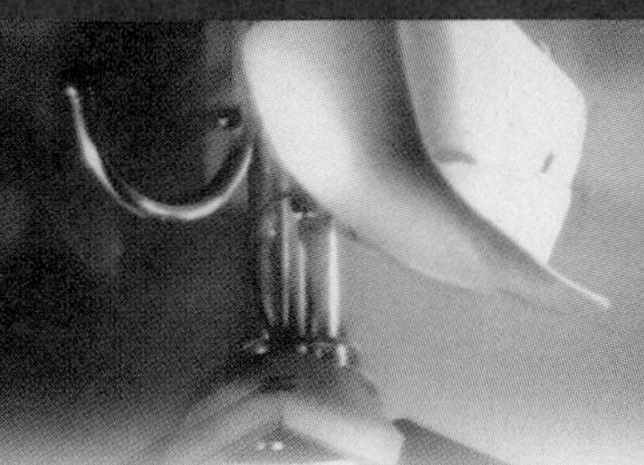

Chapter Focus

The last two components of the nursing process—implementation and evaluation—involve monitoring the client's health status, nurse- or health care provider-prescribed interventions, and client education as well as determining the effectiveness of the therapeutic regimen. This chapter focuses on the nursing management of these last nursing process components as they relate to drug therapy.

Learning Objectives

1. Identify common pharmaceutical preparations and dosage forms.
2. Identify nursing activities related to proper drug storage and distribution.
3. Describe the factors considered in establishing the dose, dosing intervals, and scheduling of medication.
4. Cite methods used to measure the correct dosage or rate of administration.
5. Differentiate between systemic effects and local effects of medications.
6. Cite the advantages and disadvantages of the various routes of medication administration.
7. Identify the landmarks for the administration of medications via the subcutaneous and intramuscular routes.
8. Identify specific procedures used to maintain client safety during the preparation and administration of medications.
9. Evaluate the effectiveness of a client's drug therapy.

Key Terms

apothecary system, p. 83
drug potency, p. 81
duration of action, p. 81
household system, p. 83
infiltration, p. 96
infusion, p. 96
injection, p. 96
latency, p. 81
maximum effect, p. 81
metric system, p. 82
therapeutic index, p. 81
time for maximum effect, p. 81
Z-track method, p. 95

IMPLEMENTATION

The implementation phase of the nursing process consists of putting goals into action. It is the actual giving of care as prescribed by the nursing care plan or nursing orders. The nurse is guided by the nursing care plan (formal or informal), with the goals (expected nursing and other outcomes) clearly in focus, and can initiate the proposed actions in an orderly way. The best chance for success lies in clear, frequent communication and collaboration with clients, because any action or outcome not viewed by clients as congruent with their own goals will decrease participation.

The implementation phase in drug therapy comprises all the steps of the act of administering medications. It includes collaborating with the prescriber and medicating clients according to the prescribers' orders using nursing judgment, preparing drugs (including performing any necessary mathematical calculations), using techniques and procedures with modifications for individual clients, being alert to errors, recording medications given, and teaching clients about their drugs. Evaluation of goals follows and, depending on the specific outcomes of care, most often relates to some aspect of drug effects. For individual clients, outcomes are measured and compared with the criteria established in the goals during the planning phase. Broader evaluation is performed through continuous quality initiative committees that critique the quality of nursing care administered to groups of clients as well as individuals. To perform all functions of the nursing process, nurses must have strong interpersonal, cognitive, and psychomotor skills. Nursing actions are the product of foundational work in the psychosocial, biologic, and physical sciences.

Drug Administration

The nursing function most closely identified with nursing by the public, and the one that carries the most legal vulnerability, is that of administering medications. This function requires much preparation, a solid knowledge base, skilled decision-making abilities, and close attention to the "Five Rights" (see Chapter 4).

Pharmaceutical Preparations

Pharmaceutical preparations are the formulations that make a drug suited to various methods of administration. They may be made up by the pharmacist but more often are prepared by the pharmaceutical company from which they are purchased. The nurse who is informed about various preparations can make more astute judgments about their individual applications and can make appropriate recommendations to the prescriber when necessary. Common preparations and their various applications are detailed in Box 5-1.

Drug Storage

The appropriate storage of drugs on the nursing unit is a nursing responsibility and usually occurs with the guidance and supervision of pharmacy staff.

The potency (strength per milligram of drug) and efficacy (maximum ability of a drug to produce a result) of drugs are affected by the way in which they are handled and stored. Proper storage of a drug is necessary to maintain drug stability. Most drugs can be stored in the medication cart, but some must be stored according to specific manufacturer's directions (on the label or package insert) to slow deterioration (e.g., live vaccines, most reconstituted drugs, and most suppositories). Many drugs change composition or potency when exposed to light, heat, moisture, or gases in the environment. The *United States Pharmacopeia Dispensing Information (USP DI)* (1999) has defined the nomenclature used in instructions for the prevention of changes from heat:

- Freeze: below −20° to −10° C (−4° to 14° F)
- Store in a cold place: temperature no higher than 8° C (46° F)
- Refrigerate: 2° to 8° C (36° to 46° F)
- Warm: any temperature between 30° to 40° C (86° to 104° F)
- Avoid excessive heat: temperature no higher than 40° C (104° F)

Most drugs may be stored at room temperature, which is considered to be between 20° and 25° C (68° and 77° F). Brief deviations from these temperatures are acceptable, such as 15° C and 30° C (59° and 86° F) (*Quality Review,* 1999).

Medication refrigerators should be used solely for the storage of drugs and related necessities and should be cleaned out regularly; expired drugs or drugs belonging to discharged clients should be returned to the pharmacy. To ensure a more constant cool temperature, medications should be stored within the refrigerator—not on the door shelves or within the freezer compartment. At least one thermometer should be kept inside to monitor temperature maintenance.

The use of amber-colored containers protects some medications (e.g., furosemide [Lasix] and nitroglycerin) against deterioration by light. This fact and its significance should be pointed out to clients who are self-medicating and who might otherwise transfer medications to a different container (to take to work, on vacation, and the like). Storage in a closed cabinet or other dark place should also be advised. If it is feasible, clients should be given information about how to tell if their medication has deteriorated. They should also be told that the medication needs to be replaced if storage requirements have not been maintained or if the appearance or effects of the medication have changed.

Certain drugs given intravenously are significantly sensitive to light: amphotericin B (Fungizone), B-complex vitamins, cisplatin (Platinol), daunorubicin (Cerubidine), doxorubicin (Adriamycin), and nitroprusside (Nipride). These medications should be checked for visible signs of deterioration, such as color change, precipitation, or gas formation. Deterioration may neutralize the drugs or make them toxic, and this can occur without any warning signs. Nitroprusside (Nipride) and amphotericin B (Fungizone) solutions for infusions should be kept covered with foil or an amber plastic

BOX 5-1
Common Drug Preparations and Their Applications

Preparations for Oral Use

Liquids

Aqueous solutions—substances dissolved in water and syrups
Aqueous suspensions—solid particles suspended in liquid
Emulsions—fats or oils suspended in liquid with an emulsifier
Spirits—alcohol solution
Elixirs—aromatic, sweetened alcohol and water solution
Tinctures—alcohol extract of plant or vegetable substance
Fluidextracts—concentrated alcoholic liquid extract of plant or vegetables
Extracts—syrup or dried form of pharmacologically active drug, usually prepared by evaporating solution

Solids

Capsules—soluble case [usually gelatin] that contains liquid, dry, or beaded drug particles
Tablets—compressed, powdered drug(s) in small disk
Troches/lozenges—medicated tablets that dissolve slowly in mouth
Powders/granules—loose or molded drug substance for drug administration, with or without liquids

Preparations for Parenteral Use

Ampules—sealed glass container for liquid injectable medication
Vials—glass container with rubber stopper for liquid or powdered medication
Cartridge/Tubex—single-dose unit of parenteral medication to be used with a specific injecting device

Intravenous Infusions (Suspended on Hanger at Bedside)

Glass bottles, flexible collapsible plastic bags, and semirigid plastic containers in sizes from 150 to 1000 mL—used for continuous infusion of fluid replacement with or without medications
Intermittent IV infusions—usually a secondary IV setup of a small plastic or glass bottle (volume between 50 to 250 mL) to which medication is added; runs as a "piggyback" and is hung separately from the primary IV infusion via a secondary administration tubing set, usually for a period of 20 to 120 minutes; the primary IV solution is run during the time between medication doses
Heparin lock or angiocath—a port site for direct administration or intermittent IV medications without the need for a primary IV solution

Preparations for Topical Use

Liniments—liquid suspensions for lubrication that are applied by rubbing
Lotions—liquid suspensions that can be protective, emollient, cooling, astringent, antipruritic, cleansing, etc.
Ointment—semisolid medicine in a base for local protective, soothing, astringent, or transdermal application for systemic effects [e.g., nitroglycerin, scopolamine, estrogen]
Paste—thick ointment primarily used for skin protection
Plasters—solid preparations that are adhesive, protective, or soothing
Creams—emulsions that contain an aqueous and an oily base
Aerosols—fine powders or solutions in volatile liquids that contain a propellant
Transdermal patches—patches containing medication that is absorbed continuously through the skin and acts systemically

Preparations for Use on Mucous Membranes

Drops—aqueous solutions with or without a gelling agent to increase retention time in the eye; used for eyes, ears, or nose
Instillations of an aqueous solution of medications—usually for topical action but occasionally used for systemic effects, including enemas, douches, mouthwashes, throat sprays, and gargles
Aerosol sprays, nebulizers, and inhalers—deliver aqueous solutions of medication in droplet form to the target membrane, such as the bronchial tree (e.g., bronchodilators)
Foams—powders or solutions of medication in volatile liquids with a propellant, such as vaginal foams for contraception
Suppositories—usually contain medicinal substances mixed in a firm but malleable base (cocoa butter) to facilitate insertion into a body cavity (e.g., rectal or vaginal)

Miscellaneous Drug Delivery Systems

Intradermal implants—pellets containing a small deposit of medication; are inserted in a dermal pocket; designed to allow medication to leach slowly into tissue; usually used to administer hormones such as testosterone or estradiol
Micropump system—a small, external pump that is attached by belt or implanted to deliver medication via a needle in a continuous, steady dose (e.g., insulin, anticancer chemotherapy, and opioids)
Membrane delivery systems—drug-laden membranes that are instilled in the eye to deliver a steady flow of medications (e.g., pilocarpine or corticosteroids)

bag (not a brown paper bag, which is not light protective) while being administered by continuous IV infusion. Unless freshly prepared, all the other solutions should also be kept covered.

Tight lids can prevent the drug form or its active constituents from degrading or changing by preventing the exchange of moisture or gases within the container.

The expiration dates printed on drug labels mean simply that the drug contained is probably at its peak effectiveness until some point in time past that date. Because quality controls in drug production are subject to error rates similar to all other control programs, pharmaceutical companies tend to estimate these expiration dates somewhat conservatively. Thus the drug is not instantly rendered useless or harmful by that date, but the effectiveness of the therapy may be gradually diminished and the drug may produce inadequate or occasionally even toxic results some time after the printed date. The nurse should not administer doses from an outdated lot of drug or container; a fresh supply must be obtained.

Certain precepts should guide the way in which clients' drugs are stored, distributed, and managed. Health care agencies have developed policies that, with some variations, support these precepts as rules for client protection and prevent nurses from making errors. In addition, rational nursing judgments must enter into decision making; such judgments allow a departure from these rules as a wise and necessary choice, but these should never be undertaken lightly. It should also be a practice to consult other expert personnel or authorities.

The following are additional guidelines for handling medications and are not necessarily listed in order of importance:

1. All medicines should be kept in a special place, which may be a cart or room. This area should not be freely accessible to the public.
2. Narcotic drugs and those dispensed under special legal regulations must be kept in a locked box or compartment (many states require double locks) and accounted for at the end of each shift. Another nurse must attest to any dose that is wasted or discarded by initialing such a notation.
3. Each client's medicines are kept in a designated drawer of the medication cart. The nurse must be careful to keep the client's medicines in the right area and must make certain that the medicines are returned to the pharmacy when the client leaves the hospital.
4. If stock supplies are maintained, they should be arranged in an orderly manner. Preparations for internal use should be kept separate from those for external use.
5. Some preparations, such as serums, vaccines, certain suppositories, certain antibiotics, and insulin, may need to be refrigerated.
6. The labels of all medicines should be clean and legible. If they are not, they should be sent to the pharmacist for relabeling. *Nurses should not label or relabel medicines.*
7. Bottles of medicines should always be stoppered and protected from light, heat, and high humidity as necessary.

Many IV drugs require a diluent to dissolve the medication, which then can be added to a larger volume of solution for administration. The storage times for such medications can vary, depending on the following:

1. The expiration date on the fresh package of medication stored under the specific instructions of the manufacturer
2. The expiration time period allotted for the dissolved medication
3. The expiration time period allotted for the dissolved medication added to a larger volume of solution

To obtain accurate information for an individual drug, the nurse should refer to the package insert or the *USP DI.* Table 5-1 illustrates differing storage requirements and expiration times within the same drug classification (cephalosporin antibiotics).

Preparation of the Dose

Technically, written medical orders are the only legal means for the administration of medications by nurses. Written orders constitute permanent legal records of the prescriber's plans and can be submitted as evidence in litigation. Because nurses are held legally accountable for every dose of medication they administer, they must routinely ensure that (1) each order is appropriate, accurate, and complete; and (2) the order is followed unerringly to completion, or the prescriber is consulted as to why it was not completed. The free flow of communication between prescriber and nurse is crucial to fulfillment of this responsibility. Nurses must be ready to consult with the prescriber as necessary to clarify, understand, or suggest medication therapy as needed. Professional nurses must develop assertiveness if they are to obtain an appropriate position of strength within the health care system to promote their clients' best interests while achieving equity for their own contributions.

What is the process by which a prescriber's order is translated into the administration of a medication? The order is first transcribed by a unit secretary, nurse manager (or nursing care coordinator), or primary nurse from an order sheet onto the Kardex or medication administration record (MAR) (Figure 5-1); this entire process may also be computerized. In many health agencies the prescriber places the medication order into a computer that requisitions the drug from the pharmacy, and the order is automatically transcribed directly onto a computerized MAR from which the nurse prepares the medication. Accuracy in transcription of the medication order to the MAR is essential. If a unit secretary has processed a handwritten order, it should be verified by a nurse, who can better relate the medication to the client and the diagnosis. To prevent error, the nurse must check the dosage of the medication and the age of the client, check for drug interaction possibilities and allergies, and ensure the completeness and clarity of the order

TABLE 5-1 Storage Requirements and Expiration Times of Selected Intravenous Drugs

Drug	Stability After Reconstitution: Room Temperature*	Refrigeration*	If Frozen*
cefamandole (Mandol)	24 hours	96 hours	6 months
cefazolin sodium (Ancef, Kefzol)	24 hours	10 days	12 weeks
cefoperazone sodium (Cefobid) and parenteral solution used	24 hours	5 days	3-5 weeks, depending on concentration
sterile cefoxitin sodium (Mefoxin)	24 hours	7 days	At least 30 weeks, depending on method of preparation
cefotetan for injection (Cefotan)	24 hours	96 hours	1 week

Information from *United States Pharmacopeia Dispensing Information (USP DI): Drug information for the health care professional* (19th ed.). (1999). Rockville, MD: United States Pharmacopeial Convention.

*Recommended temperatures: room temperature, 20° to 25° C (68° to 77° F); refrigeration, 2° to 8° C (36° to 46° F); frozen, −20° to −10° C (−4° to 14° F).

(Box 5-2). Whatever the question concerning the prescriber's order, legally it can be clarified only with the prescriber who has written the order. Verifying an order with the physician or nursing colleague who happens to be present in the clinical or home setting does not suffice.

In the hospital or extended care facility, the institution's pharmacy department supplies the drug. When the supply arrives, it is appropriately stored in an individual client's own medication box or in the drawer of a medication cart. In the home, a local pharmacy or mail order pharmaceutical supplier may supply the drug to the client or client's family, with the nurse administering the medication as scheduled.

Because of space limitations, prescribers, pharmacists, and nurses rely on pharmacologic abbreviations or symbols for communication. These abbreviations are often from Latin and are universally used. Abbreviations are a key to communication in the busy health field and should be learned. Table 5-2 includes the most commonly used abbreviations, as well as some symbols common to clinical practice. Although apothecary symbols are sometimes used, they are often misinterpreted and may be used incorrectly. The pharmacist or nurse should convert the apothecary measure to a metric measure when transcribing the medication order. Prescribers should be encouraged to use the metric system to avoid errors.

A number of prescribers also use abbreviations for ordering specific medications (Table 5-3). Because of the danger of misinterpretation, variant or nonstandard abbreviations should not be used. The nurse should review the approved abbreviation listing for the specific health agency.

When transcribed, the prescriber's order must contain all the elements described in Chapter 4. It must contain the *full name* of the client (and bed location, such as "Room 212, Bed A"); the *date* the order was written; the *medication name, dosage, route of administration,* and *frequency of administration;* and, according to agency policy, the *name* or *initials* of the nurse responsible for the transcription or computer entry.

BOX 5-2

Checking Transcription

Which Medication?

Is it quinine sulfate (a medication for leg cramps) or quinidine sulfate (a cardiac depressant)? Pentobarbital or phenobarbital? Digoxin or digitoxin? Ornade or Orinase? Decadron or Doriden?

Which Dose?

Is it a loop of an f, g, or q, or another zero?

Vital signs q 4 h
Gentamycin 60 mg IV 6 h

Anything Missing?

Does Halcion i HS mean 0.125 mg or 0.25 mg?

Types of Drug Delivery Systems

There are several approaches to distributing and dispensing drugs to clients in an institutional setting: the floor stock system, unit dose drug distribution, or a combination of these. In the floor stock system, all medications except those infrequently used are stored in bulk in the medication room of the nursing unit. The floor stock system is rarely used because of (1) the increased potential for medication errors caused by the large array of stock medications from which

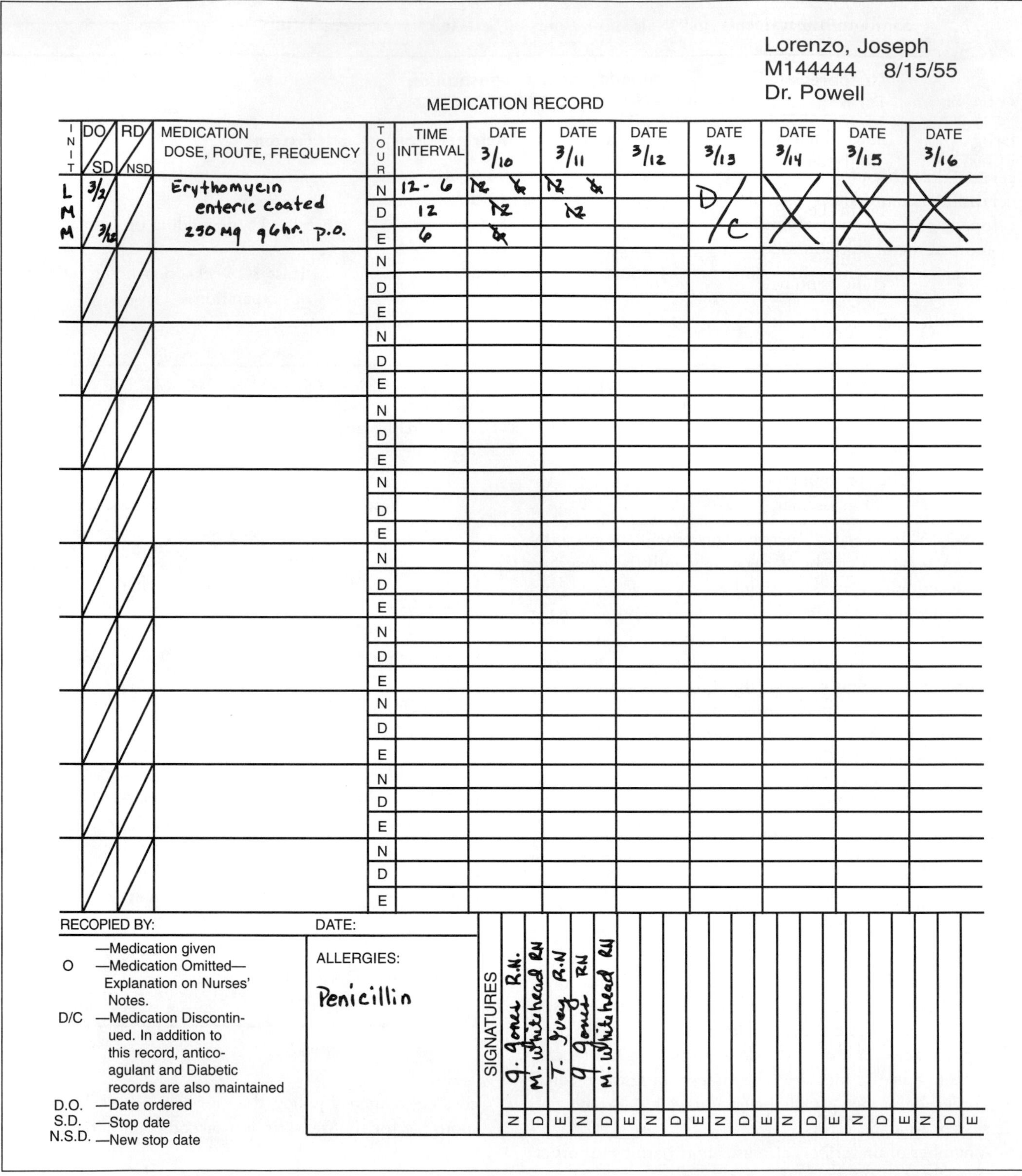

Lorenzo, Joseph
M144444 8/15/55
Dr. Powell

MEDICATION RECORD

INIT	DO / SD	RD / NSD	MEDICATION DOSE, ROUTE, FREQUENCY	HOUR	TIME INTERVAL	DATE 3/10	DATE 3/11	DATE 3/12	DATE 3/13	DATE 3/14	DATE 3/15	DATE 3/16
L	3/2		Erythomycin	N	12 - 6	12 6	12 6		D/C	X	X	X
M	3/12		enteric coated	D	12	12	12					
M			250 mg q6hr. p.o.	E	6	6						
				N								
				D								
				E								
				N								
				D								
				E								
				N								
				D								
				E								
				N								
				D								
				E								
				N								
				D								
				E								
				N								
				D								
				E								
				N								
				D								
				E								
				N								
				D								
				E								
				N								
				D								
				E								

RECOPIED BY: DATE:

—Medication given
O —Medication Omitted—Explanation on Nurses' Notes.
D/C —Medication Discontinued. In addition to this record, anticoagulant and Diabetic records are also maintained
D.O. —Date ordered
S.D. —Stop date
N.S.D. —New stop date

ALLERGIES:
Penicillin

SIGNATURES
N: J. Jones R.N.
D: M. Whitehead RN
E: T. Ivey R.N
N: J. Jones RN
D: M. Whitehead RN
N D E N D E N D E N D E N D E N D E N D E

Figure 5-1 Sample medication administration record. In many health care agencies, this form has been computerized.

to choose, (2) the financial loss caused by misplaced or forgotten charges and expired drugs to be returned, (3) the need for frequent total drug inventories, and (4) the storage problems inherent in crowded medication rooms. Therefore this system is more costly and less safe for the client.

The national norm for institutions is unit dose dispensing of most if not all prescribed medications. With this system, single-dose packages of drugs are dispensed. For example, each oral dose may be a tablet encased in a blister pack or in a paper tear-off strip of tablets. This packaging is said to

TABLE 5-2 Common Abbreviations and Symbols Related to Medication Administration*

Abbreviation	Unabbreviated Form	Meaning
ac	ante cibum	before meals
ad lib	ad libitum	freely
AM	ante meridiem	morning
bid	bis in die	twice each day
c̄	cum	with
caps	capsule	capsule
cc, cm^3	cubic centimeter	cubic centimeter (mL)
clt	client	client
D/C or DC	discontinue	terminate
elix	elixir	elixir
g, gm	gram	1000 milligrams
gr	grain	60 milligrams
gtt	guttae	drops
h, hr	hora	hour
hs	hora somni	at bedtime
IM	intramuscular	into a muscle
IV	intravenous	into a vein
IVPB	IV piggyback	secondary IV line
kg	kilogram	2.2 pounds
KVO	keep vein open	very slow infusion rate
Ⓛ	left	left
L	liter	liter
μg, mcg	microgram	one millionth of a gram
mg	milligram	one thousandth of a gram
mEq	milliequivalent	the number of grams of solute dissolved in one milliliter of a *normal* solution
min or m	minim	minim (1/15 or 1/16 mL)
ml, mL	milliliter	one thousandth of a liter
ng	nanogram	one billionth of a gram
ō	no or none	no or none
OD	oculus dexter	right eye
OS	oculus sinister	left eye
os	os	mouth
OTC	over-the-counter	nonprescription drug
OU	oculus uterque	each eye
pc	post cibum	after meals
PM	post meridiem	after noon
PO	per os	by mouth, orally
prn	pro re nata	according to necessity
pt	patient	patient
q	quaque	every
qd	quaque die	every day
qh	quaque hora	every hour
q4h, $q4^{\circ}$	every 4 hours	every 4 hours around-the-clock
qid	quater in die	four times each day
qod	quaque altera die	every other day
qs	quantum satis	sufficient quantity
®	right	right
℞	recipe	take
s̄	sine	without
SL	sub lingua	under the tongue
SOS	si opus sit	if it is necessary, one dose only
ss	semisse	a half
stat	statim	at once
SC, SQ	subcutaneous	into subcutaneous tissue
tbsp	tablespoon	tablespoon (15 mL)
tid	ter in die	three times a day
TO	telephone order	order received over the telephone
tsp	teaspoon	teaspoon (4 or 5 mL)
U	unit	a dose measure for insulin, penicillin, heparin
VO	verbal order	order received verbally
i, ii	one, two	one, two (as in "gr i," "gr ii,")
ʒ	dram	4 or 5 mL
℥	ounce or fluid-ounce	ounce (30 milliliters)
×	times	as in two times a week
$>$	greater than	greater than
$<$	less than	less than
=	equal to	equal to
↑, ↗	increase or increasing	increase or increasing
↓, ↙	decrease or decreasing	decrease or decreasing

*It is recommended that certain abbreviations be abandoned if they are found to be confusing.

be the safest and most economical method of drug distribution. However, in many instances drug wastage occurs in long-term care settings in which the drugs are issued in 30-day blister packages; these packages must be discarded when the drug is discontinued for the client—even if only a few of the total doses have been administered. The regulations governing this practice are being reviewed in many states.

The advantages of using the unit dose system far outweigh the disadvantages. The most important advantages

TABLE 5-3 Abbreviations for Specific Medications

Abbreviation	Definition
ACTH	adrenocorticotropic hormone
ASA	acetylsalicylic acid (aspirin)
DES	diethylstilbestrol
DM	dextromethorphan
D_5W	5% dextrose in water
D_5S	5% dextrose in normal saline
DSS or DOSS	dioctyl sodium sulfosuccinate
DW	distilled water
EC	enteric-coated
ETH-C	elixir terpin hydrate with codeine
Fe	iron
5-FU	5-fluorouracil
FUDR	floxuridine
HC	hydrocortisone
HCTZ	hydrochlorothiazide
INH	isoniazid
K	potassium
KCl	potassium chloride
LOC	laxative of choice
MOM	milk of magnesia
6-MP	6-mercaptopurine
MS	morphine sulfate
Na	sodium
NS	normal saline
NSAID	nonsteroidal antiinflammatory drug
NTG	nitroglycerin
PAS	para-aminosalicylic acid
PB	phenobarbital
PCN	penicillin

are increased medication safety and decreased errors, because drug computations are largely eliminated. The drug is already properly labeled and does not need to be prepared. All the nurse needs to do is deliver the package to the client; it is opened at the bedside and administered. This system may permit clients to check on their own drugs and be assured that they are receiving the proper medication and the proper dose. Unit dose packaging also decreases the chances of deterioration and, in most instances, clients can be given financial credit for drugs that are not used. Disadvantages include increased cost to set up the system and the need for additional pharmacy personnel to fill new orders and resupply the client's units every 24 hours. Because the drugs are not immediately available on the unit, the administration of new and stat medication orders may be delayed while the medication order is sent to the pharmacy, filled, and delivered back to the nurse. However, the safety features of the unit dose system far outweigh any temporary inconvenience.

Strip packages make narcotic counting more convenient for nurses, because all packages in the strip are numbered. This also prevents the contamination caused by pouring narcotic tablets into the hands for counting—a grossly improper technique. Prefilled unit dose disposable syringes are also available.

Unit dose dispensing systems in hospitals, rehabilitation centers, or extended care facilities may be centralized, decentralized, or a combination of both. In the centralized system, the pharmacist and pharmacy are located in a central area from which drugs are distributed to client care areas. In the decentralized system, clinical pharmacists and satellite pharmacies are located in client care areas, and drugs are prepared and distributed to clients from those particular areas. In the combined system, medications are prepared in a central area, and clinical pharmacists are assigned to various client care areas to oversee drug therapy, thus providing safer and more controlled drug ordering and drug distribution.

In the home setting the nurse is not usually administering drugs to multiple clients. In this case the individual drugs for the client are kept in a common container or may be in a blister pack.

Role of the Clinical Pharmacist

A present trend in drug delivery is toward more extensive use of clinical pharmacists stationed in nursing areas to work closely with prescribers, nurses, therapists, and dietitians. Because pharmacists are educated in the compounding, dispensing, and control of drugs, they can be an invaluable resource for assistance in solving pharmacologic problems in the institutional or community setting. Nurses often consult them about medication administration methods, dosages, drug identification, and secondary effects. Health care professionals from all disciplines consult with clinical pharmacists with questions relating to drug therapy. Today's health care system demands more of this type of interdisciplinary collaboration and shared expertise for the benefit of all, especially the client.

Many pharmacies can have special "clean rooms" and specially filtered air for compounding various parenteral solutions. A pharmacist or supervised designee may be responsible for putting all additives into IV solutions and checking all such solutions for compatibility reactions.

Role of the Nurse

Regardless of any changes in ordering, distributing, or administering drugs, nurses share in the responsibility for their clients' medication safety. This is true whether they practice in a home, a primary health care setting, or an institution. Advanced technology and the availability of more potent drugs make it crucial for the nurse to be better informed about drugs and their actions. Nurses must observe clients and their response to drug therapy, determine whether prn orders are to be given, and consult with prescribers about withholding, discontinuing, or changing drugs. They must continue to obtain histories, teach clients about medications and their effects, work collaboratively with pharmacists, and work with clients to plan the management of drug therapy in the home setting.

Preparing to Administer Drugs

Doses, Dosing Intervals, and Scheduling

Understanding the rationale for selecting a particular dose and frequency of administration requires a basic understanding of the drug in question. Within limits, increasing a dose or frequency of administration increases the pharmacologic effect, but it can also increase the risk of side effects/adverse reactions. The various relationships involved can be represented as follows:

Optimal doses → Dose-response relationship
Optimal frequencies → Time-response relationship

The variables to deal with in *dose-response* relationships are defined as follows:

Drug potency: absolute amount of drug required to produce a desired effect

Therapeutic index: relative margin of safety; the ratio of lethal dose to effective dose

Maximum effect: greatest response possible regardless of dose given

Time-response relationships deal with the following variables:

Latency: time necessary for therapeutic effect

Time for maximum effect: time after administration for the effect of the drug to peak

Duration of action: length of time of a drug effect

These last variables are affected by the route of administration used, the pharmacokinetics involved, and the biorhythms of the individual client.

Doses are given at appropriate intervals to avoid wide fluctuations in the serum concentration of a drug and to avoid drug accumulation and toxicity. If the interval is too short, drug accumulation with the potential for toxicity will occur. If it is too long, serum concentration will drop because the drug continues to be excreted and not replaced. Drugs with very short half-lives do not accumulate and therefore need to be given frequently to achieve a steady state (see Chapter 3 for a discussion of drug half-life). Drugs with very long half-lives are often given once a day.

Dosing relationships are interpreted on the basis of a normal curve in drug studies. Doses and dosing intervals are derived for treating the ideal "average" person in a population. Although dosing intervals have been studied statistically, drug therapy regimens must be reassessed continually for individual needs. Some people will always fall outside the "average" range in responding to a drug. In addition, dosing intervals may be modified in consideration of client convenience and their effect on the client's management of the therapeutic regimen.

The time for administering routine medications may be determined by agency policy. For example, qid drugs may be given at 10 AM, 2 PM, 6 PM, and 10 PM, or at 9 AM, 1 PM, 5 PM, and 9 PM, and so forth. Special units, such as pediatrics, have other medication hours to coincide with the special needs of their clients. In the home the client may determine the times as long as the timing of the doses maintains therapeutic drug blood levels and client safety. Depending on the pharmacokinetics of the drug, client convenience, and the need to avoid mealtimes or other activities that might interfere with drug administration, nurses may choose autonomously to vary the administration times (but not the intervals)—if the decision is based on solid rationale (Box 5-3). For example, calcium supplements might be given at bedtime rather than at 9 AM on a daily schedule because calcium is better absorbed at night. Drugs administered once daily can usually be given according to a flexible schedule, perhaps just before or after a treatment that would interfere with a dosing time, such as a client's trip off the nursing unit to the physical therapy department or radiology department. At home, clients are encouraged to take their medications at the same time each day. This helps to establish a daily pattern and enhances adherence to the drug regimen.

BOX 5-3

Examples of Clinical Implications of Drug Dosing

Blood levels of steroids administered between 7:30 AM and 8:30 AM most closely match levels as they would occur normally. Permanent night shift workers would be exceptions.

Antibiotics should be administered around-the-clock to achieve a steady state in the bloodstream.

Anticoagulant doses should be titrated with tests of the client's own partial thromboplastin time or a similar determination.

Diuretics should not be administered late in the day or before appointments, when urinary urgency would be inconvenient for the client.

Drugs should be administered as close to the time indicated as possible, but obviously a nurse practicing within an institutional setting cannot medicate each of a group of assigned clients at exactly the same time. Agency policies may vary but usually stipulate administration within ½ hour before or after the indicated time. Exempt from this flexibility are stat or one-time-only drug orders, such as those given before diagnostic procedures or surgery, and those medications administered at more frequent intervals, such as every 2 hours or every 4 hours.

Drug effects are monitored by the prescriber and the nurse according to either direct assessment (subjective, by observation for clinical responses) or indirect assessment (objective, by serum concentrations of the drug or by relevant laboratory values). Because of their unique presence and expertise, nurses are most capable of assisting the prescriber in making keen assessments of clients' responses.

Dosage Measurement

If the drug is formulated in units that are multiples of the prescribed dose (tablet or liquid), the computation to determine the correct dosage is simple. However, dosage calculations are necessary if the drug does not come in units that are multiples of the prescribed dose, if the drug must be dissolved in water, or if the order is written in the apothecary system and the drug is available only in metric units.

For certain therapies, flow rate calculations are necessary to set the proper amount for the desired dose effect. IV infusions necessitate careful calculations of flow rate. (A simple formula for IV flow rate calculation is found in Exercise 9 later in this chapter.) IV therapies should be ordered by the prescriber in definitive amounts and rates. IV fluids can be adjusted to deliver the number of drops per minute that will provide the prescribed total amount over the prescribed time. The prescribed drops per minute are calculated from the total volume of solution to be infused, the total number of minutes the solution is to be infused, and the drop factor (number of drops per milliliter that the tubing setup delivers—this number varies among tubing manufacturers and is found on the back of the tubing box). The IV flow rate is then regulated by counting drops in the drip chamber of the tubing or by programming the infusion pump or controller. Details of regulating by manual clamps may be found in a basic nursing text such as Potter and Perry (1997). Infusion controllers and pumps are discussed later in this chapter.

Most dosage calculations deal with computing the number of tablets to give or with changing from one unit of measurement to another. A dosage problem may be as simple as giving 400 mg of ibuprofen µmotrin) from a container of 200 mg tablets. It is almost as easy to figure out how many milliliters of morphine sulfate to give if the container is labeled "15 mg = 1 mL" and the order reads "10 mg morphine sulfate SC." Calculating dosages becomes more complex when the units of measurement in the medication order must be converted to the units in which the drug is available.

Three systems of measurement are currently in use for administering medications: the metric system (the most widely adopted and the most convenient), the apothecary system (which has been nearly phased out), and the household system (the least accurate and not widely used except in the home setting).

Metric System. The **metric system** of weights and measures was invented by the French at the end of the eighteenth century. Toward the end of the nineteenth century the Bureau of Weights and Measures was formed and given the challenge to develop metric standards for international use. The United States joined the worldwide trend toward adoption of the metric system with the enactment of the Metric Conversion Act of 1975.

The basic metric units of measurement are the meter, the liter, and the gram. The *meter* is the unit for linear measurement, the *liter* for capacity or volume, and the *gram* for weight. A meter is a little longer than a yard; a liter is a little more than a quart; and a gram is a little more than the weight of a steel paper clip.

The metric system is a decimal system; the basic units can be divided or multiplied by 10, 100, or 1000 to form secondary units that differ from each other by 10 or some multiple of 10. The names of the secondary units are formed by joining Greek or Latin prefixes to the names of the primary units (Table 5-4). Moving the decimal point to the left makes subdivisions of the basic units, and multiples of the basic units are indicated by moving the decimal point to the right.

TABLE 5-4 Metric Prefixes, Meanings, and Relationships

Prefix	Meaning
Giga	Billions
Kilo*	Thousands
Hecto	Hundreds
Deka	Tens
Base units of meter, liter, gram	One unit
Deci	Tenths
Centi*	Hundredths
Milli*	Thousandths
Micro*	Millionths
Nano*	Billionths

*Prefixes most commonly encountered in nursing.

The meter is the unit from which the other metric units are derived. Centimeters and millimeters are the common linear measures used in health-related work. Measurement of the size of body organs is made in centimeters and millimeters, and the sphygmomanometer used to measure blood pressure is calibrated in millimeters of mercury. There are approximately 2.5 cm (25 mm) in 1 inch.

The liter is the unit of capacity or volume and is equal to approximately 1000 cc or 1000 mL. Fractional parts of a liter are usually expressed in milliliters or cubic centimeters. For example, 0.6 L would be expressed as 600 mL or 600 cc. Multiples of a liter are similarly expressed; 2.4 liters would be 2400 mL or 2400 cc. The abbreviation *cc* is in the process of being dropped and is considered obsolete; according to the National Bureau of Standards, either ml or mL may be used.

The gram is the metric unit of weight used in weighing drugs and various pharmaceutical preparations. The approved abbreviation for gram is g; G is no longer approved as the abbreviation because it conflicts with the abbreviation for the prefix *giga*. Gm is also not approved by the National Bureau of Standards.

As a review of Table 5-4 indicates, a decigram is 10 times greater than a centigram and 100 times greater than a milligram. To change decigrams to centigrams, one multiplies by 10; to change decigrams to milligrams, one multiplies by 100. To change milligrams to centigrams, one divides by 10; to change milligrams to decigrams, one divides by 100; to change milligrams to grams, one divides by 1000; and so forth.

The style of notation proposed as the International System of Units from the National Bureau of Standards is rec-

TABLE 5-5 Approximate Equivalents of Common Metric, Apothecary, and Household Weights and Measures

Metric	Apothecary	Household
Weight		
1 kg*	2.2 pounds	
1000 mg = 1 gram*	gr xv	
60 mg* (occasionally seen as 65 mg)	gr i	
30 mg	gr ss (one half)	
1 μg (mcg) = 0.001 mg		
Volume		
	4 quarts	1 gallon
1000 mL* = approximately 1 liter = 1000 cc	Approximately 1 quart	1 quart
500 mL	Approximately 1 pint (½ quart)	16 ounces
240 or 250 mL	℥ viii (8 fluidounces)† = approximately ½ pint	1 cup or 1 glass
30 mL* = approximately 30 cc	℥ i (1 fluidounce)	2 tablespoons
Approximately 16 mL = approximately 16 cc	ʒ iv (4 fluidrams)	1 tablespoon
4 to 5 mL	ʒ i (1 fluidram)	1 teaspoon
1 mL* = approximately 1 cc	Minims xv or xvi	Minims cannot be compared with drops

*These equivalents may be committed to memory for ready application to dosage problems.
†Note the small difference in the symbols for fluidounce and fluidram.

ommended except when it conflicts with proper English language norms:

- Units are not capitalized (gram, not Gram).
- Periods are not used with abbreviations of units (mL, not m.L. or mL.).
- A single space should be left between the quantity and the symbol (24 kg, not 24kg).
- Except in the apothecary system, only decimal notations should be used, not fractions (0.25 kg, not ¼ kg).
- Numerical quantities less than 1 should have a zero placed to the left of the decimal point (0.75 mg, not .75 mg).
- Abbreviations should not be pluralized (kg, not kgs).

Nurses need to have the metric system and its styles of notation as part of their knowledge base to use not only in preparing medications but also in interpreting laboratory data (some are reported in milliliters, others in deciliters or nanograms, and so forth), weighing clients (kilograms instead of pounds), and figuring flow rates of IV infusions. (Refer to Table 5-2 as necessary.)

Until the metric system is fully accepted in clinical practice, nurses may need to deal with all three systems of measurement: metric, apothecary, and household. The nurse can memorize a few crucial relationships. These data can then be readily inserted where applicable as part of a formula or as half of the ratio-and-proportion equation often used for dosage calculation. A suggested practical list of equivalents that nurses should know is presented in Table 5-5.

Apothecary System. Only a few medications are now available in units of the **apothecary system.** This system is less convenient and less precise than the metric system. In response to a survey, most nurses said they rarely (42%) or never (19%) see a drug ordered in the apothecary system (Cohen, 1993). However, unfamiliarity with the apothecary system may lead to dosing errors. The basic unit of weight is the *grain*; this weight is derived from the age-old standard of the weight of a single grain of wheat, which is now variously accepted as equivalent to approximately 60 or 65 mg (60 mg is the more widely accepted of the two). Other units of weight commonly used in the apothecary system are the fluidram, the fluidounce, and the pound.

The basic unit of fluid volume is the *minim* and is approximately equal to the volume of water that would weigh a grain; this amount is very small—approximately 0.05 or 0.06 mL. Other volume measures, which may also be considered household measures, are the pint and the quart.

In written prescriptions using the apothecary system, the placement of abbreviations and the type of numerals used follow a more complex arrangement than in the metric system. In the apothecary system the abbreviation is placed before the numeral. Whole numerical quantities usually are expressed in Roman numerals (e.g., gr x for 10 grains). Fractional quantities are usually expressed with Arabic numerals rather than with decimals (e.g., gr ¼, not gr 0.25, for one-quarter grain).

Household Systems. Measurements in the **household system** include the glass, cup, tablespoon, teaspoon, and drops; pints and quarts are often included in this system and in the apothecary system. The number of people receiving their care at home has increased as a result of shortened hospital stays, correspondingly lengthened convalescence at home, and an increasing older population. Because standardized measurements of household equipment usually do not exist in the home, the home health nurse may not have access to accurately calibrated measuring devices. For example, the average teacup or coffee cup can hold from 5 to 9 ounces or more—not the accepted 8 ounces or half pint. The average household teaspoon can hold 4 to 5 mL or more of liquid medication rather than the standard 5 mL. A drop and a minim *cannot* be considered equivalents, because drop size varies with the viscosity of the medication, even when measured with an approved dropper. Therefore any listing of household measurements on a table of equivalent measures must be considered only an approximation.

Depending on the situation (e.g., medicating infants) and the need for precise dosing, the household system of measurement may or may not be adequate. Clients may need to obtain precise measuring instruments from the local pharmacy or the home health nurse for medication administration at home. Most liquid medications are now packaged with measuring devices that are calibrated with both metric and household measurements.

Dosage Calculation

Challenges to the mathematical skills of nurses occur infrequently in the administration of medications. An equation can be set up to apply what the nurse has learned about a few crucial equivalents and how that relates to what needs to be solved—all in a logical sequence or relationship. Calculators may not be appropriate in the nursing unit because they tend to have exasperating battery failures or to "disappear" from busy hospital units and nursing homes. It is more reliable to develop and maintain a basic competence in mathematical calculations. Following are some typical exercises accompanied by explanations and answers. These exercises assume a working knowledge of decimals, fractions, and a ratio-and-proportion approach to problem solving. If you are used to working with another method that works as well, use it instead; just check your answers and rationale with the following.

Exercises

1. If a drug is ordered in units different from the units on hand, the order must be mathematically translated into the units available. Thus if the medication order is written in terms of milligrams and the client's drug is supplied in grams, the needed dose must be translated into grams.
Question: A drug is ordered to be given in the amount of 1500 mg. How many grams would you give?
Answer: Knowing that there are 1000 mg in a gram, set up the ratio in logical sequence. The logic of the relationships ("this is to this as that is to that") remains constant in a ratio-and-proportion approach; the relationship set down first in the equation does not matter. Some people first set down (on the left side of the equation) the relationship between what has been ordered or what information is wanted and the unknown quantity, or x. On the right side of the equation they set down the known equivalents, the conversion factors, or the "givens." Once set up, the equation is solved by multiplying the means (the middle adjacent numbers) by the extremes (the numbers on each end):

$$1500\text{ mg}: x = 1000\text{ mg}: 1\text{ g}$$
$$1000x = 1500$$
$$x = \frac{1500}{1000} = 1.5\text{ g}$$

An alternate arrangement is

$$\frac{1500\text{ mg}}{x} = \frac{1000\text{ mg}}{1\text{ g}}$$

Then cross multiply so that

$$1000x = 1500 \times 1$$
$$1000x = 1500$$
$$x = \frac{1500}{1000}$$
$$x = 1.5\text{ g}$$

Question: A dose of 30 mL of cough syrup is ordered to be given qid. The label on the bottle of medication states that it contains a total of 240 mL. How many doses of medication are available?
Answer: $30\text{ mL}: 1\text{ dose} = 240\text{ mL}: x\text{ doses}$

$$240 = 30x$$
$$x = \frac{240}{30} = 8\text{ doses or a 2-day supply}$$

Question: 10 mEq of potassium chloride (KCl) is to be added to an IV infusion solution. KCl is available for this application in vials of 40 mEq/20 mL. How many milliliters would you give?
Answer: Again set up the equation in logical sequence, possibly starting with the desired ingredient and the unknown quantity.

$$10\text{ mEq}: x = 40\text{ mEq}: 20\text{ mL}$$
$$40x = 200$$
$$x = \frac{200}{40} = 5\text{ mL}$$

2. Sometimes medication for injection comes in powdered or concentrated liquid form and must be dissolved (reconstituted) or diluted before it can be injected. Most often the label of the drug container has directions regarding how much and what type of diluent (dissolving or diluting solution) should be added by needle and syringe. Labels for drugs that are to be reconstituted will indicate the concentration of drug per mL that results if the reconstitution directions are followed. The label contains all the nurse needs to know to determine the amount to give.
Question: A certain antibiotic has been ordered "750 mg IV." The drug comes in a 10-g multiple-dose vial (there is more than enough of the drug in the vial for one dose) in powdered form. The label reads, "Add 7.2 mL sterile water or sodium chloride solution for injection to yield 10 mL of 1g per 1 mL reconstituted drug." After the diluent has been added, how many milliliters would you give?
Answer: 10 mL now contains 10 g; thus 1 mL equals 1 g. You should already know or be able to refer to a listing of standard equivalents to find out that 1 g equals 1000 mg. You may then start the equation by setting down the relationship between what you want to give and the volume that contains it. Then follow the same sequence of relationship

on the other side of the equation, which indicates what is available in which volume.

$$750 \text{ mg: } x = 1000 \text{ mg: } 1 \text{ mL}$$
$$1000x = 750$$
$$x = \frac{750}{1000} = 0.75 \text{ mL}$$

Whenever a drug appears in concentrated form (powder or liquid), the same mathematical approach can be used after the appropriate diluent has been added and well dispersed or dissolved—no matter what the volume of the finished solution. NOTE: Do not fall into the trap of including the amount of *diluent* anywhere in your equation.

3. *Question:* The quantity of a certain medication is ordered as "gr xv," and the tablets on hand are in gr v dose. How many tablets should be given?
Answer:
$$\text{gr } 15: x = \text{gr } 5:1 \text{ tablet}$$
$$5x = 15$$
$$x = \frac{15}{5} = 3 \text{ tablets}$$

4. *Question:* A client's medication has been ordered based on body weight. If the client weighs 150 pounds, how many kilograms is that?
Answer: You need to know that 1 kg is equal to 2.2 pounds.
$$150 \text{ lb: } x = 2.2 \text{ lb: } 1 \text{ kg}$$
$$2.2x = 150$$
$$x = \frac{150}{2.2} = 68.2 \text{ kg}$$

5. *Question:* Atropine sulfate gr 1/150 is ordered. How many tablets would you give if the available supply were in tablets of 0.2 mg?
Answer: First you need to know that 1 grain is equivalent to 60 mg; then you can find how many milligrams are equivalent to gr 1/150. Second, you need to find out how many tablets provide the milligram equivalent of gr 1/150.
$$\text{gr } 1/150: x(\text{mg}) = \text{gr } 1:60 \text{ mg}$$
$$x = 60(1/150)$$
$$x = \frac{60}{150} = 0.4 \text{ mg}$$
The second step may certainly be performed without pencil and paper, but it is more likely to be accurate if not calculated in the head.
$$0.4 \text{ mg: } x = 0.2 \text{ mg: } 1$$
$$0.2x = 0.4$$
$$x = \frac{0.4}{0.2} = 2 \text{ tablets}$$

6. *Question:* You may also be confronted with the reverse of the preceding question. How many grains would you give if 0.6 mg scopolamine has been ordered?
Answer:
$$0.6 \text{ mg: } x \text{ (gr)} = 60 \text{ mg: gr } 1$$
$$60x = 0.6$$
$$x = \frac{0.6}{60}$$
$$x = \text{gr } 0.01 = \text{gr } 1/100$$

7. *Question:* Codeine gr ss is ordered; how many milligrams would you give?
Answer: You need to know that the symbol "ss" indicates the quantity one half.
$$\text{gr } \frac{1}{2}: x \text{ (mg)} = \text{gr } 1:60 \text{ mg}$$
$$x = 60 \ (1/2)$$
$$x = \frac{60}{2} = 30 \text{ mg}$$

8. *Question:* The client is to take 6 ounces of magnesium sulfate solution, and the calibrations on the available measuring device are in milliliters. How many milliliters would you give?
Answer: You need to know that 1 ounce is equivalent to 30 mL.
$$6 \text{ oz: } x \text{ (mL)} = 1 \text{ oz: } 30 \text{ mL}$$
$$x = 60 \times 30$$
$$x = 180 \text{ mL}$$

9. Although some practitioners may not technically consider IV infusions to be medications, we will practice figuring IV infusion rates here.
The amount of IV solution to be infused during a given length of time is the IV flow rate. It is dictated by the prescriber's order, which should give the total amount of fluid and the number of milliliters that should be infused over each 1-hour period or less, or the number of drops per minute that should be infused. However, some prescribers write IV orders that give only the total volume of solution to be infused (e.g., 1000 mL) over a longer period (e.g., 8 hours). If the order does not specify the rate of flow in drops per minute, the following formula may be used to figure this out:
$$\frac{\text{Total number of milliliters to be infused}}{\text{Total number of minutes infusion is to run}} \times \text{Drop factor} = \text{Rate in drops per minute}$$
Question: If an order is given for 1000 mL D_5W to run for 8 hours and the drop factor is 10 drops per milliliter for the particular tubing used (other types deliver 15 drops or 60 drops—often used to infuse children), how fast should the IV infusion be set to run?
Answer:
$$\frac{1000 \text{ mL}}{480 \text{ min}} \times 10 = \frac{100}{48} \times 10$$
$$= 20.8 \text{ drops (gtt)/min}$$
$$= 21 \text{ gtt/min}$$

A bit more challenging are some of the calculations involved with IV rates for infusion pumps. These pumps are often used for giving drugs whose dosages must be calculated more closely.
Question: Dopamine 400 mg is ordered to be added to 250 mL D_5W for infusion at a rate of 350 μg/min. It is to be regulated by a volumetric infusion pump that is calibrated to deliver the fluid in units of milliliters per hour. At how many milliliters per hour should the pump be set?
Answer: Here you are asked to convert the "language" of one flow rate to the language of another. First, you need to know that 1 μg is equal to 0.001 mg, so:
$$350 \ \mu\text{g: } x = 1 \ \mu\text{g: } 0.001 \text{ mg}$$
$$x = 350 \times .001$$
$$x = 0.350 \text{ mg or } 0.35 \text{ mg}$$

Thus 0.35 mg is being infused every minute. Now you need to calculate the rate per hour. That is, if 0.35 mg is infused every minute, how many milligrams will be infused per hour?

$$x: 60 \text{ min} = 0.35 \text{ mg}: 1 \text{ min}$$
$$x = 60 \times 0.35$$
$$x = 21 \text{ mg}$$

Now convert to milliliters per hour:

$$21 \text{ mg}: x \text{ (mL)} = 400 \text{ mg}: 250 \text{ mL}$$
$$400x = 21 \times 250 = 5250$$
$$x = \frac{5250}{400} = 13.125 \text{ or } 13 \text{ mL/hr}$$

10. *Question:* 30 mg of a drug for three-times-a-day dosing has been ordered for a child who weighs 15 kg and is 90 cm tall. The recommended 24-hour total pediatric dose is 90 to 150 mg/m^2. Is the ordered dose safe or unsafe for this child? Refer to the West nomogram (see Figure 7-1).
Answer: According to the nomogram, a line drawn from points indicating 90 cm and 15 kg crosses the body surface area (BSA) column at the 0.62 point. This means that the child's body surface area is about 0.62 m^2. Multiply 0.62 by each of the numbers indicating the drug's range of safety to see if the ordered 24-hour dose is within that range.

Some rules of thumb will become more important as the metric system predominates:

- Place a zero to the left of the decimal point when there is no integer in the decimal.
- Carry out problems to the hundredths place, and then round off only in the final answer.
- Use judgment in rounding off numbers. The smaller the answer (the lower the number), the more significant the relative change in the answer made by rounding off.

Many excellent nursing texts are available for developing and practicing the arithmetic skills necessary in the administration of medications. (See the Bibliography at the end of this chapter.) Much more practice is necessary than is presented here for introductory purposes.

Procedures and Techniques of Administration

Accurate and full identification of the client before the administration of each dose of medication ensures that the right person gets the right medication. Using the client's full name on all paperwork and in all references helps prevent mix-ups, as does being alert to similarities in names and geographically separating people with similar names within institutional settings. Nurses should not rely on memory to identify clients. *Checking the client's name on the wristband or name tag* against the name on the accompanying medication sheet is the *most reliable* mode of identification. Asking the client his or her name and comparing it with the name on the medication Kardex, computer sheet, or MAR is not foolproof. For example, a client may give his name as "James" or "Santiago" (first name), and then be given medication intended for "Mr. James" or "Mr. Santiago" (last name). Checking the client's name by calling it out and waiting for a corroborating answer is particularly risky; clients have been known to answer to almost any name when in a sleepy state. Relying on names on bed tags or labels is dangerous because clients are often away from their beds; a bed can be inadvertently occupied by another client who is in a groggy state after returning, for example, from a laboratory test. Asking a family member is not foolproof either; a distraught family member may respond inappropriately.

Again, the *surest* way to identify a client before giving medication is to *check the wristband or identifying tag*. In an institutional setting, medications should not be administered to any client not wearing an identification band or tag. Each institution has a policy for replacing identification bands or tags inadvertently removed or lost, and this policy should be complied with and the band or tag restored before any medications are administered. An exception might be an emergency, in which a delay might be detrimental. However, even in an emergency the client's identity should be verified by some method before drug administration.

Before administering medications, the nurse must also make sure the drug order has not been changed in any way (e.g., discontinued or dosage changed) from what appears on the medication sheet or MAR. It is also wise to check the MAR to see that the dose about to be given has not already been given by someone else caring for the client (such as another nurse or nursing student). Individual agency policies spell out the checking procedure to be used; these policies should be followed routinely to avoid error.

The following are recommended guidelines for distributing or administering drugs to clients:

1. When preparing or giving medicines, concentrate your whole attention on what you are doing. Do not permit yourself to be distracted while working with medicines.
2. Make certain that you have a written order for every medication for which you assume the responsibility of administration. (Verbal and telephone orders should be written out and signed by the prescriber as soon as possible. These types of orders should be used only in limited circumstances—not for the convenience of the prescriber.)
3. Make certain that the data on the medication computer sheet or MAR corresponds exactly with the prescriber's written order and with the label on the client's medicine container. Do not decipher illegible orders or make assumptions. Do not accept incomplete orders. Question the use of nonstandard abbreviations and symbols, and do not use them yourself.
4. Make a habit of reading the label on the medicine container and comparing it with the MAR carefully at least three times: first, when removing the drug from the supply drawer or medication cart; second, when placing the medication in a soufflé cup, ounce cup, or syringe; and third, just before administering it to the client, before the container is discarded. Never give a medicine from an unlabeled container or from one that has an illegible label.

5. Look up information on all new or unfamiliar drugs before administering them. When administering a drug for the first time, read the package insert carefully for specific instructions.
6. If you must calculate the dose for a client from the preparation on hand and you are uncertain of your calculation, verify your work on paper by having some other responsible person—an instructor, nurse in charge, or pharmacist—check it. In some hospitals another nurse routinely verifies certain drug doses (e.g., insulin). It is highly unusual for more than two units of a single drug to be administered in a single dose. Therefore double check a calculation whenever the result calls for more than two units (e.g., tablets, vials) of a drug to make a dose.
7. Measure quantities as ordered using the proper equipment: graduated containers for milliliters, fluidounces, or fluidrams; minim glasses or calibrated syringes for minims; and droppers for drops. When measuring liquids, hold the container so that the line indicating the desired quantity is on a level with the eye. The quantity is read when the lowest part of the concave surface of the fluid (meniscus) is on this line.
8. Dosage forms such as tablets, capsules, and pills should be handled so that the fingers do not come into contact with the medicine. Use the cap of the container to guide or lift the medicine into the medicine glass or container you will be taking to the bedside of the client. Administer the medication with water (8 ounces).
9. Avoid wasting medicines. Medicines tend to be expensive; in some instances a single capsule may cost the client several dollars. Dropping medicine on the floor is one way of being wasteful. When preparing medications, work over a clean and dry counter workspace.
10. When pouring liquid medicines, hold the bottle so the liquid does not run over the side and obscure the label. This is known as "palming the label." Wipe the rim of the bottle with a clean piece of paper tissue before replacing the stopper or cover.
11. Always prepare an IV admixture before labeling the container, and verify the dose on the emptied additive container when labeling the IV container.
12. When preparing an injection, always label the syringe immediately. Keep the vial with the syringe, and do not rely on memory to determine what solution is in which syringe.
13. Never administer a medication prepared by another person. In doing so, you accept the responsibility for accuracy, dose, correct medication, and so forth. If the person who prepared the medication has made an error, you are accountable for any harm done to the client.
14. Positively identify the client by comparing the wristband and the name on the MAR.
15. If a client expresses doubt or concern about a medication or the dose of a medication, reassure the client as well as yourself by rechecking to make certain there is no error; do this *before* administering the medication. You may need to recheck the order, the label on the medicine container, or the client's chart. The astute and caring nurse also recognizes that a client who refuses medication has the right to do so and that this behavior is giving a message about expressed or unexpressed feelings. The understanding nurse is not content to simply chart that the client refused his or her medication. Clients should be able to talk about whatever feelings caused the behavior or their concerns about the medication. This helps clients feel that their concern is important and understood and, depending on the reasons, will be appropriately addressed.
16. Assist weak or impaired clients to take their medications, and do so as patiently and unhurriedly as possible. Taking a small sip of water before taking a tablet assists with swallowing solid forms of medications.
17. Many liquid medicines should be diluted with water or another liquid. This practice is especially desirable if the medicine has a bad taste. Exceptions to this rule include cough medicines that are given for a local effect in the throat. Unless the client is allowed only limited amounts of fluid, he or she (in the sitting position) should be supplied with at least 8 ounces *(glassful) of water* for swallowing solid forms such as tablets or capsules. This facilitates dissolution and reduces gastric irritation, if any. Esophageal erosion caused by an adherent tablet or pill has been reported when inadequate amounts of water were given. Having the client sit upright after taking oral medications also helps medication pass into the stomach. Some medications may be crushed (others may not) and mixed with a small amount of jam to make them easier to swallow and more palatable.
18. *Remain with the client until the medication has been taken.* Most clients are very cooperative about taking medicines when the nurse brings them. However, sometimes clients are more ill than they appear, and such clients have been known to hoard medicines until they have accumulated a lethal amount and then take the entire amount, with fatal results. In some instances clients may be permitted to keep certain medicines (e.g., nitroglycerin and antacids) at their bedsides (with a prescriber's order) and take them as necessary.
19. If the client is receiving the first dose of an IV medication, especially antibiotics, stay for at least 5 minutes and monitor closely for adverse effects.
20. Do not leave a tray or cart of medicines unattended. If you are in a client's room and must leave, take the tray of medicines with you. Similarly, do not leave the medication cart unattended in the hall; either

lock the cart in the hallway or take it into the client's room with you.

21. Record the administration of each dose on the MAR as soon as possible. Never chart a medicine as having been given until it has been administered. Nursing students should check the MAR before giving a medication. MARs should document all medications, including prn ones, one-time-only medications, and special drugs (e.g., heparin), in one place to allow the nurse to consider incompatibilities and/or duplications of similar drugs. The name of the drug, the dosage, the time of administration, and the route of administration should be noted on the medication record in the chart. The site of injection is always included when recording parenteral medications. The client's response to the medication, both adverse and intended, should be recorded in the progress notes or nursing notes.
22. Always verify a drug's route of administration. Sometimes preparations for a specific route of administration may be used for another route. For example, Mycostatin suppositories developed for vaginal use may be used as an oral troche for an oral yeast infection; some parenteral preparations may be diluted for oral use, such as vancomycin when indicated for pseudomembranous colitis. To prevent the accidental parenteral injection of this type of oral preparation, oral drugs are not put in syringes used for injection. Oral syringes that cannot accommodate a needle should be used.
23. Within an institutional setting, any unused medication should be returned to the pharmacy. Institutional policy and, in some states, the law requires the unused portion to be credited to the client's account. If the medication can be used for another client, the pharmacy will verify that it has been stored correctly and relabel it.
24. Borrowing medications from one client's supply for another client is not appropriate and leads to dosing errors. Only medications issued by the pharmacy and labeled for a specific client should be used for that client, except in the case of a stock medication kept on the nursing unit. If the facility has a unit dose system, unpackaged or "loose" medications are never administered. Medications brought into the hospital by a client should be sent back home with a family member or, if they are to be used in the institutional setting, sent to the hospital pharmacy to be verified and relabeled.

All medicine containers and trays should be scrupulously clean, and water supplied to the client with the medicine should be fresh. Carelessly prepared medicines and a lack of consideration in the way a medicine is handed to a client can convey a demeaning or insulting message, whether intended or not.

When administering medicine with an unpleasant taste, it is better to admit that it may be unpleasant than to make a client feel that his or her reaction is grossly exaggerated or silly. The nurse can attempt to improve the taste by diluting the medicine (if possible) or by offering chewing gum or hard candy immediately after administering the medicine.

If an injection is likely to sting or hurt, it is honest to tell the client beforehand. The client who is told is also more likely to deal with the pain more effectively than one who is not told. It is better to tell a child just before the injection rather than much beforehand so there is little time for the child to anticipate and grow anxious, thereby actually increasing the pain.

The route of administration is determined by the physical and chemical properties of the drug, the condition or status of the client, the desired action of the drug, its speed of absorption, and the rapidity of response desired. As a rule, drugs are administered for either local or systemic effects (see Chapter 3). Some drugs given locally may produce both local and systemic effects if they are partly or entirely absorbed; some drugs are applied for local absorption (i.e., transdermally) yet are targeted solely for systemic effect, such as nitroglycerin (Transderm-Nitro), fentanyl (Duragesic), and scopolamine (Transderm-Scop). A drug may be injected into a joint cavity and have little or no effect beyond the tissues of that structure.

There is an increasing awareness that many more substances are absorbed through the skin than previously believed. Incidents of toxicity in infants exposed to topically applied dermal medications are increasing. These drugs include boric acid, iodides, hexachlorophene, corticosteroids, and rubbing alcohol. Care is advised in the use of any drug topically applied to an infant's skin.

Administration for Local Effects

Application to Skin. Medications are applied to the skin primarily for the following effects:

1. *Astringent:* to constrict or draw together; this substance may result in vasoconstriction, tissue contraction, and decreased secretions and sensitivity
2. *Antiseptic* or *bacteriostatic:* to inhibit the growth and development of microorganisms
3. *Emollient:* to soothe and soften to overcome dryness and hardness
4. *Cleansing:* to remove dirt, debris, secretions, or crusts

These medications may be applied in the form of a lotion, tincture, ointment or cream, foam, wet dressing, bath, or soak. The effectiveness of medicinals applied to the skin for local effect is limited by the fact that, to protect the internal body environment, highly specialized layers of skin resist the penetration of many (but not all) foreign substances. Topical absorption is increased when the skin is thin or macerated, when drug concentration is increased, when contact of the drug with the skin is prolonged, or when the drug is combined with a solvent-penetrant such as dimethyl sulfoxide [DMSO]. (See Chapter 66 for information on dermatologic drugs and Chapter 67 for information on debriding agents.)

Application to Mucous Membranes. Drugs are well absorbed across mucosal surfaces, and therapeutic effects are easily obtained. However, mucous membranes are highly selective in their absorptive capacity and vary in sensitivity. To produce the same effect, a drug applied to the oral (buccal or sublingual) mucosa may be twice as concentrated as that applied to the nasal mucosa, and the concentration of the same drug may be reduced one fourth to one half for application to delicate membranes of the eye or urethra. Aqueous solutions are quickly absorbed from mucous membranes; oily liquids are not. Oily preparations should not be applied to nasal or respiratory mucosa by sprays or nebulae because the droplets of oil may be carried to terminal portions of the respiratory tract and be retained there, causing lipid pneumonia.

The respiratory mucosa may be medicated by means of inhalation or insufflation. The inhalation method uses sprays or nebulae whereby the drug is sprayed in the nose or throat by a nebulizer; aerosols are delivered by a flow of air or oxygen under pressure to disperse the drug throughout the lower respiratory tract. In the insufflation method a fine powder is blown or sprayed. Drugs administered by means of inhalation or insufflation tend to produce both a local respiratory and a systemic effect. The respiratory mucosa offers an enormous surface of absorbing epithelium. The drug is instantaneously absorbed (1) if the drug is volatile and can be absorbed chemically, and (2) if there is more in the inspired air than in the blood. This fact is of significance in emergencies. Amyl nitrite and oxygen are examples of volatile and gaseous agents given by inhalation.

Drugs in suppository form can be used for their local effects on the mucous membranes of the vagina, urethra, or rectum. Packs and tampons may be impregnated with a drug and placed in a body cavity; these are used particularly in the nose, ears, and vagina. Drugs may also be painted or swabbed on a mucosal surface, instilled (e.g., a vaginal douche), or administered via irrigation.

Administration for Systemic Effects

Drugs that produce a systemic effect must be absorbed into the bloodstream and carried to the cells or tissues capable of responding to them. The route of administration used depends on the nature and amount of drug to be given, the desired rapidity of effect, and the general condition of the client. Routes selected for systemic effect include the following: dermal, oral, sublingual, rectal, and parenteral (injection). Routes of parenteral administration include intradermal (or intracutaneous), subcutaneous, intramuscular, intravenous, intraspinal (or intrathecal), epidural, and sometimes intraarticular, intracardiac, intrapericardiac, intraosseous, and intraperitoneal.

Application to Skin. Now that microquantitative assay capabilities make possible precise unit doses using transdermal modes, topical applications of some medications can be administered in patch form for systemic effect. Nitroglycerin (Nitrodisc, Nitro-Dur, Transderm-Nitro), which is used to treat anginal pain, is available in small unit-dose adhesive bandages that slowly release the medication over a 24-hour period. Some bandages use a semipermeable, rate-controlling membrane placed next to the skin; others disperse the nitroglycerin evenly throughout a gel matrix. See Figure 29-2 for a diagram of some transdermal patches. Motion sickness is treated with scopolamine (Transderm-Scop); the duration of effect of one application behind the ear is approximately 3 days. Fentanyl (Duragesic), an analgesic, is also available in a transdermal system to provide continuous release of the potent opioid for 72 hours. Clonidine, estrogen, and nicotine are other medications available in patch form. The nurse should apply the patch over a clean, dry, and hair-free area; the application sites should be rotated.

Oral Administration. Oral administration is the safest, most economical, and most convenient way of giving medicines. It is the preferred route unless some distinct advantage is to be gained by using another way. Most drugs are absorbed from the small intestine; only a few are absorbed from the stomach and colon. This explains the ineffectiveness of cathartics and enemas in removing most toxins and overdoses in cases of poisoning.

The effects of orally administered drugs are slower in onset and more prolonged but are less potent than those of parenterally administered drugs. Therefore when a steady state in pharmacokinetics is desired, it is often more closely approached with oral than with parenteral administration. The parenteral route may be used when rapid, high doses are needed as loading doses or in emergencies. If carefully tailored to individual needs, strategies for wise pain management can exploit the characteristics of the oral and parenteral routes for analgesics. For clients with low-level pain or chronic pain, the oral route for analgesics can be more successful than other routes in promoting a steady state (fewer oscillations) of pain relief. Acute pain may submit to an initial dose of analgesic by the parenteral route, followed by oral doses.

Altered effects from oral administration may result from (1) variation in absorption as a result of drug composition, gastric or intestinal pH and motility, food content, or a pathologic condition within the gastrointestinal tract; or (2) alteration of the drug resulting from its retention, inactivation, or biotransformation in the liver.

Disadvantages of the oral administration of certain drugs are that (1) they may have an objectionable odor or taste or be bulky to swallow; (2) they may irritate the gastric mucosa, causing nausea and vomiting; (3) they may be aspirated by a seriously ill or uncooperative client; (4) they may be destroyed by digestive enzymes; and (5) they may be inappropriate for some clients, such as those who must be given nothing by mouth.

Sublingual Administration. Drugs given sublingually are placed under the tongue, where they should be retained until they are dissolved and absorbed. The thin epithelium and rich network of capillaries on the underside of the tongue permit both rapid absorption and rapid drug action. There is greater potency than with oral administration, because the drug gains access to the general circulation without initially entering the portal circulation of the liver or being affected by gastric and intestinal enzymes. Many of the same effects apply to buccal administration, whereby a tablet is held in the mouth in the pocket between the gums and the cheek for local dissolution and absorption.

The number of drugs that can be given sublingually is limited (e.g., nitroglycerin tablets). The drug must dissolve readily and the client must be able to cooperate. He or she must understand that the drug is not to be swallowed and that taking a drink or falling asleep must be avoided until the drug has been absorbed. However, usually little harm is done if a sublingual drug is inadvertently swallowed; the effects may be neutralized or delayed slightly.

Rectal Administration. Rectal administration of certain preparations can be used advantageously when the stomach is nonretentive or traumatized, when the medicine has an objectionable taste or odor, or when the medicine can be changed by digestive enzymes. It is also a reasonably convenient and safe method of giving drugs when the oral method is unsuitable, such as when the individual is either a small child (or infant) or is unconscious. Rectal administration is contraindicated if the anal area is irritated or if diarrhea, rectal bleeding, or hemorrhoids are present.

Use of the rectal route avoids irritation of the upper gastrointestinal tract (although aminophylline suppositories often irritate the rectal mucosa) and may promote higher bloodstream drug titers because venous blood from the lower part of the rectum does not initially traverse the liver before entering the general circulation. The suppository is often superior to the retention enema because, with the suppository, the drug is released at a slow but steady rate to ensure a protracted effect. One disadvantage of the retention enema is unpredictable retention of the drug; another is that some of the fluid may pass above the lower rectum and be absorbed into the portal circulation. Administering an evacuant enema before administering a rectal medication is usually advisable to ensure that there is no fecal bulk in the rectum to obstruct free flow of the medicated enema or the action of a suppository. The amount of solution that can be given rectally is usually small.

Refrigerated suppositories will soften and cannot be inserted if they are handled or carried in the pocket for even a brief period. Cold running water will restore rigidity to suppositories. To be retained for effective therapy, suppositories and enema tubing must be inserted beyond the internal anal sphincter (2 to 3 inches). The dose of a drug in suppository form cannot be divided by cutting the suppository in sections because the active drug constituent may not be evenly distributed throughout the suppository.

Parenteral Administration. Strictly speaking, parenteral administration means administration by any route other than oral and thus can technically be defined to include topical or inhalation administration. In practical usage, however, parenteral usually means administration by the use of a needle (Table 5-6).

Parenteral administration of drugs includes all forms of drug injection into body tissues or fluids using a syringe and needle or catheter and container (Figures 5-2 and 5-3). Drugs given parenterally must be sterile, readily soluble and absorbable, and relatively nonirritating. Because the parenteral administration of drugs can be hazardous, several precautions are required: (1) aseptic technique must be used to avoid infection, and (2) accurate drug dose, proper rate of injection, and proper site of injection are essential to avoid harm such as lipodystrophy (atrophy or hypertrophy of subcutaneous fat tissue), abscesses, necrosis, skin slough, nerve injuries, prolonged pain, or periostitis. *An injected drug is irretrievable,* and an error in dose or method or site of injection is not easily corrected.

There are several differences between drugs given parenterally and drugs administered orally. The following is true of parenteral drugs: (1) the onset of drug action is more rapid (except as noted previously), (2) the dosage is often smaller because of the lack of a hepatic first-pass effect, and (3) the cost of drug therapy may be greater. Parenteral administration requires specialized knowledge, aseptic technique, and manual skill to ensure safety and therapeutic effectiveness. The nurse may perform most methods of parenteral administration, but some are usually performed only by a physician or other health care provider with advanced educational preparation. The nurse should know and adhere to agency policy. Clients and family members may also learn to administer injections.

Intradermal Injection. An intradermal or intracutaneous injection is made into the upper layers of the skin, almost parallel to the skin surface (Figure 5-4). The amount of drug given is small, and absorption is slow. This method is advantageous in testing for allergic reactions and for giving small amounts of a local anesthetic. In a test for allergic reactions, minute amounts of the solution to be tested are injected just under the outer layers of the skin. The medial surface of the forearm and the skin of the back are commonly used sites. These injections are best made with a fine, short needle (26- or 27-gauge) and a small-barrel syringe (such as a tuberculin syringe) (Figure 5-5).

Subcutaneous Injection. Small amounts of drug in solution are given subcutaneously, usually by means of a 25-gauge (or thinner) needle and syringe. The greater the number of the gauge of the needle, the finer the needle. The needle is inserted through the skin with a quick movement, but the injection is made slowly and steadily (Figure 5-6). To make sure that a blood vessel has not been entered, the nurse should slightly withdraw the plunger of the syringe before injecting the drug. If a blood vessel has been entered, the medication may take on a pinkish tinge close to the needle hub, or a small amount of blood may enter the syringe. In this case the needle and the medication-filled syringe should be withdrawn and discarded and a new syringe prepared. The angle of insertion should usually be 45 to 60 degrees, but it can be any angle from 30 to 90 degrees, depending on needle length and depth of fat pads.

Needle insertion should be made into the fat pads of the abdomen, the outer surface of the upper arm, the anterior surface of the thigh or, occasionally, the lower abdominal

TABLE 5-6 Guidelines for Parenteral Drug Administration

Route	Common Areas	Region	Needle Sizes*	Volume Injected (mL)		Examples of Medication Given by This Route
				Average	Range†	
Intradermal (intracutaneous)	Skin (corium)	Inner aspect of mid-forearm or scapula	26 or 27 gauge × 3/8 inch	0.1	0.001 to 1.0	Tuberculin, allergens, local anesthetics
Subcutaneous	Beneath the skin	Lateral upper arms, thighs, abdominal fat pads (except the 1-inch area around umbilicus and tissue over bone), upper back, upper hips	25 to 27 gauge 1/2 to 5/8 inch‡	0.5	0.5 to 1.5	Epinephrine (non-oily), insulin, some narcotics, tetanus toxoid, vaccines, vitamin B_{12}, heparin
Intramuscular	Gluteus medius	Dorsogluteal area	20 to 23 gauge × 1½ to 3 inches‡	2 to 4	1 to 5	Most IM and Z-track injections
	Gluteus minimus	Ventrogluteal area	20 to 23 gauge × 1½ to 3 inches‡	1 to 4	1 to 5	All IM medications
	Vastus lateralis	Anterolateral midthigh	22 to 25 gauge × 5/8 to 1 inch‡	1 to 4	1 to 5	Almost all IM medications
	Deltoid	Upper arm below shoulder	23 to 25 gauge × 5/8 to 1 inch‡	0.5	0.5 to 2	Vaccines, absorbed tetanus toxoid, most narcotics, epinephrine, sedatives, vitamin B_{12}, lidocaine
Intravenous bolus	Cephalic and basilic veins	Dorsum of hand and forearm; antecubital fossa	18 to 23 gauge × 1 to 1½ inches	1 to 10	0.5 to 50 (or more by continuous infusion)	Antibiotics, vitamins, fluids and electrolytes, antineoplastics, vasopressors, corticosteroids, aminophylline, blood products

*Needles used for withdrawing medication from a container should be changed before injecting medication drawn (1) from ampules, because irritating medication may cling to needle (filter needles should be used to withdraw medication from ampules) [Meister, 1998]); and (2) from vials, because needles are dulled after insertion through rubber tops; disposable needles are thus labeled "for one-time use only."

†Administration of the largest volumes listed here should be avoided if possible by dividing the dose and using different sites or by using another route in consultation with the prescriber.

‡See text for discussion of factors influencing choice of needle length.

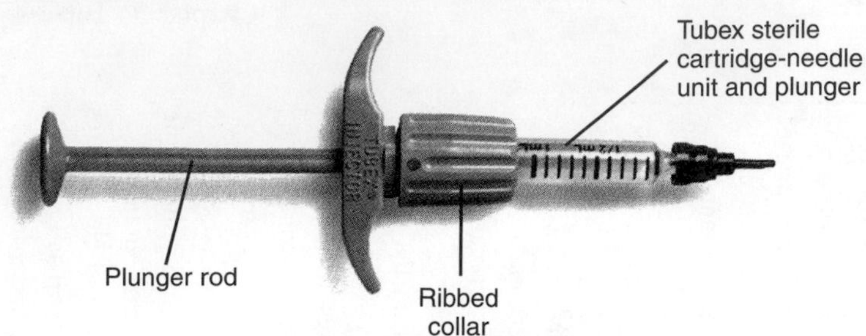

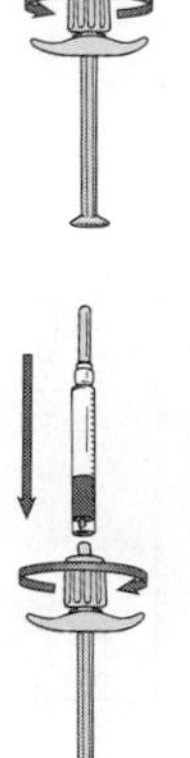

How to load

1. Turn the ribbed collar to the "open" position until it stops.

2. Hold injector with the open end up and fully insert the Tubex sterile cartridge-needle unit.

   Firmly tighten the ribbed collar in the direction of the "close" arrow.

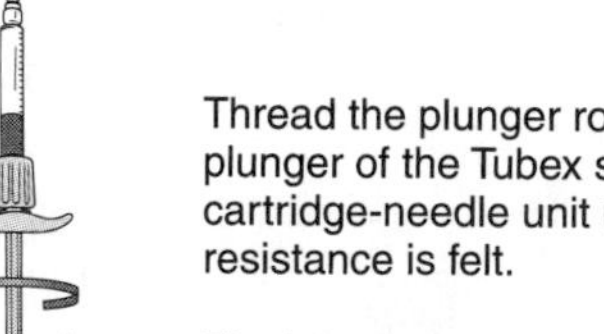

   Thread the plunger rod into the plunger of the Tubex sterile cartridge-needle unit until slight resistance is felt.

   The injector is now ready for use in the usual manner.

How to administer

Method of administration is the same as with conventional syringe. Remove needle cover by grasping it securely; twist and pull. Introduce needle into patient, aspirate by pulling back slightly on the plunger, and inject.

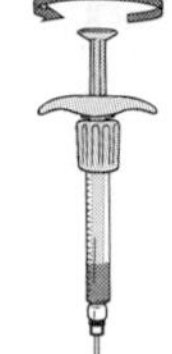

How to unload and discard used unit

1. Do not recap the needle. Disengage the plunger rod.

2. Hold the injector, needle down, over a needle disposal container and loosen the ribbed collar. Tubex cartridge-needle unit will drop into the container.

   Discard the needle cover.

   The Tubex injector is reusable; do not discard.

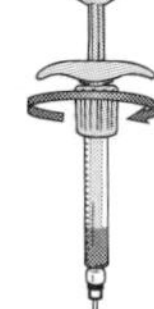

Figure 5-2 Directions for use of the Tubex closed-injection system. (Courtesy of ESI Lederle Division of American Home Products Corporation, St. Davids, PA.)

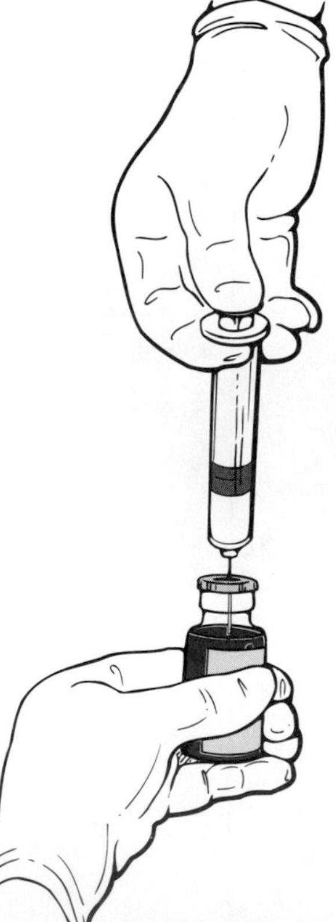

Figure 5-3 Withdrawing medication from a rubber-topped vial. To prevent a vacuum, the vial is inverted to inject a volume of air equivalent to the volume of medication to be withdrawn. If a large amount is to be withdrawn, it may be necessary (in order to be able to withdraw the liquid) to alternate actions (while the needle remains inserted) of instilling air and withdrawing medication. Another method is to use a second needle as an airway in the vial top, maintaining the tip of the medication needle within the liquid; otherwise, only air will be drawn up. Current literature is equivocal about the procedure of drawing an additional 0.1- to 0.3-mL bubble of air into the syringe after the precise medication dose has been drawn up. When injected, this bubble will rise to the top of the medication dose in the syringe to form an absorbable plug so that an irritating medication will not back up the skin track made by the needle.

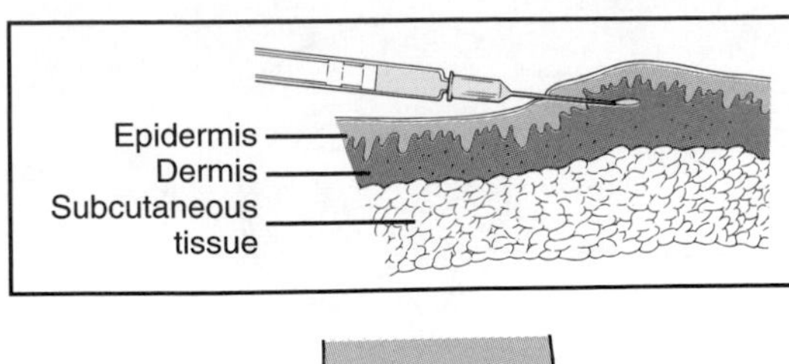

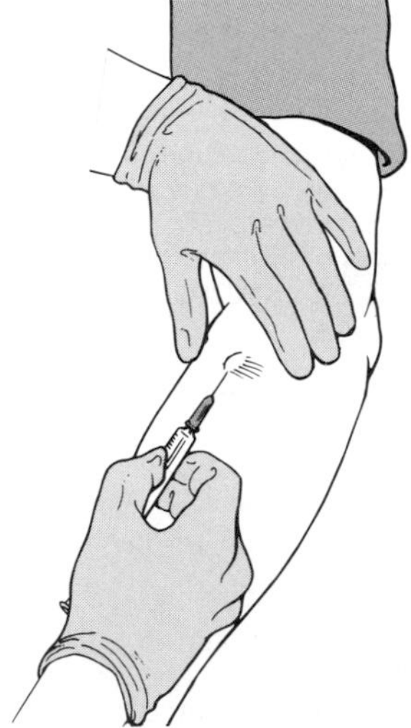

Figure 5-4 Intradermal injection. The needle penetrates the epidermis and goes into the dermis but not subcutaneous tissue. (Note that the skin is not pinched up.)

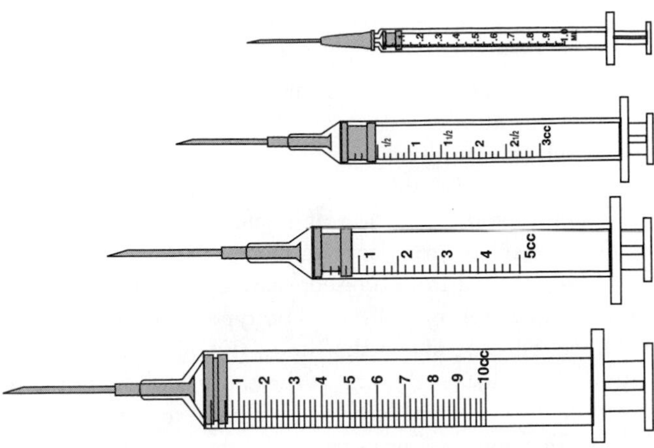

Figure 5-5 These syringes are used for accurate measurement of varying amounts of liquids and liquid medications. The uppermost syringe is known as a tuberculin syringe and is graduated in 0.01-mL increments. It is the syringe of choice for the administration of very small amounts. The 3-mL syringe is the one commonly used for giving a drug subcutaneously, intramuscularly, or intravenously; for withdrawing blood for laboratory testing; or for obtaining urine specimens from urinary catheters (20-mL syringes may be preferred for the last two uses). These syringes and needles are not drawn to scale (e.g., the tuberculin syringe is much thinner and shorter than the others).

surface for drugs such as heparin and insulin. In these locations there are fewer large blood vessels, and sensation is less keen than on the medial surfaces of the extremities. Massaging the part after injection tends to increase the rate of absorption but should be avoided after the injection of certain drugs (e.g., heparin) to minimize bruising as the drug spreads through the tissues. Disposable syringes and needles contribute to the aseptic safety of the procedure but also to cost and problems of storage and disposal. Subcutaneously injected medicines are limited to drugs that are highly soluble and nonirritating and to solutions of limited volume (ideally no more than 1 mL).

Irritating drugs given subcutaneously can result in the formation of sterile abscesses and necrotic tissue, especially if injections are made repeatedly in the same site. Care should be exercised to avoid contamination and to rotate sites. SC injections are not effective in individuals with sluggish peripheral circulation (i.e., the client in shock).

Intramuscular Injection. When a drug is too irritating to be given subcutaneously, deeper injections are made into muscular tissue, through the skin and subcutaneous tissue. However, irritation may occur with some drugs given intramuscularly. Larger doses can be given with IM injection—up to 5 mL—than with SC injection. IM absorption of drugs is delayed in circulatory collapse (i.e., shock states); in such cases the IV route should be chosen.

A drug may be given intramuscularly in an aqueous solution, an aqueous suspension, or a solution or suspension of oil. Suspensions form a depot of drug in the tissue, and slow,

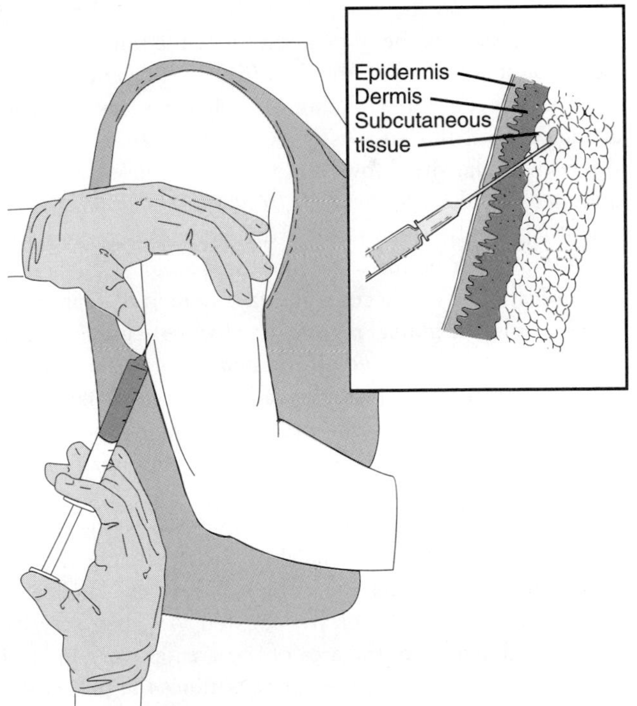

Figure 5-6 SC injection. The skin surface has been cleansed, and the syringe is held at the angle at which the needle will penetrate subcutaneous tissue. The left hand is used to pinch the arm gently but firmly. Once the needle has been inserted into the subcutaneous tissue, the solution is steadily injected. Based on the client's condition or the medication to be injected, nursing judgment may dictate a different angle or an approach different from pinching up the skin.

gradual absorption usually results; this allows the drug to act over a longer period of time. Few drugs are formulated in oil. Two disadvantages are sometimes encountered when preparations in oil are used: (1) the client may be sensitive to the oil, or (2) the oil may not be absorbed. In the latter case, incision and drainage of the oil may be necessary.

Criteria for the selection of a safe IM injection site include the distance from large, vulnerable nerves, bones, and blood vessels and from bruised, scarred, or swollen sites of previous injection or infusion. The type of needle used for IM injection depends on the site of the injection, the condition of the tissues, the size of the client, and the nature of the drug to be injected. Needles from 1 to 1½ inches in length are common. The usual needle gauge is 21 to 23. Fine needles (higher gauges) can be used for thin solutions, and heavier needles (lower gauges) for suspensions and oils. Needles for injection into the deltoid area should be ⅝ to 1 inch in length; again, the gauge depends on the material to be injected. The deltoid can readily absorb up to 2 mL of drug. The gluteals are preferred for many IM injections because of fewer nerve endings and less discomfort at this site. The needle must be long enough to avoid depositing the drug into the subcutaneous or fatty tissue. The depth of insertion depends on the amount of subcutaneous tissue and varies with the weight of the client.

It is essential to locate the appropriate landmarks that limit the areas safe for injections (Figure 5-7 and Table 5-6). IM injections may be given into clearly defined areas of musculature such as the gluteal region of the buttocks (provides slowest absorption), the deltoid area, the ventrogluteal area, and the anterolateral thigh. At first it seems to most nursing students that the fleshy part of the buttock is a logical intramuscular site. However, it is not because the sciatic nerve lies underneath, centrally, and runs diagonally; permanent leg paralysis can result if this nerve is damaged. Every attempt must be made to avoid this area.

There are now two acceptable ways to map the appropriate IM sites in the gluteal region. The formerly used method of dividing the gluteus medius into imaginary quadrants and injecting into the upper outer quadrant is out of favor because it does not necessarily prevent an injection into the sciatic nerve, especially if the nerve runs abnormally in an individual.

The nurse can best locate the *dorsogluteal* site (the muscle underneath is the gluteus medius) by asking the client to lie face down and exposing the entire area so the landmarks and injection site can be clearly located. An imaginary diagonal line drawn from the area of the greater trochanter of the femur to the posterior iliac spine outlines the proper site for this injection. The injection should be given at any point between that imaginary straight line and below the curve of the iliac crest (see Figure 5-7, *A*).

The *ventrogluteal* site can be made accessible with the client in a supine, prone (which is awkward), or side-lying position. This site is used for IM injections in children and adults and could be used more often than it is. To locate this site on the right side, the nurse should palpate for the right greater trochanter with the left palm, point the left index finger to the anterior superior iliac spine, and extend the middle finger toward the iliac crest. The injection should be made in the center of the V formed between the index and middle fingers (see Figure 5-7, *B*). The right hand is used to detect landmarks in the left hip.

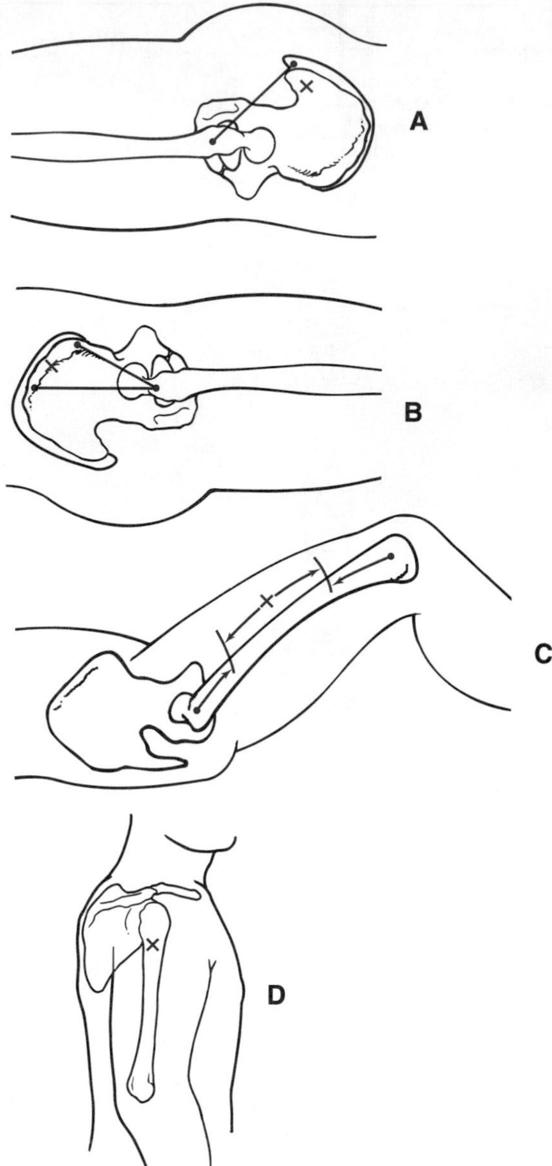

Figure 5-7 IM injection. **A,** Dorsogluteal site. This site is located anterior to the diagonal line from the trochanter to the posterior iliac spine. An injection near the middle of the buttocks may result in injury to the sciatic nerve. The needle is inserted with a quick, firm movement, entering perpendicular to the skin. The solution is injected slowly and steadily after aspiration to make certain the needle is not in a blood vessel. **B,** Ventrogluteal IM injection site. The V fans out from the greater trochanter between the anterior iliac spine and iliac crest. The injection site (**X**) is centered at the base of the triangle. **C,** Vastus lateralis (midlateral thigh) IM injection. This site lies a handbreadth below the greater trochanter, a handbreadth above the knee, and halfway between the front and side of the thigh. **D,** Mid-deltoid IM injection site. This site lies below the acromion and lateral to the axilla.

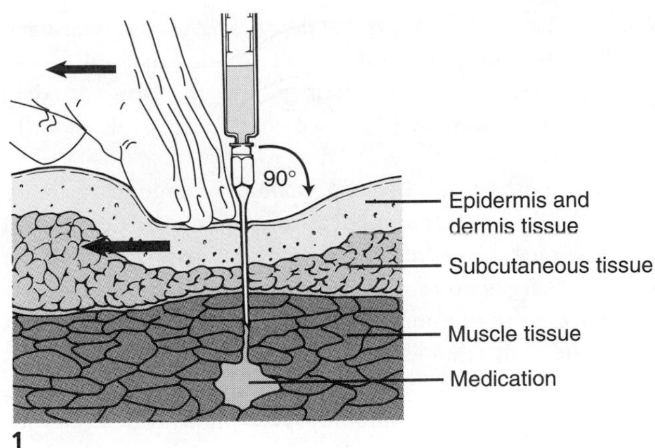

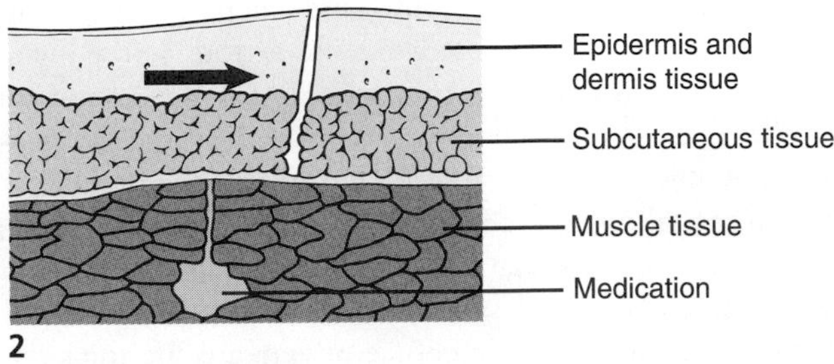

Figure 5-8 Z-track IM injection method. This method is useful for administering medications known to cause pain or permanent staining of superficial tissues. *1*, The skin is stretched to one side and the medication is injected as usual, perpendicular to the skin surface. *2*, The needle is removed and the skin allowed to return to a resting position, sealing off the deposited medication from the track made by the needle. With this method, the site is not massaged.

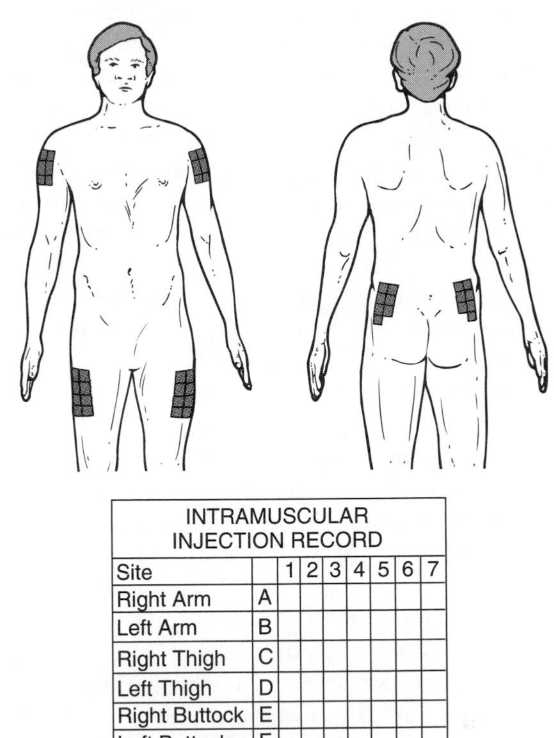

INTRAMUSCULAR INJECTION RECORD

Site		1	2	3	4	5	6	7
Right Arm	A							
Left Arm	B							
Right Thigh	C							
Left Thigh	D							
Right Buttock	E							
Left Buttock	F							

Figure 5-9 Anatomic chart for the rotation of IM injections. The chart may be kept with the MAR, nursing Kardex, or care plan to provide a reference for the nurse administering the medication.

Either of these two gluteal sites is preferred for the **Z-track method,** an injection method useful for administering medications known to cause pain or permanent staining of superficial tissues (Figure 5-8).

The *mid-deltoid* area is the muscular area in the arm formed by the rectangle bounded on the top by the edge of the shoulder and on the bottom by the beginning of the axilla (see Figure 5-7, *D*). The deltoid muscle has a considerably higher blood flow than the other IM injection sites; for rapid onset, this is the area of choice for many small-volume (2 mL or less) medications.

The *vastus lateralis* is a muscular area in the upper outer leg. The potential site for injection is within a long rectangular area just lateral to the frontal plane of the thigh. Its top boundary is located approximately one handbreadth below the greater trochanter, and the bottom boundary is located approximately one handbreadth above the knee (see Figure 5-7, C). This area can accommodate the same volumes of medication as the gluteus medius and is distant from any major blood vessels or nerves. However, an injection here may be more painful than in the buttocks.

Relaxation and comfort may be enhanced during an IM injection into the gluteal muscles if the client lies in a prone position with a pillow under the legs just below the knees, using a toes-in position (to relax the buttocks) or putting the toes of both feet together. The side-lying position is an alternative. To prevent local postinjection complications (e.g., discomfort, scars, abscesses), no two injections should be made in the same spot during a course of treatment. Injection sites should be rotated, and the site for each IM injection should be recorded on the clinical record (Figure 5-9).

When administering an IM injection, one hand holds the needle and syringe assembly as if it were a dart while the other hand stretches taut the skin of the injection site. The nurse can test the sensitivity of the area by tapping it with the fingers. If the muscle mass underlying the injection site is inadequate to accommodate the length of the needle, the muscle may be pinched up before needle insertion. The injection should be made *perpendicular to the skin surface,* from a distance of about 2 inches, in one quick motion. If possible, the needle should not be inserted to its full depth; a small portion should be left accessible above the skin so it can be retrieved if it breaks (a very rare event).

To prevent the unintended deposit of medication into the bloodstream instead of muscle tissue (also very unusual), it is necessary to make certain the needle is not in a blood vessel. This is accomplished by pulling out the plunger slightly after placing the needle in the tissue (termed "aspiration"). If the needle is in a blood vessel rather than in tissue, the medication may have a slight pinkish tinge close to the needle hub, or a small amount of blood may enter the barrel of the syringe. If this is the case, the needle and the medication-filled syringe should be withdrawn and discarded and a new syringe prepared. In certain instances, inadvertent intravessel administration of oily or particulate medicines or killed bacteria can result in a serious emergency.

Contrary to popular belief, needle puncture of the skin is not always the prime source of discomfort associated with injections, although a dull needle (e.g., one that has been inserted through a vial's rubber stopper) will certainly contribute to pain. In addition, it is not the length of the needle that causes pain, but the diameter; a 3-inch needle will hurt no more than a ⅝-inch needle if the diameter is similar. Except for the psychologic aspect of anxiety about needles, most injection pain is thought to occur from stretching of tissue (pain receptors in the flesh) as it accommodates the volume of the drug; from irritation from the drug itself; from unsteadiness in the injector's technique, which results in jiggling of the needle during overly slow insertions; during aspiration; while the injector is reaching for the antiseptic swab at completion; or from wet antiseptic on the skin during insertion. Discomfort as the injection is completed can be prevented by quickly withdrawing the needle in the same angle as insertion while applying firm pressure to the injection site with an antiseptic swab. Massaging the site (except after the injection of iron dextran products and others) disperses the medication and may also reduce any discomfort.

Intravenous Injection/Intravenous Infusion. When an immediate effect is desired, when for any reason a drug cannot be injected into other tissues, or when absorption may be inhibited by poor circulation, the drug may be given directly into a vein as an intravenous **injection** (the act of forcing a liquid into the body by means of a syringe) or as an intravenous **infusion** (the introduction of a substance directly into a vein by means of gravity flow). The terms *injection* and *infusion* also refer to the substances so administered. These methods require skill and asepsis, and the drugs used in these methods must be highly soluble and capable of withstanding sterilization.

These methods are of great value in emergencies. In addition, the dose and amount of absorption can be determined with accuracy. However, the rapidity of absorption and the fact that there is no recall once the drug has been given are dangers worthy of consideration. From this standpoint it is one of the least safe methods of administration. Precautions must be taken to prevent extravasation, or leakage, of the drug or fluids into surrounding tissue **(infiltration).**

With an IV injection ("IV push"), a comparatively small amount of solution (also referred to as a bolus) is given by means of a syringe into IV tubing, into a heparin lock, or directly into a vein over a 1- to 7-minute period. Before injection, the drug is dissolved in a suitable amount of normal (physiologic) saline solution or some other isotonic solution. The injection may be made into the median basilic or median cephalic vein at the bend of the elbow (Figure 5-10), or into the basilic, dorsal metacarpal, and cephalic veins of the forearm and dorsal surface of the hand (Figure 5-11). Factors that determine the choice of vein are the thickness of the skin over the vein, the closeness of the vein to the surface, the presence of a firm support (bone) under the vein, and the need to use a larger vein for concentrated or irritating substances. The veins in the antecubital fossa are readily accessible, but the veins of the back of the hand are

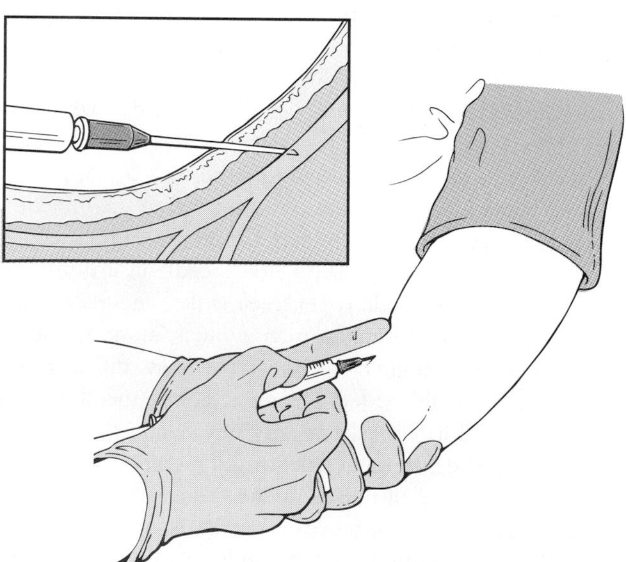

Figure 5-10 IV injection. A tourniquet is placed on the upper arm. The skin is cleansed with a solution of alcohol, and the thumb of the left hand holds the skin taut. The withdrawal of blood indicates that the needle is in the vein. The tourniquet is released and the solution is injected slowly and steadily.

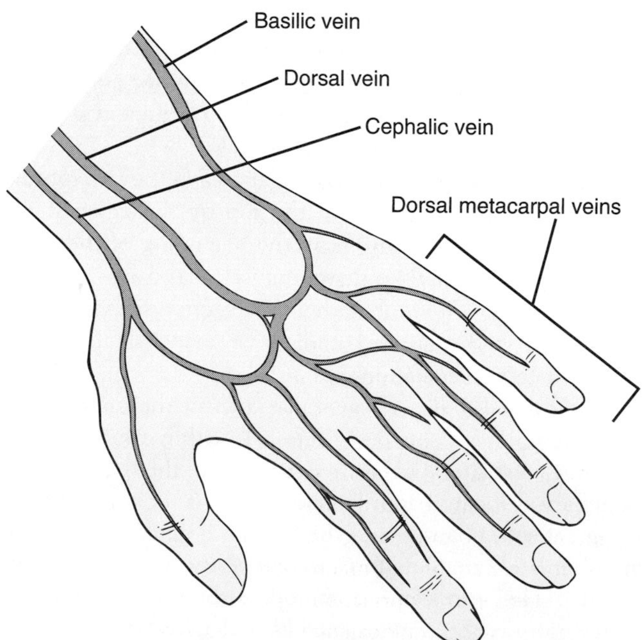

Figure 5-11 The major sites for IV injection in the hand include the basilic, dorsal metacarpal, and cephalic veins. These vessels are fairly easy to locate. As the cephalic and basilic veins traverse the forearm, they branch into other vessels that also are easily accessible for IV injections.

also sometimes used for infusions. Leg veins are avoided because of their potential for phlebitis.

A vein that is normally distended with blood is much easier to enter than a partially collapsed vein. A tourniquet is drawn tightly around the extremity proximal to the IV site to distend the vein, air is expelled from the syringe, and the needle is introduced pointing proximally, bevel up. A few drops of blood aspirated into the syringe indicate that the needle is in the vein; the tourniquet is then removed and the solution is injected slowly. As in all types of injections, the needle, syringe, and solution must be sterile; the hands must be scrupulously washed and gloved; and antiseptic must be applied to the insertion site and allowed to dry.

An IV bolus dose is the method of choice for rapidly administering drugs in an emergency because it is a reliable way to achieve optimal drug blood levels rapidly. It is also the way to administer certain IV medications that may be incompatible in solution: digoxin (Lanoxin), diazepam (Valium), furosemide (Lasix), diazoxide (Hyperstat), certain anticancer drugs, and diagnostic agents in dye form. A 20-gauge needle is commonly used for IV push or bolus doses. Many drugs given intravenously must be given slowly to avoid cardiac, neurologic, or respiratory changes. It is necessary for the nurse to know the appropriate IV dosage rate to avoid a potentially fatal problem.

With an IV infusion a larger amount of fluid is given (usually to adults), starting with 1 L. The solution flows by gravity from a graduated glass bottle or plastic bag through tubing, a connecting tip, and a needle or catheter into a vein, or it may be infused with an IV controller or pump.

The rate of administering fluids (with or without other additives) by IV infusion may be regulated in one of two basic ways. One is by a simple *roller clamp* on the tubing, which can be manually adjusted to deliver the number of drops per minute that will provide the prescribed total amount over the prescribed time. (See the formula for calculating IV flow rate, which was discussed in Exercise 9 earlier in this chapter.)

Another way to make infusions run more precisely is to use IV controllers and pumps. Such instrumentation can be used in situations that require more accurate titration of infusion fluids or nutrients than is provided by hand-adjusted roller clamps, which can allow up to a 5% error in flow rate within the first 15 minutes of flow and other variations thereafter. Most instrumentation to regulate infusions consists of various applications of either infusion controllers or infusion pumps. These small, boxlike devices are attached to IV poles. Pressure on the infusion tubing regulates the rate of IV flow to ensure automatic delivery of solutions at preselected rates or volumes. **CAUTION**: For instruments that can accommodate either macrodrip or microdrip tubing, the tubing must be appropriate for the drop factor used to calculate drop rate. A rate calculated on the basis of microdrip tubing but accidentally administered by macrodrip could seriously overdose or overhydrate a client.

There are many infusion pumps and controllers on the market, and manufacturers produce new models frequently. Infusion controllers are useful in 80% to 85% of cases calling for IV therapy. They work simply by using the force of gravity. Controllers are not capable of delivering rates with the accuracy of infusion pumps in special situations in which increases in back pressure are transmitted to the fluid in the tubing (e.g., arterial infusions, a restless child, a woman in labor). However, unlike infusion pumps, infusion controllers will not pump fluid into interstitial tissue if the infusion needle infiltrates.

There are at least two types of infusion pumps, both of which deliver infusion fluids under positive pressure: (1) nonvolumetric ("infusion pumps"), which measure fluid volume delivery by drop rate (not as accurate because drop volume may vary); and (2) volumetric ("volume pumps"), which can measure very precisely even smaller volumes of infusion solution by milliliter per hour. This latter pump is especially useful for small children, total parenteral nutrition, and the administration of potent drugs by continuous IV infusion (such as streptokinase, dopamine, or nitroglycerin). Alarm readout messages (e.g., "fix me") may be displayed on the front panel of the instrument.

Similar infusion pumps are made by several different manufacturers and use various physical principles to sense pressures and amount of pump fluid and to read out flow-rate settings and other measures. Their capabilities include greater accuracy than other modes of infusion delivery systems and alarms to warn of blocked tubing, air in the tubing, or empty solution containers. These features sound ideal but, as with all mechanical devices, infusion pumps are subject to malfunction; nurses need to be continually watchful to ensure reliability of these devices. They also need to maintain personal contact with the purpose of it all—the client. Currently there is a growing body of literature regarding this type of equipment. Its intricacy presents nurses with still another challenge, although not an insurmountable one. (See the excellent Bibliography at the end of this chapter for more information.)

IV infusions are most commonly given to relieve tissue dehydration, to restore depleted blood volumes, to dilute toxic substances in the blood and tissue fluids, to supply electrolytes or drugs, to provide an IV line if an emergency is anticipated, or to provide a fluid challenge to evaluate kidney function.

The fluid is usually given slowly to prevent a reaction or fluid overload, which may impair cardiac or pulmonary function, especially in older adults or in those with cardiac disease. Eight hours are usually required for every 1000 mL of fluid, depending on the condition of the client and the nature of and reason for the solution. This rate is slower in children and is determined by age, weight, and urinary output.

A number of commercial solutions are used in IV replacement therapy. Some solutions contain not only salts of sodium and potassium but also salts of calcium and magnesium. Vitamins are also added to IV fluids when necessary. (See Unit 19 for a discussion of various IV infusion solutions and parenteral nutrition, and Chapter 31 for a discussion of blood products.)

Total parenteral nutrition (TPN) or hyperalimentation is the infusion of an individual's total basic nutritional need via an infusion catheter into a large central vein and/or into a peripheral one. The choice of site depends partly on the potential of the medium to cause phlebitis. Fat emulsions have a much lower potential for causing phlebitis than the hypertonic dextrose solutions used for TPN.

Whole blood and blood products are given intravenously to restore depleted blood volume and blood constituents. Blood products should be introduced through IV tubing that has been primed with a normal saline infusion solution rather than a dextrose solution, which would cause "stickiness" of red blood cells and cause them to clump artificially, possibly clogging the needle or causing hemolysis. Inserting an 18-gauge or larger needle when the infusion of blood products is expected helps minimize trauma to blood cells. Tubing should also incorporate a filter to trap cell particles and clumped cells to prevent them from circulating or clogging the needle.

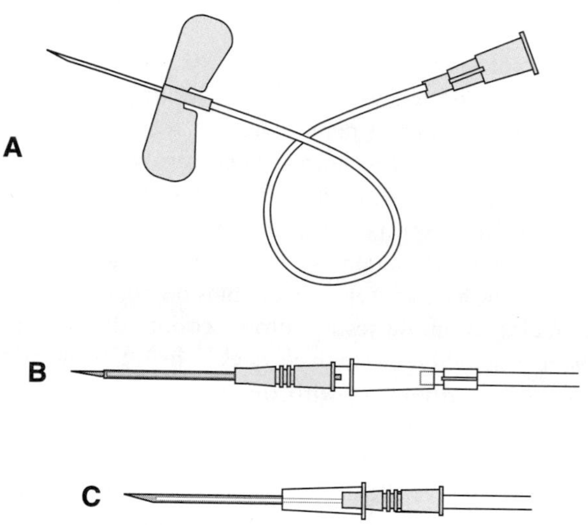

Figure 5-12 IV needles. **A**, Butterfly needle. **B**, Over-needle catheter. **C**, Cannula (through-the-needle catheter).

Some drugs, such as antibiotics, are administered by intermittent infusion (known as "IV piggyback" [IVPB] or "IV rider" in some parts of the United States). They are given via a setup that is secondary to the primary IV infusion and hung in tandem and connected to the primary setup.

Most intermittent diluted drug infusions are meant to have a total infusion time of 20 or 30 minutes to 1 hour, depending on factors such as the amount of diluent required and the potential for vein wall irritation by the drug.

The presence of particulate matter (which can consist of tiny chunks of rubber stoppers or glass slivers from ampules) in IV infusion solutions is disturbingly common. Such matter can be introduced during manufacture, during changing of the solution bottle, or during administration of a medication. The resulting potential for phlebitis is high. Therefore it is recommended that in-line filtering devices be used for all IV therapy. Optimal filtration is provided by 0.22-μm filters; most organisms, except certain strains of *Pseudomonas* and the viruses, are filtered out by 0.45-μm in-line filters. To prevent the injection of larger particles, disposable needles with 5-μm filters can be used to draw medication up.

For peripheral IV therapy, stainless steel scalp-vein needles ("butterfly needles") produce lower rates of infection and phlebitis, but plastic catheters (over-needle catheters) or cannulas (through-the-needle catheters) tend to decrease the incidence of infiltration and work best when an infusion needle will be in place for a long period (Figure 5-12). The advantages and disadvantages of each type of needle must be weighed at the time of insertion (Table 5-7).

Central venous infusion is the administration of fluid through an IV catheter placed in a central vein. The catheter tip rests in the superior vena cava if the subclavian vein and internal and external jugular veins are cannulated; the catheter tip rests in the inferior vena cava if the femoral vein is cannulated. With peripheral central venous therapy, the

TABLE 5-7 Intravenous Needles in Common Use by Nurses

IV Needle	Length of Needle	Length of Tubing	Indication
Wing-tip or scalp-vein needle (E-Z Set or butterfly)	½ to 1¼ inches (1.3 to 3.1 cm)	3 to 12 inches (7.5 to 30 cm)	Client in stable condition; IV fluids or medications of short duration; intermittent IV push injections, indefinite period of time; pediatric scalp vein (see Figure 5-12)
Over-the-needle catheter (Abbocath, Jelco, or Angiocath)	Varies	1¼ to 5½ inches (3.1 to 13.8 cm); 1¼ to 2 inches (3.1 to 5 cm) most commonly used	Client in unstable condition (needs large volume replacement); only poor veins are available; caustic medications are to be administered
Through-the-needle catheter (Intracath)	1½ to 2 inches (3.8 to 5 cm)	8 to 36 inches (20 to 90 cm)	Client has poor venous access; long-term IV therapy; extremely caustic medications (continuous chemotherapy, total parenteral nutrition)

central catheter is inserted in a peripheral vein, usually the basilic or cephalic vein, and the distal end of the catheter rests in the superior vena cava. Central venous infusion is used when poor venous access prohibits the use of peripheral veins or when irritating solutions must be infused directly into a large central vein to avoid phlebitis. Central IV devices are inserted by physicians for either short-term or long-term use. For short-term use, the central venous catheter has multiple lumens to allow simultaneous administration of more than one solution. Catheters for long-term use are more flexible and less thrombogenic but must be surgically implanted. These catheters are for long-term central access for the infusion of fluids, antibiotics, parenteral nutrition, chemotherapy, and home IV therapy.

Although starting infusions and drawing blood were traditionally the responsibility of physicians, most nurses today perform these functions, especially in critical care areas. Probably one of the most effective approaches is the preparation of IV teams whose sole job is to maintain, remove, and replace IV needles, catheters, and so forth. Such teams may prove to be a mixed blessing, however, because although such teams become very proficient at their job, they also may serve to further fragment a client's care.

Table 5-8 lists data to assess for IV needle site complications and suggests concomitant nursing interventions.

Epidural Injection. Epidural analgesia is being used increasingly for the management of acute and chronic pain. For this route of drug administration, the physician implants an epidural catheter beneath the client's skin with its tip in the epidural space, which lies just outside the subarachnoid space in which the cerebrospinal fluid (CSF) circulates. The drug bypasses the blood-brain barrier and diffuses into the CSF. This route of administration works well for narcotic analgesics such as morphine, fentanyl (Sublimaze), and hydromorphone (Dilaudid), administered either by IV bolus dose or by continuous infusion because opiate receptors are found along the spinal cord, which allows the drugs to produce localized analgesia without loss of motor function. Once the epidural catheter is in place, the nurse is responsible for monitoring the infusion and the client's status relative to it.

To prepare the infusion device, the nurse should follow the manufacturer's instructions and the policies of the health care agency; the drug concentration and infusion rate is checked against the prescriber's order. The nurse should ensure that the client understands the procedure and that an appropriate consent form has been completed. The nurse assists with insertion of the epidural catheter and labels the tubing as "epidural infusion" to avoid confusion with other infusion lines in which drugs might be administered. To prevent migration of the catheter, it is taped securely, and the symbols on the catheter that indicate the extent of tubing inserted are monitored. Oxygen, an intubation set, resuscitation equipment, naloxone (Narcan) 0.4 mg IV, and ephedrine 50 mg IV should be on hand for emergency use. The client should have peripheral IV access (IV infusion or heparin lock) to permit immediate access for the administration of emergency drugs. The client should be instructed to report pain using a pain scale from 0 to 10 (see Chapter 14, Nursing Management: Pain Therapy).

The nurse should assess the client's respiratory rate and blood pressure every 2 hours for the first 8 hours, every 4 hours for the first 24 hours, and then once a shift according to the client's condition, as prescribed, or according to

TABLE 5-8 Common Intravenous Needle Site Complications

Needle Site Data	Infiltration	Clot Over Needle Opening or Obstruction	Phlebitis	Infection at Site of Needle Insertion
Color	Pale	No change	Red	Red over site
Temperature	Cool to cold	No change	Warm to hot	Warm at site
Swelling	Rounded	None	Cordlike vein path	Small amount at site
Pain	Yes, usually	None	Yes	None usually
Flow	Slowed or stopped	Slowed or stopped	No change or may be slowed	No change
Nursing actions	Tourniquet proximally (flow continues—infiltration) Lower bottle (blood in tubing—no infiltration) Discontinue IV Restart IV at another site or call IV team	Check for infiltration Reposition arm Raise IV container, close clamp, coil tubing, release quickly Restart IV at another site or call IV team	Discontinue IV *usually* Contact prescriber Resite IV to another area/call IV team Note irritating solution (Valium, Keflin, KCl running too fast) Warm compresses; elevate and immobilize part	Do not discontinue IV until IV team advice has been sought or prescriber has been notified (it may be the only vein available for essential infusion)

agency policy. The prescriber is notified if the client's respiratory rate is less than 10 per minute or if the systolic blood pressure is less than 90 mm Hg. The client's level of sedation, mental status, and pain relief are assessed every hour initially until the client reports adequate pain control, then every 2 to 4 hours. The prescriber is notified if the client becomes extremely drowsy or experiences other adverse effects such as nausea and vomiting, pruritus, urinary retention, or unrelieved pain. Strength and sensation in the lower extremities are assessed every 2 to 4 hours. The dosage may need to be decreased if deficits occur. Because drugs administered by the epidural route diffuse slowly, the client is monitored for adverse effects for 12 hours after the infusion is discontinued.

The dressing over the catheter site is changed every 24 to 48 hours, and the infusion tubing is changed every 48 hours, as needed, or according to the policies of the health care institution. The nurse should observe the catheter insertion site for redness and swelling. Headache as a complication can be minimized by having the client lie flat and maintain an adequate fluid intake. If epidural analgesia is to be used at home, the client/caregiver must be willing and capable of managing the therapy. The client must avoid using alcohol and street drugs, because these substances potentiate the effects of the opiates.

Intrathecal Injection. Intrathecal (into a sheath) injection is also known as intraspinal, subdural, subarachnoid, or lumbar injection. The technique is the same as that required for a lumbar puncture. Nurses do not usually directly administer drugs intraspinally, but they may be required to fill the drug reservoir of an implanted intraspinal delivery system. The nurse needs to be specially trained, and the manufacturer's instructions should be followed closely.

In addition, drugs are occasionally administered by intracardiac, intrapericardiac, intraventricular, intraperitoneal, intraarticular, and intraosseous injections; however, state regulation and institutional policy may not allow nurses to administer drugs by these routes.

Special Situations

Swallowing Difficulty. The following suggestions are for clients who have difficulty swallowing oral medications. If the cause is a diminished swallow reflex, the drug should be given by another route after consultation with the prescriber:

1. Have the client drink some water *just before* taking the medication and drink only a small amount *with* the medication. At least 240 mL of liquid should be taken after the drug. Clients are capable of taking fluids more easily if they are in Fowler's position (upright sitting position).
2. Instruct the client to place the tablet at the midpoint of the tongue and toss it back to the throat with the water. If the client is hemiplegic, place the tablet on the unaffected side of the tongue for swallowing.
3. The client may also chew a small amount of food and then place the tablet in the mouth to be swallowed with the food.

If the head is tipped slightly forward, the act of swallowing follows more naturally; choking is more likely when the head is tilted back. Massaging the laryngeal prominence (Adam's apple) or the area just under the chin may facilitate initiation of the mechanical act of swallowing.

Medications may be crushed unless they are enteric-coated or sustained-action forms. Box 5-4 lists medications that should not be crushed. Capsules may also be opened and the contents sprinkled on a small portion of easy-to-swallow food such as applesauce or a gelatin dessert. The client should be told about this procedure and instructed to eat the medicated contents first so that very little remains unadministered if the rest of the food is refused. This approach should be used cautiously on children because the particular food may be rendered distasteful and be rejected by the child in the future.

Medications may be liquefied for drinking by adding water, or they may be administered by instillation into the mouth next to the cheek by a large syringe (with or without a short tubing attached).

Suggestions for Clients with a Tracheostomy Tube in Place. The tube should have a cuff, which should be inflated whenever any substance is taken by mouth; this prevents the substance from accidentally entering the lungs. If an external attachment is in place to allow the client to talk, a one-piece tracheostomy tube should be substituted before inflating the cuff. To perform this procedure, the tracheostomy is suctioned, and the nurse ensures that the cuff is inflated. The client should sit upright. After the client swallows the medication, suctioning is performed and the cuff is deflated. If the client coughs or chokes, the procedure is immediately stopped and is resumed when the client indicates that it is all right to continue. Large tablets or capsules are never used.

Suggestions for Administering Medications to Clients with a Nasogastric or Gastrostomy Tube. The procedure for administering tube feedings is followed, with these additional precautions:

1. Check placement of the tube before giving medications or tube feedings. Consider the tube's placement in relation to drug absorption. If the tube is placed in the duodenum or jejunum and the drug is absorbed in the stomach, consult with the pharmacist before administering the medication.
2. Give medications and tube feedings at separate intervals to avoid potential drug-food interactions. If the drugs are to be ingested on an empty stomach, hold the tube feeding for an appropriate time before and after the medication.
3. If drugs must be administered with a feeding, assess for potential drug-food interactions (penicillin G, phenytoin [Dilantin], and most tetracyclines), just as would be done with any oral drugs. Administer the medications before the tube feeding.
4. Check with the pharmacy for the availability of liquid preparations of the client's medications. Liquids are always preferable to crushing tablets. If tablets must

BOX 5-4

Medications That Should Not Be Crushed

The following is a partial listing of drugs that should not be crushed.* It is suggested that if a liquid dosage form of the medication is available, it should be used instead of a crushed tablet whenever possible. In general, coated tablets should not be crushed because the coating has been applied for a specific reason, such as (1) to prevent stomach irritation (e.g., Dulcolax Tablet); (2) to prevent destruction by stomach acids (e.g., Ananase); (3) to produce a prolonged or extended effect (e.g., Dimetapp); or (4) to avoid an unwanted reaction (e.g., chloral hydrate in capsule has a very bitter taste and Povan tablets will stain the mouth red; Kaon tablets may produce a burning effect on sensitive mucosa).

Albendazole tablet	Donnatal Extentab	Ferro Grad-500 Tab	Quinidex Extentab
Allerest capsule	Drixoral tablet	Inderal LA	Slow K tablet
Artane Sequel	Dulcolax tablet	Isordil sublingual	Sudafed 12-hour capsule
ASA Enseals	Ecotrin tablet	Kaon tablet	Teldrin capsule
Azulfadine EN-tabs	E-Mycin tablet	Nitroglycerin tablet	Theo-Dur tablet
Betapen-VK	Entozyme tablet	Norpace CR	Trental tablet
Compazine Spansule	Feosol tablet	Ornade Spansule	
Diamox Sequel	Feosol Spansule	Quinaglute Dura-tab	

Although pharmaceutical manufacturers develop new drugs and reformulate existing ones, some common terms attached to a drug name may indicate a sustained-release form of a drug, which consequently should not be crushed:

Bid: Lithobid, Pavabid
Dur: Theo-Dur
LA (long-acting): Inderal LA, Inderide LA
SA (sustained-action): Peritrate SA
SR (sustained-release): Pronestyl SR, Ritalin SR

*From *Mosby's GenRx.* (1999). St. Louis: Mosby.

be crushed, flush the tubing before and after the medication to prevent the drug from sticking to the inside of the tube. (See Box 5-4 for cautions about tablet crushing.)

5. Flush the feeding tube with 20 to 30 mL of tepid water before administering the medication; repeat the flushing after administering the medication to clear it from the tube. If administering more than one drug, give each separately with a 5- to 10-mL rinse between doses.
6. After administration, position the client upright; in addition, turn the client slightly to the left if the medication is for local effect in the stomach (e.g., antacids). Have the client remain in this position for a time.

Alternative Drug Delivery Systems

Innovative advances in scientific technology and computerization provide impetus for the development of increasingly sophisticated drug delivery systems, particularly in the treatment of diabetes mellitus and cancer. Examples of these technologies include implanted drug deposits and needle-syringe pump assemblies.

Implanted capsules of a progestin hormone, levonorgestrel (Norplant System), are being used for contraceptive efficacy. Implantation takes 15 minutes and is immediately effective. The contraceptive effects are said to last 5 years.

Small pumps weighing approximately one-half pound are now available as portable infusion systems for continuous drug treatment of certain clients with type I diabetes or cancer. The systems currently approved and in use usually consist of a battery, a programmable electronic "brain," an electric motor and pump, and a syringe, all of which are detachable as a unit from the small needle kept in place either in subcutaneous abdominal or thigh tissue (for diabetes), or by Silastic catheter inserted into an artery supplying the malignant tumor. These programmable pumps allow for various flow rates and have an on-off feature. They appear to be quite efficient for clients with varying clinical needs. Some systems are designed to be worn externally over clothing, stored in a pocket, or suspended from a belt or a neck chain (Figures 5-13 and 5-14). The Sof-set cannula procedure is illustrated in Figure 5-15.

Preventing and Reporting Errors

It may help to be aware of some of the pitfalls regarding medication administration. Box 5-5 recounts actual errors related to medication administration and calls attention to some common but careless nursing acts.

To prevent the medication administration errors described in Box 5-5, the recommended guidelines presented on pp. 86 to 88 should be followed. The nurse should refuse to allow a drug to be administered against good nursing

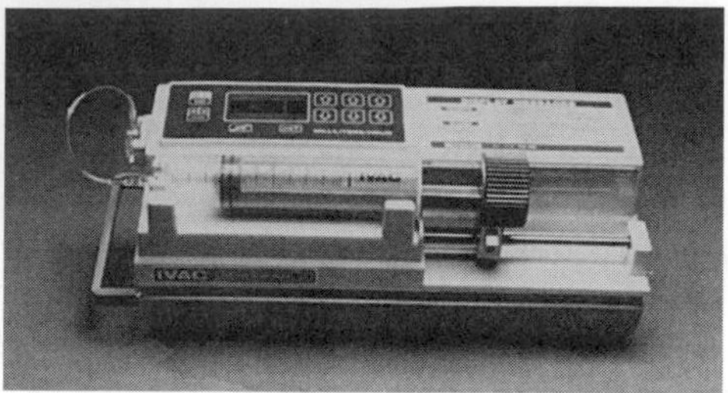

Figure 5-13 Microcomputer-controlled, larger-volume syringe pump for use when medication or fluids of up to 50 mL need to be administered with accuracy and at a constant rate.

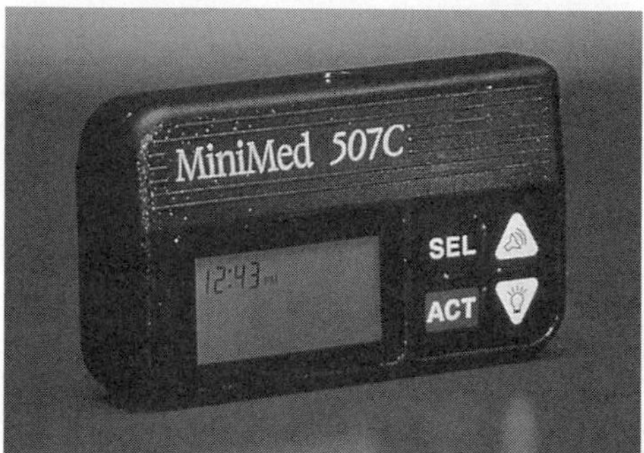

Figure 5-14 MiniMed Insulin Syringe. This pump (MiniMed 507C Insulin Pump) is one of the smallest and lightest available—it weighs only 3.5 ounces. The pump is easy to wear under clothing, carry in pockets, or attach to belts. Its features include a water-resistant package, a long battery life (monthly change of batteries), and an alarm system to warn the user of an occlusion, an empty syringe, a runaway infusion, or a low or depleted battery. The unit can be programmed for 48 basal variation rates in 24 hours, thus providing flexibility for the user. A 24-hour hotline is available to answer any questions on diabetes and the pump battery. (Courtesy of MiniMed, Inc., Sylmar, CA.)

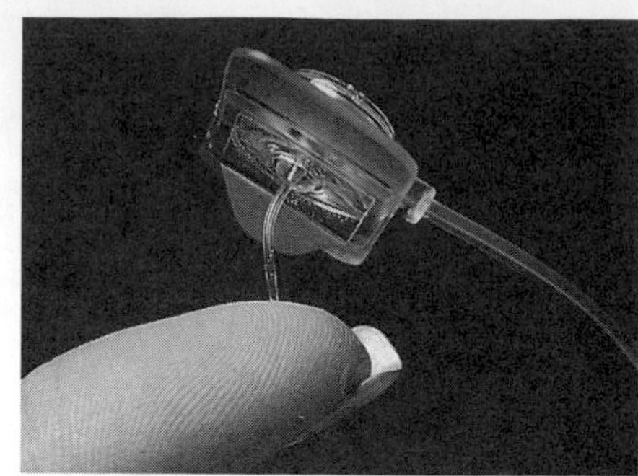

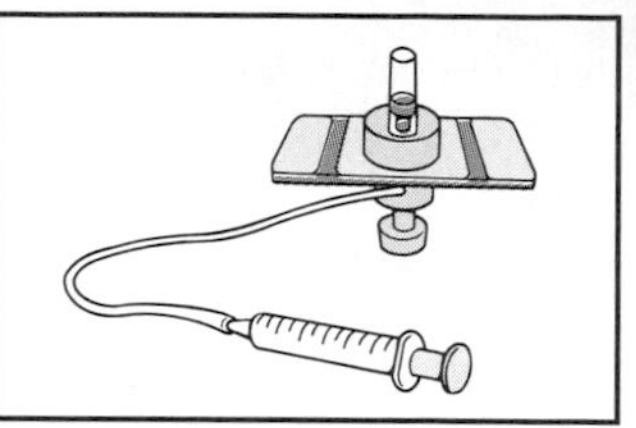

1. Fill syringe and Sof-set

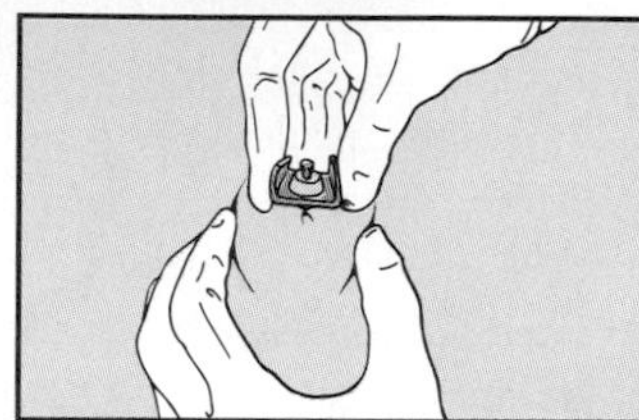

2. Cleanse and pinch skin

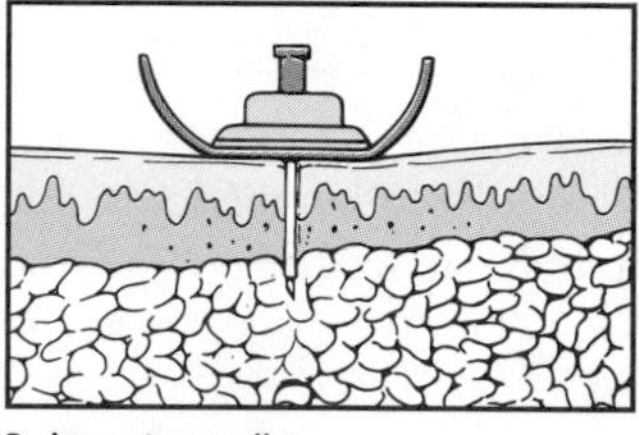

3. Insert needle

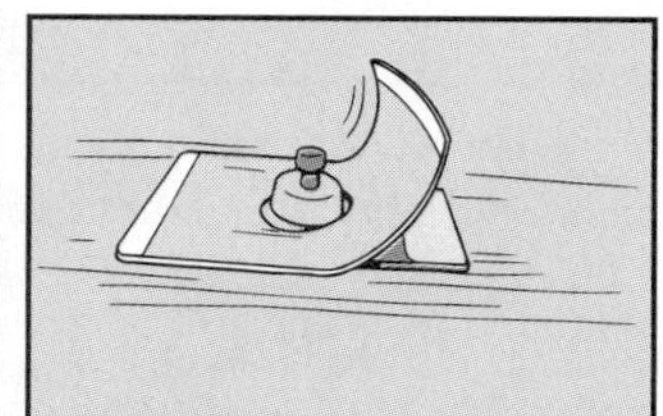

4. Place tape over Sof-set

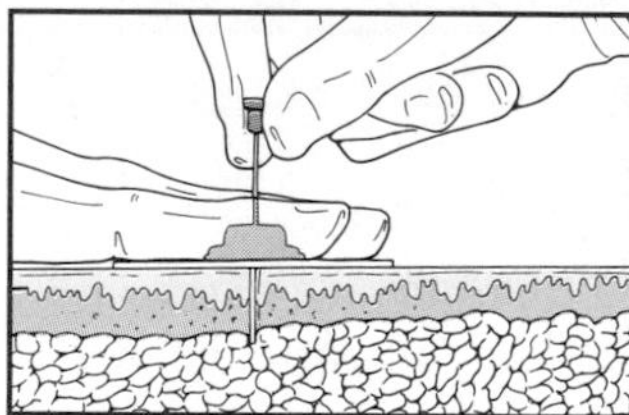

5. Remove introducer needle

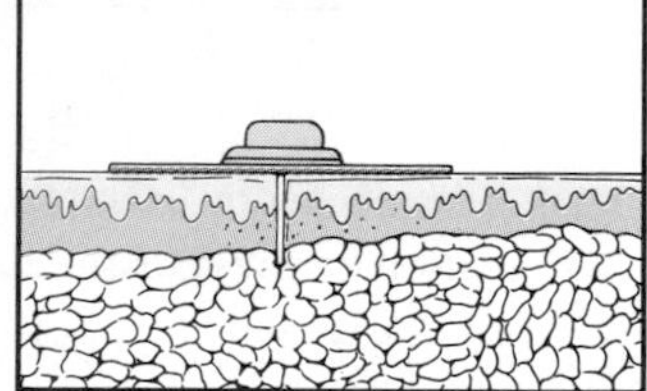

6. Begin pumping

Figure 5-15 The Sof-set infusion set consists of a soft Teflon cannula and tubing that is inserted by needle; the needle is then withdrawn so the pump can operate without one. This product has a special adhesive dressing that inhibits bacterial growth. (Courtesy of MiniMed, Inc., Sylmar, CA.)

judgment. Mistakes seem to breed other errors. It is axiomatic that when one thing goes wrong in a client's care, other mishaps generally follow. No one knows why. Stay alert! Question! Learn!

Medication errors are a significant problem in the delivery of health care (Box 5-6). In 1991, drug-related malpractice in the United States accounted for approximately 10% of all cases. Researchers predict that more than 770,000 hospital clients alone will experience an adverse drug event each year; of these, almost half are preventable (Fiesta, 1997). However, only about 1 in a 100 of these adverse events actually results in harm to the client (Bates, 1996). Most successful litigation against nurses concerns the administration of medications. There are many types of medication errors—omission, unauthorized dose, wrong dose, wrong route, wrong rate, wrong dosage form, wrong time, wrong preparation, and incorrect administration technique—with wrong dose heading the list. Many computer programs for updating dosage calculation skills now exist, and more are on the way. Innumerable helpful instructional materials, including programmed learning texts, are available; some are listed at the end of the chapter. All personnel who must calculate dosages should be alert for gaps in their mathematical competence. Double-checking calculations with others when uncertain and maintaining proficiency by practice are practical, professionally necessary actions (Cohen & Cohen, 1996; Bayne & Bindler, 1997).

To err is human. However, to admit the possibility of error and one's susceptibility is essential. To safeguard the client as well as one's reputation and psyche, the first step in a suspected medication error is to backtrack and double-check all actions or computations to see if an error occurred. Although Hackel, Butt, and Banister (1996) found that medication errors are underreported by nurses, it is essential for the client that errors be reported. The next step requires the most accountability—consulting the instructor or superior to inform him or her and to gain perspective and objective support. The client's prescriber should also be informed.

BOX 5-5

Errors Related to Medication Administration

1. *Not knowing why a medication is to be administered.* This type of error caused one nurse to irrigate a client's bladder with a topical astringent-antiinflammatory agent (Burow's solution) instead of with the genitourinary antibiotic irrigant distributed by a manufacturer of a similar name. In another instance, a nurse delayed giving a dose of medication essential to recuperation after cancer chemotherapy because she believed it to be "just a vitamin" instead of folinic acid.
2. *Not identifying clients by their wristbands.* This type of error caused several nurses to give medication to the wrong individual in the right beds. One of the nurses even asked a client his name, which turned out to be similar to another client's. One nurse called out her client's name, and the wrong person responded. The result was the same—all of them received the wrong medication.
3. *Not checking with the prescriber.* This type of error caused one nurse to give her client 30 mL of Milk of Magnesia every hour rather than every night because she misinterpreted the "qn" (an unacceptable abbreviation) order for "qh." Another nurse gave 2.5 mg of digoxin instead of 0.25 mg; the order was wrong, but the nurse did not recognize that it was excessive. As a result, the client received a toxic dose of medication.
4. *Storing vials with a similar appearance in the same area.* Because of this type of error, the nurse gave a neuromuscular blocker instead of the flu vaccine. The nurse admitted to not reading the label (Cohen, 1996).
5. *Poor handwriting.* Because of this type of error, a nurse administered Ritalin (methylphenidate) sent by the pharmacy instead of ritodrine (Yutopar). Neither the pharmacist nor the nurse questioned why the client would be receiving a CNS stimulant during her sixth month of pregnancy (Cohen, 1997b)
6. *Not investigating a questionable dose.* A client's daughter questioned an insulin dose of 60 U, but the nurse did not investigate. The dose was actually 6 U, and the client died (Cohen, 1997a).
7. *Knowledge and performance deficits.* Three Colorado nurses were indicted on charges of negligent homicide in a drug error that resulted in the death of a neonate. Knowledge deficits (not being familiar with the drug) and performance deficits (fatigue, use of a complex technique, and being interrupted while preparing medications) were considered to be the cause of the error (Smetzer, 1998).

BOX 5-6

Medication Errors in the United States

A recent study at the University of California determined that the numbers of Americans who have died from medication errors has sharply increased between 1983 and 1993. An analysis of all U.S. death certificates coded as medication errors in the database of the Department of Health and Human Services National Center for Health Statistics determined that inpatient deaths increased 2.4-fold and outpatient deaths increased 8.5-fold in that time period. These increases were not related to an increased number of prescriptions, which grew only 1.4-fold for the same time period. The authors suggest that the increased deaths may be the result of recent changes in U.S. health care—with more medications being taken by clients in their homes rather than being given by health care professionals in a controlled setting—or the result of a declining continuity and quality of relationships between provider and client.

To assist in determining the issues involved in medication errors, the National Coordination Council for Medication Reporting & Prevention (NCC MERP), a council of 17 organizations, has developed a new taxonomy that provides a uniform framework for consistent reporting and analysis to aggregate data from many health care organizations. This taxonomy has eight major categories of medication error information: client information, the error event, the client outcome, product information, the personnel involved, the type of error, causes of the error, and any contributing factors. Potential causes of medication errors are included in the taxonomy, such as confusion over brand or generic drug names, confusion over manufacturers' labels or cartons, and unclear package inserts. Human factors in the process include lack of knowledge, miscalculation of the dosage, computer glitches, drug preparation errors, and transcription errors. NCC MERP also takes note of stress, fatigue or lack of sleep, and confrontational or intimidating behaviors as other human factors in medication errors. Other factors that could contribute include lighting, noise level, interruptions and distractions, staffing, training, policies, and client counseling.

Over time the NCC MERP analysis will contribute much data that will be useful in decreasing the disturbing rate of medication errors. In the meantime, the significance of the medication error issue emphasizes the need for nurses to continue to be knowledgeable about the drugs they administer; skillful in administration techniques, client teaching, and counseling; and careful in monitoring client care and evaluating their own practice.

- What situations have you observed in your clinical practice that might contribute to medication errors?
- What steps would you take to minimize error in those situations?

Actions to correct the effects of the drug and to normalize the client's condition follow. The client and family should then be informed. If intentional concealment occurs, punitive damages may be awarded; intentional acts are not covered by malpractice insurance (Fiesta, 1998). Precise, objective documentation of the event and the circumstances is made both on the chart and on a special form called an incident report. This report is an intraagency communication that is analyzed by the agency's risk management personnel to develop procedures for preventing the same or similar incidents.

Monitoring

Although evaluation is considered to be the final step of the nursing process, this text presents a cluster of nursing actions to be included in monitoring the client for therapeutic effect and the occurrence of adverse drug reactions. These actions fall within the implementation activities of the nursing process related to drug therapy The nurse constantly monitors the client to assess the progress toward the outcome criteria for the pharmacologic therapies and to assess the client's response to the pharmacologic interventions. Such monitoring is important, because approximately 30% of hospitalized clients experience an adverse drug reaction, and as many as 1.5 million persons are hospitalized because of an adverse drug reaction.

Adverse reactions might be related to an underlying condition of the client (medical condition, age, childbearing status), other drugs that the client might be taking, and side effects/adverse reactions of the drug itself. O'Donnell (1992) divides these reactions into two broad categories. The first of these, type A, has predictability; if the properties of the drug are known, the nurse has a fair idea of the type of reaction that may occur. Most of these reactions relate to the mechanism of action of the drug and are often dose dependent. Examples of type A reactions are the orthostatic hypotension with volume depletion that can occur with furosemide (Lasix), a powerful diuretic, or the overgrowth of nonsusceptible organisms that can occur with ampicillin, an antibiotic. Type B reactions are not as predictable as type A reactions. Anaphylaxis is a classic example of a type B reaction; it is unusual, unexpected, life-threatening, and occurs even when a normal therapeutic dose is administered.

Early recognition of adverse drug reactions is important so that therapy can be altered as quickly as possible to prevent or minimize injury to the client; therapy is altered by decreasing the dosage or discontinuing the drug, administering an antidote or symptomatic treatment, or both. In addition, the nurse documenting the reaction in the clinical records should alert other caregivers. The client is advised to alert future caregivers and to carry a medical information wallet card or wear a MedicAlert bracelet warning others that he or she has had an adverse reaction to a specific drug.

The nurse should be alert for adverse drug reactions if the client evidences clinical or laboratory findings that are not typical of the client's disease, if a pathologic sign or symptom occurs at a site that is not involved with the condition being treated, or if a pathologic process occurs that is not in keeping with the condition being treated. If the client exhibits any of these signs or symptoms, the nurse should review the medication record to see if they are related to one or more of the client's drugs. Issues to be considered in determining causality are: (1) *temporal relationship* (Did the reaction occur at a reasonable time after the drug was administered?); (2) the presence of a positive *dechallenge* (Did the client's reaction diminish or resolve after the drug was discontinued?); (3) the presence of a positive *rechallenge* (Did the client's reaction return when the drug was administered again?); and (4) *lack of a confounding effect* (Can the reaction be explained by a concurrently administered drug or the client's clinical condition?).

Therapeutic drug monitoring requires that the nurse understand the mechanism of action of the drug in relation to the client's health status in order to clinically determine whether the drug is effective. Clinical indicators should be monitored at appropriate intervals to assess drug efficacy. For example, in an acute asthmatic episode the nurse monitors vital signs, breath sounds, skin color, sputum, and signs of respiratory dysfunction such as irritability, stridor, nasal flaring, and retractions. A beta$_2$-agonist drug administered as a bronchodilator is evaluated as effective if respiratory and pulse rate decrease toward a more normal rate and if the client experiences less wheezing and irritability, is relaxed, and expends less effort with the respiratory process. Other signs of respiratory dysfunction also diminish within minutes. In another example, hemoglobin concentration should increase by approximately 0.1 g/dL daily within 2 weeks of starting oral iron therapy for iron deficiency anemia in a client who is not actively bleeding.

Therapeutic drug monitoring may entail determining blood drug levels to determine effective drug dosages and to prevent adverse reactions related to toxicity. This is particularly important with drugs such as cardiotonics, anticonvulsants, and others, in which the margin of safety within the therapeutic range is narrow. Blood samples may be obtained at the drug's peak level (the highest concentration) and/or at the trough/residual level (the lowest concentration) after a steady state of the drug has been reached in the client. Steady state is generally reached after four to five half-lives of a drug. Peak levels are useful when testing for toxicity, and trough levels are useful to demonstrate the maintenance of a satisfactory therapeutic level. Different laboratories use different units for reporting test results and normal ranges.

Some drugs have organ-specific or system-specific adverse or toxic effects, or potential complications, to which the nurse should be particularly alert. For example, clients receiving drugs that have the potential complication of hepatotoxicity need to be monitored for symptoms of hepatic dysfunction such as anorexia, indigestion, malaise, jaundice, petechiae, ecchymoses, dark urine, clay-colored stools, and increased bleeding tendencies. There is little evidence that drug-induced liver damage can be diagnosed routinely by performing frequent liver function studies before symptoms develop (American Medical Association, 1995). Liver function tests (serum bilirubin, alkaline phosphatase [ALP], alanine aminotransferase [ALT or SGPT], lactate dehydrogenase [LDH]) or a prothrombin time test may be ordered as part of a baseline assessment before the drug regimen is started or if clinical symptoms of hepatic dysfunction appear.

On the other hand, the development of drug-induced nephrotoxicity is usually subtle, and kidney damage may occur before symptoms such as insufficient urine output (>30 mL/hr), elevated blood pressure, and dependent edema become evident. When a nephrotoxic drug is given in higher doses or for prolonged periods, routine urinalyses and serum creatinine determinations are helpful in the early detection of toxicity. (See Chapter 36 [Boxes 36-1 and 36-2] for formulas for estimating renal impairment from serum creatinine.)

Many drugs cause blood dyscrasias, a pathologic condition in which any of the constituents of the blood are abnormal in structure, function, or quality. This condition may be caused by a hemolytic effect, in which there is premature destruction of the red blood cells. It may also be caused by bone marrow depression that results in the decreased manufacture and maturation of red blood cells, most white blood cells, and platelets. Some drugs inhibit platelet aggregation, putting the client at risk for bleeding. In addition to monitoring the client's hematology laboratory reports for these abnormalities, the nurse must have astute assessment skills. Anemia is evidenced by lower than normal levels of hemoglobin, hematocrit, and red blood cells, as well as by a change in the size and hemoglobin content of the red blood cells; it may also be noted by fatigue, exertional dyspnea, dizziness, headache, insomnia, pallor, confusion, and cardiac changes in the later stages. Leukopenia, an abnormal decrease in white blood cells to fewer than $5000/cm^3$, is evidenced by fatigue, pallor, weight loss, easy bruising, fever, bone or joint pain, and repeated infections. Thrombocytopenia, a reduction in the number of platelets, may be evidenced as bleeding from small capillaries, such as easy bruising, bleeding gums, nosebleeds, hematuria, melena, or rectal bleeding.

Some drugs, particularly the antihypertensives and central nervous system (CNS) depressants, also cause hypotension. This may be evidenced as an abnormally low blood pressure when a client assumes a standing posture. Having the client come to an upright position in slow stages may prevent this effect. Lying, sitting, and standing blood pressures help in monitoring the client's vasomotor status.

Some drugs affect electrolyte balances, particularly potassium, which results in either hypokalemia or hyperkalemia. This may occur because the drug contains potassium or because it affects the excretion of potassium, either enhancing its loss from the body or causing it to be retained or spared. The nurse needs to monitor both the serum electrolytes and the clinical symptoms of the appropriate electrolyte imbalance.

There are many adverse neurologic effects of drugs. Some drugs cause CNS depression, which results in dizziness, drowsiness, hypotension, and confusion and progresses to respiratory depression, coma, and death. Other drugs cause CNS stimulation, resulting in nausea, nervousness, tremor, tachycardia, extra systoles, increased blood pressure, diuresis, and visual disturbances. In addition to the drugs known as anticholinergics, many other drugs have anticholinergic effects. This means the client should be monitored for dry mouth, constipation, urinary retention, confusion, and delirium. Adverse neurologic effects may also be peripheral; drugs with this effect are said to be neurotoxic. The early signs of such neurotoxicity are paresthesia (tingling, a "pins and needles" feeling, numbness), motor weakness, limb pain, and decreased deep tendon reflexes. Ototoxicity is the result of a drug's harmful effect on the eighth cranial nerve or on the organs of hearing and balance. The loss of hearing may be reversible or irreversible, and ataxia may also occur.

The nurse needs to remain vigilant in the ongoing monitoring of the client's health status by direct observation and by evaluation of laboratory and diagnostic tests in relation to drug therapy.

Client Teaching

Updating clients, keeping them informed about their treatment, and providing other necessary information should be an ongoing activity that occurs naturally during any interaction with clients. In any nursing process, teaching should be a part of the plan. The plan may be formal (e.g., a diabetic teaching program), or it may be a simple impromptu discussion based on a question raised by the client.

A strong rationale for teaching clients comes from the many state nurse practice acts that define teaching as a necessary part of nursing, thereby giving it the power of a state mandate: one could be sued for not teaching clients. Although teaching-learning interactions between the client and nurse are among the most necessary and professionally demanding, teaching clients is not as visible as bathing them, measuring their vital signs, or giving them injections. Consequently, teaching may not be seen as important enough to be noted in nursing progress notes. Accreditation agencies, such as the Joint Commission on Accreditation of Health Care Organizations (JCAHO), recognize the importance of client teaching and look for such documentation during their inspection visits to evaluate agencies that provide health care.

Successful client learning has a direct bearing on successful convalescence at home. Clients need to learn the following about their medications: the names of the medications (should be written down), what they are for, how to recognize the proper effects (in very specific ways), some of the major secondary effects (those that are expected and tolerable, and those that represent toxicity), which symptoms require prescriber notification, ways to prevent or minimize side effects/adverse reactions, what to do if they miss a dose, how to store the medication, how to take it (e.g., with meals), and whom to call if there is a problem. Clients can be expected to forget many of the instructions; a printed fact sheet or checklist to take home will be helpful to many clients and should augment the verbal explanation. (See Chapter 10 for further discussion of this essential role of nursing.)

Recording Drug Administration

Recording the administration of each dose of medication as soon as possible after it is given provides a documented record if there is any question as to whether the client received the dose. If the administration is not documented, the client may inadvertently receive a second dose from another nurse or nursing student. The busy nurse who "double-pours" (prepares two doses at one time—a "sloppy" practice) may also be tempted to record the second dose at the same time the first dose is recorded. Medications should not be recorded (charted) before they are actually given because something may occur to prevent that dose from being administered; as a result, the client would go unmedicated. The medication record, which is a legal document, would need to be corrected carefully and an incident report filed.

Several different forms are used to record the medications for each client. These forms usually include areas to note each medication's name, date, dose, route, and time of administration, as well as the initials of the administering nurse (see Figure 5-1). Extra notations may be added in certain instances. For example, when digoxin is given, the apical and radial pulses taken just before administration are noted (e.g., "AP, 78; RP, 76"). If the pulses are found to be outside the normal limits established by that agency, the medication should not be given, the record should be marked "held" and initialed, and the prescriber should be consulted. Clients also have the right to refuse treatment, including medications; despite teaching and counseling, they sometimes do. "Refused" is then noted in the appropriate spot on the medication record, with the reason for the client's refusal. A medication may also be recorded as "discarded" or "wasted" if only part of it was administered and the rest had to be discarded (as in a prefilled syringe), or if the medication was dropped or contaminated. If the medication is a controlled substance, its reason for disposal must be documented and fully witnessed; the signatures of two nurses are required on the narcotic record.

Routine (or continuous) daily medications are recorded on the MAR. Once-only, loading doses, prn medications, and stat medications should be recorded on the same MAR. Administration of a controlled substance is recorded both on the MAR and on that particular drug's control sheet in the "narcotic book," which includes a running tally of the balance of the controlled substance. A notation is made in the progress notes of the client's chart relating to the assessment of the need for any prn medication and the evaluation of the client's response to the prn medication at an appropriate time interval.

The potential for error in drug administration is almost limitless. Some significant mistakes can be rectified if discovered and acted on quickly. Courts tend to look more kindly on the nurse if an error is properly reported and the appropriate actions are taken. Courts generally recognize that nurses are human and that there is the potential for error in clinical practice.

EVALUATION

Evaluation, the final step in the nursing process, facilitates the delivery of high-quality nursing care in regard to pharmacotherapeutics. While planning nursing care and establishing goals, the nurse determines what type of evaluation will occur and when and how it will be performed. Clear and specifically stated goals or outcome criteria make it easy to determine whether the intended outcomes have been achieved or to what degree they have been achieved. Evaluation includes both subjective and objective data. When evaluating nursing care for a client undergoing drug therapy, the nurse looks at the nursing outcomes and other outcome criteria for the specific nursing diagnoses/collaborative problems. In general, an evaluation of drug therapy includes the following areas:

1. Therapeutic response to the drug
2. Nontherapeutic responses to the drug, such as side effects, or adverse reactions related to the administered drug itself, the client's health status, or concurrent drug therapy
3. Level of client's knowledge related to the medication regimen
4. Client's ability to manage the therapeutic regimen (self-medication)

In evaluating a therapeutic response, the nurse must have a clear understanding of the therapeutic goals. Evaluation may center on a reduction of symptoms, decreased frequency of recurrences, enhanced organ function, elimination of infection, or a multitude of other goals. Clinical observation of the client and monitoring of the appropriate laboratory studies is essential. Evaluation examines a drug's therapeutic response but is also directed toward detecting any response that may be attributed to the drug. The outcome criteria to be evaluated may also relate to the absence of any side effects or adverse reactions. An awareness of the pharmacology of the drug used and any potential effects guides this evaluation. For example, outcome criteria related to the therapeutic response for the anticonvulsant phenytoin (Dilantin) are that the client will demonstrate the following: (1) an absence of or decrease in the frequency or severity of seizures, (2) maintenance of therapeutic serum levels of the drug, and (3) an absence of side effects/adverse reactions such as ataxia, slurred speech, mental confusion, drowsiness, nystagmus, diplopia, or gingival hyperplasia.

The nurse will need to determine if educational goals are being met. Often, clients can report back what they have been told yet remain unable to apply this knowledge. Asking hypothetical questions and observing return demonstrations are helpful techniques for evaluating learning. Examples of outcome criteria for client teaching are that the client will do the following:

- State the correct name of the medication
- Identify the medication by its color and shape
- Describe the therapeutic purpose of the medication
- Describe the common side effects and how to minimize them
- Identify at least three adverse reactions to the drug for which consultation should be immediately sought with the prescriber or other health care professional
- List other drugs that have the potential to interact with the medication
- Demonstrate the proper administration of the medication
- Demonstrate any monitoring techniques associated with the drug, for example, pulse and blood pressure measurements and daily weights

In addition, the nurse needs to evaluate whether the client can effectively manage the therapeutic medication regimen in the home environment. Effective management of the therapeutic regimen refers to following the prescribed regimen correctly. This means that, in addition to the outcome criteria for educational goals, the client will do the following:

- State an intent to practice the self-medication behaviors needed to recover from the illness and prevent a recurrence or complications
- Report less anxiety related to fear of the unknown, fear of loss of control, or misconceptions about his or her medications
- Describe the disease process, causes and factors contributing to symptoms, and the medication regimen for disease and symptom control
- Describe strategies to address complications of the medication regimen should they arise
- Discuss situations that can challenge continued successful management of the medication regimen

Research indicates that at least one fourth of all outpatients fail to follow their prescribed drug therapy correctly. The inability to accomplish any of the previously mentioned outcome criteria indicates ineffective management of the therapeutic regimen. Other behaviors might also be indicators:

- Does the client or family/caregiver continue to speak of nonparticipation in the regimen?
- Have partially used or unused prescriptions been observed?
- Is there persistence or progression of the underlying condition even though the regimen prescribed is an appropriate one?
- Have undesired effects of the drug gone unreported to the health care provider?

In addition to the evaluation by the individual nurse or nursing team of the client's progress toward the goals and expected outcomes of nursing care, health care agencies evaluate the process of medication administration as an important aspect of nursing care provided by that agency. Standards by which to evaluate care are developed from within the health care organization and may also be suggested by external organizations. JCAHO is an organization that offers voluntary accreditation to health care agencies throughout the United States on the basis of standards that are "recognized as representing a contemporary national consensus on quality patient care that reflects changing health care practices and current health care delivery trends" (Joint Commission on Accreditation of Health Care Organizations, 1990). Within the JCAHO standards for nursing services regarding policies and procedures, guidelines are set forth concerning medication administration; this is done in an effort to ensure safe nursing practice. These guidelines stipulate that the nursing department or service of a health care organization have policies and procedures to govern medication administration and that these "should specify, in accordance with applicable law and regulation and pertinent medical staff rules and regulations, who may give orders for drugs; who may accept verbal orders for drugs and when the orders must be authenticated by the prescribing practitioner; who may verify orders for drugs and how this must occur; who may supervise the administration of medications; and who may administer these medications, which medications they may administer, and how these individuals are to be supervised, if necessary" (JCAHO, 1986). These policies and procedures serve to protect both the client and the nurse by stating the roles and responsibilities of all members of the health care team for the administration of medications. Nursing practice can then be evaluated to determine whether the care provided to clients was in keeping with the policies and procedures of the agency.

The following are suggested indicators for evaluating the administration of medications as part of the nursing quality monitoring process, which may also be known as Total Quality Management (TQM) or Continuous Quality Improvement (CQI):

1. The drug is administered in the ordered dose.
2. The drug is administered by the ordered route.
3. The drug is administered by the ordered site.
4. The drug is administered at the ordered rate.
5. The drug is administered in the ordered drug form.
6. The drug is administered by the ordered schedule.
7. The drug is administered using the correct technique.

These indicators may be incorporated into a process of monitoring and evaluation by which nursing professionals examine the care they provide, determine possibilities for improvement of their practice, and take necessary action.

SUMMARY

The implementation phase of the nursing process with regard to drug therapy begins when the nurse acts to attain the goals established as described in Chapter 4. Nursing interventions are directed at the actual administration of drugs, which includes the preparatory steps as well as the subsequent recording of drug administration.

The traditional Five Rights—to ensure the right client, the right medication, the right route, the right dose, and the right time—continue to be reliable criteria for competent, safe, and individualized medication administration. The right documentation is also essential. For nurses who are eager to provide high-quality care and have penetrating questions, some of the theoretical bases for the selection of drug doses and dosing intervals have been included in this chapter. Also presented are typical types of dosage calculations that sometimes challenge nurses—even those who have been practicing for a long time. The answers to and the explanations of these calculations are included. Common drug routes and sites have been detailed and illustrated.

The evaluation of nursing functions in medication administration includes, but is not limited to, a critique of one's own techniques. The environment should be made conducive to high-quality care by the nurse's efforts toward thoughtful and safe medication administration. Enough time must be set aside, and double-checking calculations should be routine. Careful identification of clients is essential to ensure that the right person receives the medication as intended. Because nurses are in the position of being on the client care scene and of taking care of clients as no one else does, they are uniquely placed to detect even subtle secondary drug effects, interactions, or incompatibilities.

Preventing errors in medication administration is crucially important to nurses because it is an area fraught with much potential for irreversible harm to clients. Alert attention to all the details of medication administration, including client comments, must be maintained so that safety is not compromised and clients obtain the most beneficial effects of their drug therapy. Recording a drug dose is the final act of communication; it signifies that the drug was given and ensures accountability by the nurse who "signs for it."

In short, the actual act of administering medications—the implementation or intervention phase of the nursing process—demands a solid knowledge base, well-practiced skills, commitment to continuous learning, and intense, unremitting concentration to sustain the best interests of the client. The potential for error is rife; medication administration cannot be a casual act or the risk will escalate.

Evaluation of therapeutic effects and secondary effects, effective management of the prescribed regimen, and client learning follows the implementation phase of the nursing process. This step allows the nurse to determine if nursing outcomes and other outcome criteria were met and measures the effectiveness of nursing care.

Critical Thinking Questions

1. As a student, what restrictions are placed on your role in the administration of medications? How will you respond to a prescriber who gives you a verbal order for a medication at the client's bedside?
2. You are preparing a client medication with which you are not familiar. You search through the drug references on the unit, but information about the drug cannot be found. What actions should be taken?
3. A hospitalized client expresses curiosity after observing that his medications are administered "in little packages" rather than the "childproof" containers that he is used to receiving from his pharmacy. How would you compare the advantages and disadvantages of the medication delivery systems for your client?
4. If one of the adverse effects of the drug you were administering were bone marrow depression, what laboratory results would you monitor to evaluate your client's drug therapy?

Collaborative Learning Activities

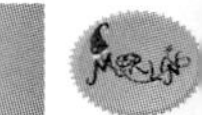

For Collaborative Learning Activities, go to mosby.com/MERLIN/McKenry/.

CASE STUDY

For a Case Study that will help ensure mastery of this chapter content, go to mosby.com/MERLIN/McKenry/.

BIBLIOGRAPHY

American Medical Association. (1995). *Drug evaluations: Annual 1995*. Chicago: Author.

Anderson, K.N., Anderson, L.E., & Glanze, W.D. (Eds.) (1998). *Mosby's medical, nursing, & allied health dictionary*. (5th ed.). St. Louis: Mosby.

Bates, D.W. (1996). Medication errors. How common are they and what can be done to prevent them? *Drug Safety, 15*(5), 303-310.

Bayne, T. & Bindler, R. (1997). Effectiveness of medication calculation enhancement methods with nurses. *Journal of Nursing Staff Development, 13*(6), 293-301, 324.

Carpenito, L.J. (2000). *Nursing diagnosis: Application to clinical practice*. (8th ed.). Philadelphia: J.B. Lippincott.

Cohen, M.R. (1993). What you said about the apothecary system. *Nursing, 23*(7), 56-58.

Cohen, M.R. (1996). Medication errors. *Nursing, 26*(2), 16.

Cohen, M.R. (1997a). Medication errors. *Nursing, 27*(4), 18.

Cohen, M.R. (1997b). Medication errors. *Nursing, 27*(9), 22.

Cohen, M.R. & Cohen, H.G. (1996). Medication errors: Following a game plan for continued improvement. *Nursing, 26*(11), 34-37.

Covington, T.R. (1996). *Handbook of nonprescription drugs*. Washington, D.C.: American Pharmaceutical Association.

Fiesta, J. (1997). Law for the nurse manager. Legal update-1996. Part 2. *Nurse Manager, 28*(6), 16-19.

Fiesta, J. (1998). Legal aspects of medication administration. *Nursing Management, 29*(1), 22-23.

Hackel, R., Butt, L., & Banister, G. (1996). How nurses perceive medication errors. *Nursing Management, 27*(1), 31, 33-34.

Hardman, J.G. & Limbird, L.E. (1996). *Goodman & Gilman's The pharmacological basis of therapeutics*. (8th ed.). New York: McGraw-Hill.

Hicks, W. (1995). Taking the right approach to a drug error. *Nursing, 25*(3), 72.

Joint Commission on Accreditation of Healthcare Organizations. (1990). *Committed to quality: An introduction to the joint accreditation of healthcare organizations*. Oakbrook Terrace, IL: Author.

Joint Commission on Accreditation of Healthcare Organizations (1986). *A guide to JCAHO nursing services standards.* Chicago: Author.

Lilley, L.L. & Guanci, R. (1994). Getting back to basics. *American Journal of Nursing, 94*(9), 15-16.

Loeb, S. (Ed.). (1993). *Giving drugs by advanced techniques.* Springhouse, PA: Springhouse.

McConnell, E.A. (1998). Clinical do's and dont's. Giving medication through an enteric feeding tube. *Nursing, 28*(3), 66.

McFarland, G.K. & McFarland, E.A. (1997). *Nursing diagnosis & intervention: Planning for patient care.* (3rd ed.). St. Louis: Mosby.

Medication errors: Help new nurses avoid making errors. (1993). *Nursing, 23*(3), 66.

Meister, F.L. (1998). Ask the experts. *Critical Care Nurse, 18*(4), 97.

Mosby's GenRx. (1999). St. Louis: Mosby.

National Bureau of Standards, U.S. Department of Commerce. (1977). *The international system of units (SI).* Special Pub No 330.

O'Donnell, J. (1992). Understanding adverse drug reactions. *Nursing, 22*(12), 48.

Potter, P.A. & Perry, A.G. (1997). *Fundamentals of nursing: Concepts, process and practice.* (4th ed.). St. Louis: Mosby.

Quality review: A publication of the USP practitioners' reporting network. (1999). (http://www.usp.org/pubs/review/rev___040c.htm)

Smetzer, J.L. (1998). Lesson from Colorado: Beyond blaming individuals. *Nursing Management, 29*(6), 49-51.

United States Pharmacopeia Dispensing Information (USP DI): Drug information for the health care professional (19th ed.). (1999). Rockville, MD: United States Pharmacopeial Convention.

6 Cultural and Psychologic Aspects of Drug Therapy

Chapter Focus

Health beliefs and treatment outcome are strongly influenced by a client's cultural background, ethnic practices, psychologic beliefs, and traditions. Effective caring for clients from different cultural groups requires an understanding of the predominant ethnic-specific influences and an assessment of the individual client to determine how those cultural influences affect health needs. Because nearly 2000 cultures and subcultures exist, it is impossible for the nurse to have a working knowledge of all of them. Instead, nurses and other health care professionals should study the predominant cultural groups in their communities. This chapter focuses on certain health beliefs and practices related to pharmacology.

Learning Objectives

1. Discuss the influence of culture and psychologic beliefs on drug therapy.
2. Discuss on a symbolic level what drugs mean to clients.
3. Identify situations in which placebos are appropriately used.
4. Differentiate between the advantages and disadvantages of self-treatment using herbal and non-prescription medications.

Key Terms

cultural background, p. 111
health beliefs, p. 111
placebo, p. 120

The **cultural background** of a client is a set of learned values, beliefs, customs, and behaviors of the client; cultural background influences health beliefs and various practices that relate to pharmacology. **Health beliefs** are perceptions of susceptibility to a disease or condition, the consequences of contracting the disease or condition, the benefits of care and barriers to preventive behavior, and the internal or external stimuli that result in appropriate health behaviors. The health beliefs of an individual influence the management of and response to drug therapy. Some similarities exist across cultures in the way the use of drugs is perceived; a primary goal of the appropriate use of medications is to achieve optimal health. Although most individuals share common views regarding life patterns, significant differences occur in values, beliefs, and attitudes. Clients bring to health settings cultural and psychologic differences in perceptions of masculine and feminine roles, in rural and urban backgrounds, in ethnic groups, and in social classes that influence drug use. The literature from transcultural nursing and anthropology (see the Bibliography at the end of this chapter) provides valuable insights into various health care beliefs and practices.

In addition, there is a fundamental difference between the health beliefs of health care providers and the health beliefs of clients. Although each person enters the health professions with culture-bound definitions of health and illness, these ideas change as the person is socialized into the "health care provider culture." This creates a schism between the provider and the recipient of health care. Comprehensive and appropriate health care be provided only if health care providers become more sensitive to the traditional health beliefs and practices of clients (Spector, 1991).

Increased cultural awareness takes on even greater importance when the demographic changes occurring in North America are considered. According to the 1990 U.S. census, whites comprised 80.3% of the population. The ethnic/racial minorities constituted 16.8% of the population in 1980 and 19.7% in 1990. The distribution of those minorities by percentage are as follows: black, 12%; Spanish origin, 8.9%; Asian and Pacific Islander, 2.9%; American Indian, Eskimo, and Aleut, 0.8%; other races, 4%. The numbers of the adult and older adult populations have increased the most, with the 25-to-44 age-group growing from 63 million in 1980 to 80.8 million in 1990. The 65-and-over population has increased from 26.3 million to 31.2 million persons, or from 11.4% to 12.6% of the total population. The median age of the total population increased from 30.0 years in 1980 to 32.9 years in 1990. According to the 1986 census in Canada, the total population was 23,941,000, with 11% being age 65 or over. The dominant ethnic groups at that time were the British (34%) and the French (24%), with 5% of the population being a British-French mixture. Sixteen percent of the population in Canada was Asian, 3% was black, and 6% was aboriginal Canadians (Communication Division of Statistics, 1992). Canadians are living longer and having fewer children. As the twenty-first century begins, significant changes are occurring in the population of the United States and Canada. The white majority is shrinking and aging, and the black, Hispanic, Asian, and Native American populations are young and growing.

Because of these demographic changes, the nurse's practice will be increasingly concerned with the care of older and ethnic populations. To meet this challenge, the nurse needs to better understand the different health and illness perspectives of these groups. This chapter examines the cultural and psychologic aspects of drug therapy; the special needs of older adults are addressed in greater detail in Chapter 8. Administering medications effectively and teaching clients self-administration requires an understanding of the predominant cultural influences within the community, a knowledge base of the psychologic aspects, and an assessment of the individual client to determine how these factors influence health needs.

CULTURAL INFLUENCES ON HEALTH CARE

Published anthropologic and transcultural studies have offered nurses extensive information on assessing the effect of cultural influences on their clients. Creative cultural measures for improved therapeutics and comfort are available in numerous books and research articles (Andrews & Boyle, 1995; Baker, 1997; Geissler, 1994; Leininger, 1991; Pachter, 1994; Seto, Mokuau, & Tsark, 1998; Spector, 1991). The nurse needs to remember that each cultural group has different cultural attitudes toward health, health care, and illness; in addition, within each of these groups exist widely varying health and illness beliefs and practices.

Dr. M. Leininger (1978), a nurse-educator credited as the major voice of the transcultural impetus in nursing, has suggested asking questions such as the following to assess a client's cultural influences: "Could you tell me about yourself and your family?" "How do you keep well?" "What made you become ill?" The client is also likely to respond more readily to therapy if the nurse treats this information with respect and incorporates some of its important aspects into the nursing care plan. Feelings and beliefs will be more openly discussed if the nurse has gained the confidence of the client and family. Box 6-1 provides a comprehensive guide to the assessment of cultural manifestations.

If an illness is mild, the person self-treats the symptoms or, as is often the case, does nothing; gradually the symptoms disappear. If the illness is more severe or is of longer duration, the assistance of a healer of one type or another, usually a physician, is sought. Many cultural groups avoid standard Western medicine until herbal or home remedies are totally ineffective or the illness becomes acute. Such groups may also use both traditional and Western remedies concurrently to validate each other or to enhance the therapy. Haitian, Hispanic, Cuban, Vietnamese, Samoan, Jamaican, Chinese, Native American, and other clients generally follow this practice. Nurses should be aware of any reluctance to seek standard medical care. Such individuals

BOX 6-1

Guide for the Assessment of Cultural Manifestations

I. Brief history of the origins of the cultural group, including location
II. Value orientations
  A. World view
  B. Code of ethics
  C. Norms and standards of behavior (authority, responsibility, dependability, competition)
  D. Attitudes toward the following:
    1. Time
    2. Work vs. play/leisure
    3. Money
    4. Education
    5. Physical standards of beauty, strength
    6. Change
III. Interpersonal relationships
  A. Family
    1. Courtship and marriage patterns
    2. Kinship patterns
    3. Childrearing patterns
    4. Family function
      a. Organization
      b. Roles and activities (sex roles, division of labor)
      c. Special traditions, customs, ceremonies
      d. Authority and decision making
    5. Relationship to community
  B. Demeanor
    1. Respect and courtesy
    2. Politeness, kindness
    3. Caring nature
    4. Assertiveness vs. submissiveness
    5. Independence vs. dependence
  C. Roles and relationships
    1. Number and types
    2. Functions
IV. Communication
  A. Language patterns
    1. Verbal
    2. Nonverbal
    3. Use of time
    4. Use of space
    5. Special usage: titles and epithets, forms of courtesy in speech, formality of greetings, degree of volubility vs. reticence, proper subjects of conversation, impolite speech
  B. Arts and music
  C. Literature
V. Religion and magic
  A. Type (modern vs. traditional)
  B. Tenets and practices
  C. Rituals and taboos (e.g., fertility, birth, death)
VI. Social systems
  A. Economics
    1. Occupational status and esteem
    2. Measures of success
    3. Value and use of material goods
  B. Politics
    1. Type of system
    2. Degree of influence in daily lives of populace
    3. Level of individual/group participation
  C. Education
    1. Structure
    2. Subjects
    3. Policies
VII. Diet and food habits
  A. Values (symbolism) and beliefs about foods
  B. Rituals and practices
VIII. Health and illness belief systems
  A. Values, attitudes, and beliefs
  B. Use of health facilities (popular vs. folk vs. professional sectors)
  C. Effects of illness on the family
  D. Health/illness behaviors and decision making
  E. Relationships with health practitioners
  F. Biologic variations

From Andrews, M.M. & Boyle, J.S. (1995). *Transcultural concepts in nursing care* (2nd ed.). Philadelphia: J.B. Lippincott.

should be counseled on appropriate ways in which to seek health care when the need arises.

African Americans

Although a number of blacks have emigrated voluntarily from Africa and the various islands of the West Indies during this century, the majority of African Americans are descendants of the Africans brought to America as slaves. Brought to this continent against their will, those of African heritage endured overwhelming hardships and inhumane treatment during slavery but in most circumstances maintained a family and community awareness (Gutman, 1976). After the Civil War, those in the South were overtly segregated and lived in conditions of hardship and poverty; the people who migrated to the North were subjected to the poverty, racism, and covert segregation of urban life (Bullough & Bullough, 1982). The nurse who wants to integrate traditional health and illness beliefs with modern practice needs to appreciate the historic problems of the African-American community (Spector, 1991).

Traditional beliefs about health and illness stem from the African origins of African descendants. Life was considered a process rather than a state and could be influenced by other forces. When healthy, one was in harmony with nature; illness was a state of disharmony. In traditional African belief there was no separation of mind, body, and spirit (Jacques, 1976). Disharmony or illness was the result of the activity of demons and evil spirits; the goal of prevention was to ward off these spirits, and the goal of therapy was to remove them from the body of the ill person. Several traditional practices were used to meet these goals. Voodoo, a belief system evolved from ancient West African practices, reached its height in Louisiana in the mid-1800s. Although there is little evidence that voodoo is practiced today, many people continue to fear voodoo and believe in it to some extent. In this belief system many illnesses were the result of a "hex" placed on a person. Gris-gris, usually oils or powders, were used as symbols of voodoo to prevent illness or to cause illness in others. Gris-gris are available today and can be purchased in many American cities, particularly cities with significant Haitian populations, such as Miami.

Many individuals of African descent believe in the power of healers. These healers may rely on the strong religious faith of the people and use prayer and the laying on of hands, or they may be more traditional healers and use herbs and roots in the treatment of illness. (See Table 6-1 for additional cultural values and culture care meanings and action modes for the African-American culture.) Advertisements for both types of practitioners are commonly found in African-American community newspapers.

Some individuals of African descent are practicing Muslims and maintain a highly structured lifestyle based on religious beliefs. Muslims believe in self-help and the need for self-discipline, and they highly value life and good health. This belief system fosters the effective management of a therapeutic regimen. Dietary restrictions are similar to a kosher diet—abstinence from pork or pork products, as well as from beans (e.g., black-eyed, kidney, and lima beans), which are considered to be for animal consumption (Spector, 1991). Alcohol ingestion is not permitted because it is believed to cause illness. Because pork consumption is prohibited, a Muslim who has diabetes should not be administered pork insulin. As with other religions, Islam has various sects that differ in the strictness of their practices.

The practices for health promotion and the treatment of illness in the African-American community are varied and abundant. Proper diet, rest, and a clean environment are believed to be important for health maintenance. Herb teas and laxatives may be used to keep the body working well. Amulets or bracelets may be worn to protect the wearer from harm; during nursing care precautions should be taken so these items are not removed. In addition to prayer and the laying on of hands, "rooting" may be used as folk medicine. In "rooting" the healer or "root man" determines the cause of the illness and then prescribes a therapeutic regimen of substances and practices. Because "rooting" is a practice derived from voodoo, it is essential to obtain a healer who is stronger than the originator of the "hex" or the cause of illness; the more prestigious the healer, the stronger the medicine. There are also a variety of home remedies, which are passed from one generation to the next. Remedies for colds and congestion include the following: hot lemon water with honey; hot toddies of tea, honey, lemon, and an alcoholic beverage; the ingestion of Vicks Vaporub mixed with sugar; and a body rub with white high-proof rum. The health practices of each client should be determined so the prescribed therapeutic regimen can be individualized to meet that client's needs.

For a number of reasons folk medicine continues to be used even when African Americans live close to local health services. According to Spector (1991), African Americans may perceive their interaction with the health care system as a degrading and humiliating experience. Although a health care provider may not intend to be patronizing or demeaning, the client may feel insulted. Those who use clinics may have long waits and lose time at work, and those who are indigent cannot afford health insurance or the high cost of health care. Although these issues could apply to any health care recipient, "the inherent racism within the health system cannot be denied" (Spector, 1991).

Hispanic Americans

Hispanic Americans have their origins in Cuba, Mexico, Puerto Rico, any Central or South American country, or Spain. Mexican Americans constitute the largest group of Hispanic Americans, and their number is rapidly rising because of high birth rates and immigration.

Some Mexican Americans consider health to be the consequence of good luck, whereas others see it as being the result of good behavior. One is expected to maintain health by acting, eating, and working appropriately. Prayer, the wearing of amulets, and herbs and spices are used to prevent illness. Poor health is perceived as a change of luck, an imbalance in the body, or the result of some misdeed (Table 6-1).

According to Spector (1991), the causes of illness can be grouped into five major categories: imbalance in the body, dislocation of parts of the body, magic causes outside the body, strong emotional states, and "envidia" (envy). Imbalance in the body relates to the four aspects of the body: blood, which is hot and wet; yellow bile, which is hot and dry; phlegm, which is cold and wet; and black bile, which is cold and dry. According to the "imbalance" theory, equilibrium can be regained if cold remedies or foods are taken for "hot" illnesses and vice versa. However, perceptions of what foods or medications are hot or cold may vary from client to client because these terms do not refer to temperature but are qualities assigned to particular substances. It is best to consult with the client for specifics once it is determined that the imbalance theory is part of the client's health belief system.

"Empacho" is an example of a dislocation of a part of the body being a cause of illness. Symptoms of abdominal discomfort, pain and cramping, are thought to be caused by a ball of food clinging to the wall of the stomach and are treated by massaging the spine while prayers are spoken. Although this practice is helpful in many cases, as with many folk practices it may delay the client from seeking

TABLE 6-1 Cultural Values and Culture Care Meanings and Action Modes for Selected Groups

Cultural Values	Culture Care Meanings and Action Modes
Anglo-American Culture (Mainly Middle and Upper Classes in the United States)	
1. Individualism—focusing on a self-reliant person	1. Alleviation of stress
2. Independence and freedom	Physical means
3. Competition and achievement	Emotional means
4. Materialism (things and money)	2. Personalized acts
5. Technology dependence	Doing special things
6. Instant time and actions	Giving individual attention
7. Youth and beauty	3. Self-reliance (individualism)
8. Equal sex rights	Reliance on self
9. Leisure time (highly valued)	Reliance on self (self-care)
10. Reliance on scientific facts and numbers	Becoming as independent as possible
11. Less respect for authority and older adults	Reliance on technology
12. Generosity in time of crisis	4. Health instruction
	Teach us how "to do" this care for self
	Give us the "medical" facts
Mexican-American Culture*	
1. Extended family	1. Succorance (direct family aid)
2. Interdependence with kin and social activities	2. Involvement with extended family ("other care")
3. Patriarchal (machismo)	3. Filial love/loving
4. Less value of exact time	4. Respect for authority
5. High respect for authority and older adults	5. Mother as care decision maker
6. Religion (many Roman Catholics)	6. Protective (external) male care
7. Native foods for well-being	7. Acceptance of God's will
8. Traditional folk-care healers for folk illnesses	8. Use of folk-care practices
9. Belief in hot-cold theory	9. Healing with foods
	10. Touching
Haitian-American Culture†	
1. Extended family as support system	1. Involve family for support (other care)
2. Religion—God's will must prevail	2. Respect
3. Reliance on folk foods and treatments	3. Trust

Modified from Leininger, M.M. (1991). *Culture care diversity and universality: A theory of nursing.* New York: National League for Nursing Press.
*These findings were from Leininger's transcultural nurse studies (1970, 1984) and other transcultural nurse studies in the United States during the past two decades.
†These data were from Haitians living in the United States during the past decade (1981-1991).

medical attention for serious illnesses. "Mal ojo" (evil eye), an example of an illness caused by magic, has symptoms of malaise, lethargy, and headaches and is thought to be the result of being excessively admired by another. The remedy is to locate the admirer to provide care for the affected individual. "Susto" is a state of depression caused by a strong emotional state of fright. This illness involves the loss of soul, which leaves the body and wanders freely. A "curandero," or folk healer, is required to coax the soul back into the body. "Envidia," or envy, as a cause of illness is part of a more universally held belief in peasant cultures of "limited good"—material wealth or achievement comes at the expense of the rest of the community because there is only a certain amount of "good" available. Misfortune, or ill health, is therefore the result of the envy and resentment of neighbors.

The services of a curandero may be sought and religious rituals may be practiced (e.g., lighting candles, praying, and visiting shrines). Curanderismo is a relatively well-documented form of holistic folk medicine (Kiev, 1968; Saunders, 1958). Kay (1977) reported that a third of her interviewees used the services of a curandero, as well as local health services. Curanderos prescribe specific herbs to take in teas, which are usually determined by the content of the affected individual's dreams. Therapies by the curandero include support for the religious practices, massage, and "cleansings" such as the passing of an unbroken egg or small bundles of herbs over the body of the

TABLE 6-1 Cultural Values and Culture Care Meanings and Action Modes for Selected Groups—cont'd

Cultural Values	Culture Care Meanings and Action Modes
Haitian-American Culture†—cont'd	
4. Belief in hot-cold theory 5. Male decision maker and direct caregivers 6. Reliance on native language	4. Succorance 5. Touching (body closeness) 6. Reassurance 7. Spiritual healing 8. Use of folk food, care rituals 9. Avoidance of evil eye and witches 10. Speaking the language
African-American Culture‡	
1. Extended family networks 2. Religion (many are Baptists) 3. Interdependence with "blacks" 4. Daily survival 5. Technology (e.g., radio, car) 6. Folk (soul) foods 7. Folk healing modes 8. Music and physical activities	1. Concern for my "brothers and sisters" 2. Being involved with church as center of community 3. Giving presence (physical) 4. Family support and "get togethers" 5. Touching appropriately 6. Reliance on folk home remedies 7. Reliance on "Jesus to save us" with prayers and songs
North-American Indian Culture§	
1. Harmony between land, people, and environment 2. Reciprocity with "Mother Earth" 3. Spiritual inspiration (spirit guidance) 4. Folk healers (shamans) (the circle and four directions) 5. Practice of culture rituals and taboos 6. Rhythmicity of life with nature 7. Authority of tribal elders 8. Pride in cultural heritage and "nations" 9. Respect and value for children	1. Establishing harmony between people and environment with reciprocity 2. Actively listening 3. Using periods of silence ("Great Spirit" guidance) 4. Rhythmic timing (nature, land and people) in harmony 5. Respect for native folk healer, carers, and curers (use of circle) 6. Maintaining reciprocity (replenish what is taken from Mother Earth) 7. Preserving cultural rituals and taboos 8. Respecting elders and children

‡These findings were from Leininger's study of two southern U.S. villages (1980-1981) and from a study of one large northern urban city (1982-1991) along with other studies by transcultural nurses.
§These findings were collected by Leininger and other contributors in the United States and Canada during the past three decades. Cultural variations among all nations exist, and so these data are some general commonalities about values, care meanings, and actions.

client. Curanderos are well respected within the Mexican-American community and usually maintain a personal relationship with the client. Mexican Americans may expect to have such a relationship with their health care providers, which may not be met within the established health care system (Spector, 1991) and may account for the continued popularity of curanderismo as a health care modality.

Language and poverty continue to be barriers for many Hispanic Americans in receiving appropriate health care. Despite the fact that Spanish-speaking individuals are one of the largest minority groups, there still are inadequate numbers of Spanish-speaking health care providers. This discrepancy will be remedied when more Hispanic Americans are recruited into the health field and when more health care providers learn to speak Spanish (Spector, 1991).

Asian Americans

Although the Asian American community includes people whose origins are in Japan, Korea, Hawaii, Vietnam, and the Philippines, this discussion will focus on Chinese Americans, who constitute the majority of Asian Americans.

Medicine has been a recorded science in China since the Emperor Huang-ti's writings, *Huang-ti Nei Ching* (The Yellow Emperor's Classic of Internal Medicine), in 1628. Within these writings the universe is seen as an indivisible entity in which man must adapt to the order of nature. This universe has two basic components, yin and yang, which are in opposition as well as in unison. Yang is the male force, a positive energy that creates light, warmth, and fullness. Yin is female, a negative energy representing darkness, cold, and emptiness. Illness is caused by an imbalance of yin and yang. If yin is too strong, one is nervous, apprehensive, and catches colds easily. Yang must be nurtured because it protects the body against outside forces. The inside of the body is yin, and the outside is yang. The five solid organs, which collect and store secretions—the liver, heart, spleen, lungs, and kidneys—are yin. The six hollow organs, which excrete—the gallbladder, stomach, large intestine, small intestine, bladder, and lymph nodes—are yang. The organs have a complex interrelationship that maintains the balance and harmony of the body (Chang, 1991).

Traditionally, illness was prevented by wearing amulets to ward off evil spirits, or jade charms, which were believed to bring health. The individual is expected to practice moderation, balancing the yin and yang aspects of the body and taking foods and herbs as supplements to maintain that balance (Louie, 1990). The healer in Chinese medicine is the physician, who in ancient times was responsible for not only curing disease but also preventing it. In fact, physicians were paid only when the client was healthy. In the event of illness, physicians were not paid and had to provide the necessary medicines. The traditional Chinese physician uses inspection, particularly of the tongue, from which more than 100 conditions can be determined, and palpation of many different pulse types, in which there are 15 ways of characterizing (Spector, 1991).

The three primary methods of traditional Chinese healing are acupuncture, moxibustion, and herbal remedies, the purpose of which is to restore the balance of yin and yang. Acupuncture, a practice that has been mainstreamed into allopathic medicine, is a method of producing analgesia or altering the function of a body system by inserting fine, wire-thin needles into the skin at specific sites on the body along a series of lines called meridians. Precise puncture points along the meridians are identified in terms of yin and yang, as well as for specific symptoms and diseases. Whereas acupuncture is perceived as a cold treatment, moxibustion is based on the therapeutic value of heat and is used for an excess of yin. In moxibustion, pulverized wormwood is heated and placed on the skin over specific meridian points (Spector, 1991).

The purpose of herbal remedies prepared according to specific prescriptions by Chinese herbalists is to restore the balance of yin and yang. In China these folk remedies usually consist of a single dose of a liquid preparation; therefore taking tablets or capsules on a regular schedule could be confusing to the older Chinese client. This may be why this group prefers teas and topical remedies.

For Chinese Americans, barriers to health care relate to language difficulties and poverty, as with other minorities; barriers may also include their beliefs regarding medical practices. Although immunization and the use of x-ray studies are accepted, intrusive practices such as blood drawing and surgical procedures are seen as contrary to having respect for an intact body (Spector, 1991).

Hospital food is seen as alien and increases the client's sense of social isolation. Even the common practice of leaving ice water at the client's bedside for the administration of medications is questionable because many Chinese and Chinese Americans believe that cold drinks are unhealthy for the sick; they may therefore avoid this fluid intake. This preference, as well as any food preferences, should be discussed with the individual; if medically acceptable, hot tea or other substitutes should be provided. If appropriate, the family should be encouraged to supply the client with his or her preferred foods.

Native Americans

Culturally, the Native Americans' belief system of being in harmony with nature or of maintaining a balance between the body, the mind, and the environment is crucial to health maintenance (Williams & Ellison, 1996). Illness is perceived as being out of balance because of ill spirits, not following traditional beliefs, or a disruption in nature (see Table 6-1). Because Native Americans do not ascribe to the germ theory, the cause of the illness must be traced back to an action or lack of action on the part of the client, which may not be known to the individual (Wauneka, 1990). Recovery therefore is based on diagnosing the problem and reestablishing the harmony or balance with nature. These are just some of the beliefs held by Native Americans; each tribe (there are well over 200) has specific ideas and practices related to health and illness.

The medicine man is the traditional healer of Native Americans and is considered to be wise in the ways of nature and able to seek out the spiritual causes of illness. For diagnosis, the medicine man may use meditation (or, in the case of the Navaho, sandpainting, in which the shape of the painting determines the illness and its treatment); stargazing, in which the color emanating from the star determines the cause and prognosis of the illness; and listening, in which the divination is heard rather than seen (Wyman, 1966).

Treatments used by medicine men include massage, the application of heat, sweatbaths, total immersion in water as an act of purification, and the use of herbal remedies. Because of the belief in harmony with nature, herbs are specifically prescribed and carefully prepared, and meticulous attention is given to the timing and the procedures used for gathering them (Spector, 1991). Again, the personal bond between the healer and client is strong, which is why folk medicine continues to be popular.

The difference between what the health care provider and the Native American client believe to be the cause of the illness can constitute a barrier to health care for Native Americans (Mercer, 1996; Sanchez, Plawecki, & Plawecki, 1996). In addition, differences in communication styles may lead to misunderstanding. The questioning involved in taking a health or drug history may be seen as intrusive as well as a demonstration of incompetence because Native Americans believe the diagnosis should be made through observation of nonverbal communication. In most Western cultures maintaining direct eye contact during communication is seen as demonstrating interest in the client; however, this practice may be considered inappropriate by many Native Americans. Because Native Americans have maintained their rich history through an oral tradition, note taking is not viewed favorably; the nurse should rely on memory rather than on notes when in the client's presence.

■ ■ ■

In addition to the various cultural groups briefly discussed, there are white ethnic communities to be served by the health care delivery system. To describe the health beliefs and practices of all the various cultures is beyond the scope of this text. The student is advised to seek additional information from the current journals and references cited in the Bibliography of this chapter. The nurse should gain knowledge of the various cultural groups within the local area of clinical practice. Local hospitals and other health care settings often hold conferences and maintain reference sources of relevant cultural material for the local communities.

Dietary concerns are also strongly intertwined with cultural beliefs. Many ethnic groups (Italian, Mexican, Cuban, and others) believe that their own foods hasten the recovery process. Therefore one major way in which many private and some public hospitals have recognized the cultural differences in health care is in offering ethnic meals as alternatives to the standard fare. Discussing food preferences and preferred methods of preparation with clients is often very important for their well-being.

In addition, the nurse should be aware of possible cultural influences on the medicating behaviors of clients. Such information may be used to guide the nurse to ask the right questions during the initial history, to be aware of possible reasons for ineffective management of a therapeutic drug regimen, and to help identify specific areas needing additional client teaching.

The client is always the ultimate source of information on the specific ways in which culture affects the client's participation in health care (Holroyd, Katie, Chun, & Ha, 1997; Wright, Cohen, & Caroselli, 1997). Nurses need to be sensitive to the client's life experiences and adapt their nursing care accordingly. The nurse should be aware of two dangerous misperceptions: (1) ethnocentrism, the belief that the health care provider's ethnic group is superior to other cultures or ethnic groups; and (2) client stereotyping, the assumption that all persons from a particular culture or ethnic group will have the same response to the same or a similar situation (Villarruel, 1995). These are mistaken beliefs. Ethnocentrism can interfere with the provision of health care to individuals from groups other than the provider, and client stereotyping may limit the provider's objectivity and ability to provide nursing care.

Within each cultural or ethnic group can be a wide range of different responses to the administration of medications and management of the therapeutic regimen. An understanding of the potential cultural or ethnic patterns of a client is helpful as a starting point in caring for the individual, as long as stereotypical conclusions are avoided (Salerno, 1995).

ETHNIC AND RACIAL DIFFERENCES IN DRUG RESPONSE

In addition to differences in health beliefs, values, and attitudes, pharmacologic research in the last 15 years has uncovered significant differences among racial and ethnic groups in their metabolism rates, clinical drug responses, and side effects to drugs. A new field, pharmacogenetics, has evolved to study the genetic influence on drug response that may occur from inherited metabolic defects or deficiencies. This emerging area of clinical investigation is leading to new, clinically relevant information about drug responses in ethnic and racial minorities (Levy, 1993). Nurses need to be aware of these differences to better monitor the drug therapy of clients from culturally diverse populations. These differences, where documented by research, will be discussed throughout the text.

Analgesics

Some individuals have an inadequate analgesic response to codeine because of a genetic alteration in debrisoquine-sparteine polymorphism, an enzyme responsible for metabolizing codeine to morphine. Approximately 5% to 10% of the population are poor metabolizers. When Chinese participants were compared with Caucasians in a study using codeine as the analgesic for pain, the Chinese participants were found to be less able to metabolize codeine and required increased dosage adjustments to achieve a therapeutic effect (Levy, 1993).

The debrisoquine-sparteine metabolic path is important for the metabolism of cardiac antidysrhythmics, antidepressants, beta-blocking agents, neuroleptics, and opioids. Therefore persons who are extensive metabolizers (metabolize at a high rate) may produce multiple chemical substances at the enzyme site that clinically may result in an increase in drug interactions. The drugs capable of producing this type of effect in extensive metabolizers include quinidine (Quinaglute), propafenone (Rythmol), flecainide (Tambocor) and metoprolol (Lopressor). Alternately, poor metabolizers may have a variety of drug responses such as prolonged drug effects or toxicity to thioridazine (Mellaril), isoniazid (INH), sulfapyridine, and codeine (Meyer, 1992).

Cardiovascular Medications

The debrisoquine-sparteine polymorphism is also an important pathway for a number of cardiac medications. It has been reported that individuals of African descent are less responsive to beta-blocking agents, especially propranolol (Inderal), nadolol (Corgard), and atenolol (Tenormin). Labetalol (Normodyne), a combination drug with alpha- and beta-blocking properties, is equally effective in Caucasians and individuals of African descent.

TABLE 6-2 Ethnic and Racial Differences in Response to Central Nervous System Agents

Comparison Groups	Drug Class Example	Clinical Response
Chinese/whites	Benzodiazepines (diazepam, alprazolam)	Chinese require lower doses; more sensitive to the sedative effects
Chinese/whites and Hispanics/Anglos	Antidepressants (imipramine, desipramine, amitriptyline, clomipramine)	Chinese and Hispanics require lower doses; side effects greater in Hispanics
Asians/whites	Neuroleptics (e.g., haloperidol)	Asians require lower doses
Asian Indians/whites	Analgesics (e.g., acetaminophen, codeine)	Asian Indians have greater clearance rates
Chinese/whites	Analgesics (e.g., morphine)	Chinese less sensitive to cardiovascular and respiratory effects but more sensitive to gastrointestinal side effects
Asians/whites	Alcohol	Asians more sensitive to side effects
Native Americans/ whites	Alcohol	Native Americans have faster metabolism and less tolerance

From Levy, R.A. (1993). *Ethnic and racial differences in response to medicines: Preserving individualized therapy in managed care pharmaceutical programs.* Reston, VA: National Pharmaceutical Council.

In general, individuals of African descent respond better to diuretics than to beta-blockers if only one agent is used. Even among the beta-blocking agents, responses vary widely between racial or ethnic groups. For example, Chinese persons are considerably more sensitive than Caucasians to the effects of the beta-blocker propranolol (Inderal) (Zhou, Adedoyin, & Wilkinson, 1990). It was reported that Chinese persons may be twice as responsive to the effects of propranolol on blood pressure and heart rate and also have a greater atropine-induced increase in heart rate than the Caucasian population in comparative studies (Levy, 1993).

Plasma renin levels may also be important in determining a person's response to the beta-blocking agents; Caucasians usually have higher levels than individuals of African descent, and this may contribute to the racial difference in drug response (Levy, 1993).

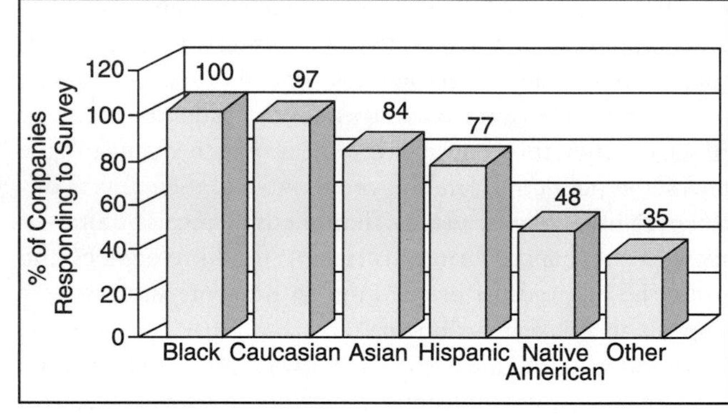

Figure 6-1 Percentage of companies (of those responding to the Pharmaceutical Manufacturers Association survey) that include different racial groups in their drug trials.

Central Nervous System Agents

A comparative study between Chinese and Caucasian subjects indicated that the Chinese participants required lower doses of benzodiazepines (diazepam [Valium], alprazolam [Xanax]), tricyclic antidepressants, atropine, and propranolol (Inderal) (Levy, 1993). When the doses were comparable to those of the Caucasians, an increase in side effects occurred in the Chinese subjects. Table 6-2 gives a summary of ethnic and racial differences in response to central nervous system (CNS) agents.

▪ ▪ ▪

As a result of pharmacologic research conducted over the last two decades, more consideration is being given to the need to individualize drug therapy for special population groups. When testing and evaluating new drugs, the vast majority of drug manufacturers now include ethnic and racial minorities within the clinical trial groups. A survey by the Pharmaceutical Manufacturers Association revealed that 79% of pharmaceutical companies collect data on race, and the majority (67%) are making extra efforts to include racial minorities in their clinical trials (Edwards, 1991). All of the companies (100%) responding to the survey include African Americans in their trials, and more than three quarters also include Asians (84%) or Hispanics (Figure 6-1). This effort is likely to reveal additional drug actions and side effects specific to minority groups and may also lead to the discovery of therapies that are of specific advantage to minorities (Levy, 1993).

PSYCHOLOGIC ASPECTS

In addition to its pharmacodynamic action, every drug administered to a client has a symbolic meaning and a potential psychologic effect. A drug not only alters the function or structure of some part of the body but also may influence the behavior, sense of well-being, and mental state of the client. The psychologic responses of clients to symbolism may mimic pharmacologic reactions, adverse effects, or even allergic reactions. A profound reaction may even be observed in clients receiving placebos.

Medications tend to be more effective when individuals believe in their capacity to get well, when they have a strong desire to get well, and when they believe that the health care personnel expect the medication to be effective and say so. Clients' past and present conditioning to drugs, illness, hospitals, nurses, and other health personnel, as well as their health goals, are determinant factors in the response to drugs. Nurses must remember that among the major deterrents to successful drug therapy are divergent goals of the client and the health care personnel. An accurate appraisal of the client's goal in seeking health advice and therapy is important to planning and implementing an effective plan of care.

Symbolic Meaning of Drugs to Clients

Medications may be a symbol of help to the client. This meaning is strengthened and drug effectiveness is enhanced when prescribers and nurses suggest to a client that a particular drug will be helpful or beneficial. Repeated suggestions to the client that the drug is beneficial further reinforce the therapeutic value. This effect is similar to the relief that a mother's kiss brings to her child's pain; the assurance given by the kiss makes the child feel better. Investigations of the effects of drugs on the mind has resulted in the conclusion that some drugs are effective only in the presence of an appropriate mental state.

Drugs may also be viewed as symbols of danger. Clients who are using their illness to meet a need for dependence may interpret a cure as a serious threat to their emotional security. Taking medication may also be objectionable if there is a strong need to exhibit an image of independence; adverse reactions may even result. The client may complain of dry mouth, nausea, vomiting, palpitation, fatigue, and other vague feelings of discomfort. The individual may resist taking the medication, refuse to have the prescription refilled, or even throw the drug away.

Many people have ambivalent feelings about taking medications. An expressed desire to regain health may coexist with an unconscious reluctance to give up the secondary gains of the sick role, which can include extra attention and freedom from responsibilities. To retain these benefits, individuals may report secondary drug effects or find reasons why they cannot take the medication.

Clients may harbor unsubstantiated notions about medications. Some may believe a medication is too strong or not needed any longer and therefore may refuse to take the drug, decrease its dose at any one time, or decrease the number of times it is taken. This behavior may be suspected when a drug known to be effective for a specific condition is ineffective in a particular client with that condition.

A client who believes the drug is too weak may take the drug too often, request the drug more often than prescribed, or continue drug therapy for longer than prescribed. However, medications such as analgesics may be inadequately prescribed or administered, thus resulting in this type of behavior. Therefore the drug therapy itself should be reviewed first to eliminate the possibility of undertreatment by the professional staff. Some clients who are self-medicating will increase the amount of drug taken, believing that "if one pill is good, two will be better," and overdose themselves. When the drug therapy as prescribed is determined to be appropriate, the reasons for this behavior should be sought and addressed.

Some fantasies concerning resistance evolve from fears. Individuals tend to fear radioactive drugs such as phosphorus-32 or iodine-131 and to fear dependence on drugs that have antidepressant, analgesic, or sedative effects. Although few people today believe in cure-all remedies, some have blind faith in a certain medication and prefer taking that drug rather than making an alteration in their lifestyle.

Clients who believe they are allergic to a certain drug, for real or imagined reasons, are likely to react with fear or panic when administration of that drug is contemplated. A detailed personal history and (when possible) tests for drug allergy should be used to corroborate or refute the client's belief. Rejecting a client's claim of an allergic response without evidence is an unwise assessment of data and is negligent to say the least.

The extent, duration, and intensity of the client's response to medication is influenced by several factors, including the following: the route of administration of a drug, the financial cost of treatment, and the client's conscious and unconscious attitudes toward illness, drugs, physicians, nurses, and other health care providers. Certain medications used in the usual dosages may not be effective when a client is angry, resentful, or hostile.

The illness itself may also affect a client's emotional response to a drug. When the illness is short, the recovery complete, and the medical and drug expense not too great, the client tends to have a positive reaction to drugs, hospitals, and health and nursing personnel. Strong negative reactions toward drugs or health personnel result when clients are falsely reassured of a quick and complete recovery, when drugs are ineffective and/or expensive, or when symptoms of allergy, side or toxic effects, or overdose occur. Preparing clients for the realistic limitations of drugs, for side and adverse effects, and for drug expense tends to create reasonable expectations.

With any chronic illness, a client may suddenly rebel against ill health and resist therapy with life-sustaining medications. When this occurs, clients may be testing to see if they are really dependent on the drugs, or they may be attempting a real or symbolic act of self-destruction. A stressful event or decision may be the root cause of this behavior.

Exploring the client's underlying fears and concerns is essential, and support, caring, and objective assistance in coping is necessary.

To avoid causing the client unnecessary concern or to deflect time-consuming questions, many health care providers are reluctant to present any negative aspects when teaching clients about drugs. A clear, nonthreatening explanation about the purpose of the medication and its effects (including the most common side effects reported) is only the most basic of explanations required by the client. Most clients prefer knowing the potential risks of drug therapy. This knowledge also tends to increase their participation and to engender trust. Litigation could ensue if clients suffer harm from unrecognized secondary effects of a drug because they were not informed. However, the nurse should be aware that some people do not want to know the details of their treatment and that some are very suggestible.

It is important to *listen intently to what the client says* about the medication, the feelings associated with it, and the condition for which it has been prescribed. With this information the health care provider can begin to see the situation from the client's point of view and develop an understanding of the client's motivation to seek health care. Does the individual see the treated condition as a physical threat? How much of a threat? How susceptible is the condition to treatment? How much control does the client want to exert over the condition? How probable is it that such control will reduce the threat adequately? Until these concerns and other personal factors are at least briefly explored, the success of treatment is uncertain.

Effects of Drugs on the Mind

Many common drugs have a secondary effect on the client's CNS and result in altered thought processes and sensory-perceptual alterations. Drugs may interfere with judgment, mood, sense of values, motor ability, and coordination. Certain antihistamines used to treat allergies may decrease alertness and cause drowsiness, depression, and predisposition to accidents. Antihypertensive agents may cause depression. Barbiturates and tranquilizers may induce inattentiveness and confusion and reduce initiative. Drug-induced depression calls for discontinuing or decreasing the dosage of the offending drug. Clients should be monitored for self-destructive tendencies—the pharmacologic literature has abundant examples of clients with drug-induced depression who have attempted suicide.

Placebo Therapy

In the past when a physician had no medicine to offer a client who expected treatment, a "sugar pill," or **placebo**, was given to placate the sick individual. A placebo is any treatment—a medication, a surgical or diagnostic procedure, or a nursing action—that elicits a client's response simply because of its intent rather than its known active properties. A placebo is most often a formulation of a pharmacodynamically inert substance such as lactose or sugar, distilled water, normal saline, or a very small dose of a substance such as a vitamin. In medicine, placebos are used in one of two ways. In experimental drug studies, placebos are used as a simulated medication given to a control group (e.g., before the approval of the drug by the Food and Drug Administration [FDA]). More rarely, placebos are used to satisfy a client's demand for a particular medication when, in the considered judgment of the prescriber, withholding a dose will impede psychologic or physical health.

The nurse should be aware that pain relief with administration of a placebo does not mean the client did not have real pain. Studies on effective clinical responses of pain to a placebo indicate that a physiologic response does indeed occur. Endogenous substances called endorphins are stimulated and released by the brain, which interact with the opioid receptors in the body to reduce pain; the effect produced is similar to the effect achieved by an opioid analgesic. Various other stimuli such as vigorous exercising and jogging may also increase the release of these chemicals in the brain. Such evidence indicates that a client's response to a placebo is therefore physical and not mental as previously believed.

The placebo response may result from objective physiologic and biochemical changes in the body as well as a change in the client's subjective complaints. This response can vary considerably from one client to another, but in published studies it is reported to be fairly consistent, with approximately 20% to 40% of clients experiencing a placebo response (Katzung, 1998).

"The use of a placebo for the treatment of pain to distinguish psychic and real pain is a deceptive practice that should be avoided" (Salerno & Willens, 1996). The guidelines of the American Pain Society (1992) discourage the use of placebos in the assessment of pain and state that "the deceptive use of placebos and the misinterpretation of the placebo response to discredit the client's pain report are unethical and should be avoided."

SELF-TREATMENT

Public interest in self-care management is at an all-time high and is exemplified by the numerous self-care books and clinics that now abound. One of the most effective and inexpensive ways to counteract rising health care costs may be through expanded, educated self-care management. Many people who visit a health care provider have already started a self-treatment plan. If these people were also helped to learn when to seek medical supervision and how to follow treatment advice wisely, they would have a still greater potential for regaining good health.

With their commitment to collaboration with the client to further health, nurses can educate clients; pharmacists, physicians, nurse practitioners, and many other health care professionals can also work to educate clients. Consumer information pamphlets abound; they are printed by the FDA and others—in large type for the visually impaired, or in various languages—and they offer valuable advice about drug interactions, health foods, and nonprescription pain relievers. Health information, some reliable, some unreliable, is available on the Internet. Clients should be encouraged to obtain Internet information only from government sources, recognized health organizations, and health science schools.

Development of the science of public health has led to the realization that the state of a nation's health does not depend exclusively on the interplay between professional medical practice on the one hand and bacteria, malignancy, and other causes of disease on the other. The influence of the individual's personal attempts at self-treatment or at lifestyle alterations on community health is often ignored or underestimated.

Drugs sold without prescription can induce sleep or wakefulness, relieve pain or tension, or supply the body with vitamins and minerals. Remedies can be purchased for symptoms affecting any part of the body. Sales of prescription and nonprescription (over-the-counter [OTC]) drugs have made the pharmaceutical industry a continually growing, multibillion dollar industry. Concern regarding the use of home remedies and self-medication is not new but continues to be a controversial subject (see Chapter 11).

Self-Treatment Using Herbal Remedies

Treating illness with a natural remedy, such as herbal products, is common in many cultures and dates back to the earliest records of humankind. The idea that a simple herbal or folk medicine can cure or prevent many health problems is believed and practiced in many societies today. Although some of the prominent medications used today originated from plant sources (e.g., digitalis from foxglove and vincristine or vinblastine from periwinkle), home brewing such plants can be extremely dangerous.

The use of herbals, or the back-to-nature movement, has largely evolved from the frequent warnings issued about food additives, preservatives, or products that are said to contain cancer-causing substances. This movement has spawned a multi-million dollar enterprise that no longer appeals only to specific cultural or ethnic groups but is widespread in the general population. This trend is demonstrated by the proliferation of health food stores, natural organic vegetables, and pharmacies and other outlets that sell organic vitamins, cosmetics, and other products. Although herbal remedies may be perceived as helpful, they are not regulated by the FDA. Therefore there are some concerns about the use of these products: adulteration of these products with harmful substances, the lack of determination of the active ingredients in each dose, and the lack of standardization of the medication from dose to dose. Chapter 12 examines self-medication with nontraditional remedies in greater detail.

Self-Treatment Using Nonprescription Drugs

Advantages. The individual has a right to practice self-medication. Throughout history the public has searched for medicines to relieve ailments and has tried almost every natural material known in the battle against pain, discomfort, and disease. That the public is health conscious is evident by the number of OTC and nonprescription drugs available. Many ailments are minor and temporary, and the client wants to eliminate discomfort as quickly as possible. Minor ailments do not always require the expertise of a prescriber, but because many nonprescription drugs can interact with prescription drugs, it is best to check with a prescriber or pharmacist. Minor complaints can be successfully treated by self-medication. Indeed, if individuals sought medical advice for every minor ailment (colds, headaches, minor wounds, temporary gastrointestinal upsets, or minor burns), health care providers would be unable to attend to individuals who need professional health care. However, self-medication can be harmful if misused or abused. Box 6-2 lists the general benefits and risks of OTC medications. The risks associated with the use of nonprescription drugs can be reduced by professionally implemented client teaching.

Disadvantages. Most preparations available before the twentieth century were either harmless vegetable concoctions or narcotic-laced nostrums. Modern chemistry and pharmacology produced literally thousands of preparations for self-medication. Some are quite effective for certain minor ailments, some are potentially dangerous, and some are worthless. Generally speaking, Americans are overmedicated. Americans have developed a casual attitude toward drug use and often believe every discomfort or disorder requires chemical treatment.

Today, OTC drugs can be bought in drugstores, supermarkets, restaurants, and vending machines. Widespread sales promotion via the media encourages self-medication. Because the hazards are generally insufficiently detailed in advertisements and commercials, persistent abuse of medications, and the resultant toxic effects, are fairly common. Many drugs tested and found to be harmless can actually cause serious secondary effects. Aspirin may upset the gastrointestinal tract or cause bleeding; one 325-mg tablet of aspirin impairs platelet aggregation to some extent for up to 1 week.

Serious, complex problems can develop from the overuse of vitamins and minerals (e.g., vitamin A or D overdose). Habitual use of mineral oil may prevent the absorption of fat-soluble vitamins or cause colon atony so that the treatment perpetuates constipation. Few established dosage limits exist for the use of OTCs by women who are pregnant or breastfeeding, and the effects on the fetus and neonate may be extremely harmful. Therefore *no drug of any sort should be taken by a pregnant or breastfeeding woman until a health care provider is consulted.* Many OTC drugs are intended only for adults, not for children; the dosage should not simply be altered for administration to children.

In addition, *a health care provider should be consulted before a client takes any drug that may have caused a previous allergic reaction.* Often a surprising lack of critical judgment is used when evaluating a newly marketed drug. Typically there is an initial overreaction, especially to a new OTC medication or to a well-marketed prescription drug—a "honeymoon phase" occurs in which the agent is introduced with fanfare and used and prescribed somewhat casually for a time. When long-term results become apparent and newly discovered secondary reactions are reported, the reputation of the drug suffers for a while, and its use may be overcautiously controlled. After another time period, use again builds to a more moderate level as the prescribers and the public recognize that judicious use under specified circumstances is the rational approach.

Habitual self-medication with nonprescription drugs may mask a serious condition, prevent diagnosis, endanger the individual's life, or create long-term, expensive medical problems. Health care providers have an obligation to understand how taking medication "fits" with clients' understandings, attitudes, and lifestyles. Box 6-2 outlines how to understand and explore the risk-to-benefit ratio when consumers are contemplating the use of nonprescription drugs. An additional factor for consideration is the influence that culture has on self-treatment behaviors.

Cultural Influences on Self-Treatment Behaviors

Although research on the use of medications in various ethnic-cultural groups is limited, an awareness of the meaning of specific terms or health care perceptions of an individual cultural group is crucial in the health care setting. Gaston-Johansson, Albert, Fagan, & Zimmerman (1990) studied the use of language or pain terms commonly used by Hispanic Americans, Native Americans, African Americans, and others and concluded that the word descriptors used (e.g., pain, ache, and hurt) were similar in clients with different cultural backgrounds.

DeSantis (1989) performed a descriptive survey of 30 Cuban and 30 Haitian immigrant mothers to study their health care orientations, that is, their different concerns about types of illnesses, the meanings attached to signs and symptoms, typical therapy management groups, and their use of the biomedical health care system. For a sick child, home remedies such as teas, herbs, warm oil rubs, and castor oil were generally tried first. A sick child with an illness believed to be caused by a supernatural power (spells or evil spirits) would be taken to a voodoo priest or priestess; the traditional physician would be consulted for the treatment of natural disease states (fever, bronchitis, impetigo). DeSantis reported that, unlike Cuban mothers, Haitian mothers did not mention OTC medications, nor did they identify by name any prescribed medications that were used for their children. This finding was similar to the results reported by Salerno et al. (1985).

Salerno et al. (1985) performed a descriptive survey study of the four predominant cultural groups in Miami (i.e., Hispanics, Haitians, African Americans, and Caucasians).

BOX 6-2

General Benefits and Risks of Over-the-Counter Medications

Benefits

The occasional use of certain simple preparations can be highly effective for specified minor, usually self-limiting conditions.

The cost is low in relation to prescription drugs, and the cost of a visit to the health care provider is eliminated.

The client regains some control over personal health care.

Directions and some possible secondary effects are listed on the label.

The condition is immediately treatable. OTC medications are as accessible as the nearest store supply, and a wait for a health care provider's appointment is eliminated.

Risks

Treatment depends on client judgment in distinguishing between a minor condition and a major, more complex one and in selecting the appropriate medication.

The signs and symptoms of a serious condition may be masked by the medication.

In the long run, costs may be higher if a serious condition progresses while being improperly treated.

Substances taken as OTC drugs are not always viewed as "drugs" with the potential for harm, and therefore dosing may be exceedingly casual.

In addition to the active ingredient, available combination preparations very often contain useless or harmful stimulants or depressants (caffeine or alcohol) and allergy-producing preservatives.

Professional advice to integrate the drug into an overall plan (e.g., to prevent interactions) is absent unless all drugs are obtained from one source that keeps a drug profile on clients.

The dosage may be too low to be effective, risking decisions by the client to overdose or delay needed professional treatment.

Many clients do not read labels; most label print is too small for easy reading, even with glasses, by those with failing eyesight.

Professional follow-up for other conditions may be avoided unknowingly.

Self-treatment with OTC drugs promotes the idea that there is a "magic bullet" for every ailment, major or minor, and that no discomfort should be tolerated.

OTC drug containers are especially vulnerable to criminal package tampering if they are kept accessible on shelves or are not in tamper-proof containers.

This study reviewed the factors that influenced the older adults in these groups when choosing and using OTC substances. An added feature was the development of a Self-Medicating Behavior Safety Scale (SMBSS), which included a numerical value for safety. The pharmacist investigator reviewed all questionnaires and extracted data to determine whether there was any difference between the cultures in regard to the potential for the misuse or abuse of OTC medications. The following data were extracted from this study:

1. Haitian older adults reported the highest number of health problems, but Caucasian subjects reported use of the greatest number of OTC products. The mean OTC product usage per group was Caucasian, 7.4; African American, 4.4; Haitian, 5.8; and Hispanic, 2.4. Despite this result, caution should be used in applying self-reported health information. The nurse should be aware of the "yea-saying" tendencies of minority groups when they are asked about their health or health care attitudes; their answer is often an effort to please a member of the dominant group and/or health care provider. This behavior is much more likely in minorities of Spanish heritage than in others. Lopez-Aquires et al. (1984) advise caution when using the traditional measure of self-reported health perceptions among Hispanics because their findings indicate that they significantly underestimate their objective health problems and conditions.
2. The ability to read and understand the label of a typical OTC cold medicine was tested on all individuals, and the findings here were particularly alarming. More than 50% of the subjects could not read or comprehend the package label. This high incidence has explicit implications for all health care personnel working with older adults. Many older clients may need help in choosing an appropriate OTC medication and specific instructions concerning the proper way to take the medication.
3. The influencing factors reported to affect the selection of OTC products were significantly different in the four groups. All groups relied highly on the suggestions of others, including professionals, but the Caucasians reported a high reliance on reading materials, television, radio, and self-knowledge in choosing OTC products.
4. The most common types of OTC medications used by all groups were gastrointestinal products (antacids, antidiarrheals, and laxatives) and analgesics (aspirin and acetaminophen). Caucasian subjects reported a high use of vitamins, whereas Haitians reported a high use of herbals and teas. The latter was not a major report from the other groups. This finding is not surprising, however, because Scott (1978) reported that many Haitians self-treat with herbs and home remedies before seeking orthodox health care.
5. Statistics concerning forgetfulness in taking medications were also significant among all four groups. Each group reported that memory was the most common system used to remember to take a medication.
6. The evaluation of the abuse and misuse of nonprescribed medications was largely dependent on the items listed in the SMBSS. This scale ranged from 1 to 15, with 15 [100%] being the highest and safest score possible. Although the researchers reported no differences among the four groups studied, the group mean was only 8.4. The lowest score for safety, 7.6 (51%), was reported by the Haitian group; 8.03 by Caucasians; 8.63 by Hispanics; and 10.9 (73%) by African Americans. The overall findings were in the low to low-average range of safety for all four groups.

   Approximately 56% of all subjects in the study used OTC medications inappropriately. The Caucasian group, at 81% inappropriate usage, was the highest. This was mainly demonstrated in the inappropriate use of vitamins and health food products, with doses exceeding the FDA's U.S. recommended daily allowances (RDAs) and, in some instances, approaching megadoses (Covington, 1996). Specific examples included the following:

   For example, one individual believed all OTC substances were "foods" and not only consumed large amounts of such products but also advised all her friends to do the same. Another interviewee reported taking vitamin K tablets to treat "blood spots" or "skin bruises." All four groups offered many unapproved indications as reasons for consuming nonprescribed substances. Examples included taking vitamin C "to help the eyes" or "whenever it rains"; Milk of Magnesia tablets "whenever dizzy"; Pepto Bismol for "hard stools"; Alka-Seltzer for "throat allergies"; Bufferin for "indigestion or greasy food"; and aspirin "to clean out the stomach" or "for heat in the stomach." Although some expressions were endemic to a specific culture, the basic need for guidance and valid professional advice was evident.
7. Other potentially dangerous situations noted included a number of drug-drug interactions, the use of an OTC sympathomimetic in hypertensive persons, and the use of alcohol by clients taking aspirin, nitrates, antihypertensives, and CNS depressants. Many participants were not aware of the possible interactions or the alternate methods available (spacing drugs apart with antacids) used when using such medications. Foreign drugs were being taken along with American medications. Duplicate consumption of the same medications under different names was identified in several instances. (See Chapter 11 for additional information on OTC medications.)

SUMMARY

Medications tend to be more effective when clients believe in their own capacity to get well and in the drug itself. A client's response to drug therapy is influenced by past and present experiences with drugs, illness, hospitals, nurses, and other health care personnel, as well as their own health beliefs and practices. Assessing all of these factors is most important in planning and implementing an effective care plan.

Health beliefs and treatment outcome are strongly influenced by a client's cultural background, ethnic practices, beliefs, and tradition. Providing effective care to clients from different cultural groups requires an understanding of the predominant ethnic-specific influences and an assessment of individual clients to determine how those cultural influences affect health needs. There are also significant differences among racial and ethnic populations in terms of drug metabolism rates, clinical drug responses, and side effects to drugs.

Because many clients avoid standard American medicine until either their home remedies or OTC self-treatments become totally ineffective or they become acutely ill, it is essential that the nurse be aware of alternative practices and be prepared to counsel and support clients on appropriate methods to use in seeking health care. Although self-treatment using nonprescription drugs has its advantages for the treatment of minor complaints, consumers need a greater awareness of the risks of such medications. Clients should be reminded that nonprescription drugs are not curative but offer only symptomatic relief and that a health care provider should be seen when treated conditions are persistent or recurrent or when unusual reactions occur.

Critical Thinking Questions

1. What personal experiences or client experiences with drug therapy can you think of that relate to the expectations of a drug's effect on symptoms?
2. What do you think are your health beliefs related to the use of medications?
3. Under what circumstances would it be appropriate to administer a placebo? What would you say to a client if you were about to administer a placebo and he or she asked what the medication was?
4. How would you respond to a client who is requesting information on the advisability of self-medicating with OTC preparations?

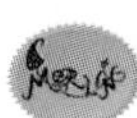

Collaborative Learning Activities

For Collaborative Learning Activities, go to mosby.com/MERLIN/McKenry/.

CASE STUDY

For a Case Study that will help ensure mastery of this chapter content, go to mosby.com/MERLIN/McKenry/.

BIBLIOGRAPHY

American Nurses Association. (1991). *Position statement on cultural diversity in nursing practice.* Kansas City, MO: Author.

American Pain Society. (1992). *Principles of analgesic use in the treatment of acute pain and cancer pain* (3rd ed.). Skokie, IL: Author.

Anderson, K.N., Anderson, L.E., & Glanze, W.D. (Eds.) (1998). *Mosby's medical, nursing, & allied health dictionary* (5th ed.). St Louis: Mosby.

Andrews, M.M. (1999). How to search for information on transcultural nursing and health subjects: Internet and CD-ROM resources. *Journal of Transcultural Nursing, 10*(1), 69-74.

Andrews, M.M. & Boyle, J.S. (1995). *Transcultural concepts in nursing care* (2nd ed.). Philadelphia: J.B. Lippincott.

Baker, C. (1997). Cultural relativism and cultural diversity: implications for nursing practice. *Advances in Nursing Science, 20*(1), 3-11.

Brink, P.J. (Ed.). (1990). *Transcultural nursing*. Prospect Heights, IL: Waveland Press.

Bullough, V.L. & Bullough, B. (1982). *Health care for other Americans.* New York: Appleton-Century-Crofts.

Caudle, P. (1993). Providing culturally sensitive health care to Hispanic clients. *Nurse Practitioner, 18*(12), 40, 43-44, 46.

Chang, K. (1991). Chinese Americans. In J.N. Giger & R.E. Davidhizar (Eds.), *Transcultural nursing: Assessment and intervention.* St Louis: Mosby.

Communication Division of Statistics (1992). *Canada year book 1992.* Ottawa: Publications Division, Statistics Canada.

Covington, T.R. (Ed.). (1996). *Handbook of nonprescription drugs.* Washington, D.C.: American Pharmaceutical Association.

DeSantis, L. (1989). A profile of cultural diversity in nursing practice. *Florida Nurse, 37*(9), 15.

Edwards, L. (1991). Most major companies test medicines in women, monitor data for gender differences. In *New Medicines in Development for Women*. Pharmaceutical Manufacturers Association.

Gaston-Johansson, F., Albert, M., Fagan, E., & Zimmerman, L. (1990). Similarities in pain descriptions of four different ethnic-culture groups. *Journal of Pain Symptom Management, 5*(2), 94.

Geissler, E.M. (1994). *Pocket guide to cultural assessment.* St Louis: Mosby.

Germain, C.P. (1992). Cultural care: A bridge between sickness, illness, disease. *Holistic Nursing Practice, 6*(3), 1-9.

Giger, J.N. & Davidhizar, R.E. (Eds.) (1999). *Transcultural nursing: Assessment and intervention* (3rd ed.). St. Louis: Mosby.

Gordon, S.M. (1994). Hispanic cultural health beliefs and folk remedies. *Journal of Holistic Nursing, 12*(3), 307-322.

Gutman, H.G. (1976). *The black family in slavery and freedom, 1925-1975.* New York: Pantheon.

Holroyd, E., Katie, F.K.L., Chun, L.S., & Ha, S.W. (1997). "Doing the month": an exploration of postpartum practices in Chinese women. *Health Care for Women International 18*(3), 301-313.

Jacques, G. (1976). Cultural health traditions: A black perspective. In M. Branch & P.P. Paxton (Eds.), *Providing safe nursing care for ethnic people of color.* New York: Appleton-Century-Crofts.

Katzung, B.G. (1998). *Basic and clinical pharmacology* (7th ed.). Norwalk, CT: Appleton & Lange.

Kay, M.A. (1977). Health and illness in a Mexican American barrio. In E.H. Spicer (Ed.), *Ethnic medicine in the Southwest.* Tucson: University of Arizona press.

Kiev, A. (1968). *Curanderismo: Mexican-American folk psychiatry.* New York: The Free Press.

Koerner, J. (1992). Culturally competent nursing. *Quality Assessment Quarterly,* Summer, 2.

Leininger, M. (1978). *Transcultural nursing: Concepts, theories, and practices.* New York: John Wiley & Sons.

Leininger, M. (1991). *Culture care diversity and universality: A theory of nursing.* New York: National League for Nursing.

Levy, R.A. (1993). *Ethnic and racial differences in response to medicines: Preserving individualized therapy in managed care pharmaceutical programs*. Reston, VA: National Pharmaceutical Council.

Lopez-Aqueres, W., Kemp, B., Plopper, M., Staples, F.R., & Brummel-Smith, K. (1984). Health needs of the Hispanic elderly. *Journal of American Geriatric Society*, 32(3), 191-198.

Louie, T.T. (1990). Explanatory thinking in Chinese Americans. In P.J. Brink (Ed.), *Transcultural nursing*. Prospect Heights, IL: Waveland Press.

Lynch, E.W. (1992). The importance of cross-cultural effectiveness. *Caring*, 11(10), 14-19.

Mercer, S.O. (1996). Navaho elderly people in a reservation nursing home: admission predictors and culture care practices. *Social Work: Journal of the National Association of Social Workers*, 41(2), 181-189.

Meyer, U.A. (1992). Drugs in special patient groups: Clinical importance of genetics in drug effects. In K.L. Melmon, H.F. Morrelli, B.B. Hoffman, & D.W. Nierenberg (Eds.), *Clinical pharmacology: Basic principles in therapeutics* (3rd ed.). New York: McGraw-Hill.

Pachter, L.M. (1994). Culture and clinical care: Folk illness beliefs and behaviors and their implications for health care delivery. *JAMA: Journal of the American Medical Association*, 271(9), 690-694.

Rawl, S.M. (1992). Perspectives on nursing care of Chinese Americans. *Journal of Holistic Nursing*, 10(1), 6-17.

Salerno, E. (1995). Drug update: Race, culture and medications. *Journal of Emergency Nursing*, 21(6), 560-562.

Salerno, E. & Willens, J.S. (1996). *Pain management handbook*. St Louis: Mosby.

Salerno, E., Rics, D.N., Sank, J., West, E., & Currier, M. (1985). Self-medicating behaviors. *Florida Journal of Hospital Pharmacy* 5(3):13.

Sanchez, T.R., Plawecki, J.A. & Plawecki, H.M. (1996). The delivery of culturally sensitive health care to Native Americans. *Journal of Holistic Nursing*, 14(4), 295-307.

Saunders, L. (1958). Healing ways in the Spanish Southwest. In E.G. Jaco (Ed.), *Patients, physicians, and illness*. Glencoe, IL: Free Press.

Scott, C.S. (1978). Health and healing practices among five ethnic groups in Miami, Florida. In E. Bauwens (Ed.), *The Anthropology of Health*. St Louis: Mosby.

Seto, D., Mokuau, N. & Tsark, J.U. (1998). The interface of culture and rehabilitation for Asian and Pacific Islanders with spinal cord injuries. *SCI Psychosocial Process*, 10(4), 113-119.

Spector, R.E. (1991). *Cultural diversity in health and illness*. (3rd ed.). Norwalk, CT: Appleton & Lange.

United States Department of Commerce, Bureau of the Census. (1992). *Population profile of the United States*. Washington, DC: U.S. Government Printing Office.

Villarruel, A.M. (1995). Mexican-American cultural meanings, expressions, self-care and dependent-care actions associated with experiences of pain. *Research in Nursing and Health*, 18(5), 427-436.

Wauneka, A.D. (1990) Helping a people to understand. In P.J. Brink (Ed.), *Transcultural nursing*. Prospect Heights, IL: Waveland Press.

Williams, E.E. & Ellison, F. (1996). Culturally informed social work practice with American Indian clients: Guidelines for non-Indian social worker. *Social Work: Journal of the National Association of Social Workers*, 41(2), 147-151.

Wright, F., Cohen, S., & Caroselli, C. (1997). Diverse decisions: How culture affects ethical decision making. *Critical Care Nursing Clinics of North America*, 9(1), 63-74.

Wyman, L.C. (1966). Navaho diagnosticians. In Scott, W.R. & Volkart, E.H. (Eds.). *Medical Care*. New York: John Wilcy & Sons.

Zhou, H.H., Adedoyin, A. & Wilkinson, G.R. (1990). Differences in plasma binding of drugs between Caucasians and Chinese subjects. *Clinical Pharmacology Therapeutics*, 48, 10.

7 Maternal and Child Drug Therapy

Chapter Focus

The effects of pharmaceutical agents vary in clients of different ages. The reasons for these variations are complex. Understanding the rationale behind these effects will help the nurse to administer medications safely and to evaluate the responses to these drugs appropriately. The client's age might also determine special techniques of administering medication to provide greater safety for the client.

This chapter and Chapter 8 discuss special factors relating to the dosing and administration of medications in childbearing clients, neonates (birth to approximately 1 month of age), infants (1 month to 2 years), children, and older adults. Because medication use in the adult is discussed throughout this text, a special chapter devoted to this topic is unnecessary.

Learning Objectives

1. Discuss special considerations for drug administration to childbearing or breastfeeding women.
2. Calculate pediatric dosages using body weight and body surface area methods.
3. Identify the preferred intramuscular injection sites in the infant or child.
4. Describe pharmacokinetic alterations related to childbearing clients, breastfeeding clients, or children.
5. Administer medications safely and accurately to childbearing clients, breastfeeding clients, or children.

Key Terms

carcinogenic, p. 129
fetal alcohol syndrome, p. 129
mutagenic, p. 129
teratogenic, p. 127

The human life span is a continuum in which development, maturity, and degeneration occur without any distinct demarcation. However, individuals mature and decline and/or have special needs at different ages, at different rates, and under different circumstances. These factors affect the client's response to drug therapy in characteristic ways. Therefore nursing management of drug therapy needs to be based on both physiologic and psychosocial development levels.

CHILDBEARING CLIENTS

Any substance ingested or absorbed by a pregnant woman is likely to reach the fetus by way of maternal circulation or to be transferred to the breastfed neonate by way of breast milk if the substance is in a sufficient concentration and is well distributed. Therefore drugs taken by the mother can cause serious harm to the fetus or neonate. No drug is known to be absolutely safe for the developing embryo, but some oral medications that are inactivated in the mother's stomach or are not absorbed by the maternal gastrointestinal tract are assumed to be relatively safe. However, the effects of many drugs and other substances on the fetus are unknown.

Considerations for drug therapy in the childbearing client center on the risk-benefit ratio. This ratio is evaluated on the basis of the mother's condition and the effect of the drug(s) on the mother and the developing fetus or nursing infant. In some instances prescription and over-the-counter (OTC) drugs taken during pregnancy have resulted in fetal drug toxicity and teratogenicity (the ability to cause fetal abnormalities). Although the possible effect of some medications taken during pregnancy is known, new medications, different drug combinations, or a deficiency in metabolism in the fetus may change a drug previously known to be safe into a hazardous one. The period of greatest danger for drug-induced developmental defects is the first trimester of pregnancy. Therefore self-treatment of minor illnesses is discouraged during pregnancy, and women should be instructed to keep a complete record of all medications consumed during pregnancy (Bobak, Lowdermilk, & Jensen, 1995). Because of their risk for pregnancy, this same self-medication counseling should also be provided to all women of childbearing age who are either not using or are considering not using contraception.

Pregnant women take an average of four or more drugs (other than vitamins) during their pregnancy, and the fetal effects of these drugs are unknown. This topic is therefore of utmost concern during the parenting stage of life. Nurses are commonly required to provide accurate information with rationales, discuss available health care options, and support parents' decisions during the childbearing process. Nurses should ensure that the information is current and based on evidence and that the woman understands that the baseline risk for **teratogenic** (causing fetal defects) effects in pregnancy is approximately 3%—even in the absence of any known teratogenic exposure (Katzung, 1998). Health care providers and parents alike may need to make difficult choices on the basis of the benefit-to-risk ratio, which is determined by maternal medication regimens, the benefits to the mother, and the risks to the fetus or neonate. This dilemma illustrates the absolute necessity for nurses to be knowledgeable about medications and highly skilled at retrieving information from reliable sources. Parents should make the final care decisions regarding care on the basis of informed, sensitive input from all appropriate health care professionals.

Drug Transfer to the Fetus

Pharmacokinetics

There are multiple physiologic changes related to pregnancy that affect pharmacokinetics. Pregnancy does not seem to have much effect on drug absorption from the gastrointestinal tract, but protein binding is decreased for some substances, which increases the amount of drug available for placental transfer. Biotransformation of drugs in the liver is probably delayed in pregnancy, but renal excretion may be more rapid because renal blood flow dramatically increases glomerular filtration rate (see Chapter 3).

The placenta plays a role in protecting the fetus from drugs in the maternal circulation. At the placental interface, the transfer of drugs and other substances occurs primarily by simple diffusion and partly by active transport. Transfer across the placenta depends on the chemical properties of the drug: its molecular weight, protein-binding capabilities, chemical configuration, and lipid solubility. The potential for transfer to the fetus is proportional to the period of time the drug remains in the maternal bloodstream. Transfer is greater during late gestation because of enhanced uteroplacental blood flow, increased placental surface at the interface, thinner membranes separating maternal blood flow and placental capillaries, and an increased proportion of free drug available to the circulation. Pathologic processes in the placenta, such as inflammation, degeneration, or partial separation, can alter blood flow and thus drug transfer. In addition, the placenta itself is a site of drug metabolism. It converts some drugs (e.g., phenobarbital) to harmless metabolites, but it may create toxic metabolites and increase drug toxicity for other drugs (e.g., ethanol). By whichever mechanism, drug transfer can result in significant fetal drug effects (see Fetal Drug Effects, p. 128).

The traditional concept of the placenta being a completely protective barrier to circulating substances must be discarded. Many drugs are transferred across the placenta, but not all are dangerous. Most drugs that cross the placenta stabilize in the fetus at a level between 50% and 100% of the maternal level. Some drugs (e.g., diazepam and local anesthetics) stabilize at levels even higher than those of the mother's. However, continued exposure of the fetus to a drug is more important than the rate of placental transport. Table 7-1 lists drugs associated with neonatal withdrawal symptoms (Levy & Spino, 1993).

TABLE 7-1 Drugs Associated with Neonatal Withdrawal Symptoms

	Withdrawal Symptoms	
	General	**Central Nervous System**
Alcohol	Irritability, poor sleep pattern, diaphoresis	Crying, hyperactivity, increased sensitivity to sound, hypertonicity, tremor, seizures
Cocaine	Tremulousness, poor sleep pattern	Hypotonia, hyperreflexia
Antihistamines		
diphenhydramine (Benadryl)	Tremulousness	
hydroxyzine (Atarax, Vistaril)	Irritability	Hyperactivity, tremor, jitteriness, shrill cry, hypotonia, seizures
Barbiturates		
amobarbital (Amytal) ethchlorvynol (Placidyl) phenobarbital, secobarbital (Seconal)	Irritability, poor sleep pattern, diaphoresis, skin abrasions	Excessive crying, hyperreflexia, increased sensitivity to sound, hypertonicity, tremor, seizures
Benzodiazepines		
chlordiazepoxide (Librium)	Irritability	Tremors
diazepam (Valium)	Hypothermia	Hyperactivity, hypotonia, hypertonia, apnea/tremor, hyperreflexia
Opiates		
codeine heroin meperidine (Demerol) methadone morphine pentazocine (Talwin)	Irritability, wakefulness, yawning, tearing, fever, diaphoresis, skin excoriations, voracious sucking, poor sleep pattern, hypothermia Respiratory symptoms (stuffy/runny nose, sneezing, tachypnea, respiratory alkalosis), gastrointestinal symptoms (hiccups, salivation, vomiting, diarrhea, failure to thrive)	Coarse tremors, seizures, twitching Hyperactivity (high-pitched cry), hypertonicity Hyperreflexia, increased sensitivity to sound, photophobia, apneic spells
propoxyphene (Darvon)	Irritability, fever	Hyperactivity, tremor, high-pitched cry

Modified from Levy, M. & Spino, M. (1993). Neonatal withdrawal syndrome: Associated drugs and pharmacologic management. *Pharmacotherapy, 13*(3), 202-211.

Fetal Drug Effects

Drugs crossing the placenta enter the fetal circulation via the umbilical cord. Approximately 40% to 60% of umbilical venous blood enters the fetal liver; the rest directly enters the fetal circulation. A drug passing through the fetal liver may be partially metabolized before entering the fetal circulation. In addition, a large proportion of the blood returning to the placenta from the fetus may be shunted through the placental tissue, back to the umbilical vein, and into the fetus again.

The effects of drugs in the fetus may be more significant and prolonged than in the mother because of (1) probable immature enzyme drug metabolizing systems or an absence of such systems, and (2) slower excretion rates. In the fetus, drug excretion is accomplished by the kidneys. Waste products are excreted into the amniotic fluid, which is reabsorbed by the mother or swallowed by the fetus. Thus the immature or underdeveloped physiologic mechanisms of the fetus may result in altered drug responses and perhaps toxicity.

Occasionally, various fetal complications such as anemia and syphilis exposure are actively treated by drugs in utero. Corticosteroids are used to stimulate fetal lung maturation when a premature birth is expected (Katzung, 1998). The chosen routes of drug delivery have been either a passive, transplacental approach or direct instillation into the amniotic fluid.

It continues to be well documented that the administration of various drugs before delivery or the continued use of abuse drugs throughout pregnancy may have toxic and harmful effects on the newborn. The embryo or fetus runs the risk of developing the usual side or toxic effects, just as the mother does. For example, if the mother consumes alcohol, barbiturates, or narcotics, the neonate at birth may have withdrawal symptoms: hyperactivity, crying, irritability, seizures and, perhaps, sudden death. (See Table 7-1 for a list of drugs that can cause symptoms of withdrawal.)

Medications may be lethal or teratogenic, **mutagenic** (causing genetic mutation), or **carcinogenic** (causing or accelerating the development of cancer). An example of a carcinogenic effect is the precancerous or cancerous cell changes discovered in youths whose mothers took the hormone diethylstilbestrol (DES) during pregnancy.

Every embryo undergoes a series of precisely programmed steps from cell proliferation, differentiation, and migration to organogenesis. The critical periods for drug effects on the fetus are (1) the first 2 weeks of rapid cell proliferation, when exposure to drugs can be lethal to the embryo, and (2) the third through the tenth weeks of pregnancy, when the axial skeleton, muscles, limbs, and organs are developing most rapidly. Figure 7-1 illustrates the critical periods of human development.

Indirectly, teratogenic drugs may interfere with the passage of oxygen and nutrition through the placenta and affect the most rapidly metabolizing fetal tissues. More directly, some drugs may alter the normal processes of differentiation of fetal development, such as vitamin A analogue (isotretinoin). Deficiencies of crucial substances appear to play a role in some fetal abnormalities. This may be demonstrated by the fact that an increased intake of folic acid during pregnancy appears to reduce the incidence of neural tube defects, such as spinal bifida.

An unfortunate example of a teratogenic effect is the hypnotic drug thalidomide, which caused abnormal limb development (phocomelia) in many children whose mothers received the drug during pregnancy, especially between the third and sixth week of pregnancy. When it was administered beyond the tenth week of pregnancy (after the rapid development of the skeleton) physiologic or behavioral alterations and delays in growth were more likely.

Cocaine abuse by pregnant women has resulted in frequent miscarriages, fetal hypoxia, and low-birth-weight infants. Cocaine exposure in utero has caused fetal tremors, fetal strokes, and an increase in stillbirth rates. Exposed infants are also at high risk for developing congenital heart disease, skull defects, and other congenital malformations. At birth the newborn may exhibit symptoms of withdrawal: increased irritability, increased respiratory and heart rates, diarrhea, irregular sleeping patterns, and poor appetite. Long-term behavioral patterns of infants born to cocaine-abusing women, such as poor attention spans and a decrease in organizational skills, have been reported (Hall et al., 1990). In a number of instances the legal system or the courts have intervened to protect the unborn fetus or to punish the mother of a child born with medical complications resulting from cocaine abuse.

In certain situations drugs are necessary during pregnancy and breastfeeding. Some maternal conditions (e.g., hypertension, epilepsy, diabetes, and infection) seriously jeopardize both mother and fetus if left untreated. Although authoritative literature and drug package inserts routinely warn that drugs have not been tested for use in pregnancy, during breastfeeding, or for infants, much empiric and some research data are accumulating. The Food and Drug Administration (FDA) rates drugs according to their safety for use during pregnancy. This rating is discussed in Chapter 2 and is included in the discussion of specific drugs throughout this text.

A major issue regarding the use of drugs during pregnancy and the neonatal period involves the legal and ethical problems associated with drug research experiments during pregnancy; these problems contribute to the lack of information in this area. Although fraught with ethical dilemmas, well-controlled research is undeniably needed. Nurses are in a good position to participate in this important research, and they should do so.

Certain categories of drugs are expressly contraindicated during pregnancy or are used only when the risk-benefit situation has been carefully considered and thoroughly discussed with the client. Drugs with reported teratogenic effects are listed in Table 7-2. Some drugs considered relatively safe during pregnancy, depending on the situation, are listed in Table 7-3.

Drug use during pregnancy should be severely curtailed and limited to situations in which the life of the pregnant women or the fetus would be in jeopardy without drug treatment. The following variables should be considered when drug therapy is considered necessary:

1. Maternal dosage, maternal volume of distribution, and metabolic clearance rate of the mother, all of which are factors that determine the dose that reaches the embryo or fetus
2. Fetal gestational age at time of exposure
3. Duration of therapy planned
4. Fetal and maternal genotypes
5. Other drugs being administered concurrently

Doses, dosing intervals, and treatment durations should be adjusted carefully by the prescriber to avoid harmful effects.

Excessive maternal intake of alcohol, especially at or near the time of conception, is associated with **fetal alcohol syndrome (FAS)**, which produces congenital anomalies and both growth and mental retardation (Box 7-1). Other very common, potentially dangerous substances during pregnancy include extended-release aspirin (pregnancy category D), parenteral vitamin A (category X), and nicotine chewing gum and nicotine transdermal systems (category X and category D, respectively) (*United States Pharmacopeia Dispensing Information*, 1999).

A problem with drug use is that the effects on the embryo may occur before the woman is aware she is pregnant. Women of childbearing age who are not using contraceptives and who are sexually active should be prescribed drugs carefully and should be instructed to use OTC medications cautiously. Education and prevention are considered the best therapy.

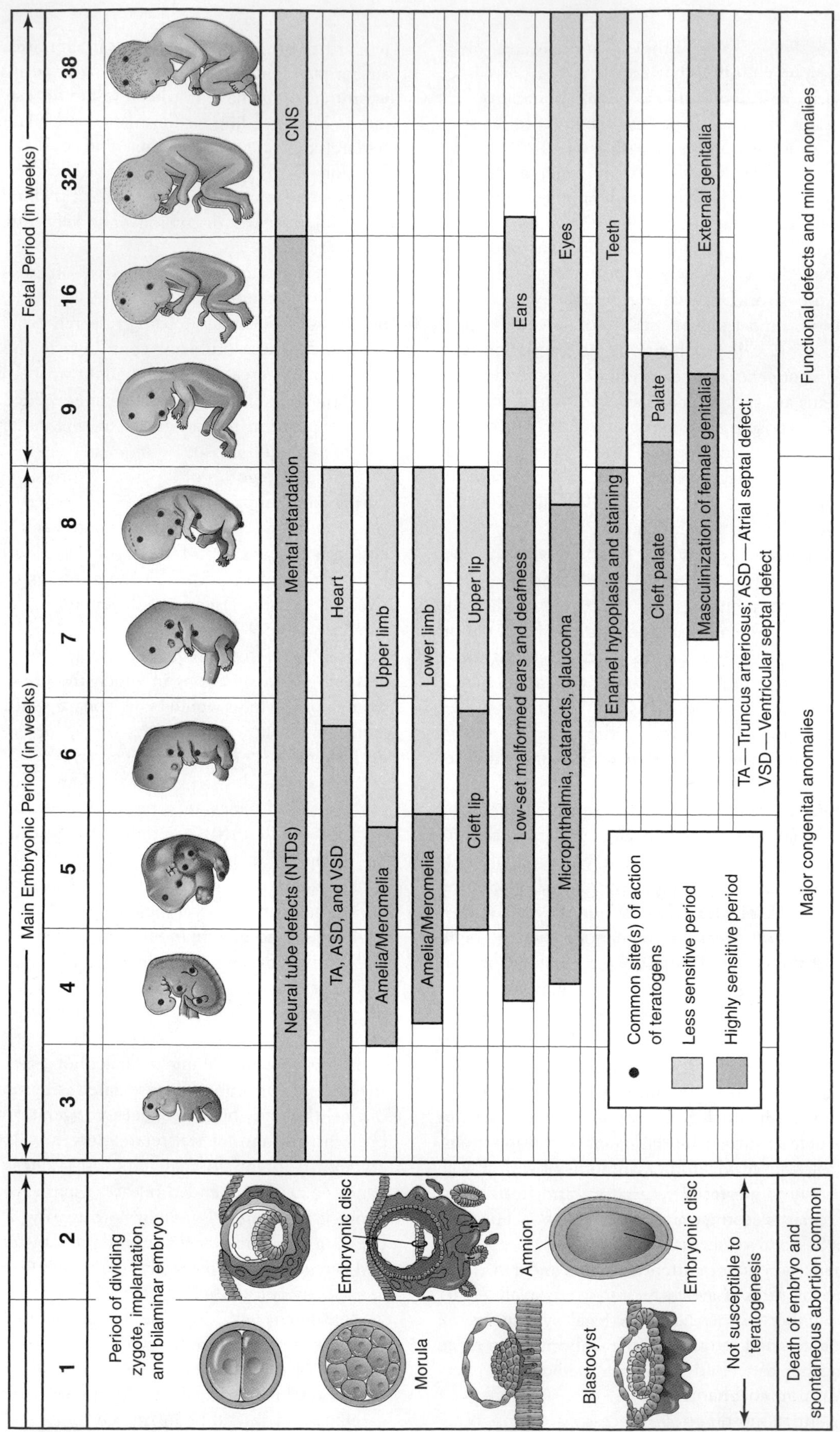

Figure 7-1 Schematic illustration of the critical periods in human prenatal development. (Modified from Moore, K.L, & Persaud, T.V.N. [1998]. *The developing human: Clinically oriented embryology* [6th Ed.]. Philadelphia: W.B. Saunders.)

TABLE 7-2 Drugs with Reported Teratogenic Effects

Drug	Critical Time Period of Pregnancy	Potential Defect
alcohol, chronic use	<12 weeks	Heart defects, CNS abnormalities
	>24 weeks	Developmental delay, low birth weight
acitretin (Soriatane)	All trimesters	Anophthalmia, heart defects, microcephalus, skeletal and/or connective tissue malformations
androgens	>10 weeks	External female genitalia masculinization
angiotensin-converting enzyme (ACE) inhibitors	All, especially second and third trimester	Renal dysgenesis, defects in skull ossification
carbamazepine	<30 days after conception	Spina bifida
cigarettes	<20 weeks	Miscarriage
	>20 weeks	Low birth weight and perhaps delay in development
cocaine	Second and third trimester	Abruptio placentae
	Third trimester	Premature labor and delivery, intracranial bleeding
diethylstilbestrol (DES)	All trimesters	Vaginal adenosis, vaginal carcinoma, uterine abnormalities, male infertility
isotretinoin (Accutane)	All trimesters	Hydrocephalus, CNS abnormalities, fetal death
lithium	<3 months	Ebstein's anomaly
methotrexate	6-9 weeks after conception	Skull ossification defect, limb and craniofacial defects
phenytoin (Dilantin)	All trimesters	Cleft palate, cleft lip, heart abnormalities, fetal anticonvulsant syndrome*
tetracycline	All trimesters	Stained teeth, bone growth defect
vaccines (measles, mumps, rubella)	First trimester	Spontaneous abortions, premature births, possible congenital defects
valproic acid	All trimesters	Spina bifida, fetal anticonvulsant syndrome*
vitamin A (high doses and parenteral)	All trimesters	Fetal abnormalities, including urinary tract malformations, growth retardation
warfarin	All trimesters	Fetal hemorrhage, optic atrophy, brain abnormalities

Information from Jennings, J.C. (1996). Guide to medication use in pregnant and breastfeeding women. *Pharmacy Practice News, 23*(4), 10; Katzung, B.G. (1998). *Basic & clinical pharmacology* (7th ed.). Stamford, CT: Appleton & Lange; and *United States Pharmacopeia Dispensing Information (USP DI): Drug information for the health care professional* (19th ed.) (1999). Rockville, MD: United States Pharmacopeial Convention.
*Mental and prenatal growth deficiency, microcephaly, fingernail hypoplasia, and craniofacial defects.

Nursing Management

Medication Administration with Childbearing Clients

Most nursing goals related to medication administration should be aimed at ensuring that parents know that any foreign substance absorbed by the mother may have lifelong effects on the child and family. A balance must be maintained between protecting the individual while promoting the role and formation of the family. To accomplish these goals, be an advocate for the client, establish an environment conducive to the exchange of information, and minimize the parents' feelings of guilt or fear associated with drug administration and the potential impact on the unborn. The following information should be conveyed to the family:

1. Both the potential harm to the unborn child resulting directly from substances to which the mother is exposed and the potential risks and benefits to both mother and child if treatment is not begun must be weighed. These decisions must be made with the prescriber whenever exposure to an unfamiliar substance or drug is contemplated.
2. OTC medications and other common substances such as aspirin, high-dose or multiple vitamin supplements, alcohol, caffeine, and nicotine may have detrimental effects on the fetus.
3. An obstetrician or pediatrician should evaluate any prescription written by a professional who is not a specialist in the care of pregnant women or nursing mothers. The specialist may need to change the prescription to a safer drug or dosage.
4. Close health care supervision is essential if the mother is exposed to a questionable substance. If there is high risk for fetal or infant injury, the parents need ongoing support as they endure the sometimes long wait for manifestation of the effects. If birth defects or toxic effects are present or if invasive diagnostic tests or a therapeutic abortion is to be performed, objective

TABLE 7-3 Some Drugs Considered Relatively Safe for Use in Pregnancy

Agent	Recommendations and Cautions*
Analgesics	
acetaminophen (Tylenol)	Considered safest analgesic during pregnancy
Antiasthmatics	
cromolyn sodium (Intal)	Relatively safe
metaproterenol (Alupent) (aerosol)	Relatively safe for mild, intermittent episodes; avoid oral form
theophylline (Theo-Dur)	Relatively safe if blood levels are closely monitored
Anticoagulants	
heparin	For use during first trimester; use caution if given during last trimester
Anticonvulsants	
phenobarbital	Can cause malformations; for use only if necessary to maintain seizure control; if given during pregnancy, monitor neonate during first 24 hours for neonatal coagulation defect (bleeding)
Antidiabetics	
insulin	Relatively safe; drug of choice
Antiemetics	
pyridoxine (Vitamin B_6)	Relatively safe for morning sickness
prochlorperazine (Compazine)	For use as necessary for severe nausea or vomiting
trimethobenzamide (Tigan)	
cyclizine (Marezine)	
meclizine (Antivert)	
Antihypertensives	
methyldopa (Aldomet)	Safest of antihypertensives during pregnancy (especially as substitute for diuretics in pregnancy for diastolic blood pressure >110 mm Hg in the third trimester)
hydralazine (Apresoline)	Safest for hypertensive crises in pregnancy
Antiinfectives	
cephalosporins	Safe during pregnancy
erythromycin (E-Mycin)	For use as substitute for penicillin hypersensitivity
metronidazole (Flagyl)	Not to be used during first trimester
miconazole (Monistat)	Relatively safe
penicillin and derivatives	Relatively safe
Antituberculosis Drugs	
rifampin (Rifadin)	Relatively safe
ethambutol (Myambutol)	
Cardiac Glycosides	
digoxin (Lanoxin)	Relatively safe; maternal plasma levels should be closely monitored

*Recommendations are likely to change; therefore manufacturers' package inserts should always be consulted. No drugs are known to be absolutely safe during pregnancy. The risks and benefits of using many substances, including most drugs not on this list, should be carefully considered by the obstetrician. See drug monographs for specific drug information; see also the Bibliography for sources of information about drugs in this table.

psychologic intervention may help parents endure this critical period.

CHILDREN

Neonates

Newborns require special considerations because they lack many of the protective mechanisms that allow older children and adults to be relatively resistant to all types of stressors. Their skin is thin and permeable, their stomachs lack acid, and their lungs lack much of the mucus barrier. Neonates regulate body temperature poorly and become dehydrated easily. Their liver and kidneys are immature and cannot manage foreign substances as well as older children and adults. Specific factors affecting medication use in neonates are listed in Table 7-4.

Breastfed Infants

Almost all forms of drugs in the maternal circulation can be readily transferred to the colostrum and breast milk. Because

BOX 7-1

Alcohol and the Childbearing Client: Fetal Alcohol Syndrome

Many people do not consider alcohol to be a drug; thus it may be overlooked as being hazardous if used during pregnancy. The teratogenic effects of intrauterine alcohol exposure on the fetus are well documented. Heavy use of alcohol by the childbearing client has been associated with the following effects:

- Facial: ptosis, strabismus, myopia, cleft lip or palate
- CNS: retardation, impaired coordination, increased irritability during infancy, hyperactivity in childhood
- Growth: slowed
- Cardiac: murmurs, tetralogy of Fallot
- Muscular: hernias of the groin, umbilicus, or diaphragm

Although a direct relationship between the quantity of alcohol consumed and the severity of FAS has not been identified, it appears that the fetus is at greatest risk when alcohol consumption is in excess of the liver's capability to detoxify it. The exact mechanism of FAS has not been identified, but studies indicate that counseling to eliminate maternal alcohol intake has a beneficial effect on the health of both the mother and infant. It has been recommended that women discontinue alcohol use at least 3 months before becoming pregnant (Wong, 1997).

The nurse must be aware of clients who are at risk of FAS and be prepared to provide client education, counseling, and referral (Briggs, 1995; Wong, 1997).

drugs or their biotransformed products are handled by different pathways in the infant and the fetus, the impact of maternal medications on the infant is probably different from (probably less than) the impact on the fetus. This difference can guide the health care professional in prescribing medications for the breastfeeding woman. Typical nontherapeutic outcomes in the breastfed infant are signs of the drug's usual side effects or toxic effects.

Adverse reactions may also occur, such as allergic sensitization to penicillin or gray-brown stains of later-erupting teeth as a result of tetracycline therapy of more than 10 days' duration. Most drug products that reach the neonate via the breast milk have undergone maternal biotransformation and are probably less than the original dose. However, immaturity of the neonate's hepatic and renal systems may limit the capacity for further metabolism and excretion.

Data about an infant's capabilities for drug absorption, digestion, distribution, metabolism, and excretion are scant and conflicting. In general, the proved benefits of continuing breastfeeding must be weighed on an individual basis against the risks of maternal medication to the infant (Banta-Wright, 1997). The mammary glands are a relatively insignificant route for maternal drug excretion and the drug level in breast milk is usually less than the actual maternal dose, and the infant's actual dose depends largely on the volume of milk consumed. Thus a single measurement of a drug in human milk will not accurately reflect the total dose received by the infant.

The concentration of the drug in maternal circulation depends on the relationship of several factors: dosing and route of administration, distribution, protein binding, and maternal metabolism and excretion. The mammary alveolar epithelium consists of a lipid barrier with water-filled pores; thus it is more permeable to drugs during the colostrum stage of milk production—during the first week of life.

Drug factors that enhance drug excretion into milk are nonionization, low molecular weight, fat solubility, and concentration. Drug distribution and the absorptive processes of the infant's gastrointestinal tract are estimated to be similar to those in the adult, which means that lipid-soluble substances are well absorbed. The infant's age (thus the amount of drug-containing milk consumed) and the relative immaturity of the infant's important organs has a significant effect on the outcome. The following factors are also relevant: (1) if the drug is fat soluble, it may be more highly concentrated in breast milk at the end of feedings and at midday; (2) because the infant's total serum protein is lower in comparison to the adult's, more free drug may be available to the circulation; (3) metabolic reactions in the infant's liver are slower than in the older child's, and therefore drug biotransformation may likewise be delayed; and (4) drug excretion is delayed in the neonate because it occurs mainly via the kidneys, where immature glomerular filtration rates and tubular functioning are maintained for several months. The extreme variability among drug effects and infants' capabilities makes it difficult to decide whether or not the mother should take a drug and whether or not she should breastfeed.

If human milk contains small, fixed amounts of substances absorbed by the mother, it is usually recommended that breastfeeding be temporarily interrupted (usually for 24 to 72 hours) and the breasts pumped to remove drug-containing milk. Less often, it is advisable to cease breastfeeding altogether. Dosages and routes may also be changed. It is recommended that certain drugs be avoided while breastfeeding (Box 7-2).

Drug effects may be minimized by substituting formula for the midday breastfeeding, because that feeding is highest in fat content and thus is more likely to contain higher amounts of fat-soluble drug products. Breastfeeding mothers who must take medications can take the medication immediately *after* breastfeeding so as much time as possible elapses and the drug can reach a relatively low concentration before the next feeding. Drugs considered relatively safe during breastfeeding are summarized in Table 7-5.

Therapy with radioactive substances is of short duration; if a diagnostic radioisotope test is to be performed, breastfeeding is interrupted until all radiation is absent from milk samples. Breastfeeding will probably be terminated whenever the drug is so potent that minute amounts may profoundly affect the infant, when the drug has high allergenic potential, when the mother's renal function decreases

TABLE 7-4 Physiologic Processes Affecting Medication Use in Neonates

Physiologic Process	Neonate	Type of Drugs Affected
Absorption		
Gastric pH	Increases to 6 to 8 for first 24 hours; then achlorhydria usually occurs for 10-15 days	Acid-labile drugs, such as oral penicillin, are better absorbed. Oral forms of phenobarbital or phenytoin have reduced bioavailability.
Gastric emptying time	Prolonged, usually 6 to 8 hours	Oral absorption of penicillin is increased; absorption of phenytoin and phenobarbital is decreased.
Distribution		
Total body water (TBW) content	75% to 79%	Average adults have approximately 60% TBW and 25% to 45% fat. There are vast differences in drug distribution across the age span.
Adipose (fat) content	5% to 12%	Water-soluble drugs have a larger volume of distribution in newborns, whereas fat-soluble drugs have considerably less. Drug dosage adjustments are largely based on this factor.
Protein binding	Decreased	Highly protein-bound drugs require dosage adjustments to avoid toxicity due to increased free drug concentrations in the plasma.
Metabolism		
Liver metabolism	Decreased	Potent or potentially toxic drugs requiring liver metabolism are slowly metabolized; lower dosages are necessary for such drugs, especially chloramphenicol (Chloromycetin) and theophylline (Theo-Dur), among others.
Microsomal enzymes	Low	
Excretion		
Glomerular filtration	Decreased	Drugs excreted by filtration or secretion will accumulate in the neonate; dosage adjustments are necessary, especially with aminoglycosides and digoxin [Lanoxin].
Tubular secretion	Decreased	

(which augments drug excretion into breast milk), or when serious pathologic conditions require prolonged administration of high doses of the drug.

Changes in the activity levels of the fetus or nursing infant signal dangerous effects resulting from drug administration. Parents should be taught how to assess and report unusual fetal inactivity or infant apathy.

Both health care professionals and clients place a high value on the use of pharmaceuticals to treat minor illnesses. However, many illnesses are self-limited or cause only minor discomforts that end or decrease without medication or with nondrug alternatives (e.g., relaxation techniques rather than tranquilizers). The risk-to-benefit effect of any medication should consider the physiologic, physical, and psychologic effects of therapy on both the mother and the child (Schou, 1998).

Another possibility is to delay the mother's pharmacologic therapy until the infant is weaned or to select another drug that can meet the therapeutic goal without interfering with breastfeeding. The age and maturity of the child must also be considered, because the ability of a drug to cause harmful effects diminishes as an infant develops physiologically. The frequency of feedings should also be considered. An infant who depends on breast milk for total nutrition will receive higher doses of drugs than an infant who breastfeeds only once or twice a day and receives other forms of nourishment.

Nonbreastfed Infants

Infant formula feeding is used for the following situations:

1. The mother chooses not to breastfeed.

   or

2. The mother is advised not to breastfeed because of illness or disease.

   or

3. The infant has special formulation needs.

Commercial formulas prepared from nonfat cow's milk are available and are generally divided into two categories: general purpose formulas and special purpose infant formulas. Select formulas from each category are listed in Table 7-6.

Infant formulas contain essential and minor trace elements as found in human breast milk, plus the three sources of calories (protein, carbohydrate, and lipids) in a balanced proportion to promote growth. Many formulas contain vitamins and minerals, and usually the vitamin K in these formulas is more than is contained in breast milk. Vitamin K is

BOX 7-2

Drugs Contraindicated During Breastfeeding

The American Academy of Pediatrics committee on drugs has suggested that the following drugs be avoided by women who are breastfeeding:
amphetamines
bromocriptine (Parlodel)
chloral hydrate (Aquachloral Supprettes)
chloramphenicol (Chloromycetin)
cocaine
cyclophosphamide (Cytoxan)
cyclosporine (Sandimmune)
diazepam (Valium)
doxorubicin (Adriamycin)
ergotamine (Ergostat)
gold salts
heroin
iodine (radioactive)
lithium (Lithobid)
marijuana
methotrexate
nicotine (smoking)
propylthiouracil

included because it reduces the risk of hemorrhagic disease in the infant. Cow's milk differs from human milk in protein content. The protein (80%) in cow's milk is casein, whereas human milk contains whey protein (70%). Human milk protein (whey) is richer in immunoglobulins, albumin, lysozyme, amylase, transaminase, protease, and lipases; casein provides lesser amounts of these ingredients. Although the protein in many infant formulas is of a higher quality than cow's milk, some infant formulas may contain bovine whey, a protein that contains beta-lactoglobulin. This substance contributes to the development of cow's milk allergies.

Infants can absorb 20% to 50% of the iron they need from breast milk, whereas the iron from infant formulations is only minimally absorbed (4% to 7%). The reason for this difference in absorption is unknown. The FDA has issued recommendations that all infant formulations contain at least 0.3 to 0.5 mg/L (the lowest iron level found in human milk) and that the iron be in a bioavailable form. Infants at risk for iron deficiency should be given supplements containing 1 to 2 mg/100 kcal of iron, or approximately 6 to 12 mg/L. Most iron-supplemented infant formulas today contain 12 or 13 mg/L (Sagraves, Kamper, & Doerr, 1996).

Drug Administration in Children

Administering medications to children requires special knowledge and approaches. The dosage of a medication may be prescribed, but it is the nurse's responsibility to know the safe dosage range of any medication administered to children. Usually, the most reliable pediatric dosage information is that provided by the manufacturer in the package insert. However, many times such information is not included from the manufacturer, even though studies have been published in the medical literature; this reflects the reluctance of the manufacturers to label their products for pediatric use (Katzung, 1998). A standard medication dosage is nearly nonexistent in pediatrics (Box 7-3); medications are usually ordered according to the weight or body surface area of the child. Some pharmaceutical companies continue to supply medications in a standard adult-dose strength, and the nurse must be able to calculate the correct pediatric dosage before administering the medication.

A nurse calculating dosages of digitalis, insulin, barbiturates, and narcotics should have the calculations and the prepared medication dose checked by a nurse or pharmacist before administering the drug. Pediatric dosages are often minute, and thus a slight calculation error may result in a greater proportional error.

Weight as a Basis. The following is a formula for calculating estimated safe dosages based on weight alone (Clark's rule). Because this formula is based on weight alone, it is an imprecise calculation for children and is not often used.

$$\frac{\text{Average adult dose} \times \text{Weight of child in pounds}}{150}$$

Example: How much acetaminophen (Tylenol) should a 1-year-old child weighing 21 pounds receive if the average adult dose is 10 grains?

Answer:

$$\frac{10\ (\text{grains}) \times 21\ (\text{weight in pounds})}{150} = \text{gr } 1\tfrac{2}{5}$$

Calculating the pediatric dosage on the basis of weight alone implies that the pediatric client is a small adult, which is not true. The physiologic differences between infants and adults definitely affects the amount of drug needed to produce a therapeutic effect. For example, an infant's body composition is approximately 75% water (adults have 50% to 60%), and infants have a smaller fat content than adults. Therefore water-soluble drugs are generally administered in larger doses (in proportion to body weight) to infants and children than to adults. A good example of this is the water-soluble drug gentamicin, an IV antibiotic. The following are recommended dosages from *United States Pharmacopeia Dispensing Information (USP DI)* (1999): older neonates and infants, 2.5 mg/kg every 8 to 16 hours; children, 2 to 2.5 mg/kg every 8 hours; and adults under 60 kg, 1.5 mg/kg every 12 hours.

Rules based on weight, such as Clark's rule, are generally taught and used by students in clinical areas to assess pediatric dosages; this rule has limited usefulness as a guide. For the approximately 75% of drugs that have no established dosage for children, Clark's rule to calculate the pediatric dosage as a fraction of the average adult dosage is really too imprecise. Determining pediatric drug dosages by body surface area is considered more accurate. However, Clark's rule

TABLE 7-5 Drugs Considered Relatively Safe During Breastfeeding

Agent	Recommendations and Precautions*
Analgesics	
acetaminophen	Relatively safe
butorphanol	With usual dosages, drug levels in breast milk are usually low
codeine	
meperidine	
morphine	
propoxyphene	
Antiinfectives	
cefadroxil	Low concentrations distributed into breast milk, no problems reported
cefazolin	
cefoxitin	
ceftriaxone	
isoniazid	Relatively safe
ethambutol	No problems reported
Cardiovascular Drugs	
digoxin	Safe if maternal serum levels are closely monitored
guanethidine	Safe in recommended dosages
methyldopa	Distributed in breast milk; no documented problems in humans
propranolol	Relatively safe at lower maternal dosages (higher drug levels in breast milk than in maternal bloodstream because of high lipid solubility of drug)
Diuretics	
spironolactone	Safe
thiazides	May suppress lactation; avoid in first month of lactation
Bronchodilators	
cromolyn sodium	Observe for infant irritability or insomnia
theophylline	
Antidiabetics	
insulin	Safe; not distributed in breast milk
Thyroid Drugs	
thyroid hormones	Relatively safe if monitored for thyroid function and response
Gastrointestinal Drugs	
antacids	Relatively safe
cisapride	
laxatives (except cascara and danthron)	
Air pollutants	Have not been found in human milk
Vaccines	
RhoGAM	Considered safe

*Recommendations may change over time; therefore manufacturer's package inserts should always be consulted by pediatricians and nurses. Most substances should be avoided during the period of breastfeeding. (Details about specific drugs are located under relevant chapter headings in this text.) Consult Bibliography for sources of information.

may be used (mg/kg) when the dosage according to body surface area has not been established.

Body Surface Area as a Basis. Years ago it was suggested that drug dosages be calculated on size or on the proportional amount of body surface area (BSA) to weight. Although prescribers continue to use weight as the basis for calculating drug dosages and BSA for calculating fluid requirements, most clinicians advocate using BSA for determining drug dosages for adults and children. Prescribers usually carry a simple slide rule or nomogram, such as the

TABLE 7-6 Selected Examples of Infant Formulas

Product Name/Manufacturer	Indications/Special Features
General-Purpose Formulas	
Enfamil (Mead Johnson)	Supplement to breastfeeding
Good Start (Carnation)	
PediaSure (Ross)	
Special-Purpose Formulas	
Alimentum Liquid (Ross)	Severe food allergies, protein sensitivity or maldigestion, or fat malabsorption; corn and lactose free
Isomil Liquid & Powder (Ross)	Infants and children who are allergic to cow's milk, lactose deficient, or galactosemic; lactose free
Phenex-1 Powder (Ross)	Infants with phenylketonuria (PKU)
Pregestrimil Powder (Mead Johnson)	Severe malabsorption disorders
ProSobee (Mead Johnson)	Infants with family history of allergies; lactose, milk, and sucrose free
Infant Formulas with Iron	
Enfamil with Iron (Mead Johnson)	
Similac with Iron (Ross)	
SMA Iron Fortified (Mead Johnson)	
Lofenalac Powder (Mead Johnson)	Low phenylalanine plus iron

West nomogram (Figure 7-2) to make rapid BSA conversions from weight and height. It is believed that the larger amount of total body water (TBW) in children—as well as the percentage of water in body weight and the part of that percentage formed by extracellular water—accounts for the fact that children tolerate or require larger dosages of some drugs on a mg/m^2 basis.

As a relationship between height and weight, BSA can provide a more precise guide to the maturity of the child's organs and metabolic rate of functioning for effective pharmacokinetics. The dosage should be tailored to the individual child according to the amount of medication per square meter of BSA. The following is the BSA rule for pediatric dosages:

$$\text{Approximate pediatric dose} = \frac{\text{Child's BSA in square meters (from nomogram)} \times \text{Adult dose}}{1.73}$$

For example, using Figure 7-2, a child with a height of 34 inches and a weight of 10 kg would be considered to have a BSA (m^2) of 0.5. The dosage calculation would be as follows:

$$\text{Child's approximate dose} = \frac{0.5 \times \text{Adult dose}}{1.73}$$

The following sources are recommended for students who are uncertain about dosage: the drug monograph in a package insert, *USP DI*, *American Hospital Formulary Service*

BOX 7-3

Pediatric Drug Labels

Before 1997 many drugs were released without pediatric dosage information. Earlier FDA regulations requested that drug manufacturers add more complete pediatric dosing information on their drug products, but this was voluntary. In 1997, with a concern that more medical treatments should be available for children, the FDA required pediatric-use information for drugs that might offer improved therapy for children as compared to existing drug therapies. The difference now is that this information is required so physicians and other prescribers and health care providers have the most current scientific information available for making appropriate medical decisions related to safe pediatric drug use (FDA, 1999).

Critical questions that need answers to ensure safe pediatric drug use include the following:

- Are there data about the pediatric use of this drug as the result of well-designed, controlled studies?
- If so, what was the dosage and method of administration?
- What was the age of the youngest child or infant who received the drug?
- Were any side or adverse effects reported? What was the frequency of such effects?

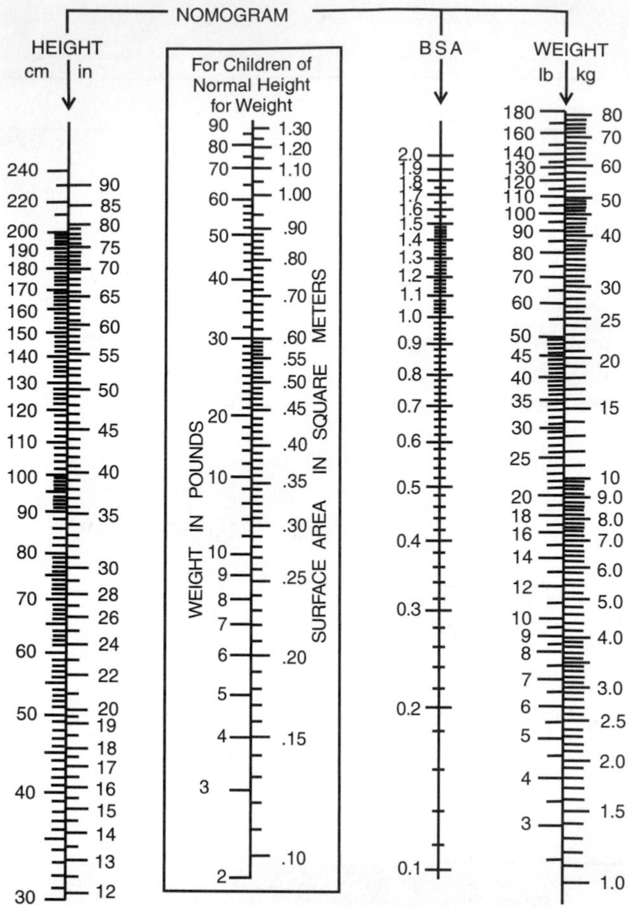

Figure 7-2 BSA is indicated where the straight line that connects height (on the left) and weight (on the right) intersects the BSA column or, if client is above average size, from weight alone (enclosed area). (Modified from data of E. Boyd by C. D. West; from Behrman, R. E., & Vaughan, V. C. [Eds.] [2000]. *Nelson's textbook of pediatrics* [16th Ed.]. Philadelphia: W.B. Saunders.)

(AHFS) Drug Information, pediatric drug handbooks, or consultation with a pharmacist.

BOX 7-4

Drug Administration Guidelines for Children

1. Parents are often good sources of information about successful methods or vehicles of giving medications to their children.
2. Try to avoid putting medications in essential foods such as milk, cereal, or orange juice, because the child may refuse to accept that food in the future.
3. Never underestimate a child's reactions. The taste of the medication may not need to be disguised.
4. A sip of cold fruit juice, ice chips, a frozen fruit bar, or a mint-flavored substance before and after the administration of an unpalatable medicine may effectively dull its taste.
5. Sugarless vehicles should be used to disguise the taste of medications given to children who have diabetes or are following a ketogenic diet.
6. Jam and syrup are ideal for suspending drugs that do not dissolve easily in water.
7. Because fruit syrups are usually acidic, they should not be used for medicines that react in an acid medium (e.g., sodium bicarbonate, soluble barbiturates, and penicillin).
8. Elixirs have an alcohol base that, when undiluted, may cause the child either to refuse them or to cough and choke; they may also cause a drug-drug interaction. Small amounts of water added to elixirs of phenobarbital or chloral hydrate occasionally help.
9. Nursing time can be saved by recording the most successful method of administering medications and pertinent nursing orders on the child's care plan. This notation also saves the child frustration, fear, and anxiety.

Nursing Management

Medication Administration in Children

Although the previously discussed rules have been devised for converting adult dosage schedules to schedules for infants and children, it must be emphasized that *no rules or charts are adequate to guarantee safety of dosage at any age, particularly in the neonate.* No method takes into account all variables, particularly individual tolerance differences. Astute, accurate nursing observations of how individual children react to drugs can assist in monitoring drugs and dosages.

Administering medications to infants and children is both challenging and frustrating. Giving injections skillfully will enhance safety and help to gain a child's cooperation. A sound knowledge of growth and development also provides the nurse with information about how a child might be approached, whether reasoning will help or hinder the process, and whether assistance will be needed. The principles of safe administration of medication apply to all age-groups, but children differ from adults, and the nurse has added responsibilities when administering a medication to a child (Box 7-4).

Ideally, a child will cooperate more readily with a nurse once a positive relationship has been established. The child may also more easily accept the discomforts of injections and of some oral medications from a nurse who is associated with daily hygiene, feeding, holding, play, and happy times. In addition, the nurse will feel less guilty when the child associates the nurse with pleasure and comfort most of the time and with discomfort only when it is necessary in order for the child to get well.

When a child is afraid or anxious, his or her natural response is to strike out at the frustration or avoid it. By accepting this behavior as a natural response, the nurse will be able to deal with it and to be honest when a medication or procedure will be unpleasant or painful. Truthful explanations are essential with children. They have a right to an explanation of any procedure that concerns them. The timing and type of explanation should be geared to the child's ability to perceive and understand. For the child 2 years of age or younger very simple explanations such as "I have some medicine for you to drink" or "I have an injection to give you, and it will hurt a little" are sufficient. Young children may be less resistant to injectable medications if a parent holds and comforts them. In an ambulatory care setting, it is best to have the child all dressed and ready to leave before administering immunizations and other injectables. A brief exposure of the appropriate injection site to determine landmarks, a quick injection, and then an exit from the facility will decrease the child's association of the discomfort of an injection with the clinical setting.

Long explanations to children under 5 years of age do little more than prolong the anticipation and increase anxiety or fear. Telling 4-year-old children to stop kicking, hitting, or performing any other avoidance behavior only conveys to them that they are not understood and that they will receive little or no help with their feelings of frustration about being medicated. Providing the preschool-age child opportunities at play (e.g., to give a doll an "injection" [empty syringe without a needle] or "drops") affords an important outlet and allows the child to work through the trauma of the experience.

Many children are courageous, or like to be considered so, and therefore appealing to their courage is sometimes effective. Children 4 years old or over may choose to hold their own medicine cup or drink unassisted and to take pills from the container without any assistance from the nurse. Children of this age are motivated by social reinforcers, such as being praised for their cooperation or being told that "your job is to stay very still," which enhance their self-esteem and feelings of competence. Helping the child to identify what he or she can do during the procedure will help him or her to cope. Because of the sense of achievement that follows, children may want to save the medicine cups to show their parents. Box 7-5 lists developmental perspectives for administering medications.

■ **Oral Medications.** Success in administering oral medications usually requires a kind but firm approach and a positive attitude. Certainty that the child will take the medicine should be reflected in the nurse's choice of words and tone of voice. The nurse might say, "Jimmy, it's time to take your yellow medicine" or "Do you want to take your pill now or with your Jell-O?" Such statements indicate that the child is expected to cooperate and also allow him or her some control over the situation. An unwise approach that conveys doubt on the nurse's part might be "I have your yellow pill, Jimmy. Will you take it for me, please?"

Nurses should be aware of how a medicine tastes so that they can answer questions such as, "Does it taste bad?" or "Will it burn my mouth?" A helpful reply would be, "It tastes like cherry to me. Tell me what it tastes like to you." Often the child will accept the suggestion to taste and find out. However, if the medication has an unpleasant taste, attempting to deceive or lie is as futile and destructive with a child as it is with an adult.

Medications that have a disagreeable taste should be disguised if at all possible. Small amounts of syrup, jam, fruit, and some fruit juices are suitable sweet vehicles for less palatable drugs. Some pills can be crushed and suspended in small amounts of these substances as long as the two substances are compatible. Infants and children swallow many liquid medications more readily if mixed with a sweet substance or diluted with a small amount of water. (If large amounts of water or other substances are used and the child refuses to take all of the mixture, it is difficult to estimate how much medication the child received.) Fortunately, many drugs are available as palatable syrups or in a suspension form well suited for administration to infants and children. Suspensions should be thoroughly agitated to ensure that doses are not offered in unequal concentrations.

To prevent aspiration, exercise caution when giving oral medications to children. Medications must be given to infants slowly and in small amounts to avoid choking. Liquid medications may be administered via a nipple, plastic medicine cup, plastic dropper, or plastic syringe without the needle. Water should be rinsed through the inside of these containers *first* to prevent the medication from sticking, which can cause an inaccurate dose. Glass cups, droppers, or syringes should be avoided because of the obvious danger of them breaking in the child's mouth. A dropper or syringe is best suited for placing a liquid medication along one side of an infant's tongue. Older infants and toddlers seem to prefer taking their medications from a plastic medicine cup. Children are less likely to aspirate the medication if they are held or placed in a sitting position than if they lie on their backs.

When administering a medication with a dropper or syringe, the nurse may purse the infant's lips with one hand to keep the medicine from running out of the mouth. Droppers and syringes used for medication should be kept clean, should be reserved for only one client's use, and should be rinsed or washed before being returned to the medication bottle.

If the child refuses to cooperate even after being given explanations and encouragement, the nurse may need to ask whether the child will take the medication alone or will need the nurse to give it. Physical coercion is seldom necessary; if used, it should be mild, quick, and firm, because aspiration is a danger. The nurse must not combine force with anger or resort to force when one nurse has been unable to administer the medication. Careful consideration should be given to factors such as the following: Why does the child resist? Does the child disapprove of only one nurse? Have past experiences with medications given at home or in the hospital frightened the child? Will forcing a medication cause a struggle that will negate the effects of a drug given for sedation? If mild restraint is necessary, explain to the child that this form of treatment is necessary. The child will not cooperate if force is seen as a punishment for an inability to cooperate; often the child loses confidence in all personnel.

BOX 7-5

Developmental Perspectives for Administering Medications

General Interventions

Always come prepared for the procedure with all necessary equipment and assistance.

For in-hospital administration, ask the parent and/or child if the parent should or should not remain for the procedure.

Assess comfort methods appropriate for preadministration and postadministration.

Infants

Perform the procedure swiftly, then offer comfort measures (e.g., parent holding, rocking, cuddling, soothing).

Allow self-comforting measures (e.g., use of pacifier, fingers in mouth, self-movement).

Toddlers

Offer a brief, concrete explanation of procedure, and then perform it.

Accept aggressive behavior (within reasonable limits) as a healthy response.

Provide comfort measures immediately after the procedure (e.g., touch, holding).

Help the child to understand the treatment and his or her feelings through playing with puppets or hospital equipment, such as a syringe and water.

Provide for ways to release aggression with play, such as hammering or water play.

Preschoolers

Offer a brief, concrete explanation.

Provide comfort measures after the procedure (e.g., touch, holding).

Accept aggressive responses and provide outlets for them.

Make use of magical thinking; use "ointments" or "special medicines" to make the discomfort go away.

The role of the parent is very important for comfort and understanding.

School-Aged Children

Explain the procedure, allowing for some control over body and situation.

Provide comfort measures.

Explore feelings and concepts through therapeutic play, drawings of own body and self in the hospital, and the use of books and realistic hospital equipment.

Set appropriate behavior limits (e.g., okay to cry or scream but not to bite).

Provide activities for releasing aggression and anger.

Use this opportunity to teach about the relationship between the medication and body function and structure (e.g., what a seizure is and how medication helps prevent the seizure).

Offer the complete picture (e.g., need to take medication, relax with deep breaths, medication will help prevent pain).

Adolescents

Prepare in advance for the procedure.

Allow for expression in a way that does not cause the adolescent to "lose face," such as giving the adolescent time alone after the procedure and giving him or her time to discuss the discomfort if he or she wants to verbalize feelings.

Explore current concepts of self, hospitalization, and illness and correct any misconceptions.

Encourage self-expression, individuality, and self-care.

Encourage participation in the procedure to the extent agreed on in advance. Increased participation should be discussed after the procedure.

Modified from Blaber, M. (1990). Related to nursing intervention in pain. *Newington Children's Hospital Manual for Global Pediatric Nursing Assessment* (unpublished).

■ **Topical Medications.** Children have a large skin surface area in proportion to total body weight. Their skin, especially the skin of neonates, is particularly thin and permeable and has limited protective oil.

Although adults absorb much more medication through intact skin than was previously believed, the child is at even more risk for systemic medication administration. The discovery that hexachlorophene can cause encephalopathy in newborns and that topically applied boric acid can cause systemic poisoning testifies to the hazard of applying drugs to children's skin, especially for contact that is prolonged or is over broken skin areas. Plain soap and water, not medicated dressings, may be the preferred treatment for abrasions or open lesions.

■ **Subcutaneous Injections.** There are wide variations in the amounts of subcutaneous fat in children. Neonates have a proportionately smaller amount, with body fat increasing slightly to 23% by 1 year of age. From 1 to 5 years of age the amount of body fat drops to between 8% and 12%; it climbs to approximately 20% when the child reaches 10 years of age. Lipid-soluble drugs have an affinity for fat tissue; less subcutaneous fat means that lower dosages of fat-soluble drugs (e.g., diazepam and barbiturates) are necessary to maintain blood levels. In addition, less subcutaneous tissue for injections may be available. An alternate route may need to be selected—oral, IM, or IV.

■ **Intramuscular Injections.** The principles and techniques of administrating IM injections in children are similar to those for adults.

Most authorities believe that the risk of sciatic nerve injury is too great to warrant the use of the gluteal site for administration. The sciatic nerve is the largest nerve in the body; its normal pathway is the hollow midway between the ischial tuberosity and the greater trochanter, and it is covered by the gluteus maximus muscle. This pathway varies a great deal from individual to individual. In addition, the small size of the gluteal mass in the infant or neonate and the potential neurotoxicity of many drugs enhance the possibility of iatrogenic trauma secondary to IM injections. Trauma of this type is the leading cause of sciatic neuropathy in infancy. A lesion at this level of the sciatic nerve is usually tragically associated with marked permanent disability.

The younger the child, the less muscle tissue available for IM injections. If repeated injections are necessary, the available sites may become overused, inflamed, or dystrophic; the nurse is therefore required to make a concerted effort to develop systematic plans for rotating sites and inform the rest of the staff about them, or to consult with the prescriber about changing to an oral or IV dosage form. The vastus lateralis muscle is the site of choice for IM injections in children under 3 years of age because it is well developed at birth (see Chapter 5 and Figure 5-7, *C*). The ventrogluteal site is preferred for children over 3 years of age who have been walking for a year or two (see Figure 5-7, *B*). The dorsogluteal muscles should not be used for injections in children under 4 to 6 years of age if other IM sites are available, nor should they be used for any injections until the younger child has been walking for at least 1 year. The deltoid muscle is not used for children under 5 years of age because of its underdevelopment.

For injection into the left gluteal muscles, the thumb is placed on the trochanter, and the middle finger is placed on the iliac crest. The index finger is placed midway between the thumb and middle finger, and this indicates the area safe for injection. Infants should receive no more than 0.5 mL in each injection site; small children can tolerate a volume of 1 mL at each site. Instead of holding the skin taut, as for adults, the muscle mass should be pinched up to prevent the needle from striking deeper-lying structures such as nerves, bones, or blood vessels. The IM injection is made at a 90-degree angle to the top of the massed flesh. Preferred needle sizes for pediatric IM injections are 25- to 27-gauge and ½ to 1 inch in length. A 21- or 22-gauge needle may be preferred when administering a viscous medication such as procaine penicillin.

In the interest of safety, the child should usually be restrained for an injection, and the injection is given rapidly.

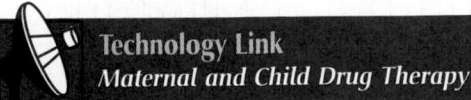

Technology Link
Maternal and Child Drug Therapy

CD-ROM Resources

Mosby's Pediatric Patient Teaching Guides (ISBN 1-556-64456-6)

Mosby, Inc., 11830 Westline Industrial Drive, St. Louis, MO 63146; (800) 426-4545; www.mosby.com.

Video Resources

Neonatal Emergencies, Series #3, Video Package (Mosby), ISBN 0-8151-2370-1
- Video 1: *Respiratory Emergencies,* ISBN 0-8151-2372-8
- Video 2: *Cardiovascular Emergencies,* ISBN 0-8151-2372-6
- Video 3: *Gastrointestinal Emergencies,* ISBN 0-8151-2376-0

Neonatal Infectious Disease, Series #2, Video Package (Mosby), ISBN 0-8151-2357-4
- Video 1: *Bacterial Sepsis,* ISBN 0-8151-2358-2
- Video 2: *Meningitis,* ISBN 0-8151-2359-0
- Video 3: *Perinatal Infections,* ISBN 0-8151-2360-4

Whaley & Wong's Pediatric Nursing Videotape Series (Mosby), ISBN 0-8151-6943-4
- *Communicating with Families and Children,* ISBN 0-8151-7050-5
- *Pain Assessment and Management,* ISBN 0-8151-7052-1
- *Growth and Development,* ISBN 0-8151-7053-X
- *Medications and Injections,* ISBN 0-8151-7055-6
- *Family-Centered Care,* ISBN 0-8151-7056-4
- *Pediatric Assessment,* ISBN 0-8151-7057-2

Web Resources

A Guide to Children's Medication (American Academy of Pediatrics) (www.aap.org/family/medications.htm/)

This site has a guide to children's medications—prescription and over-the-counter—the most common children's medications, how to read labels, and tips on the administration of various drug therapies.

ADP—Alcohol, Other Drugs and Pregnancy (www.adf.org.au/adp/index.html/)

This site from the Australian Drug Foundation covers pregnancy and drugs, such as alcohol, tobacco, cannabis, analgesics, LSD, and other drugs.

About Kids Health (www.kidshealth.org)

This is the largest and most visited site on the Web, providing approved health information for children, teens, and parents. It provides accurate, up-to-date information about medications and children in its medical library.

For additional WebLinks, a free subscription to the "Mosby/Saunders ePharmacology Update" newsletter, and more, go to mosby.com/MERLIN/McKenry/.

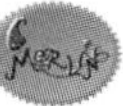

Two or more persons should be available for children over 4 years of age, even children who promise to "hold still." An extra sterile needle may be carried in a pocket in case the first needle becomes contaminated when a child moves unexpectedly. Asking the child to wiggle the toes may distract his or her attention from the injection. Because children enjoy trying out each other's beds, the identifying wristband must be checked to ensure proper client identification before giving each medication.

▪ Rectal Administration. Several drugs, such as sedatives, aspirin, and antiemetics, are available in suppository form. The rectal route is often advised when oral administration is difficult or contraindicated. Many children perceive use of the rectal route as an extreme invasion of their bodies or anticipate pain as a result. It may help to let them participate (e.g., to insert the suppository). Suppositories made with a cocoa butter base melt rapidly at normal body temperature, releasing the drug for absorption. After inserting a suppository into an infant, the buttocks should be held or taped together for 5 to 10 minutes to relieve pressure on the anal sphincter and thereby help ensure retention and absorption of the medication. Infants and children with diarrhea may easily expel suppositories with explosive stools. Similarly, if a child has constipation or a rectum full of stool, the suppository will be surrounded with stool and has little chance of being absorbed.

Health care professionals often divide suppository doses by cutting them. This is dangerous practice because all of the medication might be contained in one area of the suppository. If divided doses must be administered, the pharmacist should be contacted for alternate product advice and guidance.

▪ Nose Drops, Eardrops, and Eyedrops. Because of the danger of aspiration, aqueous preparations of nose drops are the only safe preparations to use. Many nose drop preparations contain vasoconstrictors, and prolonged or excessive use may be harmful. Infants are nose breathers, and nasal congestion will inhibit their sucking. For this reason, nose drops, if necessary, should be instilled 20 minutes to ½ hour before feedings. The following procedures are used when instilling *nose drops* (Figure 7-3):

1. Hold the infant in your arm and allow the head to fall back over the edge of your arm, or place a small pillow under the shoulders and allow the head to fall back over the edge of the pillow.
2. Place your free arm so the forearm is around the far side of the child's head, stabilizing the head between your forearm and your body. Use your hand to stabilize the arms and hands.
3. With your free hand you can instill the prescribed drops with minimum struggle and maximum accuracy.

Before the initial administration of a course of therapy with *eardrops,* assess whether the child has excessive cerumen. If so, it may be necessary to consult with the prescriber about removing it with cerumen softeners or irrigation before instilling the eardrops. Instilling eardrops requires knowledge of anatomic structure, because the shape of the auditory canal of a young child differs from that of an adult. Figure 7-4 illustrates the administration of eardrops. After instillation, gently massaging the area immediately anterior to the ear will facilitate the entry of the drops deeper into the ear canal.

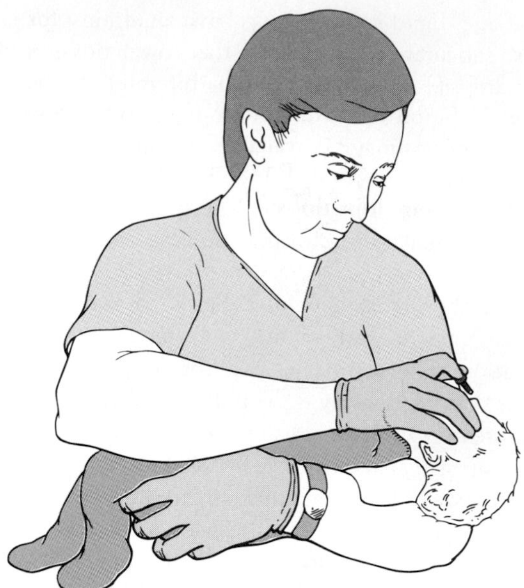

Figure 7-3 Administration of nose drops.

Eyedrop instillation in children is performed in the same way as with adults except that the head may be stabilized by an assistant. Depending on the child's age, he or she may be asked to look up so that the cornea reflex is diminished, and the dropper should be introduced from the side. The lower lid is retracted, and the drops are instilled into the conjunctival sac. Many eyedrops cause a burning sensation for a few seconds, so if both eyes are to be medicated it is wise to do the second instillation quickly—before the child begins to blink and tear as a reaction to the burning sensation in the first eye. Mild pressure for 30 seconds over the inner canthus next to the nose prevents premature drainage of the medication away from the eye (see Box 43-1).

Aqueous preparations of nose drops, eardrops, and eyedrops may support the growth of bacteria and fungi. For this reason small volumes of such medications are ordered and should be used for only *one* individual (not shared by family members). The dropper (especially eyedroppers) should not be permitted to become contaminated by touching anything but the medication. To avoid forming a medium for microbiologic growth, the dropper should never be inverted so that medication or water runs into the rubber bulb. A dropper from one medication should not be used to measure and administer another type of medication because droppers are not standardized—not all droppers are manufactured to deliver drops of the same volume. The viscosity of drugs also varies, which affects drop size.

Eyedrops and eardrops are more comfortably tolerated if they are warmed (if not contraindicated) before instillation. To do this, warm water is run over the side of the bottle

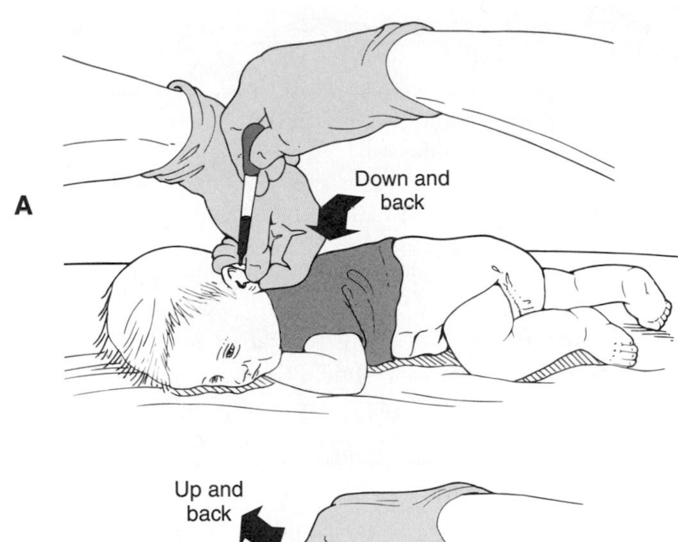

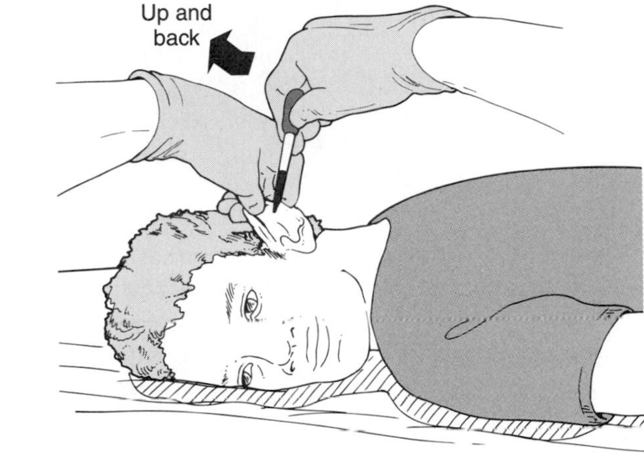

Figure 7-4 Administration of eardrops. The infant or child is positioned on the side of the unaffected ear. **A,** To administer eardrops to infants and children under 3 years of age, the nurse pulls the pinna down and back. **B,** To administer eardrops to children older than 3 years (and to adults), the nurse gently pulls the pinna up and back. The nurse should stabilize his or her hand on the client's head for safety and instill the prescribed number of drops. The drops are directed toward the ear canal to avoid hitting the tympanic membrane, which can cause pain. The client should remain in position for 5 to 10 minutes. To prevent nausea or vertigo, otic drugs should be warmed before being instilled.

BOX 7-6

IV Drug Administration in Children

1. IV drug therapy should be used only if other channels of drug administration are impractical. Pediatric nurses who are skilled in giving medications to children via other routes may be able to influence prescribers' decisions regarding successful routes of drug administration.
2. For small infants a scalp vein or a superficial vein of the wrist, hand, foot, or arm may be most convenient and most easily stabilized. Scalp veins are the most frequent sites for infant infusions; because these veins have no valves, infusions may be in either direction. Older children may receive infusions through any accessible vein.
3. An IV infusion or injection that is too rapid may cause "speed shock," with a rapid fall in blood pressure, respiratory irregularity, blood incoagulability, and even death. Preventive measures include use of the minidropper (note that the milliliter per hour in the order translates to the drops per minute with this tubing), calibrated volume control chambers, and infusion pumps.
4. Total parenteral nutrition (TPN) solutions are usually infused into the vena cava or innominate or subclavian veins approached via the external or internal jugular veins. The inferior vena cava is occasionally entered via the femoral vein.
5. Once a drug is injected intravenously, the action of the drug is relatively irreversible.
6. Drugs must be properly diluted. Too much emphasis cannot be placed on this caution. **Give the smallest possible dose at the slowest possible rate.**

without the label, or the bottle is immersed in some warm water in a medicine cup. Carrying the bottle in a pocket for half an hour or so also takes the chill off the drops.

■ **Intravenous Medications.** The use of IV drug therapy is widespread on most pediatric services for several reasons. In children with vomiting and diarrhea, medications given by mouth may be vomited, and precious time in drug management is lost. Because these children may have poor absorption of drugs and fluids as a result of dehydration or peripheral vascular collapse, drugs administered via the IM route may be equally ineffective (see the Case Study box on p. 144). Premature infants are at risk for necrotizing enterocolitis (NEC) and death when administered feedings or oral drugs that have an osmolality greater than that of body fluids. Elixirs of theophylline, phenobarbital, calcium, digoxin, and dexamethasone have osmolalities 10 times greater than body fluids and have been implicated in causing NEC, and analysis shows that the contained additives actually raise the medication's osmolality. Therefore it may be preferable to give premature or physiologically distressed neonates certain high-osmolality drugs by IV administration.

The suggestions in Box 7-6 may be helpful to pediatric nurses responsible for the administration of IV drugs (see also Chapter 5). Most older children may be given fluids or drugs intravenously following the same principles and techniques used for adults. The younger and smaller the child, the narrower the margin for error.

Neonates, infants, and children must be adequately restrained so the infusion needle or catheter is not dislodged or pulled out once it is in place. The following hints may be helpful to the nurse caring for a client receiving IV therapy (Figure 7-5):

1. The needle or catheter should be fixed with plastic tape.

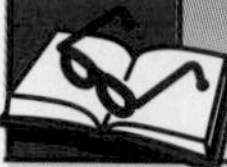

Case Study *Obstructive Airway Disease in a Child*

Timmy, a 4-year-old child with reversible obstructive airway disease, is admitted to the emergency department with bilateral wheezing and moderate respiratory distress. He has received two aerosol treatments but continues to be in moderate distress with continued wheezing. An IV bolus of aminophylline has been ordered to be followed by a continuous IV infusion of aminophylline.

1. What factors should be considered in selecting the IV route for drug administration in the child?
2. What measures should the nurse use to maintain the integrity of the IV infusion?
3. Timmy is to be discharged on oral theophylline. The appropriate dose of oral theophylline for a child Timmy's age is 16 mg/kg. Calculate the dose for Timmy, who weighs 42 pounds. Convert his weight in pounds to kilograms.
4. Given that Timmy is developmentally appropriate for his chronologic age, what should the nurse teach Timmy's parents about administering this oral medication?

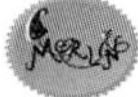

For answer guidelines, go to mosby.com/MERLIN/McKenry/.

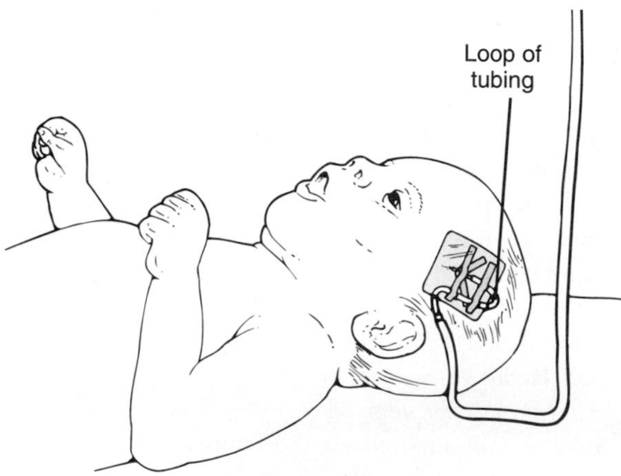

Figure 7-5 Securing a scalp vein infusion for infants.

2. Securing a loop of tubing directly above the needle to the tape relieves tension from the needle should sudden movement pull it.
3. Most children move about or are restless. Therefore, if the IV site is in the arm, it is necessary to support the limb with a padded arm board and immobilize the site of IV therapy. Support should extend to the joints above and below the site (with arm boards or IV boards).
4. If the infusion bottle is too high, the pressure in the vein increases, causing fluid to seep into the surrounding tissues.
5. Specific classifications of medications must be administered over a specific time period and require the use of an electronic medication pump or infusion device.

■ **Other Factors Influencing Drug Dosages.** Again, the dosage of most agents is related to the child's age, weight, and height. A child's body systems grow and develop at varying rates, which makes for unpredictable primary and secondary effects in pediatric medication administration. One example of secondary effects specific to children is discoloration of teeth and depression of enamel growth with the administration of tetracycline liquid medications in children under 8 years of age. Although this adverse reaction is well documented, the drug is still being prescribed for this age-group, according to the FDA. Children receiving long-term adrenocortical steroids experience impaired skeletal growth.

Individual variations are noted in children's responses to digitalis, insulin, opiates, and oral enzyme products; doses require careful titration. Paradoxic responses are noted with a few drugs; the responses may be directly opposite to those expected in adults. Excessive reactivity to atropine by infants may be related to immaturity of the central nervous system (CNS). Because of the complex medicolegal issues involved in experimentation on children, many drugs that are safe and effective for adults have not been tested for use with children, nor have dosages been established.

SUMMARY

Nursing management of the administration of medications to clients of different age-groups requires that the nurse be knowledgeable about growth and development and about the various effects of pharmaceutical agents on clients of different ages. Understanding the rationale behind these effects will help the nurse to administer medications safely and to evaluate client responses appropriately, regardless of the client's age. Childbearing clients, neonates, infants, and children have unique needs related to the accurate and safe administration of medications—needs that are based on their unique physiologic and psychosocial development.

Critical Thinking Questions

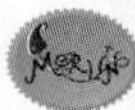

1. Select one drug, such as phenytoin or warfarin, and discuss the potential risks to the fetus or breastfeeding child in relation to needed benefits to the mother.
2. Ms. Leverett, a nursing student, is assigned to care for Sally, a 3-year-old, and Loretta, an 8-year-old, who are sharing the same hospital room. From a

developmental perspective, how will her approach to the two children differ when it comes to administering medications?

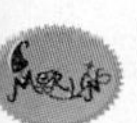

Collaborative Learning Activities

For Collaborative Learning Activities, go to mosby.com/MERLIN/McKenry/.

BIBLIOGRAPHY

American Hospital Formulary Service. (1999). *AHFS drug information '99*. Bethesda, MD: American Society of Hospital Pharmacists.

Anderson, K.N., Anderson, L.E., & Glanze, W.D. (Eds.) (1998). *Mosby's medical, nursing & allied health dictionary* (5th ed.). St Louis: Mosby.

Banta-Wright, S. (1997). Minimizing infant exposure to and risks from medications while breastfeeding. *Journal of Perinatal & Neonatal Nursing, 11*(2), 71-86.

Bobak, I.M., Lowdermilk, D.L., & Jensen, M.Dd. (1995). *Essentials of maternity nursing* (4th ed.). St Louis: Mosby.

Briggs, G.G. (1995). Teratogenicity and drugs in breast milk. In L.Y. Young, & M.A. Koda-Kimble (Eds.), *Applied therapeutics: The clinical use of drugs* (6th ed.). Vancouver: Applied Therapeutics.

Chi, J. (1992). FDA tries again for improved pediatric labels: Will it work? *Hospital Pharmacy Report, 6*(12), 9.

Drug Facts and Comparisons. (2000). St Louis: Facts and Comparisons.

Food and Drug Administration. (1999). FDA proposes to require pediatric data prior to drug and biologic product approvals. (http://www.hhs.gov/news/press/1997pres/970813b.html [4/26/1999]).

Hall, W.C., Talbert, R.L. & Ereshefsky, L. (1990). Cocaine abuse and its treatment. *Pharmacotherapy, 10*(1), 47.

Jennings, J.C. (1996). Guide to medication use in pregnant and breastfeeding women. *Pharmacy Practice News, 23*(4), 10.

Katzung, B.G. (1998). *Basic & clinical pharmacology* (7th ed.). Stamford, CT: Appleton & Lange.

Keene, E.F. (1993). Another way to administer antiepileptic medications in infants and children. *MCN, 18*(6), 270.

Levy, M. & Spino, M. (1993). Neonatal withdrawal syndrome: Associated drugs and pharmacologic management. *Pharmacotherapy, 13*(3), 202-211.

Pray, W.S. (1993). Infant formulas and nutrition. *US Pharmacist, 18*(3), 29.

Sagraves, R., Kamper, C., & Doerr, J. (1996). Infant formula products. In T.R. Covington (Ed.), *Handbook of nonprescription drugs* (11th ed.). Washington, D.C.: American Pharmaceutical Association.

Schou, M. (1998). Treating recurrent affective disorders during and after pregnancy. What can be taken safely? *Drug Safety, 18*(2), 143-152.

United States Pharmacopeia Dispensing Information (USP DI): Drug information for the health care professional (19th ed.). (1999). Rockville, MD: United States Pharmacopeial Convention.

Wong, D.L. (1997). *Whaley & Wong's Essentials of pediatric nursing* (5th ed.). St Louis: Mosby.

8 Drug Therapy for Older Adults

Chapter Focus

Older adults represent the fastest growing population in the United States and Canada. An understanding of the physiologic changes that occur with the aging process will help the nurse in safely administering, teaching, and monitoring drug regimens. The goal of drug treatment is to develop strategies to treat or alter a disease process and, if possible, to restore function to older adults. Many of the medication-related problems reported in older adults are preventable, and the nurse and all health care professionals play a vital role in preventing these adverse drug effects.

Learning Objectives

1. Discuss factors that promote drug misuse in older adults.
2. Describe the alterations in pharmacokinetics and pharmacodynamics related to aging.
3. Identify the risk factors for ineffective management of the medication regimen by the older adult.
4. Manage effectively the administration of medications for older adults.

Key Terms

polypharmacy, p. 147

Although the older adult population represents only approximately 13% of the population in the United States and Canada today, the following has been reported:

- They consume 37% of all prescribed drugs and 50% of all over-the-counter (OTC) medications (Trends & Analysis, 1995; Why Senior Care Pharmacy?, 1999).
- Persons over 60 years of age represent 51% of the deaths and 39% of the hospitalizations that result from adverse drug reactions (ADRs).
- Older adults experience more drug-related incidents than other age-groups (25% of all admissions from a nursing home setting to a hospital are drug related) (Trends & Analysis, 1995).
- Approximately 28% of all hospitalizations for older adults are the result of an ADR.
- In older adults receiving five or more different medications, 36% have an ADR, 63% need prescriber intervention, 10% result in an emergency department visit, 11% require admission to a hospital and—the most important statistic of all—95% of the ADRs were predictable and therefore preventable (Why Senior Care Pharmacy?, 1999).

It has been projected that more than 20% of the population will be 65 years or older by the year 2030 (Trends & Analysis, 1995). Because older adults are the most rapidly increasing segment of the population, an understanding of age-related alterations in pharmacokinetics and pharmacodynamics is necessary. The increased incidence of chronic diseases in older adults often results in an increase in the number of prescriptions, OTC medications, and home remedies (prescribed or self-selected). The age of specialization has in some ways added to this problem, with multiple health care providers usually prescribing a variety of medications—often without discontinuing the drugs the client is currently taking. This practice, the indiscriminate use of numerous medications concurrently, is often referred to as **polypharmacy** (Jones, 1997).

Polypharmacy can be a dangerous practice that may increase the risk of drug interactions and adverse reactions and the need for, or prolonging of, hospitalization. Jinks and Fuerst (1995) report that, in 1985, ADRs in older adults resulted in 243,000 hospitalizations, 32,000 hip fractures, and 163,000 cases of drug-induced mental alterations or impairments. Although the magnitude of problems caused by polypharmacy is enormous, it is often overlooked as being the causative factor. It is important for health care providers to realize that the vast majority of undesirable drug effects resulting from polypharmacy are *preventable.*

To minimize the risks associated with the use of multiple medications and ADRs in this population, the health care provider needs to provide continuous drug regimen monitoring, with a primary goal of reducing or eliminating inappropriate medications and improving the client's quality of life.

PHYSIOLOGIC CHANGES OF AGING

Older adults undergo a variety of physiologic changes that may increase their sensitivity to drugs and drug-induced disease (Figure 8-1). The loss of body weight in many older adults may require initiating therapy at a lower adult dosage or reevaluating dosages of medications already in use. The criterion for dosages should be shifted from age to weight. Even though some older adults weigh no more than the average large child, and some weigh a lot less, they are prescribed the larger "adult" dosages; this practice is not correct.

Pharmacokinetics are altered in older adults because reduced gastric acid and slowed gastric motility results in unpredictable rates of drug dissolution and absorption (Box 8-1). Changes in absorption may occur when acid production decreases and alters the absorption of weakly acidic drugs such as barbiturates. However, few studies of drug absorption have shown clinically significant changes occurring with advanced age.

Changes in body composition have been noted in older adults and include an increased proportion of body fat and decreased total body water, plasma volume, and extracellular fluid. An increased proportion of body fat increases the body's ability to store fat-soluble compounds such as phenothiazines and barbiturates and thus increases the accumulation of those drugs. Reduced lean body mass

BOX 8-1

Potential Altered Pharmacokinetics in Older Adults

Absorption

Increase in gastric pH
Altered gastric emptying and intestinal blood flow
Decrease in first-pass metabolism in the liver

Distribution

Altered body composition (decrease in lean body mass, increase in adipose [fat] stores)
Decrease in total body water
Decrease in serum albumin
Decrease in blood flow and cardiac output

Metabolism

Decrease in phase I metabolic reactions
Decrease in enzymatic activity (cytochrome P-450 system)
Decrease in hepatic blood flow and drug metabolism

Excretion

Decrease in renal function (with most persons, a loss of 10% of renal function per decade after age 50)

Modified from Trends & Analysis (1995). Long-term care of elderly patients: Chronic disease comorbidity and other considerations. *Consultant Pharmacist, 10*(6), 583-593.

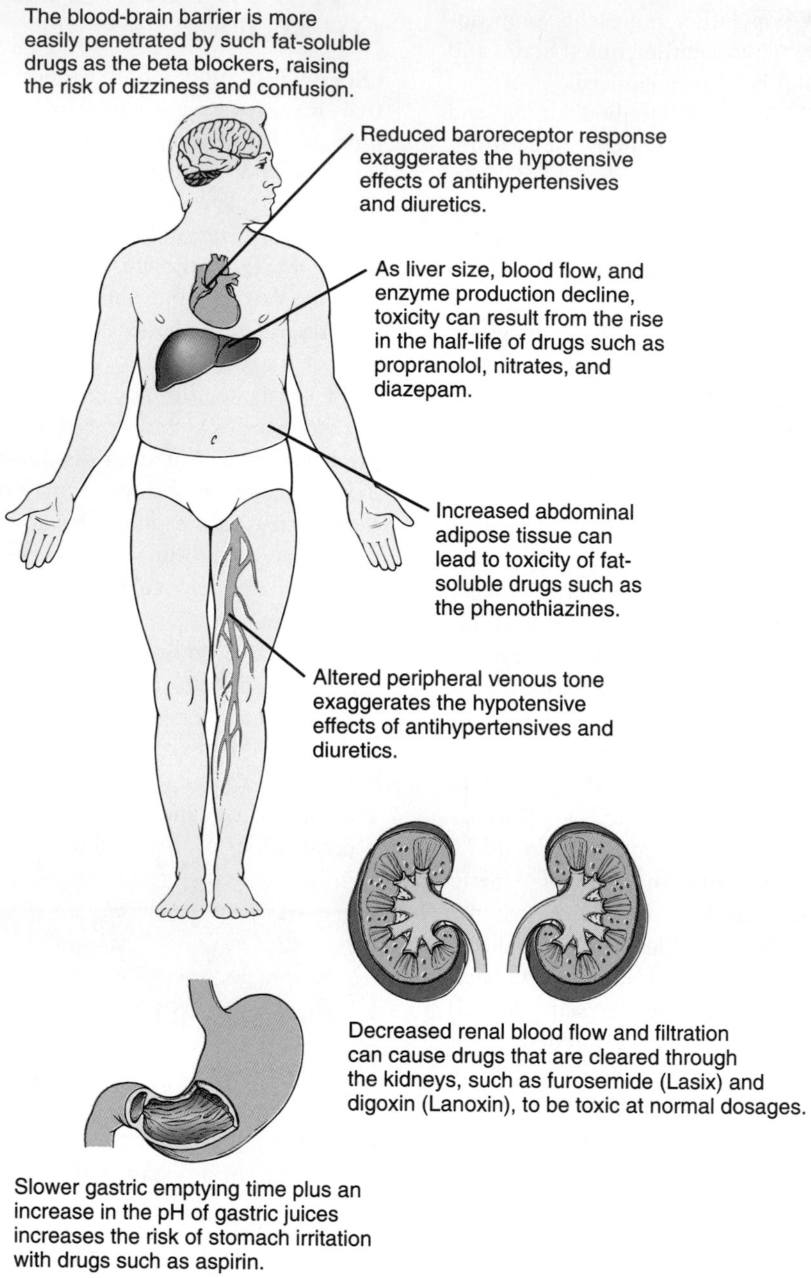

The blood-brain barrier is more easily penetrated by such fat-soluble drugs as the beta blockers, raising the risk of dizziness and confusion.
Reduced baroreceptor response exaggerates the hypotensive effects of antihypertensives and diuretics.
As liver size, blood flow, and enzyme production decline, toxicity can result from the rise in the half-life of drugs such as propranolol, nitrates, and diazepam.
Increased abdominal adipose tissue can lead to toxicity of fat-soluble drugs such as the phenothiazines.
Altered peripheral venous tone exaggerates the hypotensive effects of antihypertensives and diuretics.
Decreased renal blood flow and filtration can cause drugs that are cleared through the kidneys, such as furosemide (Lasix) and digoxin (Lanoxin), to be toxic at normal dosages.
Slower gastric emptying time plus an increase in the pH of gastric juices increases the risk of stomach irritation with drugs such as aspirin.

Figure 8-1 How physiologic changes increase sensitivity to drugs and drug-induced disease.

affects drug distribution by decreasing the volume in which the drug circulates, thereby causing higher peak levels. The risk of toxicity with hydrophilic or water-soluble drugs increases as total body water decreases. Digoxin (Lanoxin), theophylline (Theo-Dur), and the aminoglycosides are examples of hydrophilic drugs that may accumulate and result in an adverse reaction or toxicity.

Decreased serum albumin for highly protein-bound drugs may lead to increased amounts of free drug in the circulation. Warfarin (Coumadin), phenytoin (Dilantin), and diazepam (Valium) are a few examples of highly protein-bound drugs.

Drug metabolism in the liver is also affected by aging. Medications that undergo phase I metabolism (reduction, oxidation, hydroxylation, or demethylation) may have a decreased metabolism, whereas phase II (glucuronidation, acetylation, conjugation) is not affected by aging. Thus nitrates, barbiturates, propranolol (Inderal), and lidocaine may have decreased hepatic metabolism in older adults (Jinks & Fuerst, 1995).

Disorders common to older adults, such as congestive heart failure (CHF), may impair liver function and influence biotransformation by decreasing the metabolism of drugs and increasing the risk of drug accumulation and toxicity. Renal function may be impaired because of a loss of

BOX 8-2

How to Assess the "At-Risk" Older Adult

1. Interview the client to obtain a complete drug history. Carefully question him or her about disease states, illnesses, current use of medications (e.g., prescribed, OTC, home remedies, herbals, vitamins), drug allergies (description of allergy, time it occurred, intervention used, outcome), and any troubling side effects/adverse reactions.
2. Make a list of the name, strength, and directions of each medication (prescribed and OTC) taken by the client. Include prn medications, especially if the client reports taking them one or more times per week.
3. Identify all prescribers for this client. This information may be obtained by client interview and should be verified by checking prescription labels.
4. Prescription bottles may also provide additional information to review. For example, check the name(s) of the pharmacy (or pharmacies) that have dispensed medications to the person. If more than one pharmacy is involved, determine the reason why.
5. Check all prescription and OTC drug containers for expiration dates. Ask the client for permission to destroy any expired medications because they have the potential of being ineffective or causing harm.
6. Question clients on their self-medication practices: How do they remember to take their scheduled medications? Do they ever forget to take a dose and, if so, what do they do? Have they ever deliberately stopped their medication (if yes, obtain an explanation why)? Such information will help in evaluating compliance and in determining if the medications are being consumed safely according to the prescribed schedule.
7. Determine whether the client has any limitations that may impair the safe self-administration of medication. Examples include physical impairment, memory loss, health or cultural beliefs, financial constraints, and a lack of social support.

nephrons, decreased blood flow, and decreased glomerular filtration rate. A reduction in renal function is also secondary to CHF. Decreased renal clearance may cause increased plasma drug concentrations and longer half-lives of drugs and active metabolites that the kidney usually excretes. Drugs that are highly dependent on the kidneys for excretion include the aminoglycosides, ciprofloxacin (Cipro), digoxin (Lanoxin), lithium (Eskalith), and numerous other drugs (Jinks & Fuerst, 1995).

Therefore careful monitoring of drug regimens is crucial, especially for older adults. Box 8-2 describes how to assess the "at-risk" older adult.

ALTERATIONS IN PHARMACOKINETICS

It has been estimated that 70% to 80% of all adverse drug reactions in older adults are dose-related. The physiologic changes previously discussed may result in a decrease in drug metabolism, distribution in the body, and renal excretion. The higher blood and tissue levels of potent medications may result in an increased incidence of adverse drug reactions. The half-life of diazepam (Valium) increases from 20 hours in a 20-year-old to 90 hours in individuals in their 80s because of the increase in drug volume in the body of the older adult.

The previously described aging process does not necessarily affect all older adults. For example, with drugs primarily excreted by the kidneys, reduced or impaired renal function may result in drug accumulation and perhaps toxicity. However, up to one third of older adults have little or no "age-related renal insufficiency" (McCue et al., 1993).

ALTERATIONS IN PHARMACODYNAMICS

Changes in target organ or receptor sensitivity in older adults may result in a greater or lesser drug effect at these sites. The reason for this alteration is unknown but may be due to a decrease in the number of receptors at the site or to an altered receptor response to the medication. Older adults often exhibit a decreased response to beta agonists and antagonists, but they have a greater response (central nervous system [CNS] depression) with benzodiazepines, such as diazepam (Valium) (Erwin, 1997). It has also been reported that the muscarinic receptors in the cortex tend to decrease with aging, and therefore older adults are often very sensitive to anticholinergic medications. The anticholinergic side effects of confusion, dry mouth, blurred vision, constipation, and urinary retention are often noted (Lucas, Noyes, & Stratton, 1995). (See Chapter 21 for additional information on anticholinergic drugs.)

There is also believed to be a loss in responsiveness or an age-related decline in beta-adrenergic receptors and dopamine receptors in older adults. The number of receptors may vary or the alteration may be in different areas of the aging body, which may result in altered drug responses or an increased risk for drug-induced Parkinson's disease (Lucas et al., 1995).

In summary, older adults are perceived to have a greater sensitivity to drugs, especially to medications that act on the CNS. If monitoring and dosage adjustments are not instituted, they may encounter more adverse reactions than occur in younger persons.

INEFFECTIVE MANAGEMENT OF THE SELF-MEDICATION REGIMEN

The numerous factors that complicate drug therapy regimens may result in improper self-medication, errors in administration, and therapeutic failure (Box 8-3). Detecting medication misuse is an important function of the health care provider, because appropriate interventions may reverse this outcome. A variety of situations may result in medication misuse, which leads to the following questions:

1. Does the risk or cost of one or more of the drugs in the client's drug regimen outweigh the benefits? Benefits may be viewed as physiologic responses or as psychologic and economic considerations.
2. What is the older adult's or primary caregiver's knowledge of the prescribed therapy? Does the client follow a specific medication schedule (by times or hours) and keep track of all medications taken daily? Does the client or primary caregiver know the name of and use for each of the medications? Can they explain the instructions from the label on each bottle? (See Chapter 10 for a detailed discussion of client education.)
3. Can the client open the child-resistant caps on his or her medications? Is the client aware that he or she can receive regular caps if requested from the pharmacist?
4. Is the client having any difficulty taking the medication, perhaps needing a change in dosage form to facilitate swallowing (e.g., from tablet to liquid)?
5. Is the client exhibiting drug side effects or adverse reactions? Such reactions are often overlooked, and the prescriber may prescribe a new medication for the symptoms rather than discontinue the offending medication.

Behavioral and mental changes are very common symptoms of medication misuse, and therefore the nurse should constantly compare the client's current function with his or her past performance. Consultation with a family member or caregiver is essential. Confusion, increased irritability, disorientation, and agitation are just a few of the changes often caused by medications (Miller, 1995). Physical problems such as increased weakness, falls, and a decrease in physical activity may also be caused by a variety of prescribed medications. Although most individuals can identify an acute drug reaction if it occurs after the start of a new medication, the slower-evolving side effects are often more difficult to identify. At times the prescriber may discontinue a potential offending drug and observe the client to see if the side effects are alleviated. The prescriber may discontinue a drug that has a long duration of action and substitute a drug that has a shorter duration of action. This, too, helps in preventing the cumulative or additive effects of medications, especially the CNS-acting drugs (e.g., hypnotics, antianxiety agents, antidepressants, narcotics, and tranquilizers).

BOX 8-3

Factors That May Complicate Drug Therapy in Older Adults

Older adults:

- Are living longer
- May have one or more chronic diseases
- May receive prescriptions from two or more prescribers
- Undergo physiologic changes that may result in the following:
  - Altered pharmacokinetics
  - Altered pharmacodynamics
- May have altered thought processes such as confusion, memory loss
- May have impaired physical mobility related to arthritis, fatigue
- May have sensory-perceptual alterations such as impaired vision or hearing
- May have limited income, which may affect the continuity of drug therapy
- On the average, use more prescription and OTC drugs than the general population
- May experience polypharmacy, which has resulted in an increase in the reports of drug interactions, side effects, and adverse reactions

MEDICATIONS IN OLDER ADULTS

The potent medications available to treat older adults often have a narrow index between effectiveness and toxicity. A study of more than 6000 persons age 65 years or older living in the community indicates that physicians prescribe inappropriate medications for at least 25% of the older adult population (Willcox, Himmelstein, & Woolhandler, 1994). Table 8-1 summarizes inappropriate drugs for older adults. This list of potentially inappropriate medications was derived from a previously published list (Beers et al., 1991) and was limited to drugs that should be avoided entirely in older adults. For example, the three long-acting benzodiazepines (diazepam [Valium], chlordiazepoxide [Librium], and flurazepam [Dalmane]) have been associated with daytime sedation and an increased risk of falls, whereas the antidepressant amitriptyline (Elavil) has been reported to cause the most anticholinergic and orthostatic hypotensive side effects as compared with other drugs in this category. Therefore prescribing such medications for older adults increases the risk of inducing side effects, adverse drug reactions, and perhaps injury.

Table 8-2 is a list of commonly prescribed medications for older adults and includes the most commonly reported side effects or adverse reactions. "Although all systems are altered by the aging process, the CNS and the cardiovascular system appear to be the most affected" (Lucas et al., 1995). To reduce the potential for adverse effects, it has been recommended that CNS-acting medications be reduced to approximately 50% of the usual adult recommended dosage (Lucas et al., 1995). The potential for drug-induced adverse effects declines if the prescriber titrates slowly to the therapeutic effect.

Avorn and Gurwitz (1995) report that nursing home residents receive more medications than do noninstitutionalized older adults. The use of inappropriate medications (see Table 8-1) has also been documented in this setting. Prolonged use of oral antibiotics, short-acting benzodiazepines, and histamine-2 antagonists, as well as high dosages of iron products, histamine-2 antagonists, and antipsychotic medications were also reported. Inappropriate prescribing of psychotropic medications in long-term facilities has resulted in federal legislation Omnibus Reconciliation Acts (OBRA) that has established guidelines for the proper use of such medications in older adults. (See Chapter 19 for additional information.)

The primary responsibility of a health care provider is to reduce or eliminate the potentially adverse risk factors associated with various drug regimens. This can be accomplished with a thorough assessment of the client's health status, current medication regimen, and environmental factors that would influence the accurate and safe administration of medication by the client or the client's caregivers, as well as implementation of the appropriate interventions, client education, and counseling. (See Chapters 4, 5, 6, and 10 for more information.)

A study involving the assessment and monitoring of an older adult hospital population by a multidisciplinary team (physician, geriatric nurse specialist, home care nurse, pharmacist, social worker, dietitian, and physical therapist) reported a significant decrease in hospital readmissions and mortality rates as compared with a control group of participants (62 persons in the study group, 58 persons in the control group). Each team member evaluated each person in the experimental group, made recommendations in the chart, forwarded the recommendations to the client's primary physician, and continued to monitor each person throughout the study. The control group did not receive recommendations or any subsequent visits. After 6 months, the experimental group demonstrated a reduced mortality rate (6% of

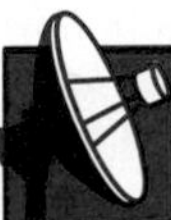

TechnologyLink
Drug Therapy for Older Adults

Video Resources

Geriatric Symptom Assessment and Management, ISBN 0-8151-1227-0

Mosby, Inc., 11830 Westline Industrial Drive, St. Louis, MO 63146; (800) 426-4545; www.mosby.com.

Module 1: *Symptom Assessment Framework Video and Workbook Package*, ISBN 0-8151-2692-1

Module 2: *Cardiopulmonary Video and Workbook Package*, ISBN 0-8151-2693-X

Module 3: *Gastrointestinal Video and Workbook Package*, ISBN 0-8151-2694-8

Module 4: *Neuromuscular and Urinary Video and Workbook Package*, ISBN 0-8151-2695-6

Web Resources

AgeNet—Geriatric Health (www.agenet.com/index.asp/)

This site serves as a bridge between adult children and their aging parents. It provides a wide range of information that includes drugs, health, legal data, insurance, finances, and product availability for older adults, as well as support for the caregiver.

National Institute on Aging (NIA) (www.nih.gov/nia/)

The NIA is a division of the National Institutes of Health. The NIA site offers information on research, funding, training, and health.

Nursing Home Info—The Nationwide Nursing Home Directory (www.nursinghomeinfo.com/)

This site offers information on nursing homes, including facilities by state and how to select a nursing home, assessment tips, financial information, and information on assisted living.

The Novartis Foundation for Gerontology (www.healthandage.com/)

This site is for both professionals and older adults. It provides health news and medical information.

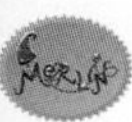

For additional WebLinks, a free subscription to the "Mosby/Saunders ePharmacology Update" newsletter, and more, go to mosby.com/MERLIN/McKenry/.

TABLE 8-1 Inappropriate Drugs for Older Adults

Category	Drug Examples
Analgesics	propoxyphene (Darvon) pentazocine (Talwin)
Antidiabetics	chlorpropamide (Diabinese)
Antidepressants	amitriptyline (Elavil)
Antiemetics	trimethobenzamide (Tigan)
Antihypertensives	propranolol (Inderal) methyldopa (Aldomet) reserpine (Serpasil)
Hypnotics/sedatives	diazepam (Valium) chlordiazepoxide (Librium) flurazepam (Dalmane) meprobamate (Miltown) pentobarbital (Nembutal) secobarbital (Seconal)
Muscle relaxants	cyclobenzaprine (Flexeril) methocarbamol (Robaxin) carisoprodol (Soma) orphenadrine (Norflex)
Nonsteroidal antiinflammatory drugs (NSAIDs)	indomethacin (Indocin)
Platelet inhibitors	dipyridamole (Persantine)
Peripheral vasodilators (dementia therapy)	cyclandelate (Cyclospasmol) isoxsuprine (Vasodilan)

TABLE 8-2 Commonly Prescribed Medications in Older Adults

Medication	Common Side Effects/Adverse Reactions
Aminoglycoside antibiotics (e.g., gentamicin)	Ototoxicity (hearing impairment or loss), renal impairment or failure
Analgesics, opioids (morphine and others)	Confusion, constipation, urinary retention, nausea, vomiting, respiratory depression
Anticholinergics, antispasmodics, especially antihistamines, antiparkinsonian drugs, atropine	Blurred vision, dry mouth, constipation, confusion, urinary retention, nausea, delirium
Anticoagulants (heparin, warfarin [Coumadin])	Bleeding episodes, hemorrhage, increase in drug interaction potential
Antihypertensives	Sedation, orthostatic hypotension, sexual dysfunction, CNS alterations, nausea
Aspirin, aspirin-containing products	Tinnitus, gastric distress, ulcers, gastrointestinal bleeding
Digoxin [Lanoxin], digitalis preparations, especially at higher dosages	Nausea, vomiting, cardiac dysrhythmias, visual disorders, mental status changes, hallucinations
Diuretics (e.g., thiazides, furosemide [Lasix])	Electrolyte disorders, rash, fatigue, leg cramps, dehydration
Hypnotics/sedatives (e.g., flurazepam [Dalmane], triazolam [Halcion])	Confusion, daytime sedation, gait disturbances, lethargy, increased forgetfulness, depression, delirium
H_2 receptor antagonists (e.g., cimetidine [Tagamet], ranitidine [Zantac])	Confusion, depression, mental status alterations
Nonsteroidal antiinflammatory drugs (NSAIDs)	Gastric distress, gastrointestinal bleeding, ulceration
Psychotropics (neuroleptic agents)	Sedation, confusion, hypotension, drug-induced parkinsonian effects, tardive dyskinesia
Tricyclic antidepressants (e.g., amitriptyline [Elavil], doxepin [Sinequan])	Confusion, cardiac dysrhythmias, seizures, agitation, anticholinergic effects, tachycardia, and other effects

BOX 8-4

Over-the-Counter Drug Use by Rural Older Adults

Moore and Johnson (1993) used a multiple-choice/fill-in-the-blank questionnaire to examine the OTC drug–taking practices of noninstitutionalized older adults (100 rural and 100 urban adults over the age of 65). Participants answered questions about the number and names of the OTC drugs used, the frequency with which they were taken, the degree of their dependence on these drugs for daily functioning, and the occurrence of side effects related to their use.

Both urban and rural older adults used OTC drugs daily, with 14% of urban older adults and 27.3% of rural older adults using four or more medications. Individuals in both groups also took prescription drugs every day, with 62% of the rural and 50% of the urban subjects responding that they combined them with OTC drugs on a daily basis. Thirty-nine percent of the rural and 18% of the urban participants said that they could not perform their daily living activities without the OTC drugs.

The findings indicate that rural older adults are more likely to engage in self-diagnosis and self-treatment of their health problems. This may be the consequence of geographic and physical isolation and the fact that many rural areas are medically underserved. The implications for nursing are that older adults, particularly those in rural areas, require additional education regarding responsible drug use and that nurses need to maintain an awareness that older adults may be using multiple medications.

Critical Thinking Questions

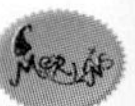

- What ways could be used to disseminate information regarding the safe use of OTC medications to the older adults in a rural community?
- As a community health nurse, what steps would you take with your individual clients in their home settings to ensure that they take their medications safely and accurately?

Case Study *Polypharmacy in Older Adults*

Walter Smith is an 86-year-old divorced man who lives alone in a public housing project for older adults. He describes himself as a loner and expresses a great deal of pride at being independent his entire life. He weighs 138 pounds and is 5 feet 10 inches tall. He has very poor vision and hearing.

Mr. Smith was admitted to the hospital after a fall in which he received scalp lacerations. He was alert and well-read but was quite suspicious of the health care providers. Mr. Smith was diagnosed with hypertension, arteriosclerotic heart disease, atrial fibrillation, eczematous dermatitis of his legs, and a urinary tract infection. He spent 3 days in the hospital and was discharged on the following medications:

betamethasone valerate (Valisone) cream 0.1% to legs twice daily
digoxin (Lanoxin) 0.125 mg daily
furosemide (Lasix) 20 mg daily
atenolol (Tenormin) 60 mg daily
isosorbide dinitrate (Isordil) 5 mg four times daily
ferrous sulfate (Feosol) 200 mg two times daily
vitamin C 100 mg daily
trimethoprim and sulfamethoxazole (Bactrim DS) two times daily
propoxyphene and acetaminophen (Darvocet-N) 100 mg four times daily as needed

Before this hospitalization, Mr. Smith relied heavily on self-care and self-medication. He resumed his self-care regimen after discharge, consuming large quantities of natural vitamin and mineral supplements and using Corn Huskers Lotion on his legs. One week after discharge, the visiting nurse found that Mr. Smith had fallen twice during the week but had sustained only minor bruises. He was weak, and although he was oriented to place and person, he was uncertain of the time and showed memory loss and some incoherence in thought processes. He had trouble describing his medications but complained they were expensive and caused him to experience incontinence. His blood pressure was 98/64 mm Hg.

The nurse convinced Mr. Smith to visit a health care provider he knew and liked. The provider was tolerant of Mr. Smith's need to remain in his home and perform his health practices. Mr. Smith insisted on using the Corn Huskers Lotion instead of the "too expensive" cream. The prescriber agreed to this change and in addition was able to reduce Mr. Smith's medications to digoxin (Lanoxin) 0.125 mg daily, isosorbide (Isordil) 5 mg qid, and triamterene/hydrochlorothiazide (Dyazide) 1 capsule daily. Mr. Smith agreed to take his heart medications and to use fewer of his nonprescription vitamins and minerals.

1. Why is polypharmacy a common problem with older adults?
2. What assessment data should the nurse obtain to understand the client's beliefs and practices regarding medications?
3. How might the following have contributed to the confusion experienced by Mr. Smith?
   a. Effects of age-related changes in circulatory, renal, and hepatic function on the drugs taken.
   b. The specific actions or adverse effects of the following drugs:
      Lanoxin
      Lasix
      Tenormin
      Darvocet-N
4. What factors affected Mr. Smith's ability and willingness to carry out the medication regimen?

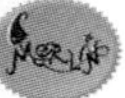

For answer guidelines, go to mosby.com/MERLIN/McKenry/.

persons died, compared with 21% of persons in the control group) and persons in this group were more actively involved in the daily activities necessary for independence (Practice Trends, 1993). These results indicate the benefits of a thorough assessment and close monitoring of older adults.

Ideally the prescriber individualizes and simplifies drug therapy for the client (Gambert, Grossberg, & Morley, 1994). Keeping medications to a minimum with the least frequent dose administration necessary will help to reduce the potential for drug interactions and also improve the client's ability to manage the drug regimen effectively (Box 8-4). The nurse should be an advocate for simplification of the client's medication regimen (see the Case Study box above).

■ Nursing Management

Medication Administration for Older Adults

Older adults are at risk for toxicity because of the effects of drugs in the aging body, variables of drug administration, and the effects of polypharmacy. Nurses must make every attempt to simplify the drug therapy plan in view of the effects just outlined and because of the multiplicity of drugs prescribed for older adults and the older adult's potential for occasionally unreliable memories and senses, inadequate financial status, and propensity for developing adverse secondary effects to drugs. Medications should be suspected as the cause whenever there is a change in an older adult's behavior, particularly restlessness, irritability, and confusion. Alterations in thought processes may be the earliest signs of drug toxicity. Nursing assistants, home health aides, family caregivers, and others should be encouraged to report to a nurse any change in the client's behavior. Often what passes for senility is drug-induced lethargy or confusion.

In the administration of medications, the older adult may have special needs as discussed in Chapter 5. Older adults often have dry mucous membranes, which impede swallowing, and thus water should be offered both before and after oral medications (if the client's condition permits). Older adults should be positioned so that gravity can assist the drug through the esophagus and minimize the possibility of aspiration. Because of diminished sensation, the client may be unaware that the tablet is stuck between the lip and gum, so the client should be asked for permission to examine his or her mouth to ensure that the medication has been swallowed. Some older adults may have slowed reflexes and a reduced understanding of treatment. It helps to organize the dispensing of medication so that enough time is allowed for clients who require more time and assistance with medications, possibly by medicating them last to prevent being rushed.

With older adults, the selection of sites for injectable medications may present the nurse with a challenge. Because muscle mass declines with age, there may be fewer suitable sites for IM injection than in younger individuals, and palpating to detect muscles of adequate body and size requires more skill and effort. On the other hand, decreased sensory perception, including pain perception, may make injections less painful.

Physical problems may often interfere with the ability of older adults to comply with prescribed drug regimens. Some may be unable to read labels or locate drugs because of failing eyesight; others, such as clients with arthritis, may have difficulty opening bottles (particularly childproof containers) or handling small pills; and clients with hearing impairments may not hear all of the instructions. The logistics and economic cost of obtaining drugs may be a deterrent to complying with therapy. Multiple-drug therapy may simply be too complex for the client to manage without assistance. The nurse can simplify drug administration and scheduling as much as possible. Dosage schedules and calendars often help the forgetful client. Drug packaging that is easy to use and is clearly labeled, as well as printed directions and drug information, help to ensure compliance in older adults.

The older adult's functional capabilities must be assessed to determine the educational requirements for safe and accurate self-administration of medications in the home (Isaac, Tamblyn, & the McGill-Calgary Drug Research Team, 1993) (Box 8-5). The nurse's creativity and skill are essential in devising teaching plans to enhance client compliance with the home medication regimen (see Chapter 10). Discuss prescription and OTC medications with clients and their family and caregivers; clients and caregivers should be able to describe in detail how and when they take all medications. Nurses should frequently reassess the effectiveness of the management of the therapeutic regimen as the older adult's functional capacity changes (Cohn, Taylor, & Messina, 1995).

BOX 8-5

Client Education for Medication Administration

1. Review all medications with the client or caregiver to determine drug effectiveness and side effects/adverse reactions.
2. Have the client (or the caregiver) repeat the name and use for each medication plus the dosing instructions. If necessary, clarify the information.
3. Perform a functional assessment to determine if the client needs a compliance aid or a memory cue to take medications. If a caregiver is not available, determine if one is necessary.
4. Provide a written medication schedule in large print for the client, which will enhance independent, effective management of therapeutic regimen.
5. If the drug regimen is complicated, discuss possible changes (simplification) with the prescriber. Then recommend ways the client may be able to manage the drug regimen.

The most important part of the nursing process for older adults may be the nurse's ability to communicate patience, warmth, and understanding and to treat older adults as persons having dignity and the ability to reason, to feel, and to contribute.

SUMMARY

As the older adult population within the Western world increases, both proportionately and in numbers, it becomes of greater importance to ensure their well-being. The tendency toward polypharmacy in this population requires that the nurse be more astute in assessment, intervention, teaching, and counseling. All older adults have unique physiologic and psychosocial needs. The nursing management of medication administration to older adults requires that the nurse be knowledgeable about the various pharmacokinetic and pharmacodynamic effects of pharmaceutical agents in this population. Understanding the rationales behind these effects will help the nurse to administer medications safely and to evaluate client responses appropriately, regardless of the client's age.

Critical Thinking Questions

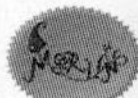

1. In the Moore and Johnson (1993) study of OTC medication use by older adults, one of the participants

stated, "I've been taking care of myself, wife, and kids all of my life. I ran this ranch year-round, even when snow was everywhere and the wind blew so hard a body could hardly stand. Why would I drive 112 miles just to see a doctor and get some pills when I can go to the store 20 miles down the road and get some that do the trick just as good?" What approach would you use to provide information about the safe use of OTC medications with this client?

2. Mr. Holmes is an 81-year-old client of a home health agency in a rural area of western Massachusetts. He lives alone and still drives himself for shopping, health care provider visits, and other errands. Describe the assessment required to determine if Mr. Holmes is at risk for ineffective management of his medication regimen.

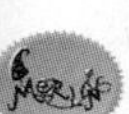

Collaborative Learning Activities

For Collaborative Learning Activities, go to mosby.com/MERLIN/McKenry/.

CASE STUDY

For a Case Study that will help ensure mastery of this chapter content, go to mosby.com/MERLIN/McKenry/.

BIBLIOGRAPHY

American Hospital Formulary Service. (1999). *AHFS drug information '99*. Bethesda, MD: American Society of Hospital Pharmacists.

Anderson, K.N., Anderson, L.E., & Glanz, W.D. (Eds.) (1998). *Mosby's medical, nursing & allied health dictionary* (5th ed.). St Louis: Mosby.

Avorn, J. & Gurwitz, J.H. (1995). Drug use in the nursing home. *Annuals of Internal Medicine, 123*(3), 195-204.

Beers, M.H., Ouslander, J.G., Rollingher, I., Reuben, D.B., Brooks, J., & Beck, J.C. (1991). Explicit criteria for determining inappropriate medication use in nursing homes. *Archives of Internal Medicine, 151*:1825-1832.

Cohn, V.S., Taylor, S.G., & Messina, C.J. (1995). Older adults and their caregivers: The transition to medication assistance. *Journal of Gerontological Nursing, 21*(5), 33-38.

Erwin, W.G. (1997). Geriatrics. In J.T. DiPiro, R.L. Talbert, G.C. Yee, G.R. Matzke, B.G. Wells, & L.M. Posey (Eds.), *Pharmacotherapy* (3rd ed.). Norwalk, CT: Appleton & Lange.

Isaac, L.M., Tamblyn, R.M., & the McGill-Calgary Drug Research Team (1993). Compliance and cognitive function: A methodological approach to measuring unintentional errors in medication compliance in the elderly. *Gerontology, 33*(6), 772-781.

Gambert, S.R., Grossberg, G.T., & Morley, J.E. (1994). How many drugs does your aged patient need? *Patient Care, 28*(6), 61-66, 69-72.

Jinks, M.J. & Fuerst, R.H. (1995). Geriatric drug use and rehabilitation. In L.Y. Young, & M.A. Koda-Kimble (Eds.), *Applied Therapeutics: The Clinical Use of Drugs* (6th ed.). Vancouver, WA: Applied Therapeutics.

Jones, B.A. (1997). Decreasing polypharmacy in clients most at risk. *AACN Clinical Issues: Advanced Practice in Acute & Critical Care, 8*(4), 627-634.

Kovach, L.J. (1992). Polypharmacy in the elderly. *Pharmacy & Therapeutics Journal, 17*(11), 1709.

Lucas, D.S., Noyes, M.A. & Stratton, M.A. (1995). Principles of geriatric pharmacotherapy. *Clinical Consultant 14*(5):1-8.

McCue, J.D., et al. (1993). *Geriatric drug handbook for long term care.* Baltimore: Williams & Wilkins.

Melmon, K.L., Morrelli, H.F., Hoffman, B.B., & Nierenberg, D.W. (Eds.). (1992). *Melmon's & Morrelli's Clinical pharmacology: Basic principles in therapeutics* (3rd ed.). New York: McGraw-Hill.

Miller, C.A. (1995). Medications that may cause cognitive impairment in older adults. *Geriatric Nursing, 16*(1), 47.

Moore, J.F. & Johnson, J.E. (1993). Over-the-counter drug use by the rural elderly. *Geriatric Nursing, 14*(4), 190-191.

Pollow, R.L., Stoller, E.P., Forster, L.E., & Duniho, T.S. (1994). Drug combinations and potential for risk of adverse drug reaction among community-dwelling elderly. *Nursing Research, 43*(1), 44-49.

Practice Trends (1993). Geriatric assessment reduces mortality, *American Pharmacist. NS33*(7), 10.

Trends & Analysis (1995). Long-term care of elderly patients: Chronic disease comorbidity and other considerations, *Consultant Pharmacist. 10*(6), 583-593.

United States Pharmacopeia Dispensing Information (USP DI) (1999). *USP DI: Drug information for the health care professional* (19th ed.). Rockville, MD: United States Pharmacopeial Convention.

Why Senior Care Pharmacy? (1999). *ASCP Update, 10*, 5.

Willcox, S.M., Himmelstein, D.U., & Woolhandler, S. (1994). Inappropriate drug prescribing for the community-dwelling elderly. *JAMA, 272*(4), 292-296.

9 Substance Misuse and Abuse

Chapter Focus

Despite concerted efforts to educate the public, the misuse and abuse of drugs and alcohol in North American society are widespread. Because of the scope of the problem, this issue has moved to the forefront of health care. No matter what the health care delivery setting, the nurse must be able to recognize and assist clients with substance abuse problems.

Learning Objectives

1. Describe the scope of substance abuse.
2. Cite etiologic factors of substance abuse.
3. Identify the pharmacologic basis of physical drug dependence and tolerance.
4. Describe the pathophysiologic changes characteristic of chronic substance abuse.
5. Identify the signs, symptoms, and treatment for the overdose of commonly abused drugs.
6. List the street names for commonly used drugs.
7. Discuss nursing management of the care of clients who abuse drugs and other substances.

Key Terms

abstinence or withdrawal syndrome, p. 164
Drug Abuse Warning Network (DAWN), p. 159
drug misuse, p. 157
hallucinogen, p. 163
metabolic (pharmacologic) tolerance, p. 160
physical dependence, p. 160
pK_a, p. 175
psychologic dependence or addiction, p. 157
receptor site (tissue) tolerance, p. 160
substance abuse, p. 157
tolerance, p. 160

All prescribed or self-administered drugs have the potential to be misused or abused. One example of drug misuse by a prescriber is the prescribing of drugs without adequate exploration of the client's presenting complaint. Another example is prolonged and unsupervised administration of drugs for symptomatic relief. In general, **drug misuse** refers to the nonspecific or indiscriminate use of drugs, including alcohol. **Substance abuse** refers to self-medication or self-administration of a drug in chronically excessive quantities, resulting in physical and/or psychologic dependence, functional impairment, and deviation from approved social norms.

Psychologic dependence or addiction is a behavioral pattern characterized by drug craving, out-of-control drug use, overwhelming concern with obtaining a drug supply, personal and legal problems, denial, and continued use of the drug despite personal and legal difficulties. Most important, the use of the drug does not improve the person's quality of life.

SUBSTANCE ABUSE

Substance abuse is neither a new nor a recent phenomenon. It has been known throughout history as one expression of an individual's search for the relief of physical, psychologic, social, and economic problems. Contemporary substance abuse has attained prominence as an issue with moral, legal, religious, social, psychologic, and medical implications. Substance abuse is not confined to any particular socioeconomic, cultural, or ethnic group. It is a major medical, social, economic, and interpersonal problem that affects individuals across the life span and from all economic backgrounds and urban and rural settings (Cronk & Sarvela, 1997).

In the United States, drug and alcohol abuse in the workplace has been estimated to cost businesses up to $100 billion a year (Malatestinic & Jorgenson, 1991). Figure 9-1 illustrates the recent increases in substance use among adolescents. The impact that alcohol and substance abuse have on society is tremendous. For example, alcohol plays a role in the following societal problems:

- 40% of assaults reported and at least one third of all rape and child abuse cases are alcohol related.
- Nearly 50% of prisoners state being under the influence of alcohol when they committed their crimes.
- Half of all US traffic accidents and nearly 80% of accident fatalities that occur between 8 PM and 4 AM involve alcohol-impaired drivers.
- In one rural state, alcohol was present in 35% of suicides, 63% of homicides, and 49% of unintentional injury fatalities (Baldwin & Cook, 1995).

In 1984 Bissell and Haberman studied alcoholism and the use of other drugs with alcohol in professionals, including doctors, nurses, dentists, attorneys, social workers, and college women. After following a group of approximately 400 professionals for 5 to 7 years, they found that alcoholism or alcohol abuse with other drugs was usually identified as a problem during the first 15 years of professional practice.

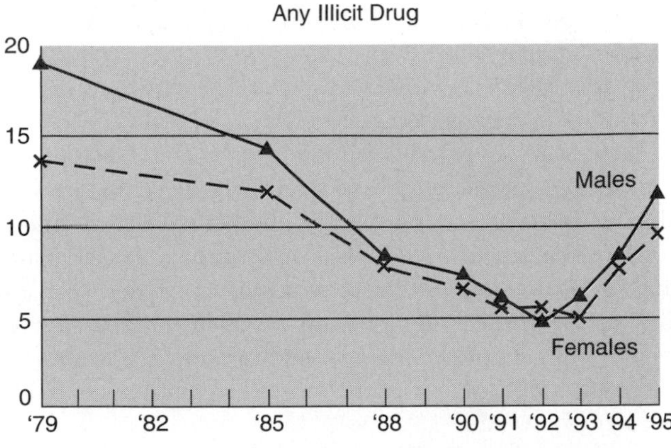

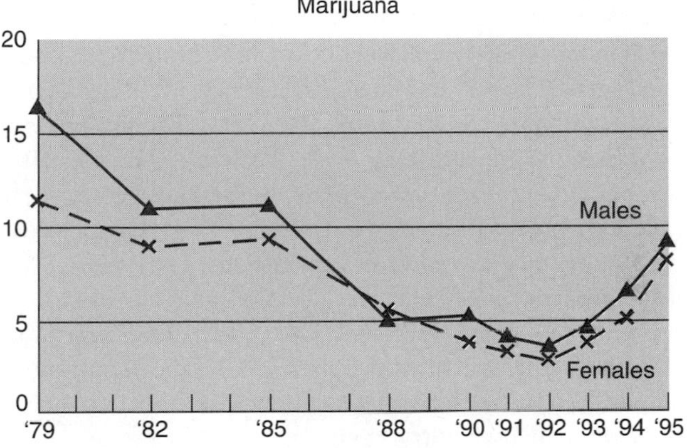

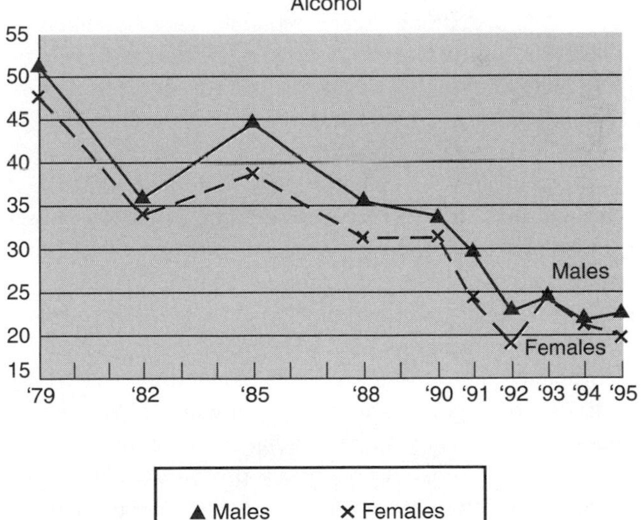

Figure 9-1 Recent increases in substance abuse among adolescents. (Redrawn from Office of Applied Studies, Substance Abuse and Mental Health Services Administration [1997]. *Substance abuse among women in the United States.* Rockville, MD: Department of Health and Human Services.)

The combination of alcohol and other drugs was quite prevalent, especially with physicians and nurses. This group reported the greatest addiction to hard narcotics, with the narcotic of choice being meperidine (Demerol) because of its ready availability in their workplace and also because it produces less pupillary constriction than the other opioids. Most physicians and nurses stated obtaining their drugs through professional channels. Many started with legitimate drugs prescribed for stress or a painful condition such as back pain. Another study of nearly 2000 chemically dependent health care professionals found that those who abused medications generally used more than four substances (Gallegos et al., 1988).

Recent work by Trinkoff and Storr (1998) examined the prevalence of past-year substance use among registered nurses by specialty. Of the 4438 nurses responding, the prevalence of past-year substance use for all substances combined was 32%. For marijuana/cocaine use, the prevalence was 4%; for prescription drugs, 7%; for cigarette smoking, 14%; and for binge drinking, 16%. Rates varied by specialty, with oncology nurses reporting the highest past-year prevalence for combined substances (42%), followed by psychiatry (40%) and emergency and adult critical care (both 38%). The highest prevalence of marijuana/cocaine use was found with emergency and pediatric critical care nurses (7%) followed by adult critical care nurses (6%). Prescription drug use was less varied across specialties, with oncology, rehabilitation, and psychiatry having the highest prevalence of use. Psychiatry had the highest prevalence of cigarette smoking (23%), followed by emergency and gerontology (both 18%); pediatric critical care nurses were least likely to smoke (8%). Binge drinking was high among oncology, emergency, and adult critical care nurses. In general, substance use among nurses occurred at rates comparable to rates in the general population.

Although many nurses find it difficult to believe that their colleagues may be substance abusers, the American Nurses Association has publicly recognized substance abuse as a problem among nurses (American Nurses Association, 1984). Substance abuse is estimated to involve 6% to 8% of the 1.9 million nurses in the United States (Stammer, 1988).

Although the substances most commonly abused by health care professionals are prescription drugs (opioids and benzodiazepines), alcohol, and tobacco, the choice of drug and route of administration vary by profession. Nurses and physicians are more apt to abuse injectable drugs, pharmacists often use multiple oral drugs, dentists have a problem with nitrous oxide addiction, and anesthesiologists and nurse anesthetists commonly abuse fentanyl (Sublimaze) or similar products (Baldwin & Cook, 1995).

Career pressures and easy accessibility to drugs place health care professionals at greater risk for substance abuse. Impaired health care professionals constitute a hazard to their clients' and their own well-being; therefore these problems cannot be ignored, overlooked, or left unreported. It is vital that health agencies be alert to suspected substance abusers on their staffs. Many agencies and most states have mandatory reporting of, as well as active rehabilitation programs for, impaired health care professionals.

Substance abuse (alcohol and drugs) is considered a "handicap," and such employees may be protected by state and federal employment discrimination laws. The Rehabilitation Act (29 USC, Section 706[7][B]) states that employers are required to employ these individuals if they can properly perform their job functions and are not a threat to safety or property. Many health care facilities and other businesses have established employee assistance programs to help impaired employees with rehabilitation.

DRUG TESTING

In an effort to identify persons with alcohol- and drug-related problems, many businesses, government agencies, and health-related facilities perform drug analysis or urine drug tests on their employees under specified conditions. Drug screens may also be part of a preemployment physical examination. A number of testing procedures are available, and it is important to know the analytic techniques used and the purpose and limitations of any tests performed. Urine testing for specific drugs may detect substances used days or even a week before the test (Table 9-1). Such tests give evidence only of use or of prior exposure to a drug; they are not indicative of the individual's pattern of substance abuse or degree of drug dependency.

Initial positive tests should be confirmed with more specific and accurate tests because false-positive and false-negative results may occur. A second test specific for the agent reported in the screening test is necessary to ensure accuracy. The health care providers interpreting the tests should be familiar with drugs known to cross-react or give a

TABLE 9-1 Time vs. Drug Detection in Urine

Drug	Detection in Urine (days)*
Alcohol	Less than 1 day
Amphetamines	Up to 1 day
Barbiturates	Up to 1 day
Benzodiazepines	Up to 2 days
Cocaine	Up to 2 days
Methadone	Up to 3 days
Marijuana	
Single use	Up to 6 days
Chronic use	Up to 29 days
Opioids	
Short acting	Up to 1 day
Phencyclidine	Up to 6 days
Phenobarbital	Up to 6 days

Information from Baldwin, J.N. & Cook, M.D. (1995). Issues: Psychoactive substance use disorders. In L.Y. Young & M.A. Koda-Kimble (Eds.), *Applied therapeutics: The clinical use of drugs* (6th ed.). Vancouver, WA: Applied Therapeutics.

*Chronic high doses may extend the time intervals.

false-positive result with the test in use. For example, diphenhydramine (Benadryl) may test positive in urine for methadone, and phenylpropanolamine (Dexatrim) has been reported to test positive for amphetamines. An alternate, more specific drug test can be ordered if the individual reports taking such medications.

It is beyond the scope of this chapter to explore all aspects of substance abuse in depth. Rather the focus is on the actions of drugs and on the treatment of substance abuse. To achieve a more holistic frame of reference, the nurse is urged to investigate independently other aspects of the complex phenomenon of substance abuse.

ETIOLOGIC FACTORS

A characteristic common to most drugs that cause dependence is that they are initially taken because the individual believes a desirable pharmacologic effect will result. The person who is dependent on a drug has found something that provides relief from personal problems, and the drug generally is used as a maladjustive coping mechanism or, as evidence of the nursing diagnosis, ineffective coping. Because very few drugs or substances without central nervous system (CNS) effects are abused, one of the predominant factors contributing to substance abuse appears to be intrapsychic—a desire to alter one's state of mind. This desire may arise from a number of factors such as curiosity, boredom, peer pressure, multiple and diverse alienation, hedonism (pleasure-seeking behavior), affluence, and the attention paid to substance abuse by the mass media. More individual or subjective reasons are personal inadequacy or failure, conflicts terminating in tension, feelings of shame, and a predisposition to depression, which may lead to emotional and behavioral problems. All or any combination of these factors may lead to misuse of drugs and substances. The characteristics of substance abuse are listed in Box 9-1.

More specifically, some psychologic hypotheses have been advanced in relation to persons prone to use drugs as escape mechanisms. Persons with potentially drug-dependent predispositions are described as having a strong psychologic dependence, a low threshold of frustration, a fear of failure, and feelings of inadequacy. Other authorities dispute the "addiction-prone" personality hypothesis and maintain that everyone has the potential to become dependent on something.

BOX 9-1

The Four Characteristics of Substance Abuse

1. Altered state of consciousness
2. Development of tolerance
3. Rapid onset of action of desired effects
4. Possible abstinence syndrome if drug is discontinued abruptly after extended period of use

In 1990 the American Society of Addiction Medicine (ASAM) described alcoholism and other chemical dependencies as "primary, chronic, relapsing diseases with genetic, psychosocial, and environmental factors influencing their development and manifestations" (Baldwin & Cook, 1995). Treatment centers have evolved to address the biopsychosocial factors associated with substance abuse.

Although all drugs have some abuse potential, the more commonly abused chemically active substances are the xanthines and caffeine, which are found in coffee, tea, chocolate, and colas (see Chapter 18). Although the lay public rarely perceives these substances as drugs, they do produce mild stimulant and euphoric effects, and their use may lead to physical dependence. Nicotine and ethyl alcohol (ethanol) are the most commonly misused and abused drugs, and physical and psychologic dependence may result. Other CNS drugs such as anticholinergics, steroids, amphetamines, pentazocine (Talwin), and levodopa (Larodopa) may induce altered states of perception, thought, and feelings and drug-induced psychoses as a result of prolonged and concentrated therapeutic use or abuse. Few drugs without CNS effects are misused or abused.

This chapter will review the drugs most commonly reported to the **Drug Abuse Warning Network (DAWN)** as being involved in drug-abuse–related episodes resulting in death. DAWN is a federal agency that monitors the data on medical and psychologic problems associated with drug use and changing patterns of substance abuse. Table 9-2 lists the top 15 drugs detected by medical examiners in deaths due to substance abuse by gender. Table 9-3 lists selected drugs commonly abused and symptoms of their abuse.

Substance abuse may take several forms:

1. *Experimental abuse* occurs when individuals use drugs in an exploratory way, after which they accept or reject continuing use of the drugs.
2. *Social-recreational substance abuse* may occur only in social contexts. The drugs commonly abused in social situations are alcohol, marijuana, cocaine, nicotine, and caffeine.
3. *Episodic substance abuse* refers to the periodic abuse of a drug.
4. *Compulsive substance abuse* is characterized by irrational, irresistible, or compelling abuse of a drug.
5. *Ritualistic substance abuse* may be related to religious practices.

Polydrug or multiple substance abuse is common. Marijuana, alcohol, and other depressants are often used together and in conjunction with CNS stimulants. Heroin may be used with cocaine, and pentazocine (Talwin) may be used with tripelennamine (PBZ), alcohol, or other depressants.

Cocaine (especially crack cocaine) became popular in the 1980s. Its abuse was seen fairly often but initially was somewhat curtailed by its high cost. According to emergency department statistics, cocaine use increased in the 1990s; its use was reported in 37% of emergency department drug episodes involving men and in 18% of drug episodes involving women.

TABLE 9-2 Top 15 Drugs in Substance Abuse Deaths by Gender*

Males	Females
1. Heroin/morphine/ opioids	1. Cocaine
2. Cocaine	2. Heroin/morphine/ opioids
3. Alcohol in combination	3. Alcohol in combination
4. Codeine	4. Codeine
5. Marijuana/hashish	5. Diphenhydramine (Benadryl)
6. Diazepam (Valium)	6. Diazepam (Valium)
7. Methamphetamine/ speed	7. Amitriptyline (Elavil)
8. Methadone	8. Acetaminophen (Tylenol)
9. Amphetamines	9. D-propoxyphene (Darvon, Darvocet N)
10. Diphenhydramine (Benadryl)	10. Nortriptyline (Aventyl, Pamelor)
11. Amitriptyline (Elavil)	11. Methadone
12. Quinine	12. Methamphetamine/ speed
13. D-propoxyphene (Darvon, Darvocet N)	13. Marijuana/hashish
14. Acetaminophen (Tylenol)	14. Fluoxetine (Prozac)
15. Nortriptyline	15. Hydrocodone

Information from Drug Abuse Warning Network (DAWN). (1999). *Drug Abuse Warning Network. Emergency Department Data. Office of Applied Studies, Substance Abuse and Mental Health Services Administration.* Rockville, MD: Department of Health and Human Services.
*Trade names are in parentheses; many of these products are also available under other trade or generic names. Statistics are based on drug-induced or drug-related episodes caused by an illegal drug or the nonmedical use of a legal drug that contributed to the individual's death.

The 1980s also documented the development of synthetic "designer drugs" produced by illegal laboratories or chemists. The molecular structure of a controlled substance is modified to produce a new variant that mimics the effects of the original drug. The types of drugs most commonly modified and sold are analogues of meperidine (Demerol), fentanyl (Sublimaze), and MDMA (3, 4-methylenedioxymethamphetamine, also known as "ecstasy") from the illicit psychedelic agent MDA (3,4-methylenedioxyamphetamine). When "designer drugs" are identified, the Drug Enforcement Administration (DEA) enacts regulations to ban them. Until it is banned, such a substance is legal to make, sell, and use. Once a substance is outlawed, underground chemists often make a new, legal variation of the product, which is sold until a ban against it is established. Therefore "designer drugs" are constantly changing and should be considered potentially dangerous substances. Contaminants have been identified in these products, and overdoses and deaths have been reported with their use.

PHARMACOLOGIC BASIS OF DEPENDENCE AND TOLERANCE

Psychologic and physical dependence on a drug can exist independently or simultaneously. Both psychologic and physical dependence can potentially lead to compulsive patterns of drug use in which the user's lifestyle is focused on procurement and administration of the drug. However, unlike psychologic dependence, **physical dependence** is an adaptive state that occurs after prolonged use of a drug. Discontinuation of the drug causes physical symptoms that are relieved by readministering the same drug or a pharmacologically related drug. Several hypotheses attempt to explain the pharmacologic basis of the physiologic adaptation that occurs in tolerance and physical dependence.

Tolerance is the tendency to increase drug doses to maintain the effect formerly produced by a lower dose. Tolerance may exist with either psychologic or physical dependence and may be viewed in two ways. **Receptor site (tissue) tolerance** is a form of adaptation in which the effect produced depends both on the concentration of the drug and on the duration of exposure. The clinical effect of the drug is reduced as the duration of exposure continues because of changes in the number or function of receptors. **Metabolic (pharmacologic) tolerance** refers to an aspect of drug disposition. Prolonged exposure to a drug can change the body's metabolic response to the drug, increasing drug clearance with repeated ingestion. For example, with prolonged exposure to barbiturates, steady-state blood concentrations fall progressively with continued administration of the same dose. This may be attributed to the inducing effect of the barbiturates on hepatic microsomal enzymes, which increases barbiturate metabolism.

PATHOPHYSIOLOGIC CHANGES

Physical and psychologic dependence on drugs is often associated with debilitated physical states caused by extensive abuse of the drug, which often results in malnutrition, dehydration, and hypovitaminosis. Respiratory complications such as pneumonia, pulmonary emboli, and abscesses are often associated with neglect, debilitation, and the respiratory depression produced by CNS depressants. The IV administration of illicit drugs often leads to a high incidence of sepsis, hepatitis, infective endocarditis, and acquired immunodeficiency syndrome (AIDS) as a result of using contaminated equipment. Alcohol and drug use also increase risk behaviors associated with accidents and the contraction of sexually transmitted diseases (O'Hara, Parris, Fichtner, & Oster, 1998). Cellulitis, sclerosis of the veins, phlebitis, and skin abscesses may occur. Death from accidental overdose is common.

Overdose is a particularly significant potential danger because illegal drugs are notoriously unreliable in regard to the

TABLE 9-3 Selected Drugs Commonly Abused and Symptoms of Abuse

Drug Category	Street Names	Methods of Use	Symptoms of Use	Hazards of Use
Marijuana/Hashish	Pot, grass, reefer, weed, Colombian, hash, hash oil, sinsemilla, joint	Most often smoked; can also be swallowed in solid form	Sweet, burnt odor Neglect of appearance Loss of interest, motivation Possible weight loss	Impaired memory, perception Interference with psychologic maturation Possible damage to lungs, heart, and reproductive and immune systems Psychologic dependence
Alcohol	Booze, hooch, juice, brew	Swallowed in liquid form	Impaired muscle coordination, judgment	Heart and liver damage Death from overdose Death from car accidents Addiction
Stimulants				
Amphetamines*				
Amphetamine	Speed, uppers, pep pills, Bennies	Swallowed in pill or capsule form, or injected into veins	Excess activity Irritability; nervousness Mood swings Needle marks	Loss of appetite Hallucinations, paranoia Convulsions, coma
Dextroamphetamine	Dexies			
Methamphetamine	Moth, crystal Black beauties			
Cocaine	Coke, snow, toot, white lady, crack, ready rock	Most often inhaled (snorted); also injected or swallowed in powder form; smoked	Restlessness, anxiety Intense, short-term high followed by dysphoria	Intense psychologic dependence Sleeplessness, anxiety Nasal passage damage Lung damage Death from overdose
Nicotine	Coffin nail, butt, smoke	Smoked in cigarettes, cigars, and pipes; snuff; chewing tobacco	Smell of tobacco High carbon monoxide blood levels Stained teeth	Cancers of the lung, throat, mouth, esophagus Heart disease, emphysema
Depressants				
Barbiturates	Barbs, downers	Swallowed in pill form or injected into veins	Drowsiness Confusion Impaired judgment Slurred speech Needle marks Constricted pupils	Infection after parenteral use Addiction with severe life-threatening withdrawal symptoms Nausea Death from overdose
Pentobarbital	Yellow jackets			
Secobarbital	Red devils			
Amobarbital	Blue devils			
Opioids	Dreamer, junk	Swallowed in pill or liquid form, injected	Drowsiness Lethargy Needle marks Loss of appetite	Loss of appetite Addiction with severe withdrawal symptoms
Dilaudid, Percodan				
Demerol, Methadone		Injected into veins, smoked		
Morphine		Swallowed in pill or liquid form		
Heroin	Smack, horse			
Codeine	Schoolboy			

Information from Doering, P.L. (1999). Substance-related disorders: Overview and depressant, stimulants, and hallucinogens. In J.T. DiPiro, R.L. Talbert, G.C. Yee, G.R. Matzke, B.G. Wells, & M.L. Posey (Eds.), *Pharmacotherapy: A pathophysiologic approach* (4th ed.). Stamford, CT: Appleton & Lange; O'Brien, C.P. (1996). Drug addiction and drug abuse. In J.G. Hardman & L.E. Limbird (Eds.), *Goodman & Gilman's The pharmacological basis of therapeutics* (9th ed.). New York: McGraw-Hill; and NIDA (1999). Commonly abused drugs, street names for drugs of abuse, National Institute on Drug Abuse (www.nida.nih.gov/DrugsofAbuse.html [2/28/2000]).

*Includes look-alike drugs resembling amphetamines that contain caffeine, phenylpropanolamine (PPA), and ephedrine.

Continued

TABLE 9-3 Selected Drugs Commonly Abused and Symptoms of Abuse—cont'd

Drug Category	Street Names	Methods of Use	Symptoms of Use	Hazards of Use
Hallucinogens				
PCP (phencyclidine)	Angel dust, killer weed, hog, dust, Love Boat	Most often smoked; can also be inhaled (snorted), injected, or swallowed in tablets	Slurred speech, blurred vision, incoordination Impaired memory, perception Confusion, agitation Aggression	Anxiety, depression Death from accidents Death from overdose
LSD	Acid, cubes, purple haze	Injected or swallowed in tablets		
Mescaline	Mesc, cactus	Usually ingested in natural form	Dilated pupils Delusions, hallucinations	Breaks from reality Emotional breakdown
Psilocybin	Magic mushrooms		Mood swings	Flashback
Inhalants Gasoline Airplane glue Paint thinner		Inhaled or sniffed, often with use of paper or plastic bag or rag	Poor motor coordination Impaired vision, memory and thought processes Abusive, violent behavior	High risk of sudden death Drastic weight loss Brain, liver, and bone marrow damage
Nitrites Amyl Butyl	Poppers, locker room, rush, snappers	Inhaled or sniffed from gauze or ampules	Slowed thought Headache	Anemia, death by anoxia

Information from Doering, P.L. (1999). Substance-related disorders: Overview and depressant, stimulants, and hallucinogens. In J.T. DiPiro, R.L. Talbert, G.C. Yee, G.R. Matzke, B.G. Wells, & M.L. Posey (Eds.), *Pharmacotherapy: A pathophysiologic approach* (4th ed.). Stamford, CT: Appleton & Lange; O'Brien, C.P. (1996). Drug addiction and drug abuse. In J.G. Hardman & L.E. Limbird (Eds.), *Goodman & Gilman's The pharmacological basis of therapeutics* (9th ed.). New York: McGraw-Hill; and NIDA (1999). Commonly abused drugs, street names for drugs of abuse, National Institute on Drug Abuse (www.nida.nih.gov/DrugsofAbuse.html [2/28/2000]).

TABLE 9-4 Common Drug Groups That Are Abused

Drug(s) Abused	Signs and Symptoms
Cannabis drugs	Tachycardia and postural hypotension, conjunctival vascular congestion, distortions of perception, dryness of mouth and throat, possible panic
Cocaine	Increased stimulation, euphoria, increased blood pressure and heart rate, anorexia, insomnia, agitation; in overdose, increased body temperature, hallucinations, seizures, death
Opiates	Depressed blood pressure and respirations; fixed, pinpoint pupils; depressed sensorium; coma; pulmonary edema
Barbiturates and other general CNS depressants	Depressed blood pressure and respirations, ataxia, slurred speech, confusion, depressed tendon reflexes, coma, shock
Amphetamines	Elevated blood pressure, tachycardia, other cardiac dysrhythmias, hyperactive tendon reflexes, pupils dilated and reactive to light, hyperpyrexia, perspiration, shallow respirations, circulatory collapse, clear or confused sensorium, possible hallucinations, paranoid feelings
Hallucinogenic agents	Elevated blood pressure, hyperactive tendon reflexes, piloerection, perspiration, pupils dilated and reactive to light, anxiety, distortion of body image and perception, delusions, hallucinations

potency of their active ingredient. The drugs are commonly adulterated (mixed) with various substances such as active substances (e.g., amphetamines, benzodiazepines, hallucinogens) and inactive substances (e.g., lactose, sugars) by the time they reach the user. The risk of toxicity and death exists if an individual who has been using adulterated drugs unknowingly receives pure or stronger drugs. Overdose may also occur when an individual who has been withdrawn from drugs for some time (and has thereby lost accumulated tolerance) injects the previous usual dose, which now is in excess of the tolerance level.

As a consequence of all these factors, the life expectancy of persons who are psychologically dependent on drugs is generally lower than that of nondependent individuals. Table 9-4 presents common drug groups that are abused, along with the signs and symptoms of acute intoxication.

CULTURAL ASPECTS OF SUBSTANCE ABUSE

In various societies certain drugs are accepted as legal and useful, and other drugs may be banned or considered illicit. For example, alcohol, caffeine, and nicotine are widely accepted and commonly used substances in the United States, Canada, and parts of Western Europe. Amphetamines are the major drugs of abuse in Japan, where increases in personal productivity are desired. Cannabis is considered a legal drug in the Middle East, but alcohol is usually forbidden. Some Native American tribes use peyote, a **hallucinogen** (a drug that causes auditory or visual hallucinations), for religious services. In general, such hallucinogens have no accepted therapeutic use in the United States. In the high-altitude areas of the South American Andes mountains (e.g., Peru), coca leaves are brewed as a tea or chewed to decrease the sensation of hunger, increase work performance, and increase a sense of well-being.

The use and acceptance or rejection of a substance depend on the society and its subgroups. When drug substances are considered illicit or illegal and are in short supply, non–law-abiding persons may be motivated to produce and/or sell the banned substances. This activity is usually extremely profitable.

TYPES OF DRUGS MOST COMMONLY ABUSED

Opioids (Heroin/Morphine and Other Agonist Opioids)

Opioids are one of the most commonly abused types of drugs and often are listed in the top five for drug-related emergency department episodes. The pharmacologic types of drugs from natural sources (opiate) include the opium alkaloids (heroin, morphine), the semisynthetic group (hydromorphone [Dilaudid], oxymorphone [Numorphan]), and the synthetic group (meperidine [Demerol], levorphanol [Levo-Dromoran], methadone [Dolophine]). Heroin, D-propoxyphene (Darvon), oxycodone (Percodan, Percocet), and morphine are the opioids most often abused. The term *opioid* is preferred because it refers to both natural and synthetic products that have morphine-like effects.

Mode of Administration. In general, the opium derivatives can be administered percutaneously (absorbed through the mucous membranes) by sniffing (*snorting*), by SC injection (*skin popping*), or by direct IV injection (*mainlining*). The rate of absorption is correspondingly increased, with mainlining producing almost immediate drug effects.

Mechanism of Action and Effects. Opium derivatives are CNS depressants that probably act on the sensory cortex, on higher centers, and on the thalamus. These drugs do not produce hallucinogenic or psychotomimetic effects. They are particularly likely to lead to physical and psychologic dependence because they can relieve pain; change or elevate mood; relieve tension, fear, and anxiety; and produce feelings of peace, euphoria, and tranquility. Rapid IV injection produces warm, flushing sensations described as being similar to sexual orgasm followed by a soothing state that seems to be best characterized as a state of complete drive satiation. An individual who is "high" on opioids feels no need to satisfy drives for basic biologic needs and is often described as being "on the nod"—drowsy, content, and euphoric.

Acute Overdose. Acute overdose of opioid substances may result in severe pulmonary edema and respiratory depression. These outcomes are dose dependent and are related to the degree of individual tolerance. What constitutes a lethal dose depends on the individual's tolerance for the drug. Symptoms of overdose occur rapidly in most individuals (see Table 9-4).

Opioid toxicity is manifested in various ways, such as slow, shallow breathing; cold, clammy skin; severe hypoxia (American Hospital Formulary Service, 1999); mixed overdose conditions; or severe acidosis. Miosis (pinpoint pupils) are common with most opioids, but mydriasis (dilated pupils) may occur with meperidine overdose. Bradycardia, hypotension, muscle spasm, lethargy, respiratory depression, and urinary retention may also occur, but the toxic effects of meperidine may be more excitatory, causing significant tachycardia (Sinatra & Savarese, 1992). The presence of thrombophlebitis, scarred veins, and puckered scars from SC injections may help identify the client with opioid toxicity. Opioids tend to delay motility and gastric emptying time; reviving the client may increase peristalsis and further increase absorption of oral forms of the drug, producing a coma cycle. Chronic abuse may result in abscesses, cellulitis, endocarditis, glomerulonephritis, encephalopathy, tetanus, and thrombophlebitis. These conditions are caused by a spectrum of factors that range from injection technique to adulterants in the substance of abuse.

The treatment of choice for acute overdose of opioids is administration of an antagonist (e.g., naloxone) and respiratory support (see the Management of Drug Overdose box on p. 164).

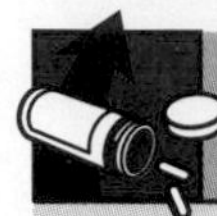

Management of Drug Overdose
Opioids

General Approach

- Provide symptomatic and basic supportive care of airway, breathing, and circulation (the "ABCs"). Maintain cardiac output, blood pressure, urinary output, and peripheral perfusion.
- If oral opioids were consumed and the client is not lethargic or unresponsive, empty stomach by emesis or gastric lavage.

Specific Approach

- If apnea is present, maintain a patent airway, using assisted or controlled respiration and oxygen as necessary.
- When the triad of miotic pupils, coma or stupor, and bradypnea (respirations slowed to a rate of 4 to 6 per minute) appears, the administration of naloxone (Narcan) is indicated and will help to differentiate narcotic poisoning from other conditions.
- Naloxone, a pure narcotic antagonist, reverses opioid toxicity. The usual adult dose is 0.4 to 2 mg IV, which may be repeated at 2- to 3-minute intervals if necessary. Larger doses may be required to treat acute overdoses of butorphanol (Stadol), nalbuphine (Nubain), propoxyphene (Darvon and Darvocet products), and pentazocine (Talwin). Failure to respond to high doses of a narcotic antagonist may indicate a mixed substance overdose or involvement of a nonopiate substance.
- Support blood pressure and maintain respirations after the client responds to naloxone (Narcan). Blood and urine samples should be examined with a multiple drug screen to aid in diagnosis. A positive response to naloxone is characterized by dilation of the pupils (if previously miotic) and an increase in respiratory function, blood pressure, and cardiac rate.
- Children with a known or suspected narcotic overdose may receive 0.01 mg/kg of naloxone (Narcan) as the first dose. (Dilute naloxone with sterile water for injection.) If the child does not respond to the first dose, additional IV doses at 2- to 3-minute intervals may be administered.
- Naloxone reverses apnea and coma within minutes and should be titrated to the client's arousal with a respiratory rate in a range of 10 to 20 breaths per minute. Continued client monitoring is necessary because additional naloxone (IV bolus or IV infusion) is often necessary to prevent the reemergence of opioid toxicity.

Physical Dependence and Acute Abstinence Syndrome. Physical dependence on opioids usually is described in relation to heroin or morphine, but the other derivatives manifest similar symptoms. Physical dependence is evident in the marked tolerance that develops with continued use of the drug and in the symptoms of **abstinence or withdrawal syndrome** experienced by a chemically dependent person who is suddenly deprived of the substance of abuse.

Persons dependent on heroin or morphine often feel satiated, and therefore physical, emotional, and social deterioration commonly occur. The individual may feel little need for food and may become grossly malnourished and weak. A preoccupation with obtaining the drug makes participation in the usual social and vocational aspects of life difficult if not impossible. As the drug craving grows, tolerance to the drug also increases, and eventually the motivation for using the drug becomes oriented more to the avoidance of withdrawal symptoms and less to the achievement of euphoria.

In a client who is physically dependent on opioids, the use of naloxone to produce an abrupt and complete reversal of the narcotic effects may precipitate an acute abstinence or withdrawal syndrome. Although opioid abstinence syndrome may be reversed by administration of an opioid, doing so in a drug-dependent client is prohibited by law except if he or she has been admitted to the hospital for an emergency procedure or is being detoxified or maintained in an approved federal drug treatment program. Methadone is usually considered the drug of choice in the treatment of this clinical condition.

Withdrawal Symptoms. The initial withdrawal symptoms are related to the half-life of the opioid being used. Symptoms of withdrawal from heroin are autonomic in origin and appear within 8 hours after the last dose in physically dependent individuals. These symptoms are less life threatening than those of other substances of abuse and are manifest as restlessness, chills and hot flashes, restless sleep, piloerection on the skin (which gives rise to the term *cold turkey*), rhinorrhea, drowsiness, lacrimation, and mydriasis during the first 24 hours. These symptoms become more severe as withdrawal progresses, and additional symptoms may include sneezing, yawning, generalized anxiety, abdominal cramps, lower back pain, lower extremity cramps, vomiting, diarrhea, anorexia, diaphoresis, muscular twitching, insomnia, elevated pulse rate, elevated blood pressure, elevated temperature, and a craving for the drug. Occasionally withdrawal symptoms are severe enough to result in cardiovascular collapse.

Depending on the drug used, abstinence syndrome develops within 2 to 48 hours and peaks at 72 hours. Withdrawal that is left untreated may continue for up to 7 to 10 days, after which the physical dependence of the body on the presence of opioids is eventually lost. Psychologic dependence continues for a longer period; some authorities claim it continues forever.

Treatment of Opioid Dependence

Withdrawal Programs. In general, opioid withdrawal is difficult, and repeated relapses may be expected. Abrupt and complete withdrawal (cold turkey) can be accomplished, but this procedure is dangerous (especially in clients with a co-existing medical illness) and inhumane and should generally be avoided. Therapeutic withdrawal from an opioid may be somewhat more comfortably achieved by successively tapering the drug's dosage over a period of several days.

The choice of withdrawal program is partly influenced by the following factors: the client's physical condition, the duration of drug dependence, the type and amount of drug being taken, motivations for substance abuse and withdrawal, and whether the individual is also dependent on other drugs, such as alcohol. Depending on these factors, opioid withdrawal may in some instances need to be accomplished in a hospital with close medical supervision.

In identifying the criteria for evaluating opioid withdrawal, it should be noted that recovery from morphine-type dependence is not equated with cure. Therapeutic programs should continue regardless of repeated relapses to substance abuse. Progress in withdrawal may be indicated by progressively longer periods of abstinence from opioids without resorting to the use of other psychoactive drugs or alcohol and by the client's growing confidence in the ability to function effectively without drugs.

Therapeutic Community Programs. The ultimate goal of using any medication to treat dependency is to provide relief from the compulsive craving for the drug of abuse. To achieve rehabilitation, the individual needs to turn to more than just another prescribed or illicit medication. He or she also needs human dignity, sincerity, compassion, warmth, self-respect, and hope with positive reinforcement. To achieve independence and become a self-sustaining, productive member of the community, he or she must be provided with emotional and social support. Many treatment programs do not effectively address these human resources, and failures have resulted.

Because persons withdrawing from drugs often cannot make the transition easily, groups of persons who have decided to abstain from drug use can meet or live together in an attempt to support and guide one another. Therapeutic community programs such as Phoenix House and halfway houses have been established to include group psychotherapy and self-help approaches. Ultimately, an individual should emerge from such a program with sufficient personal growth and appropriate support systems to be able to manage life satisfactorily without resorting to substance abuse.

Methadone Detoxification and Withdrawal. A currently preferred method of withdrawal is substitution of methadone. Methadone is a synthetic opioid analgesic that, by virtue of cross-tolerance, permits effective substitution of methadone dependence for heroin dependence. Its effectiveness against heroin dependence results from its ability to forestall the euphoriant effects of heroin and the craving for the drug without producing the deleterious physical and mental effects. When properly administered, methadone allows the individual to function adequately without intellectual or emotional impairment.

For adults in detoxification, methadone is taken orally in 15- to 40-mg doses per day, titrated according to client response, until withdrawal symptoms are controlled. Methadone therapy is initiated empirically according to client symptoms. As a general guide, 1 mg of methadone is substituted for 20 mg of meperidine, 4 mg of morphine, or 2 mg of heroin (Baldwin & Benson, 1995). (For a review of recommended dosages and dosage adjustments, see current substance abuse references or the references cited in this chapter.)

Regular administration of methadone results in the development of tolerance to methadone and cross-tolerance to heroin. The client does not experience an opioid-induced "rush" and euphoria unless a dose that exceeds the tolerance level is administered. The nurse should be aware that some clients might exaggerate their withdrawal symptoms to obtain more methadone. Supportive psychologic or psychiatric counseling of clients being treated with methadone may relieve some of the burdens that led to drug dependence. During this phase the methadone may be gradually withdrawn, usually at a rate of 20% reduction or 5 mg in daily doses.

Methadone maintenance programs are controversial and are not always successful. Previous opioid abusers who are unable to negotiate life in a drug-free state may revert to their former dependence or alternative substance abuse or may return to the methadone therapy detoxification.

Methadone Maintenance. Maintenance methadone treatment programs in the United States require licensing and approval from both the Food and Drug Administration (FDA) and the state. The ultimate goal of these programs is complete withdrawal from drug dependency, but some clients continue taking methadone for an extended time. Methadone programs can include psychologic, vocational, and rehabilitation services in addition to medical support. Approved methadone programs are required to comply with all the requirements in the Federal Methadone Regulations.

Admittance to a methadone maintenance program usually requires evidence of current dependence on morphine-type drugs and at least a 1-year history of opioid dependence. Nurses should be aware that addicts hospitalized with medical conditions other than addiction might require pharmacologic support with methadone or opioids during their stay. Because a cross-tolerance to opioids is common, these clients usually require higher analgesic doses to control pain. Verification of enrollment in an approved methadone maintenance program is usually required in order to continue methadone during the hospital stay. The hospital pharmacist should be consulted on the regulations and for assistance in such matters.

The nurse should also be aware that treatment centers vary in their methods and drugs used for opioid withdrawal. Some treatment centers report having accomplished withdrawal from opioids through the use of clonidine (Catapres), whereas others maintain that methadone is the drug of choice.

Methadone dependence does occur. The withdrawal symptoms are less severe but last for a longer period. Methadone withdrawal programs generally include supplemental rehabilitation techniques such as vocational and social rehabilitation. Theoretically, an individual can be withdrawn from methadone maintenance after he or she has functioned free from other opioids for a sufficient period, secured steady employment, and readjusted his or her lifestyle.

Additional Agonist Analgesics

Levomethadyl Acetate Treatment. Levomethadyl acetate (Orlaam) is a longer-acting alternative to methadone and is for use only in approved opioid treatment programs. It is similar to methadone and has a longer duration of action. It is usually given three times a week, such as Monday, Wednesday and Friday. This product can be dispensed only through approved opioid addiction treatment programs, and it should never be given daily. Because federal regulations do not allow take-home doses of Orlaam, clients who are ill or require hospitalization are usually transferred to methadone on a temporary basis (Baldwin & Benson, 1995; *United States Pharmacopeia Dispensing Information*, 1999).

Heroin Maintenance. Diacetylmorphine (heroin), a Schedule I drug (see Chapter 2), is a substance with no accepted medical use in the United States. It has been banned because of its high potential for abuse and because of the increasing number of heroin addicts. Today it remains one of the top drugs abused in the United States and often is used in combination with cocaine.

Although most countries have banned heroin use, it is legal in Belgium, Canada, and England; it is rarely used in Belgium and Canada. Physicians are permitted to prescribe heroin and other opioids for persons with a history of intractable dependence, thereby maintaining them and preventing withdrawal symptoms. Prescriptions are issued through designated hospitals or clinics.

The approval of heroin as an analgesic for intractable pain has been proposed and denied numerous times in the United States. Pharmacologically, heroin is a pro-drug—it is converted in the liver to morphine. Opponents of heroin legislation state that legalized heroin is unnecessary because morphine and other opioids are available in the United States (Lipton, 1993).

Clonidine Treatment. Clonidine (Catapres), a sympatholytic antihypertensive, decreases sympathetic outflow from the CNS by stimulating $alpha_2$ receptors in the brain. This produces a decrease in peripheral resistance, heart rate, and blood pressure. Clonidine is also under investigation for relief of the symptoms of acute drug withdrawal (e.g., opioids, nicotine, alcohol) and as an aid in detoxification. Withdrawal symptoms may be caused by hyperactivity of the noradrenergic pathways of the brain. The nurse should be aware that it takes 2 to 3 days to reach a peak effect when clonidine transdermal patches are used, which is often too late to treat the worst effects of opioid withdrawal. The tablet dosage form offers a quicker and more easily titratable method of preventing or reducing unwanted effects.

A clonidine dosage of 5 μg/kg/day, increasing to 17 μg/kg/day as necessary, has been used to prevent withdrawal syndrome. The dosage is individualized according to the client's tolerance and the quantity and type of opioid agonist used. The daily dose is administered in equally divided doses over a 24-hour period for approximately 10 days; it is then reduced by 50% on days 11, 12, and 13 and discontinued on day 14 (*USP DI*, 1999).

The sedative and hypotensive effects of clonidine limit its clinical usefulness, and extremely close supervision of the client is necessary to monitor side effects, adverse reactions, and any manipulation of the dosage by the client. The nurse should withhold the dose of clonidine and consult the prescriber if the client's blood pressure is less than 90 mm Hg systolic or 60 mm Hg diastolic. This detoxification process eliminates physical dependence on opioids; nonpharmacologic intervention can be used to address the remaining psychologic dependence.

Other Analgesics

pentazocine [pen taz′ oh seen] (Talwin)

Pentazocine (Talwin) 60 mg IM is considered approximately equivalent to 10 mg IM of morphine. Sharp increases in the incidence of pentazocine substance abuse led the DEA to place it in Class IV under the Controlled Substances Act. The potential for pentazocine to produce psychologic and physical dependence is significant even in low doses; infants born to women who are pentazocine dependent experience withdrawal immediately after birth. Pentazocine can cause psychotomimetic reactions such as visual hallucinations, feelings of depersonalization, and nightmares.

The CNS effects of pentazocine are similar to those of the opioids and include analgesia, sedation, and respiratory depression (reversed by naloxone [Narcan]). In high doses pentazocine causes increases in blood pressure and heart rate. Lung problems in pentazocine abusers have been reported when tablets are crushed, dissolved, and administered intravenously. This may be due to the talc binders and other particulate matter in tablet dosage forms. The use and reuse of cotton as a filter may result in "cotton fevers," a type of allergic reaction caused by tiny cotton fibers. This syndrome occurs within 30 minutes of the injection, with the client experiencing increased heart rate, hypotension, increased sweating, shaking chills, and fever. These symptoms often resolve in approximately 4 to 24 hours without treatment, but the health care provider should be aware that sepsis, embolism, and other complications are possible. Other potential effects include seizures and ulceration and severe sclerosis of the skin and subcutaneous tissue and muscles caused by SC or IM injections. The combination of pentazocine with other CNS depressants such as barbiturates and alcohol may be lethal.

The abuse of pentazocine (Talwin) and tripelennamine (PBZ) first appeared in the late 1960s to early 1970s as a result of shortages or the high cost of heroin in large metropolitan areas. Substance abusers report that tripelennamine is used to increase the onset of action and prolong the duration of the euphoria produced by pentazocine. This combination is known as *Ts and blues* (*T* for Talwin and *blue* for the color of the generic tablet of tripelennamine). Ts and blues are oral tablets that are crushed together, dissolved, and injected either through a cotton filter intravenously (like heroin) or subcutaneously. Abscesses and necrotic tissue that require hospitalization and grafting have resulted.

To discourage abuse, oral pentazocine now contains naloxone with a brand name of Talwin-Nx. The addition of naloxone has no effect on the analgesic properties of oral pentazocine, but if this combination is administered intravenously, the naloxone nullifies or cancels the rush effect of the injected "Ts and blues" combination.

Treatment of pentazocine dependence is gradual reduction of the drug in a controlled environment. The psychotomimetic effects should be observed closely in a controlled environment because they may persist for 5 to 7 days.

propoxyphene [proe pox' i feen] (Darvon, Novopropoxyn 🍁)

The use of propoxyphene products in excessive doses, either alone or in combination with other CNS depressants (including alcohol), is a significant cause of drug-related deaths. Because an overdose of propoxyphene may result in fatality, intensive supportive and symptomatic therapy must be instituted immediately.

Clients should be warned not to take propoxyphene in doses higher than those recommended by the manufacturer. The judicious prescribing of propoxyphene is essential for the safe use of this drug. With clients who are depressed or suicidal, consideration should be given to the use of nonnarcotic analgesics.

Because of its depressant effects, propoxyphene should be prescribed with caution for those whose medical condition requires the concomitant administration of sedatives, tranquilizers, muscle relaxants, antidepressants, or other CNS depressant drugs. Clients should be cautioned against the concomitant use of propoxyphene products and alcohol because of the potentially serious CNS additive effects of these agents. Deaths have occurred as a consequence of the accidental ingestion of excessive quantities of propoxyphene alone or in combination with other drugs. Propoxyphene-related deaths have occurred in individuals with previous histories of emotional disturbances or of misuse of tranquilizers, alcohol, and other CNS depressant drugs.

The clinical effects of an acute propoxyphene overdose are similar to acute opioid toxicity—coma, respiratory arrest, pulmonary edema, circulatory collapse, and death. Grand mal seizures have also been reported. Propoxyphene is metabolized in the liver to norpropoxyphene, which may be responsible for some of its toxicity. Toxic propoxyphene serum levels are between 0.6 and 10 μg/ml; lethal levels are reportedly more than 10 μg/ml (AHFS, 1999).

Norpropoxyphene has a smaller CNS depressant effect than propoxyphene but has a greater anesthetic effect on the myocardium—similar to that of amitriptyline and antidysrhythmic drugs such as lidocaine and quinidine. Electrocardiographic monitoring is essential in the management of overdose. The manufacturer recommends contacting a poison control center in all suspected overdose cases for the most current treatment of the overdose.

Propoxyphene has also been abused by parenteral administration of the oral dosage form. Propoxyphene napsylate (Darvon-N, Darvocet-N) is considered a less toxic propoxyphene formulation because of its delayed absorption orally and its relative insolubility in water. Thus the napsylate dosage form has less abuse potential than propoxyphene hydrochloride.

Propoxyphene is pharmacologically related to the opioids; therefore naloxone may reverse the signs of toxicity. Propoxyphene overdose may be accompanied by seizures and require anticonvulsants, and emergence from a coma may require the use of restraints before administering naloxone because of the client's disorientation, agitation, and confusion. Clients need psychologic and emotional support during this time. A quiet, calm environment with reduced sensory stimulation may reduce disorientation and agitation. The nurse should use a simple, direct approach and communicate with reality orientation and reassurance.

Alcohol

Although there are many different types of alcohols, the term *alcohol* usually refers to ethyl alcohol. Methyl, propyl, butyl, and amyl alcohols are examples of other alcohols that are very toxic when taken orally.

ethyl alcohol (ethanol)

Ethyl alcohol is the only alcohol used extensively in medicine and in alcoholic beverages. It is colorless and mixes readily with water; because it lowers surface tension, it is a good solvent for a number of substances. Ethyl alcohol is also referred to as grain alcohol and is the product of the fermentation of a sugar by yeast. Many over-the-counter (OTC) "nighttime" cough and cold remedies contain alcohol (up to 25%, or 50 proof) with antihistamines and may be abused because of their considerable sedative potential. Table 9-5 lists the ethyl alcohol content of various OTC preparations.

Therapeutically, ethyl alcohol has been used as a cardiac disease preventative, an appetite stimulant for clients with poor appetite during periods of convalescence and debility, and as a hypnotic for older persons who do not tolerate other hypnotics.

Mechanism of Action. Ethyl alcohol may have either a local or a systemic action.

Local Effect. Ethyl alcohol denatures proteins by precipitation and dehydration, which may be the basis for its germicidal, irritant, and astringent effects. It irritates denuded skin, mucous membranes, and subcutaneous tissue. SC injection of ethyl alcohol may cause considerable pain and sloughing of tissues. When injected into or near a nerve, it may cause nerve degeneration and anesthesia.

Systemic Effect. Contrary to popular belief, ethyl alcohol is not a stimulant but a CNS depressant. What sometimes appears to be stimulation results from the depression of the higher faculties of the brain and represents the loss of inhibitions acquired by socialization.

Alcohol is thought to interfere with the transmission of nerve impulses at synaptic connections, but how this is accomplished is not known. It causes progressive and continuous depression of the CNS, the sequence being cerebrum, cerebellum, spinal cord, and medulla. Its action is compa-

TABLE 9-5 Ethyl Alcohol Content of Over-the-Counter Preparations

Medicinals	Alcohol Content (%)	Alcohol Proof
Cough-Cold Preparations		
Ambenyl-D	9.5	19
Comtrex Maximum	10	20
Vicks 44	10	20
NyQuil	10	20
Benadryl	0	0
Benylin Expectorant	0	0
Naldecon DX and EX	0	0
Triaminic	0	0
Mouthwash Preparations		
Cepacol	14.5	29
Listerine	26.9	53.8

Information from *Nonprescription products: formulations & features '97-'98.* (1997). Washington, D.C.: American Pharmaceutical Association.

TABLE 9-6 Content of Ethyl Alcohol in Various Beverages

Beverages	Alcohol Content (%)	Alcohol Proof
Beer	4	8
Wine (red/white)	12	24
Brandy	30-45	60-90
Whiskey, vodka	45	90
Martini, Manhattan	30	60
Daiquiri, Alexander	15	30

Information from Hinds, M. (Ed.). (1985). How much blood alcohol content per drink? *Informed Families of Dade County, 26*(6), 1.

rable to that of the general anesthetics except that the excitement stage is longer and definite toxic symptoms are present when the anesthetic stage is reached. The margin between the anesthetic stage and the fatal dose is a narrow one.

The action of alcohol varies with the individual's tolerance, the presence or absence of extraneous stimuli, the rate of ingestion, and the gastric contents. Small or moderate quantities produce a feeling of well-being, talkativeness, greater vivacity, and increased confidence in mental and physical power. There is a general loss of inhibitions. The finer powers of discrimination, insight, concentration, judgment, and memory are gradually dulled and lost. Large quantities may cause excitement, impulsive speech and behavior, laughter, hilarity and, in some persons, pugnaciousness; others may become melancholy or unduly sentimental. Table 9-6 lists the content of ethyl alcohol in various beverages.

The effects of large quantities of alcohol become apparent when the individual attempts to operate machinery such as an automobile. Visual acuity (especially peripheral vision) is diminished, reaction time is slowed, judgment and self-control are impaired, and the individual tends to be complacent and pleased with himself or herself. Drivers under the influence of alcohol take chances they would never take ordinarily. This leads to disaster, as accident statistics reveal.

An individual who is intoxicated usually becomes ataxic, mutters incoherently, has disturbance of the special senses, is often nauseated, may vomit, and may eventually lapse into stupor or coma. The respiratory neurons are usually not depressed except by large doses of alcohol.

Cardiovascular. Alcohol depresses the vasomotor neurons in the medulla and causes dilation of the peripheral blood vessels, especially those of the skin. This causes a feeling of warmth. Heat is lost from the interior, which accounts for the fact that an intoxicated person may freeze to death more quickly than a nonintoxicated person. Alcohol also depresses the heat-regulating mechanism.

Small doses of alcohol (10 to 25 mL) produce an insignificant increase in pulse rate, which is caused mainly by the effect of excitement and reflex on the gastrointestinal tract. Larger doses (more than 25 mL) produce the same effect but may be followed by lowered blood pressure caused by the effect on the vasoconstrictor neurons. Chronic alcoholism may result in cardiomyopathy, hypertension, and a variety of cardiac dysrhythmias, especially atrial fibrillation and flutter. However, epidemiology studies report that light to moderate consumption of alcohol (up to 2 drinks per day) reduces the risk for myocardial infarction and cardiac death (Jungnickel & Hunnicutt, 1995).

Gastrointestinal. The effect of alcohol on the function of the digestive organs depends on the presence or absence of gastrointestinal disease, the degree of alcohol tolerance, the concentration of the alcohol, and the type and amount of food present. Small doses of alcohol stimulate the secretion of gastric juice that is rich in acid. Salivary secretion is also reflexively stimulated. Large and concentrated doses of alcohol tend to inhibit secretion and enzyme activity in the stomach, but the effect in the intestine seems to be negligible. Chronic alcohol ingestion causes pancreatitis and hepatic cellular damage, which results in fibrosis and scarring, cirrhosis, and/or hepatitis. In addition, gastritis, nutritional deficiencies, and other untoward results have been observed when large quantities of alcohol are ingested over a prolonged period (Box 9-2).

Pharmacokinetics. Alcohol does not require digestion before absorption. A small amount is absorbed in the stomach, and most is absorbed in the small intestine. Approximately 90% of the alcohol is metabolized in the liver. Alcohol dehydrogenase, the liver enzyme, oxidizes alcohol (ethanol) to acetaldehyde; acetaldehyde oxidizes to acetic acid, which is buffered to acetate that eventually oxidizes to carbon dioxide and water. Approximately 90% to 98% of ethanol is metabolized (oxidized) in the liver, with the remainder primarily excreted by the lungs and kidneys. As plasma ethanol levels increase, the hepatic alcohol dehydrogenase pathway becomes saturated, resulting in an increase

BOX 9-2

Organ Transplantation in People with Unhealthy Lifestyles

Organ transplantation is a widely accepted treatment option in the United States for individuals with end-stage renal, heart, or liver disease. Because most grafts that fail do so in the first year, success rates for transplantation are reported as the percentage of functioning grafts 1 year after transplant. The success rate for heart transplants is between 80% and 85% and for liver transplants between 70% and 80%. With kidney transplants, approximately 75% are functioning after 5 years (Thomas, 1993). Noncompliance with medications and appointments significantly increases the risk of rejection (DeGeest et al., 2000).

With rising health care costs the economics of transplantation is called into question. When the cost analysis for kidney transplantation is calculated by comparing the cost of transplantation with the cost of 5 years of hemodialysis (the alternative to transplantation), transplantation is seen as more cost-effective. Such calculations are not possible for heart and liver transplantation because no other treatment is available for end-stage heart and liver disease—the alternative is death.

With organ transplantation established as a cost-effective and desirable treatment for people with end-stage disease, how are these limited resources allocated? The debate over the rationing of health care is ongoing and increasing. To allocate scarce donor organs is to make judgments about the worthiness of the potential recipients. It would seem that the rationing of donor livers already exists—only 10% of liver transplants are performed on recovering alcoholics, even though alcoholism is the leading cause of liver failure in the United States. The position taken to limit transplantation for alcoholics (even those who are "dry") is that the donor organ is a nonrenewable resource that should be reserved for those whose disease was not a result of their behavior. The argument that survival rates will be lower in recovering alcoholics has been disproved. DeGeest and others (2000) have profiled heart transplant recipients to allow the identification of clients at risk for appointment and medication noncompliance–associated late acute rejection episodes. Fifty-seven percent of the appointment noncompliers experienced one or more late acute rejection episodes, compared to 2% of the appointment compliers.

Critical Thinking Questions

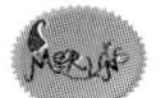

- What factors might be involved in the selection process for liver transplantation in recovering alcoholics?
- Would the situation be different for heart transplantation to individuals with unhealthy lifestyles of smoking, overeating, and not exercising?
- If noncompliance is a critical behavioral risk factor in the occurrence of late acute rejection episodes in heart transplant clients, would it be justified to assess this risk in potential transplant recipients given the limited resources available?
- What is the nurse's role in giving comprehensive and individualized care to people in stigmatized groups?

Data from Thomas, D.J. (1993). Organ transplantation in people with unhealthy lifestyles. *AACN Clinical Issues: Advanced Practice in Acute and Critical Care, 4*(4), 665-668; and DeGeest, S., Dobbels, F., Martin, S., Willems, K., & Vanhaecke, J. (2000). *Progress in Transplantation 10*(3): 162-168.

in the unmetabolized alcohol ratio. Chronic alcohol use may result in hyperlipidemia, fatty deposits in the liver and, ultimately, alcoholic cirrhosis.

Alcohol produces an increased flow of urine because of the increase in fluid intake. Alcohol also acts as a diuretic through CNS depression and inhibition of the release of antidiuretic hormone (ADH). If the individual has preexisting renal disease, the kidney may be further damaged. Large and concentrated doses of alcohol are thought to injure the renal epithelium.

After absorption, alcohol is distributed in every tissue of the body in approximately the same ratio as its water content. Therefore a rough estimate of the quantity consumed may be obtained from an analysis of the blood (Table 9-7).

Health care professionals should be aware of the approximate total amount of alcohol in different beverages: 12 ounces of beer = 4 ounces of wine = 1 ounce of whiskey. Therefore alcohol abuse can occur with any alcoholic beverage, depending on the quantity consumed.

Drug Interactions. Alcohol is the most commonly used and abused drug in North America. Because of its associated medical conditions, alcohol dependence is often seen by health care providers, occurring in 15% to 20% of primary care and hospital clients (Mayo-Smith, 1997). It interacts with many prescription and OTC drugs, resulting in serious adverse reactions that lead to emergency department admission or even death. The magnitude of this potential interaction is enormous. Most people, professionals and laypersons alike, may not be fully cognizant of some of the most significant alcohol-drug interactions (Table 9-8).

Alcohol Abuse

The typical signs of alcohol abuse are changes in drinking patterns, such as the need for early morning drinking, drinking alone, hiding partial or full liquor bottles, or the need to have a drink before performing a potentially stressful event (e.g., job interview, keeping an appoint-

TABLE 9-7 Concentration of Alcohol in Blood and Related Clinical Observations

Stage	Blood Alcohol (mg/dL)	Clinical Observations
Subclinical	30-100	Slight evidence of performance deterioration possible, such as motor function, coordination, personality or mood, and mental acuity
Emotional instability	100-200	Decreased inhibitions; emotional instability; slight muscular incoordination; slowing of responses to stimuli
Confusion	200-300	Disturbance of sensation; decreased pain sense; staggering gait; slurred speech
Stupor	300-400	Marked decrease in response to stimuli; muscular incoordination approaching paralysis
Coma, death	Over 400	Complete unconsciousness; depressed reflexes; subnormal temperature; anesthesia; impairment of circulation; possible death

TABLE 9-8 Selected Significant Alcohol-Drug Interactions

Substances Interacting with Alcohol	Mechanism	Possible Effect(s)
I. antihistamines antidepressants opioid analgesics sedative-hypnotics antianxiety agents antipsychotic drugs	Additive	Enhanced CNS depressant effects
II. disulfiram (Antabuse) cefamandole and some other second- and third-generation cephalosporins chlorpropamide (Diabinese) and other oral antidiabetic agents to varying degrees griseofulvin (Fulvicin) metronidazole (Flagyl) procarbazine (Matulane)	Inhibition of aldehyde dehydrogenase in metabolism of alcohol, leading to acetaldehyde accumulation (disulfiram or a "disulfiram-type reaction")	Most severe effects seen with disulfiram and alcohol: flushing, stomach pain, head throbbing, increased heart rate, hypotension, sweating, nausea, and vomiting With antidiabetic agents: mild to severe hypoglycemia
III. phenytoin (Dilantin)	Increase or decrease in liver metabolism	With chronic alcohol abuse: possible decrease in anticonvulsant effect caused by increased metabolism With acute alcohol use: a possible decrease in metabolism, causing increased serum levels of phenytoin and toxicity
IV. salicylates	Additive	Increased gastrointestinal irritability and bleeding
V. nitrates nitroglycerin	Additive	Vasodilation leading to hypotension, syncope

ment); personality changes; family discord; job absenteeism; personal appearance neglect; poor eating habits; memory lapses; and blackouts. Table 9-9 provides an overview of the psychophysiologic effects of various levels of blood alcohol concentration, and Table 9-10 lists the clinical manifestations and suggested drug treatment of alcohol withdrawal.

The major objectives for the treatment of alcohol withdrawal include a quiet environment, monitoring of health status, symptom relief, prevention or treatment of complications, and the development of long-term rehabilitation plans. Supportive care includes fluid and electrolyte replacement, adequate nutrition, thiamine to prevent the development of Wernicke's encephalopathy, and anticonvulsant

TABLE 9-9 Psychophysiologic Effects of Various Levels of Blood Alcohol Concentration

BAC (mg%)*	Psychophysiologic Effect
20	Light and moderate drinkers begin to feel some effects. Approximate BAC is reached after one drink.†
40	Most people begin to feel relaxed.
60	Judgment is mildly impaired. People are less able to make rational decisions about their capabilities (e.g., driving skills).
80	Definite impairment of muscle coordination and driving skills occurs. Person is legally drunk in some states.
100	Clear deterioration of reaction time and control is observed. Person is legally drunk in most states.
120	Vomiting occurs unless this level is reached slowly.
150	Balance and movement are impaired. Equivalent of one-half pint of whiskey is circulating in the bloodstream.
300	Many people lose consciousness.
400	Most people lose consciousness, and some die.
450	Breathing stops; person eventually dies.

From Lewis, S.L., Heitkemper, M.M., & Dirksen, S.R. (2000). *Medical-surgical nursing: Assessment and management of clinical problems.* St. Louis: Mosby.

*Blood alcohol concentration (BAC) is generally recorded in milligrams of alcohol per deciliter (mg/dl) of blood, or milligrams percent (mg%). BAC is determined by how much alcohol is consumed, how fast it is consumed, and the person's weight.

†One drink is 12 ounces of beer, 5 ounces of wine, or 1 ounce of distilled spirits, which provide the same amount of alcohol.

TABLE 9-10 Clinical Manifestations of Alcohol Withdrawal with Suggested Drug Treatment

Clinical Manifestations	Medications
Gross tremors	Benzodiazepines (e.g., chlordiazepoxide [Librium])
Seizures	Thiamine (prevention of Wernicke's encephalopathy)
Hallucinations	Multivitamins (folic acid, B vitamins)
Delirium tremens (DTs)	Phenytoin (Dilantin)—for seizures or past history of seizures
Minor withdrawal syndrome:	Magnesium sulfate (if serum magnesium is low)
Tremulousness, anxiety	Temazepan (Restoril)
Increased heart rate	Haloperidol (Haldol) for hallucinations
Increased blood pressure	For DTs: may need IV fluids (do not overhydrate), cooling blanket, well-lighted quiet room, consistent staff, frequent vital signs, check for hypoglycemia, assessment of any other health problems
Sweating	
Nausea	
Hyperreflexia	
Insomnia	
Major withdrawal (DTs):	
Disorientation	
Visual/auditory hallucinations	
Increased hyperactivity without seizures	

From Lewis, S.L., Heitkemper, M.M., & Dirksen, S.R. (2000). *Medical-surgical nursing: Assessment and management of clinical problems.* St. Louis: Mosby.

medications if necessary. A sedative drug such as a long-acting benzodiazepine may be necessary for severe withdrawal reactions; its dosage can then be tapered and discontinued (Mayo-Smith, 1997). In selected persons, beta-adrenergic blocking agents or clonidine may be used to reduce the sympathetic manifestations of alcohol withdrawal such as increased anxiety, tachycardia, hypertension, and tremors.

Toxic Alcohols

Isopropyl alcohol and methyl or wood alcohol are toxic when taken internally. When some alcoholic individuals are unable to purchase ethanol (ethyl alcohol), they substitute agents such as isopropyl (rubbing) alcohol, methyl alcohol (antifreeze), or any available substance that might prevent alcohol withdrawal. This is a dangerous practice that can cause severe poisoning and death.

isopropyl alcohol

A clear, colorless liquid with a characteristic odor, isopropyl alcohol compares favorably with ethyl alcohol in its antiseptic action. It has been recommended for skin disinfection and for rubbing compounds and lotions used on the skin. Its bactericidal effects are said to increase as its concentration approaches 100%.

methyl alcohol (wood alcohol, methanol)

Methyl alcohol is a CNS toxin if taken orally. Intoxication does not occur as readily as with ethyl alcohol unless large amounts are consumed. Methyl alcohol is oxidized in the tissues to formic acid, which is poorly metabolized; this is the basis for the development of a severe acidosis.

Symptoms of methyl alcohol poisoning include nausea and vomiting, abdominal pain, headache, dyspnea, blurred vision, and cold, clammy skin. Symptoms may progress to delirium, convulsions, coma, and death. In nonfatal cases the individual may become blind or suffer from impaired vision. Treatment is directed toward the relief of acidosis because this symptom seems to be related to the severity of the visual symptoms. Large amounts of sodium bicarbonate may be needed to treat acidosis successfully. One dose of 60 mL of methyl alcohol has been known to cause permanent blindness. Fluids containing methyl alcohol usually bear a "Poison" label.

Drugs Used in the Treatment of Chronic Alcoholism

disulfiram [dye sul′ fi ram] (Antabuse)

Disulfiram is used to sensitize an individual to alcohol by inducing an unpleasant alcohol-disulfiram reaction. This reaction begins with flushing of the face and develops into intense vasodilation of the face, neck, and upper body. Hyperventilation and increased pulse rate may occur. Nausea occurs in 30 to 60 minutes along with facial pallor, hypotension, and copious vomiting. There is usually an intense feeling of discomfort, a pulsating headache, palpitations, dyspnea, syncope, and a constrictive feeling in the neck. The reaction lasts from 30 minutes to several hours—as long as the alcohol is being metabolized. It is then followed by drowsiness and sleep. (See Table 9-8 for a list of other drugs that have been reported to cause a disulfiram-type reaction when taken with alcohol.)

Mechanism of Action. Disulfiram inhibits the enzyme aldehyde dehydrogenase. As a result, acetaldehyde cannot be converted to acetate. Acetaldehyde then accumulates and causes the unpleasant toxic effects. Disulfiram has few effects unless the person ingests alcohol.

Pharmacokinetics. Disulfiram is metabolized in the liver. The initial effect may be delayed from 3 to 12 hours because of drug storage in adipose tissue. Studies indicate that up to 20% of a dose remains in the body for up to 6 days. Elimination is via the kidneys, with smaller amounts excreted in the feces and lungs. Because of slow and incomplete absorption and elimination, the effects persist up to 2 weeks after therapy is discontinued. Clients should be instructed not to ingest any alcohol-containing substance during this time.

Dosage and Administration. Initially the client is given up to 500 mg PO daily for 7 to 14 days; the maintenance dosage is 250 mg PO daily.

▪ Nursing Management

Disulfiram Therapy

▪ **Assessment.** The client's history should be reviewed for conditions in which particular caution should be used for disulfiram therapy, such as allergic eczematous contact dermatitis, cardiovascular disease, diabetes mellitus, epilepsy, hypothyroidism, and severe pulmonary insufficiency; a disulfiram-alcohol reaction may worsen these conditions. Behavioral toxicity may be precipitated in clients with psychosis or depression. There is a higher rate of hepatotoxicity in clients with existing hepatic dysfunction. Sensitivity to disulfiram, rubber, pesticides, and fungicides should be ascertained. The use of disulfiram should be carefully considered during pregnancy. It must be ascertained that the client has not ingested alcohol in any form (e.g., beverages, vinegars, sauces, OTC preparations, liniments, colognes, and aftershave lotions) or been treated with paraldehyde in the 12 hours before beginning a disulfiram regimen.

Because of the unpleasant reaction the client will experience with the ingestion of alcohol, the client's level of understanding of the purpose, procedure, and consequences of disulfiram therapy should be determined before treatment commences. Written client consent should be obtained before beginning disulfiram therapy.

Review the client's current medication regimen for the risk of significant drug interactions, such as those that may occur when disulfiram is given concurrently with the following drugs:

Drug	Possible Effect and Management
alcohol	Will result in a disulfiram-alcohol reaction if alcohol is consumed during or within 2 weeks of disulfiram therapy.
anticoagulants	Increased anticoagulant effects; dosage adjustments may be necessary; monitor closely for untoward bleeding.
anticonvulsants, phenytoin (Dilantin), hydantoins	Increased serum levels of hydantoins; monitor serum levels before and during concurrent drug therapy because dosage adjustments may be necessary.
benzodiazepines	Decreased plasma clearance of benzodiazepines metabolized by oxidation, resulting in increased CNS depressant actions. Oxazepam (Serax), alprazolam (Xanax), or lorazepam (Ativan) may be used for benzodiazepine therapy because they are metabolized by glucuronidation.

Drug	Possible Effect and Management
isoniazid (INH)	Increased CNS side effects; disulfiram dosage may need to be reduced or stopped; monitor closely for ataxia, insomnia, dizziness, irritability.
metronidazole (Flagyl)	Confusion and psychotic episodes; this combination should be avoided. Metronidazole should not be administered concurrently or during the 2 weeks after disulfiram therapy.
paraldehyde	Inhibition of acetaldehyde dehydrogenase may occur, resulting in increased blood levels of paraldehyde and acetaldehyde.
tricyclic antidepressants	Coadministration may result in acute organic brain syndrome; monitor for irritability, personality changes, confusion, and other mental changes.
warfarin	Increased anticoagulant effect of warfarin. Monitor prothrombin time and adjust warfarin dosage as necessary.

A complete blood count (CBC), blood chemistry profile, and liver function studies should be performed as a baseline assessment before therapy begins. The nature of the client's support services should also be determined.

■ **Nursing Diagnosis.** The following selected nursing diagnoses/collaborative problems may be identified with a client receiving disulfiram: risk for injury related to adverse drug reactions, a preexisting condition that contraindicates or requires the cautious use of disulfiram, or the occurrence of a disulfiram-alcohol reaction (nausea and vomiting, blurred vision, confusion, dizziness, tachycardia, flushing of the face, diaphoresis, headache, dyspnea and, rarely, seizures, chest pain, loss of consciousness, or death); disturbed sleep pattern related to the CNS effects of the drug (drowsiness); impaired comfort (headache, rash, stomach discomfort); imbalanced nutrition: less than body requirements related to gustatory alterations (metallic or garlic-like taste in the mouth); disturbed thought processes related to a psychotic reaction (mood or mental changes); ineffective sexuality patterns related to decreased sexual ability in men; and the potential complications of peripheral neuritis (numbness, tingling, or weakness in the hands and feet), optic neuritis (change in vision), encephalopathy (mental changes), and hepatitis (abdominal discomfort, jaundice, dark urine, light stools).

■ **Implementation**

■ ***Monitoring.*** The effectiveness of disulfiram therapy is monitored by assessing the client's abstinence from alcohol use. The client should be observed for visual disturbances and eye pain, which might indicate optic neuritis. Tingling or numbness of the hands or feet may indicate the development of peripheral neuritis. Jaundice may indicate a drug-induced hepatotoxicity.

A transaminase test for liver function is recommended 10 to 14 days into disulfiram therapy and every 6 months during therapy, along with a CBC and blood chemistry profile to monitor for adverse reactions to the drug. Serum cholesterol concentrations may increase with disulfiram dosages of 500 mg/day.

■ ***Intervention.*** Provide support to assist the client in achieving the goal of abstinence. Psychotherapy aimed at mental and social rehabilitation should accompany disulfiram therapy. Refer to an appropriate support group in planning for discharge.

In instances of a severe alcohol-disulfiram reaction, supportive measures need to be instituted to restore the blood pressure and treat the client for shock. This type of reaction lasts until the alcohol is metabolized—usually 30 minutes to several hours depending on the amount of alcohol ingested, the dose of disulfiram, and the time since its last administration. Administer oxygen and monitor potassium levels and electrocardiogram (ECG) tracings (AHFS, 1999).

Ensure safety precautions such as assistance with transferring and ambulating if the client has the CNS effect of drowsiness.

■ ***Education.*** Caution the client that ingesting any form of alcohol while taking disulfiram, and for up to 14 days after the last dose, will cause a very unpleasant response—dizziness, syncope, nausea and vomiting, headache, chest pain, dyspnea, palpitations, tachycardia, profuse sweating, facial flushing, and blurred vision. If the response is severe, seizures, unconsciousness, heart attack, and death can result. The extent of the reaction depends on the dose of the drug and the amount of alcohol ingested.

All foods and liquid medications should be checked for the presence of alcohol. Alcohol is available in prescription drugs, OTC drugs, liquid cough-cold analgesic products, foods, flavoring, mouthwashes, salad dressings, vinegars, and other such products. The client should be warned of possible interactions and the need to check all liquids for alcohol. Topical lotions with a high alcohol content should be used cautiously.

The client should wear Medic Alert identification while taking the drug and should alert any health care professionals providing care. Identification cards describing the most common symptoms of the alcohol-disulfiram reaction are available from the manufacturer.

Caution the client against driving or operating any hazardous equipment if drowsiness occurs. A slight metallic or garlic-like taste may occur for the first few weeks of therapy. Alert the client that many drug-induced reactions subside after approximately 2 weeks of therapy. The client should consult with the health care provider at 6-month intervals for blood studies or if any of the following occur: chest pain, respiratory difficulty, jaundice, or the ingestion of alcohol.

■ **Evaluation.** The client will abstain from alcohol, experience no disulfiram-alcohol reactions, demonstrate no adverse reactions to disulfiram, verbalize content taught about the drug, and self-administer the drug safely and accurately when managing his or her own medication regimen.

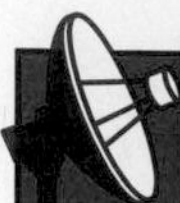

TechnologyLink
Substance Misuse and Abuse

Video Resources

Mosby's Nursing Care of the Client With Substance Abuse Videotape Series, Vol. 1-6 (ISBN 0-8151-5994-3)

Mosby, Inc., 11830 Westline Industrial Drive, St. Louis, MO 63146; (800) 426-4545; www.mosby.com.

Dual Diagnosis, ISBN 0-8151-6000-3

Substance Abuse in Families, Children and Adolescents, ISBN 0-8151-5999-4

Substance Abuse in Chemical Dependency Treatment Centers, ISBN 0-8151-5997-8

Substance Abuse in Perinatal Care, ISBN 0-8151-5998-6

Substance Abuse in the Community, ISBN 0-8151-5996-X

Substance Abuse in the Hospital, ISBN 0-8151-5995-1

Mosby's Psychiatric Nursing Videotape Series, Volume 4: *Substance Abuse,* ISBN 0-8151-8573-1; Mosby, Inc.

Web Resources

About—Substance Abuse (substanceabuse.about.com/health/substanceabuse/)

This site offers a variety of resources on substance abuse, such as articles, netlinks, newsletter, drug information, search tools, related forums, and frequently asked questions.

American Outreach Association Educational Material for Children (www.americanoutreach.org/index.htm)

This site provides educational material for children, parents, and teachers regarding substance abuse.

National Council on Alcohol and Drug Dependence (NCADD) (www.ncadd.org/)

This organization offers education and information on alcohol and drug abuse, a list of prevention and treatment programs in the United States, publications, and other resources.

The National Center on Addiction and Substance Abuse at Columbia University (www.casacolumbia.org/)

This site reviews the social and economic costs of substance abuse; reviews what works for prevention, treatment, and law enforcement; lists research programs; and more.

National Institute on Drug Abuse (NIDA) (www.nida.nih.gov/)

This organization provides research, training, and information on the prevention and treatment of drug abuse.

U.S. Department of State, International Information Programs (usinfo.state.gov/topical/global/drugs/)

This site provides global and local information on publications, policy, and resources on narcotics and the drug trade. It also lists prevention, treatment, education, and research programs.

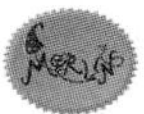

For additional WebLinks, a free subscription to the "Mosby/Saunders ePharmacology Update" newsletter, and more, go to mosby.com/MERLIN/McKenry/.

Central Nervous System Stimulants

The primary CNS stimulants abused in the United States include cocaine and amphetamine products, especially methamphetamine.

Cocaine

Although classified as a controlled substance, cocaine is an alkaloid related to the belladonna alkaloids. Topically it has the therapeutic effects of local anesthesia and vasoconstriction; thus it has limited use in a few selected surgical procedures, such as nasal surgery.

Cocaine is a very dangerous substance with a high amount of financial, psychologic, and physical control over the user. The abuse of this substance has reached epidemic levels. In Canada and the United States it is one of the most commonly mentioned drugs resulting in emergency department visits, second only to alcohol in combination with other substances (Drug Abuse Warning Network, 1999). It has been estimated that 3 million Americans are regular users of cocaine (Scott & Gabel, 1995).

Cocaine is a very potent, short-lived CNS stimulant; it is a highly addicting and potentially lethal drug. As a social-recreational drug of abuse, it is popular for its euphoric effects. It also produces increased energy like the amphetamines and may lead to a similar psychotic state with strong elements of paranoia.

The purity of the illicitly produced drug varies greatly because it is often diluted or cut with agents such as amphetamines, boric acid, quinine, mannitol, procaine, and lidocaine. The vasoconstricting effect of cocaine may be responsible for limiting its own absorption. Multiple drugs are often taken with or after cocaine, such as alcohol (84% of users), marijuana (98% of cocaine addicts), heroin, barbiturates, benzodiazepines, and phencyclidine (PCP) (Scott & Gabel, 1995).

Routes of Administration. Cocaine may be taken by sniffing (snorting) the white, fluffy crystalline powder (which resembles snow, hence its street name), by direct IV injection, or by smoking the converted base form called "freebase" or crack (transalveolar route). In the United States, cocaine is usually found as the hydrochloride (HCl) salt or in the base form. Cocaine HCl is water soluble and thus can be inhaled (snorted) or injected intravenously. It may be inhaled from a small spoon, rolled dollar bills, a lengthened fingernail, or various other inhalation devices. Sniffing causes vasoconstriction, which limits the amount of cocaine absorbed from the nasal mucosa into the systemic circulation; more intense effects are derived from freebase or crack cocaine.

Freebase and crack cocaine (minus the HCl salt) are essentially the same free alkaloid base; the difference between them is that different solvents are used in the manufacturing process (Scott & Gabel, 1995). Freebase is dangerous to make (ether and ammonia are involved) and dangerous to use. The freebase form is heat resistant, which lends itself to smoking in any form, including "coke pipes." Smoking freebase cocaine produces a more intense effect and is dangerous because of the possibility of administering an excessive dose. The freebase solvents are flammable and may explode during the process, causing further harm to the user.

When dried, freebase cocaine looks like rocks; when smoked, it makes a cracking sound. Therefore the street names of freebase cocaine include "rock," "crack," "gravel," and "readyrock." Freebase cocaine has largely been replaced by crack cocaine, which produces a fast and very intense effect. Crack cocaine is a freebase, but it is made without any volatile chemicals. It has become popular because of its availability in smaller amounts at a much lower cost than freebase cocaine and because its use does not require any elaborate paraphernalia. The cocaine market has thus become affordable to all economic groups.

Pharmacokinetics. Cocaine is rapidly metabolized in the liver; the cocaine abuser may need to use the drug every half hour or less to maintain the high. Cocaine serum levels are not proportional to toxicity, and the elimination half-lives by oral, intranasal, and IV routes are similar (50, 80, and 60 minutes, respectively). Cocaine stimulation of the CNS initially affects the intellect (cognition) and behavior (affective domain).

At this time there is no absolute level that is lethal. In determining fatal reactions, the rapidity of the increase in blood level may be as important as the peak blood concentration. Factors other than blood concentration must be examined, including tolerance, reverse tolerance, previous history of cocaine abuse, individual susceptibility, the presence of other drugs, and medical problems associated with cocaine abuse.

The initial symptoms of cocaine use are restlessness, mydriasis, hyperreflexia, vasoconstriction, tachycardia, hypertension, hallucinations, nausea, vomiting, and muscle spasms. These symptoms may be followed by respiratory failure, convulsions, coma, and circulatory collapse. In chronic abusers, a toxic cocaine psychosis (similar to paranoid schizophrenia) is often found and is characterized by hallucinations and paranoid delusions. Skin eruptions (with itching and compulsive scratching) caused by self-inflicted skin irritation are also commonly observed. Energetic individuals may be prone to outbursts of violent behavior. Blood in the nose and a perforated nasal septum are often seen in individuals who chronically snort cocaine.

The medical complications associated with cocaine abuse are numerous and vary with the type of cocaine used and the route of administration. Many body systems are affected, including cardiovascular (hypertension, tachycardia, myocardial infarction, dysrhythmias, thrombosis, and sudden death); respiratory (pulmonary abscesses, lung infections, pulmonary edema and hemorrhage, and pneumonitis); renal (rhabdomyolysis—the release of skeletal muscle contents into the plasma, which results in generalized muscle aches and pains and, in one third of the reports, acute renal failure); and neurologic (seizures, stroke, and intracranial hemorrhage). Psychiatric conditions (psychosis, suicide, delirium, and clinical depression) may occur, as well as miscellaneous other conditions such as septicemia, hepatitis, and human immunodeficiency virus (HIV) infection.

Cocaine is particularly dangerous in pregnant women. It has been associated with an increased risk of stillbirth, preterm labor, and neonatal complications such as congenital malformations, cerebral infarction and hemorrhage, and sudden infant death syndrome. Neonatal complications include acute withdrawal symptoms (increased irritability, tremors, abnormal reflexes, tachypnea, and poor eating and sleeping patterns) and neurobehavioral delays during the first year of life. Such infants may also be susceptible to cocaine-induced seizures, cerebral infarction, and potentially a variety of other complications (Young, Vosper, & Phillips, 1992). Such effects have resulted in child-abuse convictions for mothers who used cocaine while pregnant (Schydlower, 1990). (See the Management of Drug Overdose box on p. 176.)

Amphetamine Products

Amphetamine abuse has been reported for more than 50 years. After declining for a while, its use has now increased (see Table 9-2). It has been estimated that 3 million Americans used these drugs for nonmedical purposes in 1992 (Scott & Gabel, 1995). (See Table 9-3 for street names of and additional information about amphetamines.)

Chemically, amphetamines are similar to the natural catecholamines, epinephrine, norepinephrine, and dopamine. They can activate catecholamine receptor sites to increase stimulation and therefore have been classified as sympathomimetic agents. In addition, they increase the release of natural catecholamines and block their reuptake into the neurons, which results in the induction of an artificial "fight-or-flight" response (Scott & Gabel, 1995).

Oral amphetamines are absorbed from the gastrointestinal tract and concentrate in the brain, kidneys, and lungs. They are metabolized in the liver and excreted via the kidneys. Amphetamines are a basic drug with a **pK_a** (the point at which half the drug amount in the body is ionized and half is nonionized) of 9.9; therefore a urine pH of 7 or more extends the half-life to approximately 20 hours. A urine pH of 5 reduces the half-life to 5 to 6 hours. Persons who abuse amphetamines are usually aware of the prolonged effect they can achieve by alkalizing their urine. Prescribers are also aware that acidifying the urine to a pH of 4.5 to 5.5 will enhance amphetamine excretion.

Effects. The amphetamines are usually abused because they produce mood elevation, reduction of fatigue, and a

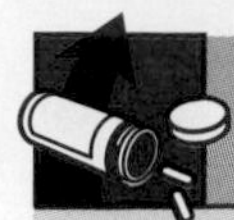

Management of Drug Overdose
Cocaine

General Approach

- Provide symptomatic and basic supportive care of airway, breathing, and circulation (the ABCs).
- Establish an IV line using an isotonic or hypotonic solution for the administration of the medications necessary to treat the adverse effects induced by cocaine.
- Continuously monitor client's vital signs and core body temperature.
- Avoid or reduce sensory stimulation because it may provoke or worsen agitation and paranoid behavior.

Specific Approach

Treat medical complications as necessary:

- For metabolic acidosis, administer sodium bicarbonate.
- For hyperthermia, use external cooling measures such as sponging with cold water, or use a cooling blanket.
- For seizures, administer diazepam (Valium), lorazepam (Ativan), phenobarbital (Luminal), phenytoin (Dilantin), or thiopental (Pentothal) intravenously as necessary.
- For cardiac dysrhythmias, administer propranolol (Inderal), labetalol (Normodyne), phentolamine (Regitine), or lidocaine as necessary.
- For hypertension, administer phentolamine (Regitine), labetalol (Normodyne), verapamil (Isoptin), or nitroprusside as indicated.
- Monitor and treat other side effects/adverse reactions as necessary.

sense of increased alertness. They do not create extra physical or mental energy but instead promote the expenditure of present resources, often to the point of hazardous fatigue. IV injection of amphetamines results in marked euphoria—an orgasmic feeling known as a "rush" that is accompanied by a sense of great physical strength and clear thinking. The person feels little or no need for rest, sleep, or food and may continually engage in vigorous activity that the user may perceive as exhilarating and creative. To an observer, however, the individual appears inefficient and is performing repetitious behaviors, which is common during an amphetamine high.

Termination of the drug's effect may result from exhaustion, fright, or an inability to obtain more drug. Drug withdrawal is followed by long periods of sleep, and on awakening the individual often feels hungry, extremely lethargic, and profoundly depressed. This phenomenon is known as "crashing." Suicide risk is quite possible during this period.

The stimulant properties of amphetamines can cause dramatic cardiorespiratory effects such as tachycardia, dyspnea, chest pain, and hypertension. The person may panic because these signs and symptoms are also those of a myocardial infarction. To deal with these disturbing symptoms, individuals often use depressants or "downers" such as large amounts of alcohol, marijuana, benzodiazepines, barbiturates, or heroin to offset the overstimulation effect (Scott & Gabel, 1995).

Acute toxic amphetamine effects can be very serious. In addition to the signs and symptoms mentioned previously, seizures and circulatory collapse have been reported. According to Scott and Gabel (1995), "fatal intoxication usually is preceded by hyperpyrexia, convulsion, and shock." Detoxification and the use of conventional therapies for medical complications are necessary in the treatment of the acute toxicity.

Amphetamines are also said to be psychotomimetic, but there is conflicting evidence regarding the cause of amphetamine psychosis. Is the psychosis caused by heavy use of amphetamines, or is the user perhaps also mentally ill? Or are some of the symptoms (paranoia, aggression, delusions of persecution, hallucinations) secondary to the insomnia (sleep deprivation) induced by prolonged amphetamine abuse?

The health care professional should be aware that the use of amphetamines (especially methamphetamine) is on the increase, with much of it being made by illicit laboratories in the United States. Crystal methamphetamine (known as "ice" or "crystal meth") is gaining popularity because a high usually results in less than a minute when these crystals are heated and the vapor inhaled (Scott & Gabel, 1995). In some instances individuals who use oral amphetamine also smoke methamphetamine concurrently to vastly increase the intensity of effect. Methamphetamine serum levels after smoking produce elevated plasma levels and a high that can persist for 12 hours (with a half-life of approximately 12 hours), whereas the smoking of freebase cocaine rapidly peaks and is rapidly eliminated because it has a half-life of approximately 1 hour. The toxicity resulting from the combination of smoking and oral administration produces an enhanced and potentially dangerous effect. (See the Management of Drug Overdose box on p. 177.)

Preparations. Chemically, there are three types of amphetamines—salts of racemic amphetamines, dextroamphetamines, and methamphetamines—all of which vary in their degree of potency and peripheral effects. Dextroamphetamine is said to have the fewest peripheral effects, such as hypertension and tachycardia.

Cannabis Drugs (Marijuana/Hashish)

The cannabis drugs are derived from the leaves, stems, fruiting tops, and resin of both female and male hemp plants (*Cannabis sativa*). The potency of the active ingredient, tetrahydrocannabinol (THC) is greatest in the flowering tops of the plant and seems to vary according to the climatic conditions under which the plant is grown. In North America the plants grow wild or are illegally cultivated; their potency therefore varies. The only legal cultivation in the United

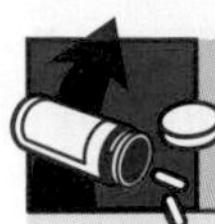

Management of Drug Overdose
Amphetamines

General Approach

- No specific antidote is available to treat amphetamine overdose.
- Psychotic symptoms usually occur within 36 to 48 hours after a single large overdose. These symptoms usually clear in approximately 1 week.
- Treatment is mainly supportive and symptomatic.

Specific Approach

- If a large overdose is discovered within 1 hour in a conscious, nonconvulsant client, vomiting or gastric lavage may be used and followed with a saline cathartic.
- The person should be closely monitored because of the potential for hypertension, hyperpyrexia, and seizures.
- To increase renal excretion of amphetamines, an osmotic diuretic such as mannitol with a urinary acidifier (ammonium chloride) may be necessary.
- After the acute episode, the amphetamine abuser will need intensive counseling, and perhaps desensitization techniques, on a long-term basis to overcome the craving and relapses common with the abuse of this stimulant drug.

States and Canada is that by the government for research purposes.

Both the availability of more potent species and varieties of marijuana and the increase in use among young adolescents (12 to 14 years of age) require a new attitude of concern toward the substance. The potency of THC in marijuana varies, with the typical leaf containing 3%. When carefully cultivated, imported marijuana may contain 6% to 10% THC (Jungnickel, 1995). Marijuana grown under scientifically controlled conditions is often much more potent than the domestic variety smoked in the past.

Preparations. Marijuana and hashish are the most common forms of cannabis in use. *Hashish* refers to the powdered form of the plant's resin, which contains 7% to 12% THC (Jungnickel, 1995). Other forms of cannabis used in such countries as Jamaica, Mexico, Africa, India, and the Middle East include *ganja, bhang,* and *charas,* which corresponds to American marijuana. *Kif* is used in Morocco, whereas in South Africa a cannabis drug called *dagga* is often used.

Marijuana plants contain hundreds of different chemicals. Approximately 100 chemicals have been isolated and are generally termed *cannabinoids.* Of these, only THC (delta-9-tetrahydrocannabinol) and CBD (cannabidiol) have been studied in humans to identify their pharmacologic effects. Although many questions remain unanswered, it is believed the major psychoactive ingredient in cannabis is THC.

Dronabinol (Marinol or THC) and nabilone (Cesamet) are synthetic cannabinoids available for the treatment of cancer chemotherapy–induced nausea and vomiting that is not responsive to standard therapies. Both products have a high potential for abuse and are therefore closely regulated under the Federal Controlled Substances Act (Schedule II).

Mode of Administration. Cannabis drugs may be absorbed when administered by oral, subcutaneous, or pulmonary routes, but they are most potent when inhaled. Either the pure resin or the dried leaves of the cannabis plant may be smoked in pipes or cigarettes (joints). Because the smoke is acrid and irritating, some users prefer to smoke marijuana through a water pipe. The smoke is inhaled deeply and retained in the lungs as long as possible to achieve maximal saturation of the absorbing surface. Powdered hashish and marijuana may also be mixed with foods, a mode of administration that delays the drug's absorption. The effects sought by individuals who use this substance are mental relaxation and euphoria. The sedative-hypnotic effects of smoking are rapid and generally last 2 to 3 hours, whereas the effects of the orally ingested drugs may not begin for several hours. Hashish oil injected intravenously has a high incidence of mortality.

Mechanism of Action. All of the cannabis drugs seem to act as CNS depressants. They depress higher brain centers and consequently release lower centers from inhibitory influences. Although some controversy exists regarding their classification, the cannabis drugs are not narcotic derivatives but are legally classified as controlled substances. They are more commonly classified as sedative-hypnotic-anesthetics or psychedelic (capable of altering perception, thought, and feeling) drugs. Like the sedative-hypnotics, they appear to depress the ascending reticular activating system. As the dose increases, their effects proceed from relief of anxiety, disinhibition, and excitement to anesthesia. If the dose is high enough, respiratory and vasomotor depression and collapse may occur.

Pharmacokinetics. The peak plasma level of THC after smoking one marijuana cigarette is reported to occur within minutes. THC is metabolized in the liver, with the major route of elimination being bile and feces. Only trace amounts of the unmetabolized THC are detected in the urine.

Marijuana may affect the metabolism of other drugs in the liver or compete with other drugs for protein-binding sites in the plasma; ethyl alcohol, barbiturates, amphetamines, cocaine, opiates, and atropine are some of the reportedly affected drugs.

Effects. The potency of marijuana varies with plant strain and cultivation, but the cigarettes usually produce moderate to intense psychopharmacologic effects that peak in 15 minutes and last 1 to 4 hours. The drug has intoxicating, mind-altering properties. It induces an anxiety-free state characterized by a feeling of well-being. Perceptions of time and space are distorted. Ideas flow freely and disconnectedly; interruptions in thought that are blanks or gaps similar to an epileptic absence may occur. The individual may experience palpitations, loss of concentration, lightheadedness, and floating sensations followed by weakness, tremors, postural hypotension, incoordination, and ataxia. Hallucinations can occur with high doses of the drug.

Dissociative phenomena are also reported; research suggests that impaired decision making and psychometric performance are related to marijuana use. The drug experience is highly subjective; the novice may not perceive the presence of an altered state of consciousness until sensitized to it by colleagues. Factors that influence the psychologic and behavioral effects of marijuana include drug dose, the user's personality, the user's expectations of the effects of the drug, the environment, social influences, and life experiences.

The side effects of marijuana use include immediate tachycardia and delayed bradycardia, delayed hypotension, conjunctival vascular congestion (red eyes), dry mouth and throat, delayed gastrointestinal disturbances, possible vasovagal syncope, and enhanced appetite and flavor appreciation. The more serious side effects are psychologic and include fear, panic (especially among first-time or naive users), paranoia, disorientation, memory loss, confusion, and a variety of perceptual alterations. Marijuana has been known to precipitate acute psychotic reactions and toxic psychoses in poorly organized personalities. The incidence of adverse reactions appears to be highest in novice users of the drug.

Withdrawal Symptoms. Physiologic withdrawal symptoms have been reported with discontinued use of marijuana. Minor discomfort may pass in several days, but insomnia, anxiety, irritability, and restlessness may persist for weeks. Craving for the drug can recur intermittently for months after the drug is stopped. In general, nonpharmacologic interventions and an exercise program are preferred over substitution of another drug product.

BOX 9-3

Classification of Benzodiazepines

Short-Acting (Half-life Less Than 24 Hours)

alprazolam (Xanax)
bromazepam (Lectopam 🍁)
clonazepam (Klonopin)
lorazepam (Ativan, Apo-Lorazepam 🍁)
nitrazepam (Mogadon 🍁)
oxazepam (Serax, Ox-Pam 🍁)
temazepam (Restoril)
triazolam (Halcion)

Long-Acting (Half-life Longer Than 24 Hours)

chlordiazepoxide (Librium, Novo-Poxide 🍁)
clorazepate (Tranxene)
diazepam (Valium, Apo-Diazepam 🍁)
flurazepam (Dalmane, Novoflupam 🍁)
halazepam (Paxipam)
ketazolam (Loftran 🍁)
prazepam (Centrax)
quazepam (Doral)

Central Nervous System Depressants

Barbiturates and Nonbarbiturates

Reports of the use and abuse of barbiturates and nonbarbiturate sedative-hypnotics have declined greatly in recent years, probably as a result of the availability of newer agents that have greater safety and effectiveness profiles. It has been suggested that treatment of abuse and addiction to these agents should be similar to the interventions reviewed for alcohol and benzodiazepine abuse (O'Brien, 1996). (See Table 9-3 for barbiturate information.)

Benzodiazepines (diazepam, alprazolam, lorazepam)

Benzodiazepines are commonly prescribed for anxiety or insomnia. Although they are not considered street or illegal drugs, misuse, abuse, and drug dependency have been reported, especially with diazepam (Valium), alprazolam (Xanax), and lorazepam (Ativan).

Benzodiazepine withdrawal syndrome is more likely to occur if the drug has been taken regularly for more than 3 months, if the drug dose consumed was higher than recommended, if clients have a history of substance abuse or passive and dependent personality traits, or if the drug is discontinued abruptly. Withdrawal symptoms from short-acting benzodiazepines occur within 1 to 2 days and from long-acting benzodiazepines in 5 to 7 days. Symptoms include increased anxiety and irritability, twitching, aching, muscle weakness, tremors, headache, nausea, anorexia, depression, lethargy, blurred vision, sleep disturbance, hypersensitivity to stimuli (light, touch, sound), and hyperreflexia. Delirium, psychosis, and convulsions are rare but have been reported.

Management of benzodiazepine dependence should include gradual drug withdrawal. If the individual is dependent on a short-acting benzodiazepine, a switch to a long-acting benzodiazepine is recommended for the withdrawal process. Withdrawal symptoms occur more frequently and are more severe in individuals who suddenly withdraw from short-acting benzodiazepines, whereas the use of a long-acting benzodiazepine is associated with less prominent withdrawal symptoms (Box 9-3). In general, a 10% to 25% reduction in the benzodiazepine dosage every 1 to 2 weeks is recommended. Titration schedules and dosage reductions may vary, but the time frame is usually within 1 to 4 months. In very difficult withdrawals, the addition of the anticonvulsant carbamazepine (Tegretol) or the beta-adrenergic blocker propranolol (Inderal) may help to reduce withdrawal symptoms (Grimsley, 1995).

Flumazenil (Romazicon) is a benzodiazepine receptor antagonist that is administered intravenously for the treatment of benzodiazepine toxicity. Although it appears to have no pharmacologic effects of its own, it has been reported to be associated with seizures, cardiac dysrhythmias, and other serious adverse reactions in clients receiving benzodiazepines or in those with mixed drug overdoses (particularly with tricyclic antidepressants). Therefore in high-risk clients the smallest effective dose should be used with close monitoring (*Drug Facts and Comparisons*, 2000). (See Chapter 16 for benzodiazepine pharmacokinetics, additional pharmacologic information, treatment of benzodiazepine overdose, and nursing management of benzodiazepine therapy.)

Nonopioid Analgesics (acetaminophen, aspirin, ibuprofen)

Acetaminophen (Tylenol), aspirin, and ibuprofen (Motrin) are OTC drugs readily available in many outlets in the United States and Canada. These same ingredients may also be contained in additional combination formulations and sold with or without a prescription. Thus the potential for intentional and nonintentional drug overdose exists with this category of drugs.

Overdoses from nonopioid analgesics are commonly seen in emergency departments. Covington (1996) reports that 66% of OTC analgesic overdose reports in the United States are associated with acetaminophen, with ibuprofen and aspirin accounting for 19% and 15%, respectively. Approximately 58% of the overdoses occur in children under 6 years of age. (See Chapter 11 for additional information on this drug category.)

Hallucinogens

Classifications of the most common hallucinogenic agents include lysergic acid diethylamide or lysergide (LSD) and its variants, mescaline, psilocybin, and phencyclidine (PCP). The term *entactogen* is also used to refer to substances that have mind-altering effects (Jungnickel, 1995). A number of psychoactive hallucinogenic drugs have been used as adjuncts to religious services or were used experimentally on college campuses in the 1960s. LSD, dimethyltryptamine (DMT), PCP, mescaline, psilocybin, and MDMA (3, 4-methylenedioxymethamphetamine, also known as ecstasy) are examples of the drugs that can produce distortions in perception or thinking at very low doses (Box 9-4). The use of most of these drugs declined in the 1970s to 1980s, with the exception of PCP; the use of hallucinogens has increased again in the 1990s (Kaufman & McNaul, 1992).

LSD (lysergide)

LSD is a very potent and illicit hallucinogen that is usually available in doses of approximately 200 μg. It causes a central sympathomimetic effect within 20 minutes of oral administration—hypertension, dilated pupils, hyperthermia, tachycardia, and enhanced alertness. The psychoactive effects occur in approximately 1 to 2 hours and have been described as heightened perceptions, distortions of the body, and visual hallucinations. The effect on mood is unpredictable and ranges from euphoria to severe depression and panic.

BOX 9-4

Hallucinogens

MDA An amphetamine-type drug similar in structure to MDMA; destroys serotonin-producing neurons in the brain.

MDMA (ecstasy, Adam, XTC) A stimulant-hallucinogenic used largely by college students; evidence indicates it can destroy dopamine neurons in the brain; high doses or chronic use may lead to Parkinson's symptoms and, eventually, paralysis.

MPPP (meperidine analogue) Synthesis usually produces a toxic byproduct, MPTP, which has caused permanent, irreversible Parkinson's disease in users.

Information from Hall, I.N. (1989). U.S. illicit drug production booming. *Street Pharmacology, 12*(Spring), 4.

Unpleasant experiences with LSD are rather common. Clinically, evidence of impaired judgment in the toxic state is common and well known; such behavior is demonstrated, for example, by LSD users attempting to stop traffic with their bodies. Altered states of consciousness may cause psychosis or trigger a latent psychosis into activity. Feelings of acute panic and paranoia during a toxic LSD psychosis can result in homicidal thoughts and actions. Toxic delirium, with altering and alternating levels of consciousness, follows toxic psychosis; the experience generally resolves in a stage of exhaustion in which the user feels "empty," is unable to coordinate thoughts, and is depressed. Suicide is a definite risk during this time.

Significant unfavorable reactions induced by LSD include prolonged, delayed, and recurrent reactions such as depression and long-term schizophrenic or psychotic reactions. Recurrent reactions have been described as flashback phenomena and refer to the transient, spontaneous repetition of a previous LSD-induced experience that is unrelated to renewed administration of the drug. Flashbacks occur in 15% to 77% of LSD users. A bad "trip" (anxiety or panic reaction) on LSD is likely to be a paranoid experience, and tendencies toward violence can be characteristic of LSD intoxication.

The treatment for bad trips has not changed over the years. A "talk-down" approach in a quiet, relaxed environment is often used. This helps to reassure the individual that he or she is safe and that the drug effects will dissipate in a few hours. If talking down cannot help the panic, then drug therapy with an oral benzodiazepine such as diazepam (Valium) might be considered. The use of phenothiazines, especially chlorpromazine (Thorazine) is avoided because such agents can potentiate the panic reaction, induce postural hypotension, and perhaps induce anticholinergic toxicity. In any case, the administration of medication is recommended only as an adjunct to crisis intervention psychotherapy, which consists of directing the person's attention away from perceptions that produce panic and providing reassurance that the experience will dissipate and that no permanent harm has been done. Flashbacks are treated as acute drug-induced episodes (Jungnickel, 1995).

The practice of administering massive doses of tranquilizers, applying restraints, and isolating such individuals should be avoided. The client's dramatically heightened awareness of the environment and distorted perceptions may render these measures traumatic rather than therapeutic.

Pregnant women should be especially cautioned against taking LSD. Because lysergic acid is the base of all ergot alkaloids, it has uterine stimulant properties that can adversely affect a pregnancy.

mescaline [mes' kah leen]

Mescaline is the chief alkaloid extracted from mescal buttons (flowering heads) of the peyote cactus; it produces subjective hallucinogenic effects similar to those of LSD. It is usually ingested in the form of a soluble crystalline powder that is either dissolved into teas or capsulated. The usual dose of mescaline is 300 to 500 mg.

Prodromal abdominal pain, nausea, vomiting, and diarrhea characterize the effects of mescaline doses up to 500 mg, and these are followed by vivid and colorful visual hallucinations. After oral ingestion, a syndrome of sympathomimetic effects is encountered and includes anxiety, hyperreflexia, static tremors, and psychic disturbances with vivid visual hallucinations. The half-life of mescaline is approximately 6 hours, and it is excreted in the urine.

psilocybin [sye loh sye' bin]

Psilocybin is a drug derived from Mexican mushrooms and produces subjective hallucinogenic effects similar to those of mescaline but of shorter duration. A hallucinogenic dysphoric state begins within 1/2 to 1 hour after the ingestion of 5 to 15 mg psilocybin. A dose of 20 to 60 mg may produce effects lasting 5 or 6 hours. The mood is pleasant to some users, and others experience apprehension. The individual using psilocybin has poor critical judgment capacities and impaired performance ability. Hyperkinetic compulsive movements, laughter, mydriasis, vertigo, ataxia, paresthesia, muscle weakness, drowsiness, and sleep are also seen.

PCP (phencyclidine)

PCP is a hallucinogen with a history of the most serious adverse reactions; more suicides, assaults, and murders appear to result from its use. It was developed in the late 1950s as an anesthetic for dissociative anesthesia, a cataleptic state in which the person appears to be awake but is detached from the surroundings and unresponsive to pain. The drug was withdrawn from human use after hallucinogenic effects were noted in clients emerging from this anesthetic. It is, however, used in veterinary practice, and this use is the origin of one of its street names, "hog" (Katzung, 1997).

Pharmacokinetics. PCP is rapidly metabolized in the liver to inactive metabolites. The ingestion of large amounts results in high concentrations of the unmetabolized drug in urine. PCP is lipophilic and has a half-life of 1/2 to 1 hour in small doses and from 1 to 4 days in larger doses. The pK_a of the drug is 8.5. The "ion trapping" of the drug into extravascular areas, which are more acidic than the serum, is thought to be a major cause of prolonged toxicity. Recirculation of the drug, secretion into the acidic gastric fluid, and reabsorption in the small intestine may also account for the prolonged toxicity and offers a key to the management of the toxicity of overdose. These observations have led to treatment using urine acidification with diuresis and continuous gastric drainage in severe intoxication to enhance elimination. Urinary excretion is enhanced when the urine is acidified with ascorbic acid to a pH of 5.5 or less. The fact that PCP may be found in adipose tissue may indicate that the long-term effects are related to its lipophilic nature. PCP is possibly released during a nutritional fast, and the resulting symptoms are interpreted as a flashback.

Effects. In humans, the common peripheral signs of PCP use include flushing, profuse sweating, nystagmus, diplopia, ptosis, analgesia, and sedation. Other effects of PCP are as follows:

- A state similar to alcohol intoxication with ataxia and generalized numbness of the extremities
- Psychologic effects that usually proceed in three stages:
  - Change in body image and feelings of depersonalization
  - Perceptual distortions (visual or auditory)
  - Discomforting feelings of apathy, estrangement, or alienation
- Disorganization of thought and derealization that is greater than with LSD
- Impairment of attention span, motor skills, and sense of body boundaries, movement, and position
- Hallucinations that can recur unpredictably for days, weeks, or months

PCP is similar to ketamine in producing stages of anesthesia. In addition, excitation, paranoid behavior, self-destructive acts (because the sensation or feeling of pain is absent), horizontal and vertical nystagmus, tachycardia, hypertension, seizures, increased reflexes, muscle rigidity, respiratory depression, and coma with open eyes may ensue. PCP is a strong sympathomimetic and hallucinogenic dissociative anesthetic agent. Because the drug is now classified as a controlled substance, penalties for illegal manufacture have been enacted and enforced.

Some investigators claim that the effects of PCP mimic schizophrenia more accurately than those of other psychotomimetics or hallucinogenics. Like the symptoms of schizophrenia, the effects of PCP are reduced by sensory deprivation. Currently no chemical antidote exists for inhibiting the effects of PCP. Keeping the user quiet and away from sensory stimuli may decrease the intensity of some of the effects.

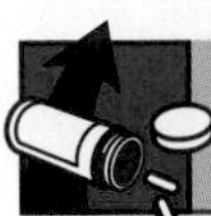

Management of Drug Overdose
PCP

General Approach

- The clinical symptoms and signs of PCP intoxication are dose related. The waxing and waning of these signs may be related to the pharmacokinetics of enteric reabsorption of the alkalized (nonionized) PCP with the recirculation and redistribution of the agent, as described earlier.
- The health care professional should be aware of these signs because this time period constitutes the greatest threat for both the client and the health care professional.
- The client often has alternating periods of paranoia, assaultiveness, terror, and hyperactivity followed by a calm demeanor, blank stare, or withdrawn period.
- During the first 10 days after ingestion, the health care professional should never assume that the calm states are permanent. During the acute intoxication phase, the patient is unable to process incoming sensory stimuli.

Specific Approach

- Treatment is primarily symptomatic.
- Keep patient in a dark room with minimal sensory stimulation and protection from self-inflicted injury. Do not attempt to talk down the PCP-anxious individual because it may provoke more serious anxiety or agitation.
- Diazepam (Valium) or haloperidol (Haldol) have been used for their antianxiety and antipsychotic effects, respectively.
- Urine acidification will enhance the excretion rate of PCP. Cranberry juice is commonly used to acidify the urine for this purpose.
- The use of PCP causes a wide range of subjective effects that require careful monitoring of the patient. Be aware that prolonged and severe behavioral disturbances may progress to respiratory and cardiovascular emergencies as serum levels of the drug change.

Toxic Effects. The pressor effects of PCP may cause hypertensive crisis, intracerebral hemorrhage, convulsions, coma, and death. (See the Management of Drug Overdose box above.)

Inhalants

Volatile hydrocarbons and aerosols are other substances of abuse. Representatives of this group include toluene, xylene, benzene, gasoline, paint thinner, typewriter correction fluid, lighter fluid, airplane glue, and nitrous oxide.

Volatile hydrocarbons are often used as propellants in aerosol products. When sniffed (inhaled), these agents may produce a rapid general CNS depression with marked inebriation, dizziness, floating sensations, exhilaration, and intense feelings of well-being that are at times exhibited as reckless abandon, disinhibition, and feelings of increased power and aggressiveness similar to those seen with alcohol intoxication. Inhalation may result in bronchial and laryngeal irritation, transient euphoria, headache, giddiness, vertigo, ataxia, and renal tubular acidosis, especially with glue sniffing. At high doses, confusion, coma, and blood dyscrasia occur. Depression may follow these early excitatory effects.

Chronic toluene abuse leads to hepatic and renal toxicity, and death from cardiac dysrhythmia and respiratory failure has been reported. Recovery from lower doses may be seen in 15 minutes to a few hours. Inhalant use is no longer limited to young children and preteens. Inhalants are widely used in the 12-to-17 age-group, with equally common use by both sexes (Neumark, Delva, & Anthony, 1998). The nurse in the pediatric setting may be the first health care professional to become aware of a problem with inhalants in a child or adolescent.

Butyl nitrite is a clear, yellow liquid sold as a room deodorizer under trade names such as Rush, Bolt, and Bullet. This substance is sold in drug paraphernalia shops and adult bookstores and by mail order. The opened container is placed under the nose; the individual inhales deeply and becomes dizzy, feels faint, and possibly loses consciousness. This rush lasts less than 1 minute and may include a headache, perspiration, and flushing, all caused by rapid vasodilation. It strongly resembles the effects achieved from amyl nitrite (a prescription smooth muscle relaxant and vasodilator). Amyl nitrite is sometimes abused to heighten a sexual orgasm in both partners. Both butyl nitrite and amyl nitrite lower blood pressure and reduce the heart's oxygen consumption. They diminish sexual inhibition and by their physiologic action may prolong sexual intercourse (Katzung, 1997).

Inhaled nitrite abuse has been implicated as being associated with or as being a contributory factor in the development of opportunistic infections and Kaposi's sarcoma in immunosuppressed homosexuals. The nitrites themselves are not considered a major risk factor, but individuals who use amyl nitrite and other nitrite products tend to have more sexual partners and could be at a higher risk of developing such infections (AHFS, 1999).

The development of tolerance also occurs with inhalants. For example, persons starting with one tube of sniffing glue per day may eventually increase to three, four, or more tubes per day to maintain the effect. In economically depressed populations, inhalants are often the first drug of abuse used.

Anabolic (Androgenic) Steroids

Anabolic-androgenic steroids are synthetic formulations produced from testosterone, the male hormone. Young

BOX 9-5

Major Effects of Anabolic Steroids

Androgen-Type Effects

Increased growth and development of the seminal vesicles and prostate gland
Increased body and facial hair
Increased production of oil from the sebaceous glands
Deepening of the voice
Increased sexual interest and desire
Enhancement of abstract and spatial dimension thinking ability
Increased aggression

Anabolic-Type Effects

Increased organ and skeletal muscle mass
Increased calcium in bones
Increased retention of total body nitrogen
Increased hemoglobin concentration
Increased protein synthesis

Information from Council on Scientific Affairs. (1990). Medical and nonmedical uses of anabolic-androgenic steroids. *JAMA, 264*(22), 2923.

people take these agents to increase strength and body weight, to look good, and to improve their chances of winning in sports (Faigenbaum, Zaichkowsky, Gardner, & Micheli, 1998). Box 9-5 lists the major effects of anabolic steroids. The Council on Scientific Affairs (1990) reported that men and women of all ages who are involved in athletic activity use anabolic steroids. Use is estimated in up to 80% of weight lifters and bodybuilders, and its use overall in competitors is approximately 50%. The abuse of these drugs is widespread and has been documented in young school-age students, in older persons, and in both males and females.

Since 1984 many organizations have publicly denounced or banned the use of anabolic steroids, including the American College of Sports Medicine, the American Medical Association, the National Collegiate Athletic Association, the International Olympic Committee, and the US Powerlifting Federation. Many states have also passed laws to ban or limit the selling of such products (Council on Scientific Affairs, 1990).

Nevertheless the debate continues over the use of steroids. Anabolic steroids have been prescribed, especially for underweight persons and for athletes seeking an edge in the competitive field. Many steroidal preparations are available and are used orally and parenterally. Athletes often use the drugs in amounts far in excess of the recommended dosages. This misuse led to the withdrawal of anabolic steroid products from the market in 1982. "Stacking" drugs or taking multiple anabolic steroids at one time is practiced by a number of athletes. This usually includes taking very large doses of the steroids on an 8-week cycle schedule while following a regular strenuous exercise program (perhaps on isolated muscle groups) and consuming a high-protein diet. The long-term effects of such a schedule have not been studied, but documented short-term effects include increased aggressive behavior and some masculinization in females.

BOX 9-6

Major Adverse Reactions to Anabolic Steroids

Females

Oily skin; acne
Decrease in breast size, ovulation, lactation, or menstruation
Hoarse and deep voice tone (usually irreversible)
Clitoral enlargement
Unusual hair growth and/or male-type baldness (usually irreversible)

Males

Prepuberty
Increased size of penis, number of erections, and secondary male characteristics
Postpuberty
Priapism (continuing erections), difficult/increased urination
Increased breast size (gynecomastia)
Testicular atrophy, oligospermia, impotence

Both Sexes

Hypercalcemia
Edema of the feet or legs
Jaundice, liver impairment
Liver carcinoma (rare)
Urinary calculi
Hypersensitivity
Insomnia
Iron deficiency anemia
Nausea, vomiting, anorexia, stomach pains

The disqualification of Olympic athletes for using steroids, in addition to the many undesirable and harmful effects reported from their usage, has led to an increase in the regulation of this category of drugs. In 1991 all anabolic steroids were placed in the Schedule III controlled substances category. Some states have even further restricted the availability of these drugs for nontherapeutic usage or are considering doing so (Surface, 1991). The general public should be informed of the serious health problems associated with short-term and long-term consumption of anabolic steroids (Box 9-6).

■ Nursing Management

Substance Misuse and Abuse

Because substance abuse transcends the boundaries of economics, social class, race, and ethnic background, all clients have the potential to abuse substances or be affected by someone who does. Great diversity exists among substances that may be abused and the manner in which they are abused. The role of the nurse may involve prevention, detection, treatment, and rehabilitation. Preventive nursing roles both inside and outside the health agency environment include the following (ANA, 1987):

- Education on addiction as it is manifested in relation to a substance or behavior, including the recreational misuse of substances such as alcohol and drugs
- Identification of individuals at high risk for the development of addictions, such as children of alcoholics and individuals who have been involved in a wide range of drug experimentation
- Identification of early signs and symptoms of addiction
- Activities to effect social change, such as networking and supporting legislation and policy directed toward reducing the incidence of addiction and its consequences to society
- Use of knowledge about alcohol, tobacco, food, and drug use and abuse in the comprehensive health teaching of clients receiving nursing care
- Use of knowledge of compulsive and dependent behaviors as the basis for health maintenance teaching

Health care providers, including nurses, have a high rate of substance abuse and related problems. Nurses must be aware of the potential for drug or substance abuse among themselves and other health care providers and be alert to recognize and deal with this problem should it arise. Many health care agencies and most states and provinces have substance abuse rehabilitation programs specifically for health care professionals.

Although the nurse plays an essential role in the prevention of substance abuse, many times the initial contact with the client is in the acute setting during acute drug intoxication and withdrawal. Signs of acute intoxication differ according to the substance abused and may have various manifestations. In addition, identification of the problem may be complex if multiple drugs are used.

Alcohol and drug overdose and intoxication may be life threatening. The immediate goals are to stabilize and maintain vital functions and minimize damage. Supportive treatment is combined with specific treatment once the drug has been identified. This is a time of acute psychologic stress for the client, and the nurse must remember to treat the whole client, not just a physiologic system. It is also a time of crisis during which the client and family may be especially receptive to intervention and long-term treatment of the problem.

Each nurse must evaluate his or her own feelings about and responses to substance abuse. Some nurses tend to react with disgust or disdain; this type of behavior often increases a client's low self-esteem and results in ineffective lectures and scare tactics. Another common response of the nurse is that of "enabler"—someone who shields the client from the consequences of substance abuse or unintentionally encourages continued substance abuse. The most effective response is to recognize and confront the problem directly. Nurses must acknowledge that substance abuse often results in death if left untreated. Appropriate treatment can often help these individuals overcome their problems and restore them to productive lives without dependence on harmful substances or drugs. Simply addressing the problem and providing an avenue for assistance can often begin the process of recovery, which might not start then but months or years later.

In 1978 the National Nurses Society on Addictions (NNSA) developed a position statement on the role of the nurse in alcoholism treatment. This statement can be used to consider concerns related to substance abuse in general. The five areas of nursing interventions addressed were (1) identification of the problem with alcohol, (2) communication about the problem, (3) education regarding alcohol use, abuse, and alcoholism, (4) counseling the alcoholic individual, family, and significant others, and (5) referral for treatment and aftercare (Bennett & Woolf, 1991). This approach is not limited to alcohol abuse but is also useful for intervention with clients abusing other substances.

■ **Assessment.** Assessment includes both physical and psychologic signs and symptoms of substance abuse. Observe closely both verbal and nonverbal responses to questions because an element of denial may often be ascertained in clients who abuse substances. The client's nonverbal responses may provide additional information and either contradict or reinforce what is verbally stated.

Physical assessment includes assessing vital signs, pupillary signs, and skin (especially for needle marks or "tracks" and abscesses that are often seen with injected substance abuse), as well as collecting data on nutrition, elimination, and sleep patterns. Diagnostic tests may be used to detect drugs or their metabolites in the blood or urine. Be aware of the possibility of false-positive results.

Past medical history of the client may include prior treatment of substance abuse or a history of drug-related illness such as hepatitis, abscesses, or bacterial endocarditis. Alcohol-related problems should be considered in clients with any of the following medical diagnoses: cellulitis, gastritis, ulcers, pancreatitis, cirrhosis, pneumonia, tuberculosis, peripheral neuropathy, seizure disorders, cerebellar degeneration, depression, suicide attempt, injuries from accidents or victimization, anemia, or malnutrition (Zahourek, 1986). A thorough drug history for current or past use of OTC, prescribed, or social/recreational drugs should be obtained and should include the frequency, magnitude, and circumstances of drug use and abuse, as well as the development of withdrawal symptoms if drug use was stopped.

Table 9-11 uses Gordon's Function Health Patterns to provide examples of selected clinical data that may indicate substance abuse. A further assessment is needed if a cluster of data indicates possible substance abuse.

One of the simplest and most widely used screening tools is the CAGE questionnaire (Mayfield, McLoed, & Hall, 1974; Zahourek, 1986; Iber, 1991). It was designed for use with alcohol addiction but can be modified for substance

TABLE 9-11 Nursing Assessment for Substance Abuse

Functional Health Pattern	Client Data That May Indicate Substance Abuse
Health perception–health management	Choices of daily living that are ineffective for meeting the goals of a treatment or prevention program
	Leaving the hospital against medical advice
	Stated desire to decrease substance use
	Boasting of ability to tolerate large amounts of substances
	Frequent changing of health care providers
	Appearance older than stated age
Nutritional-metabolic pattern	Malnutrition
	Irregular meal pattern
	Poor dental hygiene
	Frequent heartburn, anorexia, nausea
	Skin lesions (rash, ulcers, bruises, needle marks)
Elimination pattern	Recurrent diarrhea
	Chronic constipation
Activity-exercise pattern	Fatigue, decreased energy
	Loss of interest in non–substance seeking activities
	Poor hygiene
	Smelling of alcohol or other substances
	Heavy smoking
Sleep-rest pattern	Insomnia
	Diminished response to sleep or pain medication
Cognitive-perceptual pattern	Mental confusion
	Memory loss
	Poor judgment
	Diminished reality testing
	Blackouts
	Hallucinations
	Seizures
Self-perception–self-concept pattern	Denial of problem
Role-relationship pattern	Social life that revolves around substance use
	Poor fiscal management
	Marital problems
	Neglect of vulnerable individuals in home
	Verbalized inability to meet role expectations
	Unemployment or excessive absenteeism from work
	Repeated minor injuries on and off the job
Sexuality-reproductive pattern	Impotence
Coping–stress tolerance pattern	Binge drinking/drug bingeing
	Negative behaviors: hostility, aggression, lying, paranoia
	Depression
	Chronic complaints of anxiety/stress
	Frequent hospitalization
	Suicide attempts
Values-belief pattern	Lack of belief in future
	Lack of realistic goals
	Lack of belief system (religious or philosophical)

Modified from Bennett, E.G. & Woolf, D.S. (1991). *Substance abuse: Pharmacologic development and clinical perspectives* (2nd ed.). Albany, NY: Delmar Publishers.

abuse. It can be verbally incorporated into the process of taking every client's history by asking the following:

- Have you ever felt the need to Cut down your drinking (use of drugs)?
- Have you ever felt Annoyed by criticism of your drinking (drug use)?
- Have you ever had Guilt feelings about drinking (drug use)?
- Have you ever taken a morning Eye opener (required a drug fix to get on with your day's activities)?"

This assessment addresses common reactions to abuse, including concern for harm, hypersensitivity to criticism, perception of guilt in the harm the abuse does to others, and the occurrence of habituation or tolerance that requires a repeated dose to prevent early withdrawal symptoms (Iber, 1991).

■ **Nursing Diagnosis.** The following selected nursing diagnoses/collaborative problems may be identified in a client with substance abuse problems: deficient knowledge related to denial of problem, misinformation from associates, or no experience with substance abuse; ineffective coping related to lack of support from others, inadequately learned coping behaviors, or a social life that revolves around substance use; risk for self-directed/other-directed violence related to social isolation, hopelessness, or depression; ineffedctive health maintenance related to substance dependency, inadequate diet, poor lifestyle habits, impaired perception, poverty, inability to communicate needs, or denial of a need for change; ineffective therapeutic regimen management related to lack of resources (financial, social, personal), deficient knowledge, denial of substance abuse, mistrust of health personnel, or powerlessness; and the potential complication of withdrawal syndrome.

■ **Implementation**

■ ***Monitoring.*** Assessment of the effectiveness of the client's therapy is focused on how the client has tolerated the withdrawal period and developed new coping strategies. After the withdrawal period, the client must decide to remain drug free and maintain a healthy lifestyle. Relapses may occur and should not be viewed as the nurse's failure; the goal of treatment is longer and longer periods of sobriety/substance-free status and shorter and less frequent relapses. Participation by the client in long-term support from the appropriate agencies is essential in helping to remain drug free. Ultimately the decision to use and abuse drugs remains with the client.

■ ***Intervention.*** Physical and/or psychologic withdrawal symptoms may follow the abrupt cessation of drug or substance use. Interventions include monitoring vital signs, administering medications (if prescribed for treatment of withdrawal), and providing supportive nursing care. Clients who abuse substances often have nutrition deficiencies and other health problems, which should be corrected. Promotion of adequate nutrition, safety, rest, and orientation are general nursing interventions during this time. Rehabilitation begins during the withdrawal period and is continued in an attempt to avoid relapse.

Use a straightforward and receptive approach with clients who are abusing substances. Therapeutic communication should be focused on increasing self-esteem and confronting manipulative behavior while teaching effective coping mechanisms and problem solving. A client cannot restructure a manner of thinking, feeling, and acting until he or she achieves a new image. Many individuals who abuse substances suffer from the deprivation of basic needs such as physical closeness and emotional openness, which may in part be caused by the dissolution of basic family relationships. Such deprivation affects individual needs and the expectations of what one is entitled to in these meaningful relationships. A lack of fulfillment of these needs leads to a pronounced disequilibrium. Substance abuse affects all members of the family. Family members often enable the alcoholic or substance abuser to continue the abuse pattern by denying the problem. An open, caring, nonjudgmental discussion of the problem with the client and family members can have a positive effect on client outcomes.

A multidisciplinary approach is often best for these clients because they commonly have many health, personal, and social problems that must be addressed. Referral to appropriate agencies (e.g., Alcoholics Anonymous, Alateen, Cocaine Anonymous, Narcotics Anonymous, Al-Anon, Rational Recovery, and Adult Children of Alcoholics) will assist in the follow-up care of these clients and their family members and will provide much needed support and encouragement.

■ ***Education.*** Assist the client in developing effective coping mechanisms and "nondrug strategies" to deal with stress. Information should be provided in a factual, nonjudgmental way. Education of the client and family should include content about drugs and abused substances, such as signs and symptoms, effects on the body, progression of the condition, health problems associated with substance abuse, and psychosocial effects of substance abuse. General treatment options and the types and location of specific treatment facilities within the community should be discussed.

■ **Evaluation.** The client will experience minimal or no effects of withdrawal, verbalize an understanding of substance abuse and treatment, evidence positive coping without abused substances, experience no violent behaviors, demonstrate improvements in health maintenance, and successfully manage the therapeutic regimen.

SUMMARY

Although substance abuse is not a new phenomenon, the dimension of the problem for society is great. Substance abuse is a common denominator across cultural, ethnic, and socioeconomic populations and affects every aspect of life. As a consequence, the nurse needs to be familiar with drugs that have a potential for abuse—not only in their therapeutic use but also in their street forms. This knowledge will enhance the nursing role for the prevention, detection, treatment, and rehabilitation of clients with substance abuse.

The etiology of substance abuse for any given client may vary. The drug must produce a desired effect for it to cause dependence. Currently the commonly abused drugs are opioids and related compounds; antianxiety agents; amphetamines, cocaine, and other CNS stimulants; cannabis; hallucinogens and other mood modifiers; inhalants; and anabolic steroids. In addition, multiple drug use is common, and psychologic and physical dependence can exist independently or simultaneously.

Opioids are some of the most commonly abused drugs. Therefore the nurse should be alert to opioid abuse in the general population, as well as in the health professions. Because the "high" from opioids is characterized by complete drive satiation, the client may exhibit malnutrition and other signs of neglect from ignoring basic biologic needs. Acute overdose of opioids with miotic pupils, stupor, and respiratory depression is considered to be a medical emergency; symptoms may be reversed by adequate amounts of naloxone (Narcan), a narcotic antagonist. Treatment of opioid dependence may involve withdrawal with supportive therapy, methadone detoxification and withdrawal, or clonidine treatment followed by either a methadone maintenance program or a therapeutic community program.

Other forms of analgesics such as pentazocine (Talwin) and propoxyphene (Darvon) tend to be abused based on access, fashion, and availability of other substances on the street.

Alcohol is the most common substance of abuse. The ingestion of alcohol does not carry with it the social stigma attached to the abuse of other drugs. However, the chronic abuse of alcohol causes physiologic damage to every body system; its therapeutic use is quite limited. Disulfiram (Antabuse) is used to sensitize the individual to alcohol by causing such an unpleasant response—nausea, headache, palpitations, dyspnea, and intense discomfort—that the use of alcohol is no longer desired.

Benzodiazepines are the antianxiety agents most abused, generally as the result of overprescribing to women and older adults.

Amphetamines and cocaine are the most commonly abused CNS stimulants. Because cocaine is available as "crack" at a much lower cost than other drugs, it is becoming increasingly popular and is much more of a health problem with its strong physical and psychologic dependence.

Cannabis drugs are increasingly being used by young teenagers for recreation to produce an anxiety-free state of relaxation and a sense of well-being. Studies indicate that impaired decision making, apathy, and memory loss are related to cannabis use. Psychologic and physical dependence develop with chronic use.

Psychedelic drugs and inhalants are also substances for abuse because of their mind-altering properties. Anabolic steroids are abused by individuals who want to improve their appearance or performance in sports.

The nurse has an important role in preventing substance abuse because of his or her knowledge and extent of contact with individuals of all ages and circumstances. Assessment for the detection of substance abuse and intervention in an acute overdose or withdrawal situation are performed in a straightforward and receptive manner. Because of the multiplicity of problems in clients who abuse substances, the nurse may be part of a multidisciplinary team in the provision of support.

Critical Thinking Questions

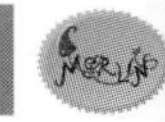

1. Jane Parker is a receptionist for the executive office suite of a large manufacturing firm. She is single, attractive, and enjoys an active social life. A few months ago she began attending parties where cocaine was being used, and she began using cocaine to "fit in" with the crowd. Her co-workers have noticed that she has become edgy, has lost weight, and has been unable to concentrate on her work. One of the executives sends Jane to the company nurse because she "does not look well." As the company's occupational nurse, how could you intervene with Ms. Parker? What activities could the company undertake as part of a substance abuse prevention program?
2. Ronald Taylor, age 72, is brought to the hospital after falling off his roof while doing home repairs. He is taken to surgery for an open reduction of a fractured femur. On the third day of hospitalization, Mr. Taylor becomes increasingly irritable and refuses to participate in his physical therapy. He indicates that he wishes to sign himself out of the hospital. The nurse notes from Mr. Taylor's past medical history that he has sustained multiple injuries as the result of minor automobile and home accidents. The nurse begins to consider that Mr. Taylor might abuse alcohol. Why would that be a consideration at this time? As the nurse in question, how will you intervene?

Collaborative Learning Activities

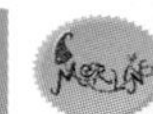

For Collaborative Learning Activities, go to mosby.com/MERLIN/McKenry/.

CASE STUDY

For a Case Study that will help ensure mastery of this chapter content, go to mosby.com/MERLIN/McKenry/.

BIBLIOGRAPHY

American Hospital Formulary Service. (1999). *AHFS drug information '99*. Bethesda, MD: American Society of Hospital Pharmacists.

American Nurses Association. (1984). *ANA cabinet on nursing practice: Statement on scope of addiction nursing practice*. Kansas City: Author.

American Nurses Association, Drug and Alcohol Nursing Association, and National Nurses Society on Addictions. (1987). *The care of clients with addictions: Dimensions of nursing practice*. Kansas City: Author.

Anderson, K.N., Anderson, L.E., & Glanz, W.D. (Eds.). (1998). *Mosby's medical, nursing & allied health dictionary* (5th ed.). St. Louis: Mosby.

Antai-Otong, D. (1995). Helping the alcoholic patient recover. *American Journal of Nursing, 95*(8), 22-29.

Baldwin, J.N. & Benson, B. (1995). Depressant and inhalant use. In L.Y. Young & M.A. Koda-Kimble (Eds.), *Applied therapeutics: The clinical use of drugs* (6th ed.). Vancouver, WA: Applied Therapeutics.

Baldwin, J.N. & Cook, M.D. (1995). Issues: Psychoactive substance use disorders. In L.Y. Young & M.A. Koda-Kimble (Eds.), *Applied therapeutics: The clinical use of drugs* (6th ed.). Vancouver, WA: Applied Therapeutics.

Bennett, E.G. & Woolf, D.S. (1991). *Substance abuse: Pharmacologic development and clinical perspectives* (2nd ed.). Albany, NY: Delmar Publishers.

Bissell, C. & Haberman, P.W. (1984). *Alcoholism in the professions*. Oxford: Oxford University Press.

Burns, C.M. (1993). Assessment and screening for substance abuse: Guidelines for the primary care nurse practitioner. *Nurse Practitioner Forum, 4*(4), 199-206.

Caulker-Burnett, I. (1994). Primary care screening for substance abuse. *Nurse Practitioner, 19*(4), 42, 44-48.

Council on Scientific Affairs. (1990). Medical and nonmedical uses of anabolic-androgenic steroids. *JAMA, 264*(22), 2923.

Covington, T.R. (Ed.) (1996). *Handbook of nonprescription drugs* (11th ed.). Washington, DC: American Pharmaceutical Association.

Cronk, C.E. & Sarvela, P.D. (1997). Alcohol, tobacco and other drug use among rural/small town and urban youth: A secondary analysis of the monitoring the future data set. *American Journal of Public Health, 87*(5), 760-764.

DeGeest, S., Dobbels, F., Martin, S., Willems, K., & Vanhaecke, J. (2000). *Progress in transplantation 10*(3): 162-168.

Drug Abuse Warning Network (DAWN). (1999). *Drug Abuse Warning Network. Emergency Department Data. Office of Applied Studies, Substance Abuse and Mental Health Services Administration*, Rockville, MD: Department of Health and Human Services.

Drug Facts and Comparisons. (2000). St. Louis: Facts and Comparisons.

Faigenbaum, A.D., Zaichkowsky, L.D., Gardner, D.E., & Micheli, L.J. (1998). Anabolic steroid use by male and female middle school students. *Pediatrics, 101*(5), E6.

Gallegos, K. et al. (1988). Substance abuse among health professionals. *Maryland Medical Journal, 37*(3), 191-196.

Gordon, M. (1987). *Manual of nursing diagnosis 1986-1987*. New York: McGraw-Hill.

Grimsley, S.R. (1995). Anxiety disorders. In L.Y. Young, & M.A. Koda-Kimble (Eds.), *Applied therapeutics: The clinical use of drugs* (6th ed.). Vancouver, WA: Applied Therapeutics.

Hall, I.N. (1989). U.S. illicit drug production booming. *Street Pharmacology, 12*(Spring), 4.

Henderson, G.L., Hoffman, R.S., Kulig, K.W. (1992). Street and designer drugs. *Patient Care, 26*(18), 118-124, 129-132, 135-136, 143-144, 146, 148-150,153-154, 157.

Hinds, M. (Ed.). (1985). How much blood alcohol content per drink? *Informed Families of Dade County, 26*(6), 1.

Hughes, T.L. & Smith, L.L. (1994). Is your colleague chemically dependent? *American Journal of Nursing, 94*(9), 31-35.

Iber, F.L. (Ed.). (1991). *Alcohol and drug abuse as encountered in office practice*. Boca Raton, FL: CRC Press.

Jungnickel, P.W. (1995). Entactogen and phencyclidine abuse. In L.Y. Young & M.A. Koda-Kimble (Eds.), *Applied therapeutics: The clinical use of drugs* (6th ed.). Vancouver, WA: Applied Therapeutics.

Jungnickel, P.W. & Hunnicutt, D.M. (1995). Alcohol abuse. In L.Y. Young & M.A. Koda-Kimble (Eds.), *Applied therapeutics: The clinical use of drugs* (6th ed.). Vancouver, WA: Applied Therapeutics.

Katzung, B.G. (1997). *Basic & clinical pharmacology* (7th ed.). Norwalk, CT: Appleton & Lange.

Kaufman, E. & McNaul, J.P. (1992). Recent developments in understanding and treating drug abuse and dependence. *Hospital & Community Psychiatry, 43*(3), 223-236.

Lipton, A.G. (1993). The argument against therapeutic use of heroin in pain management. *American Journal of Hospital Pharmacists, 50*(5), 996-998.

Long, M.C. (1993). Overview of substance abuse: Implications for the primary care nurse practitioner. *Nurse Practitioner Forum, 4*(4), 191-198.

Malatestinic, W.N. & Jorgenson, J.A. (1991). Dealing with substance abuse in the workplace. *Hospital Pharmacist, 26*(1), 102-105.

Mayfield, D., McLoed, G., & Hall, P. (1974). The CAGE questionnaire: Validation of a new alcoholism screening instrument. *American Journal of Psychiatry, 131*, 1121.

Mayo-Smith, M.F. for the American Society of Addiction Medicine Working Group. (1997). Pharmacological management of alcohol withdrawal: A meta-analysis and evidenced-based practice guideline. *JAMA, 278*(2), 144-151.

Milzman, D.P. & Soderstrom, C.A. (1994). Substance use disorders in trauma patients: Diagnosis, treatment, and outcome. *Critical Care Clinics, 10*(3), 595-611.

Navarra, T. (1995). Enabling behavior: The tender trap. *American Journal of Nursing, 95*(1), 50-52.

Neafsey, P.J., Fisk, N.B., & Williams, C.A. (1993). Updating the critical care nurse on alcohol and other drug abuse. *Critical Care Nurse, 13*(5), 98-101, 103-107.

Neumark, Y.D., Delva, J., & Anthony, J.C. (1998). The epidemiology of inhalant drug involvement. *Archives of Pediatrics & Adolescent Medicine, 152*(8), 781-786.

O'Brien, C.P. (1996). Drug addiction and drug abuse. In J.G. Hardman & L.E. Limbird (Eds.), *Goodman & Gilman's The pharmacological basis of therapeutics* (9th ed.). New York: McGraw-Hill.

Office of Applied Studies, Substance Abuse and Mental Health Services Administration. (1997). *Substance use among women in the United States*. Rockville, MD: Department of Health and Human Services.

O'Hara, P., Parris, D., Fichtner, R.R., & Oster, R. (1998). Influence of alcohol and drug use on AIDS risk behavior among youth in dropout prevention. *Journal of Drug Education, 28*(2), 159-168.

Schydlower, M. (1990). Current issues affecting drug-exposed infants and their mothers. *Healthcare Executive Currents*, Special Issue, *34*(1), 2.

Scott, D.M. & Gabel, T.L. (1995). Central nervous system (CNS) stimulant abuse. In L.Y. Young & M.A. Koda-Kimble (Eds.), *Applied therapeutics: The clinical use of drugs*. Vancouver, WA: Applied Therapeutics.

Sees, K.L. & Clark, H.W. (1993). Opioid use in the treatment of chronic pain: Assessment of addiction. *Journal of Pain & Symptom Management, 88*(5), 257-264.

Sinatra, R.S. & Savarese, A. (1992). Parenteral analgesic therapy and patient-controlled analgesia for pediatric pain management. In R.S. Sinatra, A.H. Hord, B. Ginsberg, & L. Preble (Eds.), *Acute pain: Mechanism and management*. St. Louis: Mosby.

Stammer, M.E. (1988). Understanding alcoholism and drug dependency in nurses. *Quality Review Bulletin, 14*(3), 75-80.

Surface, R.E. (Ed.) (1991). Drug information: Anabolic steroids now Schedule III. *The White Sheet, 25*(3), 3.

Thomas, D.J. (1993). Organ transplantation in people with unhealthy lifestyles. *AACN Clinical Issues, 4*(4), 665-668.

Trinkoff, A.M. & Storr, C.L. (1998). Substance use among nurses: Differences between specialties. *American Journal of Public Health, 88*(4), 581-585.

United States Pharmacopeia Dispensing Information (USP DI): Drug information for the health care professional (19th ed.). (1999). Rockville, MD: United States Pharmacopeial Convention.

Wadler, G.I. (1994). Drug use update. *Medical Clinics of North America, 78*(2), 439-455.

Watling, S.M., Fleming, C., Casey, P., & Yanes, J. (1995). Nursing-based protocol for treatment of alcohol withdrawal in the intensive care unit. *American Journal of Critical Care, 4*(1), 66-70.

Young, S.L., Vosper, H.J., & Phillips, S.A. (1992). Cocaine: Its effects on maternal and child health. *Pharmacotherapy, 12*(1), 2-17.

Zahourek, R.P. (1986). Identification of the alcoholic in the acute care setting. *Critical Care Quarterly, 8*(4), 1-10.

10 CLIENT EDUCATION FOR SELF-ADMINISTRATION OF MEDICATION

Chapter Focus

Effective management of a therapeutic regimen requires a major commitment by the client and the family or caregiver. A well-planned teaching program can provide the information needed to accurately self-manage medications in the home setting. It can also decrease the number of complications arising from medications by preparing the client to recognize the early signs and symptoms of adverse reactions and to report them to the prescriber. Therefore the nurse needs to be not only knowledgeable in pharmacologic content but also skilled in client education.

Learning Objectives

1. Assess a client and family regarding the need and readiness to learn how to administer medications.
2. Write measurable objectives for the client who is learning to self-administer medications.
3. Discuss at least three teaching techniques that may increase a client's knowledge of medications.
4. Identify four or more safety precautions necessary for clients in self-administering medications.
5. Document the client's and the family's learning, including content, method, and progress toward learning goals.
6. Identify the nursing diagnoses of deficient knowledge, noncompliance, and ineffective therapeutic regimen management as they relate to self-administration of medications.
7. Identify factors that affect client compliance in the self-administration of medications.

Key Terms

compliance, p. 195
ineffective therapeutic regimen management, p. 195
knowledge deficit, p. 195
locus of control, p. 193
noncompliance, p. 195
therapeutic seeding, p. 198

Nurses have been teaching their clients since the beginning of this discipline. However, in the last three decades an increasing emphasis has been placed on the role of nurses in supporting clients' abilities for self-care, adaptation to illness, and high-level wellness. Various factors are responsible for this change in emphasis. A growing consumer awareness of health issues and services has made the client much more of a participant in his or her own health care than in the past. The client is more apt to request information. Nurses have responded by promoting the client's active involvement in planning and implementing nursing care. In 1972 the American Hospital Association published "A Patient's Bill of Rights," which gave formal recognition to the client's right to know about his or her health status, treatments, alternative methods of treatment, and continuing care requirements. Client education is being recognized as one way of making possible a shorter length of hospital stay. A shorter length of hospital stay has been an important factor in the economic climate since the development of a prospective payment system for health care by the Health Care Financing Administration in 1983, the advent of diagnosis-related groups (DRGs), the development of managed care, and the increasing growth of health maintenance organizations (HMOs), which continue to shorten lengths of stay.

Technology has both extended life expectancy and increased the number of chronically ill individuals. Many older adults or debilitated clients require health teaching to enable them to remain independent. Since 1976 the Joint Commission for the Accreditation of Healthcare Organizations (JCAHO) has required evidence in the client's clinical record that specific instructions were provided to the client and his or her family regarding medications, diet, and follow-up care. Nurse practice acts have set guidelines and developed standards for the nurse's role in health education. There have been successful lawsuits alleging that nurses provided less than adequate health teaching. All of these factors have reinforced the importance of the nurse's participation in client education.

Client education is a process that helps people to learn and incorporate health-related behaviors into everyday life. Learning is defined as a change in behavior, and nurses assist individuals in changing their behavior. Nurses provide health-related information and teach in a way that ensures the client's compliance with a therapeutic regimen. At no time is this more important than when educating clients in the self-administration of prescription medications. Misuse and noncompliance with drug regimens have been well documented (Charonko, 1992; Gullickson, 1993; Proos et al., 1992; Shea, Misra, Erlich, Field, & Francis, 1992; Wainwright & Gould, 1997). Although a number of factors determine whether or not clients will adhere to a medication regimen, clients must be provided with accurate information on which to base their behaviors.

One of the current trends is to relegate counseling about proper medication administration to the community pharmacist. Many clients have difficulty with this process because of the lack of privacy and the busy environment of the pharmacy setting. Some health care providers are concerned because the pharmacist does not have access to the client's medical history. Johnson, Butta, Donohue, Glenn, & Holtzman (1996) found that only 44% of families were counseled about their child's medication by their pharmacist. Their recommendation was for health care professionals engaged in the client's care to teach the client and/or family safe and accurate medication administration.

The teaching-learning process may be structured along the lines of the nursing process with the first step being assessment—the gathering of facts and information that will assist the nurse in meeting the client's and family's needs for learning. Planning, the next step in the process, begins as soon as a learning need has been identified, with goals being written as outcomes for the client's learning. The implementation phase is the actual communication of information. Evaluation focuses on the client's behaviors and attitudes as a measure of whether or not the client has achieved the learning objectives.

ASSESSMENT

A thorough assessment of the client is essential for educating about medications in the most efficient and effective way. Realistic goals for a client's medicating behaviors are the result of the nurse's accurate assessment. The nurse should conduct a comprehensive assessment regarding the client's response to illness. A comprehensive assessment includes determining the client's competence in self-care and mobility, nutritional status, sleep patterns, and social support mechanisms. The data collected should describe factors influencing the client's ability, motivation, and interest in following health advice. The client's cultural perspectives, health beliefs, and attitudes need to be included in the assessment. All of these factors influence the teaching-learning process for the self-administration of medications. Not all clients need to know everything about their medications, nor are all clients ready to learn about them. However, Czar and Engler (1997) found that content about medications was ranked as one of the three most important learning needs of clients during hospitalization and follow-up clinic visits.

Assessing a client's learning needs means ascertaining what the client already knows: "What medications are you presently taking?" "What is each medication for?" "How often and how much of each medication should you be taking?" "What are the side effects of each drug?" "Which of these side effects should you report to your prescriber?" (See Chapter 4 for a medication history form.) If the client knows the answers to these questions, the objective for learning may have been met.

Research by Petrie, Weinman, Sharpe, & Buckley (1996) suggests that clients focus their ideas about illness on five themes, which health psychologists call illness perceptions:

1. **Identity**: the label the client uses to describe the illness and the symptoms that he or she views as being part of the disease

2. **Cause:** personal ideas about the cause of the illness
3. **Time line:** how long the client believes the illness will last
4. **Consequences:** the expected effects and outcomes of the illness
5. **Cure or control:** how the client recovers from or controls the illness

Although the research of Petrie et al. examined client participation in rehabilitation regimens following myocardial infarction, their findings could relate to adherence practices with medication regimens. Clients who strongly believed that their illnesses were amenable to cure or control were more likely to participate in rehabilitation programs (adhere to a medication regimen). Clients who anticipated that their illness would have major consequences on their life were slower to recover. Client beliefs may not correspond to professional views of the illness, and health care professionals may not be aware of these differences. The client's meaning or perception of his or her illness experience is very influential in determining the client's participation with the medication regimen. It is essential that the nurse assess the client's perceptions of illness.

The nurse also needs to determine a point of reference for learning by validating the client's present level of knowledge. New information is easier to absorb when it can be related to what the client already knows. For example, when teaching about nitroglycerin (an antianginal medication), the nurse might ask the client what he or she understands about the diagnosis of angina. The nurse can discuss the therapeutic action of the nitroglycerin by using the words the client used to describe his or her condition. A baseline of data must be determined to evaluate what knowledge the client has gained by comparing what was known before and after the learning process.

The nurse needs to be aware of any incorrect knowledge or misunderstanding the client may have. The client's health information may be a collection of folklore, hearsay, handed-down family experience, advertising claims, and misconceptions. Incorrect information needs to be identified and dealt with before the teaching of the correct material can be initiated. The Cultural Considerations box on p. 192 describes a study by Lile and Hoffman (1991) that provides examples of medication-taking beliefs and behaviors.

Because of shortened hospital stays, instruction must sometimes be limited to survival content—only the most important information (Proos et al., 1992). What will the client need to know about what to do when he or she returns home? What must the client learn to survive until additional information can be obtained? Does the client know whom to call if additional information is needed? Although many nurses prefer to teach some pharmacokinetics of the client's drug as a foundation for the self-administration of medications, the anxiety and health status of the client sometimes preclude that depth of explanation. Clients who have undergone ambulatory surgery are discharged after having received an array of medications before and during their surgical procedures; as a result, they may have a decreased ability to understand and process information (Jones, 1995). The types of agents commonly used in these settings (e.g., benzodiazepines, opioid analgesics, and anticholinergics) have been shown to impair the ability of clients to process and recall information (Kerr et al., 1991; Barbee, 1993).

A client can become easily overwhelmed by highly technical content and lose the essential information needed to take the drug safely and accurately. However, some clients may ask for additional technical information. Hospitalized clients tend to focus on the issues related to hospitalization (e.g., how to administer the insulin injection) rather than on long-term dietary management of their diabetes mellitus. Clients in ambulatory care may have difficulty absorbing all they need to understand about their medications in the brief time of a typically scheduled visit. In-home assessments are beneficial for assessing the client's adherence to the prescribed medication regimen (Der, Rubenstein, & Choy, 1997).

Not all clients are ready to learn. During an assessment, the nurse needs to consider the client's current emotional state, adaptation to the illness, level of maturity, and expectations. A client's emotional state influences his or her perspective on the world and readiness to learn. Smith (1989) found that clients' feelings of satisfaction not only correlated with current compliance but also predicted future compliance, indicating a readiness to participate in their own care. Mild anxiety may stimulate the client to learn, whereas severe anxiety may shorten the attention span and be incapacitating.

Many factors affect the client's readiness to learn (Petrie et al., 1996) (Box 10-1). A client goes through various stages in adapting to illness or injury, including developing awareness, reorganization, resolution, and identity change. During the assessment the nurse should be aware of the client's stage of adaptation. Understanding the client's coping strategies will prevent the nurse from attempting to teach information that the client is not ready to learn. Anger, fear, and mistrust of health care personnel may also impede readiness for learning.

Clients who lack functional literacy (lack the ability to read well enough to understand and use information as in-

BOX 10-1

Factors Affecting Readiness to Learn

Pathophysiologic: severity of illness, pain, fatigue, sensory deprivation, physical disabilities
Treatment-related: complexity of regimen
Situational: illiteracy, language differences, ineffective coping patterns, financial concerns, home environment
Maturational: family roles and relationships, health maintenance practices

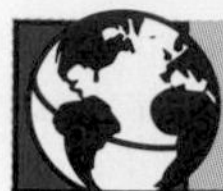

Cultural Considerations
Medication Taking by Frail Older Adults in Two Ethnic Groups

Drug therapy is a complex and dangerous area of medical intervention with the older adult population. Many older adults use large quantities of both prescription and OTC medications with little understanding of the potential health risk. Lile and Hoffman (1991) investigated the medication-taking behaviors of Hispanic and Anglo noninstitutionalized, frail older adults in the Las Cruces, New Mexico area.

The sample of 20 (10 Anglo, 10 Hispanic) consisted of subjects attending senior citizen community centers, those waiting to see doctors in the office, and some individuals at home. Six men and 14 women participated, and the age range was 70 to 90 years. The median age of the Anglo group was 81 years, and median age of the Hispanic group was 85.5 years. The educational level ranged from less than high school (55%) to college graduates (5%). The majority of Anglo subjects had an annual income between $10,000 and $20,000, and the majority of Hispanic subjects had an annual income less than $10,000.

An interview schedule containing 20 items was used to facilitate data collection related to the medication-taking behaviors of the participants. The tool focused on prescription and OTC medications, current home remedies, factors influencing the purchase of OTC drugs, difficulties with taking the medications, adverse reactions to the drugs, methods of record keeping, and money spent on medications. The tool was translated into Spanish for Hispanic subjects and then retranslated into English to determine accuracy. The interview was administered by a trained bilingual registered nurse.

The findings revealed that the subjects used cardiovascular drugs (Anglos, 80%; Hispanics, 90%), diuretics (Anglos, 40%; Hispanics, 10%); and antianxiety drugs (both groups, 40%). Thirty percent of the Hispanic group used drugs for the treatment of diabetes, which is prevalent in their ethnic group; no one in the Anglo group used these drugs. Both groups used respiratory drugs (20%) and laxatives (40%). OTC acetaminophen and aspirin were used by 70% in the Anglo group and by 80% in the Hispanic group. A variety of other prescription and nonprescription drugs were used by both groups. Anglo subjects used home remedies such as warm milk, beer, and bourbon for sleep and raspberry tea for hypertension. Hispanic subjects used prunes as a laxative, mustard weed for an upset stomach, and herbal teas for sleep and as diuretics.

The investigators reported that Hispanic subjects were three times more likely to be influenced by television in making OTC drug purchases, whereas 60% of the Anglo group were influenced by family in their OTC purchases. Interestingly, as opposed to 10% of the Anglo group, 70% of the Hispanic group shared or gave their medications to others, and 20% borrowed drugs from others.

Both groups expressed concern for the difficulty involved in taking their medications. Although the drug labels were written in English, 90% of the Hispanic subjects and 50% of the Anglo subjects had difficulty reading them. Forty percent of the Hispanic subjects and 10% of the Anglo subjects admitted to having difficulty understanding the labels. Fifty percent of the Anglo subjects had difficulty opening the drug containers. Most were able to administer their own medications (Anglos, 90%; Hispanics, 60%); the rest depended on family members or others to assist.

These findings indicate that noninstitutionalized, frail older adults in both ethnic groups are at risk for injury because of their medication-taking behaviors.

Critical Thinking Questions

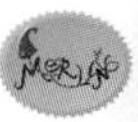

- What are the implications of the results of this study for the community?
- What are the implications for nursing?

tended), as well as those who have a language barrier, are also at risk for not following a medication regimen. Language barriers exist not only when there are differences in the primary language spoken by the health care provider and the client, but also when health care providers use unfamiliar medical terminology when describing disease processes and medical interventions. When questioned about understanding, the client will most likely indicate an understanding of the material, even if it is not understood. This response may be due to an inadequate vocabulary or an inability to explain what is not understood (Hussey, 1991). Clients from other cultures may indicate understanding as a sign of respect. For example, in Asian cultures it is respectful to smile and nod one's head to a person of authority, regardless of the level of understanding. In these instances the nurse may enlist the assistance of the client's support system—the individuals or group that provide comfort, aid, and information to help him or her cope with life. The support system can consist of family, friends, and members of the community and church or religious groups.

Whenever possible, nurses should learn the language of the clients with whom they are interacting. If that is not practical, nurses should learn key phrases related to greetings and the health care services provided. Interpreters can also be used, but they should understand health care terminology, have training in transcultural interpretation, know the language of both the health care provider and the client, and respect both cultures (Wenger, 1993).

If at all possible, the nurse should avoid using family members or visitors as interpreters because the shared information sometimes includes sensitive material. Family members or visitors may modify the interpretation to protect the client from information they believe will cause cultural strain or difficulty for the client and family (Wenger, 1993).

Tripp-Reimer & Afifi (1989) offer the following guidance for working with clients when there is a language barrier:

- Speak slowly (plan the teaching session to last at least twice as long as a typical session).
- Make the sentence structure simple (use active, not passive, voice; use a straightforward subject-verb pattern).
- Avoid technical terms (e.g., use "heart" rather than "cardiac"), professional jargon, and American idioms ("red tape").
- Provide instructional material in the same sequence in which the client should carry out the plan.
- Do not assume you have been understood. Ask the client to explain the protocol; optimally, if appropriate, obtain a return demonstration.

Although these guidelines are suggested for clients with a language barrier, they hold true for most clients.

Nonverbal communication is also important in teaching across cultures. Unspoken cues such as eye contact, distance between speakers, body movements, touch, and silence have cultural components. In general, Caucasians value direct eye contact when speaking. Eye contact provides feedback to ensure understanding of what has been communicated. In some other cultures (e.g., Native American, Asian, and African), direct eye contact is considered disrespectful. Diverting the eyes downward and to one side of the speaker indicates that a person is listening intently. Nurses need to be observers of nonverbal communication and learn what these cues mean from the client's cultural perspective (Wenger, 1993).

A cultural assessment should be conducted to elicit the client's beliefs, values, and attitudes about health, illness, medications, and the client role (see Chapter 6). Care should be negotiated between the client and nurse until an agreement is reached for a culturally appropriate and acceptable intervention. Only then will culturally appropriate teaching and learning take place (Wenger, 1993).

The manner in which a client perceives his or her ability to change or control his or her life has an impact on his or her willingness or ability to adhere to a medication regimen. **Locus of control** concerns how a client perceives his or her ability to influence or control his or her life along an internal-external continuum. At one end of the continuum a client is internally (self) oriented; at the other end a client is externally (others- or fate-) oriented about his or her health behaviors. Clients with an internal locus of control are more apt to be health oriented and adhere to a medication regimen. Locus of control may be assessed by listening to client's statements, such as "I forgot to take my medication" (internal locus) rather than, "My husband didn't remind me to take my medicine" (external locus). In one instance the client assumes accountability for the actions, and in the other the responsibility is placed elsewhere.

BOX 10-2

Erickson's Stages of Development

Infant (birth to 1 year of age): Trust vs. mistrust. Infant learns to trust self, others, and the environment; learns to love and be loved.

Toddler (1 to 3 years of age): Autonomy vs. shame and doubt. Toddler learns independence; learns to master the physical environment and maintain self-esteem.

Preschooler (3 to 6 years of age): Initiative vs. guilt. Preschooler learns basic problem solving; develops conscience and sexual identity; initiates and imitates activities.

School-age child (6 to 12 years of age): Industry vs. inferiority. School-age child learns to do things well; develops a sense of self-worth.

Adolescent (12 to 18 years of age): Identity vs. role confusion. Adolescent integrates many roles into self-identity through role models and peer pressure.

Young adult (18 to 45 years of age): Intimacy vs. isolation. Young adult establishes deep and lasting relationships; learns to make commitment as spouse, parent, partner.

Middle-aged adult (45 to 65 years of age): Generativity vs. stagnation. Adult learns commitment to community and world; is productive in career, family, civic interests.

Older adult (over 65 years of age): Integrity vs. despair. Older adult appreciates life role and status; deals with loss and prepares for death.

The nurse should assess the client's level of development because this will affect the ability to make decisions, to assume responsibility for the result of those decisions, and to manage life. If the client's developmental stage is not accurately assessed, the nurse may misdirect goals and inhibit client learning. The physical, emotional, and psychologic stages of development and related developmental tasks have been described by Erickson and other researchers. Box 10-2 describes Erickson's stages of development.

All individuals pass through the same predictable life stages, but passage through these stages occurs at different rates. Some individuals are ready to accept adult responsibilities at age 18; others may be well past 35 before they are ready to accept responsibility for themselves and others. Although movement through these stages is sequential, clients can fluctuate among stages, often in response to stress. Stressors such as illness and hospitalization may cause the client to regress temporarily to an earlier stage. The client needs to be addressed at his or her current developmental stage rather than at the developmental stage expected for the client's chronologic age. Table 10-1 summarizes changes related to aging and the educational strategies to address them. These changes are important in deciding whether the

TABLE 10-1 Educational Strategies for Common Changes Related to Aging

Changes Related to Aging That May Influence Learning	Educational Strategy
Altered Thought Processes	
Slowed cognitive functioning Decreased short-term memory Decreased ability to think abstractly Decreased ability to concentrate Increased reaction time (slower to respond)	Slow pace of presentation. Provide smaller amounts of information at one time. Repeat information frequently. Use examples to illustrate information. Decrease external stimuli as much as possible. Allow more time for feedback. Use a variety of methods, such as audiovisuals and practice sessions. Provide written instructions for home use.
Altered Sensory-Perceptual Status	
Hearing	
Decreased ability to distinguish sounds (e.g., words beginning with S, Z, T, D, F, and G) Decreased conduction of sound Loss of ability to hear high frequency sounds	Speak distinctly. Sit on side of learner's "best" ear. Do not shout; speak in a normal voice, but lower its pitch. Face the client so that lipreading is possible. Use visual aids to reinforce verbal instruction. Reinforce teaching with easy-to-read materials. Decrease extraneous noise.
Vision	
Decreased visual acuity Decreased ability to read fine detail Decreased ability to discriminate among blue, violet, and green; all colors tend to fade, with red fading the least Thicker and yellower lenses of eyes; with decreased accommodation Smaller pupils; decreased amount of light reaching retina	Ensure that glasses are clean and in place. Use printed material with large print. Use high-contrast materials, such as black on white. Avoid the use of blue, violet, and green in type or graphics; use red instead. Use nonglare lighting and avoid contrasts of light (e.g., darkened room with single light).
Decreased depth perception	Adjust teaching to allow for the use of touch to gauge depth.
Decreased peripheral vision	
Touch and vibration	
Decreased sense of touch	Increase time for the teaching of psychomotor skills, repetitions, and return demonstrations.
Decreased sense of vibration	Teach client to palpate more prominent pulse sites (e.g., carotid and radial arteries).

Modified from Weinrich, S.P. et al. (1989). Continuing education: adapting strategies to teach the elderly. *Journal of Gerontological Nursing, 15*(11), 17.

client can self-administer medications accurately (Drake & Romano, 1995). In some instances responsibility for the administration of medications may need to be delegated to a caregiver.

The nurse also needs to consider modifying the teaching plan for clients with vision and hearing impairments. Instructions in large print and pill containers with the days of the week printed in Braille are two modifications that may be considered for the visually impaired client. Written instructions are imperative for the hearing impaired; the nurse should try to keep all written communication simple and straightforward. If the client with a hearing impairment can read lips or speech, the nurse should make sure to support this activity.

The assessment for teaching-learning is similar to other types of nursing assessment; it is continuous and involves observation, listening and questioning, and other communication skills. The assessment phase can be used to establish rapport and gain the mutual nurse-client respect necessary for the teaching-learning process. Because nurses are seen as having a position of power in relation to the client, they must recognize the need to initiate the educational process.

When the client perceives an attitude of sincerity, integrity, and warmth in the nurse, the milieu is set for the client to feel free to ask questions and to discuss all matters, regardless of how personal those issues may be.

NURSING DIAGNOSIS

Three of the most common nursing diagnoses in relation to clients and the self-administration of medications are deficient knowledge, noncompliance, and ineffective therapeutic regimen management. **Deficient knowledge** is the state in which the individual has a deficiency in cognitive knowledge or psychomotor skills regarding the condition or treatment plan; this is somewhat different from noncompliance. **Noncompliance** is the state in which an individual or group desires to comply but is prevented from doing so by factors that deter adherence to health-related advice given by health care professionals (Carpenito, 2000). **Ineffective therapeutic regimen management** is a pattern of regulating and integrating into daily living a program for treating illness and the sequelae of illness that is unsatisfactory for meeting specific health goals (Carpenito, 2000). These three nursing diagnoses are not always listed for each drug as it is discussed in the text. However, *all clients undergoing drug therapy, whether administered by the client or a health care provider, should be assessed for the nursing diagnoses of risk for deficient knowledge, noncompliance, and ineffective therapeutic regimen management.* Any of these nursing diagnoses might appear in the same fashion: the client's inability to administer medications safely and accurately, a return of the client's symptoms or the occurrence of complications, or inappropriate behavior related to the therapeutic regimen.

Interventions to enhance compliance and effective therapeutic regimen management focus on client concerns or health beliefs (e.g., concern over possible adverse reactions or the cost of the drug), and they are distinctly different than teaching for deficient knowledge. Teaching for deficient knowledge is appropriate when the assessment clearly identifies that the client does not have sufficient or accurate information about the medication regimen and that the deficiency is interfering with the client's ability to self-administer medications. The client may request information, verbalize a misconception, or state the problem (e.g., "I don't understand. . . ."). With noncompliance or ineffective therapeutic regimen management, the client may fail to keep appointments or demonstrate an inability to set or keep mutually agreed on goals. The nurse may be aware of previous appropriate health education from the clinical record or may have performed the teaching and determine that the client did not seem to integrate the content into health-related behaviors. The issue then becomes a matter of noncompliance or ineffective therapeutic regimen management rather than deficient knowledge.

When care is mutually planned by the nurse and client, noncompliance is minimized. **Compliance** is the degree to which clients take medication instructions seriously, concur with them, and follow through. This term can have an offensively controlling ring to it, implying that the prescriber directs the client, who must follow those directions. Some practitioners prefer the term *adherence,* or *effective management of the therapeutic regimen.* However, because compliance is the standard accepted term, it is used here; but "concurrence with therapy" and "adherence to instructions" are synonymous terms.

Why do clients seek medical care and then not follow through with the suggested medication plan at home? There are many reasons—some personal, some social, some psychologic, some cultural. Everyone is potentially noncompliant, whether or not they intend to be. Medication compliance has been estimated to vary between 13% and 93% (Bond & Hussar, 1991; Harvey & Plumridge, 1991). Some clients never fill the prescription, most take them at unscheduled times, and many stop taking the medication early.

The consequences of not following the medication plan include inexplicable medication failures with continuing symptoms or overdoses. Medications not used may be kept and taken inappropriately later, when the potency and chemical activities may have changed. When confronted with apparent medication failures, prescribers tend simply to increase the drug dosage or change medications instead of investigating for noncompliance with the therapeutic plan.

The following are examples of situations known to foster noncompliance or ineffective management of the therapeutic regimen:

1. The client is chronically ill or is undergoing prolonged therapy. In chronic illness, symptoms tend to grow worse and then improve in a cyclic fashion. Clients often do not see any clear causal relationship between taking or not taking the prescribed medication and the waxing and waning of symptoms. It has been shown that routinely reviewing medications with clients and inquiring how they are taken at home will dramatically increase compliance. When appropriate, it should be stressed to the client that the medication will need to be taken indefinitely and should not be precipitously discontinued.
2. The client is relatively asymptomatic or feels better. Reasons for needing to take all of the drug should be explained. For example, many people are not aware that organisms mutate and that antibiotic medications should be completed as prescribed to ensure their eradication in the first place.
3. The medication is expensive or inconvenient to obtain. Prescriptions purchased by generic name and further explanations of the importance of the medication (i.e., the consequences of not taking the drug) may be effective in remotivating the client.
4. The medication instructions are complex and not easily understood. "Take with meals" may mean twice a day to the person who always skips breakfast or before or after meals for others. Written instructions with a sample of the drug taped to them may assist as a reminder when the client is home and has forgotten what was heard in the office or in the

hospital when being discharged (Martens, 1998; McKenry, 1999).

5. The medication is unwieldy to take because the bottle cap is difficult for arthritic hands or because there are complicated mixing or measuring directions. Measuring cups or droppers can be offered, and the client should be told that easy-to-remove caps can be requested when the medicine is purchased.
6. The medicine tastes unpleasant or must be taken at inconvenient times (e.g., during sleep hours, at work) or too many times a day to be feasible. The medication can be mixed with or taken with various liquids that are both pleasant and compatible. After consultation with the prescriber, medication prescriptions can often be changed to higher doses given less frequently or to a sustained-action form if available and if feasible.
7. The therapeutic plan contains many different medications, and the drug-taking schedule is complicated. Occasional systematic review of the medications by the prescriber and the nurse, especially in home health care, is necessary to see if the client still needs all of them and to simplify the care plan (Drake & Romano, 1995). Confrontation of the client's habits is necessary when medication containers that should be empty remain full. Written schedules with sample drugs attached are helpful. Small medication boxes with separate compartments for each dosing time are available at pharmacies. The nurse may suggest that the client keep the medication near equipment used at a specific time each day (e.g., a coffee cup or the kitchen table) or associate taking the medication with a specific routine activity (e.g., walking the dog or watching the television news).
8. Many people wait more than an hour to be seen by their prescriber in the office or clinic setting. Waiting longer than this has been correlated with a distinct drop in following the prescriber's medication instructions. Often the wait is unavoidable, but the situation can be improved if the practitioner is empathic.
9. The client does not understand or accept the illness or disorder, or the explanation of the illness or treatment plan does not fit the client's concepts of illness, health care, or health. Typical of the factors that influence attitudes toward treatment are the extent to which clients believe that (1) they are susceptible to the illness, (2) the illness is serious, and (3) they will benefit from taking action. *Therefore giving information is not the entire answer.* It helps to seek the active participation of the client in the health and nursing process and to show interest in and respect for client ideas, feelings, and beliefs.
10. The client and health care practitioners perceive the problems or goals in divergent ways, yet do not effectively communicate this (Britten, 1996).
11. The medication is seen as an artificial additive or contaminant to the body or as a crutch on which dependence should be limited.
12. Side effects are severe or interfere with functioning in daily activities.
13. The client has problems with memory or confusion or has visual or hearing impairments.

The specific nursing diagnosis selected for a particular client will depend on the nurse's astute assessment of the individual situation with the client and family.

PLANNING

The next part of the teaching-learning process is planning, which begins once a learning need has been identified. The learning needs are discussed; planning the objectives is a mutual undertaking between the nurse, the client and, where appropriate, the family. The learning objectives for the client's ability to self-medicate are goals or expected outcomes that should result from the teaching-learning interactions. The teaching plan needs to be included in the written plan of care whether it is a standardized one generated as part of a protocol or is a unique one developed specifically for a client with complex learning needs. The written plan should include the topic, who initiates teaching and when, who reinforces teaching and when, educational materials given, and a comments section for documenting client/caregiver response (Weaver, 1995).

In order for the teaching plan objectives to clarify what is to be learned and how that learning will be evaluated, the objective should contain a verb that is measurable (Box 10-3). Although the nurse would like the client to "know" about his or her medications, "understand" how the medication relates to the illness, and "comprehend" what action to take if an

BOX 10-3

Examples of Measurable and Nonmeasurable Verbs

Measurable Verbs

describe	administer	stand
discuss	demonstrate	walk
identify	perform	has an increase in
list	self-administer	has a decrease in
relate	exercise	has an absence of
state	cough	
verbalize	sit	

Nonmeasurable Verbs

accept	feel	think
appreciate	know	understand

How will you know that the client understands? What behaviors need to be evident for you to observe that he or she appreciates (or accepts, etc.)?

adverse reaction occurs, these verbs are not appropriate for writing goals because they are neither easily interpreted nor measurable. Terms such as "define," "list," "identify," and "state" are measurable, have fewer interpretations, and are therefore more useful in evaluating the achievement of goals for learning. The following are examples of statements that include measurable verbs:

The client will:

State the major action of digoxin.

Identify at least three adverse reactions to digoxin that should be reported to the prescriber.

List the signs and symptoms of hypoglycemia (e.g., tachycardia; palpitations; cool, clammy skin; diaphoresis; irritability; tiredness; hunger; numbness; and blurred vision).

Goals need to be realistic with regard to the client's achievements. They can be determined only by assessing with the client his or her ability to achieve the expected outcomes.

IMPLEMENTATION

The most difficult steps of the teaching-learning process have been completed once a learning need has been identified and the expected outcomes have been agreed on by the client and the nurse. The implementation phase consists of conveying the specific information required by the objectives.

Instructional sessions about medications should be integrated throughout the extent of nurse-client interactions and not saved for the day of discharge from the health agency. Short encounters staggered over the course of the client's length of stay enhance learning because it takes place in small incremental steps rather than in one overwhelming session. One of the most appropriate times to teach the client about medications is as they are being administered. This dialogue will help the client to cue in specific medications at certain times of the day and at particular intervals.

The practice of manual skills is rather straightforward, such as the manipulation of a syringe and vial to self-administer insulin. Nurses are familiar with the practices of demonstration and return demonstration, but variations exist that can conserve time. A nurse may draw up the insulin and ask the client to complete the injection, may ask the client to direct the procedure, or may coach the client through the procedure. Equipment may be left with the client to allow for practice time without the nurse's presence before a return demonstration is scheduled. Such equipment should be labeled as "practice equipment," and the client should be instructed that this material is contaminated and should not be used on himself or herself.

The communication of ideas is more complex but just as necessary. Ideas are more easily understood if they are organized in a logical order and if they move from simple to complex. For example, it is helpful for clients to know the therapeutic effect of a drug before learning about its side effects/adverse reactions. Ideas need to be practiced, too. The application of information is important for clients. Knowing what to do is more helpful than reciting the symptoms of digoxin toxicity. Clients should be asked questions such as, "What will you do if you take your pulse and the rate is below 60 beats per minute?"

Providing the client with scenarios in which decisions must be made regarding lifestyle and medications is beneficial. For example, a client who takes disulfiram (Antabuse), a drug that causes vomiting when alcohol is ingested, could be asked, "Suppose you're having dinner at a friend's home and you're asked to have a drink. How will you respond?" The client can demonstrate commitment to a medication regimen if he or she is able to state to the nurse and family how he or she intends to manage a medication that needs to be taken four times a day within a schedule that includes home, office, and business travel. Coudreaut-Quinn, Emmons, & McMurrow (1992) report that a self-medication program while the client is still in the hospital can increase adherence to a medication regimen.

The client should be encouraged to plan for the administration of medications and the incorporation of this activity into his or her lifestyle. Written instructions are particularly helpful for the client to refer to once discharged from the health care setting (Figure 10-1). Medication schedules have proven to be particularly helpful in assisting clients with adherence to a medication regimen (see the Nursing Research box on p. 199). A medication calendar may be made by obtaining a calendar with space enough to write in the names of the drugs and the times of the day they should be taken. The medications can be checked off on the calendar as they are taken, and the client will have a home medication record. This method is particularly helpful with clients who are concerned that they may forget or for those clients trying to establish a routine for taking their medications. Having an alarm clock next to the calendar so that it may be reset for the next dose helps to decrease the anxiety related to forgetting a dose. The client should be given written information about the medication, including its name, its purpose, its appearance, directions for taking it, the time to take it, what action to take if a dose is missed, and any special precautions related to the drug. The side effects/adverse reactions should also be written, along with the symptoms that should be reported and to whom they should be reported. In addition to providing information regarding the client's specific medication regimen, the nurse should take the opportunity to educate the client as a consumer of drugs (Box 10-4).

The nurse should develop a repertoire of approaches and materials to be used for client teaching. A nurse who relies solely on the client's hearing is not encouraging an optimal learning experience. The nurse should include as many of the client's senses in the learning experience as possible. For example, in teaching about medications while administering them, the nurse allows the client to hear the reason the drug is indicated for the condition. The pill can also be seen and felt by the client and tasted while taken. During recent years the amount of health teaching materials and the variety of media have proliferated. Audiovisual and other materials

MEDICATION CAUTIONS

☐ 1. Avoid alcoholic beverages while taking this medication.

☐ 2. Swallow these tablets. Do not chew them. Do not take if coating is cracked.

☐ 3. Do not drive a car or operate machinery if this medication makes you drowsy. If you have to drive home, wait until you get home to take your first dose.

☐ 4. Do not allow this medication to contact the skin, eyes, or clothing.

☐ 5. Take this medication on an empty stomach either 1 hour before meals or 2 hours after meals. You may drink water.

☐ 6. Do not take this medication with fruit juice.

☐ 7. Take this medication _______ hour(s) before meals.

☐ 8. Limit caffeine use.

☐ 9. Do not take this medication with milk or milk products. You may drink water or juice.

☐ 10. Take this medication with at least 8 ounces of water.

☐ 11. Take this medication with food to avoid upset stomach.

☐ 12. This medication may discolor the urine or stools.

☐ 13. Do not take this medication with antacids.

☐ 14. Do not take aspirin with this medication.

☐ 15. Do not take mineral oil with this medication.

☐ 16. Take orange juice, bananas, and other foods high in potassium while taking this medication.

☐ 17. Avoid tyramine-rich foods such as cheese, pickled herring, and wine while taking this medication.

☐ 18. Count your pulse (by feeling at the wrist) each time before taking this medication. If it is less than 60 beats a minute, do not take the dose. Contact the prescriber.

☐ 19. Check with your prescriber before taking any other medications (even over-the-counter medications).

☐ 20. Do not take this medication if pregnant or breastfeeding or if you have ever had an allergic reaction to it. Instead, contact prescriber for instructions.

☐ 21. Do not take this medication if you have the following medical problems or symptoms:
____
____
____

Figure 10–1 Example of a general medication instruction sheet for the client, which may be individualized by indicating specific instructions appropriate to the client's therapeutic regimen.

such as pamphlets and videotapes can show the client settings and situations that are beyond the ability of the nurse to present at the bedside, in the clinic, or in the home setting. Computer-generated instructions as part of a standard teaching plan (Weaver, 1995), as well as computer-assisted instructions for some clients (Tibbles, Lewis, Reisine, Rippey, & Donald, 1992), have demonstrated success.

These useful supplements should be used by the nurse to enhance the teaching process. With increasingly short lengths of stay in hospitals or brief encounters in the office, clinic, or home, these adjuncts become more important to include in the nurse's scope of teaching techniques. Materials should be selected according to the appropriateness of content, accuracy, simplicity, and appeal for the client. However, they should never replace individualized instruction, because the client may overlook needed information or be overwhelmed by a comprehensive audiovisual presentation. These various media techniques should facilitate the nurse's role as a teacher rather than act as substitutes.

Bille (1981) recommends the process of **therapeutic seeding** as a teaching approach when clients are unable to express learning needs or concerns. This technique involves mentioning ideas to clients, allowing time to pass so the client has a chance to think about the idea, then reintroducing the idea. On the second opportunity the client may more easily identify the concept and see it as a learning need. For example, an older female client who has received a prescription for conjugated estrogens may not identify any drug-related learning needs at that time. On the next visit, the nurse may use therapeutic seeding with a statement such as, "Ms. Ackerman, many women who take this medication have expressed concerns about its adverse effects. What concerns do you have about the medication?" If the client states, "I'm not concerned about that," she may be saying, "I'm not ready to hear that information yet." Referring to the comment on the next visit may prepare the way for discussing possible adverse reactions and what symptoms to report to the prescriber. Therapeutic seeding allows the client more of an opportunity to negotiate the teaching-learning program.

Practical information about prescription drugs is available to consumers from the American Medical Association, package inserts produced by the pharmaceutical houses, some health care providers, the *United States Pharmacopeia Dispensing Information* (*USP DI*, Volume 2: *Advice for the Patient*), or *Mosby's Pharmacology Patient Teaching Guides*. Most printed information includes the drug's purpose, possible side effects/

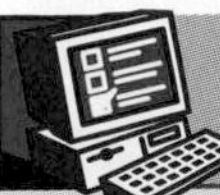

Nursing Research

The Effects of Medication Education on Adherence to Medication Regimens in an Older Adult Population

Citation: Esposito, L. (1995). The effects of medication education on adherence to medication regimens in an elderly population. *Journal of Advanced Nursing, 21*, 935-943.

Abstract: The population of individuals over age 65 is increasing rapidly, and a third of all prescriptions are being written for this population. As a result, the numbers of older adults hospitalized annually for adverse drug reactions are increasing. Improving the effective management of the therapeutic regimen in older adults would decrease the cost and increase the quality of health care by decreasing the risk of hospitalization for such reactions. The purpose of this study was to evaluate educational protocols to see which is more effective in increasing medication compliance rates within an older adult population.

Clients participating in the study were age 65 or older; hospitalized for at least 24 hours; oriented to time, place, and person; discharged to home; able to self-administer medications or take them with minimal assistance; and able to complete a mini-mental test with a score of 23 or higher to screen for dementia and to determine cognitive functioning. Mini-mental test scores, education levels, and age were similar in all groups.

The participants were randomized into four intervention groups. Group 1 (n = 11) received the medication information usually distributed by the study site institution. This included a medication fact sheet and a discharge instruction sheet indicating the date of return visit; special instructions related to diet, activity, dressings, and treatments; when to call the doctor; and medications prescribed by the doctor (name, dose, and frequency of dosage). Group 2 (n = 8) received the medication fact sheet and 30 minutes of verbal instruction. Group 3 (n = 10) received a medication schedule written in large dark lettering. This schedule included the name of the medicine, the color of the pill, the dose, a list of side effects, a dosage schedule, and the reason for each medication. Group 4 (n = 14) received the same medication schedule and 30 minutes of verbal instruction.

Visits were made to the clients' homes three times: 2 weeks, 1 month, and 2 months after discharge. At each visit, pill counts were performed and compared with medication orders, and clients gave self-reports on how they administered their medications and on whether they missed or increased any doses. Reasons for noncompliance were recorded, and it was determined whether the client had received any medication education other than that from the investigator.

An evaluation of the results from the three follow-up visits showed groups 3 and 4 had fewer medication errors than groups 1 and 2. Adherence scores in groups 1 and 2 exhibited increased changes in the follow-up visits when compared with groups 3 and 4. Involvement in home health services did not seem to effect the rate of error in the medication regimen. Individuals in this study reported forgetting to take their medication as the primary reason for noncompliance. The groups with the medication schedule (groups 3 and 4) did have a decreased incidence of medication error compared with those in groups without a schedule. However, given the sample size of this study (n = 42), further research is needed to provide more evidence of the benefits of medication schedules as compared with other education protocols.

Critical Thinking Questions

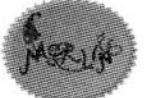

- The clients in group 1, which had the highest error rate, also had a slightly higher medication complexity index. How might this contribute to higher error rates?
- Given the rationale cited by these participants for noncompliance, what would be the advantage of a medication schedule?
- What could you generalize from these results?

adverse reactions, and the best way to take the drug. More than 1000 common drugs are listed annually in the *USP DI*, which is geared partly to those who dispense or administer prescriptions and partly to those who take them. *USP DI: Advice for the Patient*, offers jargon-free guidelines for safe and informed self-administration of prescription drugs by generic name. The *USP DI* information is available to consumers from their health practitioners or pharmacists, who can reproduce for distribution a limited number of pages from the Advice section.*

The client and family need to be active members of the team, especially since much of the convalescent care is shifting from hospital to home. They need to be encouraged to participate whenever and wherever possible in all aspects of the client's care. Family members may be responsible for changing dressings, taking care of drains and IV lines, running complex equipment, and administering IM and IV medications. The client's family may be of great support not only in providing assistance but also in easing the transition to home.

The nurse needs to identify which family members are supportive and can assume the ongoing responsibility for care, including the administration of medications. In a crisis, family members tend to gather around the client but may normally live at some distance or return to a daily work

*The *USP DI* is available for purchase from Micromedex, P.O. Box 564, Williston, VT 05495-0564; or use the toll-free number: (800) 877-6209. Students and faculty receive a discount.

BOX 10-4

Guidelines for Educating Clients as Consumers of Drugs

1. Be aware that, like prescription medications, OTC medications are truly drugs and deserve the same care in use.
2. Identify some types of medications that are considered useful for home treatment (see Chapter 11).
3. Advise the client about safety precautions:
   a. Make sure all medications, including OTC medications, have clear and understandable labels.
   b. Heed instructions and explain warnings on labels, such as "Do not drive or operate machinery while taking this medication" or "Discontinue use if rapid pulse, dizziness, or blurring of vision occurs" (see Figure 10-1).
   c. Drink 1 to 2 ounces of water before taking solid dosage forms; this hastens their movement to the stomach. Whenever possible, drink a full glass of water to assist in their dissolution.
   d. Check all medications periodically for expiration dates and for deterioration. Discard outdated or deteriorated medications.
   e. Discard unused portions of drugs; do not share these with friends or family, even if they appear to have symptoms like your own. Do not even save them for yourself without asking a prescriber.
   f. Keep all medications out of children's reach, and never refer to medications as "candy" to induce children to take the medication. A childproof cap may serve only to slow a child down.
   g. Do not take any medication in the dark.
   h. Do not mix medications in one container. Store drugs in the original container with the original label. Keep the container tightly capped.
   i. If you suspect a mistake or overdose, call your local Poison Control Center, prescriber, or pharmacist. Have the medication container at hand.
   j. Learn both the generic and brand or trade names of prescribed drugs. Learn the appearances of your drugs.
   k. Tell the prescriber and pharmacist about any allergies or other conditions you have, any previous unusual reactions, a current pregnancy, or if you are breastfeeding.
   l. Take the medication precisely as directed and for the length of time prescribed. Ask your health care practitioner or consult the *USP DI* about what to do if one dose of the medication is omitted. Do not just stop the medication on your own.
4. Instruct that nonprescription drugs do not usually cure a condition but instead make the symptoms bearable. Treated conditions that persist, recur, or produce unusual reactions should be evaluated by a health care provider.
5. Counsel and instruct the client, when appropriate, about alternate nursing therapies or therapies that accompany drug taking (e.g., instruct about increasing fluids, activity, and roughage to reduce a laxative habit).
6. Warn about certain drugs that can produce physical and psychologic dependence (e.g., analgesics, stimulants, and laxatives).

schedule when the client is ready to return home. The nurse must ensure that the appropriate family members are taught to provide the ongoing care. If the family will not be in attendance at home, it may be more appropriate to provide information to the client's friends, neighbors, or paid care providers regarding the medications.

Although there may be many opportunities to teach family members, the nurse may need to schedule an appointment with them to ensure that they are present to learn the medication regimen and other discharge instructions. The assistance of family members needs to be actively sought and encouraged; some may be hesitant because they are unsure of the part they are to play in the client's care.

Successful teaching programs with clients and families include the following: (1) positive reinforcement or praise for desired behaviors; (2) feedback about progress toward goals; (3) individualization, whereby learning needs are determined for the specific client and the pace of teaching is mutually negotiated; (4) facilitation, in which the nurse assists the client to take action, such as making personalized medication schedules; and (5) relevance, making sure that the content and teaching-learning methods are meaningful for the client. The nurse should attempt to incorporate these issues into each of the teaching sessions.

There is no single best way to educate clients about self-administering medications. Using the same approach each time does not take into account the data gathered from the client in the assessment phase of the teaching-learning process. Assessing each individual's learning needs in order to develop the best teaching approach results in the most effective use of nursing resources. Given the seriousness of client's nonadherence to medication regimens, additional efforts need to be directed toward developing and testing innovative approaches to assist clients in following treatment prescriptions.

EVALUATION

Evaluating whether client education has taken place is essential. Some nurses may consider the teaching process complete after handing out a brochure or showing a videotape. However, the emphasis should be on the client's response—behavioral changes, knowledge, and skills gained as a result of the method and content of the teaching-learning process. The evaluation process should involve assessing the client's progress toward specific goals for self-administration of medication, as well as the response to the teaching-learning process.

DOCUMENTATION

Documentation is the final step in the process of client teaching for the self-administration of medications. Unfortunately, JCAHO has found the lack of documentation of the client's and family's knowledge of self-care to be one of the most common nursing deficiencies cited during accreditation audits. Documentation related to education about medications should contain at least three items: the specific content, the method of teaching, and the evaluation of learning.

Although the nursing care plan contains the specific learning goals agreed on by the nursing team and the client, the narrative documentation following the teaching-learning process should indicate the specific content that was covered. This information needs to be recorded in such a way that any other nurse will know enough about what was taught to be able to continue the teaching from that point. The following are appropriate examples: "The need for taking a pulse before a digoxin dose was discussed," "The client was cautioned not to take antacids with the tetracycline," or "The side effect of furosemide, hypokalemia and its symptoms, were discussed." A common error of documentation is the statement "Medications taught," particularly in a setting where the client may have a polydrug regimen, such as in home health care. The following questions are raised: What medications? What about them? What dosing schedule? What side effects/adverse reactions? What special precautions? Such vague documentation does not support the provision of skilled nursing care and in the home health care setting may provide justification for nonreimbursement for nursing care. Because clients are transitioned from one health care setting to another more often in today's health care environment, documentation becomes even more important. Such data allows the nurse within the client's next health care setting to provide continuity of instruction without repeating previous information or omitting essential learning.

Documenting the method of instruction allows the next nurse to know which teaching techniques were successful for the client's learning. Although "taught" is the most common verb used, it does not explain what or how the material was covered. More appropriate words are "discussed," "demonstrated," or "a specific piece of literature was reviewed and given to the client." Documentation may also include the client's characteristics as a learner and any barriers to learning that may have been determined. Recording the "teaching" part of the teaching-learning process leads then to the most important part—recording the "learning" of that process.

Many health care agencies that use a clinical pathway approach to the provision of care and its documentation have also developed teaching pathways to provide a comprehensive approach to client education for specific disease or procedure populations. These teaching pathways serve as a guide to teaching and identifying learning objectives along a designated time line, and they provide consistent documentation (Sciartelli, 1995).

Recording an evaluation of the client's and/or family's learning indicates the achievement of, or progress toward, the learning goals originally established by the client and the nurse. The evaluation documentation includes a description of what occurred, the client's response to the teaching-learning encounter (using his or her own words and behaviors), and the observable or measurable activities of the client and family that would indicate that the instructions were understood. Documentation, as the final step of the teaching-learning process, is essential in recording the client's progress.

SUMMARY

Medications tend to be more effective when clients believe in the drug and in their capacity to get well. Their past and present conditioning to drugs, illness, hospitals, nurses, and other health care personnel, as well as their own health beliefs and practices, influence their response to drug therapy. An accurate assessment of these factors is most important in order to plan and implement an effective care plan.

The three most common nursing diagnoses related to the self-administration of medications for which the client is at risk are deficient knowledge, ineffective therapeutic regimen management, and noncompliance. These problems need to be resolved so that the client may accurately and safely self-administer medications.

From the onset of drug therapy, the client should be advised of the purpose of the medication and any possible side effects/adverse reactions. All information should be presented in a nonthreatening and straightforward manner. It is important to listen to what the client has to say about the medication, the feelings associated with the drug and whether these feelings are based on fear or anxiety, and the perception of the condition for which the drug has been prescribed.

Client education plays an important role when the individual needs to follow a prescribed medication plan after discharge. Routinely reviewing medications with clients and inquiring about how medications are taken at home have been shown to increase compliance with a medication plan.

The nurse should make sure that the client thoroughly understands the medication instructions. Written schedules and instructions will remind clients when they are at home and may have forgotten what they heard in the office or on discharge from the hospital.

Documentation of the teaching-learning process for self-administration of medications needs to include content, method, and the client's and the family's progress in relation to the planned objectives for learning.

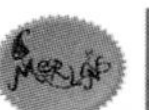

Critical Thinking Questions

1. What type of strategies would you use to determine the educational needs of a client who will eventually self-administer medications at home?
2. If your contact time with a client is limited (e.g., an emergency department setting), what are the most essential elements to get across to the client?
3. How would you differentiate between the nursing diagnoses of deficient knowledge and ineffective therapeutic regimen management if you ascertained that the client was not taking his or her medications as prescribed?
4. How would you assess the learning needs of and develop a teaching plan for an older adult? A client with a language barrier?

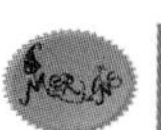

Collaborative Learning Activities

For Collaborative Learning Activities, go to mosby.com/MERLIN/McKenry/.

BIBLIOGRAPHY

Barbee, J.G. (1993). Memory, benzodiazepines, and anxiety: Integration of theoretical and clinical perspectives. *Journal of Clinical Psychiatry, 54* (suppl), 86-97.

Bille, D.A. (Ed.). (1981). *Practical approaches to patient teaching*. Boston: Little, Brown & Co.

Bond, W.S. & Hussar, D.A. (1991). Detection methods and strategies for improving medication compliance. *American Journal of Hospital Pharmacy, 48*, 1978-1988.

Britten, D.M. (1996). Lay views of drugs and medicine: Orthodox and unorthodox accounts. In S.J. Williams & M. Calnam (Eds.), *Modern medicine: Lay perspectives and experience*. London: U.C.L. Press.

Carpenito, L.J. (2000). *Nursing diagnosis: Application to clinical practice* (8th ed.). Philadelphia: J.B. Lippincott.

Charonko, C.V. (1992). Cultural influences in "noncompliant" behavior and decision making. *Holistic Nursing Practice 6*(3), 73-78.

Coudreaut-Quinn, E.A., Emmons, M.A., & McMurrow, M.J. (1992). Self-medication during inpatient psychiatric treatment. *Journal of Psychosocial Nursing, 30*(12), 32-36.

Craig, C. (1995). Teaching food-drug interactions. *Journal of Psychosocial Nursing, 33*(2), 44-46.

Czar, M.L., & Engler, M.M. (1997). Perceived learning needs of patients with coronary artery disease using a questionnaire assessment tool. *Heart Lung, 26*(2), 109-117.

Der, E.H., Rubenstein, L.Z., & Choy, G.S. (1997). The benefits of in-home pharmacy evaluation for older persons. *Journal of the American Geriatrics Society, 45*(2), 211-214.

Drake, A.C. & Romano, E. (1995). Protect your older patient from the hazards of polypharmacy. *Nursing, 25*(6):34-39.

Esposito, L. (1995). The effects of medication education on adherence to medication regimens in an elderly population. *Journal of Advanced Nursing, 21*, 935-943.

Gullickson, C. (1993). Client-centered drug choice: An alternative approach to managing hypertension. *Nurse Practitioner, 18*(2), 30-41.

Harvey, L.J. & Plumridge, R.J. (1991). Comparative attitudes to verbal and written medication information among hospital outpatients. *DICP, 25*, 925-928.

Hussey, L.C. (1991). Overcoming the clinical barriers of low literacy and medication noncompliance among the elderly. *Journal of Gerontology Nursing, 17*(3), 27.

Johnson, K.B., Butta, J.K., Donohue, P.K., Glenn, D.J., & Holtzman, N.A. (1996). Discharging patients with prescriptions instead of medications: Sequelae in a teaching hospital. *Pediatrics, 97*(4), 481-485.

Jones, L.A. (1995). Patient information issues in the ambulatory surgery setting. *Today's OR Nurse, 17*(2), 9-12.

Kerr, B., Hill, H., Coda, B., Calogero, M., Chapman, C.R., Hunt, E., Buffington, V., & Mackie, A. (1991). Concentration-related effects of morphine on cognition and motor control in human subjects. *Neuropsychopharmacology, 5*, 157-166.

Lile, J.L. & Hoffman, R. (1991). Medication-taking by the frail elderly in two ethnic groups. *Nursing Forum, 26*(4), 19-24.

Martens, K.H. (1998). An ethnographic study of the process of medication discharge education (MDE). *Journal of Advanced Nursing, 27*(2), 341-348.

McKenry, L.M. (1999). *Mosby's patient guide to medications*. St. Louis: Mosby.

Petrie, K.J., Weinman, J., Sharpe, N., & Buckley, J. (1996). Role of patient's view of their illness in predicting return to work and functioning after myocardial infarction: Longitudinal study. *British Medical Journal, 312*(7040), 1191-1194.

Proos, M., Reiley, P., Eagan, J., Stengrevics, J., Castile, J., & Arian, D. (1992). A study of the effects of self-medication on patients' knowledge of and compliance with their medication regimen. *Journal of Nursing Care Quality*, Special Report, 18-26.

Redman, B.K. (1997). *The practice of patient education*. (8th ed.). St. Louis: Mosby.

Sciartelli, C.H. (1995). Using a clinical pathway approach to document patient teaching for breast cancer surgical procedures. *Oncology Nursing Forum, 22*(1), 131-137.

Shea, S., Misra, D., Erlich, M.H., Field, L., & Francis, C.K. (1992). Correlates of nonadherence to hypertension treatment in an inner-city minority population. *American Journal of Public Health, 82*(12), 1607-1612.

Smith, C.E. (1989). Overview of patient education: opportunities and challenges for the twenty-first century. *Nursing Clinics of North America, 24*(3), 583-587.

Tibbles, L., Lewis, C., Reisine, S., Rippey, R., & Donald, M. (1992). Computer assisted instruction for preoperative and postoperative patient education in joint replacement surgery. *Computers in Nursing, 10*(5), 208-212.

Tripp-Reimer, T. & Afifi, L.A. (1989). Cross-cultural perspectives on patient teaching. *Nursing Clinics of North America, 24*(3), 613-619.

United States Pharmacopeia Dispensing Information (USP DI): Advice for the patient (19th ed.) (1999). Rockville, MD: United States Pharmacopeial Convention.

Wainwright, S.P. & Gould, D. (1997). Non-adherence with medications in organ transplant patients: A literature review. *Journal of Advanced Nursing, 26*(5), 968-977.

Weaver, J. (1995). Patient education: An innovative computer approach. *Nursing Management, 26*(7), 78-83.

Wenger, A.Z. (1993). Teaching families from diverse cultural backgrounds. *Neonatal Network, 12*(1), 69-70.

11 Over-the-Counter Medications

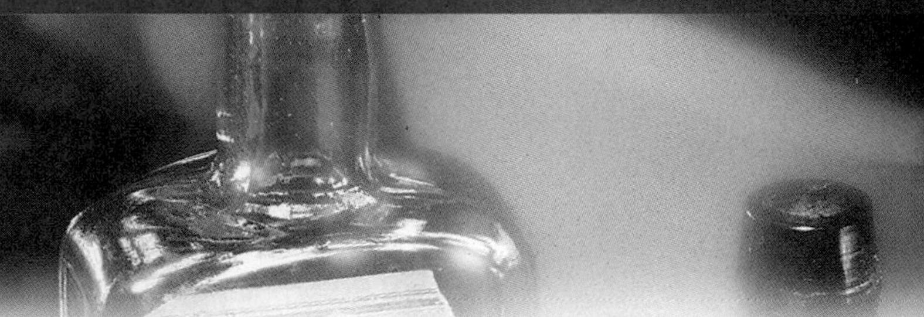

Chapter Focus

Over-the-counter (OTC), or nonprescription, drugs are medications that can safely be used to self-treat minor illnesses without the supervision of a licensed health care practitioner—provided that consumers follow the directions on the package. Because OTC drugs are widely available and commonly used by clients, nurses need to obtain information about their use as part of every drug history. Nurses' knowledge of nonprescription drugs should be as thorough as their knowledge of prescription drugs so they can provide client education regarding potential drug-drug interactions, expected outcomes of their use, and other issues related to OTC drugs. Collaboration with a pharmacist is recommended.

Learning Objectives

1. Compare and contrast the strength, dosing, and other recommendations for prescription and OTC (nonprescription) drugs.
2. Discuss issues related to drug marketing, safety, selection, storage, and administration of OTC medications by the client.
3. Advise the client on the safe self-administration of selected OTC preparations (e.g., analgesics, antacids, laxatives, cough-cold preparations) as they become available.

Key Terms

analgesic, p. 208
antacid, p. 213
antihistamine, p. 225
constipation, p. 215
diarrhea, p. 221
dysmenorrhea, p. 228
laxative, p. 215
perceived constipation, p. 215
premenstrual syndrome, p. 228

Key Drugs [✔]

acetaminophen, p. 208
aspirin, p. 210

Over-the-counter (OTC), or nonprescription, medications are used by the general public to self-treat minor illnesses. Such preparations are readily available in pharmacies, supermarkets, and other nonpharmacy outlets for selection by individuals who want to avoid the time and expense associated with going to a prescriber. The Nonprescription Drug Manufacturers Association reports that Americans visit their physicians for only 10% of their illnesses and injuries, and the Health Care Financing Administration (HCFA) states that 6 out of every 10 medications purchased are OTC medications. OTC drugs have a tremendous market; it has been estimated that more than 300,000 such products are available in the United States. These products contain between 700 and 1000 active ingredients (Burns, 1991; Zimmerman, 1993). When used wisely, they result in time and money savings for the individual and, ultimately, a reduction in overall health care costs. A good example of these cost savings is the use of hydrocortisone cream, a product commonly used to treat rash and pruritus. When the cream became available as an OTC preparation, it was estimated to have saved Americans more than one billion dollars over a 3-year period when compared with the medical model of physician visits, prescriptions, and other related costs (Burns, 1991).

Although OTC medications are generally considered to be safe and effective for consumer use, problems can result. Self-medication requires a self-diagnosis of the signs and symptoms of a clinical condition. In general, the public may consider most illnesses to be minor. However, if a potentially serious condition is self-treated with an OTC medication, the condition may be masked, and professional help for appropriate treatment is delayed (Covington, 1996). In addition, OTC drugs may contain potent chemicals, many of which used to be prescription drugs. The trend in the 1990s was to transfer more and more prescription medications to OTC status. The health care professional should be aware that many OTC products (new and old) are capable of producing both desired and undesirable effects, drug interactions, and drug toxicity. This potential problem has been recognized by a current pharmacy law (Omnibus Budget Reconciliation Act, or OBRA), which mandates that OTC drugs be considered an important part of the client's medical record (Fitzgerald, 1994).

Although the Food and Drug Administration (FDA) issued regulations that require OTC package labeling to be stated in terms that are likely to be read and understood by the average consumer, many consumers believe the labels are confusing; often the print is too small to read. Approximately 35% of Americans read at a 6th to 10th grade level, and an estimated 20% are considered functionally illiterate (i.e., read below a 5th grade level) (Covington, 1996). Therefore OTC labeling that is difficult to understand and apply may result in unsafe or improper medication use. This chapter reviews the regulatory difference between a prescription and an OTC drug and discusses the process involved in changing a drug from prescription to OTC status. General considerations on drug marketing, consumer education for the safe administration of OTC drugs, and selected major OTC drug categories are also discussed.

The FDA regulates and makes decisions about the safety and effectiveness of a drug, the classification of a product as a prescription or an OTC drug, and the information printed on the drug labels. Drug substances are subjected to regulation, review, and various study requirements before being released with FDA approval and may be monitored afterward to a limited extent. Medications not considered safe enough for the general public to use without medical supervision are restricted to prescription status only. OTC drugs are defined as safe and effective drugs for self-treatment by the public, assuming that good manufacturing practices are followed by the manufacturer and that label directions are followed by the consumer.

At one time many OTC drugs were being marketed without the more current standards of proof of documented safety and effectiveness, in 1972 the FDA established a number of OTC expert advisory panels to review drug categories and make recommendations to the FDA. As a result of this review, many ingredients used in OTC products were removed from the market, including aphrodisiacs, hair growers, hexachlorophene products, and others. These drugs were found to be either ineffective, dangerous, or both. In 1991 the FDA established an OTC Drugs Advisory Committee to assist in review and evaluation and to advise the FDA Commissioner on its findings and recommendations. The Committee may also suggest prescription drugs to change to OTC status on the basis of expert findings that the medication is safe and effective for general public use.

The definitions for OTC drug safety and effectiveness include the following:

- *Safety:* The drug product has a low incidence of severe side effects and a low potential for harm, assuming that proper instructions and adequate warnings are given on the label.
- *Effectiveness:* When properly used, the drug ingredient will provide relief of the minor symptom or illness in a significant portion of the population.

CHANGING A DRUG FROM PRESCRIPTION TO OVER-THE-COUNTER STATUS

Over the years the FDA has approved nearly 600 prescription drugs for OTC availability (Lipinsky, 1999). Approximately one third of all new OTC drugs released between 1975 and 1994 were previously prescription medications (Jacobs, 1998). With some products a lower strength of the active ingredient was required in the OTC product, and with others the same strength as the prescription drug was released in an OTC form. Ibuprofen (Motrin) was released in a 200-mg strength as an OTC drug; the higher dose tablet strengths, 400 or 800 mg, still require a prescription. The lower strength of ibuprofen is considered to be safe and effective for the self-treatment of a minor illness if the label

TABLE 11-1 Prescription Drugs That Have Been Reclassified as Over-the-Counter Drugs

Ingredient (Prescription Name)	OTC Name (examples)	Principal Use
brompheniramine (e.g., Dimetane)	Dimetane, Bromphen	Antihistamine
clemastine (Tavist)	Tavist	Antihistamine
chlorpheniramine (e.g., Chlor-Trimeton)	Chlor-Trimeton, Aller-Chlor	Antihistamine
cimetidine (Tagamet)	Tagamet HB	Heartburn, acid indigestion relief
clotrimazole (e.g., Lotrimin)	Lotrimin AF, Mycelex	Antifungal
diphenhydramine (Benadryl)	Benylin Cough, Diphen Cough	Cough suppression
diphenhydramine (Benadryl)	Nytol, Sominex	Sleeping aid
famotidine (Pepcid)	Pepcid AC	Heartburn, acid indigestion
hydrocortisone (e.g., Cort-Dome)	Cortizone, Dermolate	Topical for itching and rash relief
ibuprofen (Motrin)	Advil, Nuprin	Analgesic
ketoconazole	Nizoral	Dandruff shampoo
loperamide (e.g., Imodium)	Imodium A-D, Kaopectate II	Antidiarrheal
miconazole (Monistat)	Micatin	Antifungal
nicotine polacrilex	Nicorette	Smoking cessation
nicotine transdermal	Nicotrol, Nicoderm CQ	Smoking cessation
nizatidine (Axid)	Axid AR	Heartburn, acid indigestion relief
pyrantel (Antiminth)	Reese's Pinworm	Pinworm remedy
sodium fluoride	Fluorigard, ACT	Dental rinse
tioconazole	Vagistat-1	Anticandidal

instructions are followed. Use of higher strength ibuprofen requires medical supervision and a prescription because it has the potential to cause serious side effects/adverse reactions. Table 11-1 provides examples of prescription drugs that have been reclassified as OTC drugs.

DRUG MARKETING

In contrast to prescription drugs, OTC medications may be marketed without FDA approval. Monographs of information developed by the OTC drug review identified specific drugs "generally recognized as safe and effective" (GRASE). Any drug manufacturer may produce such products for marketing without prior government approval. The manufacturer has flexibility in package labeling. Although the use of certain approved terminology is required (e.g., heartburn, acid indigestion, and sour stomach for antacids), other terms that have not been approved may also be used as long as they are not false or misleading.

In contrast to prescription medications, no regulations require that adverse reactions to an OTC product be reported. The manufacturer may substitute one GRASE ingredient in an OTC preparation for another GRASE ingredient without changing the name of the OTC drug and without indicating the change to the public with a warning on the package or label. The only method of determining the ingredients in a product is to check the label before each purchase (Covington, 1996).

Another important concept to understand is the difference between drug potency and drug effectiveness. As defined in Chapter 5, drug potency is the amount of drug required to produce a desired effect. When drug manufacturers claim their product is more potent than another product, they usually mean that a smaller quantity of the drug is necessary to produce the same effect as the comparison drug. This does not mean the *more potent drug is also the more effective drug* (unless greater effectiveness has been proven and clearly stated)—it refers only to the amount of drug necessary to produce a desired effect. This terminology is often used and may be misleading if health care providers or consumers do not understand the difference between potency and effectiveness.

OTC analgesics have a number of extra-strength dosage forms that imply greater potency than the regular strength of the same brand or the competitor's usual adult strength (usually 500 mg compared with 325 mg of analgesic). However, if a more potent drug does not have documented proof of greater effectiveness when compared with an equivalent dose of the second drug, then there is no advantage to a "more potent" medication. When the only difference is drug strength, the therapeutic effect expected with either drug is the same; the potential disadvantages in using a more potent drug may include increased costs, side effects, and unknown long-term effects.

CONSUMER EDUCATION FOR OVER-THE-COUNTER DRUGS

Nurses have a major role in the education of consumers for the accurate and safe self-administration of OTC medications. Although many of these medications are also found in care settings in which the role of the nurse is to administer such drugs, it is important to maintain a familiarity with OTC medications to best advise clients for safe self-treatment of minor illnesses. The following information about OTC preparations should be shared with clients as an aspect of health promotion in both formal and informal instructional situations. Such teaching is applicable to almost any setting in which the nurse interacts with clients.

OTC drugs have the image of being very safe and thus not requiring the special precautions necessary to take a prescription drug safely. Nothing could be farther from the truth. As with prescription drugs, OTC products have the potential for being misused, abused, and inducing side effects/adverse reactions. They also may be very dangerous if taken in certain concurrent disease states or if taken concurrently with other drugs, food, or alcohol. The health care professional needs to be aware of this information before administering or advising about an OTC preparation.

Product ingredients have either proven or questionable effectiveness; a careful check of ingredients is necessary to select the appropriate product in a specific drug category. The consumer should be encouraged to select the proper ingredient for treating the client's specific symptom. Combination products may contain substances that are not necessary for the person's symptoms. If the individual has an adverse reaction to the combination drug, it would be difficult to determine the responsible ingredient. In addition, many different products may have the same active ingredients that may or may not differ in strength, dosage form (liquid, tablet, capsule), or combination. If the ingredients are not carefully checked, an accidental overdose is possible by taking the same ingredient in a number of different products.

Having the same ingredients in different preparations may allow for product substitution. For example, thousands of antacid products are available throughout the United States that primarily contain only four or five recognized active ingredients; many OTC antacids are therefore duplicate preparations. The generic product is often as effective as the advertised product, and there is usually little if any advantage in purchasing the more expensive item.

Consumers should check the selected product for tampering. Most products are now packaged in tamper-resistant or tamper-evident packaging, which allows the consumer to detect signs of tampering. If the package is suspect, it should be taken to the pharmacist or store manager. The expiration date should also be checked to ensure that it has not passed.

Consumers should read labels very carefully if they have ever had an allergic or unusual response to any medication, food, or other substance (e.g., yellow dye or sulfites) to ensure that such an ingredient is not included. Caution should be used if the individual is on a special diet, (e.g., low-sugar or low-sodium), because many OTC drugs contain more than their active ingredients, and many liquid preparations contain alcohol. A woman who is pregnant or breastfeeding should not take OTC medications without first consulting her health care provider. Individuals with underlying medical conditions such as hypertension or diabetes should read labels carefully to assess whether the medication may be contraindicated with their condition.

BOX 11-1

Situations and Conditions That Require Evaluation by a Physician or Other Health Care Provider

Before purchasing OTC medications, the following situations or conditions should be evaluated by a physician or other health care provider:

- Child is under 6 months old.
- Infant has had diarrhea for more than 24 hours.
- The woman is pregnant.
- The individual has any of the following:
  - An oral temperature >39.8°C (102°F) or a fever lasting more than 2 days
  - Cold or influenza symptoms lasting more than 1 week
  - Vomiting for more than 12 hours
  - Severe abdominal pain or cramps
  - Redness or swelling in a painful site
  - Difficulty breathing
  - A sudden, severe headache, slurred speech, and confusion
  - Visual changes or eye pain
  - Recurrent or persistent pain or fever
  - Severe sore throat lasting more than 2 days
  - Diarrhea lasting more than 2 days
  - Consumption of three or more alcohol-containing beverages daily

The above are selected general guidelines; the nurse should be aware that other criteria may also be applied.

OTC medications are just that, medications that should be reported to any health care provider when a drug history is being obtained. Instructions and warnings on the label are to be followed carefully. The individual should be advised to consult with a pharmacist before purchasing an OTC medication if he or she has medical condition(s), is not familiar with the proper way to select an individual product based on ingredients and cost, if the package instructions seem unclear, or if the current problem for which he or she is self-medicating is persistent and requires a referral from a health care provider. Additional situations and conditions that require evaluation by a physician or other health care provider are summarized in Box 11-1. A health care provider should be consulted if the symptoms for which the OTC drug is being taken are not relieved in an appropriate time interval as indicated on the label.

Unless instructed otherwise, both prescription and OTC medications should be stored in closed containers in a cool, dry place and out of the reach of children. They should not be stored in the bathroom, near sinks, or in damp places because heat, moisture, and strong light may cause deterioration or a loss of medication potency.

All solid-dose medications (tablets and capsules) should be taken with a full glass of water (8 ounces). The individual should be advised to sit up for approximately 15 to 30 minutes after taking the solid-dose medication to help reduce the potential for esophageal irritation or injury. Drinking a small amount of water before taking a tablet or capsule is very helpful for individuals with problems of dry mouth or minor problems in swallowing. If the drug is a long-acting medication, it should be swallowed whole. If the medication is in liquid form, the specially marked measuring spoon or other device provided by the manufacturer should be used to measure each dose accurately.

SELECTED OVER-THE-COUNTER DRUG CATEGORIES

The following sections review the most common OTC drug categories: analgesics, antacids, laxatives, antidiarrheals, cold-cough preparations, and products related to women's health. The following sections include a review of the ingredients in each category, as well as the mechanism of action, indications, pharmacokinetics, warnings, drug interactions, and specific tips on the proper and safe use of the individual product.

This information should assist the nurse in identifying and evaluating the multitude of OTC medications on the market. By understanding the basic information presented in this chapter and checking package ingredients, a safer and more logical approach to product selection can be made. The nursing management of the client receiving any of these OTC medications is discussed in the chapters that present these same drugs in their prescription status.

Analgesics

Pain is one of the most common and feared symptoms known to humans. For minor pain such as headache, toothache, muscle and joint aches, swelling (inflammation), and fever, many people can obtain relief fairly inexpensively with an OTC medication. **Analgesic** is the term used to describe a drug that relieves pain.

OTC analgesics have different therapeutic effects, side effects, drug interactions, and other characteristics, and in the following sections they are divided into the three major OTC categories available: acetaminophen, aspirin, and the nonsteroidal antiinflammatory drugs (NSAIDs). (See Chapter 14 for additional information on analgesics, especially the prescription analgesics.)

acetaminophen [a seat a min′ oh fen]

Many brand name products of acetaminophen are available and include Tylenol, Anacin-3, Feverall Sprinkle, Liquiprin, Panadol, and Tempra. The mechanism of action for acetaminophen is primarily inhibition of prostaglandin synthesis in the central nervous system (CNS) and, to a lesser degree, blockage of the generation of peripheral pain impulses. Acetaminophen is equivalent to aspirin as an analgesic and antipyretic agent but does not have antiinflammatory effects. Acetaminophen has been used to treat mild forms of arthritis (osteoarthritis), but aspirin or the NSAIDs are preferred for treating moderate to severe arthritis, especially rheumatoid arthritis (Box 11-2).

Acetaminophen offers several advantages over aspirin, which include the following:

- It may be used by people who are allergic to aspirin.
- It rarely causes abdominal upset, tinnitus, or gastric bleeding (inhibition of platelet aggregation), which are reported more often with aspirin.
- It may be used by clients taking anticoagulant medications.
- It may be used by children with colds and influenza symptoms because, unlike aspirin, it has not been associated with Reye's syndrome (Box 11-3).

Acetaminophen taken orally is rapidly absorbed and reaches peak serum levels in ½ to 1 hour; its half-life is 2 to 3 hours. It is metabolized in the liver and excreted by the kidneys.

Side effects/adverse reactions are rare with acetaminophen, although in some instances nausea and rash have occurred. The drug should be discontinued and a health care provider contacted immediately if any of the following oc-

BOX 11-2

Common Types of Arthritis

Osteoarthritis or degenerative joint disease is a common form of arthritis, affecting 85% of persons over 70 years old. Symptoms may start in the fifth or sixth decade of life. Unlike rheumatoid arthritis, which is an inflammatory disease, osteoarthritis is the result of a deformation or mismatched joint surfaces. Symptoms include joint stiffness that usually lasts only a few minutes after initiating joint movement and perhaps an aching pain in weight-bearing joints. Early disease stages may respond to local heat and nonprescription analgesics. Later stages may require orthopedic or other interventions.

Rheumatoid arthritis usually occurs between 30 and 70 years of age and more often in women than in men. Early symptoms may include feelings of fatigue and weakness, joint pain and stiffness and, several weeks later, joint swelling. The joints are inflamed (warm, red, swollen) and often are limited in range of motion. Rheumatoid arthritis is a progressive disease that leads to joint deformity. Aspirin and aspirin-type products (NSAIDs) are usually necessary to reduce inflammation around the joints. Heat therapy, weight control, and exercise may also be helpful.

For a Concept Map on osteoarthritis, go to mosby.com/MERLIN/McKenry/.

BOX 11-3

Acetaminophen and Aspirin Over-the-Counter Warnings

General Precautions for Both Analgesics

- Individuals should consult with the prescriber before taking any analgesic if they are allergic to an analgesic or have had a severe allergic analgesic reaction such as asthma, swelling, hives, rash, and other symptoms.
- Individuals should avoid taking analgesics if they have kidney disease or liver damage, are pregnant or breastfeeding, have taken the analgesics for pain for more than 10 days (in an adult) or 5 days (in a child) or for fever for 3 days, if pain increases or the painful site is inflamed, if new symptoms develop, or if a sore throat is very painful or lasts more than 2 days.
- If stomach distress occurs, the analgesic should be taken after meals or with food.

Special Dosing Information: Aspirin

- Children and teenagers (under 17 years of age) should avoid using aspirin to treat fever or symptoms of a viral infection, especially influenza or chickenpox, without prescriber approval. The use of aspirin for viral illnesses in children may cause a very serious condition known as Reye's syndrome. Symptoms include severe vomiting, weakness, and stupor that may progress to coma, convulsions, and even death.
- Aspirin use should be discontinued at least 5 to 7 days before a scheduled surgery.
- Aspirin products should never be put directly on a tooth or gum surface, because they can burn the tissues and cause injury.
- Aspirin that has a strong, vinegar-like odor should not be taken; such an odor indicates that the aspirin is deteriorating.
- The prescriber should be informed about an individual who has an aspirin or salicylate allergy, asthma, nasal polyps, anemia, gout, ulcers or ulcer symptoms, or hemophilia or other bleeding problems.

cur: an allergic-type reaction (hives, pruritus, respiratory difficulties), blood in the urine or stool, severe pain in the side or lower back, or unusual bleeding, bruising, weakness, or tiredness.

An overdose of acetaminophen can cause serious damage to the liver and kidneys (see Chapter 14 for management of an acetaminophen overdose). The maximum daily acetaminophen dose for adults is 4 g; for children, the single dose is 40 to 480 mg depending on age and weight, with no more than 5 doses being given in 24 hours (Insel, 1996).

Prescription and OTC drug interactions with acetaminophen include the following:

Drug	Possible Effect and Management
alcohol	Increased possibility of hepatotoxicity, especially chronic alcoholism, if more acetaminophen is taken than recommended on the label or if acetaminophen is taken over a long period. Avoid alcoholic beverages when taking acetaminophen.
anticoagulants such as warfarin (Coumadin) and heparin	High doses and frequent use of acetaminophen may increase the anticoagulant action of these drugs, increasing the risk of bleeding. Occasional use of acetaminophen in persons taking anticoagulants is usually not a problem.
prescription drugs containing acetaminophen (e.g., Tylenol with codeine, Darvocet, Percocet)	Combined use may result in an acetaminophen overdose. (See Chapter 14 for symptoms and treatment of an acetaminophen overdose.)
other OTC drugs that contain acetaminophen	Use of two or more OTC products containing acetaminophen may result in an acetaminophen overdose.

OTC acetaminophen is available in powder, tablet, chewable tablet, liquid, drops, and suppository dosage forms. The usual adult dosage is 325 to 650 mg every 4 hours, or 325 to 500 mg every 3 hours, or 650 to 1000 mg every 6 hours when needed. The usual pediatric dosage is 10 to 15 mg/kg body weight every 4 to 6 hours as needed.

Acetaminophen Combinations

Analgesic combinations of acetaminophen with other ingredients are also available as OTC products. At one time combination products were thought to be stronger because of the extra ingredients and also were thought to have fewer side effects because the dose of each ingredient was usually less than the full dose of a single ingredient alone. This reasoning is now outdated and highly questionable. Most combination products offer little advantage over acetaminophen or aspirin alone.

The more common combinations include acetaminophen combined with salicylates (aspirin, salicylamide), with a salicylate and caffeine, or with an antacid (sodium bicarbonate, calcium carbonate, or "buffered"). Box 11-4 lists acetaminophen and aspirin formulations.

Salicylates, salicylamide, and aspirin are from the salicylate drug family and have analgesic, antipyretic, and antiinflammatory effects. The antiinflammatory effect depends on the amount of salicylates in the product; because the combination doses of aspirin are usually low, they are not recommended to treat severe inflammation or severe arthritic

BOX 11-4

Acetaminophen and Aspirin Formulations*

- Acetaminophen with salicylates
  acetaminophen with salicylates (Gemnisyn)
  acetaminophen and salicylamide (Duoprin)
- Acetaminophen with aspirin/salicylate and caffeine
  acetaminophen, aspirin, salicylamide, and caffeine (Saleto; Tri-Pain)
  acetaminophen, aspirin, and caffeine (Goody's Extra Strength Tablets, Duradyne, Excedrin Extra-Strength)
  acetaminophen, salicylamide, and caffeine (Rid-A-Pain Compound; S-A-C)
- Aspirin/salicylates combined with caffeine
  aspirin and caffeine (Anacin and others)
- Acetaminophen combinations with antacid
  buffered acetaminophen, aspirin, and caffeine (Gelpirin, Supac, Buffets, Vanquish)
  buffered acetaminophen, aspirin, and salicylamide (Presalin)
  acetaminophen, sodium bicarbonate, and citric acid (Bromo-Seltzer)
  acetaminophen with calcium carbonate (Extra Strength Tylenol)
- Aspirin/salicylates with antacid (buffering agents)
  aspirin, sodium bicarbonate, citric acid (Alka-Seltzer Original, Alka-Seltzer Flavored, Alka-Seltzer Extra Strength†)
  aspirin, aluminum hydroxide, magnesium hydroxide (Arthritis Pain Formula, Magnaprin, Maprin)
  aspirin, calcium carbonate, magnesium carbonate, magnesium oxide (Bayer Plus Buffered Aspirin and Bayer Plus, Extra Strength Buffered Aspirin)
  aspirin, magnesium oxide (Buffaprin, Buffaprin Extra, Buffasal, Buffasal Max, Buffinol)
  aspirin, calcium carbonate, magnesium oxide, magnesium carbonate (Bufferin Tri-Buffered, Bufferin Arthritis Extra Strength, Tri-Buffered)
- Enteric-coated or delayed-release aspirin (e.g., Ecotrin, Bayer 8-hour, Extra Strength Bayer Caplets)

*_Extra strength_ usually refers to 500 mg analgesic as compared with 325 mg in regular strength products.
†The primary difference between the Alka-Seltzer products is taste and 500 mg aspirin in the extra-strength product compared with 325 mg in the other two products.

pain. Salicylamide is also considered to be much less effective than either acetaminophen or aspirin. In addition, the FDA has stated that salicylamide lacks documented proof of being effective as an analgesic or antipyretic.

Caffeine and analgesic combinations may enhance or produce better pain relief than the individual analgesic alone. Although some studies report that caffeine-analgesic combinations may provide better pain relieving effects, the FDA indicates a lack of sufficient proof (*United States Pharmacopeia Dispensing Information*, 1999).

The addition of an antacid buffer to acetaminophen or aspirin is also of questionable benefit. The addition of an antacid is unnecessary if the acetaminophen causes little if any stomach upset. The addition of an antacid is also questionable if the purpose is to avoid gastric distress caused by the other ingredients (aspirin or salicylates), because studies have indicated no difference between buffered and unbuffered tablets in the production of gastric damage. It appears that the amount of antacid or buffering agent added in the tablets may not be sufficient to produce this protective effect.

A more rapid absorption of the analgesic may occur if the buffer hastens drug dissolution; this explains why effervescent antacid preparations (e.g., Alka Seltzer, Bromo Seltzer) are more rapidly absorbed. In general, liquid dosage forms are faster and better absorbed. However, evidence is lacking that such products produce more rapid or more effective analgesia than the tablet dosage form, especially when the tablets or capsules are taken with a full glass of water (8 ounces). The nurse should be aware that effervescent medications usually contain a large amount of sodium, which must be avoided in persons with cardiac problems or renal failure (Lipman, 1996).

In summary, combination analgesic products are no more effective and often are more expensive than either acetaminophen or aspirin alone. The health care provider should also be aware that acetaminophen is often included in numerous products that contain more than one ingredient, such as cold, cough, allergy, menstrual or premenstrual, and sleeping aid products.

aspirin [as′ pir in]

Aspirin available as an OTC product includes ASA, acetylsalicylic acid, Bayer, Ecotrin, Norwich, St. Joseph, and many other commercial products. The mechanism of action for aspirin and the NSAIDs is inhibition of prostaglandin synthesis in both the central and peripheral nervous system. (See Chapter 14 for additional information on analgesics and NSAIDs.)

Aspirin has analgesic, antipyretic, antiplatelet, and antiinflammatory effects. It is indicated for the treatment of pain, fever, rheumatic fever, rheumatoid arthritis, and osteoarthritis, as well as for the prevention of myocardial infarction or reinfarction and the prevention of platelet aggregation in ischemia and thromboembolism. The advantages of aspirin over acetaminophen include its antiinflammatory effects and its effectiveness in preventing myocardial infarction and thrombus formation.

When taken orally in tablet form, aspirin is rapidly absorbed and reaches a peak serum level within 1 to 2 hours (more rapidly with liquid preparations); the peak antirheumatic effect occurs in 2 to 3 weeks. Tissue and blood esterases hydrolyze aspirin to acetic acid and salicylate; salicylates are then metabolized in the liver and excreted primarily by the kidneys.

Common side effects/adverse reactions include stomach irritation, cramps or discomfort, heartburn or indigestion, and nausea or vomiting. Taking aspirin with a full glass of water helps to reduce these effects. Less common or rare adverse reactions include severe abdominal pain, blood in stools, tinnitus, hematemesis, allergic reaction, confusion, weakness, flushing, visual disturbances, severe nausea or vomiting, and gastric ulcers. (See the Management of Drug Overdose box in Chapter 14 for clinical management of aspirin overdose.)

Prescription and OTC drug interactions with aspirin include the following:

Drug	Possible Effect and Management
alcohol, NSAIDs, and corticosteroids	Increased risk of gastrointestinal side effects, such as irritation, bleeding, and ulceration. Avoid taking aspirin concurrently with these substances.
anticoagulants (e.g., warfarin [Coumadin] and heparin), thrombolytic agents, antibiotics (carbenicillin [Geopen] cefamandole [Mandol], cefoperazone [Cefobid], cefotetan [Cefotan] plicamycin [Mithracin] ticarcillin [Ticar], and anticonvulsants (e.g., divalproex [Depakote] valproic acid [Depakene]	Can increase anticoagulant effects, resulting in increased risk of bleeding and hemorrhage. Avoid taking aspirin concurrently with these drugs.
furosemide (Lasix)	Increased risk for hearing loss, especially if high doses of aspirin or salicylates are consumed routinely. Limited, intermittent use may not be problematic.
methotrexate (Mexate)	May increase methotrexate plasma levels, leading to severe systemic toxic effects. Avoid taking salicylates while taking this drug.
probenecid (Benemid), sulfinpyrazone (Anturane)	Concurrent administration decreases the effect of antigout medications. Avoid using aspirin or salicylates if taking these medications.
sulfonylureas (oral antidiabetic drugs)	May increase therapeutic and side effects of the antidiabetic agents, especially when large doses of aspirin/salicylates are taken. Avoid taking aspirin/salicylates concurrently.
vancomycin (Vancocin)	Increased potential for hearing loss, which can progress to deafness. Avoid taking aspirin/salicylates concurrently.
Antacid-analgesic combinations:	The same drug interactions as listed above plus the following:
bismuth subsalicylate (Pepto Bismol)	Taking large, repeated doses of this product with frequent use of aspirin products increases the risk of toxicity (overdose). If taking this product for traveler's diarrhea or chronic diarrhea, be careful or avoid taking additional aspirin-containing products.
bulk-forming laxatives (Metamucil, Perdiem, and others)	These products may reduce the absorption and effect of aspirin/salicylates. Take these products 2 hours apart from aspirin/salicylates.
ketoconazole (Nizoral)	Antacids or buffering agents may increase stomach acidity, which reduces the absorption and effectiveness of ketoconazole. Buffered aspirin products should be taken at least 3 hours before or after ketoconazole.
oral tetracycline (Achromycin V)	Antacids and the magnesium in some salicylate medications can interfere with the absorption of tetracyclines. To reduce this effect, take the aspirin/salicylate preparation 3 to 4 hours apart from the tetracycline.

In addition to the interactions previously noted, *enteric-coated aspirin products* may interact with the following:

antacids or H_2-blocking agents such as cimetidine (Tagamet), ranitidine (Zantac), nizatidine (Axid), and famotidine (Pepcid)	The increase in gastric pH produced by these drugs may cause enteric-coated tablets to dissolve early, thus losing the benefit of the enteric coating in the stomach.

In addition to the interactions previously noted, the following interactions might occur with *caffeine* in analgesic medications:

other caffeine products, appetite suppressants, theophylline, pemoline (Cylert), selegiline (Eldepryl), tranylcypromine (Parnate), fluoxetine (Prozac), methylphenidate (Ritalin), sertraline (Zoloft), and sympathomimetics in oral, inhaled, and injectable dosage forms	An increase in CNS stimulation effects occur, such as nervousness, tremors, increased irritability, insomnia, and possibly cardiac dysrhythmias. Reducing or avoiding caffeine-containing products can reduce this effect.
lithium	Caffeine may increase lithium excretion from the body, which results in a reduction of lithium effects. Reduce or avoid the use of caffeine-containing products.

Drug	Possible Effect and Management
monoamine oxidase (MAO) inhibitors such as tranylcypromine (Parnate), procarbazine (Matulane), and possibly selegiline (Eldepryl)	May result in an increase in CNS stimulating effects (see p. 211), hypertension, and dangerous cardiac dysrhythmias. Avoid the use of large amounts of caffeine-containing products.

Aspirin products are available in tablet, chewable tablets, chewing gum tablets, extended-release tablets, and suppository dosage forms. The usual adult dosage is one to two regular-strength tablets (325 to 650 mg) every 4 hours or 500 to 1000 mg extra-strength tablets every 6 hours as needed. The adult maximum OTC aspirin dosage is 4 g/day. The pediatric dosage is 1.5 g/m^2/day in 4 to 6 divided doses. The nurse should check package labels for further dosing information.

Aspirin Combinations

Pain-relieving combinations of aspirin and other ingredients are available without a prescription. As with acetaminophen, aspirin/salicylates have been combined with acetaminophen, caffeine, and antacids (buffering agents); therefore the same comments regarding acetaminophen combinations also apply to aspirin combinations. (See Box 11-4 for examples of acetaminophen and aspirin formulations.)

Nonsteroidal Antiinflammatory Drugs

The NSAIDs and aspirin have analgesic, antipyretic, and antiinflammatory effects. Unlike aspirin, all NSAIDs were prescription drugs before being approved by the FDA for the change to OTC status. Currently, ibuprofen (e.g., Advil, Motrin IB), naproxen (Aleve), and ketoprofen (Actron, Orudis KT) are available as OTC products, and the manufacturers of other NSAIDs are expected to seek OTC approval in the near future.

With NSAIDs, the difference between the prescription and OTC medications is the strength of the product. Prescription strengths for ibuprofen tablets are 300 mg, 600 mg, and 800 mg, whereas the OTC product is 200 mg. Prescription strengths for naproxen tablets are 250 mg, 375 mg, and 500 mg, whereas the OTC product is 200 mg. Ketoprofen prescription strengths are 25 mg, 50 mg, 75 mg, and a 200 mg extended-release dosage form, whereas the OTC product is 12.5 mg. Again, OTC strengths are considered to be safe and effective for consumer use without professional supervision, assuming the label instructions and warnings are closely followed. The higher strength products require a prescription in the United States because of their potential side effects/adverse reactions.

The mechanism of action for the NSAIDs is inhibition of cyclooxygenase, which results in a decreased synthesis of prostaglandins. This decrease in prostaglandins may be responsible for both the therapeutic and the adverse reactions associated with this drug category. (See Chapter 14 for more information.)

Ibuprofen, naproxen, and ketoprofen are well absorbed orally. If gastric distress occurs, the medication should be taken with food or an antacid. The onset of action is ½ hour for ibuprofen, 1 hour for naproxen, and unknown for ketoprofen. The peak effect is 2 to 4 hours for ibuprofen, ½ to 2 hours for ketoprofen capsules, 6 to 7 hours for ketoprofen extended-release capsules, and 2 to 4 hours for naproxen. The duration of action is 6 hours for ibuprofen, up to 7 hours for naproxen, and not available for ketoprofen (*Drug Facts and Comparisons*, 2000; *USP DI*, 1999). The metabolism of NSAIDs is primarily hepatic, with excretion by the kidneys.

The usual adult dosage for ibuprofen is one tablet (200 mg) every 4 to 6 hours when necessary. If the pain or fever does not respond to one tablet, two may be taken. The maximum dosage is 6 tablets in 24 hours without prescriber approval.

The usual adult dosage for ketoprofen is one tablet (12.5 mg) every 4 to 6 hours. A second dose may be taken if pain or fever does not improve within 1 hour. No more than 2 tablets may be taken in any 4- to 6-hour period, or more than 6 doses in 24 hours. Ketoprofen is not administered to children under 16 years of age.

The usual adult dosage for naproxen is one tablet (200 mg) every 8 to 12 hours when necessary. Some persons may need 2 tablets initially and then one 12 hours later. No

BOX 11-5

Over-the-Counter Nonsteroidal Antiinflammatory Drug Warnings

General Precautions

- With NSAIDs, individuals should contact the prescriber if they have a severe allergic reaction to any analgesic (e.g., asthma, swelling, hives, rash, or any other reaction), because the NSAIDs are capable of causing similar reactions.
- Individuals should avoid taking NSAIDs with any other OTC analgesics (acetaminophen, aspirin, or other NSAIDs).
- Individuals should avoid taking NSAIDs for more than 10 days for pain or for more than 3 days for fever, if painful area is inflamed, if pregnant or breastfeeding, if new symptoms occur or current symptoms worsen, or if abdominal pain occurs. They should contact the prescriber for advice.
- Individuals should not use NSAIDs during the last 3 months of pregnancy, because it may adversely affect the fetus or result in complications during delivery.
- Alcohol (especially 3 or more drinks daily) and many other medications may result in adverse drug interactions. Individuals should review all medications with the prescriber or pharmacist before taking an NSAID.

more than 3 tablets may be taken in 24 hours. Older adults should not take more than 2 tablets in 12 hours, and children under 12 years of age should not take this product.

The side effects/adverse reactions of the NSAIDs are primarily gastrointestinal distress (nausea, vomiting, diarrhea, cramps, gas), gastric ulcers, and bleeding. (See Chapter 14 for additional side effects/adverse reactions and drug interactions.) Box 11-5 presents warnings for OTC NSAIDs.

Antacids

Various medical conditions, overeating, or eating certain foods may result in stomach upset, gas, heartburn, and indigestion. **Antacids** are drugs that buffer, neutralize, or absorb hydrochloric acid in the stomach, and they are commonly used for these conditions. It is estimated that Americans spend one billion dollars annually on antacids (Cornacchia & Barrett, 1993). Antacids buffer or neutralize hydrochloric acid in the stomach, increasing gastric pH. The major ingredients in antacids include aluminum salts, calcium carbonate, magnesium salts, magaldrate (aluminum-magnesium combination), and sodium bicarbonate. Simethicone may be added to these preparations as a defoaming or anti-gas agent. (See Chapter 41 for additional information on antacids.)

In general, antacids have a rapid onset of action. A small amount of absorbable antacid is absorbed systemically (15% to 30%), but the remainder is broken down via the digestive process and excreted in the feces. Long-term use of antacids or their use in the presence of impaired renal function may result in increased adverse reactions from metal ion absorption, especially the absorption of calcium carbonate or magnesium hydroxide. Table 11-2 lists the side effects/adverse reactions of the antacids.

TABLE 11-2 Antacids: Side Effects/Adverse Reactions

Name	Side Effects/Adverse Reactions*
Aluminum	Constipation (reduced by using combination products with magnesium)
aluminum carbonate gel (Basaljel)	Phosphate depletion via feces (including weakness, apnea, hemolytic anemia, tetany)
aluminum hydroxide (AlternaGEL, Alu-Cap, Amphojel)	Delay in gastric emptying
aluminum/magnesium compounds (Aludrox, Gaviscon, Maalox, Mylanta)	Concretions (intestinal and renal)
	Encephalopathy from aluminum intoxication
	Bone demineralization (osteomalacia, osteoporosis)
Bicarbonate	Systemic alkalosis or sodium overload (elevated plasma pH and carbon dioxide, anorexia, mental confusion)
sodium bicarbonate (Alka-Seltzer, Instant Metamucil)	Gastric acid hypersecretion ("acid rebound")
	Enhanced effects of amphetamines, quinidine, quinine
Calcium	Milk-alkali syndrome (including metabolic alkalosis, anorexia, nausea, vomiting, confusion, hypercalcemia, possible renal impairment)
calcium carbonate (Tums)	Increased potential for calcium stone formation
	Nephrocalcinosis
	Gastric acid hypersecretion ("acid rebound")
	Antagonism of digitalis preparations
	Elevated serum and urine calcium levels
	Kidney failure
	Constipation
	Decreased phosphate levels (if dietary phosphate intake is low)
Magnesium	Diarrhea (reduced by using combination products with aluminum)
magnesium hydroxide (Milk of Magnesia)	Decreased potassium levels (hypokalemia)
magnesium trisilicate	Increased magnesium levels (hypermagnesemia) in clients with renal failure or severe kidney impairment, which causes low blood pressure, nausea, vomiting, respiratory depression, CNS depression, coma
Sodium	Sodium overload or systemic alkalosis
sodium bicarbonate	Salt and water retention (causing edema, ascites, effusion, hypertension)
	Metabolic alkalosis
	Milk-alkali syndrome (see Calcium)
	Gastric acid hypersecretion ("acid rebound")

*Chronic, high-dose use.

Dosage and Administration. The amount of antacid necessary to neutralize hydrochloric acid depends on the individual, the condition being treated, and the buffering capability of the preparation used. The acid-neutralizing property of antacids varies for the individual client. Antacids taken before meals have a duration of action of approximately 30 minutes. If the antacid is taken after meals, the duration may be prolonged up to 3 hours. Duodenal ulcers, Zollinger-Ellison syndrome, and other hypersecretory conditions may require 80 to 160 mEq of the acid-neutralizing effect per dose (*USP DI*, 1999); for pain relief, the dose of antacids should provide 40 to 80 mEq of the neutralizing effect (Pinson & Weart, 1996). Antacids are not very effective for the treatment of gastric ulcers (Brunton, 1996). Table 11-3 summarizes the acid-neutralizing capacity of antacids.

Liquid and powder dosage forms of antacids have been found to be more effective than the tablet dosage forms. Most tablets require chewing before swallowing to be effective. Most antacids contain 10 mg or less of sodium per recommended adult dose. Clients on sodium-restricted diets should read the ingredient listings carefully. Examples of antacids containing more than 10 mg per recommended adult dose (Pinson & Weart, 1996) include the following:

Alka-Seltzer Extra Strength	588 mg sodium/tablet
Alka-Seltzer Original	567 mg sodium/tablet
Bellans	144 mg sodium/tablet

The maximum dosages listed on the packages should be followed. Many individuals exceed the FDA recommendations, which increases the potential for many of the potential side effects/adverse reactions.

Pregnancy Safety. Antacids are generally considered safe for use in pregnancy if prolonged or high doses are avoided.

Antacid Combinations

Although there are numerous antacid preparations on the market, the magnesium-aluminum combinations (e.g., Gelusil, Maalox, Mylanta) are the antacids most commonly selected by individuals and recommended by health care professionals. The recommendation for an antacid should be based on its ingredients relative to the client's health status. Combination antacids have been formulated to reduce the

TABLE 11-3 Antacids: Acid-Neutralizing Capacity

Antacid	Primary Ingredients	Acid-Neutralizing Capacity	Dose to Neutralize 80 mEq HCl
Liquid Preparations		**mEq/5 mL**	**mL needed**
Gelusil	Aluminum hydroxide, magnesium hydroxide, simethicone	12	33
Maalox	Aluminum hydroxide, magnesium hydroxide	13.3	30
Maalox Plus Extra Strength	Aluminum hydroxide, magnesium hydroxide, simethicone	29	14
Mylanta	Aluminum hydroxide, magnesium hydroxide, simethicone	12.7	31
Mylanta Double Strength	Aluminum hydroxide, magnesium hydroxide, simethicone	25.4	16
Riopan Plus Suspension	Magaldrate, simethicone	15	27
Tablet Preparations		**mEq/tablet**	**Approximate Number of Tablets Needed**
Gelusil	Aluminum hydroxide, magnesium hydroxide, simethicone	11	7
Maalox	Aluminum hydroxide, magnesium hydroxide	8.5	9
Maalox Plus	Same as Maalox, plus simethicone	10.6	7
Mylanta	Aluminum hydroxide, magnesium hydroxide, simethicone	11.5	7
Mylanta Gelcaps	Same as Mylanta, but double strength	23	3.5
Riopan Plus	Magaldrate, simethicone	13.5	6
Rolaids	Calcium carbonate, magnesium hydroxide	7.5	10.5
Tums	Calcium carbonate	10	8

Information from *United States Pharmacopeia Dispensing Information (USP DI): Drug information for the health care professional* (19th ed.) (1999). Rockville, MD: United States Pharmacopeial Convention.

risk of diarrhea or constipation as a side effect. The antacid combination Gaviscon deserves particular attention because of its uniqueness and widespread use.

antacid combination plus alginic acid (Gaviscon)

Gaviscon forms a viscous cohesive foam that floats on the surface of the stomach contents, neutralizing stomach acid. The foam is caused by the alginic acid contained in the product; the other ingredients are aluminum hydroxide, magnesium trisilicate, and sodium bicarbonate. This foam helps to protect the sensitive mucosa from irritation because the foam precedes the stomach contents into the lower esophagus when reflux occurs.

Antiflatulents

simethicone [si meth′ i kone] (Phazyme, Mylanta Gas)

Simethicone, a defoaming agent, relieves flatulence by dispersing and preventing gas retention, which involves the formation of mucus-surrounded gas pockets in the gastrointestinal tract. Gas retention is a problem in conditions such as air swallowing, diverticulitis, functional dyspepsia, peptic ulcer, postoperative gaseous distention, and spastic or irritable colon.

Simethicone tablets are taken four times daily, chewed thoroughly after meals and at bedtime, and as needed for flatulence. Antacid liquid combination products also often contain simethicone.

Laxatives

Laxatives are given to induce defecation and may be classified according to their source, site of action, degree of action, or mechanism of action. Figure 11-1 and Table 11-4 summarize the traditional laxatives that can be bought without a prescription.

One of the major indications for the use of laxatives is constipation. **Constipation** is difficult fecal evacuation as a result of hard stool and perhaps infrequent movements. The primary causes of constipation are reviewed in Chapter 41. Failure to respond to the normal defecation impulse, insufficient time to permit the bowel to produce an evacuation, inadequate fluid and dietary fiber intake, sedentary habits, and insufficient exercise may be factors in the development of constipation. Constipation is also a side effect of many medications such as antacids, diuretics, morphine, tricyclic antidepressants, codeine, aluminum hydroxide, and anticholinergics.

Laxatives are also used to keep the stool soft when it is essential to avoid the irritation or straining that accompanies the passage of a hardened stool. Such indications might include rectal disorders, irritated polyps in the bowel, hemorrhoidectomy, perianal abscess, the recovery phase of a myocardial infarction or cerebrovascular accident, or the repair of a hernia. Saline laxatives are routinely used to expel parasites and toxic anthelmintics and to secure a stool specimen to be examined for parasites.

Laxatives should not be taken if the individual is experiencing undiagnosed abdominal pain because it may be due to an inflammatory disorder of the alimentary tract, such as appendicitis, typhoid fever, and chronic ulcerative colitis. If an inflamed appendix causes the pain, a laxative may bring about a rupture of the appendix by increasing intestinal peristalsis. Laxatives should be taken with caution after some surgical procedures (e.g., repair of the perineum or rectum (at least for a time), during pregnancy and breastfeeding, by clients with severe anemia, and by debilitated clients. Other conditions in which caution is needed include chronic and spastic constipation.

Perceived constipation is a nursing diagnosis, the state in which an individual makes a self-diagnosis of constipation and ensures a daily bowel movement through use of laxatives, enemas, and suppositories. In this instance, laxatives may be misused and abused to meet the client's perception of a normal bowel elimination pattern (Box 11-6). Consumer education should be focused on the lifestyle changes necessary to promote a normal bowel elimination pattern for individuals with constipation and perceived constipation.

Because constipation is common in children, parents need to be informed about the problems associated with the indiscriminate use of laxatives. In children, emotions, environmental changes (new home, new school, new friends), dietary changes, and febrile illnesses may contribute to or cause constipation. Adding or increasing fluids, vegetables, fruits, and bran products may be very helpful. Malt soup extract is often suggested for infants up to 2 months old. For older children, glycerin suppositories or docusate sodium (Colace) may be appropriate.

BOX 11-6

Laxative Abuse

Regular or excessive use of laxatives usually leads to laxative abuse. This syndrome takes several years to develop and often goes undiagnosed. It is often reported among older adults.

Laxative abuse may occur in conjunction with eating disorders such as bulimia or anorexia. Symptoms are similar to other disease states such as nephritis, diabetes insipidus, ulcerative colitis, or Addison's disease. The major complaints on hospital admission are diarrhea and abdominal cramps. More often than not, clients deny excessive laxative use.

If chronic laxative abuse is not detected and the client is not weaned off the laxative, permanent bowel damage, osteomalacia, and electrolyte imbalance may occur.

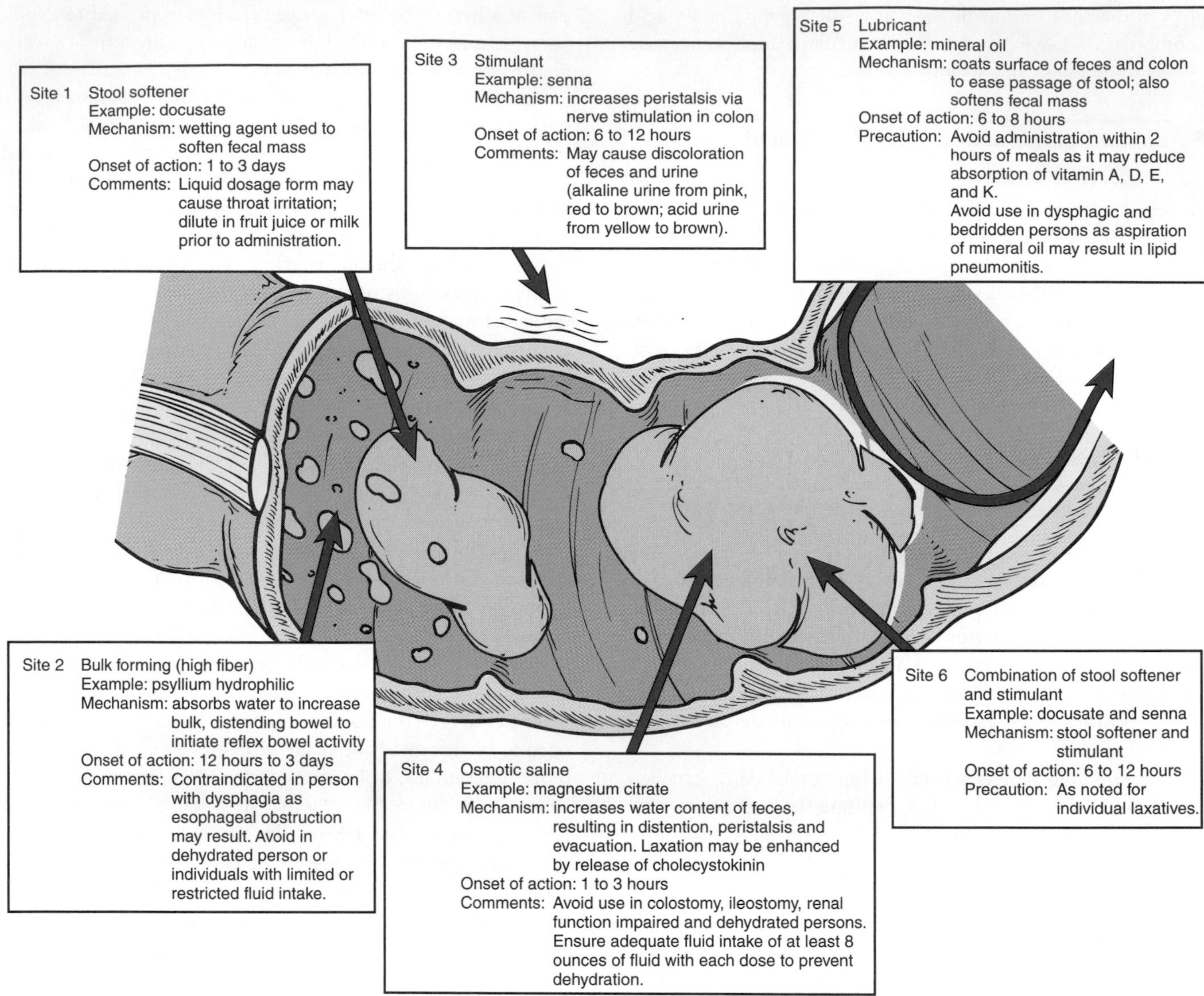

Site 1 Stool softener
Example: docusate
Mechanism: wetting agent used to soften fecal mass
Onset of action: 1 to 3 days
Comments: Liquid dosage form may cause throat irritation; dilute in fruit juice or milk prior to administration.
Site 3 Stimulant
Example: senna
Mechanism: increases peristalsis via nerve stimulation in colon
Onset of action: 6 to 12 hours
Comments: May cause discoloration of feces and urine (alkaline urine from pink, red to brown; acid urine from yellow to brown).
Site 5 Lubricant
Example: mineral oil
Mechanism: coats surface of feces and colon to ease passage of stool; also softens fecal mass
Onset of action: 6 to 8 hours
Precaution: Avoid administration within 2 hours of meals as it may reduce absorption of vitamin A, D, E, and K.
Avoid use in dysphagic and bedridden persons as aspiration of mineral oil may result in lipid pneumonitis.
Site 2 Bulk forming (high fiber)
Example: psyllium hydrophilic
Mechanism: absorbs water to increase bulk, distending bowel to initiate reflex bowel activity
Onset of action: 12 hours to 3 days
Comments: Contraindicated in person with dysphagia as esophageal obstruction may result. Avoid in dehydrated person or individuals with limited or restricted fluid intake.
Site 4 Osmotic saline
Example: magnesium citrate
Mechanism: increases water content of feces, resulting in distention, peristalsis and evacuation. Laxation may be enhanced by release of cholecystokinin
Onset of action: 1 to 3 hours
Comments: Avoid use in colostomy, ileostomy, renal function impaired and dehydrated persons. Ensure adequate fluid intake of at least 8 ounces of fluid with each dose to prevent dehydration.
Site 6 Combination of stool softener and stimulant
Example: docusate and senna
Mechanism: stool softener and stimulant
Onset of action: 6 to 12 hours
Precaution: As noted for individual laxatives.

Figure 11-1 Classification of laxatives according to site of action.

Older adults may have an increased incidence of constipation because of multiple illnesses that require a variety of medications, the aging process with its associated decline in physiologic functions, and a progressive decrease in physical activity (see the Special Considerations for Older Adults box on p. 218). An increase in fluid intake, a moderate exercise program (if permitted), and an increase in the intake of bran products, vegetables, and fruit will help to correct this problem. Laxative abuse is often reported with this age-group. Because there may be many factors contributing to constipation, a complete and thorough history by the health care professional is necessary.

Constipation is commonly reported during pregnancy. It is usually caused by colon compression as a result of the increase in the size of the uterus or a decrease in muscle tone and peristalsis. Vitamins containing iron and calcium are often prescribed for pregnant women, and such products tend to produce constipation. Laxatives used in pregnancy should be limited to emollients or bulk-forming laxatives. Most of the other laxatives have the potential for undesirable effects—castor oil may induce premature labor, mineral oil may decrease the absorption of fat-soluble vitamins, and osmotic agents may induce dangerous electrolyte alterations. Pregnant women should be advised about proper diet, adequate fluid intake, appropriate exercise programs, and the importance of discussing the problem with her nurse-midwife or physician.

In addition to treating constipation, laxatives may be administered within a health care agency setting for a variety of purposes, such preparing for surgery, treating cases of food and drug poisoning, and promoting the elimination of an offending substance from the gastrointestinal tract. Saline cathartics are considered useful for this purpose. (See Chapter 41 for additional information on the nursing management of laxative therapy.)

Saline Laxatives

Saline laxatives are soluble salts that are only slightly absorbed from the alimentary canal. Because of their osmotic effect of drawing water in the small intestine, they retain

TABLE 11-4 Laxatives: Over-the-Counter Varieties

	Contact Stimulant	Osmotic Saline	Stool Softener Surfactant or Wetting Agent	High-Fiber and Bulk-Forming Agent	Lubricant
Disadvantages with repeated, frequent (long-term) administration	Watery stools, gripping	Watery stools, cramps	Unreliable results, may contribute to liver toxicity	Obstruction of narrowed lumen, some difficulty in chewing and swallowing	Anal leakage, lipid pneumonia
Increases rate of transit in small bowel?	Yes	Yes	Yes	Yes	Unknown
Causes net secretion of water and electrolytes in small bowel?	Yes	Yes	Yes	Yes	No
Inhibits absorption in small bowel?	Yes	Yes	Yes	Yes	Yes
Increases mucosal permeability in small bowel?	Yes	Not studied	Yes	Not reported	Not reported
Causes mucosal damage in small bowel?	Yes	Not studied	Yes	Not reported	Not reported
Acts only in colon (not small bowel)?	No	No	No	No	Yes
Indicated for long-term treatment?	No	No	No	Probably	No
Examples of type	Anthraquinone, bisacodyl, phenolphthalein, castor oil, danthron	Magnesium salts, milk of magnesia, sodium salts, glycerin	D-S-S, Colate, Docusate	Methylcellulose, karaya gum, sodium CMC, malt soup extract, psyllium seed, agar, Plantago bran (unprocessed), polycarbophil	Mineral oil
Physical or chemical property responsible for action	Irritates mucosal surface to stimulate or increase intestinal motor function or activity	Hyperosmolar ingredients trap water in intestinal lumen; hypertonicity of colon increases liquid in colon; hyperosmotic or saline	Changes surface tension of fecal mass; provides increased penetration of colonic water; penetrates and softens fecal mass by wetting agents	Absorbs water on surface; increases soft fecal mass; adds bulk and moisture to feces, causing distention and elimination	Coats over fecal mass, which passes with ease; lubricates gastrointestinal tract and softens feces

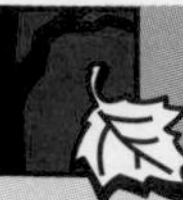

Special Considerations for Older Adults
Nonpharmacologic Laxative Therapy

Many adults often use and/or abuse laxatives because they believe that regularity implies a daily bowel movement (Longe & DiPiro, 1999). The nursing diagnosis of perceived constipation is a common finding in older adults.

To reduce the potential for chronic laxative use and/or dependency, the client should be taught nonpharmacologic measures, such as increasing fluid intake to 6 to 8 glasses of water/day if permitted and tolerated. Also recommended is a regular exercise routine, such as a daily walk or active and passive exercise for bedridden clients.

The nurse should obtain a dietary and laxative history from the client. Consistent intake of low-fiber diets or a regular intake of foods that tend to harden stools (e.g., processed cheese, hard-boiled eggs, liver, cottage cheese, high-sugar foods, and rice) may result in constipation.

High-fiber or high-residue diets and adequate fluid intake accelerate food transport time in the gastrointestinal tract and exert a mild laxative effect.

High-fiber foods include orange juice with pulp, fresh oranges, bran or whole grain cereals, whole grain or bran breads, leafy vegetables, and fresh fruits. Prunes, bananas, figs, and dates are high in dietary fiber, and prunes also contain a laxative substance that stimulates intestinal motility pharmacologically.

Fiber supplements should be avoided in nonambulatory clients or in clients with a restricted or limited fluid intake. Bulk or fiber laxatives are also contraindicated in fecal impaction.

and increase the water content of feces. The water in the intestinal lumen produces fluid accumulation and distention, which leads to peristalsis and the eventual evacuation of bowel contents. The result is a fecal mass of liquid or semiliquid stools. The laxative effect may be enhanced by the intestinal release of cholecystokinin (CCK). Diarrhea is created in the small intestine to overcome constipation in the colon. Laxation may occur in 30 minutes to 3 hours.

The saline laxatives are the laxative of choice for securing a stool specimen for examination, for fecal impaction, for use with certain anthelmintics, and in some cases of food and drug poisoning.

Phosphate enemas are useful as preparations for a barium enema. When the goal is merely to empty the intestine, magnesium sulfate, sodium phosphate, or milk of magnesia is effective. Milk of magnesia (magnesium hydroxide) is the mildest of the salines and is often the cathartic of choice for children. Sodium salts are contraindicated for those on a sodium-restricted diet, and magnesium and potassium salts are contraindicated in clients with renal disease.

The intestinal membrane is not entirely impermeable to the passage of saline laxatives, and electrolyte disturbances have been reported with their long-term daily use. Some saline laxatives find their way into the general circulation only to be excreted by the kidney, in which case they act as saline diuretics. Hypertonic saline solutions in the bowel may result in so much fluid loss that little or no diuretic effect is possible. Some saline laxatives contain up to 1 g or more of sodium per dose. Some ions may have a toxic effect if they accumulate in the blood in sufficient quantity in clients with impaired renal function. This may occur with magnesium ions if a solution is retained in the intestine for a long time or if the client suffers from renal impairment. Magnesium acts as a depressant of the central nervous system and neuromuscular activity.

The following salts, when taken for their laxative effect, are usually taken orally. Some of them may be given rectally as an enema. The salts tend to have a rapid action, especially if ingested before breakfast. They may be taken at bedtime with food for early morning evacuation (food delays the effect). Clients sometimes complain of gaseous distention after taking saline laxatives. All preparations should be dissolved and accompanied by a liberal (8 ounce) intake of water, because the salts do not readily leave the stomach and may cause vomiting if not well diluted.

When a salt such as magnesium sulfate is taken, it should not only be dissolved in an adequate amount of water and taken on an empty stomach but also disguised in fruit juice, plain water (chilled), citrus-flavored carbonate beverage, or chipped ice to increase palatability.

magnesium sulfate [mag nee′ zee um] (Epsom salt)

Magnesium sulfate occurs as a crystal or white powder that is readily soluble in water. It has a bitter saline taste. The usual dose for laxative effect is 15 g in 8 ounces of water. Children over 6 years of age are given 5 to 10 g in 4 ounces of water.

magnesium hydroxide (Milk of Magnesia, MOM)

Magnesium hydroxide is also used as an antacid. It reacts with hydrochloric acid in the stomach to form magnesium chloride, which is responsible for the laxative effect. The usual dose for adults is 30 to 60 mL with additional liquids; children 1 to 12 years of age receive 7.5 to 30 mL.

magnesium citrate solution

Magnesium citrate solution is not very soluble, and therefore a relatively large dose is necessary. It is not unpleasant to take because it is carbonated and flavored. The usual dose is 240 mL for adults and 50 to 100 mL for children 6 to 12 years of age.

TABLE 11-5 Stimulant Laxatives

Name	Therapeutic Effect (hours)	Stool Consistency	Remarks
bisacodyl (Dulcolax)	6-10	Soft	Not to be taken with or within 1 hour of ingestion of milk or antacids to prevent premature dissolving of enteric coating and gastrointestinal irritation
castor oil (Neoloid emulsion, castor oil)	2-6	Watery	Chilling and mixing with fruit juice or carbonated drinks increases palatability
cascara sagrada	6-10	Soft, formed	Gives a yellowish brown color to acid urine and a reddish color to alkaline urine
senna (X-Prep, Senokot)	6-12	Soft	As with cascara, crude senna may cause urine discoloration

effervescent sodium phosphate

Sodium phosphate is made effervescent by the addition of sodium bicarbonate and citric and tartaric acids. The usual dose is 10 g. A concentrated aqueous solution of sodium biphosphate and sodium phosphate is available as a laxative under the name of Fleet Phospho-Soda. The usual oral adult dose is 20 to 45 mL mixed with one-half glass of cold water. Children 6 to 9 years of age are given 5 mL, and children over 10 years of age receive 10 mL, diluted in 4 ounces of water. Sodium phosphate is also marketed in a disposable enema unit for rectal administration.

Stimulant (Contact) Laxatives

Stimulant laxatives are used in preparation for barium enemas, in some cases of acute constipation, and before a proctologic examination.

With the exception of bisacodyl (Ducolax), the principal members of the stimulant laxatives (cascara, senna, rhubarb, and aloe) are botanical glycoside drugs obtained from the bark, seed pods, leaves, and roots of a number of plants. These laxatives are absorbed and later secreted to produce stimulation and peristalsis in the intestines. Their exact mechanism of action is unknown.

The stimulant laxatives usually act in 6 to 8 hours. Their primary effect is on the small and large intestines, which explains their tendency to produce cramping. Aloe and rhubarb are almost obsolete because of their irritating properties.

The side effects of stimulant laxatives include abdominal cramping, nausea, diarrhea, and flatulence. Adverse reactions that should be reported to a health care provider include allergic reactions, esophageal or intestinal obstruction, change in heart rate, disorientation, cramping of muscles, increased weakness, and skin rash. Senna, cascara sagrada, and aloe are passed through the breast milk, initiating laxation in the nursing infant. Their occasional use should be restricted to 1 week because long-term abuse may lead to a poorly functioning large intestine. The contact stimulant laxatives may also lead to mucus secretion and fluid evacuation.

Table 11-5 compares the stimulant laxatives in use today. Laxatives are habit forming and should be used judiciously.

bisacodyl [bis a koe′ dill] (Dulcolax)

Bisacodyl is a relatively nontoxic laxative agent that reflexively stimulates peristalsis on contact with the mucosa of the colon. Bisacodyl has been successful in the treatment of various types of constipation. It is widely used in larger doses for cleansing the bowel before some surgeries and before proctoscopic and roentgenographic examinations.

Bisacodyl has an insoluble coating that was formulated to dissolve in intestinal fluids; when released, this substance produces stimulating effects on the colon. It should not be chewed, crushed, or taken with milk or antacids because it can have an irritating effect on the stomach that might manifest as severe abdominal cramps. If antacids are to be taken, they should be taken at least several hours apart from the bisacodyl.

The oral adult dose is 2 to 3 tablets (10 to 15 mg). The tablets produce bowel evacuation in 6 to 8 hours, and suppositories and enemas act within 15 to 60 minutes. The suppositories may cause a burning sensation and proctitis.

cascara sagrada [kas kar′ a]

Cascara sagrada used to be one of the most extensively used laxatives and is considered to be the mildest laxative of this group. It acts mainly on the small and large intestine. The active ingredients reach the large intestine through of the bloodstream and by passage along the alimentary tract. Bowel evacuation occurs in approximately 8 hours. The client should be informed that cascara sagrada may discolor urine to pink, red, violet, or brown depending on urinary pH.

Aromatic cascara fluidextract contains 18% to 20% alcohol. Each milliliter represents 1 g of cascara sagrada. The usual dose is 5 mL (range 5 to 15 mL) for adults and 1 to 3 mL for infants up to 2 years of age. Cascara is also available in tablet form.

senna [sen′ a] (Senexon, Senokot)

Senna is obtained from the dried leaves of the Cassia plant. It produces a thorough bowel evacuation in 6 to 12 hours, which may be accompanied by abdominal pain or gripping. Senna resembles cascara but is more powerful. It is also found in proprietary remedies such as Fletcher's Castoria and Black Draught. Senna tea is an infusion of senna leaves made by adding a teaspoonful of leaves to a cup of hot water.

A powdered concentrate of senna (X Prep Liquid) is said to contain the desirable laxative components but to be free of the impurities that cause cramping. This compound is sold under the name of Senokot (tablets, syrup, granules, and suppositories). The usual adult dosage of Senokot is 2 tablets, 10 to 15 mL of the syrup, or 1 teaspoon of the granules twice daily. For children over 6 years of age, the dosage is 1 tablet twice daily.

castor oil [kas′ tor]

Castor oil is obtained from the seeds of the castor bean. It is a bland, colorless, emollient glyceride that passes through the stomach unchanged. As with other fatty substances, it slows the emptying of the stomach. For this reason it is usually given when the stomach is empty. In the small intestine the oil is hydrolyzed by pancreatic lipase to glycerol and a hydroxy fatty acid, (ricinoleic acid). This hydroxy fatty acid is responsible for irritation of the bowel, especially the small intestine. Its irritating effect causes the rapid propulsion of contents from the small intestine, including any of the oil that may have escaped hydrolysis.

A therapeutic dose of castor oil will produce several copious semiliquid stools in 2 to 6 hours and therefore should not be taken at bedtime. The fluid nature of the stool is caused by the rapid passage of fecal content rather than by a diffusion of fluid into the bowel. This drug is excreted into the milk of nursing mothers.

Castor oil is used much less often today, but it may be used to prepare certain clients for a roentgenographic examination of the abdominal viscera. The usual adult dose of castor oil is 15 to 60 mL PO. The dose for children 2 years of age and older is 5 to 15 mL.

phenolphthalein [fee nole thay′ leen] (Ex-Lax, Phenolax)

Phenolphthalein is a synthetic stimulant laxative that has been available for many years but was banned by the FDA in 1997. The OTC products containing this ingredient have been reformulated with a safer ingredient. Consumers should check ingredient labels and avoid purchasing any product that may still contain phenolphthalein.

Bulk-Forming Laxatives

Bulk-forming laxatives include polycarbophil (Mitrolan) and other natural or semisynthetic cellulose derivatives such as psyllium (Metamucil) and methylcellulose (Citrucel). Hydrophilic colloids stimulate peristalsis by swelling, increasing bulk, and modifying the consistency of the stool. This mechanism of laxative action is normal stimulation and is one of the least harmful. These drugs do not interfere with food absorption but can cause esophageal obstruction, fecal impaction, or obstruction if not administered with sufficient fluids (8 ounces of water or juice).

The effect of bulk-forming laxatives may not be apparent for 12 to 24 hours, and their full effect may not be achieved until the second or third day after administration. Some prescribers maintain that bran and dried fruits (e.g., prunes, prune juice, and figs) exert the same effect, and they prefer to suggest these foods rather than the bulk-forming laxatives.

Bulk-forming laxatives are used in irritable bowel syndrome, diverticular disease, and postpartum constipation. Because of the altered bulk consistency, they have been found to be useful in the treatment of diarrhea. The side effects are minimal, with the most commonly reported effects being flatulence and bulky stools.

polycarbophil calcium [pol i kar′ boe fil] (Mitrolan)

Polycarbophil is used to normalize stools both in diarrhea and in constipation by restoring the normal moisture level and by providing bulk in the intestinal tract. In diarrheal conditions the intestinal mucosa is unable to absorb excess fecal water. Polycarbophil absorbs water (up to 60 times its weight) by forming a gel in the intestinal lumen, thus creating formed stools. In cases of constipation, polycarbophil retains water in the lumen.

Polycarbophil has a low sodium content, and each tablet contains 150 mg of calcium. The maximum dose of calcium recommended by the FDA is much higher than the 1800 mg a client would receive by taking the maximum daily dose of 12 tablets. Nevertheless, clients with hypercalcemia or clients susceptible to hypercalcemia should not take this product without prior consultation with their prescriber (Curry & Tatum-Butler, 1996).

psyllium [sill′ i yum] (Metamucil, Konsyl)

Psyllium hydrophilic mucilloid is a powder that contains approximately 50% powdered mucilaginous portion (outer epidermis) of psyllium seeds and approximately 50% dextrose or sucrose. This mixture is used to treat constipation because it promotes the formation of a soft, water-retaining gelatinous residue in the lower bowel within 12 to 72 hours. It also has a demulcent effect on inflamed mucosa. The dosage is 4 to 7 g administered one to three times daily.

Sugar-free Metamucil contains aspartame (Nutra-Sweet). Clients following a phenylalanine-restricted diet should not take products containing aspartame.

Lubricant Laxatives

mineral oil

Mineral oil (liquid petrolatum, MO) is a mixture of liquid hydrocarbons obtained from petroleum; it is not digested, and absorption is minimal. Mineral oil penetrates and coats the fecal mass and also prevents excessive absorption of water.

Mineral oil is especially useful when it is desirable to keep the feces soft and when straining must be reduced, such as in the prevention of hemorrhoidal tearing or after abdominal surgery, rectal operations, hernia repair, eye surgery, aneurysm, or myocardial infarction. It is also indicated for clients who have chronic constipation because of prolonged inactivity, such as clients with orthopedic conditions.

Some health care providers object to the use of mineral oil on the basis that it impairs the absorption of the fat-soluble vitamins A, D, E, and K. Gastric emptying time is delayed if mineral oil is taken with meals. Another objection to its use is that in large doses it tends to leak or seep from the rectum, which may cause anal pruritus and interfere with the healing of postoperative wounds in the region of the anus and perineum. This leakage is often an embarrassment to the client.

Although the absorption of mineral oil is limited, prolonged use may cause a chronic inflammatory reaction in tissues where it is found. Indiscriminate use by older adults or weak individuals should be discouraged because of the increased potential for aspiration leading to lipid pneumonia.

The concurrent use of mineral oil with fecal moistening agents should be avoided because the moistening agents increase the absorption of mineral oil. The dose ranges from 15 to 45 mL for adults and from 5 to 15 mL for children over 6 years of age.

Emollient or Fecal Moistening Agents

Emollient or fecal moistening agents include stool softeners and surfactants. They decrease the consistency of stools by reducing surface tension; this allows water to penetrate the feces. They are commonly used for the treatment of hard or dry stools.

docusate or dioctyl sodium sulfosuccinate
[dok′ yoo sate] (Colace, Doxinate)
docusate calcium (Surfak)
docusate potassium (Dialose)

Docusate acts like a detergent; it permits water and fatty substances to penetrate and be well mixed with the fecal material. It may also inhibit water absorption from the bowel and stimulate water secretion into the gastrointestinal tract. In this way it promotes the formation of soft-formed stools and is useful in the treatment of constipation. Formed stools are usually excreted in 1 to 3 days.

Docusate agents are indicated for clients with rectal impaction, hemorrhoids, chronic constipation, postpartum constipation, and painful conditions of the rectum and anus, as well as for persons who should avoid straining during defecation (e.g., after rectal surgery or myocardial infarction). Docusate may be useful for immobile clients, especially children. It is said to have a wide margin of safety and few potential adverse reactions. All of the following dosages should be given with a full glass of water:

- *docusate sodium:* Adults and children over 12 years, 50 to 500 mg PO daily; children 6 to 12 years, 40 to 120 mg daily
- *docusate calcium (Surfak):* Adults, one capsule (50 to 240 mg) PO daily
- *docusate potassium (Dialose):* Adults, 100 to 300 mg daily; children over 6 years, 100 mg at bedtime

hyperosmotic suppository

Glycerin suppositories are available in adult, child, and infant sizes. The suppositories are osmotic agents that absorb water, lubricate, and increase stool bulk. They may also promote peristalsis through local irritation of the mucous membrane of the rectum. The dosage is 3 g for adults and 1 to 1.5 g for children under 6 years of age; the suppository is held high in the rectum for 15 minutes. Evacuation occurs 15 to 60 minutes after insertion.

Antidiarrheal Agents

The term **diarrhea** describes the abnormal passage of stools with increased frequency, increased fluidity, or increased weight, as well as with an increase in stool water excretion. Diarrhea is acute when it is of sudden onset in a previously healthy individual, lasts approximately 3 days to 1 to 2 weeks, is self-limiting, and resolves without sequelae. Morbid and mortal consequences are seen in malnourished populations, older adults, infants, and debilitated persons. (See the Special Considerations for Children box on p. 222).

Chronic diarrhea lasts for more than 3 to 4 weeks, with the recurring passage of diarrheal stools, fever, anorexia, nausea, vomiting, weight reduction, and chronic weakness. It is the result of multiple causative factors (Box 11-7). Chronic diarrhea necessitates definitive treatment directed to the organic cause or causes, which can vary from psychogenic to neoplastic origins.

This section focuses on the OTC drugs that have a direct pharmacologic effect on the gastrointestinal tract. The drugs providing symptomatic therapy do not alter the pathophysiology of diarrhea and do not prevent electrolyte and fluid loss. The antidiarrheal agents diminish stool water by inhibiting intestinal fluid secretion or by increasing intestinal fluid absorption. Although these drugs decrease the number, consistency, and fluidity of the stool, there is no absolute clinical evidence that the client experiences an effective antidiarrheal therapeutic benefit. However, the bothersome symptoms that interrupt daily routines are relieved.

See Chapter 41 for additional information on the nursing management of antidiarrheal therapy.

Special Considerations for Children
Over-the-Counter Medications for Diarrhea

Diarrhea is a common problem in children and may be due to a variety of causes, such as intestinal disease, infection, a congenital disorder, and food or formula intolerance. In some instances it may be secondary to antibiotic use.

Persistent diarrhea can lead to water and electrolyte imbalance. In infants or very young children it can cause cardiovascular collapse and death. Therefore rehydration and correction of electrolyte disturbances is critical in the treatment of diarrhea.

Although hospitalization may be necessary in severe dehydration, milder cases are often treated with oral replacement therapy with products such as PediaLyte and InfaLyte. When Gatorade or a similar product is used, the preparation should be diluted to half-strength with water. Be aware, however, that glucose concentrations over 5% can cause osmotic diarrhea.

The use of any OTC antidiarrheal products is not usually recommended for preschool children without the specific advice of a physician. Package labeling often provides age-specific dosage instructions; follow such instructions carefully or, preferably, consult first with the prescriber.

Information from Olds, S.M. (1995). *The one-minute counselor: A pharmacist's guide to pediatric diarrhea and constipation.* Washington, D.C.: American Pharmaceutical Association.

Adsorbents

Adsorbents act by coating the walls of the gastrointestinal tract, absorbing the bacteria or toxins causing the diarrhea, and passing them out with the stools. Examples of OTC drugs in this class are activated charcoal, aluminum hydroxide, bismuth salts, attapulgite, kaolin, and pectin. Attapulgite, activated charcoal, polycarbophil, and bismuth salts are the gastrointestinal adsorbents in clinical use today. The bismuth salts are used as adsorbent, astringent, and protective agents.

Adsorbent preparations are usually taken after each loose bowel movement until the diarrhea is controlled. Constipation may develop because of the large amounts of adsorbent products that must be used. A caution with all the adsorbents is that they may interfere with the absorption of a wide range of nutrients and medications given concurrently (e.g., digoxin [Lanoxin], clindamycin [Cleocin]). This interference may be decreased by administering the adsorbent at least 2 hours before or after a drug, except when the adsorbent is used to inactivate a drug or a specific poison in overdose situations.

bismuth subsalicylate [biz′ muth] (Pepto-Bismol)

Bismuth subsalicylate is an antidiarrheal agent, weak antacid, and antiulcer medication. It has several actions, including (1) inhibition of gastrointestinal secretions (i.e., it stimulates the absorption of fluid and electrolytes in the intestine), (2) inhibition of the synthesis of prostaglandins that produce intestinal inflammation and hypermotility, and (3) suppression of the growth of *H. pylori.* Bismuth subsalicylate is the only bismuth preparation available in the United States (Pinson & Weart, 1996; *USP DI,* 1999).

Administered orally, more than 90% of bismuth subsalicylate is absorbed; it is bound to plasma proteins and excreted by the kidneys. Because bismuth subsalicylate is a salicylate and may be taken in large amounts to control diarrhea, it enhances the effects of oral anticoagulants, resulting in increased bleeding time and excessive bruising. Methotrexate may be displaced from its protein binding sites, leading to methotrexate toxicity. Probenecid, an antigout agent, promotes the renal excretion of uric acid. The uricosuric effects of probenecid can be inhibited when combined with bismuth subsalicylate.

Bismuth salicylate may antagonize the effects of sulfonylurea hypoglycemic agents and could require a change in the dosage of the hypoglycemic agent. The nurse should be aware of possible salicylate toxicity when persons taking large amounts of aspirin daily also take bismuth salicylate in large doses. Bismuth salicylate also has the potential for drug interactions if taken with oral anticoagulants, methotrexate, or any other drug that interacts with aspirin. The suspension of bismuth salicylate contains 130 mg of salicylate in 15 mL; the original tablet contains 102 mg, and the caplets and cherry-flavored tablets contain 99 mg of salicylate (Longe, 1996).

The usual adult dosage of bismuth subsalicylate is 30 mL or two tablets chewed or dissolved every 30 to 60 minutes (up to eight doses in 24 hours).

activated charcoal (Charcoaid)

Activated charcoal is used for the relief of intestinal gas, diarrhea, and gastrointestinal distress associated with indigestion. It acts as an adsorbent for toxic substances, irritants, and gas. It may also adsorb medications, nutrients, and enzymes.

Activated charcoal is administered as two capsules every 30 to 60 minutes as needed, with up to eight doses (16 Charcocaps) for the treatment of diarrhea symptoms. Tablets may be chewed or dissolved in the mouth and followed by water.

attapulgite (Kaopectate)

Attapulgite, a hydrated magnesium aluminum silicate, is a gastrointestinal adsorbent and protective agent that has replaced the kaolin-pectin in Kaopectate. Kaolin and pectin are being reviewed by the FDA, and currently the evidence for kaolin is better than the combination of kaolin and pectin for the treatment of acute, nonspecific diarrhea (Longe, 1996). Attapulgite is also being reviewed for both safety and efficacy. The nurse should watch for labeling changes on these products in the future.

BOX 11-7

Causes of Acute and Chronic Diarrhea

Causes of Acute Diarrhea

Bacterial

1. Invasive organisms
   a. *Campylobacter fetus* (jejuni)
   b. *Clostridium difficile*
   c. *Escherichia coli* (enteropathogenic)
   d. *Salmonella*
   e. *Shigella dysenteriae*
   f. Staphylococci
2. Noninvasive toxigenic organisms
   a. Cholera (*Vibrio cholerae*) enterotoxin
   b. *E. coli* (enterotoxigenic) toxin
3. Food poisoning (toxin mediated)
   a. *Bacillus cereus*
   b. *Clostridium perfringens*
   c. *Salmonella*
   d. *Staphylococcus aureus*

Viral

1. Adenoviruses
2. Coxsackievirus
3. Coronaviruses
4. Echoviruses
5. Norwalk agents
6. Rotaviruses

Protozoal

1. Amebic dysentery (*Entamoeba histolytica*), amebiasis
2. Giardiasis (*Giardia lamblia*)

Nutritional

1. Allergy
2. Ingestion without discretion (spices, fats, roughage, seeds, preformed toxin)
3. Enteral nutrition

Other

1. Bile acids
2. Carcinoma
3. Diverticulitis
4. Fatty acids
5. Neurogenic condition
6. Psychogenic condition
7. Radiation therapy
8. Regional and ulcerative colitis
9. Stress

Causes of Chronic Diarrhea

1. Addison's disease
2. Diabetic enteropathy/neuropathy
3. Iatrogenic conditions
   a. Bacterial overgrowth
   b. Postsurgical conditions
4. Inflammatory bowel disease
   a. Chronic ulcerative and granulomatous colitis
   b. Crohn's enteritis
5. Irritable bowel syndrome
6. Malabsorption syndrome
7. Pancreatic adenoma—nongastrin secreting (e.g., syndrome of watery diarrhea-hypokalemia-achlorhydria [WDHA])
8. Pancreatic insufficiency
9. Thyroid condition—hyperthyroidism
10. Tumors
    a. Carcinoma of colon and rectum
    b. Intestinal condition
    c. Lymphoma
    d. Polyposis
    e. Villous adenoma
11. Other
    a. Blind loops, ileostomy, colostomy
    b. Carcinoid syndrome
    c. Enteritis
    d. Gardner's syndrome
    e. Gastrointestinal hormones
    f. Gluten enteropathy
    g. Zollinger-Ellison syndrome
    h. Many other conditions

Synthetic Opioids

loperamide [loe per′ a mide] (Imodium)

Loperamide is a synthetic OTC opioid that decreases gastrointestinal motility by inhibiting propulsive movements in the gut. It produces a direct musculotropic effect that decreases hyperperistalsis, slows passage of intestinal contents, and allows reabsorption of water and electrolytes, resulting in a reduction in stool frequency.

Loperamide is indicated for the treatment of acute nonspecific and chronic diarrhea. Peak plasma levels after administration occur in 5 hours with the capsule dosage form or in 2.5 hours with the oral liquid; the half-life ranges from 9 to 14 hours, with a duration of action up to 24 hours. Loperamide is metabolized in the liver and excreted both fecally and by the kidneys.

Side effects are usually minimal and include dizziness, dry mouth, and skin rash. Drug-induced gastrointestinal side effects are difficult to separate from those of the diarrhea itself (epigastric pain, abdominal cramps, nausea, vomiting, and anorexia).

The usual adult OTC dosage is 4 mg (two tablets) initially, followed by 2 mg after each loose stool, not to exceed 8 mg/day for more than 2 days.

Cough-Cold Preparations

In 1990 it was estimated that more than $10 billion was spent on OTC medications; of this amount, nearly $3 billion was used to buy cough, cold, and influenza preparations (Popovich, Newton, & Pray, 1992). Table 11-6 describes the major differences between colds, allergic rhinitis, and influenza (flu). This section will describe the symptoms of these conditions and the medications used to treat coughs and colds, such as antitussives, antihistamines, expectorants, and decongestants. Many cough-cold products contain a combination of ingredients, some of which are subtherapeutic dose combinations or are unnecessary for the particular symptoms they are purported to treat. Such preparations are not considered rational and may not be safe and effective.

Some combination products are very useful, but they should be selected carefully according to the presenting symptoms. In general, cough-cold preparations that contain analgesic and antipyretic agents should be avoided. The routine use of such products may mask a fever secondary to a bacterial infection, and it would be difficult to determine the causative ingredient of any side effects/adverse reactions. The American Academy of Pediatrics Committee on Drugs has recommended against the use of combination cold-cough preparations (Tietze, 1996). Products that do not provide full information on the label, such as the strength and/or amount of each ingredient, should also be avoided. It is difficult to evaluate such products when essential information is missing. Information on selecting a combination product is provided later in this chapter.

Coughing is defined as a protective reflex for clearing the respiratory tract of environmental irritants, foreign bodies, or accumulated secretions and therefore should not be depressed indiscriminately. The afferent impulses that arise from irritated pharyngeal and laryngeal tissues initiate the central cough reflex. A productive cough occurs when irritants or secretions are removed from the respiratory tract and in general should not be suppressed because it helps to clear the airways. A nonproductive cough that is dry, irritating, frequent, and prolonged should be treated because it can be exhausting, painful, and taxing to the circulatory system and the elastic tissue of the respiratory system, particularly in older adults and young children.

Treatment of a cough is secondary to treatment of the underlying disorder. Antitussives should not be taken in situations in which the retention of respiratory secretions or exudates could be harmful. The therapeutic objective is to decrease the intensity and frequency of the cough yet permit adequate elimination of tracheobronchial secretions and exudates.

Drugs act either by suppressing the cough center in the medulla or by lessening irritation of the respiratory tract peripherally. Intake of fluids and inhalation of fully water-saturated vapors (steam) should be stressed as one of the most important means of producing increased amounts of mucus and thinning such secretions.

Antitussives

The primary OTC cough suppressant agents that affect the cough center centrally are codeine and dextromethorphan. Diphenhydramine (Benadryl), which is an antihistamine, and benzonatate (Tessalon) also have antitussive effects. Benzonatate is a prescription drug in the United States and is reviewed in Chapter 39; diphenhydramine is reviewed in the antihistamine section of this chapter.

Although codeine is included in selected combination products, dextromethorphan is the preferred antitussive agent in OTC preparations. Codeine is an effective antitussive, but because it is an opioid many laws govern its use as a nonprescription drug. The amount of codeine permitted in OTC products is also limited because codeine has a higher potential for misuse and abuse than other products. Dextromethorphan has no addictive properties and works centrally to raise the coughing threshold. It also has fewer side effects (drowsiness and gastric distress) than codeine. As an antitussive, 8 to 15 mg of codeine is considered equivalent to 15 to 30 mg of dextromethorphan (*Drug Facts and Comparisons*, 2000).

TABLE 11-6 Colds, Allergic Rhinitis, and Influenza: Major Differences

Signs or Symptoms	Common Cold	Allergic Rhinitis	Influenza
Fever	Rare	Absent	Common; sudden onset; may range from 102° to 104° F
Aches and pains	Slight	Absent	May be severe
Sneezing	Usual	Common	Infrequent
Pruritus	Absent or rare	Common	Absent
Cough	Mild-moderate	Uncommon	Common
Headaches	Rare	Can occur	Prominent
Cause	Usually viruses	Usually allergens	Usually viruses
Occurrence	Anytime	Usually seasonal	Anytime
Complications	Sinus congestion, earache	Uncommon	Bronchitis, pneumonia

dextromethorphan [dex troe meth or' fan] (Sucrets Cough Control and others)
dextromethorphan combinations
benzocaine (Spec-T Anesthetic, Vicks Cough Silencers, and others)

Dextromethorphan is well absorbed orally and has an onset of action between 15 and 30 minutes and a duration of activity up to 6 hours. The side effects are minimal with the usually recommended doses. Nausea, mild dizziness, and drowsiness have been reported.

Significant drug interactions have been reported with CNS depressants and MAO inhibitor medications. The former may result in enhanced CNS depressant effects, and concurrent use with MAO inhibitors may result in increased excitability, tremors, sedation, severe hypertension, intracranial bleeding, hyperpyrexia, and psychosis. Persons taking a MAO inhibitor should not take dextromethorphan.

The dosage for adults and children 12 years and older is 10 to 20 mg PO every 4 hours or 30 mg every 6 to 8 hours, up to a maximum of 120 mg/day. For children 6 to 12 years, the recommended dosage is 5 to 10 mg every 4 hours up to a maximum of 60 mg/day; for children 2 to 6 years, 2.5 to 5 mg every 4 hours to a maximum of 30 mg/day. Dextromethorphan is not recommended for use in children under 2 years of age. Pregnancy safety has not been established.

Many other products have been used as antitussive agents in various preparations, but the FDA advisory review panel on nonprescription cold, cough, allergy, bronchodilator, and antiasthmatic products has indicated that more evidence is needed to prove their effectiveness. Some of the products in this category include noscapine, beechwood creosote, elm bark, cod liver oil, horehound, and others.

Antihistamines

Antihistamines are drugs that compete with histamine for its receptor sites. Two histamine receptors, H_1 and H_2, have been discovered. The antihistamines related to cold and allergy symptoms, such as diphenhydramine (Benadryl), chlorpheniramine (Chlor-Trimeton), and others, are H_1 receptor antagonists; the H_2 receptor antagonists related to the symptoms of gastric hyperacidity, such as cimetidine (Tagamet), ranitidine (Zantac), and others, are discussed in Chapter 41.

Antihistamines prevent the physiologic histamine effects of sneezing, increased nasal secretions, and itching and watering eyes by preventing histamine from reaching its site of action. The antihistamines of the H_1 type have the greatest therapeutic effect on nasal allergies, particularly on seasonal hay fever and colds with histamine-like symptoms. In allergies, they relieve symptoms better at the beginning of the hay fever season than during its height but fail to relieve the asthma that often accompanies the hay fever. Antihistamines are palliative agents. Their action is comparatively short-lived and provides only symptomatic relief.

Many OTC preparations contain antihistamines, and some contain two or more. Antihistamines may be used in a variety of OTC medications, including antitussive agents, cough-cold products, sleep-inducing products, oral analgesic products, menstrual formulations, and many others. For example, diphenhydramine depresses the cough center in the medulla of the brain (antitussive effect), has antihistamine effects (blocks H_1 receptors), central antimuscarinic effects (antiparkinsonian action), and sedative-hypnotic effects, and it is used to prevent or treat the nausea and vomiting associated with motion sickness. Consumers should check the ingredients of all medications they buy, consume, or administer. Individuals often experience unwanted side effects or an accidental overdose because the same product is available in several different medications they are consuming; unfortunately, this fact is often overlooked in a community setting.

Currently available OTC antihistamines include the following:

- brompheniramine [brome fen ir' uh meen] (Dimetane, generics)
- chlorpheniramine [klor fen ir' uh meen] (Aller-Chlor, Chlor-Trimeton, and others)
- diphenhydramine hydrochloride [dye fen hye' dra meen] (AllerMax, Benadryl Allergy, and others)
- phenindamine [fen in' da meen] (Nolahist)
- pyrilamine [peer il' uh meen] (generics available)

The primary difference between the OTC and prescription antihistamines is the strength of the product. For example, OTC chlorpheniramine is 4 mg, whereas the prescription products are 8 mg, 12 mg time-release, and injectable dosage forms.

The absorption of oral doses of antihistamines is good, with an onset of action within 15 to 60 minutes. The time to peak effect can vary with each individual preparation. For example, brompheniramine has a peak effect in 3 to 9 hours, chlorpheniramine within 6 hours, and diphenhydramine in 1 to 4 hours. The duration of action also varies, with brompheniramine 4 to 8 hours, chlorpheniramine 4 to 8 hours, diphenhydramine 6 to 8 hours, and pyrilamine 8 hours. These agents are primarily metabolized in the liver and excreted by the kidneys.

The most commonly reported OTC antihistamine side effects include constipation, decreased sweating, difficulty in initiating the urinary stream (older males), sedation, visual disturbances, photosensitivity, nausea or vomiting, and a dry mouth, nose, or throat. Less commonly reported effects are orthostatic hypotension, headaches, anxiety, weakness of the hands or feet, sore mouth and tongue, abdominal pain or increased excitability, and muscle cramps. Rarely reported adverse reactions include glaucoma or eye pain in susceptible persons (persons with a predisposition to angle-closure glaucoma), skin rash, and confusion, especially in older adults who have taken high doses. Figure 11-2 shows a comparison of selected antihistamines, efficacy, and side effects.

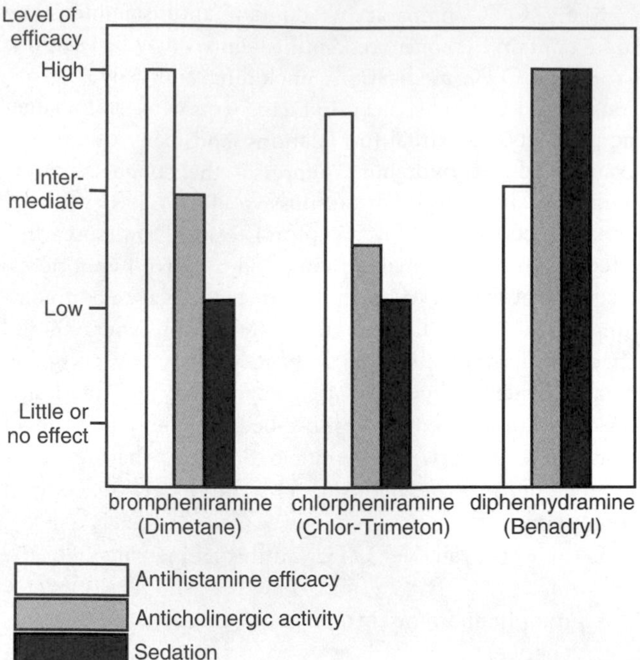

Figure 11-2 Comparison of efficacy and side effects of selected antihistamines.

Expectorants

Expectorants are substances that reduce the viscosity of secretions, thus promoting the ejection of mucus or other exudates from the lungs, bronchi, and trachea. In OTC preparations the only expectorant with evidence of safety and effectiveness is guaifenesin (Robitussin). Many other expectorants such as ammonium chloride, iodides, and terpin hydrate are listed as Category III—they are safe but have not proven to be effective (Tietze, 1996). Table 11-7 lists selected cough-cold combinations.

Decongestants

Decongestant agents are vasoconstricting agents used to shrink engorged nasal mucous membranes in mild upper respiratory tract infections. In OTC products, they are available in oral and nasal preparations.

The oral agents are sympathomimetic amines, and their vasoconstricting properties are not limited to the nasal mucosa. They can also elevate blood pressure in individuals with hypertension, induce cardiac stimulation and dysrhythmias in some people and, depending on the sympathomimetic amine, may increase blood glucose in individuals with diabetes. For this reason, warnings on the labels instruct consumers with hypertension, hyperthyroidism, diabetes mellitus, or ischemic heart disease to contact their prescriber before using the product. Reported side effects/adverse reactions include CNS stimulation or nervousness, insomnia, restlessness, dizziness, headaches, and increased irritability.

Three agents (phenylephrine, phenylpropanolamine, and pseudoephedrine) have been classified as Category I—they are safe and effective if the label instructions are followed. These ingredients are often incorporated in combination products for their decongestant effects.

Many drugs are used exclusively as nasal vasoconstrictors or topical decongestants. Because of their wide popular use and lack of serious hazard (when used topically), a large number of preparations have been provided by the pharmaceutical industry for direct sale to the public. The FDA advisory review panel has recommended the following topical nasal decongestant products as safe and effective: ephedrine 0.5%; naphazoline (Privine) 0.05%, 0.025%; oxymetazoline (Afrin, Dristan) 0.05%, 0.025%; phenylephrine (Neo-Synephrine) 0.125%, 0.25%, 1%; and xylometazoline (Otrivin) 0.1%, 0.05%. Table 11-8 lists the recommended dosages for topical nasal decongestant products and oral decongestant products. These drugs are adrenergic agents that act on the alpha receptors of blood vessels in the nasal mucosa to produce vasoconstriction and therefore a decrease in mucosal swelling. Some nasal decongestant products (those containing ephedrine, epinephrine, metaproterenol, and others) also possess beta-stimulating effects, which may cause CNS stimulation and perhaps the adverse reaction of vasodilation after vasoconstriction.

Nasal decongestant drugs are used to shrink engorged mucous membranes of the nose and to relieve nasal stuffiness. However, consumers tend to use them excessively or too frequently. Excessive use may result in "rebound" engorgement or swelling of the mucous membranes and a paradoxical bronchospasm. Sprays and nose drops are beneficial when used judiciously. However, if an infection is present, there is always the possibility that nasal sprays or drops will spread the infection deeper into the sinuses or to the middle ear. Additives such as preservatives, antihistamines, and detergents are sometimes included in a decongestant preparation. In some cases, reactions may be caused by the additive rather than by the decongestant.

Selection of Combination Cough-Cold Preparations

Combination OTC products require careful selection because some of these multidrug formulations contain unnecessary drugs. As previously mentioned, combinations that contain an analgesic or antipyretic agent should be avoided for several reasons. First, there is the risk of masking a bacterial infection. Second, a fixed amount of analgesic or antipyretic is taken with other ingredients on a regular basis, whether needed or not. Third, it would be difficult to identify the offending agent if a side effect/adverse reaction occurs. If an analgesic/antipyretic is necessary, the proper dose should be selected and administered separately.

When only one drug effect is necessary (e.g., a nasal decongestant, an expectorant, or an antihistamine effect), a therapeutic dose of that single drug entity should be taken. If the individual has several symptoms that need to be addressed, selection of a combination product should be limited to addressing just those symptoms, with few if any ad-

TABLE 11-7 Selected Cough-Cold Combinations

Brand Name	Ingredients	Pharmacologic Effect
Robitussin	guaifenesin	Expectorant
Robitussin A-C	guaifenesin, codeine	Expectorant, cough suppressant
Robitussin-CF	guaifenesin, phenylpropanolamine, dextromethorphan	Expectorant, decongestant, and cough suppressant
Robitussin-DM	guaifenesin, dextromethorphan	Expectorant, cough suppressant
Robitussin-PE	guaifenesin, pseudoephedrine	Expectorant, decongestant
Robitussin Night Relief	pyrilamine, pseudoephedrine, dextromethorphan, acetaminophen	Antihistamine, decongestant, cough suppressant, analgesic, alcohol free
Robitussin Night-Time Cold Formula	doxylamine, pseudoephedrine, dextromethorphan, acetaminophen	Antihistamine, decongestant, cough suppressant, analgesic
Benylin Expectorant	guaifenesin, dextromethorphan	Expectorant, cough suppressant, alcohol and sugar free
Cheracol Syrup	guaifenesin, codeine	Expectorant, cough suppressant, contains alcohol (4.75%)
Cheracol D Cough Solution	guaifenesin, dextromethorphan	Expectorant, cough suppressant, contains alcohol (4.75%)
Cheracol Plus Syrup	chlorpheniramine, phenylpropanolamine, dextromethorphan	Antihistamine, decongestant, cough suppressant, contains alcohol (8%)

Information from *United States Pharmacopeia Dispensing Information (USP DI): Information for the health care professional* (19th ed.). (1999). Rockville, MD: United States Pharmacopeial Convention.

TABLE 11-8 Topical/Oral Nasal Decongestants: Dosages

Drug/Strength	Adults	Children (6 to 12 years)
ephedrine, 0.5% (in Va-Tro-Nol and others)	2-3 drops q4h	1-2 drops q4h
naphazoline (Privine and others)		
0.05%	1-2 drops/spray q6h	Not recommended
0.025%	—	1-2 drops q6h
oxymetazoline (Afrin, Allerest, Dristan Long-Lasting, and others)		
0.05%	2-3 drops 2 times daily	Same as adults
phenylephrine (Neo-Synephrine and others)		
1%	1-2 drops/spray q4h	Not recommended
0.25%	Same as 1%	1-2 drops q4h
xylometazoline (Otrivin)		
0.1%	2-3 drops/spray q8-10h	Not recommended
0.05%	Same as 0.1%	2-3 drops/spray q8-10h
Oral Nasal Decongestants (Usually Combined with Other Drug Products)		
phenylephrine	10 mg q4h	5 mg q4h
phenylpropanolamine	25 mg q4h	12.5 mg q4h
pseudoephedrine	60 mg q6h	30 mg q6h

ditional substances. For example, for cough suppressant and expectorant effects, an OTC product that contains guaifenesin and dextromethorphan (Robitussin DM and many others) may be selected. To treat allergy, nasal congestion, sneezing, and rhinorrhea, an antihistamine and decongestant combination is used, such as triprolidine and pseudoephedrine (Actifed), chlorpheniramine and phenylpropanolamine (e.g., Allerest), or many others. For nasal or sinus congestion alone, an oral or a nasal decongestant may be selected, such as pseudoephedrine (Sudafed) or oxymetazoline [Afrin, Allerest]). (See Table 11-7 for selected cough-cold combinations.)

Women's Health Over-the-Counter Drugs

Women may have a broad range of medical problems, which includes nearly all of the diseases that affect men as well as many additional disorders and/or conditions. From puberty, women may encounter dysmenorrhea and premenstrual syndrome, pregnancy, fertility and family planning, menopause, and osteoporosis, as well as the gynecologic issues of yeast infections, pelvic inflammatory disease, urinary tract infections, bacterial vaginosis, and the various cancers that primarily affect women, such as cervical, endometrial, ovarian, and breast cancer. Many of the pharmacologic treatments for these disorders are discussed in the appropriate chapters throughout this text. This chapter specifically addresses the OTC drugs that women may select for self-treatment before visiting their health care provider (e.g., dysmenorrhea and premenstrual treatments, vaginal products, and contraceptives).

Drugs for Dysmenorrhea and Premenstrual Syndrome

Hormonal changes during the menstrual cycle may affect the physical and emotional symptoms that women experience during a month. Although most women have mild symptoms, some experience symptoms severe enough to compromise their ability to function. The majority of women with premenstrual syndrome and dysmenorrhea use OTC preparations. (See Chapter 51 for an overview of the menstrual cycle and Chapter 52 for discussion of the hormones and drugs that affect the female reproductive system.)

Dysmenorrhea

Dysmenorrhea is pain that usually occurs before or during menses and is believed to be due to uterine contractions and ischemia caused by the release of prostaglandins from the endometrium. This type of dysmenorrhea is also known as primary dysmenorrhea because of its association with the ovulatory cycle. Secondary dysmenorrhea or acquired dysmenorrhea is a painful menses caused by other reproductive problems, such as fibroid tumors, endometriosis, pelvic lesions, or an infection, all of which require intervention and treatment by a health care provider.

Approximately 10% of women with primary dysmenorrhea experience lower abdominal cramps and pain that impairs their functioning for up to 3 days a month. Other symptoms may include headache, nausea, increased irritability, depression, nervousness, fluid retention, constipation or diarrhea, and frequent urination. The most effective pharmacologic treatment is the use of the NSAIDs (prostaglandin inhibitors) discussed earlier in this chapter. Mild symptoms of dysmenorrhea are treated with acetaminophen or aspirin and the application of a heating pad or local heat to the abdomen or lower back; moderate to severe primary dysmenorrhea may require an NSAID such as ibuprofen, naproxen, or ketoprofen.

Individuals should not receive an NSAID if they are allergic to aspirin or NSAIDs or have a condition that is contraindicated for NSAID use, such as peptic ulcers, gastritis, bleeding problems, asthma, or renal impairment. The individual's current drug regimen should be reviewed for potential drug duplication and drug interactions before using an NSAID (Covington, 1996; Fankhauser, 1996).

In addition to the NSAIDs, a number of OTC menstrual products are available (see Table 11-9). The primary ingredients in these products are acetaminophen for pain, a mild diuretic such as pamabrom or caffeine for fluid accumulation, and pyrilamine (an antihistaminic, antipruritic agent). Pamabrom is a theophylline derivative used for diuresis and is used in dosages of 50 mg four times daily. Caffeine is a xanthine that promotes diuresis by inhibiting the reabsorption of sodium and water in the renal tubules. The dosage to produce this effect is 100 to 200 mg every 3 to 4 hours (Shimp & Fleming, 1996). However, large doses of caffeine can cause gastrointestinal irritation, nervousness, irritability, tachycardia, anxiety, and insomnia. Tolerance to the diuretic effect may also occur. Individuals should avoid products containing caffeine if they have a history of peptic ulcer disease or insomnia or are taking other caffeine-containing foods, beverages, or medications (e.g., xanthine, theophylline).

Many other medications have been evaluated for the treatment of dysmenorrhea and premenstrual syndrome but have not been classified in Category I (safe and effective). These include the smooth muscle relaxants, antihistamines, sympathomimetics, and herbal preparations (Shimp & Fleming, 1996).

Premenstrual Syndrome

Premenstrual syndrome (PMS) refers to the physical and mood changes that some women experience in the luteal phase of the menstrual cycle—usually the week before menstruation. Symptoms include abdominal bloating, headache, irritability, fatigue, fluid retention, weight gain, and breast tenderness, which may be related to estrogen causing a fluid retention effect in the body. The exact cause of PMS is unknown, but theories include alterations in estrogen and progesterone, dysfunction of the serotonin system, endorphin withdrawal, deficiencies of vitamin (B_6) and other minerals (magnesium, calcium, zinc), and other systemic abnormalities (Fankhauser, 1996). This condition usually improves and/or disappears within a few hours of the onset of menses (Covington, 1996).

There is no single treatment for PMS. The treatment is usually dependent on the symptoms that are present. For example, reducing salt intake or taking a mild diuretic may be helpful for edema. For increased irritability, avoiding caffeine products such as coffee, tea, colas, and chocolate may be helpful. Some of the products listed in Table 11-9 may also be tried.

TABLE 11-9 Over-the-Counter Menstrual Products

Product	Ingredient*	Indications
Bayer Select Aspirin Free Menstrual	acetaminophen 500 mg pamabrom 25 mg	Analgesic Diuretic
Midol Menstrual Maximum Strength Multisymptom Formula	acetaminophen 500 mg caffeine 60 mg pyrilamine maleate 15 mg	Analgesic Diuretic Antihistamine, antipruritic
Midol PMS Maximum Strength Multisymptom Formula	acetaminophen 500 mg pamabrom 25 mg pyrilamine 15 mg	Analgesic Diuretic Antihistamine, antipruritic
Midol PMS Multisymptom Formula	Same as Midol PMS	
Midol Teen Multisymptom Formula	acetaminophen 400mg pamabrom 25 mg	Analgesic Diuretic
Pamprin Multisymptom Formula	acetaminophen 500 mg pamabrom 25 mg pyrilamine	Analgesic Diuretic Antihistamine, antipruritic
Premsyn PMS	Same as Pamprin Multisymptom	

Information from American Pharmaceutical Association. (1996). *Nonprescription products: Formulations & features* '96-'97. Washington, D.C.: Author.
*Check package for ingredients as formulations may change without notification.

Vaginal Products

Vaginal OTC preparations include antifungal, feminine hygiene (antimicrobial), and lubricating products.

Drugs for Vaginal Infections

Vaginal infections primarily include bacterial vaginosis (noninflammatory infection), candidal vulvovaginitis, and trichomoniasis. *Bacterial vaginosis* is the most prevalent vaginal infection occurring in women of childbearing age. This infection has been referred to as nonspecific vaginitis, *Haemophilus* vaginitis, and *Gardnerella* vaginitis, and it usually results in an increase in anaerobe bacteria (*Peptostreptococcus, Bacteroides*) and a decrease in *Lactobacillus*. The classic symptom is a vaginal discharge with a fishy odor.

Trichomoniasis is caused by *Trichomonas vaginalis* and is considered to be a sexually transmitted disease (STD). It affects young women with symptoms usually during or after menstruation, but up to 50% of women can be asymptomatic. Symptoms include a white (or yellow, gray, green), foamy vaginal discharge that may have an odor. Other symptoms may include stomach pain and pruritus (Shimp & Fleming, 1996).

Candidal vulvovaginitis is a fungal vaginal infection most often caused by *Candida albicans*. Symptoms may include a thick white discharge, vaginal erythema, and intense pruritus. The absence of an offensive discharge odor is helpful in distinguishing a candidal infection from other vaginal infections. Women are more susceptible to this infection during pregnancy, during infection with human immunodeficiency virus (HIV), during the use of estrogen-containing oral contraceptives, with diabetes, or following treatment with a broad-spectrum antibiotic or immunosuppressant agent.

The usual treatment involves prescription drugs such as metronidazole vaginal gel (MetroGel-Vaginal) and clindamycin (Clcocin) vaginal cream for bacterial vaginosis. Oral metronidazole is often used to treat trichomoniasis. Treatment of candidal vaginal infections requires the use of antifungal agents.

The OTC antifungal vaginal agents are primarily the imidazole derivatives and include butoconazole (Femstat 3 vaginal cream), miconazole (Monistat 7 cream and suppository), and clotrimazole (Femizole-7, Gyne-Lotrimin, Mycelex-7, and others) (American Pharmaceutical Association, 1996). These products are considered to be equivalent and effective and in general lack any major adverse effect. They produce their effect by inhibiting the cytochrome P-450 enzymes in the fungal cell membrane, which results in decreased synthesis of fungal ergosterol. The reduction of ergosterol results in an increase in methylated sterols that cause damage and in the loss of normal fungus membrane function.

OTC antifungal vaginal agents are minimally absorbed, and the side effects include vaginal burning, itching, and irritation in approximately 7% of women (Shimp & Fleming, 1996). If the rare adverse reactions of abdominal cramps, headache, hives, urticaria, and allergic reactions occur, the woman should stop using the medication and contact her health care provider. A provider's evaluation is necessary if no improvement is noted after 3 days of therapy, if the symptoms are not completely resolved after the course of therapy, or if the symptoms return within 2 months of treatment.

Contraceptives

The most effective form of birth control is oral contraceptives (see Chapter 52). Nonprescription contraceptive approaches include a variety of natural family planning approaches (e.g., rhythm method, basal body temperature method), condoms (female and male), diaphragms, and spermicides. Spermicides are the only pharmacologic agents in this group, and the following discussion is limited to them.

Spermicides are vaginal contraceptives that use a surface-active agent to immobilize sperm. The majority of OTC products contain nonoxynol-9 (Delfen, Emko, Encare, K-Y Plus and many others); only a few products contain octoxynol-9 (Ortho-Gynol). These agents are available in jelly, cream, film, foam, and suppository dosage forms:

1. *Jelly and creams.* If the vaginal cream or jelly is to be used without a diaphragm, a product with a high spermicide concentration should be selected. Creams are better lubricants, whereas the gel product is usually less messy. These agents are effective immediately after application and are usually effective for approximately 60 minutes. It is recommended that douching be delayed for at least 8 hours after intercourse to give the spermicide time to produce its effect on sperm. Allergic reactions are rare with these products.
2. *Foam.* Foam contraceptives are more effective alone than the other topical vaginal contraceptives because they adhere better and are more evenly distributed to the cervix and vaginal walls (Parent-Stevens & Lourwood, 1996). This dosage form is often used as a backup method or in combination with other contraceptives (oral, condoms, intrauterine devices). Women should be advised to follow labeled directions closely because they vary from product to product. Foams are effective immediately, are similar to the creams and jellies, and may be inserted up to 1 hour before coitus. It is also recommended that douching be delayed for at least 8 hours after intercourse.
3. *Suppositories.* A vaginal suppository is inserted high in the vagina approximately 10 to 15 minutes before coitus. The suppository is activated by moisture in the vaginal tract and in general is not recommended because of its low efficacy.
4. *Film.* A vaginal film is placed near the cervix, where it is activated by vaginal secretions. It should be inserted approximately 5 minutes before intercourse and is effective for approximately 2 hours.

Spermicides have a high failure rate, especially during the first year of use. The vaginal foam appears to be the most effective spermicide. The efficacy of the product is increased if used in combination with a condom or diaphragm (Parent-Stevens & Lourwood, 1996).

SUMMARY

OTC, or nonprescription, drugs are medications that are safe for self-treating the symptoms of minor self-limiting illnesses without the supervision of a health care practitioner. Because these drugs are widely used and readily available, the nurse should be knowledgeable about a client's OTC drug practices and the drugs themselves. In addition to acquiring the skill to elicit information about such practices during the client's drug history, the nurse's knowledge of OTCs will assist in the guidance of clients on the safe self-administration of these medications. The most commonly used types of OTC medications are analgesics, antacids, laxatives, cough-cold preparations, antidiarrheals, and products for women.

Clients should be instructed to review the labels of OTC medications carefully before selection to ensure that the ingredients have proven to be safe and effective and are also safe for them to use (check warnings and contraindications). The nurse should advise the client to follow dosing instructions carefully and to be aware that many OTC medications do not contain a list of possible drug interactions. Clients taking prescription drugs should consult with their prescriber before taking any OTC medication. OTC preparations that are used wisely can effectively treat many symptoms at a cost savings to the individual and the health care delivery system.

Critical Thinking Questions

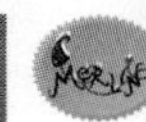

1. One of the home health aides at the health care agency comes to you and indicates that her two children are home from school with colds. She asks your advice about treating them with OTC preparations. How will you respond?
2. Paul Taylor, age 55, comes to the health center for symptoms of an upper respiratory infection. Mr. Taylor, a client with moderate hypertension, has had his blood pressure well controlled with his antihypertensive drug regimen for more than 3 years, but on this visit you find it to be elevated above his usual level. What information should be elicited from Mr. Taylor?

Collaborative Learning Activities

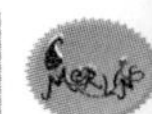

For Collaborative Learning Activities, go to mosby.com/MERLIN/McKenry/.

BIBLIOGRAPHY

Anderson, K.N., Anderson, L.E., & Glanz, W.D. (Eds.) (1998). *Mosby's medical, nursing, & allied health dictionary* (5th ed.). St. Louis: Mosby.

American Pharmaceutical Association. (1996). *Nonprescription products: Formulations & features '96-'97.* Washington, D.C.: Author.

Burns, J. (Ed.). (1991). OTC drugs can be a low-cost alternative: The value of pharmaceuticals, *Business & Health Special Report.* Montvale, NJ: Medical Economics Publishing.

Brunton, L.L. (1996). Agents for control of gastric acidity and treatment of peptic ulcers. In J.F. Hardman & L.E. Limbird (Eds.), *Goodman & Gilman's The pharmacological basis of therapeutics* (9th ed.). New York: McGraw-Hill.

Carpenito, L.J. (2000). *Nursing diagnosis: Application to clinical practice* (8th ed.). Philadelphia: J.B. Lippincott.

Cornacchia, H.J. & Barrett, S. (1993). *Consumer health: A guide to intelligent decisions*. St. Louis: Mosby.

Covington, T.R. (1996). Self-care and nonprescription pharmacotherapy. In T.R. Covington (Ed.), *Handbook of nonprescription drugs* (11th ed.). Washington, DC: American Pharmaceutical Association.

Curry, Jr. C.E., & Tatum-Butler, D. (1996). Laxative products. In T.R. Covington (Ed.), *Handbook of nonprescription drugs* (11th ed.). Washington, D.C.: American Pharmaceutical Association.

Drug Facts and Comparisons. (2000). Philadelphia: J.B. Lippincott.

Fankhauser, M.P. (1996). Treatment of dysmenorrhea and premenstrual syndrome. *Journal of the American Pharmaceutical Association, NS36*(8), 503-513.

Fitzgerald, W.L. (1994). Legal control of pharmacy services. In OBRA '90: *A practical guide to effecting pharmaceutical care*. Washington, D.C.: American Pharmaceutical Association.

Food and Drug Administration. (1997). *HHS News: FDA proposes ban on OTC sale of laxative ingredient*, August 29, 1997, Washington, D.C.: Department of Health and Human Services, Food and Drug Administration (http://www.fda.gov/bbs/topics/NEWS/NEW00589.html [8/9/98]).

Insel, P.A. (1996). Analgesic-antipyretic and anti-inflammatory agents and drugs employed in the treatment of gout. In J.F. Hardman & L.E. Limbird (Eds.). *Goodman & Gilman's The pharmacological basis of therapeutics* (9th ed.). New York: McGraw-Hill.

Jacobs, L.R. (1998). Prescription to over-the-counter drug reclassification. *American Family Physician* (home.aafp.org/afp/980501ap/jacobs.html [2/29/2000]).

Lipinsky, M.S. (1999). The "prescription to OTC switch" movement: Its effects on antifungal vaginitis preparations. *Archives of Family Medicine*, 8(4), 297-300.

Lipman, A.G. (1996). Internal analgesic and antipyretic products. In T.R. Covington (Ed.). *Handbook of nonprescription drugs* (11th ed.). Washington, D.C.: American Pharmaceutical Association.

Longe, R.L. (1996). Antidiarrheal products. In T.R. Covington (Ed.). *Handbook of nonprescription drugs* (11th ed.). Washington, D.C.: American Pharmaceutical Association.

Longe, R.L. & DiPiro, J.T. (1999). Diarrhea and constipation. In J.T. DiPiro, R.L. Talbert, G.C. Yee, G.R. Matzke, B.G. Wells, & L.M. Posey (Eds.), *Pharmacotherapy: A pathophysiologic approach* (4th ed.). Stamford, CT: Appleton & Lange.

Newton, G.D., Pray, W.S., & Popovich, N.G. (1996). New OTC drugs and devices: A selected review. *Journal of the American Pharmaceutical Association, S36*(2), 108-116.

Parent-Stevens, L. & Lourwood, D.L. (1996). Contraceptive methods and products. In T.R. Covington (Ed.), *Handbook of nonprescription drugs* (11th ed.). Washington, D.C.: American Pharmaceutical Association.

Pinson, J.B. & Weart, C.W. (1996). Acid-peptic products. In T.R. Covington (Ed.). *Handbook of nonprescription drugs* (11th ed.). Washington, D.C.: American Pharmaceutical Association.

Popovich, M.G., Newton, G.D., & Pray, W.S. (1992). New OTC drugs: A selected review. *American Pharmacy, NS32*(2), 26-38.

Shimp, L.A. & Fleming, C.M. (1996). Vaginal and menstrual products. In T.R. Covington, (Ed.). *Handbook of nonprescription drugs* (11th ed.). Washington, D.C.: American Pharmaceutical Association.

Smith, E.A. (1998). Rx-to-OTC: To switch or not to switch? *Drug Topics Supplement*. June, 24s, 26s.

Tietze, K.J. (1996). Cold, cough, and allergy products. In T.R. Covington (Ed.), *Handbook of nonprescription drugs* (11th ed.). Washington, DC: American Pharmaceutical Association.

United States Pharmacopeia Dispensing Information (USP DI): Drug information for the health care professional (19th ed.) (1999). Rockville, MD: United States Pharmacopeial Convention.

United States Pharmacopeia Dispensing Information (USP DI): Advice for the patient (19th ed.) (1999). Rockville, MD: United States Pharmacopeial Convention.

Zimmerman, D.R. (1993). *Complete guide to nonprescription drugs* (2nd ed.). Detroit: Gale Research.

12 Complementary and Alternative Pharmacology

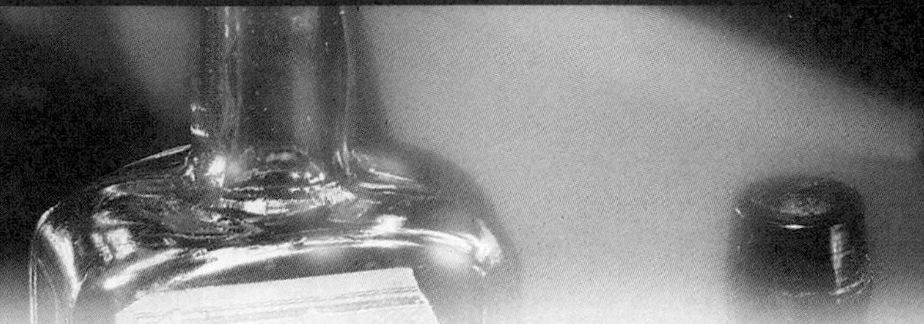

Chapter Focus

Today, one in three clients within the "mainstream" health care delivery system uses an alternative therapy. In a 1998 survey, approximately 60 million Americans reported having taken botanical supplements (Eisenberg et al., 1998). Individuals are taking an increasingly proactive approach to promoting their own health and treating their own medical conditions. Seven of every ten clients who use alternative therapies do so without the physician's knowledge (Anderson, 1996). Health care professionals should be knowledgeable about alternative options to help guide the client through the array of options and use those that may be of benefit (Liebert, 1994). This chapter will provide an understanding of the most common complementary and alternative substances taken to prevent and/or treat disease.

Learning Objectives

1. Differentiate between allopathic medicine and complementary and alternative therapies.
2. Describe the role of the National Center for Complementary and Alternative Medicine in evaluating complementary and alternative therapies.
3. Discuss the advantages and disadvantages of complementary and alternative therapies.
4. Discuss specific complementary and alternative therapies that might help or harm.
5. Provide consumer information for clients taking complementary and alternative therapies.

Key Terms

Treating illness with a natural remedy, such as herbal products, dates back to the earliest records of humankind. All cultures have long histories of folk medicine that include the use of plants and other substances. Throughout history people have methodically and scientifically collected information on herbs and other medicinal materials and have maintained well-defined pharmacopeias. Many remedies of scientific medicine were derived from the herbal lore of native people well into the twentieth century. As medicine evolved in North America, plants continued to be a mainstay of rural medicine. Until the 1940s, textbooks of pharmacognosy—books that characterize plants as proven-by-use medications—contained hundreds of medically useful comments about barks, roots, berries, twigs, and flowers. Many drugs used today, such as aspirin, vincristine, curare, and ergot, are of herbal origin.

As twentieth century technology advanced and created an increasing admiration for technology, simple plant and water mixtures and other folk remedies were discarded by allopathic medicine. **Allopathic medicine** is the dominant medical culture of the Western world, a system of medical therapy in which a disease or abnormal condition is treated with active interventions, such as medical or surgical treatment, intended to bring about effects opposite from those produced by the disease or condition. Many therapies that fall outside of this scientific type of medicine are now considered alternative therapies. **Complementary and alternative therapies** are considered to encompass all health systems, modalities, and practices that are not intrinsic to the politically dominant health system. Although many modalities are considered complementary or alternative (e.g., massage, acupressure, bioelectromagnetic applications), the content of this chapter will focus on herbs and other substances taken to promote health, prevent illness, relieve symptoms, and cure disease.

In general, the Food and Drug Administration (FDA) considers herbal remedies to be worthless or potentially dangerous and allows them to be marketed only as food supplements (Snider, 1991). Yet a growing number of Americans are again becoming interested in herbal and other remedies. This may result from the increasing availability of herbs and other remedies in health food stores, the increasing cost of pharmaceutical drugs, and the increasing willingness of people to self-treat or to supplement allopathic medicine.

Homeopathy is a system of therapeutics based on the theory that "like cures like"—if a large amount of medicine produced symptoms of a disease, then a small amount may reduce those symptoms. Only the smallest amount of the drug necessary to control the symptoms is prescribed, and only one drug is prescribed at a time. In France, 32% of all physicians regularly prescribe homeopathic remedies, and 68% of all French citizens believe them to work (*Journal of the National Association of Registered Druggists*, 1992). One in five physicians in Germany and 42% of all physicians in the United Kingdom use remedies that would be considered alternative (*NARD J*, 1992).

Mainstream medical practitioners in North America are trained to prescribe medicines whose composition is well defined and whose safety and efficacy have been established in scientifically designed tests and trials. Physicians who have spent years studying physiology and biochemistry tend at best to be uneasy about substances such as herbs, enzymes, and extracts from plant and animal sources. Although traditional healers, homeopathic physicians, and non-Western medical practitioners have administered many of these substances for years to hundreds of thousands of sick people, the composition can vary enormously and may not be as effective for some individuals as for others.

Most alternative therapies have little scientific data to support their claims. Until recently, the research that has been done has been performed in Europe, India, China, and Japan, where herbal and other alternative therapies are more widely accepted.

In the last 20 years considerable interest has been growing in complementary and alternative approaches to mainstream medicine. As public interest has grown, some allopathic prescribers are beginning to become interested in learning about alternative treatments and determining what complementary and alternative treatment entails, what benefits are claimed, the potential risks, and the physiologic effects of the ingredients. Some prescribers are attempting to submit such substances to the same rigorous study as other pharmaceutical agents.

To support this interest, the Office of Alternative Medicine (OAM) was established at the National Institutes of Health (NIH) in 1992 and became the National Center for Complementary and Alternative Medicine (NCCAM) in 1999. The role of this agency has been "to facilitate the evaluation of alternative medical treatment modalities for the purpose of determining their effectiveness and to help integrate effective treatments into the mainstream medical practice" (McDowell, 1994). Part of the problem lies in determining which therapies are considered alternative. This would include any health practice "that does not have sufficient documentation in the United States to show that (1) it is safe and effective against specific diseases and conditions; (2) it is not generally taught in medical schools; and (3) it is generally not reimbursable for third party insurance billing" (McDowell, 1994). The NCCAM is attempting not to be exclusionary in nature. It is considering a broad interpretation of alternative therapies including "approaches from nutritional and lifestyle changes to hypnotherapy, acupressure, chelation therapy, and bioelectromagnetic applications such as magnetoresonance spectroscopy and blue light treatment" (McDowell, 1994).

In 1998, while still the OAM, the agency established eight specialty research centers in the United States for health issues such as cancer, substance abuse, rehabilitation, cardiovascular disease, pediatrics, and women's health. Of the grant awards since 1993, the topic of modality and the frequency of 75 grant awards are as follows: acupuncture (20), herbal therapy (12), massage therapy (5), spirituality (4), imagery (4), hypnosis (3), electrical therapy (3), yoga

Product (listed alphabetically)	Ginseng per capsule*	Ginsenosides per capsule†	Concentration† (percentage ginsenoside)
American Ginseng	250 mg	12.8 mg	
Ginsana (extract)	100	3.0	
Herbal Choice Ginseng-7 (extract)	100	6.5	
KRG Korean Red Ginseng	518	11.5	
Natural Brand Korean Ginseng	648	23.2	
Naturally Korean Ginseng	648	2.3	
Nature's Resource Ginseng	560	10.7	
Rite Aid Imperial Ginseng	250	0.4	
Solgar Korean Ginseng (extract)	520	10.6	
Walgreen's Gin-zing (extract)	100	7.6	

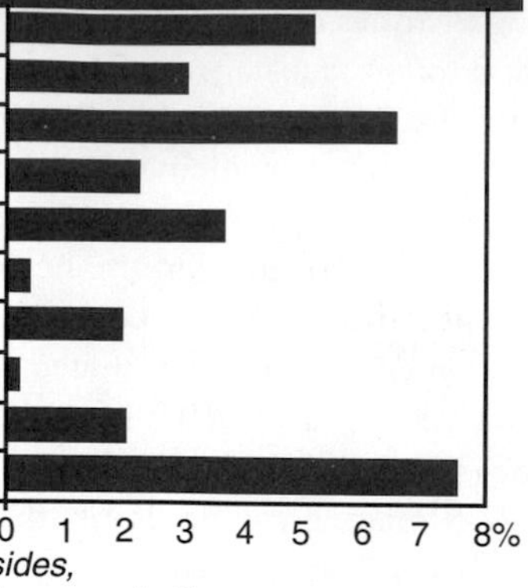

** According to label*
† Based on six major ginsenosides. Estimates for two other ginsenosides, if added, would boost totals only slightly and not change variation in concentrations.

Figure 12-1 Variations of total "ginsenoside" in 10 brands of ginseng. The amounts of ginseng found in the products in this chart were learned as a result of Consumers Union's test, not as reported by the manufacturers or distributors. ("Herbal Roulette." Copyright 1995 by Consumers Union of U.S., Inc. Yonkers, NY 10703-1057, a nonprofit organization. Excerpted with permission from the November 1995 issue of *Consumer Reports* for educational purposes only. No commercial use or photocopying is permitted. To subscribe, call (800) 234-1645 or visit www.ConsumerReports.org.)

(3), homeopathy (2), Ayurvedic therapy (2), biofeedback (2), dance/movement therapy (2), and one each for enzyme therapy, antihepatitis plants, music therapy, energetic therapy, tai chi, manual palpation, macrobiotics, acumoxa, therapeutic touch, antioxidants, intercessory prayer, self-care, and qi gong.

The NCCAM serves as a clearinghouse of information for the alternative health community by sponsoring research and programs for grant writing and clinical research and by maintaining a network within the NIH and other government agencies for collaboration. Although the NCCAM cannot serve as a referral agency or advise individual clients, it does provide information about specific therapies. It provides contact names for organizations that represent different types of treatments and individual fact sheets on issues and events.

As a result of the establishment of a federal office for alternative therapy, the allopathic medical community is reconsidering its position toward understanding the alternative therapies and their benefits. According to Daly (1995), 28 U.S. medical schools now offer 45 courses in alternative therapy, and both Harvard University and Columbia University have established centers for the study of complementary and alternative therapies. Nurses should also have an understanding of these alternative modalities so they can respond to clients' questions or direct clients to appropriate sources of information. Given the range of alternative therapies, this chapter will consider only alternative pharmacology, and only the most commonly used substances will be discussed.

Clients who do wish to use alternative therapy need to be aware that currently there is no guarantee about these medications. Under the Dietary Supplement Health and Education Act of 1994, a new category of substances has been created that is distinct from food or drugs. This category includes vitamins, herbs, amino acids, and any other substance sold as a supplement before October 15, 1994. Manufacturers of these remedies are not required to test for standardization, safety, or efficacy, which is routine for regular drugs. As a consequence, there is no way to be sure of the following: (1) the active ingredients, whatever they might be, have actually ended up in the pills or other dosage form; (2) the ingredient is in a form usable by the body; (3) the dosage is appropriate; (4) there are no other ingredients in the pills; (5) the pills are safe; or (6) the next bottle of pills will have the same ingredients. Figure 12-1 illustrates the lack of standardization of ginseng, one of these alternative products.

This lack of standardization also applies to home preparation of herbal remedies. The efficacy of herbal preparations depends on the ailment and the quality and dose of the preparation used. Efficacy cannot be determined with the home preparation of herbs because the quality and dose of the preparation is unknown.

There is also concern that complementary and alternative therapies may be harmful. Their use may delay the individual from seeking medical consultation for a condition that warrants allopathic medicine. There is also concern that the preparations have no efficacy and so are a waste of effort and money or that they may actually be toxic. Some Chinese herbal medications have been found to be contaminated with a variety of substances: undeclared prescription drugs such as nonsteroidal antiinflammatory drugs (mefenamic acid, phenylbutazone), benzodiazepines, anticholinergics, corticosteroids, or ephedrine (Gertner, Marshall, Filandrinos, Potek, & Smith, 1995; Nelson, Shih, & Hoffman, 1995; Goldman & Myerson, 1991); aconitine (a family of plants that have medicinal and poisonous properties); heavy metals (lead) (Chan, Chan, Tomlinson, & Critchley, 1993); benzaldehyde (a solvent used in the synthesis of dyes and perfumes); and other deleterious substances (Gorey, Wahlqvist, & Boyce, 1992). Table 12-1 lists the 20 most popular Asian patent medicines that contain toxic ingredients.

TABLE 12-1 The 20 Most Popular Asian Patent Medicines That Contain Toxic Ingredients

Product Name	Manufacturer	Toxic Ingredients
Ansenpunaw Tablets	Chung Lien Drugs Works Hankow, China	cinnabar (mercury chloride)
Bezoar Sedative Pills	Lanzhou Fo Ci Pharmaceutical Factory Lanzhou, China	cinnabar 2% or 10%
Compound Kangweiling	Wo Zhou Pharmaceutical Factory Zhe Jiang, China	centipede (Scolopendra) 10%
Dahuo Luodan	Beijing Tung Jen Tang Beijing, China	centipede (Scolopendra)
Danshen Tabletoco	Shanghai Chinese Medicine Works Shanghai, China	borneol
Fructus Persica Compound Pills	Lanzhou Fo Ci Pharmaceutical Factory Lanzhou, China	cannabis indica seed*
Fuchingsung-N Cream	Tianjin Pharmaceutical Corporation Tianjin, China	fluocinolone acetonide* (topical corticosteroid)
Kwei Ling Chi	Changchun Chinese Medicines & Drugs Manufactory Chang Chun, China	cinnabar
Kyushin Heart Tonic	Kyushin Seiyaki Company, Ltd. Tokyo, Japan	toad venom, borneol
Laryngitis Pills	China Dzechuan Provincial Pharmaceutical Factory Chenhtu Branch	borax 30%, toad-cake 10%
Leung Pui Kee Cough Pills	Leung Pui Kee Medical Factory Hong Kong	Dover's powder (opium powder)*
Lu-Shen-Wan	Shanghai Chinese Medicine Works Shanghai, China	toad secretion
Nasalin	Kwangchow Pharmaceutical Industry Company Kwangchow, China	centipede 5%
Nui Huang Chieh Tu Pien	Tung Jen Tang Beijing, China	Borneo camphor
Nui Huang Xiao Yan Wan Bezoar Antiphlogistic Pills	Soochow Chinese Medicine Works Kiangsu, China	realgar 19.23% (arsenic disulfide, used in pyrotechnics)
Pak Yuen Tong Hou Tsao Powder	Kwan Tung Pak Yuen Tong Main Factory, Hong Kong	scorpion 10%
PoYing Tan Baby Protector	Po Che Tong Poon Mo Um Hong Kong	camphor 20%
Superior Tabellae Berberini HCl	Min-Kang Drug Manufactory I-Chang, China	berberini HCl*
Watson's Flower Pagoda Cakes	A.S. Watson & Company, Ltd. Hong Kong	piperazine phosphate*
Xiao Huo Luo Dan	Lanzhou Fo Ci Pharmaceutical Factory Lanzhou, China	aconite 42%

Modified from the Oriental Herb Association, State of California Department of Health Services, January 28, 1992.
*Requires a prescription.

REMEDIES THAT MIGHT HELP

The substances discussed in the following paragraphs have reasonably strong evidence of beneficial physiologic effects and are the subject of further research. This information is not a recommendation for their use. Some substances, such as ginger, are considered innocuous, but none should be relied on for regular medical therapy. All clients should discuss their use of complementary and alternative therapies with their prescriber. As with any other drug, these substances should be discussed within the context of a health history.

Astragalus *(Astragalus membranaceus [huanqi])*. Astragalus, an herb, is used as a tonic and for the treatment of colds and influenza. The herbal medicine is derived from the root of the nontoxic Chinese species. Traditional Chinese physicians consider this plant to be a true tonic that helps strengthen debilitated people and increases resistance to disease. In contemporary Chinese medicine *Astragalus* is a chief component of combination therapy to restore immune function in oncology clients undergoing chemotherapy and radiation (Oubre, 1995). Pharmacologic studies in the West support the immune system–enhancing effects of *Astragalus* (Smee et al., 1996; Weil, 1995). In vitro and in vivo studies of *Astragalus membranaceus* show that it contains active compounds that increase phagocytic activity, stimulate interferon production, and potentiate the effects of biologic response modifiers such as recombinant interleukin (Chu, Wong, & Mavaligit, 1988b). In addition, in vivo animal studies have demonstrated that substances isolated from this herb can reverse immune suppression (Calis et al., 1997; Yoshida, Wang, Liu, Shan, & Yamashite, 1997; Chu, Wong, & Mavaligit, 1988a). Chu and his colleagues at M.D. Anderson Medical Center isolated an important immune-enhancing fraction that they labeled fraction 3 (F3), composed largely of polysaccharides (Oubre, 1995). At present, more research is being performed in relation to the therapeutic effects of *Astragalus*.

***Echinacea* (Purple Cornflower).** *Echinacea*, an herb, is used as a general immunity booster. It was one of the most popular plant drugs in North America until the advent of sulfa drugs in the 1930s, and it has remained an active part of folk medicine. In Europe, clinicians use *Echinacea* preparations as preventatives and treatments for colds and flu. In more than 350 studies, most of them conducted in Europe, *Echinacea* seems to stimulate the immune system nonspecifically rather than act against specific organisms. A critical review of five of these studies by Melchart et al. (1995) identified only three randomized, placebo-controlled clinical trials of monopreparations (i.e., preparations in which *Echinacea* was not combined with other substances). Two of these studies determined that an extract of the root of the plant had a positive effect on the symptoms of upper respiratory tract infections, and the other study demonstrated a slight reduction in the risk of infection. There are an additional 15 randomized trials of antineoplastic therapies in the treatment and prevention of infections or in the reduction of undesirable effects; 13 of these studies claim to have positive results (Melchart et al., 1995). Melchart (1995) believed that the use of *Echinacea* would continue to be based on subjective experience until the problems of dose-response relationships and the influence of application schedules have been resolved. More recent studies continue to support the immune-stimulating efficacy of *Echinacea* (Burger, Torres, Warren, Caldwell, & Hugues, 1997; See, Broumand, Sahl, & Tilles, 1997).

In laboratory tests, *Echinacea* increased the number of immune system cells and developing cells in bone marrow and lymphatic tissue, and it seemed to speed their development into immunocompetent cells (Stimpel, Proksch, Wagner, & Lohmann-Matthes, 1984). It speeds the release of these cells into circulation so that more are present in blood and lymph, and it increases their phagocytosis rate (Coeugniet & Elek, 1987). A few controlled studies suggest that it can increase resistance to upper respiratory infections, probably by stimulating white blood cells, and can help to prevent skin photodamage from UVA/UVB radiation by protecting collagen from free radical–induced degradation (Facino et al., 1995). In view of the lack of toxicity data, excessive use of *Echinacea* should be avoided (Newall, Anderson, & Phillipson, 1996).

Echinacea is contraindicated for progressive diseases such as infectious or autoimmune diseases, including tuberculosis, lupus, multiple sclerosis, acquired immunodeficiency syndrome (AIDS), and infections with human immunodeficiency virus (HIV). The herb may also interfere with immunosuppressive therapy.

Feverfew *(Tanacetum parthenium)*. Feverfew has been used for the treatment of headaches since the first century. Parthenolide is considered to be the active component of feverfew for the treatment of migraines. Depending on geographic location, the parthenolide content of feverfew has been found to be highly variable or absent (Awang, 1989). To ensure uniformity of dose, the Canadian government requires a minimal level of 0.2% parthenolide for feverfew products when they are submitted for a Drug Identification Number, along with certification of botanical identity; the French government requires 0.1%. However, in the United States, all herb products sold before the passage of the Dietary Supplement Health and Education Act of 1994 are "grandfathered" in as dietary supplements (Foster, 1995). Heptinstall et al. (1992) found that none of the North American products tested contained as much as 0.1% parthenolide—if it was detected at all. It is essential that only products in which the parthenolide has been assayed or standardized be used. The recommended daily dose is 125 mg of dried leaves that contain a minimum parthenolide content of 0.2%.

Drug trials conducted to demonstrate the efficacy of feverfew use only feverfew capsules of known parthenolide content. In a 1988 study conducted at the University Hospital in Nottingham, England, treatment with feverfew was clearly associated with a reduction in migraines and associated vomiting attacks, with a trend toward a reduction in migraine severity (Berry, 1994; Murphy, Heptinstall, & Mitchell, 1989). Results of a study that investigated the usefulness of feverfew in treating rheumatoid arthritis were less encouraging; feverfew provided no additional benefit when added to existing NSAID therapy (Pattrick, Heptinstall, & Doherty, 1998).

Feverfew appears to be well tolerated, but no long-term clinical toxicity studies have been conducted. Mouth ulcers, swelling of the lips and tongue, and digestive disturbances have been reported with the chewing of fresh leaves of feverfew, particularly in those who do so for the prevention or treatment of migraine (Johnson, Kadam, Hylands, & Hylands, 1985).

Garlic *(Allium sativum [da suan])*. Garlic has long been used as a flavoring in many of the world cuisines and as a substance with healing properties in many folk medicine traditions. Recent research indicates that garlic may have a wide range of health benefits, enough to justify its use as a general tonic (Craig, 1997; Weil, 1995).

Garlic has far-reaching effects on the cardiovascular system. It is used primarily to decrease serum cholesterol levels. As Warshafsky, Kamer, & Sivak reported in the *Annals of Internal Medicine* (1993), a metaanalysis of the controlled trials of garlic to reduce hypercholesteremia showed a significant reduction in total cholesterol levels. The best available evidence suggests that garlic, in an amount approximating ½ to 1 clove per day, decreased total serum cholesterol levels by approximately 9% in the groups of individuals studied. However, in a multicenter, randomized, placebo-controlled trial, Isaacsohn et al. (1998) found that garlic powder was ineffective in lowering cholesterol levels in clients with hypercholesteremia. In the same type of study, Berthold, Sudhop, and von Bergmann (1998) found the same thing with garlic oil.

Garlic lowers blood pressure like the antihypertensive drugs but without causing the impotence, headache, and other effects that these drugs may have (Brody, 1994). One of the therapeutic actions of garlic includes inhibition of platelet aggregation, which reduces the clotting tendency of blood and may prevent heart attacks and stroke. Das, Khan, & Sooranna (1995) found this effect to be dose dependent. This effect may account for the many reports in the literature related to garlic and an increased risk of bleeding in persons undergoing surgery (German, Kumar, & Blackford, 1995; Burnham, 1995; Petry, 1995). Clients who are taking drugs with anticoagulant effects (e.g., warfarin and aspirin) should be cautioned about garlic dietary supplements.

Garlic also acts as an antiinfective, counteracting the growth of many types of bacteria that cause disease in humans (Farbman, Barnett, Bolduc, & Klein, 1993). There is also interest in garlic for its antiviral activity. In one study, Guo et al. (1993) evaluated the in vitro antiviral activity of garlic extract on human cytomegalovirus (HCMV), and a dose-dependent inhibitory effect was evident. The effect was stronger with pretreatment with garlic extract and persisted after the extract was removed. Their recommendation for the clinical use of garlic extract against HCMV was that it be used persistently and that prophylactic use is preferable in immunocompromised individuals. Again, further research is required before the antiviral activity of garlic can be substantiated.

Recent in vitro and in vivo models have been used to test the chemical constituents of garlic for their inhibiting effects on carcinogenesis, and the results have varied. In some studies it appears that, in addition to stimulating the immune system, garlic blocks the formation of carcinogens in the gut and protects DNA from damage by other carcinogens (Weil, 1995). After reviewing the strengths and weaknesses of 60 of these studies, Dorant, van den Brandt, Goldbohm, Hermus, and Sturmans (1993) concluded in the *British Journal of Cancer* that laboratory experiments and epidemiologic studies have not provided conclusive evidence of the preventive activity of garlic. However, the data that are available warrant further research into the possible role of garlic in the prevention of cancer in humans.

The major component of garlic is alliin; when garlic is crushed, alliin is converted to allicin, the pharmacologically active ingredient. Alliin must be converted to allicin to be effective. Because alliin is unstable in gastric fluid, the best commercial preparations are enteric-coated or capsule forms. The recommended daily dose of alliin is approximately 8 mg, the equivalent of one clove of garlic.

Ginger *(Zingiber officinale [sheng jiang]).* Like garlic, ginger is a culinary spice. It has been used for medicinal purposes since ancient times. Ginger is recommended to stimulate digestion and to relieve nausea and aches and pains. It improves the digestion of protein, strengthens the mucosal lining of the upper gastrointestinal tract (and therefore protects against ulcers), and has a wide range of action against intestinal parasites (Weil, 1995). Phillips, Ruggier, & Hutchinson (1993) studied 120 women presenting for elective laproscopic gynecologic surgery on a day-stay basis and found the incidence of nausea and vomiting to be similar in subjects given metoclopramide (Reglan) and ginger (27% and 21%, respectively) and less than in subjects who received a placebo (41%); there was no difference in the requirements for postoperative analgesia, recovery time, and time until discharge. These antiemetic effects are not associated with gastric emptying (Phillips, Hutchinson, & Ruggier, 1994). The antiemetic properties of ginger may be considered as an alternative for treating the nausea and vomiting of pregnancy (Aikins-Murphy, 1998), but its antiemetic efficiency as an adjunct to cancer chemotherapy is controversial (Sharma, Kochupillai, Gupta, Seth, & Gupta, 1997; Arfeen et al., 1997). The use of ginger as a prophylactic remedy for motion sickness is also controversial (Wood et al., 1988).

No side effects have been noted with therapeutic doses, but the potential to inhibit clotting does exist (Lumb, 1994). There is evidence that ginger modulates the synthesis of eicosanoid (prostaglandins, thromboxanes, and leukotrienes) in ways that reduce abnormal inflammation and clotting. It may be as effective as some of the NSAIDs while also protecting the stomach lining rather than damaging it as the NSAIDs sometimes do. The antiinflammatory effects of ginger may have an inhibitory effect on skin tumor promotion (Katiyar, Agarwal & Mukhtar, 1993; Park, Chun, Lee, Less, & Surh, 1998). Recent research indicates that it also has a hypolipidemic effect (Bhandari, Sharma, & Zafar, 1998).

Ginger comes in a variety of forms, from fresh rhizome to candied pieces to encapsulated dried, powdered ginger. The average dose is 2 to 4 g. It is considered to be nontoxic, but some individuals may experience heartburn if large amounts of raw ginger are taken on an empty stomach; it should be taken with food. There is some controversy about the use of ginger in pregnancy because of its abortifacient effects, but this effect has not been documented in humans. A recent review of the literature found no reason for contraindicating ginger during pregnancy when it is taken at the usual therapeutic dose.

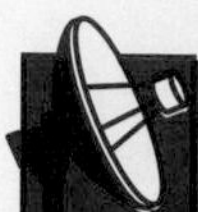

TechnologyLink
Complementary and Alternative Pharmacology

Web Resources

Alternative Health News Online (www.altmedicine.com/)
This site presents alternative and traditional health news, such as news on diet and nutrition, mind/body connections, Web links for nonconventional approaches, and more.

Alternative/Complementary Medicine (wellweb.com/AlternativeComplementary_Medicine.htm)
This site includes three major "Sections" on alternative and complementary medicine, conventional medicine, and nutrition and fitness, along with links to a variety of specialized "Centers" (cancer, diagnostic tests, heart, impotence, and more).

National Center for Complementary and Alternative Medicine (nccam.nih.gov)
This site is a division of the National Institutes of Health, whose mission is to evaluate alternative treatments and their effectiveness. This organization facilitates research in this area but does not make referrals.

Ask Dr. Andrew Weil (www.pathfinder.com/drweil/)
This site, offered by a well-known alternative medicine expert, includes a question-and-answer library, a self-help section, information on recipes, a healing center, information on sexual health, and more.

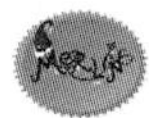

For additional WebLinks, a free subscription to the "Mosby/Saunders ePharmacology Update" newsletter, and more, go to mosby.com/MERLIN/McKenry/.

Ginkgo *(Ginkgo biloba L.).* The *G. biloba* leaf, its extract, or purified mixtures of ginkgolides are contained in many herbal preparations. It has been suggested that ginkgo is effective in the treatment of arterial insufficiency in the brain and extremities, allergic responses, and memory impairment. Clinical data based on double-blind clinical trials using matched client groups with peripheral arterial insufficiency have demonstrated the clinical efficacy of a standardized extract of *G. biloba.* Significant improvements in pain-free walking time and maximum walking distance were achieved (Pizzorno & Murray, 1985). Vorberg (1985) studied 112 individuals with a mean age of 70.5 years who were experiencing chronic cerebral insufficiency. They were treated as outpatients with *G. biloba* leaf standardized extract at 120 mg/day in an open 1-year trial. The results demonstrated a statistically significant regression of major symptoms, including vertigo, headache, tinnitus, short-term memory, and vigilance and mood disturbance. During the trial no changes were noted for heart rate or blood pressure, and the blood concentration of cholesterol and triglycerides remained unchanged. In addition, no significant side effects or interactions with existing medications, including cardiac glycosides and antidiabetic preparations, were noted.

In animal studies ginkgolides competitively inhibit the binding of platelet-activating factor (PAF) to its membrane receptor (Hosford & Braquet, 1990). In human studies antagonism of the effects of PAF was found to significantly inhibit wheal and flare responses in a double-blind, placebo-controlled cross study (Chung, 1987) and to be effective in both the early and late phase of airway hyperactivity in a double-blind, randomized cross-over study (Braquet, 1987). The clinical data based on trials with small numbers of clients indicate that the use of ginkgo is promising and that further clinical trials need to be undertaken.

Ginkgo leaf extract is usually well tolerated. Mild gastrointestinal disturbances may be minimized by slowly titrating the ginkgo dose. Contact with and ingestion of the fruit pulp has produced severe allergic reactions and should not be handled or ingested. The seed of the plant also causes severe adverse reactions when ingested. Ginkgo products are usually standardized at 24% flavonoids and 6% terpenes. The daily dose of standardized ginkgo leaf extract is 120 to 160 mg.

Ginseng Root *(Panax schinseng [ren shen]).* The Chinese have used ginseng for more than 3000 years as a tonic, a restorative, and a specific treatment for several ailments. Ginseng has been subjected to extensive study in recent years. In a review of recent advances in ginseng research, Liu and Xiao (1992) indicated that ginseng has a wide range of pharmacologic actions. It acts on the central nervous system (Lim et al., 1997), cardiovascular system (Kim, Chen, & Gillis, 1992), and endocrine secretion; promotes immune function and metabolism; possesses biomodulation action (Watanabe et al., 1991); and promotes antistress activity (Bhattacharya & Mitra, 1991).

In a multicenter, two arm, randomized, placebo-controlled, double-blind study, Scaglione, Cattaneo, Alessandria, & Cogo (1996) found an increased immune response following a vaccination against influenza. The study participants were followed for a 3-month period, and the ginseng group experienced significantly fewer cases of influenza and the common cold—15 of 114 were affected, whereas 42 of 113 in the placebo group were affected. Yun and Choi (1995) examined the preventive effect of ginseng intake against various types of cancers using a case-control study of 1987 pairs. Individuals taking ginseng had a decreased risk for most cancers compared with those who didn't take ginseng; this decrease was dose related (i.e., there was a decrease in risk with increasing frequency and duration of ginseng intake). In 1993 Saita et al. isolated an antitumor substance called panaxynol from ginseng and found that it inhibited the growth of various types of cultured tumor cell lines in a dose-dependent manner. Tomoda et al. (1993) found immunologic activity in other derivatives of ginseng. Other researchers have documented the cancer-inhibiting effects of ginseng (Xiaoguang et al., 1998; Sohn, Lim, Lee, Lee, & Kim, 1993; Tode et al., 1993), as well as its antiulcer effects (Sun, Matsumoto, & Yamada, 1992). Song et al. (1997) believe that ginseng may have the potential to be a promising natural medicine in conjunction with other forms of treatment for cystic fibrosis clients with chronic *Pseudomonas aeruginosa* lung infection. They found that treatment with ginseng reduced bacterial load and lung pathology in chronic *P. aeruginosa* pneumonia in laboratory rats. However, despite its reputation as a tonic, Engels and Wirth (1997) conducted a randomized, double blind, placebo-controlled trial and were unable to demonstrate any ergogenic effect to improve submaximal and maximal performances as a result of taking ginseng.

Ginseng may potentiate the action of monoamine oxidase (MAO) inhibitors; it should not be taken with stimulants, including coffee, or during treatment with hormones, especially estrogens and corticosteroids (Newall et al., 1996). Because ginseng has a history of being adulterated or mislabeled, some adverse reactions may be due to contaminants; individuals who experience adverse reactions should discontinue its use. Headache may be the result of extremely high doses of ginseng. Individuals with hypertension should not use ginseng.

Green Tea *(Camellia simensis).* In general, tea is one of the most popular beverages consumed worldwide. Many individuals consume green tea as a refreshing beverage as well as a tonic. Studies in Japan, where green tea is the national beverage, indicate an inverse association between the consumption of green tea and various serum markers, which shows that green tea may act protectively against cardiovascular disease and liver disorders (Imai & Nakachi, 1995). Green tea improves the risk factors for heart disease by hypolipidemic and antioxidant mechanisms and possibly has a fibrinolytic effect (Vinson & Dabbagh, 1998; Yang & Koo, 1997). Many laboratory studies have demonstrated the inhibitory effects of green tea preparations and tea polyphenols against tumor formation and growth (Imai, Suga, & Nakachi, 1997; Dreosti, Wargovich, & Yang, 1997); skin carcinogenesis and tumor progression (Wang et al., 1994; Katiyar et al., 1993; Wang et al., 1992b); lung tumorigenesis (Xu, Ho, Amin, Han, & Chung, 1992; Wang et al., 1992a); and small bowel and liver cancers (Khan, Katiyar, Agarwal, & Mukhtar, 1992). This inhibitory activity is believed to be mainly a result of the antioxidative and possible antiproliferative effects of polyphenolic compounds in green tea. Polyphenolic compounds suppress the activation of carcinogens and trap genotoxic agents. A large population-based, case-control study of esophageal cancer in urban Shanghai suggested a protective effect of green tea consumption (Gao et al., 1994). The effect of tea consumption on cancer is likely to depend on the causative factors of the specific cancer. Further laboratory and epidemiologic study is required to determine the relationship between green tea consumption and human cancer risk (Yang & Wang, 1993).

Hawthorn *(Crataegus oxyacantha).* Hawthorn grows as a spiny tree or shrub with thorny, branching stems. Both its blossoms and its berries are used for their therapeutic properties. Hawthorn had a long history of use in Europe before being introduced to this country in the nineteenth century. Since then it has been used as a folk remedy, primarily as a cardiac tonic and a mild diuretic. Its therapeutic properties have long been recognized in Europe. This acceptance has been supported by a 4-year study of hawthorn commissioned by the German Federal Ministry of Health. The study concluded that hawthorn increases cardiac contractility and the rate of blood flow. It was also found to increase both coronary and myocardial circulation by its dilation effect on the coronary arteries. After taking hawthorn, individuals report a reduction in the number of angina attacks as well as symptom relief (Loew, 1999). In the United Kingdom clinicians use hawthorn for its mild antihypertensive effect in clients with hypertension (Hoffman, 1995). In these individuals, hawthorn inhibits angiotensin-converting enzyme (ACE), increases the contractility of the heart, and confers a mild diuretic action. If clients also take beta-blockers for their hypertension, which reduce cardiac output, the inotropic effects of hawthorn may cause a slight increase in blood pressure.

Hawthorn has been used in combination with digitalis, enhancing the effects of the cardiac glycosides found in digitalis. The dose of digitalis may be decreased if used in conjunction with hawthorn. Individuals with mild to moderate congestive heart failure may benefit from hawthorn alone. Because of a lack of data, hawthorn cannot be seen as a substitute for the more powerful prescription drugs, but it may complement them and enhance their activity. Clients currently taking cardiac drugs should discuss the use of hawthorn with their prescriber before taking the drug.

Milk Thistle *(Silybum marianum).* Milk thistle is used to prevent the liver from damage by a variety of toxins. It protects against genomic injury, increases hepatocyte protein growth, and decreases the activity of tumor promoters (Flora, Hahn, Rosen, & Benner, 1998). Standardized extracts of milk thistle concentrate silymarin, a substance that apparently prevents the membrane of undamaged liver cells from letting toxins enter. Human trials for the treatment of hepatitis and cirrhosis have been "encouraging" (Weil, 1995). Recent research indicates that milk thistle may also have some anticancer effects in human prostate carcinoma (Zi, Grasso, Kung, & Agarwal, 1998) and breast cancer (Zi, Feyes, & Agarwal, 1998). There are no documented contraindications or interactions with other remedies. Although there are no known serious side effects, a mild laxative effect is occasionally reported.

St. John's Wort *(Hypericum perforatum).* St. John's wort, a flowering perennial plant, has been used medicinally for hundreds of years and has most recently been identified as an effective treatment for mild to moderate depression. Extract of hypericum, the reference substance for pharmaceutical standardization, is widely used in Europe, especially Germany. It has been used for excitability, neuralgia, and specifically for menopausal neurosis (Newall et al., 1996). A recent overview and meta-analysis of randomized clinical trials from 1979 to 1996 concluded that such extracts are more effective than a placebo for the treatment of depressive disorders; however, it is not known whether they are more effective for certain disorders than others (Linde, Ramirez, Mulrow, Pauls, & Weidenhammer, 1996). Since that study, others have concluded that St. John's wort has results equivalent to those of many antidepressant drugs and has a much more favorable incidence of side effects (Cott & Fugh-Berman, 1998; Miller, 1998; Wheatley, 1997). Additional trials should be conducted to investigate the long-term side effects and relative efficacy of different preparations and doses.

Delayed hypersensitivity or photodermatitis has been documented for St. John's wort following the ingestion of an herbal tea made from the leaves (Newall et al., 1996). Individuals taking this herb should be warned to avoid direct sunlight and to wear sun protective lotion of SPF 15. In view of the lack of toxicity data and documented photosensitizing activity, excessive use of St. John's wort should be avoided.

Shark Cartilage. Shark cartilage is one of the most controversial subjects of current medical debate. Although it has been suggested to have antineoplastic properties and is presently in FDA clinical trials with terminally ill individuals in New Jersey, shark cartilage is becoming more widely known as a treatment for osteoarthritis and rheumatoid arthritis. Researchers have been unable to determine the exact therapeutic agent in shark cartilage, but most agree that the primary antiinflammatory components are mucopolysaccharides (complex carbohydrates). Two of these mucopolysaccharides, chondroitin sulfates A and C, have long been used by nutrition medicine practitioners to fight inflammation and enteritis. The naturally occurring forms of these compounds in shark cartilage are more effective than the synthetically refined mucopolysaccharides. When combined with the angiogenesis inhibition properties attributed to these proteins, shark cartilage may not only provide inflammation relief but also inhibit the vascularization of joint cartilage that is associated with advanced cases of osteoarthritis and rheumatoid arthritis. This action, inhibiting the formation of new blood vessels, is the basis for the alleged anticancer activity of shark cartilage (Sculti, 1994).

Shark cartilage has been deemed nontoxic by the FDA and is sold as a food supplement in the United States. There are major differences in the available dosage forms—tablets, capsules, caplets, soft gelcaps, powders, and liquids. More than 40 different brand name products of shark cartilage are sold directly to consumers in the United States and Canada. Many manufacturers claim their products have advantages in terms of purity, source, or manufacture, but there is no industry standard. Many formulations contain binders or fillers; consumers should seek a product that is 100% pure shark cartilage. Even at that, bioavailability studies of shark cartilage components are lacking and the recommended dose is unsubstantiated. In general, pure shark cartilage contains approximately 35% protein, 50% minerals (60% of which is calcium and phosphorus in a 2:1 ratio), 8% carbohydrates (mainly present as mucopolysaccharides), 7% water, and less than 1% fat. The protein strands are thought to contain the active antiangiogenic components (Holt, 1995).

Although the dosage is unsubstantiated, most providers familiar with shark cartilage agree that it is effective when taken orally, three times daily, in equal amounts, and approximately 15 to 30 minutes before meals. Each gram of dried powdered shark cartilage may be mixed in a blender with 2 ounces of nonacidic fruit juice or nectar to make it more palatable. The capsules can be taken with water. The side effects seem to be limited to nausea related to its fishy taste. Because of the material's antiangiogenetic effect, children, pregnant women, and those who have experienced a recent myocardial infarction should not take shark cartilage. It should be discontinued 3 months before and after any surgical procedure (Sculti, 1994).

Valerian *(Valeriana officinalis)*. Valerian, an herb, is used for sleep problems and probably has mild sedating and tranquilizing effects. The medicinal use of this plant has been recorded since ancient Greek and Roman times. Although it is an attractive plant with pink and white flowers, even the Roman physician Galen noted its objectionable odor. Valerian is used extensively in Europe, where it is accepted by allopathic medicine (Ravitzky, 1994).

The root and the rhizome of the plant are used for therapeutic effect. The root contains the volatile oil (valerenic acid) and valepotriate fractions, which have a calming effect (Jellin, Batz, & Hitchens, 1999). Many studies have demonstrated that valerian not only eases the trouble of falling asleep but also improves the quality of sleep during the night. It seems to offer the benefit of a good night's sleep without the grogginess that accompanies some over-the-counter sleep medications. However, valerian has not been found to have any effect on objective measures such as electroencephalogram (EEG) sleep parameters (Newall et al., 1996). Unlike some other sedatives, valerian seems to have none of the dependency risk; there is no synergistic effect when taken concurrently with alcohol or prescription drugs. However, individuals taking benzodiazepine and other sedative drugs may want to avoid consuming valerian.

It is recommended that the root be chopped into small pieces and steeped until cool before drinking (1 teaspoon of root for each cup of liquid). One to three cups may be consumed each day. Valerian is also prepared in capsule and tincture forms for dosing. It is considered to be nontoxic even when taken over long periods.

REMEDIES THAT MIGHT HARM

Some herbal remedies can be harmful, and the nurse should be familiar with the more toxic agents. Table 12-2 lists selected unsafe herbs that should not be formulated and used as food, beverage, or medication. Table 12-3 lists herbal teas and the potential harmful effects associated with their use. Other remedies that might be harmful are discussed in the following sections.

TABLE 12-2 Selected Unsafe Herbs

Botanical Name	Common Names	Comments
Arnica montana	Arnica flowers, wolf's bane, mountain tobacco, *Flores Arnicae*	Extracted substances affect heart and vascular systems; extremely irritating and can induce toxic gastroenteritis, nervous system disturbances, extreme muscle weakness, collapse and, perhaps, death
Artemisia absinthium	Wormwood, absinthe, madderwort, absinthium, mugwort	Contains a narcotic poison (oil of wormwood); can cause nervous system damage and mental impairment
Atropa belladonna	Belladonna, deadly nightshade	Considered a poisonous plant that contains the toxic alkaloids of atropine, hyoscyamine, and hyoscine; anticholinergic symptoms range from blurred vision, dry mouth, and inability to urinate to unusual behaviors and hallucinations
Aesculus hippocastanum	Buckeye, horse chestnut, aesculus	Contains coumarin glycoside, aesculin; may interfere with normal blood clotting; a toxic plant
Conium maculatum	Hemlock, conium, spotted hemlock, spotted parsley, St. Bennet's herb, spotted cowbane, fool's parsley	Contains toxic alkaloid coniine and perhaps four other related alkaloids
Lobelia inflata	Lobelia, Indian tobacco, wild tobacco, asthma weed, emetic weed	Toxic plant that contains lobeline plus other alkaloids; excessive use of plant or its leaves or fruit extracts can result in severe vomiting, pain, sweating, paralysis, decreased temperature, collapse, coma, and death
Vinca major *Vinca minor*	Periwinkle, vinca, greater or lesser periwinkle	Contain toxic alkaloids (vinblastine, vincristine) that are cytotoxic and may cause liver, kidney, and neurologic damage

Information from Tyler, V.E. (1993). *The honest herbal* (3rd ed.). New York: Pharmaceutical Products Press.

TABLE 12-3 Herbal Teas and Toxic Reactions

Herbal Tea	Proposed Usage	Potential Toxic Effect
Chamomile	Appetite stimulant, anodyne, carminative, antispasmodic	Can cause skin rash and severe hypersensitivity reactions, including anaphylaxis, in persons allergic to ragweed, chrysanthemums, etc.
Hydrangea	Kidney stones, diuretic	Some species contain cyanide-producing compounds, especially when smoked; may make users very ill
Mistletoe	Parasitic American mistletoe stimulates smooth muscles, increasing blood pressure and GI contractions European mistletoe has opposite effect; it lowers blood pressure and is antispasmodic	More than 200 species available with toxic proteins; can be poisonous; avoid use
Rue	Antispasmodic, calmative, abortifacient, insect repellent	Contains coumarin derivatives; external use can cause skin blisters and photosensitization; internal use can cause gastric upset and toxicity
Shave grass or horsetail plants	Diuretic	Contains silica and glycosides; when consumed by horses and other grazing animals, anorexia, loss of muscle control, excitability, diarrhea, seizures, coma, and death may occur

Information from Tyler, V.E. (1993). *The honest herbal* (3rd ed.). New York: Pharmaceutical Products Press; Nightingale, S.L. (1993). From the Food and Drug Administration: Public warning about herbal products. *JAMA, 269*(3), 328.

Chaparral. Chaparral, a desert shrub, is sold as a tea, tablet, and capsule for its antioxidant properties. Chaparral was removed from the FDA's "generally recognized as safe" list in 1970 after animal studies revealed damage to kidney and lymph organs. Four reports of liver toxicity occurred in 1992, which prompted the FDA to warn against the use of any product containing chaparral (News you can use, 1995). In addition to these U.S. cases, three cases have been reported in Canada (Food and Drug Administration, 1993). The National Nutritional Foods Association has asked its member companies not to carry these products, but chaparral is still being sold and sometimes is an ingredient in combination products.

Comfrey. Comfrey, an herb, is sold as a tea, tablet, capsule, tincture, poultice, and lotion. It has been linked to a number of cases of liver impairment, and studies with animals demonstrate injury to lung, kidney, and gastrointestinal tissue. Australia, Canada, Germany, and the United Kingdom restrict the availability of comfrey.

Ephedra *(ma huang)*. Ephedra is promoted for energy boosting and weight control. It contains the sympathomimetic drugs ephedrine and pseudoephedrine, both of which cause vasoconstriction and may increase blood pressure and cause cardiac dysrhythmias. These drugs are contraindicated for clients with angle-closure glaucoma, thyroid disorders, diabetes, hypertension, and angina. Ohio has restricted the use of over-the-counter ephedrine products, including ma huang, and a number of state drug regulators have requested the FDA to limit it to prescription use only.

Lobelia (*Lobelia inflata* [Indian Tobacco]). The lobelia leaf yields lobeline sulfate, which acts like nicotine and so may be used as anti-tobacco therapy. It acts as an agonist at nicotine receptors both peripherally and centrally. Lobelia produces behavioral stimulation and depression, cardiac acceleration, peripheral vasoconstriction, and elevated blood pressure. It is contraindicated for use in individuals with unstable cardiovascular conditions such as angina, dysrhythmias, postmyocardial infarct, and hypertension.

Yohimbe *(Corynanthe yohimbe)*. Yohimbe is a plant product made from the bark of an African tree; it is generally touted as an aphrodisiac for men. Its active ingredient, yohimbine, is used for the treatment of erectile impotence, but neither the United States nor Canada include that as an indication for its use in its package labeling. In some individuals it has caused increased blood pressure and heart rate, dizziness, headache, irritability, or nervousness. Documentation of the usefulness of yohimbe to treat impotence is inconclusive; it is likely unsafe (Jellin, Batz, & Hitchens, 1999).

CONSUMER EDUCATION FOR COMPLEMENTARY AND ALTERNATIVE THERAPIES

Complementary and alternative remedies will continue to be used because of strong traditions and because of the desire of client to increase a sense of control to improve their well-being.

The nurse must recognize and clarify his or her own values. This awareness will prevent the nurse from imposing his or her own health beliefs onto the client and family. The nurse needs to self-educate himself or herself with scientific proof, including clinical studies, to discuss with the clients. The nurse can then assist the client and family to explore their values and beliefs. This will help the client to make the "right" decisions and will help the nurse to better understand and support the client's choices. The nurse may then incorporate the reasonable components of alternative therapy into the client's therapeutic regimen.

If a client takes or wishes to take a complementary or alternative remedy, he or she should consult with his or her primary health care provider about the benefit or harm that might occur as a result of taking the substances. This would prevent the client from delaying contact with a caregiver because of the use of an alternative therapy. The prescriber could also provide information on the efficacy of the particular remedy. This consultation would be especially important if the client is taking prescription medications. Any of the complementary and alternative medications may interact with the client's current medication regimen by enhancing or inhibiting its effects or by combining for a toxic effect. Pregnant and breastfeeding women should not take any alternative remedies without the prescriber's approval.

Just as with OTC drugs, complementary and alternative remedies should be considered as medications, and information related to their use should be shared as current medications in the client's health history. Providers should proactively question clients about the use of complementary and alternative remedies, and the answers should be documented in their health record.

The client should be counseled about lifestyle changes that may be more effective than complementary and alternative remedies in accomplishing therapeutic goals. For example, if the client wishes to lower serum cholesterol levels, a low-fat, high-fiber diet and exercise may be more effective and less expensive than garlic supplements. Just as with allopathic medications, the therapeutic outcome is enhanced by supportive behavioral changes.

Just as with OTC medications, the client should use single-agent products. This provides for more effective evaluation of the remedy's therapeutic effect and also minimizes the adverse responses that may occur as a result of ingesting multiple substances. If the client experiences an adverse reaction, determination of the causative agent is easier. The nurse should make sure that all ingredients and the dose of each are listed on the product label. The product should also be evaluated for standardization; this increases the chance that the contents of the remedy will be consistent from dose to dose.

If a serious toxicity is suspected, the client should be able to provide a sample of the remedy for chemical analysis. Clients should be encouraged to purchase products with labels that show the scientific name of the herb, the name and address of the manufacturer, a lot number, the date of manufacture, and an expiration date. This will provide valuable information if there is an adverse reaction. Health care providers should report serious adverse reactions involving herbal remedies to the FDA MedWatch Program (800-332-1088).

Labels should be well read and warnings on the package heeded. Parents need to be cautioned to keep these substances out of the reach of children. The client needs to be knowledgeable about the expected actions of the medication; if these actions do not occur in a reasonable time, the drug should be discontinued. Objective criteria should be determined with the client so that measurable progress or lack of progress can be documented to decrease the power of suggestion regarding the therapeutic effects of the drug (e.g., weekly weights in the case of weight loss medications). Adverse reactions should also be known, and the client should discontinue the drug and notify a physician if there is a problem.

Clients should be cautioned that commercially available alternative medications may be adulterated because they do not undergo standardized testing for safety and efficacy by the FDA. The role of the nurse is to educate clients regarding the appropriate use or possibly hazardous misuse of complementary and alternative remedies.

SUMMARY

Many complementary and alternative remedies have been promoted on the basis of anecdotal accounts—sometimes for hundreds of years—from people who indicate that a particular substance has kept them well or cured their illness. There is no way of knowing what might have been the result if the individual had not taken the remedy; many illnesses are self-limiting, and the placebo effect cannot be discounted. Many of these remedies show promise for further research. Until the same rigorousness of randomized, double-blind trials is applied to complementary and alternative remedies, consumers need to remain cautious about their use.

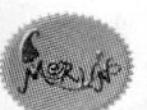

Critical Thinking Questions

1. How would the cautions previously discussed regarding complementary and alternative remedies differ from the adverse reactions of allopathic medicines?

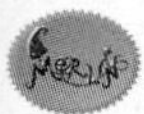

Collaborative Learning Activities

For Collaborative Learning Activities, go to mosby.com/MERLIN/McKenry/.

CASE STUDY

For a Case Study that will help ensure mastery of this chapter content, go to mosby.com/MERLIN/McKenry/.

BIBLIOGRAPHY

Aikins-Murphy, P. (1998). Alternative therapies for nausea and vomiting of pregnancy. *Obstetrics & Gynecology, 91*(1), 149-155.

Anderson, L.A. (1996). Concern regarding herbal toxicities: Case reports and counseling tips. *Annuals of Pharmacotherapy, 30*, 79-80.

Arfeen, Z., Owen, H., Plummer, J.L., Ilsey, A.H., Sorby-Adams, R.A., & Doecke, C.L. (1995). A double-blind randomized controlled trial of ginger for the prevention of post-op nausea and vomiting. *Anesthesia & Intensive Care, 23*(4), 449-452.

Awang, D.V.C. (1989). Feverfew. *Canadian Pharmacological Journal, 122*(5), 266-270.

Berry, M. (1994). Feverfew. *Pharmacological Journal, 253*, 806-808.

Berthold, H.K., Sudhop, T., & von Bergmann, K. (1998). Effect of a garlic preparation on serum lipoproteins and cholesterol metabolism: a randomized controlled trial. *Journal of the American Medical Association, 279*(23), 1900-1902.

Bhandari, U., Sharma, J.N., & Zafar, R. (1998). The protective action of ethanolic ginger (Zingiber officinale) extract in cholesterol fed rabbits. *Journal of Ethnopharmacology, 61*(2), 167-171.

Bhattacharya, S.K. & Mitra, S.K. (1991). Anxiolytic activity of Panax ginseng roots: An experimental study. *Journal of Ethnopharmacology, 34*(1), 87-92.

Braquet, P. (1987). The ginkgolides: potent platelet-inactivating factor antagonists isolated from *Ginkgo biloba L.*: Chemistry, pharmacology and clinical application. *Drugs of the Future, 12*, 643-699.

Brody, J.E. (1994, July 27). Personal health: Modern doctors confirm the ancient wisdom that garlic has many benefits. *New York Times*.

Burger, R.A., Torres, A.R., Warren, R.P., Caldwell, V.D., & Hughes, B.G. (1997). Echinacea-induced cytokine production by human macrophages. *International Journal of Immunopharmacology, 19*(4), 371-379.

Burnham, B.E. (1995). Garlic as a possible risk for postoperative bleeding. *Plastic Reconstructive Surgery, 96*(2), 483-484.

Calis, I., Yuruker, A., Tasdenir, D., Wright, A.D., Sticher, O., Luo, Y.D., & Pezzuto, J.M. (1997). Cycloartane triterpene glycosides from the roots of *Astragalus melanophrurius*. *Planta Medica, 63*(2), 183-186.

Chan, T.Y., Chan, J.C., Tomlinson, B., & Critchley, J.A. (1993). Chinese herbal medicines revisited: A Hong Kong perspective. *Lancet, 342*(8886-8887), 1532-1534.

Chu, D.T., Wong, W.K., & Mavaligit, G.M. (1988a). Immunotherapy with Chinese medicinal herbs. I. Immune restoration of local xenogeneic graft-versus-host reaction in cancer patients by fractionated Astragalus membranaceous in vitro. *Journal of Clinical Laboratory Immunology, 25*, 119-123.

Chu, D.T., Wong, W.K., & Mavaligit, G.M. (1988b). Immunotherapy with Chinese medicinal herbs. II. Reversal of cyclophosphamide-induced immune induced suppression by administration of fractionated Astragalus membranaceous in vivo. *Journal of Clinical Laboratory Immunology, 25*, 125-129.

Chung, K.F. (1987). Effect of a ginkgolide mixture (BN 52063) in antagonizing skin and platelet responses to platelet activating factor in man. *Lancet, I*, 248-251.

Coeugniet, E.G. & Elek, E. (1987). Immunomodulation with Viscum album and Echinacea purpurea extracts. *Onkologie, 10*(3 suppl), 27-33.

Cott, J.M. & Fugh-Berman, A. (1998). Is St. John's wort (Hypericum perforatum) an effective antidepressant? *Journal of Nervous & Mental Disease, 186*(8), 500-501.

Craig, W.J. (1997). Phytochemicals: guardians of our health. *Journal of the American Dietetic Association, 97*(10 Suppl 2), S119-204.

Daly, D. (1995). Alternative medicine courses taught at U.S. medical schools: An ongoing listing. *Journal of Alternative & Complementary Medicine, 1*(2), 205-207.

Das, I., Khan, N.S., & Sooranna, S.R. (1995). Potent activation of nitric oxide synthase by garlic: A basis for its therapeutic applications. *Current Medical Research & Opinion, 13*(5), 257-263.

Dorant, E., van den Brandt, P.A., Goldbohm, R.A., Hermus, R.J., & Sturmans F. (1993). Garlic and its significance for the prevention of cancer in humans: A critical review. *British Journal of Cancer, 67*(3), 424-429.

Dreosti, I.E., Wargovich, M.J., & Yang, C.S. (1997) Inhibition of carcinogenesis by tea: The evidence from experimental studies. *Critical Reviews in Food Science & Nutrition, 37*(8): 761-770.

Eisenberg, D.M., Kessler, R.C., Foster, C., Norlock, F.E., Calkins, D.C., & Delbanco, T.L. (1993). Unconventional medicine in the United States: Prevalence, costs, and patterns of use. *New England Journal of Medicine, 328*(8), 246-252.

Eisenberg, D.M., Davis, R.B., Ettner, S.L., Appel, S., Wilkey, S., Van Rompay, M., Kessler, R.C. (1998). Trends in alternative medicine use in the United States, 1990-1997: Results of a follow-up national survey. *Journal of the American Medical Association, 280*(18), 1569-1575.

Engels, H.J. & Wirth, J.C. (1997). No erogenic effects of ginseng (Panax ginseng C.A. Meyer) during graded maximal aerobic exercise. *Journal of the American Dietetic Association, 97*(10), 1110-1115.

Facino, R.M., Carini, M., Aldini, G., Saibene, L. Pietta, P., & Mauri, P. (1995). Echinacoside and caffeoyl conjugates protect collagen from free radical-induced degradation: a potential use for Echinacea extracts in the prevention of sun photodamage. *Planta Medica, 61*(6), 510-514.

Farbman, K.S., Barnett, E.D., Bolduc, G.R., & Klein, J.O. (1993). Antibacterial activity of garlic and onions: A historical perspective. *Pediatric Infectious Disease Journal, 12*(7), 613-614.

Fletcher, D.M. (1992). Unconventional cancer treatments: Professional, legal, and ethical issues. *Oncology Nursing Forum, 19*(9), 1351-1354.

Flora, K., Hahn, M., Rosen, H., & Benner, K. (1998). Milk thistle (Silybum marianum) for the therapy of liver disease. *American Journal of Gastroenterology, 93*(2), 139-143.

Food and Drug Administration (1993). From the Food and Drug Administration. *JAMA, 269*(3), 328.

Foster, S. (1995). Feverfew: When the head hurts. *Alternative & Complementary Therapies, 1*(5), 335-337.

Gao, Y.T., McLaughlin, J.K., Blot, W.J., Ji, B.T., Dai, Q., & Fraumenti, J.F. Jr. (1994). Reduced risk of esophageal cancer associated with green tea consumption. *Journal of the National Cancer Institute, 86*(11), 855-858.

German, K., Kumar, U., & Blackford, H.N. (1995). Garlic and the risk of TURP bleeding. *British Journal of Urology, 76*(4), 518.

Gertner, E., Marshall, P.S., Filandrinos, D., Potek, A.S., & Smith, T.M. (1995). Complications resulting from the use of Chinese herbal medications containing undeclared prescription drugs. *Arthritis & Rheumatism, 38*(5), 614-617.

Goldman, J.A. & Myerson, G. (1991). Chinese herbal medicine: Camouflaged prescription antiinflammatory drugs, corticosteroids, and lead. *Arthritis & Rheumatism, 34*(9), 1207.

Gorey, J.D., Wahlqvist, M.L., & Boyce, N.W. (1992). Adverse reaction to a Chinese herbal remedy. *Medical Journal of Australia, 157*(7), 484-486.

Guo, N.L., Lu, D.P., Woods, G.L. Reed, E., Zhou, G.Z., Zhang, L.B., & Waldman, R.H. (1993). Demonstration of the antiviral activity of garlic extract against human cytomegalovirus in vitro. *Chinese Medical Journal, 106*(2), 93-96.

Heptinstall, S., Awang, D.V., Dawson, B.A., Kindack, D., Knight, D.W., & May, J. (1992). Parthenolide content and bioactivity of feverfew: Estimation of commercial and authenticated feverfew products. *Journal of Pharmacy Pharmacology, 44*, 391-395.

Herbal roulette. (1995). *Consumer Reports, 60*(11), 698-705.

Hoffman, D. (1995). Hawthorn: The heart helper. *Alternative & Complementary Therapies, 1*(3), 191-192.

Holt, S. (1995). Shark cartilage and nutriceutical update. *Alternative & Complementary Therapies, 1*(6), 414-416.

Hosford, D. & Braquet, P. (1990). Antagonists of platelet-activating factor; Chemistry, pharmacology, and clinical applications. *Progress in Medicinal Chemistry, 27*, 325-380.

Hun, J.H., Wen, T.C., Matsuda, S., Tanaka, J., Maeda, N., Peng, H., Aburaya, J., Ishihara, K., & Sakanaaka, M. (1997). Protection of ischemic hippocampal neurons by ginsenoside Rb1, a main ingredient of ginseng root. *Neuroscience Research*, 28(3), 191-200.

Imai, K. & Nakachi, K. (1995). Cross sectional study of effects of drinking green tea on cardiovascular and liver diseases. *British Medical Journal, 310*(6981), 693-696.

Imai, K., Suga, K., & Nakachi, K. (1997). Cancer-preventive effects of drinking green tea among a Japanese population. *Preventive Medicine, 26*(6), 769-775.

Isaacsohn, J.L., Moser, M., Stein, E.A., Dudley, K., Davey, J.A., Liskov, E., & Black, H.R. (1998). Garlic powder and plasma lipids and lipoproteins: A multicenter, randomized, placebo-controlled trial. *Internal Medicine, 158*(11), 1189-1194.

Jellin, J.M., Batz, F., & Hitchens, K. (1999). *Pharmacist's letter/prescriber's letter natural medicines comprehensive database.* Stockton, CA: Therapeutic Research Faculty.

Johnson E.S., Kadam, N.P., Hylands, D.M., & Hylands, P.J. (1985). Efficacy of feverfew as a prophylactic treatment of migraine. *British Medical Journal, 291*, 569-573.

Journal of National Association of Registered Druggists. (1992). Real medicine or snake oil? *Journal of National Association of Registered Druggists, 115*(2), 17-20.

Katiyarr, S.K., Agarwal, R., & Mukhtar, H. (1996). Inhibition of tumor promotion in SENCAR mouse skin by ethanol extract of Zingiber officiale rhizomes. *Cancer Research, 56*(5), 1023-1030.

Katiyar, S.K., Agarwal, R., & Mukhtar, H. (1993). Protection against malignant conversion of chemically induced benign skin papillomas to squamous cell carcinomas in SENCAR mice by a polyphenolic fraction isolated from green tea. *Cancer Research, 53*(22), 5409-5412.

Khan, S.G., Katiyar, S.K., Agarwal, R., & Mukhtar, H. (1992). Enhancement of antioxidant and phase II enzymes by oral feeding of green tea polyphenols in drinking water to SKH-1 hairless mice: Possible role in cancer prevention. *Cancer Research, 52*(14), 4050-4052.

Kim, H., Chen, X., & Gillis, C.N. (1992). Ginsenosides protect pulmonary vascular endothelium against free radical–induced injury. *Biochemistry & Biophysiology Research Communication, 189*(2), 670-676.

Liebert, M.A. (1994). From the publisher: Introducing alternative & complementary therapies. *Alternative & Complementary Therapies, 1*(1), ix.

Lim J.H., Wen, T.C., Matsuda, S., Tanaka, J., Maeda, N., Peng, H., Aburaya, J., Ishihara, K., & Sakanaka, M. (1997). Protection of ischemic hippocampal neurons by ginsenoside Rb1, a main ingredient of ginseng root. *Neuroscience Research, 28*(3), 191-200.

Liu, C.X. & Xiao, P.G. (1992). Recent advances on ginseng research in China. *Journal of Ethnopharmacology, 36*(1), 27-38.

Linde, K., Ramirez, G., Mulrow, C.D., Pauls, A., & Weidenhammer, D.M. (1996). St. John's wort for depression: An overview and meta-analysis of randomised clinical trials. *British Medical Journal, 313*, 253-258.

Loew, D. (1999). Phytogenic drugs in heart diseases exemplified by Crataegus. *Wiener Medizinische Wochenschrift, 149*(8-10), 226-228.

Lumb, A.B. (1994). Effect of dried ginger on human platelet function. *Thrombosis & Haemostasis, 71*(1), 110-111.

McDowell, B. (1994). Institutional profile: The National Institutes of Health Office of Alternative Medicine: Evaluating research outcomes. *Alternative & Complementary Therapies, 1*(1), 17-25.

Melchart, D., Linde, K., Worku, F., Sarkady, L., Holzmann, M., Jurcic, K., & Wagner, H. (1995). Results of five randomized studies on the immunomodulary activity of preparation of Echinacea. *Journal of Alternative & Complementary Medicine, 1*(2), 145-160.

Miller, A.L. (1998). St. John's wort (Hypericum perforatum): Clinical effects on depression and other conditions. *Alternative Medicine Review, 3*(1), 18-26.

Murphy, J., Heptinstall, S., & Mitchell, J.R.A. (1989). Randomized, double-blind, placebo-controlled trial of feverfew in migraine prevention. *Lancet,* 2(8604), 189-192.

Nelson, L., Shih, R., & Hoffman, R. (1995). Aplastic anemia induced by an adulterated herbal medication. *Journal of Clinical Toxicology, 33*(5), 467-470.

Newall, C.A., Anderson, L.A., & Phillipson, J.D. (1996). *Herbal medicine: A guide for health care professionals.* London: The Pharmaceutic Press.

News you can use. (1995). *Alternative & Complementary Therapy, 1*(5), 342.

Nightingale, S.L. (1993). From the Food and Drug Administration: Public warning about herbal products. *JAMA, 269*(3), 328.

Oubre, A. (1995). Social context of complementary medicine in Western society. Part II: Traditional Chinese medicine and HIV illness. *Journal of Alternative & Complementary Medicine, 1*(2), 161-185.

Park, K.K., Chun, K.S. Lee, J.M., Less, S.S., & Surh, Y.J. (1998). Inhibitory effects of (6)-gingerol, a major pungent principle of ginger, on phorbol ester-induced inflammation, epidermal ornithine decarboxylase activity and skin tumor promotion in ICR. *Cancer Letters, 129*(2), 139-144.

Pattrick, M., Heptinstall, S., & Doherty, M. (1998). Feverfew in rheumatoid arthritis: A double-blind controlled study. *Annals of Rheumatic Disease, 48,* 547.

Petry, J.J. (1995). Garlic and postoperative bleeding. *Plastic Reconstructive Surgery, 95*(1), 213.

Phillips, S., Hutchinson, S., & Ruggier, R. (1994). Zingiber officinale does not affect gastric emptying rate: A randomised, placebo-controlled, crossover trial. *Anaesthesia, 48*(5), 393-395.

Phillips, S., Ruggier, R., & Hutchinson, S. (1993). Zingiber officinale (ginger)—an antiemetic for day case surgery. *Anaesthesia, 48*(8), 715-717.

Pizzorno, J.E. & Murray, M.T. (1985). *A textbook of natural medicine.* Seattle: John Bastyr College Publications.

Ravitzky, M. (1994). Valerian: Nature's antianxiety agent. *Alternative & Complementary Therapy, 1*(1), 48-49.

Saita, T., Katano, M., Matsunaga, H., Yamamoto, H., Fujito, H., & Mori, M. (1993). The first specific antibody against cytotoxic polyacetylenic alcohol, panaxynol. *Chemical & Pharmaceutical Bulletin, 41*(3), 549-552.

Scaglione, F., Cattaneo, G., Alessandria, M., & Cogo, R. (1996). Efficacy and safety of standardized Ginseng extract G115 for potentiating vaccination against influenza syndrome and protection against the common cold. *Drugs Under Experimental and Clinical Research, 22*(2), 165-172.

Sculti, L. (1994). Arthritis benefits from shark cartilage therapy. *Alternative & Complementary Therapy, 1*(1), 35-37.

See, D.M., Broumand, N., Sahl, L., & Tilles, J.C. (1997). In vitro effects of echinacea and ginseng on natural killer and antibody-dependent cell cytotoxicity in healthy subjects and chronic fatigue syndrome or acquired immunodeficiency syndrome patients. *Immunopharmacology, 35*(3), 229-235.

Sharma, S.S., Kochupillai, V., Gupta, S.K., Seth, S.D., & Gupta, Y.K. (1997). Antiemetic efficiency of ginger (Zingiber officinale) against cisplatin-induced emesis in dogs. *Journal of Ethnopharmacology, 57*(2), 93-96.

Smee, D.F., Sidwell, R.W., Huffman, J., Higgins, J.W., Kende, M., & Veobiscar, A.J. (1996). Antiviral activities of tragacanthin polysaccharides on Punta Toro virus infections in mice. *Chemotherapy, 42*(4), 286-293.

Snider, S. (1991). Beware the unknown brew: Herbal teas and toxicity. *FDA Consumer,* May, 31-33.

Sohn, H.O., Lim, H.B., Lee, Y.G., Lee, D.W., & Kim, Y.T. (1993). Effect of subchronic administration of antioxidants against cigarette smoke exposure in rats. *Archives of Toxicology, 67*(10), 667-673.

Song, Z., Johansen, H.K., Faber, V., Moser, C., Kharazini, A., Rygaard, J., & Hoiby, N. (1997). Ginseng treatment reduces bacterial load and lung pathology in chronic Pseudomonas aeruginosa pneumonia in rats. *Antimicrobial Agents & Chemotherapy, 41*(5), 961-964.

Stimpel, M.A., Proksch, A., Wagner, H., & Lohmann-Matthes, M.L. (1984). Macrophage activation and induction of macrophage cytotoxicity by purified polysaccharide fractions from the plant Echinacea purpurea. *Infection Immunology, 46*(3), 845-849.

Sun, X.B., Matsumoto, T., & Yamada, H. (1992). Anti-ulcer activity and mode of action of the polysaccharide fraction from the leaves of Panax ginseng. *Planta Medica, 58*(5), 432-435.

Tode, T., Kikuchi, Y., Hirata, J., Kita, T., Imazumi, E., & Nagata, I. (1993). Inhibitory effects by oral administration of ginsenoside Rh2 on the growth of human ovarian cancer cells in nude mice. *Journal of Cancer Research & Clinical Oncology, 120*(1-2), 24-26.

Tomoda, M., Hirabayashi, K., Shimizu, N., Gonda, R., Ohara N., & Takada, K. (1993). Characterization of two acidic polysaccharides having immunological activities from the root of Panax ginseng. *Biological & Pharmaceutical Bulletin, 16*(1), 22-25.

Tyler, V.E. (1993). *The honest herbal* (3rd ed.). New York: Pharmaceutical Products Press.

Vinson, J.A. & Dabbagh, Y.A. (1998). Effect of green and black tea supplementation on lipids, lipid oxidation and fibrinogen in the hamster: Mechanisms for the epidemiological benefits of tea drinking. *Federation of European Biochemical Societies Letters, 433*(1-2), 44-46.

Vorberg, G. (1985). *Gingko biloba* extract (GBE): A long-term study on chronic cerebral insufficiency in geriatric patients. *Clinical Trials Journal, 22,* 149-157.

Wang, Z.Y., Huang, M.T., Lou, Y.R., Xie, J.G., Reuhl, K.P., Newmark, H.L., Ho, C.T., Yang, C.S., & Conney, A.H. (1994). Inhibitory effects of black tea, green tea, decaffeinated black tea, and decaffeinated green tea on ultraviolet B light-induced skin carcinogenesis in 7,12-dimethylbenz[a]anthracene-initiated SKH-1 mice. *Cancer Research, 54*(13), 3428-3435.

Wang, Z.Y., Hong, J.Y., Huang, M.T., Reuhl, K.R., Conney, A.H., & Yang, C.S. (1992a). Inhibition of N-nitrosodiethylamine- and 4-(methylnitroamino)-1-(3-pyridyl)-1-butanone-induced tumorigenesis in A/J mice by green tea and black tea. *Cancer Research, 52*(7), 1943-1947.

Wang, Z.Y., Huang, M.T., Ho, C.T., Chang, R., Ma, W., Ferrero, T., Reuhl, K.R., Yang, C.S., & Conney, A.H. (1992b). Inhibitory effect of green tea on the growth of established skin papillomas in mice. *Cancer Research, 52*(23), 6657-6665.

Warshafsky, S., Kamer, R.S., & Sivak, S.L. (1993). Effect of garlic on total serum cholesterol: A meta-analysis. *Annals of Internal Medicine, 119*(7 Pt 1), 599-605.

Watanabe, H., Ohta, H., Imamura, L., Asakura, W., Matoba, Y., & Matsumoto, K. (1991). Effect of Panax ginseng on age-related changes in the spontaneous motor activity and dopaminergic nervous system in the rat. *Japanese Journal of Pharmacology, 55*(1), 51-56.

Weil, A. (1995). *Spontaneous healing: How to discover and enhance your body's natural ability to maintain and heal itself.* New York: Alfred A. Knopf.

Wheatley, D. (1997). LI 160, an extract of St. John's wort, versus amitriptyline in mildly to moderately depressed outpatients: A controlled 5-week clinical study. *Pharmacopsychiatry, 30*(Suppl 2), 77-80.

Wood, C.D. et al. (1988). Comparison of efficacy of ginger with various antimotion sickness drugs. *Clinical Research Practitioners Drug Regulatory Affairs, 6*, 129-136.

Xiaoguang, C., Hongyan, L., Xiaohong, L., Zhaodi, F., Yan, L., Lihua, T., & Rui, H. (1998). Cancer chemopreventive and therapeutic activities of red ginseng. *Journal of Ethnopharmacology, 60*(1), 71-78.

Xu, Y., Ho, C.T., Amin, S.G., Han, C., & Chung, F.L. (1992). Inhibition of tobacco-specific nitrosamine-induced lung tumorigenesis in A/J mice by green tea and its major polyphenol as antioxidants. *Cancer Research, 52*(14), 3875-3879.

Yang, T.T. & Koo, M.W. (1997). Hypocholesterolemic effects of Chinese tea. *Pharmacological Research, 35*(6), 505-512.

Yang, C.S. & Wang, Z.Y. (1993). Tea and cancer. *Journal of the National Cancer Institute, 85*(13), 1038-1049.

Yoshida, Y., Wang, M.Q., Liu, J.N., Shan, B.E., & Yamashite, J. (1997). Immunomodulating activity of Chinese medicinal herbs and Oldenlandia diffuse in particular. *International Journal of Immunopharmacology, 19*(7), 359-370.

Yun, T.K. & Choi, S.Y. (1995). Preventive effect of ginseng intake against various human cancers: A case-control study on 1987 pairs. *Cancer Epidemiological Biomarkers & Previews, 4*(4), 401-408.

Zi, X. & Agarwal, R. (1999). Silibinin decreases prostate-specific antigen with cell growth inhibition via G1 arrest, leading to differentiation of prostate carcinoma cells: implications for prostate cancer intervention. *Proceedings of the National Academy of Sciences of the United States of America, 96*(13), 7490-7495.

Zi, X., Feyes, D.K., & Agarwal, R. (1998). Anticarcinogenic effect of a flavonoid antioxidant, silymarin, in human breast cancer cells MDA-MB 468: induction of G1 arrest through an increase in Cip1/p21 concomitant with a decrease in kinase activity of cyclin-dependent kinases and associated cyclins. *Clinical Cancer Research, 4*(4), 1055-1064.

Zi, X., Grasso, A.W., Kung, H.J., & Agarwal, R. (1998). A flavonoid antioxidant, silymarin, inhibits activation of erbB1 signaling and induces cyclin-dependent kinase inhibitors, G1 arrest, and anticarcinogenic effects in human prostate carcinoma DU145 cells. *Cancer Research, 58*(9), 1920-1929.

13 Overview of the Central Nervous System

Chapter Focus

The nervous system coordinates all body functions, and its activities allow the individual to adapt to the internal and external environment. Because of the complexity of this system, the monitoring of pharmacologic interventions can be challenging. Knowledge of the anatomy and physiology of the central nervous system provides a foundation for sound clinical decision making in this area.

Learning Objectives

1. Identify the major components of the central nervous system.
2. Describe the functions of the components of the central nervous system.
3. Identify the structure and function of the blood-brain barrier.
4. Describe three major functional systems of the central nervous system.
5. Describe the function of the common neurotransmitter substances.

Key Terms

acetylcholine, p. 254
blood-brain barrier, p. 252
brainstem, p. 250
catecholamines, p. 254
cerebellum, p. 250
cerebrum, p. 248
endorphins, p. 254
extrapyramidal system, p. 253
hypothalamus, p. 249
limbic system, p. 253
midbrain, p. 250
neurons, p. 251
pons, p. 250
reticular activating system, p. 253
synapse, p. 251
thalamus, p. 249

The nervous system consists of the central nervous system (CNS) and the peripheral nervous system (PNS) (Figure 13-1). The PNS is discussed in Chapter 20. This chapter reviews the primary areas of the CNS and focuses on the specific areas affected by drug therapy.

The CNS is composed of the brain and spinal cord and essentially controls all functions in the body. When a drug is described as having a central action, it means that it has an action on the brain or the spinal cord. The PNS is the network that transmits information to and from the CNS and alerts the CNS to internal and external changes such as muscle tension, blood vessel alterations, pain, fever, sound, smell, taste, touch, and sight. This information is integrated, and instructions are then relayed to the appropriate cells or tissues for producing the necessary actions and environmental adjustments. Information concerning these actions and adjustments is fed back into the CNS. This constant feeding of information into the CNS permits continuous adjustments in the instructions sent to various tissues to ensure effective control of body functions.

BRAIN

The brain can be physically divided in various ways. A simplified approach is to divide it into its major components—cerebrum, thalamus, pineal body, hypothalamus, midbrain, pons, medulla oblongata, and cerebellum (Figure 13-2). The following sections discuss the major areas of the brain affected by specific drug therapies.

Cerebrum. The **cerebrum,** the largest and uppermost section of the brain, is the highest functional area of the brain. Memory storage and sensory, integrative, emotional, language, and motor functions are controlled in this area. The cerebrum consists of two hemispheres (right and left) and the corpus callosum, the nerve tissues that connect the right and left hemispheres. The outer surface of the cerebrum is the cerebral cortex or gray matter of the brain; this surface covers the four lobes into which each hemisphere is divided. These lobes are named for the bones of the skull under which they lie—frontal, parietal, occipital, and temporal. The frontal lobe contains the motor and speech areas. The sensory cortex is located in the parietal lobe, the visual cortex in the occipital lobe, and the auditory cortex in the temporal lobe. Association areas lie near these lobes and act in conjunction with them. In addition, large parts of the cortex are concerned with higher mental activity—reasoning, creative thought, judgment, and memory. These attributes are unique to humans and separate them from other animals.

Drugs that depress cortical activity may decrease the acuity of sensation and perception, inhibit motor activity, decrease alertness and concentration, and even promote drowsiness and sleep. Drugs that stimulate the cortical areas

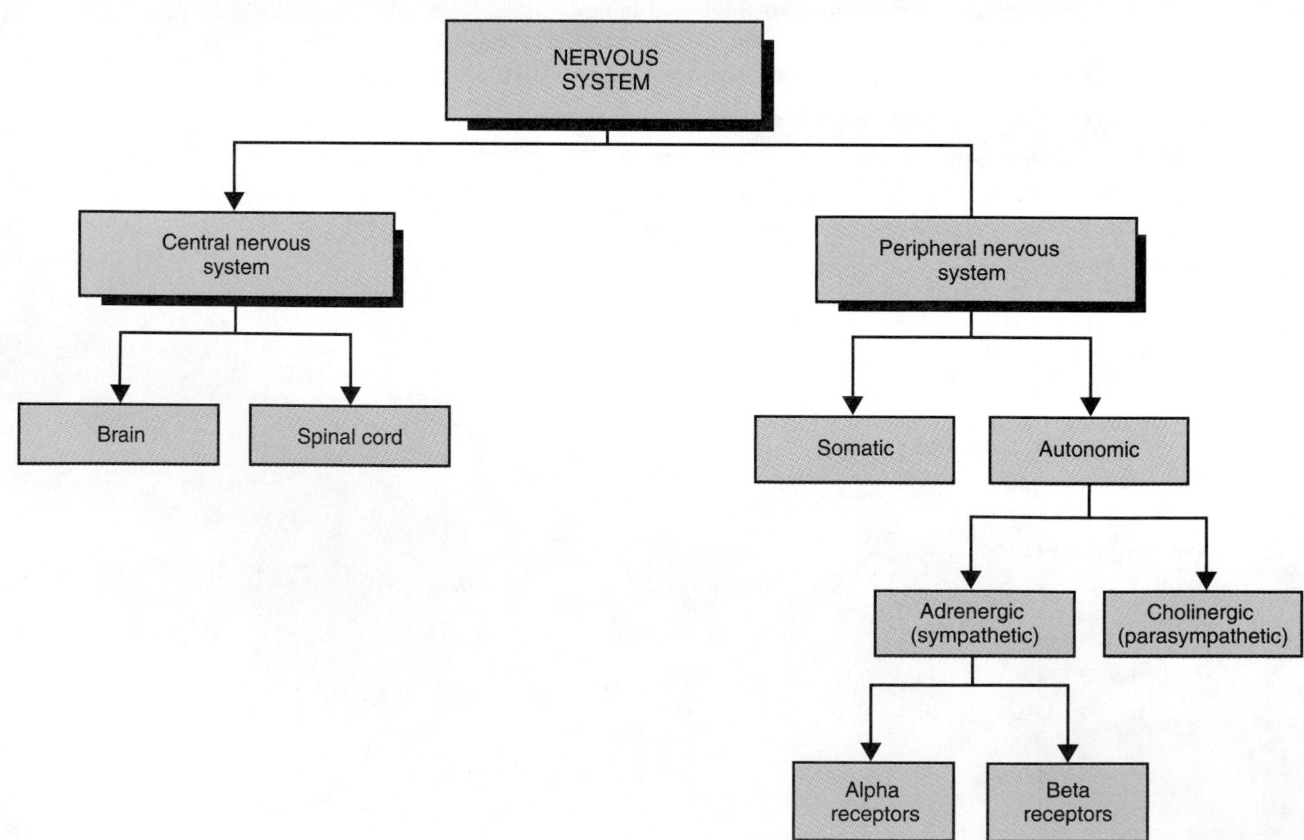

Figure 13-1 Overview of the nervous system.

may cause more vivid impulses to be received and greater awareness of the surrounding environment. Increased muscle activity and restlessness may also occur. The specific response brought forth by a drug depends to a large extent on the personality of the individual, his or her emotional and physiologic state, the specific attributes of the drug, and a host of other factors.

Thalamus. The **thalamus** is composed of sensory nuclei and serves as the major relay center for impulses to and from the cerebral cortex. It also registers sensations such as pain, temperature, touch, and other sensory impulses and relays this information to the cerebrum.

The thalamus enables the individual to have impressions of pleasantness or unpleasantness, and it also appears to play a part (with the reticular activating system) in arousal or alerting signals. (See Reticular Activating System, p. 253.) Drugs that depress cells in various portions of the thalamus may interrupt the free flow of impulses to the cerebral cortex. This is one way in which pain may be relieved.

Pineal Body. The pineal body resembles a small pinecone and appears to be involved in regulating the human body's biological clock. It also produces hormones, such as melatonin. The secretion of melatonin is inhibited by sunlight and has been related to sleep and mood disorders.

Hypothalamus. The **hypothalamus** provides a major link between the mind and the body. It lies below the thalamus and is vital for maintaining many body functions and the well-being of the individual. Functions of the hypothalamus include regulation of body temperature, carbohydrate and fat metabolism, and water balance; it is also believed that the appetite center and pleasure or reward centers are located here. There is evidence that a center for sleep and wakefulness also exists within the hypothalamus. Some of the sleep-producing drugs are thought to depress hypothalamic centers.

As part of its integrative role in neurohormonal regulation, neurons in the hypothalamus release hormones that affect the anterior pituitary gland. Growth hormone, hormones that affect sexual glands or functions, thyroid hormones, and the adrenal cortex hormones are under the control of the hypothalamus.

The hypothalamus, along with other specific areas of the brain, is also involved with the control of emotions. Drugs may affect these functions of the hypothalamus. An example is the use of antidepressants to treat the symptoms of depression. The action of tricyclic antidepressants on the hypothalamus often reverses the symptoms of weight loss, anorexia, decreased libido, and insomnia associated with

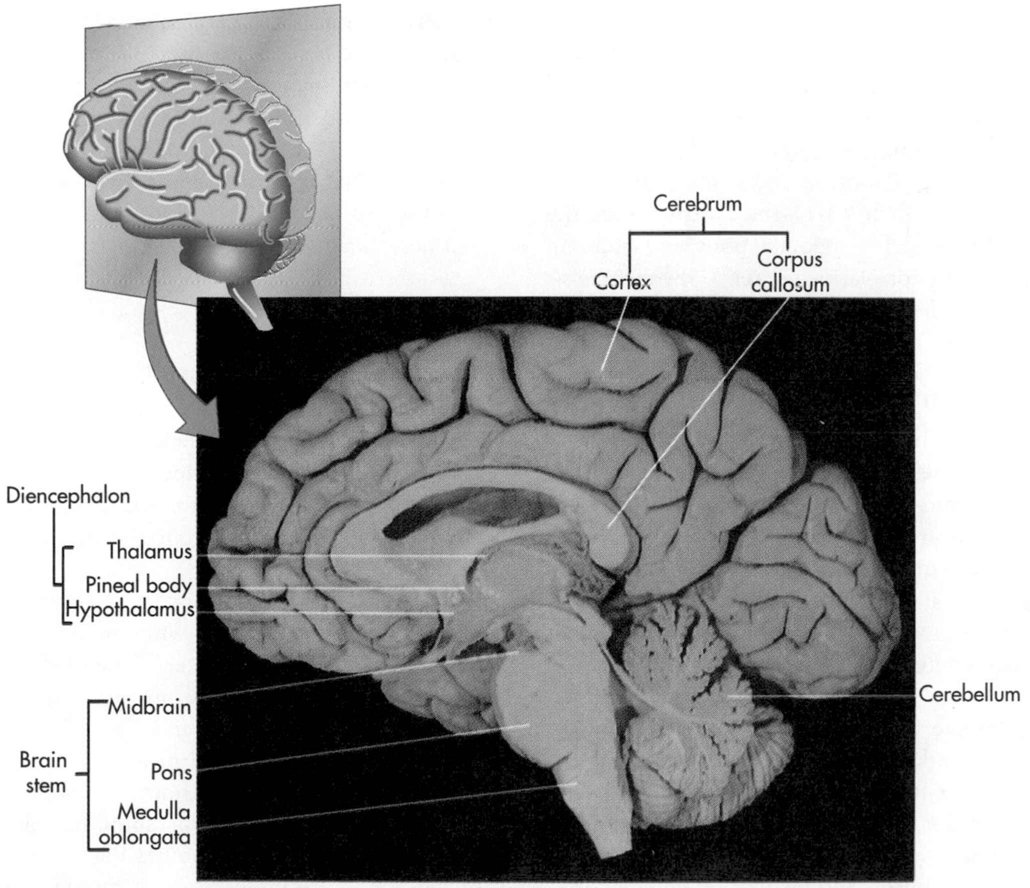

Figure 13-2 Divisions of the brain. (From Patton, K.T., & Thibodeau, G.A. [2000]. *The human body in health and disease* [2nd ed.]. St. Louis: Mosby.)

TABLE 13-1 Cranial Nerves

Cranial Nerve	Type of Nerve	Function*
I Olfactory	Sensory	Smell
II Optic	Sensory	Sight
III Oculomotor	Motor	Movement of eye and eyelid muscles, pupillary constriction
IV Trochlear	Motor	Eye muscle movement for downward and inward motion of eye
V Trigeminal	Motor	Chewing, lateral jaw movement
	Sensory	Sensations of the face, scalp, oral cavity, teeth, and tongue
VI Abducens	Motor	Eye movements
VII Facial	Motor	Facial expressions
	Sensory	Taste
VIII Acoustic	Sensory	Hearing, equilibrium
IX Glossopharyngeal	Motor	Swallowing, salivation
	Sensory	Taste, throat sensations
X Vagus	Motor	Voice production, swallowing, decrease in heartbeat, increased peristalsis
	Sensory	Gag reflex; sensations of throat, larynx, and abdominal viscera
XI Spinal accessory	Motor	Head and shoulder movements
XII Hypoglossal	Motor	Tongue movements

*Drug effects, toxicity, or both have been reported to affect various cranial nerve functions. For example, ototoxicity (damage to cranial nerve VIII) has been reported with aminoglycoside antibiotics. Vincristine, an antineoplastic agent, may produce ptosis (cranial nerve III), trigeminal neuralgia (cranial nerve VII), facial palsy (cranial nerve V), and jaw pain. Because various medications have the potential to affect the cranial nerves adversely, students should be familiar with the functions of the cranial nerves.

depression. Other psychotherapeutic agents may cause a number of hypothalamic side effects, including breast engorgement, lactation, amenorrhea, appetite stimulation, and alterations in temperature regulation.

Brainstem. The **brainstem** is composed of the midbrain, pons, and medulla oblongata and is the source of 10 of the 12 cranial nerves (Table 13-1); the exceptions are the olfactory and optic nerves. The medulla, pons, and midbrain contain many important correlation centers (gray matter), as well as ascending and descending pathways (white matter). The **midbrain** contains nerve tracts to and from the cerebrum and serves as a relay station from higher areas of the brain to lower centers. It is the source of the third (oculomotor) and fourth (trochlear) cranial nerves; some optic fibers are also located here. The **pons** is the source of the fifth, sixth, seventh, and eighth cranial nerves. It also contains a center that controls involuntary respiratory regulation. Drugs also affect the midbrain and pons as the reticular activating system is stimulated or depressed. The medulla oblongata contains the vital centers: the respiratory, vasomotor, and cardiac centers. Such centers are referred to as vital because they are necessary for survival. Other essential functions also originate here, such as vomiting, hiccuping, sneezing, coughing, and swallowing reflexes.

If the respiratory center is stimulated by a drug, it will discharge an increased number of nerve impulses over nerve pathways to the muscles of respiration. If it is depressed, it will discharge fewer impulses, and respiration will be correspondingly affected. Other centers in the medulla that respond to certain drugs are the cough center and the vomiting center.

Cerebellum. The **cerebellum,** located in the posterior cranial fossa behind the brainstem, contains centers for muscle coordination, equilibrium, and muscle tone. It receives afferent impulses from the vestibular nuclei and the cerebrum, and it plays an important role in the maintenance of posture and voluntary muscular activity. Drugs that disturb the cerebellum or vestibular branch of the eighth cranial nerve cause dizziness and loss of equilibrium.

SPINAL CORD

The spinal cord, a center for reflex activity, also functions in the transmission of impulses to and from the higher centers in the brain and may be affected by the action of drugs. Ascending sensory tracts conduct impulses up from the peripheral nerves to the brain, and descending motor tracts conduct impulses down from the brain to the peripheral nerves.

A cross section of the spinal cord reveals an internal mass of gray matter enclosed by white matter (Figure 13-3). The butterfly-shaped gray matter is divided into sections, or horns; the afferent (sensory) nerve fibers are located in the dorsal or posterior horn, and the efferent (motor) nerve fibers exit from the ventral or anterior horn. When a pain impulse reaches the dorsal horn, the impulse is transmitted along special tracts (lateral spinothalamic tract) to the thalamus, which then distributes the message to other areas of the brain. The brain responds by means of the descending efferent fiber pathways to inhibit or modify other incoming pain stimuli. (See Chapter 14 for further discussion of the gate control theory.) Small doses of spinal stimulants

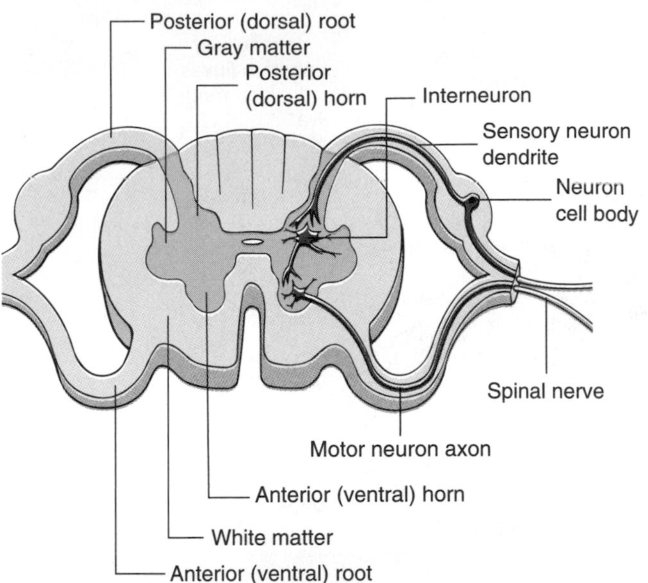

Figure 13-3 Cross section of the spinal cord.

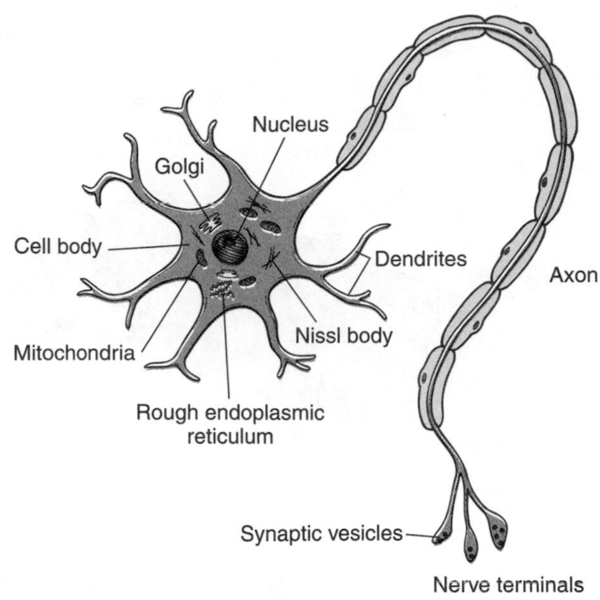

Figure 13-4 Structural components of neurons.

may increase reflex excitability; larger doses may cause convulsions.

CELL TYPES

The two major cell types in the CNS are glial cells and neurons. The functions of the glial cells are not fully understood, but recent studies indicate they are composed of many types of neurotransmitter receptors and ion channels. It is possible that this type of network serves to support and assist neurons in the transfer and integration of information in the CNS (Wingard, 1991).

Neurons have four basic parts: dendrites, cell body, axon, and axon or nerve terminals (Figure 13-4). The cell body contains the nucleus (genetic information) and the ribosomes, Nissl substance, and endoplasmic reticulum necessary for protein synthesis. The Golgi complex stores, processes, and concentrates the protein, and the mitochondria in the cell body and dendrites provide the production of energy necessary for protein synthesis and lipid metabolism.

Dendrites also contain some neurotransmitter vesicles; thus incoming messages from other neurons are received in the dendrites, processed in the cell body, transported in the axon, and exit via the axon terminal. This process of conveying messages from one cell body to another usually involves electrical or chemical transport of the message across a **synapse,** the junction point between neurons or between a neuron and an effector organ. Most information transmitted in the CNS is the result of alterations in electrical currents. The following paragraphs provide a brief summary of this process; more detailed information can be found in a current anatomy and physiology text.

The electrical properties of nerve cells are generated by various ions, pumps, and channels located in the cell membrane. A nerve cell in the resting state is illustrated in Figure 13-5. A membrane difference or potential is caused by changes in the concentration of sodium, potassium, and chloride ions. Pumps are capable of actively moving charged ions from one side of the membrane to the other side, and channels are membrane pores that allow specific ions to pass from one side of the membrane to the other.

In the resting state, sodium and chloride are found in large amounts outside the cell, and potassium is in high concentration inside the cell. These concentration gradients (the resting membrane potential) are stabilized and maintained by the sodium-potassium ATPase (adenosinetriphosphatase) pump, which trades three sodium ions from the intracellular fluid for two potassium ions from the extracellular fluid. The movement and concentration of these ions in and around the cell are the primary determinants that affect the membrane potential of the nerve cells.

During rest or after an electrical potential, potassium ions selectively flow to outside the nerve cell, which allows sodium (positive ions) to enter the nerve cell. This action alters or reduces the membrane potential; as the sodium influx increases, the cell depolarizes. Depolarization results in the opening of more sodium channels; this allows more sodium to flow into the cell and causes further depolarization of the nerve cell. This reduction in membrane potential generates an action potential as a result of the changes illustrated in Figure 13-6.

Drugs can act directly on the ion channel or via receptors that affect ion channels. For example, general anesthetics and ethanol bind to specific receptors, which effectively reduces sodium influx to prevent regeneration of action potentials and conduction of nerve impulses. The action of the sodium-potassium pump on cardiac cells is discussed in the cardiac glycoside section in Chapter 25.

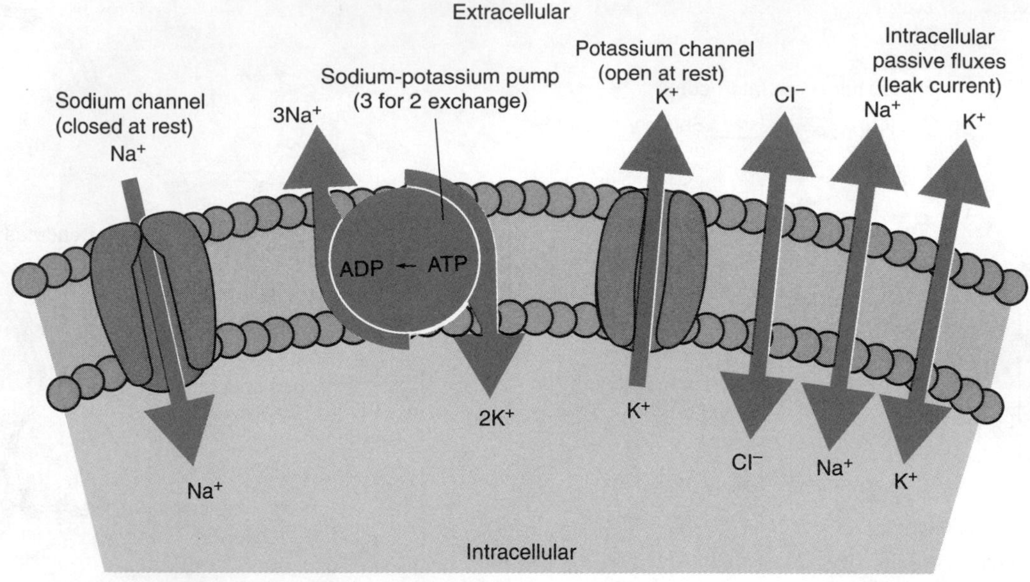

Figure 13-5 A nerve cell in the resting state.

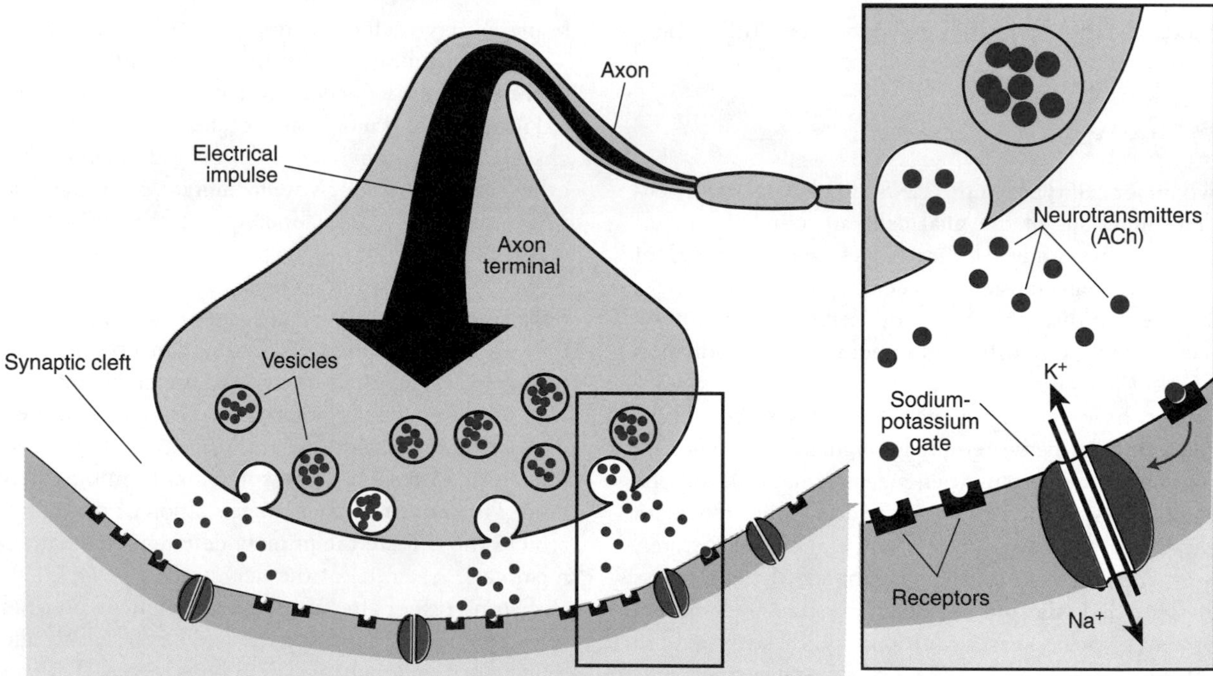

Figure 13-6 Nerve cell depolarization. In the resting state, intracellular sodium concentration is lower than extracellular sodium concentration; this gradient is regulated by the sodium-potassium ATPase pump. Electrical impulses release neurotransmitters that alter the membrane potential of the nerve cell. The sodium-potassium gate opens during cell depolarization, resulting in an increased influx of sodium ions into the cell. The sodium channels are inactivated (gate is closed) to start the beginning of the repolarization phase. (See text for further information.)

BLOOD-BRAIN BARRIER

The **blood-brain barrier** is actually a covering of nerve cells (astrocytes) that encircle the capillary walls of the brain. This covering prevents the passage of many drugs or large molecules into the brain, but it does allow small molecules (e.g., water, alcohol, oxygen, and carbon dioxide), glucose, gases, and lipid-soluble substances to penetrate. Such selective processing allows the brain a degree of security against the toxic effects of some drugs on the CNS. However, the permeation of such substances across the blood-brain barrier increases with large doses or in instances of meningeal inflammation. Current research is studying methods to increase the permeability of the blood-brain barrier to specific therapeutic agents, such as antibiotics or antineoplastic agents needed to treat a localized brain infection or brain tumors.

FUNCTIONAL SYSTEMS OF THE CENTRAL NERVOUS SYSTEM

The three major functional systems of the CNS that are affected by select drug or chemical administration are (1) the reticular activating system, (2) the limbic system, and (3) the extrapyramidal system.

Reticular Activating System. The **reticular activating system (RAS)** is a diffuse system of nuclei in the brainstem that permits two-way communication among the spinal cord, thalamus, and cerebral cortex. The following are the primary functions of the RAS:

1. A consciousness and arousal effect
2. An alerting mechanism
3. A filter process that allows for concentration

When stimulated, the gray matter of the pons and the midbrain transmits impulses to the thalamus, which further transmits the impulse to various areas of the cerebral cortex. This results in consciousness or awakening and possibly an arousal effect. Arousal reactions require an external signal, such as a pain stimulus, an alarm clock, or bright lights. The cerebral cortex may signal the RAS or vice versa, but the end result is activation of both areas that may lead to the additional transmission of impulses throughout the body (e.g., skeletal muscle activation). Inactivation of the RAS results in sleep, whereas injury or disease may produce a lack of consciousness or a comatose state.

The primary function of the alerting mechanism is self-preservation (e.g., waking up at night because of a chilly sensation). Once awakened, the individual can assess the situation and discover the reason for awakening, such as the blanket on the bed having fallen to the floor. In this situation the sensation of feeling chilly has activated the RAS and caused the awakening, but the situation must be assessed to determine why the chilliness occurred.

The filter mechanism of the RAS allows for a decrease in the perception of monotonous stimuli that usually surrounds everyone. It permits an individual to concentrate on a specific stimulus at a given time. For example, at a large party where nearly everyone is talking at the same time, a functioning RAS allows an individual to focus on a single conversation or person of interest by filtering out all other conversations. In other words, it permits selective concentration.

Many drugs act on the RAS. Anesthetics dampen its activity and induce sleep, whereas amphetamines stimulate or activate it. Lysergic acid diethylamide (LSD), and certain other hallucinogenic agents may act on the RAS by interfering with its ability to filter out stimuli; a person taking this substance is therefore bombarded by all types of wanted and sometimes unwanted stimuli. In contrast, it is a proposed theory that chlorpromazine (Thorazine) stimulates the activity of the RAS and reinstates the activity of the filtering process, thus making it useful for reducing hallucinations in clients who are psychotic and in individuals experiencing an untoward reaction to LSD.

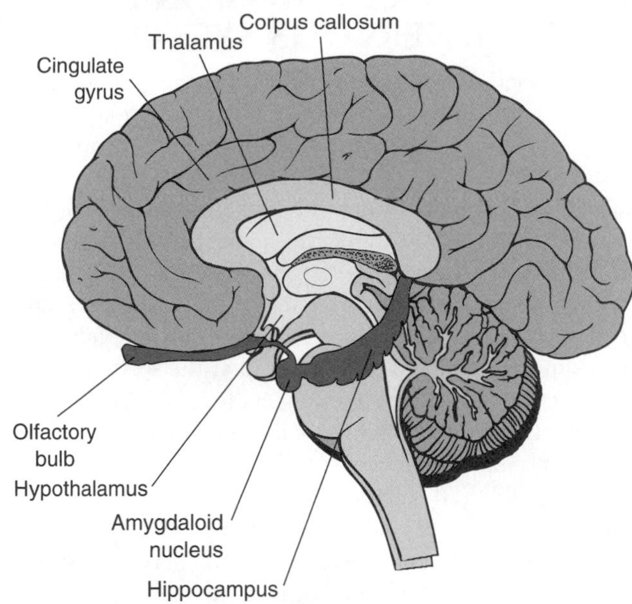

Figure 13-7 The limbic system.

Limbic System. The **limbic system** is a border of subcortical structures that surround the corpus callosum (Figure 13-7). This system forms a ring around the top of the brain stem and consists of the portions of the brain remaining after the cerebral hemispheres and cerebellum have been removed.

The limbic system is extremely complex in its functioning. The emotions of anger, fear, anxiety, sexual feelings, pleasure, and sorrow are related to the limbic system. It may work with or inhibit other parts of the brain such as the ce rebral cortex, brainstem, or hypothalamus to normalize expressions of emotions, influence their ultimate expression to other than normal, or affect the biologic rhythms, sexual behavior, and motivation of an individual. Learning and memory have been associated with the hippocampus, a component of this system.

Drugs that affect the limbic system are the benzodiazepines, meprobamate, and morphine. The benzodiazepines and meprobamate (Miltown) are believed to suppress the limbic system, which prevents it from stimulating the reticular activating system and thus results in drowsiness and sleep, especially in clients with anxiety. Morphine is thought to alter subjective reactions to pain in addition to abolishing pain stimuli received by special areas within the limbic system.

Extrapyramidal System. The **extrapyramidal system** is a somatic motor pathway located in the CNS that affects skeletal muscles. This system is associated with posture and the coordination of muscle group movements. Antipsychotic agents that block dopamine receptors may produce side effects or adverse reactions related to this system. (See Chapter 19 for further discussion of these effects.)

SYNAPTIC TRANSMISSION IN THE CENTRAL NERVOUS SYSTEM

As mentioned previously, the synapse is the junction point between two neurons or between a neuron and an effector organ. There is evidence that the transmission of impulses at synapses in the CNS is humoral, occurring through a neurotransmitter secretion. When a neurotransmitter is released, it either stimulates or inhibits the activity of the postsynaptic neurons.

Inhibition of motor neuron activity may be presynaptic or postsynaptic. Studies indicate that presynaptic inhibition occurs in the brain and is widespread at the spinal level, affecting transmission in afferent fibers from skin and muscle. The function of presynaptic inhibition is probably to suppress weak inputs that would otherwise cause unnecessary responses. With this modulation of nerve impulses, less transmitter substance is liberated. The net effect is a limiting or "inhibiting" of impulses to postsynaptic nerve fibers. Inhibition is important for orderly function.

Postsynaptic inhibition may be the result of changes in the membrane permeability of the postsynaptic cells caused by the release of chemical transmitters from presynaptic nerve endings. Upper motor neurons are scattered throughout the cerebral cortex, and a number of them are located in the motor cortex. Approximately three fourths of the nerve fibers from these motor neurons cross to the opposite side at the level of the medulla, descend to the spinal cord, and synapse with interneurons, which in turn synapse with the lower motor neurons. Almost all motor neurons of one side are controlled by the motor cortex of the other side. Therefore injury to the motor cortex of the right side of the brain causes paralysis on the left side of the body (left hemiplegia). Although systems other than the upper and lower motor neuron systems are concerned with voluntary movement, the lower motor neurons form the common final pathway for stimuli for voluntary movement.

Some of the neurotransmitters that are discussed in the following sections are acetylcholine, the catecholamines (dopamine, norepinephrine, and epinephrine), serotonin, and neuroactive peptides (enkephalins, endorphins, and dynorphins).

Acetylcholine. **Acetylcholine** is the best known chemical transmitter of nerve impulses. Not all parts of the CNS contain acetylcholine. Areas with high concentrations of acetylcholine are the motor cortex, thalamus, hypothalamus, and anterior spinal roots; very low concentrations are found in the cerebellum, optic nerves, and dorsal roots of the spine. Acetylcholine can cause cardiac inhibition, vasodilation, gastrointestinal peristalsis, and other parasympathetic effects.

The lower motor neurons release acetylcholine at the neuromuscular junction, causing contraction in striated (voluntary) muscle. The concentration of acetylcholine must be high because a large number of muscle fibers must respond synchronously for striated muscle contraction to occur and because acetylcholine is very rapidly destroyed by the enzyme cholinesterase.

Catecholamines and Related Substances. Dopamine, norepinephrine, and epinephrine (which are neurotransmitters of the **catecholamine** subclass, a group of sympathomimetic compounds) and the amine neurotransmitter serotonin (5-hydroxytryptamine) are synthesized, stored, and metabolized in the brain. They act directly on sympathetic effector cells by binding to receptors. These substances do not easily penetrate the blood-brain barrier, but their precursors do. The effect of injected catecholamines on the CNS is slight in comparison with the effect on the autonomic nervous system. An increase in catecholamines and serotonin causes cerebral stimulation. Drugs such as reserpine that release catecholamines and reduce amine concentration in the brain have a depressing or sedative action. Methyldopa lowers the levels of serotonin and norepinephrine; this, too, has a cerebral depressing effect.

Special staining techniques indicate that there are adrenergic (sympathomimetic) and serotoninergic tracts within the CNS. Dopamine is especially concentrated in the basal ganglia. The low level of dopamine at this site in individuals suffering from Parkinson's disease led to the use of its precursor, L-dopa, as a therapeutic approach; in many cases the results have been good.

Neuroactive Peptides. Neuroactive peptides may be considered neuromodulators, neurohormones, or neurotransmitters. Studies indicate that a peptide may affect neuronal activity by increasing or decreasing the synthesis, release, or breakdown of neurotransmitters, neurohormones, or neuromodulators. The parenteral or intracerebral injection of these components causes potent behavioral effects. A number of these peptides exist in tissues other than the CNS, primarily in the cells of the gastrointestinal tract.

Enkephalins, endorphins, and dynorphins are three major polypeptides that are found in the brain and have opioid activity. The concept of internal opiates or natural painkillers developed after studies indicated that enkephalins may bind to the same neuroreceptor membranes as morphine. Enkephalins behave as inhibitory neurotransmitters, allowing modification and control of the perception and emotional aspect of pain. To do this, enkephalins may block opiate receptors in the dorsal horn of the spinal cord by blocking the release of substance P. Substance P, a transmitter of pain impulses in the nerve fibers, has been proposed to be a transmitter for the primary afferent sensory fibers.

Endorphin (from "endogenous morphine") is a general term that includes many peptides in the brain that suppress pain. These peptides are also found in the pituitary gland, the intermediate lobe, and the corticotropin cells of the adenohypophysis. Subgroups of endorphins have been isolated and identified, including beta-endorphin, an analgesic substance that is much more potent than enkephalin.

Technology has shown that the brain, pituitary gland, and gastrointestinal tract each have enkephalins and beta-endorphins. These peptides are not found in the same cells. The brain cells containing beta-endorphin are different from those that contain enkephalins.

Dynorphin is an endorphin found in the pituitary gland, hypothalamus, and spinal cord. It is the most potent pain-relieving substance discovered; dynorphin is 50 times more potent than beta-endorphin and 200 times more potent than morphine.

Naloxone, a potent opioid antagonist, reverses the analgesic effect of narcotics. Animal studies demonstrate that if naloxone is administered after enkephalins or endorphins are given, the analgesic effect produced by the polypeptides will be reversed. Endorphin release in the body is higher after acupuncture and transcutaneous electrical nerve stimulation, and both effects may be reversed by the use of naloxone.

It has been proposed that the analgesic response associated with the use of a placebo may result from an increased release of endorphins in the body. From peptide research may come pain relievers with fewer side effects and minimal to no addiction potential. An increased understanding of mental disorders and addiction mechanisms may also be gained from this research.

SUMMARY

The CNS is composed of the brain and the spinal cord and essentially controls all of the functions of the body. The CNS integrates information received from the peripheral nervous system concerning the internal and external environment of the body and then sends messages to produce the adjustments necessary for maintaining homeostasis.

The cerebrum is the highest functional area of the brain. Drugs that affect the cerebral cortex may decrease mental acuity, consciousness, and motor function by their depressive action or increase muscle activity and restlessness through their stimulating effects. The thalamus relays impulses to the cerebral cortex and also registers pain, temperature, touch, and other sensory impulses. The hypothalamus is a major link between the nervous system and the endocrine system. The origins of 10 of the 12 cranial nerves and the involuntary respiratory center are found in the brainstem.

The RAS, limbic system, and extrapyramidal system are the three major functional systems of the CNS. The RAS is responsible for consciousness, filtering, and alerting to stimuli; the limbic system, for learning and memory and for the emotions of anger, fear, anxiety, pleasure, and sorrow; and the extrapyramidal system, for muscle coordination.

The passage of many drugs into the brain is prohibited by the blood-brain barrier. The respiratory centers, as well as the centers for coughing and vomiting in the brainstem, are highly sensitive to drugs. Medications that disturb the cerebellum cause dizziness and loss of balance. Drugs may also affect the spinal cord, which transmits impulses to and from the brain. The RAS, limbic system, and extrapyramidal system may also be affected by medications.

Neurotransmitters affect the postsynaptic neurons to increase or decrease their activity. The most important of the neurotransmitters are acetylcholine, the catecholamines, serotonin, and the neuroactive peptides. Neurobiologic research is currently demonstrating the increasing importance of understanding more about these substances and, in general, the CNS.

Critical Thinking Questions

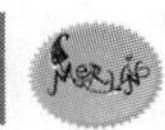

1. Harry Green was accidentally struck on the head with a golf club and became unconscious. When he regained consciousness, he was unable to recall what had occurred during the 15 minutes before he was struck. Why could that occur?
2. Delores Lightfoot sustained a head injury in an automobile accident. The physician suspects there may be injury to the cerebellum. What symptoms would Delores most likely exhibit if there were cerebellar injury?
3. How do neurotransmitters function in synaptic transmission?

Collaborative Learning Activities

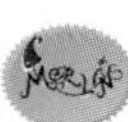

For Collaborative Learning Activities, go to mosby.com/MERLIN/McKenry/.

BIBLIOGRAPHY

Anderson, K.N., Anderson, L.E., & Glanz, W.D. (Eds.) (1998). *Mosby's medical, nursing & allied health dictionary* (5th ed.). St. Louis: Mosby.

Barker, E. (1994). *Neuroscience nursing*. St. Louis: Mosby.

Katzung, B.G. (1997). *Basic & clinical pharmacology* (6th ed.). Norwalk, CT: Appleton & Lange.

McCance, K.L. & Huether, S.E. (1998). *Pathophysiology: The biological basis for disease in adults and children* (3rd ed.). St. Louis: Mosby.

Melmon, K.L., Morrelli, H.F., Hoffman, B.B., & Nierenberg, D.W. (Eds.) (1992). *Melmon and Morrelli's Clinical pharmacology: Basic principles in therapeutics* (3rd ed.). New York: McGraw-Hill.

Seeley, R.R., Stephens, T.D., & Tate, P. (1996). *Anatomy and physiology* (3rd ed.). St. Louis: Mosby.

Thibodeau, G.A. & Patton, K. (1999). *Anatomy and physiology* (4th ed.). St. Louis: Mosby.

Van Wynsberghe, D., Noback, C.R., & Carola, R. (1995). *Human anatomy and physiology* (3rd ed.). New York: McGraw-Hill.

Wingard, L.B. et al. (1991). *Human pharmacology*. St. Louis: Mosby.

14 Analgesics

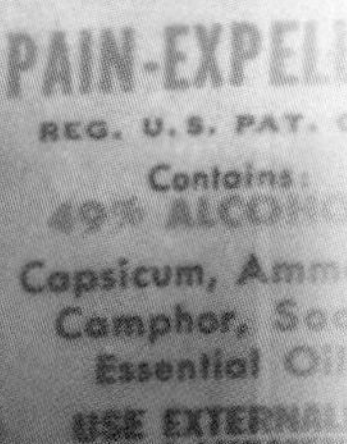

Chapter Focus

Pain is a paradox. It is a sufficiently universal occurrence—everyone experiences pain occasionally in a lifetime. However, everyone's experience is unique and subjective. Only the client is an expert on his or her pain. Because the pain experience is so common with clients, nurses need to be knowledgeable about pain and skillful in interventions to prevent and relieve it.

Learning Objectives

1. Describe the physiology, characteristics, and types of pain.
2. Discuss the myths that interfere with pain management.
3. Discuss special considerations for opioid use during pregnancy, labor, delivery, and breast-feeding.
4. Discuss special considerations for opioid use in children and older adults.
5. Describe the nurse's role in opioid therapy.
6. Differentiate among the opioid analgesics, antagonists, and agonist-antagonist agents.
7. Describe the relationship between prostaglandin synthesis and nonsteroidal antiinflammatory drug effects in inflammation.
8. Discuss the pharmacokinetics, side effects/adverse reactions, and drug interactions of nonsteroidal antiinflammatory drugs.
9. Implement a plan of care for individual clients who require the administration of opioid analgesics, opioid antagonists, and nonsteroidal antiinflammatory drugs.

Key Terms

abstinence syndrome, p. 275
acute pain, p. 259
analgesic, p. 257
chronic pain, p. 259
equianalgesic, p. 281
gate control theory, p. 260
neuropathic (deafferentation) pain, p. 260
nociceptive pain, p. 259
opioid, p. 258
opioid agonist-antagonist, p. 269
physical dependence, p. 257
prostaglandin, p. 259
somatic pain, p. 259
three-step analgesic ladder, p. 270
tolerance, p. 257
visceral pain, p. 259

Key Drugs [✔]

morphine, p. 270
naloxone, p. 284
pentazocine, p. 287

Pain is one of the most common problems that afflict human beings. It is more distressing and disabling than nearly any other client symptom (Salerno, 1996). This is unfortunate because the potent **analgesics** (pain-relieving drugs) currently available are safe and effective when properly selected and applied according to the pharmacokinetics of the drug and the individual client's response. This chapter reviews the primary fears or myths that interfere with pain management, pain components and concepts, and analgesic pharmacology (opioid and nonopioid).

ISSUES AFFECTING PAIN MANAGEMENT

Addiction or Tolerance

The greatest abuse with opioid analgesics is not inducing addiction but the *fear* of inducing addiction. Health care providers and the general public are overly concerned about the potential of inducing addiction with the use of opioid analgesics for the treatment of pain. This is unfortunate because addiction is very rare in clinical practice, and the fear of inducing addiction or even respiratory depression in a client with severe pain is not an acceptable reason for undertreatment of pain (Salerno, 1996). "Pseudoaddiction" refers to clients who are inadequately treated for pain and, as a result, develop a pattern of drug-seeking behaviors to achieve pain control (Weissman & Haddox, 1989). This pattern is often mistaken for opioid addiction (Agency for Health Care Policy and Research, 1994).

Studies have reported a minimal risk for addiction in hospitalized persons receiving opioids at regular intervals. Porter and Jick (1980) reviewed approximately 40,000 hospital charts and reported that nearly 12,000 clients had received opioid analgesics. In this group only four cases of addiction were documented in clients with no previous history of substance abuse. Another study of more than 10,000 hospitalized individuals with burns reported no cases of opioid- or iatrogenic-induced addiction (Watt-Watson & Donovan, 1992). Thus psychologic dependence (addiction) is a rare complication of opioids.

Tolerance, or the need to increase the dosage of an analgesic to maintain the desired effect, is another concern in practice. Tolerance is not usually seen in opioid-naïve clients (clients who have never used opioids before) with severe acute or chronic pain resulting from a physical cause such as trauma, tumor growth, and postsurgical pain. An increase in pain in such individuals is usually a result of disease progression or complications. Persons in pain respond differently to analgesics than do drug-seeking individuals who crave opioids for an euphoric effect. Physical or psychologic dependence should not be confused with tolerance (AHCPR, 1994). **Physical dependence** is an altered physiologic condition in a long-term drug user in which consistent use of the drug is required to avoid withdrawal symptoms.

Fear of Inducing Respiratory Depression

An additional fear of health care professionals is the risk of inducing respiratory depression with the use of opioids. However, with careful assessment, prescribing, and monitoring, the potential for this adverse effect is low (Box 14-1). Very large amounts of opioids are often necessary to control pain in clients who have advanced cancer or are terminally ill. Clients with cancer may be titrated to large amounts of opioids to control pain without producing the adverse effects of respiratory depression or excessive sedation. Pain specialists believe this to be the result of selective tolerance, a tolerance to some of the effects of the drug (e.g., respiratory depression) without interfering with the analgesic effects of the drug (AHCPR, 1994; Foley, 1991).Therefore the client in true pain may have opioid dosages increased until pain control is achieved (Gossel & Wuest, 1993). Significant respiratory depression is rarely seen in this population because the dosage of medication has been titrated to meet an individual's requirement.

Biases of Health Care Professionals

Another area of concern is the influence of personal biases on the administration of pain medications. McCaffery and Ferrell (1992) have raised the question of gender effect and bias in pain management. It was reported that nurses generally believe there to be a difference between male and female pain sensitivity, pain tolerance, and distress. This belief can influence the nurse's assessment of the client's pain and the amount of drug used in treatment, which in turn can lead to undertreatment of pain in women.

In 1994 Cleeland et al. studied pain treatment in approximately 1300 outpatients with metastatic cancer; these outpatients came from 54 cancer treatment centers that ranged from university cancer centers to community-based hospitals and oncology programs. The study outcome indicated the following: (1) women were at a greater risk for being undermedicated for pain, especially women under the age of 50; (2) older adults over 70 years of age (both sexes) often received less potent pain medication, even with reports of significant pain; (3) clinics that service predominantly minority populations were nearly three times more likely to undertreat pain compared with nonminority cen-

BOX 14-1

Time Required to Produce Maximum Respiratory Depression with Opioid Analgesics

Route of Administration	Approximate Times
Intravenous (IV)	Within 7 minutes
Intramuscular (IM)	Within 30 minutes
Subcutaneous (SC)	Within 90 minutes

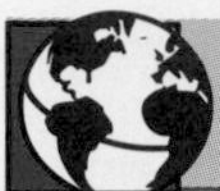

Cultural Considerations
Culture and Pain: A Mesoamerican Perspective

Culture has been identified as a factor that influences a person's reaction to pain. Research in the area of pain and culture has not established a clear link between cultural meanings and attitudes associated with pain and pain behaviors. The purpose of the ethnohistoric study by Villarruel and Ortiz de Montellano (1992) was to explore the beliefs related to the experience of pain within ancient Mesoamerica. Six themes regarding the cultural meaning of pain emerged from this study, and they have relevance in contemporary Mesoamerican cultures, specifically Mexican Americans:

1. Pain was an accepted, anticipated, and necessary part of human life.
2. Humans had an obligation to the gods, and to the community of man, to endure pain in relation to the performance of duties.
3. The ability to endure pain and suffering stoically was valued.
4. The type and amount of pain a person experienced were in part predetermined by the gods.
5. Pain and suffering were viewed as a consequence of immoral behavior.
6. Specific methods of pain alleviation were directed toward maintaining balance within the person and the surrounding environment.

These findings serve as a benchmark from which to understand Mexican-American meanings, expressions, and care associated with pain. Villarruel and Ortiz de Montellano indicate that previous studies have identified specific Mexican-American cultural responses to pain that fall within the themes emerging from this study. However, additional research is needed to determine how these ancient beliefs have evolved and are more specifically expressed in contemporary cultures.

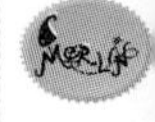

Critical Thinking Questions

- How transferable are findings of ethnohistoric study to contemporary times? Can you identify other historic beliefs about illness that have contemporary relevance?
- Given the six themes identified above, how might these beliefs influence the behavior of a client experiencing pain?

ters; (4) there was a vast discrepancy between the physician's and the individual cancer client's estimate of pain severity; and (5) more than half of the clients in this study had pain, with 62% reporting that pain interfered with their daily functioning.

Studies and research have identified the problems associated with inadequate cancer pain management, and the Agency for Health Care Policy and Research (AHCPR) has issued Clinical Practice Guidelines for Acute Pain Management and Cancer Pain Management (AHCPR, 1992; AHCPR, 1994) to help correct this problem.* However, additional studies are needed in the area of sex, age, and ethnic and cultural biases in pain management (see the Cultural Considerations box above).

Fear of Legal Regulation of Opioids

Opioids are natural or synthetic agents that have a morphine-like effect. Because they have the potential for abuse and illegal diversion, federal and state laws strictly monitor and regulate their availability, prescription, and use. Although the intent of federal law is not to interfere with the appropriate prescribing of these substances, many states have enacted laws or regulations that limit, restrict, and closely monitor opioid prescribing. As a result, many prescribers are reluctant to prescribe opioids for fear of prosecution and suspension or the loss of their professional licenses. Such regulations have resulted in undertreatment of pain, even in clients with severe cancer pain (AHCPR, 1994).

Need for More Potent Analgesics

During the past decade or two, congressional legislation for the approval of heroin (diacetylmorphine) for intractable pain has been proposed and denied. Proponents of this bill have used the argument that heroin is an alternate therapy comparable to other opioids and that it might be useful for persons in intolerable pain because of its analgesic and euphoric effects. Some advocates believe it is more potent, faster acting, and produces a more prolonged analgesic and euphoric effect than other analgesics (McCarthy & Montagne, 1993). Opponents of heroin state that it is unnecessary because the opioids currently available, if properly prescribed, are sufficient for the treatment of intractable pain.

Pharmacologically, heroin is a prodrug; that is, it is converted in the liver to morphine and morphine metabolites when administered orally or intravenously. Although rapid IV injection of heroin crosses the blood-brain barrier faster than morphine to cause the euphoric or high effect, a potentially clouded sensorium is generally undesirable clinically. Most seriously ill persons want pain relief but also want to be able to communicate with their health care providers, friends, and family.

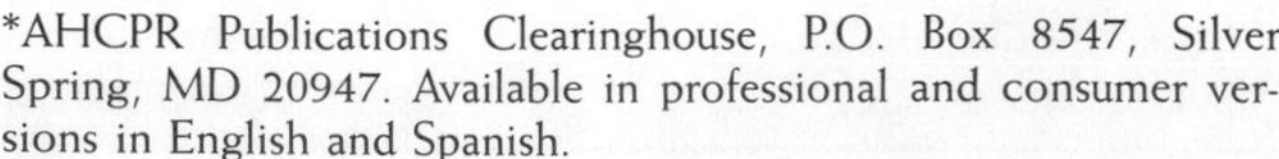

*AHCPR Publications Clearinghouse, P.O. Box 8547, Silver Spring, MD 20947. Available in professional and consumer versions in English and Spanish.

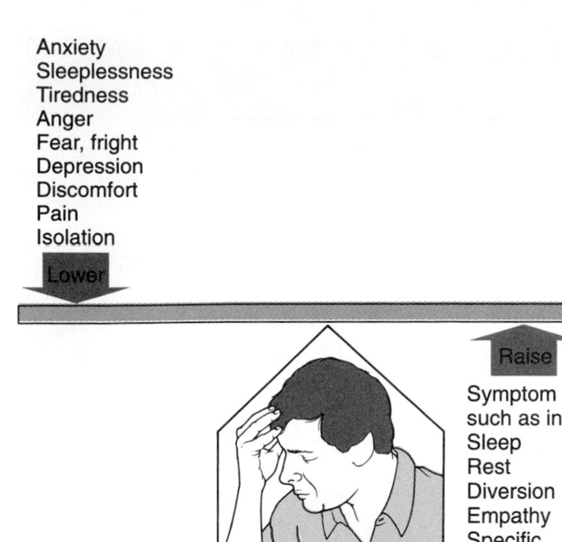

Figure 14-1 Factors affecting the pain threshold.

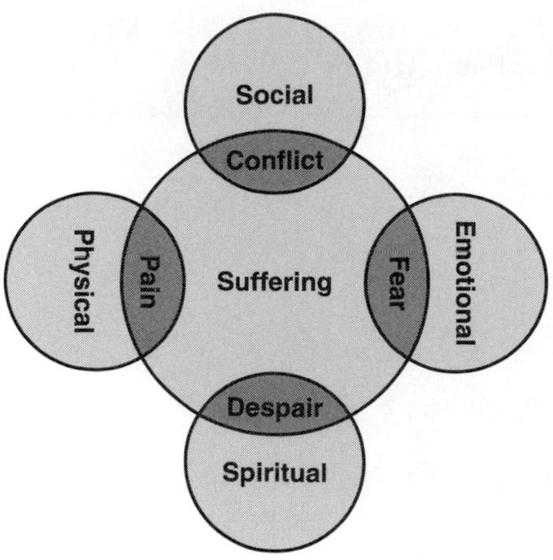

Figure 14-2 Education model illustrating pain and suffering. (From Welk, T.A. [1991.] An educational model for explaining hospice services. *American Journal of Hospice & Palliative Care,* 8[5], 14-17.)

Although heroin is legitimately available in Belgium, Canada, and England, it is rarely used in Belgium and Canada. Heroin is a popular illegal drug of abuse, so an additional fear in legalizing it is that it may result in an increased risk for drug diversion, pharmacy burglaries, and crime. If heroin offers few (if any) advantages over the already marketed opioids, then, as Dr. A.G. Lipman (1993) has succinctly stated, ". . . legalization of heroin is not in the public interest."

COMPONENTS AND CONCEPTS OF PAIN

Because of its highly subjective nature, pain is difficult to define. Pain can be viewed as having two components: (1) the physical component or the sensation of pain, and (2) the psychologic component or emotional response to pain. The physical component of pain involves the nerve pathways and the brain. The psychologic component or the emotional response to pain is the product of factors such as the individual's anxiety level, previous pain experience, age, sex, and culture.

A relatively constant pain threshold exists in all persons under normal circumstances. For example, heat applied to the skin at an intensity of 45° to 48° C will initiate a sensation of pain in almost all individuals. However, pain tolerance—the point beyond which pain becomes unbearable—varies widely among individuals and under different circumstances in a single individual. Figure 14-1 shows the factors that affect the pain threshold.

Welk (1991) has described an educational model that illustrates pain and suffering and the various issues that influence suffering in a terminally ill client (Figure 14-2). As noted from this model, physical pain is only part of the suffering model and is not interchangeable with suffering. A person may be suffering without physical pain or may have physical pain without suffering. Suffering involves multiple issues that prevent a person from living without fear, such as physical pain, emotional fear (e.g., fear of the unknown, fear of dying, fear of dying alone), social conflict (e.g., conflicts with family and friends), and spiritual despair (not necessarily religious, a spiritual dimension to meet an individual client's need). Other persons with persistent, chronic pain may also have factors other than physical pain involved. These factors are often addressed by interdisciplinary teams in hospices and pain management programs.

Pain Classification

Pain can be classified in various ways. For example, it may be acute or chronic. **Acute pain**, the presence of severe discomfort or an uncomfortable sensation, has a sudden onset and usually subsides with treatment. Examples of acute pain include the pain of myocardial infarction, appendicitis, and kidney stones. **Chronic pain**, such as that which accompanies cancer and rheumatoid arthritis, is a persistent or recurring pain that continues for more than 6 months. Chronic pain can be difficult to treat (Table 14-1).

Pain may also be classified as visceral, somatic (nociceptive), or neuropathic (deafferentation). **Visceral pain** originates in smooth musculature or sympathetically innervated organ systems. This pain is often difficult to localize because it is dull and aching and may also be referred (i.e., felt at a site distant from its origin). An example of referred pain is the pain of a myocardial infarction that is felt initially in the arm. **Somatic pain**, or **nociceptive pain**, arises from the activation of nociceptors in the skeletal muscles, fascia, ligaments, vessels, or joints. This pain is usually localized, constant, and may be described as aching or throbbing (Patt, 1993). Somatic pain responds best to nonsteroidal antiinflammatory drugs (NSAIDs), whereas visceral pain usually responds well to opioid analgesics.

Direct cancerous infiltration of the bone causes a somatic pain mediated by prostaglandins. **Prostaglandins** are

TABLE 14-1 Pain: Acute vs. Chronic

	Acute Pain	Chronic Pain
Onset	Usually sudden	Longer duration
Characteristics	Generally sharp, localized; may radiate	Dull, aching, persistent, diffuse
Signs and symptoms		
Physiologic response	Increased blood pressure and heart rate, sweating, pallor	Often absent
Emotional response	Increased anxiety and restlessness	Client may be depressed, withdrawn, expressionless, and exhausted
Therapeutic goals	Relief of pain Sedation often desirable	Prevention of pain Sedation usually unwanted
Drug administration		
Timing	As needed or on request often adequate	Regular preventive schedule
Dosage	Standard dosages are often adequate	Individualize according to client response
Route	Usually parenteral	Oral

hormone-like, unsaturated fatty acids that act on local target organs to affect vasomotor tone, capillary permeability, smooth muscle tone, platelet aggregation, endocrine and exocrine functions, and the autonomic and central nervous systems. They have been referred to as tissue hormones because they are secreted in many different tissues and perform their activity only within a short distance—usually to other cells within the same tissue. They are rapidly metabolized in the bloodstream, and therefore circulating prostaglandin levels are low. At least 16 prostaglandins have been identified and produce a variety of diverse effects. For example, prostaglandin F is involved in the reproductive system and causes uterine muscle contractions; they have been used to induce labor.

Prostaglandins and leukotrienes (biologically active compounds that occur naturally in leukocytes and are found in the lungs, mast cells, leukocytes and platelets) are also mediators of allergic and inflammatory reactions (i.e., redness and heat in an inflamed area, swelling, and pain). Therefore the cancer-induced somatic bone pain mediated by prostaglandins may present as a persistent ache that diffuses widely over the affected areas and is usually unrelated to position or activity. In some persons it may appear as an intermittent piercing pain localized to a small area, which may be related to position, weight bearing, and activity (Kinzbrunner & Salerno, 1994).

Whereas nociceptive (somatic) pain is usually the result of direct stimulation of intact afferent nerve endings, **neuropathic (deafferentation) pain** is caused by peripheral nerve injury and not stimulation. This pain is called paresthesia and is described as a burning, shooting, and/or tingling sensation. It is often associated with dysesthesia, a common effect of spinal cord injury that also includes numbness. This type of pain caused by cancer tumor invasion or treatment-induced nerve damage may be accompanied by sympathetic nervous system dysfunction. Neuropathic pain responds less well to opioid analgesics and often requires adding an adjunct medication (e.g., anticonvulsant, tricyclic antidepressant) to the client's drug regimen.

Pain may also have psychogenic origins. Psychiatric illness or psychosocial issues (e.g., anxiety and depression, fear of dying) have been known to cause severe somatic pain. In such cases, drug therapy alone does not usually bring relief; psychotherapy is indicated.

The great variation in the pain experience has prompted research and has led to the proposal of several theories of pain transmission and pain relief. The **gate control theory** proposed by Melzack and Wall (1965) attempts to explain modulations in the pain experience (Figure 14-3). This theory proposes that a mechanism in the dorsal horn of the spinal cord (the "spinal gate") can alter the transmission of painful sensations from the peripheral nerve fibers to the thalamus and cortex of the brain, where they are recognized as pain. The "spinal gate" is closed by large-diameter, low-threshold afferent fibers (the fast-acting A-delta fibers) and is opened by small-diameter, high-threshold afferent fibers (the slower-acting C fibers). Descending control inhibition from the brain further influences the "gate." Thus the stimulation of large-diameter fibers will "close the gate" to stop the perception of slower-acting painful stimuli (Warfield, 1993). It is on this theory that many nondrug regimens for pain relief are based, including massages or the use of counterirritants. It is also a foundation of the Lamaze method of "natural childbirth."

Pain Management

Although proper pain management techniques are available, the wide institution or application of such approaches has been slow. The foreword of the AHCPR publication on acute pain management (1992) states the following:

> Unfortunately, clinical surveys continue to indicate that routine orders for intramuscular injections of opioid "as needed"—the

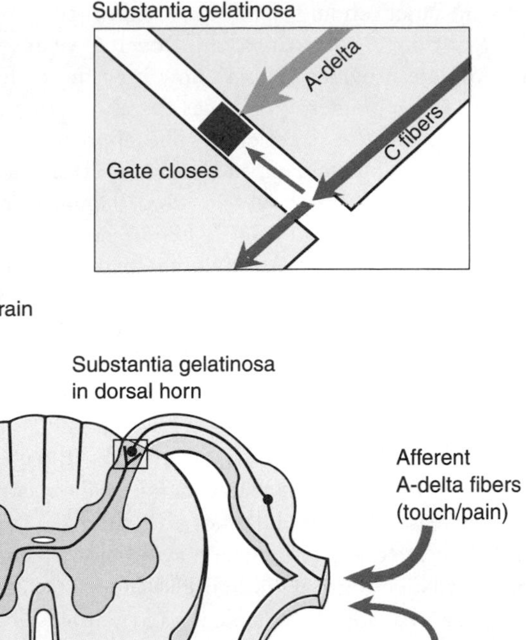

Figure 14-3 Gate control theory. Activity from A delta (large afferent) fibers excites activity in the substantia gelatinosa, thus closing the gate to C fibers, the pain-stimulating fibers.

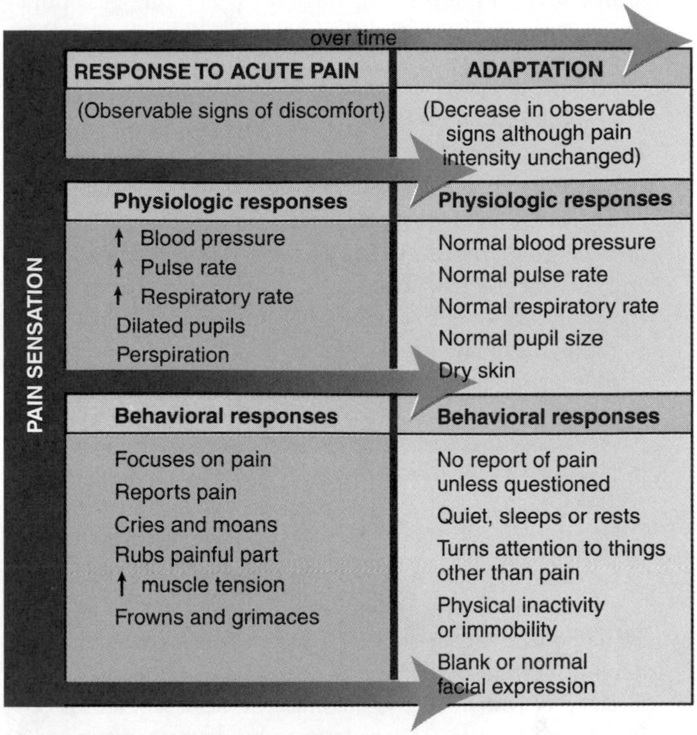

PAIN SENSATION — over time

RESPONSE TO ACUTE PAIN	ADAPTATION
(Observable signs of discomfort)	(Decrease in observable signs although pain intensity unchanged)
Physiologic responses	**Physiologic responses**
↑ Blood pressure ↑ Pulse rate ↑ Respiratory rate Dilated pupils Perspiration	Normal blood pressure Normal pulse rate Normal respiratory rate Normal pupil size Dry skin
Behavioral responses	**Behavioral responses**
Focuses on pain Reports pain Cries and moans Rubs painful part ↑ muscle tension Frowns and grimaces	No report of pain unless questioned Quiet, sleeps or rests Turns attention to things other than pain Physical inactivity or immobility Blank or normal facial expression

Figure 14-4 Acute pain model vs. adaptation. (Information from McCaffery, M., & Pasero, C. [1999]. *Pain: Clinical manual for nursing practice* [2nd Ed.]. St Louis: Mosby.)

standard practice in many clinical settings—fail to relieve pain in about half of postoperative clients. Postoperative pain contributes to client discomfort, longer recovery periods, and greater use of scarce health care resources and may compromise client outcomes.

In the United States, cancer is diagnosed in more than a million persons each year and is the reason for 20% of all reported deaths (AHCPR, 1994). Pain is a common symptom identified in persons with cancer, with 20% to 50% reporting pain at the time of diagnosis and approximately 33% reporting pain during therapy (Hammack & Loprinzi, 1994). In the general population, Gu and Belgrade (1993) reported that nearly 35% of hospitalized medical inpatients identified pain as their major complaint. The undertreatment with analgesics of clients in pain is well documented in the literature (Cleeland et al., 1994; Zhukovsky, Gorowski, Hausdorff, Napolitano, & Lesser, 1995).

Although several major reasons for the undertreatment of pain were reviewed earlier in this chapter, the nurse should be aware that a major difference exists in the expression of pain in a client with acute pain as compared with a client with chronic, severe pain. The latter person experiences an adaptation process; thus there may be a decrease or absence of the observable signs and symptoms, even in a client with very severe pain. McCaffery and Pasero (1999) have described the differences in both behavioral and physiologic responses to pain (Figure 14-4).

Undertreatment of pain resulted in a court awarding a multimillion dollar settlement to the family of a nursing home resident because his pain was mismanaged by the nurses and he died an unnecessarily painful death (Cushing, 1992). Despite health care providers being both legally and morally responsible for pain relief, undertreatment or the improper use of analgesics continues to be a major problem in both acute and chronic pain settings. Extensive information about the proper treatment of pain is available and should be used in practice today (Salerno & Willens, 1996).

Opioid Use in Pregnancy, Labor, and Delivery

Most women experience pain during labor. Ideally the analgesic used should provide pain relief without interfering with labor and also without increasing the risk or danger to the mother or fetus. Currently there is no ideal analgesic available for use during pregnancy, and therefore the prescriber should carefully choose the analgesic based on the individual and the prevailing conditions.

Opioid analgesics may increase or decrease the time of labor, and the primary concern with their use is neonatal respiratory depression. These agents cross the placenta to enter fetal circulation, and therefore the dose administered to the mother should be sufficient to reduce the pain and discomfort to a level that can be tolerated by the woman but not large enough to cause respiratory depression in either the mother or fetus. The IV route is the preferred method of drug administration, and meperidine is the drug most commonly used. In a primigravida (a woman who is pregnant for the first time) the analgesic medication is usually not administered until the contractions occur approximately every 2 to

3 minutes and the cervix is dilated (3 to 4 cm). A multiparous woman might receive the analgesic slightly earlier (McCombs, 1993).

Although meperidine is commonly prescribed for pain during pregnancy, ". . . it is not recommended as a first-line opioid for any type of pain, including perinatal pain" (McCaffery & Pasero, 1999). Morphine and fentanyl are the most commonly prescribed opioids for newborns. The nurse must be aware that although morphine causes more sedation and has less risk of causing chest wall rigidity than fentanyl, the pharmacokinetics of morphine are significantly different in the preterm and term neonate. The preterm neonate has a longer elimination half-life than term neonates, and term infants (less than 4 days old) have an elimination half-life that is seven times higher than in older infants. Dosage adjustments are necessary to avoid drug accumulation and toxicity. McCaffery and Pasero (1999) have a guideline chart for health care professionals on morphine and fentanyl infusion rates for preterm, term, and older infants.

Naloxone (Narcan), an opioid antagonist, should be available to treat the mother or neonate if excessive central nervous system depression occurs. If an opioid is administered to a woman who is nursing, the next scheduled feeding should be 4 to 6 hours later to minimize the amount of drug passed on to the infant.

A second concern with the use of opioids during pregnancy (particularly in an addicted woman) is that these agents may lead to physical drug dependence in the fetus and cause severe withdrawal reactions in the neonate after birth. Pregnant women enrolled in methadone maintenance programs may present with fetal distress syndrome in utero and often deliver an underweight baby.

Opioid Use in Children

Children are also untreated or inadequately treated for pain. They suffer needlessly because of the many myths and misconceptions about pain and pain management in this population. The assessment of pain in a young child is more difficult and should be based on thorough knowledge of the pain-producing procedure or event and the child's nonverbal behavior. Even when children have the ability to verbalize their feelings, they are often reluctant to express pain, fearing the results (diagnostic test, examination, or injection) may be more painful. Young children are unable to make the connection between the immediate pain from the injection and the pain relief experienced later. Their reaction to the injection may interfere with nursing judgment, resulting in no medication and unnecessary pain for the child (Waters, 1992).

The health care provider should consider giving pain medication to a child for the same circumstances in which it would be given to an adult. In children under 2 years of age with observably increased irritability, anorexia, and loss of interest in play and in whom the assessment of whether the problem is "merely" irritability or pain is unclear, the decision to medicate appropriately is justified. Medicating in this instance should lead to a more comfortable, less anxiety-ridden child. In a child over 2 years of age, the health care provider should know how the child's age and stage of development influences the ability to perceive and communicate the experience. The approach to the child should be individualized, and the child's words and gestures for communication should be used. Figure drawings may help the child to point out "where it hurts." More graphic scales may be used with children to rate the intensity of their pain (Figure 14-5). Other signs of discomfort, such as restlessness, decreased activity, anorexia, whining, and crying, should be assessed. The parents are to be consulted regarding the child's pain status, because they are most familiar with the child.

As with adults, pain is best managed if the child is given medication early rather than when the pain becomes severe. To decrease the possibility of the child denying pain to avoid an injection, the nurse may administer analgesics by an alternative route. Children find suppositories and liquid formulations more acceptable than injections. The nurse can assist the child in associating the medication with pain relief by indicating that it will make him or her "feel better." The nurse must check to see if the medication has been effective and remind the child that he or she probably "feels better" because of the medication. Guidelines for the administration of injections to the child are found in Chapter 7. Table 14-2 lists dosing data for opioid analgesics in infants, children, and adolescents.

Opioid Use in Older Adults

Analgesic dosing in older adults usually requires dosage and dosing interval adjustments according to the client's therapeutic response and the development of undesirable side effects (increased pain, confusion, excessive untoward CNS effects, respiratory depression). Older adults reportedly have enhanced medication responses and may not tolerate side or adverse drug effects as well as younger clients. Older adults often have multiple medical problems and may have additional medications prescribed for them (polypharmacy). Thus it is important to carefully assess, evaluate, and closely monitor the older adult to reduce the potential for undertreatment or overtreatment and adverse effects. Height, weight, and body surface area are not accurate measurements for dosing analgesics in older adults.

Older adults often report pain differently than younger persons, often because of physiologic, psychologic, and cultural differences (AHCPR, 1992). Cognitive impairment, dementia, and confusion may add to the barriers for pain assessment. Because traditional approaches are limited in this population, pain assessment and management require close supervision and the monitoring of daily functioning and quality of life as outcomes. In the past, lower dosages of analgesics were often recommended for older adults, but this approach should not be the rule. Although age is not a significant factor in determining analgesic dosage, it is important in establishing the frequency of drug dosing.

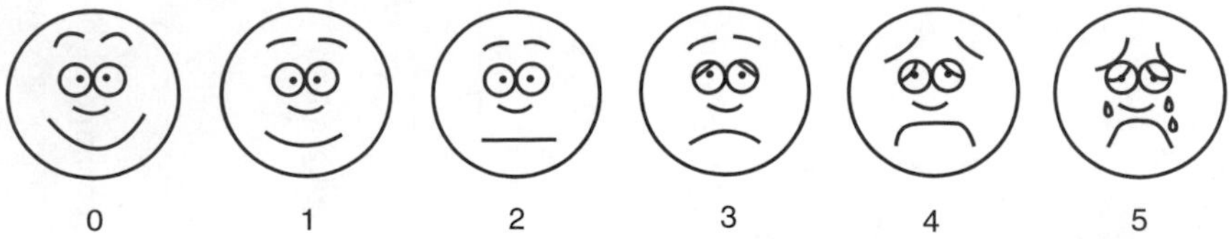

0 1 2 3 4 5

1. Explain to the child that each face is for a person who has no pain (hurt, or whatever word the child uses) or has some or a lot of pain.
2. Point to the appropriate face and state, "This face is ..."
   0-"very happy because he doesn't hurt at all."
   1-"hurts just a little bit."
   2-"hurts a little more."
   3-"hurts even more."
   4-"hurts a whole lot."
   5-"hurts as much as you can imagine, although you don't have to be crying to feel this bad."
3. Ask the child to choose the face that best describes how much pain he has. Be specific about which pain (e.g., "shot" or incision) and what time (e.g., now? earlier? before lunch?).

Figure 14-5 Scale for rating the intensity of pain with pediatric clients. (Modified from Wong, D. [1999]. *Whaley & Wong's Nursing care of infants and children* [6th Ed.]. St Louis: Mosby.)

Because liver or kidney impairment may reduce drug clearance, less frequent drug dosing may be necessary. Both dosage and drug frequency should be carefully titrated to the individual's response to the analgesic medication. The presence of adverse effects influences drug dosage and drug frequency.

Specific analgesics that may be considered inappropriate for use in older adults include propoxyphene (Darvon products), pentazocine (Talwin) (Beers et al., 1992; Wallace, 1994; Willcox, Himmelstein, & Woolhandler, 1994), and meperidine (Demerol) (Wallace, 1994). It is generally believed that these agents are more toxic in older adults; much safer analgesics are available.

The aging process may also influence the route of analgesic administration. Older adults may have a diminished circulatory process, which results in slower absorption of drugs administered intramuscularly or subcutaneously. Administering additional doses in such a situation may result in unpredictable or increased drug absorption, which increases the potential for adverse reactions.

Careful nursing care should be used in working with older adults who are experiencing pain. Older adults may be less likely to ask for pain medication because they accept pain as a part of old age, do not want to be a "bother," or deny discomfort as a cultural and ethnic issue. Nonverbal communication, such as irritability, anorexia, decreased activity, a tendency to cry easily, or object gripping, should be carefully assessed. Decreased activity resulting from pain increases the risk of complications of immobility. The stress of the pain experience leads to fatigue and anxiety and reduces the older adult's diminished physical and psychologic resources. Because an older adult may be taking many drugs concurrently, health care providers should be aware of specific drug interactions with analgesic therapy.

■ Nursing Management

Pain Therapy

Nurses must use all of their skills to successfully manage the care of clients who are experiencing pain. The nurse often initiates or coordinates the implementation of pain management.

■ **Assessment.** Accurate pain assessment is based on both subjective and objective information. Because "pain" cannot be observed (it is a perception, not an object), the nurse must assess the client's physical and psychologic signs and symptoms. Each person perceives and reacts to pain differently on the basis of physical, emotional, and cultural influences. In particular, a client's cultural background affects the manner in which pain is communicated. In addition, the perception of pain is unique for each individual; there is the capacity to respond differently to the same noxious stimulus. A given pain stimulus will not necessarily produce the same amount of pain for all clients. Children generally experience less pain when receiving injections by using a simple coping strategy (e.g., squeezing a hand in proportion to the pain they feel) or by being actively involved in selecting the site or cleaning the site with an alcohol swab (McGrath, 1990). Nurses should not assess pain by the presence or absence of any individual behavior such as crying or moaning but should evaluate the totality of signs and symptoms that the client presents and evaluate each episode of pain as unique.

The assessment of pain requires careful documentation as a baseline for the nurse to select appropriate nursing inter-

TABLE 14-2 Dosing Data for Opioid Analgesics

Drug	Approximate Equianalgesic Dosage		Recommended Starting Dosage (Adults More Than 50 kg Body Weight)		Recommended Starting Dosage (Children and Adults Less Than 50 kg Body Weight)*	
	Oral	Parenteral	Oral	Parenteral	Oral	Parenteral
Opioid Agonist						
morphine†	30 mg q3-4h (around-the-clock dosing) 60 mg q3-4h (single dose or intermittent dosing)	10 mg q3-4h	30 mg q3-4h	10 mg q3-4h	0.3 mg/kg q3-4h	0.1 mg/kg q3-4h
codeine‡	130 mg q3-4h	75 mg q3-4h	60 mg q3-4h	60 mg q2h (IM/SC)	1 mg/kg q3-4h§	Not recommended
hydromorphone† (Dilaudid)	7.5 mg q3-4h	1.5 mg q3-4h	6 mg q3-4h	1.5 mg q3-4h	0.06 mg/kg q3-4h	0.015 mg/kg q3-4h
hydrocodone (in Lorcet, Lortab, Vicodin, others)	30 mg q3-4h	Not available	10 mg q3-4h	Not available	0.2 mg/kg q3-4h§	Not available
levorphanol (Levo-Dromoran)	4 mg q6-8h	2 mg q6-8h	4 mg q6-8h	2 mg q6-8h	0.04 mg/kg q6-8h	0.02 mg/kg q6-8h
meperidine (Demerol)	300 mg q2-3h	100 mg q3h	Not recommended	100 mg q3h	Not recommended	0.75 mg/kg q2-3h
methadone (Dolophine, others)	20 mg q6-8h	10 mg q6-8h	20 mg q6-8h	10 mg q6-8h	0.2 mg/kg q6-8h	0.1 mg/kg q6-8h

oxycodone (Roxicodone, also in Percocet, Percodan, Tylox, others)	30 mg q3-4h	Not available	10 mg q3-4h	Not available	0.2 mg/kg q3-4h§	Not available
oxymorphone† (Numorphan)	Not available	1 mg q3-4h	Not available	1 mg q3-4h	Not recommended	Not recommended
Opioid Agonist-Antagonist and Partial Agonist						
buprenorphine (Buprenex)	Not available	0.3-0.4 mg q6-8h	Not available	0.4 mg q6-8h	Not available	0.004 mg/kg q6-8h
butorphanol (Stadol)	Not available	2 mg q3-4h	Not available	2 mg q3-4h	Not available	Not recommended
nalbuphine (Nubain)	Not available	10 mg q3-4h	Not available	10 mg q3-4h	Not available	0.1 mg/kg q3-4h
pentazocine (Talwin, others)	150 mg q3-4h	60 mg q3-4h	50 mg q4-6h	Not recommended	Not recommended	Not recommended

From Agency for Health Care Policy and Research, Public Health Service. (1992). *Clinical practice guideline: Acute pain management: operative or medical procedures and trauma.* AHCPR Pub No 92-0032. Rockville, MD: Department of Health and Human Services.

NOTE: Published tables vary in the suggested dosages that are equianalgesic to morphine. Clinical response is the criterion that must be applied for each client; titration to clinical response is necessary. Because there is not complete cross tolerance among these drugs, it is usually necessary to use a lower than equianalgesic dosage when changing drugs and to retitrate to response.

CAUTION: Recommended dosages do not apply to clients with renal or hepatic insufficiency or other conditions affecting drug metabolism and kinetics.

*CAUTION: Dosages listed for clients with body weight less than 50 kg cannot be used as initial starting dosages in babies less than 6 months of age. Consult the AHCPR's *Clinical Practice Guideline: Acute Pain Management: Operative or Medical Procedures and Trauma* for recommendations on the management of pain in neonates.

†For morphine, hydromorphone, and oxymorphone, rectal administration is an alternate route for clients unable to take oral medications. However, equianalgesic dosages may differ from oral and parenteral dosages because of pharmacokinetic differences.

‡CAUTION: Codeine doses above 65 mg often are not appropriate due to diminishing incremental analgesia with increasing doses but continually increasing constipation and other side effects.

§CAUTION: Doses of aspirin and acetaminophen in combination opioid-NSAID preparations must also be adjusted to the client's body weight.

Date ____________

Client's Name ____________ Age ______ Room ______

Diagnosis ____________ Physician ____________

Nurse ____________

I. Location: Client or nurse mark drawing

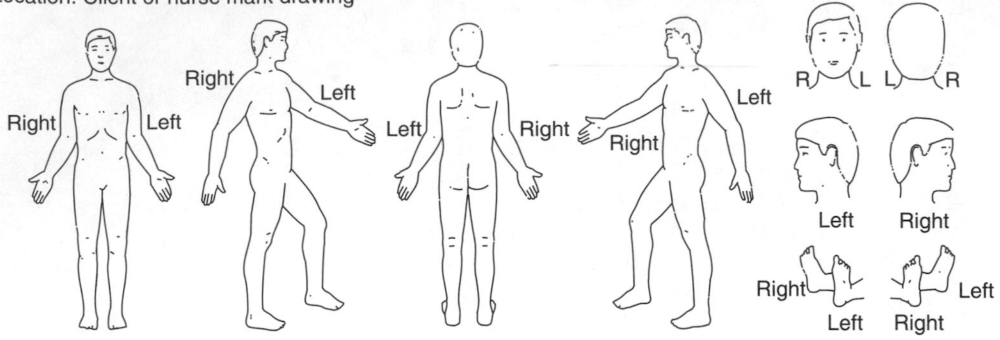

II. Intensity: Client rates the pain. Scale used ____________

Present: ____________

Worst pain gets: ____________

Best pain gets: ____________

Acceptable level of pain: ____________

III. Quality: (Use client's own words, e.g., prick, ache, burn, throb, pull, sharp) ____________

IV. Onset, duration variations, rhythms: ____________

V. Manner of expressing pain: ____________

VI. What relieves the pain? ____________

VII. What causes or increases the pain? ____________

VIII. Effects of pain: (Note decreased function, decreased quality of life)

Accompanying symptoms (e.g., nausea) ____________

Sleep ____________

Appetite ____________

Physical activity ____________

Relationship with others (e.g., irritability) ____________

Emotions (e.g., anger, suicidal, crying) ____________

Concentration ____________

Other ____________

IX. Other comments: ____________

X. Plan: ____________

Figure 14-6 Pain assessment tool from M. McCaffery and A. Beebe. (From McCaffery, M. & Pasero, C. [1999]. *Pain: Clinical manual for nursing practice* [2nd ed.]. St. Louis: Mosby.)

ventions and to evaluate the effectiveness of nursing care. Figure 14-6 is an example of a tool from McCaffery and Pasero (1999) that illustrates the essential components for the assessment of pain. It is necessary to determine the location of the client's pain. For example, postoperative discomfort cannot be assumed to be "incisional" pain when it is possible that the client may be experiencing pain related to other conditions such as deep vein thrombosis or myocardial infarction. It is vital that the assessment be described in the client's own words, both in terms of the quality of the pain (sharp, dull, burning, radiating, stabbing, or cramping) and what seems to intensify or relieve it. The nurse can then determine the client's manner of expressing pain and its effects.

Although a complete pain assessment tool such as the one in Figure 14-6 may not be available in all health care agencies, many agencies use scales to rate the intensity of pain. Figure 14-7 illustrates a number of these scales. If printed scales are not available, ask the client to rate the pain on a scale of 0 (no pain) to 10 (unbearable pain); this will provide consistency for the assessment of the client's perception of the pain. In addition, having the client rate the pain at an appropriate time interval after administering an analgesic allows for evaluation of the effectiveness of the medication and for titration of the dosage to achieve adequate pain relief without adverse reactions.

Pain may bring forth many emotions from the client, such as fear, anger, or impatience. There are a number of

I. Pain Intensity Scales

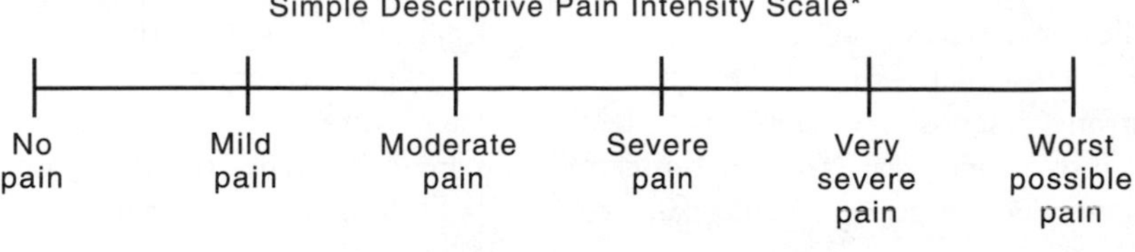

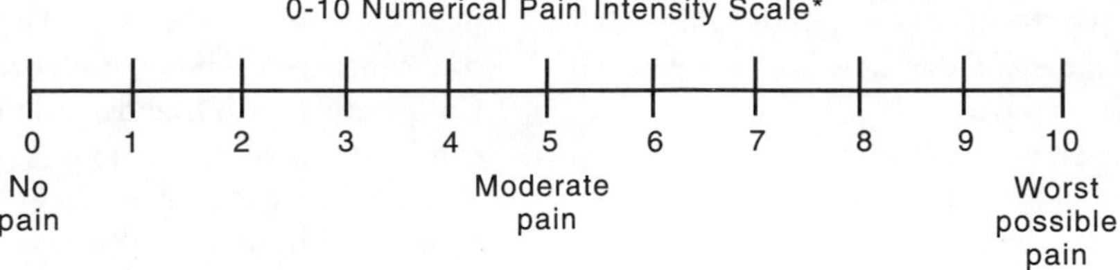

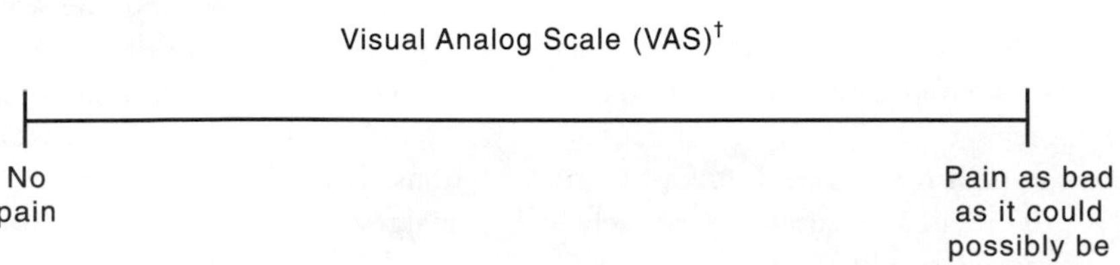

II. Pain Distress Scales

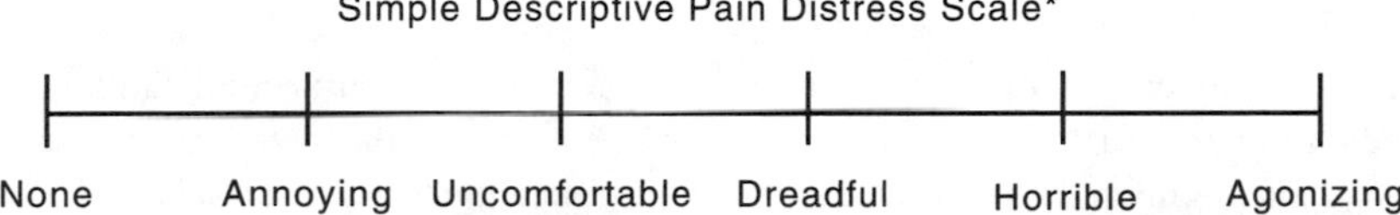

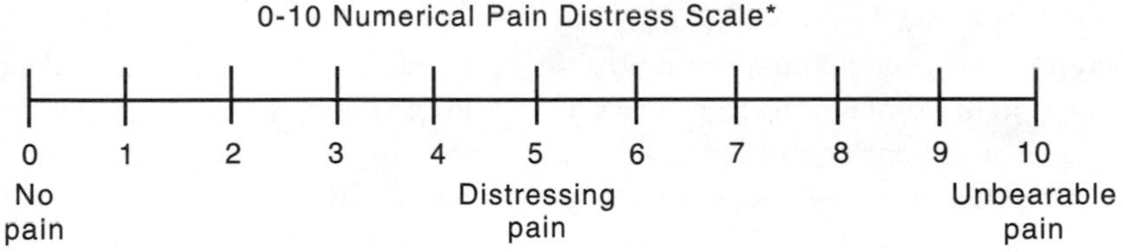

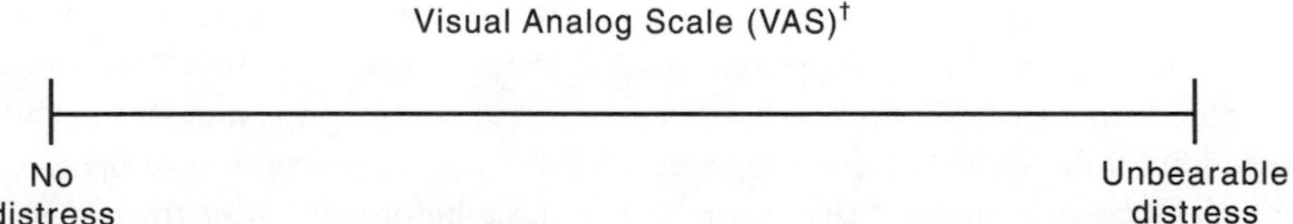

Figure 14-7 Scales for rating the intensity and distress of pain. *If used as a graphic rating scale, a 10-cm baseline is recommended. †A 10-cm, baseline is recommended for VASs.(From Acute Pain Management Guideline Panel [1992]. *Acute pain management: Operative or medical procedures and trauma. Clinical practice guideline.* AHCPR Pub. No. 92-0032. Rockville, MD: Agency for Health Care Policy and Research, Public Health Service, US Department of Health and Human Services.)

physiologic responses to pain; these are usually sympathetic in nature and include increased blood pressure, pulse, or respirations; sweating; pallor; restlessness; or agitation.

■ **Nursing Diagnosis.** The client should be assessed for the following nursing diagnoses: anxiety, disturbed sleep pattern, activity intolerance, fear, fatigue, self-care deficit, social isolation, ineffective coping, acute pain, or chronic pain.

■ **Implementation**

■ ***Monitoring.*** Observe the client's response to the analgesic, and record the degree and duration of pain relief and any adverse effects that may occur.

■ ***Intervention.*** All clients in pain should receive nursing care directed toward reducing the perception of and reaction to pain and toward enhancing the analgesic effect of medications. The nurse often has significant influence over pain medication through prn (when needed) prescribing of analgesic medications. As previously mentioned, the greatest abuse of analgesics is underutilization, which results in failure to adequately relieve or control pain. Analgesics should be used before the pain reaches peak intensity and painful events occur. A prn order can be used preventively if the nurse meticulously assesses the client's needs. For acute, intermittent pain, the appropriate dose of analgesic with a rapid onset of action should be used, with dosing on an as-needed or prn basis. If the order is for "q4h prn" and the nurse determines that the pain will be fairly constant for the next 24 hours, the drug may be given at 4-hour intervals and documented in the medication record to be given every 4 hours around-the-clock. This regimen in no way exceeds what the prescriber has specified as long as the nurse monitors the client for signs that the frequency or the dose should be decreased (e.g., respiratory depression or confusion). With this strategy, the blood levels of the analgesic remain steady, and therefore there should be no pain breakthrough. An alternate method of maintaining serum levels of the analgesic is the use of a patient-controlled analgesic (PCA) infusion pump. The PCA pump provides consistent pain relief, allows the client to participate more freely in his or her care and, it is hoped, helps the client to recover more quickly. The client's anxiety level should be reduced, because he or she knows when the next dose is being administered. For chronic, continuous pain, the appropriate dosage of analgesic is titrated to the client's needs. The analgesic should have as long a duration as feasible and be given on an around-the-clock basis to prevent the return of pain. Breakthrough pain should be medicated using appropriate medications on a prn basis.

Nonpharmacologic forms of interventions can serve as adjuncts to analgesic therapy. It is well known that anxiety exacerbates pain and causes muscle tension. Relaxation techniques can be effective in reducing the amount of pain experienced. Simple methods that promote comfort, such as a quiet, pleasant environment or proper body position, may prove very effective. Rhythmic breathing, counting, and purposeful relaxation of muscle groups are among the techniques that nurses can teach clients. More advanced methods include guided imagery, therapeutic touch, biofeedback, and hypnosis. An example of a highly successful relaxation technique for pain control is the psychoprophylactic or "Lamaze" method of rhythmic breathing and focusing to blunt the perception of pain during labor and delivery. These same techniques are useful for the management of many other types of acute pain.

Shifting the client's focus of attention away from the painful stimulus is known as distraction. This technique greatly improves the client's ability to cope with chronic pain. Clients may even find they have developed the ability to distract themselves without realizing it. Watching television, visiting with friends, walking, or working on a project can be effective distractions.

Stimulating the client's skin (cutaneous stimulation) has been found to be very effective in pain management. Nurses have used cutaneous stimulation for years in the form of massage, stroking, and the application of heat and cold. With transcutaneous electrical nerve stimulation (TENS), a small electrical current is applied to skin areas over nerves or around surgical incisions; it works very well in select situations. TENS has been shown to cause the release of natural analgesic substances (endorphins) and to interfere with pain impulse conduction (see the discussion of gate control theory, p. 260).

Always remember to question the client about past methods of pain relief. Reinforcing these methods and supplementing them with new techniques often reduces the need for pain-relieving medications.

■ ***Education.*** Instructing clients in various techniques for relieving pain themselves is an important part of pain therapy, especially in chronic pain. The nurse can work with the client to determine a method for dealing with pain. The nurse may know many techniques for dealing with pain and can teach them to the client (e.g., splinting an abdominal incision with a pillow to reduce the discomfort of coughing). Clients given drugs pain relief should be informed of the purpose of the medication. Analgesic effects may be enhanced by positive suggestion. Clients who self-administer pain-relieving medications should be taught the adverse effects, proper dosage, drug or food interactions, correct administration, and safe storage of medications.

■ **Evaluation.** After the implementation of pain relief therapy, an evaluation of effectiveness must be made. Assessment once again evaluates the physiologic responses and the client's perception of pain. Rating the pain using a pain scale before and after treatment serves to document the response to treatment. In evaluating analgesic drug therapy, the nurse looks at several parameters, including compliance with therapy and the development of addiction, dependence, tolerance, or adverse effects.

OPIOID ANALGESICS

Receptor Classification

The term *agonist* means "to do," and the term *antagonist* means "to block." Opioids are classified as agonist, partial agonist, or agonist-antagonist medications. An agonist drug binds with the receptor(s) to activate and produce the maximum response of the individual receptor, whereas a partial agonist produces a partial response. An **opioid agonist-antagonist** drug produces mixed effects, acting as an agonist at one type of receptor and as a competitive antagonist at another receptor (Figure 14-8). A review of select opioid receptor responses is presented in Table 14-3.

The mechanism of action for opioids is related to their binding to specific opioid receptors inside and outside of the central nervous system (CNS) (AHCPR, 1994). The primary opioid receptors concentrated in the CNS are mu (μ), kappa (κ), delta (δ), and sigma (σ) receptors. Analgesia is associated with the first three receptors. Research on the delta receptor is limited, and therefore the primary analgesic receptors at this time are the mu and kappa receptors. The sigma receptors are primarily associated with psychotomimetic or unwanted effects, such as dysphoria (depression and anguish), hallucinations, and confusion.

The agonist analgesics (e.g., morphine, hydromorphone) activate both the mu and kappa receptors, and the agonist-antagonist agents (butorphanol, nalbuphine, and pentazocine) activate kappa receptors (agonist) and block or have minimal effects on the mu receptors (antagonist). The agonist-antagonist drugs, especially pentazocine, may induce the undesirable effects associated with sigma receptor activity.

In addition to producing analgesia, opioids are capable of altering the perception of and emotional responses to pain because the receptors are widely distributed in the CNS, especially in the spinal and medullary dorsal horn, limbic system, thalamus, hypothalamus, and midbrain. Pain perception is inhibited when these areas are stimulated

TABLE 14-3 Selected Opioid Receptor Responses

Receptor	Medication Examples	Response
mu	Strong agonist: morphine, hydromorphone Partial agonist: buprenorphine Weak agonist: meperidine	Supraspinal analgesia, euphoria, respiratory depression, sedation, constipation, urinary retention, drug dependence
	Antagonist: naloxone, opioid agonist-antagonist	Reversal of opioid effects; acute withdrawal induced in opioid dependency
kappa	Agonist: pentazocine, morphine, nalbuphine, butorphanol Little or no activity: levorphanol, methadone, meperidine	Spinal analgesia, sedation
	Antagonist: naloxone, buprenorphine	Reversal of opioid effects; acute withdrawal induced in opioid dependency

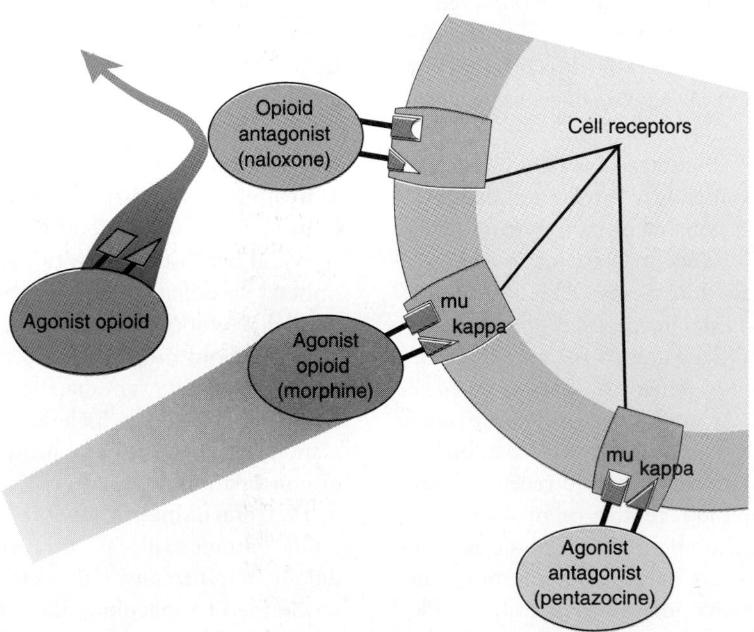

Figure 14-8 Receptor interactions of opioids.

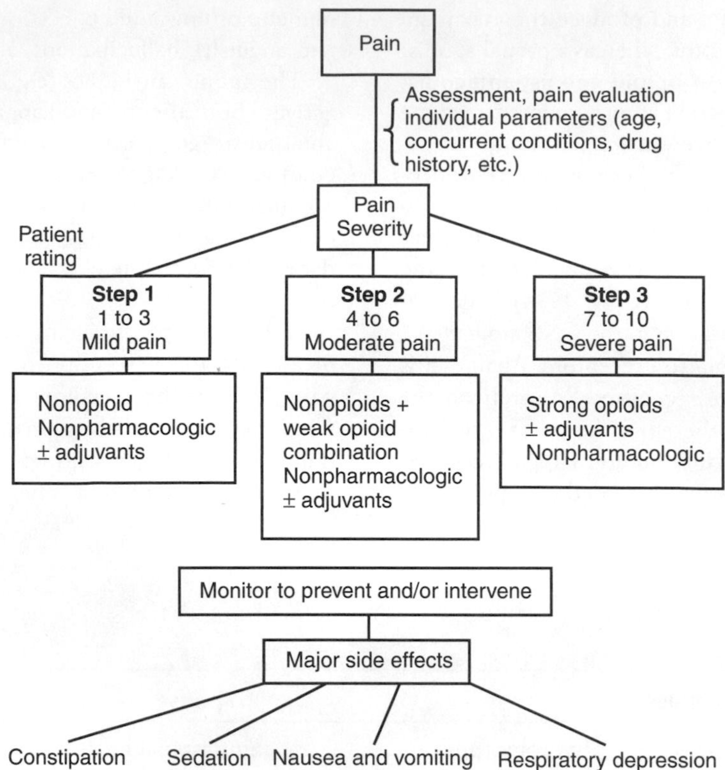

Figure 14-9 Pharmacologic flow chart for the management of pain. (From Salerno, E. & Willens, J.S. (1996). *Pain management handbook: An interdisciplinary approach*. St. Louis: Mosby.)

(Willens, 1996), and this enhances the analgesic effect of morphine.

Agonist Opioids

morphine [mor′ feen]

Morphine is the prototype agonist opioid. It is still obtained from opium poppy because of the difficulty encountered in synthesizing morphine in the laboratory. Many analgesics are available now, but none has been proved to be clinically superior to morphine. In fact, all new analgesics are compared with morphine, the analgesic standard, for potency and for side effects/adverse reactions. The World Health Organization (WHO) recommends a **three-step analgesic ladder** approach to the management of cancer pain, using nonopioid analgesics initially and progressing to stronger analgesics in the second and third steps (AHCPR, 1994). Morphine and other agonist opioids are used in step three, the treatment of severe pain. See Figure 14-9 for a pharmacologic flow chart for the management of pain.

Mechanism of Action. As mentioned previously, morphine produces its potent analgesic effects by combining with receptor sites in the brain called opioid receptors (see the previous discussion of opioid receptors on pp. 268-269).

Indications. The analgesic effect of morphine is indicated for the treatment of severe pain. Although morphine is considered the drug of choice for cancer pain (AHCPR, 1994), it has additional pharmacologic effects that are useful in treating symptoms other than pain. For example, small doses of morphine may depress the cough center, and this secondary effect is useful in certain situations. Therefore morphine may be used in clients with lung cancer to treat pain aggravated by coughing or to treat an unproductive, nagging cough. For persons with a cough caused by a cold, less potent and potentially safer medications, such as the nonopioid antitussive dextromethorphan, should be used.

Another indication for morphine therapy is in the treatment of acute pulmonary edema secondary to left ventricular heart failure. The peripheral vasodilation effect of morphine on the veins and arteries can be very useful in decreasing heart workload, resulting in enhanced cardiac function and a reduction of lung fluid. Morphine is effective in treating myocardial infarction because it does not significantly alter heart rate and blood pressure at the usual dosages and because it has a calming effect along with the peripheral vasodilation effect, which may result in a decrease in cardiac workload (Salerno & Willens, 1996).

The opioid drugs also act centrally and locally to alter intestinal motility (antidiarrheal effect). The gastrointestinal effects of morphine include a decrease in peristalsis and glandular secretions, which usually result in the side effect of constipation.

Pharmacokinetics. Morphine may be administered orally, intramuscularly, intravenously, subcutaneously, epidurally, intrathecally, and rectally. Tables 14-4 and 14-5 describe the pharmacokinetics and dosage and administration of morphine. Morphine is distributed widely in body tissues.

TABLE 14-4 Selected Opioid Dosage Forms: Pharmacokinetics

Drug/Dosage Form	Onset of Action (minutes)	Peak Effect (minutes)	Duration of Action (hours)
codeine			
Oral	30-45	60-120	4
IM	10-30	30-60	4
SC	10-30	—	4
hydrocodone (Hycodan)			
Oral	10-30	30-60	4-6
hydromorphone (Dilaudid)			
Oral	30	90-120	4
IM	15	30-60	4-5
IV	10-15	15-30	2-3
SC	15	30-90	4
Rectal	Not available	Not available	6-8
levorphanol (Levo-Dromoran)			
Oral	10-60	90-120	6-8
IM	Not available	60	6-8
IV	Not available	Within 20	6-8
SC	Not available	60-90	6-8
meperidine (Demerol)			
Oral	15	60-90	2-4 (usually 3)
IM	10-15	30-50	2-4 (usually 3)
IV	1	5-7	2-4 (usually 3)
SC	10-15	30-50	2-4 (usually 3)
methadone			
Oral	30-60	90-120	4-6*
IM	10-20	60-120	4-5*
IV	—	15-30	3-4
morphine			
Oral			
Solution,† syrup,‡ tablets	10-30	60-120	4-5
Extended-release tablets§	—	—	8-12
IM	10-30	30-60	4-5
IV	—	20	4-5
SC	10-30	50-90	4-5
Epidural‖	15-60	—	Up to 24
Intrathecal‖	15-60	—	Up to 24
Rectal¶	20-60	—	4-5
oxycodone			
Oral	Not available	60	3-4
Controlled release	Not available	3-4	12
oxymorphone (Numorphan)			
IM	10-15	30-90	3-6
IV	5-10	15-30	3-4
SC	10-20	Not available	3-6
Rectal	15-30	120	3-6
propoxyphene (Darvon)			
Oral	15-60	120	4-6

*With active metabolites and continuous dosing, half-life and duration of action may increase to 22 to 48 hours.
†Roxanol, MSIR, Statex Drops.
‡Morphitec, M.O.S.—available in Canada.
§MS Contin, Roxanol SR.
‖Duramorph (preservative-free).
¶RMS suppositories.

TABLE 14-5 Morphine Dosage and Administration

Route	Adult Dosage
IV	4-10 mg diluted in 4-5 mL sterile water administered slowly
IM	5-20 mg q4h
SC	5-20 mg q4h
Epidural	1-5 mg initially; assess in 1 hour; if inadequate for pain relief, increments of 1-2 mg may be administered; 10 mg in 24 hours maximum
Intrathecal	0.2-1 mg as single dose only; repeated administration by this route not recommended
Oral (individualized)	Initially 10-30 mg q4h for morphine sulfate syrup, oral solution, and tablets; may be increased according to pain severity and client's response
Rectal suppositories	20-30 mg rectally q4-6h

It is metabolized in the liver primarily to morphine-3-glucuronide (M3G) and morphine-6-glucuronide (M6G), an active metabolite, and it is excreted primarily via the kidneys.

Side Effects/Adverse Reactions. The most commonly reported side effects of morphine and the other opioids include vertigo, faintness, and light-headedness, which occur most often in ambulatory clients. Fatigue, sleepiness, nausea and vomiting, increased sweating, constipation, and hypotension may also occur. Less common side effects include dry mouth, headache, anorexia, abdominal cramping, nervousness, increased anxiety, mental confusion, urinary retention or painful urination, visual disturbances, and nightmares. With epidural administration, pruritus is common.

Among the more serious adverse reactions reported are seizures (particularly with meperidine and propoxyphene), tinnitus, jaundice (hepatic toxicity), pruritus, skin rash or facial edema (allergic reaction), breathing difficulties, respiratory depression, excitability (paradoxical reaction seen mainly in children), confusion, and tachycardia (*United States Pharmacopeia Dispensing Information,* 1999). The Management of Drug Overdose box at right discusses the treatment of an opioid overdose.

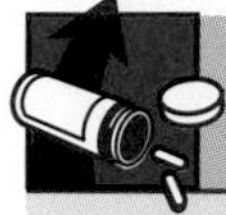

Management of Drug Overdose
Opioids

- Emesis or gastric lavage is used to empty the stomach if an oral opioid overdose occurs. If respiratory depression or any other life-threatening adverse effect is present, the treatment for these effects takes precedence.
- For respiratory depression, establish a patent airway and controlled respiration. Administer naloxone (Narcan) to reverse the opioid-induced respiratory depression and sedation by displacing the opioids at the receptor site. In opioid-dependent individuals, naloxone can also induce acute drug withdrawal. The IV route of administration is the preferred method of administering naloxone, with its effects being seen within 2 minutes. It can also be given intramuscularly or subcutaneously, but the onset of action is then seen within 2 to 5 minutes.
- Naloxone is shorter acting than most opioids and therefore must be administered by continuous infusion or by repeated injections (intramuscularly or subcutaneously) to prevent the recurrence of respiratory depression. (See the drug monograph on naloxone, p. 284, for additional information.)

Continuous Infusion of Opioids

Continuous infusion of opioids may be used when other routes of administration have failed to provide satisfactory pain relief, such as for clients with severe pain unrelieved by oral, rectal, or intermittent parenteral opioid dosing. IV opioids are helpful for the short-term treatment of severe pain (e.g., pain management in the postoperative period) or when other routes of administration may be inappropriate, such as in clients with intractable vomiting or when severe local bruising follows an IM or SC injection.

Before starting the pump infusion, the nurse should obtain a baseline blood pressure and respiratory rate, rhythm, and depth. All previous medication orders for pain are discontinued. The solution is administered using a microdrip infusion set and infusion control pump. Figure 14-10, *A*, shows a portable wrist model of a PCA unit commonly used in a hospital setting, most often after surgery. This pump allows the client to receive a predetermined IV bolus (a quantity of drug introduced into a vein at one time) of an analgesic (usually morphine) by striking the syringe pump mechanism. Thus the client can control the administration of the analgesic. The prescriber orders the predetermined analgesic dose and a set lockout interval of 5 to 20 minutes. The pump is then calibrated to deliver the ordered dose whenever the client activates the button. The lockout

A

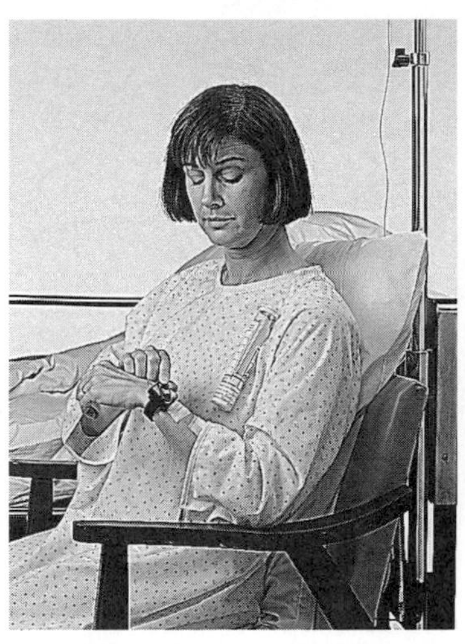

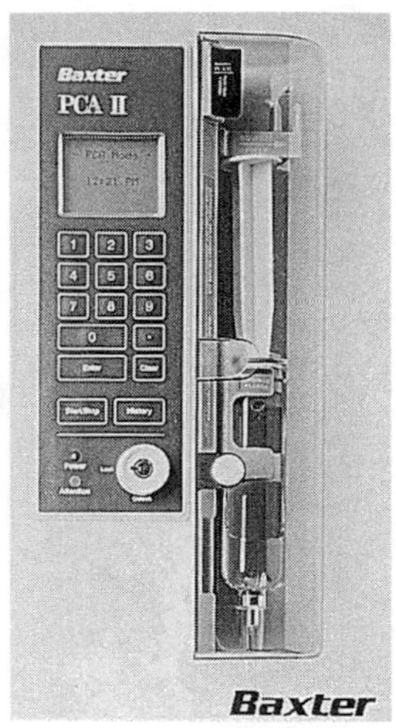

B

Figure 14-10 Examples of continuous infusion pumps. **A**, Portable wrist model. **B**, PCA pump is designed for client- or clinician-activated medication delivery. (Courtesy Baxter Healthcare Corporation, Deerfield, IL.)

mechanism prevents an inadvertent overdose or excessive analgesic administration by the client. This pump can also record the number of times the button is struck and the total cumulative dose delivered. Figure 14-10, *B*, illustrates a pump that may be programmed for continuous administration, client-activated delivery, or clinician-activated delivery. The pump also records all bolus attempts, successful and unsuccessful, made by the client. Thus the nurse and the prescriber are able to evaluate the appropriateness of the medication therapy and determine when the client is not receiving adequate medication. Because it is lightweight (approximately 15 ounces) and easily worn, it does not impair ambulation in mobile clients.

The initial infusion rate is determined by the client's current pain treatment requirements and degree of pain control. Adjustments to the initial infusion rate are based on objective and subjective evidence of pain relief and side effects. The client should be monitored for potential respiratory depression every hour for the first 4 hours and routinely thereafter. If the client's respiratory rate falls below the established limit, the nurse should reduce the rate of flow, notify the prescriber, and have naloxone (an opioid antagonist) ready to administer. Mechanical ventilation may be preferred to naloxone to relieve the respiratory depression, because naloxone will also diminish the client's pain relief.

Duramorph, a preservative-free morphine sulfate solution, is commonly prescribed for IV, epidural, or intrathecal use. The risk of inducing respiratory depression is reportedly greater with the intrathecal route than with epidural administration (*USP DI*, 1999). Although nurses do not usually administer drugs intraspinally, they may be required to fill the drug reservoir of an implanted intraspinal delivery system. Special training of the nurse is required, and the manufacturer's directions should be followed closely.

■ Nursing Management

Opioid Therapy

■ **Assessment.** A thorough assessment regarding the location, severity, quality, and intensity of the client's pain needs to be accomplished to establish a baseline for management of the client's condition. It is necessary to individualize the drug dose and its frequency according to the potency and duration of action of the specific drug used, the severity of pain, the use of a pain scale, the condition of the client, other medications that the client is receiving concurrently, and the client's response to the analgesic regimen (see the assessment discussion under Nursing Management: Pain Therapy, p. 263).

The client should be assessed for preexisting conditions that would be worsened by the use of opioids and therefore for which opioids are contraindicated: hypersensitivity to the prescribed drug; acute respiratory depression; or diarrhea associated with pseudomembranous colitis caused by cephalosporins, lincomycins, penicillins, or poisoning. For epidural or intrathecal administration, contraindications include coagulation defects (uncontrollable CNS hemorrhage may result) or infection at or near the site of administration (infection may spread into the CNS). Opioids should be used with extreme caution in conditions such as acute bronchial asthma or any respiratory impairment or chronic disease, increased intracranial pressure (may increase), or severe inflammatory bowel disease (risk of toxic megacolon). See the Pregnancy Safety box on p. 274 for the Food and Drug Administration's (FDA's) pregnancy safety classifications of analgesics.

Pregnancy Safety
Analgesics

Category	Drug
B	diclofenac, flurbiprofen, ketoprofen, nalmefene, naloxone, naproxen, oxycodone
C	auranofin, aurothioglucose, buprenorphine, codeine, dezocine, diflunisal, etodolac, fentanyl, hydrocodone, hydromorphone, ketorolac, mefenamic acid, morphine, nabumetone, naltrexone, opium, oxaprozin, pentazocine, tolmetin
Unclassified	butorphanol, fenoprofen, indomethacin, levorphanol, meclofenamate, meperidine, methadone, nalbuphine, oxymorphone, penicillamine, piroxicam, propoxyphene, sulindac, tiaprofenic acid

Review the client's current medication regimen for the risk of significant drug interactions, such as those that may occur when opioids are given concurrently with the following drugs:

Bold/color type indicates the most serious interactions.

Drug	Possible Effect and Management
alcohol or other CNS depressants	May result in enhanced CNS depression, respiratory depression, and hypotension. Reduce dosage of one or both drugs and monitor closely for decreased respiratory rate and blood pressure, slowed reflexes, and drowsiness.
buprenorphine (Buprenex)	**May result in additive effect of respiratory depression if given concurrently with low dosages of mu receptor agonists or with kappa receptor agonist. Avoid concurrent usage. Buprenorphine has partial agonist effects on the mu receptor. If given before or after an opioid agonist, it may reduce the analgesic effects of the opioid.**
carbamazepine (Tegretol)	**Concurrent use with propoxyphene may result in decreased metabolism and increased carbamazepine serum concentration, thus increasing the potential for toxicity. Avoid concurrent drug administration.**
monoamine oxidase (MAO) inhibitors (furazolidone [Furoxone], procarbazine [Matulane])	**Test dose with one fourth of the dose of morphine (or any prescribed opioid analgesics) to ascertain compatibility of the medications. There is a possibility of inducing excitability, hypertension, or hypotension; increased sweating; convulsions; respiratory depression; fever; and cardiac dysfunctions. Therefore it is usually recommended that caution be taken and reduced dosages of opioids be prescribed for clients receiving MAO inhibitors. Concurrent administration with meperidine has resulted in very severe and, at times, fatal reactions. The effects include sudden excitation, increased sweating, rigidity, very severe hypertension (or hypotension in some persons), coma, seizures, hyperpyrexia, and collapse. The use of meperidine is contraindicated in any clients who are receiving or who have received a MAO inhibitor within 2 to 3 weeks** *(USP DI,* 1999).
naloxone (Narcan)	Will produce withdrawal symptoms in clients who are dependent on opioid medications. Avoid concurrent administration in clients receiving opioids therapeutically.
rifampin (Rifadin)	May increase methadone metabolism and so may precipitate withdrawal symptoms in clients being treated for opioid dependence. Methadone dosage adjustment may be required.
zidovudine (AZT)	**Morphine may decrease clearance of zidovudine. Concurrent use should be avoided because toxicity of one or both drugs may occur.**

■ **Nursing Diagnosis.** In many instances, the nursing diagnoses indicated in the Nursing Care Plan on p. 275 may be overcome with appropriate nursing care.

■ **Implementation**

■ ***Monitoring.*** Observe the client's response to the analgesic, and record the degree and duration of pain relief and any adverse effects that may occur. Vital signs, particularly respiratory rate, should be obtained and recorded before morphine sulfate is given. Morphine can cause respiratory depression; if the client's respiratory rate is less than 12 per minute, the dose may need to be withheld or decreased. In addition, monitor the client's orientation, reflexes, bilateral grip strength, level of consciousness, pupil size, bowel sounds, urinary output, and liver and kidney function tests. The nurse's assessment is important information and is required by the prescriber to determine the possibility of adverse drug reactions in the client. Signs of opioid overdose are cold and clammy skin, drowsiness, dizziness, restlessness and mental confusion, miosis (pinpoint pupils), and decreas-

Nursing Care Plan
Selected Nursing Diagnoses Related to Opioid Therapy

Nursing Diagnosis	Outcome Criteria	Nursing Interventions
Ineffective airway clearance related to cough reflex suppression	Evidence of good pulmonary ventilation Absence of rhonchi	Reposition the immobile client frequently. Teach turning, coughing, and deep breathing.
Ineffective breathing pattern: hypoventilation related to CNS depressant effects of drug	Respiratory rate 16-20 breaths/min Absence of cyanosis	Assess respiratory rate before administering each dose; if below 12 breaths/min, hold dose. Administer oxygen. Elevate head of bed. Have narcotic antagonist and respiratory support systems nearby during IV administration.
Risk for deficient fluid volume related to nausea and/or vomiting	Absence of and/or decrease in nausea and/or vomiting	Administer prescribed antiemetics. Administer oral analgesics with food. Reduce noxious environmental stimuli. Apply cool cloth to the face. Provide small, frequent meals.
Constipation	Evidence of client's normal bowel patterns	Assess client's bowel status. Increase fluid consumption. Instruct in high-fiber diet. Encourage ambulation. Obtain an order for a stool softener and/or a bulk-forming laxative. Provide relaxed environment for elimination.
Urinary retention	Evidence of urinary status without urgency and/or retention	Increase fluid intake to approximately 2500 mL daily unless contraindicated. Administer sitz bath. Provide relaxed environment for elimination. Suggest a dosage reduction or switch to alternative therapy.
Risk for injury related to sensory-perceptual alterations	Absence of injury	Assist in ambulation. Caution against driving and other hazardous activities. Caution against taking alcohol and other CNS depressants concurrently.

ing pulse rate and blood pressure. Oral and injectable opioid analgesics produce unacceptable or undesirable effects such as nausea and vomiting, constipation, urinary retention, cough reflex suppression, and CNS effects.

Tolerance is another undesirable effect of narcotic analgesics. An increase in dosage may be needed to obtain the same degree of analgesic effectiveness. A lack of reliable data has led to many misconceptions about tolerance. For example, tolerance is sporadic and unpredictable and does not always occur. One client may take the same dosage of the same opioid for years and never need an increase, whereas another client with similar pain problems may require periodic increases. In the majority of clients with genuine pain who receive opioids in therapeutic dosages, the dependence liability is relatively uncommon; most clients do not report euphoria or psychologic dependence. Tolerance in clients needing pain relief (not tolerance in clients who take drugs for pleasure) is managed by gradually decreasing the dosage when an analgesic effect is achieved. Once pain is controlled (e.g., the tumor that is causing the pain is removed), a lower dosage will maintain the analgesic effects. The need for an increase in the analgesic dosage will usually be a result of the disease process or progression. Assess for pupillary constriction. As the drug is eliminated from the body, the pupils return to normal. Continued constriction of the pupils with an early return of the symptoms for which the medication was administered may indicate a developing tolerance—the drug has not yet been eliminated from the body but has diminished effectiveness.

Abrupt withdrawal of opioid analgesics after prolonged use and physical dependence may result in abstinence syndrome. **Abstinence syndrome** is a collection of symptoms: restlessness, chills and hot flashes, piloerection ("goose bumps"), rhinorrhea ("runny nose"), drowsiness, lacrimation (tearing of the eyes), mydriasis (dilation of the pupils), sneezing, yawning, generalized anxiety, abdominal cramps, lower back pain, lower extremity cramps, anorexia, vomiting and diarrhea, sweating, muscular twitching, and a craving for the drug. Decreasing the dosage of the medication gradually as the severity of the pain decreases may diminish the development of withdrawal symptoms.

BOX 14-2

Epidural Analgesia

Epidural analgesia is a therapeutic modality that offers an alternative to traditional methods of pain control. It can be administered as an intermittent injection or a continuous infusion of opiate into the epidural space. The nursing management of clients receiving epidural analgesia to manage postoperative pain is an essential for client comfort and safety. In general, the client should understand the purpose and the benefits of epidural analgesia and provide consent to the modality before surgery.

With the client in a side-lying position, the epidural catheter is inserted most commonly at the L2 level by the anesthesiologist. Once the catheter is tested for placement, it is stabilized with an occlusive dressing. It should be taped in such a manner that the tubing does not pull or kink. The anesthesiologist should be notified if the catheter becomes dislodged or the dressing becomes loose or wet. The catheter may be connected to a continuous infusion or capped and should be carefully labeled "for epidural use only." Because some preservatives might be toxic to neural tissue, medications for epidural use must not contain preservatives.

Although rare, respiratory depression can occur with the administration of spinal opiates. The respiratory status of the client receiving intermittent epidural analgesia should be monitored once each hour for the first 12 hours or until the respiratory rate exceeds 12 breaths/min, then every 2 hours for 12 hours, and then every 4 hours for the duration of therapy. With continuous infusion of the analgesic agent, the client should be monitored every hour for the first 24 hours or until the respiratory rate is greater than 12 breaths/min, then once every 4 hours for the duration of therapy. Clients with low respiratory rates should be monitored as necessary.

Naloxone is usually kept in the immediate client environment according to agency policy. The anesthesiologist is called immediately if respiratory depression occurs. Naloxone 0.4 mg IV is usually ordered, but this dose may also reverse the analgesic effect of the opiate, and the client will experience pain.

Pruritus is experienced by approximately one third of all clients receiving spinal opioids. Although the mechanism is unclear, this reaction is believed to occur when epidural opiates produce sensory sensations that are interpreted by the sensory cortex as itching. Low doses of naloxone are administered to relieve the pruritus without concomitant reversal of analgesia. Nausea and vomiting may also be an issue with some clients. Fluid balance monitoring and the assessment of bladder distention should be maintained while the client is receiving epidural analgesia to detect any urinary retention that may occur.

Using a pain scale, the client's level of comfort should be assessed every 2 to 4 hours for the first 24 hours after surgery. Supplemental parenteral analgesics may be required for "breakthrough" pain. Assess the level of consciousness every 2 hours for the first 24 hours and then every 4 hours for the duration of therapy. Some agencies require a motor and sensory assessment at least every 8 hours and before ambulation. Blood pressure and pulse should be determined before ambulating the client for the first time.

Instruct the client to notify the nurse if pain is experienced and if increased drowsiness and/or leg numbness and weakness occur. Epidural analgesia is not usually continued past the fifth postoperative day.

Modified from Keeney, S.A. (1993). Nursing care of the postoperative patient receiving epidural analgesia. *MEDSURG Nursing*, 2(3), 191-196.

■ ***Intervention.*** Preventive pain treatment with analgesics involves frequent administration on a regular fixed-time interval in anticipation of pain. Analgesics are to be given before the client anticipates the recurrence of pain or before the pain reaches an intensity that makes the client feel a loss of control. The client should actively participate in the pain treatment process with trust and confidence and be able to assist in planning a schedule of pain medication based on lifestyle. A fixed-time schedule of administration decreases suffering until the next scheduled dose because a blood level of the analgesic is reached to control the client's pain. If the fixed-time schedule is inappropriate, it is the nurse's responsibility to teach the client to request medication before the pain becomes severe. Often clients are unaware that they need to ask for pain medication, because none of their other medications may be on a demand schedule.

Encourage the client's and family's belief in the pain-treatment process and willingness to participate in its reinforcement. Combinations of optimal doses of NSAIDs and opioid agonists indicated for pain may permit lower dosages of the opioid agonist. A stepped-care or flow chart approach (see Figure 14-9) is the optimal plan to follow because it uses nonopioid analgesics and progresses to other stronger analgesics to manage the client's pain with the most effective dosage.

To achieve the best analgesic effect after administering the medication, provide comfort measures such as reducing environmental stimuli, assisting the client to a comfortable

BOX 14-3

Intraspinal Analgesia

Another type of analgesic therapy—continuous intraspinal morphine infusion—reduces the client's pain without diminishing CNS functioning. An implantable infusion device is connected to an implantable catheter that is placed in the epidural and intrathecal space. The system administers the medication continuously and is refilled by injection through a septum into a central chamber of the device. In the home setting the client and family are taught how to care for the device and how to evaluate the response to the therapy. The device is usually refilled every 2 weeks by a home health care nurse. Study is continuing with this unique method of pain control, which promises relief for clients with intractable pain while increasing quality of life.

BOX 14-4

Analgesic Equivalency Chart

All analgesics are compared with 10 mg IM morphine to determine an analgesic dosage equivalent. Equianalgesic information, that is the dose of one drug that produces approximately the same analgesic effect as the dose of another drug, is very useful information for the health care professional, who is considering drug alternatives.

Analgesic	IM dose (mg)	Oral dose (mg)
morphine	10	20-60*
hydromorphone	1.5	7.5
oxycodone	Not available	15-30
levorphanol	2	4
methadone	10	20
meperidine	75	300

Suppository Dosage Form

Hydromorphone, 3 mg, is approximately equivalent to 1.5 mg IM dose.

Morphine, 10-30 mg, is considered equivalent to the oral dosage.

Individualize dosage according to patient response.

Oxymorphone, 5-10 mg, is approximately equivalent to 1 mg of IM oxymorphone.

*For a single dose or intermittent use. Chronic administration may decrease oral dose to 20 or 30 mg equivalent.

position, and massaging the client's back. These and other nonpharmacologic measures for pain (e.g., relaxation techniques and cutaneous stimulation) may be used concurrently and considered as substitutes for pharmacologic interventions with some clients. If CNS effects occur, the client's safety should be maintained (e.g., assisted ambulation).

Injection sites should be rotated to prevent induration and abscess. Oral, IV, or other routes of administration should be considered if an analgesic medication is required for more than 2 weeks. Epidural or intrathecal administration may be considered for prolonged pain relief (Boxes 14-2 and 14-3). Naloxone must be on hand when a narcotic is administered by the epidural, intrathecal, or IV route, because the risk of respiratory distress significantly increases with these routes of administration. Clients in shock may have impaired tissue perfusion, and therefore repeated IM or SC administration of opioids may result in an overdose when the client's circulation is restored.

Morphine sulfate intensified oral solution (Roxanol, 20 mg/mL) comes with a specific calibrated dropper; no other dropper should be used for dosing. The medication is diluted in 30 mL or more of fluid or semisolid food. Make sure the entire dose is removed from the dropper.

When the prescriber changes the client's medication from one route of administration to another, check the dosage against the Analgesic Equivalency Chart (Box 14-4).

Other side effects/adverse reactions of opioid therapy can be managed with nursing actions as discussed in the Nursing Care Plan on p. 275.

■ ***Education.*** Because orthostatic hypotension (a form of low blood pressure that occurs when a person stands) can occur in an ambulatory client, the client should be cautioned about rising quickly from a supine position. The client should be instructed to have assistance, if necessary, if he or she wishes to ambulate. Opioids can also impair mental and physical abilities, so caution should be exercised when the drug is prescribed for ambulatory clients or for anyone who will be driving a car or operating any type of machinery. The client should be instructed to increase daily fluid intake to minimize the constipating effects of opioids and to take a stool softener or mild laxative if necessary.

A client taking opioids needs to be reminded that the combination of ethanol and the normal dosage of the drug can render him or her incapable of normal functioning. Instruct the client to alert the prescriber to other drugs being taken concurrently. The dosage may be altered by a prescriber if a client is taking other opioid analgesics, CNS depressants, cyclic antidepressants, neuroleptics, anxiolytics, ethanol, or sedative-hypnotics, because the combination of any of these can produce CNS depression.

Roxanol is the most convenient method of receiving oral morphine but requires careful instruction of the client. Because it is a controlled substance, the client should be instructed to prevent theft by drug-dependent individuals.

■ **Evaluation.** Because opioid analgesics are often used inappropriately, be aware of and report any instances of suspected abuse. Some health professionals are not well versed in pain control, and therefore nurses should take the initiative in reversing the undertreatment of clients in pain. Educating others within the clinical setting is important in promoting comfort for the client. The client should report pain relief after administration of the drug, the respiratory status should be within the normal limits, and other adverse responses to the drug (e.g., CNS depression, urinary retention, and constipation) should not occur.

Opium Preparations

Opium contains several alkaloids, including morphine and small amounts of codeine and papaverine. The effects of opium result from the presence of morphine in the preparations. The mechanism of action and pharmacokinetics are the same as or similar to morphine.

Opium tincture contains 10 mg morphine/mL and is used as an antidiarrheal agent. When diluted, it is used for the treatment of neonatal opioid dependence.

Camphorated tincture of opium (paregoric) contains 2 mg morphine/5 mL. It is an antidiarrheal agent. In some instances it has been used to treat neonatal opioid dependence, but this use is controversial. Paregoric contains camphor, which can cause serious toxicity, including seizures and respiratory depression; it also contains benzoic acid, which can displace bilirubin from albumin. Both substances may enhance the typical problems seen in opioid-dependent infants (e.g., convulsions and hyperbilirubinemia); therefore many prescribers seem to prefer the use of diluted opium tincture to paregoric.

Opium alkaloids hydrochloride injection (Pantopon) contains 10 mg morphine/mL. This product is available only in Canada. Number 15A opium and belladonna suppositories (B&O Supprettes) contain 30 mg powdered opium (10% morphine and other alkaloids) and 16.2 mg powdered belladonna alkaloid (the principal belladonna alkaloids are atropine and scopolamine). Number 16A contains 60 mg powdered opium and 16.2 mg belladonna extract. The preparations are used to relieve moderate to severe pain reported with ureteral spasms and have also been prescribed for breakthrough pain between injections of opioids. (See Morphine, p. 270, for side effects/adverse reactions and significant drug interactions.)

The adult dosage for opium tincture is 0.3 to 1 mL PO four times daily, to a maximum of 6 mL daily. The dosage for camphorated tincture of opium (paregoric) is 5 to 10 mL PO one to four times daily, with a maximum of 10 mL four times daily. The paregoric dosage for children 2 years and older is 0.25 to 0.5 mL/kg body weight one to four times daily.

▪ Nursing Management

Opium Preparation Therapy

In addition to the following discussion, see Nursing Management: Opioid Therapy, p. 273. Opium tincture may be diluted with water for administration; the solution will become milky. Other liquid forms of opioids may be given with fruit juice to increase their palatability. If opium tincture is given as an antidiarrheal, its effectiveness is monitored by checking the frequency and character of stools. If rectal suppositories are being used to administer opioids, the rectum should be emptied first to enhance absorption of the drug.

codeine [koe′ deen] (Paveral)

Codeine is available in sulfate and phosphate salts and is marketed as oral tablets, oral solution, and injectable dosage forms. Codeine is absorbed well after either oral or parenteral administration and is excreted by the kidneys. Oral administration is used for analgesic, antitussive, and antidiarrheal effects. Codeine may also be injected for the treatment of mild to moderate pain. See Tables 14-2 and 14-4 for a pharmacokinetic overview and dosing data for opioid analgesics.

▪ Nursing Management

Codeine Therapy

In addition to the following discussion, see Nursing Management: Opioid Therapy, p. 273. Oral codeine should be administered with milk or food to reduce any gastrointestinal distress. Codeine has been added to cough elixirs because it acts as a cough suppressant. Encourage fluid hydration, which helps to liquefy sputum and reduces the constipating effects of codeine.

hydrocodone bitartrate [hye droe koe′ done] (Vicodin, Hycodan)

Hydrocodone is marketed in combination with homatropine in the United States. In Canada, Hycodan consists of hydrocodone bitartrate only. Although the product name is similar in both countries, the formulation is not identical. Hydrocodone bitartrate is used as an analgesic and antitussive. See Tables 14-2 and 14-4 for additional information.

hydromorphone [hye droe mor′ fone] (Dilaudid, Dilaudid HP)

Hydromorphone is a semisynthetic opioid that has a faster onset of action but a shorter duration of action than morphine. It is prescribed for its analgesic and antitussive effects. See Tables 14-2 and 14-4 for additional information.

meperidine [me per′ i deen] (Demerol, Pethidine)

Meperidine is an effective analgesic for short-term use but is considered "the least potent of the common opioid analgesics, and is administered in the largest doses" (Mather & Denson, 1992). A commonly prescribed opioid, it has a pharmacologic profile similar to morphine, with the following noted differences:

1. Meperidine is less apt to release histamine or to increase biliary tract pressure than morphine; thus it is often prescribed for clients with acute asthma, biliary colic, and pancreatitis (Sinatra & Savarese, 1992).
2. Its duration of action is shorter than morphine; thus a more frequent dosing schedule is necessary (see Table 14-4).
3. Meperidine has poor oral bioavailability. Achieving an analgesic equivalency approximate to a 75-mg IM

dose requires an oral dose of 300 mg (*USP DI*, 1999). Because the largest oral form of meperidine marketed is a 100-mg tablet, this preparation is often prescribed in dosages that are less effective than the injectable dosage form. See Table 14-2 for dosing data.

4. Meperidine is metabolized in the liver to normeperidine, a CNS neurotoxic metabolite. Normeperidine has a half-life between 15 and 20 hours in persons with normal renal function. Prolonged administration, the use of high dosages of meperidine, or the use in older adults or in clients with impaired renal or hepatic function has resulted in normeperidine-induced CNS toxicity. This neurotoxicity may produce significant mood changes such as sadness, anger, restlessness and apprehension, increased irritability, nervousness, tremors, agitation, quivering, convulsions, and myoclonus (American Hospital Formulary Service, 1999; AHCPR, 1994). Neurotoxicity has also been reported in clients with sickle cell anemia, burn injuries, or cancer who had normal renal and hepatic function but were receiving repeated large doses of meperidine (AHFS, 1999).

   Although the use of meperidine for only a few days may generally result in mild and tolerable problems, it should be avoided in clients who require prolonged usage or high-dose therapy or who have renal or liver dysfunction. The Nursing Research box at right discusses research on the postoperative use of meperidine. The nurse should be aware that naloxone (opioid antagonist) antagonizes meperidine but not normeperidine and may in some instances cause further CNS excitation and seizures. Management of normeperidine toxicity includes stopping meperidine and substituting an alternate opioid such as morphine. An anticonvulsant may be used if seizures occur.

5. Meperidine produces a vagolytic effect, which results in significant tachycardia. Therefore its use should probably be avoided or closely monitored in clients with dysrhythmias or myocardial infarction.

The drug interaction table on p. 274 should be reviewed, especially for concurrent use of MAO inhibitors with meperidine. Very severe, unpredictable life-threatening reactions may result.

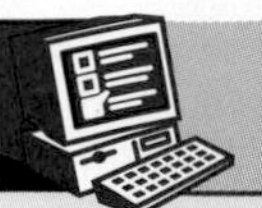

Nursing Research
Postoperative Use of Meperidine

Citation: McDonald, D.D. (1993). Postoperative narcotic analgesic administration. *Applied Nursing Research, 6*(3), 106.

Abstract: Administration of a narcotic analgesic is an integral part of nursing care for postoperative clients. However, moderate to severe pain remains the norm for most hospitalized clients. Undertreatment of pain appears to be the most common explanation for the frequency and severity of pain experienced by postoperative clients. The purpose of this study was to describe the types and amounts of narcotic analgesics administered postoperatively to clients by nurses.

The postoperative administration of narcotic analgesics was examined with 180 uncomplicated adult appendectomy clients. Narcotic analgesic dosages were transcribed from the hospital records of these clients for the entire postoperative period. Equianalgesic dosages were calculated so that all medications were comparable with meperidine. Eighty-three percent (n = 150) of the clients received meperidine. Clients who received meperidine were given significantly more narcotic analgesics than those who received morphine sulfate. A greater amount of narcotic analgesics received by clients was significantly related to increases in the length of stay. Meperidine and Tylenol #3 (acetaminophen with codeine phosphate) comprised the analgesics significantly associated with length of stay. These findings suggest a need to reexamine the current use of meperidine in postoperative analgesia.

Critical Thinking Questions

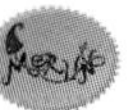

- What is specific about the pharmacokinetics of meperidine that might have contributed to this finding?
- Within the data of this research was a finding that eight people received no narcotic analgesic at all. How might this result occur?
- What other factors might result in the association between meperidine and extended length of hospital stay for clients?

■ Nursing Management
Meperidine Therapy

■ **Assessment.** The administration of meperidine is contraindicated in the following situations: clients with severe dysfunction of the liver because the drug is inactivated in the liver; with head injury and increased intracranial pressure because it may mask neurologic parameters; and with chronic obstructive pulmonary disease because it may result in respiratory depression and shock. Respiratory depression occurs as with morphine but is of shorter duration. Meperidine causes CNS excitation that ranges from irritability to seizures. When administered with a phenothiazine such as promethazine (Phenergan), which also lowers the seizure threshold, the client is at higher risk for seizures. Meperidine should be used with caution in clients who have atrial flutter or other supraventricular tachycardia, because meperidine may increase ventricular response through vagolytic action. Meperidine is not administered for chronic pain because of its short duration of action. It may be given orally but is more effective when given intramuscularly.

A thorough assessment of the client's pain regarding location, severity, and quality needs to be performed as discussed under Nursing Management: Opioid Therapy, p. 273.

■ **Nursing Diagnosis.** In addition to the nursing diagnoses considered under Nursing Management: Opioid Therapy (p. 273), clients are at risk for impaired skin integrity (fibrotic areas) related to IM administration and for disturbed sensory perception, such as restlessness, agitation, and hallucinations, related to CNS stimulation.

■ **Implementation**

■ ***Monitoring.*** Vital signs should be monitored and recorded before and after the administration of meperidine, because it may cause tachycardia and hypotension. Observations for behavioral change are indicated. Other observations of the client are the same as discussed for morphine.

■ ***Intervention.*** Consult a specific reference before mixing meperidine in solution with another medication, because meperidine tends to be physically and chemically incompatible with a wide range of substances.

Tissue irritation is common with the administration of IM meperidine. Clients often experience muscle damage, poor absorption, and pain during injection. The rotation of injection sites is essential. Meperidine is diluted for IV administration, but this is not the recommended route of administration. IV administration needs to be titrated for the client's response because of its respiratory depressant effects.

The dosage of meperidine should be gradually tapered because abstinence symptoms such as nausea, vomiting, and diarrhea may occur. Such symptoms should be reported to the prescriber so that the dosage can be adjusted.

■ ***Education.*** Client teaching is the same as for the client education discussed in the section on morphine, p. 270. (See also the Case Study box below.)

■ **Evaluation.** The expected outcome of meperidine therapy is the same as for morphine.

methadone [meth' a done] (Dolophine, Methadose)

Methadone is an effective analgesic with properties similar to morphine (with the exception of its extended half-life). The duration of action for methadone is usually listed at 4 to 6 hours, but with repeated oral dosing the half-life may extend from 22 to 48 hours (perhaps even longer in older adults and in clients with renal dysfunction). This extended half-life is not related to its analgesic effect. To control pain, methadone is administered every 6 to 8 hours based on the individual's response. See Table 14-2 for dosing information.

Because of its extended half-life, methadone is approved by the FDA for use in detoxification and maintenance treatment programs approved by the various states. In Canada, it is available through specially authorized physicians. Oral administration is preferred for detoxification and required for maintenance programs. Methadone dependence is substituted in individuals who are physiologically dependent on heroin, opium, or other opioids. (See Chapter 9 for information on methadone treatment programs.)

The mechanism of action and the pharmacokinetics of methadone are similar to that of morphine (see Table 14-4). Side effects/adverse reactions are also similar to those for morphine, although the miotic and respiratory depressant effects of methadone may be present for more than 24 hours. Excessive sedation is reported in some clients following a regular dosing schedule.

■ Nursing Management

Methadone Therapy

See also Nursing Management: Opioid Therapy, p. 273.

■ **Assessment.** When a client is receiving methadone for the treatment of heroin abuse, be aware of possible outside sources of OTC drugs (liquid cough preparations with alcohol) and alcohol (alcohol or alcohol beverages brought in

Case Study *Pain Management*

Daniel Watkins is a 53-year-old man who was admitted to the hospital for severe abdominal pain. A bowel resection was performed to relieve an obstruction. By his fourth postoperative day he is ambulating and tolerating oral intake. He has been taking both injections and oral medications for pain. The following medications are currently ordered:

meperidine, 50-75 mg IM q4h prn for pain
Tylox, one or two capsules PO q4h prn for pain
Tylenol, 650 mg PO q4h prn for headache and fever

Mr. Watkins is complaining of pain around his incision after a dressing change and removal of surgical drains. He is very anxious and upset and is requesting pain medication. He had his last dose of meperidine 6 hours ago. He took one capsule of Tylox 2 hours ago for mild pain after ambulating.

1. What assessment data does the nurse need in order to decide how to intervene at this time?
2. The nurse decides to administer meperidine 50 mg IM. What assessment should be performed to monitor for adverse reactions to the meperidine?
3. What should the nurse document in the client's chart about the pain management?
4. Mr. Watkins complains that the drugs do not always help when he has severe pain. What is the nurse's appropriate action for this situation?
5. What measures can the nurse teach Mr. Watkins to promote more effective pain management?
6. What medication would be most appropriate for the nurse to administer when Mr. Watkins complains of a headache?

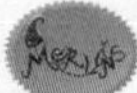

For answer guidelines, go to mosby.com/MERLIN/McKenry/.

by friends and family). These substances may potentiate the action of methadone.

■ **Implementation**

■ ***Monitoring.*** Although most adverse effects dissipate in the first 3 weeks of methadone therapy, constipation and diaphoresis may persist.

■ ***Intervention.*** An overdose of methadone can cause extreme respiratory depression. Naloxone should be readily available for IV administration. The antagonist action of naloxone is only 1 to 3 hours, but the action of methadone is 36 to 48 hours or more; thus repeated doses of naloxone for up to 8 to 24 hours may be required to treat respiratory depression.

When methadone is used for detoxification and maintenance therapy, it is administered as an oral liquid. If dispersible tablets are used, they are dissolved in 120 mL of water or citrus-flavored solution such as Tang, Kool-Aid, or fruit juice. Dissolution takes a minute or so and may be enhanced by using cold and/or acidic solvents. If the concentrated oral solution is used, it should be diluted in at least 90 mL of solution to enable the complete dose to be received. It has also been used for pain management in terminally ill clients.

■ ***Education.*** Methadone is commonly given on an outpatient basis for withdrawal from heroin or morphine-like drugs. Clients should be cautioned about operating a car or other potentially dangerous equipment, because mental and physical abilities may be impaired. Orthostatic hypotension is a common side effect and can last for several weeks. Clients should be instructed to rise slowly from a recumbent position and to sit or lie down in the event of dizziness or faintness.

■ **Evaluation.** If methadone is administered for detoxification, the client will demonstrate effective management of the therapeutic regimen by remaining free of the abused substance and by participating in psychiatric, social, and vocational rehabilitation programs. If pain management is the goal of methadone therapy, the client will experience pain relief without the adverse effects of therapy, such as constipation, confusion, or respiratory depression.

levorphanol [lee vor′ fa nole] (Levo-Dromoran)

Levorphanol is an opioid analgesic used for moderate to severe pain. This drug has a longer analgesic duration of effect than morphine or meperidine (AHFS, 1999) and a half-life of 11 to 16 hours (*Drug Facts and Comparisons*, 2000). Therefore a drug accumulation and overdose may result from doses that are too large or are administered too frequently, chronic dosing of children or small adults, or even the use of average dosages in medically compromised clients. (See Tables 14-2 and 14-4 for additional information.)

The actions of levorphanol are identical to morphine, but the effective dosage is one-fourth to one-fifth that of morphine. Note, too, that the duration of action is 6 to 8 hours and will accumulate in the body and place the client at risk for respiratory depression if administered with the frequency of other opioids. (For nursing management of levorphanol therapy, review Nursing Management: Opioid Therapy, p. 273.)

oxycodone [ox i koe′ done] (Roxicodone, OxyIR)

Oxycodone is approximately 10 times more potent than codeine. It is available alone (Roxicodone, Oxy IR), in combination with aspirin (Percodan) or acetaminophen (Percocet, Roxicet ◆), and in extended-action dosage form (Oxycontin ◆). (See Tables 14-2 and 14-4 for additional information.) The suppository dosage form is not available in the United States but is available in Canada. (Review Nursing Management: Opioid Therapy, p. 273.)

oxymorphone [ox i mor′ fone] (Numorphan)

Oxymorphone is pharmacologically similar to morphine, with a few exceptions. In equianalgesic dosages, oxymorphone usually causes more nausea, vomiting, and psychic effects (euphoria) than morphine; it may also be less constipating and cause less suppression of the cough reflex than morphine. Oxymorphone is a potent analgesic used for moderate to severe pain, preoperative medication, obstetric analgesia, and as adjunct therapy for the treatment of anxiety caused by dyspnea that results from pulmonary edema associated with left ventricular failure. It is available in parenteral and rectal suppository dosage forms. (See Tables 14-2 and 14-4 for additional information.)

■ **Nursing Management**

Oxymorphone Therapy

Oxymorphone should be given with milk or meals to decrease the incidence of gastrointestinal distress. It tends to cause more nausea and vomiting than **equianalgesic** (producing approximately the same degree of analgesia) dosages of morphine sulfate. Oxymorphone suppositories need to be stored in the refrigerator but protected from freezing.

fentanyl [fen′ ta nil] (Sublimaze, Innovar, Duragesic)

Fentanyl is an opioid analgesic available in a preservative-free solution (Sublimaze), in combination with droperidol (Innovar), and as a topical transdermal patch (Duragesic). Fentanyl solution and fentanyl with droperidol are used parenterally (IV) for analgesia as a premedication, as an adjunct to anesthesia, and in the immediate postoperative period. Parenteral administration of fentanyl should be restricted to those experienced with this product and with the management of fentanyl-induced respiratory depression. Fentanyl and the fentanyl derivative sufentanil (Sufenta) may cause rigidity of muscle in the chest wall if given rapidly in large doses; this reaction requires supportive respiratory ventilation and perhaps a rapid-acting muscle relaxant. Respiratory depression is dose related (*USP DI*, 1999). (See also Appendix G.)

Fentanyl is metabolized in the liver and excreted in urine. Drug interactions and side effects/adverse reactions are similar to the other opioids. The patch system is available in 25, 50, 75, and 100 μg/hr dosage forms. The manufacturer publishes an equianalgesic potency chart and a morphine-to-fentanyl conversion chart that should be used to determine the fentanyl dosage.

▪ Nursing Management
Fentanyl Transdermal System

In addition to the following discussion, see Nursing Management: Opioid Therapy, p. 273.

▪ Assessment. In opioid-naïve clients, in older adults (60 years of age and older), and in cachectic or debilitated clients, the starting dose should not be higher than 25 μg/hr. This product is used in the management of chronic pain as an alternative to the other opioids, especially for clients who have difficulty swallowing or complying with a schedule of oral medications.

▪ Implementation

▪ *Monitoring.* Monitor respiratory status and keep naloxone and resuscitative equipment available.

▪ *Intervention.* Remove the transdermal system from the package immediately before applying. Use water to clean the skin area before application. Do not use soap, oils, lotions, alcohol, or other products because they may alter the absorption of this product. Apply the medication to a dry, flat (hairless) area of the upper torso (front or back). Do not apply to skin that is burned, cut, irritated, very oily, or recently shaved. If the skin area is hairy, cut the hair with scissors. Hold the patch in place for 10 to 20 seconds to be sure it is securely fastened to the client. Then check the patch to make certain skin contact is complete and the edges of the system adhere to the skin. Wash hands after applying the patch. Use large amounts of water in washing, especially if the gel accidentally comes in contact with your skin. Avoid using soap, alcohol, or any other solvent. The patch releases fentanyl continuously by absorption through the skin, which aids in controlling pain around-the-clock for 72 hours.

After application, fentanyl is absorbed and concentrated in the upper layers of skin. Serum levels increase slowly and usually reach a plateau between 12 and 24 hours. During the initial application of the patch, it is recommended that a short-acting analgesic be prescribed for the first 20 to 24 hours, because peak serum levels usually occur between 24 and 72 hours. Thereafter the person should have an order for a short-acting opioid for breakthrough pain.

The average half-life of fentanyl is 17 hours (range is 13 to 22 hours). Because it may take as long as 6 days to reach steady-state levels of a new dose, dosage adjustments after the initial 72-hour change should be instituted on an every-6-day schedule.

If another system is required after 72 hours, apply it to a new site. Withdraw the drug gradually. Because the serum level of fentanyl decreases slowly, give half the equianalgesic dose of the new analgesic 12 to 18 hours after removal.

▪ *Education.* Instruct the client to dispose of the system by folding the adhesive sides together and flushing the system down the toilet.

▪ Evaluation. The expected outcome of fentanyl therapy is that the client will experience pain relief without experiencing breakthrough pain or any adverse reactions to the drug.

propoxyphene [proe pox′ i feen] (Darvon)
propoxyphene napsylate combinations (Darvocet-N)

Propoxyphene is a synthetic analgesic that is structurally related to methadone and is indicated for the treatment of mild to moderate pain. Controlled studies have reported that propoxyphene 65 mg is equivalent to or less effective than acetaminophen 650 mg, aspirin 650 mg, codeine 32 mg, pentazocine (Talwin) 30 mg, or meperidine (Demerol) 50 mg (McCaffery & Beebe, 1989). When combined with aspirin or acetaminophen, propoxyphene combinations usually provide more analgesia than either medication alone.

Propoxyphene binds to opioid receptors and produces an analgesic effect similar to codeine and the opioids. The hydrochloride dosage form is more rapidly absorbed than the water-insoluble napsylate formulation, but peak serum levels are approximately equivalent. The bioavailability of propoxyphene hydrochloride 65 mg is equivalent to that of propoxyphene napsylate 100 mg. The duration of action is 4 to 6 hours. Propoxyphene crosses into the CNS and is believed to cross the placenta.

Metabolism occurs mainly in the liver, where approximately one fourth of the dose is metabolized to norpropoxyphene, a toxic metabolite with a half-life of 30 to 36 hours (*USP DI*, 1999). This toxic metabolite may cause seizures and cardiotoxicity (Abramowicz, 1998). Propoxyphene is also more apt to cause convulsions than most of the other opioid analgesics. (See Table 14-4 for pharmacokinetic information.)

The usual adult dosage for propoxyphene and propoxyphene napsylate is one tablet or capsule every 4 hours when needed. The pediatric dosage has not been established.

▪ Nursing Management
Propoxyphene Therapy

Propoxyphene should be used with caution in clients with a history of excessive alcohol intake, and it is contraindicated in clients who are suicidal or prone to addiction. Preparations containing propoxyphene taken in excessive doses or in combination with alcohol or other CNS depressants are a major cause of drug-related deaths. Ambulatory clients should be cautioned about driving a car or operating dangerous machinery, because judgment may be impaired.

Opioid-Like Analgesics

tramadol [tram′ a dole] (Ultram ◆)

Tramadol is a central-acting synthetic analgesic that is not chemically related to the opioids. This product appears to bind to the mu opioid receptors and also inhibits the re-

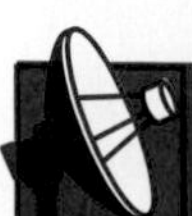

TechnologyLink
Analgesics

Web Resources

American Chronic Pain Association (www.theacpa.org)
A support system that provides education and self-help group activities for persons with chronic pain.

International Association for the Study of Pain (www.halcyon.com/iasp/)
This site is maintained by a multidisciplinary association devoted to the research and control of pain.

Mayo Clinic (www.mayohealth.org/)
This site offers a wide variety of medical information. A pain management search on this site provides a long list of articles on pain.

National Hospice and Palliative Care Organization (www.nhpco.org)
This organization is devoted to improving end-of-life care. The site provides information on hospices in the United States, educational and conference programs, and more.

Roxane Laboratories Pain Institute (www.roxane.com/)
This commercial site is replete with information on new findings, lecture seminar announcements, hospice nursing, and a database on cancer pain and palliative care.

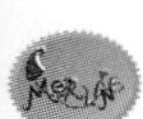

For additional WebLinks, a free subscription to the "Mosby/Saunders ePharmacology Update" newsletter, and more, go to mosby.com/MERLIN/McKenry/.

uptake of norepinephrine and serotonin. It is indicated for the treatment of moderate to moderately severe pain.

Tramadol was initially believed to have less potential for respiratory depression and drug dependency than the opioids. However, in 1996 the manufacturer sent a letter to professionals to warn them of potential seizures, anaphylactoid reactions, and substance abuse associated with tramadol (FDA News and Product Notes, 1996). Therefore this product is not recommended for use in persons with a history of opioid allergy, dependence, or a past or present history of addiction.

Tramadol is well absorbed orally with an onset of action within 60 minutes, a peak effect in 2 hours, and a half-life of approximately 6 to 7 hours. It is metabolized in the liver to inactive and active metabolites and is primarily excreted in urine. The usual adult dosage is 50 to 100 mg every 6 hours. The maximum daily dose is 400 mg.

■ Nursing Management

Tramadol Therapy

Because of the risk of altered breathing patterns (respiratory depression), the administration of tramadol is contraindicated for clients experiencing acute intoxication with alcohol, sedatives, opioids, psychotropic drugs, or other central-acting analgesics. Clients with a history of or active substance abuse or dependence issues have the potential for substance abuse. Sensitivity to opioids or to tramadol itself would also be a contraindication. The risk-benefit of tramadol should be considered for clients with seizures, respiratory depression, or hepatic or renal impairment.

Review the client's current medication regimen for the risk of significant drug interactions, such as those that may occur when tramadol is given concurrently with the following drugs:

Drug	Possible Effect and Management
Bold/color type indicates the most serious interactions.	
alcohol, anesthetics, and CNS depressants	Concurrent administration with tramadol may result in an increase in CNS depressant effects. An increased risk of seizures may result if tramadol is given with fluoxetine, sertraline, or a tricyclic antidepressant. A dosage reduction is highly recommended.
carbamazepine (Tegretol)	Increases the metabolism of tramadol; a dosage increase in tramadol may be necessary.
MAO inhibitors; furazolidone (Furoxone), procarbazine (Matulane), phenelzine (Nardil), tranylcypromine (Parnate)	**MAO is necessary for serotonin metabolism, but tramadol inhibits the reuptake of serotonin. Serotonin is suspected to be responsible for the toxic effects of tramadol; therefore concurrent use may lower the seizure threshold and result in an increase in toxic effects. If drugs are administered concurrently, monitor closely.**

See also Nursing Management: Opioid Therapy, p. 273.

OPIOID ANTAGONISTS

Naloxone, naltrexone, and nalmefene are opioid antagonists; they competitively displace the opioid analgesics from their receptor sites, thus reversing their effects. Nalmefene is a chemical analogue of naltrexone and at full dosages has a longer duration of action than naloxone. Nalmefene and naloxone are administered parenterally, whereas naltrexone is available as an oral dosage formulation.

Antagonists block the subjective and objective opioid effects and can precipitate withdrawal symptoms in individuals who are physically dependent on opioids. These products are used to reverse the adverse or overdose effects of the opioids (codeine, diphenoxylate, fentanyl, heroin, hydromorphone, levorphanol, meperidine, methadone, morphine, oxymorphone, opium derivatives, and propoxyphene) and the partial agonists (agonist-antagonist drugs such as butorphanol, nalbuphine, and pentazocine).

Respiratory depression induced by nonopioids (e.g., barbiturates), CNS depression, or disease progression does not usually respond to antagonist drug therapy. It has also been reported that larger drug dosages are necessary to antagonize the effects of buprenorphine, butorphanol, nalbuphine, and pentazocine. However, a buprenorphine overdose may not respond to the opioid antagonists or, at best, may only partially respond (*USP DI*, 1999).

In an opioid analgesic overdose, naloxone and naltrexone reverse respiratory depression, sedation, miosis (constriction of pupils), and euphoric effects; they may also reverse the psychotomimetic effects of the agonist-antagonist analgesics (pentazocine and others). The drugs are believed to work at all three receptor sites, but their greatest activity is at the mu receptors.

Side effects/adverse reactions include nausea, vomiting, dizziness, hypertension, tachycardia, sweating, nervousness, abdominal cramps or pain, headache, weakness, joint and muscle pain, insomnia, hallucinations, confusion, mood alterations, tinnitus, and fever.

nalmefene [nal′ mah feen] (Revex)

Nalmefene has an onset of action of 2 to 5 minutes (IV) or 5 to 15 minutes (IM or SC). Time to peak levels is 90 minutes by SC injection and 2.3 hours by IM injection; therefore the time to peak effect and duration of action is dependent on the dose and route of administration. Nalmefene is metabolized in the liver and excreted primarily by the kidneys.

The adult dose to manage an opioid overdose is 0.5 mg/70 kg of body weight (IV); a second dose of 1 mg/70 kg can be given 2 to 5 minutes later. To reverse postoperative opioid depression, the dosage is 0.25 μg/kg (IV) at 2- to 5-minute intervals, as necessary.

naloxone hydrochloride [nal oks′ one] (Narcan)

Naloxone is inactivated orally but is very effective parenterally. Its onset of action is 1 to 2 minutes (IV) and 2 to 5 minutes (IM or SC). The half-life is between 60 and 100 minutes. Duration of action depends on the dose administered and the route of administration. Usually the IM dose results in a prolonged effect. Naloxone is widely distributed throughout the body and also crosses the placenta. It is metabolized in the liver and excreted via the kidneys.

The adult dose of naloxone is 0.4 to 2 mg as single dose or 0.1 to 0.2 mg for postoperative opioid depression. For continuous infusion, 2 mg of naloxone may be diluted in 500 mL of normal saline or 5% dextrose injection. Because naloxone is shorter acting than most opioids, repeat naloxone injections or continuous infusion is necessary to prevent the recurrence of respiratory depression.

naltrexone [nal trex′ one] (ReVia)

Naltrexone is indicated for adjuvant treatment in detoxified, opioid-dependent clients. Absorption is rapid, but it undergoes an extensive first-pass metabolism in the liver to the major metabolite 6-beta-naltrexol, which also has opioid antagonist effects. Peak serum concentration is reached in 1 hour; the elimination half-life for naltrexone is 4 hours, and approximately 13 hours for the metabolite. The duration of action is dose dependent. Excretion is via the kidneys.

Treatment with naltrexone is started cautiously—usually 25 mg PO with close monitoring for withdrawal signs and symptoms for approximately 1 hour. The balance of the daily dose is given if no withdrawal effects occur. The maintenance dosage is usually 50 mg PO daily.

■ Nursing Management

Opioid Antagonist Therapy

Nurses administer opioid antagonists for the emergency treatment of opioid overdose and for maintenance therapy of former opioid-addicted individuals. The nurse must have an understanding of opioid analgesics and opioid antagonists to provide nursing care to these clients.

■ **Assessment.** A baseline assessment should include hepatic function studies for naltrexone, as well as the status of the symptoms for which the opioid antagonist is being administered.

Clients should be observed carefully. Abrupt and complete reversal of opioid effects will produce an acute abstinence syndrome in clients who are physically dependent. Therefore opioid antagonists should either not be administered or administered with extreme caution if the client is known or suspected to be physically dependent on opioids (including newborns of dependent mothers). Naloxone should be used with caution in clients with preexisting ventricular irritability because ventricular tachycardia and fibrillation may occur. Naltrexone is contraindicated in clients with acute hepatitis or hepatic failure because there is an increased risk of hepatotoxicity.

■ **Nursing Diagnosis.** The client who is receiving nalmefene or naloxone is at risk for the following nursing diagnoses/collaborative problems: impaired comfort related to withdrawal symptoms (anxiety, irritability, body aches, diarrhea, tachycardia, runny nose, sweating, yawning, anorexia, nausea, vomiting, trembling, shivering); and the potential complication of decreased cardiac output related to the cardiovascular effects of the drug (tachycardia, hypotension, hypertension). In addition to these symptoms, the neonate may also experience convulsions with naloxone.

With naltrexone, impaired comfort may be a concern as described above, with additional symptoms (abdominal cramping, headache, joint and muscle pain). The client may also experience impaired skin integrity (rash occurs in 1% to 10% of clients), constipation (up to 10%), and sexual dysfunction (in men). Although the symptoms of body aches, abdominal discomfort, nausea and vomiting, lethargy, and anxiety may be the same as for withdrawal, these symptoms may disappear with continued use.

■ **Implementation**

■ ***Monitoring.*** Continued nursing observation is necessary for the client who has responded to naloxone; doses should be repeated as necessary because the duration of action of some opioids exceeds the duration of action of naloxone. Monitor closely for airway obstruction and maintain suction equipment at the bedside until the client is recovered. Monitor vital signs, particularly respirations, at least every 5 minutes until the client is stable. Respiratory rate should increase within 1 to 2 minutes of the first dose. The IV infusion rate of administration should be titrated according to the client's response. An intensive care unit is probably the most appropriate place for this client until the effects of the drug have completely abated. Clients should be observed for a day or longer, regardless of the apparent recovery.

With naltrexone, monitor hepatic studies monthly for the first 6 months and periodically after that. Naltrexone should be discontinued if significant hepatic abnormalities occur.

■ ***Intervention.*** In addition to opioid toxicity, one of the major indications for naltrexone is the treatment of opioid dependency and addiction. It should be used as an adjunctive measure to a comprehensive drug rehabilitation program involving counseling and psychotherapy. Naltrexone therapy should not be instituted until the client has been completely detoxified as evidenced by being opioid free for 7 to 10 days, by the absence of withdrawal symptoms, and by abstinence verification via a negative urinalysis for opioids or a naloxone challenge test. If an opioid analgesic is required in an emergency situation for a client receiving naltrexone therapy, its administration should be accomplished in a hospital setting where careful monitoring is available. Because high doses of analgesic are required to overcome the effects of naltrexone, the client will be at risk for prolonged respiratory depression and circulatory collapse. Naltrexone does not cause physical or psychologic dependence.

A naloxone challenge test is commonly performed before naltrexone therapy to verify abstinence from opioids. This test should not be performed in the presence of withdrawal symptoms (body aches, diarrhea, gooseflesh, sneezing and runny nose, irritability, diaphoresis, trembling and weakness, abdominal cramping, tachycardia, nausea and vomiting) or opioids in the urine. If administered intravenously, an initial dose of 0.2 mg is given and the client is observed for 30 seconds for withdrawal symptoms. If no symptoms occur, an additional 0.6 mg may be administered, and the client is observed for 20 minutes. If administered subcutaneously, 0.8 mg is given, and the client is observed for 45 minutes. If withdrawal symptoms occur, the test should be repeated at 24-hour intervals until the absence of opioid dependence is confirmed. It should be remembered that naloxone has no effect on respiratory depression caused by non-opiate drugs. If the client has taken multiple drugs, naloxone will reverse only the opioids.

It is recommended that naloxone not be mixed with other agents because it becomes unstable. After dilution, any unused solution should be discarded after 24 hours. Additional resuscitative measures such as oxygen and mechanical ventilation should be available when necessary to counteract opioid overdose.

■ ***Education.*** When opioid antagonists are used in emergency treatment, client education should be focused on assisting the client to cope with the immediate situation. Instructions should be given to keep the client informed about what is to occur and to help the client cooperate with treatment procedures, even when the client appears unresponsive. Discussing the dangers of substance abuse or dependence may be appropriate at some time after emergency treatment. Compliance with long-term naltrexone therapy is improved if someone other than the client (health care provider or family member) administers the naltrexone.

With naltrexone, stress to the client the importance of regular visits to the prescriber for hepatic function studies to detect hepatotoxicity, the need to maintain other parts of the rehabilitation program (e.g., counseling sessions, support group meetings), the need to notify other health care providers of naltrexone use, and the need to carry identification indicating the use of this drug. Alert the client not to take opioid medications for pain relief, diarrhea, or cough because they will not be effective. Warn the client not to take large doses of opioids to overcome the effects of the drug, because doing so may result in coma and death. The drug should not be shared with others, including those dependent on opioids.

■ **Evaluation.** After the administration of antagonists, evaluation takes place to help identify the development of opioid withdrawal syndrome in the client with possible opioid dependence. Follow-up evaluations are needed to reinforce and ensure compliance when naltrexone is used for maintenance of the opioid-free state in clients formerly addicted to opioids.

With the use of nalmefene and naloxone in the reversal of opioid toxicity, respiratory rate and volume will increase to normal parameters for the client, and blood pressure will return to normal if it has been depressed.

OPIOID AGONIST-ANTAGONIST AGENTS

Although the exact mechanism of action of the opioid agonist-antagonist agents is unknown, these agents have both agonist and antagonist effects on the opioid receptors. For example, buprenorphine (Buprenex) is a partial agonist at the mu receptors. Butorphanol (Stadol), nalbuphine (Nubain), and pentazocine (Talwin) produce agonist effects at the kappa and sigma receptors and may displace agonists (opioids) from their mu receptor sites, thus inhibiting their effects and perhaps inducing a drug withdrawal reaction in clients who are physically dependent on agonist opioids. Dezocine (Dalgan) is a partial agonist at the mu receptor and has some effect at the sigma receptors after high doses. In general, these drugs are less potent analgesics and have a lower dependency potential than opioids, and withdrawal symptoms are not as severe as those reported with the opioid agonist medications.

The opioid agonist-antagonist agents have pharmacokinetics, adverse effects, and significant drug interactions similar to morphine. Table 14-6 lists pharmacokinetics, equivalency, and dosing of the agonist-antagonist agents.

butorphanol tartrate (byoo tor′ fa nole) (Stadol)

Butorphanol tartrate is indicated for the treatment of moderate to severe pain and as an anesthetic adjunct. It is administered parenterally (IM or IV) and as a nasal spray.

▪ Nursing Management

Butorphanol Therapy

In addition to the following discussion, see Nursing Management: Opioid Therapy, p. 273.

▪ **Assessment.** Use caution when administering butorphanol as a preoperative medication for hypertensive clients, because it may increase blood pressure. It should not be administered to clients with acute myocardial infarction because the cardiovascular effects tend to increase the workload on the heart. However, butorphanol may be used with clients with gallbladder disease or gallstones because biliary spasm has not been reported.

If the client is suspected of being physically dependent on narcotics, butorphanol should not be given until the person is detoxified. Because butorphanol is a narcotic agonist-antagonist, it would counteract only the effects of the original narcotic, set up a need for a dosage increase, and precipitate an abstinence syndrome.

Butorphanol may elevate cerebrospinal fluid (CSF) pressure; therefore it should be used with caution in clients with head injuries or preexisting increased CSF pressure. Because butorphanol is metabolized in the liver, it should be given with caution to clients with compromised or impaired renal or hepatic function. Because of decreased metabolism of the drug in the liver, side effects and greater activity may result.

The safety of using butorphanol in pregnancy before the labor period has not been established. The safety to the mother and fetus after the administration of butorphanol during labor has been established, with clients experiencing no adverse effects other than those observed with commonly used analgesics. This drug should be used with caution in women delivering premature infants. It is also passed on in breast milk.

TABLE 14-6 Agonist-Antagonist: Pharmacokinetics, Equivalency, and Dosage

Drug	Equivalent Dose* (mg)	Onset (minutes)	Peak (minutes)	Duration (hours)	Half-life (hours)	Usual Dosage
buprenorphine (Buprenex)						
IV	0.3	<15	<60	6	2-3	0.3 mg q6h
IM	0.3	15	60	6	2-3	
butorphanol (Stadol)						
IV	2	2-3	30	2-4	2-4	0.5-2 mg q3-4h
IM	2	10-30	30-60	3-4	2-4	
nasal spray	—	15	30-60	4-5	3-6	1 mg spray in nostril q3-4h
dezocine (Dalgan)						
IV	10	<15	—	2-4†	2	2.5-10 mg q2-4h
IM	10	<30	60-120	2-4†	2	
nalbuphine (Nubain)						
IV	10	2-3	30	3-6	5	10 mg q3-6h
IM	10	<15	60	3-6	5	
SC	10	<15	—	3-6	5	
pentazocine (Talwin)						
PO	180	15-30	60-90	3	2-3	50 mg PO or 30 mg parenteral q3-4h
IM	60	15-20	30-60	2-3	2-3	
IV	60	2-3	15-30	2-3	2-3	
SC	60	15-20	30-60	2-3	2-3	

*Equivalent to dose of 10 mg morphine IM.
†Dose dependent.

Review the client's current medication regimen for the risk of significant drug interactions, such as those that may occur when butorphanol is given concurrently with following drugs:

Drug	Possible Effect and Management
Bold/color type indicates the most serious interactions.	
alcohol or CNS depressants	May increase the potential for CNS depression, respiratory depression, and hypotension. Monitor closely for adverse effects because one or both drugs may need to be reduced.
buprenorphine (Buprenex)	**May reduce the therapeutic effects of butorphanol, nalbuphine, or pentazocine at the kappa receptors. Increased respiratory depressant effects may occur when buprenorphine is given with low doses of other mu receptor agonists or kappa receptor agonists. Avoid concurrent administration.**
MAO inhibitors	Use opioid analgesics (other than meperidine) cautiously in reduced dosages. For safety's safe, one fourth of the usual analgesic dose should be given to determine the client's response to this combination.
naltrexone (Narcan)	The use of naltrexone will precipitate withdrawal symptoms in clients who are dependent on butorphanol. It will also negate any therapeutic use of the drug.

■ **Nursing Diagnosis.** The client receiving butorphanol therapy is at risk for injury related to the CNS effects of the drug and pain related to the underlying condition and the ineffectiveness of the drug.

■ **Implementation**

■ ***Monitoring.*** Monitor for pain relief. Butorphanol tartrate can cause respiratory depression if the dose exceeds 4 mg as a single dose. If the usual IM dose of 2 mg is insufficient to relieve the client's pain, the dose can be increased by 1 to 4 mg every 3 to 4 hours. It is important for the nurse to assess the client's response to this medication and to be aware of any signs of respiratory depression. These could be changes in rate, depth, or regularity of respiratory rate. Monitor for adverse CNS reactions (e.g., confusion and vertigo), fluctuations in blood pressure, and bowel function for constipation.

■ ***Intervention.*** The SC route is not recommended; do not use rapid IV administration. Ensure that naloxone and resuscitative equipment are in the immediate environment. Provide for the client's safety.

■ ***Education.*** Instruct the client to change positions slowly and to avoid activities that require concentration and alertness. Instruct in measures to prevent constipation such as a high fiber diet and adequate hydration, even though butorphanol is not as constipating as other opioids. Butorphanol also has a lower risk of dependence, and the withdrawal symptoms are not as severe as with the opioid agonists.

■ **Evaluation.** The expected outcome of butorphanol therapy is that the client will have relief from pain without experiencing any adverse effects.

dezocine [dez′ oh seen] (Dalgan)

Dezocine, a potent parenteral opioid agonist-antagonist comparable to morphine in analgesic potency, onset, and duration of action, is indicated for the treatment of pain. It is administered parenterally (IM or IV).

An additive CNS depressant effect may occur when dezocine is used concurrently with other CNS depressants. It is suggested that the dosage of either or both drugs be reduced.

Side effects/adverse reactions include nausea, vomiting, drowsiness, injection site reactions, dizziness, increased sweating, chills, hypotension or hypertension, chest pain, dry mouth, constipation, muscle pain or cramps, increased anxiety, crying spells, headaches, respiratory depression, urinary retention, and delirium.

For the nursing management of dezocine therapy, see Nursing Management: Opioid Therapy, p. 273.

pentazocine [pen taz′ oh seen] (Talwin)

The analgesic pentazocine is not indicated for pain caused by acute myocardial infarction because of its effects on cardiac function. It increases cardiac workload by increasing systemic and pulmonary arterial pressure, systemic vascular resistance, and left ventricular end-diastolic pressure. It also has a higher incidence of psychotomimetic side effects than the majority of other analgesics, thus limiting its usefulness, especially in terminally ill clients or in clients who are already anxious or fearful.

In the United States, pentazocine tablets are combined with naloxone (Narcan) because of the high incidence of pentazocine abuse. Naloxone taken orally is not pharmacologically active, but if this combination is dissolved and injected, naloxone will block the effects of pentazocine that lead to abuse. Significant drug interactions are the same as those for butorphanol. SC administration is to be avoided because of tissue damage at the injection sites; IM sites should be routinely rotated for the same reason.

For the nursing management of pentazocine therapy, see Nursing Management: Opioid Therapy, p. 273.

nalbuphine [nal′ byoo feen] (Nubain)

Nalbuphine, an analgesic for moderate to severe pain, is also used preoperatively as an adjunct to anesthesia and for obstetric analgesia. Drug interactions are similar to butorphanol.

For the nursing management of nalbuphine therapy, see Nursing Management: Opioid Therapy, p. 273.

buprenorphine [byoo pre nor′ feen] (Buprenex)

Buprenorphine dissociates very slowly from the mu receptor; thus it reduces or blocks the effect of concurrent or subsequent dosing with opioid agonist drugs. It can precipitate withdrawal symptoms if administered to persons who are physically dependent on opioids. Respiratory depression and other adverse effects of this drug are often difficult to reverse because naloxone is not very effective in treating buprenorphine-induced adverse effects. Doxapram, a respiratory stimulant, is recommended when naloxone is ineffective, but assisted ventilation may be necessary (*USP DI*, 1999).

Review the client's current medication regimen for the risk of significant drug interactions, such as those that may occur when buprenorphine is given concurrently with the following drugs:

Drug	Possible Effect and Management
Bold/color type indicates the most serious interactions.	
other CNS depressants or MAO inhibitors	May result in increased CNS depressant effect, respiratory depression, and hypotension. Monitor closely because one or both drugs may need to be decreased by the prescriber.
opioid analgesics	**The therapeutic effects of the opioid may be reduced. In clients with physical opioid dependence, withdrawal symptoms may be precipitated by the coadministration of buprenorphine. Avoid this combination.**

For the nursing management of buprenorphine therapy, see Nursing Management: Opioid Therapy, p. 273.

NONOPIOID ANALGESICS

The nonopioid analgesics are effective for mild to moderate pain; they are often combined with opioid analgesics to enhance the control of severe pain. In combination with a weak opioid, they correspond to step 2 in Figure 14-9. The major drugs in this classification include acetaminophen, aspirin, NSAIDs, and the adjunct analgesics. These agents are used for the treatment of mild to moderate pain, fever, and inflammation caused by rheumatoid arthritis, osteoarthritis, and various other acute and chronic musculoskeletal and soft tissue inflammations. The NSAIDs are also used to treat metastatic bone pain, usually in combination with an opioid analgesic (Twycross, 1994). The over-the-counter (OTC) dosage forms of these preparations are discussed in Chapter 11. (See the Special Considerations for Children box above.)

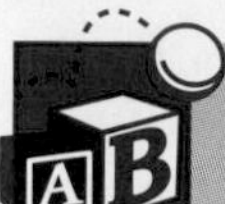

Special Considerations for Children
Managing Pain in Children

Acetaminophen (e.g., Tylenol) is usually the drug of choice for children with mild to moderate pain and fever. It is available in liquid, tablet, and capsule dosage forms. If necessary, tablets may be crushed and mixed with food or liquid.

Acetaminophen may be administered with food or milk. However, it should not be administered with a high-carbohydrate meal, which may decrease drug absorption (Miller & Fioravanti, 1997).

Avoid the use of aspirin and other salicylates in young children, especially if they have a varicella infection, influenza, or flu-like symptoms, because of the increased risk of Reye's syndrome.

An opioid may be necessary for severe pain in children. The combination of an opioid with a nonopioid often reduces the amount of opioid necessary to control the pain (McCaffery & Portenoy, 1999).

Aspirin (acetylsalicylic acid) may also be prescribed to reduce the risk of transient ischemic attacks (TIAs), myocardial infarcts, and stroke.

Aspirin and the NSAIDs peripherally inhibit the cyclooxygenase (COX) enzyme (the first enzyme in the prostaglandin pathway), which results in a reduction of the synthesis and release of prostaglandins. Two forms of COX have been identified: COX-1 and COX-2. COX-1 is found primarily in the blood vessels, stomach, and kidneys, whereas COX-2 is activated by inflammation induced by the cytokines and inflammatory mediators. The cause of the adverse gastrointestinal (GI) and renal toxicity is believed to be secondary to the inhibition of COX-1, whereas COX-2 inhibition produces the beneficial effects reported with this drug classification.

Aspirin affects both COX-1 and COX-2, causing an irreversible inhibition of cyclooxygenase activity; the NSAIDs produce reversible, competitive inhibition of cyclooxygenase (Insel, 1996). Nabumetone (Relafen) is an exception; it is a pro-drug that is inactive when ingested and is converted in the liver to its active compound, which then primarily inhibits COX-2 (Davis, 1998). Thus nabumetone is reported to be less likely to cause GI bleeding or ulcers (Insel, 1996). Two agents released in 1999, celecoxib (Celebrex ◆) and rofecoxib (Vioxx ◆), are selective COX-2 inhibiting agents. These drugs are indicated for the treatment of rheumatoid arthritis and osteoarthritis; rofecoxib is also approved for the treatment of acute pain in adults. Their major advantage over the NSAIDs are that they are much less apt to inhibit COX-1 (the cyclooxygenase that protects the stomach) and therefore should be much less ulcerogenic (Arthritis, 1998).

Salicylates also block the generation of pain impulses and may have a central analgesic action in the hypothalamus. The NSAIDs are effective analgesics for pain induced by in-

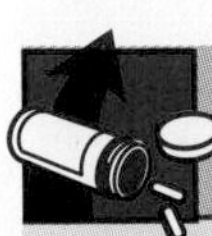

Management of Drug Overdose
Acetaminophen

- Early symptoms: Sweating, anorexia, nausea or vomiting, abdominal pain or cramping and/or diarrhea. Symptoms usually occur 6 to 14 hours after ingestion and last for approximately 24 hours.
- Late symptoms: Abdominal area may exhibit swelling, tenderness, or pain 2 to 4 days after ingestion (hepatotoxicity).
- Treatment: Gastric lavage or emesis. Start acetylcysteine administration as soon as possible. Determine acetaminophen serum levels 4 hours or more after ingestion. Hepatotoxicity is possible if serum acetaminophen is more than 150 μg/mL at 4 hours, 100 μg/mL at 6 hours, 70 μg/mL at 8 hours, 50 μg/mL at 10 hours, or 3.5 μg/mL at 24 hours. Administer acetylcysteine orally as soon as possible, within 24 hours of ingestion (see *USP DI* for dosage instructions).
- Perform liver, renal, and cardiac function tests. Institute supportive measures as indicated.

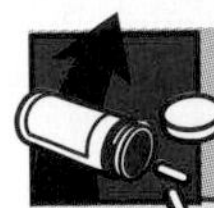

Management of Drug Overdose
Aspirin

- The treatment of an aspirin overdose may include gastric lavage or emesis followed by the administration of activated charcoal. Close monitoring is necessary to institute appropriate nursing or medical interventions such as correcting hyperthermia, fluid and electrolyte imbalance, acid-base imbalances, hyperglycemia, or hypoglycemia (especially in children).
- Serum salicylate levels are monitored until the concentration is lowered to a nontoxic level. For example, a salicylate concentration of 500 μg/mL (50 mg/dL) 2 hours after ingesting large amounts of aspirin indicate a serious toxicity; a serum level of 800 μg/mL (80 mg/dL) is potentially fatal. Prolonged monitoring of salicylate serum levels is indicated in situations of massive salicylate overdose.
- Serum levels are not reliable for measuring degree of toxicity following the consumption of large amounts of delayed-release formulations.
- Exchange transfusion, hemodialysis, peritoneal dialysis, or hemoperfusion may be necessary in severe salicylate overdoses.

flammation. These agents also inhibit leukocyte migration and the release of lysosomal enzymes, which contributes to their antiinflammatory effect.

Aspirin also inhibits the formation of platelet aggregation in the blood vessels by inhibiting prostacyclin. Prostacyclin is a platelet aggregation (reversible) inhibitor in blood vessels. Both effects may be dose dependent. Prescription salicylates include controlled-release aspirin 800 mg (ZORprin), salsalate (Disalcid and others), choline magnesium trisalicylate (Trilisate), and magnesium salicylate (Magan). Salsalate is converted to salicylate during absorption from the GI tract and in the liver. Both salsalate and choline magnesium trisalicylate have the advantage of producing little, if any, adverse GI effects, and they do not affect platelet aggregation. The analgesic effects of salsalate are equivalent to aspirin. The magnesium from these combination agents may be absorbed, which may result in systemic toxicity in clients with renal impairment.

Acetaminophen appears to produce its analgesic effect by inhibiting prostaglandin synthesis in the CNS (predominant effect) and peripherally. Although the exact mechanisms of action are unknown, the antiinflammatory effects are minimal. The antipyretic effect for these non-opioid analgesic agents is mediated centrally via the hypothalamus. (See the Management of Drug Overdose boxes above.)

NONSTEROIDAL ANTIINFLAMMATORY DRUGS

Approximately 20 different NSAIDs are now available in the United States. Although aspirin is also an NSAID, the term *NSAID* most commonly refers to the newer aspirin substitutes on the market. Aspirin and the OTC NSAIDs are reviewed in Chapter 11. The NSAIDs have analgesic, antipyretic, and antiinflammatory effects, and the indications for each NSAID may vary according to specific testing and clinical data submitted to the FDA for approval.

The NSAIDs inhibit cyclooxygenase and prevent the synthesis of prostaglandins and thromboxane, which are responsible for the therapeutic effects and some of the adverse reactions of this drug classification (Figure 14-11). The nurse should be aware, however, that the inflammatory process has a purpose in the body; it attempts to neutralize, destroy, or prevent the dissemination of toxic or foreign substances. The cardinal signs of inflammation that result include swelling, pain, redness, and heat at the site. By interfering with prostaglandin synthesis, the NSAIDs tend to reduce the inflammatory process and ultimately provide pain relief. It is quite possible that other, currently unknown actions may also contribute to the therapeutic effects of these medications.

The NSAIDs are indicated for the treatment of acute or chronic rheumatoid arthritis, osteoarthritis, ankylosing spondylitis, and other rheumatic diseases; mild to moderate pain, especially when the antiinflammatory effect is also desirable (such as after dental procedures, obstetric and orthopedic surgery, and soft tissue athletic injuries); gouty arthritis; fever; nonrheumatic inflammation; and dysmenorrhea. Refer to a current package insert or *USP DI* for a listing of approved and investigational use of NSAIDs. The primary NSAIDs include the following:

Acetic acids

diclofenac [dye kloe′ fen ak] (Voltaren, Voltaren-SR)
etodolac [ee toe′ doe lak] (Lodine)
indomethacin [in doe meth′ a sin] (Indocin)
ketorolac [kee′ toe role ak] (Toradol)

nabumetone [na byoo′ me tone] (Relafen ◆)
sulindac [sul in′ dak] (Clinoril)
tolmetin [tole′ met in] (Tolectin)

Fenamates

meclofenamate [me kloe fen am′ ate] (Meclomen)
mefenamic [me fe nam′ ik] (Ponstel)

Oxicams

piroxicam [peer ox′ i kam] (Feldene)
meloxicam [mel ox′i kam] (Mobic)

Propionic acids

fenoprofen [fen oh proe′ fen] (Nalfon)
flurbiprofen [flure bi′ proe fen] (Ansaid)
ibuprofen [eye byoo proe′ fen] (Motrin, Advil)
ketoprofen [kee toe proe′ fen] (Orudis)
naproxen [na prox′ en] (Naprosyn)
oxaprozin [ox a proe′ zin] (Daypro)

Combination Drug

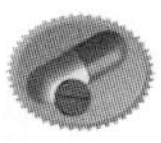
diclofenac and misoprostol [dye kloe′ fen ak and mye soe prost′ ole] (Arthrotec)

Salicylates (which would also include aspirin, salsalate, and others):

diflunisal [dye floo′ ni sal] (Dolobid)

These NSAIDs have the same general pharmacokinetics. Oral absorption of these drugs is very good. Food may delay absorption but has not been proven to significantly change the total amount absorbed. Protein binding is high (greater than 90%). Sulindac is an inactive substance (prodrug) that is converted by the liver to an active sulfide metabolite. Most of these agents are metabolized by the liver and excreted by the kidneys. (See Table 14-7 for specific pharmacokinetics, usual adult dosage, dosing recommendations, and comments.)

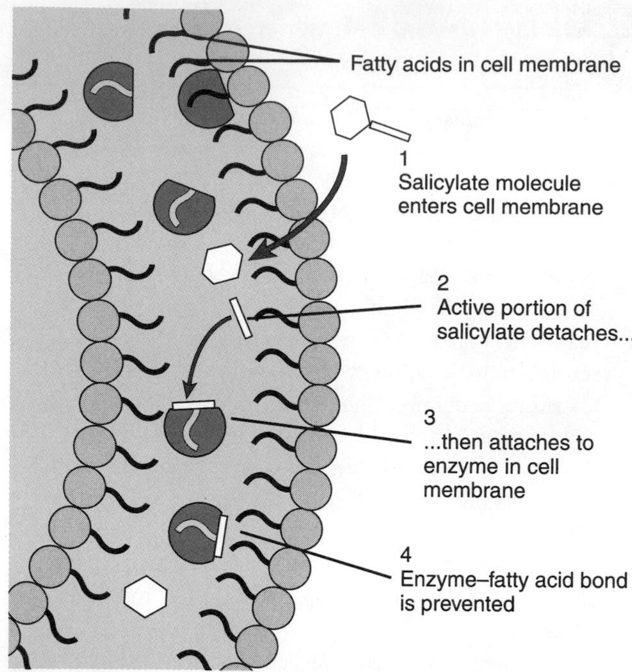

Figure 14-11 Inhibition of prostaglandin production. Inflammatory diseases and local injuries often lead to an increased production of prostaglandins. NSAIDs act peripherally by entering the cell membrane (*1*); the active portion (salicylate) detaches (*2*) and attaches to the enzyme (cyclooxygenase) in the cell membrane (*3*). This new complex (*4*) cannot react with fatty acids to induce prostaglandin synthesis, thus reducing inflammation and pain in the affected area.

■ Nursing Management

NSAID Therapy

■ **Assessment.** Establish the client's allergies before administering NSAIDs. The anaphylactoid reaction may be life threatening in individuals with a documented history of allergy or hypersensitivity to aspirin. Clients with the triad of aspirin allergy, nasal polyps, and bronchospastic disease may experience bronchospasm, leading to respiratory failure with the use of NSAIDs. Clients sensitive to one NSAID may be sensitive to any of the other NSAIDs. The NSAIDs are contraindicated in individuals when the drugs have caused asthmatic symptoms, rhinitis, urticaria, nasal polyps, angioedema, or bronchospastic events. Diclofenac is contraindicated for clients with a history of or active blood dyscrasias or bone marrow depression because these conditions will be precipitated or worsen.

NSAIDs are to be used with caution in older adults, who are more prone to the upper gastrointestinal, hepatic, or renal effects of these agents. For indomethacin, older adults may start with less than half the adult dosage. (See the Special Considerations for Older Adults box on p. 293.)

The NSAIDs should be used cautiously in individuals with preexisting hepatic impairment. Prudent long-term management for clients should include liver enzyme determinations for a baseline level and periodic monitoring. Cautious use in individuals with impaired renal function is required; creatinine clearance should be closely monitored in these clients. A reduced dosage should be used in clients with diminished renal function to prevent drug accumulation. Cautious use is also required for clients with inflammatory or ulcerative disease of the small or large bowel, hemophilia or other bleeding problems (increased risk of bleeding as a result of platelet aggregation inhibition), or stomatitis

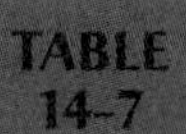

TABLE 14-7 Nonsteroidal Antiinflammatory Drugs: Pharmacokinetics, Dosing, and Comments

NSAID	Onset of Action (hours)	Half-life (hours)	Usual Adult Dosage (mg/day)	Comments*
Acetic Acids				
diclofenac (Voltaren)	0.5	1.2-2	50 mg 3 or 4 times daily	Has less effect on platelet aggregation that most other NSAIDs (*USP DI,* 1999). Used to treat arthritis, pain, primary dysmenorrhea, and acute gout attacks
etodolac (Lodine)	0.5	6-7	200, 300, or 400 mg 3 or 4 times daily	Has uricosuric effects. Gastrointestinal distress and ulceration reported less often (Insel, 1996).
indomethacin (Indocin)	0.5	4-6	25 or 50 mg 2 to 4 times daily	Higher risk for GI effects and renal function impairment than other agents. Used cautiously in persons with epilepsy, depression and Parkinson's disease because it may aggravate these conditions
ketorolac (Toradol)	IM: 10 minutes (dose dependent)	PO: 4 IM: 6	30 mg IM/IV q6h, then 10 mg PO q4-6h	Should not be given by any route for longer than 5 days. Increased risk of GI bleeding and other severe effects with duration of treatment. Do not give preoperatively or intraoperatively if bleeding control is necessary. Severe allergic reactions or anaphylaxis may occur with first dose
nabumetone (Relafen)	—	22	500, 750, or 1000 mg daily (hs) or in two divided doses	Pro-drug (inactive); converted to active metabolite (6-MNA) in liver. Absorption increased by food and milk. Has lower reports of GI ulceration and bleeding than other NSAIDs
sulindac (Clinoril)	—	8	150-200 mg 2 times daily	Renal calculi and biliary obstruction containing sulindac metabolites is reported, but it is less likely than most NSAIDs to cause renal toxicity.
tolmetin (Tolectin)	—	5	400 mg 3 times daily	High evidence of anaphylactic reactions and may also cause serum sickness or flu-like syndrome (*USP DI,* 1999).
Fenamates				
meclofenamate (Meclomen)	1	2-3	50 mg 3 or 4 times daily	Less effect on platelet aggregation than most other NSAIDs Used cautiously in persons on sodium-restricted diet (*USP DI,* 1999)
mefenamic acid (Ponstel)	—	2	250 mg q6h	Less effect on platelet aggregation but can prolong prothrombin time. Used for short-term treatment of pain and dysmenorrhea; also for acute gouty attacks and vascular headaches

CAP, Capsule; *ERC,* extended-release capsules; *ERT,* extended-release tablets.
*All oral NSAIDs should be taken with 8 ounces of water with the person remaining upright for at least 15 to 30 minutes afterward (*USP DI,* 1999).

Continued

TABLE 14-7 Nonsteroidal Antiinflammatory Drugs: Pharmacokinetics, Dosing, and Comments—cont'd

NSAID	Onset of Action (hours)	Half-life (hours)	Usual Adult Dosage (mg/day)	Comments*
Oxicams				
piroxicam (Feldene)	2-4	24	20 mg daily or 10 mg 2 times daily	Contraindicated in renal impairment. May cause flu-like syndrome. May accumulate in older women (*USP DI,* 1999).
Propionic Acids				
fenoprofen (Nalfon)	—	3	300-600 mg 3 or 4 times daily	Contraindicated in persons with renal impairment. Food decreases absorption and peak serum levels; therefore is administered 30 minutes before or 2 hours after meals unless GI distress occurs, then administered with milk.
flurbiprofen (Ansaid)	—	5.7	100 mg daily 2 or 3 times daily	Similar to other agents in this category. Currently under study in transdermal patch to treat soft tissue lesions (Insel, 1996)
ibuprofen (Motrin, Advil)	0.5	2	300-800 mg 3 or 4 times daily	Available in tablet, liquid, and OTC form. May decrease blood glucose levels (*USP DI,* 1999). Incidence of GI side effects less than with aspirin (Insel, 1996)
ketoprofen (Orudis)	—	CAP: 1.6 ERC: 5.4 ERT: 3-4	25-75 mg 3 or 4 times daily	Can cause fluid retention and increase in creatinine levels, especially in older adults and in persons receiving diuretics. Monitor renal function closely (Insel, 1996)
naproxen (Naprosyn)	1	13	250, 375, or 500 mg 2 times daily	Available in liquid, tablet, and extended-release tablets. Use tablets and liquid with caution in persons on sodium-restricted diet (*USP DI,* 1999)
oxaprozin (Daypro)	—	21-25	600 mg 1 or 2 times daily	Has a long half-life that accumulates with chronic dosing; half-life may be 40-60 hours or more, which increases with age (Insel, 1996). Discontinued at least 1-2 weeks before elective surgery because it has greater tendency to cause perisurgical bleeding (*USP DI,* 1999)
Salicylates				
diflunisal (Dolobid)	1	8-12	250-500 mg 2 times daily	Higher risk of causing renal impairment but less apt to cause antiplatelet effect than other NSAIDs (*USP DI,* 1999). Does not have any antipyretic effects (Insel, 1996)

CAP, Capsule; *ERC,* extended-release capsules; *ERT,* extended-release tablets.
*All oral NSAIDs should be taken with 8 ounces of water with the person remaining upright for at least 15 to 30 minutes afterward (*USP DI,* 1999).

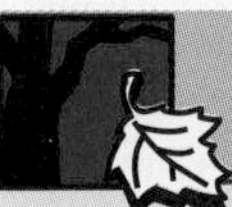

Special Considerations for Older Adults
Nonsteroidal Antiinflammatory Drugs

Among individuals taking NSAIDs, the incidence of perforated peptic ulcers and/or bleeding is more common in older adults than in younger adults, with serious consequences occurring more often in this older age-group.

Clients with renal impairment may be at increased risk for NSAID-induced liver or renal toxicity and often require a dosage reduction to prevent drug accumulation.

Clinicians have recommended that clients 70 years or older be started at one-half the usual adult dosage with close monitoring and careful dosage increases. The dosage increase should be based on the client's therapeutic response and lack of signs and symptoms of toxicity. Specific drug warnings include the following:

1. Flurbiprofen (Ansaid) may result in elevated peak serum levels in women between 74 and 94 years of age. This serum level has not been documented in older men (*USP DI*, 1999). Therefore older women may need a lower dosage to produce a therapeutic response.
2. Indomethacin (Indocin) is responsible for a higher incidence of CNS side effects, especially confusion, in older adults.
3. The use of naproxen (Naprosyn) administration in older adults results in a higher proportion of unbound (free) naproxen, which may not be reflected by the total serum level. The steady-state concentration of unbound naproxen may be nearly double that of a younger adult, which may result in an increase in side/adverse/toxic effects, even with a normal serum level range. The nurse should be aware of this potential because the prescriber may need to be notified about the possible need for a dosage reduction (*USP DI*, 1999).

(may mask the symptoms of blood dyscrasias). In addition, indomethacin is to be used cautiously in clients with mental depression and other psychiatric problems because they may be aggravated. Sulindac may cause renal calculi in clients with a history of kidney stones; adequate hydration and cautious use is necessary. For clients with a history of or active anal or rectal bleeding, hemorrhoids, inflammatory lesions of the anus or rectum, or proctitis, rectal forms of the NSAIDs may reactivate or exacerbate the condition.

Review the client's current medication regimen for the risk of significant drug interactions, such as those that may occur when NSAIDs are given concurrently with the following drugs:

Drug/Herb	Possible Effect and Management
Bold/color type indicates the most serious interactions.	
anticoagulants, oral (coumarin or indanedione, heparin or thrombolytic agents)	May increase the risk of GI ulcers or hemorrhage. Avoid concurrent drug administration. If administered, monitor closely for signs of these effects. Coumarin or indanedione anticoagulants may be displaced from protein-binding sites, resulting in an increased risk of bleeding episodes. Monitor closely with laboratory coagulation testing. Platelet inhibition may be dangerous for individuals receiving anticoagulant or thrombolytic agents. Avoid concurrent drug administration if possible. If an NSAID is necessary, the usual dosages of diclofenac, diflunisal, meclofenamate, and mefenamic acid are reportedly less likely to significantly affect platelets (*USP DI*, 1999). With concurrent therapies, monitor closely for potential serious side effects.
antihypertensives, diuretics (especially triamterene [Dyrenium])	Flurbiprofen, indomethacin, ibuprofen, naproxen, oxaprozin, and piroxicam may reduce the effectiveness of antihypertensive agents. Monitor antihypertensive effects closely whenever an NSAID is used concurrently. Concurrent use of an NSAID and a diuretic may result in a decrease in diuretic, natriuretic, and antihypertensive diuretic effects. Diflunisal has not been reported to decrease the effectiveness of furosemide, but it is reported to increase the serum level of hydrochlorothiazide and decrease the hyperuricemic response to hydrochlorothiazide or furosemide. May increase the risk of inducing renal failure in some clients. Triamterene and indomethacin reportedly caused acute renal failure or renal function impairment; therefore this drug combination should be avoided.
cefamandole (Mandol), cefoperazone (Cefobid), cefotetan (Cefotan), plicamycin (Mithracin), or valproic acid (Depakene)	These drugs may cause a decrease in prothrombin blood levels and an inhibition of platelet aggregation. Concurrent administration with an NSAID may increase the risk for bleeding episodes, GI ulceration, and hemorrhage. Avoid concurrent administration if possible.
cyclosporine (Sandimmune), gold compounds, nephrotoxic drugs	Concurrent use with NSAIDs may result in increased serum levels of cyclosporine and possibly gold compounds, resulting in an increased potential for nephrotoxicity. Concurrent use of nephrotoxic drugs and NSAIDs may also increase the risk for nephrotoxicity. Monitor closely.
herbals (feverfew, garlic, ginger, ginkgo, gossypol)	May cause GI distress and antiplatelet effects. Monitor closely—avoid concurrent use if possible.
lithium (Lithane)	Diclofenac, ibuprofen, indomethacin, naproxen and piroxicam may decrease excretion

Continued

Drug/Herb	Possible Effect and Management
lithium (Lithane)—cont'd	of lithium, which may result in an increased lithium serum level and toxicity. Thus the possibility of inducing this effect with the other NSAIDs exists. Monitor lithium serum levels and clinical symptoms of lithium for toxicity during concurrent therapy and after the NSAID is discontinued.
methotrexate (Mexate)	**Concurrent use of methotrexate with low to moderate dosages of an NSAID may result in methotrexate toxicity. Adjust methotrexate as necessary according to methotrexate serum levels and the client's renal function. This reaction can be severe and even fatal; therefore close monitoring is necessary.**
administration of two NSAIDs concurrently, especially diflunisal (Dolobid) and indomethacin (Indocin) or aspirin	**May increase the risk of gastrointestinal side effects, such as duodenal ulcers or hemorrhage. These combinations should be avoided.**
probenecid (Benemid)	May result in an increase in serum levels of the NSAIDs and an increased risk of toxicity. Concurrent use with ketoprofen is not recommended. If probenecid is given with an NSAID, monitor closely, because a decrease in NSAID dosage may be indicated.
zidovudine (AZT)	**When given concurrently with indomethacin, a decrease in the metabolism of zidovudine may result, leading to increased serum levels and toxicity. It is also possible that an increase in indomethacin serum levels and toxicity may occur. Avoid concurrent use of these medications.**

A baseline assessment should include the client's blood pressure, temperature, pulse, respirations, adventitious lung sounds, orientation, complete blood count (CBC), clotting times, renal and hepatic function tests, stool guaiac. A detailed description of the client's pain should also be included.

■ **Nursing Diagnosis.** Clients receiving NSAID therapy have the potential for the following nursing diagnoses: constipation or diarrhea; impaired comfort related to ineffective dosage of the NSAID, gas, mild stomach distress, or skin rash; disturbed sensory perception as evidenced by visual changes, tinnitus, or dizziness; excess fluid volume (periorbital edema, peripheral edema, respiratory rales); ineffective protection related to hypoprothrombinemia; and ineffective health maintenance related to insufficient knowledge of contraindications, potential hazards, or signs and symptoms of bleeding. The potential complications of convulsions, acute renal failure, hemorrhage, and gastrointestinal ulcers and perforation exist with the administration of NSAIDs. (See the Nursing Care Plan on p. 295 for selected nursing diagnoses related to the administration of nonsteroidal anti-inflammatory analgesics.)

■ **Implementation**

■ ***Monitoring.*** The client's pain and mobility of affected areas should be monitored periodically.

Clients require close monitoring of their prothrombin time if they are receiving concomitant anticoagulant therapy or if they have other intrinsic hemostatic coagulation defects. Clients taking two or more NSAIDs should have hematologic determinations only if symptoms of blood dyscrasias occur.

Precipitation of acute renal failure may occur in clients with preexisting diminished sodium excretion, congestive heart failure, cirrhosis, hypertension, or renal disease.

Eye problems that surface during therapy should be handled by an ophthalmologic examination, and drug therapy should be discontinued until evaluation has ruled out the drug therapy as a causal agent.

Monitor fluid intake and output and other symptoms of fluid volume excess (weight gain, edema, increase in blood pressure) with the administration of diclofenac, fenoprofen, flurbiprofen, indomethacin, ketoprofen, nabumetone, naproxen, and tolmetin. In addition, clients taking indomethacin need to be monitored periodically for confusion, mood changes, and hallucinations.

■ ***Intervention.*** Doses may be taken 30 to 60 minutes before meals or 2 hours postprandially to reach a blood level more readily. Administer the doses with a full glass of water, and have the client remain in an upright position for 15 to 30 minutes to minimize the risk of tablets becoming lodged in the esophagus, which may cause esophageal irritation. Administration with a meal followed by a full glass of water will also help to prevent gastric upset. Indomethacin may be taken with antacids to prevent gastric irritation, but it should not be mixed directly with antacids or other medications. Indomethacin suppositories need to remain in the rectum to be effective.

Ketorolac is the first injectable analgesic NSAID reported to have an efficacy comparable to morphine and meperidine without the undesirable side effects/adverse reactions. It has no respiratory depression effects and produces far fewer CNS side effects compared with the opioids. It is currently reported to have little or no potential for abuse or addiction and therefore no special handling procedures are required by the federal government. Ketorolac is indicated for the short-term management of pain but should not be used for the long-term treatment of chronic rheumatic disease or as an obstetric preoperative medication or obstetric analgesic.

Be aware that headache and drowsiness occur in approximately 15% of individuals taking fenoprofen.

Mefenamic acid is not administered for more than 7 days.

■ ***Education.*** Clients who are self-managing their NSAID therapy should be made aware of the need for periodic de-

Nursing Care Plan

Selected Nursing Diagnoses Related to the Administration of Nonsteroidal Antiinflammatory Drugs

Nursing Diagnosis	Outcome Criteria	Nursing Interventions
Risk for impaired comfort related to CNS, GI, dermatologic effects	Absence of dizziness and changes in sensorium	Institute safety measures if CNS symptoms develop.
	Absence of GI symptoms: nausea, and vomiting, abdominal pain or cramps, indigestion	Administer with food or after meals. Provide small, frequent meals. Caution against alcohol ingestion.
	Absence of rash, hives, pruritus, and SLE-type syndrome	Provide comfort measures to reduce pain, inflammation, and other dermatologic effects. Report adverse symptoms to the prescriber. Institute emergency procedures if severe adverse symptoms occur.
Risk for injury related to CNS, GI, and sensitivity effects	No occurrence of injury symptoms	Assist client with ambulation. Caution against driving and other hazardous activities. Advise against alcohol ingestion. Report sore throat, fever, rash, itching, sudden weight gain, edema of ankles and fingers, changes in vision, epigastric pain ("heartburn") and black, tarry stools.
Deficient knowledge related to drug therapy	Self-administers drug with accuracy and safety Relates signs and symptoms of side effects/adverse reactions and those to report to prescriber	Instruct client in name and dosage of drug and its relationship to client's own condition. Avoid concurrent use of OTC medications and steroids. Teach signs and symptoms of side effects/adverse reactions and how to prevent or minimize them as in the interventions above.

SLE, Systemic lupus erythematosus.

terminations of white blood cell counts (WBCs), hemoglobin, and/or hematocrit.

A woman who is pregnant or intends to become pregnant while using an NSAID should notify her health care provider, because these drugs may interfere with maternal and infant blood clotting and prolong the duration of pregnancy and parturition. There is an increase in the incidence of stillbirths and neonatal deaths in humans. If the mother intends to breastfeed, she should be made aware of the fact that salicylates are detected in the breast milk and are cleared from the body more slowly by infants. See the Pregnancy Safety box on p. 274 for the FDA classification of the various NSAIDs.

Clients who are receiving anticoagulant drugs or have a clinical problem such as erosive gastritis, ulcers, bleeding disorders, mild diabetes, or gout should be warned to discuss NSAID use with their prescriber. The effect of edema caused by these agents should be considered in individuals with diseases such as congestive heart failure and hypertension.

The client who omits a scheduled dose should not double the next dose but should resume the usual dosing interval. The analgesia provided by NSAIDs is subject to a ceiling effect; higher than recommended dosages may not provide more therapeutic effect in the treatment of pain not associated with inflammation.

Discuss with the client the most common side effects and adverse reactions, which are not always an indication of excessive dosage and should be reported to the prescriber. Clients should be told to notify their prescriber immediately if a skin rash, itching, visual disturbances, edema, persistent headache or heartburn, or dark stools occur. A therapeutic alternative may need to be evaluated. Some individuals experience drowsiness and dizziness and should be cautioned about performing tasks with which the drug would interfere. The problem of morning stiffness in affected joints may be overcome by taking the last dose as late as possible in the evening.

Because photosensitivity occurs with diflunisal and ibuprofen, advise the client to wear sunscreen and avoid the use of sunlamps and prolonged exposure to the sunlight. Alcoholic beverages produce a synergistic effect with NSAIDs in causing gastrointestinal bleeding.

The client should be cautioned not to use any OTC analgesics concurrently with NSAIDs unless specifically recommended by the prescriber. Compliance may be an issue

Case Study *The Client Taking NSAIDs*

Rita Amherst is a 35-year-old woman who has had vague aches and pains along with malaise for the past 8 months. In recent months she has noticed that her finger joints have been somewhat swollen and painful. Her left knee also began to stiffen several weeks ago, but she attributed this to a recent fall. She went to her primary care provider, who examined her and referred her to a rheumatologist. He had an outpatient diagnostic workup performed. Rita has no history of serious medical illness.

Rita is placed on a regimen of aspirin 1 g PO qid; the dosage is to be increased until antiinflammatory effects are seen. She is also placed on diflunisal to reduce the acute inflammatory process.

1. What two actions of NSAIDs seem to be most responsible for their therapeutic effects?
2. For what interaction should Rita be monitored while taking aspirin concurrently with diflunisal?
3. What are some of the most commonly observed side effects of diflunisal?
4. Why is it important for Rita to contact her prescriber if she suspects she is pregnant?

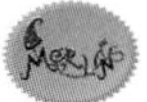

For answer guidelines, go to mosby.com/MERLN/McKenry/.

for some NSAIDs because the time until effectiveness is lengthy (e.g., 2 weeks with indomethacin).

Ibuprofen is available without prescription in the 200 mg strength for self-medication. Clients using ibuprofen as an OTC medication should be instructed to report to their health care provider if their symptoms do not improve, if fever persists for more than 3 days, or if swelling or redness occurs in the painful area. (See the Case Study box above.)

■ **Evaluation.** The expected outcome of NSAID therapy is that the client will report increased comfort and increased range of motion and ability to perform activities of daily living. There will be a decrease in or an absence of joint swelling, redness, and warmth. If administered as an antipyretic, the client's temperature will be within normal limits. The client will not experience any untoward effects of NSAID therapy.

THROMBOXANE A_2

Thromboxane A_2 (TXA_2) is a potent vasoconstrictor that stimulates additional platelet aggregation. Inhibiting TXA_2 formation will decrease platelet aggregation. Aspirin inhibits thromboxane synthetase, thereby preventing prostaglandin formation. Aspirin irreversibly blocks prostaglandin synthetase, whereas the other NSAIDs are primarily reversible inhibitors (*USP DI*, 1999).

OTHER DRUGS

Other products, such as the antimalarial agents (see Chapter 61), gold salts, and penicillamine, are also used to treat inflammation in clients who have not responded to or cannot tolerate salicylates or NSAIDs. Two new drugs, leflunomide (Arava) and etanercept (Enbrel), are available for the treatment of rheumatoid arthritis. In addition, adjuvant analgesic medications are added to opioid medications to enhance analgesia.

Although in use for more than 50 years in the treatment of rheumatoid arthritis, gold compounds are generally much slower acting and more toxic than other products. Therefore they are reserved for individuals who demonstrate continued or increased disease activity while receiving conservative therapy.

auranofin [au rane′ oh fin] (Ridaura)
aurothioglucose suspension [aur oh thye oh gloo′ kose] (Solganal)
gold sodium thiomalate injection (Myochrysine)

Although the exact antiinflammatory mechanism of action is unknown, auranofin, aurothioglucose suspension, and gold sodium thiomalate injection appear to suppress the synovitis of the acute stage of rheumatoid disease. Proposed mechanisms of action include the inhibition of sulfhydryl systems, various enzyme systems, suppression of the phagocytic action of macrophages and leukocytes, and an alteration of immune response.

Gold products are indicated for the treatment of rheumatoid arthritis; aurothioglucose and gold sodium thiomalate are used to treat juvenile arthritis.

The onset of action after oral administration is 3 to 4 months; with parenteral administration, 6 to 8 weeks. The half-life of oral gold is 21 to 31 days in blood and 42 to 128 days in body tissues. Auranofin is rapidly metabolized, but the metabolism of aurothioglucose and gold sodium thiomalate is unknown. Excretion is primarily by the kidneys.

With auranofin the more common side effects include abdominal distress or pain, gas, diarrhea, nausea, and vomiting. These effects are rare with the other gold products. The most common adverse reactions include a sore, irritated tongue or gums (less with auranofin), an allergic skin reaction, and mouth ulcers or fungus.

The adult dosage for auranofin is 6 mg daily; the maximum dosage is 9 mg/day. The pediatric dosage has not been determined. The adult dosage for aurothioglucose suspension and gold sodium thiomalate injection is 10 mg IM the first week, which increases weekly according to the manufacturer's schedule until a total dose of 800 mg to 1 g has been reached. The maintenance dosage is 25 to 50 mg IM every 2 to 4 weeks according to the manufacturer's schedule. In children 6 to 12 years of age, the initial dosage is 2.5 mg IM the first week and increases weekly according to schedule until the total dose of 200 to 250 mg has been reached. The maintenance dosage for children is 6.25 to 12.5 mg IM every 3 to 4 weeks. The adult dosage of gold sodium thiomalate is 10 mg the first week, 25 mg the second week, then 25 to 50 mg a week thereafter. The gold sodium thiomalate pediatric dosage is 10 mg IM the first week, then 1 mg/kg (up to 50 mg/dose) following the adult recommendations for weekly intervals.

■ Nursing Management

Gold Therapy

■ **Assessment.** A baseline assessment should include the extent of joint involvement, discomfort and mobility, and hepatic and renal function values, WBC, platelet count, and urinalysis. Clients should be assessed for sensitivity to gold and other heavy metals, because they may also be intolerant to gold salts. Clients with a history of bone marrow dysplasia or other severe hematologic disorders, exfoliative dermatitis, necrotizing enterocolitis, or pulmonary fibrosis may experience a recurrence of the condition. Gold therapy is used with caution in clients with renal dysfunction, severe debilitation, Sjögren's syndrome in rheumatoid arthritis (an immunologic disorder characterized by deficient moisture production of the lacrimal, salivary, and other glands), inadequate cerebral or cardiovascular circulation, systemic lupus erythematosus, urticaria, eczema, colitis (especially for auranofin), or blood dyscrasias.

The risk for very serious kidney or blood adverse reactions is increased when gold compounds are given concurrently with penicillamine. Administration of this combination should be avoided.

■ **Nursing Diagnosis.** Assessment of the client receiving gold compounds should include consideration of the following nursing diagnoses/collaborative problems: impaired skin integrity related to pruritus (auranofin, 17%), rash (auranofin, 24%), and exfoliative dermatitis; ineffective protection related to leukopenia, thrombocytopenia, and anemia; impaired comfort as evidenced by numbness and tingling of the hands and feet (peripheral neuritis), abdominal cramps (auranofin, 14%), metallic taste, and conjunctivitis (auranofin); deficient fluid volume related to anorexia, nausea, and vomiting (auranofin, 10%); impaired oral mucous membrane as evidenced by glossitis, gingivitis, or stomatitis (auranofin, 13%); disturbed thought processes related to CNS effects as evidenced by confusion and hallucinations; diarrhea (auranofin, 47%); disturbed sensory perception (visual) related to iritis or corneal ulcers; and the potential complications of allergic reaction, hepatitis, and renal toxicity.

■ **Implementation**

■ ***Monitoring.*** Platelet counts, WBCs, and urinalyses should be completed periodically during therapy (urinalysis before every injection and platelets and WBCs before every second injection). All three should be accomplished monthly with auranofin therapy. In addition, renal and hepatic function studies are required before and periodically during the course of auranofin therapy.

Glossitis, gingivitis, and stomatitis may result from gold compound therapy. Because these conditions may cause a lack of appetite, the client's nutritional status should be monitored. Skin symptoms such as itching and rash are quite common with auranofin. Gastrointestinal symptoms such as abdominal cramps and diarrhea are quite common. Both should be reported promptly to the prescriber.

■ ***Intervention.*** Therapy is often begun with the concurrent administration of NSAIDs during the first few months of gold therapy (until it becomes effective). If the client experiences mild adverse symptoms, gold therapy is discontinued until the symptoms have resolved and is then reinstituted at a lower dosage. Adverse responses such as anaphylaxis, angioedema, and syncope may result after an injection; emergency equipment should be available. If the client experiences a severe reaction, gold therapy is discontinued and not restarted.

To administer the IM injection, shake the vial vigorously and warm it to body temperature to ease drawing the suspension into the syringe. An 18-gauge, 1½-inch needle should be used to deposit the gold deep into the muscular tissue of the upper quadrant of the gluteal region; a 2-inch needle may be used for clients who are obese. With parenteral forms of the medication, there is the possibility of a nitritoid reaction after the injection (hypotension, flushing, light-headedness, and fainting) and joint pain for 1 to 2 days after an injection.

■ ***Education.*** Advise clients that dental work should not be undertaken if the administration of gold compounds has had a leukopenic or thrombocytopenic effect. Instruct the client about appropriate oral hygiene, including gentle toothbrushing and flossing and avoiding the use of toothpicks.

Encourage effective self-management of the therapeutic regimen; relief from symptoms may not occur for 3 to 6 months. Regular visits to the health care provider are necessary to monitor progress.

Caution the client that exposure to sunlight may aggravate gold-induced dermatitis or cause a rash. Alert the client that side effects may occur even after the discontinuation of gold compounds.

■ **Evaluation.** After 2 to 6 months of successful gold therapy, the client will report increased comfort and an increased range of motion and ability to perform activities of daily living. There will be a decrease in or absence of joint swelling, redness, and warmth. The client will not experience any untoward effects of gold therapy.

penicillamine [pen i sill′ a meen] (Cuprimine, Depen)

Penicillamine is a *chelating agent* for heavy metals such as mercury, lead, copper, and iron. This medication makes such metals more soluble so the kidneys can readily excrete them.

The mechanism of action as an antirheumatic agent is unknown, although lymphocyte function is improved and IgM rheumatoid factor and immune complexes located in the serum and synovial fluids are reduced. The relationship of these effects to rheumatoid arthritis is unknown.

Penicillamine is indicated for the prophylaxis and treatment of Wilson's disease (a rare inherited disorder that causes copper to accumulate in the body); the treatment of rheumatoid arthritis (especially for individuals with severe arthritis who have not responded to other therapies); and the treatment of cystinuria.

The most common side effects include anorexia, diarrhea, loss of taste, nausea, vomiting, and abdominal pain. Adverse reactions reported include allergic reactions and stomatitis.

The adult dosage of penicillamine as a chelating agent is 250 mg PO four times daily. The dosage as an antirheumatic agent is 125 or 250 mg PO daily; this is increased if necessary at 2- to 3-month intervals, up to a maximum of 1.5 g/day. The dosage as an antiurolithic agent is 500 mg PO four times daily. For infants over 6 months of age and young children, the chelating dosage is 250 mg daily and is administered in fruit juice; the pediatric dosage for the antirheumatic agent has not been determined.

■ Nursing Management

Penicillamine Therapy

In addition to the following discussion, see Nursing Management: NSAID Therapy, p. 290.

■ **Assessment.** Because penicillamine is chemically related to penicillin, determine the client's allergy to penicillin before the first dose. Use with caution in clients with hepatic or renal dysfunctions.

■ **Implementation**

■ ***Monitoring.*** If penicillamine is given as an antirheumatic, monitor the client's joint involvement, pain, and mobility.

For clients with Wilson's disease, 24-hour urinary copper analyses are recommended to determine optimum penicillamine dosages. For clients developing moderate proteinuria, 24-hour urinary protein determinations are recommended at 1- to 2-week intervals. Obtain urinalyses and complete blood and platelet counts and hemoglobin determinations twice a month for the first 6 months and each month thereafter to monitor for toxicity. Hepatic function studies should be completed every 6 months for the first 18 months of therapy to monitor for toxic hepatitis. For clients with cystinuria, x-ray examinations for renal calculi should be performed on an annual basis.

■ ***Intervention.*** Administer the drug on an empty stomach at least 1 hour apart from any other drug, food, antacid, or milk. If the course of therapy is interrupted, it needs to be restarted at a low dosage and gradually increased to the appropriate dosage to prevent adverse reactions. The penicillamine dosage should be reduced to 250 mg daily if the client is going to have surgery because of the effects of the drug on collagen and elastin, which results in increased skin friability. The usual dosage should not be resumed until wound healing is complete.

If penicillamine is administered for cystinuria, the client should be undergoing a high fluid intake, especially at night when the urine is more acidic and concentrated; 500 mL at bedtime and 500 mL once in the middle of the night is adequate. The greater the fluid intake, the lower the therapeutic dose of penicillamine.

Pyridoxine 250 mg daily is recommended for clients with impaired nutrition because penicillamine increases the requirement of this vitamin.

■ ***Education.*** The client should be encouraged to comply with the medication regimen because an interruption in the medication for even a few days may cause a sensitivity reaction when it is restarted. Long-term compliance may be especially difficult for clients with rheumatoid arthritis because an improvement in the status of their illness may require 2 to 3 months of therapy.

If administered for Wilson's disease, the dosage is calculated on the basis of the urinary copper excretion; the objective is to maintain a negative copper balance. The client should be advised that a low copper diet is necessary. This means omitting mushrooms, chocolate, dried fruit, nuts, shellfish, liver, molasses, and broccoli. Suggest the use of distilled water, because most tap water flows through copper pipes.

Alert the client that taste may be impaired. The ability to taste may be enhanced by administering 5 to 10 mg of copper daily, except for individuals with Wilson's disease, in whom copper intake is restricted.

■ **Evaluation.** The expected outcome of penicillamine therapy is that the client with Wilson's disease will experience increased urinary copper excretion with a 24-hour urine specimen, hepatic and renal function studies within normal limits, and a reduction or absence of neurologic symptoms. If penicillamine is administered as an antiurolithic, the client will not show evidence of any cystine calculi.

leflunomide [leh floo′ no myde] (Arava) **etanercept** [et ah ner′ sept] (Enbrel)

Leflunomide and etanercept are two new breakthrough drugs for the treatment of rheumatoid arthritis (RA). These agents are disease-modifying agents that actually slow the joint destruction produced by rheumatoid arthritis. Leflunomide is an immunomodulator and reduces the synthesis and mobilization of immune cells that attack the joints, whereas etanercept inhibits the tumor necrosis factor (TNF). Etanercept is a biologic response modifier; that is, it appears to bind excess TNF (inactivating it in an antibody-type reaction) and may also inhibit the binding of TNF to cell receptors, thus blocking the inflammatory effects of TNF (Davis, 1998). Leflunomide appears to be equivalent in action to methotrexate, and etanercept is reported to be more effective than methotrexate with less adverse effects (*Pharmacist's Letter,* 1998). Etanercept can be used alone or in combination with methotrexate.

The side effects/adverse reactions of leflunomide (Arava) include headache, dizziness, pruritus, rash, alopecia, diarrhea, nausea, cough, bronchitis, back and stomach pain, and elevation of liver enzymes. Rifampin has been reported to increase serum concentrations of leflunomide. Leflunomide is contraindicated for clients who have hepatic disease and during pregnancy (FDA category X) because it can cause birth defects. The adult dosage of leflunomide is 100 mg/day for 3 days; the maintenance dosage is 20 mg/day.

The side effects/adverse reactions of etanercept (Enbrel) include redness at the injection site and mild upper respiratory tract symptoms. The usual adult dosage is 25 mg SC twice a week. Children should be current with all immunization doses before etanercept therapy is started. Although it is not known whether the drug interferes with the immunologic response to vaccines, live virus vaccines should not be administered while a child is taking etanercept. The drug is packaged with its own diluent and should be administered as soon as possible after reconstitution.

ADJUVANT MEDICATIONS

Adjuvant (coanalgesic) medications are used in combination with other analgesics to enhance pain relief or to treat symptoms that exacerbate pain; in some instances they are used alone to treat specifically identified pain. The NSAIDs are often listed with the adjuvant analgesics but, with this exception, the primary indications for adjuvant medications are not for the treatment of pain. Nevertheless, these agents have been reported to have an analgesic effect in some pain conditions.

Adjuvant analgesic medications include a variety of medications such as anticonvulsants, antidepressants, antihistamines, corticosteroids, local anesthetics, antidysrhythmics, psychostimulants, clonidine, and capsaicin. Anticonvulsants, antidepressants, anesthetics, and antidysrhythmics are often prescribed for the treatment of neuropathic pain. They are often used in combination with opioids for cancer-associated nerve pain (AHCPR, 1994; Salerno, 1996).

Corticosteroids are beneficial for cancer pain that originates in a fairly restricted area, such as in the intracranial region, alongside a nerve root, or in pelvic, neck, or hepatic areas. Dexamethasone is prescribed for an increase in intracranial pressure and for relief of pain caused by pressure on a nerve. Corticosteroids may also relieve pain by suppressing the release of prostaglandins and thus inhibiting the inflammatory process.

The antihistamine hydroxyzine (Vistaril) is reported to have some analgesic properties (Haddox, 1992). It also has anxiolytic and sedative effects, which may be useful in some clients. Psychostimulants such as methylphenidate (Ritalin) and dextroamphetamine (Dexedrine) potentiate opioid analgesia and also help to increase alertness or reduce persistent, opioid-induced sedation in some clients. The analgesic effects are postulated to occur centrally and in the descending spinal inhibitory pathways. Opioid-induced cognitive impairment in clients with cancer or acquired immunodeficiency syndrome (AIDS) has improved with the administration of a psychostimulant drug (Bruera & Watanabe, 1994).

BOX 14-5

Bladder Pain

Pentosan polysulfate sodium (Elmiron) is a semisynthetic, heparin-like derivative used to treat bladder pain or discomfort from interstitial cystitis. This product is a weak anticoagulant and fibrinolytic with an unknown analgesic mechanism of action. It has been postulated that pentosan adheres to the bladder wall mucosa to prevent irritating substances in the urine from reaching bladder cells.

Pharmacokinetically, pentosan is administered orally, has an elimination half-life of approximately 5 hours, is metabolized primarily in the liver and spleen, and is excreted in urine. The side effects/adverse reactions include urinary frequency, alopecia, diarrhea, nausea, headache, dyspepsia, and stomach distress (incidence of 4% or less). The recommended dosage is 100 mg tid, 1 hour before or 2 hours after meals (*Drug Facts and Comparisons*, 2000).

Information from *United States Pharmacopeia Dispensing Information (USP DI): Drug information for the health care professional* (19th ed.) (1999). Rockville, MD: United States Pharmacopeial Convention.

The usual approach to opioid-induced persistent sedation is to reduce the opioid dosage and increase daily drug frequency. The opioid should be switched if the client does not respond appropriately with this method. If the sedation problem persists with these alternative strategies, a psychostimulant may be added to the opioid regimen (AHCPR, 1994).

Additional useful adjuvant analgesics include clonidine (Catapres, epidural Duraclon) and capsaicin. Clonidine is a centrally acting, alpha$_2$-adrenergic agonist that has been used for the treatment of pain associated with reflex sympathetic dystrophy (Rauck, Eisennach, Jackson, Young, & Southern, 1993), diabetic neuropathy, postherpetic neuralgia, spinal cord injury, phantom pain, and pain in cancer clients who are opioid tolerant (Portenoy, 1993). Box 14-5 provides information on bladder pain.

Capsaicin, an alkaloid found in chili peppers, is formulated into a topical cream (Zostrix) that is indicated for the treatment of neuralgia and arthritic pain. On application it causes an initial release and then a depletion of substance P from nerve fibers, which results in a decrease in pain transmission (Salerno, 1996). (See the Bibliography for additional information on adjuvant medications.)

SUMMARY

Pain continues to be a worldwide health problem. It disables and distresses more people than any other symptom and is probably the most common reason for seeking health care.

Few things that a nurse does are more important than alleviating pain. The delicate task of balancing the therapeutic relief of analgesics against their toxicity continues to be a challenge for nurses. The attitudes, fears, and biases of clients, families, and caregivers contribute to the unnecessary undertreatment of pain. The nurse must have skill and knowledge to assess accurately and intervene effectively in the relief of the pain of the clients in his or her care.

Morphine and other opioid agonists were the earliest substances used for pain relief and are still among the more effective. However, the nurse needs to be alert to the toxic symptoms resulting from inappropriate use of these analgesics. Naloxone, nalmefene, and naltrexone are opioid antagonists used for the reversal of opioid toxicity. Opioid agonist-antagonists are also used for pain relief.

NSAIDs are used to treat the signs and symptoms of inflammation, fever, and pain. Since the mid 1970s these aspirin substitutes have become quite popular for the treatment of mild to moderate pain and for the antiinflammatory treatment of arthritis. Although widely available, these agents are not without adverse GI, hepatic, and renal effects. Gold compounds, also used in the treatment of arthritis, are much slower acting and much more toxic than the NSAIDs.

Critical Thinking Questions

1. Tyrone Scali, age 42, has come to the emergency department after a fall while playing tennis. The health care provider diagnoses a sprained ankle, wraps his ankle with an elastic bandage, and advises him to elevate the ankle and keep it at rest. Aspirin 650 mg PO every 4 hours prn for pain is prescribed. Before instructing Mr. Scali regarding his aspirin therapy, you review his health history. What data would you be looking for which might contraindicate the use of aspirin for Mr. Scali?
2. Sarah Smith, age 53, has just returned to the general surgical unit from the postanesthesia recovery unit after having a thyroidectomy. Her physician has prescribed morphine 10 mg IM every 4 hours prn for postoperative pain. She is requesting pain medication for "a stabbing pain in her throat." What assessments will be critical before an analgesic is administered?
3. Robert Staysa, age 85, has osteoarthritis that is causing pain in his back, hips, and knees. His physician prescribes ibuprofen 400 mg PO qid. Why would the physician prescribe ibuprofen rather than a low-dose opioid analgesic? Given his age, Mr. Staysa is most at risk for what adverse reaction of NSAID therapy?
4. Jessie Holstein, age 72, is receiving auranofin for her rheumatoid arthritis. Why would gold salts rather than NSAIDs be used for clients with arthritis? While reviewing Mrs. Holstein's blood work, you notice that her platelet count is 155,000/mm^3. What action do you take?

Collaborative Learning Activities

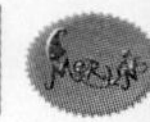

For Collaborative Learning Activities, go to mosby.com/MERLIN/McKenry/.

CASE STUDY

For a Case Study that will help ensure mastery of this chapter content, go to mosby.com/MERLIN/McKenry/.

BIBLIOGRAPHY

Abramowicz, M. (1998). Drugs for pain. *The Medical Letter on Drugs and Therapeutics, 40*(1033), 79-84.

Agency for Health Care Policy and Research (AHCPR), Public Health Service. (1992). *Clinical practice guideline: Acute pain management: Operative or medical procedures and trauma.* Rockville, MD: Department of Health and Human Services.

Agency for Health Care Policy and Research (AHCPR), Public Health Service. (1994). *Clinical practice guideline: Management of cancer pain.* Rockville, MD: Department of Health and Human Services.

American Hospital Formulary Service. (1999). *AHFS: Drug information '99.* Bethesda, MD: American Society of Hospital Pharmacists.

Anderson, K.N., Anderson, L.E., & Glanze, W.D. (Eds.) (1994). *Mosby's medical, nursing, and allied health dictionary* (4th ed.). St. Louis: Mosby.

Arthritis. (1998). *Pharmacist's Letter, 14*(2), 68-69.

Beers, M.H., Ouslander, J.G., Fingold, S.F., Morgenstern, H., Reuben, D.B., Rogers, W., Zeffren, M.J., & Beck, J.C.. (1992). Inappropriate medication prescribing in skilled-nursing facilities. *Annals of Internal Medicine, 117*(8), 680-684.

Bobak, I.M. & Lowdermilk, D.L. (1995). *Maternity nursing* (4th ed.). St Louis: Mosby.

Bruera, E. & Watanabe, S. (1994). Psychostimulants as adjuvant analgesics. *Journal of Pain & Symptom Management, 9*(6), 412-415.

Cleeland, C.S., Gonin, R., Hatfield, A.K., Edmonson, J.H., Blum, R.H., Stewart, J.A., & Pandya, K.J. (1994). Pain and its treatment in outpatients with metastatic cancer. *New England Journal of Medicine, 330,* 592-596.

Covington, T.R. (Ed.). (1996). *Handbook of nonprescription drugs* (11th ed.). Washington, DC: American Pharmaceutical Association.

Cushing, M. (1992). Pain management on trial. *American Journal of Nursing, 92*(2), 21-22.

Davis, W.M. (1998). A pharmacist's guide to anti-inflammatories. *Drug Topics, 142*(23), 89-96.

Drug Facts and Comparisons. (2000). St. Louis: Facts and Comparisons.

Eisenberg, D.M., Davis, R.B., Ettner, S.L., Appel, S., Wilkey, S., VanRompay, M., & Kessler, R.C. (1998). Trends in alternative medicine use in the United States, 1990-1997: Results of a follow-up national survey. *Journal of the American Medical Association, 280*(18), 1569-1575.

FDA News and Product Notes (1996). *Ultram Formulary, 31,* 450.

Foley, K.M. (1991). The relationship of pain and symptom management to patient requests for physician-assisted suicide. *Journal of Pain & Symptom Management, 6*(5), 289-297.

Gossel, T.A. & Wuest, J.R. (1993). Control of chronic cancer pain. *Florida Pharmacy Today, 57*(4), 21.

Gu, X. & Belgrade, M.J. (1993). Pain in hospitalized patients with medical illnesses. *Journal of Pain & Symptom Management, 8*(1), 17-21.

Haddox, J.D. (1992). Neuropsychiatric drug use in pain management. In Raj, P.P. (Ed.). *Practical management of pain* (2nd ed.). St. Louis: Mosby.

Hammack, J.E. & Loprinzi, C.L. (1994). Use of orally administered opioids for cancer-related pain. *Mayo Clinic Proceedings, 69*, 384-390.

Insel, P.A. (1996) Analgesic-antipyretic and antiinflammatory agents and drugs employed in the treatment of gout. In J.G. Hardman & L.E. Limbird (Eds.), *Goodman & Gilman's The pharmacological basis of therapeutics* (9th ed.). New York: McGraw-Hill.

Keeney, S.A. (1993). Nursing care of the postoperative patient receiving epidural analgesia. *MEDSURG Nursing, 2*(3), 191-196.

Kenyon, J. (Ed.) (1993). Fear of adverse effects should not hinder opioid use. *Drugs Therapy Perspectives, 1*(6), 13.

Kinzbrunner, B. & Salerno, E. (1994). *Vistas pain management formulary.* Miami: Vistas Healthcare Corporation.

Lipman, A.G. (1993). The argument against therapeutic use of heroin in pain management. *American Journal of Hospital Pharmacy, 50*(5), 996.

Mather, L.E. & Denson, D.D. (1992). Pharmacokinetics of systemic opioids for the management of pain. In R.S. Sinatra, A.H. Hord, B. Ginsberg, & L.M. Preble (Eds.). *Acute pain.* St Louis: Mosby.

McCaffery, M. & Beebe, A. (1989). *Pain: Clinical manual for nursing practice.* St. Louis: Mosby.

McCaffery, M. & Ferrell, B. (1992). Pain control decisions. *Nursing, 22*(8), 48.

McCaffery, M. & Pasero, C. (1999). *Pain: Clinical manual for nursing practice* (2nd ed.). St. Louis: Mosby.

McCaffery, M. & Portenoy, R.K. (1999). Nonopioids. In M. McCaffery & C. Pasero (Eds.), *Pain: Clinical manual* (2nd ed.). St. Louis: Mosby.

McCarthy, R.L. & Montagne, M. (1993). The argument for therapeutic use of heroin in pain management. *American Journal of Hospital Pharmacy, 50*(5), 992.

McCombs, J. (1993). Therapeutic considerations during pregnancy and lactation. In J.T. DiPiro, R.L. Talber, G.C. Yee, G.R. Matzke, B.G. Wells, & L.M. Posey (Eds.), *Pharmacotherapy: A pathophysiologic approach* (2nd ed.). Norwalk, CT: Appleton & Lange.

McDonald, D.D. (1993). Postoperative narcotic analgesic administration. *Applied Nursing Research, 6*(3), 106.

McGrath, P.A. (1990). *Pain in children: Nature, assessment, and treatment.* New York: Guilford Press.

Melzack, R. & Wall, P.D. (1965). Pain mechanisms: A new theory. *Science, 150*, 971-979.

Miller, S. & Fioravanti, J. (1997). *Pediatric medications: A handbook for nurses.* St. Louis: Mosby.

North American Nursing Diagnosis Association. (2001). *Nursing diagnoses: Definitions & classification 2001-2002.* Philadelphia, PA: Author.

Patt, R.B. (1993). Classification of cancer pain and cancer pain syndromes. In R.B. Patt (Ed.), *Cancer pain.* Philadelphia: J.B. Lippincott.

Patt, R.B. (1996). Using controlled-release oxycodone for the management of chronic cancer and noncancer pain. *American Pain Society Bulletin, 6*(4), 1-6.

Peat, S. (1995). Providing pain relief for the surgical patient. *Care of Critical Illness, 11*(1), 16-19.

Pharmacist's Letter (1998). Rheumatoid arthritis. *Pharmacist's Letter,* 14(9), 49-54.

Physicians' Desk Reference. (1999). Oradell, NJ: Medical Economics.

Portenoy, R.K. (1993). Adjuvant analgesics in pain management. In D. Doyle, G.W.C. Hanks, & N. MacDonald (Eds.). *Oxford textbook of palliative medicine.* New York: Oxford University Press.

Porter, J. & Jick, H. (1980). Addiction rare in patients treated with narcotics. *New England Journal of Medicine, 302*, 123.

Rauck, R.L., Eisennach, J.C., Jackson K., Young, L.D., & Southern, J. (1993). Epidural clonidine treatment for refractory reflex sympathetic dystrophy. *Anesthesiology, 79*(6), 1163-1169.

Rheumatoid arthritis. (1998). *Pharmacist's Letter, 14*(9), 49-54.

Salerno, E. (1996). Pharmacologic approaches. In E. Salerno & J.S. Willens (Eds.), *Pain management handbook.* St. Louis: Mosby.

Salerno, E. & Willens, J.S. (1996). *Pain management handbook.* St Louis: Mosby.

Sinatra, R.S. & Savarese, A. (1992). Parenteral analgesic therapy and patient-controlled analgesia for pediatric pain management. In R.S. Sinatra, A.H. Hord, B. Ginsberg, & L.M. Preble (Eds.), *Acute pain.* St. Louis: Mosby.

Twycross, R. (1994). *Pain relief in advanced cancer.* Edinburgh: Churchill Livingstone.

United States Pharmacopeia Dispensing Information (USP DI): Drug information for the health care professional (19th ed.) (1999). Rockville, MD: United States Pharmacopeial Convention.

Villarruel, A.M. & Ortiz de Montellano, B. (1992). Culture and pain: A Mesoamerican perspective. *Advances in Nursing Science, 15*(1), 21.

Wallace, M. (1994). Assessment and management of pain in the elderly. *MEDSURG Nursing, 3*(4), 293-298.

Warfield, C.A. (Ed.). (1993). *Principles and practice of pain management.* New York: McGraw-Hill.

Waters, L. (1992). Pharmacologic strategies for managing pain in children. *Orthopedic Nursing, 11*(1), 34.

Watt-Watson, J.H. & Donovan, M.I. (1992). *Pain management: Nursing perspective.* St. Louis: Mosby.

Weissman, D.E. & Haddox, J.D. (1989). Opioid pseudoaddiction: An iatrogenic syndrome. *Pain, 36*(3), 363-366.

Welk, T.A. (1991). An educational model for explaining hospice services. *American Journal of Hospice Palliative Care, 8*(5), 14-17.

Willcox, S.M., Himmelstein, D.U., & Woolhandler, S. (1994). Inappropriate drug prescribing for the community-dwelling elderly. *JAMA, 272*(4), 292-296.

Willens, J.S. (1996). Introduction to pain management. In E. Salerno & J.S. Willens (Eds.), *Pain management handbook.* St. Louis: Mosby.

World Health Organization. (1989). *Freedom from pain cancer pain: Educational lecture for health care professionals.* Geneva: Author.

Zhukovsky, D.S., Gorowski, E., Hausdorff, J., Napolitano, B., & Lesser, M. (1995). Unmet analgesic needs in cancer patients. *Journal of Pain & Symptom Management, 10*(2), 113-119.

15 Anesthetics

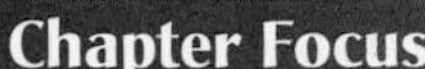

Chapter Focus

Advances in modern surgical technique would not be possible without the developments that have occurred in anesthesia. Anesthetic agents prevent the pain that would otherwise be experienced during surgery. These agents protect the client from the trauma of surgical pain and provide the surgeon the time and exposure to the surgical field necessary to accomplish sophisticated procedures. Nursing during the perioperative period involves three distinct phases: preoperative, intraoperative, and postoperative. Although the care the nurse provides in each of these phases varies in its approach, the ultimate goal is the safety and well-being of the client.

Learning Objectives

1. Describe common general anesthetic agents.
2. Identify the significant physiologic changes observable in the client at each stage of anesthesia.
3. List the common drugs that interact with anesthetic agents and the possible result of concomitant use.
4. Identify disease and risk factors that can alter the response to anesthesia.
5. Discuss nursing measures to prevent or treat common postoperative complications.
6. Discuss the use and side effects of local anesthetics.
7. Apply the nursing process to the client receiving general or local anesthetic agents.

Key Terms

balanced anesthesia, p. 303
caudal anesthesia, p. 322
conduction anesthesia, p. 322
dissociative anesthesia, p. 314
general anesthesia, p. 303
infiltration anesthesia, p. 322
local anesthesia, p. 317
neurolepsis, p. 315
neuroleptanalgesia, p. 314
neuroleptanesthesia, p. 312
regional anesthesia, p. 317
saddle block, p. 322
spinal anesthesia, p. 322

Key Drugs [✔]

halothane, p. 309

Anesthetic drugs are central nervous system (CNS) depressants used to induce a loss of sensation, especially the sensation of pain. There are two major categories of anesthesia: general and regional (local). General anesthesia induces a state of unconsciousness and varying amounts of analgesia, amnesia, muscle relaxation, and loss of reflexes (sensory and autonomic). This state is achieved with IV or inhalation routes of drug administration. Regional or local anesthesia blocks pain sensations in specific areas of the body without loss of consciousness. In general, the effect of regional anesthesia is related to the target nerve and its distribution in the body, whereas local anesthesia is a blockade of the nerves in the infiltrated tissues. Local anesthesia may be achieved topically or by setting up a field block in an area that encircles the surgical field (infiltration anesthesia). Spinal, epidural, caudal, and nerve block anesthesia have been referred to as both regional and local anesthesia.

GENERAL ANESTHESIA

General anesthesia is the absence of sensation and consciousness and is induced by inhalation or IV injection of various anesthetic agents. It is an important mode of therapy, especially for surgical procedures. A general anesthetic alters the CNS to produce varying degrees of analgesia, depression of consciousness, skeletal muscle relaxation, and reflex reduction.

MECHANISM OF ACTION

At concentrations that produce anesthesia, general anesthetics affect all excitable tissues of the body. They vary widely in their individual effects and in the concentration necessary for each to produce a given state of anesthesia. Although many theories of anesthesia have been proposed, none satisfactorily explains the basic mechanisms of action. Indeed, different anesthetics may have different modes of action, and no single theory may suffice.

The pattern of depression is similar for all general anesthetics—irregular and descending. The medullary centers are depressed last, which is fortunate because these are the vital centers concerned with heart action, blood pressure, and respiration. Initially, an anesthetic produces a loss of the perception of sight, touch, taste, smell, awareness, and hearing. Unconsciousness is usually produced. The two classes of general anesthetics are inhalation anesthetics (gases or volatile liquids) and IV agents.

A combination of drugs is necessary to produce all of the desired effects sought with anesthesia. Analgesia, muscle relaxation, unconsciousness, and amnesic effects are not produced safely by a single anesthetic. **Balanced anesthesia** involves the induction of anesthesia with a combination of drugs, each for its own specific effect, rather than with a single drug that has multiple effects. For example, anesthesia may be induced by premedicating with a short-acting barbiturate or benzodiazepine and then with an opioid analgesic and a skeletal muscle relaxant, followed by an anesthetic gas administered by the anesthetist. The specific drugs and dosages depend on the procedure being performed, the physical condition of the client, and the client's response to the medications. The advantage of balanced anesthesia is a lower reported incidence of postoperative nausea, vomiting, and pain.

STAGES OF GENERAL ANESTHESIA

General anesthesia generally consists of four stages, which vary with the choice of anesthetic, speed of induction, and skill of the anesthetist. Not all stages occur with all anesthetics. The current practice of administering an IV anesthetic before administering an inhalation anesthetic promotes rapid transition from consciousness to surgical anesthesia, and the early stages of anesthesia are not seen. However, if the drug is given slowly enough, all stages are usually observed. All stages are most easily seen when an inhalation anesthetic is used as the only anesthetic. The four stages are described in the following paragraphs.

Stage 1: Analgesia. This stage begins with the onset of anesthetic administration and lasts until loss of consciousness. Smell and pain are abolished before consciousness is lost. Vivid dreams and auditory or visual hallucinations may be experienced. Speech becomes difficult and indistinct. Numbness spreads gradually over the body, and the body feels stiff and unmanageable. Hearing is the last sense lost.

The nurse should maintain a quiet and tranquil environment for the client because even low voices and equipment sounds may be interpreted as excessively loud and may be counterproductive to the anesthetic. Before the anesthetic is administered, restraining straps are placed on the client, and the client is covered for warmth and modesty.

Stage 2: Excitement. During this stage, reflexes are still present and may be exaggerated, particularly with sensory stimulation such as noise. The client may struggle, shout, laugh, swear, or sing. Autonomic activity, muscle tone, eye movement, and rapid and irregular breathing increase. Irregular respirations may cause uneven absorption of the anesthetic; a period of apnea followed by a few deep breaths may produce a high concentration of anesthetic in the blood. Vomiting and incontinence sometimes occur in this stage. The client should not be touched during this stage except to restrain him or her for safety reasons.

Stage 2 varies greatly with individuals and depends on (1) the amount and type of premedication, (2) the anesthetic agent used, and (3) the degree of external sensory stimuli. Since the advent of balanced anesthesia, the signs and duration of this stage have been reduced. Stages 1 and 2 constitute the *stage of induction.*

Stage 3: Surgical Anesthesia. This stage is divided into four planes of increasing depth of anesthesia. Which plane a client is experiencing is determined by the character of the respirations, eyeball movement, pupil size, and the degree to which reflexes are present. As the client moves into plane one, the respiratory irregularities of the second stage usually disappear and respirations become full and regular. Respiration becomes shallower and more rapid as anesthesia deepens. Increased abdominal breathing follows paralysis of the intercostal muscles; finally, only the diaphragm is active. A loss of reflexes occurs in a cephalocaudal direction—from the head downward. The eyelid reflex is lost and the eyeballs, which initially exhibit a rolling movement, gradually move less and then cease to move. If the pupils were reflexively dilated in the second stage, they normally now constrict to their approximate size in natural sleep; their reaction to light becomes sluggish. The pupils dilate as plane 4 is approached.

The client's face is calm and expressionless and may be flushed or even cyanotic. The musculature becomes increasingly relaxed as the reflexes are progressively abolished. Most abdominal surgery cannot be performed until the abdominal reflexes are absent and the abdominal wall is soft. Body temperature is lowered as the anesthetic state continues. The pulse remains full and strong. Blood pressure may be elevated slightly, but in plane four the blood pressure drops and the pulse weakens. The skin, which was warm, now becomes cold, wet, and pale.

Most surgical procedures are performed in plane two or in the upper part of plane three. The anesthetist closely monitors each phase of anesthesia and gives approval to begin the procedure when the client has reached the appropriate plane for surgery. This approval is obtained before preparing the skin, surgically draping the client, and proceeding with surgery.

Stage 4: Medullary Paralysis (Toxic Stage). This stage is characterized by respiratory arrest and vasomotor collapse. Respiration ceases before the heart action. This stage may be reversed by reducing the gaseous agent to lighten the anesthetic state.

The nurse is part of the surgical team in providing resuscitative measures; the necessary drugs, equipment, and supplies; and other assistance as necessary.

SIGNIFICANT DRUG INTERACTIONS

Among the dangers facing a surgical client is an unexpected drug interaction that occurs during preparation or during anesthesia. Anesthetists must always be familiar with the interactions between anesthetic drugs and the maintenance drug therapies used in a wide range of illnesses. A serious drug interaction may be underway before surgery, and the surgical anesthesia may complicate the interaction. A critical analysis of the client's drug regimen (prescribed, over-the-counter, and alternative/complementary medications) should be performed in relation to the anesthetic drugs and preanesthetic drugs to be used.

Although it is the anesthetist's responsibility to obtain the preoperative drug history, the nurse should also be aware of all the medications the client consumed in the 2- to 3-week preoperative period. Various pharmacologic classes of medication may result in adverse reactions in clients anesthetized for surgery. For example, *anticoagulants* such as heparin and coumarin are usually discontinued 48 hours (aspirin, 7 days) before surgery to reduce the increased risk of hemorrhage. *CNS depressants* such as opioids and hypnotics may increase the risk of enhanced CNS-depressant effects.

Antidysrhythmics such as propranolol hydrochloride may induce decreased cardiac output, decreased heart rate, and bronchospasm. Quinidine, procainamide, and lidocaine may reduce cardiac conduction, increase peripheral vasodilation, and potentiate neuromuscular blocking agents such as tubocurarine.

Combining local anesthetic agents with *sympathomimetic* or *vasoconstrictive agents* (e.g., epinephrine, phenylephrine, or methoxamine) can cause ischemia, leading to sloughing of tissue or gangrene in fingers, toes, or other areas that have end arteries. If combined with local anesthetics, these agents should be carefully dosed and closely monitored.

Selected *antihypertensive agents* such as guanethidine (Ismelin) and methyldopa (Aldomet) deplete the synthesis or storage of norepinephrine in the sympathetic (adrenergic) nerve endings and may result in severe hypotension when combined with anesthetics and analgesics. Prescribers may consider reducing or stopping such medications before surgery.

When used as long-term therapy, *corticosteroids* usually produce adrenal gland suppression, which may result in hypotension during surgery. Because the stress of anesthesia and surgery usually increases the need for and release of endogenous corticosteroids, it is recommended that corticosteroid dosages be increased in the perioperative period.

Cholinesterase inhibitors (e.g., echothiophate iodide [Phospholine Iodide] and demecarium bromide [Humorsol]) and exposure to organophosphate insecticides may prolong succinylcholine blockade. Extended apnea and death have been reported with this combination. It is generally recommended that cholinergic eyedrops be stopped approximately 2 weeks before elective surgery.

Antibiotics—particularly aminoglycoside antibiotics (e.g., amikacin [Amikin], gentamicin [Garamycin]), clindamycin (Cleocin), tetracyclines, and polymyxin antibiotics—may potentiate the neuromuscular blocking agent or cause neuromuscular blockade. A reduction in the dosage of the neuromuscular blocking agent may be necessary, along with careful titration or careful dosing of the drug for the client (to response). Clients with myasthenia gravis, Parkinson's disease, or other neuromuscular disorders must be monitored carefully.

Many other drugs have the potential to induce an unwanted effect intraoperatively or postoperatively. Concurrent administration of various drugs with anesthetic agents requires close supervision and monitoring of the surgical client. As a general guideline, a drug that is needed for treatment preoperatively should be continued through surgery. Drugs that may be suspended temporarily without harming the client's health are discontinued before surgery for a period at least five times the half-life of the drug. Drugs having significant interactions with anesthetic agents are replaced, when possible, with an alternative medication before surgery.

SPECIAL CONSIDERATIONS

Many disease states and risk factors can alter the client's response to anesthesia. The preoperative assessment of the client's health status by the nurse includes, among other factors, acute and chronic medical conditions.

Alcoholism. Clients who are alcoholic may have a variety of associated disease states, including liver dysfunction, pancreatitis, gastritis, and esophageal varices. The anesthetic requirements for these clients may be increased because of an increase in liver-metabolizing enzymes and the development of cross-tolerance. Alcoholic clients are monitored closely during the postanesthetic period for alcohol withdrawal syndrome, because its onset may be delayed with the administration of medications for pain relief. Pharmacologic intervention with diazepam (Valium) or other agents may be required to prevent the occurrence of withdrawal symptoms.

Obesity. Clients who are overweight or obese may have cardiac insufficiency, respiratory problems, atherosclerosis, hypertension, or an increased incidence of diabetes, liver disease, or thrombophlebitis. Obtaining the desired depth of anesthesia and muscle relaxation may be a problem. With prolonged administration of fat-soluble anesthetic agents, there is delayed recovery due to the saturation of fat depots. In general, fat-soluble anesthetics, especially those with toxic metabolites such as methoxyflurane (Penthrane), should be avoided.

Smoking. Clients who smoke usually have an increasingly rigid arterial vascular system, adrenal gland stimulation, and perhaps lung disease (e.g., bronchitis, emphysema, carcinoma). Postoperative complications are therefore six times more common in smokers than in nonsmokers. Smoking also increases the client's sensitivity to muscle relaxants.

Pregnancy. See the Pregnancy Safety box below for the Food and Drug Adminstration's (FDA's) rating of anesthetic drug safety during pregnancy. Before any drug is used, the expected drug benefits should be considered against the possible risk to the fetus. Box 15-1 describes the risks of waste anesthetic gases to health care providers.

Young Age. The physical characteristics of neonates may predispose them to upper airway obstruction or laryngospasm during anesthesia induction or resuscitation. A small mandible and neck, a narrow cricoid ring, a large body water compartment with a high extracellular water turnover rate, immaturely functioning liver and kidneys, and a rapid metabolic rate all contribute to the need for careful consideration of infants or children. Drug dosages and administered fluids must be carefully calculated using the body weight or surface area of the child. Halothane and nitrous oxide are commonly used in pediatrics because the incidence of hepatitis in children is considered rare after the use of halothane. Neonates are usually more sensitive to the nondepolarizing muscle-relaxing agents.

Advanced Age. Aging results in a generalized decline in organ function (approximately 1% per year after age 30), the existence of chronic disease processes, or both. The complexity of drug treatment increases as the number and complexity of illnesses increase with age; this results in a greater potential for drug interactions and side effects. In general, an increased and prolonged drug effect is seen in older adults. Mortality rates for older adults undergoing major surgery may be 4 to 8 times higher than for younger clients.

Pregnancy Safety
Anesthetics

Category	Drug
B	enflurane, etidocaine, lidocaine, methohexital, prilocaine, propofol
C	alfentanil, bupivacaine, chloroprocaine, dibucaine, etomidate, fentanyl, mepivacaine, methoxyflurane, sufentanil, tetracaine, thiopental
Unclassified	droperidol, halothane, isoflurane, ketamine, procaine, sevoflurane

■ Nursing Management
General Anesthetics

Nursing during the perioperative period encompasses three distinct phases: preoperative, intraoperative, and postoperative. These phases are a continuum, but nursing care during each phase differs in its approach to the client and nursing care goals.

BOX 15-1

Risk of Waste Anesthetic Gases to Health Care Providers

Chronic exposure to waste anesthetic gases in the operating room may present a significant occupational health hazard to health care providers. Studies have demonstrated an increased incidence of spontaneous abortions among women exposed to nitrous oxide, as well as among the wives of men who have been exposed. In addition, neurologic, hepatic, and renal disorders have been seen in the chronically exposed. Health care providers should protect themselves by avoiding the area within a foot of the client's mouth and nose when the breath contains exhaled anesthetic agents. Health care providers should be active in establishing exposure monitoring programs to detect unsafe levels caused by faulty equipment and unsafe practices.

Preoperative Phase

One of the major responsibilities of the nurse during the preoperative period is to accomplish a focus assessment—the acquisition of selected or specific data as determined by the nurse and the client or family or as directed by the client's condition (Carpenito, 2000). Although general health data are gathered during admission of the client to the health care agency, it is important to focus on those factors that will influence the client's experience with anesthetic agents to allow optimal anesthesia to be achieved without adverse reactions.

One of these factors is the client's underlying acute and chronic conditions and the medications the client has recently taken or is currently taking. Disease states and risk factors that can alter the individual response have been discussed previously.

The nurse must also assess the client's experience with previous surgeries to allay anxiety and to identify risk factors to prevent adverse reactions, particularly malignant hyperthermia. *Malignant hyperthermia* is a condition characterized by often-fatal hyperthermia. It is important to ask if the client or a family member has ever had problems with anesthesia, because this condition is associated with an autosomal dominant trait.

If the client is hospitalized the night before surgery, sedatives or hypnotics may be administered to ensure a sound and restful sleep. The timing of the administration of this medication provides an opportunity to assess the client's emotional state regarding the anticipated surgical procedure. Many clients have anxieties regarding the experience of anesthesia, such as a fear of not waking up, having pain during surgery, talking while they are anesthetized, or having nausea and vomiting after surgery. These anxieties can be minimized if the client and family are well prepared about the perioperative routine and the anesthetic agents to be used.

The surgeon or the anesthetist can best answer questions about the rationale for a particular agent or method. Very few clients talk while anesthetized, and those who do are generally unintelligible. However, clients do have other valid concerns that need to be discussed to ensure that there is informed consent for the anesthesia. Clients can be reassured that they will have close surveillance throughout the surgical procedure and in the immediate postoperative period. Clients who persist in their fears regarding the anesthesia or the surgery need a consultation with the surgeon and/or the anesthetist before undergoing final preparation for surgery. Unless allayed, severe anxiety or fear affects both the autonomic and central nervous systems and may cause reactions that are detrimental both physiologically and psychologically. An anxious client may resist relaxation and fight the anesthetic. In such a case a greater amount of anesthetic would be required, and toxic levels of drugs might be administered inadvertently. Preoperative teaching and counseling by the nurse help in alleviating a client's anxiety. This preoperative counseling may be managed by a case manager or by preoperative visits to the hospital, particularly with day or short-stay surgeries.

In addition to the preanesthetic medications, all of the preparations required for the surgical procedure should be carefully explained to the client. Most clients are not familiar with the procedures related to the perioperative experience. Alert the client that he or she will "wake up" or recover from the anesthetic in a different place or postanesthetic recovery room (PARR). The necessity for postoperative coughing, deep breathing, frequent turning, and the use of spirometers should be taught to the client preoperatively. These activities help to prevent the postoperative complications of general anesthetics, such as hypostatic pneumonia and atelectasis. Preoperative teaching promotes cooperation when the client is asked to do these activities, which often cause discomfort after a surgical procedure.

Food is usually withheld after the evening meal, and standard procedure is to put the client on NPO status after midnight (nothing to eat or drink). This procedure helps prevent aspiration if vomiting occurs as a response to anesthesia.

Attention should be given to the client's drug history during the preoperative preparation. Withholding maintenance medications because the client is NPO for surgery has the physiologic effect of abrupt withdrawal. Therefore specific orders should be obtained from the primary prescriber regarding rescheduling the time of administration, changing the route of administration of the client's standing medications, or both. When a parenteral form of a medication is not available, a client who is NPO for surgery may sometimes be allowed to take oral medications with a small amount of water (30 to 60 mL).

In addition, as previously discussed, some medications may remain in the client's system and interact with the anesthetic to cause serious problems such as arterial hypotension and circulatory collapse or respiratory depression.

Premedicating the client is less common now than in the past. The client's age, weight, physical condition, and level of anxiety; the anesthetic method selected; and the duration and type of surgery are taken into consideration. Not including drugs in the preoperative preparation may be appropriate for some clients, whereas other clients may need aggressive pharmacologic intervention to produce the desired preoperative state. When drugs are prescribed, a combination such as morphine or meperidine (Demerol), hydroxyzine (Atarax), and atropine is generally used for the immediate preoperative preparation of the client for major surgery. In this instance, atropine is used to block the action of acetylcholine at parasympathetic nerve endings, to overcome the vagal effects of anesthesia, and to dry secretions.

Opioid analgesics, barbiturates, or benzodiazepines (the anxiolytics most commonly used) may be administered before the client is taken to surgery to promote serenity and amnesia, to smooth induction, and to decrease the amount of anesthetic required to produce anesthesia. It is important that the nurse administer the preoperative medications at the exact time ordered. If given too close to the time of administration of the general anesthetic, they may achieve their full effect during anesthesia and cause severe respiratory depression or hypotension.

Because the time needed to complete specific surgical procedures varies, it is impossible for many preoperative medications (other than the first cases of the day) to be ordered for a specific time. For cases other than the first of the day, the preoperative medication is ordered "on call" from the operating room.

All of the physical tasks involved with the client's preparation for surgery (e.g., signing surgical permits, final voiding before surgery, obtaining vital signs) should be accomplished before the preoperative medication is administered. The consent for anesthesia, surgery, or both is not considered valid if the client has received sedation before signing. Once the medication is administered, the client should be placed on bed rest with the side rails up and the call light within reach. This decreases stimulation and favors the action of the medication.

Intraoperative Phase

The nurse has a highly specialized role within the operating room. Nursing responsibilities entail the maintenance of safety, physiologic monitoring, and psychologic support of the client, but the nurse's role in relation to the administration of anesthetic agents is to support the anesthesiologist or the nurse anesthetist administering the anesthetic.

The operating room nurse should monitor for factors that may result in hypotension, nerve injury, or malignant hyperthermia. Hypotension may result from an excess of nonvolatile drugs that depress the vasomotor center. When opioids are given, the client's pain must be assessed thoroughly and the vital signs recorded. Because they may increase hypotension, these drugs should be avoided. However, severe pain can also cause hypotension. In such cases an opioid may both alleviate pain and as a result increase blood pressure.

The operating room nurse must also be on the alert for nerve injury, which may follow spinal anesthesia or malpositioning during general anesthesia. The brachial, radial, ulnar, and perineal nerves are the nerves most likely to be injured. The operating room nurse is responsible for ensuring that the client is positioned properly to prevent injury from nerve damage. Having knowledge of proper positioning for the particular surgical procedure is essential.

A rare but very dangerous adverse reaction to inhaled, fat-soluble anesthetics is malignant hyperthermia—an emergency situation in which the client's temperature suddenly escalates. The client may die if this condition is not treated appropriately and promptly. Individuals susceptible to malignant hyperthermia have an underlying muscle disorder, which is an autosomal dominant trait. The use of neuromuscular blocking agents has also been associated with this adverse reaction, especially when used with the inhalation anesthetics. The onset of this condition may be more abrupt with concurrent use of succinylcholine.

With malignant hyperthermia, body temperature may increase as much as 1° C (1.8° F) every 5 minutes, reaching reported highs of 43° C (109.4° F). Although the condition is relatively rare, occurring 1 in 50,000 surgical clients, it is a life-threatening condition with a mortality rate of 30% to 40%. The operating room team, within which the nurse has a key role, should have a preplanned course of action, including the availability of dantrolene sodium (see Chapter 23 for a thorough discussion), a complete change of anesthesia circuit, hyperventilation with 100% oxygen, methods to lower body temperature rapidly, and other symptomatic treatment. Dantrolene sodium has been used prophylactically and in the treatment of this disorder.

Nursing Role Within Intraoperative Phase. The clinical role of the nurse anesthetist, who assumes direct responsibility for the administration of anesthetics, requires a formal certification program for advanced practice of that specialty.

Postoperative Phase

The major objective of the immediate postoperative period is to help the client to recover from the effects of the anesthetic and the surgery safely, comfortably, and as quickly as possible.

■ **Assessment.** A general postoperative assessment should include the following (Beare & Myers, 1998):

1. *Airway and breathing:* adequacy of the airway and airway reflexes (gag, cough, swallow), type of airway in place, rate and quality of respiration, breath sounds, ability to cough and deep breathe, amount and method of oxygen administered and the time it was initiated
2. *Circulation:* pulse rate, peripheral pulses, blood pressure readings, cardiac monitor pattern (if applicable), skin color and temperature
3. *Metabolic state:* skin integrity and turgor, temperature, urine output, type and rate of IV fluids administered
4. *General:* location, condition, and output from drains and catheters; muscle strength and response; bowel sounds; status of the surgical incision; position of client; pain; level of consciousness; ability to communicate

■ **Nursing Diagnosis.** The client receiving a general anesthetic may experience the following nursing diagnoses/collaborative problems: ineffective airway clearance related to inadequate cough and tenacious secretions; ineffective breathing pattern related to excess or cumulative effects of drugs administered during anesthesia induction; risk for aspiration related to nausea and vomiting, gastrointestinal distention, medication and anesthesia, stimulation of the vomiting center or chemoreceptor trigger zone, or anoxia during anesthesia; pain; hypothermia; disturbed sensory perception; and the potential complications of urinary retention, abdominal distention or paralytic ileus, and shock.

■ **Implementation**

■ ***Monitoring.*** At frequent intervals that depend on the client's condition, evaluate the client's status as in the initial assessment.

■ ***Intervention.*** Neuromuscular blocking agents such as curare, succinylcholine, and D-tubocurarine can cause hypoventilation. Maintaining a patent airway until the client has fully responded is important in the postoperative period. Nursing measures include encouraging clients to deep breathe and cough frequently. A change of position to prevent pooling of pulmonary secretions can help to improve ventilation and prevent atelectasis. Most clients receiving a general anesthetic will be administered supplemental oxygen until they are fully recovered from the anesthesia. Mobilization and alternating the contraction and relaxation of muscles promote circulation.

Postoperatively, the nurse can administer a prescribed antiemetic and position the client on his or her side to prevent aspiration. Do not give the client anything by mouth until peristalsis returns. Normal bowel sounds and progression to an appropriate diet are the client outcomes sought.

Detecting impending shock early and instituting the proper therapy may prevent or at least modify its severity. The rate, volume, and rhythm of the pulse, as well as the client's color and skin temperature, should be noted. A rapid, thready, weak pulse; cyanosis or extreme pallor; cold, clammy skin; and low blood pressure are characteristic signs of shock. Checking for bleeding at the surgical site is important; hemorrhagic shock may occur if the client continues to lose blood postoperatively. Postoperative shock also may result from extensive surgical trauma, prolonged operating time, prolonged deep anesthesia, or even inadequate anesthesia.

▪ ***Education.*** Increasing numbers of surgeries are being performed at ambulatory surgical centers, and client-family teaching for the client who is returning home the same day as the surgery is necessary to help him or her recover more fully from the anesthesia and the surgery. In addition to providing specifics regarding the client's surgical procedure and its relevant postoperative care, prepare the client for experiencing some degree of psychomotor impairment and sensory-perceptual alterations during the first 24 hours following anesthesia. Caution the client against attempting tasks that require alertness and coordination, such as driving. The client should be instructed to avoid using alcohol or other CNS depressants within the first 24 hours unless prescribed by the health care provider.

▪ **Evaluation.** The client will effectively maintain his or her own airway and will have an effective cough, normal respiratory rate and depth, and normal breath sounds. Temperature, blood pressure, and pulse will be within normal limits. The client will experience no postoperative pain or an acceptable level of postoperative discomfort. The client's urinary output will be more than 30 to 50 mL/hr without complaints of urgency or bladder fullness. The client will be oriented to person, time, and place.

TYPES OF GENERAL ANESTHETICS

General anesthetics are usually divided into two groups: (1) inhalation anesthetics, which include gases and volatile liquids; and (2) IV anesthetics, which include barbiturates and nonbarbiturates.

Inhalation Anesthetics

Inhalation, or *volatile,* anesthetics are gases or liquids that can be administered by inhalation when mixed with oxygen. These can effect a concentration in the blood and brain to depress the CNS and cause anesthesia. Inhalation anesthetics have the following characteristics:

- They are complete anesthetics and thus can abolish superficial and deep reflexes.
- They provide for controllable anesthesia, because depth of anesthesia is easily varied by changing the inhaled concentration.
- Allergic reactions to these agents are uncommon.
- Rapid recovery can occur as soon as administration ceases because the anesthetic is excreted in expired air.

Ether and chloroform (as volatile liquids) and cyclopropane and nitrous oxide (as gases) were commonly used over the years, but only nitrous oxide is clinically still in use today. Chloroform is hepatotoxic, and ether and cyclopropane are highly flammable; thus these agents have been replaced by safer anesthetics. In 1956 halothane (Fluothane), a nonflammable agent, largely replaced the older volatile liquids. However, halothane has been associated with hepatic dysfunction and failure. Since then, newer less toxic volatile liquids have been developed: desflurane (Suprane), enflurane (Ethrane), isoflurane (Forane), methoxyflurane (Penthrane), and sevoflurane (Ultane).

▪ Nursing Management

Inhalation Anesthetic Agents

A physician or nurse who has specialized training in anesthetic management conducts the actual administration of general anesthesia, which is beyond the scope of this text. The general nursing measures discussed in this section focus on client care after surgery and should be followed in addition to the activities discussed under Nursing Management: General Anesthetics, p. 305.

To allay the client's fears, explain preoperatively that he or she will receive oxygen during the recovery period and be closely monitored until the anesthetic effects have completely worn off.

Monitor the client's temperature, blood pressure, pulse, and respiratory rate closely during the immediate postoperative period. The recovery phase for volatile anesthetic agents is generally short and there is no analgesia residue; thus the postoperative analgesia phase is short. Thoroughly assess the client for postoperative pain. Shivering and tremors may be observed postoperatively.

Use caution when changing the client's position during the recovery phase. In addition to vasodilation, compensatory vasoconstriction mechanisms are depressed, which may result in a significant drop in blood pressure with position changes (postural hypotension). Oxygen is administered during the immediate recovery period to compensate for the respiratory depression caused by anesthetic agents and for the increased oxygen needs of the body from shivering. Pain relief medications provide relief from immediate postoperative pain. Because of the combined effects of the CNS depressants (e.g., residual anesthetic agents and analgesics), *re-*

member that any sedative or analgesic probably needs to be decreased to one half to one fourth of the usual dose for the first dose after surgery. Measures to prevent heat loss from vasodilation include using warm blankets, covering the head with a blanket, and using a hyperthermic automatic blanket.

The client should demonstrate normal breath sounds and an effective cough and gag reflex. Vital signs should be within normal limits, and the client should be able to respond to verbal commands.

Gases

nitrous oxide [nye′ trus ok′ syde]

Nitrous oxide, an anesthetic gas, is the most commonly used agent for analgesia during dental surgery, minor surgery, and obstetric procedures. It is often combined with other anesthetics to enhance its effects and therefore is also used extensively in major surgery. It is excreted 100% unchanged through the lungs. Its few side effects primarily consist of postoperative nausea, vomiting, or delirium, and it has no known significant drug interactions. For general anesthesia, the recommended dose is 70% with 30% oxygen inhalation for induction, and 30% to 70% with oxygen for maintenance.

At the termination of anesthesia, the rapid movement of large amounts of nitrous oxide from the circulation into the lungs may dilute the oxygen in the lungs. This dilution may result in a phenomenon known as diffusion hypoxia. To prevent this the anesthetist usually administers 100% oxygen to clear the nitrous oxide from the lungs. During recovery the client should be administered humidified oxygen by mask and encouraged to breathe deeply to promote ventilation.

Volatile Liquid Anesthetics

halothane [ha′ loe thayn] (Fluothane, Somnothane ♣)

Halothane is used primarily as a general anesthetic. The pharmacokinetics of halothane and a list of its side effects/adverse reactions are detailed in Table 15-1. Postoperative nausea and vomiting may occur in many clients and may be more common if nitrous oxide is used to supplement other anesthetics. A rare complication of halothane is liver damage, or *halothane hepatitis.* Although the mechanism is not known, some experts believe the liver damage to be caused by a hypersensitivity-type reaction to a metabolite of halothane. The diagnosis is made on the clinical findings of unexplained fever, eosinophilia, rashes, and abnormal liver function tests within 2 weeks of exposure, especially after a repeat exposure. The syndrome is more common in older or obese clients and is not seen in children.

Significant Drug Interactions. Halothane is the only volatile anesthetic agent that sensitizes the myocardium. It sensitizes the myocardium to the effects of catecholamines (epinephrine, norepinephrine, or dopamine) or sympathomimetic agents (e.g., ephedrine, metaraminol). These agents may produce serious cardiac dysrhythmias in the presence of halothane. Levodopa, which pharmacologically increases the quantity of dopamine in the CNS, should be discontinued at least 6 to 8 hours before halothane is administered.

Skeletal muscle weakness, respiratory depression, or apnea (absence of respiration) may result when systemic aminoglycosides, lincomycins, polymyxins, and capreomycin (Capastat) are administered concurrently with any of the volatile anesthetics. Clients usually require mechanical ventilation. If these medications are used, the dose of the nondepolarizing neuromuscular blocking drugs should be decreased to one third or one half of the usually prescribed dose.

Dosage and Administration. See Table 15-1 for the dosage and administration of halothane.

desflurane [des floo′ rayn] (Suprane)

Released in late 1992, desflurane is an alternative to halothane and isoflurane. It produces a more rapid induction of and emergence from anesthesia than the agents in the following sections. The use of desflurane has been associated with a moderately high incidence of airway irritation, coughing, and laryngospasm. For this reason it is not indicated for anesthesia induction in children, although it is approved for anesthesia maintenance in infants and young children.

enflurane [en floo′ rayn] (Ethrane)

Enflurane is indicated for the induction and maintenance of general anesthesia. It is only slightly metabolized in the body. Its clinical effects are similar to those of halothane, but it is less potent. Enflurane may cause seizures when given at high concentrations; therefore it is not recommended for use with clients who are seizure prone, such as those with epilepsy or head injuries.

isoflurane [eye soe floo′ rayn] (Forane)

Isoflurane is indicated for the induction and maintenance of general anesthesia. It undergoes an extremely low degree of metabolism. Until the release of desflurane, isoflurane was promoted as having a more rapid action than the other inhalation agents and causing less cardiovascular depression. Nephrotoxicity is minimal with the use of isoflurane.

methoxyflurane [me thox i floo′ rayn] (Penthrane)

Methoxyflurane is used for anesthesia and analgesic effects and is a potent anesthetic agent used for obstetric analgesia. It is given in concentrations of 0.3% to 0.8%. Methoxyflurane is highly metabolized; a by-product of its metabolism is free fluoride, which is toxic to the kidney (nephrotoxic). Because of the potential for nephrotoxicity with methoxyflurane, its use is limited to minor surgical procedures and obstetrics.

TABLE 15-1 Volatile Liquid Anesthetic Agents

Agent	Pharmacokinetics			MAC (%)*	Toxicity	Side Effects/Adverse Reactions
	Absorption	Metabolism	Excretion			
halothane (Fluothane, Somnothane 🍁)	By lungs	Up to 20% by liver	60%-80% unchanged by the lungs; remainder excreted or metabolized through kidneys	0.75	May cause "halothane hepatitis" (see p. 309)	Hypotension, cardiovascular depression, lowered body temperature, respiratory depression, malignant hyperthermia Emergence delirium—shivering and trembling, confusion, hallucinations, nervousness, increased excitability
desflurane (Suprane)	By lungs	<0.2% by liver	Primarily lungs	7.3	Airway irritation, severe laryngospasm, coughing	See halothane
enflurane (Ethrane)	By lungs	Approximately 2.5% by liver	80% unchanged by lungs; remainder excreted as metabolites through kidneys	1.68		See halothane
isoflurane (Forane)	By lungs	Less than 1% by liver	Almost all through lungs: less than 1% as metabolites through kidneys	1.15		See halothane
methoxyflurane (Penthrane)	By lungs	Approximately 50% by liver	35% unchanged by lungs; remainder excreted as metabolites through kidneys	0.16	Dose-related nephrotoxicity (renal tube damage) from fluoride metabolite	See halothane
sevoflurane (Ultane)	By lungs	—	Primarily lungs	2.1	Cardiac depressant (bradycardia)	See halothane

*MAC, Minimum alveolar concentration (percent in oxygen) that prevents movement in 50% of patients exposed to painful stimuli. May need higher concentrations in some patients; in general, it is highest in very young children and lowest with increasing age, pregnancy, hypotension, or concurrent CNS depressant use.

BOX 15-2

Advantages and Disadvantages of Intravenous Anesthetics

Advantages

Rapidity with which unconsciousness is induced
Amnesic effects
Prompt recovery with minimal doses
Simplicity of administration
No irritation of mucous membranes
Use not accompanied by the hazard of fire or explosion

Disadvantages

Swelling, pain, ulceration, tissue sloughing, and necrosis if drug infiltrates into tissue
Thrombosis and gangrene if arterial injection occurs
Hypotension, laryngospasm, and respiratory failure from overdose or prolonged administration
Minimal muscle relaxation and analgesic effects

sevoflurane [sev oh floo′ rayn] (Ultane)

Sevoflurane is an inhalation general anesthetic indicated for induction and maintenance during surgery. The induction dose is individualized, but the usual adult inhalation dose is between 0.5% to 3% alone or combined with nitrous oxide. Sevoflurane was released in 1995 and has a faster uptake, distribution, and rate of elimination than isoflurane and halothane. When compared with desflurane, it has a slower uptake and distribution but a similar rate of elimination (*Drug Facts and Comparisons*, 2000).

Intravenous Anesthetics

IV anesthetic agents are used for the induction or maintenance of general anesthesia, for the induction of amnesia, and as an adjunct to inhalation-type anesthetics. They are seldom used alone for anesthesia except for short procedures such as electroconvulsive therapy, cast application or removal, and hypnosis. The major groups of IV anesthetic agents include ultrashort-acting barbiturates, nonbarbiturates, dissociative anesthetics, and neuroleptanesthetics. IV anesthetics reduce the amount of inhalation anesthetic required. They are therefore valuable in allaying emotional distress, because many clients dread having a tight mask placed over their face while they are fully conscious. Box 15-2 lists the advantages and disadvantages of IV anesthetics.

The ultrashort-acting barbiturates are the most commonly used IV anesthetics. These drugs are rapidly taken up by brain tissue because of their high solubility. For example, equilibrium between the brain and blood occurs within 1 minute after the injection of thiopental. Shortness of action results from the drug being quickly redistributed into the fat depots of the body. The amount of body fat affects drug action; the greater the amount of body fat, the briefer the effect of a single IV dose. However, with prolonged administration or large doses, prolonged drug action results in delayed recovery. This is caused by the saturation of fat depots and the slow rate of drug release (10% to 15% per hour).

■ Nursing Management

Intravenous Anesthetic Agents

In this text the nurse's role in IV general anesthetics does not include administration of the anesthetic. The focus of the role includes client care during the recovery period that follows the anesthesia.

■ **Assessment.** *Remember that the first dose of any postoperative sedative or analgesic probably needs to be one third to one fourth of the usual dose;* after that the dosage of the analgesic is titrated according to the client's needs. The nurse must assess the client's response to the analgesic and relay the information to ensure adequate medication dosage.

■ **Nursing Diagnosis.** Nursing diagnoses/collaborative problems related to the administration of IV anesthesia may include, but are not limited to, the following: ineffective airway clearance, ineffective breathing patterns, impaired gas exchange, risk for aspiration, and the potential complications of thrombophlebitis at the infusion site and decreased cardiac output.

■ **Implementation**

■ ***Monitoring.*** The client's cardiovascular and respiratory status, as well as the client's behavioral response to IV anesthetic agents, should be assessed at frequent intervals. Monitor the IV site for color, temperature, swelling, pain, and patency.

■ ***Intervention.*** Resuscitative equipment should be within the immediate environment when IV anesthetic agents are administered.

■ ***Education.*** In general, there is some impairment of psychomotor skills for 24 hours after the administration of these drugs. Instruct the client not to engage in any activities that require alertness and coordination, such as driving. Caution the client to avoid alcohol and CNS depressants for the first 24 hours after taking these drugs, except as prescribed.

■ **Evaluation.** The client will demonstrate normal breath sounds and an effective cough. Vital signs will be within normal limits, and there will be no evidence of a thromboembolic event.

Ultrashort-Acting Barbiturates

Ultrashort-acting barbiturates include thiopental sodium (Pentothal) and methohexital sodium (Brevital Sodium). The ultrashort-acting barbiturates are CNS depressants that produce hypnosis and anesthesia without analgesia. They are often combined with other drugs for muscle relaxation and analgesia in balanced anesthesia. Their exact mechanism of action for anesthesia, anticonvulsant effects, or the reduction of intracranial pressure (an indication for thiopental) is unknown, but a variety of theories have been proposed. General anesthesia with ultrashort-acting barbiturates is believed to result from suppression of the reticular activating system.

The onset of action for these barbiturates is generally rapid (20 to 60 seconds), and they have an extremely short duration. Barbiturates are distributed rapidly throughout the body and across the blood-brain barrier. They are then redistributed from the brain to other body organs, muscles, and fatty tissues. These drugs are metabolized in the liver and excreted by the kidneys.

The most common side effects during the recovery period are shivering and trembling. Nausea, vomiting, prolonged somnolence, and headache are less commonly reported. Serious adverse reactions include emergence delirium (increased excitability, confusion, and hallucinations), cardiac dysrhythmias (tachycardia, bradycardia, or myocardial depression), allergic response (bronchospasm, rash, hives, hypotension, and edema of eyelids, lips, or face), respiratory depression, and thrombophlebitis.

Careful assessment and close monitoring are required when IV barbiturates are used in combination with other CNS depressants, which may result in enhanced depression effects, as well as with diuretics, antihypertensive agents, and calcium-blocking drugs, because hypotension may occur.

Doses vary for the induction of general anesthesia and the resultant duration of action. Methohexital requires 1 to 2 mg/kg for induction and has a duration of action of 5 to 7 minutes. Thiopental is individually dosed according to the client's response.

■ Nursing Management

Ultrashort-Acting Barbiturates

IV barbiturates must be administered by personnel trained in their use and in the management of possible complications. Continuous monitoring is essential during the administration of ultrashort-acting barbiturates. Barbiturates cause depression of respiratory and cardiovascular functions, and therefore resuscitation equipment, a laryngoscope, an endotracheal tube, suction, and oxygen must be on hand.

In addition to the following discussion, see Nursing Management: Intravenous Anesthetic Agents, p. 311. The injection site should be monitored closely. Ultrashort-acting barbiturates are very alkaline and are therefore irritating to the tissues. Take care to avoid extravasation of the drug into the tissues during IV injection; pain, swelling, ulceration, and necrosis may occur. Intraarterial injection may result in tissue necrosis and gangrene.

IV barbiturates are incompatible with a wide range of solutions, including bacteriostatic diluents and lactated Ringer's solution. Consult the drug insert or a specialized reference before mixing substances. They should not be administered if they are cloudy or if there is a precipitate. Thiopental solutions should be freshly prepared and used within 24 hours.

Nonbarbiturates

Nonbarbiturate IV anesthetic agents include the benzodiazepines midazolam, diazepam, and lorazepam; the short-acting hypnotics etomidate and propofol; the opioids fentanyl, sufentanil, and alfentanil; and ketamine, a dissociative anesthetic. Several drugs may be combined to produce **neuroleptanesthesia**—a general anesthesia produced by the administration of a neuroleptic agent, a narcotic analgesic, and nitrous oxide in oxygen.

midazolam [mid′ ay zoe lam] (Versed)
diazepam [dye az′ e pam] (Valium)
lorazepam [lor az′ e pam] (Ativan)

Benzodiazepines are given intravenously as a premedication or for the induction of anesthesia. In general, these agents have a slower onset of CNS effects than the barbiturates and a more prolonged postanesthetic recovery period, and they often produce an amnesic effect. Diazepam and lorazepam are not water soluble, and thus their nonaqueous solutions may cause local irritation. Midazolam is water soluble and is less irritating locally. Midazolam becomes more lipid soluble in the body and can readily cross the blood-brain barrier.

Midazolam also causes a decrease in cerebrospinal fluid (CSF) pressure and thus may be selected for anesthesia induction in clients with intracranial lesions. Midazolam administered intravenously has a rapid onset of action (1 to 3 minutes) and a short elimination half-life (approximately 2.5 hours). It is metabolized in the liver and excreted by the kidneys.

The concurrent use of benzodiazepines with alcohol or CNS depressants may result in hypotension, respiratory depression, and possible respiratory and cardiac arrest. A reduction in drug dosage and close monitoring are indicated if such drugs are used concurrently. Debilitated clients and those 55 years and older require a smaller than normal midazolam dose administered at a slower rate (Wangaman & Foster, 1991). A current reference should be checked for dosing recommendations. If CNS depressants are used concurrently, the midazolam dose should be reduced by at least 50% and the diazepam dose reduced by 33%.

etomidate [eh toe′ mi date] (Amidate)

Etomidate is a short-acting, nonbarbiturate hypnotic used for the induction of general anesthesia. It is reported to decrease the activity of the reticular formation in the brainstem (in animals). Because it has minimal cardiac and respiratory effects, it may be advantageous for the client with impaired cardiac function, respiratory function, or both. Etomidate is used intravenously in induction of general anesthesia and also supplements subpotent anesthetic agents (nitrous oxide in oxygen) for short procedures.

Etomidate induces hypnosis within 1 minute and has a duration of action between 3 and 5 minutes. To reduce recovery time in adults, a 0.1 mg IV dose of fentanyl (Sublimaze) is administered 1 or 2 minutes before anesthesia induction, thus reducing the amount of etomidate needed. Etomidate is metabolized in the liver and excreted by the kidneys.

The side effects most commonly reported during the recovery period are nausea and vomiting; hypotension, hypertension, dysrhythmias, and breathing difficulties are reported less often. Involuntary muscle movements have been reported, especially when fentanyl is not given before induction with etomidate. Pain at the injection site is also reported. SPECIAL WARNING: Etomidate can suppress the production of steroid hormones in the adrenal gland (e.g., cortisol), which can result in temporary gland failure. Electrolyte imbalance, hypotension, and shock may result. Seriously ill or postoperative clients may need adrenal cortex supplementation.

Significant Drug Interactions. The client should be monitored for enhanced CNS depression when etomidate is given with other CNS depressants.

Dosage and Administration. See Table 15-2 for the dosage and administration of etomidate.

For the nursing management of clients receiving etomidate, see Nursing Management: Intravenous Anesthetic Agents, p. 311.

TABLE 15-2 Nonbarbiturates: Dosage and Administration

	Dosage	
Agent	**Adults**	**Children**
alfentanil (Alfenta)		
Adjunct to general anesthesia	8-20 μg (0.008-0.02 mg)/kg body weight IV initially; additional doses of 3-5 μg/kg as needed for short duration (up to 30 minutes) For induction anesthesia, may use initial dose of 130-245 μg (0.130-0.245 mg)/kg body weight	Adjunct to anesthesia: IV 30-50 μg (0.03-0.05 mg)/kg body weight initially, then 0.5-1.5 μg/kg body weight by continuous infusion
etomidate (Amidate)		
Anesthesia induction	0.2-0.6 mg/kg body weight administered over 30-60 seconds	Over 10 years: 0.2-0.6 mg/kg body weight
fentanyl (Sublimaze)		
Adjunct to general anesthesia		
Minor surgery	2 μg (0.002 mg)/kg body weight IV	Less than 2 years: no established dose
Major surgery	2-20 μg (0.002-0.02 mg)/kg body weight IV High doses used for open heart surgery, complicated neurosurgery, or orthopedic procedures (i.e., 20-50 μg [0.02-0.05 mg]/kg body weight IV)	
Primary agent in major surgery	50-100 μg (0.05-0.1 mg)/kg body weight IV given with oxygen, nitrous oxide, or both and neuromuscular blocking agent	2-12 years: 2-3 μg (0.002-0.003 mg)/kg body weight IV
Presurgical or postoperative use	0.7-1.4 μg (0.0007-0.0014 mg)/kg body weight IM	
sufentanil (Sufenta)		
Adjunct to general anesthesia	Low doses: 0.5-1 μg (0.0005-0.001 mg)/kg body weight IV initially; additional doses of 10-25 μg may be given as needed Moderate doses: 2-8 μg/kg body weight IV initially; additional doses of 10-50 μg may be given as needed	
Primary agent in major surgery	8-30 μg/kg body weight IV initially with oxygen; additional doses of 25-50 μg may be given as needed	Cardiovascular surgery: initially, 10-25 μg/kg body weight IV given with 100% oxygen. Maintenance, up to 25-50 μg IV

Information from *United States Pharmacopeia Dispensing Information (USP DI): Drug information for the health care provider* (19th ed.) (1999). Rockville, MD: United States Pharmacopeial Convention.

propofol [proe poe′ fol] (Diprivan)

Propofol is a rapidly acting, nonbarbiturate hypnotic used for the induction and maintenance of general anesthesia. It has a rapid onset of action (within 40 seconds), and the duration of effect is only 3 to 5 minutes. Its redistribution from the brain to other body tissues explains the short effect. The elimination half-life is 3 to 12 hours.

Propofol is a respiratory depressant and may produce apnea and cardiac depression depending on the dose, rate of administration, and concurrent drugs administered. Bradycardia and hypotension may also occur frequently. Nausea, vomiting, and involuntary muscle movement are commonly reported.

The nursing management of the client receiving propofol is the same as for other IV anesthetics (see Nursing Management: Intravenous Anesthetic Agents, p. 311).

fentanyl [fen′ ta nil] (Sublimaze)
sufentanil [soo fen′ ta nil] (Sufenta)
alfentanil [al fen′ ta nil] (Alfenta)

Adjunct medications for anesthesia include fentanyl (Sublimaze), sufentanil (Sufenta), and alfentanil (Alfenta). These agents have been theorized to produce their effects at the mu receptor. All three are opioid analgesics that are used for balanced anesthesia (see p. 303) and in combination with oxygen, nitrous oxide, or both for the induction and maintenance of anesthesia. When combined with an agent such as droperidol (Inapsine), which produces **neuroleptanalgesia**—an altered state of consciousness characterized by quiescence, reduced motor activity and anxiety, and indifference to surroundings—fentanyl, sufentanil, and alfentanil may be used for neuroleptanesthesia, which alters the consciousness even more (see p. 312).

The most commonly reported side effects/adverse reactions are drowsiness, hypotension, bradycardia, and respiratory depression (allergic reaction). Less common reactions are chills, nausea, vomiting, increased weakness, dizziness, constipation, depression, pruritus, muscle spasms, and increased excitability (paradoxical reaction). Convulsions are reported with fentanyl, and dysrhythmias are reported with sufentanil.

The concurrent use of fentanyl, sufentanil, and alfentanil with CNS depressants may result in an enhanced CNS depressant effect, hypotension, and respiratory depression. Dosage adjustments and careful monitoring are required. If an opioid is necessary for elective surgery, naltrexone should be stopped for several days before the scheduled operation because it blocks the effects of opioid analgesics.

Information on the dosage and administration of these drugs appears in Table 15-2. Fentanyl, sufentanil, and alfentanil all cross the blood-brain barrier and are rapidly distributed to various tissues. They are highly protein bound and have a triphasic half-life, that is, a distributive phase, a redistributive phase, and an elimination phase. All three drugs are metabolized in the liver; sufentanil may also have some intestinal metabolism. They are excreted by the kidneys.

Fentanyl produces an analgesic effect in 7 to 15 minutes when given intramuscularly or in 1 to 2 minutes when given intravenously. The rate of the loss of consciousness depends on the dosage and the rate of administration (usually 4 to 5 minutes at a rate of 0.4 mg/min IV). Its peak effect occurs at 3 to 5 minutes when given intravenously and at 20 to 30 minutes when given intramuscularly. The duration of effect is 0.5 to 1 hour IV and 1 to 2 hours IM.

Sufentanil has an immediate analgesic effect, with the time until loss of consciousness depending on the dosage and rate of administration (usually 1 to 1.6 minutes at a rate of 0.3 mg/min). The duration of action is less than 1 hour.

Alfentanil has an immediate analgesic effect and produces a peak effect in 1 to 2 minutes. The duration of action is dose dependent but is usually less than 10 to 15 minutes.

▪ Nursing Management

Fentanyl, Sufentanil, Alfentanil

Carefully monitor all clients receiving fentanyl during surgery, because respiratory depression is a side effect and all precautions need to be taken; an oral airway and oxygen should be readily available. CNS depressants can potentiate the respiratory and sedative effects of sufentanil and fentanyl, and therefore *the initial dose of any postoperative sedative or analgesic should be reduced to one third to one fourth of the usual recommended dose.* The client should be made to lie down if he or she experiences nausea, vomiting, dizziness, or syncope. (See also Nursing Management: Opioid Therapy, Chapter 14.)

Dissociative Anesthetics

ketamine hydrochloride [keet′ a meen] (Ketalar)

Ketamine is a rapid-acting nonbarbiturate IV anesthetic. It is a derivative of phencyclidine, a psychotomimetic drug of abuse. As with the barbiturates, ketamine acts on the midbrain within the reticular formation. It produces analgesia and amnesia but not muscular relaxation. The mechanism of action is not fully known. Ketamine blocks the afferent transmission of impulses associated with the affective-emotional aspect of pain perception, and it may also suppress spinal cord activity. Ketamine produces a **dissociative anesthesia,** an anesthesia characterized by analgesia and amnesia without the loss of respiratory function or pharyngeal and laryngeal reflexes. It produces a cataleptic state in which the client appears to be awake but is detached from his or her environment and is unresponsive to pain. The client's eyelids usually do not close; nystagmus (rapid, involuntary oscillation of the eyeballs) is common, and slight involuntary and purposeless movements may occur.

Ketamine increases the secretions of the salivary and bronchial glands; therefore the administration of an anticholinergic agent (e.g., atropine) may be necessary. Ketamine may increase blood pressure, muscle tone, and heart rate. Respirations are usually not depressed. After recovery, the client has no recall of events that occurred while under the influence of ketamine.

Ketamine is best suited for short diagnostic or surgical procedures that do not require skeletal muscle relaxation. It is also used to induce anesthesia before the administration of general anesthetics and as an adjunct to low-potency anesthetics, such as nitrous oxide.

When ketamine is given intravenously, the onset of anesthesia occurs within 30 seconds. When administered intramuscularly, the onset of action occurs within 3 to 4 minutes. The duration of action is 5 to 10 minutes for an IV dose of 2 mg/kg body weight or 12 to 25 minutes for an IM dose of 10 mg/kg body weight. Ketamine is metabolized in the liver. Termination of anesthetic action occurs with redistribution from the CNS and liver biotransformation. Ninety percent is excreted in the kidneys.

The most commonly reported side effects/adverse reactions of ketamine include hypertension and increased pulse rate and an emergence reaction, such as a distortion in body image, delirium, explicit dreams, illusions, and dissociative-type experiences. Flashbacks of vivid dreams with or without illusions may occur weeks later in some clients. Less commonly reported side effects include hypotension, bradycardia, respiratory depression, and vomiting. No significant drug interactions have been reported.

The recommended adult dose for anesthesia induction is 1 to 2 mg/kg body weight IV or 5 to 10 mg/kg body weight IM. The recommended rate for maintenance is 10 to 50 μg/kg body weight by infusion at a rate of 1 to 2 μg/min. As with any anesthetic, the dosage needs to be carefully assessed and individualized.

■ Nursing Management

Ketamine Hydrochloride

■ **Assessment.** Obtain a baseline assessment of the client's vital signs and mental status before ketamine administration. Ketamine is contraindicated in clients with hypertension, increased intracranial pressure, intracranial lesions, intracranial surgery, or a history of psychiatric problems or alcoholism.

■ **Nursing Diagnosis.** The following nursing diagnoses may be identified with a client receiving ketamine: risk for injury related to the drug's dissociative reaction, ineffective breathing patterns related to the respiratory depressive effects of the drug, risk for aspiration, and disturbed sensory perception (visual and auditory).

■ **Implementation**

■ ***Monitoring.*** Ketamine produces a dissociative state; the client may not appear to be asleep but is dissociated from the environment. Observe clients anesthetized with ketamine for blood pressure elevation, tachycardia, bradycardia, dreaming, delirium, hallucinations, euphoria, and increased muscle tone. Monitor cardiac status and observe for respiratory depression.

■ ***Intervention.*** Protect clients from visual, tactile, and auditory stimuli during emergence from ketamine to decrease the possibility of psychic effects. Up to 50% of unpremedicated clients report dreams and hallucinations as the medication wears off, and these can occur up to 24 hours after the administration of ketamine. Disturbing responses may be alleviated with diazepam. Keep environmental stimulation to a minimum during recovery to reduce the risk of an emergent reaction. Do not arouse these clients until they awaken on their own.

■ ***Education.*** Because of psychomotor impairment, caution the client against driving, other hazardous activities, and alcohol ingestion for at least 24 hours after recovery from ketamine.

■ **Evaluation.** The expected outcome of ketamine administration is that the client will experience effective anesthesia, and his or her safety will be maintained. The airway will be patent, and adequate ventilatory status will be maintained. Sensory-perceptual alterations will be minimized or absent.

Neuroleptanesthesia

Neuroleptanesthesia is a general anesthesia produced by combining a neuroleptic (antipsychotic) such as droperidol (Inapsine), diazepam (Valium), or ketamine (Ketalar) with a narcotic analgesic, most commonly fentanyl (Sublimaze) but sometimes meperidine (Demerol), morphine, or pentazocine (Talwin). It is used primarily for procedures that require the client's cooperation. An example of this classification is droperidol and fentanyl (Innovar injection). Innovar consists of 1 part fentanyl to 50 parts droperidol.

droperidol [droe per′ i dole] (Inapsine)

Droperidol is a neuroleptic drug with prolonged action and is used to produce neuroleptic anesthesia. The combination of droperidol and fentanyl produces **neurolepsis,** a state in which a client is neither asleep nor awake but is in a state of profound analgesia and psychomotor sedation. This state permits the client to undergo short procedures that require consciousness and cooperation (e.g., bronchoscopy, cystoscopy) without pain. Droperidol (Inapsine) is also used as a premedication for anesthesia and as an adjunct for the induction and maintenance of anesthesia. Droperidol has lost some of its earlier popularity because clinical investigation has demonstrated that depression of respiratory rate and alveolar ventilation may persist longer than the analgesic effect.

The onset of action for droperidol, when given either intravenously or intramuscularly, is between 3 and 10 minutes, with a peak effect at 30 minutes. The duration of action is 2 to 4 hours. Alteration of consciousness may persist up to 12 hours. Droperidol is metabolized in the liver and excreted by the kidneys.

The most commonly reported side effects/adverse reactions for droperidol are hypotension, hypertension, dystonia, increased hyperexcitability, anxiety, and sweating. Less commonly reported effects include bronchospasm, emergence delirium (hallucinations), chills, shivering, depression, and nightmares. Respiratory depression has been reported when the drug is used in combination with an opioid

TABLE 15-3 Droperidol: Dosage and Administration

Use	Dosage: Adults	Dosage: Children
Premedication for general anesthesia	0.5-2 mg IM given ½-1 hour before surgery	Over 2 years: 75 to 150 μg/kg ½ to 1 hour before surgery
General anesthesia adjunct		
Induction	1.25 mg IV per 20-25 pounds of body weight, or 100 to 140 μg/kg body weight Individualize dose because smaller doses have been found adequate depending on client's response	

Information from *United States Pharmacopeia Dispensing Information (USP DI): Drug information for the health care provider* (19th ed.) (1999). Rockville, MD: United States Pharmacopeial Convention.

analgesic; this can lead to respiratory arrest. Concurrent use should be avoided; if concurrent use is necessary, the dose of the opioid should be reduced to one fourth to one third of the usual dose. Concurrent use of other CNS depressants may result in enhanced CNS depressant effects.

Table 15-3 lists dosage and administration recommendations for droperidol. Droperidol is also available in combination with fentanyl (Innovar).

■ Nursing Management

Droperidol (Inapsine)

■ **Assessment.** Droperidol produces neuroleptic anesthesia. The client is usually free of pain, not necessarily asleep, easily aroused, able to cooperate, and psychologically indifferent to the environment, which is beneficial when the client must participate in the procedure. Obtain a baseline assessment of the client's vital signs and general physical status before drug administration. Droperidol should be used with caution in clients with renal, respiratory, cardiovascular, or hepatic impairment.

■ **Nursing Diagnosis.** The client receiving droperidol may have the following nursing diagnoses/collaborative problems: ineffective breathing patterns related to the respiratory depressive effects of the drug, risk for injury related to sedation, risk for aspiration, disturbed sensory perception (visual and auditory), and the potential complication of decreased cardiac output related to drug-induced hypotension.

■ **Implementation**

■ ***Monitoring.*** Assess the client frequently for any signs of respiratory depression, because increased rigidity of the respiratory muscles may result in insufficient breathing. Because droperidol has hypotensive effects, monitor the client's blood pressure until the effects of the drug have dissipated completely. Orthostatic hypotension is possible. The client may not complain of postoperative pain because droperidol alters the perception of pain. In these clients pain may manifest itself as restlessness, agitation, or any number of other nonspecific complaints.

■ ***Intervention.*** If a client who has received droperidol does experience postoperative pain, the dose of analgesic may be decreased to one third or one fourth of the usual dose. Droperidol potentiates the actions of barbiturates and narcotics, and therefore the analgesic dose is decreased until all of the droperidol is eliminated. Some alteration of consciousness may last for 12 hours after the last dose.

If the drug is given preoperatively, the client should be assisted if ambulating is necessary. Move and position the client slowly during anesthesia recovery to prevent hypotension. If hypotension is caused by hypovolemia, several approaches may need to be taken. Fluids may be ordered to treat hypotension, the client may be repositioned to improve venous return (supine with feet elevated), and a vasopressor may be given. Resuscitative equipment and a narcotic antagonist should be available in the immediate environment.

■ **Evaluation.** The expected outcome of the administration of droperidol is that the client's respiratory status and blood pressure will remain within normal limits, and sedation will be achieved. The client will recover from anesthesia without adverse reactions.

Preanesthetic Agents/Anesthetic Adjunctive Agents

Various medications are used as preanesthetic agents, or as adjuncts to anesthesia, to reduce the undesirable effects produced by apprehension or by the induction and maintenance of anesthesia. Some of the common agents are reviewed in Table 15-4. Narcotic analgesics not only reduce anxiety and provide analgesia but because of their additive effects also allow for a reduction in the dose of anesthetic administered. The administration of muscle relaxants pro-

TABLE 15-4 Preanesthetic Agents

Drug Classification	Agents Most Commonly Used	Desired Effect
Narcotic analgesics	morphine meperidine (Demerol)	Sedation to decrease tension and anxiety, provide analgesia, and decrease amount of anesthetic used
Barbiturates	pentobarbital (Nembutal) secobarbital (Seconal)	Decreased apprehension Sedation Rapid induction
Phenothiazines	promethazine (Phenergan)	Sedation Antihistaminic effects Antiemetic effects Decreased motor activity
Anticholinergics	glycopyrrolate (Robinul) atropine scopolamine	Inhibition of secretions, vomiting, and laryngospasms, plus sedation (with scopolamine)
Skeletal muscle relaxants	succinylcholine (depolarizing) (Anectine, Quelicin, Sucostrin) D-tubocurarine (nondepolarizing)	Promotion of muscular relaxation

BOX 15-3

Rapid-Acting Opioid for Use During General Anesthesia

Remifentanil (Ultiva) is a short-acting analgesic used during the induction and maintenance of general anesthesia and also for the immediate postoperative period. This drug should be administered only under the direct supervision of an anesthetist.

A mu-receptor agonist, remifentanil has a rapid onset of action, is metabolized by nonspecific esterases in blood and tissues, and lasts between 5 to 10 minutes after the drug is discontinued. To control postoperative pain, adequate analgesia should be instituted before remifentanil is discontinued (New Ultiva, 1996). Side effects/adverse reactions include hypoxia, apnea, respiratory depression, and muscle rigidity. See current reference or package insert for additional information.

vides surgeons easier access to and increased visualization of the abdominal cavity during abdominal surgery or in cases in which controlled mechanical ventilation is required. Many nondepolarizing neuromuscular blocking agents are available, including atracurium (Tracrium), cisatracurium (Nimbex), doxacurium (Nuromax), mivacurium (Mivacron), pancuronium (Pavulon), pipecuronium (Arduran), rocuronium (Zemuron), and vecuronium (Norcuron) (*Drug Facts and Comparisons,* 2000). See Box 15-3 for information about remifentanil, a rapid-acting opioid used during general anesthesia.

LOCAL ANESTHESIA

Local anesthesia refers to the direct administration of an anesthetic agent to tissues to induce the absence of sensation in a portion of the body. Unlike with general anesthesia, consciousness is not depressed. Local anesthetic agents may be applied to an area or injected into tissues, where they produce their effect in the immediate area only; hence the term *local anesthesia.* Local anesthetic drugs may also be injected around a nerve or nerve trunk (spinal, epidural) to produce anesthesia in a large region of the body. This is referred to as **regional anesthesia.**

SURFACE OR TOPICAL ANESTHESIA

The use of surface, or topical, anesthetics is restricted to mucous membranes, damaged skin surfaces, wounds, and burns. The anesthetic is applied in the form of a solution, ointment, gel, cream, or powder to paralyze afferent nerve endings and produce a loss of sensation. Topical anesthetics do not penetrate unbroken skin. Topical anesthesia is used to relieve pain and itching and to anesthetize mucous membranes of the eye, nose, throat, or urethra for minor surgical procedures. Cocaine in a 4% to 10% solution continues to be one of the most widely used agents for topical anesthesia.

Local anesthesia may also be achieved by freezing. Low temperatures in living tissues produce diminished sensation. This form of anesthesia is sometimes used for minor surgical procedures. Tissues that are frozen too intensely for too long may be destroyed. Ethyl chloride is a local anesthetic that can be used to produce this effect, but it is not used extensively.

LOCAL ANESTHETICS

Local anesthetics are used to abolish pain sensation in a particular part of the body (Tables 15-5 and 15-6). The basic mechanism of action of these drugs is unknown, but most act by stabilizing or elevating the threshold of excitation of the nerve cell membrane without affecting resting potential (blockage of sodium channels). This action is a result of the reduction of membrane permeability to all ions, thus preventing depolarization and the transmission of nerve impulses.

Table 15-6 presents some commonly used local anesthetics and their properties. Benzyl alcohol, an aromatic alcohol

TABLE 15-5 Local Anesthetics: Administration and Use

Method	Tissue Affected	Preparation Used	Examples of Drugs Used	Therapeutic Use
Topical	Sensory nerve endings in mucous membranes and dermis	Solution Ointment Cream Powder	cocaine benzocaine ethyl aminobenzoate lidocaine tetracaine bupivacaine	Relief of pain or itching Examination of conjunctiva
Infiltration	Sensory nerve endings in subcutaneous tissues or dermis	Injection	etidocaine procaine prilocaine lidocaine chloroprocaine mepivacaine	Minor surgery
Block	Nerve trunk	Injection	etidocaine procaine prilocaine lidocaine chloroprocaine mepivacaine	Dental and limb surgery Sympathetic block
Spinal (subarachnoid block)	Spinal roots	Injection	procaine tetracaine lidocaine	Abdominal surgery Surgery of the lower extremities Muscle relaxation

TABLE 15-6 Properties of Commonly Used Local Anesthetics

	Procaine	Cocaine	Benzocaine
Trade names	Novocain	—	Americaine Hurricaine
Potency	—	2-3 times that of procaine	Very low
Onset of action	2-5 minutes	1 minute	Immediate
Duration	½-1 hour	½-1 hour	15-20 minutes
Dose	0.25%-2%, depending on method of administration 10% for spinal anesthesia Not used topically	1%-4% topically	Variable 5%-20% ointment topically
Toxicity	Least toxic of all local anesthetics	More toxic than procaine when injected subcutaneously	Relatively nontoxic
Precautions	Overdose of rapid injection may cause CNS stimulation	Not recommended for infiltration, nerve block, or spinal anesthesia Repeated use causes psychologic dependence	Suitable for topical use only Sensitization may develop

of low potency, is used topically with procaine to extend procaine's duration of action. The choice of local anesthetic for a particular procedure depends on the duration of drug action desired. Table 15-7 lists short-, intermediate-, and long-acting local anesthetic drugs. Vasoconstrictors such as epinephrine and norepinephrine are used with the local anesthetic to decrease systemic absorption and prolong the duration of action of the anesthetic. They are not used for nerve blocks in areas with end arteries (fingers, toes, ears, nose, and penis) because ischemia may develop, resulting in gangrene.

A number of local anesthetic agents cannot be injected. However, because they are absorbed slowly, they can be used safely on open wounds, ulcers, and mucous membranes. Occasionally they cause dermatitis and allergic sensitization, in which case they are discontinued. The ester-type local anesthetics (cocaine, procaine, tetracaine, and benzocaine) are metabolized to para-aminobenzoic acid (PABA) metabolites, which are mainly responsible for allergic reactions in some clients. The amide anesthetics (lidocaine, mepivacaine, bupivacaine, etidocaine, prilocaine) are not metabolized to PABA derivatives, and therefore allergic reactions induced by these anesthetics are very rare (Katzung, 1997).

Topical anesthetics for skin disorders are used primarily to relieve pruritus, discomfort, pain, and soreness; the indications for mucous membranes are similar. These anesthetics are poorly absorbed through intact skin, but absorption is increased through mucous membranes and skin breaks and sores (e.g., abrasions, trauma, and ulcers); this leads to the possibility of systemic involvement. When they are used in the oral cavity (mouth and pharynx), interference with swallowing may occur and puts the client at risk for aspiration. The client is assessed for a returning gag reflex by gently touching the back of the pharynx with a tongue blade. All foods and fluid are withheld until the reflex returns.

Local anesthetics are capable of abolishing all sensation, but pain fibers are affected first, probably because they are thinner, unmyelinated, and more easily penetrated by these drugs. Loss of pain is followed in sequence by a loss of response to cold, warmth, touch, and pressure. Most motor fibers also can be anesthetized when an adequate concentration of the drug is present over a sufficient time.

Parenteral local anesthetics have complete systemic absorption, which is decreased by the addition of a vasoconstrictor such as epinephrine. The half-lives of selected anesthetics are as follows: bupivacaine, 3½ hours; etidocaine, 2¾ hours; lidocaine, 1½ hours; and mepivacaine, 2 hours. Onset of action is a function of the anesthetic technique used, the type of block desired, dosage, and the pK_a of each anesthetic (negative logarithm of ionization constant of an acid, or the pH at which equal concentrations of the acid and conjugate base forms of a substance are present). The time it takes for a drug to reach a peak concentration depends on the type of block but ranges from 10 to 30 minutes.

Reactions to Local Anesthetics

Local anesthetics produce vasodilation by acting directly on blood vessels and by anesthetizing sympathetic vasoconstrictor fibers. This action can cause rapid absorption of the drug; when the rate of absorption exceeds the rate of elimination, toxic effects can occur. Epinephrine or other vasoconstrictor drugs are used to prolong local anesthetic effects and to decrease the rate of absorption and incidence of toxic effects by allowing more time for metabolic degradation. The dosages of vasoconstrictors must be carefully determined to prevent ischemic necrosis at the injection site. Be

Lidocaine	**Tetracaine**	**Mepivacaine**
Xylocaine	Pontocaine	Carbocaine
2 times that of procaine	10 times that of procaine	2 times that of procaine
2-5 minutes	3-10 minutes	Less rapid than procaine
1-3 hours	1->3 hours	1-3 hours
0.5%-4% for injection 2% and 5% topically	1% topically 0.15%-0.25% for injection	1%-2% solution
See procaine	More toxic than procaine, but toxic effects rare because of low dose used	2 times that of procaine; less than lidocaine
Convulsions and hypotension when administered rapidly or in large doses	Drug interaction with cholinesterase inhibitors and sulfonamides	Combined with vasoconstrictor to delay drug absorption and prolong duration Avoid in pregnancy; may cause constriction of uterine artery

TABLE 15-7 Short-, Intermediate-, and Long-Acting Local Anesthetic Drugs: Pharmacokinetic Overview

Name	Metabolism	Use	Dosage and Administration
Short-Acting (1/2-1 Hour)			
procaine (Novocain)	Ester compound; same as chloroprocaine	Infiltration, nerve block, spinal anesthesia, epidural block	Usual adult dose for infiltration: 350-600 mg as 0.25%-0.5% solution Peripheral nerve block: 500 mg as 0.5%, 1%, or 2% solution Spinal and epidural dose: vary with individual client, procedure, and degree of anesthesia desired Pediatric dose: not available
chloroprocaine (Nesacaine, Nesacaine-MPF)	Ester compound; metabolized by cholinesterases in plasma and liver to a PABA compound Excretion: kidneys	Nesacaine: infiltration and regional anesthesia Nesacaine-MPF: caudal and epidural anesthesia	Usual adult dose for infiltration nerve blocks: 30-800 mg as 1% or 2% solutions, depending on site and length of surgical procedure Caudal and epidural: 40-500 mg as 2% or 3% solution, without epinephrine Usual pediatric dose for infiltration nerve blocks: up to 20 mg/kg body weight
Intermediate Duration (1-3 Hours)			
lidocaine (Xylocaine, Xylocard ♣)	Amide compound Metabolism: liver to active and toxic metabolites Excretion: kidneys	Infiltration, nerve block, spinal anesthesia, epidural block	Usual adult dose: depends on site and length of surgical procedure Pediatric dose: same as adult Lidocaine is available with and without epinephrine
mepivacaine (Carbocaine)	Amide compound; see above	Infiltration, nerve blocks, caudal and epidural block	Available alone and with levonordefrin (vasoconstrictor) Dose: depends on site and length of surgical procedure Adult maximum dose: Dental: up to 6.6 mg/kg body weight (300 mg maximum per appointment) Other uses: up to 7 mg/kg body weight Pediatric dose: up to 5 or 6 mg/kg body weight
prilocaine (Citanest, Citanest Forte)	Amide compound; see above	Local anesthesia by nerve block or infiltration in dental procedures	Available alone or with epinephrine (vasoconstrictor) Although doses vary with site and length of procedure, adult maximum doses are as follows: Dental: up to 400 mg as a 4% solution in a 2-hour period Other procedures: individualize Pediatric maximum dose: Dental: children up to 10 years, 40 mg (4% solution) maximum Other procedures: individualize
Long Duration (3-10 Hours)			
bupivacaine (Marcaine, Sensorcaine)	Amide type; see above	Infiltration, caudal anesthesia, subarachnoid block, peripheral nerve blocks	Available alone or with dextrose (Marcaine spinal) or with epinephrine Dose: varies with site, additional drugs, and length of procedure
etidocaine (Duranest)	Amide type; see above	Infiltration; peripheral nerve blocks, caudal and epidural nerve blocks	Available alone and with epinephrine Dose: varies with site and length of procedure
tetracaine (Pontocaine)	Ester compound; see above	Saddle block (low spinal), up to costal margin, spinal anesthesia	Available alone and with dextrose Dose: varies with site and length of procedure

cause local anesthetics are potentially toxic drugs, a client's age, weight, physical condition, and liver function must be taken into account in determining drug dose. Most reactions to local anesthetics result from overdose, rapid absorption into the systemic circulation, or individual hypersensitivity or allergic response.

Central Nervous System. At first the CNS may be stimulated and cause anxiety, restlessness, confusion, dizziness, tremors, and even convulsions. Depression may then occur, and unconsciousness and death may ensue.

Cardiovascular System. Myocardial depression, bradycardia, and hypotension can occur because of smooth muscle relaxation and inhibition of neuromuscular conduction. The client suddenly becomes pale, feels faint, and experiences a drop in blood pressure. Cardiac arrest can be the result of a cardiovascular reaction.

Anesthetics containing a vasoconstrictor are used with caution in clients receiving drugs that may change blood pressure, such as monoamine oxidase inhibitors, phenothiazines, and tricyclic antidepressants. Such a combination may produce severe hypotension or hypertension. Cardiac dysrhythmias occur when catecholamine vasoconstrictors (e.g., epinephrine) are used in clients receiving cyclopropane, halothane, or trichloroethylene.

Allergic Reaction. True allergic reactions are said to be uncommon. Sometimes a reaction is thought to be allergic when really it is caused by overdose. Nevertheless, allergic reactions can occur and may be relatively mild (hives, itching, skin rash) or acutely anaphylactic.

Allergic reactions are characteristically manifested by cutaneous lesions, urticaria, or edema and may result from factors such as hypersensitivity, idiosyncrasy, or diminished tolerance. These rare allergic reactions are usually limited to the ester type of anesthetics. The most important risk with local anesthetics is dose-related CNS toxicity, which may progress from sleepiness to convulsions.

Small test doses are often given to gauge the extent of the client's sensitivity to the anesthetic agent. The anesthetic agent chosen, its concentration, the rate of injection, and physical and emotional factors in the client all influence reactions to local anesthetics.

■ Nursing Management

Local Anesthetics

Unlike with general anesthetics, nurses often administer topical local anesthetic agents and therefore have a much broader role in relating to these agents.

■ **Assessment.** Assess the client for previous responses to local anesthetics and for the existence of preexisting diseases or drug allergies.

■ **Nursing Diagnosis.** The following nursing diagnoses/collaborative problems may be identified in the client receiving a local anesthetic agent: pain related to an inadequate block, risk for injury related to the loss of sensation, and decreased cardiac output related to an adverse response to the drug, and the potential complication of an allergic reaction.

■ **Implementation**

■ ***Monitoring.*** During and after the administration of a local anesthetic, monitor the client for signs of pain, allergy, or other adverse reactions. Minimal monitoring parameters for clients receiving a local anesthetic should include blood pressure, heart rate and rhythm, respiratory rate, skin condition, and mental status. It is especially important to monitor hypertension and cardiac status for dysrhythmias when a local anesthetic containing a vasoconstrictor such as epinephrine is administered.

■ ***Intervention.*** Resuscitative equipment must be available in case the client has an anaphylactic reaction. Do not use the local anesthetic solution if it is cloudy, discolored, or contains crystals. Solutions that do not contain preservatives should be discarded after the vial has been opened. Most commercial preparations of local anesthetic agents are acidic solutions. Some surgeons may adjust the pH of the solution by mixing it with sodium bicarbonate to decrease pain with infiltration. This increase in pH is also reported to make the onset more rapid and increase the duration of sensory analgesia (Watson, 1991).

Thoroughly cleanse and dry the area before applying local anesthetic ointments or creams. When the suppository form of the agent is used, chill the agent in the refrigerator 30 minutes, remove the wrapper, and moisten the suppository with water or a lubricant for insertion.

Note that local anesthetics may cause paralysis of the upper respiratory tract when used topically in the nose or throat; this may lead to aspiration. Measure the preparation accurately and apply it with a cotton swab; swishing should be used for application to the mouth and gums and gargling for application to the throat. Do not allow the local anesthetic to be swallowed unless this has been specifically cleared with the prescriber. After inducing local anesthesia of the nasopharyngeal area, test for adequacy of the client's gag reflex by touching the back of the throat with a tongue depressor or swab. To prevent aspiration, food or drink should be withheld until this reflex returns.

The client who has regional anesthesia needs to be protected from trauma to the anesthetized portion of the body because the perception of pain and pressure, the body's normal protective mechanism, has been diminished or obliterated. Pressure from side rails and other objects normally perceived and avoided by the client may cause injury.

After the use of spinal anesthetics, the client should be well hydrated and remain lying down for up to 12 hours to minimize the risk of spinal headache.

■ ***Education.*** For local anesthetics that may be self-administered, instruct the client to use the preparation exactly as prescribed—not to use more, more often, or for a longer period of time. Caution the client not to inhale while using the topical aerosol or spray dosage forms. Instruct the client in the use of the provided applicator for the rectal aerosol foam preparation. Avoid using if bleeding hemorrhoids are present.

If local anesthetic preparations are used topically in the nose or throat, instruct the client not to eat for 1 hour after administration to prevent aspiration. Because of the variability in response, each client must be able to swallow before food is offered. Advise the client not to chew gum while the anesthetic is in effect, because there is a risk of biting the tongue or buccal mucosa.

■ **Evaluation.** The expected outcome of local anesthetics is that the client will experience an effective sensory block without experiencing any adverse reactions to the drug.

ANESTHESIA BY INJECTION

Anesthesia by injection is accomplished with either infiltration or conduction (spinal, caudal, or saddle block).

Infiltration anesthesia is produced by injecting dilute solutions (0.1%) of the agent into the skin and then subcutaneously into the region to be anesthetized. The sensory nerve endings are anesthetized. Epinephrine is often added to the solution to intensify the anesthesia in a limited region and to prevent excessive bleeding and systemic effects. Repeated injections prolong the anesthesia as long as needed. This method of administration is used for minor surgery such as incision and drainage or excision of a cyst (see Table 15-7).

Conduction (block) anesthesia involves a loss of sensation, especially pain, in a region of the body. This type of anesthesia is produced by injecting a local anesthetic into the vicinity of a nerve trunk to inhibit the conduction of impulses to and from the area supplied by that nerve (the region of the surgical site). The injection may be made at some distance from the surgical site. A single nerve may be blocked, or the anesthetic may be injected where several nerve trunks emerge from the spinal cord (paravertebral block). A more concentrated solution is required because of the thickness of nerve trunk fibers. This method of anesthesia is often used for foot and hand surgery.

Spinal anesthesia is a type of extensive nerve block that is sometimes called a subarachnoid block. The anesthetic solution is injected into the subarachnoid space and affects the lower part of the spinal cord and nerve roots.

For low spinal anesthesia, the client is placed in a flat or Fowler's position. A solution with a specific gravity greater than that of the CSF is used, because the solution tends to diffuse downward. For high spinal anesthesia, Trendelenburg's position with the head sharply flexed is used along with an anesthetic solution that is of lower specific gravity than the CSF (which tends to diffuse upward) or the same specific gravity as the CSF (which may diffuse upward or downward, depending on position used). Solutions with the same specific gravity as the CSF act primarily at the site of injection.

The onset of spinal anesthesia usually occurs within 1 to 2 minutes after injection. The duration of anesthesia is 1 to 3 hours depending on the anesthetic used. Spinal anesthesia is used for surgical procedures on the lower abdomen, inguinal area, or lower extremities. It may be the method of choice for clients with severe respiratory problems or with liver, kidney, or metabolic disease. Marked hypotension, decreased cardiac output, and respiratory inadequacy tend to occur during anesthesia and are considered disadvantages of this method of anesthesia.

Headache is the most common postoperative complaint and may be accompanied by hearing or seeing difficulties. Headache may be postural and occur only in the head-up or sitting or standing position. This symptom is the result of the opening in the dura made by the large spinal needle, which may persist for days or weeks, permitting a loss of CSF and decreasing CSF pressure. These symptoms are usually alleviated when CSF pressure returns to normal. Paresthesias such as numbness and tingling may occur after spinal anesthesia; these sensations are usually limited to the lumbar or sacral areas and disappear within a relatively short time. The success and safety of spinal anesthesia depend primarily on the skill and knowledge of the anesthetist.

Caudal anesthesia is produced by injecting an anesthetic solution into the caudal canal, the sacral part of the vertebral canal containing the cauda equina (the bundle of spinal nerves that innervates the pelvic viscera). It is used in obstetrics and for pelvic or genital surgery. The advantage over spinal anesthetics is that caudal anesthetics do not have direct access to the spinal cord and medullary centers. Thus the respiratory muscles and blood pressure are not directly affected, and undesirable effects are less likely to occur.

Saddle block is sometimes used in obstetrics and for surgery involving the perineum, rectum, genitalia, and upper parts of the thighs. The client sits upright while the anesthetic is injected after a lumbar puncture. The client remains upright for a short time, until the anesthetic has taken effect. The name *saddle block* is used because the body parts that become anesthetized are those that contact a saddle when riding.

Injectable Local Anesthetics

The injectable local anesthetics are listed in Table 15-7. In general, the onset of action for an anesthetic is the result of drug concentration and the targeted nerve-tissue area. The potency and duration of anesthetic action increase with lipid solubility of the drug. Further information on metabolism, indications, and pharmacokinetics is provided in Table 15-7.

Side Effects/Adverse Reactions. The adverse reactions of injected local anesthetics generally require medical intervention. Cyanosis caused by methemoglobinemia is one of the most common adverse reactions reported with an epidural block or high spinal injection. It has been reported with all local anesthetics but is most prevalent with prilocaine (Citanest). Symptoms may include weakness, breathing difficulties, increased heart rate, dizziness, or collapse.

Other reactions reported with an epidural block or high spinal injection include diaphoresis, hypotension, bradycardia or irregular heart rate, pale skin color (cardiovascular depression), diplopia, seizures, tinnitus, increased excitability, shivering, involuntary shaking (caused by stimulation of CNS), nausea, and vomiting.

The effects most commonly reported with ester compounds include skin rash and an allergic reaction manifested by edema of the face, lip, mouth, or throat. Anaphylaxis and severe hypotension have been reported but are rare.

With central nerve block anesthesia, the most common adverse reactions are in the form of neuropathies or neurologic effects, including headaches. Other adverse reactions include paresthesia or paralysis of the lower legs, breathing difficulties, severe hypotension, bradycardia, and backache. Some clients report a reduction or loss of sexual functions, bladder control, or bowel movements.

Meningitis-type effects are most often reported with spinal anesthesia. These effects include headaches, nausea, vomiting, and a stiff or sore neck.

Allergic effects manifested by dental anesthesia are numbing or tingling of the lips and mouth and edema of the lips or mouth. Sympathomimetic or adrenergic effects are reported with epinephrine or other vasoconstrictors. These most commonly include hypertension, shaking, increased anxiety or nervousness, tachycardia, headache, and chest pain.

Significant Drug Interactions. Significant drug interactions with injectable local anesthetics are limited. However, this does not preclude a variety of unexpected responses, thus indicating the need for close observation.

Prior or concurrent administration of CNS depressant drugs may result in additive CNS depression effects. Dosages should be adjusted and monitored closely.

When combined with local anesthetics, vasoconstrictor agents such as epinephrine, norepinephrine, or phenylephrine may cause impaired circulation of the area, resulting in sloughing of tissue. Ischemia resulting in gangrene may develop if vasoconstrictor agents are used for end arteries, such as toes or fingers. Extreme caution is advised.

Dosage and Administration. See Table 15-7 for the dosage and administration of the injectable local anesthetics.

SUMMARY

Anesthetic agents are invaluable in limiting pain and suffering. These agents allow surgical procedures and other painful therapies to be performed by either altering consciousness or interfering with the conduction of impulses to the pain centers of the CNS.

There are two major categories of anesthesia: general and regional (or local). General anesthesia may be achieved either intravenously or by inhalation. Regional anesthesia is obtained by injecting an anesthetic drug near a nerve trunk or into a specific site. Local anesthesia may be accomplished with either topical application or infiltration of the surgical area. Because no anesthetic agent produces analgesia, muscle relaxation, unconsciousness, and amnesic effects with perfect safety, a combination of agents is generally used, each for its specific effect; this technique is called balanced anesthesia.

Although nurses do not administer general anesthetics unless they are certified nurse anesthetists, they may be called on to assist the physician to a degree, depending on the clinical setting. It is also necessary for the nurse to have an understanding of the effects of anesthetic agents in order to provide appropriate nursing care in the perioperative period. In the preoperative period, the emphasis of the nurse is on thorough assessment and preparation of the client to alleviate anxiety and to minimize the potential for physiologic injury intraoperatively and in the postoperative period. Immediately after surgery, the need is to help the client to recover from the effects of the anesthetic safely, comfortably, and as quickly as possible. Common postoperative complications for which the nurse should be alert are hypotension, nausea and vomiting, hypoventilation, oliguria, nerve injury, paralytic ileus, thrombosis, shock, atelectasis, hypothermia/hyperthermia, and malignant hyperthermia.

Inhalation therapy can be administered by gases or volatile liquids. Because these agents are primarily exhaled and excreted through the lungs, their anesthetic effect can be rapidly reversed if respiration is maintained satisfactorily.

IV anesthetic agents are used to induce amnesia, to induce and maintain general anesthesia, and as adjuncts to inhalation anesthetics. Because of the risk of respiratory and cardiovascular depression, the client's vital signs need to be closely monitored, and resuscitation equipment must be nearby when these agents are administered.

Neuroleptanesthesia is a type of general anesthesia that results from the combined use of a neuroleptic agent and a narcotic analgesic; it is used for procedures in which the client's cooperation is desired. Although the client can be easily aroused, he or she remains psychologically indifferent to events; however, hypotension and respiratory depression may still occur.

Consciousness is not depressed with local anesthesia, but a portion of the body is rendered insensitive to pain. Because the perception of pain and pressure is a protective mechanism of the body, the observations of the nurse are important to ensure that the client does not aspirate (if topical anesthesia has been used in the nose and throat) or that tissue damage does not occur through trauma to anesthetized parts of the body.

The role of the nurse in the administration of anesthetics is generally not a direct one but one in which assessment and protection of the client take priority.

Critical Thinking Questions

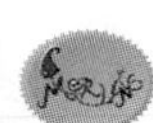

1. Mrs. Clarke, age 42, has been admitted to the hospital for an abdominal hysterectomy. While you are reviewing the preoperative routine with her on the night before surgery, she asks why she should get an injection before she goes to the operating room. How do you respond?
2. Differentiate between the different regional block anesthesias—caudal, saddle, and spinal. Under what cir-

cumstances would each be the regional block of choice?

3. What are the additional nursing observations required if a client receives a local anesthetic with epinephrine rather than one without epinephrine?

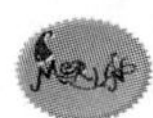

Collaborative Learning Activities

For Collaborative Learning Activities, go to mosby.com/MERLIN/McKenry/.

CASE STUDY

For a Case Study that will help ensure mastery of this chapter content, go to mosby.com/MERLIN/McKenry/.

BIBLIOGRAPHY

American Hospital Formulary Service. (1999). *AHFS drug information '99*. Bethesda, MD: American Society of Hospital Pharmacists.

Anderson, K.N., Anderson, L.E., & Glanz, W.B. (Eds.) (1998). *Mosby's medical, nursing, & allied health dictionary* (5th ed.). St Louis: Mosby.

Beare, P.G. & Myers, J.L. (1998). *Principles and practice of adult health nursing* (3rd ed.). St. Louis: Mosby.

Carpenito, L.J. (2000). *Nursing diagnosis: Application to clinical practice* (8th ed.). Philadelphia: J.B. Lippincott.

Drug Facts and Comparisons. (2000). St. Louis: Facts and Comparisons.

Katzung, B.G. (1997). *Basic and clinical pharmacology* (7th ed.). Norwalk, CT: Appleton & Lange.

Kendall, F. (1993). Documenting local anesthesia patient care. *AORN Journal, 58*(4), 715-719.

Mosby's Gen Rx. (1999). St. Louis: Mosby.

New Ultiva (1996). Letter from Glaxo Wellcome, Glaxo Wellcome Inc., #ULT037RO.

Parnass, S.M. (1993). Ambulatory surgical patient priorities. *Nursing Clinics of North America, 28*(3), 531-545.

Phillips, M. (1994). Into the land of Nod: Drugs used during anesthesia in day surgery. *Canadian Operating Room Nursing Journal, 12*(4), 5-9.

Physician's Desk Reference (1999). (50th ed.). Montvale, NJ: Medical Economics.

Smith, C.J. (1994). Preparing nurses to monitor patients receiving local anesthesia: Using the decision-making process. *AORN Journal, 59*(5), 1036-1041.

United States Pharmacopeia Dispensing Information (USP DI): Drug information for the health care provider (19th ed.) (1999). Rockville, MD: United States Pharmacopeial Convention.

Wangaman, W.R. & Foster, S.D. (1991). New advances in anesthesia. *Nursing Clinics of North America, 26*(2), 451.

Watson, D.S. (1991). Safe nursing practices involving the patient receiving local anesthesia. *AORN Journal, 53*(4), 1055.

16 Antianxiety, Sedative, and Hypnotic Drugs

Chapter Focus

Anxiety and sleep disorders are common health problems across the life span. Anxiety with apprehension, tension, or uneasiness related to anticipated danger is often a normal and beneficial response to a situation. However, excessive anxiety can interfere with daily functioning. As a group, the anxiety disorders affect approximately 15% of the population. During the course of a year, 35% of adults report episodes of insomnia, making it by far the most common sleep disorder. The antianxiety, sedative, and hypnotic drugs discussed in this chapter, along with supportive nursing care, should enable clients to increase their psychologic and physiologic comfort.

Learning Objectives

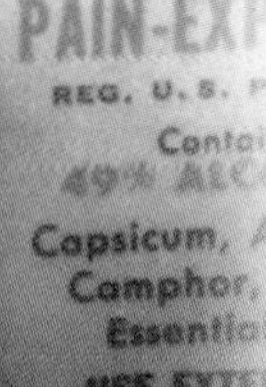

1. Describe the physiology and stages of sleep.
2. Differentiate between antianxiety, sedative, and hypnotic drug effects.
3. Discuss specific nursing interventions for the use of antianxiety, sedative, and hypnotic agents in children and older adults.
4. Identify the characteristics of commonly used benzodiazepines and barbiturates.
5. Formulate an appropriate plan of care for a specific client who requires the administration of an antianxiety, sedative, or hypnotic agent.

Key Terms

amnesic effect, p. 332
antianxiety or anxiolytic agent, p. 326
anxiety, p. 326
hypnotic, p. 326
insomnia, p. 327
non-REM sleep, p. 326
REM sleep, p. 326
sedative, p. 326

Key Drugs [✓]

diazepam, p. 338

The **antianxiety or anxiolytic agents** reduce feelings of excessive anxiety, such as apprehension, fear, nervousness, worry, or panic. **Anxiety** is a state or feeling of apprehension, uneasiness, agitation, uncertainty, and fear resulting from the anticipation of some threat or danger, usually of intrapsychic origin, whose source is generally unknown or unrecognized. It is usually a normal psychologic and physiologic response to a personally threatening situation, such as a threat to health, body, loved ones, job, or lifestyle. In general, anxiety stimulates the person to take a purposeful or deliberate action to counteract or offset the anxiety-producing state. Help is necessary when excessive anxiety interferes with daily functioning and a person is unable to cope with a persistently stressful situation. Although many nonpharmacologic modalities are available, antianxiety agents are commonly prescribed for the treatment of anxiety. (See Limbic System, Chapter 13, for information on the proposed site of action for the benzodiazepines.)

Sedatives are central nervous system (CNS) depressant drugs that were commonly prescribed before the advent of the benzodiazepine family. Their general use today has declined. **Sedatives** reduce nervousness, excitability, or irritability by producing a calming or soothing effect. **Hypnotics** are used to induce sleep. The major difference between a sedative and a hypnotic is the degree of CNS depression induced. A small dosage may be used for a sedative effect, and larger dosages may be used for hypnotic effects. Barbiturates have been used extensively as sedative-hypnotic agents but, because of their low degree of selectivity and safety, they have been largely replaced by the safer benzodiazepines.

PHYSIOLOGY OF SLEEP

Sleep is a recurrent, normal condition of inertia and unresponsiveness during which an individual's overt and covert responses to stimuli are markedly reduced. During sleep a person is no longer in sensory contact with the immediate environment and stimuli that bombard the senses of sight, hearing, touch, smell, and taste during the waking hours. Such factors no longer attract attention or exert a controlling influence over voluntary and involuntary movements or functions. It is not difficult to understand that everyone needs to escape from constant stimuli.

Research has shown that sleep is not one level of unconsciousness but consists of two basic stages that occur cyclically:

1. Non-rapid eye movement (non-REM) sleep
2. Rapid eye movement (REM) sleep

The stages of sleep are based on electrical activity that can be observed in the brain with an electroencephalogram (EEG). The EEG provides graphic illustrations of brain waves, which are an indication of the electrical activity occurring in the brain (Figure 16-1).

During sleep an individual moves through the four stages of **non-REM sleep.** These first four stages are characterized on the EEG by alpha waves, which are slow and of low amplitude; stage 4 is considered the deepest level of non-REM sleep. The individual then moves through the fifth stage of sleep, **REM sleep,** which is characterized by rapid eye movement, dreaming, and delta waves on the EEG (Figure 16-2). Alternating periods of REM and non-REM sleep occur throughout the night (McCance & Huether, 1998). It

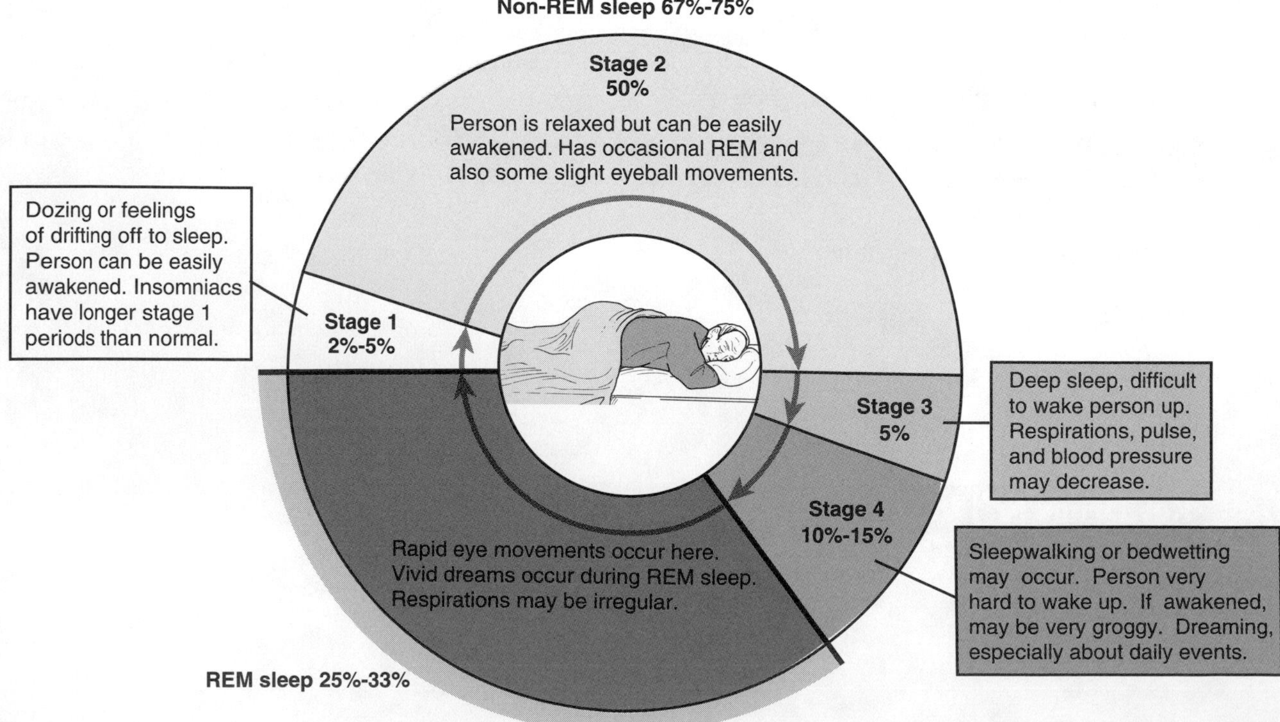

Figure 16-1 Stages of sleep.

should be kept in mind that REM sleep is not synonymous with light sleep. It takes a more powerful stimulus to arouse a person from REM sleep than from synchronous slow-wave sleep.

The dynamic physiologic equilibrium of the body continues to be maintained even during sleep. Depression of physiologic functions occurs during deep, nondreaming sleep, whereas an increase in functions occurs during dreaming. It is known that the following occurs during nondreaming sleep:

- Blood pressure falls by 10 to 30 mm Hg
- Pulse rate is slowed
- Metabolic rate is decreased
- Gastrointestinal tract activity is slowed
- Urine formation is slowed
- Oxygen consumption and carbon dioxide production are lowered
- Body temperature is decreased slightly
- Respirations are slower and shallower
- Body movement is minimal

Dreaming sleep tends to increase most of these parameters. Body movements are more noticeable—turning, jerking, moving the arms and legs, talking, crying, or laughing; eye movements are visible under the closed lids.

Sleep research indicates that there are psychologic and physiologic reasons for the body to maintain equilibrium between the various stages of sleep. Studies have shown that

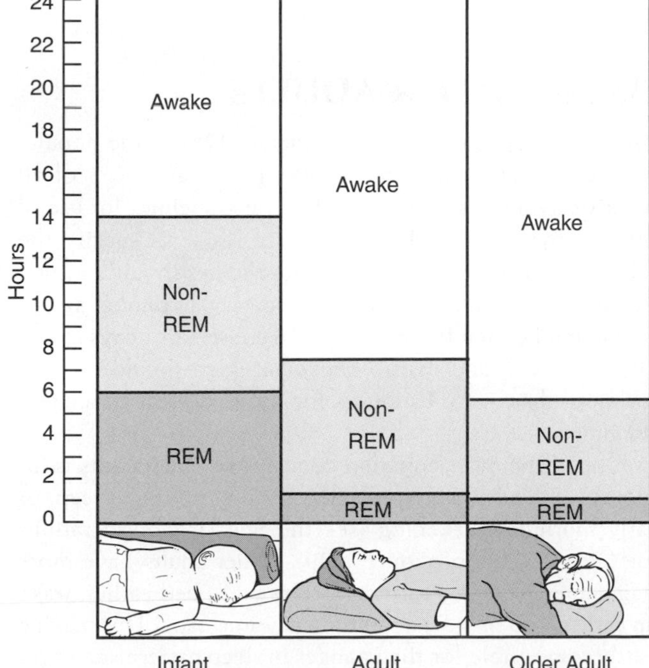

Figure 16-2 Sleep-wake cycles across the life span. Infants: approximately 40% of total sleep time is REM. Adults: 20% of total sleep time is REM. Older adults: total sleep time is slightly reduced; REM remains 20% of total. (From Beare, P.G. & Myers, J.L. [1994]. *Principles and practice of adult health nursing* [2nd ed.]. St. Louis: Mosby.)

when individuals are deprived of deep sleep, they become physically uncomfortable, tend to withdraw from their friends and society, become less aggressive and outgoing, and manifest concern over vague physical complaints and changes in bodily feelings. The overall impression made by persons deprived of deep sleep is that of a depressive and hypochondriac reaction.

Dream sleep is also important. Many psychologists and psychiatrists believe that wish fulfillment finds expression in dreams and that potentially harmful thoughts, feelings, and impulses are released through dreams so there is no interference with the functioning of the personality during waking hours.

Studies indicate that subjects deprived of dreaming sleep (awakened every time they attempt to dream, as evidenced by rapid eye movements) experienced a variety of undesirable effects afterward. During waking hours these individuals became less integrated and less effective and exhibited signs of confusion, suspicion, and withdrawal. They appeared anxious, insecure, and irritable; had greater difficulty concentrating; had a marked increase in appetite with a definite weight gain; and were introspective and unable to derive support from other people.

It is also known that the longer dream deprivation continues, the greater the increase in attempts to dream until the individual begins to dream almost on falling asleep. When subjects are finally allowed to dream, a marked increase in dreaming is noted for the entire night, and as much as 75% of the night may be spent in dreaming. This amount diminishes for each succeeding recovery night until the individual reestablishes his or her normal sleep pattern.

Research has shown that deep sleep takes priority over dreaming sleep when there has been prolonged sleep deprivation. In other words, deep sleep needs are met first, after which dreaming sleep needs are met. The body then attempts to reestablish the normal equilibrium between the sleep stages.

Each individual establishes his or her own normal sleep pattern, which may vary from night to night and is influenced by the individual's emotional and physical state. For most individuals, any disturbance in the sleep pattern will cause **insomnia** (problems in falling asleep, staying asleep, or both). Because drugs affect physical and emotional states, they also influence an individual's sleep pattern. Box 16-1 lists selected drugs that may cause insomnia.

USE IN CHILDREN

The use of antianxiety, sedative, or hypnotic agents in children is limited. Because young children are much more sensitive to the CNS depressant effects of this classification of drugs, counseling and psychotherapy are usually tried first. Paradoxical reactions (reactions contrary to the expected reaction) have been reported with the use of barbiturates in both children and older adults. These reactions include increased excitability, hostility, confusion, hallucinations, and

BOX 16-1

Drugs That May Cause Insomnia

alcohol
beta-adrenergic blocking agents (propranolol [Inderal], atenolol [Tenormin], and others)
captopril (Capoten)
CNS stimulants (caffeine, methylphenidate [Ritalin], and others)
enalapril (Vasotec)
fluoroquinolones (ciprofloxacin [Cipro], enoxacin [Penetrex], lomefloxacin [Maxaquin], norfloxacin [Noroxin], ofloxacin [Floxin])
gemfibrozil (Lopid)
levodopa (Larodopa)
levothyroxine (Synthroid)
maprotiline (Ludiomil)
methyldopa (Aldomet)
metoclopramide (Reglan)
metronidazole (Flagyl)
nicotine
nicotine gum (Nicorette)
oxybutynin (Ditropan)
protriptyline (Vivactil)
pentoxifylline (Trental)
phenylpropanolamine combinations (Contac, Dimetapp, Triaminic, and others)
pseudoephedrine combinations (Seldane-D, Sudafed, and others)
quinapril (Accupril)
theophylline (Slo-Bid, Theo-24, Theobid, and others)
thyroid

Withdrawal from CNS Depressants

alcohol
barbiturates
hypnotic drugs
triazolam (Halcion)
tricyclic antidepressants (e.g., amitriptyline [Elavil], imipramine [Tofranil], doxepin [Sinequan], and trimipramine [Surmontil])

Miscellaneous Drugs with the Potential for Inducing Insomnia

corticosteroids
MAO inhibitors
oral contraceptives
phenytoin (Dilantin)

perhaps an acute elevation of body temperature. Sedation may be indicated for particular situations if the drug and dosage are carefully selected for the individual child (e.g., for the treatment of severe anxiety associated with an acute attack of asthma, as an adjunct preanesthetic agent, or in the treatment of convulsive disorders). Close monitoring and assessment by a health care provider is required (see the Special Considerations for Children box above).

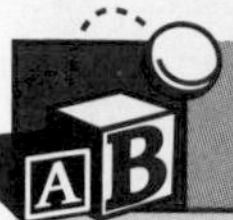

Special Considerations for Children
Antianxiety Agents and Sedatives

Young children are more susceptible to the CNS depressant effects of the benzodiazepines. In neonates, profound CNS depression may result because of the lower rate of drug metabolism by the immature liver.

Chronic use of clonazepam (Klonopin) may result in impaired physical or mental functions in the developing child, which may not become apparent until years later.

Buspirone (BuSpar) use has not been studied in persons under 18 years of age; therefore it is not recommended for use in this age-group.

Although diazepam (Valium) may be used in infants 6 months of age and older, this drug and other benzodiazepines should not be used to treat a hyperactive or psychotic child.

To reduce or minimize potential adverse CNS depressant effects, carefully follow the manufacturer's dosage instructions and, whenever possible, avoid concurrent administration of other CNS depressant types of drugs.

Monitor the child for excessive sedation, lethargy, and lack of coordination; if any of these effects are present, dosage adjustments may be necessary.

Paradoxical reactions to barbiturates have been reported in both children and older adults. (See description under Use in Children, p. 327.)

USE IN OLDER ADULTS

Although they make up approximately 12% of the population, older adults consume between 35% and 40% of all sedative-hypnotics prescribed. Federal guidelines for use of sedative-hypnotics in long-term care residents specify the following: (1) short-acting benzodiazepines should be tried before long-acting agents are used, (2) hypnotic agents should not be used for more than 10 consecutive days in any 30-day period; and (3) no benzodiazepine should be used for more than 3 to 4 months for the treatment of anxiety (Regimen, 1995).

One of the most common concerns of older adults is insomnia, difficulty falling asleep, difficulty staying asleep, or early morning awakening (see the Special Considerations for Older Adults box on p. 329). Older adults have more fragmented sleeping patterns—they go to bed earlier, wake up earlier, and may take multiple daytime naps. This may be partly responsible for the changes in sleep pattern stages reported in this age-group, such as a progressive decline in REM sleep (Gottlieb, 1990; Asplund, 1999). Age-related physiologic changes may also contribute to the reported changes in sleep patterns. Many other factors may result in sleep disturbances, such as retirement, death of a close friend or spouse, social isolation, increased use of medications, and many other issues.

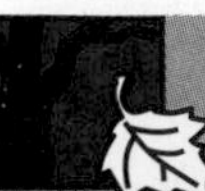

Special Considerations for Older Adults
Insomnia and Hypnotics

Sleep latency increases, and REM and stage 4 sleep may be absent in older adults. Sleep disturbance is one of the most common concerns of older adults.

Evaluate the individual for preexisting health conditions, because various illnesses such as arthritic pain, hyperthyroidism, cardiac dysrhythmia, and paroxysmal nocturnal dyspnea may alter sleep patterns.

Hypnotics should be reserved to treat acute insomnia and, when prescribed, limited to short-term or intermittent use to avoid the development of tolerance and dependency.

A hypnotic with a short duration of action is preferred. When longer-acting hypnotics are given, daytime sedation, ataxia, and memory deficits may result.

Encourage older adults to use nonpharmacologic approaches to promote sleep.

Be aware that older adults, children, and persons with CNS dysfunction may experience a paradoxical reaction (CNS stimulation) to hypnotics and antihistamines.

Common side effects with the antihistamine sleeping aids (which may be prescribed but are also usually in OTC drugs) include dizziness, tinnitus, blurred or altered vision, gastrointestinal disturbance, and dry mouth.

In one study, 430 older adults reported staying asleep as their most common sleep-related problem (Dopheide, 1995). The three most common reasons for not being able to maintain sleep were respiratory difficulties, pain, and muscle or leg cramps. Gottlieb (1990) indicates that older women report more difficulties with their sleeping patterns than do men. Older women are more apt to take hypnotic medications, and sleep deprivation in women is more likely to result in mood alterations.

Appropriate therapy for insomnia should be limited to identification of the cause and treatment of the specific problem. Careful selection of drugs and dosages is necessary to avoid producing excessive CNS depression in older adults. The aging process may be associated with physiologic alterations, including a decline in metabolism and in many organ functions, especially liver and kidney functions. Because drug half-lives may be extended, agents with shorter half-lives and no active metabolites may be safer for older adults. Older adults should be monitored for paradoxical reactions (i.e., increased excitability, rage, hostility, confusion, and hallucinations), which have been reported with the barbiturates and, in rare instances, the benzodiazepines. The appearance of such adverse reactions requires immediate discontinuance of the medication and consultation with the prescriber. (See Chapter 8 for additional information on inappropriate drug use in older adults.)

Barbiturates should be avoided in older adults because enhanced CNS depression, confusion, ataxia, and paradoxical reactions are commonly reported. The short-acting benzodiazepines are usually the agents of choice for treating insomnia in older adults and are much safer than the barbiturates, which are less effective anxiolytic and hypnotic agents. Studies have indicated that long-acting benzodiazepines are associated with a greater risk of delirium and hip fractures (Pasero, Reed, & McCaffery, 1999). Therefore oxazepam (Serax), lorazepam (Ativan), temazepam (Restoril), alprazolam (Xanax), and triazolam (Halcion), which have short to intermediate half-lives, are usually recommended for older adults who require a benzodiazepine.

It has been reported that many anxiolytic benzodiazepines may also be very effective hypnotic agents. Clients receiving a daytime benzodiazepine (e.g., alprazolam [Xanax], diazepam [Valium], or lorazepam [Ativan]) who also require temporary use of a hypnotic drug may be prescribed an equivalent hypnotic dose of the anxiolytic agent. For example, 0.5 mg alprazolam, 5 mg diazepam, and 1 mg of lorazepam are considered equivalent to 15 mg flurazepam (Dalmane), 15 mg temazepam (Restoril), or 0.25 mg triazolam (Halcion) (Crismon, 1992).

When possible, prescribers often suggest that older adults limit their intake of hypnotics to three or four times a week, which allows clients to select the nights on which they need to take their medication. This schedule usually results in enhanced effectiveness, less daytime drowsiness or sedation, and a decreased potential for inducing tolerance to the medication. Regular and careful assessment, monitoring, and reevaluation of the need for hypnotics are highly recommended.

■ Nursing Management
Sedative-Hypnotic Therapy

The following nursing management is common to all drugs prescribed for sedative-hypnotic therapy. Nursing management issues unique to specific sedative-hypnotics will be described as that drug is discussed.

■ **Assessment.** Find out the client's sleep habits and how a good night's sleep is usually ensured. A thorough sleep history is required before a regimen of medications can begin. Such a history includes the following information:

- What does the client do about environmental control, which includes ventilation, lighting, and noise?
- What does the client do about physical care? Does he or she shower or bathe or go for a walk before retiring?
- What does the client do about food? Does he or she snack before retiring?
- Does the client engage in quiet recreation, such as reading, before sleep?
- What is the client's desired sleep pattern? How does his or her current sleep pattern differ from what he or she desires?

Various problems may cause the client to have insomnia. These problems include circadian rhythm irregularities, sleep apnea, restless leg syndrome, intake of alcohol or caf-

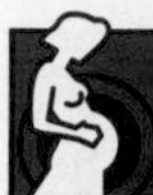

Pregnancy Safety
Antianxiety, Sedative, and Hypnotic Drugs

Category	Drug
B	buspirone, zolpidem
C	chloral hydrate, dexmedetomidine, ethchlorvynol, paraldehyde
D	alprazolam, barbiturates, halazepam, lorazepam (parenteral), midazolam (parenteral)
X	temazepam, triazolam, quazepam
Unclassified	other benzodiazepines, estazolam, meprobamate, hydroxyzine

feine, use of various medications (see Box 16-1), and poor sleep hygiene, which is characterized by irregular bedtimes, daytime napping, and strenuous exercise or heavy eating just before bedtime. If the client's disturbed sleep pattern is a result of discomfort or pain at night, an analgesic or an increased dose of analgesic may be indicated at bedtime. Joint pain or stiffness that results in insomnia will usually respond to a nonsteroidal antiinflammatory drug (NSAID) such as ibuprofen (Motrin) or naproxen (Naprosyn).

A thorough drug history should be obtained when a client is admitted to the hospital and should include the use of prescription, herbal, and over-the-counter (OTC) sleep preparations. Within the hospital environment, all sleep medications brought from home should be removed for the client's safety. Concern for sedatives and hypnotic drug interactions generally involves alcohol and other CNS depressants.

The general health status of the client should be determined because children and older adults are more sensitive to the effects of sedative-hypnotics. Clients with hepatic and renal function dysfunctions require smaller or less frequent doses. The use of these drugs should be avoided in clients who are pregnant or breastfeeding. (See the Pregnancy Safety box above for Food and Drug Administration [FDA] classifications.)

■ **Nursing Diagnosis.** The following nursing diagnoses/collaborative problems may be identified when sedative-hypnotics are administered to clients: disturbed sleep pattern related to the client's underlying problem; disturbed sensory perception (blurred vision, diplopia); disturbed thought processes (confusion); risk for injury related to the CNS effects of the drug (daytime sedation, dizziness, incoordination, ataxia, withdrawal syndrome); deficient knowledge related to sedative-hypnotic therapy; and the potential complication of paradoxical stimulation (increased irritability, hyperactivity).

■ **Implementation**

■ ***Monitoring.*** Evaluating the effectiveness of the medication may be facilitated by use of a written "sleep diary." Among the information recorded in the diary are the foods eaten and activities engaged in before sleep, bedtimes, waking times, naps, and medication administration. A review of the diary will help identify the success of therapy or areas of poor sleep hygiene. Monitor for symptoms of overdose (e.g., inappropriate sleepiness, slurred speech, confusion, and respiratory depression) and tolerance (e.g., continuing and increasing anxiety and insomnia).

■ ***Intervention.*** Because nurses are in a strategic position to influence the client's sleep through direct administration of a drug or client education, it cannot be stressed enough that caution be exercised when decisions are made about giving or repeating an hs or prn order for a sleeping medication. Immediately administering a sleeping medication when a client complains of being unable to sleep may do the client more harm than good. An assessment of the client and alternative methods of relaxing the client must be considered. Try using supportive nursing measures (e.g., a back rub, reduction of environmental stimuli, relaxation therapy, or a warm drink) either alone, before administering a hypnotic, or together with the drug.

If the client is depressed or has a history of attempted suicide, precautions should be taken to prevent him or her from hoarding sedative-hypnotics. Ensure that the client has swallowed each dose.

Many interruptions for various aspects of care can do nothing but further alter a client's sleep pattern. Every effort should be made not to disrupt a sleeping client. If at all possible, other medications are scheduled before sedative-hypnotics are given. Measure vital signs before the client falls asleep.

Because clients can become physically and psychologically dependent on sedative-hypnotic drugs, gradually taper the medications to avoid an abstinence syndrome reaction. Some hypnotics are used on a long-term basis, but this is not recommended. Intermittent nightly use of the drug is suggested to reduce or avoid the development of tolerance. For example, if the client has one or two nights of "good" sleep (as defined by the client), it may be possible to omit the drug the next night.

■ ***Education.*** Until the effects of a particular drug are known, caution the client against driving a car, operating machinery, or participating in any activity that may be dangerous. Although the client may deny feeling sleepy the next day, activity performance may show a definable impairment because serum levels of some of these drugs are retained. Alert the client to call for assistance in ambulating if required.

Clients and their families need to be taught ways to promote restful sleep without resorting to OTC sleep aids such as Sominex, Nytol, Sleep-Eze, or Unisom. Instruct the client that nonpharmacologic approaches to promote sleep will enhance the effectiveness of any agent prescribed (Box 16-2).

Explain to the client that sedative or hypnotic drugs taken in combination with alcohol, antihistamines, antianxiety agents, antidepressants, or antipsychotic agents will produce an enhanced CNS depressant effect. This combination should be avoided.

BOX 16-2

Nonpharmacologic Approaches to Promote Sleep

1. Restrict the use of caffeinated beverages or any caffeine-containing product within 8 hours of bedtime. Read labels because many OTC drugs also contain caffeine.
2. Establish set times for retiring and arising from bed. Avoid daytime napping whenever possible. Try to make the bedroom quiet and dark.
3. Avoid consuming alcohol and smoking cigarettes within 8 hours of bedtime or during the night.
4. Avoid heavy meals several hours before bedtime.
5. Avoid strenuous exercise before bedtime. Exercising during the day is recommended if physical condition permits it.
6. Relax in the evening before retiring by reading, using relaxation techniques, taking a warm bath, listening to relaxing music, or going for a pleasant walk.
7. Try not to worry if you are unable to sleep, because anxiety will add to or cause insomnia. If you cannot sleep, get out of bed and go to another room until you become sleepy.
8. Do not use the bedroom for wake-time activities, such as eating or watching television.
9. If recurrent and disturbing thoughts interfere with sleep, it may help to write them down and consider a plan of action to solve the problem.
10. Drink warm, noncaffeinated drinks, such as warm milk with honey, before bedtime. Home remedies that help induce sleep include a high-carbohydrate, low-protein snack or a few crackers or cookies with a glass of warm malted milk.

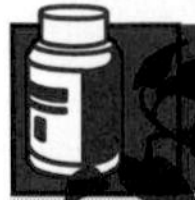

Complementary and Alternative Therapies
Kava

The kava plant is indigenous to the islands of the South Pacific and is used in that region as a ceremonial beverage to induce relaxation. Kava is one of the most popular sleeping aids in Europe; it is used orally to treat anxiety, stress, and restlessness.

The rhizome, or root, of the kava plant contains many active constituents. The kavalactones may act in the limbic system to produce the characteristic effects of kava, or GABA-A receptors may be potentiated by kava use. Some of the constituents of kava have been compared favorably with aspirin, benzodiazepines, and local anesthetics. Kava is likely to be effective for the treatment of anxiety, stress, and restlessness when taken orally in extracts containing 70% kavapyrones.

Although previously thought to be relatively safe, recent studies have shown that kava preparations can cause hepatotoxicity and liver failure with even short-term therapy. Kava can also cause drowsiness and impair the ability to drive or operate other hazardous equipment. The use of kava is contraindicated in pregnancy, lactation, and endogenous depression. The oral use of kava may cause gastrointestinal symptoms, headache, drowsiness, dizziness, and skin reactions. Because of its sedative properties, it may increase the effects of benzodiazepines, barbiturates, sedatives, and other CNS depressants.

Kava is available in capsule form in OTC oral preparations. The typical dosage for natural kava is a cup of tea three times daily; the tea is prepared by simmering 2 to 4 g of the root in 150 mL of boiling water for 5 to 10 minutes and then straining.

Information from Cirigliano, M.D. (1999). Ten most common herbs in clinical practice. In M.S. Micozzi (Ed.), *Current review of complementary medicine.* Philadelphia: Current Medicine; and Jellin, J.M., Batz, F., & Hitchens, K. (2002). *Pharmacist's letter/prescriber's letter natural medicines comprehensive database.* Stockton, CA: Therapeutic Research Faculty.

■ **Evaluation.** The expected outcome of sedative-hypnotic therapy is that the client will report feeling rested and wakeful without residual drowsiness or "drug hangover" during the daytime.

BENZODIAZEPINES

The benzodiazepines are among the most widely prescribed drugs in clinical medicine, primarily because of their advantages over the older agents (e.g., barbiturates, meprobamate, and alcohol). Their popularity probably results from their anxiolytic and hypnotic dose-related effects, which have the following advantages: (1) lower fatality rates with acute toxicity and overdose, (2) lower potential for abuse, (3) more favorable side effect/adverse reaction profiles, and (4) fewer potentially serious drug interactions reported when administered with other medications. (See the Complementary and Alternative Therapies box above.)

Mechanism of Action. Benzodiazepines do not exert a general CNS depressant effect. Instead a wide range of selectivity is seen with various members of this class. Some general pharmacologic properties of this class include muscle relaxant, antianxiety, anticonvulsant, and hypnotic effects.

At least two benzodiazepine receptors have been identified: BZ_1 and BZ_2. The BZ_1 receptors are primarily located in the cerebellum and are believed to mediate the antianxiety and sedative effects. BZ_2 receptors are found in the basal ganglia and hippocampus and are therefore associated with muscle relaxation and cognitive effects (memory and sensory functions).

Both benzodiazepines and barbiturates potentiate the effects of gamma-aminobutyric acid (GABA), the inhibitory neurotransmitter. Benzodiazepines bind to specific benzodiazepine receptors in the brain and spinal cord, which increases the effect of GABA on chloride influx and results in hyperpolarization of the cell membrane and nerve inhibition. Barbiturates increase GABA binding to receptor sites and in high concentrations may directly depress calcium-dependent action potentials and increase chloride flux without GABA. Therefore barbiturates result in a broader effect than the benzodiazepines because they also depress excitatory transmitters and nonsynaptic membranes, resulting in a more pronounced CNS depressant effect.

The limbic system, which is associated with the regulation of emotional behavior, contains a highly dense area of benzodiazepine receptors in the amygdala that appear to correspond to the specific antianxiety effects of certain drugs. Subtypes of GABA receptors have also been reported: GABA-A and GABA-B. The BZ_1 and BZ_2 receptors have been reported to be associated with the GABA-A receptor subtype. GABA-A also has binding sites for alcohol, barbiturates, and some anesthetic agents, which may explain the cross-tolerance observed with these agents (Grimsley, 1995).

Indications. The most common indications for benzodiazepines include anxiety disorders, alcohol withdrawal, preoperative medication, insomnia, seizure disorders, and neuromuscular disease. They are also used to induce amnesia during cardioversion and endoscopic procedures.

Anxiety Disorders. Alprazolam (Xanax), bromazepam (Lectopam 🍁), chlordiazepoxide (Librium), clorazepate (Tranxene), diazepam (Valium), halazepam (Paxipam), ketazolam (Loftran 🍁), lorazepam (Ativan), oxazepam (Serax), and prazepam (Centrax) are the benzodiazepines used as antianxiety agents. In addition, alprazolam (Xanax), lorazepam (Ativan—oral), and oxazepam (Serax) are used as adjunct medications to treat anxiety associated with depression.

Alcohol Withdrawal. The benzodiazepines are the drugs of choice for the treatment of acute alcohol withdrawal (Holbrook, Crowther, Lotter, Cheng, & King, 1999). The medications most often used for this syndrome are chlordiazepoxide (Librium), clorazepate (Tranxene), diazepam (Valium), and oxazepam (Serax). These drugs are very useful for the acute agitation, tremors, and other symptoms of acute alcohol withdrawal.

Panic Disorders. Alprazolam (Xanax) is approved by the FDA for the treatment of panic disorders.

Preoperative Medication. Parenteral chlordiazepoxide (Librium), diazepam (Valium), lorazepam (Ativan), and midazolam (Versed) are used preoperatively to reduce anxiety and to help induce general anesthesia; the latter three drugs may also decrease the client's memory of the procedure. These three drugs are also used for endoscopic procedures to decrease anxiety and tension and to produce an anterograde **amnesic effect**, a loss of memory about the procedure.

Sleep Disorders. Estazolam (ProSom), flurazepam (Dalmane), nitrazepam (Mogadon 🍁), quazepam (Doral), temazepam (Restoril), and triazolam (Halcion) are usually prescribed for sleep disorders such as insomnia. In general, these drugs are indicated for short-term treatment of insomnia only.

Seizure Disorders. Clonazepam (Klonopin) is available orally as an anticonvulsant (see Chapter 17). Parenteral diazepam (Valium) is indicated for intractable, repetitive seizures such as status epilepticus. To treat convulsions, oral diazepam may be used for short-term adjunct therapy (1 to 2 weeks) with other anticonvulsants.

Neuromuscular Disease. Benzodiazepines, especially diazepam (Valium), may be useful as adjunct medications for the treatment of skeletal muscle spasms caused by muscle or joint inflammation or spasticity resulting from upper motor neuron dysfunction, such as cerebral palsy and paraplegia.

Pharmacokinetics. Oral benzodiazepines are readily absorbed from the gastrointestinal tract. Clorazepate (Tranxene) and diazepam (Valium) are the most rapidly absorbed drugs in this class. The more rapidly absorbed benzodiazepines usually produce a more prompt and intense onset of action.

The more lipid soluble (lipophilic) benzodiazepines, such as diazepam (Valium), are widely distributed in the body and brain and are also highly protein bound. Benzodiazepines accumulate in the fluids and tissues of the body after multiple doses. This saturation of storage sites allows for greater blood concentration and longer action; it also accounts for the prolonged action of benzodiazepines after they have been discontinued.

The gastrointestinal tract and the liver are the sites of metabolism for either the active drug or the metabolite dosage forms of the benzodiazepines. The acid environment of the stomach is the site of conversion of clorazepate (Tranxene) to its active form, desmethyldiazepam, a long-acting metabolite (30 to 100 hours). Prazepam (Centrax) also undergoes metabolism in the stomach and liver to the active metabolite desmethyldiazepam. Chlordiazepoxide (Librium), diazepam (Valium), flurazepam (Dalmane), halazepam (Paxipam), ketazolam (Loftran 🍁), and quazepam (Doral) are converted to active metabolites, notably desmethyldiazepam, (*United States Pharmacopeia Dispensing Information*, 1999). The long-acting benzodiazepines and their active metabolites are more apt to accumulate, especially in older adults, resulting in an increased risk for falls and hip fractures (*USP DI*, 1999).

All benzodiazepines are highly protein bound and lipid soluble and are excreted by the kidney. Protein binding is reduced in newborns, alcoholic clients, and clients with cirrhosis or renal insufficiency. Oxazepam (Serax) and lorazepam (Ativan) are metabolized to inactive metabolites and thus may be preferred agents in older adults and in persons with liver disease.

The injectable benzodiazepines include chlordiazepoxide (Librium), diazepam (Valium), and lorazepam (Ativan). The onset of the anticonvulsant, antianxiety, and muscle relaxant effects of these agents after IV administration is approximately 1 to 5 minutes. Onset of action is approximately 15 to 30 minutes after IM injection. Table 16-1 gives a pharmacokinetic overview of selected benzodiazepine drugs.

Side Effects/Adverse Reactions. The most common side effects of benzodiazepines include drowsiness, hiccups (especially with midazolam [Versed]), lassitude, and loss of

TABLE 16-1 Pharmacokinetic Overview: Benzodiazepines

Name	Duration of Action	Time to Peak Plasma Concentration (hours) (oral)	Half-life (hours)*	Active Metabolites (half-life in hours)
alprazolam (Xanax)	S-I	1-2	11-16	None
chlordiazepoxide (Librium)	L	0.5-4	5-30	desmethylchlordiazepoxide (18) demoxepam (14-95) desmethyldiazepam (30-100) oxazepam (5-15)
clonazepam (Klonopin, Rivotril ♣)	S-I	1-2 (some clients from 4-8 hours)	18-50	None
clorazepate (Tranxene, Novo-Clopate ♣)	L	0.5-2	Parent drug not active	desmethyldiazepam (30-100) oxazepam (5-15)
diazepam (Valium, Apo-Diazepam ♣)	L	0.5-2	20-70	desmethyldiazepam (30-100) temazepam (9.5-12.4) oxazepam (5-15)
estazolam (ProSom)	S-I	2	10-24	None
flurazepam (Dalmane, Apo-Flurazepam ♣)	L	0.5-1	2.3	desalkylflurazepam (30-100) N-1-hydroxyethylflurazepam (2-4)
halazepam (Paxipam)	L	1-3	14	desmethyldiazepam (30-100)
ketazolam (Loftran ♣)	L	3	2	desmethyldiazepam (30-100) N-methylketazolam (34-52) diazepam (20-70)
lorazepam (Ativan, Apo-Lorazepam ♣)	S-I	1-6	10-20	None
midazolam HCl (Versed)	S	0.25-1	2.5	1-hydroxymethyl and 4-hydroxy midazolam
oxazepam (Serax, Novoxapam ♣)	S-I	1-4	5-15	None
prazepam (Centrax)	L	2.5-6 for metabolite desmethyldiazepam (single dose)	Parent drug not active	desmethyldiazepam (30-100) oxazepam (5-15)
quazepam (Doral)	L	2	39	desalkylflurazepam (30-100) 2-oxoquazepam (39)
temazepam (Restoril)	S-I	1-2	8-15	None
triazolam (Halcion)	S-I	Within 2	1.5-5.5	None

Information from *United States Pharmacopeia Dispensing Information (USP DI): Drug information for the health care professional* (19th ed.). (1999). Rockville, MD: United States Pharmacopeial Convention.
S, Short; *S-I*, short to intermediate acting; *L*, long acting.
*Elimination half-life.

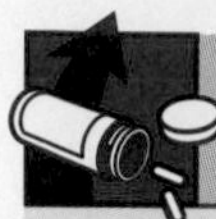

Management of Drug Overdose
Benzodiazepines

- In conscious clients, administer an emetic followed by activated charcoal to adsorb the benzodiazepine. A gastric lavage with a cuffed endotracheal tube may be used for unconscious clients.
- Ensure maintenance of an adequate airway, closely monitor vital signs, administer oxygen for depressed respirations, and promote diuresis by administering IV fluids.
- Medications that may be used include IV administration of flumazenil (Romazicon) as a benzodiazepine antagonist and vasopressors such as norepinephrine, metaraminol, or dopamine to treat hypotension. Do not use barbiturates to treat excitation effects because they may exacerbate the condition.
- Dialysis is of limited value in treating a benzodiazepine overdose.

dexterity. Less common side effects include dry mouth, nausea, vomiting, headaches, constipation, abdominal cramping, unsteadiness, dizziness, and blurred vision. The prescriber should be informed if side effects continue, increase, or disturb the client. Adverse reactions include increased behavioral problems, which are seen mostly with children (anger, decreased ability to concentrate). Neurologic reactions include insomnia, increased excitability, hallucinations, and apprehension (paradoxical reactions). In addition, the client may experience pruritus, skin rash, sore throat, elevated temperature, increased bruising or bleeding episodes, mental depression, hepatitis, confusion, mouth or throat sores, and muscle weakness. Clients using midazolam (Versed) have reported muscle tremors, tachycardia, shortness of breath, or breathing difficulties. The prescriber should be contacted if adverse reactions occur, because medical intervention may be necessary. (See the Management of Drug Overdose box above for the treatment of benzodiazepine overdose.)

Significant Drug Interactions. Significant drug interactions, such as enhanced CNS depressant effects, may occur when benzodiazepines are used in combination with alcohol and CNS depressants, opioid analgesics, anesthetics, or tricyclic antidepressants. Close monitoring is necessary because the dosage of one or both drugs may need to be adjusted. Concurrent administration of benzodiazepines with zidovudine (AZT), an antiviral drug, may inhibit zidovudine metabolism, leading to an increased potential for accumulation and toxicity. If used concurrently, the client should be monitored closely for adverse reactions.

In 1996 the manufacturers of Halcion and Xanax issued warnings that these benzodiazepines are contraindicated for use in persons receiving ketoconazole and itraconazole (Drug Product Update, 1996). Since then, nefazodone (Serzone) and drugs that significantly impair the oxidative metabolism associated with cytochrome P-450 3A (CYP 3A) have also become contraindicated (*Physician's Desk Reference*, 1999).

Dosage and Administration. See Table 16-2 for the dosage and administration of benzodiazepines.

■ Nursing Management
Benzodiazepine Therapy

Concern about the overuse or overprescribing of benzodiazepines leading to tolerance, dependency, and withdrawal problems is discussed in Chapter 9. Several general guidelines are offered to reduce the potential for substance abuse with this drug classification:

1. Benzodiazepines are antianxiety agents; they are used to control the symptoms of anxiety but are not curative agents.
2. Benzodiazepines are indicated for short-term therapy or on an as-needed basis. The dosage should be the minimum necessary to produce the desired effect. The client should be reevaluated every 2 weeks to detect the effectiveness of the medication, the need for continued therapy, or both.
3. When a benzodiazepine is being discontinued, the dosage should be tapered over 2 weeks. Severe withdrawal symptoms have been reported with abrupt discontinuation of the short-acting benzodiazepines (lorazepam [Ativan], alprazolam [Xanax]). Switching for a few weeks to a benzodiazepine that has a longer half-life before starting the tapering procedure helps to reduce more serious withdrawal symptoms, such as tonic-clonic seizures.
4. Concurrent consumption of two or more benzodiazepine agents, even for daytime anxiety and bedtime insomnia, is considered inappropriate therapy. Using one benzodiazepine to accomplish both purposes is preferred because (1) the effectiveness is usually equivalent, (2) the drug will be better tolerated and controlled by the client, and (3) the therapy is less expensive.

In addition to the following discussion, see Nursing Management: Sedative-Hypnotic Therapy, p. 329 (see also the Case Study box on p. 336).

■ **Assessment.** Initially it should be determined if the client has a hypersensitivity to any of the benzodiazepines, because there may be a cross sensitivity to other benzodiazepines. Pregnant women should usually avoid using benzodiazepines because their use in the first trimester is associated with an increased risk of congenital anomalies. Chronic use of benzodiazepines during pregnancy may result in a neonate with withdrawal symptoms. If used in the last weeks of pregnancy, these drugs may cause neonatal CNS depression or, if used just before or during labor, neonatal flaccidity. Women of childbearing age should be advised to notify the prescriber immediately if they become pregnant or intend to become pregnant

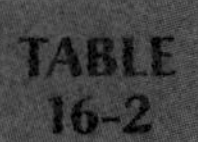

TABLE 16-2 Benzodiazepines: FDA-Approved Indications, Dosage, and Administration

Drug	FDA-Approved Indications	Dosage and Administration
alprazolam (Xanax, generic)	Anxiety, panic	*Adults:* antianxiety, 0.25-4 mg/day in divided doses. Antipanic, up to 10 mg/day. *Children up to 18 years:* not recommended.
chlordiazepoxide (Librium, generic)	Anxiety, sedative-hypnotic (alcohol withdrawal)	*Adults:* antianxiety, 5-25 mg PO 3 or 4 times daily. Alcohol withdrawal, 50-100 mg PO initially, repeat as needed up to 400 mg/day. Parenteral, 50-100 mg IM or IV 3 or 4 times daily. Preoperative, 50-100 mg IM 1 hour before surgery. *Children:* 6 years and older, 5-10 mg PO 2 or 3 times daily. Parenteral up to 12 years, dosage not established; parenteral 12 and over, 25-50 mg IM or IV.
clonazepam (Klonopin)	Seizures, panic	See Chapter 17 for information.
clorazepate (Tranxene, generic)	Anxiety, seizures, sedative-hypnotic (alcohol withdrawal)	*Adults:* antianxiety, 7.5-15 mg PO 2-4 times daily. Alcohol withdrawal, 30 mg initially, then 15 mg 2-4 times daily eventually reduced to 3.75 mg (see current reference for dosing guidelines). Anticonvulsant, 7.5-30 mg 3 times daily per recommended schedule (refer to current drug references for dosing guidelines).
diazepam (Valium, generic)	Anxiety, sedative-hypnotic, seizures, skeletal muscle relaxant	*Adults:* antianxiety, 2-10 mg PO 2-4 times daily. Sedative-hypnotic (alcohol withdrawal), 5-10 mg 3 or 4 times daily. Anticonvulsant or skeletal muscle relaxant (adjunct), 2-10 mg 3 or 4 times daily. Parenteral (IM or IV), individualized dose (usually 5 mg up to 20 mg depending on procedure). See current guidelines.
estazolam (ProSom)	Sedative-hypnotic	*Adults:* 1-2 mg PO. *Children up to 18 years:* not recommended.
flurazepam (Dalmane, generic)	Sedative-hypnotic	*Adults:* 15-30 mg PO. *Children up to 15 years:* not recommended.
halazepam (Paxipam)	Anxiety	*Adults:* 20-40 mg 3 or 4 times daily. *Children up to 18 years:* not recommended.
lorazepam (Ativan, generic)	Anxiety, sedative-hypnotic	*Adults:* antianxiety, 1-3 mg 2 or 3 times daily. Sedative-hypnotic, 2-4 mg at bedtime. Parenteral, 0.5 mg/kg IM up to maximum of 4 mg or 0.044 mg/kg or a total dose of 2 mg IV (whichever is less). *Children up to 12 years:* PO not recommended. Parenteral not recommended for children up to 18 years of age.
midazolam (Versed)	Preoperative sedation and amnesia, conscious sedation	*Doses are individualized, generally adults:* 70-80 µg/kg ½-1 hour before surgery. (See also Chapter 15.)
oxazepam (Serax, generic)	Anxiety, sedative-hypnotic	*Adults:* antianxiety, 10-30 mg 3 or 4 times daily. Sedative-hypnotic (alcohol withdrawal), 15 or 30 mg 3 or 4 times daily. *Children up to 12 years:* dosage not established.
prazepam (Centrax, generic)	Anxiety	*Adults:* 10-20 mg PO 3 times daily or 20-40 mg at bedtime. *Children up to 18 years:* dosage not established.
quazepam (Doral)	Sedative-hypnotic	*Adults:* 7.5-15 mg at bedtime. *Children up to 18 years:* dosage not established.
temazepam (Restoril, generic)	Sedative-hypnotic	*Adults:* 7.5-15 mg at bedtime. *Children up to 18 years:* dosage not established.
triazolam (Halcion)	Sedative-hypnotic	*Adults:* 125-250 µg at bedtime. *Children up to 18 years:* dosage not established.

Information from *United States Pharmacopeia Dispensing Information (USP DI): Drug information for the health care professional* (19th ed.). (1999). Rockville, MD: United States Pharmacopeial Convention.

Case Study *The Client Taking Antianxiety Agents*

Anna Smith is a 45-year-old mother of four children. She is an attractive and intelligent woman of medium build. She describes herself as being somewhat of a perfectionist and a very sensitive person. In the last few months she has become increasingly concerned with various family problems. Her 19-year-old son has dropped out of college and has developed new friends that concern her. She suspects that his behavior changes are related to drugs.

Lately she has been feeling very fatigued during the day, but she is unable to sleep at night because of "worrying" over problems. She does not believe she can talk to her husband, because he has been working long hours at his executive job and falls right to sleep as soon as he goes to bed. She tried an OTC medication (Vivarin) to get some pep but found it just made her feel jittery and nervous and made it even more difficult to get to sleep.

She went to her primary care provider, who initially prescribed diazepam (Valium) 5 mg PO tid and pentobarbital (Nembutal) 100 mg PO at bedtime. After 2 weeks' time she still had the same difficulty in sleeping and had become more depressed and irritable. She could not manage to keep the house clean because she just did not have the energy, and she had crying spells late each afternoon when no one else was home except her 4-year-old son. Her prescriber then ordered some blood tests; after ascertaining that the tests were normal, he advised Anna to see a psychiatrist. The psychiatrist prescribed alprazolam (Xanax) 0.25 mg PO tid for her anxiety and the same drug 0.25 mg, 1 or 2 tablets prn at bedtime. Over the next 4 weeks her anxiety began to decrease and she was able to sleep through the night.

1. How would benzodiazepines affect Anna's anxiety levels?
2. For what side effects/adverse reactions should Anna be monitored?
3. What are some of the important points to stress to Anna while she is taking Xanax?
4. While taking Xanax, Anna is to attend an obligatory cocktail party given by her husband's business associates. How would you advise her when she asks you, "Would it hurt if I have a cocktail or two?"

For answer guidelines, go to mosby.com/MERLIN/McKenry/.

during anxiolytic therapy; a decision about discontinuing the drug must be made.

Nursing mothers should not be given benzodiazepines. Because of their molecular size, the benzodiazepines and their metabolites probably are excreted in breast milk. This may result in sedation, feeding difficulties, and weight loss in the infant.

To preclude ataxia or excessive sedation in older adults or debilitated clients, the initial dose should be small and increments added gradually according to the response of each client. Doses of benzodiazepines sufficient to control anxiety cause unwanted drowsiness less often than equivalent doses of barbiturates or meprobamate. The benzodiazepines have a high therapeutic effectiveness and a low potential for addiction and lethality. They are generally desirable agents for anxious older adults. These drugs occasionally cause paradoxical reactions such as agitation and confusion, but these occur to a lesser degree than with barbiturates.

Careful titration to individual needs is essential in older adults. Remember that older adults are more vulnerable to the adverse effects of benzodiazepines. Excretion is delayed in this population, and thus the half-life increases. This response may allow the client to attain therapeutic blood levels with a single dose rather than with two or three doses per day. Daytime sedation can be reduced if the single daily dose is administered at bedtime. Excessive doses of benzodiazepines may result in incontinence, a loss of the ability to ambulate, or confusion in older adults who were previously continent, ambulatory, and alert.

When depression accompanies the client's anxiety, the incidence of suicidal tendencies is significant. Further protective measures may be required to avoid self-destructive acts such as a multidrug overdose. As small an amount of the drug as possible should be available to such a client at any one time. This requires accurate medical office data about prescriptions and their refill dates and ensures greater control by the prescriber or case manager.

Because of their anticholinergic effects, benzodiazepines should be used with caution in clients with angle-closure glaucoma. Their use may also result in respiratory failure in clients with severe chronic obstructive pulmonary disease. Clients with myasthenia gravis may experience an exacerbated condition with the use of benzodiazepines. CNS depression may be intensified with clients experiencing acute alcohol intoxication, coma, or shock.

A baseline assessment of the client should include a description of the client's underlying condition and CNS and mental status, as well as a complete blood count (CBC) and liver function tests. The usual precautions in treating clients with impaired renal or hepatic function should also be observed.

Dosages should be carefully determined for clients with renal impairment, especially when chlordiazepoxide (Librium) and diazepam (Valium) are administered, because active metabolites may accumulate and produce toxicity. Flurazepam (Dalmane) should be avoided, whereas other agents such as clonazepam (Klonopin), lorazepam (Ativan), oxazepam (Serax), and temazepam (Restoril) seem to pose no risk of toxicity for clients who have renal impairment.

Clients often experience a number of physical and psychiatric problems at the same time and may require treatment with several drugs. This multiple drug therapy is sometimes called "polypharmacy." Many clients benefit diagnostically and therapeutically from a health evaluation made during a drug-free period of time. However, some clients exhibit symptoms of withdrawal if abruptly withdrawn from high dosages or therapeutic dosages of benzodiazepines taken over prolonged periods. These symptoms may resemble those of the anxiety for which the drug was originally prescribed. A mild withdrawal syndrome is characterized by feelings of tension or anxiety, anorexia, gastrointestinal symptoms (e.g., diarrhea), weakness, lethargy, light-headedness, tremor, and mild numbness. Clients who exhibit moderately severe symptoms report anxiety, apprehension, restlessness, insomnia, increased frequency of dreaming, anorexia-induced weight loss, dysphoric moods, and palpitations. Rarely, clients exhibit seizures and delirium.

Withdrawal symptoms usually begin 24 to 72 hours after withdrawal. When the client is withdrawn from a short-acting benzodiazepine, symptoms peak in approximately 5 to 7 days and subside after 7 to 10 days. The withdrawal syndrome of the long-acting benzodiazepines peaks at approximately 5 days but may last 2 to 4 weeks. Administering a dose of the anxiolytic agent can relieve withdrawal symptoms. The withdrawal syndrome can be avoided by gradually tapering the dosage of the anxiolytic agent and supporting the client during this period with other anxiety-relieving techniques.

■ **Nursing Diagnosis.** Because of the CNS effects of benzodiazepine therapy, the following nursing diagnoses/collaborative problems may be identified: risk for injury related to dizziness, incoordination, and ataxia; disturbed sensory perception (blurred vision, diplopia); disturbed thought processes (anterograde amnesia, memory impairment, and vivid dreams); impaired verbal communication (slurred speech); disturbed sleep pattern (daytime sedation and hangover); and the potential complication of drug dependence. There may occasionally be an alteration in bowel function (constipation) and an alteration in urinary pattern (urinary retention). Drug-related depression is rare.

■ **Implementation**

■ ***Monitoring.*** The effectiveness of the medication as an antianxiety agent or as a sedative-hypnotic should be assessed periodically over the course of therapy. Clients receiving benzodiazepines for prolonged periods should have liver function tests, as well as periodic blood counts to monitor for neutropenia. Mental status and CNS, bowel, and urinary functioning should be monitored.

■ ***Intervention.*** Avoid IM administration because the benzodiazepines are highly alkaline and irritating to tissues, and absorption by this route is erratic. Administer IV preparations slowly because apnea, hypotension, bradycardia, and cardiac arrest have been associated with rapid administration. Arteriospasm with resultant gangrene results from accidental intraarterial, rather than IV, administration. After receiving a parenteral dose of a benzodiazepine, the client needs close observation for at least 3 hours, preferably with bed rest.

■ ***Education.*** Nonpharmacologic interventions for reducing anxiety related to the stress of everyday life should be encouraged; benzodiazepines are not indicated for the long-term management of this anxiety. Stress-reduction techniques such as self-coaching, thought stopping, guided imagery, and progressive relaxation exercises may be used as adjuncts to the benzodiazepines.

Instruct the client to avoid alcoholic beverages, sleep-inducing OTC medications, and other CNS depressants while taking benzodiazepines. Caution the client not to take more than the prescribed dosage if the medication seems less effective but to consult the prescriber. On a scheduled dosing regimen (e.g., used as an anticonvulsant rather than as a prn medication), the client should take a missed dose within 1 to 2 hours of when it should have been taken. If the dose is remembered much later, the client should skip the missed dose and continue the regimen; doses should not be doubled.

■ **Evaluation.** If a drug is being used for its antianxiety properties, the client will report an increase in psychologic and physiologic comfort and will appear to have relaxed facial expressions and body movements. Clients using a benzodiazepine for nighttime sedation will report an increase in the amount and quality of sleep and daytime wakefulness.

alprazolam [al pray′ zoe lam] (Xanax)

Alprazolam is used as an antianxiety and antipanic agent. Accumulation is minimal after multiple doses, and elimination rapidly follows termination of therapy. Reports of violent and aggressive behavior have been associated with the use of alprazolam (Glod, 1992). In some clients rapid decreases in dosage or an abrupt discontinuation of therapy has resulted in seizures, delirium, and withdrawal reactions. The risk of seizures is greatest within 1 to 3 days of abrupt discontinuation. To reduce or avoid the potential for these adverse effects, alprazolam should be gradually tapered at 3- to 5-day intervals until discontinued. (See the Cultural Considerations box on p. 338 for racial differences in the response to alprazolam.)

bromazepam [brom az′ e pam] (Lectopam 🍁)

Bromazepam is a short to intermediate half-life benzodiazepine that is used as an antianxiety agent. The client should be advised to avoid alcoholic beverages and to be aware that this product may cause drowsiness.

chlordiazepoxide [klor dye az e pox′ ide] (Librium, Libritab)

Besides its use as an antianxiety agent, chlordiazepoxide is also used as a sedative-hypnotic, an antitremor drug, an antipanic agent (parenteral), and for the relief of acute alcohol

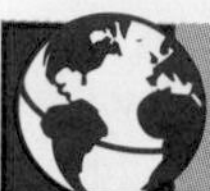

Cultural Considerations

Racial Differences in Response to Alprazolam

An awareness of the potential for unusually high plasma concentrations of some drugs in Asian clients may help nurses detect and prevent adverse drug effects. Lin et al. (1988) studied blood plasma levels of alprazolam (Xanax), a widely prescribed benzodiazepine, in 42 healthy men (14 American-born Asians, 14 foreign-born Asians, and 14 Caucasians) and found that both American-born Asians and foreign-born Asians required smaller dosages to achieve the same blood plasma levels as Caucasian subjects. In both Asian groups the drug remained in the blood for a longer time. Body heights and weights are not a factor (Kudzma, 1992).

withdrawal symptoms. It has also been used to treat tension headaches.

Parenteral IV administration is preferred to IM injection, because IM absorption is slow and erratic. IV administration should be slow, over a period of at least 1 minute. The nurse should be careful not to use the IM diluent when preparing solution for IV administration, because the IM diluent tends to form air bubbles.

When preparing a chlordiazepoxide solution for IM administration, only the manufacturer's diluent is used, and the drug is administered deeply into the muscle. Mixing the drug with sodium chloride or sterile water for injection will cause pain on injection. Solutions should be used immediately after reconstitution, and any unused solution should be discarded.

After receiving the drug parenterally, the client should rest in bed and be monitored carefully for up to 3 hours for decreases in respiratory rate, heart rate, and blood pressure. Because the long-acting metabolites remain in the bloodstream for several days, the client should be monitored for cumulative effects of the drug.

clonazepam [kloe na′ zi pam] (Klonopin, Rivotril ♣)

Clonazepam is used as an anticonvulsant and for the treatment of panic disorders. When used as an anticonvulsant, clients receiving long-term therapy should avoid abrupt withdrawal because this may result in seizures. However, tolerance develops after a few months of therapy, resulting in a loss of anticonvulsant activity in up to 30% of clients (*USP DI*, 1999). Dosage adjustments will restore the efficacy of clonazepam.

Clonazepam administered concurrently with carbamazepine may result in a decrease in the serum levels and half-life of clonazepam. Clients receiving combination anticonvulsant therapies should be monitored closely.

clorazepate [klor az′ e pate] (Tranxene, Novo-Clopate ♣)

Clorazepate is used as an antianxiety agent, sedative-hypnotic, anticonvulsant, and for the relief of acute alcohol withdrawal symptoms. When given orally, it is one of the most rapidly absorbed benzodiazepines.

✓ diazepam [dye az′ e pam] (Valium, Apo-Diazepam ♣)

Diazepam is used as an antianxiety agent, sedative-hypnotic, anticonvulsant, skeletal muscle relaxant, antitremor agent, and antipanic agent. It is also indicated for the treatment of acute alcohol withdrawal, status epilepticus, tension headache, temporomandibular joint disorders, and as a preoperative medication. Parenteral diazepam also has an amnesic indication.

IV administration should be accomplished slowly, at least 1 minute for each 5 mg, to prevent apnea, hypotension, bradycardia, or cardiac arrest. The client should be observed at bed rest for at least 3 hours after parenteral administration. IV injection should be made into a large vein, not small veins such as those found on the back of the hand and wrist.

Diazepam is not compatible with aqueous solutions. Continuous IV infusion is not recommended, because diazepam may precipitate in the infusion bag and be adsorbed by the plastic infusion bags and tubing. If direct IV injection is not possible, the drug should be slowly injected through an infusion port as close as possible to the point of the needle or cannula insertion. Glass infusion sets and polyethylene/polypropylene plastic syringes are recommended for the administration of diazepam emulsion. Diazepam emulsion should be used within 6 hours of opening the ampule, and it should not be diluted or mixed with other solutions.

The use of a topical anesthetic for the insertion of the endoscope is recommended when diazepam is administered parenterally for peroral endoscopy. Increased coughing, decreased respirations, dyspnea, hyperventilation, and laryngospasm have been known to occur; resuscitation measures to assist with respirations should be available.

Diazepam is also available in a rectal gel dosage form (Diastat) for use primarily as an anticonvulsant. A diazepam oral solution is also available (Diazepam Intensol, PMS-Diazepam ♣) (*USP DI*, 1999). This variety is very useful in helping the health care provider to select a proper diazepam dosage form for an individual client.

See Chapter 17 for the nursing management of diazepam as an anticonvulsant therapy.

estazolam [es taz′ oh lam] (ProSom)

Estazolam is similar to the other hypnotic benzodiazepines. It is indicated for the short-term treatment of insomnia. It is widely distributed in the body and easily crosses the blood-brain barrier. It has an intermediate to long half-life and is less likely to cause rebound insomnia after drug withdrawal.

flurazepam [flure az' e pam] (Dalmane, Apo-Flurazepam ♣)

Flurazepam is indicated for use only as a sedative-hypnotic. Although the sleep pattern will improve the first night, the client should be instructed that 2 to 3 nights might be required before flurazepam becomes fully effective. Elimination is slow; metabolites remain in the body several days. This may produce unwanted daytime carryover effects that result in poor coordination and drowsiness. The effects may be overcome by using lower doses and administering the medication every other evening. The client must be warned of the sustained effect of the active metabolites.

halazepam [hal az' e pam] (Paxipam)

Halazepam is indicated for use only as an antianxiety agent. It has a long half-life and active metabolites, which may be significant when multiple doses are administered. Elimination may take several days or even weeks.

lorazepam [lor a' ze pam] (Ativan, Novolorazem ♣)

Lorazepam is indicated for use as an antianxiety agent, sedative-hypnotic, amnesic, antitremor agent, adjunct skeletal muscle relaxant, anticonvulsant (parenteral only), antiemetic in cancer chemotherapy (parenteral only), and for the treatment of acute alcohol withdrawal symptoms and tension headaches.

Lorazepam must be mixed with an equal amount of a compatible diluent immediately before IV use. It may be infused directly into a vein or through IV tubing. Infusion rates are not to exceed 2 mg/min. Intraarterial injection should be avoided because it can cause arteriospasm and possible gangrene. IM lorazepam is injected undiluted into deep muscle mass.

After receiving a parenteral dose of lorazepam, the client should be observed at bed rest for at least 1 hour for decreases in respiratory rate, heart rate, and blood pressure.

The tablet dosage form may be administered orally or sublingually.

midazolam [mid' ay zoe lam] (Versed)

Midazolam is used preoperatively for sedation and amnesic effects and as an adjunct to general anesthesia. Midazolam is used only in parenteral form. Unlike diazepam (Valium), it does not cause thrombophlebitis and irritation on injection.

Dosages should be individualized according to the health status of the client. The range between therapeutic dosage and unconsciousness or disorientation is narrow, which necessitates close monitoring of the client. The client should be instructed not to engage in tasks requiring alertness (e.g., driving) for one day after administration or until the effects of midazolam have abated, whichever is longer.

IV midazolam has been associated with severe respiratory depression and arrest, especially when given concurrently with an opioid analgesic or when administered too rapidly. A warning has been issued for the IV use of this drug: it should be administered only in a hospital or ambulatory care setting that has continuous respiratory and cardiac monitoring and resuscitative drugs and equipment available.

As with diazepam (Valium), a topical anesthetic agent should be used for the insertion of the endoscopy tube when midazolam is used for peroral endoscopic procedures. Measures to support respiration (oxygen, suction airway) should be available.

oxazepam [ox a' ze pam] (Serax, Ox-Pam)

Oxazepam is indicated for anxiety associated with mental depression and for the treatment of acute alcohol withdrawal symptoms. Drug accumulation is minimal during multiple-dose therapy, and the drug is rapidly eliminated when discontinued.

prazepam [pra' ze pam] (Centrax)

Prazepam is indicated only as an antianxiety agent. It is one of the most slowly absorbed benzodiazepines after oral administration, and the accumulation of active metabolites may be significant in long-term therapy. Lethargy and increased fatigue are reported more often with prazepam than with most other benzodiazepines.

quazepam [kway' ze pam] (Doral)

Quazepam, a benzodiazepine hypnotic, has a greater affinity for the BZ_1 receptors than any of the other hypnotic benzodiazepines. Because of its extended drug half-life and active metabolites, steady-state serum levels occur between 7 and 13 days. Daytime drowsiness is more common with quazepam than with most of the other benzodiazepines, but its prolonged half-life makes rebound insomnia less likely after drug withdrawal.

temazepam [te maz' e pam] (Restoril)

Temazepam is indicated as a sedative-hypnotic. Only minimal accumulation occurs during multiple doses, and elimination is rapid when therapy is discontinued. The slow absorption pattern of temazepam means that it usually takes 1 to 2 hours to reach effective blood levels. Its effectiveness for inducing sleep can be enhanced with proper scheduling of its administration—1 to 1.5 hours before bedtime.

triazolam [trye az' oh lam] (Halcion)

Triazolam is indicated only as a sedative-hypnotic. Although anterograde amnesia may occur with any benzodiazepine, triazolam "may be associated with more frequent psychiatric disturbances than other agents in this class" (McCue et al., 1993). In several European countries the 0.5-mg dose of triazolam has been taken off the market because of the frequency of reports of amnesia and other adverse reactions. In the United States the FDA has required stronger product labeling and client information. It appears that triazolam reduces the amount of REM sleep, which may contribute to the development or exacerbation of a mental or behavior-type disorder (Jellin, 1991). Effects reported include memory impairment, confusion, depersonalization, and severe anxiety.

Paradoxical rage reactions have also been reported with the benzodiazepines. According to foreign and domestic studies, this reaction is reported more often with triazolam than with the other benzodiazepines (Crismon, 1992). The symptoms include depersonalization, increased anxiety and restlessness, agitation, paranoid behavior, rage, panic reactions, and hallucinations. This response may be dose related, because dosages in excess of 0.5 mg/day were recorded in the majority of affected individuals (Crismon, 1992).

As noted previously, the benzodiazepines have been associated with changes in cognitive function and an increased risk for falls and injuries in older adults. Altered pharmacokinetics in older adults may increase the risk for adverse reactions; thus close professional supervision along with clear guidelines for benzodiazepine use is necessary.

The package insert information for triazolam cautions the client not to take the medication for more than 7 to 10 days without prescriber consultation and to report to the prescriber any unusual thoughts or behavior. The client is advised to avoid the use of alcohol and other drugs, including OTC medications, without prescriber approval. This product should not be used when a full night's sleep is not possible, such as airline flights of less than 7 or 8 hours. Amnesic episodes caused by lack of drug elimination from the body have been reported in such situations (*Mosby's GenRx*, 1999). Although many people have taken triazolam (Halcion) without reports of adverse reactions, it may be prudent to avoid the use of this product in older adults because they generally have a higher susceptibility to memory loss and other adverse drug reactions (Sherman, 1991).

New Benzodiazepines Not Available in the United States

Several benzodiazepines currently unavailable in the United States include clobazam (Frisium), an anticonvulsant and anxiolytic similar to diazepam; and nitrazepam (Mogadon), a hypnotic used in Europe and Canada for many years. Both products have long half-lives, which increases the potential for drug accumulation and side effects. They are similar to drugs already marketed in the United States (*Drug Facts and Comparisons*, 2000). Abecarnil, a partial benzodiazepine-receptor agonist, may have a number of advantages over the currently marketed benzodiazepines. This product initially appears to have less potential for inducing sedation, drug tolerance, ataxia, amnesia, drug dependence, and abuse (Edmonds et al., 1995). A double-blind study that compared abecarnil and diazepam for the treatment of alcohol withdrawal reported similar results with both drugs, although the pharmacologic profile for abecarnil indicated a low abuse potential and fewer side effect (Anton, Kranzler, McEvoy, Moak, & Bianca, 1997). Further studies are necessary to clinically validate such claims.

Benzodiazepine Antidote

Flumazenil (Romazicon), a benzodiazepine-receptor antagonist, is indicated for the treatment of a benzodiazepine overdose or to reverse the sedative effects of benzodiazepines following surgical or diagnostic procedures. This drug will not reverse the effects of opioids or other nonbenzodiazepine drugs. Although flumazenil can reverse the sedative effects of benzodiazepines, a reversal of the benzodiazepine-induced respiratory depression has not been demonstrated (Abramowicz, 1992). Therefore hypoventilation must include the establishment of an airway, ventilation assistance, and interventions to support circulation (*USP DI*, 1999).

The mechanism of action for flumazenil is competition with the benzodiazepines at the binding site of the GABA-benzodiazepine receptor. It is administered intravenously, and antagonistic effects occur within 1 to 2 minutes; a peak effect occurs in 6 to 10 minutes, and the duration of action is approximately 1 to 3 hours, depending on the dose of benzodiazepine consumed. Because most benzodiazepines have a half-life longer than 1 hour, repeated injections of flumazenil are necessary. Flumazenil is metabolized in the liver and excreted by the kidneys.

Side effects/adverse reactions include headache, visual disturbance, excess sweating, increased anxiety, nausea, light-headedness, and pain at the injection site (which can be significantly decreased by infusing the drug through a freely running IV solution into a large vein). Flumazenil may cause convulsions in clients taking benzodiazepines to control epilepsy and in clients who have received long-term benzodiazepine therapy. Seizures have also been reported in clients who have consumed an overdose of a tricyclic antidepressant and a benzodiazepine. Cardiac dysrhythmias have also been reported with the use of flumazenil. Caution is advised when giving flumazenil to clients who are known to use benzodiazepines chronically, because moderate to severe withdrawal symptoms may be precipitated.

Reversal of benzodiazepine-induced sedation requires an initial IV dose of flumazenil, 0.2 mg injected over 15 seconds. This dose may be repeated at 1-minute intervals up to a maximum of 1 mg. The same initial dose is given for a benzodiazepine overdose, usually over 30 seconds; additional doses of 0.3 and, if necessary, 0.5 mg may be given at 1-minute intervals up to a maximum of 3 mg of flumazenil.

Nurses should refer to the current package insert for additional dosing information.

BARBITURATES

The barbiturates were once the most commonly prescribed class of medications for hypnotic and sedative effects. With only a few exceptions, they have been largely replaced by the benzodiazepines. Phenobarbital is generally considered the prototype drug for this classification.

Classification. The barbiturates are classified according to the duration of their action as long-, intermediate-, short-, and ultrashort-acting drugs. Long-acting barbiturates require more than 60 minutes for onset and peak over a period of 10 to 12 hours. Long-acting barbiturates are used for treating epilepsy and other chronic neurologic disorders, as well as for sedation in clients with high anxiety. Intermediate-acting barbiturates have an onset of 45 to 60 minutes and peak in 6 to 8 hours. Intermediate-acting barbiturates are used as sedative-hypnotics.

The short-acting drugs produce an effect (onset) in a relatively short time (10 to 15 minutes) and peak over a relatively short period (3 to 4 hours). Short-acting barbiturates are used for treating insomnia, for preanesthetic sedation, and in combination with other drugs for psychosomatic disorders. Ultrashort-acting barbiturates are used as IV anesthetics. Thiopental sodium acts rapidly and can produce a state of anesthesia in a few seconds.

Mechanism of Action. The mechanism of action for barbiturates is nonselective depression of the CNS. High doses of barbiturates may induce anesthesia. Barbiturates similar to the benzodiazepines appear to enhance systems that use GABA as an inhibitory transmitter. In addition, barbiturates may also decrease excitatory neurotransmitter effects. The ascending reticular formation receives stimuli from all parts of the body and relays impulses to the cortex (thus promoting wakefulness and alertness); barbiturate depression of the ascending reticular formation decreases cortical stimuli, thus reducing the need for wakefulness and alertness.

With barbiturates, the extent of effect varies from mild sedation to deep anesthesia, depending on the drug selected, method of administration, dosage, and reaction of the individual's nervous system. The barbiturates are not regarded as analgesics and cannot be depended on to produce restful sleep when insomnia is caused by pain. However, when a barbiturate is combined with an analgesic, the sedative action seems to reinforce the action of the analgesic and to alter the client's emotional reaction to pain.

All barbiturates depress the motor cortex of the brain when used in large doses. Phenobarbital, mephobarbital (Mebaral), and metharbital (Gemonil ♣) exert a selective action on the motor cortex even in small doses. This explains their use as anticonvulsants. Therapeutic doses have little or no effect on medullary centers, but large doses, especially when administered intravenously, depress the respiratory and vasomotor centers.

Indications. The most common indications for the use of barbiturates include adjuncts to anesthesia and treatment of seizure disorders; several are indicated for the treatment of insomnia. However, the benzodiazepine drugs have generally replaced these agents. Barbiturates are indicated for only short-term treatment of insomnia because they tend to lose their effectiveness in 14 days or fewer.

Barbiturates have been used for their sedative effects in treating anxiety and nervousness. However, for daytime use the benzodiazepines have largely replaced the barbiturates, primarily because they produce less drowsiness and ataxia.

Short-acting barbiturate anesthetics such as thiopental (Pentothal) and methohexital (Brevital) are used for selected surgical procedures, especially for those of short duration. Short-acting barbiturates such as pentobarbital (Nembutal) may be used for their preanesthetic effect to reduce anxiety and facilitate anesthesia induction. Diazepam (Valium) and other benzodiazepines are often used today for this purpose—as preanesthetic agents to help with anesthesia induction, to reduce anxiety, and to induce an amnesic effect.

Anticonvulsant. Barbiturates are also used to prevent or control convulsive seizures associated with tetanus, strychnine poisoning, meningitis, eclampsia, and epilepsy. They may be prescribed alone or in conjunction with other anticonvulsant drugs. Phenobarbital is used in the treatment of epilepsy (generalized tonic-clonic) and for seizures induced by fever. Mephobarbital (Mebaral) and metharbital (Gemonil ♣) may be alternative agents for phenobarbital.

Narcoanalysis. IV amobarbital may be used in narcoanalysis, a form of psychotherapy that helps a client to talk about suppressed feelings and events.

Hyperbilirubinemia. Although not approved for the treatment of hyperbilirubinemia, phenobarbital (oral and injectable) is often used to lower bilirubin concentrations to prevent or treat this condition in neonates and in clients with congenital nonhemolytic unconjugated hyperbilirubinemia.

Pharmacokinetics. Barbiturates are readily absorbed after oral, rectal, and parenteral administration. The soluble sodium salts are absorbed faster than the free acids. Most of the barbiturates undergo change in the liver before being excreted by the kidney. The longer-acting barbiturates are metabolized more slowly than the rapidly acting barbiturates. The slower a barbiturate is altered or excreted, the more prolonged the action. Cumulative effects result if excretion is slow and administration is prolonged.

Side Effects/Adverse Reactions. Side effects/adverse reactions of barbiturates include ataxia, drowsiness, dizziness, hangover effect, nausea, vomiting, insomnia, constipation, restlessness, faintness, headache, night terrors, hypersensitivity reaction such as skin rash, exfoliative dermatitis, sore throat, fever, edema, serum sickness, apnea, bronchospasm, urticaria, and Stevens-Johnson syndrome. Stevens-Johnson syndrome is a severe, occasionally fatal inflammatory disease of children and young adults and is characterized by fever, bullae of the skin, and ulcers of the mucous membranes of the mouth, nose, eyes, and genitalia.

Clients of any age, but especially older or debilitated clients, may exhibit confusion, disorientation, and mental depression. A paradoxical reaction (increased excitability) may occur in children, older adults, or debilitated clients. Long-term barbiturate use may result in osteomalacia and rickets (bone pain or aching, anorexia, myalgia, loss of weight). Toxic signs include very severe confusion and persistent irritability. Acute toxic effects may include bradycardia, confusion, respiratory problems (apnea, laryngospasm), ataxia, extreme weakness, and visual disturbances.

Dosage and Administration. See Table 16-3 for the dosage and administration of barbiturates.

■ Nursing Management

Barbiturate Therapy

Because of the potential for barbiturate dependence, tolerance, abuse, or misuse, the role of the nurse is essential in providing safe and effective drug therapy. In addition to the following discussion, see Nursing Management: Sedative-Hypnotic Therapy, p. 329.

■ **Assessment.** Assess and note the sleeping pattern of the client. This observation can influence the prescriber's decision about the type of barbiturate to prescribe.

Avoid giving barbiturates to clients who are hypersensitive to them or have respiratory conditions (involving dyspnea or obstruction), a previous dependency on barbiturates, or renal or hepatic impairment. Avoid giving barbiturates to children and older adults with a history of paradoxical reactions. Acute intermittent porphyria may be aggravated through barbiturate inducement of the enzyme necessary for porphyrin synthesis (molecular components of hemoglobin, myoglobin, and various enzymes).

Review the client's current medication regimen for the risk of significant drug interactions, such as those that may occur when barbiturates are given concurrently with the drugs listed below:

Drug/Herb	Possible Effect and Management
alcohol and other CNS depressants	Enhanced CNS depressant effects may result. Monitor closely for respiratory pattern changes, and perhaps decrease the dosage of one or both drugs to reduce the possibility of inducing the effect.
anticoagulants, warfarin (Coumadin)	Decrease in anticoagulant effects caused by enhanced metabolism. Prothrombin time tests may be necessary to monitor therapeutic response to the anticoagulant and to determine dosage changes of the anticoagulant.
anticonvulsants, divalproex sodium (Depakote), valproic acid (Depakene), or carbamazepine (Tegretol)	Monitor barbiturate serum levels closely because the metabolism of barbiturates may decrease, leading to elevated levels and an increase in CNS depression and neurologic dysfunction. The half-life of valproic acid may also be reduced, which would also require monitoring of blood levels and dosage adjustments. Phenobarbital may also increase valproic acid hepatotoxicity; monitor closely for jaundice, hepatomegaly, anorexia, abdominal discomfort, clay-colored stools, and dark urine. Increased metabolism of carbamazepine may occur, resulting in decreased serum levels of the drug.
contraceptives, estrogen-containing, oral	Enhanced metabolism of estrogen (particularly oral estrogen) may result in a decrease in contraceptive effects. The prescriber may need to consider a nonhormonal birth control method or progestin-only oral contraceptive.
corticosteroids	When given with barbiturates (especially phenobarbital), corticosteroids may enhance metabolism and have decreased therapeutic effects. Dosage adjustments may be necessary.
herbals (ashwagandha, calendula, hops, kava, lady's slipper, passionflower, sassafras, valerian, yerba mansa)	**May enhance sedation effects. Avoid concurrent use or monitor closely.**

A baseline assessment of the client should include a description of the client's underlying condition, mental status, blood pressure determination, and CBC and liver function studies.

■ **Nursing Diagnosis.** Because of the CNS effects of barbiturate therapy, clients are at risk for injury (drowsiness, unsteadiness), disturbed thought processes (confusion), and disturbed sleep pattern (daytime drowsiness, hangover). There may also be an alteration in bowel pattern (constipation) as a result of the drug's gastrointestinal effects. There is a risk for impaired tissue integrity (redness, swelling, pain at injection site [thrombophlebitis]) if the drug is administered intravenously. Respiratory problems may present as ineffective airway clearance or hypoventilation because of the respiratory depressant effects of barbiturates. The following potential complications exist: Stevens-Johnson syndrome, drug-induced hepatitis (jaundice), paradoxical reaction (unusual excitement), agranulocytosis (sore throat, fever), megaloblastic anemia (lethargy, weakness), thrombocytopenia (unusual bleeding or bruising), mental depression, and allergic reaction (urticaria, wheezing, or tightness in chest).

■ **Implementation**

■ ***Monitoring.*** Continuous assessment of the client is focused on detecting side effects/adverse reactions, monitoring compliance, and monitoring effectiveness of the therapy. Indicators of effectiveness include sleep time, daytime wakefulness, and client reports about feelings of rest and wakefulness. Tolerance develops to all barbiturates during long-term therapy, but it develops at unpredictable rates. The development of tolerance and possible depen-

TABLE 16-3 Selected Barbiturates: Pharmacokinetics, Indications, and Dosage

Name	Onset of Action (minutes)	Duration of Action (hours)	Indications and Dosage*
Short-Acting			
pentobarbital (Nembutal)	10-15	3-4	*Adults:* hypnotic, 100 mg PO/IV, 150-200 mg IM, or 120-200 mg rectally at bedtime. Daytime sedative, 20 mg PO or 30 mg rectally 2-4 times daily. Preoperative, 100 mg PO or 150 or 200 mg IM. Anticonvulsant, 100-500 mg IV. *Children:* sedative-preoperative, 2-6 mg/kg or maximum 100 mg/dose.
secobarbital (Seconal)	10-15	3-4	*Adults:* hypnotic, 100 mg PO, 100-200 mg IM, or 50-250 mg IV at bedtime. Daytime sedative, 30-50 mg 3-4 times daily. *Children:* daytime sedative, 2 mg/kg. Preoperative, 2-6 mg/kg or maximum 100 mg/dose given 1-2 hours before surgery.
Intermediate-Acting			
butabarbital (Butisol)	45-60	6-8	*Adults:* hypnotic and preoperative, 50-100 mg. Daytime sedative, 15-30 mg 3-4 times daily. *Children:* sedative-preoperative, 2-6 mg/kg to maximum of 100 mg/dose.
Long-Acting			
amobarbital (Amytal)	60+	10-12	*Adults:* hypnotic, 65-200 mg PO, IM, or IV at bedtime. Daytime sedative, 50-300 mg PO in divided doses or 30-50 mg IM or IV 2 or 3 times daily. Anticonvulsant, 65-500 mg IV. *Children:* sedative, 2 mg/kg PO 3 times daily. Preoperative (6 years and older), 3-5 mg/kg.
phenobarbital	60+	10-12	*Adults:* hypnotic, 100-320 mg PO or IV at bedtime. Daytime sedative, 30-120 mg PO, IM, IV in 2-3 divided doses daily. Anticonvulsant, 60-250 mg PO daily or 100-320 mg IV. *Children:* anticonvulsant, 1-6 mg/kg/day.

Information from *United States Pharmacopeia Dispensing Information (USP DI): Drug information for the health care professional* (19th ed.). (1999). Rockville, MD: United States Pharmacopeial Convention.
*Barbiturates have generally been replaced by benzodiazepines for daytime sedation and hypnotic effects. Refer to current drug references for additional information.

dence should be closely evaluated. Monitoring for paradoxical reactions, allergic reactions, or drug interactions is also essential. Function as a client advocate when evaluation suggests the need for a change in drug therapy.

■ ***Intervention.*** Be aware that long- and short-acting barbiturates may be combined in the same capsule for a client who has difficulty both in falling asleep and in remaining asleep for the desired number of hours.

To hasten the onset of sleep with oral administration, the rate of absorption may be increased by administering barbiturates well diluted or on an empty stomach.

Barbiturates are not often administered by the IV route except for anesthesia induction and control of status epilepticus. If IV barbiturates have been prescribed, dilute them according to the package insert directions and administer them slowly. If the barbiturate is to be infused in an IV solution, use an infusion control device and monitor the infusion rate closely, because rapid injection can interfere with cardiac and respiratory function. The airway should be patent and emergency resuscitative equipment should be available. For an IV injection, use the larger veins to decrease the risk of irritation. The IV site should be assessed for any signs of thrombophlebitis or extravasation.

Barbiturates may be administered rectally with a retention enema if the oral or parenteral route is undesirable.

Clients who become disoriented or confused by a barbiturate should not be restrained. They should instead be reoriented, and a calm environment should be promoted.

■ ***Education.*** Instruct the client to use the barbiturate only as directed. The client should not alter the dosage or take the drug more often or for a longer period than ordered. Barbiturates may impair mental and physical functioning. The client should avoid hazardous activities if affected by barbiturates in this manner.

Barbiturates may affect the developing fetus. If a client is pregnant or may become pregnant during therapy, she should discuss barbiturate use with her nurse-midwife, nurse practitioner, or physician. Barbiturates also pass into breast milk and may cause CNS depression of the nursing infant.

Barbiturates may cause mental or physical dependence or tolerance. Clients should consult their prescriber if they experience signs or symptoms of dependence or no longer receive the full effect of the drug.

If the client is following a scheduled dosing regimen (as when a barbiturate is used as an anticonvulsant) and misses a dose, it should be taken immediately if remembered within 1 to 2 hours of the scheduled time. The client should skip the dose if it is close to the next dose and continue with the regimen; doses should not be doubled.

Clients who are receiving long-term anticonvulsant therapy may need to increase their intake of folic acid and vitamin D. Encourage rich dietary sources of folic acid, such as spinach and other green leafy vegetables, liver, kidney, asparagus, lima beans, nuts, and whole grain cereals. Foods containing natural vitamin D are of animal origin and include saltwater fish, especially salmon, sardines, and herring; organ meats; fish-liver oils; and egg yolk.

Abrupt withdrawal from barbiturates may precipitate seizures in clients with epilepsy. Abstinence syndrome (see Chapter 9) may be seen after abrupt withdrawal of long-term therapy. Inform the client not to take any additional medications while taking a barbiturate unless the drugs have been approved by the prescriber or pharmacist. Barbiturates interact with many other drugs and alcohol, and dangerous interactions may occur.

■ **Evaluation.** If the barbiturate has been administered for sedation, the expected outcome is that the client will report feeling relaxed or sleeping well. If the indication for barbiturate use is seizures, the client will demonstrate a marked decrease or absence of seizures.

MISCELLANEOUS SEDATIVES AND HYPNOTICS

A number of antianxiety agents/sedatives and hypnotics do not fall into the previously discussed drug classes but are discussed here because they are available for client use with prescription.

Antianxiety Agents/Sedatives

buspirone [byoo spye′ rone] (BuSpar)

Buspirone is not related pharmacologically to other medications discussed in this chapter. Although it is indicated for the treatment of anxiety disorders, it is considered to be equivalent in efficacy to the benzodiazepines, with usually less sedation. The exact mechanism of action is unknown, but the drug has a high affinity for serotonin receptors and a moderate affinity for D_2 dopamine receptors in the CNS. It does not affect GABA, nor does it have any significant affinity for the benzodiazepine receptors.

Buspirone is absorbed very well but undergoes extensive first-pass metabolism in the liver. Protein binding is high (95%), and the onset of effect may take 1 to 2 weeks. Clients may not notice any effects during this time because the medication does not cause muscle relaxation or sedation. The half-life (elimination) is between 2 and 3 hours after a single 10- to 40-mg dose. Buspirone is metabolized in the liver with one active metabolite. It is excreted in the urine and feces.

Side effects/adverse reactions include headache, nausea, increased nervousness, faintness, tinnitus, abdominal distress, insomnia, nightmares, increased weakness, dry mouth, blurred vision, muscle pain or spasms, and decreased ability to concentrate. Rare adverse reactions include chest pain, tachycardia, muscle weakness, paresthesia, sore throat, elevated temperature, depression, and confusion.

The recommended dosage for adults is 5 mg PO two or three times daily, increased by 5 mg/day every 2 to 3 days, until the desired response is achieved. The maximum dosage is 60 mg/day. No dosage has been established for persons under 18 years old.

■ Nursing Management

Buspirone Hydrochloride Therapy

■ **Assessment.** The baseline assessment of the client should include the underlying condition for which buspirone is prescribed as well as the client's CNS status.

Hepatic or renal impairment is one contraindication to the use of buspirone therapy, because the drug is metabolized in the liver and mainly excreted by the kidneys. An increase in adverse reactions has been observed with the concurrent administration of erythromycin (Ilosone) or itraconazole (Sporanox). Avoid concurrent administration with monoamine oxidase (MAO) inhibitors, because severe hypertension may occur.

■ **Nursing Diagnosis.** Clients receiving buspirone are at risk for the following nursing diagnoses/collaborative problems: anxiety related to the client's underlying problem and the ineffectiveness of the drug; disturbed thought processes (confusion); risk for injury related to a drug-induced CNS response (dizziness, light-headedness); impaired comfort (headache, nausea); and the potential complication of mental depression.

■ **Implementation**

■ ***Monitoring.*** Continuous assessment should include the client's level of anxiety, mental status, neuromuscular coordination, and vital signs.

■ ***Intervention.*** Administer with food to prevent gastrointestinal distress.

■ ***Education.*** In addition to the general discussion under Nursing Management: Sedative-Hypnotic Therapy (p. 329), instruct clients to use ice chips or sugarless candies to manage the side effect of dry mouth if it occurs. Inform clients that 1 or 2 weeks of therapy may be necessary before the effects of buspirone therapy become evident. Chest pain, altered thought processes, palpitations, sensory or motor changes in the hands and feet, or fever or sore throat should be reported to the prescriber.

■ **Evaluation.** The expected outcome of buspirone therapy is that the client will report feeling less anxious and will not experience any adverse reactions to the buspirone.

hydroxyzine [hye drox′ i zeen] (Atarax, Vistaril)

Hydroxyzine, a piperazine antihistamine, is an antianxiety agent, sedative-hypnotic, antihistamine, and antiemetic. The antianxiety effect may be due to the suppression of activity in selected subcortical areas of the CNS, but its full mechanism of action is unknown. Its antihistamine and sedative effects may be due to competition with histamine at H_1 receptor sites. The antiemetic, anti–motion sickness, and antivertigo effects of hydroxyzine may be the result of central anticholinergic activity and decreased vestibular stimulation and labyrinthine function. Hydroxyzine may also have an effect on the chemoreceptive trigger zone.

Hydroxyzine is absorbed well. Onset of action occurs 15 to 30 minutes after an oral dose. The duration of effect is 4 to 6 hours when the drug is given orally, and the half-life is 20 to 25 hours. Hydroxyzine is metabolized in the liver and excreted by the kidneys.

Side effects include sedation, which usually disappears after a few days of therapy or when the dosage is reduced; and anticholinergic side effects such as dry mouth, blurred vision, and constipation. Adverse reactions are rarely reported but include skin rash and trembling or seizures (in dosages higher than recommended).

The recommended adult dosage of hydroxyzine is 25 to 100 mg PO, three to four times daily as necessary. When administered to children as an antianxiety agent or sedative-hypnotic, the dosage is 0.6 mg/kg body weight PO. For antihistaminic or antiemetic effects in adults, the dosage is 0.5 mg/kg body weight PO every 6 hours when necessary. The parenteral adult dosage is 25 to 100 mg IM every 4 to 6 hours if necessary. When used in children as an antiemetic or adjunct to narcotic medication, the dosage of hydroxyzine is 1 mg/kg body weight IM as a single dose.

■ Nursing Management

Hydroxyzine Therapy

See also Nursing Management: Sedative-Hypnotic Therapy, p. 329.

■ **Assessment.** Be aware that the antiemetic effects of hydroxyzine may mask symptoms of serious conditions that might otherwise be evidenced by nausea and vomiting, such as brain lesions, appendicitis, and other GI disorders.

The CNS depressant effects of hydroxyzine may be enhanced when given concurrently with alcohol or CNS depressants. A dosage reduction may be necessary.

■ **Nursing Diagnosis.** In addition to the anxiety related to the client's underlying condition and the ineffectiveness of the drug, the client may be at risk for the following nursing diagnoses/collaborative problems: impaired oral mucous membrane related to drug-induced dry mouth; risk of injury related to the CNS effects of the drug (dizziness, confusion, blurred vision, decreased concentration, drowsiness); and the potential complications of cardiac dysrhythmias and seizures.

■ **Implementation**

■ ***Monitoring.*** The client's level of anxiety, vital signs, and neuromuscular functioning should be monitored.

■ ***Intervention.*** Hydroxyzine is not to be administered subcutaneously, intravenously, or intraarterially because significant tissue damage may occur. It must be administered by deep IM injection; the Z-track injection is preferred.

■ ***Education.*** Clients may be instructed to use ice chips and sugarless candy or gum to manage any symptoms of dry mouth. Involuntary motor activity, such as trembling and shaking, should be reported to the prescriber; a change in medication dosage may be indicated.

■ **Evaluation.** The expected outcome of hydroxyzine therapy is that the client will state that he or she is less anxious and do not experience any adverse reactions.

dexmedetomidine [dex med i toe′ mi deen] (Precedex)

Dexmedetomidine (Precedex) is an $alpha_2$ agonist with sedative properties used to sedate intubated and mechanically ventilated patients in intensive care settings. It is administered by IV infusion at a rate of 1 μg/kg over 10 minutes initially, followed by 0.2 to 0.7 μg/kg/hr.

Hypnotics

chloral hydrate [klor al hye′ drate] (Noctec, Novo-Chlorhydrate ✤)

The CNS depressant effects produced by choral hydrate are believed to be caused by its active metabolite, trichloroethanol, but its exact mechanism of action is unknown. Chloral hydrate is indicated as a sedative and as a hypnotic. (See the Complementary and Alternative Therapies box on p. 346.)

The oral and rectal forms of choral hydrate are rapidly absorbed. The onset of action of a hypnotic dose occurs within 30 minutes, and the half-life is approximately 7 to 10 hours. It is metabolized in the liver and erythrocytes to its active metabolite, trichloroethanol; further liver metabolism is to inactive metabolites. It is excreted by the kidneys.

Side effects/adverse reactions include nausea, abdominal distress, ataxia, dizziness, drowsiness, confusion, excitability (paradoxical reaction), hallucinations, and skin rash.

The adult hypnotic dosage is 0.5 to 1 g PO or rectally 15 to 30 minutes before bedtime. The daytime sedative dosage is 250 mg three times daily, after meals. Extreme caution is used when administering chloral hydrate to children, because pediatric deaths have occurred. If the drug is administered, the child should be in a health care facility that can provide continuous monitoring (*USP DI,* 1999).

■ Nursing Management

Chloral Hydrate Therapy

See also Nursing Management: Sedative-Hypnotic Therapy, p. 329.

■ **Assessment.** The client should be assessed for medical conditions in which chloral hydrate might need to be administered with caution, such as esophagitis, gastritis, or gastric or duodenal ulcers; these conditions may be exacerbated with the oral forms of the drug. Hepatic or renal im-

Complementary and Alternative Therapies
Valerian

Valerian has been used for centuries as a sedative. It is taken orally for restlessness and insomnia and is considered likely to be effective for inducing the onset and improving the quality of sleep. Valerian does not act as a typical sleep aid in producing immediate effects; it may take 2 to 4 weeks to become effective, particularly when the sleep disorder is secondary to nervousness. The activity of valerian is thought to result from the inhibition of the enzyme system responsible for the catabolism of GABA in the brain. Increased GABA levels are associated with a decrease in CNS activity. The components of valerian may also bind to the same receptors as the benzodiazepines but with less affinity and milder effects. Theoretically, the drug may impair activities that require alertness, and the client should be so advised. Reported side effects are morning drowsiness, headache, uneasiness, ataxia, and tremor. In addition, there is the possibility that valerian could potentiate the effects of other drugs with sedative effects.

The typical dose of valerian is one cup of tea one to several times daily. The tea is prepared by steeping 2 to 3 g of the root in 150 mL of boiling water for 5 to 10 minutes and then straining the solution before consuming. The maximum daily dose is 15 grams of the root. Typically, extracts (equivalent to 2 to 3 g of the root) are taken several times daily. The tincture (1:5) is usually dosed at 15 to 20 drops in water several times daily. Alert the client that it may take 2 to 4 weeks before a significant improvement in symptoms is noted.

Information from Cirigliano, M.D. (1999). Ten most common herbs in clinical practice. In M.S. Micozzi (Ed.), *Current review of complementary medicine*. Philadelphia: Current Medicine; and Jellin, J.M., Batz, F., & Hitchens, K. (1999). *Pharmacist's letter/prescriber's letter natural medicines comprehensive database*. Stockton, CA: Therapeutic Research Faculty.

pairment should be considered, because choral hydrate is metabolized in the liver and excreted by the kidneys. There is also an increased risk of respiratory compromise in children with sleep apnea, especially in children with enlarged tonsils.

Review the client's current medication regimen for the risk of significant drug interactions, such as those that may occur when chloral hydrate is given concurrently with the following drugs:

Drug	Possible Effect and Management
alcohol or other CNS depressants	Enhanced CNS depressant effects may result. Monitor closely for respiratory depression and/or lethargy, because the dosage of one or both drugs may need to be reduced.
anticoagulants (coumarin, indanedione)	The anticoagulant may be displaced from its protein binding, especially within the first few days or weeks, leading to an enhanced hypoprothrombinemic effect. Monitor closely for bleeding tendencies.

▪ **Nursing Diagnosis.** The client receiving chloral hydrate has the potential for the following nursing diagnoses/collaborative problems: disturbed sleep pattern related to the client's underlying problem and the ineffectiveness of the drug; disturbed thought processes (confusion); impaired comfort (nausea); disturbed sleep pattern (daytime drowsiness, hangover); risk for injury related to adverse CNS reactions to the drug (dizziness, light-headedness, unsteadiness, restlessness, nervousness); and the potential complications of allergic reaction, paradoxical reaction, and convulsions.

▪ **Implementation**

▪ ***Monitoring.*** The client's sleep pattern and CNS responses to the drug should be monitored.

▪ ***Intervention.*** The chloral hydrate elixir is difficult for clients, particularly children, to ingest because of the unpleasant taste and odor. To make the elixir more palatable, mix it with fruit juice or some type of chilled fluid (e.g., ginger ale). If the client is receiving the elixir as a preoperative medication, only a small amount of liquid should be ingested; in this case a flavored extract (e.g., peppermint extract, banana extract) should be added to the elixir to make it more palatable.

Because chloral hydrate can cause gastric irritation, administer it after meals with 8 ounces of fluid (unless it is being administered as a preoperative medication). Chill suppositories in the refrigerator for ease of administration. Client safety is essential. The client should be assisted with ambulation if he or she shows signs of somnambulism, confusion, or dizziness. In addition, the prescriber should be consulted for a dosage reduction or for a change in medication for nighttime sedation.

▪ ***Education.*** Alert the client not to chew the capsule because of its unpleasant taste.

▪ **Evaluation.** As with other sedative-hypnotics, the client will report that the drug is effective in inducing nighttime sleep and daytime wakefulness without adverse effects. Client safety will be maintained.

ethchlorvynol [eth klor vi′ nole] (Placidyl)

The CNS depressant effects of ethchlorvynol are similar to those of chloral hydrate and barbiturates, but the exact mechanism of action is unknown. Ethchlorvynol is indicated for use as a sedative-hypnotic.

Absorption is good from the gastrointestinal tract. The distribution of ethchlorvynol is highly localized in lipid or fat tissues, and it has also been located in the cerebrospinal fluid, brain, bile, liver, kidneys, and spleen. It has a half-life of approximately 10 to 20 hours, an onset of action within 15 to 60 minutes, and a duration of action of approximately 5 hours. It is metabolized in the liver and excreted by the kidneys.

Side effects/adverse reactions include visual disturbances, nausea, vomiting, abdominal distress, increased weakness, facial numbness, unpleasant aftertaste, allergic reactions, paradoxical reactions (increased excitability or nervousness), and thrombocytopenia. Significant drug interactions are the same as those for chloral hydrate (see chart, left).

The sedative-hypnotic dosage for adults is 500 to 1000 mg PO at bedtime. Older adults may require lower dosages of ethchlorvynol because they are more sensitive to it. Ethchlorvynol is not available for use with children.

■ Nursing Management

Ethchlorvynol Therapy

Ethchlorvynol may produce transient giddiness and ataxia in some clients because it is absorbed rapidly. Minimize these symptoms by administering the drug with milk or food. If the client awakens in the early morning hours after a bedtime dose of ethchlorvynol, a single additional dose of 100 to 200 mg may be administered. Check to see that the dosage for older adults or debilitated clients is reduced to the smallest effective amount. The client should be instructed to report any yellowing of the skin or eyes (which might be signs of cholestatic jaundice), rash, or excessive bruising (which might indicate thrombocytopenia). (See also Nursing Management: Sedative-Hypnotic Therapy, p. 329.)

meprobamate [me proe ba′ mate] (Equanil, Miltown)

Meprobamate functions as a CNS depressant and has an unknown mechanism of action. It is indicated for use as an antianxiety agent. Absorption is good, and the half-life is approximately 10 hours. It is metabolized in the liver and excreted by the kidneys.

Side effects/adverse reactions include ataxia, drowsiness, visual disturbances, nightmares, muscle twitching, euphoria, headache, and allergic reactions. Clients taking meprobamate concomitantly with alcohol or CNS depressants may experience increased alcohol and CNS depressant effects.

The recommended adult dosage of meprobamate is 400 mg PO three or four times daily or 600 mg two times daily, up to a maximum of 2.4 g/day. Older adults may be more sensitive to this drug; their dosage should be lowered and/or they should be monitored closely. Meprobamate is not recommended for children under 6 years of age. For children 6 to 12 years old, the dosage is 100 to 200 mg PO two or three times daily. The effectiveness of meprobamate beyond 4 months of therapy has not been studied.

For the nursing management of the client receiving meprobamate, see Nursing Management: Sedative-Hypnotic Therapy, p. 329.

paraldehyde [par al′ de hyde] (Paral)

The CNS depressant effects of paraldehyde are similar to those of alcohol, barbiturates, and chloral hydrate, but the mechanism of action is unknown. Paraldehyde depresses various levels of the CNS, including the ascending reticular activating system. It is indicated as an anticonvulsant and in the past has been used as a sedative-hypnotic. The latter is no longer an approved indication because safer and more effective agents are available.

Absorption of paraldehyde is good from the gastrointestinal tract and intramuscular sites; peak serum levels are reached ½ to 1 hour after oral administration or 2½ hours after rectal administration. It has a half-life of 3 to 10 hours and is metabolized in the liver (70% to 90%), with trace amounts excreted by the kidneys. The unmetabolized paraldehyde is excreted via exhalation.

Side effects/adverse reactions include unpleasant taste, drowsiness, abdominal distress, nausea, vomiting, skin rash, muscle cramps, trembling, and confusion.

The adult anticonvulsant dosage of paraldehyde is up to 12 mL (diluted to a 10% solution) via gastric tube as needed PO every 4 hours. The rectal dosage is 10 to 20 mL. The pediatric anticonvulsant dosage is 0.3 mL/kg PO or rectally.

■ Nursing Management

Paraldehyde Therapy

■ **Assessment.** Because paraldehyde is excreted partly through the lungs and increases respiratory secretions, its administration is contraindicated in clients with bronchopulmonary disease. Oral administration is of concern in clients with gastroenteritis, because paraldehyde is a gastrointestinal irritant.

Significant drug interactions are seen when paraldehyde is used in combination with alcohol and CNS depressants (see Chloral Hydrate, p. 345). Do not give disulfiram (Antabuse) to clients receiving paraldehyde. Disulfiram decreases paraldehyde metabolism, which may lead to increased blood levels of paraldehyde and acetaldehyde.

■ **Nursing Diagnosis.** In addition to the other potential nursing diagnoses/collaborative problems for sedative-hypnotics, clients receiving paraldehyde parenterally may be at risk for impaired comfort (pain) related to the injection and for impaired gas exchange related to its effects on pulmonary capillaries.

■ **Implementation**

■ ***Monitoring.*** Monitor the client's mental status and level of consciousness. Vital signs and breath sounds should be assessed periodically in keeping with the client's status. Liver function studies should be monitored.

■ ***Intervention.*** Because paraldehyde cannot be used if the container has been open for more than 24 hours, label the container with the date and time it was opened. Do not use the drug if it is colored or has the odor of vinegar.

When giving paraldehyde orally, dilute it well in flavored syrup, iced fruit juice, or milk; the fluid should be chilled to minimize its odor and taste. Dilution also decreases gastric irritation. Administer paraldehyde in a glass container, because it reacts with plastic.

Paraldehyde will also react with plastic syringes and cause the plastic to decompose into toxic compounds. Therefore a glass syringe should be used to administer it by the IM or IV route. When administering paraldehyde by a parenteral route (rarely done), have resuscitative equipment available in the event of cardiorespiratory arrest. The client should be kept in the side-lying position to prevent aspiration of bronchial secretions, which are increased after parenteral administration of the drug.

When giving paraldehyde by the IM route, administer no more than 5 mL per injection site and rotate the sites. SC administration should be avoided because paraldehyde irritates the tissues. Rectal doses of paraldehyde should be diluted with 1 to 2 parts of olive oil, cotton-

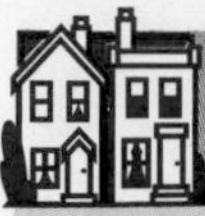

Complementary and Alternative Therapies
Melatonin

Melatonin is a hormone synthesized in the body by the pineal gland and secreted into the blood and cerebrospinal fluid. It regulates the body's circadian rhythm, endocrine secretions, and sleep patterns. After oral administration, melatonin lowers alertness, body temperature, and performance for 3 to 4 hours; it has a rapid and mild sleep-inducing effect. Melatonin formulations may be useful to treat circadian rhythm–related sleep disorders and age-related insomnia (Zisapel, 1999), but the use of melatonin for preventing jet lag needs further study (Spitzer et al., 1999). The typical dose of melatonin for insomnia is 0.3 to 5 mg at bedtime.

seed oil, or normal saline solution to prevent rectal tissue irritation.

Because paraldehyde solution is extremely volatile, avoid contact with eyes, skin, and clothing. The solution and its fumes are flammable and should be kept away from heat sources, open flames, or sparks. Ensure that the client is in a well-ventilated room, because the exhaled drug can be very pungent.

▪ ***Education.*** Prepare the client and family or caregiver for the strong unpleasant breath odor that results from paraldehyde administration, and instruct the client in oral hygiene. The client needs to be instructed to report symptoms such as yellowing of the skin or eyes, which might indicate hepatitis, and/or bloody stools, which might result from irritation of the intestinal mucosa.

▪ **Evaluation.** When paraldehyde is given as an anticonvulsant, the expected outcome is that the client will have a marked decrease or absence of seizure activity.

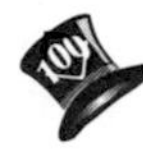

zolpidem tartrate [zole pi′ dem] (Ambien ◆)

Zolpidem tartrate is the first of a new class, nonbenzodiazepine hypnotic approved for short-term treatment of insomnia. It is more selective than the benzodiazepines in its binding to the GABA receptor. The benzodiazepines bind to omega$_1$, omega$_2$, and omega$_3$ GABA receptors, but zolpidem binds only to omega$_1$ receptors. Therefore only some of the pharmacologic properties of zolpidem are similar to those of the benzodiazepines; it lacks the anticonvulsant, muscle relaxant, and antianxiety properties associated with the benzodiazepines.

Zolpidem is rapidly absorbed orally, has a rapid onset of action, and reaches a peak serum level in ½ to 2 hours. It is metabolized in the liver into inactive metabolites and is excreted via the kidneys (48% to 67%) and feces (29% to 42%).

Side effects/adverse reactions include ataxia, depression, hypersensitivity reaction, rash, hypotension, nightmares, anterograde amnesia, drowsiness, dizziness, vertigo, dry mouth, nausea, vomiting, headache, tiredness, double vision, and diarrhea.

The adult dosage is 10 mg at bedtime. A 5 mg initial dose is recommended for older, debilitated clients and persons with hepatic insufficiency. No dosage has been established for children under 18 years old.

The client should be advised to avoid concurrent intake of alcohol and CNS depressants. It is also recommended that this medication be taken on an empty stomach, because food decreases its absorption. (See Nursing Management: Sedative-Hypnotic Therapy, p. 329.)

SUMMARY

When a client is unable to cope with a persistently stressful situation because excessive anxiety interferes with daily functioning, an antianxiety agent may be prescribed. Benzodiazepines are the most commonly used drugs in this group. Before their advent, sedatives were used to reduce nervousness or irritability by producing a soothing effect. Hypnotics are used to induce sleep. Sedatives and hypnotics differ only in the degree of CNS depression.

Benzodiazepines are among the most commonly prescribed drugs for a variety of disorders: anxiety disorders, alcohol withdrawal, preoperative medication, neuromuscular disease, and sleep and seizure disorders. Barbiturates, previously more widely used, have been largely replaced by the benzodiazepines. However, barbiturates are still indicated as hypnotic, antianxiety, anesthetic, preanesthetic, anticonvulsant, antihyperbilirubinemic, and narcoanalytic agents.

Benzodiazepines do not exert a general CNS depressant effect, and their wide range of selectivity of action allows their use for a variety of conditions—as anticonvulsants, hypnotics, muscular relaxants, and antianxiety agents. Barbiturates, on the other hand, are used for mild sedation to deep anesthesia. A barbiturate is not an analgesic, but when administered with an analgesic it reinforces analgesic effects and alters the client's emotional response to pain.

Sleep is important for humans, and both REM sleep and non-REM sleep are essential for good mental health. Antianxiety, sedative, and hypnotic drugs may be prescribed to assist with sleep.

Children and older adults are much more sensitive to the CNS depressant effects of these drugs. Children usually respond better to counseling and psychotherapy than to antianxiety agents; because of a decline in organ function, older adults are more effectively treated with shorter-acting benzodiazepines. Both groups of clients are at greater risk for paradoxical reactions than the general population.

The nurse's role in sedative-hypnotic therapy is to assess the extent of the client's sleep pattern disturbance, its cause, and the client's previous methods of coping with it. Nonpharmacologic nursing interventions to induce sleep should be used in place of or as adjuncts to a sedative-hypnotic agent. Client education should focus on good sleep hygiene and safe self-administration, emphasizing that performance may be impaired because blood levels of some of these drugs are retained. Effectiveness will be indicated by client reports of feeling rested without residual drowsiness during the day.

Although antianxiety, sedative, and hypnotic drugs create many of the same responses within the client, the nurse must be knowledgeable about the specific agents used. Because these agents exert CNS effects, the nurse needs to be aware that the client may be at risk for injury, sensory-perceptual alterations, self-concept disturbance, and further sleep pattern disturbance. The gastrointestinal effects of many of these agents may result in constipation. As with all medications, clients and their families may experience a knowledge deficit related to their drug therapy.

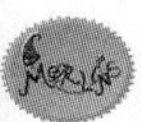

Critical Thinking Questions

1. What factors need to be included in an education plan for a client taking benzodiazepines? What if the client were a young married woman? An older adult? An Asian client? A child?
2. What nonpharmacologic nursing measures should accompany the administration of a sleep medication?
3. What actions might a nurse take if a client experiences altered comfort at night as well as insomnia?

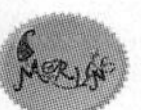

Collaborative Learning Activities

For Collaborative Learning Activities, go to mosby.com/MERLIN/McKenry/.

CASE STUDY

For a Case Study that will help ensure mastery of this chapter content, go to mosby.com/MERLIN/McKenry/.

BIBLIOGRAPHY

Abramowicz, M. (Ed.). (1992). Flumazenil. *Medical Letter, 34*(874), 66.

American Hospital Formulary Service. (1999). *AHFS drug information '99.* Bethesda, MD: American Society of Hospital Pharmacists.

Anderson, K.N., Anderson, L.E., & Glanze, W.D. (Eds.) (1998). *Mosby's medical, nursing, & allied health dictionary* (5th ed.). St. Louis: Mosby.

Anton, R.F., Kranzler, H.R., McEvoy, J.P., Moak, D.H., & Bianca, R. (1997). A double-blind comparison of abecarnil and diazepam in the treatment of uncomplicated alcohol withdrawal. *Psychopharmacology Abstract, 131*(2), 123-129.

Asplund, R. (1999). Sleep disorders in the elderly. *Drugs Aging, 14*(2), 91-103.

Crismon, M.L. (1992). Insomnia. In M.A. Koda-Kimble & L.Y. Young (Eds.), *Applied therapeutics: The clinical use of drugs* (5th ed.). Vancouver, WA: Applied Therapeutics.

DiPiro, J.T., Talbert, R.L., Yee, G.C., Matzke, G.R., Wells, B.G., & Posey, L.M. (Eds.) (1995). *Pharmacotherapy: A pathophysiologic approach* (3rd ed.). Stamford, CT: Appleton & Lange.

Dopheide, J.A. (1995). Sleep disorders. In L.Y. Young & M.A. Koda-Kimble (Eds.), *Applied therapeutics: The clinical use of drugs* (6th ed.). Vancouver, WA: Applied Therapeutics.

Drug Facts and Comparisons. (2000). St. Louis: Facts and Comparisons.

Drug Product Update. (1996). Halcion, Xanax Changes. *ASHP Newsletter, 29*(10), 5.

Edmonds, S. et al. (Eds.) (1995). Abecarnil shows promise in generalized anxiety disorder. *Drugs & Therapeutic Perspectives, 5*(12), 7-8.

Glod, C.A. (1992). Xanax: Pros and cons. *Journal of Psychosocial Nursing & Mental Health Services, 30*(6), 36-37.

Gottlieb, G.L. (1990). Sleep disorders and their management: Special considerations in the elderly. *American Journal of Medicine, 88*(suppl 3A), 29S.

Grimsley, S.R. (1995). Anxiety disorders. In L.Y. Young & M.A. Koda-Kimble (Eds.), *Applied therapeutics: The clinical use of drugs* (6th ed.). Vancouver, WA: Applied Therapeutics.

Hartmann, P.M. (1995). Drug treatment of insomnia: Indications and newer agents. *American Family Physician, 51*(1), 191-194.

Hoehns, J.D. & Perry, P.J. (1993). Zolpidem: A nonbenzodiazepine hypnotic for treatment of insomnia. *Clinical Pharmacy, 12*(11), 814-828.

Holbrook, A.M., Crowther, R., Lotter, A., Cheng, C.,& King, D. (1999). Metaanalysis of benzodiazepine use in the treatment of acute alcohol withdrawal. *Canadian Medical Association Journal, 160*(5), 649-655.

Jellin, J.M. (Ed.) (1991). Neurology/psychiatry. *Pharmacist's Letter, 7*(11), 61.

Kudzma, E.C. (1992). Drug responses: All bodies are not created equal. *American Journal of Nursing, 92*(12), 48-50.

Lammon, C.A. & Adams A.H. (1993). Recognizing benzodiazepine overdose. *Nursing, 23*(1), 33.

Lin, D.M., Lau, J.K., Smith, R., Phillips, P., Antal, E., & Poland, R.E. (1988). Comparison of alprazolam plasma levels in normal Asian and Caucasian volunteers. *Psychopharmacology Bulletin, 96*, 365.

McCance, K.L. & Huether, S.E. (1998). *Pathophysiology: The biological basis for disease in adults and children* (3rd ed.). St. Louis: Mosby.

McCue, J.D. et al. (1993). *Geriatric drug handbook for long-term care.* Baltimore: Williams & Wilkins.

Melmon, K.L., Morelli, H.F., Hoffman, B.B., & Nierberg, D.W. (1992). *Melmon's & Morelli's Clinical pharmacology: Basic principles in therapeutics* (3rd ed.). New York: McGraw-Hill.

Mosby's GenRx. (1999). St. Louis: Mosby.

Pasero, C., Reed, B.A., & McCaffery, M. (1999). Pain in the elderly. In M. McCaffery & C. Pasero (Eds.), *Pain clinical manual* (2nd ed.). St. Louis: Mosby.

Physicians' Desk Reference (53rd ed.). (1999). Montvale, NJ: Medical Economics.

Regimen: An update on long-term care drug therapy. (1995). Monitoring psychoactive drug use in nursing home patients. *Journal of the National Association of Retail Druggists, 118*(3), 1-4.

Sherman, D. (1991). Evaluation and treatment of sleep disorders. *Contemporary Long Term Care, 14*(12), 70.

Spitzer, R.L., Terman, M., Williams, J.B., Terman, J.S., Malt, U.F., Singer, F., & Lewy, A.J. (1999). Jet lag: Clinical features, validation of a new syndrome-specific scale, and lack of response to melatonin in a randomised, double-blind trial, *American Journal of Psychiatry 156*(9):1392-1396.

United States Pharmacopeia Dispensing Information (USP DI): Drug information for the health care professional (19th ed.). (1999). Rockville, MD: United States Pharmacopeial Convention.

Wong, D.L. (1999). *Whaley & Wong's Nursing care of infants and children* (6th ed.). St Louis: Mosby.

Zisapel, N. (1999). The use of melatonin for the treatment of insomnia, *Biological Signals and Receptors 8*(1-2):84-89.

17 ANTICONVULSANTS

Chapter Focus

Epilepsy is the second most common neurologic disease in North America (after stroke); it affects 1 out of 50 children and 1 out of 100 adults. As with other chronic disorders, nurses play a key role in assisting clients to manage their epilepsy effectively. This chapter provides information about anticonvulsant medications as a basis for that role.

Learning Objectives

1. Describe the international classification of epileptic seizures.
2. Identify observations to be made about a client having a seizure.
3. Discuss the nursing management for anticonvulsant therapy.
4. Identify the major anticonvulsant drug classifications, including examples of drugs and their primary methods of seizure-control activity.
5. List the common side effects/adverse reactions of anticonvulsants.
6. Implement an appropriate plan of care for a client receiving an anticonvulsant drug or drugs.

Key Terms

epilepsy, p. 351
focal seizure, p. 351
generalized tonic-clonic (grand mal) seizures, p. 351
primary (idiopathic) epilepsy, p. 352
secondary (nonidiopathic) epilepsy, p. 352
serum half-life, p. 354
status epilepticus, p. 352
toxemia of pregnancy, p. 372

Key Drugs [✔]

phenobarbital, p. 362
phenytoin, p. 358

Epilepsy is a group of chronic neurologic disorders resulting from a brain dysfunction or an abnormal discharge of cerebral neurons. This condition is characterized by sporadic, recurrent episodes of convulsive seizures, sensory disturbances, abnormal behavior, loss of consciousness, or all of these symptoms. Although nearly 70% of seizures do not have an identifiable cause (primary or idiopathic epilepsy), approximately 30% have an underlying cause (secondary epilepsy) that is treatable (e.g., head injury, cerebrovascular infarct or hemorrhage, infection, brain tumor, drug toxicity, or metabolic imbalance). The terms used to classify epileptic seizures are summarized in Box 17-1.

CLASSIFICATION OF SEIZURES

The choice of an appropriate anticonvulsant drug depends on an accurate diagnosis and a classification of the seizure type (see Box 17-1). A complete medical history, laboratory tests, a neurologic examination, and an electroencephalogram (EEG) are necessary for classification. Computerized tomography (CT) and magnetic resonance imaging (MRI) may also be used to detect anatomic defects or to locate small focal brain lesions. Identifying specific seizure types is critical to the development of a treatment plan.

TYPES OF SEIZURES

Partial simple motor epilepsy is sometimes described as a type of **focal seizure**; it is associated with irritation of a specific part of the brain. A single body part (e.g., finger or extremity) may jerk, and such movements may end spontaneously or spread over the entire musculature. Consciousness may not be lost unless the seizure develops into a generalized convulsion.

Partial complex seizures are characterized by brief alterations in consciousness, unusual stereotyped movements (e.g., chewing or swallowing movements) repeated over and over, changes in temperament, confusion, and feelings of unreality. These seizures are often associated with generalized tonic-clonic seizures and are likely to be resistant to drug therapy.

Generalized absence, simple or complex, seizures are most often seen in childhood and consist of temporary lapses in consciousness that last for a few seconds. The person does not convulse but appears to stare into space or daydream, is inattentive, and may exhibit a few rhythmic movements of the eyes (slight blinking), head, or hands. He or she may have many attacks in a single day. The EEG records a 3/sec spike wave pattern. A generalized tonic-clonic type of seizure sometimes follows an attack of generalized absence seizures. Other types of seizures may occur when the child reaches adulthood.

Generalized tonic-clonic seizures are the types most commonly seen. Such attacks may be characterized by an aura and a sudden loss of consciousness and motor control. The aura is specific to the individual—it may consist of numbness, visual disturbances, or a particular form of dizziness that warns the client of an approaching seizure. The client falls forcefully and has a series of tonic (stiffening, increased muscle tone) and clonic (rapid, synchronous jerking) muscular contractions. The eyes roll upward, the arms flex, and the legs extend. The force of the muscular contractions forces air out of the lungs, which accounts for the cry that the client may make on falling. Respirations are sus-

BOX 17-1

International Classification of Seizures

Partial Seizures

Simple (No Impairment of Consciousness)

- Motor symptoms
- Sensory symptoms (hallucinations of sight, hearing, or taste); somatosensory symptoms (tingling)
- Autonomic symptoms—autonomic nervous system responses
- Psychologic symptoms (personality changes)

Complex (Impaired Consciousness)

- Cognitive symptoms (memory impairment, confusion)
- Affective symptoms (bizarre behavioral effects)
- Psychosensory symptoms (automatisms—repetition, purposeless behaviors)
- Psychomotor symptoms (complex symptoms that may include an aura, automatism [i.e., chewing, swallowing movements], unreal feelings, bizarre behaviors, and motor seizures)
- Compound symptoms (tonic, clonic, or tonic-clonic seizures)

Partial Seizures, Secondarily Generalized

- Unilateral seizures
- Predominantly unilateral seizures

Generalized Seizures (Convulsive or Nonconvulsive)

Widespread involvement of both cerebral hemispheres

- Tonic-clonic
- Tonic (sustained contractions of large muscle groups)
- Clonic (various dysrhythmic contractions in the body)
- Myoclonic (unaltered consciousness, isolated clonic contractions)
- Absence (brief loss of consciousness for a few seconds, no confusion, EEG demonstrates 3/sec spike wave patterns)
- Atonic (head drop or falling down symptoms)

Unclassified Seizures

Available data incomplete, inadequate, or lacks classification status (such as neonatal seizures)

pended temporarily, the skin becomes diaphoretic and cyanotic, perspiration and saliva flow, and the client may froth at the mouth and bite the tongue if it gets caught between the teeth. Incontinence may occur. When the seizure subsides, the client regains partial consciousness, may complain of aching, and tends to fall into a deep sleep.

Status epilepticus is a state of acute prolonged seizure activity; it is a clinical emergency. With this condition, recurrent generalized tonic-clonic seizures last at least 30 minutes without an intervening stay of consciousness. A 10% to 20% mortality rate results from anoxia in this state. *The major cause of status epilepticus is noncompliance with the drug regimen;* other causes include cerebral infarction, central nervous system (CNS) tumor or infection, trauma, or low blood concentrations of calcium or glucose.

Mixed seizures are seen in some clients who have more than one type of seizure disorder. This is significant because different types of seizures respond specifically to certain anticonvulsant drugs. The aim of therapy is to find the drug or drugs that will control the seizures effectively with a minimum of undesirable side effects and restore physiologic homeostasis to arrest convulsive activity.

RELATIONSHIP OF AGE TO SEIZURES

There is a relationship between age and onset of an epileptic seizure state. Most clients diagnosed with epilepsy have their initial seizure before the age of 20; however, seizures may have an onset at any age in life. **Idiopathic or primary epilepsy** involves seizures that are undefined, unascertainable, or genetic in origin or cause. These types of seizures are often diagnosed between the ages of 5 and 20. Onset before or after this age period is often a result of **nonidiopathic** (identifiable, ascertainable) causes and is termed **secondary** (acquired, organic) **epilepsy.**

Neonates. Neonatal seizures occur in newborn children less than 1 month old. Among the more common causes of seizures in this age-group are congenital defects or malformation of the brain, abnormalities or infections (meningitis, encephalitis, abscess) within the CNS, hypoxia (in utero or during delivery), premature birth, and defects in metabolism. These epileptic seizures are also referred to as *secondary, organic,* or *acquired* because they originate from an identifiable preceding condition or cause.

Infants. The seizure types most commonly diagnosed in infants less than 2 years of age include generalized tonic-clonic seizures and partial seizures. The atonic epileptic seizure seen in later development (ages 2 to 5 years) may be preceded by infantile spasms before 2 years of age. The infantile spasm is not classified as a type of epileptic seizure itself. Among the more common causes of infantile seizures are those reported in the neonatal state and, additionally, injury in the perinatal period, infection, exposure to toxins (in utero caused by maternal exposure to drug use, misuse, or abuse), maternal exposure to x-rays, and postnatal trauma.

Children. The seizure types commonly diagnosed in children 2 to 5 years of age include generalized tonic-clonic seizures and atonic seizures. The causes are similar to those mentioned in neonates and infants with the addition of chronic diseases involving the CNS. The parents may wrongly believe that the child has a behavioral disorder rather than a treatable seizure disorder.

Brain tumors and vascular disease may cause seizures in children 6 years of age and older. Sometimes the convulsive seizure is associated with a brain infection, head trauma, fever, growth of scar tissue, cerebrovascular disease, the presence of a toxin or a poison, or drug withdrawal.

In children 5 to 16 years of age, the seizure types that emerge in diagnosis are absence seizures and generalized tonic-clonic seizures, which may be idiopathic in origin. Seizure types such as partial, myoclonic, and less commonly generalized tonic-clonic seizures may be caused by neurologic diseases, infection, postnatal trauma, or head trauma (accident- or sport-related).

Young Adults. Within the 16- to 25-year age-group, generalized seizures may be idiopathic in origin. Partial seizures and the less commonly seen generalized seizures may result from the use of alcohol, social/recreational drug use, drug abuse or misuse, or head injury.

Adults. In clients over 20 years of age, the seizures that emerge often are of the generalized type, which may be idiopathic. Also seen are partial seizures and less commonly generalized seizures, which may have been precipitated by trauma to the head or a tumor of the brain.

Older Adults. Persons over 60 years of age are at greater risk for seizure episodes. Osteoporosis and cerebrovascular disease are common in this population, and seizures may lead to fractures, intracranial bleeding, neurologic deficits, cognitive impairments, and severe limitations in daily functioning. Common causes of seizures in older adults include trauma, brain tumors, vascular disease, embolic stroke, and Alzheimer's disease (Rowan, 1995).

ANTICONVULSANT THERAPY

Secondary seizures usually respond to correction of the underlying condition and perhaps short-term use of anticonvulsants, but primary recurrent seizures require long-term anticonvulsant drug therapy. The primary goal of drug therapy is to control or prevent the recurrence of the seizure disorder. There is no ideal anticonvulsant drug, but the following characteristics are highly desirable:

- The drug should be highly effective but exhibit a low incidence of toxicity.
- The drug should be effective against more than one type of seizure and for mixed seizures.
- The drug should be long acting and nonsedating so that the client is not inconvenienced with the need for multiple daily drug dosing or excessive drowsiness.
- The drug should be well tolerated by the client and inexpensive, because the client may need to take it for years or for the rest of his or her life.

- Tolerance to the therapeutic effects of the drug should not develop.
- The drug should control seizures and permit the client to function effectively in any environment.

The major drugs used in the treatment of partial seizures and generalized tonic-clonic seizures are phenytoin (Dilantin), carbamazepine (Tegretol), and the barbiturates. Phenytoin is the oldest nonsedating anticonvulsant drug in clinical use and is the most commonly prescribed anticonvulsant in North America. Several more recently released miscellaneous anticonvulsants include felbamate (Felbatol), gabapentin (Neurontin), lamotrigine (Lamictal), tiagabine (Gabatril), and topiramate (Topamax). These new drugs are a welcome addition to the therapeutic options in the treatment of epilepsy, but they also create a dilemma because their individual places and their optimal use in the treatment of the various forms of epilepsy have yet to be determined (Bourgeois, 1998).

Although the exact mode and site of action of the anticonvulsant drugs are complex and incompletely understood, a major mechanism of action appears to relate to stabilization of the cell membrane by altering cation transport, especially sodium, potassium, and calcium. For example, phenytoin (a hydantoin) decreases abnormal seizure discharge by blocking sodium channels and perhaps calcium influx; phenytoin suppresses seizures by stabilizing cell membrane excitability and reducing the spread of seizure discharge. Carbamazepine also enhances inactivation of the sodium channel, which alters neuronal excitability (decreases synaptic transmission). Therefore the two main pharmacologic effects of the anticonvulsant drugs are the following:

- To increase motor cortex threshold to reduce its response to incoming electric or chemical stimulation
- To depress or reduce the spread of a seizure discharge from its focus or origin by depressing synaptic transport or decreasing nerve conduction

Anticonvulsants fall into five major classifications: hydantoins, barbiturates, succinimides, benzodiazepines, and a miscellaneous group. The miscellaneous anticonvulsants include carbamazepine (Tegretol), valproate (Depacon), primidone (Mysoline), acetazolamide (Diamox), magnesium sulfate, felbamate (Felbatol), gabapentin (Neurontin), lamotrigine (Lamictal), tiagabine (Gabatril), and topiramate (Topamax); these drugs are not chemically similar to one another (Box 17-2 and Table 17-1).

BOX 17-2

Anticonvulsant Agents for Seizure Disorders

The agents considered most effective with the least toxicity in treating seizure disorders are as follows:*

Generalized Tonic-Clonic Seizures

valproate (Depacon)
phenytoin (Dilantin)
carbamazepine (Tegretol)

Absence Seizures

ethosuximide (Zarontin)
valproate (Depacon)

Simple or Complex Partial Seizures

carbamazepine (Tegretol)
phenytoin (Dilantin)
valproate (Depacon)

Myoclonic Seizures

valproate (Depacon)
clonazepam (Klonopin, Rivotril ♣)

Information from Lott, R.S. (1995). Seizure disorders. In L.Y. Young & M.A. Koda-Kimble (Eds.), *Applied therapeutics: The clinical use of drugs.* Vancouver, WA: Applied Therapeutics.
*Listed in order of preference.

Nursing Management

Anticonvulsant Therapy

A client for whom anticonvulsants have been prescribed is treated most effectively with a holistic approach. This client has many special problems, including the fear of a sudden loss of physical and emotional control and the stigma of seizures. In recent years, emphasis has been placed on public education on epilepsy to dispel the myths associated with it. The client needs information about the seizure condition and its management, as well as psychosocial support from the nurse. The client should understand that the condition can be controlled or modified with medication. The goal is to attain maximum seizure control with minimal medication side effects. The anticonvulsant or combination of anticonvulsants prescribed depends on the type of seizure, whether the client is having more than one type of seizure, or whether the seizures are difficult to control. Finding the appropriate regimen for each client takes time.

The clinical effectiveness of anticonvulsant therapy varies with the pharmacokinetics and mechanism of action of the drug, as well as the serum levels achieved with scheduled drug dosing. Be aware that the same dose of an anticonvulsant may result in different blood levels in different clients. This variation results from a complex of interrelated factors, including individual absorption, metabolism, distribution, and excretion. These factors may be affected by genetic and/or environmental factors, concomitant ailments (e.g., renal or hepatic dysfunctions), concurrent medications, diet, individual client compliance, and physical status. The dosage of certain drugs needs to be adjusted in order to obtain optimal therapeutic effects, and this dosage may vary widely among clients.

Therapeutic dosage ranges are intended to serve merely as rough guides to therapy; they are not inflexible limits. The ranges provide a point from which the dosage of a drug may be individualized to account for the extremes in varia-

TABLE 17-1 **Pharmacokinetic Overview of Selected Anticonvulsant Drugs**

Name	Pharmacokinetics	Therapeutic Plasma Levels in Adults (μg/mL)	Serum Half-life (hours)
carbamazepine (Tegretol)	Absorption: slow and variable Metabolism: liver Excretion: urine, feces	4-12	1 dose: 25-65 Multidose: Adults 12-17
clonazepam (Klonopin, Rivotril 🍁)	Absorption: good Metabolism: liver Excretion: urine	0.02-0.08	18-50
divalproex (Depakote, Epival 🍁)	Absorption: 1-4 hours Metabolism: liver Excretion: urine, small amount from feces and lungs	50-100	6-16
ethosuximide (Zarontin)	Absorption: good Metabolism: liver Excretion: urine	40-100	Adults: 56-60 Children: 30-36
felbamate (Felbatol)	Absorption: good Metabolism: liver Excretion: urine and feces	Not determined	13-23
methsuximide (Celontin)	Absorption: good Metabolism: liver Excretion: urine	10-40	1-3 Active metabolite: 36-45
phenobarbital (Luminal and others)	Absorption: good Metabolism: liver Excretion: urine	10-40	Adults: 53-118 Children: 40-70
phenytoin (Dilantin)	Absorption: orally, slow; poor in neonates Metabolism: liver Excretion: urine and feces	10-20	Adults: 22 (range 7-42)
primidone (Mysoline, Sertan 🍁)	Absorption: good Metabolism: liver Excretion: urine	5-12	primidone: 3-24 and metabolites phenobarbital: 75-126 PEMA: 10-25
valproic acid (Depakene)	Absorption: complete and rapid Metabolism: kidney Excretion: urine, small amount from lungs and feces	50-100	Adults: 6-16

tions to response and adverse reactions. The client beginning anticonvulsant therapy should have his or her serum levels measured to establish an individual level–dose ratio. This level tends to be constant for an individual but varies considerably among clients. The time required to reach a steady serum level is usually about four to five times the half-life of a drug. A convenient time for serum level measurement is 1 month after initiating therapy, because levels measured much earlier may be lower than the steady-state level finally achieved.

The **serum half-life** of a drug (the time required for the drug serum level to drop to 50% of its initial value when no additional drug is administered) is a measure of its rate of excretion and depends on the client's age. As discussed in Chapter 3, the pharmacokinetics of a drug are affected by age. For example, drug metabolism is relatively slow in neonates, but on a mg/kg body weight basis it is higher in infants and young children than in adults. Older adults, whose metabolism is decreased, usually require a lower dosage schedule (see Chapter 8).

Women with epilepsy constitute 0.5% of all pregnancies (Nulman, Laslo, & Koren, 1999). Epilepsy may worsen during pregnancy, with status epilepticus increasing in frequency during gestation and labor. Many of the commonly used anticonvulsants are established teratogens (see the Pregnancy Safety box on p. 355). Some anticonvulsants appear in breast milk. Emotional stress (psychologic, occupational, physiologic, marital, economic) may influence seizure frequency. With proper preconceptual and perinatal management, up to 95% of pregnant women with epilepsy have been reported to have favorable outcomes (Nulman et al., 1999).

Pregnancy Safety
Anticonvulsants

Category	Drug
C	acetazolamide, carbamazepine, ethotoin, felbamate, gabapentin, lamotrigine, oxcarbazepine, phenytoin, tiagabine, topiramate, zonisamide
D	barbiturates, divalproex, paramethadione, valproate
Unclassified	clonazepam, clorazepate, diazepam, mephenytoin, primidone, succinimides

A diagnosis of epilepsy no longer implies a lifetime of drug therapy. Studies have indicated that anticonvulsant drugs may be withdrawn from selected clients who have been seizure free for at least 2 years. In long-term studies, seizures recurred in 12% to 36% of the clients monitored up to 23 years after complete drug withdrawal.

Certain risk factors help to predict which clients may experience a recurrence of seizures after drug withdrawal; such factors include an onset of seizures after 12 years of age, a family history of seizure activity, a period of 2 to 6 years before the seizures are finally controlled, a large number of seizures before control (>30) or a total of more than 100 convulsions, an abnormal EEG even with therapy, the presence of an organic neurologic disorder or moderate to severe mental retardation and, perhaps, the withdrawal from phenytoin or valproate drugs, which appears to produce a higher rate of recurrence when compared to other drugs (Lott, 1995). More than 90% of the recurrences occur within the first year of withdrawal, with most occurring during the withdrawal period or shortly thereafter (Dichter, 1992). Fewer seizures occur when the withdrawal is planned or gradual or when the dosage is reduced to minimal maintenance therapy.

■ **Assessment.** Along with a general health assessment and drug history, assessment of the client with a convulsive disorder includes data specific to the seizures. These data include the number of seizures within a specific time, precipitating events or activities, the presence of sensations or perceptions that the client experiences before a seizure (called an aura), and the character of seizures.

Assess the presence or absence of an aura and its nature. It may also be helpful to evaluate the ability of the client to describe the aura (somatic, visceral, psychic). It can also be useful to note the presence or absence of a cry. The onset of seizure should be assessed for the site of initial body movements, deviation of the head and eyes, chewing and salivation, body posture, and sensory changes.

After seizure onset, it is important to note the characteristics of the tonic and clonic phases. Characteristics include body movements as the seizure progresses, skin color, airway clearance, pupillary changes, incontinence, and the duration of each phase.

After the tonic and clonic phases, try to assess the duration of and behavior during the relaxation (sleep) phase. During the post-ictal phase, note not only its duration but also the client's general behavior, ability to remember anything about the seizure, orientation, pupillary changes, headache, and any injuries present. The duration of the entire seizure, the level of consciousness, and the length of unconsciousness (if present) should be described as accurately as possible. Often the nurse is not present when a seizure occurs; family, friends, or other witnesses may provide valuable information about the seizure.

In addition, assess the client's understanding and management of the anticonvulsant medication regimen. One of the most common causes of seizure exacerbations is the mismanagement of medications. Up to 50% of clients do not take their medications regularly (Legion, 1991). Many do not understand the concepts of steady blood levels and half-life. Some clients use the drugs as they would aspirin, taking extra doses when they are afraid they might have a seizure. Some are afraid of the harm they think their medications could cause, whereas others are concerned about becoming addicted to the drugs. Understand the client's use of medications as an attempt to gain control, and provide information to allow him or her to manage the therapeutic regimen effectively.

■ **Nursing Diagnosis.** In addition to the selected nursing diagnoses presented in the Nursing Care Plan on p. 356, the client receiving anticonvulsant therapy should be assessed for the following nursing diagnoses/collaborative problems: activity intolerance related to anticonvulsant-induced weakness; constipation or diarrhea related to gastrointestinal effects; impaired comfort related to headache, nausea, vomiting, or dermatologic effects; impaired protection related to drug-induced hematologic dysfunction; disturbed thought processes related to adverse CNS effects; disturbed body image related to hydantoin-induced enlargement of the facial features, hirsutism, alopecia, or gynecomastia (in males); excess fluid volume related to carbamazepine-induced water intoxication; risk for injury related to client's underlying seizure activity, ineffectiveness of the anticonvulsant drug, and the CNS, visual, or hypotensive effects; impaired home maintenance related to drug-imposed restrictions on driving and other activities; impaired skin integrity related to drug-induced rash; and ineffective breathing pattern (hypoventilation) related to the respiratory depressant effects of phenobarbital; and the potential complications of gingival hyperplasia (hydantoin), cognitive impairment, allergic reaction, blood dyscrasias, and hepatotoxicity.

■ **Implementation**

■ ***Monitoring.*** Therapeutic alternatives (monotherapy or polytherapy) are selected to best control the client's seizure. For many anticonvulsants, the optimal therapeutic blood levels (the level of medication needed to control seizures) are known. Therapeutic drug monitoring includes comparing the results of serum concentrations with the client's clinical response. This monitoring has reduced the need for

Nursing Care Plan

Selected Nursing Diagnoses for the Client Receiving Anticonvulsant Therapy

Nursing Diagnosis	Outcome Criteria	Nursing Interventions
Deficient knowledge related to newly prescribed or altered anticonvulsant drug therapy	The client will describe the seizure condition, how the drug therapy relates to the condition, how and when to take the medications, common drug interactions, safety precautions, common side effects and which of these warrant reporting, and storage requirements of the drugs. The client will demonstrate less anxiety related to fear of the unknown, loss of control, and misconceptions.	Assess learning needs and learning readiness. Plan with the client and family for the achievement of realistic goals. Provide information to meet outcome criteria.
Ineffective therapeutic regimen management	The client will self-administer medications safely and accurately.	Determine the client's reasons for inaccuracies of dosing and take appropriate teaching/counseling interventions. Provide needed drug information concerning rationale for the specific client's seizure status. Discuss the increased possibility of seizures with ineffective management of the regimen.
Risk for injury related to effects of anticonvulsant drug therapy	The client will maintain anticonvulsant drug therapy without untoward side effects, adverse reactions, and toxicity.	Administer drug safely and accurately. Observe the client for drowsiness, ataxia, behavioral changes, slurred speech, mental confusion, vertigo, and excessive sedation (see drug monographs for drug-specific side effects/adverse reactions). Instruct client about symptoms to be reported. Explain the importance of Medic Alert card/tag. Discourage self-altering of medication regimen. Caution against activities requiring coordination and alertness until responses to drugs are known.

polydrug anticonvulsant therapy and has added greater efficiency in drug selection for each client.

Increased anticonvulsant serum levels may signal impending toxic effects. In general, adverse reactions are more serious at higher serum levels. Maintaining a serum level within the therapeutic range is a challenge with some clients (see the Special Considerations for Children box and the Special Considerations for Older Adults box on p. 357). The challenge surfaces when other drugs are added or deleted from the client's regimen, a client mismanages the medication regimen, there is an organ system dysfunction as seen in the hepatorenal systems, or undesirable drug effects cause the client to withdraw from drug therapy. Fully informing clients about the drug therapy and the need for serum concentrations within the therapeutic range may reduce therapeutic failures caused by adverse reactions or ineffective management of the medication regimen.

The most common medical test to evaluate seizure activity is the EEG, a recording of electrical activity generated by the brain that is made by placing electrodes on the scalp. In monitoring the results of EEGs, the client's progress is indicated by decreased seizure activity of the brain. Baseline vital signs and liver function and blood studies should also be performed.

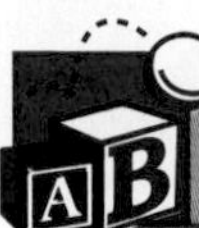

Special Considerations for Children
Anticonvulsants

Chewable phenytoin tablets are not indicated for once-daily administration.

If skin rash develops with the use of phenytoin, discontinue drug immediately and notify prescriber.

Avoid IM phenytoin injections.

Be aware that neonates whose mothers received hydantoin drugs during pregnancy may require vitamin K to treat hypoprothrombinemia.

The young client (under age 23) is more susceptible to gingival hyperplasia, especially with phenytoin or mephenytoin therapy. Gingivitis or gum inflammation usually starts during the first 6 months of drug therapy, although severe hyperplasia is unlikely in dosages under 500 mg/day. A dental program of teeth cleaning and plaque control started within 7 to 10 days of initiating drug therapy helps to reduce the rate and severity of this condition.

Coarse facial features and excessive body hair growth are more commonly reported in young clients.

Impaired school performance is reported with long-term, high-dose hydantoin therapy (especially at high or toxic serum levels).

Whenever possible, other anticonvulsants should be considered first because they are less apt to cause the adverse reactions induced by the hydantoins.

Children receiving valproate, especially those up to 2 years old or those receiving multiple anticonvulsant drugs, are at a greater risk for developing serious hepatotoxicity. This risk decreases with advancing age.

Information from *United States Pharmacopeia Dispensing Information (USP DI): Drug information for the health care professional* (19th ed.). (1999). Rockville, MD: United States Pharmacopeial Convention.

Subjective data to be obtained include the client's understanding of and reaction to the convulsive disorder and drug therapy.

■ ***Intervention.*** One of the characteristics of the anticonvulsant drugs is that either the parent drug or the active metabolite has a long serum half-life. Therefore the exact daily medication schedule is seldom critical. Administration of these drugs may be one to three times daily.

The first serum concentration after the first IV dose is half the peak value attained during long-term administration. Therefore the client can attain a steady-state serum concentration quickly if the first IV dose is twice the maintenance dose. In adults, a loading (IV) dose of phenytoin (1000 mg or 13 to 14 mg/kg body weight—more than twice the usual maintenance dose of 300 mg/half-life of approximately 24 hours) will produce a therapeutic serum concentration of 10 to 20 μg/mL. The IV route is necessary because

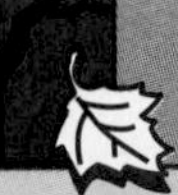

Special Considerations for Older Adults
Anticonvulsants

If skin rash develops with the use of phenytoin, discontinue drug immediately and notify the prescriber.

Debilitated clients or persons with renal or liver disease have a greater risk of developing toxicity with the anticonvulsant agents. Lower doses of the anticonvulsants will help to avoid adverse reactions.

Older adults tend to metabolize anticonvulsants more slowly; thus drug accumulation and toxicity may occur. Monitor closely because dosage adjustments (lower dosages) may be necessary.

Serum albumin levels may be lower in older adults, resulting in decreased protein binding of bound drugs, such as phenytoin and valproate. Monitor closely because lower drug dosages may be necessary.

Administer IV doses at a rate slower than the recommended rate for an adult. The rate of administration for phenytoin in older adults should be 5 to 10 mg/min, up to a maximum of 25 mg/min.

Information from *United States Pharmacopeia Dispensing Information (USP DI): Drug information for the health care professional* (19th ed.). (1999). Rockville, MD: United States Pharmacopeial Convention.

phenytoin is absorbed very slowly and erratically by the IM route—the water solubility of the drug decreases, and phenytoin crystals precipitate in the muscle. A high degree of local irritation has also been reported with IM injection.

Although anticonvulsant agents are usually given orally, there are a few parenteral forms. These are reserved for occasions in which the parenteral form is the best choice of therapy. Table 17-2 lists these conditions or situations and the parenteral drugs indicated for the treatment of each. Anticonvulsant drugs should be administered intravenously in emergency situations (e.g., status epilepticus) because of the slow absorption from the IM injection site and the low peak serum levels achieved.

Anticonvulsant drugs should be administered using as long an interval between doses as possible, depending on the half-life. In general, anticonvulsant drugs that have an elimination half-life of 24 hours or more need to be administered only once a day to maintain a therapeutic serum concentration. The daily dose may be administered at bedtime to overcome the sedation seen with peak levels of anticonvulsant drugs.

In a nonemergency situation it is best to make changes in drug therapy with one drug at a time. The nurse and the client must be aware that it takes four to five half-life intervals to achieve the total therapeutic effect of the new drug regimen each time a new anticonvulsant drug is started or the dosage of a drug is increased or decreased. This time interval allows the concentration of the new drug to reach

TABLE 17-2 Indications for Parenteral Use of Anticonvulsants

Parenteral Drug	Use
barbiturates, especially phenobarbital; also amobarbital, pentobarbital sodium, and secobarbital sodium	Eclampsia, status epilepticus, severe recurrent seizures, tetanus, convulsant drug toxicity, other convulsive states
phenytoin	Status epilepticus, seizure during neurosurgery
magnesium sulfate	Severe toxemias of pregnancy (preeclampsia and eclampsia)
benzodiazepines: diazepam, lorazepam	Status epilepticus; severe, recurrent seizures

a steady state or the drug being discontinued to decrease by 95%.

When serum levels of anticonvulsants are ordered, they should be scheduled to be measured at least 8 hours since the last dose of a once-daily medication.

▪ ***Education.*** The client undergoing anticonvulsant therapy should be encouraged to adopt a moderate lifestyle, follow an appropriate diet, and get sufficient rest and exercise. Stressful situations should be avoided; if this is not possible, the prescriber should be notified for dosage adjustments in ongoing stressful conditions. The client should be advised against drinking alcohol and taking OTC medications (see specific drugs for interactions or effects). The client should understand that some anticonvulsants take days or weeks to reach an effective level in the body. A missed dose may result in a seizure in a few days, and taking an extra dose will not prevent an impending seizure. A client who has been seizure free for some time may perceive that he or she has been "cured," but the medication should not be decreased or stopped without consulting with the prescriber.

When anticonvulsant therapy is initiated or changed, the client should avoid activities that require coordination and alertness (e.g., driving) or situations that might be hazardous (e.g., swimming or ladder climbing) until the client's response to the drug therapy has been determined.

Overdose is especially dangerous in children. Medications should be stored at home away from light and heat and out of the reach of children. Outdated and discontinued medications should be flushed down the toilet.

Suggest that family members keep a daily record of the number and types of seizures that occur during drug therapy. This is one measure of the efficacy of the medication(s) and helps the prescriber to determine if an increased dosage or an additional agent is needed.

Instruct the client and family about seizure precautions and about the importance of wearing a Medic Alert tag/card (obtainable at local pharmacy). A valuable resource for both the nurse and the client is the Epilepsy Foundation of America.*

▪ **Evaluation.** Evaluation of the client's progress on anticonvulsant therapy should be assessed in terms of achievement of the outcome criteria and the client's response to nursing interventions. As with all drugs, the client will administer the drug safely and accurately when managing his or her own medication regimen. The client will experience a decrease in or absence of seizure activity and will maintain therapeutic blood levels of the drug without experiencing any adverse reactions. Some of the behavioral and cognitive effects reported with the anticonvulsants are listed in Table 17-3.

HYDANTOINS

phenytoin [fen′ i toy in] (Dilantin ◆, Diphenylan)

The prototype hydantoin is phenytoin, which was developed from a search for an anticonvulsant that would cause less sedation than the barbiturates. Phenytoin is used for the treatment of all types of epilepsy except absence seizures. Fosphenytoin, a pro-drug of phenytoin, was formulated to avoid the problems associated with IV administration of phenytoin (i.e., pain and burning at the site of administration) (Luer, 1998). This product is rapidly converted to phenytoin in the body and has the same pharmacologic profile as phenytoin.

Two other hydantoin drugs are used for their anticonvulsant effects: ethotoin (Peganone) and mephenytoin (Mesantoin). Ethotoin and mephenytoin are usually prescribed only for those clients whose symptoms cannot be controlled with other drugs or for clients who experience adverse reactions with other anticonvulsants. Both ethotoin and mephenytoin are available only in the oral form, which limits their usefulness when a rapid response or parenteral route is needed.

Phenytoin is more effective for generalized tonic-clonic seizures than for absence seizures. It is commonly prescribed in combination with phenobarbital, and it may be prescribed for clients after brain surgery, after head trauma, and for status epilepticus to prevent seizures.

See Anticonvulsant Therapy for a complete explanation of the mechanism of action. As a group, the hydantoins act to reduce the maximum activity of brainstem centers responsible for the tonic phase of grand mal seizures. See Table 17-1 for a summary of the pharmacokinetics of phenytoin.

Side effects/adverse reactions of phenytoin include hirsutism, constipation, nausea, vomiting, drowsiness, dizziness, and gingival hyperplasia (bleeding, sensitive gum tissue or overgrowth of gum tissue).

*Epilepsy Foundation of America, 4351 Garden City Drive, Landover, MD 20785; (301) 459-3700; www.epilepsyfoundation.org.

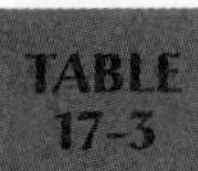

TABLE 17-3 Behavioral and Cognitive Effects of Selected Anticonvulsants

Drug	Behavioral Effects	Cognitive Effects
barbiturates, especially phenobarbital	May see paradoxical effect, especially in older adults, children, or compromised clients (e.g., increased activity or excitement, irritability, altered sleep patterns, increased tiredness)	Impaired judgment, short-term memory impairment, decreased attention span
carbamazepine	Increased irritability, insomnia, behavioral changes (especially in children), depression	Less than phenytoin, phenobarbital, or primidone
phenytoin	Fatigue, increased clumsiness, confusion, mood alterations	Decreased attention span, decreased ability to problem solve

The usual adult dosage of extended-release phenytoin is 100 mg PO three times daily. When the proper dosage is established, extended-release phenytoin capsules may be given once a day, depending on the client's tolerance. For status epilepticus, the dosage is 15 to 20 mg/kg IV at a rate of up to 50 mg/min (or in older adults, 5 to 25 mg/min). The pediatric dosage is 5 mg/kg PO in divided doses initially; the maintenance dosage is 4 to 8 mg/kg PO in two or three doses daily. For status epilepticus in children, the dosage is 15 to 20 mg/kg IV at a rate of 1 mg/kg/min, not to exceed 50 mg/min (*United States Pharmacopeia Dispensing Information*, 1999).

■ Nursing Management

Hydantoin Therapy

■ **Assessment.** The client's history should be reviewed for conditions that contraindicate the use of phenytoin, such as a known sensitivity to the drug and impaired cardiac function, because parenteral administration may affect ventricular automaticity and cause ventricular dysrhythmias. The review should also include conditions that require the cautious use of phenytoin. There is an elevated incidence of birth defects in children born to mothers who are taking phenytoin, but most deliver normal infants. The drug is excreted in breast milk. Children taking phenytoin are at higher risk for gingival hyperplasia, coarsening of the facial features, and excessive body hair growth. Because of decreased serum albumin and low protein binding, older adults have an increased possibility of experiencing toxic effects. Clients with a history of blood dyscrasias are at greater risk for serious infection, and those with porphyria may experience an exacerbation. Toxic serum concentrations of phenytoin may occur in clients with impaired hepatic and renal function as a result of altered protein binding.

There are clinically significant pharmacokinetic drug interactions among the antiepileptic drugs (Tanaka, 1999). There also exists a serious interaction between phenytoin and alcohol; a cross-tolerance to phenytoin develops in clients with epilepsy who are also heavy drinkers. Chronic alcohol use speeds up the metabolism of the drug, apparently by enzyme induction, and makes normal dosages inadequate.

Review the client's current medication regimen for the risk of significant drug interactions, such as those that may occur when hydantoins are given concurrently with the following drugs:

Drug/Herb	Possible Effect and Management
Bold/color type indicates the most serious interactions.	
alcohol, CNS depressants	May result in enhanced CNS depression. Monitor closely for respiratory depression and drowsiness.
antacids	Concurrent use may decrease the bioavailability of phenytoin; administer medications 2 to 3 hours apart.
anticoagulants, such as warfarin (Coumadin)	A decrease in metabolism may cause an increased serum level and hydantoin toxicity. The anticoagulant effect may be initially increased but decreases with continuous combined use. Monitor closely for symptoms of thromboembolism.
antifungals, such as fluconazole (Diflucan), itraconazole (Sporanox), ketoconazole (Nizoral), miconazole (Monistat)	May increase phenytoin metabolism, resulting in increased plasma levels of phenytoin and toxicity. Monitor phenytoin serum levels.
calcium	Calcium supplements or calcium sulfate may decrease phenytoin absorption by approximately 20%. Space medications 1 to 3 hours apart.
chloramphenicol (Chloromycetin), cimetidine (Tagamet), disulfiram (Antabuse), isoniazid (INH), amiodarone (Cordarone), oral anticoagulants, or sulfonamides	A decrease in metabolism may cause an increased serum level and toxicity of hydantoins. Dosage adjustments may be required.

Drug/Herb	Possible Effect and Management
corticosteroids, estrogens, or oral contraceptives	An increase in the metabolism of these drugs may result from hydantoin's induction of hepatic microsomal enzymes, which may decrease the therapeutic effects of these medications; monitor closely because dosage adjustment may be necessary. Breakthrough bleeding and increased risk of conception may occur with estrogen-containing contraceptives.
diazoxide, oral (Proglycem)	**May decrease phenytoin effects and decrease the hyperglycemic action of diazoxide. Avoid concurrent use or a potentially serious drug interaction may occur.**
felbamate (Felbatol) and fluoxetine (Prozac)	Concurrent use will increase plasma concentrations of phenytoin. Decrease in phenytoin dosage is necessary. Monitor serum levels closely and for signs of phenytoin toxicity.
ginkgo	**Contaminant in some gingko products reduces the anticonvulsant effect of phenytoin, carbamazepine, gabapentin, mephenytoin, and phenobarbital. Monitor closely.**
lidocaine, propranolol (Inderal), and possibly other beta-blocking agents	If given with IV phenytoin, additive cardiac depressant effects may occur. Hydantoins may also increase metabolism of lidocaine.
methadone	Methadone metabolism may be increased by chronic dosing of phenytoin, which may precipitate acute withdrawal reaction in clients being treated for narcotic dependence. Methadone dosages may need to be adjusted whenever phenytoin is started or discontinued.
streptozocin (Zanosar)	**Phenytoin reported to protect pancreatic beta cells from therapeutic effects of streptozocin. Avoid concurrent use or a potentially serious drug interaction may occur.**
sucralfate (Carafate)	Concurrent use may decrease absorption of hydantoin anticonvulsants. Space medications at least 2 hours apart.
valproate (Depacon)	Monitor serum levels of phenytoin (preferably unbound phenytoin) closely, because variable responses have been reported. Dosage adjustments may be necessary according to client's clinical response.
xanthines, especially theophylline	Monitor serum concentrations of both drugs. If phenytoin plasma levels are in the therapeutic range, an increase in the metabolism of xanthines (except for dyphylline) will occur. If given with xanthines, a decrease in phenytoin absorption may result; monitor closely.

■ **Nursing Diagnosis.** The following nursing diagnoses/collaborative problems may be identified in a client receiving phenytoin: risk for injury related to the client's underlying seizure activity and inadequate therapeutic serum levels of anticonvulsant medications; disturbed body image related to the coarsening of facial features, hirsutism, alopecia and, in males, gynecomastia; powerlessness related to chronicity of seizure disorder therapy; and the potential complications of cognitive impairment, blood dyscrasias, hepatotoxicity, and gingival hyperplasia.

■ **Implementation**

■ ***Monitoring.*** Monitor the effectiveness of hydantoin therapy by documenting seizure activity and the signs and symptoms of adverse responses. Monitor closely for documented drug interactions that may alter the client's response to medications. Because some drugs can impair or enhance the effects of phenytoin, monitoring drug serum levels is important for accurate dosage administration and as a mechanism of determining compliance.

Serum levels should be monitored in clients who are taking phenytoin. Peak plasma levels are usually reached in 8 to 12 hours, but it takes approximately 7 to 10 days before recommended serum levels are achieved. It is particularly important that serum levels be monitored closely in clients with renal and hepatic impairment. Clients with impaired liver function, older adults, or clients who are very ill may demonstrate early signs of toxicity. A small percentage of individuals metabolize the drug slowly because of limited enzyme availability, which may be genetically determined. The metabolism of phenytoin is dose dependent at therapeutic doses. Liver function tests and blood counts should be monitored periodically.

■ ***Intervention***

■ *Enteral Administration.* When using the suspension form of phenytoin, shake the container vigorously before measuring out the dose in a graduated or exact measuring device (oral syringe). Children and other clients with enteral tube feedings have been undermedicated and later overmedicated from the same container because of improper shaking of the container.

Oral preparations of phenytoin should be given with meals to decrease gastric distress. The appearance of side effects or adverse reactions may require nursing interventions that range from basic nursing skills to urgent consultation with the prescriber. Note that the 100-mg capsule of phenytoin sodium contains only 92% phenytoin and is not equivalent to two 50-mg phenytoin chewable tablets (Dilantin Infatabs) that contain 100% phenytoin.

■ *Nasogastric Tube Administration.* Administration of phenytoin suspension without dilution or follow-up irrigation of the nasogastric tube after the phenytoin is given prevents adequate absorption and leads to a significant decrease in plasma concentrations of phenytoin. Until further research is performed, it is recommended that the phenytoin suspension be diluted before administration and that the nasogastric tube be irrigated with 20 mL of fluid (D_5W, normal saline) before and after administration. A significant decrease in the absorption of oral phenytoin may occur when phenytoin is administered to clients receiving enteral feedings. If the client is receiving an enteral feeding, the phenytoin should be administered intravenously; if this is not feasible, serum concentrations of phenytoin should be monitored frequently. Abrupt withdrawal may precipitate status epilepticus.

■ *Parenteral Administration.* The IM route may be useful if immobilization of an extremity is impossible because of convulsions or inaccessible veins. If administration of the medication does not terminate the seizure, consult with the prescriber to consider other anticonvulsants, IV barbiturates, general anesthesia, or other measures. The IM route is not recommended for the treatment of status epilepticus because therapeutic plasma levels of phenytoin cannot be readily achieved. Because muscle tissue is more acidic than the phenytoin solution, phenytoin crystallizes when given intramuscularly. The absorption of these crystals is slow and erratic, and pain and necrosis may occur at the injection site.

Fosphenytoin, a pro-drug of phenytoin, may be used intramuscularly with little or no local irritation. Because parenteral phenytoin is an irritant to the tissues and veins and is incompatible with many solutions and medications, its use has been largely replaced by fosphenytoin (CNS Clinical Development Department, 1998). The dosing of fosphenytoin is always expressed in terms of phenytoin sodium equivalents (PEs). In the living organism, an injection of fosphenytoin sodium liberates 1 mg of phenytoin sodium; 75 mg of fosphenytoin sodium is essentially equivalent to 50 mg of phenytoin sodium. Some clients complain of burning and pain at the IV injection site, but less so than with phenytoin. Because of the alkalinity of the hydantoins, burning and pain raise suspicion of a poorly seated needle, extravasation, or a fluid load that is being infused too quickly into a small vein. Restart the infusion into a large vein, using a larger-gauge needle.

For a loading dose of fosphenytoin infusion in adult status epilepticus, the maximum administration rate should be 150 mg PE/min. Electrocardiogram (ECG) monitoring is recommended during the infusion. In general, older adults, seriously ill clients, debilitated clients, or clients with liver function impairment should receive a lower dose at a much slower rate of administration. Monitor blood pressure and cardiac function closely.

The rate and time for dilantinization, as well as the loading dose of fosphenytoin (Cerebyx), are a function of the client's clinical situation. The dose-related side effects increase with the rapidity at which the client is dilantinized to the therapeutic range. Proceeding cautiously and slowly is clinically prudent. Bilateral and vertical nystagmus develops at levels of 15 mg PE/kg body weight administered at 150 mg PE/min; tinnitus, pruritus, ataxia, drowsiness, and diplopia are also seen at this level.

With all hydantoins, monitor closely for side effects/adverse reactions. Signs of overdose or toxicity include blurred or double vision, nausea, vomiting, slurred speech, clumsiness, unsteadiness or staggering gait, dizziness, fatigue, confusion, and hallucinations.

■ ***Education.*** One of the side effects of the hydantoins is gum hyperplasia; it is therefore important that oral hygiene be emphasized. Clients should be encouraged to brush frequently, floss, and massage their gums. This tissue overgrowth is usually greater and more apparent anteriorly than posteriorly, and the client, particularly the adolescent, may have body image concerns. A program of professional dental prophylaxis and an aggressive program of plaque control by the client will minimize hyperplasia. Clients should be instructed to inform their dentist that they are taking hydantoins so that he or she can observe and monitor for periodontal problems.

Hydantoins may affect blood sugar levels. Clients who have diabetes should be instructed to report any changes in blood or urine sugar concentrations.

The client should be advised of possible skin changes. An erythematous-type rash with or without fever should be reported immediately to the prescriber. Hirsutism, or the excessive growth of body and facial hair, is reported in some clients. This alteration in body image is particularly troublesome in young women and requires supportive nursing care.

The client should be cautioned against changing drug brands, because the bioavailability of phenytoin may vary. Generic phenytoin and Dilantin (Parke-Davis) are not the same. Dilantin capsules are the only extended form of phenytoin sodium available. The extended form can be used for once-daily dosing and for clients who are stabilized on a 300-mg divided dose. All other forms of phenytoin are prompt-acting and are not intended for once-daily dosing. Generic phenytoin capsules and the chewable tablets from Parke-Davis are prompt-acting forms of the drug. It is important that this information be explained clearly to the client and family.

When discussing the appropriate means of administration of the suspension dosage form, stress to the client that very vigorous shaking of the container is mandatory before measuring out the dose in a graduated or exact measuring device (oral syringe). The hydantoins interact with a variety of drugs, and therefore clients should be cautioned against unsupervised self-administration of other drugs while taking any of the hydantoins.

Any client with epilepsy should carry an identification card or wear a Medic Alert bracelet that indicates the anticonvulsant being taken.

■ **Evaluation.** The expected outcome of hydantoin therapy is that the client will experience decreased or no seizure activity, maintain a serum level within the therapeutic range (e.g., phenytoin 10 to 20 μg/mL), demonstrate no adverse reactions to phenytoin, and administer the drug safely and accurately when self-managing the medication regimen.

fosphenytoin [foss fen′ i toy in] (Cerebyx)

Fosphenytoin is rapidly converted to phenytoin in the body and may be administered by IM and IV injection (Drug Update, 1996). Phenytoin derived from fosphenytoin has the same pharmacologic profile as phenytoin sodium. Fosphenytoin 150 mg is equivalent to 100 mg phenytoin sodium, although it may be administered at a faster rate than phenytoin (150 mg/min) (Cloyd, 1996; Bleck, 1999; *Drug Facts and Comparisons*, 2000).

For the nursing management of fosphenytoin, see Nursing Management: Hydantoin Therapy, p. 359.

mephenytoin [me fen′ i toyn] [Mesantoin]

Mephenytoin is chemically similar to phenytoin in structure, activity, and pharmacokinetics, but it is less potent as an anticonvulsant. It produces more sedation than phenytoin, but this side effect is dose related. It also has a greater potential for producing blood dyscrasias and dermatologic effects than the other hydantoins. This product is usually reserved for clients whose seizures are not controlled with safer anticonvulsants.

The usual adult dosage is 50 to 100 mg PO daily, increased weekly as necessary up to a 1.2 g/day maximum. The dosage for children is 25 to 50 mg daily.

For the nursing management of fosphenytoin, see Nursing Management: Hydantoin Therapy, p. 359.

ethotoin [eth′ oh toyn] (Peganone)

Ethotoin is similar to phenytoin but is less effective and offers little advantage over phenytoin. The side effects of ataxia, hirsutism, and gum hyperplasia are rare, and ethotoin may be substituted for phenytoin to reduce these side effects.

Ethotoin is available only for oral administration, and the dosage is individualized according to response. A maintenance dose (usually divided into four to six doses) of less than 2 g is usually not effective.

For the nursing management of fosphenytoin, see Nursing Management: Hydantoin Therapy, p. 359.

BARBITURATES

Barbiturates, especially phenobarbital, have been used for many years for the treatment of generalized tonic-clonic and partial seizures. This class of medications is relatively inexpensive, efficacious, and has a low incidence of side effects. The most commonly prescribed barbiturate is phenobarbital; mephobarbital (Mebaral) is converted to phenobarbital by metabolizing enzymes in the liver. Both phenobarbital and mephobarbital are long-acting compounds, and there is little or no advantage in using mephobarbital instead of phenobarbital, the most commonly prescribed barbiturate.

The parenteral dosage forms of amobarbital, phenobarbital, and secobarbital have been used in the emergency treatment of seizures (see Table 17-2). In general, the oral dosage forms are not indicated for the treatment of seizure disorders because of their potent sedative-hypnotic effects. See Table 17-1 for a pharmacokinetic overview of selected barbiturates.

The adverse reactions of apnea, bronchospasm, and respiratory depression may occur after rapidly administered IV injections of barbiturates. Severe withdrawal symptoms may occur in individuals who have a barbiturate dependency as a result of prolonged use at high dosages. Anxiety, trembling, nausea, vomiting, insomnia, orthostatic hypotension, seizures, hallucinations, and even death may result if the drug is withdrawn abruptly. Gradual withdrawal in a controlled setting is usually recommended for the treatment of dependence.

phenobarbital [fee noe bar′ bi tal] (Barbita, Luminal)

Phenobarbital is the prototype barbiturate for the treatment of epilepsy. Many dosage forms (tablets, elixirs, solutions, and parenteral) and strengths are available. The nurse must exercise special caution to ensure that the proper dose is given as prescribed.

Several weeks of phenobarbital therapy may be necessary to achieve the maximum anticonvulsant effects. When administered intravenously, 15 to 30 minutes are required to reach the maximum anticonvulsant effect. To avoid excessive barbiturate-induced depression, it is important to wait for the anticonvulsant effect to develop before administering additional doses. When given intravenously, phenobarbital should be administered slowly to avoid respiratory depression; a rate of 60 mg/min should not be exceeded. Resuscitative equipment should be readily available.

Seizure control and the absence of toxic effects should indicate an optimal blood concentration of phenobarbital. A serum concentration of 10 to 40 μg/mL is usually desired. The dosage and administration of phenobarbital are addressed in Table 16-3.

amobarbital [am oh bar′ bi tal] (Amytal)

Amobarbital is indicated for use as a sedative-hypnotic and anticonvulsant. Only the parenteral form is used as an anticonvulsant. IM administration of amobarbital should be deep to reduce the possibility of sterile abscesses and sloughing of tissue. When administered intravenously to an adult, the rate of injection should not exceed 100 mg/min. Parenteral solutions should be clear and without precipitates when reconstituted. The solution should be used within 30 minutes of reconstitution, because it hydrolyzes easily.

mephobarbital [me foe bar′ bi tal] (Mebaral)

Mephobarbital is a barbiturate indicated for use only as an anticonvulsant. It is available in oral dosage forms only. Therapy is usually begun with small doses and is increased over a period of 4 to 5 days until the optimal dosage has been established. Because mephobarbital is metabolized to phenobarbital, serum levels of phenobarbital may be monitored.

■ Nursing Management

Barbiturate Therapy

■ **Assessment.** Combining barbiturates with alcohol, antihistamines, antianxiety agents, antidepressants, or antipsychotic agents should be avoided because an enhanced CNS depressant effect may result.

Children and older adults may be more sensitive to barbiturates and may respond to lower dosages or may have reactions such as depression, confusion, or even excitement. These drugs should be used very cautiously in pregnant women because they can cause neonatal hemorrhage and an increased incidence of teratogenic effects. If given throughout the third trimester, physical drug dependence and withdrawal reactions have been reported in the neonate from birth to approximately 2 weeks.

Barbiturates are to be used with caution if any of the following conditions are present: hypersensitivity to barbiturates; history of substance abuse, because the client is predisposed to dependence; hepatic impairment, which would interfere with barbiturate metabolism; respiratory disease, because of the risk of ventilatory depression; or pain, because symptoms of an underlying condition may be masked. Barbiturates are contraindicated for clients with porphyria or a history of the disease because the barbiturates may increase symptoms by stimulating enzymes for porphyrin synthesis.

Review the client's current medication regimen for the risk of significant drug interactions, such as those that may occur when barbiturates, especially phenobarbital, are given concurrently with the following drugs:

Drug	Possible Effect and Management
adrenocorticoids or corticosteroids (e.g., prednisone)	The effects of these drugs may be decreased because of enhanced metabolism caused by barbiturates. Dosage adjustment may be necessary.
alcohol, anesthetics, CNS depressants (sedatives, hypnotics, narcotics)	Enhanced CNS depressant effects, respiratory depression; use extreme caution in combining such medications. Usually the dosage of one or both drugs should be reduced.
anticoagulants, such as warfarin (Coumadin)	Effects may be decreased because of enhanced metabolism produced by barbiturates. Monitor prothrombin time closely. Dosage adjustment of anticoagulants may be necessary.
carbamazepine (Tegretol)	Concurrent drug administration may result in a decrease in the serum level and half-life of carbamazepine. Monitor serum levels whenever carbamazepine is prescribed or discontinued from combination drug therapy.
contraceptives, oral, estrogen-containing	Concurrent use may result in reduced contraceptive reliability; the use of a nonhormonal method of birth control or a progestin-only oral contraceptive may be necessary.
divalproex sodium (Depakote) or valproic acid (Depakene)	Two effects may result from this combination: (1) the half-life of valproic acid may be decreased, which would require a dosage adjustment to maintain control; or (2) the metabolism of barbiturates may be decreased, which can result in elevated barbiturate serum levels and toxicity. Monitor barbiturate levels, because a dosage adjustment may be necessary. Phenobarbital may also increase the potential for valproic acid hepatotoxicity; monitor liver function studies closely.

■ **Nursing Diagnosis.** The client receiving anticonvulsant therapy with barbiturates should be assessed for the following nursing diagnoses/collaborative problems: disturbed sleep pattern (daytime sedation, hangover); risk for injury related to CNS effects of the drug (dizziness); disturbed thought processes (confusion); and the potential complications of Stevens-Johnson syndrome, blood dyscrasias, and paradoxical excitement.

■ **Implementation**

■ ***Monitoring.*** In addition to the evaluation needed for anticonvulsant therapy in general, liver and renal function are monitored (usually through blood and urine testing) during prolonged barbiturate therapy; this occurs at periodic intervals as determined by the prescriber.

Serum levels may be monitored. Optimal blood levels are determined by the client's response to seizure control and by the appearance of toxic effects.

■ ***Intervention.*** If barbiturates are administered intravenously, ensure that the airway is patent and that resuscitative equipment is readily available.

When drug therapy is initiated, the client may experience some drowsiness and dizziness. If the client is ambulatory, safety precautions should be taken until the client's response to the medication has been ascertained.

The drug dosage schedule will vary until the correct dosage maintenance level is achieved, and it is important to follow this schedule accurately. The appearance of side effects or adverse reactions may require basic nursing measures such as reassurance, safety, or comfort or may indicate the need for further consultation.

If barbiturates are used during pregnancy, consult with the prescriber to see if the client should receive vitamin K in the last month of pregnancy to prevent hemorrhagic complications of delivery and in the newborn.

■ ***Education.*** Clients undergoing barbiturate therapy should be instructed to return to their prescriber routinely for complete blood counts (CBC), blood chemistry studies, and drug blood level tests.

Clients should be cautioned to avoid driving a car or operating potentially hazardous machinery until the response to drug therapy has been determined.

Self-alteration of prescribed medications or the consumption of OTC drugs without consultation with the prescriber should be discouraged. OTC drugs may interfere

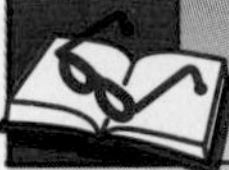

Case Study *The Client Undergoing Anticonvulsant Therapy*

Carla Blomquist, a 25-year-old school teacher, was admitted to the hospital 1 week ago to determine the cause of tonic-clonic seizures that began suddenly 2 weeks ago. Carla has no history of head trauma or recent infection. She takes no medications and her health has been very good, with no major illnesses or hospitalizations.

No cause for the seizures has been determined. Carla's blood pressure is within normal limits. All tests for space-occupying lesions and infections have proved negative, and the EEG changes are not diagnostic. However, Carla is concerned about the effects her seizures may have on her job and family life. Her health care provider has prescribed the following medications:

phenytoin (Dilantin) 100 mg PO qid
phenobarbital (Luminal) 30 mg PO tid

Her activity level has not been restricted, but she has been directed not to drive for a month. When a month has passed, she is to return to the clinic for evaluation of the medication therapy. Carla has had no seizures since beginning anticonvulsant therapy.

1. What is the major action of phenytoin? Why is phenobarbital also used?
2. What are some of the CNS effects that Carla might have in relation to taking phenytoin and phenobarbital?
3. You are discharging Carla; what instructions will enhance her ability to manage her therapeutic regimen effectively?

For answer guidelines, go to mosby.com/MERLIN/McKenry/.

with or enhance the effectiveness of the drug. CNS depression may occur if barbiturates are used in combination with alcohol. Abrupt withdrawal of the drug is contraindicated and could result in severe abstinence syndrome. The dosage should be tapered under medical supervision. (See the Case Study box above.)

Clients taking oral estrogen-containing contraceptives should be aware that concurrent use of barbiturates may result in decreased contraceptive reliability; they may wish to use a nonhormonal method of birth control or consult with their prescriber about a progestin-only oral contraceptive. Women using this drug therapy should be instructed to inform their prescriber if they become pregnant; barbiturates have been shown to cause an increase in fetal abnormalities. Barbiturates are excreted in breast milk and can cause CNS depression in the nursing infant.

▪ **Evaluation.** The expected outcome of barbiturate therapy is that the client will experience fewer seizures or remain seizure free, maintain a phenobarbital plasma concentration of 15 to 40 μg/mL, and be free of adverse reactions to the drug.

SUCCINIMIDES

The succinimides include ethosuximide (Zarontin), methsuximide (Celontin), and phensuximide (Milontin). These agents produce a variety of effects, such as increasing the seizure threshold and reducing the EEG spike-and-wave pattern of absence seizures by decreasing nerve impulses and transmission in the motor cortex.

Ethosuximide and phensuximide are indicated for the treatment of absence seizures; methsuximide is reserved for absence seizures that are nonresponsive to other medications. The pharmacokinetics of these medications are discussed in Table 17-4.

Side effects/adverse reactions of the succinimides include headache, epigastric pain, anorexia, hiccups, nausea, vomiting, rash, pruritus (possibly Stevens-Johnson syndrome), mood changes, and agranulocytosis.

The dosage of ethosuximide for adults and children 6 years and older is 250 mg PO twice daily initially, increased as necessary in 4 to 7 days; the maximum daily dose is 1.5 g. The dosage for children under 6 years is 250 mg/day initially, increased by 250 mg at 4- to 7-day intervals as necessary; the maximum daily dose is 1 g.

The dosage of methsuximide for adults is 300 mg PO daily initially, increased by 300-mg increments at weekly intervals until seizures are controlled or until a maximum daily dose of 1.2 g is reached. The dosage of methsuximide is individualized in children.

The dosage of phensuximide for adults and children is 500 mg PO two or three times daily, increased by 500 mg at weekly intervals until seizures are controlled or until a maximum daily dose of 3 g is reached.

▪ Nursing Management

Succinimide Therapy

▪ **Assessment.** In addition to obtaining a baseline assessment of the client's seizure activity, determine if the client has any preexisting health problems for which the succinimides would be contraindicated. Primarily these would be blood dyscrasias (because of the adverse hematologic effects of the drug) and hepatic and renal dysfunction (because changes may occur in these organs).

Review the client's current medication regimen for the risk of significant drug interactions, such as those that may

TABLE 17-4 Succinimides: Dosage and Administration

Drug	Adults	Children
ethosuximide (Zarontin)	Initially 250 mg PO twice daily, increased as necessary at 4- to 7-day intervals; maximum total daily dose is 1.5 g	6 years and older: follow adult schedule Up to 6 years: initial dose is 250 mg/day, increased by 250 mg at 4- to 7-day intervals; maximum total daily dose is 1 g
methsuximide (Celontin)	Initial dose is 300 mg PO daily, increased as necessary by 300-mg increments at 1-week intervals until seizures are controlled or a maximum daily dose of 1.2 g is reached	Dosage is individualized; 150-mg capsules are available for pediatric dosage adjustments
phensuximide (Milontin)	Initial dose is 500 mg PO 2 or 3 times daily, increased by 500-mg increments at 1-week intervals until seizures are controlled or a maximum daily dose of 3 g is reached	Dosage is similar to adult schedule

occur when succinimides are given concurrently with the following drugs:

Drug	Possible Effect and Management
carbamazepine (Tegretol) or phenobarbital	Results in increased metabolism of succinimide anticonvulsants and decreased serum levels. Monitor serum levels, especially when either drug is added, increased, decreased, or deleted from the drug regimen.
haloperidol (Haldol)	May change the pattern or frequency of seizures. The dosage of the anticonvulsant may need to be adjusted. Serum levels of haloperidol may be reduced, which may result in decreased effectiveness.
phenothiazines, thioxanthenes, antidepressants, loxapine (Loxitane), maprotiline (Ludiomil), or CNS depressants	May decrease the effectiveness of the anticonvulsant, enhance CNS depression, and lower the seizure threshold. Monitor closely for respiratory depression and drowsiness because dosage modifications may be necessary.
phenytoin (Dilantin)	Phenytoin serum levels may be elevated with concurrent administration of succinimides. Monitor serum levels.

■ **Nursing Diagnosis.** In addition to the nursing diagnoses/collaborative problems discussed previously for anticonvulsant therapy, the client receiving succinimide therapy has the potential for the following: ineffective protection related to the development of blood dyscrasias (agranulocytosis, thrombocytopenia); and the potential complications of Stevens-Johnson syndrome (fever, bulla on the skin, ulcers of the mucous membranes of the lips, eyes, mouth, and genitalia), and systemic lupus erythematosus (muscle aches, swollen glands, sore throat, fever, skin rash).

■ **Implementation**

■ ***Monitoring.*** In addition to monitoring the client's seizure activity, evaluate liver, renal, and hematologic studies periodically because of the possible effects of the succinimides on these systems. Report any signs of liver, kidney, or hematologic disorders to the prescriber.

■ ***Intervention.*** To decrease stomach distress, the succinimides may be taken with milk, food, or antacids.

■ ***Education.*** Although the incidence of blood dyscrasia is rare with the succinimides, when it does occur it may result in gingival bleeding, delayed healing, and an increase in the number of infections for the client. Dental work should be deferred until blood counts are within the normal range. The client may need to modify his or her dental hygiene with cautious use of toothbrushes and dental floss. The client should alert other health care providers about the succinimide regimen if surgery, dental work, or emergency medical care is required.

Caution the client about drowsiness and other possible CNS disturbances. Serum levels may be measured when dosage adjustments are made or medications are added. Explain the importance of serum levels to the client who needs to have them tested frequently. The client should be cautioned that withdrawal of the succinimides may precipitate absence seizures. Adverse personality changes can occur while taking this medication; stress to the client the importance of reporting any behavioral changes to the prescriber.

Caution any client who is taking phensuximide that the color of the urine may change to pink, red, or red-brown; this effect is harmless.

■ **Evaluation.** The expected outcome of succinimide therapy is that the client will have diminished seizures or remain free of seizures without experiencing any untoward effects.

BENZODIAZEPINES

The benzodiazepines include clonazepam (Klonopin), diazepam (Valium), clorazepate (Tranxene), and parenteral lorazepam (Ativan). These drugs appear to suppress the propagation of seizure activity produced by foci in the cortex, thalamus, and limbic areas.

Clonazepam (Klonopin) is a long-acting drug used to treat absence seizures and myoclonic seizure disorders. It has been used alone but more often is prescribed as an adjunct to other anticonvulsants in establishing seizure control. Diazepam (Valium) may be used parenterally for status epilepticus and for severe recurrent convulsive seizures. The oral dosage form of diazepam is not effective for maintenance control but has been used as an adjunctive medication for short-term treatment in convulsive disorders. Diazepam is not effective alone, and its use beyond 4 months has not been clinically evaluated (*Mosby's GenRx,* 1999).

Clorazepate (Tranxene) has been prescribed as an adjunct medication for the treatment of simple partial seizures. Although not an approved Food and Drug Administration indication, parenteral lorazepam (Ativan) has been used to treat status epilepticus (*USP DI,* 1999).

See Table 17-5 and Chapter 16 for the pharmacokinetics and side effects/adverse reactions of the benzodiazepines.

The dosage of the benzodiazepines is usually individualized for each client and is increased with caution to avoid adverse reactions. A lower dosage with a slow increase is prudent in older adults, debilitated persons, and persons taking other CNS depressant–type medications.

The adult dosage of clonazepam is 0.5 mg PO three times daily, increased 0.5 to 1 mg every third day until the seizures are controlled, side effects occur, or the maximum dosage of 20 mg/day is reached. With children less than 10 years of age or 30 kg, the initial dosage is 0.01 to 0.03 mg/kg in divided doses (three times daily). The maximum maintenance dosage for children is 0.1 to 0.2 mg/kg/day.

The adult dosage of clorazepate is 7.5 mg PO three times daily, increased if necessary by 7.5 mg/wk to a maximum of 90 mg/day. For children 9 to 12 years of age, the dosage is 7.5 mg PO twice daily, increased weekly if necessary; the maximum daily dose is 60 mg.

The adult dosage of diazepam is 5 to 10 mg IV initially, repeated in 10- to 15-minute intervals if necessary to a maximum of 30 mg. The IV drug is injected slowly, at least 1 minute for each 5-mg dose. The oral dosage is 2 to 10 mg three to four times daily. Refer to current drug references for pediatric dosing.

■ Nursing Management

Benzodiazepine Therapy

■ **Assessment.** See Chapter 16, Nursing Management: Benzodiazepine Therapy, for the detailed client assessment required before benzodiazepine therapy may be initiated.

■ **Nursing Diagnosis.** See Chapter 16, Nursing Management: Benzodiazepine Therapy, for the nursing diagnoses/collaborative problems associated with benzodiazepine therapy.

■ **Implementation.** In this chapter, discussion is limited to the use of benzodiazepines for urgent seizure control. See Chapter 16, Nursing Management: Benzodiazepine Therapy, for the general nursing management of the client receiving benzodiazepines.

■ ***Monitoring.*** Baseline vital signs should be obtained before parenteral forms of diazepam (Valium) or lorazepam

TABLE 17-5 Benzodiazepine Anticonvulsants: Dosage and Administration

Drug	Adults	Children
clonazepam (Klonopin)	Initially 0.5 mg PO 3 times daily, with increases of 0.5-1 mg every third day until seizures are controlled, side effects occur, or the maximum of 20 mg/day is reached	Under 10 years or 30 kg: initially 0.01-0.03/kg PO in divided doses (3 times daily); if necessary, increase by 0.25-0.5 mg every 3 days until seizures are controlled, side effects occur, or the maximum maintenance dose of 0.1-0.2 mg/kg is reached
diazepam (Valium)	5-10 mg IV initially; repeat at 10- to 15-minute intervals if necessary to a maximum of 30 mg; inject slowly—at least 1 minute for each 5-mg dose administered intravenously *or* 2-10 mg PO 3 or 4 times daily	1 month to 5 years: 0.2-0.5 mg by slow IV every 2-5 minutes to a maximum of 5 mg; may be repeated in 2-4 hours if necessary 5 years and older: 1 mg every 2-5 minutes by slow IV to a maximum of 10 mg; may be repeated in 2-4 hours if necessary
clorazepate (Tranxene)	Initially up to 7.5 mg PO 3 times daily; increase if necessary by 7.5 mg/wk to a maximum of 90 mg/day	9 to 12 years: up to 7.5 mg PO twice daily; increase if necessary by 7.5 mg/wk to a maximum of 60 mg daily

Information from *United States Pharmacopeia Dispensing Information (USP DI): Information for the health care professional* (19th ed). (1999). Rockville, MD: United States Pharmacopeial Convention.

(Ativan) are given. After administration, the client should be observed at bed rest for decreases in respiratory rate, heart rate, and blood pressure—at least 3 hours for diazepam and 8 hours for lorazepam.

■ ***Intervention.*** Diazepam (Valium) is insoluble in water; therefore each milliliter of the parenteral form contains 40% propylene glycol, 10% ethyl alcohol, 5% sodium benzoate, and benzoic acid as buffers, as well as 1.5% benzyl alcohol as a preservative. If this ratio is altered, the diazepam becomes insoluble. If direct IV injection is not possible, diazepam may be injected through the infusion tubing as close to the insertion point as possible. Inject slowly, at least 1 minute for each 5 mg.

Lorazepam (Ativan) must be diluted with a compatible diluent immediately before IV use. It may be infused directly into a vein or through IV tubing. Infusion rates should not exceed 2 mg/min.

Because of the short-lived effect of IV benzodiazepine administration, seizures are brought under prompt control but may recur. Be ready to readminister the drug. Benzodiazepines are not for maintenance; once seizure control is achieved, agents useful in long-term seizure control should be considered. Tonic status epilepticus has been precipitated in some clients treated with IV diazepam for absence seizure status or absence seizure variant status.

Because of the possibility of apnea and cardiac arrest, exercise extreme care when administering benzodiazepines (especially by the IV route) to older adults, very ill clients, or clients with compromised pulmonary reserve; monitor respirations every 5 to 15 minutes and before each IV dose. Resuscitative equipment should be available because of the possible occurrence of hypotension, tachycardia, and respiratory depression.

The efficacy and safety of parenteral diazepam has not been established for neonates 30 days of age or younger. Prolonged CNS depression has been reported in neonates, probably as a result of the inability to biotransform diazepam into inactive metabolites.

The benzoate in the injectable form has been reported to displace other drugs and bilirubin from the plasma protein binding sites, causing jaundice.

To minimize the occurrence of thrombophlebitis after IV injection of diazepam, the vein can be flushed with 1 mL of saline per milligram of diazepam.

If benzodiazepines are given along with a narcotic, the dosage of the narcotic should be reduced. Diazepam is a drug that may be subject to abuse by medical and nursing professionals and clients. It is a controlled drug; therefore the nurse is responsible for proper documentation of the drug's distribution and use.

■ ***Education.*** When benzodiazepines are given for treating convulsive disorders, an abrupt withdrawal of the medication can cause an increase in the frequency or severity of seizures. Clients should be instructed to take their medication as directed.

Diazepam does cross the placental barrier and has been associated with causing cleft lip in the infant. The risk-benefit ratio should be carefully considered in the client during pregnancy.

Alcohol and other CNS depressants should not be combined with benzodiazepines. Severe drowsiness, respiratory depression, and apnea may occur.

■ **Evaluation.** The expected outcome of benzodiazepine therapy is that the client will experience a decrease in the severity and frequency of seizures without experiencing any adverse reactions to the drug.

MISCELLANEOUS ANTICONVULSANTS

acetazolamide [a set a zole′ a mide] (Diamox)

Acetazolamide is a carbonic anhydrase inhibitor usually prescribed for the treatment of open-angle glaucoma. It is used in combination with other anticonvulsant agents for the treatment of absence seizures, generalized tonic-clonic seizures, mixed seizures, and myoclonic seizure patterns. The mechanism of action of acetazolamide is unknown. It has been theorized that inhibiting carbonic anhydrase in the CNS may result in an increase in carbon dioxide that slows neuronal activity. Systemic metabolic acidosis may also play a part in its action. (See Chapter 34 for the pharmacokinetics and side effects/adverse reactions of acetazolamide.)

The dosage of acetazolamide for anticonvulsant therapy in adults and children is 4 to 30 mg/kg/day PO (the initial dosage is usually 10 mg/kg/day) in four divided doses (usually 375 to 1000 mg/day).

For the nursing management of acetazolamide therapy, see Nursing Management: Anticonvulsant Therapy, p. 353, and the drug monograph in Chapter 34.

carbamazepine [kar ba maz′ e peen] (Tegretol)

The exact mechanism of action for carbamazepine is unknown, but the effects of this drug are somewhat similar to those of phenytoin. Carbamazepine is indicated in the treatment of partial seizures with complex symptoms, for generalized tonic-clonic seizures, for psychomotor seizures, and for mixed seizure patterns. This drug is also indicated in the treatment of pain associated with true trigeminal neuralgia.

See Table 17-1 for a pharmacokinetic overview of carbamazepine. Autoinduction of metabolism occurs, and the half-life decreases with repeated doses.

Side effects/adverse reactions of carbamazepine include vertigo, drowsiness, nausea, vomiting, dizziness, blurred or other visual disturbances, ataxia, confusion, muscle aches or cramps, allergic reaction, Stevens-Johnson syndrome, systemic lupus erythematosus–type syndrome, and the syndrome of inappropriate antidiuretic hormone (SIADH).

In adults, carbamazepine should be given initially at 200 mg twice daily, increased by 200 mg/day weekly in divided doses until a response is noted; the maximum dosage is 1200 mg/day, with a maintenance range of 800 to 1200 mg/day in divided doses. For children up to 6 years, the initial dosage is 10 to 20 mg/kg/day in divided doses; increase weekly if necessary up to a maximum of 100 mg/day. Maintenance usually requires between 250 and 300 mg daily to maintain the therapeutic serum level. The dosage for children 6 to 12 years is initially 100 mg twice a day; increase by 100 mg/day weekly until the desired response is obtained. Maintenance is usually between 400 and 800 mg/day in divided doses.

■ Nursing Management

Carbamazepine Therapy

■ Assessment. Carbamazepine therapy is contraindicated for clients with absence, atonic, or myoclonic seizures because of the possibility of the seizures becoming more generalized with use of the drug. There is also a risk of exacerbation of atrioventricular heart block, blood disorders, and bone marrow depression in clients with a history of these preexisting conditions. The risk-benefit ratio of carbamazepine should be considered for the client with the following health conditions: active alcoholism (potentiates CNS depression), behavioral disorders (may activate latent psychosis), cardiac damage or coronary artery disease, glaucoma (may be exacerbated), and renal or hepatic impairment. Carbamazepine is contraindicated if the client has had a sensitivity to the drug or to tricyclic antidepressants.

Review the client's current medication regiment for the risk of significant drug interactions, such as those that may occur when carbamazepine is given concurrently with the following drugs:

Bold/color type indicates the most serious interactions.

Drug	Possible Effect and Management
anticoagulants, oral warfarin (Coumadin)	Monitor for a decreased anticoagulant effect. Increased hepatic microsomal enzyme activity may increase anticoagulant metabolism, resulting in a decreased half-life and therapeutic effect. Dosage adjustments of anticoagulant may be necessary during and after treatment with carbamazepine.
anticonvulsants (hydantoin or succinimide); barbiturates; benzodiazepines metabolized by hepatic enzymes (especially clonazepam [Klonopin]), primidone (Mysoline), or valproic acid (Depakene)	Concurrent drug administration may result in increased drug metabolism and decreased serum levels and therapeutic effectiveness of these medications. Monitor blood levels whenever any of these medications are added to or discontinued in clients receiving carbamazepine, because dosage adjustments may be necessary. Valproic acid may prolong the half-life of carbamazepine.
antidepressants (tricyclic), clozapine (Clozaril), haloperidol (Haldol), loxapine, (Loxitane), maprotiline (Ludiomil), molindone (Moban), phenothiazines, pimozide (Orap), and thioxanthenes	May reduce the convulsive threshold and enhance CNS depressant effects; dosage adjustment may be necessary to control seizures and reduce side effects. Monitor closely for seizure activity.
antifungals, itraconazole (Sporanox), ketoconazole (Nizoral)	Metabolism of carbamazepine may be inhibited, resulting in increased serum levels and carbamazepine toxicity. Levels of itraconazole may be lowered and result in treatment failure.
cimetidine (Tagamet), diltiazem (Cardizem), verapamil (Calan)	May increase plasma levels of carbamazepine, which can result in toxicity. Monitor closely.
clarithromycin (Biaxin)	Concurrent use may result in elevated carbamazepine levels. Monitor serum levels closely.
corticosteroids	Concurrent administration may decrease steroidal effect because of an increase in hepatic metabolism. Monitor closely for lack of response to corticosteroid therapy; dosage adjustment may be necessary.
erythromycin	**Concurrent use may reduce carbamazepine metabolism, resulting in increased serum levels and toxicity. Avoid this combination and use a different antibiotic with clients taking carbamazepine.**
estrogen-containing contraceptives	Decrease in contraceptive reliability; clients should be advised to use a nonhormonal birth control method or to discuss the possibility of an oral progestin product with their prescriber.
felbamate (Felbatol), fluvoxamine (Luvox)	Increase in serum levels of carbamazepine; carbamazepine dosages may need to be decreased.
isoniazid (INH)	**Carbamazepine may increase liver metabolism of isoniazid, releasing an intermediate metabolite that can lead to hepatotoxicity. Isoniazid may also increase serum concentrations of carbamazepine, which may result in toxicity.**
monoamine oxidase (MAO) inhibitors	**Hypertensive crisis, elevated temperatures, severe convulsions, and even death have been reported with this combination. When switching from one therapy to another (MAO inhibitors to carbamazepine or vice versa), a drug-free interval of at least 14 days is recommended. Avoid concurrent use or a potentially serious drug interaction may occur.**
propoxyphene (Darvon, others)	May result in increased carbamazepine serum levels and toxicity. If an analgesic is necessary, it is recommended that another analgesic be selected.
quinidine	Because of increased metabolism, concurrent use may decrease the therapeutic effects of quinidine. Monitor closely for cardiac dysrhythmias; dosage adjustment may be necessary.

Drug	Possible Effect and Management
risperidone (Risperdal)	Carbamazepine will increase the clearance of risperidone and reduce its effectiveness. Monitor for increasing symptoms of psychosis if administered concurrently.

Blood studies (CBC, liver function studies, blood urea nitrates), urinalysis, physical examination, ophthalmic examinations, and ECG should be performed before beginning carbamazepine therapy.

■ **Nursing Diagnosis.** The client receiving carbamazepine therapy should be evaluated for the following nursing diagnoses/collaborative problems: risk for injury related to CNS toxicity (blurred or double vision, nystagmus); excess fluid volume related to water intoxication; impaired oral mucous membrane (dry mouth); disturbed thought processes (confusion); diarrhea; impaired comfort (headache, nausea and vomiting, aching joints and muscles); and the potential complications of Stevens-Johnson syndrome, systemic lupus erythematous–like syndrome, and blood dyscrasias.

■ **Implementation**

■ ***Monitoring.*** The level of seizure activity of the client, as well as the plasma carbamazepine concentrations, should be monitored. Weigh daily and monitor the client's intake and output to determine fluid retention. The client should be observed for any symptoms of adverse reactions to the drug.

Blood studies should be performed every 2 weeks during the second and third months and then every month while the client is taking this medication.

■ ***Intervention.*** Carbamazepine should be administered with meals to reduce gastrointestinal irritation. The importance of compliance with drug therapy should be stressed with all clients taking this drug; in clients with epilepsy, abrupt withdrawal of the drug can precipitate a seizure.

■ ***Education.*** Clients undergoing carbamazepine therapy should report to the prescriber if they experience any signs of hematologic dysfunction such as easy bruising, bleeding, sore throat or mouth, or malaise. It is not uncommon for the client to be drowsy during the initial therapy; clients should be cautioned about this so they can avoid driving a car or operating hazardous equipment.

Carbamazepine is also used specifically for the pain of trigeminal neuralgia. It should not be used as a routine analgesic.

Carbamazepine can cause breakthrough bleeding in women who are taking oral contraceptives. Women should be told that carbamazepine may interfere with the effectiveness of the contraceptive and that other birth control measures may need to be used. Because carbamazepine is excreted in breast milk, it may not be recommended for nursing mothers.

In middle-aged clients or older adults, carbamazepine may decrease salivary flow and contribute to the development of caries, periodontal disease, or discomfort. Ice chips, chewing gum, and sugarless candies may ease the discomfort caused by the dry mouth.

■ **Evaluation.** The expected outcome of carbamazepine therapy is that the client will experience decreased severity and frequency of seizures, decreased mania, or decreased pain with trigeminal neuralgia. The client will also have plasma carbamazepine concentrations of 4 to 12 μg/mL and will not experience adverse reactions to the drug.

felbamate [fel' bah mate] (Felbatol)

Felbamate is an antiepileptic used for the treatment of partial and secondary generalized seizures. It is also used as adjunct therapy for partial and generalized seizures associated with Lennox-Gastaut syndrome in children (Curry & Kulling, 1998).

The mechanism of action of felbamate is unknown, but it has some properties in common with the other anticonvulsants; it may increase seizure threshold, have an inhibitory effect on binding at the gamma-aminobutyric acid (GABA) receptors, and reduce the spread or progression of a seizure. See Table 17-1 for a pharmacokinetic profile of felbamate.

Side effects/adverse reactions include gastric distress, nausea, vomiting, taste alterations, anorexia, constipation, headache, insomnia, dizziness, fever, abnormal gait, and red-purple skin spots.

The usual dosage of felbamate for adults and children 14 years of age and older is 1200 mg/day in divided doses. Children 2 to 14 years of age receive 45 mg/kg/day or 3600 mg/day, whichever is less, in divided doses.

■ Nursing Management

Felbamate Therapy

In addition to the following discussion, see Nursing Management: Anticonvulsant Therapy, p. 353.

■ **Assessment.** Unless absolutely necessary, felbamate is contraindicated for use in clients who currently have or have a history of blood disorders, bone marrow depression, or hepatic impairment; these conditions may be exacerbated.

The baseline assessment of the client should include the status of the underlying seizure disorder, mental status, vital signs, liver function studies, serum iron concentration, and a CBC.

■ **Nursing Diagnosis.** The client receiving felbamate should be assessed for the following nursing diagnoses/collaborative problems: disturbed sleep pattern (daytime sedation); activity intolerance related to malaise and flu-like symptoms; disturbed thought processes (agitation, aggressive reactions); imbalanced nutrition: less than body requirements related to anorexia, nausea, and vomiting; constipation; and the potential complications of blood dyscrasias, hepatic dysfunction, and Stevens-Johnson syndrome.

■ **Implementation**

■ ***Monitoring.*** The value of routine monitoring of felbamate blood levels has not been established, but it may be necessary to monitor the blood levels of the client's other anticonvulsant medications because of the drug's impact on them. Monitor for signs and symptoms of side effects/adverse reactions.

▪ ***Intervention.*** Shake the oral suspension thoroughly before administering.

▪ ***Education.*** Teach the client to take felbamate as prescribed and to consult with the prescriber before taking any other medications, including OTC medications.

▪ **Evaluation.** The expected outcome of felbamate therapy is that the client will experience a decrease in the frequency and severity of seizures without experiencing adverse reactions to the drug.

gabapentin [ga ba pen′ ten] (Neurontin ◆)

Gabapentin is an antiepileptic for the treatment of adult partial seizures with or without secondary generalization. It was tested in clients with refractory partial seizures and was reported to reduce seizure frequency significantly (McLean et al., 1999). The mechanism for its anticonvulsant action is unknown.

Gabapentin is absorbed orally, distributed unbound in the circulation, and excreted by the kidneys unchanged.

Side effects/adverse reactions include drowsiness, dizziness, tiredness, ataxia, and nystagmus. The recommended adult dosage is 300 to 600 mg three times daily.

▪ Nursing Management

Gabapentin Therapy

In addition to the following discussion, see Nursing Management: Anticonvulsant Therapy, p. 353.

▪ **Assessment.** Gabapentin seems to be well tolerated, with adverse reactions that are self-limiting and mild to moderate in severity. The drug is contraindicated if the client has a sensitivity to gabapentin. Clients with impaired renal function may require dosage adjustments based on creatinine clearance.

▪ **Nursing Diagnosis.** The client receiving gabapentin should be assessed for the following nursing diagnoses/collaborative problems: disturbed sleep pattern (daytime somnolence, 19% of clients); risk for injury (dizziness, ataxia, 12.5% to 17%); fatigue (11%); and the potential complications of depression, vision disturbances, nystagmus, myalgia, tremor, and peripheral edema.

▪ **Implementation**

▪ ***Monitoring.*** Because the addition of gabapentin does not significantly alter the serum levels of other anticonvulsant medications, it is not necessary to monitor serum levels for the adjustment of concurrent anticonvulsant medications when gabapentin is added. The value of monitoring gabapentin serum levels has not been established. Dosage titration is based on clinical response.

▪ ***Intervention.*** When administered with antacids, the absorption of gabapentin is reduced. Therefore it is recommended that gabapentin be administered 2 hours after antacids. For clients who cannot tolerate oral capsules, the contents of the capsule may be sprinkled over soft foods immediately before use. The medicine degrades quickly and should be taken immediately after being prepared.

It is recommended that gabapentin be tapered over a minimum of 7 days when discontinuing its use or when switching to another anticonvulsant (*Drug Facts and Comparisons,* 2000).

▪ ***Education.*** Advise the client not to drive or operate dangerous machinery until the effects of gabapentin on him or her can be determined. Regular visits to the health care provider are essential in monitoring therapy, and adherence to the medication schedule is important. Clients taking gabapentin three times daily should not allow more than 12 hours between doses.

▪ **Evaluation.** The expected outcome is that the client will experience a decrease in the frequency and severity of seizures with the addition of gabapentin to the anticonvulsant regimen.

lamotrigine [la moe tri′ jeen] (Lamictal)

Lamotrigine is an anticonvulsant whose mechanism of action is unknown. It is believed that lamotrigine stabilizes seizures by blocking sodium channels, thus inhibiting the release of the excitatory neurotransmitters (glutamate, aspartate) believed to have a role in the development and spread of epileptic seizures (American Hospital Formulary Service, 1999). It is indicated as adjunct therapy for the treatment of partial seizures in adults (16 years and older) with epilepsy.

Lamotrigine is well absorbed orally, reaches peak serum levels in 1.4 to 4.8 hours, and has a half-life of 10 to 25 hours if taken with no other medications. If lamotrigine is administered with an enzyme-inducing anticonvulsant, the half-life is 8 to 20 hours; with valproic acid only, the half-life is 59 hours; and with both enzyme-inducing and valproic acid anticonvulsants, the half-life is 28 hours. It is metabolized in the liver and excreted primarily by the kidneys.

Side effects/adverse reactions include headache, dizziness, drowsiness, abdominal distress, ataxia, rash, and visual disturbances.

If given with enzyme-inducing anticonvulsants, the usual adult dosage of lamotrigine is 50 mg daily for 2 weeks, then 50 mg twice daily for 2 weeks. The dosage is adjusted according to the response. If lamotrigine is administered with enzyme-inducing and valproic acid anticonvulsants, the dosage is 25 mg every other day for 2 weeks, then 25 mg daily for 2 weeks. After 2 weeks, the dosage is adjusted according to client response.

▪ Nursing Management

Lamotrigine Therapy

In addition to the following discussion, see Nursing Management: Anticonvulsant Therapy, p. 353.

▪ **Assessment.** Lamotrigine is contraindicated if the client has a sensitivity to the drug. Clients with thalassemia may experience decreased erythropoiesis, and those with renal impairment may require dosage adjustments.

Review the client's current medication regimen for the risk of significant drug interactions, such as those that may

occur when lamotrigine is given concurrently with the following drugs:

Drug	Possible Effect and Management
carbamazepine (Tegretol), phenobarbital, phenytoin (Dilantin), primidone (Mysoline)	With carbamazepine, an increase in CNS adverse reactions (e.g., blurred vision, dizziness, increased excitation, ataxia) may occur. A reduction in the dosage of either drug may reduce these effects. Monitor lamotrigine serum levels closely because the clearance of it may increase with combined therapies. Monitor serum levels of other agents, because dosage adjustments may be necessary.
valproic acid (Depakene)	The half-life and serum levels of lamotrigine may be increased with this drug combination. Monitor serum levels closely because dosage adjustments may be necessary. This drug combination has also resulted in rash and tremors.

■ **Nursing Diagnosis.** The client receiving lamotrigine should be assessed for the following nursing diagnoses/collaborative problems: risk for injury related to CNS toxicity (dizziness, ataxia, confusion, depression, increased seizures, or nystagmus); disturbed sleep pattern (drowsiness); anxiety; impaired skin integrity (rash); hyperthermia; and the potential complications of vision abnormalities (diplopia, blurred vision), angioedema, blood dyscrasias, and hypersensitivity syndrome (jaundice, dark urine, flu-like symptoms, swollen lymph nodes, and fatigue).

■ **Implementation**

■ ***Monitoring.*** Seizure activity and lamotrigine serum concentrations may be monitored.

■ ***Intervention.*** Lamotrigine should be started at a low dosage and increased gradually to minimize the occurrence of skin rash. It should not be discontinued abruptly because seizure activity will increase.

■ ***Education.*** Instruct the client undergoing lamotrigine therapy to notify the health care provider if a skin rash occurs or seizure activity increases. Stress the importance of complying with the medication regimen and making regular visits to the health care provider. Instruct the client to use caution when driving or performing other hazardous activities until the effects of lamotrigine are known. Instruct the client to discuss with the health care provider the use of other medications and alcohol.

■ **Evaluation.** The expected outcome of lamotrigine therapy is that the client will experience a decrease in the frequency and severity of seizures without adverse reactions.

levetiracetam [lev eh teer ass' eh tam] (Keppra)

Levetiracetam is an anticonvulsant indicated for the treatment of partial onset seizures in adults. It is unrelated to other anticonvulsants, and its mechanism of action is unknown.

Levetiracetam is well absorbed after oral administration, and it reaches a peak level in approximately 1 hour. It is not extensively metabolized, has a half-life of 7 to 8 hours in adults, and is excreted primarily unchanged by the kidneys.

Significant side effects/adverse reactions include sedation, dizziness, asthenia, headache and, in some clients, ataxia and incoordination.

The usual adult dose is 500 mg twice daily initially, increasing by 1000 mg/day at 2-week intervals up to a maximum of 3000 mg/day (*Drug Facts and Comparisons*, 2000).

oxcarbazepine [ox car baz' i peen] (Trileptal)

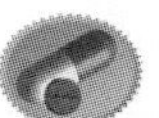

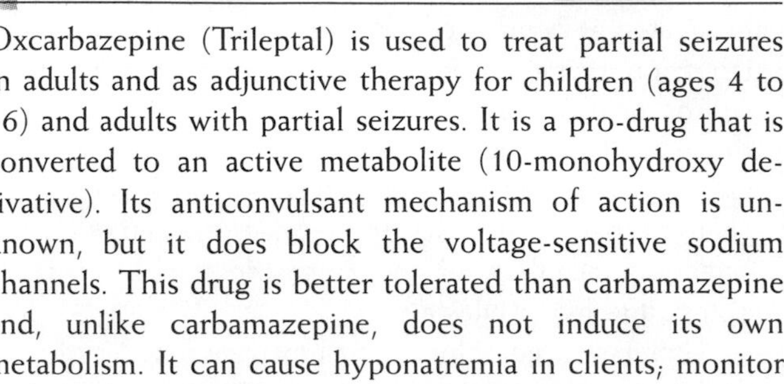

Oxcarbazepine (Trileptal) is used to treat partial seizures in adults and as adjunctive therapy for children (ages 4 to 16) and adults with partial seizures. It is a pro-drug that is converted to an active metabolite (10-monohydroxy derivative). Its anticonvulsant mechanism of action is unknown, but it does block the voltage-sensitive sodium channels. This drug is better tolerated than carbamazepine and, unlike carbamazepine, does not induce its own metabolism. It can cause hyponatremia in clients; monitor serum sodium levels. See Nursing Management: Anticonvulsant Therapy, p. 353.

primidone [pri' mi done] (Mysoline)

Primidone and its metabolites, phenobarbital and phenylethylmalonamide (PEMA), contribute to anticonvulsant activity. The mechanism of action is unknown, but primidone and its metabolites appear to have active anticonvulsant effects. Primidone is used for the control of generalized tonic-clonic (grand mal) and complex seizures. See Table 17-1 for a pharmacokinetics overview of primidone.

Side effects/adverse reactions include drowsiness, ataxia, dizziness, allergic reaction, and possibly paradoxical reactions in children and older adults.

The dosage of primidone for adults is 100 to 125 mg at bedtime for 3 days, increased by 100 or 125 mg twice daily for the fourth through the sixth day, then increased by 100 to 125 mg three times daily through day 9. On day 10, a dosage of 250 mg three times daily is established and may be altered according to the needs of the client to a maximum of 2 g/day.

For children up to 8 years, the initial dosage is 50 mg PO at bedtime for 3 days, increased to 50 mg twice daily through day 6, then increased to 100 mg twice daily through day 9. On day 10, a maintenance dosage of 125 or 250 mg three times daily is established and is adjusted according to client response.

■ **Nursing Management**

Primidone Therapy

Except for the following differences, see Nursing Management: Barbiturate Therapy, p. 363. Clients with reported reactions to barbiturates may not tolerate primidone. Concurrent administration with MAO inhibitors may prolong the effects of primidone; dosage adjustments may be necessary. Monitor closely. Shake the oral suspension well.

BOX 17-3

Toxemia of Pregnancy (Preeclampsia and Eclampsia)

Toxemia of pregnancy is a syndrome of elevated blood pressure, edema, and proteinuria and occurs in about 5% of all pregnancies in North America. The syndrome, also known as preeclampsia, is described in clinical terms because its cause is unknown.

Depending on the severity of symptoms, preeclampsia may be classified either as mild, which may be treated at home, or severe, which requires hospitalization for monitoring and treatment. Convulsions will occur if the disease progresses; the syndrome is then classified as eclampsia, which is derived from a Greek word used to describe convulsions. Sensory changes that occur in severe preeclampsia and eclampsia include headache, epigastric pain, blurred vision, and hyperreflexia.

Therapeutic goals for the treatment of toxemia of pregnancy are control of blood pressure, prevention of convulsions, maintenance of renal function, and provision of optimal conditions for the fetus. Treatment is symptomatic because the only "cure" for toxemia is delivery of the baby. Convulsions may still occur up to 48 hours after delivery, necessitating continued therapy in the immediate postpartum period.

magnesium sulfate [mag nee′ zee um]

Magnesium sulfate has a depressant effect on the CNS, which reduces striated muscle contractions. In addition, magnesium sulfate blocks peripheral neuromuscular transmission by reducing acetylcholine release at the myoneural junction, which reduces the sensitivity of the motor endplate and lowers the excitability of the motor membrane.

Magnesium sulfate has three major indications. As an anticonvulsant, it is used in the prevention and control of seizures related to acute nephritis in children and seizures related to toxemias of pregnancy (Box 17-3). As a uterine relaxant, it is used in the treatment of uterine tetany and to inhibit contractions of premature labor. Finally, it is used as replacement therapy for magnesium deficiency.

Approximately one third of dietary ingested magnesium is absorbed from the gastrointestinal tract. With IV administration, the onset of action is immediate, and the duration of action is approximately 30 minutes. With IM administration, the onset of action is approximately 1 hour, and the duration of action is 3 to 4 hours. Magnesium undergoes no metabolism and is excreted by the kidneys. (See the Management of Drug Overdose box above.)

For seizures caused by toxemia in pregnancy, the dosage is 4 to 5 g (32 to 40 mEq) IV in 250 mL of D_5W or normal saline administered over ½ hour. Administer IM doses of up to 10 g (maximum 5 g in each buttock).

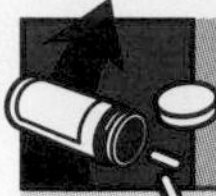

Management of Drug Overdose
Magnesium Sulfate

- Signs of hypermagnesemia, which may begin at a serum concentration at or above 5 mEq/L, include flushing, hypotension, sweating, depressed reflexes, reduced respiratory rate, hypothermia, flaccid paralysis, circulatory collapse, slowed heart rate, and CNS depression.
- Treatment includes artificial respiration and calcium gluconate IV (5 to 10 mEq of calcium) injected slowly to reverse respiratory depression and heart block. Dialysis may be necessary if renal function is reduced.

Magnesium sulfate is administered for the treatment of toxemia of pregnancy. The drug crosses the placenta, with fetal blood levels approximately equal to maternal blood levels, and produces similar effects in the neonate and in the mother. Decreased reflexes, muscle tone, blood pressure, and respiratory depression may be seen if the mother received magnesium shortly before delivery. It is recommended that magnesium sulfate not be administered during the 2 hours before delivery, if possible.

▪ Nursing Management
Magnesium Sulfate Therapy

▪ **Assessment.** Magnesium sulfate should not be used in the presence of heart block, significant heart damage, or renal failure (creatinine clearance <20 mL/min). Caution must be exercised in the presence of severe renal function impairment because of the risk of hypermagnesemia and magnesium toxicity.

Review the client's current medication regiment for the risk of significant drug interactions, such as those that may occur when magnesium sulfate is given concurrently with the following drugs:

Drug	Possible Effect and Management
Bold/color type indicates the most serious interactions.	
CNS depressants	Dosages of barbiturates, opiates, general anesthetics, or other CNS depressants should be adjusted to avoid additive CNS depressant effects.
neuromuscular blocking agents	**Excessive neuromuscular blockade has occurred when these drugs are administered with magnesium sulfate. Avoid concurrent usage.**

A baseline assessment should include blood pressure and respiratory rate determination, deep tendon reflexes, ECG for cardiac function, renal function determinations (especially urine output), and serum magnesium levels.

▪ **Nursing Diagnosis.** The client undergoing magnesium sulfate therapy should be assessed for the following nursing diagnoses/collaborative problems: risk for injury related to hypotension and electrolyte imbalances (hypermagnesemia); activity intolerance related to hypotonia; and the potential complication of cardiac dysrhythmias and respiratory paralysis.

■ **Implementation**

■ ***Monitoring.*** Monitor seizure activity. Measure vital signs every 15 minutes while the drug is administered intravenously. Respirations should be at least 16/min before each parenteral dose. Monitor intake and output; urinary output should be at least 100 mL in the 4 hours before each dose. The client must be closely monitored for the possible development of magnesium toxicity. The ECG should be monitored continuously during IV administration. Serum magnesium determinations may be obtained as clinically indicated. Normal average serum magnesium concentrations are 1.6 to 2.6 mEq/L. The following are approximate serum concentrations (mEq/L) indicative of hypermagnesemia:

- 4 to 7: therapeutic range, mild depression of deep tendon reflexes
- 5 to 10: depression of deep tendon reflexes; prolonged PQ interval or widened QRS interval on ECG
- 8 to 10: loss of deep tendon reflexes
- 10 to 13: respiratory paralysis
- 15: altered cardiac conduction
- 25: cardiac arrest

The patellar reflex or knee jerk is an indication of CNS depression from magnesium. The patellar reflex should be checked before beginning therapy and before each dose. The disappearance of the reflex indicates excessive serum levels of magnesium.

■ ***Intervention.*** Extreme care must be taken to avoid overdose and toxic serum concentrations of magnesium. IV infusions should be administered with a regulating or controlling device. A calcium salt that can be administered intravenously (calcium gluconate, calcium gluceptate, or calcium chloride) should be available when parenteral magnesium is administered.

■ ***Education.*** Alert the client to the adverse reactions to magnesium so that he or she may report them as soon as they are experienced.

■ **Evaluation.** The expected outcome of magnesium therapy is that the client will be seizure free and will not develop hypermagnesemia.

tiagabine [ti a′ ga been] (Gabatril)

Tiagabine is a GABA uptake inhibitor and is indicated as adjunct therapy in partial seizures. Oral absorption in the fasting state is rapid, with peak serum levels reached within 45 minutes. The elimination half-life is 7 to 9 hours, and a steady state is reached in approximately 2 days. This drug is metabolized in the liver and excreted in the urine and feces (*Drug Facts and Comparisons*, 2000).

Side effects/adverse reactions include stomach pain, drowsiness, weakness, memory impairment, headache, dizziness, nausea, vomiting, tremors, diarrhea, and insomnia.

The adult dosage of tiagabine is 4 mg daily initially, increased weekly by 4 to 8 mg until a therapeutic response is achieved or a total of 56 mg/day is reached. This drug should be administered in divided doses either two or four times daily.

■ Nursing Management

Tiagabine Therapy

In addition to the following discussion, see Nursing Management: Anticonvulsant Therapy, p. 353.

■ **Assessment.** Tiagabine is contraindicated for use in clients with known tiagabine sensitivity. Use with caution in clients with liver and renal function impairment or with neurologic disorders such as stroke, dementia, and Alzheimer's disease. Evaluate the client's concurrent medication regimen for significant interactions; for example, tiagabine clearance is increased by 60% in clients receiving carbamazepine, phenobarbital, phenytoin, and primidone. A baseline level of the client's seizure activity should be documented.

■ **Nursing Diagnosis.** The client undergoing tiagabine therapy should be assessed for the following nursing diagnoses/collaborative problems: risk for injury related to the CNS effects of the drug (ataxia, confusion, difficulty in concentrating, memory impairment, weakness); disturbed sleep pattern (drowsiness, insomnia); nausea; diarrhea; impaired skin integrity (rash); and the potential complications of nystagmus, flu-like syndrome, tremor, and myalgia.

■ **Implementation**

■ ***Monitoring.*** The client's seizure activity and tiagabine serum concentrations should be monitored.

■ ***Intervention.*** Tiagabine should be taken with food. The drug is not to be discontinued abruptly; the dosage should be reduced gradually.

■ ***Education.*** Stress compliance with the medication regimen and regular visits to the health care provider. Use caution when driving or performing other hazardous activities until the effects of tiagabine are known. Instruct the client to discuss with the health care provider the use of other medications and alcohol.

■ **Evaluation.** The expected outcome of tiagabine therapy is that the client will experience decreased frequency and severity or an absence of seizures without experiencing any adverse reactions to the drug.

topiramate [to pir′ a mate] (Topamax)

Although the exact mechanism of action for topiramate is unknown, it has three properties that may contribute to its anticonvulsant characteristics. First, it appears to have a sodium channel blocking action, thus blocking the repetitive depolarization of neurons; second, it potentiates the activity of the inhibitory neurotransmitter GABA; and third, it antagonizes the ability of kainate (a receptor agonist) to activate an excitatory glutamate receptor. It is indicated for adjunct therapy for adult partial onset seizures.

Topiramate is rapidly absorbed orally, has an elimination half-life of 21 hours, and reaches a steady state in approximately 4 days. It is not extensively metabolized in the body and is excreted primarily unchanged by the kidneys.

Side effects/adverse reactions include drowsiness, dizziness, ataxia, speech problems, increased nervousness, paresthesia, tremors, confusion, difficulty with concentration and memory, depression, agitation, nausea, anorexia, vision changes, weight loss, psychomotor slowing, and anxiety.

The usual adult dosage of topiramate is 50 mg/day PO initially, titrated to effectiveness. The adjunct dosage is 200 mg twice daily.

■ Nursing Management

Topiramate Therapy

In addition to the following discussion, see Nursing Management: Anticonvulsant Therapy, p. 353.

■ **Assessment.** Topiramate is contraindicated for use in clients with topiramate sensitivity and is used with caution in clients with hepatic and renal impairment.

Review the client's current medication regimen for the risk of significant drug interactions, such as those that may occur when topiramate is given concurrently with the following drugs:

Drug	Possible Effect and Management
Bold/color type indicates the most serious interactions.	
alcohol, CNS depressants	When combined with topiramate, CNS depression, cognitive impairment, and other adverse CNS effects may occur. If possible, avoid this combination.
carbamazepine (Tegretol), phenytoin (Dilantin)	Concurrent therapy may significantly decrease topiramate serum concentration (40% to 50%). Phenytoin serum levels may also increase by 25% in some clients. Monitor serum levels closely because dosage adjustments may be necessary.
carbonic anhydrase inhibitors	**Increases risk for kidney stone formation. Avoid using this drug combination.**
contraceptives, oral with estrogen	May decrease efficacy of oral contraceptives. Alternative contraceptive methods may need to be considered.

■ **Nursing Diagnosis.** The client undergoing topiramate therapy should be assessed for the following nursing diagnoses/collaborative problems: impaired verbal communication; acute confusion; risk for injury related to the CNS effects of the drug (ataxia, weakness); imbalanced nutrition: less than body requirements (anorexia, weight loss); fatigue; impaired oral mucous membrane (gingivitis); and the potential complications of vision disturbances, dysmenorrhea, renal stones, and leukopenia.

■ **Implementation**

■ ***Monitoring.*** The client's seizure status should be monitored, but serum concentrations of topiramate need to be monitored only when other drugs are added or discontinued.

■ ***Intervention.*** Dosage adjustments may be necessary if other antiepileptic drugs are started or discontinued. Topiramate should be withdrawn gradually to minimize the potential for increased seizure activity. The drug may be taken without regard to meals. Avoid breaking the tablets because of the bitter taste.

■ ***Education.*** The client undergoing topiramate therapy should be instructed to maintain an adequate fluid intake to minimize the risk of renal stone formation. Caution should be taken with activities that require alertness. The client should use alternative contraception methods if using oral estrogen-containing contraceptives.

■ **Evaluation.** The expected outcome of topiramate therapy is that the client will experience a decreased frequency and severity or an absence of seizures without experiencing adverse reactions to the drug.

valproic acid [val proe′ ik] (Depakene)
divalproex sodium [dye val′ proe ex] (Depakote ◆)
valproate [val proe′ ate] (Depacon Parenteral)

The mechanism by which valproic acid exerts its anticonvulsant effects has not been fully established. It has been proposed that its activity is related to directly or indirectly increasing or enhancing brain levels of the inhibitory neurotransmitter GABA. By competitive inhibition it may prevent the reuptake of GABA by glial cells and axonal terminals.

Valproic acid, valproate, and divalproex sodium are indicated for use as sole and adjunctive therapy in the treatment of absence seizures (including petit mal) and as adjunctive therapy in clients with multiple seizure types, including absence seizures.

See Table 17-1 for a pharmacokinetic overview of valproic acid. Chemically, valproate sodium is converted in the stomach to valproic acid, which is rapidly absorbed from the gastrointestinal tract. Divalproex sodium is a pro-drug that consists of a combination of valproic acid and valproate sodium in an enteric-coated tablet. Divalproex sodium dissociates into valproate, which is then absorbed in the small intestine. Valproate has nearly replaced the valproic acid dosage form because it produces many fewer gastrointestinal side effects. The term *valproate* has been used to reflect the presence of this drug in the body, regardless of its source (valproic acid, divalproex or valproate).

Valproate has a variable half-life of 6 to 16 hours. The time to peak serum levels varies with the dosage form: from 1 to 4 hours for capsules and syrup, from 3 to 4 hours for delayed-release capsules and tablets, and at the end of the IV infusion for parenteral administration.

Side effects/adverse reactions include tremors, mild gastric distress, diarrhea, weight gain, irregular menses, and hepatotoxicity. The adult and pediatric dosage is initially 15 mg/kg/day, increased at weekly intervals as needed. The maximum daily dose is 60 mg/kg (*Mosby's GenRx*, 1999).

■ Nursing Management

Valproic Acid Therapy

■ **Assessment.** Hepatic disease in the client contraindicates the use of valproic acid therapy, because there have been some instances of fatal hepatotoxicity with the use of this drug. It is also recommended that caution be used in clients with blood dyscrasias, organic brain disease, hypoalbuminemia, and renal function impairment. Valproic acid is excreted in breast milk and can cause CNS depression in the nursing infant. Birth defects (spina bifida) have occurred when this drug was taken during the first trimester of pregnancy. Clients taking this drug who are considering pregnancy may need to be given another anticonvulsant that has no documented risk of causing birth defects.

Review the client's current medication regimen for the risk of significant drug interactions, such as those that may occur when valproic acid and divalproex sodium (a drug that contains 50% valproic acid and sodium valproate) are given concurrently with the following drugs:

Drug	Possible Effect and Management
alcohol, anesthetics (general), CNS depressant–type drugs	May result in potentiated CNS depressant effects.
anticoagulants, warfarin (Coumadin), heparin, or thrombolytic agents	Increased risk of bleeding and hemorrhage; monitor closely for early signs if given in combination.
aspirin, dipyridamole (Persantine), or sulfinpyrazone (Anturane)	Increased risk of bleeding and hemorrhage; monitor closely; the prescriber might consider alternative therapeutic agents.
barbiturates or primidone (Mysoline)	Phenobarbital and primidone serum levels may increase, resulting in increased depression and toxicity. Monitor closely because the prescriber may need to adjust the dosage.
carbamazepine (Tegretol) and phenytoin (Dilantin)	Breakthrough seizures may occur because of decreased serum levels of carbamazepine or valproic acid. Phenytoin protein binding may be affected when combined with valproic acid; therefore monitor closely, using serum levels as a guide for dosage adjustments by the prescriber.
felbamate (Felbatol)	Concurrent administration may increase valproate plasma concentrations by 35% to 50%. Dosage adjustments may be needed when felbamate therapy is started.
lamotrigine (Lamictal)	When coadministered, the dosage of lamotrigine should be reduced. Concurrent use increases the risk of serious dermatologic reactions.
mefloquine (Lariam)	Concurrent use may result in lower valproic acid serum levels and a loss of seizure control. Monitor valproic acid levels; dosage adjustments during and after mefloquine therapy may be necessary.

■ **Nursing Diagnosis.** The client receiving valproic acid therapy has the potential for the following nursing diagnoses/collaborative problems: risk of injury related to visual effects (double vision, nystagmus); imbalanced nutrition: less than body requirements related to anorexia, indigestion, and nausea and vomiting; diarrhea; and the potential complications of hepatotoxicity, adverse ophthalmologic effects, pancreatitis (abdominal pain, nausea and vomiting), cognitive impairment, and thrombocytopenia (unusual bruising or bleeding).

■ **Implementation**

■ ***Monitoring.*** In addition to monitoring the client's seizure activity and serum valproate concentrations, observe for early signs of adverse reactions. Baseline and periodic evaluations of bleeding time, blood cell counts, and renal and hepatic function studies are recommended.

■ ***Intervention.*** These medications should be administered with or after meals to avoid gastric irritation. Avoid giving the tablet form with milk because of possible early dissolution and local irritation to the mouth and throat. The drug is available in syrup form for clients unable to swallow tablets or capsules. Divalproex sodium is prescribed for clients unable to tolerate the gastrointestinal irritation produced by valproic acid. When other anticonvulsant drugs are used in combination, the dosage of valproic acid and/or the other anticonvulsants may need to be adjusted to maintain serum levels and seizure control.

■ ***Education.*** The client should be instructed not to chew the tablet or capsule because it will irritate the mouth and throat. Combining this drug with alcohol or other CNS depressants can cause a potentiation of sedation.

Valproate from any source can cause a false-positive urine ketone test in clients with diabetes mellitus; the client should be instructed to consult the prescriber about using some other diagnostic tool for ketones. The client should be instructed to be aware of signs of decreasing mental alertness, which can occur when valproic acid is given alone or in combination with other anticonvulsants.

The client should be told to report to the prescriber if visual disturbances, rash, or diarrhea occur. Valproic acid has been shown to cause liver dysfunction; therefore the client should be instructed to report signs of liver dysfunction (e.g., spontaneous bleeding and bruising, light-colored stools, jaundice, and protracted vomiting) to the prescriber immediately. The client should undergo liver function studies at least every month during the first 6 months of therapy, when hepatotoxicity is most likely to occur.

■ **Evaluation.** The expected outcome of valproic acid therapy is that the client will experience a decrease in the frequency and severity of seizures with a predose serum valproate concentration of at least 50 μg/mL, and the client will not experience adverse reactions to the drug.

zonisamide [zo nis′ i mide] (Zonegran)

Zonisamide (Zonegran) is an adjunctive therapy drug for the treatment of partial seizures in adults. The initial dosage is 100 mg/day, which may be increased as necessary at 2-week intervals. Avoid the use of this drug in clients with sulfa allergies. Clients should be instructed to swallow the capsule whole, and women of childbearing age should use effective contraception. In addition, see Nursing Management: Anticonvulsant Therapy, p. 353.

SUMMARY

Epilepsy, a symptom of a brain disorder rather than a disease itself, occurs in only a small percentage of the population.

Epileptic seizures have various causes and are classified by symptoms. The nurse needs to be particularly observant in the assessment and documentation of seizures. The drugs used for the treatment of seizures are also varied and include barbiturates, hydantoins, succinimides, and benzodiazepines. The therapy for each client is individualized by taking into account a complex of interrelated factors, such as the pharmacokinetics of the drug in an individual, concurrent ailments and medications, diet, physical status, and compliance with the regimen. The nurse must use a holistic approach, not only to manage the client's physical symptoms but also to provide psychosocial support. For these clients, moderation in rest, exercise, diet, and avoidance of stress is important. The most common nursing diagnoses for clients receiving anticonvulsant therapy are knowledge deficit; ineffective management of therapeutic regimen; and risk for injury related to the side effects/adverse reactions of these drugs. An important evaluation factor is the effectiveness of the regimen in controlling and minimizing seizures.

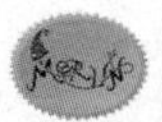

Critical Thinking Exercises

1. Why is the assessment essential in determining a therapeutic anticonvulsant medication regimen for a client? What part does the client's age play?
2. Mrs. Curtis and her husband have decided to start a family. She is 24 years of age and has been taking phenytoin since childhood for a seizure disorder; she would like to discontinue the medication before getting pregnant. What criteria will be involved in deciding to wean Mrs. Curtis from her medication?

Collaborative Learning Activities

For Collaborative Learning Activities, go to mosby.com/MERLIN/McKenry/.

CASE STUDY

For a Case Study that will help ensure mastery of this chapter content, go to mosby.com/MERLIN/McKenry/.

BIBLIOGRAPHY

American Hospital Formulary Service. (1999). *AHFS drug information '99*. Bethesda, MD: American Society of Hospital Pharmacists.

Anderson, K.N., Anderson, L.E., & Glanze, W.D. (Eds.) (1998). *Mosby's medical, nursing, & allied health dictionary* (5th ed.). St. Louis: Mosby.

Armstrong, E.P., Sauer, K.A., & Downey, M.J. (1999). Phenytoin and fosphenytoin: A model of cost and clinical outcomes. *Pharmacotherapy, 19*(7), 844-853.

Bazil, C.W. & Pedley, T.A. (1998). Advances in the medical treatment of epilepsy. *Annual Review of Medicine, 49*, 135-162.

Bialer, M., Johannessen, S.I., Kuperferberg, H.J., Levy, R.H., Loisea, P., & Perucca, E. (1999). Progress report on new antiepileptic drugs: A summary of the fourth Eilat conference (EILAT IV). *Epilepsy Research, 34*(1), 1-41.

Bleck, T.P. (1999). Management approaches to prolonged seizures and status epilepticus. *Epilepsia, 40*(suppl 1), S59-S63.

Blum, D.E. (1998). New drugs for persons with epilepsy. *Advanced Neurology, 76*, 57-87.

Bourgeois, B.F. (1998). New antiepileptic drugs. *Archives of Neurology, 55*(9), 1181-1183.

Carpenito, L.J. (2000). *Nursing diagnosis: Application to clinical practice* (8th ed.). Philadelphia: J.B. Lippincott.

Carter, J.R. (1994). The use of new antiepileptic medications in pediatric patients with epilepsy. *Journal of Pediatric Health Care, 8*(6), 277-282.

Chipps, E.M., Clanin, N.J., & Campbell, V.G. (1992). *Neurologic disorders*. St. Louis: Mosby.

Cloyd, J. (1996). Pharmacologic considerations of fosphenytoin therapy. *P & T Supplement, 21*(55), 13s-20s.

CNS Clinical Development Department, Parke-Davis Pharmaceutical Research. (1998). Clinical experience with fosphenytoin in adults: Pharmacokinetics, safety, and efficacy. *Journal of Child Neurology 13*(suppl 1), S15-S18.

Curry, W.J. & Kulling, D.L. (1998). Newer antiepileptic drugs: Gabapentin, lamotrigine, felbamate, topiramate, and fosphenytoin. *American Family Physician, 57*(3), 513-520.

Dichter, M.A. (1992). Deciding to discontinue antiepileptic medication. *Hospital Practice, 27*(20), 16.

Drug Facts and Comparisons. (2000). St. Louis: Facts and Comparisons.

Drug Update. (1996). Pharmacy News. *Journal of the American Pharmaceutical Association, NS36*(10), 566.

Elger, C.E. & Bauer, J. (1998). New antiepileptic drugs in epileptology. *Neuropsychobiology, 38*(3), 145-148.

Emilien, G. & Maloteaux, J.M. (1998). Pharmacological management of epilepsy: Mechanism of action, pharmacokinetic interactions, and new drug discovery possibilities. *International Journal of Clinical Pharmacological Therapies, 36*(4), 181-194.

Foster, S. & Tyler, V.C. (2000). *Tyler's honest herbal* (4th ed.). New York: Haworth Herbal Press.

Hardman, J.G. & Limbird, L.E. (Eds.). (1996). *Goodman & Gilman's The pharmacological basis of therapeutics* (9th ed.). New York: Macmillan.

Legion, V. (1991). Health education for self-management by people with epilepsy. *Journal of Neuroscience Nursing, 23*(5), 300.

Lott, R.S. (1995). Seizure disorders. In L.Y. Young & M.A. Koda-Kimble (Eds.), *Applied therapeutics: The clinical use of drugs*. Vancouver, WA: Applied Therapeutics.

Luer, M.S. (1998). Fosphenytoin. *Neurological Research, 20*(2), 178-182.

McLean, M.J., Morrell M.J., Willmore, L.J., Priviteria, M.D., Faught, R.E., Holmes, G.L., Magnus-Miller, L., Bernstein, P., Rose-Legatt, A. (1999). Safety and tolerability of gabapentin as adjunctive therapy in a large, multicenter study. *Epilepsia, 40*(7), 965-972.

Mosby's GenRx. (1999). St. Louis: Mosby.

Nulman, I., Laslo, D., & Koren, G. (1999). *Drugs, 57*(4), 535-544.

Physicians' Desk Reference. (1999). Montvale, NJ: Medical Economics.

Rowan, A.J. (1995). Recognition and assessment of seizure disorders in the elderly: Epidemiology, pathophysiology, and differentiation. *Consultant Pharmacist, 10*(suppl A), 4-8.

Tanaka, E. (1999). Clinically significant pharmacokinetic drug interactions between antiepileptic drugs. *Journal of Clinical Pharmacological Therapy, 24*(2), 87-92.

United States Pharmacopeia Dispensing Information (USP DI): Drug information for the health care professional (19th ed.). (1999). Rockville, MD: United States Pharmacopeial Convention.

18 Central Nervous System Stimulants

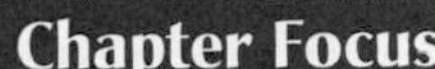

Chapter Focus

The central nervous system (CNS) stimulants may produce dramatic effects, but their therapeutic usefulness is limited because of their multiple actions and side effects. Continuous use and misuse of these drugs (especially amphetamines) can result in the development of tolerance, dependence, and abuse. Large doses of the CNS stimulants may precipitate convulsive seizures, coma, and exhaustion. Although the number of drugs that stimulate the CNS is large, only a few of these drugs are actually used for this purpose. The nurse needs to be knowledgeable about the therapeutic uses of CNS stimulant drugs as well as the nontherapeutic effects of these drugs, which are commonly abused in our society.

Learning Objectives

1. Discuss attention deficit disorder with hyperactivity and the drug treatment for this condition.
2. Define the terms *analeptic drug* and *anorexiant drug*.
3. Describe common CNS stimulant drugs and the indications for their use.
4. Identify common physical and psychologic changes attributable to CNS stimulants.
5. List caffeine-containing food and beverages, along with their approximate caffeine content.
6. Implement an appropriate plan of care for the client receiving CNS stimulant drugs.

Key Terms

amphetamines, p. 378
analeptics, p. 378
anorexiants, p. 378
attention deficit hyperactivity disorder, p. 378
narcolepsy, p. 378

Key Drugs [✔]

amphetamine, p. 381
caffeine, p. 387
methylphenidate, p. 386

The classification of a stimulant depends on where in the nervous system it exerts its major effects—on the cerebrum, the medulla and brainstem, or the hypothalamic and limbic regions. **Amphetamines** are mainly stimulants of the cerebral cortex; **analeptics** primarily affect the centers in the medulla and the brainstem; and **anorexiants** suppress the appetite, perhaps by a direct stimulant effect on the satiety center in the hypothalamic and limbic regions. Central nervous system (CNS) stimulants act by increasing neuronal discharge or by blocking an inhibitory neurotransmitter. These drugs may also affect other parts of the nervous system.

Cerebral stimulants were once commonly prescribed for obesity and to counteract an overdose of CNS depressants, but such use today is considered obsolete. Although the CNS stimulants do suppress appetite, tolerance develops to the anorexic effect usually before the weight reduction goal is reached. Treatment of severe CNS depression with stimulants is also discouraged because close monitoring and supportive measures have been found to be quite successful without producing undesirable adverse reactions. With their narrow therapeutic index between effectiveness and toxicity, CNS stimulants may induce cardiac dysrhythmias, hypertension, convulsions, and violent behavior. Thus the CNS stimulants have limited use in practice today; they are used primarily for the treatment of narcolepsy and **attention deficit hyperactivity disorder (ADHD)**.

During the past decade the prevalence of attention deficit hyperactivity disorder (ADHD) and its pharmacologic treatment has increased dramatically in the United States (Robison, Sclar, Skaer, & Galin, 1999). ADHD is a syndrome characterized by distractibility, a short attention span, impulsive behavior, hyperactivity, and learning and behavior disabilities. Improper functioning of the neurotransmitter systems (noradrenergic, dopaminergic, and serotonergic) has been implicated in this syndrome (Saklad & Curtis, 1995). Stimulant medications tend to decrease distractibility and hyperactivity, resulting in an increased attention span (Berman, Douglas, & Barr, 1999; Sunohara et al., 1999).

The onset of ADHD usually occurs between the ages of 3 and 7 years, with boys affected more often than girls by a 4 to 8 : 1 ratio (Saklad & Curtis, 1995). Professional intervention is usually unnecessary until the child enters the school setting. ADHD may persist into adulthood. In one report of young adults that had ADHD in childhood, 31% still had the full syndrome. Adults with ADHD may have a higher incidence of substance abuse, antisocial personality disorders, anxiety, and depression when compared with a control group. Children treated with stimulants were reported to have a better outcome in adulthood (Saklad & Curtis, 1995). Management of this disorder requires a behavioral modification program, with the use of pharmacologic therapy as an adjunct if necessary.

Approximately 15% to 20% of children with ADHD do not respond to stimulant drugs, or their symptoms actually increase. Antidepressant therapy (imipramine [Tofranil], desipramine [Norpramin]) should be considered for these individuals, especially if they also have symptoms of anxiety or depression. Clonidine (Catapres) has been used, especially for persons with both ADHD and Tourette's syndrome; this product should not be used for children with ADHD and depression because it can worsen the condition (Saklad & Curtis, 1995).

Although stimulant medications are available in short-acting (4-hour) and long-acting (8- to 10-hour) forms, it is general practice to establish a daily schedule using the short-acting form. The dosage required will be learned from empiric experience. For this reason the prescriber needs to work closely with the child, the parents, and school personnel in evaluating results and planning dosages.

The child's distractibility and hyperactivity must be managed during school hours. It may be equally important to contain these symptoms at other times of the day to promote the child's psychosocial development through participation in clubs, religious activities, or social events. Rather than having a continuous approach to dosing, it is more helpful to consider the child's life in 4-hour units and to provide a dose appropriate to the needs of that time block. For example, the child might take 10 mg of a short-acting stimulant at 8 AM and again at noon on a school day but add another dose at 4 PM if a music lesson is planned for that evening.

Narcolepsy is a condition characterized by excessive drowsiness and uncontrollable sleep attacks during the daytime. In addition, the client may exhibit a sleep paralysis (inability to move that occurs immediately on falling asleep or on awakening), cataplexy (stress-induced, generalized muscle weakness), and hypnagogic illusions or hallucinations (vivid auditory or visual dreams occurring at the onset of sleep). CNS stimulants are useful in controlling daytime drowsiness and excessive sleep patterns, and tricyclic antidepressants are being tested in conjunction with the stimulants for cataplexy and sleep paralysis. Box 18-1 provides information on one agent used to treat narcolepsy, modafinil (Provigil).

The mechanism of action for the cerebral stimulants (amphetamines) includes the release of norepinephrine from storage as well as direct stimulation of alpha and beta receptor sites. The CNS effects are unknown, but the primary action appears to be in the cerebral cortex and possibly the reticular activating system. Stimulation results in an increase in motor function and mental alertness, a decreased sense of fatigue, and usually a euphoric effect (American Hospital Formulary Service, 1999).

Animal studies indicate that amphetamine blocks the reuptake of dopamine and norepinephrine from the synapse, inhibits the action of monoamine oxidase (MAO), and also increases the release of catecholamines (*United States Pharmacopeia Dispensing Information*, 1999).

ANOREXIANT DRUGS

Anorexiant, or appetite-suppressant, drugs include a variety of medications that are used to treat exogenous obesity. They

BOX 18-1

Modafinil for Narcolepsy

Modafinil (Provigil) is an analeptic; it promotes wakefulness like the sympathomimetic agents (amphetamine, methylphenidate) but pharmacologically is not similar to them. Its mechanism of action is unknown.

This drug is rapidly absorbed orally and reaches peak serum levels in 2 to 4 hours. It is metabolized in the liver and excreted by the kidneys.

Modafinil is generally well tolerated. The potential side effects/adverse reactions include headache, nervousness, nausea, rhinitis, insomnia, and nervousness.

Although reported drug interactions early in the use of a product are low, the health care provider should monitor the client closely whenever multiple drug therapies are used. In addition, be aware that the effectiveness of oral contraceptives may be reduced; additional or alternative methods of contraception are recommended. Modafinil can also increase phenytoin levels when administered concurrently, so monitor closely for signs of toxicity.

The usual adult dosage is 200 mg daily, administered in the morning (*Drug Facts and Comparisons*, 2000).

BOX 18-2

Lipase Inhibitor: Orlistat (Xenical)

Orlistat (Xenical) is a reversible lipase inhibitor that controls obesity by inhibiting the absorption of dietary fats. This product forms a bond with lipase; thus the enzyme is not available to convert fat into triglycerides for absorption. The action of orlistat depends on its action in the stomach and small intestine and not on systemic absorption. Orlistat is capable of inhibiting dietary fat absorption by approximately 30%.

Clients prescribed orlistat must also be on a specific weight loss (or weight maintenance) diet. It is recommended that the client take supplements of fat-soluble vitamins, because orlistat reduces the absorption of some of these vitamins.

The side effects/adverse reactions include mainly mild and transient gastrointestinal symptoms. When taken for a year, other effects such as headache, stomach and back pain, and respiratory symptoms were reported; interestingly, however, most of these symptoms were not present in the second year of therapy (*Drug Facts and Comparisons*, 2000).

The usual adult dose is one 120-mg capsule three times daily with meals. It can be taken during a meal or up to 1 hour after a meal that contains fat.

are indirect-acting sympathomimetics and, with the exception of mazindol, they are chemically and pharmacologically amphetamine-like drugs. Their exact mechanism of action is unknown, but these agents appear to act on the satiety center in the hypothalamus and limbic areas of the brain.

Benzphetamine (Didrex), diethylpropion (Tenuate), phendimetrazine (Adphen, Bontril) and phentermine (Fastin, Phentride) mainly act on the adrenergic pathways, whereas mazindol affects both the adrenergic (norepinephrine) and dopaminergic (dopamine) pathways. The newly released drug sibutramine (Meridia) is a serotonin and norepinephrine reuptake inhibitor. Box 18-2 provides information on one lipase inhibitor, orlistat (Xenical).

Phendimetrazine affects norepinephrine and, like amphetamine, produces marked euphoria and stimulation and has an abuse potential. Phentermine and diethylpropion affect norepinephrine and produce mild euphoria, produce mild to moderate stimulation, and have a minimal abuse potential. Mazindol affects dopamine and adrenergic receptors and has the same CNS effects as diethylpropion, with a minimal abuse potential.

Anorexiants have a number of limitations, and careful selection of the clinical choices is necessary to minimize the unwanted effects. As appetite suppressants, they are recommended as an adjunct to other regimens (e.g., physical exercise, behavior modification, restriction of caloric intake). They are prescribed for a short time because tolerance to the anorectic effect may occur within a few weeks (*USP DI*, 1999).

Sibutramine (Meridia) was released in 1998 to treat obesity. This product is a serotonin and norepinephrine reuptake inhibitor, and there are specific guidelines for its use. This product must be used in conjunction with a reduced-calorie diet. The client is identified as having an initial body mass index (BMI) of at least 30 kg/m^2 or at least 27 kg/m^2 in the presence of other risk factors such as diabetes or hypertension.

Sibutramine does not increase the release of serotonin from nerve cells and therefore is less apt to induce serotonin toxicity. Serotonin toxicity is the suspected cause of the adverse cardiac reactions associated with the drugs previously withdrawn from the market, dexfenfluramine (Redux) and fenfluramine (Pondimin) (Constantine & Scott, 1997).

Pharmacokinetics. The anorexiant drugs are rapidly absorbed when taken orally, and they are lipid soluble and cross the blood-brain barrier. The immediate-release formulations usually produce their effects for 4 to 6 hours; mazindol produces its effects for 8 to 15 hours. The half-life of phendimetrazine is between 2 and 10 hours. The drugs and their metabolites are primarily excreted in urine. No pharmacokinetic data was available for sibutramine.

Side Effects/Adverse Reactions. The most commonly reported side effects of the anorexiant drugs include euphoria, increased irritability, nervousness, and insomnia. Less common side effects are visual disturbance, diarrhea or constipation, dry mouth, difficulty in urination, tachy-

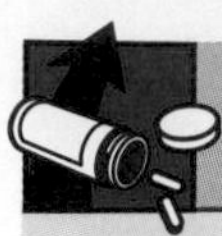

Management of Drug Overdose
Anorexiants

- There is no specific antidote for an overdose of anorexiant drugs. Institute symptomatic and supportive measures according to the requirements of the individual client.
- In general, emesis and/or the use of gastric lavage is indicated, followed by administration of activated charcoal to adsorb any remaining drug in the gastrointestinal tract.
- Excessive stimulation may be counteracted with barbiturates, chlorpromazine, or haloperidol (to decrease anticholinergic effects). Seizures may be controlled with diazepam or phenobarbital.
- Monitor vital signs and respiratory functions at frequent intervals. Closely monitor cardiac and respiratory functions. The following medications are usually used: for hypertension, IV phentolamine or nitrites; for hypotension, IV fluids; for dysrhythmias, lidocaine IV; and for tachycardia, a beta-adrenergic blocking agent.
- Urine acidification and forced diuresis are also recommended.

cardia, impotence, headaches, sweating, and nausea and vomiting.

Adverse reactions include hypertension with all stimulant drugs. Less commonly reported adverse reactions are CNS depression and confusion, allergic rashes or hives, and psychosis. (See the Management of Drug Overdose box above.)

Dosage and Administration. Table 18-1 provides the usual adult dosage and the federal Controlled Substances Act schedule for each anorexiant medication. The lower numbers on the scale of II to IV note the agents with the greatest abuse potential.

■ Nursing Management

Anorexiant Therapy

■ **Assessment.** Anorexiant drugs are used to treat the nursing diagnosis of altered nutrition: more than body requirements. Work with the client to determine the causative factors for the obesity that results from the ingestion of calories in excess of metabolic need, which can include sedentary lifestyle, lack of nutritional knowledge, or increased food intake related to stress, low self-esteem, or boredom. Nursing interventions can be planned according to the specific etiologic factor for which the anorexiant drug therapy serves as a short-term adjunct. A realistic goal for weight loss is 1 to 2 pounds per week, but clients with obesity will tend to have a greater weight loss than this, at least initially.

In general, anorexiants are contraindicated for clients with agitated states, arteriosclerotic disease, cardiovascular disease (particularly clients with dysrhythmias), cerebral ischemia, glaucoma, moderate to severe hypertension, hyperthyroidism, and psychosis; anorexiant therapy may worsen their condition. Clients who have a history of substance abuse or dependence may develop a dependence on anorexiants. Uremia may alter excretion of the drug.

Review the client's current medication regimen for the risk of significant drug interactions, such as those that may occur when anorexiants are given concurrently with the following drugs:

Drug	Possible Effect and Management
Bold/color type indicates the most serious interactions.	
alcohol	Concurrent use is not recommended, because the risk increases for adverse CNS reactions such as confusion, dizziness, and fainting.
antihypertensive agents, especially clonidine (Catapres), guanadrel (Hylorel), guanethidine (Ismelin), methyldopa (Aldomet), and Rauwolfia alkaloids	May decrease the antihypertensive effects; monitor closely.
CNS stimulants	**Combined use may result in an increase in CNS stimulant effects such as confusion, dizziness, and fainting.**
MAO inhibitors	**Avoid using concurrently or within 14 days of the administration of an MAO inhibitor, because a hypertensive crisis may result.**

Anorexiant drugs should be administered with caution to clients with diabetes, because the need for insulin may be decreased as a result of the concomitant dietary regimen. Blood and urine glucose levels should be monitored closely. General anesthetics should be administered with caution. Sensitivity to the specific drug and other sympathomimetics should be determined.

A baseline assessment should include height and weight, vital signs, lifestyle issues related to obesity, knowledge level of the therapeutic regimen, and mental status.

■ **Nursing Diagnosis.** Once the client begins anorexiant therapy, be alert for the following nursing diagnoses/collaborative problems: disturbed sleep pattern and disturbed thought processes (depression) related to CNS effects; impaired comfort related to dry mouth, rash, headache, or gastrointestinal or urinary effects; situational low self-esteem related to changes in sexual desire or decreased sexual ability; and the potential complication of altered cardiac output related to the cardiovascular effects of CNS stimulants.

■ **Implementation**

■ ***Monitoring.*** The client's weight needs to be monitored on an ongoing basis. Adverse reactions to anorexiant drugs usually relate to overstimulation such as nervousness, restlessness, insomnia, and anxiety. Blood pressure and pulse should be monitored to assess whether the client is experiencing an adverse reaction to the drug. Tolerance is a com-

TABLE 18-1 Anorexiant Medications: Adult Dosages and Controlled Substances Act Classification*

Drug	Adult Dosages	CSA Classification
benzphetamine (Didrex)	25-50 mg PO daily; increase if necessary	III
diethylpropion		
Tablets (Tenuate)	25 mg PO 3 times daily, 1 hour before meals	IV
Extended-release tablets (Tenuate Dospan, Tepanil Ten-Tab)	75 mg PO daily at midmorning	
mazindol (Mazanor, Sanorex)	1 mg PO initially, once daily before breakfast; increase if necessary	IV
phendimetrazine		
Tablets (Adphen, Bontril)	35 mg PO 2 or 3 times daily, 1 hour before meals	III
Capsules (Obalan)	35 mg PO 2 or 3 times daily, 1 hour before meals	
Extended-release (Adipost, Bontril Slow Release)	105 mg PO daily, ½-1 hour before breakfast	
phentermine		
Tablets (Phentride)	37.5 mg PO daily before breakfast	IV
Capsules (Fastin)	30 mg PO daily before breakfast	
Resin capsules (Ionamin)	15 or 30 mg PO daily before breakfast	
sibutramine (Meridia)	10 mg PO daily	IV

*CSA classification or the federal Controlled Substances Act drug schedule (II, III or IV). (See Chapter 2 for more information.)

mon occurrence with anorexiants, and the client should be assessed for the possibility of habituation and addiction.

■ ***Intervention.*** Because anorexiant drugs are to be used only for a short time, the emphasis is on a total weight reduction program that includes a suitable diet, an appropriate exercise regimen, and behavior modification related to the cause of the overeating.

Preparations administered daily should be administered in the morning to decrease insomnia. Avoid administering anorexiant drugs within 4 to 6 hours of anticipated sleep times (10 to 14 hours for extended-release or long-acting dosage forms).

After prolonged high dosages, the drug should be discontinued gradually to avoid withdrawal symptoms and a rebound increase in appetite.

■ ***Education.*** Clients undergoing anorexiant therapy should be instructed to consult the prescriber if the drug seems to be less effective than desired; they should not self-regulate the dosage. Instruct clients to avoid caffeine-containing beverages, which will increase the effects of the stimulant anorexiant drugs. Caution clients that these drugs may impair their ability to perform tasks that require physical coordination and alertness. Clients should be instructed about ways to minimize the unpleasant taste in and dryness of the mouth with mouth rinses, ice chips, chewing gum, and sugarless candies.

The client should also receive appropriate education regarding lifestyle changes, such as nutrition and exercise, to support weight loss.

■ **Evaluation.** The expected outcome of anorexiant therapy is that the client will experience decreased appetite with accompanying weight loss. The client will also be able to sleep without difficulty and will not experience any other adverse reactions to the drug.

✔AMPHETAMINES

The mechanism of action of amphetamines was reviewed earlier in this chapter. Prolonged use of amphetamines leads to the development of tolerance. Amphetamines can also produce psychologic and physical dependence if used over a long period of time. Because of their potential for abuse, amphetamines are not recommended for use as appetite suppressants. Instead they are indicated for the treatment of ADHD and in the treatment of narcolepsy.

Pharmacokinetics. Amphetamines are well absorbed and are distributed to body tissues, with especially high concentrations in the brain and cerebrospinal fluid. The half-life depends on urinary pH but, in general, is as follows: amphetamine, 10 to 30 hours; dextroamphetamine, 10 to 12 hours for adults and 6 to 8 hours for children; and methamphetamine, 4 to 5 hours. Amphetamines are metabolized in the liver and excreted by the kidneys. Excretion is pH dependent; it is increased in an acidic urine and decreased in a more alkaline urine.

The nurse should be aware that long-term amphetamine abuse can lead to chorea, a condition characterized by involuntary, purposeless, and rapid motions; this condition is mediated by alterations in the physiology of the basal ganglia. Chorea is also seen with the administration of cocaine, which reduces dopamine levels.

Side Effects/Adverse Reactions. Side effects of amphetamines include euphoria, increased irritability, nervousness, insomnia, restlessness, visual disturbance, excessive sweating, dry mouth, abdominal cramps, impotence, alterations in sexual desire, diarrhea or constipation, dizziness, anorexia, nausea or vomiting, and weight loss. Adverse reactions include tachycardia or an irregular heart rate, allergic reactions (including urticaria and hives), angina or chest pain, tremors, hyperreactive reflexes, dyskinesia, and Tourette's syndrome. Mood changes that include depression, increased agitation, and psychosis may occur with high dosages or prolonged consumption. Drug dependency and tolerance may also develop.

Dosage and Administration. See Table 18-2 and Box 18-3 for information on the dosage and administration of amphetamines.

Treatment of Amphetamine Overdose. In addition to symptomatic and supportive care as outlined in the Management of Drug Overdose box on p. 380, a saline cathartic is indicated if the client has taken the long-acting dosage form. Vital signs and respiratory functions should be monitored closely.

■ Nursing Management
Amphetamine Therapy

In addition to the following discussion, see Nursing Management: Anorexiant Therapy, p. 380.

■ **Assessment.** Be aware that amphetamines, like other CNS stimulants, should be avoided by persons with hypertension and cardiovascular disease and by those who are unduly restless, anxious, agitated, and excited. Amphetamines should be used with caution in older adults, in debilitated clients, or in clients with a history of homicidal or suicidal tendencies. Clients with bronchial asthma who are sensitive

TABLE 18-2 Amphetamines: Dosage and Administration

Drug	Adults	Children
amphetamine tablets		
Narcolepsy	5-20 mg PO 1 to 3 times daily	Up to 6 years: dosage not determined 6-12 years: 2.5 mg PO twice daily; increase by 5 mg/day at 1-week intervals until therapeutic effect or adult dosage achieved 12 years and older: 5 mg PO twice daily; increase by 10 mg/day at weekly intervals until therapeutic effect or adult dosage achieved
Attention deficit disorder	Not applicable	Up to 3 years: not recommended 3-6 years: 2.5 mg PO; increase by 2.5 mg/day at weekly intervals until therapeutic response achieved 6 years and older: 5 mg PO 1 or 2 times daily; increase by 5 mg/day at weekly intervals until therapeutic response achieved
dextroamphetamine tablets		
Narcolepsy	5-60 mg PO 1 to 3 times daily	Up to 6 years: dosage not determined 6-12 years: 5 mg PO daily; increase by 5 mg/day at weekly intervals until therapeutic effect or adult dosage achieved 12 years and older: 10 mg PO daily; increase by 10 mg/day at weekly intervals until therapeutic effect or adult dosage achieved
Attention deficit disorder	Not applicable	Up to 3 years: not recommended 3-6 years: 2.5 mg PO daily; increase by 2.5 mg/day at weekly intervals until therapeutic response achieved 6 years and older: 5 mg PO once or twice daily; increase by 5 mg/day at weekly intervals until therapeutic response achieved Dextroamphetamine extended-release capsules may be used after therapeutic dosage per day is established
methamphetamine tablets (Desoxyn), methamphetamine extended-release tablets (Desoxyn Gradumet)		
Attention deficit disorder	Not applicable	Up to 6 years: not recommended 6 years and older: 5 mg PO 1 or 2 times daily; increase by 5 mg/day at weekly intervals until therapeutic effect achieved (usually 20-25 mg/day)
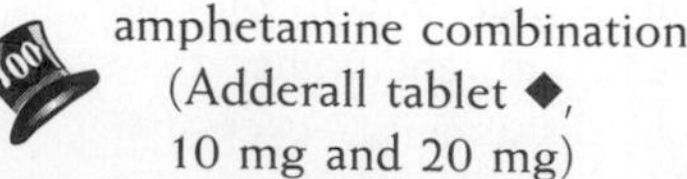 amphetamine combinations (Adderall tablet ◆, 10 mg and 20 mg)	Available in a number of different combinations (dextroamphetamine sulfate, dextroamphetamine saccharate, amphetamine aspartate, amphetamine sulfate); dosage thus varies according to age and response of individual; used to treat attention deficit disorder and narcolepsy	

to tartrazine dye should not use dosage forms that contain this dye.

Review the client's current medication regimen for the risk of significant drug interactions, such as those that may occur when amphetamines are given concurrently with the following drugs:

Drug	Possible Effect and Management
Bold/color type indicates the most serious interactions.	
antidepressants, tricyclic	May result in adverse cardiovascular effects, such as dysrhythmias, tachycardia, or severe hypertension. Monitor the pulse and blood pressure closely; dosage adjustments may be necessary. Avoid concurrent use or a potentially serious drug interaction may occur.
beta-adrenergic blocking drugs (systemic and ophthalmic)	May cause unopposed alpha-adrenergic effects and result in hypertension, bradycardia, and possible heart block. If concurrent use is necessary, labetalol, a beta-blocking agent that also has alpha-blocking effects, may reduce the risk of producing the adverse reactions. Monitor closely for dysrhythmias. Avoid concurrent use or a potentially serious drug interaction may occur.
CNS stimulants such as appetite suppressants, caffeine, methylphenidate (Ritalin), pemoline (Cylert), sympathomimetics, theophylline (Theo-Dur), amantadine (Symmetrel)	May result in an increase in adverse cardiovascular reactions, nervousness, insomnia, and convulsions. Avoid concurrent use or a potentially serious drug interaction may occur.
digitalis glycosides	May result in an increase in cardiac dysrhythmias. Avoid concurrent use or, if necessary, monitor apical pulse very closely. Concurrent use is contraindicated and not recommended because of possible serious outcome.
MAO inhibitors	Avoid concurrent use because the increased release of catecholamines, headaches, dysrhythmias, vomiting, sudden severe hypertension and, possibly, hyperpyretic crisis may result. Avoid concurrent use or a potentially serious drug interaction may occur. Do not administer concurrently or for 2 weeks after discontinuing an MAO inhibitor.
meperidine (Demerol)	Although some investigators believe the analgesic effect of meperidine might be enhanced, concurrent use should be avoided because it may result in severe respiratory depression, seizures, hyperpyrexia, severe hypotension, cardiovascular collapse, and death in some clients. Avoid concurrent use or a potentially serious drug interaction may occur.
thyroid hormones	May result in enhanced effects of thyroid hormones or amphetamines. If client has coronary artery disease, the potential for inducing coronary insufficiency is increased. Avoid concurrent use or a potentially serious drug interaction may occur.

■ **Nursing Diagnosis.** Amphetamine therapy may put the client at risk for the following nursing diagnoses: ineffective coping related to the client's underlying disorder or development of abuse problem; imbalanced nutrition: more than body requirements related to the ineffectiveness of amphetamine therapy; imbalanced nutrition: less than body requirements (particularly for children receiving amphetamine therapy for ADHD); disturbed sleep pattern related to drug-induced insomnia; disturbed thought processes related to the CNS effects of the drug; and impaired oral mucous membrane related to dry mouth.

■ **Implementation**

■ ***Monitoring.*** Assess the pulse and blood pressure of clients receiving amphetamines to monitor for adverse cardiovascular reactions to the drug. Caution should be used and the possibility of psychologic dependence and addiction considered in clients with a history of addiction to alcohol or other drugs. Evaluate for potential dependence in all clients receiving amphetamines. Their weight, dietary intake, sleep patterns, compliance with therapy, and mental status should be monitored on an ongoing basis.

BOX 18-3

Amphetamine Mixtures

Various salts of amphetamine and dextroamphetamine have been combined into a product named Adderall for the treatment of ADHD. Adderall is available in 5-, 10-, 20-, and 30-mg combinations of dextroamphetamine sulfate, dextroamphetamine saccharate, amphetamine aspartate, and amphetamine sulfate.

Manos, Short, and Findling (1999) have reported Adderall to be equivalent to methylphenidate (Ritalin) in the treatment of ADHD. Pelham et al. (1999) have concluded that a single morning dose of Adderall is equivalent to twice-daily dosing of methylphenidate, thereby eliminating the need for a mid-day drug dose in the school setting. Further studies with Adderall are suggested to determine drug dose-response and potential side effects/adverse reaction comparisons to the other CNS stimulants.

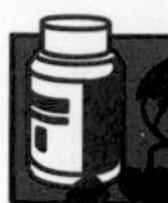

Complementary and Alternative Therapies
Ginseng

Ginseng has been one of the most widely used herbal substances for the past 2000 years. The genus name for ginseng, *Panax,* comes from a Greek word meaning "all healing," and ginseng has long been used as a general tonic to improve well-being. It has been promoted as an "adaptogen" that improves physical stamina, cognitive function and concentration, and work or athletic efficiency. It is also used as a sedative and antidepressant. These contrary activities result from differences in its active constituents, which have been identified as ginsenosides by Asian researchers and as panaxosides by Russian researchers. One constituent, ginsenoside Rg1, raises blood pressure and acts as a CNS stimulant. Ginsenoside Rg2 lowers blood pressure and acts as a CNS depressant.

Panax ginseng is considered possibly effective when taken orally to improve mental and physical ability. It may help some people by improving appetite, mental alertness, memory, and sleep pattern.

Because most of the published studies of *Panax ginseng* lack standardization or have inadequate study design and control, and because ginseng preparations vary greatly in the amount of active ingredients, there is insufficient reliable information available for the long-term use of ginseng. It is considered to be safe when used orally in recommended dosages for less than 3 months. It is likely to be *unsafe* for children, and its use is not recommended during pregnancy and lactation.

The most commonly reported side effects of ginseng are nervousness, insomnia, breast tenderness, vaginal bleeding, tachycardia, mania, headache, dizziness, rash, diarrhea, hypertension, and hypotension. Newborn deaths have been reported after the use of ginseng during pregnancy. The use of ginseng is contraindicated in clients with bleeding disorders (hemorrhage or thrombosis), insomnia, schizophrenia, diabetes, cardiac disorders, hypertension, or hypotension. Caution clients with diabetes about the hypoglycemic effects of ginseng. Theoretically, ginseng may interfere with neurotransmitters; therefore therapy with MAO inhibitors, stimulants, or antipsychotic drugs may be affected. *Panax ginseng* may decrease the effectiveness of warfarin and of hormonal therapy.

The typical oral dosage of ginseng is 0.6 to 3 g of cut or powdered root one to three times daily. A tea may also be prepared by steeping a ginseng tea bag (usually containing 1500 mg of ginseng root) or 3 g of ginseng root in 150 mL of boiling water for 10 to 15 minutes and consuming the tea one to three times daily for 3 weeks to 3 months. However, some ginseng consumers take ginseng continuously. *Panax ginseng* is also available in 100-, 250-, and 500-mg capsules; the typical dosage is 200 to 600 mg daily. (See Chapter 12 for additional information.)

Information from Cirigliano, M.D. (1999). Ten most common herbs in clinical practice. In M.S. Micozzi (Ed.), *Current review of complementary medicine.* Philadelphia: Current Medicine; and Jellin, J.M., Batz, F., & Hitchens, K. (1999). *Pharmacist's letter/prescriber's letter natural medicines comprehensive database.* Stockton, CA: Therapeutic Research Faculty.

Children receiving amphetamines for a prolonged period should have their growth carefully monitored, because these drugs are thought to inhibit growth mildly. Growth usually catches up during drug-free periods. Amphetamines should be discontinued periodically in children with ADHD to reevaluate the need for therapy; the medications should be reinstituted only if behavioral symptoms return.

▪ ***Intervention.*** To prevent insomnia, the last dose of amphetamines for the day should be administered no fewer than 6 hours before the client's bedtime (no fewer than 10 to 14 hours before bedtime if a sustained-release product is used). If before-meals dosing is prescribed, the dose should be given 30 to 60 minutes before the client's meal. Modification of diet and behavior is essential if the drug is to be successful as an anorexiant. If weight loss is not the therapeutic use, administer the drug with or after meals. Help the client to overcome a dry mouth with sugarless candy, gum, or ice chips.

After a prolonged high dosage, the medication should be gradually tapered before discontinuing to prevent withdrawal manifestations such as psychotic symptoms and lethargy. Because fatigue occurs as the effects of the drug diminish, be aware that the client will need more rest and sleep.

▪ ***Education.*** The client undergoing amphetamine therapy should be instructed not to self-regulate the dosage; the habit-forming potential of amphetamines should be stressed. If the effect of the drug seems to decrease, caution the client not to increase the dosage but to consult the prescriber. The sustained-release tablet should be swallowed whole; it should not be broken, chewed, or crushed. Inform the client of the CNS and cardiovascular side effects of the drug that need to be reported.

Clients should be cautioned that amphetamines might impair their functioning in the performance of tasks that require mental alertness and physical coordination. These drugs are commonly abused by athletes, students, and drivers for the purpose of increasing alertness but may result in an impaired ability to function. Caution the client to store the drug securely to avoid unintended use by another person.

▪ **Evaluation.** The expected outcome of amphetamine therapy is that the client will demonstrate clinical improvement. The child will have an increased attention span and decreased restlessness, be able to sleep without difficulty, and show no evidence of adverse reactions.

TABLE 18-3 Doxapram: Dosage and Administration

Indication	Adults	Children
Postanesthesia respiratory depression	Administer 0.5-1 mg/kg body weight IV; do not exceed 1.5 mg/kg as a single dose. If needed, dose may be repeated every 5 minutes up to maximum total dose of 2 mg/kg body weight.	Not recommended in children less than 12 years of age
Acute respiratory insufficiency in chronic obstructive pulmonary disease (COPD)	Administer 1 to 2 mg/min IV infusion; if necessary, administration rate may be increased to 3 mg/min. Maximum time for infusion with no additional infusions recommended is 2 hours.	—

OTHER CENTRAL NERVOUS SYSTEM STIMULANTS

doxapram [dox' a pram] (Dopram)

At low dosages doxapram stimulates respiration by acting on the peripheral carotid chemoreceptors; at higher dosages the medullary respiratory center is stimulated. This drug is used for the treatment of respiratory depression induced by a drug overdose, chronic obstructive pulmonary disease, or postanesthetic effects. (See the Complementary and Alternative Therapies box on p. 384.)

Pharmacokinetics. Doxapram is administered intravenously. It has an onset of action at 20 to 40 seconds and a peak effect at 1 to 2 minutes. The duration of action is 5 to 12 minutes. It is excreted primarily in the feces.

Side Effects/Adverse Reactions. Side effects of doxapram include urinary retention or incontinence, headache, diarrhea, dizziness, cough, hiccups, confusion, a warm or burning feeling, nausea or vomiting, and sweating. Adverse reactions include chest pains, tachycardia, extrasystoles, hemolysis, thrombophlebitis, dyspnea, and tachypnea. Signs of doxapram overdose are hypertension, convulsions, trembling, tachycardia, and increased deep tendon reflexes.

The administration of doxapram with MAO inhibitors or vasopressors may result in an increase in blood pressure or a hypertensive crisis. Vital signs should be monitored closely.

Dosage and Administration. The adult dose of doxapram for postanesthesia respiratory depression is 0.5 to 1 mg/kg body weight IV. A single dose must not exceed 1.5 mg/kg body weight. The dose may be repeated every 5 minutes up to maximum of 2 mg/kg body weight. For acute respiratory insufficiency in chronic obstructive pulmonary disease (COPD), the dose is 1 to 2 mg/min by IV infusion; the dose may be increased to 3 mg/min if necessary. The maximum infusion time is 2 hours. Table 18-3 provides additional information on the dosage and administration of doxapram.

■ Nursing Management

Doxapram Therapy

■ **Assessment.** The client's assessment should include a determination of other conditions for which the doxapram may be contraindicated, such as head trauma or seizure disorders (because of the risk of drug-induced seizures) and cardiovascular disorders (because of the vasopressor effects of the drug). Doxapram is also contraindicated if the client is experiencing incompetence of the ventilatory mechanism as a result of airway obstruction, pneumothorax, or flail chest and other respiratory diseases, because these conditions may be worsened. Doxapram has vasopressor effects, and therefore cautious use is recommended with cardiac dysrhythmias because of the risk of hypoxia and aggravation of the dysrhythmic disorder, increased intracranial pressure or cerebral edema, pheochromocytoma, or hyperthyroidism.

Obtain a baseline pulse, blood pressure, and deep tendon reflexes, and monitor those indicators at frequent intervals to avoid overdose; the rate of the infusion should be adjusted on the basis of these assessments. Arterial blood gases should be analyzed before initiation of therapy (as a baseline) and every 30 minutes during the 2-hour period of infusion to avoid the possibility of respiratory acidosis when doxapram is administered to clients with COPD.

■ **Nursing Diagnosis.** When doxapram is administered, the client is at risk for the following nursing diagnoses/collaborative problems: ineffective breathing patterns related to anesthesia-induced respiratory depression (for which the doxapram is prescribed); risk for aspiration; risk for injury related to the vasopressor effects of the drug; and the potential complication of drug-induced seizures.

■ **Implementation**

■ ***Monitoring.*** Doxapram hydrochloride has a narrow margin of safety. Observe for early signs of toxicity, such as increased blood pressure and pulse rate, dysrhythmias, dyspnea, and increased skeletal response with increased deep tendon reflexes and spasticity. Because narcosis may recur, close monitoring of the client is necessary until full alertness has been maintained for 1 hour.

■ ***Intervention.*** Before administering doxapram to clients with respiratory depression, a patent airway should be established and an adequate oxygen supply ensured in an attempt to prevent aspiration. Because IV administration tends to cause hemolysis, only diluted solutions should be administered at a slow rate of infusion. Various injection sites should be used to avoid extravasation and to decrease local tissue reaction and thrombophlebitis. Doxapram is a temporary measure to correct acute respiratory insufficiency. Mechanical assistance with ventilation is safer, more reliable, and effective for long-term (more than 2 hours) therapy.

■ **Evaluation.** The expected outcome of doxapram therapy is that the client's respirations will be within normal limits compared with baseline and that the cough and gag reflex will return. The arterial CO_2 of a client with COPD will be within normal limits as compared with baseline.

methylphenidate [meth ill fen′ i date] (Ritalin)

The mechanism of central action of methylphenidate is unknown. The pharmacologic actions are similar to those of amphetamines, with CNS and respiratory stimulation. Sympathomimetic activity is also reported. Sites of action are the cerebral cortex and subcortical areas.

Methylphenidate also appears to block the reuptake of dopamine into the dopaminergic neurons and is indicated for the treatment of ADHD and narcolepsy. In clients with ADHD, methylphenidate decreases motor activity and increases the attention span. In clients with narcolepsy it appears to stimulate the cortex and subcortex, including the thalamic area; this action increases alertness, lifts the spirits, and increases motor activity (Zeiner, Bryhn, Bjercke, Truyen, & Strand, 1999).

Pharmacokinetics. Methylphenidate is well absorbed orally. Tablets reach a peak serum concentration in 1.9 hours in children; the extended-release tablets reach peak serum concentration in 4.7 hours in children. It is metabolized in the liver and excreted by the kidneys.

Side Effects/Adverse Reactions. Side effects/adverse reactions of methylphenidate include anorexia, increased nervousness, insomnia (usually more common in children), headache, nausea, abdominal pain, drowsiness, and dizziness. Adverse reactions include hypertension, tachycardia, chest pain, trembling or uncontrolled movement of the body, rash, a fever of unknown origin, and increased bruising.

Dosage and Administration. To treat ADHD in children 6 years and older, the dosage is 5 mg twice daily (after breakfast and lunch); if necessary, this dosage is increased by 5 to 10 mg weekly, up to 60 mg/day maximum. The medication is discontinued if there is no improvement after 30 days. For adults the dosage is 5 to 20 mg two or three times daily with or after meals. The dosage for the extended-release form (Ritalin-SR) in adults is 20 mg every 8 hours one to three times daily. Table 18-4 provides additional information on the dosage and administration of methylphenidate.

■ Nursing Management
Methylphenidate Therapy

■ **Assessment.** Methylphenidate must be used cautiously in clients with epilepsy because it can lower the convulsive threshold. It is usually contraindicated for use in clients with glaucoma, motor tics other than Tourette's syndrome, anxiety, and depression because it may worsen the condition. It also should be used with caution in clients with hypertension. Some clients with Tourette's syndrome may benefit from cautious use.

The use of methylphenidate in pregnant or lactating women is not recommended and is also contraindicated in clients with glaucoma, agitation, depression, or fatigue.

Review the client's current medication regimen for the risk of significant drug interactions, such as those that may occur when methylphenidate hydrochloride is given concurrently with the following drugs (Markowitz, Morrison, & DeVane, 1999):

Drug	Possible Effect and Management
Bold/color type indicates the most serious interactions.	
other CNS stimulants	May result in additive CNS stimulation effects, causing increased nervousness, irritability, insomnia, dysrhythmias, and convulsions. Monitor apical pulse, mental status, and behaviors closely.
MAO inhibitors	**May result in hypertensive crisis. Do not give drugs concurrently or within 14 days of administration of an MAO inhibitor, or a potentially serious drug interaction may occur.**
pimozide (Orap)	**Should not be administered together. Withdraw client from methylphenidate before starting pimozide therapy. Pimozide is indicated for the treatment of tics in clients with Tourette's syndrome. Because methylphenidate may induce tics, concurrent use may mask the reason for tic development.**

TABLE 18-4 Methylphenidate: Dosage and Administration

Drug	Adults	Children
methylphenidate tablets (Ritalin)	5-20 mg PO 2 or 3 times daily with or after meals	ADHD Up to 6 years: dosage not established 6 years and older: 5 mg twice daily (after breakfast and lunch); increase if needed by 5 to 10 mg weekly up to maximum of 60 mg/day; if no improvement after dosage increases over 30 days, stop medication
methylphenidate extended-release (Ritalin-SR)	20 mg PO 1 to 3 times daily q8h	Up to 6 years: dosage not established 6 years and older: see adult dosage recommendations

A baseline assessment should include an evaluation of the child's growth and development status, complete blood counts, and blood pressure determination.

■ **Nursing Diagnosis.** Once methylphenidate therapy has begun, the client should be assessed for the following nursing diagnoses/collaborative problems: disturbed sleep pattern; disturbed thought processes (confusion); imbalanced nutrition: less than body requirements related to its anorexiant effects (especially in children); risk for injury related to its CNS effects; and the potential complications of mental depression and altered cardiac output (hypertension, tachycardia) related to the cardiovascular effects of the drug.

■ **Implementation**

■ ***Monitoring.*** Clients should be monitored for weight loss from appetite suppression. Children in particular should be assessed on a regular basis for physical growth, because normal weight gain may be suppressed. Methylphenidate must be used cautiously in emotionally unstable persons and in those with a history of drug dependence or alcoholism. Substance abusers have used it as a substitute for amphetamines. The drug should be discontinued periodically to reassess therapeutic need, which is indicated by the return of symptoms. Long-term therapy should be accompanied by repeated medical examinations and tests for complete blood counts and platelet counts.

■ ***Intervention.*** Dosages should be calculated for each client based on his or her response to methylphenidate. Extended-release dosage forms should be used only after the initial therapy has established the appropriate dosage for the client. To prevent insomnia, administer the last daily dose of the non–extended-release form several hours before bedtime.

Complete dependence on methylphenidate for the treatment of ADHD is discouraged. Other psychologic, educational, and social therapies should be used in conjunction with the drug therapy. When the symptoms of ADHD improve, it may be possible to interrupt drug therapy during times of low stress. The client may be given medication-free weekends, holidays, or vacations.

■ ***Education.*** The client undergoing methylphenidate therapy should be instructed to take the medication on an empty stomach 30 to 45 minutes before eating. Extended-release forms should be swallowed whole, not crushed, broken, or chewed.

Do not increase the dosage if the medication seems less effective. Regular visits with the client's prescriber are needed to monitor progress of the drug therapy. Withdrawal must be gradual if the client has taken large doses over an extended period. Caution clients not to stop taking the medication without checking with the prescriber, because there is a risk for depression on withdrawal. Careful supervision is therefore required during withdrawal. Tolerance and psychologic dependence have occurred with long-term use, and abnormal behavior and psychotic episodes have been observed.

■ **Evaluation.** The expected outcome of methylphenidate therapy is that the client will demonstrate clinical improvement. The child will have an increased attention span with a decreased restlessness, will be able to sleep without difficulty, and will not evidence adverse reactions.

pemoline [pem′ oh leen] (Cylert)

The mechanism of central action of pemoline is unknown. Pemoline may act by means of dopaminergic mechanisms. It is indicated for the treatment of ADHD. Pemoline has good absorption and a half-life of 12 hours. Peak serum concentration occurs in 2 to 4 hours, with the peak effect reached in 3 to 4 weeks (*USP DI,* 1999). Pemoline is partially metabolized in the liver and is excreted by the kidneys.

Side effects/adverse reactions of pemoline include anorexia, insomnia, and weight loss. Less common drug effects are dizziness, daytime sedation, irritability, depression, nausea, rash, and abdominal pain. Jaundice is a rare adverse reaction.

Signs of overdose include increased agitation, confusion, euphoria, hallucinations, severe headaches, hypertension, elevated temperatures, increased sweating, convulsions, tachycardia, dilated pupils, vomiting, and uncontrollable muscle movements of the eyes.

No significant drug interactions have been reported with pemoline.

The dosage for children younger than 6 years has not been established; the dosage for children 6 years or older is 37.5 mg PO each morning. The dosage may be increased by 18.75 mg daily at weekly intervals until a therapeutic response is noted or until a maximum of 112.5 mg/day is reached.

■ Nursing Management

Pemoline Therapy

In addition to the following discussion, see Nursing Management: Methylphenidate Therapy, p. 386. Pemoline must be used cautiously in emotionally labile clients and in clients with a history of drug dependence or alcoholism. The drug should be discontinued periodically to reassess the need for its administration, which is indicated by a return of symptoms. Caution the client that the most common side effects are insomnia and anorexia. These effects are dose related and may be decreased by a dosage adjustment by the prescriber.

The client should be prepared for an initial weight loss with a return to a normal weight curve in 3 to 6 months. Parents should be counseled that the beneficial effect of the medication may not be apparent for 3 to 4 weeks but that it is important to the success of the regimen that the drug be administered as prescribed.

caffeine [kaf feen′]

Caffeine is a stimulant found in many beverages, foods, over-the-counter (OTC) drugs, and prescription drugs (Table 18-5). It is probably the most commonly used stimulant worldwide. It has been estimated that 7 million kilograms of caffeine are consumed annually in the United

TABLE 18-5 Caffeine Content in Selected Products

Trade/Brand Name	Caffeine per Tablet/Capsule
Analgesics*	
OTC medications	
Anacin	32 mg
Cope	32 mg
Excedrin Extra Strength	65 mg
Vanquish Caplets	33 mg
Prescription medications	
Cafergot	100 mg
Fiorinal	40 mg
Wigraine	100 mg
Menstrual Medications*	
Midol Maximum	60 mg
Beverages	
Brewed coffee, automatic drip	60-180 mg/5 oz
Brewed coffee, percolator	40-170 mg/5 oz
Brewed tea, United States	20-90 mg/5 oz
Instant coffee	30-120 mg/5 oz
Instant tea	25-50 mg/5 oz
Brewed decaffeinated coffee	2-5 mg/5 oz
Chocolate milk	2-7 mg/8 oz
Soft Drinks*	
Mountain Dew	54 mg/12 oz
Coca-Cola	45 mg/12 oz
Diet Coke	45 mg/12 oz
Pepsi-Cola	38 mg/12 oz
Diet Pepsi	36 mg/12 oz
Ginger Ale	0
7-Up	0
Sunkist Orange	0

Information from American Pharmaceutical Association. (1996). *Nonprescription products: formulations and features '96-'97*. Washington, DC: Author.
*Trade or brand names.

BOX 18-4

Caffeine-Free Over-the-Counter Analgesic Medications

Aleve	Midol Menstrual
Aspergum	Motrin IB
Bayer Aspirin	Tempra
Bromo-Seltzer	Tylenol Infants
Bufferin Extra Strength	Tylenol Regular Strength
Bufferin Arthritis Strength	Tylenol Extra Strength
Liquiprin for children	

Information from American Pharmaceutical Association. (1996). *Nonprescription products: formulations and features '96-'97*. Washington, DC: Author.

States. Many persons do not consider caffeine to be a drug, but it can produce many therapeutic effects and adverse reactions. For example, a large daily intake of caffeine-containing products may increase alertness but may also induce insomnia and heart dysrhythmias in some persons, especially older adults. A withdrawal syndrome of increased irritability, headache, and increased weakness has been reported when individuals using more than 600 mg of caffeine per day (approximately 6 cups of coffee) decrease or eliminate this intake. Caffeine has also been implicated in many adverse health effects, such as cancer, fibrocystic breast disease, and birth defects.

Mechanism of Action. The mechanisms of action for caffeine were previously postulated to be an increase in cyclic adenosine monophosphate (cAMP) levels by blocking the enzyme phosphodiesterase. However, recent studies indicate that the effects of caffeine are primarily due to antagonism of the central adenosine receptors (adenosine is a neurotransmitter that is structurally similar to caffeine). Because caffeine has an effect on many body functions, both its short-term and possible long-term effects are of concern.

Central Nervous System Effects. Although all levels of the CNS may be affected, regular doses of caffeine (100 to 150 mg) stimulate the cortex to produce increased alertness and decreased motor reaction time to both visual and auditory events. Drowsiness and fatigue generally disappear. Larger doses may affect the medullary, vagus, vasomotor, and respiratory centers, resulting in slowing of the heart rate, vasoconstriction, and an increased respiratory rate. Studies attribute such effects to competitive blockade of adenosine receptors. Caffeine is still under investigation for the treatment of neonatal apnea, generally as an adjunct to nondrug measures and as an alternative to theophylline.

Analgesic Adjunct, Vascular Effect. Caffeine constricts cerebral blood vessels, resulting in decreased cerebral blood flow and oxygen tension in the brain. Thus caffeine is used in analgesic products and in combination with ergotamine to enhance pain relief and, perhaps, to hasten the onset of action. Box 18-4 lists caffeine-free OTC analgesic medications. When caffeine is given with ergotamine, the enhanced effect is believed to be the result of better absorption of ergotamine in the presence of caffeine.

Respiratory Stimulant Effects. Although the mechanism of action is not clearly defined, caffeine appears to stimulate the medullary respiratory center. Thus it may be useful for the treatment of apnea in preterm infants and for Cheyne-Stokes respirations in adults.

Cardiovascular Effects. Caffeine stimulates the myocardium, increasing both the heart rate and the cardiac output. This effect is antagonistic to that produced on the vagus center; consequently, a slight slowing of the heart may be observed in some individuals, and an increased rate may be observed in others. The latter effect usually predominates after large doses. Overstimulation may cause tachycardia and cardiac irregularities.

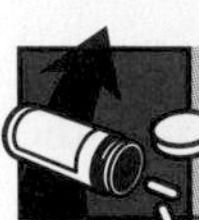

Management of Drug Overdose
Caffeine

- Institute symptomatic and supportive measures according to the requirements of the individual client.
- If treatment is started within 4 hours of overdose, induce emesis with ipecac syrup and/or gastric lavage followed by activated charcoal. A magnesium sulfate laxative (Epsom salts) should also be considered.
- Maintain fluid and electrolyte balance, ventilation, and oxygenation.
- For hemorrhagic gastritis, administer antacids and iced saline lavage; for seizures, administer IV diazepam, phenobarbital, or phenytoin.

Depending on the dose, caffeine may cause an increase in systemic vascular resistance, which can cause an increase in blood pressure. This effect may be secondary to sympathetic nervous system stimulation and blockage of adenosine-induced vasodilation.

Musculoskeletal Effects. Caffeine affects voluntary skeletal muscles to increase the contractual force and decrease muscle fatigue.

Gastrointestinal Effects. Caffeine increases the secretion of pepsin and hydrochloric acid from the parietal cells. For this reason, coffee use is restricted in clients who have a gastric or duodenal ulcer.

Renal Effects. Caffeine produces a mild diuretic effect by increasing renal blood flow and glomerular filtration rate and by decreasing the reabsorption of sodium and water in the proximal tubules.

Additional Effects. Caffeine also increases metabolic activity, inhibits uterine contractions, transiently increases glucose levels by stimulating glycolysis, and increases catecholamine levels in plasma and urine.

Indications and Pharmacokinetics. Caffeine is used in the treatment of fatigue or drowsiness and as an adjunct to analgesics to enhance pain relief. Its absorption is good, and it is distributed to all body compartments. It crosses the blood-brain barrier, enters the CNS, and crosses readily through the placenta. Caffeine is metabolized in the liver.

In adults caffeine is metabolized to theophylline and theobromine, whereas in the neonate only a small portion is metabolized to theophylline. The half-life is 3 to 7 hours in adults and 65 to 130 hours in neonates. Peak plasma levels are achieved within 50 to 75 minutes, with therapeutic plasma levels being 5 to 25 μg/mL. In adults, caffeine is excreted by the kidneys, with only 1% to 2% excreted unchanged; in neonates it is excreted by the kidneys, with approximately 85% excreted unchanged.

Side Effects/Adverse Reactions. Side effects/adverse reactions of caffeine include increased nervousness or jittery feelings and irritation of the gastrointestinal tract, resulting in nausea. More common adverse reactions in neonates include abdominal swelling or distension, vomiting, body tremors, tachycardia, jitters, or nervousness.

Signs of overdose are increased temperature, headache, increased irritability and sensitivity to pain or touch, increased urination, confusion, dehydration, abdominal pain, agitation, muscle twitching, nausea and vomiting, tinnitus, insomnia, and convulsions. (See the Management of Drug Overdose box at left.)

Dosage and Administration. The adult dosage of caffeine is 100 to 200 mg PO, repeated in 3 to 4 hours if necessary to a maximum of 1000 mg daily. The extended-release dosage form (200 to 250 mg) has the same recommendations as the tablets. Caffeine is not recommended for use in children under 12 years of age (*USP DI,* 1999).

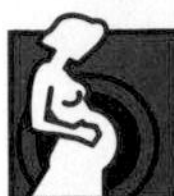

Pregnancy Safety
Central Nervous System Stimulants

Category	Drug
B	diethylpropion, doxapram, pemoline
C	amphetamines, caffeine
X	benzphetamine
Unclassified	mazindol, methylphenidate, phendimetrazine, phentermine

■ Nursing Management

Caffeine Assessment

■ **Assessment.** Assessment of caffeine intake should be a routine part of the nursing drug history. This includes caffeine intake from foods and beverages as well as from medications.

Caffeine may exacerbate gastric ulceration in peptic ulcer disease and therefore should be used with caution in clients with a history of peptic ulcers. Because of its suspected potential for causing dysrhythmias, it is recommended that clients avoid using caffeine if they have symptomatic cardiac dysrhythmias or palpitations or are in the recovery phase of acute myocardial infarctions.

The Food and Drug Administration (FDA) has warned women to avoid or to decrease caffeine consumption during pregnancy (see the Pregnancy Safety box above). Studies in humans have shown that heavy caffeine use by pregnant women may increase the risk of spontaneous abortion and intrauterine growth retardation (*USP DI,* 1999). Nurses in various settings should instruct women who are pregnant or of childbearing age to avoid drugs and sodas containing caffeine. Women who continue to drink coffee during their pregnancy should be encouraged to drink decaffeinated or instant coffee and to limit their coffee intake to 2 to 3 cups per day. Women who drink tea should decrease the brewing time or select a decaffeinated brand or herbal tea. The best solution would be to substitute fruit and vegetable juices or water for beverages that contain caffeine.

Review the client's current medication regimen for the risk of significant drug interactions, such as those that may

occur when caffeine is given concurrently with the following drugs:

Drug	Possible Effect and Management
Bold/color type indicates the most serious interactions.	
other CNS stimulants, other caffeine-containing medications or drinks	May result in increased CNS stimulation and undesirable side effects, such as increased nervousness, irritability, insomnia, dysrhythmias, and seizures. Monitor client's apical pulse and behaviors closely.
MAO inhibitors	**Concurrent use with caffeine may result in severe hypertension or dangerous dysrhythmias. A small amount of caffeine may induce an increased heart rate. Avoid concurrent use or a potentially serious drug interaction may occur.**

A baseline assessment of the infant's cardiovascular and respiratory status should be accomplished before caffeine therapy is initiated.

■ **Nursing Diagnosis.** The client taking caffeine may be at risk for the following nursing diagnoses: disturbed sleep pattern; disturbed thought processes (confusion, irritability); impaired comfort (gastrointestinal distress, headache); and ineffective therapeutic regimen management (if the client is under caffeine restrictions).

■ **Implementation**

■ ***Monitoring.*** When caffeine is administered for neonatal apnea, monitor serum caffeine levels 24 hours after the loading dose and then 1 to 2 times a week, or every 2 weeks after the infant is stabilized, to ensure therapeutic levels.

■ ***Education.*** A client who is or may become pregnant should be advised to avoid or limit her consumption of caffeine-containing foods (e.g., coffee, tea, cola drinks, cocoa, and milk chocolate) and drugs (e.g., OTC stimulants, analgesic combinations, and cold preparations). (See Table 18-5 for the caffeine content of selected products.)

Caffeine passes into breast milk and may accumulate in nursing infants. Research suggests that infants may appear jittery and have trouble sleeping when nursing mothers consume large amounts of caffeine. Breastfeeding mothers should be advised to limit their intake to one or two caffeine-containing beverages per day.

Caffeine-containing medications and beverages may interfere with sleep when taken close to bedtime. Caffeine is not intended to replace sleep and should not be used for that purpose. Clients with a hypersensitivity to caffeine should be alerted to its combination with analgesics (acetaminophen, aspirin, and phenacetin) for the treatment of headache. Because the adverse CNS reactions to the drug are increased in children, these same combination preparations should not be given to children.

The question is sometimes raised whether or not caffeine causes physical and psychologic dependence. Many persons report feeling irritable and nervous and developing a headache if they do not have their usual cup or two of coffee in the morning. This probably indicates psychologic and physical dependence. Such clients should be instructed to decrease their caffeine intake by gradually reducing the number of servings of coffee, cola, and tea or by mixing the amounts with decaffeinated preparations and gradually decreasing the proportion of the caffeinated form.

■ **Evaluation.** The expected outcome for the infant who is receiving caffeine for sleep apnea is a respiratory status within the normal limits related to the baseline. The client who is taking caffeine for other reasons will experience a restful sleeping pattern and not experience any adverse reactions to caffeine.

SUMMARY

The CNS stimulants have limited use in practice today. Although used in the past to treat obesity, their use has been discouraged because of their narrow therapeutic index and because of the rapid development of tolerance before the achievement of significant weight reduction. The prime indications for CNS stimulants are attention deficit disorder and narcolepsy. When used for their anorexiant effect, they are an adjunct to a regimen of diet and exercise. Because stimulation of the CNS occurs, clients may experience a sleep pattern disturbance, altered thought processes, sexual dysfunction, and altered comfort related to side effects such as dry mouth, headache, rash, and gastrointestinal or urinary effects. Caffeine, although not often thought of as a drug, is also a CNS stimulant, and the nurse should take an active role in educating clients about its effects.

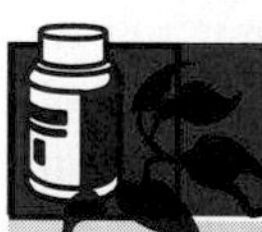

Complementary and Alternative Therapies
Chitosan

Chitosan is used as an accelerant in wound healing, as an agent in drug delivery systems, and over-the-counter as a food supplement for weight loss. It is a cationic polysaccharide obtained from the cuticle of crustacea such as crab, lobster, and shrimp, and it is similar to cellulose in its properties.

Although further independent research is required, a meta-analysis by Ernest and Pittler (1998) found that a chitosan supplement of 4 tablets per day together with a calorie-controlled diet is associated with an additional 3.28 kg weight loss over 28 days when compared with diet alone. There are also reductions in blood lipid levels and decreases in blood pressure demonstrated in the reviewed studies. However, other sources (Natural Medicines Comprehensive Database) indicate that chitosan is likely to be ineffective when taken orally for weight loss. Clients with shellfish allergies should use caution when using this agent. The ususal dosage is 4 tablets of chitosan daily.

Information from Ernst, E., Pittler, M.H. (1998). Chitosan as a treatment for body weight reduction? A meta-analysis. *Perfusion* 11:461-465; and *Prescribers' Letter,* http://www.naturaldatabase.com.

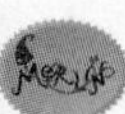

Critical Thinking Questions

1. Herbert Poulin, a client with type 1 diabetes, has been prescribed amphetamine sulfate for short-term treatment of exogenous obesity. He asks why he needs to be on a total weight reduction program in addition to anorexiant therapy. What do you tell him? What would be included in such a program? Will the amphetamine affect his management of his diabetic regimen? What other information should you provide to him?
2. The instructor of your health education class has given you the topic of caffeine habituation to present to the student group. What would you consider to be the most relevant information for your college-age group? How would you present this topic?

Collaborative Learning Activities

For Collaborative Learning Activities, go to mosby.com/MERLIN/McKenry/.

CASE STUDY

For a Case Study that will help ensure mastery of this chapter content, go to mosby.com/MERLIN/McKenry/.

BIBLIOGRAPHY

American Hospital Formulary Service. (1999). *AHFS drug information '99*. Bethesda, MD: American Society of Hospital Pharmacists.

American Pharmaceutical Association. (1996). *Nonprescription products: Formulations and features '96-'97*. Washington, DC: Author.

Anderson, K.N., Anderson, L.E., & Glantz, W.D. (Eds.). (1998). *Mosby's medical, nursing, & allied health dictionary* (5th ed.). St. Louis: Mosby.

Berman, T., Douglas, V.I., & Barr, R.G. (1999). Effects of methylphenidate on complex processing in attention-deficit hyperactivity disorder. *Journal of Abnormal Psychology, 108*(1), 90-105.

Bray, G.A. (1993). Use and abuse of appetite-suppressant drugs in the treatment of obesity. *Annuals of Internal Medicine, 119*(7), 707-712.

Constantine, L.M. & Scott, S. (1997). Just-approved antiobesity drug awaits DEA scheduling. *Pharmacy Today, 3*(12), 1.

Covington, T.R. (Ed.) (1996). *Handbook of nonprescription drugs* (11th ed.). Washington, DC: American Pharmaceutical Association.

Drug Facts and Comparisons. (2000). St. Louis: Facts and Comparisons.

Ernst, E., Pittler, M.H. (1998). Chitosan as a treatment for body weight reduction? A meta-analysis. *Perfusion 11*:461-465.

Klein, R.G. & Mannuzza, S. (1988). Hyperactive boys almost grown up: Methylphenidate effects on ultimate height. *Archives of General Psychiatry, 45*(12), 1131-1134.

Leung, A.K.C., Robinson, W.L., Fagan, J.E., & Lim, S.H. (1994). Attention-deficit hyperactivity disorder: Getting control of impulse behavior. *Postgraduate Medicine, 95*(2),153-160.

Manos, M.J., Short, E.J., & Findling, R.L. (1999). Differential effectiveness of methylphenidate and Adderall in school-age youths with attention-deficit/hyperactivity disorder. *Journal of American Academy Child Adolescent Psychiatry 38*(7), 813-819.

Markowitz, J.S., Morrison, S.D., & DeVane, C.L. (1999). Drug interactions with psychostimulants. *International Clinical Psychopharmacology, 14*(1), 1-18.

Mosby's GenRx. (1999). St. Louis: Mosby.

Pelham, W.E., Gnagy, E.M., Chronis, A.M., Burrows-MacLean, L., Fabiano, G.A., Onyango, A.N., Meichenbaum, D.L., Williams, A., Aronoff, H.R., & Steiner, R.L. (1999). A comparison of morning-only and morning/late afternoon Adderall to morning-only, twice-daily, and three times-daily methylphenidate in children with attention-deficit/hyperactivity disorder. *Pediatrics 104*(6), 1300-1311.

Prescribers' Letter, http://www.naturaldatabase.com.

Robison, L.M., Sclar, D.A., Skaer, T.L., & Galin, R.S. (1999). National trends in the prevalence of attention deficit/hyperactivity disorder and the prescribing of methylphenidate among school-age children: 1990-1995. *Clinical Pediatrics, 38*(4), 209-217.

Saklad, J.J. & Curtis, J.L. (1995). Psychiatric disorders in children, adolescents, and people with developmental disabilities. In L.Y. Young & M.A. Koda-Kimble (Eds.), *Applied therapeutics: The clinical uses of drugs* (6th ed.). Vancouver, WA: Applied Therapeutics.

Sunohara, G.A., Malone, M.A., Rovet, J., Humphries, T., Roberts, W., & Taylor, M.J. (1999). Effect of methylphenidate on attention in children with attention deficit hyperactivity disorder (ADHD): ERP evidence. *Neuropsychopharmacology, 21*(2), 218-228.

Theesen, K.A. & Stimmel, G.L. (1993). Psychiatric disorders. In J.T. DiPiro, R.L. Talbert, G.C. Yee, G.R. Matzke, B.G. Wells, & L.M. Posey (Eds.), *Pharmacotherapy: A pathophysiologic Approach* (2nd ed.). Norwalk, CT: Appleton & Lange.

United States Pharmacopeia Dispensing Information (USP DI): Drug information for the health care professional (19th ed.). (1999). Rockville, MD: United States Pharmacopeial Convention.

Zeiner, P., Bryhn, G., Bjercke, C., Truyen, K., & Strand, G. (1999). Response to methylphenidate in boys with attention-deficit hyperactivity disorder. *Acta Paediatrics, 88*(3), 298-303.

19 Psychotherapeutic Drugs

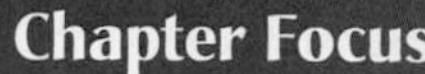

Chapter Focus

Providing nursing care for clients receiving psychotherapeutic agents can be challenging. Nursing responsibilities include not only planning, implementing, and evaluating drug therapy, but also doing so via a meaningful therapeutic relationship with the client. Whether the setting is an acute psychiatric facility, a nursing home, or a community environment, the nurse's knowledge base of psychotherapeutic drugs provides for direct care and for teaching and counseling the client and caregivers about safe and accurate self-administration of these agents.

Learning Objectives

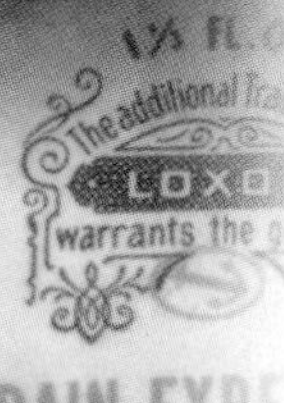

1. Discuss the use of drug therapy in psychiatry.
2. Identify the common psychotropic drugs.
3. Differentiate between the antipsychotic drugs: phenothiazine derivatives, thioxanthenes, haloperidol, molindone, loxapine, and the atypical agents.
4. Differentiate between the antidepressant drugs: tricyclic agents, second-generation agents, monoamine oxidase inhibitors, selective serotonin reuptake inhibitors, and the miscellaneous agents.
5. Discuss the use of lithium as an antimanic therapy.
6. Discuss the nursing management of the common side effects/adverse reactions of psychotherapeutic agents.
7. Implement an appropriate plan of care for clients who require the administration of psychotherapeutic agents.

Key Terms

affective disorder, p. 412
bipolar disorder, p. 413
endogenous depression, p. 413
exogenous depression, p. 413
major depression, p. 413
mania, p. 412
tardive dyskinesia, p. 402
tranquilizer, p. 398

Key Drugs [✔]

chlorpromazine, p. 398
haloperidol, p. 400
imipramine, p. 414
risperidone, p. 410

This chapter reviews the medications used to treat psychoses and affective disorders, especially schizophrenia (antipsychotic agents), depression (antidepressants), and mania (lithium and others) are reviewed in this chapter. To enhance understanding of this chapter, it is necessary to review the functional systems of the central nervous system (CNS), such as the reticular activating system (Figure 19-1), the limbic and extrapyramidal systems, and the action of acetylcholine and the catecholamines. (See Chapter 13 for a review of the physiology and functions of the various components of the CNS.) This chapter also reviews the antipsychotic agents, antidepressant therapy, and antimanic medications.

THE CENTRAL NERVOUS SYSTEM AND EMOTIONS

A holistic view of human beings and their experience no longer allows the health care practitioner to separate the functions of the mind from the functions of the body. The CNS is responsible for consciousness, behavior, memory, recognition, learning, and more highly developed attributes such as imagination, abstract reasoning, and creative thought. In addition, it serves to coordinate vital regulatory functions such as blood pressure, heart rate, respiration, salivary and gastric secretions, muscular activity, and body temperature.

The interrelationships among the various circuits in the brain produce patterns of behavior that can be modified by external situations or internal autonomic adjustments. This allows the individual to adapt to changes in both the external and the internal environments.

Autonomic Regulation

The sympathetic and parasympathetic visceral nervous systems play an important role in the production of behavior; these systems are discussed in Chapter 20. An understanding of these mechanisms is the basis for learning the actions and side effects of the drugs that affect mood and behavior.

Biochemical Mechanisms

The functions of the CNS depend on the actions of certain neurohormonal agents located in the brain and peripheral tissues. These neurohormones are stored in inactive forms; at the right moment, nerve impulses release the free forms of these neurohormones to stimulate the transmission of appropriate reactions. The neurotransmitter exerts its action by interacting with a receptor (a specialized protein), which is located on the outermost part of the postsynaptic cell and produces both electric and biochemical changes within the postsynaptic cell.

Acetylcholine, norepinephrine, and serotonin have been found in the CNS. Tyrosine and dopamine are normal constituents of the brain and are known precursors of norepinephrine synthesis. High concentrations of norepinephrine are found in the hypothalamus, medulla, limbic system, and cranial nerve nuclei. Dopamine is found in high concentrations in the striatum and caudate nucleus. It is believed that both norepinephrine and dopamine function as neurotransmitters. They exert widespread inhibitory and excitatory effects on a wide variety of centrally mediated functions such as sleep, arousal, affect, and memory. Thus some central synapses are adrenergic.

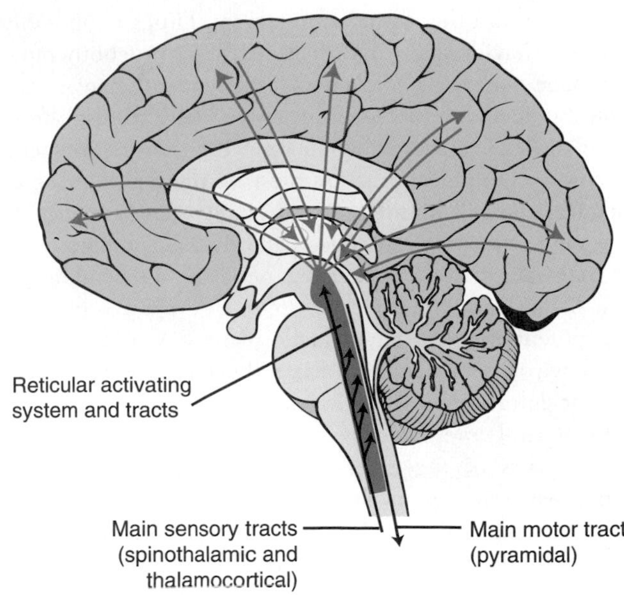

Figure 19-1 Reticular activating system.

Areas rich in serotonin include the hypothalamus, pineal gland, midbrain, and spinal cord. An alteration of serotonin levels in the nervous system is associated with changes in behavior. Many drugs mimic or block the action of serotonin on peripheral tissues and produce changes in mood and behavior, which suggests that they interfere with the action of serotonin and norepinephrine in the brain.

The relationship of dopamine to the major psychoses has received much attention. There are a variety of dopamine receptors in the brain, especially in the basal ganglia and limbic areas; D_1 and D_2 are the primary receptors involved with the antipsychotic agents. Although both receptors are involved with movement disorders in the basal ganglia, blockade of the D_2 receptors (causing supersensitivity) in animals has resulted in tardive dyskinesia. Antipsychotic agents with a low affinity for D_2 receptors, such as clozapine, are less apt to cause extrapyramidal side effects/adverse reactions (Hardman & Limbird, 1996). Further research in this area may result in the development of more specific treatment agents that produce fewer adverse reactions (Ereshefsky & Richards, 1992).

THE ROLE OF DRUG THERAPY IN PSYCHIATRY

Drugs play an important role in contemporary approaches to psychiatric care. Drug therapy reduces or alleviates symptoms and allows the client an opportunity to participate more easily in other forms of treatment. Drugs temporarily modify behavior, and other therapies (e.g., psychotherapy) can shape behavior and produce a permanent change. Any enduring effects on behavior are more likely to result from the client's concurrent interaction with the environment. Because incoming information must be translated into biochemical changes before it can affect nervous system function, environmental transactions and drugs may affect similar pathways before influencing behavior. Depending on their nature and direction, the effects of drugs can be additive, potentiating, or antagonistic (Fang & Gorrod, 1999). The environment may potentiate the effectiveness of the drug or detract from it.

In general, prescribers select psychotherapeutic agents on the basis of the diagnostic category—schizophrenia, manic-depressive syndrome, or psychoneurosis. If the client's diagnosis warrants the use of an antipsychotic agent, the prescriber will try to match the therapeutic advantages of a particular drug to the client's symptoms. Since their introduction, antipsychotic agents and other psychotropic agents have been widely prescribed and, in many instances with older adults, inappropriately used. Inappropriate prescriptions expose older adults to an increased risk of adverse or serious drug reactions or falls, which often are detrimental to the client's cognitive and functional health status (Cumming, 1998). Studies of these practices have resulted in regulations governing Medicare and Medicaid recipients in long-term care facilities.

The Omnibus Budget Reconciliation Act (OBRA) Long-Term Care Requirements Act for long-term care facilities was implemented in 1992. Although this act applies to all drugs that a client receives, surveyors at the Health Care Financing Administration (HCFA) initially focused their attention on the major CNS drug categories: antipsychotics, antianxiety agents, sedatives, hypnotics, and benzodiazepines. The purpose of this law is to review the indication, dosage (including duplicate-type drug orders), duration, and monitoring parameters to determine if the drugs are being given in the presence of side effects/adverse reactions. Surveyors may cite a facility for deficiencies in these areas (Carley, 1992).

Before antipsychotic drugs can be prescribed for a nursing home resident, an appropriate specific condition must be documented, such as schizophrenia, schizoaffective disorder, delusional disorder, psychotic mood disorder, acute psychotic episode, brief reactive psychosis, schizophreniform disorder, atypical psychosis, Tourette's syndrome, or Huntington's disease. All of these diagnoses are organic mental syndromes that have associated psychotic or agitation features. Agitation features are defined as (1) specific behaviors that can be quantitatively and objectively documented (e.g., biting, kicking, scratching) and that cause the client to present a danger to himself or others and actually interfere with the ability of the nursing staff to provide care to the client, or (2) the presence of psychotic symptoms (delusions, hallucinations, or paranoid behavior) that are not a result of a previously mentioned disorder but cause the client extreme distress (Box 19-1). To treat the symptoms of hiccups, nausea, vomiting, or pruritus, short-term therapy of 1 week is permissible.

The purpose of the OBRA regulations was to eliminate or reduce the inappropriate prescribing of these potent medications for behaviors that may be controlled by nonpharmacologic approaches. For example, insomnia, pacing, wandering, restlessness, crying spells, screaming episodes, deficient memory, uncooperativeness, nervousness, or depression would alone not warrant the use of an antipsychotic agent. For these medications to be prescribed, such symptoms would need to be associated with an appropriate diagnosis as mentioned previously. However, there is still concern for the shift to the use of newer psychotropic agents in the post-HCFA era in a population where close monitoring may not be readily available (Lasser & Sunderland, 1998).

In addition, with the care of older, frail individuals shifting to the community setting, there is concern for the lack of regulatory oversight relating to prescribing practices for this group. Golden et al. (1999) revealed a high prevalence of psychotropic medications and inappropriate drug use among older homebound residents—a group that is at the highest risk for adverse drug reactions. Psychotropic drug treatment without access to psychotherapeutic support is not appropriate for older clients in the community (Stevens, Katona, Manela, Watkin, & Livingston, 1999).

When a prescriber establishes the need for drug therapy, he or she must decide what agent or combination of agents is best suited for the client's total health needs. This requires

BOX 19-1

Positive and Negative Symptoms in Schizophrenia

Clients with schizophrenia experience a wide variety of symptoms that range from being most responsive (or positive) to least responsive (or negative) to the antipsychotic agents. Most antipsychotic agents produce an effect on the following positive symptoms: agitation, anxiety, hallucinations, poor hygiene and dress, hyperactivity, delusions, paranoia, and hostility. The negative symptoms of flat affect; social inadequacy; diminished speech patterns, judgment, and insight; and others are usually less responsive to drug therapy.

The target symptoms are used as monitoring parameters to evaluate the client's response to the medication. The atypical antipsychotic drugs such as clozapine and risperidone appear to be more effective than other neuroleptic agents in treating negative symptoms.

Information from Marken, P.A. & Stanislav, S.W. (1995). Schizophrenia. In L.Y. Young & M.A. Koda-Kimble (Eds.), *Applied therapeutics: The clinical use of drugs* (6th ed.). Vancouver, WA: Applied Therapeutics.

an intimate knowledge of the behavioral actions, pharmacologic effects, and potential adverse reactions of the agents used, as well as an awareness of the many individual and environmental factors present (Stahl, 1999). (See the Nursing Research box below and the Cultural Considerations box on p. 396.)

The additional effects or side effects profile of a drug is a useful tool in helping the prescriber select an appropriate antipsychotic agent (Table 19-1). If a drug with a strong sedation property is desired, chlorpromazine (Thorazine) or thioridazine (Mellaril) might be prescribed. If extrapyramidal side effects are troublesome, thioridazine (which has the greatest anticholinergic effect) has less potential for inducing extrapyramidal side effects. In older clients at higher risk for tardive dyskinesia (TD), the atypical antipsychotic risperidone may pose a significantly lower

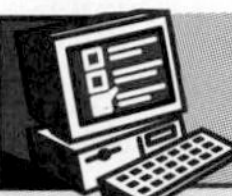

Nursing Research

Gender Differences in the Pharmacokinetics and Pharmacodynamics of Psychotropic Medications

Citation: Yonkers, K.A., Kanders, J.C., Cole, J.O., & Blumenthal, S. (1992). Gender differences in pharmacokinetics and pharmacodynamics of psychotropic medication. *American Journal of Psychiatry, 149*(5), 587-595.

Abstract: There are theoretical reasons to suggest gender-related drug effects, but there are limited clinical data to support such hypotheses for different psychopharmacologic agents. The issue discussed by Yonkers et al. is particularly important because Phase I studies, which determine therapeutic doses, have been conducted on male subjects, but women seek treatment and receive psychotropic medications more often than men. The authors concluded that there are potential gender differences in pharmacokinetics related to absorption and bioavailability, distribution, metabolism, and menstrual cycle effects, and thus empirical studies of specific drugs are required (see Yonkers et al. [1999] for the specific citations of the research reviewed).

The literature analyzing the pharmacokinetics, pharmacodynamics, and side effects of psychotropic drugs is most substantial for the antipsychotic drugs. With comparable dosing, women have been found to have higher blood levels for fluphenazine (Prolixin) and fluspirilene than men of similar weight and age. Women have had greater improvement than men after treatment with pimozide (Orap) and chlorpromazine (Thorazine). It has been hypothesized that this greater efficacy in young women is due to the presumed antidopaminergic effect of estrogen. This same protective effect for premenopausal women may hold true for antipsychotic-induced side effects—there is a higher prevalence of severe dyskinesias in young men, and the severity of TD is far greater in women over age 67. Although estrogen has not been directly tested as an antipsychotic agent in humans, age needs to be considered when looking at gender differences because of the critical interactions between gender and age.

The preponderance of evidence suggests that benzodiazepines that are conjugatively metabolized have slower elimination rates in women than in men. Oral contraceptives have been found to decrease the clearance of benzodiazepines; in women taking oral contraceptives, cognitive and psychomotor tasks were more impaired during the week they were not taking hormones, because the benzodiazepines peaked more quickly. This suggests that a change in absorption rates for the week when hormones are not being taken leads to a dose of benzodiazepines that suddenly becomes intoxicating. More studies are needed to test the physiologic response throughout the menstrual cycle.

Given the literature citing the higher prevalence of depressive disorders in women, the paucity of studies addressing gender-specific medication effects is surprising. In evaluating the efficacy of tricyclic antidepressants and MAOIs by gender in three types of atypical depression, it was found that depressed women with panic attacks had a more favorable response to MAOIs than to tricyclic antidepressants, whereas men who were more depressed and had panic attacks responded more favorably to tricyclic antidepressants. When the studies were controlled for the use of oral contraceptives, no significant gender differences were found in plasma levels of amitriptyline and nortriptyline.

Lithium carbonate has been the subject of several case reports suggesting menstrual cycle effects on serum levels. Because some women do show a phasic difference, it may be helpful to correlate lithium levels to symptoms throughout the menstrual cycle. Adverse reactions to lithium may occur with more frequency in women, particularly lithium-induced hypothyroidism.

Despite the limitations of the studies reviewed, Yonkers et al. (1992) conclude that there is evidence suggesting gender-related variations. These findings include (1) the potential for women to have higher plasma levels of psychotropic drugs (especially when given with oral contraceptives), and (2) greater efficacy of antipsychotic agents and a greater likelihood of adverse reactions, such as hypothyroidism and, in older women, TD. These suggested gender-related differences clearly require further investigation.

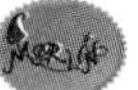

Critical Thinking Questions

- In what ways could this research influence your nursing practice in the administration of psychotropic medications?
- What instructions would you provide to Nora Parton, a 27-year-old female client who has been prescribed benzodiazepines while she is taking oral contraceptives?

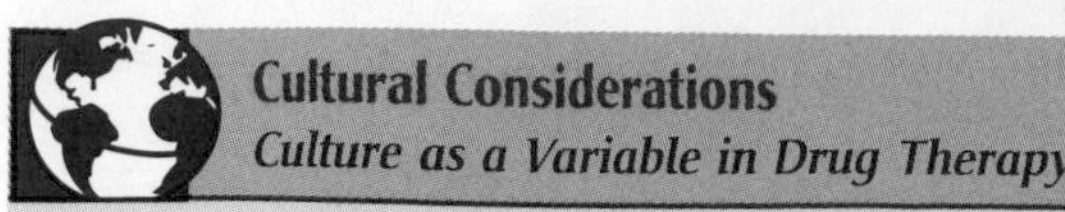

Cultural Considerations
Culture as a Variable in Drug Therapy

To deal with cultural issues in psychiatric care, attempts are usually made to promote the recognition and appreciation of cultural influences in the hope that a more sensitive and therapeutic approach may result. Keltner and Folks (1992) believe that although there has been relatively little research on the topic of culture and psychopharmacology, the work that has been published is of significance to nurses administering psychotropic agents.

Do Individuals from Varying Cultural, Ethnic, and Racial Backgrounds Respond to Psychotropic Drugs Differently?

Asians reportedly require lower dosages of drugs such as neuroleptics, tricyclic antidepressants, and lithium than do Caucasians. There are fewer studies of Hispanics and African Americans. It has been reported that Hispanic clients require lower dosages of antidepressant medications than non-Hispanics and that African Americans generally improve more rapidly with the use of neuroleptics, tricyclic antidepressants, and anxiolytics than do their Caucasian counterparts. Lithium has a significantly longer half-life in African Americans than in Caucasians or Asians.

How Can These Differences in Dosage of Psychotropics Be Explained?

Cultural, ethnic, and racial differences in drug response and metabolism have been appreciated by pharmacologists for some time. Differences in pharmacokinetics may have genetic or environmental causes. Only about 9% of African Americans and Caucasians are considered to be slow metabolizers as compared to as many as 32% of Asians. Individuals who metabolize drugs more slowly will experience a greater drug effect. There is also evidence of variability in protein binding based on ethnicity. Habits such as smoking and drinking alcohol are known to speed drug metabolism, whereas a low-protein, high-carbohydrate diet is known to slow metabolism. The fact that Caucasians and African Americans drink significantly more alcohol than Asians and eat differently may provide an environmental explanation for the greater drug response by Asians.

Do Individuals of Various Cultural Backgrounds Experience Side Effects Differently?

Asians are more sensitive than Caucasians to neuroleptics. In one study, Asian clients began experiencing extrapyramidal effects at dosages that were approximately half of those for Caucasians. At equivalent dosages, 95% of Asians experienced extrapyramidal effects, whereas only 67% of Caucasians and African Americans experienced those side effects (Lin, 1986). Hispanic clients taking tricyclic antidepressants are reported to experience side effects at half the dosages observed in white non-Hispanics (Marcos & Cancro, 1982). African Americans apparently are far more susceptible than Caucasians to tricyclic antidepressant delirium. However, one study reported no observed difference in the frequency and severity of TD among Caucasian, African-American, and Hispanic clients (Stramek et al., 1991).

Undoubtedly, psychotropic drugs help individuals from all cultural, ethnic, and racial backgrounds. However, there is growing evidence that differences do influence the course and outcome of psychopharmacologic therapy.

How would this research influence your nursing practice in administering psychotropic agents?

Modified from Keltner, N.L. & Folks, D.G. (1992). Culture as a variable in drug therapy. *Perspectives on Psychiatric Care, 28*(1), 33-36. Reprinted with permission, Nursecom, Inc.

risk for TD than the conventional neuroleptic haloperidol (Jeste et al., 1999).

Continuous nursing and medical evaluations based on observation of the client for the therapeutic and adverse effects of the drug are necessary. If anticholinergic side effects such as dry mouth, blurred vision, constipation, and urinary retention continue and are disturbing to the client, the prescriber could select an agent with less potential for inducing such effects, such as fluphenazine (Prolixin, Permitil), thiothixene (Navane), or haloperidol (Haldol).

Nurses play an important role in the evaluation and assessment of a client's response to drug therapy. They should be aware of the criteria the prescriber uses in selecting psychotherapeutic drugs and of the expected effects of the drug so they can observe and report on the client's progress. Progress is evaluated by monitoring the client's behavioral and affective responses to the medications, the client's knowledge of the drug therapy, the presence and extent of expected side effects/adverse reactions, the client's response to dosage adjustments and supportive nursing interventions, and the potential for or existence of drug or food interactions. Knowing the action of drugs also assists health care professionals in understanding the interpersonal responses that occur in the therapeutic relationship with the client.

ANTIPSYCHOTIC OR NEUROLEPTIC AGENTS

Historical Background

The population of the United States doubled between 1900 and 1950; during this time, the population in public mental hospitals quadrupled. The average length of confinement was usually years, and the trend was definitely toward an an-

TABLE 19-1 Selected Antipsychotic Agents: Potency and Major Side Effects

Chemical, Generic Name (Trade Name)	Equivalent* PO Dose (mg)	Frequency of Selected Effects and Side Effects†				
		Antiemetic	Sedation	Hypotension‡	Anticholinergic	EPS
Phenothiazines						
Aliphatic						
chlorpromazine (Thorazine)	100	3	3	3	2	2
Piperidine						
thioridazine (Mellaril)	100	1	3	3	3	1
mesoridazine (Serentil)	50	1	3	3	3	1
Piperazine						
fluphenazine (Permitil)	2	1	1	1	1	3
perphenazine (Trilafon)	10	3	1	1	1	3
prochlorperazine (Compazine)	15	3	2	1	1	3
trifluoperazine (Stelazine)	5	3	1	1	1	3
Thioxanthenes						
thiothixene (Navane)	4	—	1	1	1	3
Other Compounds						
Butyrophenone						
haloperidol (Haldol)	2	2	1	1	1	3
Dihydroindolone						
molindone (Moban)	10	—	1	1	1	3
Dibenzoxazepine						
loxapine (Loxitane)	15	—	2	2	1	3
Atypical Agents						
clozapine (Clozaril)	50	1	3	3	3	1
risperidone (Risperdal)	—	—	1	1	1	0/1

Information from *Drug Facts and Comparisons*. (2000). St. Louis: Facts and Comparisons; and *United States Pharmacopeia Dispensing Information (USP DI): Drug information for the health care professional* (19th ed.). (1999). Rockville, MD: United States Pharmacopeial Convention. *EPS*, Extrapyramidal side effects (includes akathisia, dystonia, parkinsonism, and TD); dash indicates undocumented or unknown information.
*Equivalent doses are from low potency (50 to 100 mg) to intermediate potency (10 to 49 mg) to high potency (1 to 9 mg).
†Grading: *1*, Low; *2*, moderate; *3*, high.
‡Orthostatic hypotension.

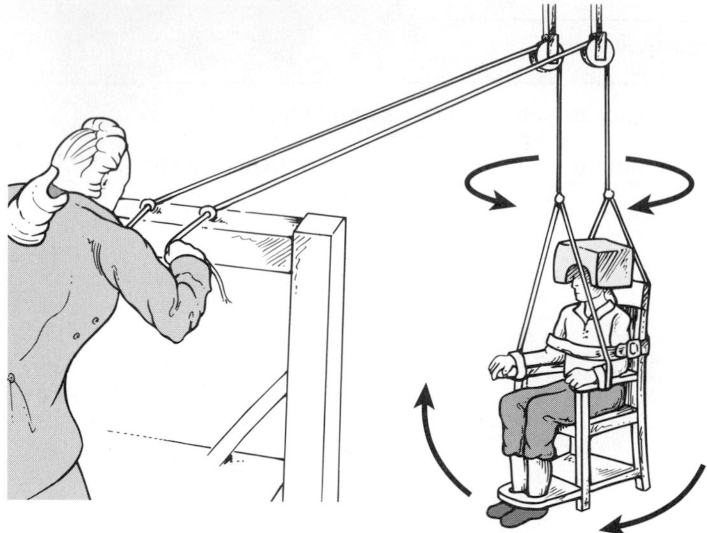

Figure 19-2 The tranquilizer or restraining chair used in the eighteenth century to "tranquilize" the agitated client.

nual increase in clients admitted to such institutions. Client and employee injuries caused by combative or abusive clients led to the common use of physical restraints and client isolation.

Before the development of the antipsychotic agents, the treatment of mentally disturbed clients consisted of either being isolated (i.e., hidden in cellars or attics in their homes) or, if they came to the attention of local authorities, being transferred to jails or homes for the insane. Actual therapies used before the advent of the antipsychotic agents were water or ice pack therapies, strait-jackets or other physical restraints, shock therapy with insulin or electricity, lobotomy, and the use of a few drugs such as paraldehyde, chloral hydrate, and the barbiturates.

Chlorpromazine (Thorazine) was the first antipsychotic agent. This phenothiazine prototype was the first **tranquilizer** (a drug prescribed to calm an agitated or anxious individual) released in the early 1950s. Dr. Benjamin Rush used the term *tranquilizer* approximately 200 years ago. Dr. Rush, an early pioneer in the mental health field and a signer of the Declaration of Independence, invented a restraining chair named the "tranquilizer chair" (Lyons & Petrucelli, 1978). This chair was modified by the addition of a pulley system; an extremely agitated client would be seated and restrained in the chair, which was then raised off the ground and rocked back and forth until the client was quieted (Figure 19-2).

Neither the tranquilizer chair nor the tranquilizing (antipsychotic) agents cure mental illness. They have been and are used to control the symptoms associated with this disease state; the chair provided physical and eventually physiologic restraints, and the antipsychotic and tranquilizing agents constitute a chemical control of the symptoms.

The use of the antipsychotic drugs proved to be a revolutionary force in the psychiatric field. The duration of institutionalization has decreased from years to months for many clients; other clients live at home and are treated at community mental health centers. The reported incidence of injuries has declined, and many large public mental health facilities have closed.

Phenothiazine Derivatives

The first phenothiazine, chlorpromazine (Thorazine), was widely accepted for the treatment of mental illness. Since its development, many other drug products have been developed, and phenothiazines are now the largest group of psychotropic agents. Phenothiazines are divided chemically into three subgroups: (1) aliphatic compounds (e.g., chlorpromazine), (2) piperidine compounds (e.g., thioridazine), and (3) piperazine compounds (e.g., fluphenazine).

Aliphatic phenothiazine derivatives include chlorpromazine (Thorazine and others), methotrimeprazine (Levoprome, Nozinan ♣), promazine (Sparine), and triflupromazine (Vesprin). Piperidine phenothiazine derivatives include mesoridazine (Serentil) and thioridazine (Mellaril, Apo-Thioridazine ♣). Piperazine phenothiazine derivatives consist of fluphenazine (Prolixin, Permitil), perphenazine (Trilafon, Apo-Perphenazine ♣), prochlorperazine (Compazine, Stemetil ♣), and trifluoperazine (Stelazine, Novoflurazine ♣). Acetophenazine (Tindal), promazine (Sparine), and triflupromazine (Vesprin) are available on the market but are not commonly used today. Table 19-2 lists the indications for and the dosage ranges of the phenothiazine derivatives.

Classification. Phenothiazines have been classified as low-potency, intermediate-potency, and high-potency drugs. The basis for classification is the quantity of medication necessary to produce an equivalent effect when compared with other agents in the same category. For example, 100 mg of chlorpromazine (Thorazine) is considered to be approximately equivalent to 50 mg of mesoridazine (Serentil) or 2 mg haloperidol (Haldol). Thus chlorpromazine is a low-potency agent, mesoridazine an intermediate-potency agent, and haloperidol a high-potency agent (see Table 19-1 for antipsychotic equivalency doses). The student is cautioned not to confuse potency with effectiveness; potency refers to the quantity of a drug necessary to produce an equivalent effect as compared with another drug in the same classification. Effectiveness measures the therapeutic response to various agents, which depending on the individual drugs being studied may range from less effective to equivalent in effectiveness to more effective.

Mechanism of Action. Although the exact mechanism of action for the antipsychotic effects is unknown, the major therapeutic effects and side effects/adverse reactions of phenothiazines are the result of dopamine blockade in specific areas of the CNS. Phenothiazines also produce an alpha-blocking effect (hypotension), inhibit or block dopamine at the chemoreceptor trigger zone (CTZ), and peripherally inhibit the vagus nerve in the gastrointestinal tract (antiemetic effect). They also produce an antianxiety effect

TABLE 19-2 Phenothiazines: Indications and Dosage Range*

Chemical Classification Generic (Trade Name)	Indication	Routes	Dosage Range (mg/24 hr) Adults	Children
Aliphatic				
chlorpromazine (Thorazine)	Antipsychotic	PO, IM, Rectal	PO 20-800	6 months and older: 0.55 mg/kg q4-6h
	Antiemetic	PO, IM, Rectal	PO 60-150	Same as above
	Hiccups or porphyria	PO, IM	PO 75-200	—
	tetanus	IM	IM 75-200	IM 0.55 mg/kg q6-8h
Piperidine				
thioridazine (Mellaril)	Antipsychotic	PO	PO 100-800	2-12 years: 0.25-3 mg/kg 4 times daily
mesoridazine (Serentil)	Antipsychotic	PO, IM	PO 30-400	<12 years: not available >12 years: see adult dosage
Piperazine				
fluphenazine (Prolixin)	Antipsychotic	PO, IM	PO 2.5-20	250-750 μg 1-4 times daily
perphenazine (Trilafon)	Antipsychotic	PO, IM	PO 8-64	<12 years: not available >12 years: see adult dosage
	Antiemetic	PO, IM	PO 8-16	<12 years: not available >12 years: see adult dosage
prochlorperazine (Compazine)	Antipsychotic	PO, IM, Rectal	PO 15-40	2-12 years: 2.5 mg PO 2-3 times daily >12 years: see adult dosage
trifluoperazine (Stelazine)	Antipsychotic	PO, IM	PO 4-40	>6 years: 1-2 mg daily

*Doses are titrated as needed and tolerated by the individual.

by depression of the brainstem reticular system. Most phenothiazines and haloperidol increase the release of prolactin, which infrequently results in breast swelling and milk secretion. Methotrimeprazine (Levoprome) is a phenothiazine with primarily analgesic and sedative effects. It is not used as an antipsychotic drug in the United States.

Indications. Various phenothiazine derivatives are used in the treatment of psychosis, nausea and vomiting, pain, and sedation, as well as adjuncts to the treatment of tetanus, acute intermittent porphyria, and intractable hiccups.

Pharmacokinetics. Phenothiazines are well absorbed orally and have an onset of action between ½ and 1 hour. The onset of action for IM phenothiazines is within 30 minutes, with the exception of the long-acting parenteral forms. The onset of antipsychotic effect is achieved gradually and usually requires several weeks, and the peak therapeutic effect occurs between 6 weeks and 6 months. The duration of action for these products ranges from 6 to 24 hours or more, depending on the dosage and frequency of drug administration. Phenothiazines are metabolized in the liver and excreted primarily by the kidneys.

Side Effects/Adverse Reactions. Side effects/adverse reactions of phenothiazines include extrapyramidal effects, such as akathisia, dystonia, drug-induced parkinsonism, and TD (Box 19-2). Boxes 19-3 and 19-4 provide a description of these disorders and their treatment.

Dosage and Administration. The dosage of phenothiazines varies according to the client, the reason for treatment, and the client's response to the medication. It is best to titrate from a low dosage and increase when necessary to produce a therapeutic response, which usually occurs within days to a couple of months. This dosage is continued for 14 days and then gradually decreased to the lowest amount that produces a therapeutic response.

When phenothiazine therapy is to be discontinued, the dosage should be gradually reduced over 2 or 3 weeks. Nausea, vomiting, dizziness, tremors, and dyskinesia have been reported when antipsychotic agents are suddenly discontinued after having been given to clients in high dosages or for a long time. (See Table 19-2 for phenothiazine indications and dosage.)

BOX 19-2

Antipsychotic Medications: Side Effects/Adverse Reactions

Side Effects*	Adverse Reactions†
More frequent: sleepiness, dizziness, dry mouth, constipation, and nasal congestion reported with aliphatic and piperidine phenothiazines and thioxanthenes; incidence is less frequent with the piperazine phenothiazines, with the exception of perphenazine	Visual changes, hypotensive episodes (more common with aliphatic and piperidine phenothiazines, thioxanthenes and, possibly, molindone)
Thioxanthenes: skin sensitivity to the sun	Dystonia and/or parkinson-type effects, including shuffle in walk, arm or leg stiffness, tremors, masklike facial expression, dysphagia, imbalance, muscle spasms or unusual twisting effects of the face, neck, or back (more common with aliphatic and piperazine phenothiazines, thioxanthenes, loxapine, molindone, risperidone, and haloperidol)
Loxapine: most common effects are blurred vision, confusion, dizziness, dry mouth, and increase in body weight	Akathisia (abnormal restlessness and agitation), increased pacing, and insomnia (more often reported with haloperidol, loxapine, thioxanthene)
Haloperidol: usually blurred vision, constipation, dry mouth, and increase in body weight	TD, a very serious adverse reaction; although rare, NMS may occur
Molindone: usually sedation, blurred vision, dry mouth, and constipation	Agranulocytosis, hypotension, tachycardia, and seizures (can occur with clozapine)
Clozapine: may cause sedation, dizziness, constipation, insomnia, headaches, tremor, and nausea	Hyperkinesia, agitation, aggressive behavior
Risperidone: nausea, dizziness, sedation, insomnia, and headache	

*If side effects continue, increase, or disturb the client, inform the prescriber.
†If adverse reactions occur, contact the prescriber, because medical intervention may be necessary.

Thioxanthenes

chlorprothixene [klor proe thix′ een] (Taractan)
flupenthixol [floo pent′ ole] (Fluanxol ♣, Fluanxol Depot ♣)
thiothixene [thye oh thix′ een] (Navane)

Thioxanthenes resemble the piperazine phenothiazines in their antipsychotic effects, including the high incidence of extrapyramidal adverse reactions (see Box 19-2). Their antipsychotic indications, side effects, precautions, and drug interactions are similar to those for the phenothiazines. Thiothixene is the drug most commonly prescribed in this category. The usual dosage of thiothixene for adults and children 12 years of age and older is 2 mg PO three times daily; an oral dosage has not been established for children up to 12 years of age. The adult parenteral dosage is 4 mg IM, two to four times daily. For the nursing management of the thioxanthenes, see Nursing Management: Antipsychotic Agent Therapy, p. 402.

Other Antipsychotic Compounds

Butyrophenone Derivatives

✔ **haloperidol** [ha loe per′ i dole] (Haldol)

The butyrophenones are structurally different from the other antipsychotic agents but have similar properties in terms of antipsychotic efficacy. Haloperidol appears to have a selective CNS effect; it competitively blocks D_2 receptors in the mesolimbic system and also causes an increased turnover of brain dopamine to produce its antipsychotic effect. It has less effect on the norepinephrine and epinephrine receptors and is associated with a significant degree of extrapyramidal effects.

Haloperidol has both antiemetic and antipsychotic effects. It is used to treat psychotic disorders, severe behavioral problems in children, and Tourette's syndrome, a rare CNS disorder that results in involuntary, rapid, and repetitive motor movements of muscle groups and is usually accompanied by involuntary vocalizations. Tourette's syndrome is more common in males, usually appearing before the age of 14, and may present initially as tics (facial grimaces and blinking). Other symptoms include vocal tics or noises, such as grunting, barking, shouting, sniffing, compulsive swearing (coprolalia), and movement disorders (involuntary, purposeless movements). The symptoms may peak and wane throughout the individual's life. The individual's intellectual functions are normal. Although there is no cure for Tourette's syndrome, haloperidol (Haldol) and pimozide (Orap) have produced dramatic improvement in some clients.

The usual adult dosage is 0.5 to 5 mg PO two to three times daily. The parenteral dosage is 2 to 5 mg IM every 2 to 4 hours initially, then every 4 to 8 hours thereafter. A dosage has not been established for children.

Very low dosages of haloperidol have been found to be useful for the treatment of severe agitation, combativeness,

BOX 19-3

Neuroleptic Extrapyramidal Adverse Reactions

Akathisia

Description

Motor restlessness is present; client is unable to sit or stand still and feels an urgent need to move, pace, rock, or tap foot.

Akathisia may also appear as apprehension, irritability, and general uneasiness and may be mistaken for agitation.

This condition is more common in females than males; it usually occurs within 5 to 30 days (up to 90 days) of starting drug therapy.

Treatment

Lower the dosage of the neuroleptic agent, switch to a different drug, or administer an antiparkinson drug, such as benztropine (Cogentin).

Dystonia

Description

Dystonia is an acute reaction that requires immediate intervention. The client exhibits muscle spasms of the face, tongue, neck, jaw, and/or back. There is hyperextension of the neck and trunk and arching of the back.

The tongue may protrude; also present are facial grimaces; exaggerated posturing of the head, neck, or jaw; and difficulty swallowing and/or talking.

The client may have a fixed upward gaze and/or eye muscle spasms. This may be accompanied by excessive salivation.

This condition commonly occurs after large doses of neuroleptics, usually within an hour up to a week of drug therapy. It occurs more often in males than females.

Treatment

Depending on the severity of the reaction, one or more of the following may be necessary: lower the neuroleptic dosage, administer benztropine (Cogentin) IM or IV, or administer diphenhydramine (Benadryl) IM.

Drug-Induced Parkinsonism

Description

Symptoms are similar to Parkinson's disease, with a shuffling gait, drooling, tremors, and increased rigidity (cogwheel). Bradykinesia (slow movements) and akinesia (immobility) are also reported.

Treatment

Add an antiparkinson drug such as benztropine (Cogentin) or diphenhydramine (Benadryl).

The prescriber may switch to a neuroleptic less likely to induce this effect, such as thioridazine (Mellaril).

Tardive Dyskinesia

Description

Oral/facial dyskinesias are present (e.g., abnormal involuntary muscle movements around the mouth, lip smacking, tongue darting, constant chewing movements, tics).

Client may also have involuntary movements of the arms or legs. This is more common in older women but has been reported in younger persons.

Treatment

Prevention is vital because the condition may be irreversible. There is no effective treatment.

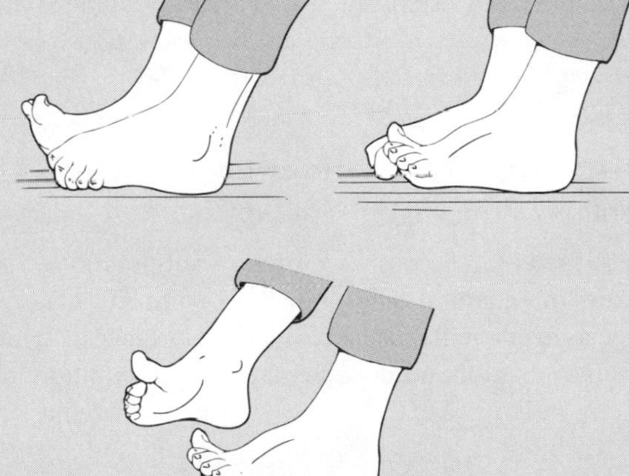

Akathisia

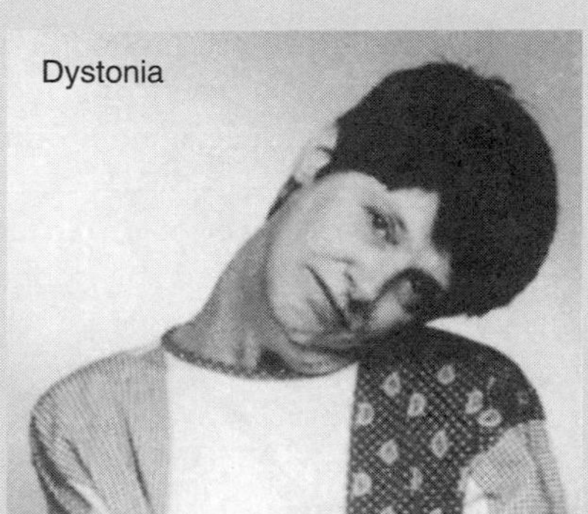

Dystonia

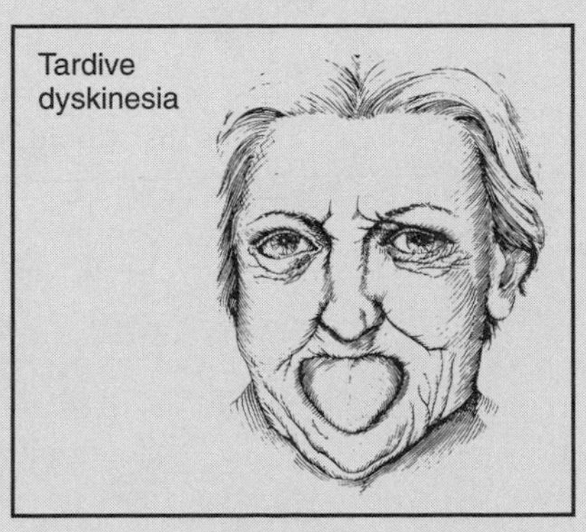

Tardive dyskinesia

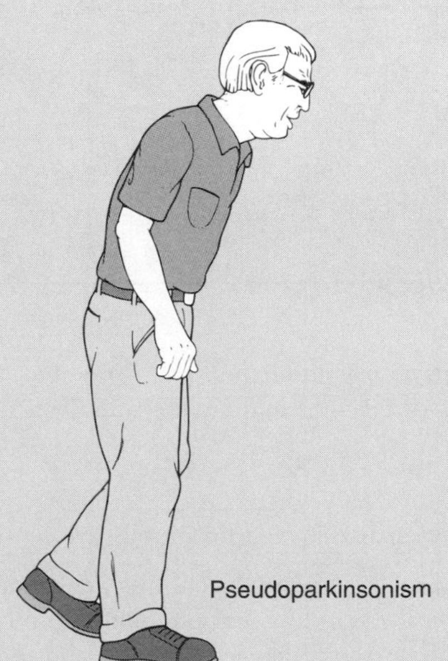

Pseudoparkinsonism

BOX 19-4

Tardive Dyskinesia

Tardive dyskinesia is a potentially irreversible neurologic disorder that primarily involves the buccolingual and masticatory muscles. This adverse reaction to the antipsychotic agents may occur within a few months or years of treatment or after these agents have been discontinued. The risk of inducing TD increases with the total dose administered and the length of treatment.

Incidence

Although 0.5% to 65% of the treated population may develop this syndrome, recent reports place the percentage of clients at risk at 10% to 20%.

Presenting Features

Facial: grimacing or scowling expression, facial tics, arching of the eyebrows

Ocular: blinking, eyelid spasms (blepharospasm)

Oral/buccal: lip smacking, lower lip thrusting, sucking, puffing of cheeks, chewing of the cheeks (the inside of the mouth should be checked for this)

Lingual/masticatory: lateral jaw movements, tongue protrusion or thrusting such as "fly catching movements," tongue in lip or cheek resulting in an observable bulge in the specific area

Systemic effects: foot tapping; rocking from side to side; arms, hands, and fingers possibly displaying a jerking and/or a writhing motion (choreoathetoid motion); pelvic thrusting motions

Treatment

Prevention is vital because the condition may be irreversible.

Early assessment and diagnosis are crucial to prevention. Decreasing or discontinuing the antipsychotic agent if possible is the recommended procedure.

At present, there is no known effective treatment for TD.

Information from *United States Pharmacopeia Dispensing Information (USP DI): Information for the health care professional* (19th ed.). (1999). Rockville, MD: United States Pharmacopeial Convention.

and psychosis in clients with dementia. In general, divided doses of 0.5 to 2 mg/day are sufficient for older adults.

Dihydroindolone Derivative

molindone [moe lin' done] (Moban)

Molindone is an antipsychotic agent that represents a new chemical class. In theory, molindone blocks dopamine receptors in the reticular activating and limbic systems, with activity similar to major tranquilizers such as the phenothiazines. As with haloperidol, molindone causes little sedation and few anticholinergic and cardiovascular adverse reactions but reportedly produces a high incidence of extrapyramidal symptoms.

Molindone is administered orally. In adults, the initial dosage is 50 to 75 mg daily in divided doses. Dosages may increase to 100 mg daily in 3 or 4 days. Dosages must be individualized to a maximum daily dose of (usually) 225 mg. The dosage for older adults is lower than for adults and is increased as necessary according to response or the development of side effects. Molindone is not recommended for children younger than 12 years of age.

Dibenzoxapine Derivative

loxapine succinate [lox' a peen] (Loxitane, Loxapac ♣)

Although structurally similar to the phenothiazines, loxapine is a member of a distinct chemical class of antipsychotic drugs—the dibenzoxapines. It causes a moderate degree of sedation and orthostatic hypotension, has few anticholinergic effects, and has a high incidence of causing extrapyramidal symptoms.

In adults, the oral dosage of loxapine (liquid or capsule) is 10 mg twice daily, increased slowly during the first 7 to 10 days as necessary. The maintenance dosage is 15 to 25 mg PO two to four times daily. The maximum dosage is 250 mg/day. For older adults, the dosage is 3 to 5 mg twice daily initially. The dosage for children younger than 16 years of age has not been established. Injectable loxapine is administered to adults at 12.5 to 50 mg IM every 4 to 6 hours as necessary, up to a maximum of 250 mg/day.

■ Nursing Management

Antipsychotic Agent Therapy

■ **Assessment.** Before starting antipsychotic drug therapy, the client should undergo a complete history and physical assessment. Of particular importance is a neurologic examination and documentation of orientation, affect, and cognition as a baseline assessment. A baseline assessment of blood pressure (sitting, standing, and lying) and pulse should be obtained. Ensure that a complete blood count (CBC) and hepatic and renal function studies have been completed before beginning antipsychotic pharmacologic therapy.

The client should also be assessed for health conditions that contraindicate the use of a particular agent or conditions that would require cautious use and special monitoring interventions.

Antipsychotic agents may cause a number of cardiovascular effects, including hypotension (caused by alpha-adrenergic blockade), tachycardia (anticholinergic effect), myocardial depressant effects, and electrocardiographic alterations that affect the ST interval and T wave and widen the QRS complex. The most cardiotoxic agents are chlorpromazine (Thorazine) and thioridazine (Mellaril). A high-

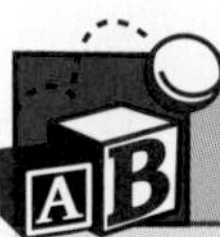

Special Considerations for Children
Psychotherapeutic Agents

Children are at a greater risk of developing neuromuscular or extrapyramidal side effects, especially dystonias. Monitor closely if antipsychotic agents are administered.

Children with chickenpox, CNS infections, measles, dehydration, gastroenteritis, or other acute illnesses will be at special risk of developing adverse reactions and possibly Reye's syndrome. Avoid the use of phenothiazine antiemetic therapy in such clients.

Tricyclic antidepressants are usually not recommended for the treatment of depression in children under 12 years of age. Some agents, such as amitriptyline (Elavil), desipramine (Norpramin), and imipramine (Tofranil) have been used in children over the age of 6 for major depressions. Several of these agents are also used in the treatment of enuresis and attention deficit disorder. Be aware that children are very sensitive to an acute overdose, which should always be considered very serious and potentially fatal. Adolescents often require a decreased dosage because of their sensitivity to this drug category.

Adverse reactions reported in children receiving the tricyclic antidepressants include changes in ECG patterns, increased nervousness, sleep disorders, complaints of tiredness, hypertension, and mild stomach distress.

Lithium may decrease the bone density or bone formation in children. If it is necessary to use lithium, monitor serum levels closely and monitor for signs of toxicity.

Information from *United States Pharmacopeia Dispensing Information (USP DI): Information for the health care professional* (19th ed.). (1999). Rockville, MD: United States Pharmacopeial Convention.

potency antipsychotic such as haloperidol (Haldol) has fewer cardiotoxic effects and therefore may be the preferred agent for clients with cardiovascular disease.

Antipsychotic agents are contraindicated in clients who are comatose or have severe cardiovascular disease or severe CNS depression. They are administered with caution to clients with active alcoholism because they may potentiate CNS depression and liver impairment and may place the client at higher risk of heat stroke. With decreased metabolism by the liver, there may be increased sensitivity to CNS effects and Reye's syndrome in children and adolescents (see the Special Considerations for Children box above). Clients with the following disorders may find their symptoms increased: blood dyscrasias, cardiovascular disease, glaucoma, Parkinson's disease, peptic ulcer, urinary retention, and chronic respiratory disorders. The thioxanthenes in particular are contraindicated in clients with blood dyscrasias and bone marrow depression. Antipsychotic drugs should be

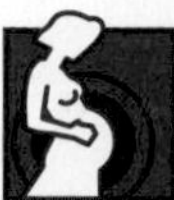

Pregnancy Safety
Psychotherapeutic Drugs

Category	Drugs
B	bupropion, clozapine, fluoxetine, maprotiline, sertraline
C	amitriptyline, amoxapine, clomipramine, desipramine, haloperidol, loxapine, mirtazapine, nefazodone, nortriptyline, olanzapine, pimozide, phenelzine, quetiapine, risperidone, trazodone, trimipramine, venlafaxine, ziprasidone
D	lithium
Unclassified	doxepin, imipramine, isocarboxazid, molindone, phenothiazines (although not recommended during pregnancy), protriptyline, thiothixene, tranylcypromine

used cautiously in clients with a history of convulsive disorders because of their action in reducing the convulsive threshold. Adequate anticonvulsant therapy needs to be maintained. The risk of administering these drugs to pregnant women should be weighed against the expected therapeutic outcome (see the Pregnancy Safety box above).

An ophthalmologic examination is recommended before the onset of antipsychotic agent therapy and includes measurement of visual acuity with and without refraction, a color vision test, a slit lamp study of the fundus, and examination of the visual fields.

Before beginning antipsychotic therapy, a drug history of the client (especially older adults) should be obtained. Older adults may experience unusual adverse drug reactions as compared with younger persons (see the Special Considerations for Older Adults Box on p. 404). Confusion, depression, and hallucinations have been reported with a wide variety of drugs in older adults, and therefore the possibility of a drug-induced effect must be addressed.

Review the client's current medication regiment for the risk of significant drug interactions, such as those that may occur when antipsychotic agents are given concurrently with the following drugs:

Drug/Herb	Possible Effect and Management
Bold/color type indicates the most serious interactions.	
alcohol, CNS depressants	May result in enhanced CNS depression, respiratory depression, and increased hypotensive effects. Monitor closely. The drug dosage should be reduced to one-fourth to one-half the usual dosage. Titrate according to client response. Concurrent alcohol use may increase the risk of inducing heat stroke. Avoid concurrent use or a potentially serious

Continued

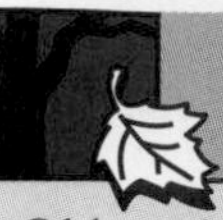

Special Considerations for Older Adults
Psychotherapeutic Agents

Older adults tend to have higher serum levels of the antipsychotic and antidepressant drugs because of changes in drug distribution resulting from a decrease in lean body mass, less total body water, less serum albumin, and usually an increase in body fat. Therefore they require a lower drug dosage and a more gradual drug dosage titration than the younger adults.

Older adults are more prone to orthostatic hypotension, anticholinergic side effects, extrapyramidal side effects, and sedation. They should be evaluated carefully before starting such potent medications; if antipsychotic agents are necessary, close supervision and prescribing of the lowest possible dosage is recommended.

In general, older adults should receive half the recommended adult dosage. Clients with organic brain syndrome should receive only 33% to 50% of the usual adult dosage, with dosage increases at 7- to 10-day periods. When clinical improvement is noted, attempts at tapering and discontinuing the drug should be instituted.

The tricyclic antidepressants may cause increased anxiety in older adults. Their use also increases the risk of inducing dysrhythmias, tachycardia, stroke, congestive heart failure, and myocardial infarction in clients with cardiovascular disease.

Lithium is more toxic in older adults; lower lithium dosages, a lower lithium serum level, and very close monitoring are critical in this age-group. Older adults are more prone to develop CNS toxicity, lithium-induced goiter, and clinical hypothyroidism than the average adult. In general, excessive thirst and the elimination of large volumes of urine may be early side effects of lithium toxicity, which is commonly seen in older adults.

Information from *United States Pharmacopeia Dispensing Information (USP DI): Information for the health care professional* (19th ed.). (1999). Rockville, MD: United States Pharmacopeial Convention.

Drug/Herb	Possible Effect and Management
alcohol, CNS depressants—cont'd	**drug interaction may occur.** Barbiturates may decrease chlorpromazine serum levels through an increase in the metabolizing enzymes in the liver. Thioridazine (Mellaril) may decrease phenobarbital serum levels. Monitor closely for loss of therapeutic effect of barbiturates, because a dosage adjustment may be necessary.
anticholinergics	Concurrent drug use may result in an increase in anticholinergic side effects.
antihypertensive agents	Concurrent drug use with the phenothiazines may result in an increase in hypotensive side effects.
antithyroid medications	Increase the risk for agranulocytosis when phenothiazines are given concurrently.
epinephrine	**Antipsychotic agents block alpha-adrenergic receptors, thus the administration of epinephrine to treat phenothiazine-induced hypotension may result in severe hypotension. With the alpha receptors blocked, epinephrine stimulates beta receptors, which can result in tachycardia and severe lowering of blood pressure. Avoid concurrent use or a potentially serious drug interaction may occur.**
extrapyramidal-inducing medications (e.g., amoxapine [Asendin], metoclopramide [Reglan], reserpine [Serpalan])	May result in increased frequency and severity of extrapyramidal effects.
guanadrel (Hylorel) or guanethidine (Ismelin)	Concurrent use with antipsychotic agents, especially loxapine and the thiothixenes, may reverse the hypotensive effectiveness of these drugs. Closely monitor the blood pressure of all clients receiving this drug combination.
levodopa (Larodopa)	Concurrent use with the antipsychotic agents may render levodopa ineffective in controlling Parkinson's disease.
lithium (Eskalith)	May decrease gastrointestinal absorption of chlorpromazine (Thorazine) by as much as 40%. Phenothiazines may increase the rate of lithium excretion in the kidneys. May result in an increase in extrapyramidal symptoms. May increase the risk of seizures, confusional states, neuroleptic malignant syndrome, and dyskinesia. Phenothiazines and molindone may mask nausea and vomiting, which are early signs of lithium toxicity. Haloperidol (Haldol) may also increase extrapyramidal side effects. Although controversial, there are reports of irreversible neurologic and brain damage when both drugs are given for periods longer than several weeks. If both drugs are given concurrently, monitor clients closely for neurologic changes, because dosage reductions may be necessary.
metrizamide (Amipaque)	**When given concurrently with phenothiazines, may lower the seizure threshold.** **Discontinue phenothiazines at least 2 days before and also for 1 day after a myelogram.**
quinidine	**When given concurrently with the thioxanthenes (chlorprothixene, thiothixene), an increase in cardiac effects may occur. Avoid concurrent use or a potentially serious drug interaction may occur.**
St. John's wort, dong quai	Increase sensitivity of phenothiazines. Monitor closely.

Drug/Herb	Possible Effect and Management
tricyclic antidepressants, monoamine oxidase inhibitors (MAOIs), and procarbazine (Matulane)	Concurrent use may increase the duration of the MAOIs and intensify the sedative and anticholinergic side effects of these medications. Metabolism of the phenothiazines and antidepressants may be inhibited. May enhance the risk of inducing neuroleptic malignant syndrome (NMS)—hyperthermia, dehydration, cardiovascular instability, hypoxemia, and muscular rigidity. Avoid concurrent use or a potentially serious drug interaction may occur.
yohimbine	May induce psychotic reactions or activate psychosis. Avoid concurrent use (Foster & Tyler, 2000).

■ **Nursing Diagnosis.** The following nursing diagnoses/collaborative problems may be identified in clients undergoing antipsychotic therapy: urinary retention related to the anticholinergic effects; impaired skin integrity (rash); ineffective protection related to bone marrow depression; and the potential complications of allergic reaction, heat stroke, hepatotoxicity, Reye's syndrome, NMS, persistent TD, and priapism. (See the Nursing Care Plan on p. 406 for a description of the more common nursing diagnoses.)

■ **Implementation**

■ ***Monitoring.*** In the past, many clients said to be resistant to antipsychotic therapy were found to be noncompliant with the prescribed therapy. Many psychotic clients deny their illness or associate the consumption of medications with dependence or weakness. Clients who are refractory to antipsychotic medications should be reviewed for the following:

- *Compliance.* The prescriber may order a plasma serum level of the medication (if such a test is available) to determine the client's reliability, or the drug order may be switched to a liquid formulation to be administered in a supervised setting.
- *Inadequate dosage.* The prescriber should adjust the dosage according to the needs of the client. An inadequate dosage or the development of drug tolerance may result in an inadequate response to the medication.
- *Questionable oral bioavailability.* Although this is not known to be a common possibility, it is a variable to consider. The prescriber may switch from an oral solid dosage form to a liquid formulation and also adjust the dosage as necessary according to the individual's response or development of side effects. Switching to another antipsychotic agent may also be considered.

Observe the client for orthostatic hypotension, especially after parenteral administration; monitor the client's blood pressure before and after injections. Alert the prescriber if orthostatic (postural) hypotension occurs and causes severe difficulties or serious hazards. The prescriber may then institute one of the following remedial measures: (1) a change to one of the phenothiazine derivatives that does not produce this side effect with such frequency, (2) a reduction of dosage, or (3) a discontinuation of medication for 24 hours with a gradual buildup of dosage as tolerated. If hypotension necessitating drug intervention occurs, norepinephrine or phenylephrine (Neo-Synephrine) may be administered. Because phenothiazines tend to reverse the vasopressor effects of epinephrine, epinephrine may not be effective in reversing hypotension.

CBCs are performed periodically. Be alert to signs of blood dyscrasias: decreased white cells, platelets, and red cells. Monitor for other symptoms of agranulocytosis such as sore throat, fever, or weakness; this usually occurs between weeks 4 and 10. The drug is usually discontinued when these symptoms appear; hold the dose and notify the prescriber as soon as possible.

Contact the prescriber about possible ocular changes, including particle deposition in the cornea and lens and pigmentary retinopathy (decreased vision, brownish coloring of vision, impaired night vision, and pigment deposits on the fundus). These changes may be related to dosage levels or therapy duration. The client following a long-term regimen or moderate- to high-dose therapy should have periodic ophthalmologic examinations.

Observe the client for neuroleptic extrapyramidal adverse reactions (see Box 19-3). In particular, monitor the client closely for early signs of TD, which usually appear as small, wormlike motions of the tongue. Because there is no known effective treatment for TD, the drug should be discontinued immediately and the prescriber notified (see Box 19-4). Monitor the client for dystonic reactions, neck spasms, eye rolling, dysphagia, and seizures.

Monitor the client for NMS (hyperthermia, dehydration, cardiovascular instability, hypoxemia, and muscular rigidity). Therapy is essentially symptomatic and supportive, and the drug is discontinued immediately.

An electrocardiogram (ECG) should be performed periodically and with every adjustment in loxapine dosage because this drug may potentiate cardiac dysrhythmias.

Because of the anticholinergic effects of the drugs, the client should be monitored for signs and symptoms of urinary hesitancy or retention, constipation, prostatic hypertrophy, narrow-angle glaucoma, or respiratory problems (e.g., intake and output for urinary retention). Hepatic function tests and urine tests for bilirubin and bile should be performed weekly during the first month of therapy to assist in the detection of cholestatic jaundice, which is more likely to occur between the second and fourth week. The client should be observed for yellow skin, nausea, flu-like symptoms, and rash. The drug should be discontinued immediately when these symptoms occur.

Monitor the client for weight gain. The antipsychotic agents may cause hypothyroidism, which is commonly manifested as weight gain.

Depression, especially if the client is not closely supervised, may account for the greater incidence of suicide in psychiatric clients undergoing drug therapy than in those receiving only institutional care. The client's emotional status should be assessed carefully because there may be a rapid mood swing from mania to depression when haloperidol (Haldol) is administered to a client with a bipolar disorder.

Nursing Care Plan
Selected Nursing Diagnoses Related to Antipsychotic Medication Administration

Nursing Diagnosis	Outcome Criteria	Nursing Interventions
Constipation related to anticholinergic effects of the drug	The client will maintain his or her usual bowel elimination pattern, select foods high in fiber from the daily menu, maintain a fluid intake of 2500 mL daily, and increase activity as allowed.	Assess client's usual bowel elimination pattern; monitor and record bowel movements. Instruct client to establish a routine for bowel elimination; select foods high in fiber; maintain fluid intake of 2500 mL/day and perform isometric abdominal strengthening exercises, unless contraindicated; increase activity as allowed.
Impaired comfort related to dry mouth	The client will maintain a healthy oral cavity as evidenced by pink, moist, intact mucosa.	Provide ice chips, sugarless candies, and frequent mouth hygiene if dry mouth occurs.
Risk for injury related to increased sensitivity to the sun, visual effects, and the development of dizziness, hypotension, akathisia, parkinsonian symptoms, extrapyramidal effects, and TD	The client will not experience sunburn, falls, or symptoms of TD.	Monitor blood pressure at appropriate intervals; keep client in recumbent position for 30 minutes after injection; provide assistance with ambulation if sedation, dizziness, orthostatic hypotension, or visual changes occur. Instruct client to change position from recumbent to upright slowly. Alert client to hypersensitivity to sun and instruct about the use of sunscreens and sunglasses. Monitor for and instruct client in the early signs of TD (facial tics, grimacing, blinking, lip smacking, tongue protrusion, writhing motions of the arms, hands, and fingers). Report immediately.
Deficient knowledge related to newly prescribed or altered psychotherapeutic agents	The client will describe his or her condition, how the drug therapy relates to the condition, how and when to take the medications, common drug interactions, common side effects and which of these warrant reporting, and storage requirements of the drug. The client will demonstrate less anxiety related to fear of the unknown, loss of control, and misconceptions.	Assess learning needs and learning readiness. Plan with the client and family for the achievement of realistic goals. Provide information to meet outcome criteria.
Ineffective therapeutic regimen management	The client will self-administer medications safely and accurately.	Determine the client's reasons for ineffective management of therapeutic regimen, and make appropriate teaching/counseling interventions. Discuss the increased possibility of the return of symptoms with ineffective management of the therapeutic regimen.

To demonstrate the efficacy or inefficacy of the drug, observe the client and note if the mental status has changed from the baseline assessment. Routine attempts at drug withdrawal should be considered for most clients receiving a psychotropic medication (Cohen-Mansfield et al., 1999).

■ ***Intervention.*** Rapid neuroleptization or high-dose antipsychotic therapy is appropriate in certain cases. For instance, aggressive treatment is used in clients with acute psychosis who may exhibit dangerous and/or destructive behaviors. IM therapy with a high-potency antipsychotic agent (e.g., haloperidol [Haldol] or thioridazine [Mellaril]) is usually given, often on an hourly schedule, until the desired effects are achieved. If a client will take an oral medication, high-dose oral therapy may be substituted. Because of the half-life of the IM doses, the first oral dose should be given 12 to 24 hours after the last IM dose.

Once a client is stabilized on antipsychotic medications, the entire daily dose may be prescribed to be given at bedtime. The long duration of action of these drugs makes a single bedtime dose feasible. This type of dosage schedule increases client compliance, lowers medication costs, decreases side effects, and decreases or eliminates the need for simultaneous hypnotic medication. This dosage schedule requires both careful drug selection and client assessment before implementation. Using a drug with a high anticholinergic potential in older adults or in clients with cardiovascular disease may result in an increased potential for cardiotoxic effects. In such cases, smaller, multiple (two or three times daily) daily doses are indicated.

Long-acting injections are often useful in antipsychotic therapy. Depot fluphenazine enanthate (Prolixin Enanthate), fluphenazine decanoate (Prolixin Decanoate), and haloperidol decanoate (Haldol Decanoate) are available for clients who are persistently noncompliant, do not understand the need for taking medications, or have a high frequency of relapses (psychotic episodes).

Fluphenazine decanoate and fluphenazine enanthate are oil preparations. They may be given intramuscularly or subcutaneously using a 21-gauge or larger needle. Fluphenazine decanoate is often a better choice than the fluphenazine enanthate because its duration of action is approximately 2 weeks longer. Clients receiving fluphenazine decanoate may exhibit a slight decrease in extrapyramidal side effects as compared with clients taking the enanthate formulation. The enanthate formulation results in a more variable fluphenazine plasma level, and thus the effect is not as prolonged as the decanoate formulation. Converting from an oral antipsychotic agent to fluphenazine decanoate is complicated, and the reader is referred to Ereshefsky and Richards (1992) for more information.

Clients being considered for haloperidol decanoate therapy should first receive oral haloperidol. Dosage and dosing interval adjustments should be carefully chosen and closely monitored. In some persons the effects of haloperidol decanoate may last up to 6 weeks.

Dosages of phenothiazines and other antipsychotic agents are individualized according to client response so that the lowest effective dosage may be used. Dosages are increased more slowly and in smaller increments for older adults or debilitated clients.

In most cases, concurrent treatment with more than one neuroleptic agent is not indicated. If the client does not respond to a particular drug, the dosage of that drug is usually increased or a different drug is prescribed. Occasionally a client may respond best to a combination of two drugs from different classes. However, the potentiation and lowered margin of safety of such combinations require greater precautions for client safety.

The administration of large doses over a prolonged time may lead to anticholinergic psychoses or TD; providing periodic "drug-free holidays" during which the client does not receive phenothiazines may prevent such adverse reactions. Because of the long elimination half-life of these drugs, "holidays" should last several weeks. Maintenance dosages should be periodically evaluated for a possible dosage reduction or the cessation of drug therapy. Clients with preexisting renal or hepatic disease may require a reduced dosage.

The oral route of administration is preferred unless the client is unable to take an oral dose. Oral forms of phenothiazines should be administered with at least 120 mL of fruit juice or other liquids or semisoft foods to decrease gastric irritation and to make the drug more palatable. The client should be informed that the medication is in the substance. Phenothiazines should not be administered concurrently with antacids or antidiarrheals; administration times should be altered to allow 2 hours between doses of these medications. Administration of the maintenance dose at bedtime facilitates sleep and decreases drowsiness during the daytime.

Fluphenazine hydrochloride (Prolixin) and perphenazine (Trilafon) oral concentrate solutions should not be mixed with fluids containing caffeine (coffee, tea, cola), tannic acid (tea), or pectinates (apple juice) because a physical incompatibility may occur. Instead, dilute the solution with at least 60 mL of lemon-lime carbonated beverage or pineapple, orange, tomato, or grapefruit juice for each 5 mL of concentrate.

A special dropper should be used for oral liquid haloperidol (Haldol) administration; a precipitate will form if it is diluted with tea or coffee. If dilution is desired, use at least 60 mL of diluent and mix it just before administration to prevent precipitation. If desired, haloperidol may be administered from a premeasured oral syringe without diluting.

When preparing phenothiazines, be aware that the injectable forms tend to be physically and/or chemically incompatible with a wide range of solutions. Check the package insert for compatibility information about the specific drugs being prepared. Avoid freezing phenothiazine solutions. Discolored solutions may be used if only slightly yellowed. The solution should not be used if marked discoloration or a precipitate is apparent. Skin and eye contact with phenothiazine solutions should be avoided because it may cause contact dermatitis and irritation. Exposed areas should be washed immediately to minimize the effect.

When given intramuscularly, antipsychotic drugs should be injected deeply and slowly into a large muscle mass (e.g., the ventrogluteal or dorsogluteal site) in divided doses of not more than 1 mL per injection site. Rotate the injection sites, and document this information. Irritation of the subcutaneous tissues can be reduced by diluting the drug with 0.9% sodium chloride injection solution and/or adding 2% procaine and by injecting the drug using the "Z-track" technique (see Figure 5-8). Massaging the injection site helps to reduce local irritation.

Some clients have been known to develop abscesses at the injection site; these are believed to result from the administration of large doses of the drug in one area. Using the IM route when administering an antipsychotic drug is usually indicated when the client refuses the tablet or concentrate form or when the most immediate effect of the drug is desired. Take care to follow safe administration technique if the client is severely agitated, combative, or struggling. Safe IM administration usually requires enough well-trained personnel to restrain the client adequately while the medication is being given.

Loxapine hydrochloride (Loxitane) may be administered orally or intramuscularly. The oral solution should be measured with the dropper provided by the manufacturer and diluted with orange or grapefruit juice just before each dose. After IM injection, the client should remain lying down for 30 minutes because of the orthostatic hypotensive effects.

IV administration of undiluted chlorpromazine (Thorazine) should be avoided. If used for direct IV administration, it should be diluted to at least 1 mg/mL and administered at a rate of 1 mg/min for adults and 0.5 mg/min for children. For IV infusion the drug should be added to 500 to 1000 mL of 0.9% sodium chloride solution and administered slowly. In both instances the client should be kept in the recumbent position to minimize hypotension.

IV administration of perphenazine (Trilafon) is limited to recumbent hospitalized adult clients and requires the availability of resuscitative equipment and drugs for the treatment of severe hypotensive episodes or extrapyramidal responses. If administered by fractional IV injection, the solution should be diluted to 0.5 mg/mL of 0.9% sodium chloride and administered slowly, 1 mg per injection, at intervals of at least 1 to 2 minutes. Blood pressure and pulse should be assessed continuously during IV administration.

For clients on high or long-term dosages, gradual reduction of the antipsychotic over several weeks will help to prevent withdrawal symptoms of nausea, vomiting, irritability, trembling, and transient dyskinetic signs. The only rationale for abrupt withdrawal is the occurrence of severe side effects/adverse reactions.

■ ***Education.*** The client who complains of dizziness, light-headedness, or palpitations may be experiencing orthostatic hypotension. This can easily be confirmed by comparing the client's blood pressure in the prone and standing positions. The client should be instructed to rise slowly from the recumbent position and to sit on the edge of the bed for a few minutes before attempting to stand. Support and reassurance may be necessary to allay the client's anxiety. Explaining orthostatic hypotension also may help him or her to understand this experience and may reduce anxiety. To minimize hypotensive episodes, clients should be encouraged to remain in a recumbent position for 1 hour after initial doses, parenterally administered doses, or large oral doses (rarely) of the phenothiazines.

Caution clients against driving, operating dangerous machinery, or performing tasks that require absolute precision, motor coordination, and mental alertness. Tolerance to drowsiness develops as therapy continues. Clients should be told that it make take several weeks before the antipsychotic medication can treat the disorder effectively.

To prevent photosensitivity, advise the client to stay out of the sun, use sunscreen lotion, or wear protective clothing to prevent solar erythema, or assist the client by providing the necessary protective measures. A dark, purplish-brown skin pigmentation induced by light (photosensitivity) has been reported in hospitalized psychiatric clients who were given large doses of phenothiazines for 3 to 10 years. Exposure to light also increases the possibility of ocular changes; therefore the client should be instructed to wear sunglasses.

Caution the client that dry mouth can be a bothersome adverse reaction to antipsychotic therapy and can contribute to the development of caries, gum disease, and oral candidiasis. The client should be instructed in the use of proper oral hygiene. Xerostomia may affect the fitting of full dentures; a referral should be made for dental care for this and other dental problems.

Long-term therapy with phenothiazines necessitates dietary increases in riboflavin. Good dietary sources of vitamin B_2 are muscle meats, organ meats, milk, eggs, leafy and yellow vegetables, and enriched cereals and breads. If the client is experiencing altered nutrition, it may be beneficial to use a vitamin supplement until adequate nutrition is ensured.

Phenothiazines affect the regulation of body temperature; clients should be cautioned to avoid extremes of environmental temperature (i.e., swimming in cold water or walking in hot, humid weather), which could lead to either hypothermia and respiratory distress or hyperthermia and heat prostration.

The client should be instructed to avoid alcohol and other CNS depressants because they increase the CNS depressant effects of the antipsychotic agents. Using these drugs concurrently with medications that cause extrapyramidal reactions will increase the frequency and severity of the extrapyramidal effects. The tablet form of molindone (Moban) contains calcium sulfate, which may impair the absorption of tetracyclines and phenytoin (Dilantin). The client should be informed about this interaction. Encourage the client to consult with the prescriber before taking any over-the-counter (OTC) drugs; this will help to prevent serious drug interactions.

With the extended-action injectable form of these drugs, the effects may last up to 6 weeks; clients should be counseled that precautions and other side effects information will apply during this time.

■ **Evaluation.** The expected outcome of antipsychotic therapy is that the client will be able to perform activities of daily living independently without experiencing adverse reactions to the drugs. In addition, the client will self-administer the medication safely and accurately.

Atypical Antipsychotic Agents

The atypical antipsychotic agents include the dibenzodiazepines (e.g., clozapine [Clozaril], olanzapine [Zyprexa] and quetiapine [Seroquel]), the benzisoxazole risperidone (Risperdal), and a diphenylbutylpiperidine analogue pimozide (Orap). These agents have diverse effects and are essentially different from the typical antipsychotic agents discussed in this chapter. They appear to have an affinity for the serotonin (5-HT_2) and dopamine receptors as well as other receptors in the body *(Drug Facts and Comparisons,* 2000).

Dibenzodiazepines

clozapine [kloz′ a peen] (Clozaril)

Clozapine is considered an "atypical" antipsychotic agent. It differs from the other neuroleptics by being active at the limbic dopamine receptors, affecting both receptors but with less affinity for D_2; thus it is less apt to induce extrapyramidal side effects. It binds more to serotonin (5-HT_2), $alpha_1$, and histamine (H_1) receptors than to dopamine receptors. Because clozapine has the potential for causing agranulocytosis, a potentially life-threatening effect, it is reserved for treatment-resistant schizophrenia or for when adverse reactions to other drugs preclude their continued use. Treatment resistance has been defined as the client not responding to an appropriate course of standard antipsychotic agents after trying at least two antipsychotic medications *(United States Pharmacopeia Dispensing Information,* 1999).

Pharmacokinetics. Clozapine is rapidly absorbed orally and is distributed extensively throughout the body, including crossing the blood-brain barrier. It reaches peak serum levels in approximately 2.5 hours; the average steady-state serum level is 319 ng/mL. The duration of action is 4 to 12 hours; it is metabolized in the liver and excreted by the kidneys (50%) and in the feces (30%).

Side Effects/Adverse Reactions. Side effects/adverse reactions of clozapine include constipation, dizziness, sedation, headache, hypersalivation, nausea, vomiting, weight gain, tachycardia, hypotension, fever, agitation, akathisia and, rarely, blood dyscrasias (agranulocytosis, leukopenia, thrombocytopenia), extrapyramidal effects, impotency, insomnia, and NMS.

Dosage and Administration. Treatment with clozapine is closely monitored, with the manufacturer recommending that only weekly supplies be dispensed and that weekly white blood cell (WBC) testing be performed. The adult dosage is 25 mg once or twice daily, increased by 25 to 50 mg/day until 300 to 450 mg/day is reached by the end of the second week of therapy. Thereafter, dosage increases should not exceed 100 mg once or twice a week. The maximum daily dose is 900 mg. *(USP DI,* 1999; *Mosby's GenRx,* 1999).

■ Nursing Management

Clozapine Therapy

In addition to the following discussion, see Nursing Management: Antipsychotic Agent Therapy, p. 402.

Clozapine is contraindicated in cases of severe CNS depression, blood dyscrasias, or a history of bone marrow depression because these conditions will be potentiated. Because of the effect of clozapine on myeloproliferation, it is essential that the client's WBC be determined at the start of therapy, at weekly intervals, and for 4 weeks after the last dose. Therapy should not be initiated if the WBC is less than $3500/mm^3$ and should be discontinued any time the WBC substantially declines from the baseline WBC or falls below $3000/mm^3$. Consideration of the risk-benefit ratio should also be given if the client has narrow-angle glaucoma, prostatic hypertrophy, intestinal hypomotility, or seizure disorders, because these conditions may be worsened.

Review the client's drug regimen. The concurrent administration of alcohol or CNS depressant drugs may enhance the CNS depressant effects of clozapine; concurrent administration of a bone marrow depressant may potentiate a myelosuppressive adverse reaction, and concurrent use with lithium increases the risk of inducing seizures, confusion, NMS, and dyskinesias. Avoid concurrent administration of these agents whenever possible. Concurrent use of hypotensive-producing medications may cause additive hypotensive effects. Tenfold serum concentrations of clozapine have been found with the concurrent use of selective serotonin reuptake inhibitors (SSRIs).

The client should be assessed for flu-like symptoms or infection. Cardiovascular effects such as tachycardia and hypotension may occur, but these may be minimized if the client is started on low dosages with gradual increments. WBC and differential counts are performed at weekly intervals and for 4 weeks after discontinuing clozapine therapy. Therapy is discontinued if the WBC is less than $3000/mm^3$ or if the granulocyte count is less than $1500/mm^3$.

In addition to the teaching included under Nursing Management: Antipsychotic Agent Therapy, p. 402, safety precautions related to hypotension should be reviewed with the client. Dose-related seizure activity has been reported with clozapine, with seizures occurring in 1% to 2% of clients receiving low doses (<300 mg/day), 3% to 4% of clients receiving moderate doses (300 to 599 mg/day), and 5% of clients receiving high doses (>600 mg/day). Clients with a history of seizures are at higher risk. Appropriate teaching and safety precautions should be taken.

Encourage the client to maintain regular visits to the prescriber for monitoring of progress and necessary blood tests. Report to the health care provider any fatigue, fever, sore throat, or other symptoms of infections because of the risk of blood dyscrasias. Contact the prescriber before resuming clozapine use if it has not been taken for 2 days.

olanzapine [oh lanz′ a peen] (Zyprexa ◆)
quetiapine [kwe tye′ a peen] (Seroquel)

Olanzapine and quetiapine are at least equal to if not more effective than the other antipsychotic agents (Buckley, 1998). They are reported to produce fewer adverse reactions (especially the extrapyramidal effects) and appear to be more effective than the other neuroleptic agents against the negative symptoms of psychosis (see Box 19-3).

Although their exact mechanism of action is unknown, their effectiveness has been proposed to result from their dopamine and serotonin type 2 blocking effects. They are antagonists at many CNS neurotransmitter receptor sites, which may be associated with their other side effects, such as sedation (histamine) and orthostatic hypotension ($alpha_1$).

Side effects/adverse reactions of olanzapine and quetiapine include dizziness, constipation, somnolence, dry mouth, gastrointestinal distress, weight gain, extrapyramidal symptoms, peripheral edema, and rash.

The usual adult dosage of olanzapine is 5 to 10 mg once daily, titrated weekly as necessary; the antipsychotic dosage range is 10 to 15 mg/day (*Zyprexa*, 1996). The usual adult dosage of quetiapine is 25 mg twice daily, increased as necessary by 25 to 50 mg; the maximum daily dose is 800 mg.

The use of olanzapine and quetiapine is of concern in clients with Alzheimer's dementia because of the increased risk of aspiration pneumonia, as well as in clients with a history of breast cancer because prolactin-dependent breast cancers may be exacerbated. (See also Nursing Management: Antipsychotic Agent Therapy, p. 402.)

Benzisoxazoles

risperidone [ris pare′ i dohn] (Risperdal ◆)
ziprasidone [zi praz′ i dohn] (Geodon)

Risperidone and ziprasidone are from a new chemical class of antipsychotic drugs that blocks both serotonin and dopamine receptors. They are indicated for the treatment of psychotic disorders and improve both the positive and negative symptoms of schizophrenia (Chengappa et al., 1999).

Risperidone taken orally reaches peak serum levels in 1 to 2 hours and is metabolized to an active metabolite in the liver (9-hydroxyrisperidone). The elimination half-life is 10 to 24 hours. Ziprasidone is highly protein bound, reaching a steady state in 1 to 3 days.

The side effects of risperidone include fatigue, cough, dry mouth, increased dreaming, nausea, weight gain, insomnia, visual changes, sexual dysfunction, anxiety, and extrapyramidal symptoms (EPS). Ziprasidone may induce sedation, respiratory disorders, EPS, and prolongation of the QT interval (arrhythmias).

The adult dosage of risperidone is 1 mg twice daily, increasing as necessary according to patient response. In older adults, the dosage is 0.5 mg twice daily. The adult dosage of ziprasidone is 20 mg twice daily with food, increasing as necessary to a maximum of 80 mg twice daily.

▪ Nursing Management

Benzisoxazole Therapy

In addition to the following discussion, see Nursing Management: Antipsychotic Agent Therapy, p. 402.

▪ **Assessment.** The risk-benefit ratio should be considered if the client has cardiovascular disease or renal or hepatic function impairment. Prolactin-dependent breast cancer and Parkinson's disease may be exacerbated. Risperidone is contraindicated in pregnancy and lactation. Clients with hypotension will experience an aggravation of their symptoms.

Drug interactions of concern in the drug history include increased CNS depression effects with alcohol and other CNS depressants; enhanced hypotensive effects with antihypertensive agents; reduced levodopa effects when given with bromocriptine (Parlodel), levodopa (Larodopa), or pergolide (Permax); increased clearance from the body when administered with carbamazepine (Tegretol); and decreased clearance if administered with clozapine (Clozaril).

A baseline assessment includes blood pressure, temperature, pulse, respirations, lung sounds, mental status, reflexes, liver and liver function studies, CBC, urinalysis, and ECG.

▪ **Nursing Diagnosis.** Clients receiving benzisoxazole therapy may experience the following nursing diagnoses/collaborative problems: anxiety; disturbed sleep pattern (insomnia or sedation); impaired comfort (headache, agitation, nausea, vomiting); constipation; and the potential complications of extrapyramidal effects and TD.

▪ **Implementation**

▪ ***Monitoring.*** If the client has difficulty with dizziness and light-headedness, measure sitting and standing blood pressures to assess for orthostatic hypotension. Monitor body temperature and notify the prescriber if the client's temperature is elevated without signs of infection. WBCs and ECGs are performed periodically. Monitor for abnormal movements to detect extrapyramidal effects and/or TD.

▪ ***Intervention.*** The dosage is increased gradually to the most effective level. Risperidone is not to be discontinued suddenly; the client should be weaned from it gradually.

▪ ***Education.*** Alert the client undergoing risperidone therapy to change positions slowly to prevent orthostatic hypotension. Provide the client with safety instructions about driving and operating hazardous equipment, and provide photosensitivity precautions. Women should practice contraception and contact the prescriber if they suspect they are pregnant or if they wish to become pregnant. Clients should report to their prescriber any symptoms of fatigue, weakness, palpitations, mouth ulcers, sore throat, or fever.

▪ **Evaluation.** The expected outcome of risperidone therapy is that client will experience a decrease of psychotic symptoms without any adverse reactions and will be able to self-administer risperidone safely and accurately.

pimozide [pi′ moe zide] (Orap)

Pimozide is indicated for the treatment of severe motor and vocal tics in clients with Tourette's syndrome who have failed to respond to haloperidol (Haldol). Although the mechanism of action is unknown, pimozide blocks dopamine in the CNS. Pimozide is administered orally, is metabolized in the liver to two major metabolites, produces a peak effect in 6 to 8 hours, and has a half-life of 29 hours. Approximately 50% is primarily excreted by the kidneys within 1 week.

The side effects/adverse reactions of pimozide include dry mouth, orthostatic hypotension, skin rash, pruritus, visual disturbances, constipation, sedation, breast soreness, possible milk secretion, akathisia, behavioral alterations, ventricular dysrhythmias, and drug-induced parkinsonian and extrapyramidal effects. With the exception of mood or behavioral changes, the adverse reactions occur most commonly during the first few days of therapy. Less common reactions include intense and irregular muscle spasms (dystonia), TD, jaundice, NMS, and blood dyscrasias.

In adults and children 12 years of age and older, the dosage of pimozide is 1 to 2 mg PO daily in divided doses. The dosage is increased gradually every other day as necessary. The dosage has not been established for children under 12 years of age. The maximum daily dose is 20 mg in divided doses.

■ Nursing Management

Pimozide Therapy

■ **Assessment.** It should be determined that the client does not have an underlying condition such as cardiac dysrhythmias or severe CNS depression; pimozide potentiates these conditions and is therefore contraindicated. The risks of cardiovascular and extrapyramidal effects are such that pimozide should not be used to treat tics other than those of Tourette's syndrome. Women with a history of breast cancer need to consider the risk-benefit ratio of the drug because the disease may be aggravated by increased serum prolactin concentrations resulting from pimozide therapy. Pimozide should not be administered in the presence of hypokalemia because of the heightened risk for ventricular dysrhythmias.

Review the client's current medication regimen for the risk of significant drug interactions, such as those that may occur when pimozide is given concurrently with the following drugs:

Drug	Possible Effect and Management
Bold/color type indicates the most serious interactions.	
alcohol, CNS depressants	May enhance CNS depressant effects. Monitor closely.
amphetamines, methylphenidate (Ritalin), pemoline (Cylert)	These drugs may cause tics and therefore should be discontinued before beginning pimozide therapy.
anticholinergic drugs	May result in enhanced anticholinergic side effects, such as dry mouth, constipation, blurred vision, and excitability.
antidepressants (tricyclic), disopyramide (Norpace), maprotiline (Ludiomil), phenothiazines, procainamide (Pronestyl), quinidine	**May enhance or potentiate cardiac dysrhythmias. Avoid concurrent use or a potentially serious drug interaction may occur.**
extrapyramidal effect–causing medications, including phenothiazines	May result in an increase in the extrapyramidal side effects of both medications. May also increase the anticholinergic and CNS depressant effects.
macrolide antibiotics, azithromycin (Zithromax), clarithromycin (Biaxin), dirithromycin (Dynabac), erythromycin (Erythrocin)	**Prolongs the QT interval; in clients with a prolonged QT interval, sudden deaths have occurred. Concurrent use is contraindicated.**
ritonavir (Norvir)	**Produces large increases in plasma concentrations of pimozide. Concurrent use is contraindicated.**

A baseline assessment of the client's behaviors, including the character and frequency of symptoms, should be recorded to enable the evaluation of client progress, the therapeutic usefulness of the pimozide therapy, and the occurrence of any adverse reaction. A baseline ECG is essential to monitor the cardiac effects of the drugs.

■ **Nursing Diagnosis.** Clients receiving pimozide therapy are at risk for the following nursing diagnoses/collaborative problems: social isolation and situational low self-esteem related to the symptoms of Tourette's syndrome and ineffectiveness of the drug; decreased cardiac output related to a prolonged QT interval (fast or irregular pulse); risk for injury related to blurred vision and orthostatic hypotension; disturbed sleep pattern (drowsiness); constipation; diarrhea; impaired oral mucous membrane (dry mouth); impaired comfort (nausea and vomiting, sore breasts, headache); disturbed thought processes (depression); and the potential complications of extrapyramidal (parkinsonian and dystonic) effects, akathisia, TD, NMS, skin discoloration, obstructive jaundice, and blood dyscrasias.

■ **Implementation**

■ ***Monitoring.*** The client's vital signs should be monitored for hypotension and dysrhythmias. Serial ECGs are measured over the course of therapy. The client should be observed carefully at least every 3 months for the early signs of TD. The client's symptoms of the underlying condition should be recorded.

■ ***Intervention.*** Periodic attempts should be made to decrease the dosage of pimozide to evaluate the status of the tic behaviors.

■ ***Education.*** Alert the client to avoid alcoholic beverages, other CNS depressants, and the macrolide antibiotics during pimozide therapy. Precautions should be taken regarding the use of hazardous equipment until the client's response to the medication has been determined. Caution the client to rise slowly from a sitting or lying position because of the hypotensive effect of the drug. Sugarless gums and candies or ice chips may be used to relieve the symptoms of dry mouth if this is of concern to the client. Advise the client to wear or carry medical identification so that other health care providers will be aware that he or she is receiving pimozide therapy. The client should consult with the prescriber before discontinuing the pimozide. Symptoms of adverse reactions to pimozide should be reviewed with the client to enable him or her to know what to report to the prescriber.

■ **Evaluation.** The expected outcome of pimozide therapy is that the client's tics will be diminished or absent, and the client will not experience any adverse reactions to the drug.

THERAPY OF AFFECTIVE DISORDERS

Defintion of Affective Disorders

Affective disorders, or mood disturbances, include depression (the most common affective disorder) and **mania** or elation. Mania is discussed later in this chapter.

Etiology of Affective Disorders

No single factor has been identified as the cause of affective disorders. Psychiatrists who believe in psychosocial factors will probe to identify stressful events or mental conflicts that preceded the onset of depression, whereas others who adhere to biologic factors tend to explain affective disorders by the monoamine theory (i.e., catecholamine [norepinephrine, dopamine, epinephrine] and indolamine [serotonin] levels in the CNS). Many practitioners today believe that both psychosocial and biologic factors lead to a common pathway that results in an affective disorder.

Many factors are involved with affective disorders, including genetics, psychosocial events (divorce, death of a mate), physiologic stress (illness, infection, childbirth), and personality traits. Any combination of these factors may also affect the biochemical mechanisms of the CNS, which lends weight to the theory that affective disorders have a common pathway.

Centrally acting monoamines, especially norepinephrine and serotonin, have been theorized to be the cause of depression and mania. A deficiency in central norepinephrine has been associated with depression, whereas an excess of norepinephrine is believed to be related to mania.

The tricyclic antidepressants may block the reuptake of one or both monoamines into the adrenergic neuron. This blockade will lead to elevated levels of norepinephrine and serotonin in the synapse areas. MAO, an enzyme found in the mitochondria of nerve cells, is responsible for metabolizing norepinephrine within the nerve. MAOIs block this enzyme, which results in increased levels of norepinephrine available for release to the synapse area.

Although the mechanism of action of many antidepressants is inhibition of the reuptake of norepinephrine or serotonin or inhibition of the MAO enzyme system, not all antidepressants have this effect. Therefore the full range of the antidepressant central activity of these medications is probably unknown (Figure 19-3).

Antidepressant Therapy

Over the years many classifications of depression have been used, such as the time of life that depression occurred (childhood, adolescence, or older adulthood), or the reason for the depression, such as exogenous (reactive) depression

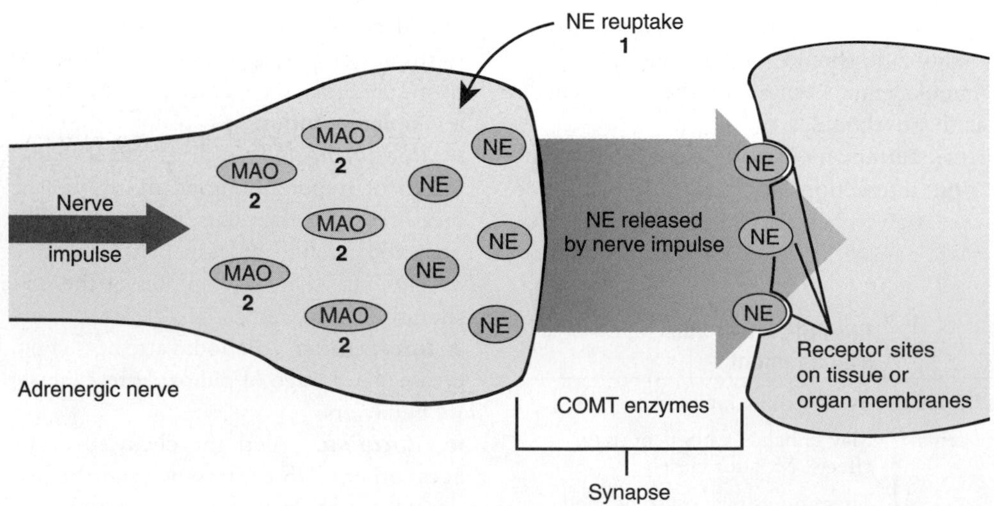

Figure 19-3 Proposed action of antidepressant drug therapy. Normally, norepinephrine (NE) is released from storage sites within the adrenergic nerve by the arrival of a nerve impulse. The released NE may be metabolized within the nerve by MAO enzymes or, after the activity of NE at the receptor sites, by catechol-O-methyltransferase (COMT) enzymes located in the synaptic cleft. Most NE is taken back into the nerve and stored by way of the reuptake mechanism. Antidepressant drug therapy: (1) tricyclic antidepressants block the reuptake of released NE and prevent it from reentering the adrenergic nerve. (2) MAOIs block MAO located on the surface of the cell mitochondria. The result is more NE available for release or available in the synapse area.

or endogenous depression. **Exogenous** (reactive or secondary) **depression** is often a person's response to a loss (a loss of pleasure or interest in activities and everyday living caused perhaps by the loss of a loved one or the presence of a debilitating illness) or disappointment (not meeting one's expectations, or the loss of a job, pet, friend). This is usually referred to as "the blues" or normal depression and it generally remits in several months without the use of antidepressant medications. The mobilization of support systems and, if necessary, psychotherapy are useful adjuncts in exogenous depression. Unipolar or **endogenous depression** is characterized by the absence of external causes. This type of depression may be caused by genetic determination and biochemical alterations (Katzung, 1998). Antidepressant medications are very useful in treating this type of depression. (See the Complementary and Alternative Therapy box below.)

The current classification of depressive disorders has eliminated the use of these terms. Instead, major affective disorders are defined as **bipolar disorders** (mixed type and manic) and **major depression** as unipolar (single episode or recurrent episodes), along with atypical affective disorders that include depression. Psychiatrists have debated over whether the new classification is an improvement over the previous types of classification, because it is important for the clinician to have a diagnostic framework from which to work.

Criteria for major depression include the presence of mood changes (sadness, despondency, anxiety, crying spells, guilt feelings, self-pity, pessimism, loss of interest in life and social activities), psychologic symptoms (low self-esteem, poor concentration, hopeless or helpless feelings, suicidal tendencies, increased focus on death), physiologic manifestations (sleep disturbances that may range from insomnia to hypersomnia, decreased interest in sex, complaints of fatigue, loss of energy, menstrual dysfunction, headaches, palpitations, constipation, loss of appetite, and weight loss or weight gain), and thinking alterations (a decrease in concentration or attention span, complaints of poor memory, confusion, delusions relating to health, persecution, or religion, and hallucinations if the client is also psychotic). Mood variations are usually diurnal and are often worse in the morning.

Measures to treat depression include electroshock therapy, psychotherapy, reduction of environmental stressors, and milieu therapy. In a number of cases, antidepressant drug therapy in combination with one or more adjunct measures is more effective than drug therapy alone.

Selection of an Antidepressant

The primary antidepressants available include the tricyclic antidepressants (TCAs), heterocyclics, SSRIs, MAOIs, and other miscellaneous antidepressants. The therapeutic response rate is similar with all antidepressants; selection often depends on the side effect profile of the individual drugs (Table 19-3).

In the past, the tricyclic antidepressants were usually the first drugs prescribed for depression. Today, second-

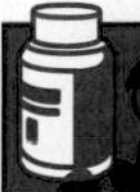

Complementary and Alternative Therapies
St. John's Wort

St. John's wort is a popular herbal preparation taken orally for anxiety, depressive moods, and menopausal mood disturbances. St. John's wort contains a number of constituents that may be responsible for its wide range of effects. Two of these constituents, Hypericin and pseudohypericin, show some activity against gram-negative and gram-positive bacteria and a wide spectrum of viruses. The anti-inflammatory effects of the topical oily Hypericum may result from its high flavinoid content. Hyperforin, another constituent, can selectively inhibit serotonin reuptake and in effect function as an SSRI; this may account for the antidepressant effects of St. John's wort. Topical hypericin preparations are used for treating contused injuries, first-degree burns, and myalgia; for relieving inflammation; and for promoting healing.

St. John's wort is considered to be effective for mild to moderate depression. Fewer side effects have been reported in clients taking St. John's wort than in those taking traditional treatments. St. John's wort is considered safe when taken in the recommended dosages. Most of its side effects are related to fatigue and photosensitivity. Caution clients to consider their response to the preparation before driving or operating other hazardous equipment, and caution them against taking other drugs with sedative properties because of additive effects. Clients should avoid excessive sun exposure and use sunscreen when exposure to direct sunlight is expected, particularly if they are light- or fair-skinned.

The various oral dosage forms of St. John's wort are prepared from the above-ground parts of the plant. The typical oral dosage is 2 to 4 g of the dried herb prepared as a tea one to three times daily by steeping in 150 mL of boiling water for 5 to 10 minutes and then straining, or 0.2 to 1 mg of total hypericin in other forms. The usual dose of the liquid extract (1:1 in 25% alcohol) or the tincture (1:10 in 45% alcohol) is 2 to 4 mL three times daily. For the treatment of mild to moderate depression, the typical dose is 900 mg/day initially, then 30 to 600 mg/day for maintenance.

Information from Cirigliano, M.D. (1999). Ten most common herbs in clinical practice. In M.S. Micozzi (Ed.), *Current review of complementary medicine.* Philadelphia: Current Medicine; and Jellin, J.M., Batz, F., & Hitchens, K. (1999). *Pharmacist's letter/prescriber's letter natural medicines comprehensive database.* Stockton, CA: Therapeutic Research Faculty.

TABLE 19-3 Side Effect Profiles of Antidepressant Medications

	Side Effect*						
	Central Nervous System			Cardiovascular			Other
Drug	Anticholinergic†	Drowsiness	Insomnia/ Agitation	Orthostatic Hypotension	Cardiac Dysrhythmia	Gastrointestinal Distress	Weight Gain (over 6 kg)
amitriptyline	4+	4+	0	4+	3+	0	4+
desipramine	1+	1+	1+	2+	2+	0	1+
doxepin	3+	4+	0	2+	2+	0	3+
imipramine	3+	3+	1+	4+	3+	1+	3+
nortriptyline	1+	1+	0	2+	2+	0	1+
protriptyline	2+	1+	1+	2+	2+	0	0
trimipramine	1+	4+	0	2+	2+	0	3+
amoxapine	2+	2+	2+	2+	3+	0	1+
maprotiline	2+	4+	0	0	1+	0	2+
trazodone	0	4+	0	1+	1+	1+	1+
bupropion	0	0	2+	0	1+	1+	0
fluoxetine	0	0	2+	0	0	3+	0
paroxetine	0	0	2+	0	0	3+	0
sertraline	0	0	2+	0	0	3+	0
MAOIs	1	1+	2+	2+	0	1+	2+

Information from Depression Guideline Panel. (1993). *Depression in Primary Care: Volume 2. Treatment of major depression. Clinical Practice Guideline #5.* Rockville, MD: Department of Health and Human Services, Public Health Service, Agency for Health Care Policy and Research. AHCPR Pub. No. 93-0551.

*0, Absent or rare; 2+, In between; 4+, relatively common.

†Dry mouth, blurred vision, urinary hesitancy, constipation.

generation drugs, the SSRIs, and the miscellaneous antidepressants are more commonly prescribed. The mechanism of action for the tricyclic and MAO antidepressants was discussed previously and illustrated in Figure 19-3. The SSRIs selectively block the reuptake of serotonin into the nerve terminal; the actions of the atypical antidepressants are less well defined.

The selection of an antidepressant is empiric and takes into consideration the side effect potential of each antidepressant compared with the medical problems of the individual client. For example, prescribers might select a sedating antidepressant (amitriptyline [Elavil], doxepin [Sinequan], or fluoxetine [Prozac]) for an agitated and depressed person or the potent blockers of norepinephrine reuptake (desipramine [Norpramin], nortriptyline [Aventyl]) for a withdrawn, depressive client. The Agency for Health Care Policy and Research (Depression Guideline Panel, 1993) has issued tables on the selection and side effect profiles of antidepressant medications (Box 19-5; see Table 19-3).

Plasma levels of the tricyclic antidepressants can vary widely between different individuals and—with the possible exception of nortriptyline (Aventyl), imipramine (Tofranil), and desipramine (Norpramin)—often do not correlate with dose or therapeutic response. Prescribers may order serum levels to monitor and help identify the noncompliant client. A low plasma level should initially indicate a need to interview the client to verify adherence to the prescribed schedule. The reason for the client's ineffective management of the therapeutic medication regimen (intolerable side effects, misunderstood directions, potential drug interactions, lack of finances to purchase medications) can then be identified and perhaps resolved (Laird & Benefield, 1995).

If compliance is verified and serum levels remain low, dosage adjustments or a switch to a different antidepressant may be necessary. If the client is nonresponsive to a predominantly norepinephrine-potentiating medication, a serotonin-potentiating agent might be indicated (Table 19-4); the individual may have biochemical differences that would indicate a trial with the opposite reuptake blocking agent.

Older adults often have reduced drug-metabolizing hepatic enzymes, and thus higher serum drug levels and a greater potential for side effects exist. Many prescribers start older adults at one-third to one-half the usual adult dosage, adjusting as necessary according to therapeutic response or the presence of undesirable side effects.

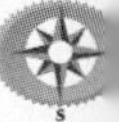

For a Concept Map on depression, go to mosby.com/MERLIN/McKenry/.

Tricyclic Antidepressants

Tricyclic antidepressants are indicated for the treatment of depression, enuresis (imipramine), and obsessive-compulsive disorder (clomipramine). They are well absorbed when given orally. The onset of antidepressant effect occurs within 2 to 3 weeks, and they are metabolized primarily in the liver and excreted by the kidneys.

BOX 19-5

Selecting Among Antidepressant Medications for Depressed Outpatients

First- and Second-Line Choices

Secondary amine tricyclics (e.g., nortriptyline, desipramine)*
Bupropion
Fluoxetine
Paroxetine
Sertraline
Trazodone

Alternative Agents for Clients with Special Presentations or Needs

Tertiary amine tricyclics (e.g., amitriptyline, imipramine)
Special considerations:
- Absence of serious medical illnesses, including cardiac disease, that preclude use
- Need for rapid sedation

MAOIs
Special considerations:
- Nonresponse or intolerance to at least one tricyclic and one heterocyclic
- Family or personal history of MAOI response
- Atypical symptom features

Selected anxiolytic medications†
Special considerations:
- Medical contraindications to antidepressant medications approved by the Food and Drug Administration (FDA)
- No adverse cardiovascular effects
- Low side-effect profile
- Substantial withdrawal with long-term use
- Limited exposure time expected (<3 months)
- No history of substance abuse
- Quick action needed

Information from Depression Guideline Panel. (1993). *Depression in Primary Care: Volume 2. Treatment of major depression. Clinical Practice Guideline, number 5.* Rockville, MD: Department of Health and Human Services, Public Health Service, Agency for Health Care Policy and Research. AHCPR Pub. No. 93-0551.

*Other first- and second-line choices are recommended for clients with dysrhythmias, cardiac conduction defects, ischemic heart disease, cardiomyopathy, or cardiac valve disease.

†Evidence is clearest for alprazolam. Not recommended in severe depressions because studies reveal reduced efficacy. Not recommended for prolonged care because studies longer than 12 weeks are not available. Not recommended when FDA-approved antidepressant medications can be used safely. For buspirone, efficacy is suggested in those with primary anxiety disorders and mild associated depressive symptoms.

NOTE: Evidence for efficacy with severely depressed inpatients is more abundant for the standard tricyclics than for newer agents.

In some instances, active metabolites produced in the liver have resulted in the marketing of new antidepressants, which are noted in parentheses in the following list:

generic (Brand name): active metabolite (Brand name if marketed)

- amitriptyline (Elavil): nortriptyline (Aventyl, Pamelor)
- amoxapine (Asendin): 7- and 8-hydroxyamoxapine
- desipramine (Norpramin): 2 hydroxydesipramine
- doxepin (Sinequan): desmethyldoxepin
- imipramine (Tofranil): desipramine (Norpramin)
- fluoxetine (Prozac): norfluoxetine

See Table 19-4 for half-lives and additional information about tricyclic antidepressants; see Table 19-3 for side effects/adverse reactions.

clomipramine [kloe mi′ pra meen] (Anafranil)

Clomipramine, an analogue of imipramine, is indicated for the treatment of obsessive-compulsive disorders. It is a potent inhibitor of serotonin reuptake, and its active metabolite inhibits norepinephrine reuptake.

Clomipramine is well absorbed orally, reaching a peak plasma level within 2 to 4 hours. It has a half-life of 19 to 37 hours and reaches steady-state levels in 1 to 2 weeks. It is metabolized in the liver and excreted by the kidneys.

The side effects/adverse reactions and drug interactions of clomipramine are similar to those of the other tricyclic agents. The initial adult dosage is 25 mg daily gradually increased as necessary and as tolerated to 100 mg (in divided doses) during the first 14 days. After 2 weeks the dosage may be increased over several more weeks if necessary to a maximum dosage of 250 mg/day. After the dosage is established, the total daily dose may be given at bedtime to reduce daytime sedation effects. In children and adolescents the initial dosage is 25 mg/day, which is increased as necessary during the first 14 days to a daily maximum of 3 mg/kg or 100 mg (whichever is the smaller dose). The dose may later be increased to 3 mg/kg or 200 mg (whichever is smaller) as necessary. Once the titrated dosage is established, the entire daily dose may be administered at bedtime.

■ Nursing Management

Tricyclic Antidepressant Therapy

■ **Assessment.** Tricyclic antidepressants should not be administered to clients who are in the acute recovery phase of a myocardial infarction. The risk-benefit ratio must be considered for clients with prostatic hypertrophy, urinary retention, or a predisposition to narrow-angle glaucoma or increased intraocular pressure, because tricyclic antidepressants possess significant anticholinergic properties; for cli-

TABLE 19-4 Pharmacology of Antidepressant Medications

Drug	Therapeutic Dosage Range (mg/day)	Average (range) of Elimination Half-lives (hour)*	Potentially Fatal Drug Interactions
Tricyclics			
amitriptyline (Elavil, Endep)	75-300	24 (16-46)	Antidysrhythmics, MAOIs
clomipramine (Anafranil)	75-300	24 (20-40)	Antidysrhythmics, MAOIs
desipramine (Norpramin, Pertofrane)	75-300	18 (12-50)	Antidysrhythmics, MAOIs
doxepin (Adapin, Sinequan)	75-300	17 (10-47)	Antidysrhythmics, MAOIs
imipramine (Janimine, Tofranil)	75-300	22 (12-34)	Antidysrhythmics, MAOIs
nortriptyline (Aventyl, Pamelor)	40-200	26 (18-88)	Antidysrhythmics, MAOIs
protriptyline (Vivactil)	20-60	76 (54-124)	Antidysrhythmics, MAOIs
trimipramine (Surmontil)	75-300	12 (8-30)	Antidysrhythmics, MAOIs
Second Generation			
amoxapine (Asendin)	100-600	10 (8-14)	MAOIs
bupropion (Wellbutrin)	225-450	14 (8-24)	MAOIs (possibly)
maprotiline (Ludiomil)	100-225	43 (27-58)	MAOIs
mirtazapine (Remeron)	15	30 (20-40)	MAOIs
trazodone (Desyrel)	150-600	8 (4-14)	—
Selected Serotonin Reuptake Inhibitors			
citalopram (Celexa)	20-40	35	MAOIs
fluoxetine (Prozac)	10-40	168 (72-360)†	MAOIs
paroxetine (Paxil)	20-50	24 (3-65)	MAOIs‡
sertraline (Zoloft ◆)	50-150	24 (10-30)	MAOIs‡
MAO Inhibitors§			For all 3 MAOIs:
isocarboxazid (Marplan)	30-50	Unknown	Vasoconstrictors‖, decongestants,‖ meperidine, and possibly other narcotics
phenelzine (Nardil)	45-90	2 (1.5-4)	
tranylcypromine (Parnate)	20-60	2 (1.5-3)	
Miscellaneous Antidepressants			
 nefazodone (Serzone ◆)	200-600	16 (11-24)	MAOIs
venlafaxine (Effexor, Effexor XR ◆)	75-225	4 (3-5)	Hypertensive crisis with MAOIs

Information from Depression Guideline Panel. (1993). *Depression in Primary Care: Volume 2. Treatment of major depression. Clinical Practice Guideline, number 5.* Rockville, MD: Department of Health and Human Services, Public Health Service, Agency for Health Care Policy and Research. AHCPR Pub. No. 93-0551.

*Half-lives are affected by age, sex, race, concurrent medications, and length of drug exposure.

†Includes both fluoxetine and norfluoxetine.

‡By extrapolation from fluoxetine data.

§MAO inhibition lasts longer (7 days) than drug half-life.

‖Including pseudoephedrine, phenylephrine, phenylpropanolamine, epinephrine, norepinephrine, and others.

ents who have a hyperthyroid condition or are taking thyroid medications, because there is a possibility of cardiovascular toxicity; and for individuals with a history of seizure disorders, because this class of drugs has been demonstrated to lower the seizure threshold.

Conditions that may be aggravated by the administration of tricyclic antidepressants are asthma, blood disorders, gastrointestinal disorders (risk of paralytic ileus), and cardiovascular disorders (risk of dysrhythmias, congestive heart failure, heart block, or stroke). Clients with active alcoholism may potentiate any CNS depressant effects of the antidepressants. Those with hepatic and renal dysfunction may experience accumulation of the drug because of the impairment in metabolism and excretion of the drug. In addition, clients with schizophrenia may have their condition activated, and clients with bipolar disorders may experience accelerated swings between mania and depression. When tricyclic antidepressants are administered to pregnant clients, the potential benefits should be weighed against the potential risks to the fetus.

A thorough drug history is required to ensure that the client does not have any drug allergies to tricyclic antidepressants, carbamazepine (Tegretol), maprotiline (Ludiomil), or trazodone (Desyrel), in which case the drug would be contraindicated. In addition, review the client's current medication regimen for the risk of significant drug interactions, such as those that may occur when tricyclic antidepressants are given concurrently with the following drugs:

Drug	Possible Effect and Management
Bold/color type indicates the most serious interactions.	
alcohol or CNS depressants	May result in enhanced CNS depressant effects; avoid concurrent use if possible, or reduce the dosage of one or both drugs and monitor closely.
antithyroid drugs	May increase risk of inducing granulocytosis. Avoid concurrent use or a potentially serious drug interaction may occur.
cimetidine (Tagamet)	May inhibit metabolism of the tricyclic agent, leading to increased serum levels and toxicity; lower tricyclic dosage by 20% to 30% and monitor closely.
clonidine (Catapres), guanadrel (Hylorel), guanethidine (Ismelin)	May decrease the antihypertensive effects of these drugs; monitor blood pressure closely because dosage changes or alternate antihypertensive agents may be necessary. Clonidine and tricyclic antidepressants may increase the risk of CNS depression; monitor closely for lethargy, confusion, and respiratory depression.
contraceptives, oral	May increase or decrease tricyclic serum levels; monitor closely for decreased therapeutic response or drug toxicity; dosage adjustments may be necessary.
extrapyramidal-inducing medications, amoxapine (Asendin), phenothiazines, haloperidol (Haldol), thioxanthenes	May increase risk and severity of extrapyramidal adverse reactions. With phenothiazines, sedative and anticholinergic side effects may be enhanced; monitor closely.
MAOIs	Should be contraindicated in outpatient settings; hypertensive crises, severely elevated temperatures, convulsions, and death have been reported with concurrent administration of MAOIs and tricyclic antidepressants. A drug-free period of at least 2 weeks from either category should be instituted before switching from one classification to the other. If concurrent use is prescribed in an inpatient setting, strict supervision and close monitoring are required because of the potentially serious adverse reactions. (See the current *USP DI* for dosing recommendations.)
metrizamide intrathecal (Amipaque)	Concurrent use of tricyclic antidepressants increases risk of inducing seizures because of a lowered seizure threshold. Discontinue tricyclic agents for at least 2 days before and 1 day after a myelogram.
sympathomimetics	May increase possibility of potentiating cardiovascular toxicities (severe hypertension, dysrhythmias, tachycardia) or severely elevated body temperatures. Avoid concurrent use or a potentially serious drug interaction may occur.

Clients must be closely assessed at the start of therapy and monitored closely throughout therapy for suicide potential. The risk of suicide increases as therapy improves the client's depressed state and energy levels increase. In addition, plasma tricyclic concentrations, ECG, complete blood counts (CBCs), tonometry examinations for glaucoma, blood pressure, pulse, and hepatic and renal function studies should be monitored.

■ **Nursing Diagnosis.** Clients receiving tricyclic antidepressants may experience the following nursing diagnoses/collaborative problems: disturbed thought processes related to the ineffectiveness of the drugs; risk for injury related to adverse CNS effects (blurred vision, confusion, tremors, hypotension, drowsiness); impaired oral mucous membrane (dry mouth); imbalanced nutrition: more than body requirements related to the appetite-stimulating effects of the drug; impaired comfort (nausea, headache); and the potential complications related to blood dyscrasias, skin photosensitivity, and the anticholinergic properties of the drug (confusion, hallucinations, blurred vision, urinary retention, constipation).

■ **Implementation**

■ ***Monitoring.*** The client's blood pressure and pulse should be monitored at appropriate intervals. Note that the possibility of suicide is inherent in any severely depressed client and persists until a significant remission occurs. The suicidal risk for clients who are taking tricyclic antidepressants is especially high; suicide attempts while taking tricyclic antidepressants are commonly seen in many emergency departments. When a client has a serious overt suicidal potential and is not hospitalized, the quantity of the tricyclic antidepressant should not exceed a 1-week supply. (See the Management of Drug Overdose box below.)

In clients with schizophrenia, activation of the psychosis may occur with the use of tricyclic antidepressants; such a reaction requires a reduction of the dosage or the addition of a major tranquilizer to the therapeutic regimen. Manic or hypomanic episodes may occur in individuals with a cyclic type of disorder. If this occurs, the tricyclic antidepressant should be discontinued until the episode is relieved and may then be reinstituted at a lower dosage if still needed in the therapy.

Use extreme caution (ECG, blood pressure and pulse monitoring, nursing observations) when administering tricyclic antidepressants to clients who have any evidence of cardiovascular disease; there is a possibility of conduction defects, dysrhythmias, myocardial infarction, cerebrovascular accidents, and tachycardia (Harrigan & Brady, 1999). The quinidine-like cardiac effects are well documented in the literature. With amoxapine (Asendin), monitor closely for early symptoms of TD.

■ ***Intervention.*** The initial dosages of tricyclic antidepressants in adolescents, older adults, and debilitated clients should be lower and increased gradually. The medication should not be withdrawn abruptly. In resistant cases of depression in adults, a dosage of 2.5 mg/kg/day or higher may need to be exceeded in the hospital. If such a dosage or higher is necessary, maintain ECG monitoring during the initiation of therapy and at appropriate intervals during stabilization of the dosage.

If the client is to be evaluated by plasma tricyclic determination because of a failure to respond to treatment, increased side effects, or questionable compliance, blood

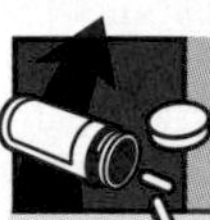

Management of Drug Overdose
Tricyclic Antidepressants

- TCA overdose can be life threatening and result in serious adverse reactions such as heart block, cardiac dysrhythmias, hypotension, seizures, coma and, in some instances, fatalities. In the United States, the third most common drug-induced death involves TCA overdoses (Montano, 1994).
- Montano (1994) also states that "70% to 80% of people who take overdoses of TCAs do not reach the hospital alive." It is therefore critically important that health care professionals know how to deal with a tricyclic overdose.

Signs and Symptoms

- The signs and symptoms of a TCA overdose may vary in severity, depending on numerous factors that include the amount ingested and absorbed, the age of the individual, and the interval between ingestion and initiation of a treatment modality. Any acute overdose or unwarranted ingestion of a TCA in children or adults must be considered serious and potentially fatal.
- CNS abnormalities include agitation, ataxia, choreoathetoid movements, drowsiness, hyperactive reflexes, muscle rigidity, restlessness, stupor, seizures, and coma. Cardiac abnormalities may include dysrhythmia, ECG evidence of impaired conduction, signs of congestive heart failure, and tachycardia. Quinidine-like adverse reactions are common in poisonings with tricyclic antidepressants.

Treatment

- Symptomatic and supportive measures are instituted according to the individual client's requirements and may include the following:
  - Emesis and/or the use of gastric lavage to empty the stomach, followed by the administration of activated charcoal to absorb any remaining drug in the gastrointestinal tract.
  - Close monitoring of cardiovascular functioning for at least 5 days. Cardiac dysrhythmias have occurred up to 6 days after massive TCA doses and may require treatment with lidocaine or phenytoin.
  - Maintenance of body temperature and respiratory and cardiac functions.
  - Physostigmine salicylate may need to be administered for all tricyclics except amoxapine. The use of this product is directed at persons with life-threatening signs such as coma with respiratory depression, very serious cardiac dysrhythmias, severe hypertension, or uncontrollable convulsions. Physostigmine salicylate is not administered for amoxapine overdoses because it has the potential to increase seizure activity.
  - Administration of anticonvulsants such as diazepam (Valium), phenytoin (Dilantin), paraldehyde, or an inhalation anesthetic to control seizures.
- Be aware that hemodialysis, peritoneal dialysis, forced diuresis, and exchange transfusions are not successful in treating a TCA overdose.

Information from *United States Pharmacopeia Dispensing Information (USP DI): Drug information for the health care professional* (19th ed.). (1999). Rockville, MD: United States Pharmacopeial Convention.

samples should be taken immediately before the first morning dose or at least 8 hours after a dose.

■ ***Education.*** During initiation or change of therapy the client should avoid activities that require coordination and alertness until his or her psychomotor response to the tricyclic antidepressant therapy has been determined.

Instruct the client to report anticholinergic effects such as blurred vision, altered thought processes, constipation, difficulty starting urinary stream, and eye pain, which may be indicative of glaucoma. The client should be advised to schedule regular appointments with the health care professional for periodic blood cell counts, glaucoma tests, and hepatic and renal function studies. Because dry mouth is a common side effect, the client should be taught appropriate oral hygiene to prevent caries and other dental problems. Breath mints may be reassuring to the client in social situations. Ice chips and sugarless candies are also helpful in promoting comfort.

Self-alteration of the prescribed medications or consumption of other medications, including OTC medications, should not occur without the prescriber's approval. Clients should be specifically instructed to avoid alcoholic beverages during the tricyclic antidepressant regimen because CNS depression may be heightened.

Orthostatic hypotension may occur. Instruct the client to come to a standing position slowly and carefully to avoid feeling faint.

Caution the client that the therapeutic response to tricyclic antidepressants is not immediate. It may be 10 to 14 days before there is a demonstrated effect and 30 days for a full effect.

Note that an emerging public health problem is tricyclic antidepressant poisoning or overdose in children. Doses in excess of 10 mg/kg body weight are potentially dangerous. The incidents are characterized as accidental because most occur when the drug is given to a household member for depression or to an enuretic child. Alert the adult family member to the possibility of accidental overdose and the need for security and administrative responsibility over the medication. There is an increasing use of these drugs in children and adolescents. The increased prescribing of TCAs for children and adolescents needs to be weighed seriously against the lethality of overdose and the availability of safer and easier ways to monitor medication use (Geller, Reising, Leonard, Riddle, & Walsh, 1999).

■ **Evaluation.** If tricyclic antidepressant therapy is successful, the client will report an improvement of depression. Clinically, the client will participate in more activities, initiate social interactions, and take more of an interest in his or her own appearance. Vital signs, ECG, and bowel elimination will be normal, and the client will not experience any adverse CNS reactions to the tricyclic antidepressants.

Second-Generation Antidepressants

The second-generation antidepressants include amoxapine (Asendin), bupropion (Wellbutrin, Wellbutrin SR ◆), maprotiline (Ludiomil), mirtazapine (Remeron), and trazodone (Desyrel). In general, these agents have fewer long-term side effects (e.g., weight gain) than the tricyclic antidepressants, and they have other advantages and disadvantages that need to be considered.

Amoxapine (Asendin), an active metabolite of loxapine (an antipsychotic agent), inhibits the reuptake of norepinephrine and is a potent dopamine-blocking agent. The latter effect may result in extrapyramidal side effects and NMS (*Drug Facts and Comparisons,* 2000). Therapeutic doses of amoxapine and maprotiline produce fewer cardiovascular side effects than the tricyclic agents (Laird & Benefield, 1995). However, an amoxapine overdose may result in seizures and status epilepticus within 12 hours of ingestion. Renal failure has also been reported with an amoxapine overdose.

The mechanism of action for bupropion (Wellbutrin) is unknown, but it weakly blocks the reuptake of dopamine, serotonin, and norepinephrine. This drug and the newer agents are used for persons who are nonresponsive to other antidepressants. Bupropion has fewer anticholinergic effects and rarely produces hypotension or sexual dysfunction, but it is reported to cause agitation, insomnia, tremors, and dose-related seizures (Abramowicz, 1994).

Maprotiline (Ludiomil) is similar to the tricyclic antidepressants except it is associated with an increased risk of skin rash (redness, swelling, pruritus) and seizures. Therapeutic daily doses of maprotiline have been reported to produce seizures in persons without any history of seizures (Wells, 1994). Therefore this product is contraindicated in anyone with a history of seizures.

Trazodone (Desyrel) is chemically different from the other antidepressants. It blocks serotonin reuptake and also produces changes in the binding at serotonin receptors. Trazodone has few if any anticholinergic effects and thus has minimal effects on cardiac conduction. The prescriber should still exercise caution in using this drug in clients with a history of cardiac disease, because several cases of ventricular dysrhythmia have been reported with its use. It can cause gastric distress and postural hypotension early in treatment, especially in older adults, as well as priapism (Laird & Benefield, 1995).

Monoamine Oxidase Inhibitors

MAOIs are indicated as second- or third-line antidepressants for the treatment of depression that does not respond to other, safer antidepressants (Depression Guideline Panel, 1993). These agents have numerous drug interactions with prescription and OTC medications, caffeine, and foods and beverages containing tyramine. The major adverse reaction with these agents is the occurrence of a sudden and possibly very severe hypertension that can progress to vascular collapse and fatality if left untreated.

MAO, an enzyme found in nerve terminals, the liver, and the brain, is necessary for the inactivation and degradation of tyramine, catecholamines, serotonin, and various medications. MAOIs interfere with this inactivation, which may result in a potentiation of vasopressor effects and serious adverse reactions.

Two types of MAO enzymes have been identified and named: MAO-A and MAO-B. MAO-A appears to have a preference for serotonin and is located throughout the body, with high concentrations located in the human placenta. MAO-B is found mainly in human platelets. Approximately equal amounts of both types are found in the liver and brain. The MAOIs currently in use are nonselective.

The MAOIs are capable of blocking or diminishing the activity of MAO, resulting in a net increase in brain amine levels. Current research indicates that the MAOIs produce desensitization of the $alpha_2$ or beta and serotonin receptors (down-regulation). During early clinical trials of MAOIs as antidepressants, orthostatic hypotension was encountered as a common but inconsistent side effect. Many MAOIs were then produced and studied specifically as antidepressant and antihypertensive agents.

The MAOIs discussed in this section are those used as antidepressants: the hydrazines—isocarboxazid (Marplan) and phenelzine (Nardil)—and the nonhydrazine, tranylcypromine sulfate (Parnate). The MAOIs are indicated primarily for resistant depression and for anxious and hostile depression, especially depression that also involves panic attacks or phobic symptoms.

MAOIs can increase the concentration of all central amines, although different effects on the individual amines are possible. For example, some MAOIs may increase dopamine or norepinephrine concentrations to a more extensive degree than serotonin concentrations, whereas other MAOIs may raise the level of serotonins to a greater degree than those of norepinephrine and dopamine. The increase in amine concentration is associated with behavioral hyperactivity (amphetamine-like psychomotor stimulation with large doses) and, in some cases, with the exacerbation of psychotic symptoms. Antiphobic and antidepressant activities are seen with lower doses. In general, these compounds are most effective in reversing the dysphoric state and its attendant vegetative disturbances in clients with depressive syndromes.

Therapeutic doses of MAOIs take from days to weeks to produce a maximal therapeutic effect. MAOIs produce an irreversible inactivation of MAO by forming a stable complex with the enzyme; recovery from the effect of MAOIs thus depends on enzyme regeneration, which may occur over several weeks. Inhibition occurs only with very high doses and may be responsible for some of the toxic effects of MAOIs.

The mechanism of action of MAOIs was discussed in the previous section. The MAOIs are well absorbed orally. In some individuals the onset of action occurs in 7 to 10 days, and it usually takes from 4 to 8 weeks of therapy to achieve the full effect. These agents irreversibly bind MAO activity; recovery may take 10 days to 2 weeks. MAOIs are metabolized in the liver and excreted primarily by the kidneys.

Side effects/adverse reactions are discussed in Table 19-3. See Table 19-4 for information on dosage and administra-

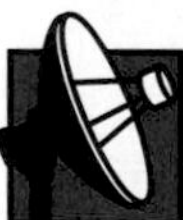

TechnologyLink
Psychotherapeutic Drugs

Video Resources

Psychiatric Emergencies Video Series, ISBN 0-8151-5699-5
Mosby, Inc., 11830 Westline Industrial Drive, St. Louis, MO 63146; (800) 426-4545; www.mosby.com.
- Module 1: *Crisis Intervention,* ISBN 0-8151-7286-9
- Module 2: *Intoxification, Abreactions, Side Effects,* ISBN 0-8151-7288-5
- Module 3: *Violence, Aggression, Suicide and Post-traumatic Stress Disorder,* ISBN 0-8151-7290-7

Mosby's Psychiatric Nursing Videotape Series, Volumes 1-6, ISBN 0-8151-8568-5
- Volume 1: *Anxiety Disorders,* ISBN 0-8151-8570-7
- Volume 2: *Major Depression,* ISBN 0-8151-8571-5
- Volume 3: *Bipolar Disorder,* ISBN 0-8151-8572-3
- Volume 4: *Substance Abuse,* ISBN 0-8151-8573-1
- Volume 5: *Dual Diagnosis,* ISBN 0-8151-8574-X
- Volume 6: *Alzheimer's Disease,* ISBN 0-8151-8575-8

Web Resources

Guide to the Mental Health Internet (www.virtualcs.com/mhi.html)
This site lists numerous resources on mental health, libraries, and seminars.

Mental Health Net (www.mhnet.org/)
A source of online mental health topics for disorders and their treatments, this site also includes professional resources and a reading room.

Internet Mental Health Schizophrenia (www.mentalhealth.com/dis/p20%2dps01.html)
This site describes schizophrenia and also includes sections on diagnosis, treatment, research, articles, books, and personal experiences.

Health Sciences Library Internet, University of Pittsburgh, Mental Health Resources (www.hsls.pitt.edu/)
This site is an online resource for the professional and the general public. It provides numerous health and mental health resources, information on federal and state grants and funds, and much more.

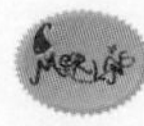
For additional WebLinks, a free subscription to the "Mosby/Saunders ePharmacology Update" newsletter, and more, go to mosby.com/MERLIN/McKenry/.

tion of the MAOIs. See also the Pregnancy Safety box on p. 403.

■ Nursing Management

MAO Inhibitor Therapy

■ Assessment. MAOIs should not be administered to clients with sensitivity to these substances, active alcoholism, congestive heart failure, pheochromocytoma (because the tumors secrete pressor substances), severe hepatic impairment (may precipitate hepatic precoma), or renal function impairment (drug may accumulate). Clients with the following conditions should consider the risk-benefit ratio of taking MAOIs: cardiac dysrhythmias, cardiovascular or cerebrovascular disease (ischemia and conduction disturbances may occur), or headaches (may mask hypertensive reaction). Clients with hypertension may experience a hypertensive crisis from dietary lapses. MAOIs may aggravate psychosis in clients with schizophrenia. Clients who have had sympathectomies may be more sensitive to the hypotensive effects of the MAOIs. Be aware that overactive, overstimulated, or agitated clients usually do not respond well to MAOIs because the drugs may cause stimulation. These drugs are also contraindicated in many other conditions.

MAOIs interact with numerous drugs, often with severe consequences; therefore it is important to complete a thorough drug history to determine any significant drug interactions. This should include the month before the administration as well as the concurrent therapy. The following effects may occur when MAOIs are administered with the following drugs:

Drug	Possible Effect and Management
Bold/color type indicates the most serious interactions.	
alcohol or CNS depressants	May enhance CNS depressive effects. If alcohol contains tyramine, a severe hypertensive reaction may result. Avoid concurrent use or a potentially serious drug interaction may occur.
local anesthetics containing epinephrine or cocaine	May result in a very severe hypertensive reaction. Cocaine should not be administered at the same time as or within 2 weeks of an MAOI. Avoid concurrent use or a potentially serious drug interaction may occur.
antidepressants, tricyclics, carbamazepine (Tegretol), maprotiline (Ludiomil), other MAOIs, furazolidone (Furoxone), selegiline (Eldepryl), or procarbazine (Matulane)	May result in severely elevated temperatures, hypertensive crises, severe seizures, and death. Avoid concurrent use or a potentially serious drug interaction may occur. Before switching from one of these medications to an MAOI or vice versa, a 2-week drug-free period should be instituted. Several studies have used tricyclic antidepressants with an MAOI for refractory depression. (See current *USP DI* for explicit instructions on proper dosing and monitoring of this combination.)
antidiabetic agents (oral or insulin)	Enhanced hypoglycemic effects have been reported. A reduction in the oral hypoglycemic agent may be required during or even after concurrent drug therapy.
bupropion (Wellbutrin)	Concurrent use increases the risk of bupropion toxicity. A 2-week interval is recommended between the discontinuance of MAOIs and the start of bupropion therapy.
buspirone (BuSpar)	May cause hypertension. Avoid concurrent use or a serious drug interaction may occur.
caffeine (e.g., drug products, coffee, tea, chocolate, cola), cyclobenzaprine (Flexeril), or other MAOIs	May result in severe cardiac dysrhythmias or hypertension. Avoid concurrent use or a serious drug interaction may occur. May result in severe hypertensive crises, convulsions, and death. A drug-free interval of at least 2-weeks is recommended to avoid this reaction.
dextromethorphan (Benylin DM, Robitussin DM)	May result in increased excitability, hyperpyrexia, and hypertension. Avoid concurrent use or a serious drug interaction may occur.
doxapram (Dopram)	Enhanced and severe hypertensive effects may result. Avoid concurrent use or a potentially serious drug interaction may occur.
fluoxetine (Prozac), paroxetine (Paxil), sertraline (Zoloft), trazodone (Desyrel)	May result in agitation, restlessness, gastrointestinal distress, or seizures and hypertensive crises. Avoid concurrent use or a potentially serious drug interaction may occur. For client safety, a drug-free period of at least 2 weeks should be instituted when switching from an MAOI to fluoxetine. When switching from fluoxetine to an MAO inhibitor, a 5-week drug-free period should be implemented.
guanadrel (Hylorel), guanethidine (Ismelin), or rauwolfia alkaloids	May result in severe hypertension. Withdraw MAOI at least 7 days before starting therapy with these agents. If an MAOI is added to a medication schedule already containing a rauwolfia alkaloid, serious CNS depression may result. If a rauwolfia alkaloid is added to a medication schedule that already includes an MAOI, hypertension and increased excitability may result. Avoid concurrent use or a potentially serious drug interaction may occur.

Continued

Drug	Possible Effect and Management
levodopa (Larodopa)	Avoid this combination. Severe and sudden hypertensive crises have been reported. Before starting levodopa therapy, the client should be withdrawn from MAOIs with a drug-free period of at least 2 to 4 weeks.
meperidine (Demerol) and perhaps other opioid narcotics	Severe hypertension, increased excitability, sweating, and rigidity have been reported with concurrent use. Hypotension, seizures, elevated temperature, respiratory depression, cardiovascular collapse, coma, and death have been reported in some individuals and may be caused by serotonin accumulation from the MAOI. Avoid concurrent use or a potentially serious drug interaction may occur. Do not use meperidine for at least 14 to 21 days after discontinuing an MAOI. Morphine and other narcotics are not reported as causing such a severe reaction, but it is recommended that the opioid dosage be reduced to one-fourth (test dose) the usual dosage. Monitor closely whenever opioids or anesthesia adjuncts (fentanyl [Sublimaze] or sufentanil [Sufenta]) are given to clients who have received MAOIs in the previous 2 or 3 weeks.
methyldopa (Aldomet)	Severe headache, hypertension, hallucinations, and increased excitability have been reported. Avoid concurrent use or a serious drug interaction may occur.
methylphenidate (Ritalin)	Concurrent use may result in a hypertensive crisis. Avoid concurrent use or a serious drug interaction may occur. A drug-free period of at least 2 weeks should be allowed before instituting methylphenidate therapy.
sympathomimetics, systemic	Direct-acting (dopamine, mephentermine, metaraminol, dobutamine, methoxamine, and phenylephrine), indirect-acting (amphetamines, phenylpropanolamine, and pseudoephedrine), or combination effects (ephedrine) should not be given during or within 2 weeks of administration of an MAOI. Severe hypertensive crisis, elevated temperatures, cardiac dysrhythmias, headaches, and vomiting have been reported. Avoid concurrent use or a serious drug interaction may occur.
tryptophan and tranylcypromine (Parnate)	May result in hyperventilation, increased temperature, shivering, disorientation, mania, or hypomania. If necessary to use both drugs, start tryptophan in low dosages and increase dosage slowly. Monitor mental status and blood pressure closely.
tyramine or high-pressor foods and beverages (see Box 19-6)	Sudden, severe hypertensive crises have been reported. Avoid concurrent use or a potentially serious drug interaction may occur. Client teaching is crucial for individuals receiving MAOIs. MAOIs and tyramine or high-pressor, amine-containing foods or beverages must be avoided during therapy and for a minimum of 2 weeks after therapy is discontinued.

A baseline assessment should include a documentation of the client's symptoms of depression, blood pressure, and renal and hepatic function studies.

■ **Nursing Diagnosis.** The client receiving MAOI therapy has the potential for the following selected nursing diagnoses/collaborative problems: disturbed sleep pattern related to CNS stimulation; activity intolerance (weakness); impaired comfort (headache, increased perspiration); diarrhea; risk for injury related to blurred vision, severe orthostatic hypotension, or weakness; excess fluid volume (edema); imbalanced nutrition: more than body requirements related to carbohydrate craving; sexual dysfunction (anorgasmia, ejaculatory disorders, impotence); and the potential complications of CNS stimulation (restlessness, twitching, agitation), hypertensive crises, hepatitis, leukopenia, and the anticholinergic effects of MAOIs (blurred vision, dry mouth, urinary retention, constipation).

■ **Implementation**

■ ***Monitoring.*** The client's statements and behaviors related to depression should be documented during MAOI therapy. Blood pressure should be monitored regularly to detect evidence of dangerous fluctuations in pressure during therapy, such as pressor amine response and orthostatic hypotension. Monitor the ECG for changes. Weigh the client biweekly and assess for pedal edema. Periodic liver function tests (bilirubin, alkaline phosphatase, or transaminase) should be performed. Darkened urine and jaundice are signs of drug-induced hepatitis and should be reported to the prescriber.

It should be noted that the suicidal tendencies present with the client's condition may compound the nursing care issues because of the delayed effect of MAOIs in relieving suicidal tendencies. This effect presents an additional risk to the client during the initial phases of drug therapy. Be alert to the possibility of any impulsive ingestion of these substances.

The risk of suicide is often higher near the end of the depressive cycle, and attention should be given to the possibility of suicidal attempts during this period. Overt client behavior may indicate a remission of depressive symptoms, but this may be caused by drug action and not by alleviation of pathologic processes. In general, antidepressants should be continued for several months after the remission of symptoms and should never be discontinued abruptly, because a relapse may occur.

■ ***Intervention.*** Note that the anorexia of a hospitalized, depressed client may prompt well-meaning family members or friends to bring in supplementary foods or a little wine to stimulate the appetite. Careful nursing observation during visiting hours and instruction of the family regarding restrictions on tyramine or high-pressor foods and beverages can prevent serious consequences. Communication with the hospital dietitian may also prevent these foods from appearing on the client's hospital menu.

MAOIs should be discontinued immediately when any adverse signs and symptoms occur. Fever should be managed by external cooling. To control severe hypertension reactions, phentolamine mesylate (Regitine) should be on hand (5 mg IV administered slowly to avoid a hypotensive effect). Oral or IV labetalol may be used, saving the phentolamine for severe or nonresponding cases.

Because MAOIs usually cause some agitation and insomnia, they are not administered late in the evening.

■ ***Education.*** Because of possible food-drug interactions, teach the client and family which foods may cause a severe reaction (Box 19-6). Tyramine-containing foods and beverages should not be ingested for at least 2 to 3 weeks after discontinuance of drug therapy. Reinstruction of the client may be necessary as the client's depression lifts or if electroshock therapy is used concomitantly with drug therapy.

Teach the client and family to recognize adverse reactions to MAOIs, to know the dietary precautions, and to understand drug effects that precipitate adverse reactions. This knowledge may avert the cardiovascular reactions. Because orthostatic hypotension is a common side effect, instruct the client to avoid syncope by coming to a sitting or lying position slowly.

Drowsiness occurs during the initiation or change of therapy, and therefore the client should be instructed to avoid activities that require coordination and alertness until the response to therapy has been determined.

The client should be alerted to the signs and symptoms of hypertensive crisis: severe headache or chest pain, increased photosensitivity, nausea and vomiting, bradycardia or tachycardia, and diaphoresis. The client should check with a physician or hospital emergency department immediately. The client should wear a medical identification band that indicates MAOI therapy and should be instructed to alert health care providers to the MAOI regimen if dental or emergency care is required.

Advise the client to observe all the rules of caution involved in MAOI therapy for at least 14 days after discontinuing the medication. The drug should be discontinued gradually and under medical supervision.

■ **Evaluation.** The expected outcome of MAOI therapy is that the client's behavior and communication will indicate an improvement of depression, and the client will not experience adverse CNS or cardiovascular symptoms.

BOX 19-6

Tyramine-Containing Substances

The tyramine content of foods varies according to the references reviewed. This variation may result from different conditions or food preparations, different food samples, or different producers or manufacturers. The major goal should be to advise the client to avoid foods and drinks with reported moderate- to high-tyramine content, such as the following:

- Cheese: aged (blue, Boursault, natural brick, Brie, Camembert, cheddar, Emmenthaler, Gruyère, mozzarella, parmesan, Romano, Roquefort, Stilton)
- Meat and fish: beef and chicken liver (unrefrigerated, fermented), caviar (fish, unrefrigerated, fermented), fish (dried), herring (dried, salted, and pickled), fermented sausages (bologna, pepperoni, salami, summer sausage), and any other unrefrigerated, fermented meats
- Vegetables: overripe avocado and overripe fava beans
- Fruit: overripe figs, bananas, and raisins
- Alcoholic beverages: red wines, especially Chianti; sherry; beer; liquors

Other foods may contain tyramine or high-pressor amines, including yogurt, sour cream, cream cheese, cottage cheese, chocolate, and soy sauce. However, these foods are reportedly less apt to cause a serious reaction when eaten in moderation and only when fresh (*USP DI,* 1999).

Selective Serotonin Reuptake Inhibitors

SSRIs are safer and as effective as the other antidepressants (Hirschfield, 1999). Fluoxetine (Prozac ◆), the first SSRI released in this category, was followed by fluvoxamine (Luvox), paroxetine (Paxil ◆), sertraline (Zoloft), and citalopram (Celexa ◆). All but fluvoxamine are used to treat depression, and fluoxetine and fluvoxamine are used to treat obsessive-compulsive disorders. Citalopram, promoted as having a better side effect profile, is a weak inhibitor of P-450 liver metabolizing enzymes but does not appear to affect the CYP3A4 liver metabolizing enzymes in vitro; it has a long half-life and is therefore administered once daily (Forest Pharmaceuticals, 1999). Unlike the tricyclic agents, which often cause weight gain, the SSRIs (with the exception of paroxetine) may cause anorexia and weight loss (*Drug Facts and Comparisons,* 2000).

When SSRIs are administered orally, peak serum levels are reached in 3 to 8 hours for fluvoxamine, 2 to 4 hours for citalopram, 2 to 8 hours for paroxetine, 4.5 to 8.4 hours for sertraline, and 6 to 8 hours for fluoxetine. The time to reach steady-state levels is 7 days or fewer for fluvoxamine, sertraline, and citalopram, whereas fluoxetine takes 28 days and paroxetine approximately 10 days. These drugs are metabolized in the liver and excreted via the kidneys and feces (*Drug Facts and Comparisons*, 2000).

See Table 19-4 for pharmacology and dosing information. See Table 19-3 for side effects and Box 19-7 for management of the serotonin syndrome.

BOX 19-7

Management of Serotonin Syndrome

Medications that affect the metabolism, synthesis, or reuptake of serotonin may result in serotonin accumulation and the serotonin syndrome (SES). This syndrome is characterized by mental status changes (confusion, restlessness, anxiety, disorientation), ataxia, myoclonus, tremors, rigidity, hypertension, and autonomic dysfunction.

Symptoms usually occur within 2 to 72 hours up to several weeks after beginning the administration of a serotonergic drug. Other causes that may cause similar symptoms need to be ruled out, such as infection, metabolic disorders, or the start or increase of a neuroleptic agent before the onset of this syndrome. The most common drug combinations that cause this syndrome include an MAOI with SSRIs, TCAs, tryptophan, lithium, or dextromethorphan.

Treatment

In mild cases, discontinue the serotonergic agent and provide supportive treatment as necessary. The symptoms may resolve within 24 hours.

Severe cases require discontinuing the offending drug and providing supportive care, but symptoms may be prolonged and, in some cases, fatal. Diazepam (Valium), propranolol (Inderal), methysergide (Sansert), cyproheptadine (Periactin), mechanical ventilation, and skeletal muscle relaxants have been used for severe cases.

Drugs That Affect Serotonin

Serotonin agonist: buspirone (BuSpar)
Inhibits serotonin metabolism: MAOIs (tranylcypromine [Parnate], phenelzine [Nardil]) and MAO-B inhibitor (selegiline [Eldepryl]).
Increases serotonin synthesis or release: methylphenidate (Ritalin), lithium, and tryptophan.
Inhibits serotonin reuptake: antidepressants such as amitriptyline (Elavil), nortriptyline (Aventyl), doxepin (Sinequan), imipramine (Tofranil), and clomipramine (Anafranil). The SSRIs include paroxetine (Paxil), fluoxetine (Prozac), sertraline (Zoloft), and fluvoxamine (Luvox). An opioid meperidine (Demerol) and miscellaneous drugs such as dextromethorphan (DM), trazodone (Desyrel), and venlafaxine (Effexor) may also cause this effect.

■ Nursing Management

Selective Serotonin Reuptake Inhibitor Therapy

■ **Assessment.** Caution is needed when administering SSRIs to clients with hepatic function impairment because the metabolism if the drug is delayed. Lower doses or less frequent dosing is recommended for clients with liver disease. Clients must be closely assessed for suicide potential at the start of and throughout therapy. A baseline measurement of weight and serum electrolytes is required if fluoxetine is administered for eating disorders.

Review client's current medication regimen for the risk of significant drug interactions, such as those that may occur when SSRIs are given concurrently with the following drugs:

Drug/Herb	Possible Effect and Management
Bold/color type indicates the most serious interactions.	
alprazolam (Xanax) and other benzodiazepines with hepatic oxidation	May prolong half-life of alprazolam; risk of injury increases because of psychomotor impairment. Concurrent administration of fluvoxamine and diazepam is not recommended.
antidepressants, tricyclic	TCA plasma concentrations increase twofold to tenfold. TCA dosage should be reduced, and TCA serum concentrations should be monitored.
astemizole (Hismanal), cisapride (Propulsid)	**Metabolism of astemizole is limited with fluoxetine, leading to increased blood levels and the risk of cardiac dysrhythmias. Concurrent use is not recommended. All of these agents are contraindicated with fluvoxamine.**
beta-blocking agents, such as metoprolol (Lopressor), propranolol (Inderal)	Increased serum concentrations of the beta blockers occur. Reduce their dosage and monitor closely for bradycardia or hypotension.
highly protein-bound medications; anticoagulants, digitalis glycosides	Increased risk of adverse reactions because the displacement of either drug can lead to increased amounts of free drug. Monitor serum drug levels and prothrombin times, and monitor client closely for toxic effects.
MAOIs	**Concurrent use is contraindicated because it may result in hyperpyretic episodes, severe convulsions, hypertensive crises, serotonin syndrome, or death.**
moclobemide (Manerex)	**Potential fatal effects due to serotonin syndrome (see Box 19-7).**
phenytoin (Dilantin), clozapine (Clozaril), theophylline (Theo-Dur)	Concurrent use may result in toxicity of these drugs; close monitoring is required.
SSRIs (other)	Increased risk of serotonin syndrome (see Box 19-7).
St. John's wort, ayahuasca	**May cause serotonin syndrome, especially with paroxetine. Herbal ayahuasca has alkaloids that have MAOI effects, which can induce serotonin syndrome. Avoid concurrent use.**

■ **Nursing Diagnosis.** Clients receiving SSRI therapy may experience the following nursing diagnoses/collaborative problems: disturbed sleep pattern (drowsiness, insomnia); sexual dysfunction (decreased libido, impotence, delayed ejaculation, anorgasmia); diarrhea; impaired oral mucous membrane (dry mouth); impaired comfort (nausea, abdominal cramps, headache); fatigue; risk for injury related to ataxia, dizziness, or vertigo; anxiety; hyperpyrexia; and the potential complications of extrapyramidal effects, dystonia, serotonin syndrome, and skin rash.

■ **Implementation**

■ ***Monitoring.*** The client's risk for suicide must be carefully assessed, especially during early treatment with SSRIs.

■ ***Intervention.*** Because of the risk for suicide, the smallest quantity needed for successful client management is usually prescribed. Do not administer an MAOI or an SSRI within 14 days of each other.

■ ***Education.*** Teach the client that 1 month or more may be necessary before antidepressant or antipanic effects are achieved; anti-obsessional effects take longer. Caution the client about driving or performing tasks that require alertness because of possible drowsiness or impaired judgment or motor skills. Check with the prescriber before discontinuing SSRI therapy; gradual reductions in dosage may be needed. The client should avoid the use of alcoholic beverages.

■ **Evaluation.** The expected outcome of SSRI therapy is that the client will report an improvement of the symptoms of depression. The client will participate in more activities, initiate social interactions, and take more of an interest in his or her surroundings and appearance.

Miscellaneous Antidepressants

Miscellaneous antidepressants include nefazodone (Serzone) and venlafaxine (Effexor). The mechanism of action for nefazodone is unknown, but it does inhibit serotonin and norepinephrine reuptake and also is a serotonin receptor antagonist. The greatest effect of venlafaxine and its active metabolite is interference with the reuptake of serotonin. It also interferes with reuptake of norepinephrine and dopamine but to a lesser degree.

Both nefazodone and venlafaxine are well absorbed orally. The half-life of nefazodone is 2 to 4 hours; the half-life of venlafaxine and its active metabolite is 3 to 5 hours and 9 to 11 hours, respectively. With both drugs, the onset of antidepressant effects requires several weeks. Both drugs are metabolized in the body and liver and excreted primarily by the kidneys.

Reported side effects with nefazodone (Serzone) include nightmares, constipation or diarrhea, sedation, dry mouth, agitation, increase in appetite and cough, insomnia, nausea, vomiting, paresthesia, peripheral edema, and tremors. Adverse reactions include ataxia, blurred vision or visual disturbances, light-headedness, skin rash, pruritus, and tinnitus.

Side effects/adverse reactions with venlafaxine (Effexor) include nightmares, anorexia, weight loss, weakness, chills, constipation or diarrhea, light-headedness, dry mouth, dyspepsia, sweating, insomnia, nausea, vomiting, abdominal gas or pain, taste alterations, tremors, rhinitis, sexual dysfunction, visual disturbances, and headaches. Some of these effects, such as sexual dysfunction, nausea, vomiting, anorexia, tremors, and chills, may be dose related.

The usual adult dosage for nefazodone is 100 mg two times daily; for venlafaxine, the usual adult dosage is 25 mg three times daily with food. Dosages may be increased according to the individual's response to and tolerance for the product. (See the Pregnancy Safety box on p. **403**.)

Antimanic Therapy

Mania is characterized by the presence of speech and motor hyperactivity, reduced sleep requirements, flight of ideas, grandiosity, elation, poor judgment, aggressiveness and, possibly, hostility. The manic state is seen with recurrent manic symptoms with little or no depression, whereas bipolar affective disorders have both an acute manic phase and a hypomanic state or alternating periods of mania and depression. Counseling, psychotherapy, and drug therapy are useful for the treatment of bipolar disorders. Although lithium is considered the drug of choice for this disorder, carbamazepine (Tegretol) and valproic acid (Depakene) have been used investigationally for persons who are unresponsive to or are unable to take lithium (*USP DI,* 1999; Love & Grothe, 1995). These agents have been approved as anticonvulsants and are reviewed in Chapter 17.

The following is a list of lithium products:

- lithium carbonate capsules (Eskalith, Carbolith ♣)
- lithium carbonate tablets (Eskalith, Lithane)
- lithium carbonate extended-release tablets (Lithobid, Eskalith CR)
- lithium citrate syrup (Cibalith-S)

The mechanism of action for lithium has not been established. It is theorized that lithium accelerates the presynaptic destruction of catecholamines (serotonin, dopamine, and norepinephrine), inhibits transmitter release at the synapse, and decreases postsynaptic receptor sensitivity with the result that the presumed overactive catecholamine systems in mania are corrected.

Sodium in the cells has been reported to increase by as much as 200% in manic clients. Lithium and sodium are both actively transported across cell membranes, but lithium cannot be pumped out of the cell as effectively as sodium. Thus lithium may stabilize cell membranes.

The third possible mechanism of action is lithium blockade of the inositol triphosphate and diphosphate system in the CNS, that is, its effects on the second messengers necessary for alpha-adrenergic and muscarinic transmission. At the current time, the latter is the most accepted theory (Katzung, 1998).

Lithium is indicated for the treatment of manic-depressive illness, and it is being investigated for other uses. With the exception of the slow-release dosage form, lithium is completely absorbed in 6 to 8 hours and has a half-life of 24 hours in adults, 18 hours in adolescents, and up to 36 hours in older adults. Time to peak serum levels is 30 minutes for syrup, 1 to 3 hours for capsules/tablets, and 4 hours for extended-release tablets. Therapeutic serum levels for the treatment of bipolar disorder are 0.8 to 1.2 mEq/L for acute mania and 0.5 to 1 mEq/L for maintenance. A clinical response is usually reported in 1 to 3 weeks. Lithium is not metabolized and is primarily excreted unchanged by the kidneys.

Side effects/adverse reactions of lithium include hand tremors (slight), thirst, nausea, increased urination, diarrhea, tachycardia, increased weakness, weight gain, respiratory difficulties (on exertion), fainting, and irregular pulse rate. Early signs of toxicity include diarrhea, anorexia, muscle weakness, nausea, vomiting, tremors, slurred speech, and drowsiness. Later signs are blurred vision, convulsions, severe trembling, confusion, ataxia, and increased urine production.

The usual adult dosage of lithium for acute mania is 300 to 600 mg three times daily, adjusted according to the client's response and tolerance up to a maximum dosage of 2.4 g/day. The maintenance dosage is 300 mg three or four times daily. Older adults usually require a lower dosage. The dosage for children up to 12 years old is 15 to 20 mg/kg in two or three divided doses, adjusted according to response.

▪ Nursing Management

Lithium Therapy

▪ **Assessment.** Lithium is contraindicated in clients with a history of leukemia because the leukemia may be reactivated. In addition, lithium may exacerbate cardiovascular disease, CNS conditions such as epilepsy and parkinsonism, and psoriasis. Severe infection with prolonged sweating, diarrhea, or vomiting may necessitate a reduction in the lithium dosage to prevent toxicity caused by dehydration. Delayed lithium excretion resulting from renal insufficiency may also lead to toxicity.

Lithium should not be administered to pregnant women during the first trimester unless the potential benefits outweigh the risks to the fetus. Lithium is excreted in the breast milk of lactating mothers in quantities sufficient to cause lithium toxicity in the child; this prohibits its use in breast-feeding mothers.

Review the client's current medication regimen for the risk of significant drug interactions, such as those that may occur when lithium is given concurrently with the following drugs:

Drug	Possible Effect and Management
Bold/color type indicates the most serious interactions.	
antiinflammatory analgesics, nonsteroidal	May decrease excretion of lithium, leading to increased lithium levels and toxicity. Monitor closely for blurred vision, confusion, and dizziness.
antithyroid drugs, calcium iodide, potassium iodide, or iodinated glycerol	May enhance the hypothyroid goitrogenic effects of lithium or these medications. Monitor closely for lethargy, intolerance to cold, and other symptoms.
chlorpromazine (Thorazine), possibly other phenothiazines	Concurrent use reduces the absorption of chlorpromazine (and possibly other phenothiazines) up to 40%. Reduced serum levels may lead to treatment failure. In addition, an increased rate of lithium excretion has been reported. Adverse reactions (especially neurotoxic and extrapyramidal reactions) and delirium are reportedly increased in older adults. Nausea, vomiting, and other signs of lithium toxicity may be masked by the phenothiazines. Monitor physical symptoms and drug serum levels closely.
diuretics	Decreases lithium excretion, resulting in an increased lithium level and toxicity. A reduction in lithium dosage may be indicated. Monitor closely (see Box 19-8 for other factors affecting lithium serum levels).
fluoxetine (Prozac)	Lithium serum levels may be altered. Monitor serum lithium levels.
haloperidol (Haldol)	Concurrent use in early therapy has been associated with irreversible neurologic toxicity and brain damage in some cases. The clients usually had organic brain syndrome or another CNS impairment. However, this interaction is controversial within the profession. Be aware that extrapyramidal signs and symptoms may be increased with this combination and that clients should be closely monitored whenever this combination is used.
molindone (Moban)	Concurrent use may result in neurotoxicity as evidenced by confusion, convulsions, delirium, or abnormal EEG changes. Avoid concurrent administration.

A baseline assessment should include documentation of the client's symptoms, weight, blood pressure, ECG, electrolyte and renal function determinations, and WBC and differential count.

▪ **Nursing Diagnosis.** The client receiving lithium therapy has the potential for the following selected nursing diagnoses/collaborative problems: diarrhea; risk for imbal-

BOX 19-8

Factors Affecting Lithium Serum Levels

Serum lithium levels are:	Excretion of lithium is:
Increased by: Diarrhea; Diuretics or dehydration; Low-salt diets; High fevers or strenuous exercise	Decreased
Decreased by: High salt intake; High intake of sodium bicarbonate; Pregnancy	Increased

anced fluid volume; impaired comfort (thirst, anorexia, nausea, vomiting); disturbed sensory perception (confusion); and the potential complications of hypovolemia, electrolyte imbalances, and seizures.

■ **Implementation**

■ ***Monitoring.*** Assess the history of manic episodes, their occurrence and degree of severity, and the cyclic appearance of the pattern. Family intervention for treatment is essential when manic-depressive symptoms appear.

Serum lithium determinations are recommended once or twice weekly during the client's manic phase and until the client is stabilized; testing is performed every 2 to 3 months while the client is in remission. Test samples are drawn just before the morning dose of lithium, when there is maximum stabilization of the serum concentrations. Serum lithium levels above 1.5 mEq/L produce toxic reactions.

Monitor the client's WBC and energy level for tiredness because of possible leukemia. Monitor the ECG for changes and the blood pressure for hypotension. Weigh the client daily and check for indicators of edema. Monitor electrolytes (hyponatremia, hypercalcemia, and hypophosphatemia) and renal and thyroid (hypothyroidism) studies. Renal function should be monitored with urinalysis, blood urea nitrogen, and serum creatinine.

■ ***Intervention.*** Administer lithium after meals to prevent laxative action and to decrease gastric upset, tremors, or weakness by prolonging the absorption rate. Dilute the syrup in juice before administration. Do not mix it with or administer it at the same time as any other medication that contains a basic form. Ensure that the client has an adequate fluid intake of 2.5 to 3 L daily and sufficient sodium intake.

■ ***Education.*** Client compliance, cooperation, and commitment to adhere strictly to all therapy are essential to lithium therapy. The family should be advised, in language they can understand, of all ramifications of therapy—including the effects related to serum level. Discuss the overt clinical signs of lithium toxicity with the client, family, or closest companion. Some of these symptoms are diarrhea, vomiting, tremors, mild ataxia, lack of coordination, drowsiness, and muscular weakness. If any of these signs appear, the client is to discontinue therapy and notify the prescriber promptly. Advise the client of facilities where prompt and accurate serum lithium determinations may be obtained.

Discuss with the client and family the importance of a normal diet because lithium decreases sodium reabsorption by the renal tubules, which may produce sodium depletion. A fluid intake of 2500 to 3000 mL daily during the initial stabilization period is essential. The client should be cautioned to avoid fluid depletion; coffee, tea, and cola intake should be limited because of the diuretic effect, and exercise, saunas, and exposure to hot weather should be avoided. The client should be advised to seek the assistance of a health care provider for illnesses that cause diaphoresis, vomiting, or diarrhea.

Advise the client that it is necessary to take the medication consistently—initially because it takes 1 to 3 weeks for improvement of the condition and thereafter even though the symptoms may abate. Assess carefully for compliance to the regimen, particularly if the client has had an increase in weight. Weight gain is a major cause of noncompliance, especially in female clients. The importance of regular visits to the prescriber for the monitoring of serum lithium levels should be stressed to the client.

Impairment of alertness may occur, so the client should be instructed to avoid activities that require coordination and close attention until the response to therapy has been determined.

■ **Evaluation.** The expected outcome of lithium therapy is that the client will demonstrate improved mental status behaviors without experiencing adverse reactions to the drug.

SUMMARY

Emotions, and therefore behaviors, are the result of a final, unified effect of the CNS, autonomic regulation, and biochemical mechanisms. Because of their ability to modify these processes, drugs are important adjuncts to the treatment of psychiatric disorders. However, it is essential that antipsychotic drugs be prescribed only for appropriate, specific disorders to assist the client to cope more effectively with the environment and better use nonpharmacologic therapies. Using these drugs as a substitute for a therapeutic milieu constitutes misuse.

Since the advent of tranquilizers in the early 1950s, institutionalization for psychiatric disorders has decreased, not only in terms of duration for the individual client but also as the sole alternative as a setting for psychiatric care. Many clients are now treated at community mental health centers as a result of the administration of psychotherapeutic agents.

Phenothiazine derivatives constitute a major group of all antipsychotic drugs. Although the exact mechanism of their antipsychotic effect is not known, a primary effect is dopamine blockade in specific areas of the CNS. A major role for nursing with the phenothiazine derivatives is the assessment of the client for the development of side effects and adverse reactions, because many of them are debilitating and irreversible. Because many clients are treated in the community, health teaching for the safe and accurate self-administration of these medications is essential. Atypical antipsychotic agents include clozapine, olanzapine, quetiapine, and risperidone. Pimozide is indicated for the treatment of severe motor and vocal tics.

Antidepressant therapy is used for the treatment of affective disorders, or mood disturbances, with tricyclic antidepressants being used for major depressions, the MAOIs for atypical depressions, and the SSRIs for depressions without producing as many adverse reactions as the other antidepressants. Lithium is considered the drug of choice for bipolar affective disorders. There is no ideal psychotherapeutic agent, because all of them produce undesirable side effects or adverse reactions. The nurse's teaching role is important for safe and accurate self-administration of these agents and for the assessment of the untoward effects of the drugs.

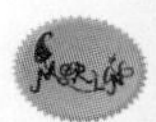

Critical Thinking Questions

1. Mrs. Thomas, age 84, has been admitted to an extended-care facility and has become increasingly combative over the first 3 days. One of the nursing assistants has indicated that she does not want to be assigned to care for Mrs. Thomas because she is afraid of her. As the nurse on the unit, you must decide whether or not Mrs. Thomas meets the criteria that must be met before an antipsychotic can be prescribed to a resident in an extended-care facility. What do you do?
2. Barbara Walton has a manic-depressive disorder for which she has been prescribed lithium 300 mg PO two times daily. On a recent visit to the clinic, her lithium blood level was 1.7 mEq/L. What action should you take?
3. Mr. Shapiro has had his depression treated unsuccessfully with tricyclic antidepressants. The prescriber is going to try to treat him with MAOIs. During the drug history, Mr. Shapiro lists the following dietary intake for the previous day: breakfast—black coffee, bran cereal with skim milk and a sliced banana on top; lunch—diet soda, bologna sandwich, and potato chips from the local lunch wagon; and dinner—salad, spaghetti, a little red wine, and garlic bread. He also stopped on the way home from work and had "a couple of beers with the guys." What instruction will you provide to assist Mr. Shapiro in managing his therapeutic regimen effectively?

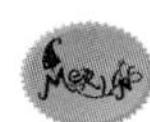

Collaborative Learning Activities

For Collaborative Learning Activities, go to mosby.com/MERLIN/McKenry/.

CASE STUDY

For a Case Study that will help ensure mastery of this chapter content, go to mosby.com/MERLIN/McKenry/.

BIBLIOGRAPHY

Abramowicz, M. (Ed.). (1994). Drugs for psychiatric disorders. *Medical Letter, 36*(933), 89-96.

American Hospital Formulary Service. (1999). *AHFS drug information '99.* Bethesda, MD: American Society of Hospital Pharmacists.

Anderson, K.N., Anderson, L.E., & Glanze, W.D. (Eds.) (1998). *Mosby's medical, nursing, and allied health dictionary* (5th ed.). St. Louis: Mosby.

Bhatia, S.C. & Bhatia, S.K. (1999). Depression in women: Diagnostic and treatment considerations. *American Family Physician, 60*(1), 225-234, 239-240.

Blin, O. (1999). A comparative review of the new antipsychotics. *Canadian Journal of Psychiatry, 44*(3), 235-244.

Bond, W.S. (1991). Ethnicity and psychotropic drugs. *Clinical Pharmacy, 10,* 467-470.

Brown, C.S. & Bryant, S.G. (1992). Major depressive disorders. In M.A. Koda-Kimble & L.Y. Young (Eds.). *Applied therapeutics: The clinical use of drugs* (5th ed.). Vancouver, WA: Applied Therapeutics.

Buckley, P.F. (1999). The role of typical and atypical antipsychotic medications in the management of agitation and aggression. *Journal of Clinical Psychiatry, 60*(suppl 10), 52-60.

Buckley, P.F. (1998). Novel antipsychotics and patient care in state hospitals. *The Annals of Pharmacotherapy, 32* (9), 906-914.

Casey, D.E. (1999). Tardive dyskinesia and atypical antipsychotic drugs. *Schizophrenic Research, 35*(suppl 35), S61-S66.

Carley, M. (1992). Unnecessary drug requirements. *Contemporary Long Term Care, 15*(12), 68.

Chengappa, K.N., Sheth, S., Brar, J.S., Parepally, H., Marcus, S., Gopalani, A., Palmer, A., Baker, R.W., & Schooler, N.R. (1999). Risperidone use at a state hospital: A clinical audit 2 years after the first wave of risperidone prescriptions. *Journal of Clinical Psychiatry, 60*(6), 373-378.

Cohen-Mansfield, J., Lipson, S., Werner, P., Billig, N., Taylor, L., & Woosley, R. (1999). Withdrawal of haloperidol, thioridazine, and lorazepam in the nursing home: A controlled, double-blind study. *Archives of Internal Medicine, 159*(15), 1733-1740.

Cumming, R.G. (1998). Epidemiology of medication-related falls and fractures in the elderly. *Drugs Aging, 12*(1), 43-53.

Depression Guideline Panel (1993). *Depression in primary care: Volume 2. Treatment of major depression. Clinical practice guideline #5.* Rockville, MD: Department of Health and Human Services, Public Health Service, Agency for Health Care Policy and Research. AHCPR pub. no. 93-0551.

Drug Facts and Comparisons. (2000). St. Louis: Facts and Comparisons.

Edwards, J.G. & Anderson, I. (1999). Systematic review and guide to selection of selective serotonin reuptake inhibitors. *Drugs, 57*(4), 507-533.

Ereshefsky, L. (1999). Pharmacologic and pharmacokinetic considerations in choosing an antipsychotic. *Journal of Clinical Psychiatry, 60* (suppl 10), 20-30.

Ereshefsky, L. & Richards, A.L. (1992). Psychoses. In M.A. Koda-Kimble & L.Y. Young (Eds.). *Applied therapeutics: The clinical use of drugs* (5th ed.). Vancouver, WA: Applied Therapeutics.

Fang, J. & Gorrod, J.W. (1999). Metabolism, pharmacogenetics, and metabolic drug-drug interactions of antipsychotic drugs. *Cellular Molecular Neurobiology, 19*(4), 491-510.

Forest Pharmaceuticals. (1999). Celexa (citalopram HBr). *Formulary, 34*(6), Rev 4/99.

Foster, S., Tyler, V.E. (2000). *Tyler's honest herbal* (4th ed.). New York: Haworth Herbal Press.

Geller, B., Reising, D., Leonard, H.L., Riddle, M.A., & Walsh, B.T. (1999). Critical review of tricyclic antidepressant use in children and adolescents. *Journal of the American Academy of Child and Adolescent Psychiatry, 38*(5), 513-516.

Generali, J.A. (1996). Serotonin syndrome. *Facts and Comparisons Drug Newsletter, 15*(10), 76-77.

Golden, A.G., Preston, R.A., Barnett, S.D., Llorente, M., Hamdan, K., & Silverman, M.A. (1999). Inappropriate medication prescribing in homebound older adults. *Journal of the American Geriatric Society, 47*(8), 948-953.

Hardman, J.G. & Limbird, L.E. (Eds.). (1996). *Goodman and Gilman's The pharmacological basis of therapeutics* (9th ed.). New York: Macmillan.

Harrigan, R.A. & Brady, W.J. (1999). ECG abnormalities in tricyclic antidepressant ingestion. *American Journal of Emergency Medicine, 17*(4), 387-393.

Hirschfield, R.M. (1999). Efficacy of SSRIs and newer antidepressants in severe depression: Comparison with TCAs. *Journal of Clinical Psychiatry, 60*(5), 326-335.

Jeste, D.V., Lacro, J.P., Bailey, A., Rockwell, E., Harris, M.J., & Caligiuri, M.P. (1999). Lower incidence of tardive dyskinesia with risperidone compared with haloperidol in older patients. *Journal of American Geriatric Society, 47*(6), 716-719.

Kando, J.C., Yonkers, K.A., & Cole, J.O. (1995). Gender as a risk factor for adverse events to medications. *Drugs, 50*(1), 1-6.

Katzung, B.G. (1998). *Basic and clinical pharmacology* (7th ed.). Norwalk, CT: Appleton & Lange.

Keltner, N.L. & Folks, D.G. (1993). *Psychotropic drugs*. St. Louis: Mosby.

Keltner, N.L. & Folks, D.G. (1992). Culture as a variable in drug therapy. *Perspectives on Psychiatric Care, 28*(1), 33-36.

Laird, L.K. & Benefield, W.H. (1995). Mood disorders I: Major depressive disorders. In L.Y. Young & M.A. Koda-Kimble (Eds.), *Applied therapeutics: The clinical use of drugs* (6th ed.). Vancouver, WA: Applied Therapeutics.

Lasser, R.A. & Sunderland, T. (1998). Newer psychotropic medication use in nursing home residents. *Journal of American Geriatric Society, 46*(2), 202-207.

Lin, T. (1986). Multiculturalism and Canadian psychiatry: Opportunities and challenges. *Canadian Journal of Psychiatry, 31*(7), 681.

Love, R.C. & Grothe, D.R. (1995). Mood disorders II: Bipolar affective disorders. In L.Y. Young & M.A. Koda-Kimble (Eds.), *Applied therapeutics: The clinical use of drugs* (6th ed.). Vancouver, WA: Applied Therapeutics.

Lyons, A.S. & Petrucelli, R.J. (1978). *Medicine: An illustrated history*. New York: Harry N. Abrams.

Marcos, L. & Cancro, R. (1982). Pharmacotherapy of Hispanic depressed patients: Clinical observations. *American Journal of Psychotherapy, 36*, 505.

Marken, P.A. & Stanislav, S.W. (1995). Schizophrenia. In L.Y. Young & M.A. Koda-Kimble (Eds.), *Applied therapeutics: The clinical use of drugs* (6th ed.). Vancouver, WA: Applied Therapeutics.

Medicare and Medicaid (1989). *OBRA requirements for long-term care facilities*. Section 483.60 Level A Requirement: Pharmacy services; Section 483.10 Level A Requirement: Resident rights; Section 483.20 Level A Requirement: Resident assessment; Section 482.25 Level A Requirement: Quality of care and interpretive guidelines. Washington, DC: Health Care Financing Administration.

Montano, C.B. (1994). Recognition and treatment of depression in a primary care setting. *Journal of Clinical Psychiatry, 55*(12 suppl), 18.

Mosby's GenRx. (1999). St. Louis: Mosby.

Physician's Desk Reference (53rd ed.). (1999). Oradell, NJ: Medical Economics.

Stahl, S.M. (1999). Selecting an atypical antipsychotic by combining clinical experience with guidelines from clinical trials. *Journal of Clinical Psychiatry, 60*(suppl 10), 31-41.

Stevens, T., Katona, C., Manela, M., Watkin, V., & Livingston, G. (1999). Drug treatment of older people with affective disorders in the community: Lessons from an attempted clinical trial. *International Journal of Geriatric Psychiatry, 14*(6), 467-472.

Stramek R. et al. (1991). Prevalence of tardive dyskinesia among three ethnic groups of chronic psychiatric patients. *Hospital & Community Psychiatry, 42*, 590.

United States Pharmacopeia Dispensing Information (USP DI): Drug information for the health care professional (19th ed.). (1999). Rockville, MD: United States Pharmacopeial Convention.

Wells, B.G. (Ed.). (1994). *Therapeutic options in the treatment of depression: A special report*. Washington, DC: American Pharmaceutical Association.

Wintz, C.J. (1998). Nursing management of psychotropic drug reactions. *Nursing Clinics of North America, 33*(1), 217-231.

Yonkers, K.A., Kanders, J.C., Cole, J.O., & Blumenthal, S. (1992). Gender differences in pharmacokinetics and pharmacodynamics of psychotropic medication. *American Journal of Psychiatry, 149*(5), 587-595.

Zal, H.M. (1994). Depression in the elderly: Differing presentations, wide choice of therapies. *Consultant 34*(3), 354-356, 358, 361.

Zyprexa. (1996). Package insert. Eli Lilly Industries, #PV2960.

20 Overview of the Autonomic Nervous System

Chapter Focus

The autonomic nervous system (ANS) regulates the functions of internal viscera such as the heart, blood vessels, digestive organs, and reproductive organs; therefore a functional knowledge of this system is essential. An understanding of this chapter will allow the nurse to predict general responses to a variety of stimuli, explain responses to changes in the environment, understand symptoms that result from ANS dysfunction, and know how drugs affect the ANS.

Learning Objectives

1. Describe the reflex control system.
2. Explain the major differences between the parasympathetic and sympathetic divisions of the autonomic nervous system.
3. Name the primary neurotransmitters for the parasympathetic and sympathetic divisions of the autonomic nervous system.
4. State the primary disposition of the neurotransmitters following release from their respective nerves.
5. Identify the three basic characteristics of the autonomic nervous system.

Key Terms

adrenergic, p. 432
autonomic nervous system, p. 431
catecholamine, p. 436
cholinergic, p. 432
feedback control mechanism, p. 431
muscarinic (M) receptors, p. 435
neuroeffector junction, p. 432
neurohumoral transmission, p. 432
neurotransmitter, p. 432
nicotinic (N) receptors, p. 435
reflex arc, p. 431
somatic nervous system, p. 438
synaptic junction, p. 432

The **autonomic nervous system** (ANS) functions primarily as a regulatory or self-governing system for maintaining the internal environment of the body at an optimal level (homeostasis). This system automatically controls the function of smooth muscle, cardiac muscle, and glandular secretions, which interact in many vital physiologic tasks. Digestion of a meal, maintenance of the pressure of circulating blood, and many other processes are internally regulated by the ANS.

REFLEX CONTROL SYSTEM

The nervous system is the important control and communication system within the body. It collects information about conditions inside and outside of the body. The simplest means by which the nervous system responds to environmental change is through the action of the reflex arc. The **reflex arc** is the automatic motor response to sensory stimuli. In any reflex a nerve fiber conducts a nerve impulse; these impulses form the basis of communication of information through the nervous system.

The reflex arc consists of two major functional processes: sensory input and motor output. The first component of the reflex arc is the receptor, which detects environmental changes such as temperature, pressure in blood vessels, and distention in the viscera. These changes are responsible for producing a stimulus in the receptor. Information from the sensitized receptor is transmitted as a nerve impulse along the afferent neuron to the central nervous system (CNS), the site of integration. The CNS then issues instructions as an altered motor nerve impulse along the efferent neuron to the effector, which produces the appropriate movements of muscles and glands.

The information carried *to* the CNS (sensory input) and instructions sent *from* the CNS (motor output) constitute a **feedback control mechanism.** Information fed back to the CNS from a receptor is modulated so that nerve impulses may vary in frequency and pattern according to the degree of activity required of the effector. The control of visceral function is involuntary; the feedback mechanism must include all the components of a control system essential for performing the reflex act. Therefore reflex action functions as a feedback mechanism, operating from a receptor to an effector. Its purpose is to prevent extreme changes in function that may create a disturbance in the internal environment.

A good example of feedback control is the blood pressure–regulating reflex. Again, the sequence of events follows the pattern of the reflex arc. The carotid sinus in the carotid artery and the aortic sinus in the aortic arch serve as pressure receptors (baroreceptors) that are highly sensitive to stretch; the degree of wall stretching is determined by the amount of pressure within these vessels. Any increase in blood pressure stimulates the baroreceptors, and this information is conveyed as nerve impulses along the afferent neuron to the vasomotor center in the medulla.

The medulla is the CNS site for integration of blood pressure regulation. After the appropriate neuronal connections have been made, a decrease in sympathetic discharge is conducted along the efferent neuron to the effectors, which produces relaxation of arteriolar smooth muscles. This relaxation causes dilation of the arteries and a reduction in blood pressure. This is only a partial explanation of blood pressure regulation, because a decrease in arterial pressure produces the opposite response in the same neuronal pathway. In addition, this control mechanism operates in coordination with cardiac function.

CLASSIFICATION OF THE NERVOUS SYSTEM

The nervous system is classified on the basis of the reflex arc. The two main divisions are the CNS and the peripheral nervous system (PNS). The CNS consists of the brain and spinal cord and performs the important integrative functions from the peripheral sources. The PNS has two divisions: (1) the somatic nervous system, which innervates voluntary or skeletal muscles; and (2) the ANS, which influences the involuntary activities of smooth muscles, cardiac muscles, and glands. The afferent fibers of both systems are the first link in the reflex arc; they carry sensory information to the CNS. After integration at various levels in the brain, the outflow from the CNS is conducted along either the somatic efferent system or the autonomic efferent system. Both of these systems constitute the final link in the reflex arc (Figure 20-1).

Several centers in the CNS integrate all activities of the ANS. There is evidence that the hypothalamus, in particular, performs such integrating activities. It contains centers that regulate body temperature, water balance, and carbohydrate and fat metabolism. It also integrates mechanisms concerned with emotional behavior, the waking state, and sleep. A series of "vital centers" in the medulla oblongata, including the vasomotor center, respiratory center, and car-

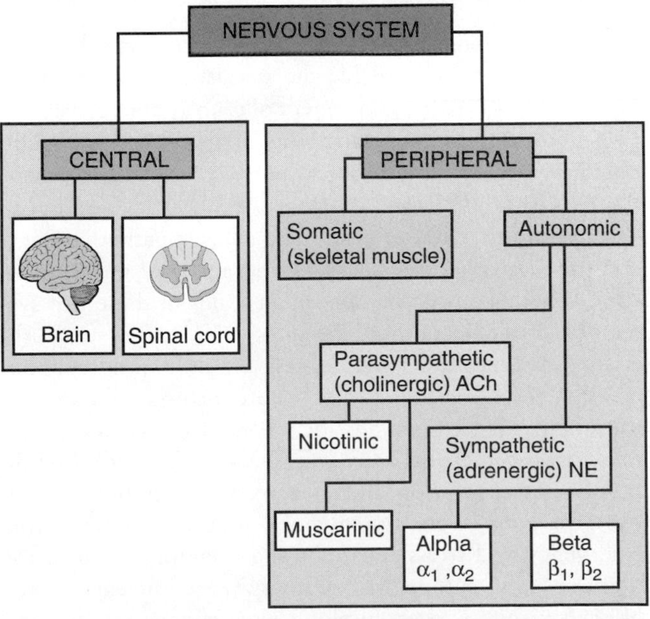

Figure 20-1 Divisions of the nervous system.

BOX 20-1

Autonomic Nervous System Terminology

Over the years various terms have been used to describe the division of the ANS. The anatomic names are sympathetic and parasympathetic; the corresponding functional terms, which relate to the primary neurotransmitters for each system, are adrenergic and cholinergic, respectively. In general, these terms are used interchangeably (i.e., sympathetic or adrenergic and parasympathetic or cholinergic nervous systems). It is important to understand the terms *parasympathomimetic* and *sympathomimetic*, which means to mimic or produce an effect similar to the activation of either system. The terms *parasympatholytic* or *sympatholytic* imply a blocking of the effects normally seen when either system is activated. The term *anticholinergic* is synonymous with the term *parasympatholytic*.

Anatomic Name	Functional Name	Primary Neurotransmitter
Sympathetic	Adrenergic	Norepinephrine
Parasympathetic	Cholinergic	Acetylcholine

diac center, integrate the control of the life-essential activities of blood pressure, respiration, and cardiac function, respectively. The midbrain, limbic system, cerebellum, and cerebral cortex are involved in the control of the ANS and the physiologic functions regulated by it.

DIFFERENCES BETWEEN THE PARASYMPATHETIC AND SYMPATHETIC NERVOUS SYSTEMS

The ANS is organized into two subdivisions: (1) the parasympathetic system and (2) the sympathetic system (Box 20-1). The anatomic arrangement of each system consists of two motor nerves, a preganglionic nerve and a postganglionic nerve; a ganglion (group of nerve cell bodies) connects the two neurons (Figure 20-2).

Physiologic Differences. The parasympathetic system and the sympathetic system innervate many of the same organs simultaneously; the opposing actions of these two systems balance one another. The parasympathetic system, otherwise known as the system of rest and digestion, functions mainly to conserve energy and restore the body resources of the organism. Its functions include cardiac deceleration, a rise in gastrointestinal activity associated with increased digestion and absorption, and an increase in excretion. In contrast, the sympathetic system mobilizes the organism during emergency and stress situations and therefore is called the "fight or flight" system. Its functions involve the expenditure of energy and increases in blood sugar concentration, heart activity, and blood pressure (Table 20-1).

Anatomic and Pharmacologic Differences. The preganglionic fibers of the parasympathetic (cholinergic) system emerge with cranial nerves III, VII, IX, and X and at the sacral spinal levels from about S3 through S4. The tenth cranial nerve, or vagus nerve, has extensive branches that supply fibers to the heart, lungs, and almost all of the abdominal organs.

The sympathetic (adrenergic) system is also called the thoracolumbar system because its preganglionic fibers originate in the spinal cord from the thoracic segment at level T1 to the lumbar segment at level L2 (Figure 20-3 and Table 20-2).

NEUROHUMORAL TRANSMISSION

There is general agreement that information in the nervous system is transmitted both electrically and chemically. This phenomenon occurs because nerve cells have two special characteristics: (1) they can conduct electrical signals, and (2) they have intercellular connections with other nerve cells and with innervated tissues such as muscles and glands. The passage of a nerve impulse or an action potential along a nerve fiber or a muscle fiber is called conduction. The presence of a specific chemical at the intercellular connections determines the type of information a neuron can receive and the range of responses it can yield in return. The passage of a nerve impulse across a synaptic or neuroeffector junction with the use of a chemical is called **neurohumoral transmission.**

Although each nerve fiber may conduct an impulse along the neuron, it is solely the chemical substance called the **neurotransmitter** or neurohormone that permits the action potential of a neuron to cross (1) the **synaptic junction** from one neuron to another neuron, or (2) the **neuroeffector junction** from a neuron to an effector organ. In this mechanism the arrival of an action potential at a nerve terminal starts the release of the neurotransmitter. This hormone or mediator then acts as a messenger by which nerve cells communicate information to the structures they innervate. The neurotransmitter exerts its influence primarily at the junctional spaces (synaptic junction or neuroeffector junction) to facilitate the transmission of impulses to their final destination. Many drugs may also act selectively at these junctions.

Types of Neurohumoral Transmission

The neurohormones acetylcholine and norepinephrine are responsible for neurohumoral transmission. Nerves that contain acetylcholine are called **cholinergic** neurons and are involved in cholinergic transmission. Nerves that contain norepinephrine or epinephrine (from the adrenal medulla) are known as **adrenergic** neurons and are associated with adrenergic transmission.

In neurohumoral transmission the sequence of events includes (1) biosynthesis, (2) storage, (3) release, (4) action, and (5) inactivation of the mediator (Figures 20-4 and 20-5).

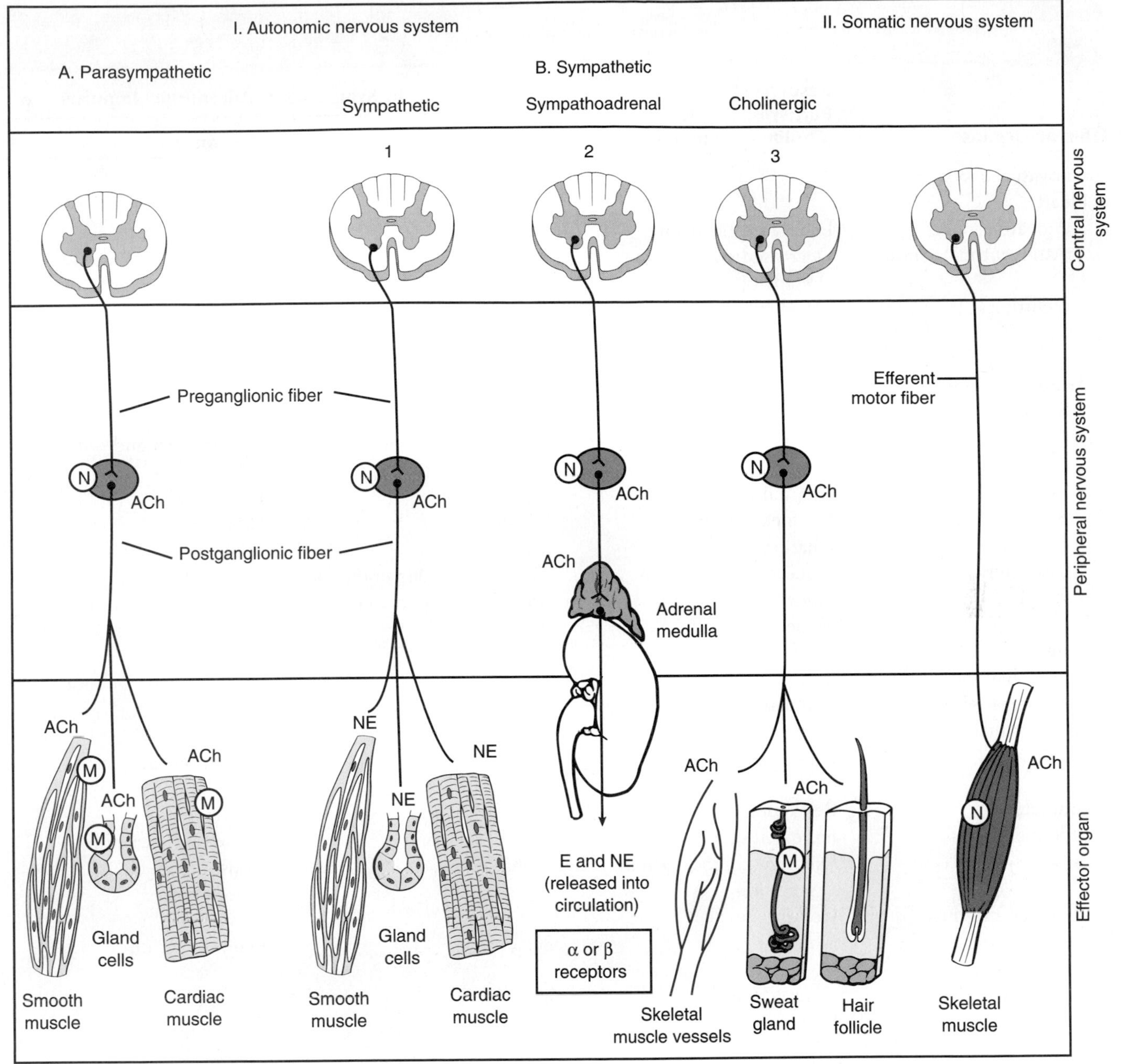

Figure 20-2 Schema of receptor sites for neurohumoral transmission. I, Autonomic nervous system, where preganglionic fibers of both parasympathetic and sympathetic nerves synapse in the ganglia. II, Somatic motor nervous system. *N*, Nicotinic sites; *M*, muscarinic sites; *ACh*, acetylcholine; *E*, epinephrine; *NE*, norepinephrine.

Many autonomic drugs affect one of these individual events, and it is essential to understand the basic mechanisms involved in this complicated process. These drugs have been useful in treating many persons afflicted with autonomic disorders.

Cholinergic Transmission

Synthesis and Storage. Acetylcholine is synthesized in the cytoplasm of the nerve terminal. Once synthesized, the acetylcholine is stored in packets called synaptic vesicles or granules, which are located in the nerve terminal (see Figure 20-4, *A*, 2). The formula for cholinergic transmission is as follows:

$$\text{Acetyl coenzyme A} + \text{Choline} \underset{\text{Acetylcholinesterase}}{\overset{\text{Choline acetylase}}{\rightleftarrows}} \text{Acetylcholine} + \text{Coenzyme A}$$

Release and Action. The arrival of an action potential at the nerve ending causes the vesicle to approach the

TABLE 20-1 Effector Organ Responses to Autonomic Nerve Impulses

Effector Organs	Response to Parasympathetic (Cholinergic) Impulses	Response to Sympathetic (Adrenergic) Impulses	
		Receptor	Response
Cardiovascular system			
Heart			
Sinoatrial node	Decreased heart rate	Beta$_1$, beta$_2$	Increased heart rate
Atrioventricular node	Decreased conduction velocity	Beta$_1$, beta$_2$	Increased automaticity and conduction velocity
Ventricles	No innervation	Beta$_1$, beta$_2$	Increased force of contraction and conduction velocity
Arterioles (smooth muscle)			
Coronary	Dilation	Alpha$_1$, alpha$_2$, beta$_2$, dopaminergic	Constriction and dilation
Skin and mucosa	Dilation	Alpha$_1$, alpha$_2$	Constriction
Skeletal muscle	No innervation	Cholinergic	Dilation
Cerebral	Dilation	Alpha$_1$	Slight constriction
Mesenteric	None	Alpha, beta$_2$, dopaminergic	Constriction and dilation
Renal	None	Alpha, beta$_2$, dopaminergic	Constriction and dilation
Veins	None	Alpha, beta$_2$	Constriction and dilation
Lung			
Bronchial muscle	Bronchoconstriction	Beta$_2$	Relaxation (bronchodilation)
Bronchial glands	Stimulation	Alpha$_1$, beta$_2$	Inhibition
Gastrointestinal tract			
Motility	Increased motility	Alpha, beta$_2$	Relaxation (decreased motility)
Sphincters	Relaxation	Alpha	Contraction
Exocrine glands	Increased secretion	—	Decreased secretion
Salivary glands	Dilation: copious, watery secretion	Alpha	Constriction: thick, viscous secretion
Gallbladder and ducts	Contraction		Relaxation
Kidney	None	Beta$_2$	Renin secretion
Urinary bladder			
Detrusor muscle	Contraction	Beta$_2$	Relaxation
Sphincter	Relaxation	Alpha$_1$	Contraction
Eye			
Radial muscle Iris	Contraction of sphincter muscle (miosis, pupillary constriction)	Alpha$_1$	Contraction of radial muscle (mydriasis)
Ciliary muscle	Contracted for near vision	Beta$_2$	Relaxation for far vision
Liver	Glycogen synthesis	Alpha, beta$_2$	Glycogenolysis, gluconeogenesis
Pancreas	Secretion	Alpha	Decreased secretion
Skin	None	Beta$_2$	Increased secretion
Sweat glands	No innervation	Cholinergic	Increased sweating
Pilomotor muscle	No innervation	Alpha$_1$	Contraction (gooseflesh)
Lacrimal glands	Increased secretion	Alpha	No innervation
Nasopharyngeal glands	Increased secretion		No innervation
Male sex glands	Erection	Alpha$_1$	Ejaculation

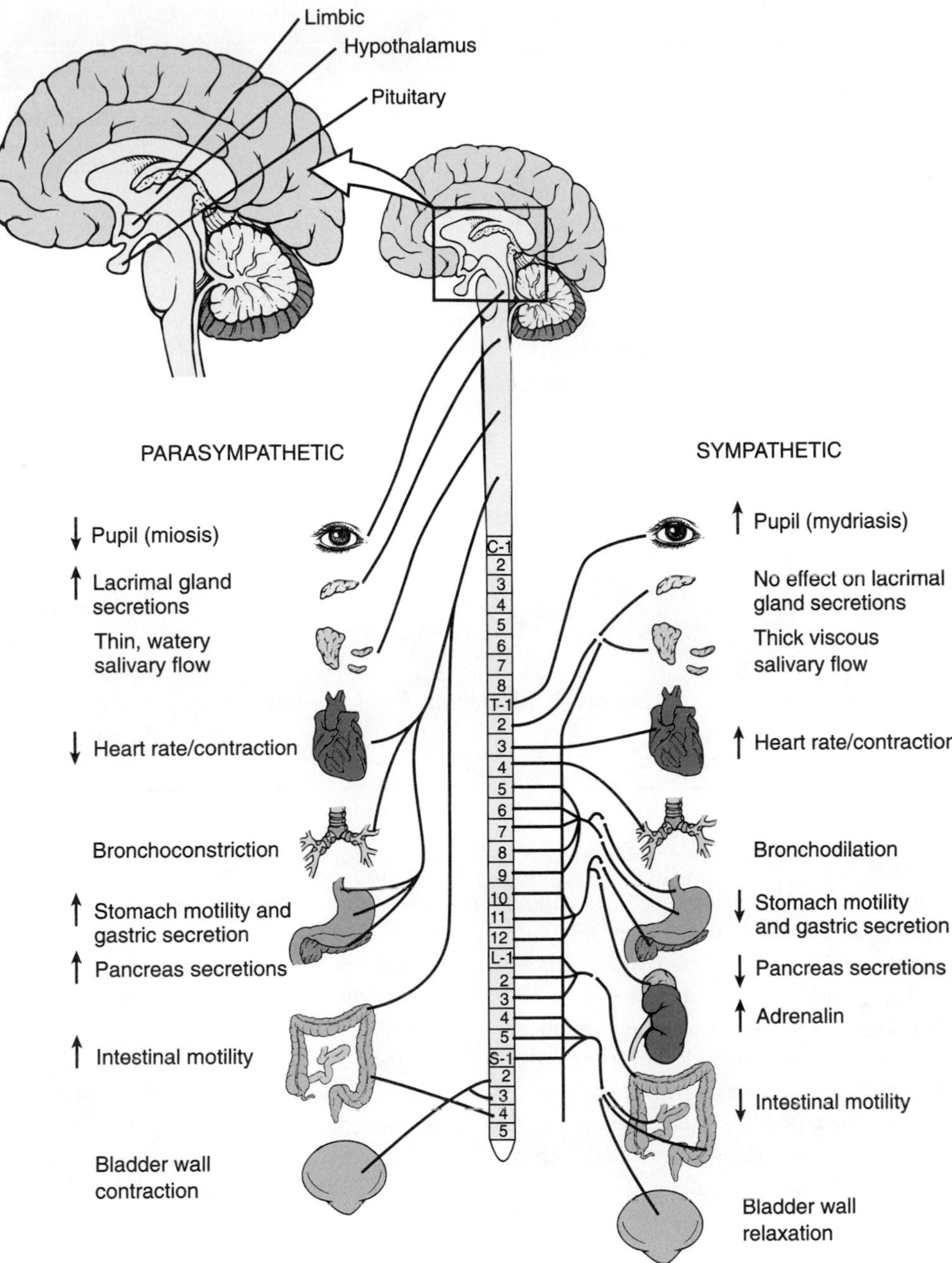

Figure 20-3 Diagram of the autonomic nervous system.

membrane and release the acetylcholine molecules into the synaptic cleft or space. Calcium ions must be present foran efficient release. Once free, the acetylcholine diffuses across the synaptic or junctional cleft and attaches itself to specialized receptors (postjunctional sites) on the membrane of the next neuron or neuroeffector. The binding of acetylcholine to the receptor increases the permeability of the membrane to sodium and potassium ions; the depolarizing action that results leads to the excitation or inhibition of neural, muscular, or glandular activity (see Figure 20-4, *A*, 3).

Cholinergic Receptors. The cholinergic receptor sites that are stimulated by acetylcholine are either nicotinic or muscarinic. **Nicotinic (N) receptors** appear in the ganglia of both the parasympathetic and sympathetic fibers, the adrenal medulla, and the skeletal (striated) muscle supplied by the somatic motor system. **Muscarinic (M) receptors** (postganglionic sites) are located in the smooth muscle, cardiac muscle, and glands of the parasympathetic fibers and the effector organs of the cholinergic sympathetic fibers. N and M receptors are shown in Figure 20-2.

Inactivation. Once acetylcholine has exerted its effect on the postjunctional sites, the excess amount is inactivated rapidly by the enzyme acetylcholinesterase. The metabolites formed in this reaction are chemically inactive and are the same compounds from which acetylcholine is formed. Inactivation of this neurohormone is shown as a reverse action in the preceding formula (see Figure 20-4, *A*, 5).

TABLE 20-2 Differentiating Characteristics Between the Parasympathetic and Sympathetic Nervous Systems

Characteristic	Parasympathetic Nervous System	Sympathetic Nervous System
Origin	Craniosacral	Thoracolumbar
Structure innervation	Cardiac muscle Smooth muscle Glands Viscera	Cardiac muscle Smooth muscle Glands Viscera
Ganglia	Near the effector (vagus, atria of heart)	Near CNS
Length of fibers	Preganglionics (long) Preganglionics (short)	Postganglionics (short) Postganglionics (long)
Ratio of preganglionics to postganglionics	Branching is minimal (1:2); very discrete, fine responses	High degree of nerve branching (1:11, 1:17)
Response	Discrete	Diffuse
Ganglion transmitter	Acetylcholine	Acetylcholine
Transmitter substance (postganglionic nerve endings)	Acetylcholine	Norepinephrine (most cases); epinephrine and norepinephrine (adrenal medulla) Acetylcholine for sweat glands and blood vessels of skeletal muscles
Blocking drugs (postganglionic nerve endings)	Cholinergic blocking agents (atropine)	Adrenergic blocking agents Alpha: phentolamine Beta: propranolol

Adrenergic Transmission

The term **catecholamine** refers to a group of chemically related compounds: norepinephrine (noradrenaline), epinephrine (adrenaline), and dopamine. All of these compounds are involved in some aspect of adrenergic transmission.

Synthesis and Storage. The catecholamines produced by the sympathetic nervous system include norepinephrine and epinephrine. The complex pathway for the synthesis of these neurotransmitters is mediated by different enzymes located in the postganglionic nerve terminals and in the chromaffin cells of the adrenal medullary glands.

The formation of norepinephrine is initiated by tyrosine, an amino acid derived from proteins in the diet. When tyrosine enters the cytoplasm of the nerve terminal, it is converted into dopa, which in turn is decarboxylated into dopamine. Dopamine is taken up into the storage vesicles, or granules, where it is transformed into the neurotransmitter norepinephrine by the enzyme dopamine β–hydroxylase. Figure 20-5, *1* shows the steps of the process of synthesis for adrenergic transmission.

In the adrenal medullary gland, the enzyme methyltransferase converts norepinephrine to epinephrine. On stimulation, both epinephrine and norepinephrine are released from the adrenal medulla and are carried by the circulation to all parts of the body.

Release. The arrival of an action potential at the nerve terminal of the postganglionic fibers causes the vesicles to fuse with the cell membrane and release the stored supply of norepinephrine into the junctional cleft. Calcium ions must be present to enhance the release of norepinephrine from the vesicles. The free form of norepinephrine then diffuses across the cleft to the receptor sites on the postjunctional membrane of neuroeffector cells (smooth muscle, cardiac muscle, or glands) (see Figure 20-5, *3*).

Action. Once the norepinephrine combines with either the alpha or beta receptor sites on the membrane of the neuroeffector cells, a series of chemical and electrical events produces either an excitatory or an inhibitory effect. The alpha receptor activation is primarily responsible for an excitatory response, although it results in intestinal relaxation. By contrast, beta receptor activation is usually inhibitory except in the myocardial cells, where norepinephrine produces an excitatory effect.

Adrenergic Receptors. The adrenergic receptor sites that are stimulated by the endogenous catecholamines—norepinephrine, epinephrine, and dopamine—are classified as alpha and beta receptors. Both classes have two subtypes. The alpha receptors are identified by neuronal location: (1) $alpha_1$ sites are located on the postsynaptic effector cells, and (2) $alpha_2$ sites appear on the presynaptic nerve terminals, controlling the amount of norepinephrine release that operates through a negative feedback mechanism. By contrast, the beta receptors are designated by organ location: (1) $beta_1$ receptors are located primarily in the heart, and (2) $beta_2$ receptors appear in the smooth muscle of the bronchioles, arterioles, and various other visceral organs in the body. At least five types of dopamine receptors have been identified in the CNS. D_1 and D_2 receptors are associated with the antipsychotic medications and movement disorders, such as Parkinson's disease. Stimulation of D_2 recep-

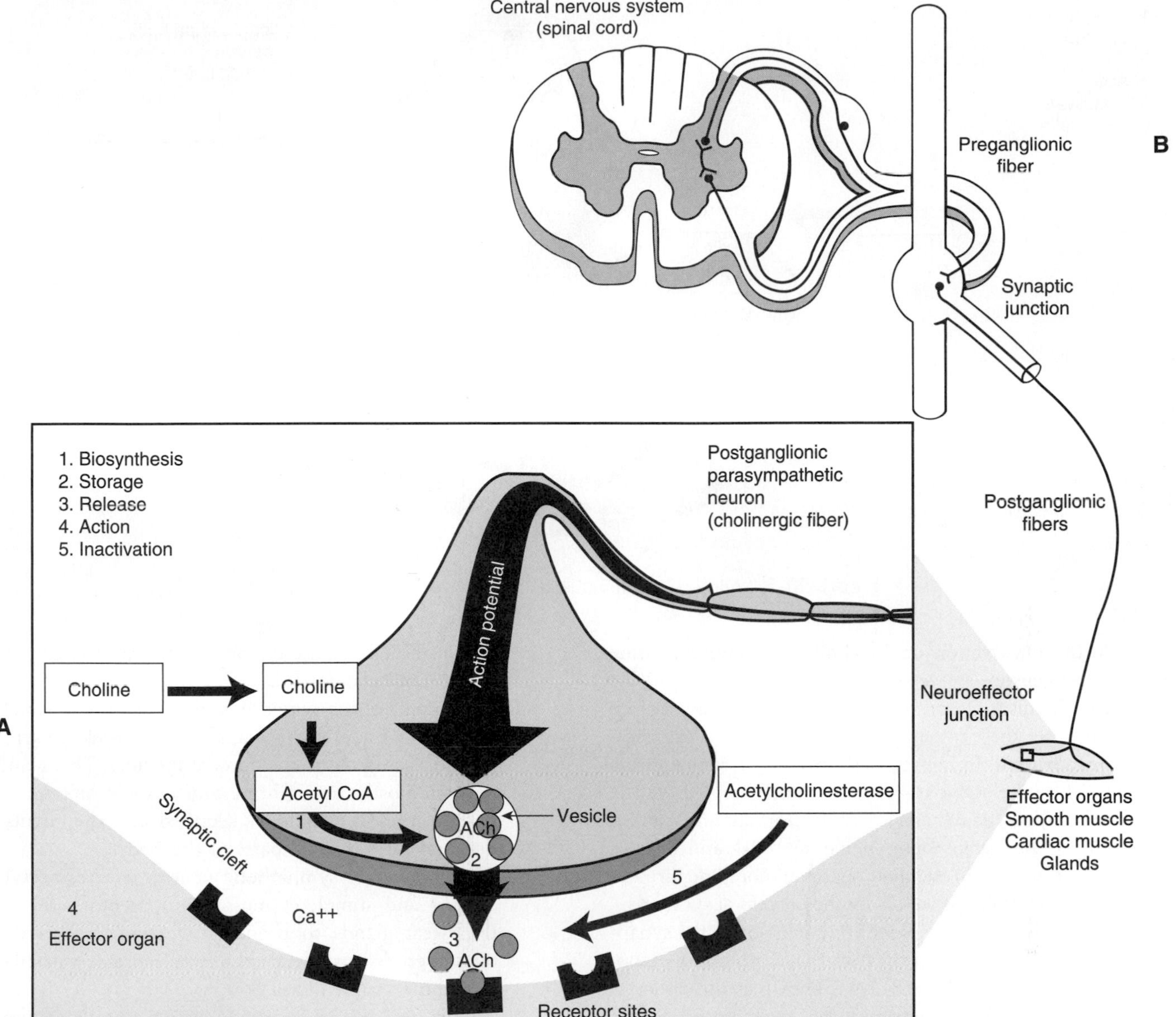

Figure 20-4 A, Cholinergic transmission. Schematic diagram of parasympathetic postganglionic neuron, showing steps in cholinergic transmission at the neuroeffector junction. *1*, Biosynthesis of acetylcholine *(ACh)*: Choline is taken up by the nerve terminal and interacts with acetyl coenzyme A to synthesize ACh. *2*, Storage: Following synthesis, ACh is stored in the vesicle until the arrival of a nerve impulse. *3*, Release: An action potential of the nerve terminal causes the vesicle to attach itself to the membrane and release ACh. The neurohormone then diffuses across the synaptic cleft and combines with the receptors on the effector cell. *4*, Action: The interaction of ACh with the receptor sites results in a motor response. *5*, Inactivation of ACh: At the synaptic cleft, ACh is hydrolyzed by the enzyme acetylcholinesterase. **B**, Schematic representation to show the relationship between a neuron in the CNS, a neuron in a peripheral ganglion, and an effector organ supplied by the parasympathetic nerve.

tors is primarily responsible for antiparkinson drug activity; the D_1 receptors may play a similar but smaller role in this area.

Inactivation. Once norepinephrine has performed its adrenergic function, its action must be rapidly stopped to prevent prolongation of its effects, which could lead to a loss of regulatory control of visceral function. The inactivation of norepinephrine occurs by (1) enzymatic transformation, (2) reuptake of the norepinephrine into nerve terminals, and (3) diffusion.

Catecholamines are metabolized by two enzymes, monoamine oxidase (MAO) and catechol O-methyltransferase (COMT). MAO, which is stored in the mitochondria of sympathetic neurons, metabolizes free norepinephrine within the cytoplasm of the nerve terminal. COMT, which is located outside the neuron or at the synaptic cleft, partici-

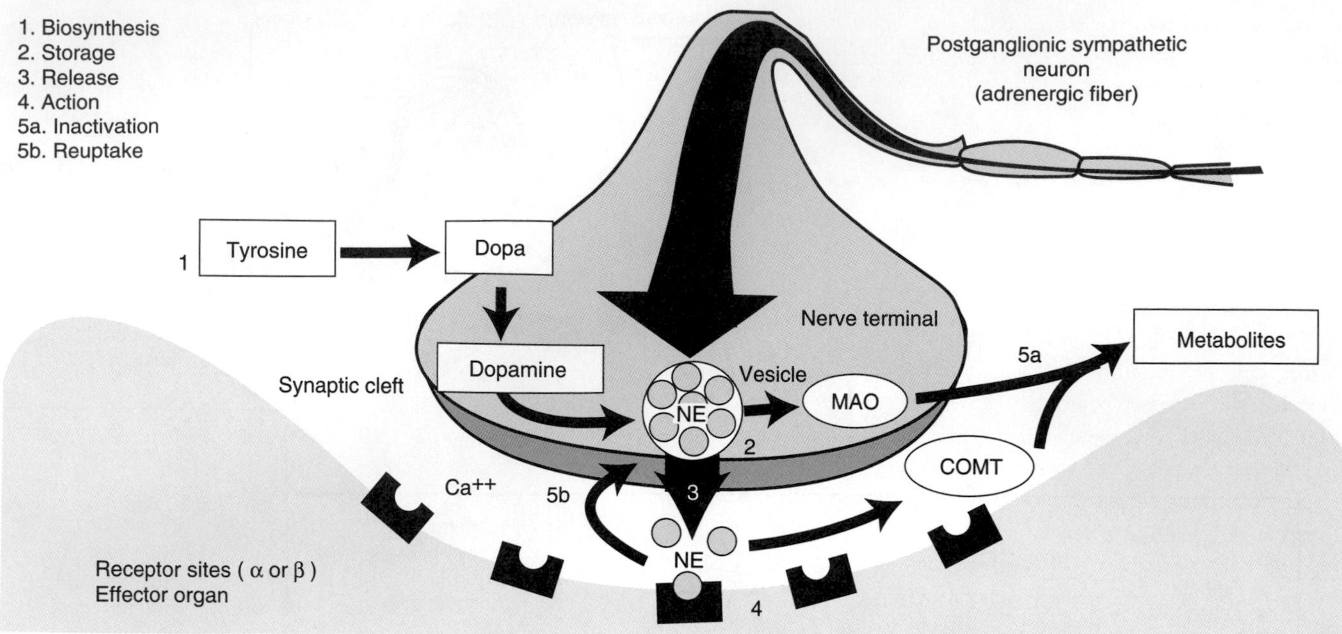

Figure 20-5 Adrenergic transmission at the neuroeffector junction.

pates in the inactivation or metabolism of norepinephrine outside the neuron.

The mechanism of norepinephrine reuptake plays a more significant role than enzymatic transformation in catecholamine inactivation. In the reuptake process, norepinephrine is removed by the active transport ("amine pump") from the junctional sites (synaptic and neuroeffector junctions) and is returned to the sympathetic nerve terminal and storage vesicles. In this way, an adequate supply of norepinephrine is provided by reuptake, as well as by the process of synthesis.

A small portion of norepinephrine released at the synaptic cleft may be picked up by the circulation and metabolized elsewhere in the body. This is known as the diffusion process. Figure 20-5, *5* portrays the steps in adrenergic transmission.

General Actions of Autonomic Transmitters

The location and chemical differences between the autonomic transmitters were identified many years ago. In the ANS, all of the preganglionic fibers originate in the CNS and synapse with the ganglia of the postganglionic fibers. The terminals of all the preganglionic fibers release acetylcholine and interact with nicotinic receptors in the membrane of the postganglionic fibers or the adrenal medulla.

In the parasympathetic system the terminals of the postganglionic fibers also release acetylcholine and interact with muscarinic receptors in the membrane of the smooth muscle, cardiac muscle, and glands.

There are three different types of postganglionic neurons in the sympathetic nervous system:

1. The sympathetic neuron, the major type, releases norepinephrine and activates either alpha or beta receptors in the membrane of the smooth muscle, cardiac muscle, and glands.
2. An example of the sympathoadrenal neuron, in which the preganglionic fiber synapses with a modified sympathetic ganglion, is the adrenal medulla. This gland releases mostly epinephrine and a small amount of norepinephrine, which are secreted into the circulation and carried to all parts of the body.
3. The cholinergic sympathetic neuron releases acetylcholine and stimulates muscarinic receptor sites on the sweat glands to produce sweating and on the blood vessels in skeletal muscle to increase vasodilation and enhance blood flow.

In the **somatic (sensory) nervous system** a single neuron, the efferent (motor) fiber, releases acetylcholine and interacts with the nicotinic sites on the skeletal muscle membrane. The autonomic drugs play an important role by enhancing or inhibiting physiologic activity at these sites of neurohumoral transmission (see Figure 20-2 and Table 20-2).

SUMMARY

A basic knowledge of the anatomy and physiology of the ANS is essential to the nurse's understanding of the pharmacology of autonomic drugs. This knowledge will help the nurse to predict the effects of drugs that stimulate or block autonomic function.

The primary function of the ANS is to control and integrate the many physiologic tasks necessary to preserve internal homeostasis, emergency mechanisms, and repair. Its activities are integrated by a number of centers within the CNS: the hypothalamus, medulla oblongata, midbrain, limbic system, cerebellum, and cerebral cortex. The ANS innervates the smooth muscles, cardiac muscles, and glands. It is composed of two divisions: parasympathetic and sympathetic. The actions of the parasympathetic and sympathetic divisions oppose and balance each other:

1. Although both systems are present in the body, only one is predominant at any given time.
2. If an ANS function is blocked, the opposite effect will take precedence.
3. Drugs are available to stimulate or block either system.

The functions stimulated by the parasympathetic system are chiefly those concerned with digestion, excretion, near vision, cardiac deceleration, and anabolism. The functions stimulated by the sympathetic system are primarily those concerned with the expenditure of energy and are called into play by physical or emotional stress.

Nerve impulse transmission is caused by the activity of chemical substances called neurotransmitters: acetylcholine and the catecholamines (norepinephrine and epinephrine). Nerve fibers that synthesize and liberate acetylcholine are known as cholinergic fibers; those that synthesize and secrete norepinephrine and epinephrine are called adrenergic fibers.

Critical Thinking Questions

1. Your client's blood pressure has suddenly dropped. How would the sympathetic reflexes that control blood vessels respond (1) to a sudden decrease in blood pressure or (2) to a sudden increase in blood pressure?
2. Clients with diabetes mellitus may develop autonomic neuropathy (i.e., degeneration of the ANS nerves). Which parts of the ANS are involved with the following symptoms:
   a. Lack of pain with a heart attack
   b. Constipation
   c. Impotence
   d. Decreased pupillary response to light

Collaborative Learning Activities

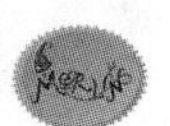

For Collaborative Learning Activities, go to mosby.com/MERLIN/McKenry/.

BIBLIOGRAPHY

Anderson, K.N., Anderson, L.E., & Glanze, W.D. (Eds.) (1998). *Mosby's medical, nursing, & allied health dictionary* (5th ed.). St. Louis: Mosby.

Guyton, A.C. (1990). *Textbook of medical physiology* (8th ed.). Philadelphia: W.B. Saunders.

Hardman, J.G. & Limbird, L.E. (Eds.) (1996). *Goodman & Gilman's The pharmacological basis of therapeutics* (9th ed.). New York: McGraw-Hill.

McCance, K.L. & Huether, S.E. (1998). *Pathophysiology: The biological basis for disease in adults and children* (3rd ed.). St. Louis: Mosby.

Thibodeau, G.A. & Patton, K.T. (1996). *Anatomy and physiology* (3rd ed.). St. Louis: Mosby.

VanWynsberghe, D., Norback, C.R., & Carola, R. (1995). *Human anatomy and physiology* (3rd ed.). New York: McGraw-Hill.

21 Drugs Affecting the Parasympathetic Nervous System

Chapter Focus

The parasympathetic component of the autonomic nervous system innervates various organs and acts on the heart, gastrointestinal tract, urinary bladder, and respiratory tract. In conjunction with the sympathetic component of the autonomic nervous system, the parasympathetic system works to control body functions that occur without conscious thought. Drug therapy associated with this system can influence autonomic processes by mimicking acetylcholine at receptor sites, or it can inhibit the breakdown of acetylcholine at these same sites, prolonging its action. In either case, the nurse needs to be knowledgeable about the drugs related to the parasympathetic nervous system because they are used across a wide variety of human conditions.

Learning Objectives

1. Explain the difference between the muscarinic and nicotinic actions of acetylcholine.
2. Describe the side effects/adverse reactions of cholinergic, cholinergic blocking, and synthetic antispasmodic agents.
3. Describe the physiologic effects of the belladonna alkaloids.
4. List the physiologic effects of nicotine.
5. Describe the use of ganglionic blocking drugs.
6. Implement the nursing management for the care of clients receiving agents that affect the parasympathetic nervous system.

Key Terms

Key Drugs [✓]

Autonomic Drugs

Autonomic drugs may mimic, intensify, or block the effects of the parasympathetic and sympathetic divisions of the autonomic nervous system. They are divided into the following groups:

1. **Cholinergic (parasympathomimetic)** drugs (e.g., bethanechol) act like mediators of the parasympathetic nervous system.
2. **Cholinergic blocking (parasympatholytic, anticholinergic,** or **antimuscarinic)** drugs (e.g., atropine) block the action of the parasympathetic nervous system.
3. **Adrenergic (sympathomimetic)** drugs (e.g., norepinephrine) act like mediators of the sympathetic nervous system.
4. **Adrenergic blocking (sympatholytic)** drugs (e.g., propranolol, a beta-blocking agent) block the action of the sympathetic nervous system.

CHOLINERGIC DRUGS

As discussed in Chapter 20, acetylcholine plays an important role in the transmission of nerve impulses in both the parasympathetic and sympathetic divisions of the autonomic nervous system.

Acetylcholine has two major actions on the nervous system: (1) it has stimulant effects on the ganglia, adrenal medulla, and skeletal muscle; and (2) it has stimulant effects at postganglionic nerve endings in cardiac muscle, smooth muscle, and glands. The first action resembles the effects of nicotine, such as tachycardia, elevated blood pressure, and peripheral vasoconstriction; this is referred to as the **nicotinic effect** of acetylcholine. The second action of acetylcholine at the postganglionic nerve endings is like that of muscarine (an alkaloid obtained from the toadstool *Amanita muscaria*)—intense vomiting, diarrhea, nervousness, severe stomach pains, labored respiration, slow and irregular pulse, delirium and even fatality. Symptoms will mimic an intense parasympathetic stimulation. This is referred to as the **muscarinic effect** or cholinergic effect of acetylcholine (Table 21-1; see Figure 20-2 for a review of nicotine and muscarinic sites).

Although acetylcholine is important physiologically, it has no therapeutic value because (1) its actions are very brief because of rapid hydrolysis by acetylcholinesterase, and (2) no selective purpose can be achieved through its use, because it has several sites of action.

Cholinergic drugs are agents that bring about effects in the body similar to those produced by acetylcholine. These agents are also called parasympathomimetics because they mimic the action produced by stimulation of the parasympathetic nervous system.

Cholinergic fibers are widespread; they are present in the heart, spleen, uterus, vas deferens, colon, and vessels of the skin and muscles. Cholinergic fibers are probably present in many more tissues of the body. Parasympathetic innervation predominates in the gastrointestinal tract; it stimulates both motor and secretory action.

Cholinergic drugs may be obtained from natural (plant) or synthetic sources. The synthetic drugs are more stable and have a more selective action on particular organs. The

TABLE 21-1 Acetylcholine: Sites for Muscarinic and Nicotinic Actions

Site	Muscarinic Action*	Nicotinic Action
Cardiovascular system		
Blood vessels	Dilation	Constriction (With large doses after atropine)
Heart rate	Slowed	Increased (With large doses after atropine)
Blood pressure	Decreased	Increased (With large doses after atropine)
Gastrointestinal system		
Tone	Increased	Increased
Motility	Increased	Increased
Sphincters	Relaxed	—
Glandular secretions	Increased salivary, lacrimal, intestinal, and sweat secretion	Initial stimulation, then inhibition of salivary and bronchial secretions
Skeletal muscle	—	Stimulated
Autonomic ganglia	—	Stimulated
Eye	Pupil constriction Decreased accommodation	—
Blocking agent	Atropine	Tubocurarine
Remarks	Above effects increase as dosage increases	Increased dosage inhibits effects and causes receptor blockade

*Usual sites for therapeutic effects.

TABLE 21-2 **Prominent Cholinergic and Anticholinesterase Drugs**

Generic Name	Usual Adult Dosage (24 hours)	Usual Route of Administration
ambenonium (I) (Mytelase)	5 mg 3 to 4 times daily	Oral
bethanechol (D) (Urecholine)	10-50 mg 3 to 4 times daily 5 mg 3 to 4 times daily	Oral SC
isoflurophate (I) (Floropryl)	Thin strip (0.5 cm) of 0.025%, variable instructions	Topical (eye) ointment
neostigmine bromide (I) (Prostigmin)	15 mg q3-4h	Oral
neostigmine methylsulfate (I) (Prostigmin)	0.5 mg (dose variable)	IM or SC
physostigmine (I) (Eserine)	1 drop, 0.25%-0.5% solution 2 or 3 times daily	Topical (eye)
physostigmine (I) (Antilirium)	0.5-2 mg (maximum)	IM or IV
pilocarpine (D)	1 drop, 0.5%-4% solution 4 times daily	Topical (eye)
pyridostigmine (I) (Mestinon)	Highly variable	Oral

D, Direct acting; *I*, indirect acting.

two groups of cholinergic drugs available are (1) direct acting, and (2) indirect acting. **Direct-acting cholinergic drugs** combine directly with the cholinergic receptors in postsynaptic membranes innervated by parasympathetic neurons and evoke effects similar to those produced by acetylcholine. By contrast, instead of producing a direct effect on receptors, **indirect-acting cholinergic drugs** act primarily on the enzyme inhibiting the action of cholinesterase (acetylcholinesterase), which normally degrades acetylcholine. This results in an accumulation of acetylcholine at all sites where it is liberated (see Figure 20-4, *A, 5*). By rendering this enzymatic action ineffective, the anticholinesterase drugs cause a prolonged and intensified cholinergic response at the various effector sites.

Cholinergic drugs may be used in the following situations:

1. To stimulate the intestine and bladder postoperatively, thus increasing peristalsis and urination
2. To lower intraocular pressure in clients with glaucoma
3. To promote salivation and sweating
4. To terminate curarization (neuromuscular blockade used as an adjunct to general anesthesia)
5. To treat myasthenia gravis symptomatically*

The therapeutic effectiveness of cholinergic drugs depends primarily on their muscarinic action, but some of them also possess nicotinic action. Nicotinic action usually requires doses much larger than those used therapeutically. However, some drugs may exhibit more nicotinic than muscarinic effects (see Table 21-1).

*Cholinergic, but not parasympathomimetic, actions involve the somatic nervous system, which innervates skeletal muscle.

The ideal cholinergic or anticholinesterase drug would do the following:

1. Mimic or inhibit the effect of acetylcholine on a particular structure or organ
2. Be effective when administered orally
3. Be more stable and less easily inactivated than the drugs now available
4. Produce a therapeutic effect with minimal side effects

Although these ideal drugs are not yet available, progress is being made in this direction. Cholinergic drugs used primarily to lower intraocular pressure include pilocarpine and carbachol and are discussed in Chapter 43. Table 21-2 lists the prominent cholinergic and anticholinesterase drugs.

Direct-Acting Cholinergic Drugs (Choline Esters)

Drugs that are chemically similar to the neurotransmitter acetylcholine include bethanechol, carbachol, and methacholine. All compounds in this group are quaternary amines and therefore are poorly absorbed orally. Their actions are comparable to but longer acting than the physiologic mediator acetylcholine. The side effects of these drugs are a consequence of parasympathetic stimulation and include bradycardia, hypotension, sweating, salivation, vomiting, diarrhea, and intestinal cramps.

bethanechol chloride [be than′ e kole] (Urecholine, Duvoid ♣)

Bethanechol is a synthetic choline ester with actions similar to those of acetylcholine. It produces the effects of stimulation of the parasympathetic nervous system. It has predomi-

TABLE 21-3 Drugs Affecting the Parasympathetic Nervous System: Side Effects/Adverse Reactions

Drugs	Side Effects/Adverse Reactions
Cholinergic	
bethanechol (Urecholine, Duvoid ✤)	Abdominal pains or upset, increased salivation, sweating, nausea or vomiting, flushed skin, blurred or disturbed vision, unsteadiness, headache, and diarrhea.
Anticholinergic	
atropine scopolamine	Inhibition of sweating; constipation; dry mouth, throat, and skin; blurred vision; urinary retention; headache; photophobia; drowsiness; weakness; nausea or vomiting; urticaria; dermatitis and eye pain from increased intraocular pressure. In addition, euphoria, amnesia, and insomnia are reported more often with scopolamine. Dilated and fixed pupils have been reported on the side where the transdermal disk is applied. To avoid extensive neurologic examinations, unconscious individuals appearing with the above symptoms should be checked first for the use of a disk behind the ear. If the disk is removed, this syndrome usually abates within 2 weeks.
Synthetic Antispasmodics	
clidinium (Quarzan) dicyclomine (Bentyl, Antispas) glycopyrrolate (Robinul)	Abdominal distention; headache; dizziness; constipation; nausea; vomiting; sedation; dry mouth, nose, throat, and skin; blurred or disturbed vision; dysuria; weakness; hypotension; decreased sexual ability.
Ganglionic Blocking Agents	
trimethaphan camsylate (Arfonad)	Side effects are dose related: anorexia, nausea, vomiting, constipation, dilated pupils, dry mouth, impotency, pruritus, hives, hypotension, tachycardia, angina, urinary retention.

nant muscarinic action with particular selectivity on the detrusor muscle of the urinary bladder and smooth muscle of the gastrointestinal tract. Hence contraction of the smooth muscle of the bladder is sufficiently strong to initiate micturition and empty the urinary bladder. In the gastrointestinal tract the drug stimulates gastric motility, increases gastric tone, and often restores impaired peristaltic activity of the esophagus, stomach, and intestine. It also promotes defecation. Unlike acetylcholine, bethanechol is not destroyed by cholinesterase, and therefore its effects are more prolonged than that of the natural neurotransmitter. Therapeutic test doses in normal human subjects have demonstrated little effect on heart rate, blood pressure, or peripheral circulation.

In general, bethanechol has been replaced by more effective drugs, but it is available in the United States for the treatment of postoperative and postpartum nonobstructive urinary retention and for neurogenic atony of the urinary bladder associated with retention. Although not indicated on its U.S. product labeling, it has also been used to relieve postoperative abdominal distention and gastric atony or stasis and reflux esophagitis associated with decreased pressure of the lower esophageal sphincter.

Despite being poorly absorbed from the gastrointestinal tract, bethanechol is effective orally. It is widely distributed to organs innervated by the parasympathetic nervous system. Onset of action is within 30 to 90 minutes of oral administration, the peak effect is within 1 hour, and the duration of action is up to 6 hours, depending on the dose administered. If administered subcutaneously, the onset of action is within 5 to 15 minutes, the peak effect is within 15 to 30 minutes, and the duration of action is approximately 2 hours. The route of excretion is currently unknown.

Table 21-3 lists the side effects/adverse reactions of bethanechol.

The oral dosage of bethanechol for adults is 10 to 50 mg three to four times daily; the oral dosage for children is 0.6 mg/kg body weight in 3 or 4 divided doses per day. The parenteral dosage for adults is 5 mg SC three or four times daily when needed; for children, *SC use only,* 0.2 mg/kg body weight in 3 or 4 divided doses per day.

■ Nursing Management
Bethanechol Therapy

■ **Assessment.** Bethanechol should not be used after gastrointestinal anastomosis or bladder surgery until healing has occurred. Its risk-benefit ratio should be considered in the presence of a peptic ulcer (increase in gastric acid secretion may aggravate ulcer), peritonitis, gastrointestinal or urinary obstruction, or an inflammatory disease of the gastrointestinal tract, when increased muscular activity might be harmful. It is also used with caution during pregnancy or in clients with coronary disease and hyperthyroidism (increased risk of atrial fibrillation), hypotension (may decrease blood pressure), bradycardia (may slow heart rate), or asthma (may cause bronchospasm). Sensitivity to bethanechol would preclude its use.

Review the client's current medication regimen for the risk of significant drug interactions, such as those that may occur when bethanechol is given concurrently with the following drugs:

Drug	Possible Effect and Management
Bold/color type indicates the most serious interactions.	
other cholinergic or anticholinesterase medications	Enhanced cholinergic effects and perhaps toxicity. Avoid this combination of medications (see Table 21-3).
ganglionic blocking agents	May result in severe abdominal distress followed by a precipitous fall in blood pressure. Avoid concurrent use or a potentially serious drug interaction may occur.
procainamide or quinidine	Cholinergic effects may be antagonized. Monitor closely for dry mouth, urinary retention, blurred vision, confusion, and ataxia.

The client's vital signs, as well as a description of the symptoms for which bethanechol is being prescribed, should be obtained as a baseline assessment before therapy is initiated.

■ **Nursing Diagnosis.** The client receiving bethanechol should be assessed for the following nursing diagnoses/collaborative problems: impaired comfort related to belching or parasympathetic stimulation (headache, increased salivation or sweating, nausea, vomiting, nervousness, flushing of the skin, and abdominal discomfort); diarrhea; impaired urinary pattern (frequency related to the effects of the drug or retention related to the ineffectiveness of the drug); risk for injury related to blurred vision, change in near or distant vision, or orthostatic hypotension; and the potential complications of bronchoconstriction (shortness of breath, wheezing, tightness in chest) and seizures.

■ **Implementation**

■ ***Monitoring.*** Observe the client closely for side effects/adverse reactions of bethanechol. Monitor vital signs and check respirations carefully for 30 to 60 minutes after an SC injection. Keep a dose of atropine available in a syringe to counteract severe side effects. Evaluate the effectiveness of the drug by monitoring intake and output, or residual urine volumes if applicable, when administering bethanechol for postoperative urinary retention. If the bladder sphincter fails to relax as the urinary bladder contracts in response to bethanechol administration, urine may be forced up the ureter into the kidney. If the client has bacteriuria, this reflux of urine into the kidney may cause a kidney infection. Intake and output must be carefully monitored in these clients. Box 21-1 describes the use of bethanechol in rehabilitation settings with clients who have a neurogenic bladder.

■ ***Intervention.*** Administer bethanechol on an empty stomach to minimize the possibility of nausea and vomiting. Parenteral bethanechol is to be administered only subcutaneously. Do not administer it intramuscularly or intravenously, because severe symptoms of cholinergic overstimulation (flushing of the skin, headache, severe hypotension, hypothermia, bradycardia, nausea and vomiting, abdominal cramps, bloody diarrhea, shock, or cardiac arrest) may occur.

■ ***Education.*** Instruct the client to move slowly from a lying to a sitting or standing position because orthostatic hypotension is a common side effect of bethanechol.

■ **Evaluation.** The expected outcome of bethanechol therapy is that the client will be able to urinate without experiencing retention and without experiencing any adverse reactions to the drug.

BOX 21-1

The Use of Bethanechol with Clients Having a Neurogenic Bladder

Bethanechol is used as an adjunct therapy in clients with chronic neurogenic bladder. After several baseline measurements of residual urine volume, the adult client is administered 5 mg of bethanechol chloride subcutaneously every 4 hours. The client is asked to void 12 hours after the first dose of bethanechol, and a residual urine volume is measured. If the amount of residual urine is less than the baseline volume, the drug is continued for another 24 hours. At that time the effectiveness of the drug is again evaluated with another residual urine volume measurement. If the amount is still less than the baseline volume, the drug is continued for another 24 to 48 hours on an "every 4 hours" schedule. After that period, the dosage should be decreased to 2.5 to 5 mg every 4 hours. When the residual urine is less than 50 mL, the dosage is changed to an oral form, 50 mg every 4 hours. According to the client's response, the dosing interval may be gradually increased and the dose decreased.

Indirect-Acting Cholinergic Drugs

The indirect-acting cholinergic drugs are anticholinesterases or cholinesterase inhibitors; they prolong the effect of acetylcholine by inhibiting the action of the enzyme cholinesterase. Anticholinesterase agents (e.g., neostigmine, physostigmine) exert their influence on both muscarinic and nicotinic sites. They are used in the treatment of myasthenia gravis and glaucoma (see Chapters 23 and 43, respectively). They are also used postoperatively for urinary retention and gastrointestinal ileus (Ponec, Saunders, & Kimmey, 1999). Physostigmine salicylate is used for overdose and anticholinergic substance toxicity. (See Chapter 19 for a discussion about the treatment for tricyclic antidepressant overdose.)

Myasthenia gravis is a condition characterized by weakness of the skeletal muscles innervated by the somatic efferent fibers. This disease affects cholinergic transmission, and the anticholinesterase drugs are used because they elevate the concentration of acetylcholine at the myoneural junctions. The prolonged activity of the neurohormone at these sites results in a dramatic increase in muscle strength and function. A more extensive discussion of myasthenia gravis and its treatment is found in Chapter 23. (See also Figure 20-2 for receptor sites for neurohumoral transmission.)

CHOLINERGIC BLOCKING DRUGS: MUSCARINIC BLOCKING DRUGS

The cholinergic blocking (parasympatholytic) drugs have many important uses in medicine. More specifically, these agents are called antimuscarinic drugs because they block the muscarinic effects of acetylcholine. When the nerve fiber is stimulated, the acetylcholine liberated from the terminal is unable to bind to the receptor site and fails to produce a cholinergic effect. Therefore these agents also are referred to as anticholinergic drugs. (See Figure 20-2 for muscarinic sites.)

Belladonna Alkaloids

The best known antimuscarinic or anticholinergic drugs are the belladonna alkaloids. The major drugs in this class are atropine, hyoscyamine, and scopolamine (Table 21-4). A number of plants belonging to the potato family *(Solanaceae)* contain similar alkaloids. *Atropa belladonna* (deadly nightshade), *Hyoscyamus niger* (henbane), *Datura stramonium* (jimsonweed or thorn apple), and several species of *Scopolia* also contain belladonna alkaloids. The principal alkaloids of these plants are atropine, scopolamine (hyoscine), and hyoscyamine. Atropine is the prototype of the antimuscarinic drugs. It has been in use for more than half a century and continues to be a popular drug because of its therapeutic effectiveness.

TABLE 21-4 Selected Anticholinergic Agents Containing Specific Alkaloids*

Alkaloid Formation†	Trade Name
hyoscyamine	Anaspaz
	Cystospaz
	Cystospaz-M
	Levsin
scopolamine	Buscopan ♣
	Transderm-Scop
	Transderm-V ♣
atropine, hyoscyamine, scopolamine, and phenobarbital	Barbidonna
	Barophen
	Donnatal
	Donnatal Extentabs
atropine and phenobarbital	Antrocol
belladonna and butabarbital	Butibel
belladonna and phenobarbital	Chardonna-2
hyoscyamine and phenobarbital	Levsin-PB

*Specific alkaloids include the active alkaloids of belladonna, such as hyoscyamine, atropine, and scopolamine.
†The alkaloid formulation lists the active ingredients as marketed under the various trade names. Individual salts, strengths, and dosing intervals may vary according to the manufacturer's instructions.

atropine sulfate [a' troe peen] (Atropine, Isopto-Atropine)

Mechanism of Action. As a competitive antagonist, atropine acts by occupying the muscarinic (M) receptor sites, thereby preventing or reducing the muscarinic response of acetylcholine (see Figure 20-2). The drug-receptor complex is formed at the neuroeffector junctions of smooth muscle, cardiac muscle, and exocrine glands.

Atropine has very little effect on the actions of acetylcholine at nicotinic receptor sites. At autonomic ganglia, where transmission normally involves the action of acetylcholine, relatively high doses of atropine are required to produce even a partial block. At the neuromuscular junctions of the somatic nervous system, where the receptors are exclusively nicotinic, extremely high doses of atropine are required to produce any degree of block. See Figure 20-2 for nicotinic sites on the ganglia or parasympathetic and sympathetic nerve divisions, and for nicotinic sites on effector organs (skeletal muscle) of the somatic motor system.

Atropine can produce a wide range of pharmacologic effects because a vast distribution of parasympathetic cholinergic nerves normally exists in the body. Furthermore, drug activity is dose dependent. Small doses depress salivary and bronchial secretions and sweating. Large doses dilate the pupils, inhibit accommodation of the eyes, and increase heart rate by blocking vagal effects of the heart. Larger doses inhibit micturition and decrease the tone and motility of the gut by inhibiting parasympathetic control of both the urinary bladder and the gastrointestinal tract. Still larger doses are required to inhibit gastric secretion and motility.

Pharmacologic Properties

Effects on the Eye. With atropine, the pupil is dilated (mydriasis), and the ciliary muscle (muscle of accommodation) is relaxed (cycloplegia). The sphincter muscle of the iris and the ciliary muscle are both innervated by cholinergic nerve fibers and therefore are affected by atropine. Because the sphincter muscle is unable to contract normally, the radial muscle of the iris causes the pupil to dilate.

Pupil dilation may reduce the outflow of aqueous humor, causing a rise in intraocular pressure. This is a hazardous situation for clients with glaucoma (angle closure). These effects in the eye are brought about by both local and systemic administration of atropine, although the usual single therapeutic dose of oral or parenteral atropine has little effect on the eye. Photophobia occurs after the pupil is dilated; when the drug has reached its full effect, the usual reflexes to light and accommodation disappear.

Ophthalmic preparations should be included in the review of the client's current medications because an ophthalmic preparation may cause systemic effects (*United States Pharmacopeia Dispensing Information,* 1999). The systemic absorption of ophthalmic medications resulting in undesirable side effects or adverse reactions has been reported with atropine and a number of other eye preparations.

Effects on the Skin and Mucous Membranes. Because the sweat glands of the skin are supplied by sympathetic cholinergic nerves, atropine decreases or abolishes their activity. This causes the skin to become hot and dry. Furthermore, the flow of secretions from glands lining the respiratory tract is reduced and, as a result, drying of the mucous membranes of the mouth, nose, pharynx, and bronchi occurs. Clients who have been given atropine, particularly for preoperative preparation, often describe having a dry mouth and thirst.

Effects on the Respiratory System. Secretions of the nose, pharynx, and bronchial tubes are decreased with the use of atropine. The muscles of the bronchial tubes relax, and the airway widens to ease breathing. Atropine and scopolamine are less effective than epinephrine as bronchodilators and are seldom used for asthma.

Effects on the Cardiovascular System. When low doses of atropine are given or an IV dose is administered slowly, the cardiac rate is temporarily and slightly slowed because of the central action of the drug on the cardiac center in the medulla (paradoxical bradycardia). Larger IV doses given rapidly will block the vagal effect on the sinoatrial node and atrioventricular junction and increase heart rate.

Atropine has little or no effect on blood pressure when given in therapeutic doses. This is expected because most vascular beds lack significant cholinergic innervation. Large (and sometimes ordinary) doses cause vasodilation of vessels in the skin of the face and neck. This may result from a direct dilator action or from histamine release. Reddening of the face and neck is seen, especially after large or toxic doses.

Effects on the Gastrointestinal Tract. It appears that the amount and character of gastric secretion are little affected by atropine given in ordinary therapeutic doses. The secretion of acid in the stomach is presumably less under vagal control than under hormonal or chemical control. The effect of atropine on the secretion of the pancreas and intestinal glands is not therapeutically significant. Atropine and other belladonna alkaloids decrease tone and peristalsis in the stomach and small and large intestines. Atropine does not affect the secretion of bile but exerts a mildly antispasmodic effect in the gallbladder and bile ducts.

Effects on the Urinary Tract. Atropine relaxes the ureter, especially when it has been in a state of spasm. Therapeutic doses decrease the tone of the fundus of the urinary bladder. Atropine relaxes a hypertonic detrusor muscle. It also causes constriction of the internal sphincter, which can produce urinary retention.

Effects on the Central Nervous System. Atropine has prominent effects on the central nervous system (CNS) and in large doses causes excitement and maniacal behavior. These behavioral effects suggest the existence of important cholinergic pathways and receptors within the CNS.

Small or moderate doses of atropine have little or no cerebral effect. Large or toxic doses cause restlessness, wakefulness, and talkativeness. This condition may develop into delirium and, finally, stupor and coma. The exalted, excited stage has sometimes been called a "belladonna jag." A rise in temperature is sometimes seen, especially in infants and young children. This is probably the result of suppression of sweating rather than action on the heat-regulating center.

Atropine has been used to diminish tremor in Parkinson's disease, perhaps because of its reduction in cholinergic synaptic transmission. Therapeutic doses of atropine stimulate the respiratory center and make breathing faster and sometimes deeper. When respiration is seriously depressed, atropine is not always reliable as a stimulant; in fact, it may deepen the depression. Large doses stimulate respiration but can also cause respiratory failure and death.

Small doses of atropine stimulate the vagus center in the medulla, causing primary slowing of the heart. The vasoconstrictor center is stimulated briefly and then depressed. Because depression follows soon after stimulation, atropine has been called a borderline stimulant of the CNS.

Topical Effects. There is a slight amount of absorption when atropine or belladonna is applied to the skin, especially if it is an alcoholic preparation or in the form of a transdermal patch.

Indications. Atropine is indicated for the treatment of irritable bowel syndrome, spastic biliary tract disorders, and genitourinary disorders. It is also used as an antidote for cholinergic toxicity from excessive amounts of cholinesterase inhibitors, muscarinics, or organophosphate pesticide poisoning. Atropine is also used to treat sinus bradycardia and Parkinson's disease, to prevent excessive salivation and respiratory tract secretions as a preanesthetic agent, as an adjunct medication for peptic ulcers, and for gastrointestinal radiography.

Pharmacokinetics. Atropine is readily absorbed with oral and parenteral administration; it is also absorbed from the mucous membranes. After oral administration, the maximum effect is reached within 1 hour; the duration of action is 4 to 6 hours. It is widely distributed in body fluids and easily passes the placental barrier to the blood of the fetus and the blood-brain barrier. Atropine is metabolized primarily in the liver; approximately 30% to 50% is excreted unchanged in the urine.

Side Effects/Adverse Reactions. See Table 21-3 for the side effects/adverse reactions of atropine.

Dosage and Administration. The oral anticholinergic dosage of atropine sulfate for adults is 0.3 to 1.2 mg every 4 to 6 hours. The dosage for children is 0.01 mg/kg PO (not to exceed 0.4 mg) every 4 to 6 hours. The oral dose for adults to prevent excessive salivation and respiratory tract secretions in anesthesia is 2 mg. The dose should be titrated as necessary to the client's response or to the appearance of side effects.

The parenteral anticholinergic dosage for adults is 0.4 to 0.6 mg IM, IV, or SC every 4 to 6 hours. The pediatric anticholinergic dose is 0.01 mg/kg SC (not to exceed 0.4 mg); the pediatric dose may be repeated every 4 to 6 hours if necessary. The parenteral dosage for adults to treat bradycardia (dysrhythmia) is 0.4 to 1 mg IV every 1 to 2 hours, up to a maximum of 2 mg; the pediatric dosage for dysrhythmia is 0.01 to 0.03 mg/kg IV.

See Chapters 41 and 43 for additional atropine preparations.

■ Nursing Management

Atropine Therapy

In addition to the following discussion, see Nursing Management: Anticholinergic Therapy, Chapter 23.

■ **Assessment.** Use atropine with caution in older adults and in children under 6 years of age because they are more susceptible to adverse reactions such as excitement, sleepiness, or confusion. Toxicity may occur in older adults even when the drug is prescribed within the normal adult dosage range. Sensitivity to the drug should be determined.

Anticholinergics should be used with caution in individuals over 40 years of age because of the risk of precipitating undiagnosed glaucoma. The use of atropine (or belladonna alkaloids) should be avoided in clients with a medical history of severe cardiac disease or tachycardia (increases heart rate), reflux esophagitis (decreased gastrointestinal motility promotes gastric retention), obstructive disease states in the gastrointestinal tract or intestinal atony (decreased motility may result in obstruction), urinary retention (aggravates symptoms), prostatic hypertrophy (aggravates symptoms), or myasthenia gravis (aggravates condition by inhibition of acetylcholine). Do not use in clients with open-angle glaucoma (mydriatic effect increases intraocular pressure), ulcerative colitis, or renal or hepatic disease (increases effects of drug). Administer systemic forms carefully to clients with chronic pulmonary disease because bronchial secretions may be sufficiently decreased to result in bronchial plugs. Use with caution in infants, blondes, clients with Down's syndrome, and children with spastic paralysis and brain damage; these individuals tend to be more sensitive to the effects of the drug.

Review the client's current medication regimen for the risk of significant drug interactions, such as those that may occur when atropine and other belladonna alkaloids are given with the following drugs:

Drug	Possible Effect and Management
antacids or antidiarrheal agents	May reduce absorption and therapeutic effectiveness of atropine. Space medications at least 2 to 3 hours apart.
other anticholinergics	Increase in anticholinergic effects reported. Monitor for symptoms such as decreased perspiration, dry mouth, blurred vision, and confusion, because a dosage adjustment may be necessary.
ketoconazole (Nizoral)	Increase in gastrointestinal pH by atropine may result in reduced absorption of ketoconazole. Atropine should be administered preferably 2 hours after ketoconazole.
potassium chloride, especially wax matrix formulations	Increased contact with gastrointestinal tract may result in mucosal irritation and lesions. Liquid formulations of potassium should be considered as a replacement for the wax matrix formulation in this situation.

Obtain a baseline assessment of the client's vital signs and urinary and bowel status. For older adults and debilitated clients, a mental status assessment is helpful in determining if the client is experiencing any drowsiness or CNS stimulation as a result of the drug. A baseline ECG is required if the drug is used as an antidysrhythmic. A baseline intraocular pressure determination is indicated for clients undergoing long-term therapy.

■ **Nursing Diagnosis.** The client receiving atropine therapy is at risk for the following nursing diagnoses/collaborative problems: hyperthermia related to the suppression of sweat gland activity; risk for injury related to blurred vision, dizziness, or light-headedness; impaired tissue integrity (irritation at injection site); disturbed thought processes (confusion, agitation); impaired comfort related to dry mouth or increased sensitivity of the eyes to light; urinary retention related to the anticholinergic effects of the drug; constipation related to decreased motility of the gastrointestinal tract; and the potential complications of allergic reaction and decreased cardiac output related to the ineffectiveness of the drug.

■ **Implementation**

■ ***Monitoring.*** Monitor the client's pulse, which is a sensitive indicator of the response to atropine. Be alert to any change in blood pressure, temperature, and respiration, particularly after IV administration. ECG recordings are monitored when atropine is used for dysrhythmias. Notify the prescriber of any significant changes. Observe older adults for excitement, agitation, and delirium. Assess for constipation, dryness of mouth and, in older men, urinary retention. Because of the mydriatic effects of atropine, intraocular pressure determinations should be performed at regular intervals for clients undergoing extended atropine therapy.

■ ***Intervention.*** Administer oral preparations 30 to 60 minutes before meals. Administer antacids or antidiarrheal medications 2 to 3 hours after administering atropine. Have physostigmine on hand to treat atropine overdose.

■ ***Education.*** Inform the client of the possible side effects of atropine. Advise the client about the use of sugarless gum and candy, ice, or saliva substitutes to relieve dry mouth. Instruct the client to avoid alcohol and other CNS depressants while taking atropine.

The decreased salivary flow produced by atropine use promotes caries, buccal candidiasis, and periodontal disease. Therefore counsel the client involved in long-term use to follow a consistent dental hygiene program, including semiannual visits to the dentist.

Instruct the client to avoid being exposed to high environmental temperatures, exercising in warm, humid weather, or taking prolonged hot baths. These activities may lead to heat stroke. Children are especially at risk for increased body temperature in hot weather. The client should report any fever to the prescriber because the medication may need to be discontinued.

Inform the client using an ophthalmic preparation that his or her vision will be impaired for a few days. The client should protect his or her eyes by wearing dark glasses. The client's ability to judge distance will also be impaired; therefore he or she should avoid driving a car or operating machinery. Signs of local irritation or follicular conjunctivitis may occur after prolonged periods of ophthalmic therapy; in such cases the drug should be discontinued.

■ **Evaluation.** The expected outcome of atropine therapy is that the client's ECG will indicate a correction of underlying dysrhythmia without any tachycardia. The client will not experience any adverse reactions to the atropine (e.g., constipation or urinary retention). If the drug is taken for an ophthalmic condition, the client will experience therapeutic mydriasis without systemic adrenergic-like effects.

scopolamine [skoe pol′ a meen] (Transderm-Scop, Transderm-V ♣)
scopolamine hydrobromide

See the preceding discussion of atropine for the mechanism of action of scopolamine. The peripheral effects of scopolamine are similar to atropine, but the CNS effects are different. At therapeutic doses it depresses the CNS and causes drowsiness, euphoria, memory loss, relaxation, sleep, and relief of fear. It does not increase blood pressure or respiration.

Scopolamine is used in the treatment of irritable bowel syndrome, renal and ureteral colic, and dysrhythmias induced during surgery because of increased vagal stimulation. Because of its depressant action on vestibular function, it is used for motion sickness to prevent nausea and vomiting. It is used as an adjunct medication with general anesthesia to check secretions, to prevent laryngospasm, and for its sedative (twilight sleep) and amnesic effects.

The pharmacokinetics of scopolamine are the same as for atropine. The transdermal dosage form produces its antiemetic effects for up to 72 hours.

See Table 21-3 for the side effects/adverse reactions of scopolamine.

An oral dosage form is not available in the United States. The parenteral dose in adults for use as an anticholinergic and an antiemetic is 0.3 to 0.6 mg as a single dose. As an adjunct to anesthesia or for sedation-hypnosis, 0.6 mg IM, IV, or SC is administered three or four times daily. For amnesia, 0.32 to 0.6 mg IM, IV, or SC is administered. Older adults are more sensitive to scopolamine; if it is used, doses smaller than the adult doses are recommended. When used as an antiemetic in children, 6 μg (0.006 mg)/kg IM, IV, or SC is administered as a single dose. To reduce excess salivation during anesthesia, various IM doses are recommended according to age; see current drug references.

For antiemetic or antivertigo effects in adults, a transdermal patch is placed behind the ear to produce an effect for 72 hours. For an antiemetic effect, it should be applied 4 hours before the desired effect is required. Older adults are more sensitive to this drug at the adult dosage; monitor closely for hyperpyrexia, confusion, blurred vision, and ataxia. The transdermal patch is not recommended for children.

■ **Nursing Management**

Scopolamine Therapy

In addition to the following discussion, see Nursing Management: Atropine Therapy, p. 447. The concurrent use of scopolamine with alcohol and other CNS depressants may result in increased CNS depression effects. Monitor closely for drowsiness and altered thought processes.

For the transdermal application of scopolamine, instruct the client to wash and dry hands before and after apply ing the patch. It is to be applied to the hairless skin area behind the ear; it is not to be applied over abrasions or rashes. Alert the client that drowsiness and dilated pupils (photophobia and blurred vision) may occur; if they occur, tasks such as driving or mowing the lawn may be hazardous.

If scopolamine has been administered as part of a preoperative medication for a day stay or ambulatory procedure, caution the client before discharge about the effects on memory and motor tasks. These effects may persist for a few hours.

Urinary Anticholinergic Agents

Bladder control and urinary incontinence are major issues that affect quality of life in older adults. Commonly used anticholinergic medications include oxybutynin (Ditropan) and tolterodine (Detrol ◆, Detrol LA). Although both drugs produce anticholinergic side effects (e.g., dry mouth, blurred vision, changes in mental status, constipation), Detrol appears to have greater affinity for bladder receptors and therefore may produce fewer side effects/adverse reactions.

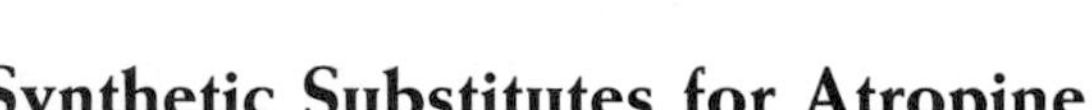

Synthetic Substitutes for Atropine

The usefulness of atropine is limited by the fact that it is a complex drug that affects a number of organs or tissues simultaneously. When administered for its antispasmodic effects, it also produces prolonged effects in the eye, causing dilated pupils and blurred vision. It also causes dry mouth and possibly a rapid heart rate. When the antispasmodic effect is desired, other effects become side effects that may be distinctly undesirable.

A large number of drugs have been synthesized in an effort to capture the antispasmodic effect of atropine without producing its other effects. These drugs are often used to relieve hypertonicity and hypersecretion in the stomach.

Many products are marketed as antispasmodic and anticholinergic agents, but their formulations are either modifications of a belladonna alkaloid or include one or more of the natural alkaloids as their active ingredients. The pharmacologic properties are therefore similar to the previously reviewed substances and are not repeated here (see Table

21-4). The more commonly used or newer systemic agents—dicyclomine (Bentyl), glycopyrrolate (Robinul), and clidinium bromide (Quarzan)—are discussed in the following sections.

dicyclomine [dye sye' kloe meen] (Bentyl, Bentylol ♣, and others)

Dicyclomine produces a direct effect on smooth muscle, resulting in decreased tone and motility of the gastrointestinal, biliary, and urinary tracts. It appears to produce the typical anticholinergic (antimuscarinic) effect only when administered in large doses. Dicyclomine is indicated for the treatment of irritable bowel syndrome.

Little has been determined about the pharmacokinetics of this product. It is rapidly absorbed after oral or parenteral administration; approximately 50% of the dose is excreted by the kidneys and the other 50% in the feces. The half-life is 1.8 hours initially and 9 to 10 hours for the second phase.

See Table 21-3 for the side effects/adverse reactions of dicyclomine.

The oral dosage of dicyclomine for adults is 10 to 20 mg three or four times daily. The dosage may be adjusted according to response, up to a maximum of 160 mg/day. Dicyclomine is not recommended for children under 6 months of age; for children 6 months to 2 years of age, 5 to 10 mg PO (syrup available) may be administered three or four times daily, with adjustments as necessary. For children 2 years of age and older, 10 mg PO may be given three or four times daily, with adjustments as necessary. The parenteral dosage for adults is 20 mg IM every 4 to 6 hours. Do not administer dicyclomine intravenously. A parenteral dosage has not been established for children.

■ Nursing Management

Dicyclomine Therapy

In addition to the following discussion, see Nursing Management: Atropine Therapy, p. 447. The significant drug interactions with antacids and antidiarrheal agents, other anticholinergics, ketoconazole (Nizoral), and potassium chloride are the same as for atropine. Dicyclomine injections should be given only intramuscularly.

Administer oral preparations with food or milk to minimize gastric distress. The syrup form may be diluted with equal parts of water to make administration easier. When administering the parenteral form, ensure that the client is lying or sitting down because some temporary lightheadedness may be experienced. Alert the client that blurred vision may occur and should be reported to the prescriber. When prescribed as adjunct therapy for peptic ulcers and other gastrointestinal disorders, the client should experience relief from gastrointestinal pain.

glycopyrrolate [gly koe pye' roe late] (Robinul, Robinul Forte)

Glycopyrrolate is a synthetic anticholinergic product with effects similar to atropine. Unlike atropine, it is unable to cross lipid membranes (e.g., blood-brain barrier) easily and thus has minimal CNS side effects. It also appears to be less likely to produce pupillary or ocular eye effects.

Glycopyrrolate is indicated as an anticholinergic (antimuscarinic) to prevent or reduce hypersecretion induced during anesthesia, reduce the dysrhythmias induced during anesthesia, and prevent or reduce toxicities induced by cholinesterase inhibitors (neostigmine or pyridostigmine).

Glycopyrrolate is administered orally, intravenously, intramuscularly, or subcutaneously. The onset of action of an IV dose occurs within 1 minute. The onset of action is 15 to 30 minutes for IM or SC routes. Vagal blocking action lasts from 2 to 3 hours, whereas the antisialagogue effect (the inhibition of the flow of saliva) may last up to 7 hours. Glycopyrrolate is excreted by the kidneys.

See Table 21-3 for the side effects/adverse reactions of glycopyrrolate. The significant drug interactions are the same as for atropine.

The adult oral dosage of glycopyrrolate to treat peptic ulcer is 1 to 2 mg two or three times daily and, when necessary, 2 mg at bedtime; the dosage is then reduced to 1 mg twice daily or adjusted according to the client's response and tolerance. Older adults may be more sensitive, and a lower dosage schedule should be considered. The dosage has not been established for children.

The parenteral anticholinergic adult dosage for peptic ulcer is 0.1 to 0.2 mg IM or IV every 4 hours if needed, up to a maximum of 4 doses per 24 hours. To prevent or reduce excessive salivation and respiratory tract secretions or gastric hypersecretory situations during anesthesia, 4.4 μg/kg body weight is given parenterally 30 to 60 minutes before anesthesia induction. For dysrhythmias during anesthesia or surgery, 0.1 mg IV is given at 2- to 3-minute intervals as needed. As a cholinergic adjunctive medication, glycopyrrolate 0.2 mg IV is given for each 1 mg of neostigmine or 5 mg of pyridostigmine and may be administered in the same syringe.

Parenteral dosages of glycopyrrolate for children with a peptic ulcer have not been determined. To prevent or reduce excessive salivation and respiratory tract secretions or gastric hypersecretory situations in children during anesthesia, 4.4 to 8.8 μg/kg body weight IM is given 30 to 60 minutes before anesthesia induction. For children with dysrhythmias during anesthesia or surgery, 4.4 μg/kg body weight IV is given every 2 or 3 minutes as necessary. As a cholinergic adjunctive medication with children, glycopyrrolate 0.2 mg IV is given for each 1 mg of neostigmine or 5 mg of pyridostigmine and may be administered in the same syringe.

■ Nursing Management

Glycopyrrolate Therapy

Alert the client to have periodic ophthalmic examinations for intraocular pressure. Intraocular pressure may become elevated because of mydriasis produced by the drug. Blurred vision should be reported to the prescriber. When contemplating mixing glycopyrrolate in a syringe with other drugs, consult the package insert, because the drug is unstable at a pH higher than 6 and forms a precipitate when combined with some other agents. For additional information, see Nursing Management: Atropine Therapy, p. 447.

clidinium [kli di′ nee um] (Quarzan)

Clidinium is a synthetic product related to the belladonna alkaloids, especially atropine. It competitively antagonizes acetylcholine at the postganglionic parasympathetic receptor sites in both smooth muscles and the secretory glands, thus reducing gastrointestinal motility and gastric acid secretion. Ganglionic blockade may be produced if high doses of clidinium are given. Unlike atropine, clidinium produces few, if any, CNS side effects or alterations on the eye.

Clidinium is indicated as an adjunctive treatment for peptic ulcers. The onset of action occurs within 1 hour following oral absorption; the duration of action lasts up to 3 hours. Clidinium is metabolized in the liver and excreted primarily by the kidneys.

See Table 21-3 for side effects/adverse reactions.

The oral dosage of clidinium for adults is 2.5 to 5 mg three or four times daily, before meals and at bedtime. Adjust the dosage according to individual response. The dosage for older adults is 2.5 mg PO three times daily, before meals. The pediatric dosage has not been determined.

▪ **Nursing Management**

Clidinium Therapy

The significant drug interactions are the same as for atropine. Administer ½ to 1 hour before meals to enhance absorption. The client should undergo periodic intraocular pressure determinations, because the mydriatic effect of the drug increases intraocular pressure. Blurred vision may occur and should be reported to the prescriber. For further nursing management, see Nursing Management: Atropine Therapy.

flavoxate [fla vox′ ate] (Urispas)
oxybutynin [ox i byoo′ ti nin] (Ditropan)
tolterodine [tol ter′ o deen] (Detrol)

These anticholinergic drugs are used to treat urologic disorders. Flavoxate is indicated for treatment of dysuria, urinary frequency, nocturia, and incontinence. Oxybutynin is primarily indicated for bladder instability due to uninhibited and reflex neurogenic bladder. Tolterodine is used for overactive bladder, with symptoms of urinary urgency, frequency, or urge incontinence. Flavoxate and oxybutynin have a direct and indirect anticholinergic effect on urinary tract smooth muscle; they relax smooth muscles in the urinary tract. In addition, flavoxate has some local anesthesic and analgesic properties. Tolterodine is a muscarinic receptor antagonist.

The adult oral dosage of flavoxate is 100 to 200 mg three or four times daily; for oxybutynin, 5 mg two to four times daily; and for tolterodine, 2 mg twice daily initially, lowered to 1 mg twice daily according to response.

Nursing management is as for atropine therapy, p. 447.

GANGLIONIC DRUGS

The major neurotransmitter of all autonomic ganglia is acetylcholine. Because postganglionic fibers produce specific effects on smooth muscle, cardiac muscle, and glands (see Figure 20-2), nonselective drugs that stimulate or block reactions in this area can produce a broad range of pharmacologic effects. This section will address drugs that affect nicotinic or cholinergic receptor sites on the autonomic ganglia, which are (1) ganglionic stimulating drugs and (2) ganglionic blocking drugs.

GANGLIONIC STIMULATING DRUGS

Nicotine

Nicotine is a liquid alkaloid and is freely soluble in water. It turns brown on exposure to air and is the chief alkaloid in tobacco. Nicotine has no therapeutic use but is of great pharmacologic interest and toxicologic importance. Its use in animal experiments has helped to increase understanding of the autonomic nervous system. Nicotine is readily absorbed from the gastrointestinal tract, respiratory mucous membrane, and skin. Nicotine is the addictive component of tobacco. Many drugs are reported to interact with nicotine.

Pharmacologic Effects

Nicotine may produce a variety of complex and often unpredictable effects in the body. Many actions are dose related, with generally small doses inducing activation or stimulation and larger doses producing a decreased or depressed response. Because nicotine acts on multiple systems, the ultimate response may be the sum of its stimulation and depressant actions.

Nicotine temporarily stimulates all sympathetic and parasympathetic ganglia in the autonomic nervous system. This is followed by depression, which tends to last longer than the period of stimulation. Its effects on skeletal muscle are similar to its effects on the ganglia—a depressant phase follows stimulation. During the depressant phase nicotine exerts a curare-like action on skeletal muscle.

Nicotine stimulates the CNS, especially the medullary centers (respiratory, emetic, and vasomotor). Large doses may cause tremors and convulsions. Stimulation is followed by depression. Death may result from respiratory failure, although it may be caused more by the curare-like action of nicotine on nerve endings in the diaphragm rather than by action on the respiratory center.

The actions and effects of nicotine on the cardiovascular system are complex. Heart rate is commonly slowed at first but later may be accelerated above normal. Nicotine usually produces an increase in heart rate and blood pressure; in general, the cardiovascular effects result from stimulation of the sympathetic ganglia and adrenal medulla along with the release of catecholamines from the sympathetic nerve endings (Taylor, 1996). Nicotine also has an antidiuretic action. Repeated administration of nicotine causes tolerance.

Toxicity

Nicotine has both short- and long-term toxic effects that are extremely important to the health care professional. Nicotine toxicity has resulted from the misuse of insecticides

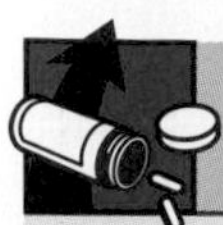

Management of Drug Overdose
Nicotine

Signs and Symptoms

- Increased saliva flow, nausea and vomiting, abdominal cramps, diarrhea, confusion, cold sweat, headache, fainting, hypotension, tachycardia, prostration and collapse; convulsions may occur; death usually results from respiratory failure.

General Approach

- *Nicotine gum.* To decrease absorption, induce vomiting in the conscious client with ipecac syrup. If the client is unconscious, a gastric lavage is followed by an activated charcoal suspension left in the stomach. A saline laxative will aid in elimination from the gastrointestinal tract.
- *Transdermal system.* Remove the patch and flush the area with water. Do not use soap because it may enhance nicotine absorption. If the patch was swallowed, an activated charcoal suspension is administered and repeated for as long as the patch is in the gastrointestinal tract. To increase the passage of the patch, a saline laxative or sorbitol may be added to the first activated charcoal dose.

Specific Approach

- Treat medical complications as necessary, as shown by the following examples:
  Provide respiratory support and interventions for respiratory failure
  Treat hypotension and cardiovascular collapse aggressively
  Use anticonvulsants (diazepam or barbiturates) for convulsions
  Use atropine for excessive bronchial secretions
- Closely monitor and treat other side effects/adverse reactions as necessary.

containing nicotine, which at times has led to the death of farmworkers. Because nicotine is a major ingredient in tobacco products, both acute toxicity (with the ingestion of such products by small children) and chronic toxicity are well documented.

Tobacco Smoking and Nicotine

The burning of tobacco can generate approximately 4000 compounds in a gaseous and particle phase, plus 60 carcinogens (Environmental Tobacco Smoke, 1998). Gas phase substances include carbon monoxide, carbon dioxide, hydrogen cyanide, ammonia, volatile nitrosamines, and many other substances. The particulate phase contains mainly nicotine, water, and tar. Known carcinogens such as tar, formaldehyde, hydrogen cyanide, benzene, carbon monoxide, and others have been identified as etiologic factors in a variety of neoplastic diseases (e.g., cancer of the bladder, lung, buccal cavity, esophagus, and pancreas). Other smoking-related illnesses include pulmonary emphysema, chronic bronchitis, coronary heart disease, and myocardial infarction. Chronic dyspepsia may develop in heavy smokers, and clients with a gastric ulcer are usually advised to avoid smoking. Of considerable importance is the fact that smokers absorb sufficient nicotine to exert a variety of effects on the autonomic nervous system. Box 21-2 provides a discussion of nurses and smoking.

In general, nicotine is believed to be a contributing factor in peripheral vascular disease such as thromboangiitis obliterans (Buerger's disease). It may cause spasms of the peripheral blood vessels, thus reducing blood flow through the affected vessels. Vasospasm in the retinal blood vessels of the eye is thought to cause serious vision disturbances and is associated with tobacco smoking.

Passive smoking (involuntary smoking, secondhand smoke) refers to the inhalation of cigarette smoke by nonsmokers. Even though this exposure is less concentrated than inhaled smoke, the health risks and/or harmful effects to the nonsmoker can be significant. Reports from the U.S. Surgeon General and the Expert Committee on Passive Smoking indicate that (1) environmental smoke can cause lung cancer in healthy nonsmokers, (2) children of smoking parents often have a greater incidence of respiratory tract symptoms and infections than children from a nonsmoking family, (3) environmental smoke may be a risk factor in cardiac disease, and (4) studies have linked environmental smoke exposure to cancers other than lung cancer (Environmental Tobacco Smoke, 1998).

BOX 21-2

Nurses and Smoking

Besides having the most prolonged contact with clients and their families, nurses have the knowledge and skills to teach them about the hazards of smoking. It is also important that nurses be role models as nonsmokers if they are to contribute to a change in the public's smoking behaviors.

An effective program of smoking cessation should incorporate acceptance, support, specific information, and regular opportunities for monitoring progress. Even a minimal-contact smoking cessation program, including a brief practitioner consultation with self-help manuals conducted in health care settings, produces significant reductions in cigarette smoking. Parents who smoke can be reminded not to smoke in their home or car because of the negative health consequences of secondhand smoke for children. Education for children can assist them in making the decision not to smoke.

Besides educating and counseling clients and their families about the benefits of smoking cessation, nurses can participate in community antismoking activities. Such activities include supporting smoking cessation programs in the workplace, advocating for clean indoor air acts, supporting legislation that impacts tobacco prevention, and teaching health education courses in schools.

In addition, the fetus of a mother who smokes may have a low birth weight and increased congenital abnormalities. Children of parents who smoke have an increased incidence of sudden infant death syndrome, an increased incidence of otitis media, respiratory infections and allergic reactions, and an increased likelihood of becoming smokers. A special effort should be made to assist women to stop smoking, particularly during the childbearing years. Smoking by women is still prevalent and may be higher and even increasing within some cultural groups (see the Cultural Considerations box below).

nicotine gum (Nicorette)
nicotine transdermal systems (Habitrol, Nicoderm, Nicotrol, Prostep)
nicotine nasal spray (Nicotrol NS)

Nicotine is available in a resin (chewing gum), transdermal systems (patches), and nasal sprays for use in smoking cessation programs. The nicotine resin in the form of chewing gum provides a source of nicotine for the nicotine-dependent client who is undergoing acute cigarette withdrawal. When the client has a strong urge to smoke, he or she chews a stick of gum to relieve the physical symptoms of nicotine withdrawal. The number of pieces of gum chewed is gradually reduced over a 2- to 3-month period. (See the discussion of the pharmacologic effects of nicotine for the mechanism of action.)

Nicotine gum is indicated for the adjunct treatment of nicotine dependence. It is absorbed through the buccal mucosa at a rate slower than if inhaled while smoking. It is metabolized primarily by the hepatic route, with smaller amounts metabolized in the kidney and lung. The half-life is 1 to 2 hours. Elimination is primarily renal, with 10% excreted unchanged and the remainder excreted as metabolites; the drug is excreted in breast milk.

Various nicotine transdermal systems (patches) are also available to aid the client in withdrawing from smoking. Table 21-5 lists the available products and dosage forms.

TABLE 21-5 Nicotine Transdermal Systems

Brand Name	Dosage per Patch*	Recommended Duration of Use
Habitrol	21 mg/24 hr	3-8 weeks
	14 mg/24 hr	2-4 weeks
	7 mg/24 hr	2-4 weeks
Nicotrol	15 mg/16 hr/day	6-8 weeks
	10 mg/16 hr/day	2 weeks
	5 mg/16 hr/day	2 weeks
Nicoderm	21 mg/24 hr	6 weeks
	14 mg/24 hr	2 weeks
	7 mg/24 hr	2 weeks
Prostep	22 mg/24 hr	4-8 weeks
	11 mg/24 hr	2-4 weeks

*Dosage for clients who weigh more than 100 pounds, smoke more than 10 cigarettes per day, and do not have cardiovascular disease.

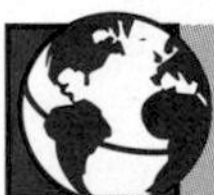

Cultural Considerations

Prevalence of Cigarette Smoking in Hispanic Women of Childbearing Age

Because of the relationship between maternal smoking and poor perinatal outcome, the prevalence of cigarette smoking in women of childbearing age is of importance. A secondary analysis of Hispanic Health and Nutrition Examination Survey data was conducted to determine the prevalence and degree of cigarette smoking among large probability samples of Cuban-American, Mexican-American, and Puerto Rican women of childbearing age. Percentages, means, and 95% confidence intervals were used to determine age-adjusted and age-specific rates for each Hispanic group.

Age-adjusted smoking prevalence rates were 23.2%, 22.6%, and 33.5% for Mexican Americans, Cuban Americans, and Puerto Ricans, respectively. Age-specific rates indicated that all Puerto Rican women under the age of 40, Mexican-American women in their forties, and Cuban-American women in their thirties had smoking prevalence higher than the national average for women. The high fertility rates for Hispanic women and the high prevalence rates of smoking for subgroups of Hispanic women support the need for smoking behavior interventions. Puerto Rican women in their twenties are of particular concern because of their high smoking prevalence (42.2%) in conjunction with their high fertility rate (Puerto Rican women in their twenties account for 61% of the births to all Hispanic women).

Although most Hispanic women are relatively light smokers, prevention and cessation interventions need to be developed for Puerto Rican women of childbearing age who demonstrated high smoking prevalence. Because of the diversity among different Hispanic groups, campaigns and interventions need to include strategies that are sensitive to the various social, educational, economic, and cultural situations.

Critical Thinking Questions

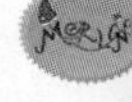

- What are some considerations related to cigarette smoking and concepts of behavior change that might be relevant for young Hispanic women?
- What factors would be useful in planning and implementing smoking cessation interventions for Hispanic women of childbearing age?

Information from Pletsch, P.K. (1991). Prevalence of cigarette smoking in Hispanic women of childbearing age, *Nursing Research* 40(2), 103.

Three of the patches (Habitrol, Nicoderm, and Prostep) are worn for 24 hours a day; Nicotrol was formulated to be worn for 16 hours a day. The latter patch was designed to mimic the individual's natural smoking pattern, which usually produces higher nicotine serum levels during the day and lower nicotine levels overnight. Theoretically, a decrease in nicotine serum levels during the night will not affect the client's sleeping patterns. A potential disadvantage is that this drug-free period may result in an early morning craving for a cigarette. To achieve long-term smoking abstinence, any of these four products should be used in conjunction with a behavioral modification program. The Nursing Research box below discusses current research related to the use of nicotine patches.

Nicotine nasal sprays administer 1 mg of nicotine per two sprays to the nasal membrane. The spray is comparable in efficacy to the gum and patches but has a faster onset of action. The client should be instructed to stop smoking before using the spray and to not use any other nicotine products while using this product. The Food and Drug Administration (FDA) recommends that the spray be used for at least 3 months but no longer than 6 months because it is possible to become dependent on the spray (New Drugs/Drug News, 1996).

Side Effects/Adverse Reactions. Side effects/adverse reactions include belching, fast heartbeat, mild headache, increased appetite, increased mouth watering, sore mouth or throat, constipation, coughing, dizziness or lightheadedness, dry mouth, hiccups, hoarseness, loss of appetite, irritability, indigestion, and difficulty in sleeping. Transdermal patches may cause pruritus and/or erythema under the patch, a generalized rash, nausea, dizziness, myalgias, coughing, difficulty in sleeping, and nightmares. Adverse reactions with nicotine gum include injury to the mouth, teeth, or dental work. Early signs of overdose are nausea and vomiting, severe increased watering of the mouth, severe abdominal pain, diarrhea, cold sweat, severe headache, severe dizziness, disturbed hearing and vision, confusion, and severe weakness. Advanced signs of overdose include faint-

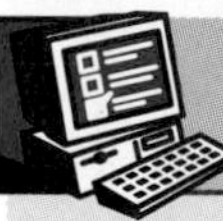

Nursing Research

Systematic Review of Nicotine Replacement Therapy

Citation: Silagy, C., Mant, D., Fowler, G., & Lancaster, T. (2001). Nicotine replacement therapy for smoking cessation (Cochran Review). In *The Cochran Library,* Issue 1. Oxford: Update Software.

Abstract: This critical review of the literature includes 100 studies. Smoking cessation rate in the intervention and control groups in those studies were identified from the published reports at 6 or 12 months. To summarize the data from a clinical perspective, the number of smokers who needed to be treated in order to produce one successful quitter at 12 months was calculated across the studies.

The results are as follows: All of the commercially available forms of nicotine replacement therapy (NRT) (nicotine gum, transdermal patch, nicotine nasal spray, nicotine inhaler, and nicotine sublingual tablet) are effective as part of a strategy to promote smoking cessation. NRT increases quit rates approximately 1.5- to 2-fold regardless of setting. The use of NRT should be preferentially directed to smokers who are motivated to quit and have high levels of nicotine dependence. There is little evidence about the role of NRT for individuals smoking fewer than 10 to 15 cigarettes/day. The choice of which form of NRT to use should reflect client needs, tolerability, and cost considerations. Patches are likely to be easier to use than gum or nasal spray in primary care settings. Eight weeks of patch therapy is as effective as longer courses, and there is no evidence that tapered therapy is better than abrupt withdrawal. Wearing a patch only during waking hours is as effective as wearing it for 24 hours per day. If gum is used, it may be offered on a fixed dose or on an ad lib basis. For highly dependent smokers who failed with 2-mg gum, 4-mg gum should be offered. There is no current evidence to suggest that routine use of a nicotine patch in doses higher than 22 mg/24 hours or of combinations of different forms of NRT are more effective in achieving long-term abstinence than standard-dose monotherapy. The effectiveness of NRT appears to be largely independent of the intensity of additional support to the smoker. Because all the trials of NRT reported so far have included at least some form of brief advice to the smoker, this represents the minimum of what should be offered to ensure its effectiveness. Provision of more intense levels of support, although beneficial in facilitating the likelihood of quitting, is not essential to the success of NRT. There is minimal evidence that a repeated course of NRT in smokers who have relapsed after recent use of nicotine patches will result in a small additional probability of quitting. NRT does not lead to an increased risk of adverse cardiovascular events in smokers with a history of cardiovascular disease. Finally, marketing claims by manufacturers of NRT products should reflect these points and avoid the possible misunderstanding by health professionals and members of the public that any of these products alone offer a magical cure for the smoking habit.

Critical Thinking Questions

- Given this critical review of the literature for evidenced-based practice, what assessments of your client would you complete before starting smoking cessation therapy?
- Based on you assessment, what NRT would you recommend and why?

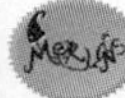

For answer guidelines for these ***new Critical Thinking Questions,*** go to mosby.com/MERLIN/McKenry/.

ing, hypotension, difficulty breathing, convulsions, and a fast, weak, or irregular pulse.

Dosage and Administration. With the chewing gum, 2 mg PO is administered and repeated as needed to curb the client's urge to smoke, up to a maximum of 30 pieces of gum per day. The client should chew the gum intermittently and very slowly when he or she has the urge to smoke. Most clients require approximately 10 pieces of gum per day during the first month of treatment. Transdermal patches are reapplied every 24 hours, except in the case of Nicotrol, which is worn for 16 hours each day. With the nasal spray, 1 to 2 mg/hr is administered initially; 1 mg of nicotine is delivered with two sprays, one in each nostril; the maximum dosage is 5 mg/hr or 40 mg/day.

■ Nursing Management

Nicotine Replacement Smoking Cessation Therapy

■ **Assessment.** A baseline assessment of the client's smoking history should be performed and cardiovascular status should be assessed before the initiation of therapy. Before beginning nicotine therapy, it should be determined that the client does not have severe angina pectoris, severe cardiac dysrhythmias, or a myocardial infarction; these conditions will be worsened by the action of catecholamine on the heart (increased heart rate and blood pressure). Temporomandibular joint disorder might be aggravated by the chewing of nicotine gum. Other disorders that require the cautious use of the gum are type 1 diabetes mellitus (increases serum concentrations of insulin); hypertension, hyperthyroidism, or vasospastic diseases (increases heart rate and blood pressure); dental problems; or esophagitis, inflammation of the mouth, or peptic ulcer (may exacerbate the condition). Chronic nasal disorders are a contraindication to the nasal spray form of the drug. Nicotine smoking cessation therapy is contraindicated in pregnant women because it may cause fetal harm. Sensitivity to nicotine should also be determined.

Review the client's current medication regimen for the risk of significant drug interactions, such as those that may occur when nicotine is given concurrently with the following drugs:

Drug	Possible Effect and Management
acetaminophen, caffeine, oxazepam (Serax), pentazocine (Talwin), propanolol (Inderal), propoxyphene (Darvon), theophylline (Theo-Dur)	Smoking increases drug metabolism, which may result in lower blood levels of these medications. Thus some clients may require higher or more frequent drug dosing. Smoking cessation will generally reverse this effect.
adrenergic agonists or blocking agents, catecholamines, cortisol	Smoking and nicotine increase cortisol and catecholamine levels; therefore therapy with the adrenergic agonists or blocking agents may necessitate a dosage adjustment based on the individual's response.
furosemide (Lasix)	A decrease in diuretic effect and cardiac output has been reported when used in combination with nicotine (smoking). These effects may be reversed if the client stops smoking.
insulin	Smoking cessation may result in an increased insulin effect; a dosage reduction may be necessary. Monitor closely for symptoms of hypoglycemia.

■ **Nursing Diagnosis.** The client participating in nicotine replacement smoking cessation therapy is at risk for the following nursing diagnoses: injury to mouth, teeth, or dental work related to viscosity of the gum; impaired comfort related to headache, increased watering of the mouth, jaw muscle ache, fast heartbeat, or a sore throat or mouth; ineffective health maintenance related to negative health habits; impaired skin integrity related to localized reaction to the transdermal patch; disturbed sleep pattern (insomnia); and disturbed thought processes (unusual irritability).

■ Implementation

■ ***Monitoring.*** Assess the client's tolerance of smoking cessation. Observe the client for symptoms of nicotine toxicity (see the Management of Drug Overdose box on p. 451).

■ ***Intervention.*** Over the course of therapy, the dose delivered by the transdermal system may be adjusted approximately every 2 weeks. The client should be weaned from the nasal spray gradually; it is not to be used for more than 3 months.

■ *Education*

■ *Gum.* The client is instructed to chew one piece of nicotine gum slowly for approximately 30 minutes when he or she has the urge to smoke. At that point most of the nicotine has been released. The amount of nicotine released depends on the rate of chewing and the amount of time the saliva is in contact with the gum. Instruct the client not to chew more than 30 pieces in a day. The number of pieces of gum chewed should be reduced each day over a 2- to 3-month period. The gum should be carried at all times during therapy. Using the gum for more than 3 months is not advised and may indicate its use as a substitute for the maintenance of nicotine dependency. A gradual withdrawal program should be instituted after 6 months of use.

Because the viscosity of nicotine gum is greater than regular chewing gum, it may cause damage to dentures, inlays, fillings, and natural teeth. Excessive chewing may lead to some temporomandibular joint discomfort. Have the client use sugarless hard candies between doses of gum to meet the need for oral stimulation and to relieve oral discomfort. Instruct the client to discontinue use and to consult with the health care provider or dentist if the gum sticks to dental work. The client should not smoke while being treated with nicotine gum.

Nicotine gum should be combined with a supervised program for smoking cessation that includes education, counseling, and psychologic support (Johnson, Budz, Mackay, & Miller, 1999). Nicotine replacement products should not be used during pregnancy.

Because an overdose of nicotine can be fatal, particularly in small children, the gum should be kept out of the reach of children. Many pieces chewed at once or in rapid succession may lead to an overdose in an adult; however, the consequences of overdose may be mitigated by the early nausea and vomiting that generally occur with excessive nicotine intake.

■ *Transdermal System.* The client should be instructed to place the patch on a nonhairy, clean, dry, and intact area of the front or back torso or the outer aspect of the upper arm. The patch should be removed from its sealed pouch just before application or it will lose efficacy.

The protective liner is removed from the sticky side of the patch; touching this side of the patch as little as possible, the patch is applied to the selected skin site. The patch is pressed to the skin with the palm of the hand for approximately 10 seconds to ensure that it sticks well, especially around the edges. The previously used patch is folded in half with the sticky side together and is placed in the newly opened pouch of the replacement patch. The pouch is thrown in the trash, away from children and pets. Nicotine can be very toxic, and the patches contain enough nicotine to poison children and pets. If a child plays with a patch, take it away from him or her and contact a poison control center or health center immediately.

Washing hands immediately after patch application is essential because the nicotine on the hands could get into the eyes and cause irritation. The client should apply a new patch every 24 hours, at approximately the same time each day, selecting a different site. Water will not harm the patch; the client may swim, shower, or use a hot tub while wearing a patch. If it should come off, a new patch is to be applied to a new site. In this case the patch may be changed to continue the client's usual 24-hour schedule. Clients should be alerted that the skin under the patch may redden but should not stay red for more than a day after the patch is removed. If the patch site becomes swollen or very red, patches should be discontinued and the prescriber should be consulted.

Nicotine has been linked with low-birth-weight infants and a decrease in fetal breathing movements, possibly as the result of decreased placental perfusion. Therefore women of childbearing age should be advised to use effective birth control to avoid pregnancy while taking nicotine-based products.

■ **Evaluation.** Evaluating the client's progress toward smoking cessation should occur at least monthly, and the efficacy of the gum or the transdermal systems in the therapy program should be determined. Treatment should be discontinued if the client is still smoking after 6 months of gum therapy or 4 weeks of transdermal patch therapy, because the client is unlikely to quit on this attempt. With successful nicotine therapy, the client is no longer smoking and denies any adverse reactions to the drug.

GANGLIONIC BLOCKING DRUGS

Ganglionic blocking drugs block the action of acetylcholine on the ganglion cells by competing with acetylcholine at the synapse of the autonomic ganglia. This results in reduced impulse transmission from preganglionic to postganglionic fibers in both sympathetic and parasympathetic nerves. A blockade of sympathetic ganglia abolishes vasoconstrictor tone; the blood vessels dilate and arterial blood pressure falls (antihypertensive effect).

The methonium derivatives were introduced in 1950, with hexamethonium chloride becoming the drug of choice in managing severe and malignant hypertension. Despite the difficulties in managing individuals receiving hexamethonium because of its erratic absorption and action and severe side effects, its use demonstrated that severe hypertension could be controlled.

The two available ganglionic blocking agents are mecamylamine hydrochloride (Inversine tablets) and trimethaphan camsylate (Arfonad injection). Since 1961 the ganglionic blocking agents have been rarely used; newer antihypertensive drugs with more selective action and fewer severe side effects are preferred. Nevertheless, the student should be aware of these products because some prescribers may select trimethaphan as an alternative for clients resistant to the effects of sodium nitroprusside. Other prescribers may use trimethaphan for the treatment of a hypertensive crisis in individuals with an acute dissecting aortic aneurysm. Mecamylamine has many side effects and is not considered a first-line drug in the treatment of hypertension; the nurse is referred to the package insert or the current *United States Pharmacopeia Dispensing Information (USP DI)* for additional information on this product.

trimethaphan camsylate [trye meth' a fan] (Arfonad)

Trimethaphan camsylate is used in the treatment of hypertension and is administered by IV infusion. It is also used to produce controlled hypotension during surgery. The onset of action is immediate, and the duration of effect is 10 to 15 minutes. Metabolism probably occurs with pseudocholinesterase. The drug is excreted mostly unchanged by the kidneys.

See Table 21-3 for side effects/adverse reactions of trimethaphan camsylate.

The normal adult dosage for a hypertensive emergency is initially 0.5 to 1 mg/min by IV infusion, with dosage adjustments made as necessary. The maintenance dosage is 1 to 5 mg/min by IV infusion. To control blood pressure during surgery, 3 to 4 mg/min is administered initially and is adjusted as necessary. The maintenance dosage is 0.3 to 6 mg/min by IV infusion.

Because older adults may be more sensitive to trimethaphan, a lower dosage with close monitoring of blood pressure is indicated. With children, the dosage is 0.05 to 0.15 mg/kg/min initially administered by IV infusion and adjusted according to individual response.

■ Nursing Management

Trimethaphan Camsylate Therapy

For a detailed discussion of the nursing management of the client receiving antihypertensive agents, see Chapter 27.

▪ **Assessment.** Use trimethaphan with caution in children and older adults, who tend to be more sensitive to its hypotensive effects. The risk-benefit ratio of its use should be determined for clients with Addison's disease, anemia, asphyxia and hypovolemic shock (may increase hypoxia), diabetes, hepatic disease (may decrease hepatic perfusion and worsen condition), renal disease (may increase the effects of the drug), respiratory insufficiency (hypoxemia may be aggravated), cardiovascular or cerebrovascular insufficiency (ischemia may be aggravated by hypotension), and for clients taking other antihypotensive or steroid medications. The client's baseline blood pressure should be assessed.

Review the client's current medication regimen for the risk of significant drug interactions, such as those that may occur when trimethaphan is given concurrently with the following drugs:

Drug	Possible Effect and Management
Bold/color type indicates the most serious interactions.	
ambenonium (Mytelase), neostigmine (Prostigmin), or pyridostigmine (Mestinon)	The antimyasthenic effects of these drugs will be blocked, which may result in increased weakness and an inability to swallow. Avoid concurrent use or a potentially serious drug interaction may occur.

▪ **Nursing Diagnosis.** The client receiving trimethaphan camsylate therapy should be assessed for the following nursing diagnoses/collaborative problems: impaired comfort related to nausea and vomiting, dry mouth, itching, and anginal pain; constipation; risk for injury related to blurred vision, weakness, and orthostatic hypertension; and the potential complications of hypoventilation (respiratory depression), paralytic ileus (with IV use over 48 hours), and urinary retention.

▪ **Implementation**

▪ ***Monitoring.*** Clients receiving trimethaphan camsylate should be in an intensive care setting for appropriate monitoring. Emergency equipment should be available in the event of respiratory arrest. Monitor the client's blood pressure and respiratory function at frequent intervals. Monitor intake and output because renal blood flow may be reduced or urinary retention may occur.

▪ ***Intervention.*** The solution should be diluted and administered by an infusion pump or microdrip regulator to ensure a precise regulation of flow rate. The prepared IV solution is stable at room temperature for 24 hours. Oral antihypertensive therapy should be started as soon as possible because a pseudotolerance to the drug may occur in some individuals.

The client should be in a supine position to avoid cerebral anoxia. Oxygen therapy should be instituted while the client is receiving trimethaphan. Assist the client with activities of daily living if trimethaphan-induced weakness is an issue. Antiemetics may be used to mitigate nausea caused by the drug. If used for controlled hypertension during surgery, the drug should be discontinued before the wound is closed to allow the client's blood pressure to return to normal.

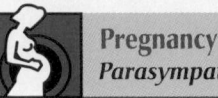

Pregnancy Safety
Parasympathetic Drugs

Category	Drugs
B	flavoxate, glycopyrrolate, oxybutynin
C	atropine, bethanechol, scopolamine, tolterodine
D	nicotine, trimethaphan
Unclassified	clidinium, dicyclomine

▪ ***Education.*** Alert the client to change positions cautiously because orthostatic hypotension is possible. Ice chips and sugarless candies can be used to alleviate dry mouth.

▪ **Evaluation.** With successful trimethaphan therapy, the client's blood pressure will be within normal limits without the client experiencing adverse reactions to the drug.

SUMMARY

Drugs that mimic, intensify, or inhibit the effects of the parasympathetic and sympathetic divisions of the autonomic nervous system are known as the autonomic drugs. They are grouped as cholinergic, cholinergic blocking, adrenergic, and adrenergic blocking drugs. The cholinergic (parasympathomimetic) drugs have nicotinic effects that stimulate the ganglia, adrenal medulla, and skeletal muscle, as well as muscarinic effects that stimulate the postganglionic nerve endings in glands and in cardiac and smooth muscle. They are used primarily to stimulate the intestine and bladder postoperatively, to terminate curarization, to lower intraocular pressure, to promote salivation and sweating, to dilate peripheral blood vessels, and to treat myasthenia gravis symptomatically.

Anticholinergic (parasympatholytic) drugs block the muscarinic effects of acetylcholine, which can produce a wide range of pharmacologic effects. They are used to treat illnesses in which spasm is a component, such as irritable bowel syndrome, spastic biliary disorders, and urinary disorders. Because anticholinergics decrease respiratory secretions, they are administered as a preanesthetic drug and to control the excessive salivation of some disorders, such as Parkinson's disease.

The ganglionic drugs are either ganglionic-stimulating or ganglionic-blocking drugs. Nicotine is a ganglionic-stimulating drug. It has no therapeutic use, but the nurse should be knowledgeable about its effects for health teaching purposes. In the 1950s, ganglionic-blocking drugs were used for the management of severe and malignant hypertension, but their use has been limited since the 1960s with the advent of more selective and effective antihypertensive drugs.

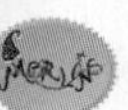

Critical Thinking Questions

1. Nurses in schools and other community agencies are well placed to serve as consultants and counselors to students and to be advocates for smoking cessation. Because children relate better to the present rather than the future consequences of their activities, what would you share with a class of fourth graders about the immediate physiologic consequences of smoking?
2. Harry Johnson is receiving atropine 0.4 mg PO every 4 hours as part of his treatment for irritable bowel syndrome. He complains of heat intolerance, dry mouth, and constipation. How will you explain these symptoms to him? What instruction will you provide to assist him in managing his therapeutic regimen effectively?

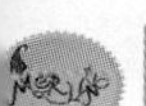

Collaborative Learning Activities

For Collaborative Learning Activities, go to mosby.com/MERLIN/McKenry/.

CASE STUDY

For a Case Study that will help ensure mastery of this chapter content, go to mosby.com/MERLIN/McKenry/.

BIBLIOGRAPHY

Abramowicz, M. (Ed.). (1992). Nicotine patches. *Medical Letter, 34*(868), 37.

American Hospital Formulary Service. (1999). *AHFS drug information '98*. Bethesda, MD: American Society of Hospital Pharmacists.

Anderson, K.N., Anderson, L.E., & Glanze, W.D. (Eds.). (1998). *Mosby's medical, nursing, & allied health dictionary* (5th ed.). St. Louis: Mosby.

Andrews, J. (1998). Optimizing smoking cessation strategies. *Nurse Practitioner, 23*(8), 47-48, 51-52, 57-58.

Environmental Tobacco Smoke. (1998). Cancer Facts, 3.90; (From rex.nci.nih.gov/INFO_CANCER/Cancer_facts/Section3/FS3_90.html (5/5/98).

Hardman, J.G. & Limbird, L.E. (Eds.). (1996). *Goodman and Gilman's The pharmacological basis of therapeutics* (9th ed.). New York: McGraw-Hill.

Holdcroft, C. (1992). Efficacy of transdermal patches for nicotine replacement and smoking cessation. *Nurse Practitioner, 17*(7), 46.

Johnson, J.L., Budz, B., Mackay, M., & Miller, C. (1999). Evaluation of a nurse-delivered smoking cessation intervention for hospitalized patients with cardiac disease. *Heart Lung, 28*(1), 55-64.

Martin, J. (1998). Nurses important in tobacco use prevention, control. *Nebraska Nurse, 31*(13):18.

New Drugs/Drug News. (1996). Nasal spray smoke cessation approved. *P&T: Pharmacy & Therapeutics, 21*(6), 303.

Ponec, R.J., Saunders, M.D., & Kimmey, M.B. (1999) Neostigmine for the treatment of acute colonic pseudo-obstruction. *New England Journal of Medicine, 341*(3), 137-141.

Silagy, C., Mant, D., Fowler, G., & Lancaster, T. (2001). Nicotine replacement therapy for smoking cessation (Cochran Review). In *The Cochran Library*, Issue 1. Oxford: Update Software.

Taylor, P. (1996). Agents acting at the neuromuscular junction and autonomic ganglia. In J.G. Hardman & L.E. Limbird (Eds.), *Goodman & Gilman's The pharmacological basis of therapeutics* (9th ed.). New York: McGraw-Hill.

United States Pharmacopeia Dispensing Information (USP DI): Drug information for the health care professional (19th ed.). (1999). Rockville, MD: United States Pharmacopeial Convention.

22 Drugs Affecting the Sympathetic (Adrenergic) Nervous System

Chapter Focus

Adrenergic receptors regulate cardiac, arteriolar, bronchial, and gastrointestinal smooth muscle. Pharmacologic intervention related to these receptors is commonplace and varied. The management of clients receiving drugs that affect the sympathetic, or adrenergic, nervous system challenges nurses daily.

Learning Objectives

1. Discuss the three types of adrenergic drugs.
2. Differentiate between alpha$_1$-, alpha$_2$-, beta$_1$-, and beta$_2$-adrenergic effects.
3. Describe the effects of the three naturally occurring catecholamines on the body.
4. List common adrenergic drugs and blocking agents, their effects, and the side effects/adverse reactions.
5. Implement the nursing management of the care of clients receiving adrenergic and adrenergic-blocking drugs.

Key Terms

alpha-adrenergic blocking agents, p. 478
beta-adrenergic blocking agents (commonly called "beta blockers"), p. 483
calorigenic effect, p. 462
dromotropic effect, p. 461
inotropic effect, p. 461
sympathomimetic drugs, p. 459

Key Drugs [✔]

dopamine, p. 471
epinephrine, p. 462
norepinephrine, p. 467
propranolol, p. 483

ADRENERGIC DRUGS

Sympathomimetic drugs are medications that enhance or mimic the effects of sympathetic nerve stimulation. These drugs are designed to produce actions similar to those of the neurotransmitters, such as increased cardiac output, vasoconstriction of arterioles and veins, regulation of body temperature, bronchial dilation, and a variety of other effects. (See Chapter 20 for additional information on adrenergic effects.) The sympathomimetic drugs are also called adrenergic drugs and are of three types: (1) direct-acting, (2) indirect-acting, and (3) dual-acting (direct and indirect) agents.

Direct-Acting Adrenergic Drugs

Catecholamines

The three naturally occurring catecholamines in the body—dopamine, norepinephrine, and epinephrine—are synthesized by the sympathetic nervous system. Dopamine is a precursor of norepinephrine and epinephrine, but it also has a transmitter role of its own in certain portions of the central nervous system (CNS). (For more information on adrenergic transmission, see Figure 20-5 and the discussion in Chapter 20.)

Epinephrine is primarily an emergency hormone, whereas norepinephrine is an important transmitter of nerve impulses and is an intermediary in epinephrine biosynthesis. In the sympathetic nervous system the adrenergic effector cells contain two distinct receptors: alpha (α) and beta (β) receptors. Catecholamines that depend on their ability to interact *directly* with the adrenergic receptors are called *direct-acting* drugs. The response of these agents is mediated by directly stimulating the adrenergic receptors.

There is evidence that the alpha receptors appear in two primary locations. The alpha$_2$ receptors are found on the presynaptic nerve terminals, platelets, and smooth muscle and thus are called presynaptic (prejunctional) receptor sites. The presynaptic receptor controls the *amount* of transmitter released per nerve impulse; this can be regulated by a feedback mechanism. When the concentration of transmitter released from the nerve terminal into the synaptic cleft reaches a high level, the presynaptic receptors are stimulated, which prevents further release of the transmitter. This type of feedback prevents excessive and prolonged stimulation of the postsynaptic cell. The postsynaptic receptors, which are located on the effector organs, are known as alpha$_1$ receptors (in the eye, arterioles, veins, male sex organ, and bladder).

The beta receptors are subdivided on the basis of their responses to drugs. Beta$_1$ receptors are located mainly in the heart, whereas beta$_2$ receptors mediate the actions of catecholamines on smooth muscle, especially bronchioles and arterial smooth muscle.

Norepinephrine acts mainly on alpha receptors, causing vasoconstriction. Epinephrine acts on both alpha and beta receptors to produce a mixture of vasodilation and vasoconstriction. Isoproterenol, a synthetic catecholamine, acts only on beta receptors. Table 22-1 provides an overview of receptor sensitivity.

The most important alpha-adrenergic activities in humans are the following:

1. Vasoconstriction of arterioles in the skin and splanchnic area, resulting in a rise in blood pressure
2. Pupil dilation
3. Relaxation of the gut

TABLE 22-1 Overview of Adrenergic Receptor Stimulation

Receptor	Effect	Location
Alpha$_1$	Contraction or vasoconstriction of peripheral blood vessels Dilation (contraction) of pupil Increased contractility of heart	α_1: Vascular smooth muscle; Pupil (dilator muscle); Heart
Alpha$_2$	Limit or control of transmitter release Aggregation of platelets Contraction of smooth muscle	α_2: Smooth muscle; Presynaptic adrenergic & cholinergic nerve terminals; Platelets
Beta$_1$	Increased acceleration of heart rate (chronotropic) Increased contractility of heart (inotropic)	β_1: Heart
Beta$_2$	Dilation of bronchial smooth muscle Relaxation of uterus Activation of glycogenolysis	β_2: Liver; Bronchial smooth muscle; Uterus

TABLE 22-2 **Adrenergic Receptor Stimulation**

Effector Organs	Receptor Type	Adrenergic Response
Heart		
Cardiac muscle (atria, ventricles)	β_1	Increased force of contraction (inotropic action)
Sinoatrial node	β_1	Increased heart rate (chronotropic action)
Atrioventricular node	β_1	Increased automaticity and conduction velocity; shortened refractory period (chronotropic action)
Blood vessels		
Arterioles		
Coronary	α_1, β_2, dopaminergic	Constriction, dilation*
Cerebral	α_1	Constriction
Pulmonary	α_1, β_2	Constriction,* dilation
Mesenteric visceral	α_1, β_2	Constriction,* dilation
Renal	α_1, β_2, dopaminergic	Constriction,* dilation
Skin, mucosa	α_1, α_2	Constriction
Skeletal muscle	α, β_2	Constriction, dilation
Veins	α_1, β_2	Constriction, dilation
Lung		
Bronchial smooth muscle	β_2	Bronchodilation
Bronchial glands	α_1, β_2	Inhibition
Gastrointestinal tract		
Smooth muscle (motility, tone)	α_1, α_2, β_2	Decreased
Sphincter	α_1	Contraction
Secretion	?	Inhibition
Gallbladder and ducts	—	Relaxation
Liver	β_2	Glycogenolysis
Spleen capsule	α_1, β_2	Contraction,* relaxation
Pancreas: insulin secretion	α_2	Decreased
Adipose tissue	β_1	Lipolysis
Urinary bladder		
Detrusor muscle	β_2	Relaxation
Sphincter	α_1	Contraction
Kidney ureter	α_1	Contraction
Kidney secretion (renin)	β_1	Increased
Uterus		
Pregnant	α_1	Contraction
Nonpregnant	β_2	Relaxation
Sex organs, male	α_1	Ejaculation
Skin		
Pilomotor muscles	α_1	Contraction
Sweat glands	α_1, cholinergic	Increased secretion
Eye		
Radial muscle, iris (pupil size)	α_1	Contraction—pupil dilation (mydriasis)
Ciliary muscle	β_2	Relaxation for far vision

*Predominant response.

Beta-adrenergic activity includes the following:

1. Cardiac acceleration and increased contractility
2. Vasodilation of arterioles supplying skeletal muscles
3. Bronchial relaxation
4. Uterine relaxation

The effects of both alpha and beta stimulation result from a summation of action where they are interrelated. That is, a change in blood pressure depends on the degree of vasoconstriction in the skin and splanchnic area *and* the extent of vasodilation in skeletal muscles, along with changes in heart rate. Large arteries and veins contain both alpha and beta receptors; the heart contains only beta receptors (Table 22-2).

Specific drugs are available to stimulate or block alpha and beta receptors. With the exception of central alpha$_2$ receptors, these agents work at peripheral autonomic sites.

As catecholamines, norepinephrine and epinephrine are important neurohormones in neural and endocrine integration. They are always present in arterial blood, but the amount varies widely during any one day. Certain physiologic stimuli such as stress and exercise significantly increase blood levels of catecholamine. Studies indicate that the major sources of circulating norepinephrine are stimulated sympathetic nerve endings. Organs such as the heart and blood vessels receive a large fraction of blood and possess large numbers of sympathetic nerve endings; thus they contain the greatest amount of catecholamines. The number of sympathetic nerve endings or adrenergic nerves to various organs determines the magnitude of response of these organs to increased levels or injections of catecholamines.

Pharmacologic Effects

Catecholamines produce a variety of physiologic responses.

Cardiac. The pharmacologic effects of the catecholamines are essentially a result of their direct effect as agonists on specific alpha and beta receptors (β_1 and β_2). Epinephrine increases heart rate, stroke volume, and cardiac output, whereas norepinephrine does not alter cardiac output and may even slightly decrease heart rate and cardiac output. This effect of norepinephrine is believed to result from its potent vasoconstriction action, which increases resistance to the ejection of blood from the heart. The increased work of the heart to move the blood against increased pressure is "pressure work" rather than "volume work."

Thus the effects of epinephrine and norepinephrine are approximately equivalent on beta$_1$ receptors, but norepinephrine is a more potent agonist at alpha receptors (vasoconstriction), with little effort on beta$_2$ receptors (vasodilation). Epinephrine is a potent stimulant of alpha and beta receptors, but its peripheral resistance effects may vary depending on the dose and the ratio of alpha to beta receptor response in various areas.

A significant increase in myocardial contraction (positive **inotropic effect**) is the result of the increased influx of calcium into cardiac fibers. Strong myocardial contractions result in more complete emptying of the ventricles and an increase in cardiac work and oxygen consumption. Strong contractions brought about by isoproterenol and epinephrine also increase cardiac output or volume.

Norepinephrine, with its predominantly alpha-adrenergic activity, may not produce as severe a tachycardia as epinephrine. The increased vasoconstriction and increased blood pressure may cause a reflex bradycardia. Isoproterenol usually produces a tachycardia, since its direct and reflex effects act in the same direction. Dosage and client variables affect these responses.

An increase in atrioventricular conduction (positive **dromotropic effect**) is another physiologic response. Because epinephrine increases atrioventricular conduction, some cardiologists use it in the treatment of heart block.

Catecholamines may also produce spontaneous firing of Purkinje fibers, which may cause them to exhibit pacemaker activity. This effect may cause ventricular extrasystoles and increase the susceptibility of ventricular muscle to fibrillation. These effects are more likely to occur with epinephrine than norepinephrine.

Vascular. The vascular effects of the catecholamines depend on the dose and the vascular bed affected. Low doses of epinephrine may decrease total peripheral vascular resistance and decrease blood pressure. In large doses epinephrine activates alpha receptors in the greater peripheral vascular system, which increases resistance and increases blood pressure. Norepinephrine elevates blood pressure by increasing peripheral resistance and decreasing blood flow through the skeletal muscles.

Norepinephrine, a vasoconstrictor, increases total peripheral resistance. Isoproterenol is not a vasoconstrictor but a pure vasodilator; epinephrine is both a vasoconstrictor and vasodilator, with vasodilation being greater in its overall net effects. For example, during great stress the release of epinephrine from the adrenal medulla constricts blood vessels in the skin and splanchnic areas but dilates those of the skeletal muscles, thus shunting blood to the areas needed for "fight or flight" responses.

Renal artery constriction and resistance is greater with epinephrine than with norepinephrine. In large doses epinephrine may actually stop blood flow through some nephrons and stimulate the release of antidiuretic hormone (ADH), thereby reducing urinary excretion.

Central Nervous System. In sufficient amounts, epinephrine and isoproterenol can lead to alertness, tremulousness, respiratory stimulation, and anxiety. Norepinephrine is less likely to cause anxiety and tremulousness. The beneficial cerebral effects from epinephrine and norepinephrine in cases of hypotension are thought to result from increased systemic pressure with a resultant improvement in cerebral blood flow.

Smooth Muscle. In general, the catecholamines relax nonvascular smooth muscles. When the smooth muscle of the gastrointestinal tract is relaxed, the amplitude and tone of intestinal peristalsis are reduced. Theoretically this may slow the propulsion of food and gastrointestinal emptying. This effect is rare in humans with therapeutic doses of catecholamines.

In some situations the smooth muscle of some organs reacts like vascular smooth muscle and contracts. For example, the radial and sphincter muscles of the iris contract, and the smooth muscle of the lids may contract, giving rise to the widened, staring eyes seen in sympathetically stimulated individuals.

In the urinary bladder, epinephrine causes trigone and sphincter constriction and detrusor relaxation with a delay in the desire to void.

Respiratory. Catecholamines dilate bronchial smooth muscle. Isoproterenol is a more active bronchodilator than epinephrine, whereas epinephrine is a stronger bronchodilator than norepinephrine.

Glandular. As a rule, sympathomimetics decrease secretion and produce a dry mouth. However, epinephrine may increase the amount of viscid saliva excreted. Catecholamines may produce local sweating on the palms of the hands and in the axillary and genital areas. The exact mechanism for these effects is not clear.

Metabolic. Epinephrine inhibits insulin secretion. Catecholamines have antagonistic effects on gluconeogenesis, and they decrease liver and skeletal muscle glycogen and increase lipolysis in adipose tissue. The result of these effects is a rise in blood sugar and an increase in free fatty acids. Thus there can be an abundant supply of fuel and energy in response to stress ("fight or flight" response) (Figure 22-1).

Catecholamines also have a **calorigenic effect** (capable of generating heat, which increases oxygen consumption) resulting from the sum of the preceding effects. The action of norepinephrine in relation to these effects is weaker than that of epinephrine or isoproterenol.

epinephrine [ep i nef′ rin] (Adrenalin)

Epinephrine is available in solutions for inhalation and nebulization, parenteral administration, and ophthalmic administration. Many bronchodilator aerosols are available over-the-counter (OTC) in solutions containing up to 1% of the epinephrine base.

Inhalation dosage forms include the following:

- epinephrine inhalation aerosol (Bronkaid Mist, Bronkaid Mistometer ♣)
- epinephrine bitartrate inhalation aerosol (Asthma-Haler, Medihaler-Epi)
- racepinephrine inhalation solution (AsthmaNefrin, Vaponefrin)

Parenteral dosage forms and ophthalmic solutions include the following; ophthalmic epinephrine is discussed in Chapter 43:

- epinephrine injection (Adrenalin, EpiPen Auto-Injector)
- sterile epinephrine suspension (Sus-Phrine)

Mechanism of Action. Epinephrine is a direct-acting catecholamine that is naturally released from the adrenal medulla in response to sympathoadrenal stimulation. It also is prepared synthetically. Epinephrine stimulates alpha and beta receptors. Its primary action is on the beta receptors of the heart, the smooth muscle of the bronchi, and the blood vessels. The $beta_1$ action stimulates the heart by increasing heart rate, the force of myocardial contraction, and cardiac output. The $beta_2$ action on the smooth muscle of the bronchioles produces bronchodilation, thereby increasing tidal volume and vital capacity of the lung. Stimulation of the alpha receptors constricts the arterioles of the bronchioles and inhibits histamine release, thus reducing nasal congestion and edema. In contrast, $beta_2$-adrenergic activity of the smooth muscle of arterioles causes vasodilation.

Another effect of epinephrine is alpha activity, which results in contraction of the radial muscle in the iris ($alpha_1$), causing dilation of the pupil (mydriasis). Constriction of the blood vessels in the skin is also activated by alpha activity. The detrusor muscle in the urinary bladder contains beta receptors and is relaxed by epinephrine (see Table 22-2).

Indications. Epinephrine is used in the following situations:

1. For symptomatic treatment of bronchial asthma and other obstructive pulmonary diseases that cause bronchospasm, such as chronic bronchitis and emphysema.
2. For symptomatic relief of acute hypersensitivity reactions. It is indicated in the emergency treatment of acute anaphylactic shock and severe acute reactions to drugs, animal serums, insect stings, and other allergens to relieve bronchospasm, urticaria, hives, angioneurotic edema, and swelling of nasal mucosa. Pulmonary congestion is also alleviated by the constriction of mucosal blood vessels.

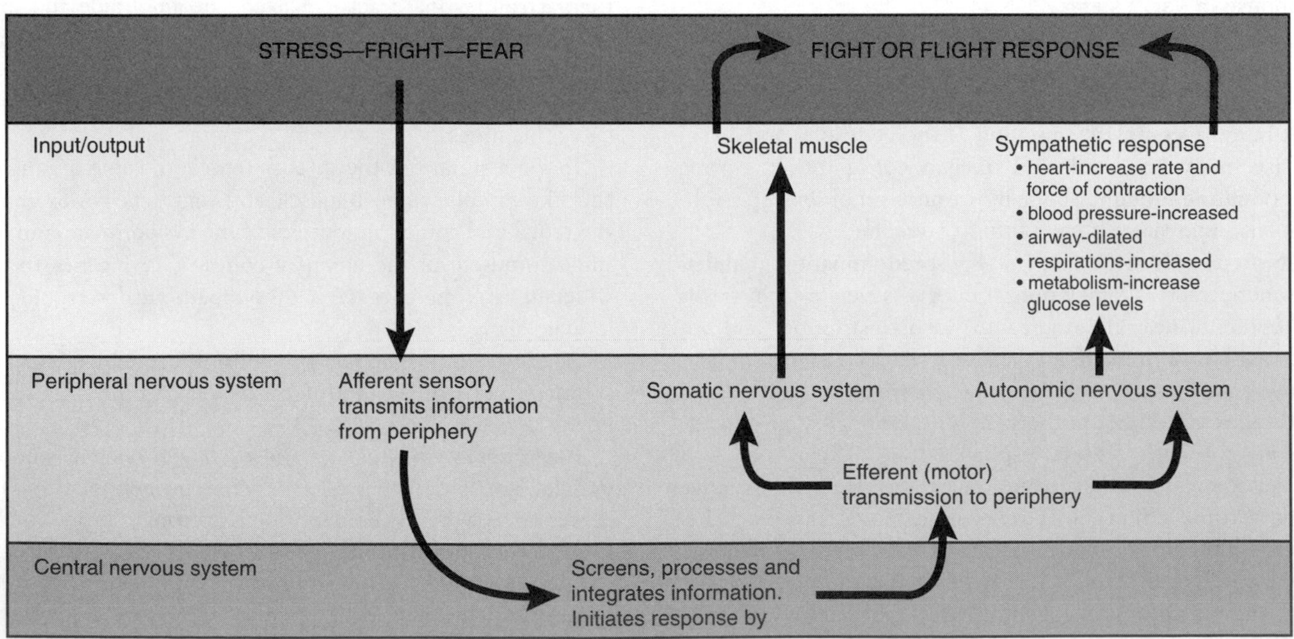

Figure 22-1 Nervous system response to severe fright or stress.

3. As an adjunct with local anesthetics. Concurrent administration of epinephrine with local anesthetics reduces circulation to the site, which results in a slowing of vascular absorption. This promotes a local effect of the anesthetic and also prolongs its duration of action, thus reducing the risk of anesthetic toxicity.
4. As a hemostatic agent to control superficial bleeding from arterioles and capillaries in the skin, mucous membranes, or other tissues.
5. In ocular surgery to control bleeding, induce mydriasis and conjunctival decongestion, and decrease intraocular pressure.
6. To treat cardiac arrest or cardiac standstill. On occasion it may be given by intracardiac injection in acute attacks of ventricular standstill, after physical measures and electrical defibrillation have failed.

Pharmacokinetics. Epinephrine should not be given orally because it is rapidly metabolized in the mucosa of the gastrointestinal tract and liver; serum levels achieved with this route would be inadequate. It is well absorbed following IM or SC injection.

Epinephrine has a rapid onset of action, from 3 to 5 minutes after inhalation or between 6 and 15 minutes after SC injection. The duration of action of epinephrine is 1 to 3 hours by inhalation and from 1 to 4 hours after IM or SC injection. In severe anaphylaxis, asthma, or cardiac arrest, epinephrine doses may need to be repeated every 5 to 20 minutes, depending on the dose used and the client's response. Epinephrine is metabolized in the liver and excreted by the kidneys.

Side Effects/Adverse Reactions. Side effects/adverse reactions of epinephrine include increased nervousness, restlessness, insomnia, tachycardia, tremors, sweating, increased blood pressure, nausea, vomiting, pallor, weakness and, with inhalation devices, bronchial irritation and coughing (with high doses), dry mouth and throat, headaches, and flushing of the face and skin.

Dosage and Administration. See Table 22-3 for the dosage and administration of epinephrine.

■ Nursing Management

Epinephrine Therapy

■ **Assessment.** Before epinephrine is administered, the client should be assessed for preexisting health conditions for which the drug may be contraindicated or a higher level of caution may be indicated, such as asymmetric septal hypertrophy, tachycardia, or pheochromocytoma (a vascular tumor of the adrenal medulla characterized by hypersecretion of epinephrine and norepinephrine). This drug should not be used by individuals with narrow-angle glaucoma, traumatic or hemorrhagic shock (increases myocardial oxygen demand), or organic brain damage.

Use epinephrine with caution in older adults and in those with cardiovascular disease, hypertension, hyperthyroidism, or psychosis because the drug may worsen the underlying condition. Pulmonary edema, which can be fatal, may occur because of peripheral constriction. Use epinephrine with caution in clients with bronchial asthma or emphysema who also have degenerative heart disease. Clients with coronary insufficiency may develop anginal pain. Clients with diabetes mellitus may require a higher insulin dosage because of epinephrine-induced hyperglycemia.

Epinephrine should be administered with great caution to clients who are pregnant. Epinephrine is known to cross the placenta, and although appropriate human studies have not been conducted to demonstrate the teratogenic effects seen in rat studies, it may cause anoxia in the fetus. If administered during labor, it may delay the second stage because of the relaxation of uterine muscles. Epinephrine can cause acceleration of the fetal heart rate when given parenterally to maintain maternal blood pressure during delivery; it is contraindicated if the maternal blood pressure is greater than 130/80 mm Hg.

Review the client's current medication regimen for the risk of significant drug interactions, such as those that may occur when epinephrine is given concurrently with the following drugs:

Drug	Possible Effect and Management
Bold/color type indicates the most serious interactions.	
anesthetics (e.g., cyclopropane, halothane [Fluothane], enflurane [Ethrane], isoflurane [Forane], trichloroethylene)	May sensitize the heart, increasing the risk of severe dysrhythmias. Monitor closely because a reduction in epinephrine (sympathomimetics) is usually necessary.
anesthetics (local parenteral)	Reduced blood supply may result in ischemia and gangrene when used in end artery areas such as fingers, toes, or penis. Use very cautiously in such areas and monitor closely.
beta-adrenergic receptor blocking agents, including ophthalmics	**The therapeutic effects of both agents may be inhibited. With bronchodilators having both alpha-and beta-stimulating effects (epinephrine), stimulation of alpha receptors with beta-receptor blockade may result in hypertension and severe bradycardia with possible heart block. Avoid concurrent use or a serious drug interaction may occur. However, concurrent use of ophthalmic betaxolol, levobunolol, or timolol with ophthalmic epinephrine may have a therapeutic additive effect in lowering intraocular pressure** (*United States Pharmacopeia Dispensing Information*, 1999).
digitalis glycosides	**Digitalis sensitizes the myocardium to the effects of epinephrine; the additive effect of the catecholamine may precipitate ectopic pacemaker activity. Caution is recommended if concurrent use is necessary.**
ergotamine or ergoloid mesylates (Hydergine)	**Concurrent use may produce severe hypertension, peripheral vascular ischemia, and gangrene. Avoid concurrent use or a serious drug interaction may occur.**

Continued

TABLE 22-3 Epinephrine: Dosage and Administration

Indication	Adults	Children
Parenteral		
Bronchodilator	0.2-0.5 mg SC every 20 minutes, up to 3 doses as needed.	0.01 mg/kg SC every 15 minutes for 3 or 4 doses, or every 4 hours if needed.
Anaphylaxis	0.3-0.5 mg IM, SC repeated every 10-20 minutes as needed for up to 3 doses.	0.01 mg/kg SC repeated every 15 minutes for up to 3 doses.
Cardiac stimulant	IV or intracardiac injection 0.1-1 mg (base) diluted to 10 mL with sodium chloride injection given to restore myocardial contractility. After intracardiac administration, external cardiac massage should be applied to enhance drug entry into coronary circulation. May repeat every 5 minutes if needed.*	0.005-0.01 mg/kg IV or intracardiac injection; repeat every 5 minutes or follow with IV infusion at an initial rate of 0.001 mg/kg/min.
Anesthetic (local) adjunct	Intraspinal 0.2-0.4 mg added to anesthetic spinal mixture. With local anesthetic: 1:200,000.	See adult dosage.
Auto-injection		
Auto-injector for emergency self-treatment of anaphylaxis (EpiPen Auto-Injector)	Available in 0.5 mg/mL and 1 mg/mL.	
Suspension (Sus-Phrine)		
Bronchodilator	0.5 mg SC initially, followed by 0.5-1.5 mg q6h as necessary.	0.025 mg/kg SC. May be repeated in 6 hours. If child weighs 30 kg, maximum single dose is 0.75 mg.
Inhalation		
Bronchodilator 1:100 (1%) solution	Proper dose automatically dispensed by metered nebulizer. Allow 1-5 minutes between inhalations. Use fewest possible inhalations.	
Topical		
Nasal decongestant	1-2 drops (0.1% solution) q4-6h.	
Antihemorrhagic	0.002%-0.1% (1:50,000 to 1:1000) solution of epinephrine applied locally.	

*If IV access cannot be achieved, epinephrine may be administered by an endotracheal tube.

Drug	Possible Effect and Management
tricyclic antidepressants, maprotiline (Ludiomil), monoamine oxidase (MAO) inhibitor antidepressants, doxapram, or cocaine	Concurrent use may result in dysrhythmias, tachycardia, hypertension, or hyperpyrexia. Avoid concurrent use or a serious drug interaction may occur.

A baseline assessment of the client's cardiopulmonary status should be obtained by electrocardiogram (ECG), blood pressure, and auscultation of heart and lung sounds.

■ **Nursing Diagnosis.** Because of the CNS effects of dizziness or light-headedness, nervousness or restlessness, trembling, and insomnia, the client with epinephrine therapy should be evaluated for the nursing diagnoses of impaired comfort, disturbed sleep pattern, anxiety, disturbed thought processes, and risk for injury. There also may be impaired comfort resulting from the gastrointestinal, respiratory, and local effects of the drug. Evaluate for ineffective airway clearance related to the client's preexisting health status to determine the effectiveness of the drug. The cardiovascular effects—headache, hypertension, palpitations, tachycardia, flushing of the face—may indicate the complication of altered cardiac output.

■ **Implementation**

■ ***Monitoring.*** Assess the client's vital signs and auscultate the heart and lungs periodically. During IV administration of epinephrine, monitor vital signs and observe ECG results continuously until stabilized. Depending on the client's condition, interarterial blood pressure, central venous pressure, pulmonary artery pressure, and pulmonary capillary wedge pressure may also be monitored. Monitor urine flow and for signs of excess fluid volume such as peripheral edema, sudden weight gain, and distended neck veins. Monitor serum potassium levels because of the risk of hypokalemia. Because epinephrine increases blood glucose levels, observe individuals with diabetes for loss of diabetic control.

■ ***Intervention.*** Avoid epinephrine overdose, particularly inadvertent IV administration of the usual SC doses, which may cause extreme hypertension. Cerebrovascular hemorrhage may result, particularly in older adults. Read the labels very carefully; ophthalmic, nasal, and topical solutions of epinephrine must not be injected.

Store medication in a tight, light-resistant container at a temperature between 15° and 30° C (59° and 86° F). Do not use if the solution is pink or brown in color or contains a precipitate. This color change is caused by oxidation of the drug; multiple-use vials in which air is injected to withdraw the solution are more prone to this change.

■ *Parenteral Administration.* Carefully recheck the strength, dosage, expiration date, and route of administration of the solution. Avoid medication errors by not confusing the 1 : 100 solution with the 1 : 1000 solution. Overdose has resulted in fatalities. Use a small syringe (tuberculin syringe) to ensure accuracy in measuring the parenteral injection. Aspirate the syringe before parenteral injection (SC and IM) to prevent IV injection, which can result in sudden hypertension. Intraarterial injection is contraindicated because the marked vasoconstriction that results may cause gangrene. Injection sites need to be rotated because repeated local injections may result in necrosis secondary to the vasoconstricting effects of the drug. Massaging the injection site will promote absorption of the drug. Because of this vasoconstriction, epinephrine should not be administered intramuscularly into the buttocks; the presence of the anaerobic organism *Clostridium welchii* and reduced oxygen tension within the tissues as a result of the administration of epinephrine creates the potential for gas gangrene.

The use of sterile epinephrine in a suspension allows the parenteral injection to be effective up to 10 hours; inject the suspension promptly after withdrawing it from the vial to prevent the solution from settling. A 1 : 1000 solution must be diluted with a 10-mL sodium chloride injection before IV or intracardiac administration.

Epinephrine may be administered intracardially in emergency situations; this type of administration should be performed by team members who have experience with this technique. If the client is intubated, the drug can be injected directly into the bronchial tree via the endotracheal tube at the same dose as for IV administration.

■ *Inhalation.* Epinephrine and other beta-adrenergic agents may be used interchangeably; allow 4 hours between doses when changing from one to another. Do not administer the doses concurrently.

■ *Nasal Administration.* To prevent epinephrine from entering the throat, instill nose drops with the head low and in the lateral position. Rinse the nose dropper with hot water to prevent contamination of medication.

■ ***Education.*** Instruct the client to take the medication exactly as prescribed and, if required, to take it around-the-clock. Caution the client against the repeated or prolonged use of epinephrine, which can cause *tolerance* or "epinephrine fastness." The effectiveness of the drug usually returns if withheld 12 hours to several days. The client should avoid self-medicating with any OTC preparations without consulting with prescriber. The client should contact the prescriber if he or she experiences tachycardia, shortness of breath, or chest pain.

■ *Emergency Auto-Injection.* Remind the client that epinephrine requires a prescription. Instruct the client to consult the prescriber or pharmacist before taking any OTC drug concurrently with epinephrine. Using a placebo trainer, review with the client in detail the operation of the EpiPen Auto-Injector (Grouhi, Alshri, Hummel, & Roifman, 1999). The package insert *must* be read carefully. Remind the client that the auto-injector contains the drug that the client injects intramuscularly in the anterolateral region of the thigh or the deltoid part of the arm. Instruct the client not to inject the drug into the buttocks because of the increased risk of infection resulting from fecal contaminants on the skin.

Emphasize the importance of keeping epinephrine on hand in case of emergency and of storing the drug in a dark, cool place to prevent deterioration. Supplies should be rotated so the client uses the oldest supplies first. Caution the client to check the auto-injector to make sure the solution is neither brown in color nor contains a precipitate; in such cases, the drug must be discarded.

■ *Inhalation.* Teach the client how to use the metered dose nebulizer (see the box in Chapter 38 on p. 715). Instruct the client to measure his or her pulse rate before inhalation therapy. Allow 2 minutes between doses, and do not administer it more frequently than required to relieve symptoms. Excessive repeated use may cause paradoxical bronchospasm. To prevent drug tolerance, caution the client not to overuse the drug.

Instruct the client to notify the prescriber if symptoms are not relieved with the usual dosage, because this may be an indication of worsening bronchospasm that requires reassessment of therapy. The prescriber should also be notified if the pulse rate increases more than 20 to 30 beats/min. The client may expect the symptoms to be relieved in 20 minutes. Instruct the client to rinse his or her mouth with water to prevent mucosal absorption of drug. Teach clients with a history of allergic reaction or bronchial asthma how to self-inject epinephrine subcutaneously in case of emergency.

■ *Nasal Administration.* Inform the client that nasal administration of epinephrine may produce a stinging sensation. Forewarn the client that rebound congestion may occur with prolonged use, which may cause rhinitis. Nose drops should not be used for more than 3 to 5 days.

■ *Ophthalmic Administration.* Alert the client that lightheadedness, increased perspiration and heart rate, trembling, and pallor are signs of systemic absorption. These symptoms may be avoided by limiting the amount of epinephrine that enters the systemic circulation through the proper instillation of eyedrops. Instruct the client to create a pocket for the solution by gently pinching the skin below the lower eyelid and pulling it away from the eye. Place a drop of the solution into the pocket and hold it open for 1 or 2 seconds to allow the solution to settle. Have the client look down and then gently release the lower eyelid. Press just under the inner corner of the eye for 1 minute. This obstructs the nasolacrimal duct and minimizes the absorption of the drug into the bloodstream.

Administer epinephrine at bedtime or following a miotic to minimize discomfort, blurred vision, and sensitivity to light caused by mydriasis.

Instruct the client to discontinue epinephrine and notify the prescriber if signs of allergy develop (itching, edema of lids, discharge from lids). Advise the client that headache and stinging of the eyes may occur after initial administration but that these symptoms disappear with continued drug use. Notify the prescriber if these symptoms persist; they may be controlled with a lower dosage. Recommend to the client that intraocular pressure determinations should be scheduled periodically.

The client should be alerted that brownish pigment deposits caused by oxidation of the drug may occur in the eyelids and conjunctiva or may appear as large dark casts in the lacrimal sac or nasolacrimal duct after long-term use of epinephrine. These deposits, which may be mistaken as foreign objects in the eye, may be removed by irrigation. Instruct clients who wear soft contact lenses to consult with the prescriber regarding the concurrent use of ophthalmic epinephrine instillation, because the medication may discolor the lenses.

■ **Evaluation.** The expected outcome of epinephrine therapy is that the client's symptoms will be relieved, vital signs will be within the normal range, and the client will not experience any adverse reactions to the drug.

isoproterenol hydrochloride [eye soe proe ter′ e nole] (Isuprel)
isoproterenol sulfate (Medihaler-Iso)

Isoproterenol, a synthetic catecholamine, is a nonselective beta-adrenergic drug and stimulates $beta_1$- and $beta_2$-adrenergic receptors. $Beta_1$ receptor activity produces an increase in the force of myocardial contraction and heart rate. The $beta_2$ receptor response of the smooth muscle of the bronchi, skeletal muscle, gastrointestinal tract, and blood vessels of the splanchnic bed causes a relaxation of these organs. More important, isoproterenol can greatly relax the smaller bronchi and may even dilate the trachea and main bronchi. This drug also stimulates insulin secretion and releases free fatty acid.

Hemodynamically, the $beta_1$ activity of the heart increases cardiac output and venous return to the heart. Peripheral vascular resistance is reduced, and in normal individuals a significant drop in blood pressure may occur with excessive dosage.

Isoproterenol relieves bronchospasm associated with bronchial asthma, pulmonary emphysema, and bronchitis. Isoproterenol may also be used as a cardiac stimulant in cardiac arrest, Adams-Stokes syndrome, atrioventricular (AV) block, and carotid sinus hypersensitivity. It may be used as adjunct therapy in the treatment of cardiogenic shock. However, isoproterenol is no longer used routinely as an inotropic agent. It has been replaced in most clinical settings by newer agents that are less prone to induce ischemia or dysrhythmias (*USP DI*, 1999).

Isoproterenol is readily absorbed when given parenterally or by inhalation. The absorption of sublingual isoproterenol is erratic and unreliable. Its duration of action is usually up to 2 hours after oral inhalation or SC administration and less than 1 hour after IV administration. Isoproterenol is metabolized in the gastrointestinal tract, liver, and lungs and is excreted in the urine.

The side effects/adverse reactions of isoproterenol are similar to epinephrine except that inhalation and sublingual dosage forms may induce a pink to red discoloration of saliva (an expected alteration).

■ **Dosage and Administration**

■ ***Bradycardia.*** The dosage for adults with heart block, Adams-Stokes attacks, and cardiac arrest is by IV injection of diluted isoproterenol, 1 mL of 1:5000 solution diluted with 10 mL of sodium chloride or 5% dextrose injection. The initial dosage is 0.02 to 0.06 mg (1 to 3 mL of diluted preparation) with a follow-up dosage range of 0.01 to 0.2 mg (or 0.5 to 10 mL of diluted solution). Refer to a current drug reference (e.g., package insert, *USP DI*) for dosing by IV infusion, intracardiac administration, IM, or SC. The dosage for children has not been determined and is individualized by the prescriber.

■ ***Inhaler.*** Follow the individual manufacturer's instructions carefully when administering isoproterenol by inhalation. In general, one inhalation is administered with a metered dose nebulizer; this may be repeated in 1 to 5 minutes if necessary. Doses may be repeated four to six times daily. When treating acute asthma in children, an oral inhalation of a nebulized solution (0.05 to 0.1 mg/kg, up to 1.25 mg diluted) is administered over 10 to 20 minutes; this may be repeated in 4 hours if necessary.

■ Nursing Management

Isoproterenol Therapy

■ **Assessment.** Use isoproterenol with great caution in clients with cardiovascular disorders such as angina, dysrhythmias, coronary insufficiency, and hypertension (condition may be worsened); hyperthyroidism (adverse reaction more apt to occur); pheochromocytoma; diabetes (drug-induced hyperglycemia may occur); or sensitivity to sympathomimetic amines. Excessive use may decrease effectiveness.

A review of the client's current medication regimen will detect any possible drug interactions. With the exception of the local-parenteral anesthetic interactions, the drug interactions with isoproterenol are similar to those listed under epinephrine. In addition, avoid the concurrent administration of epinephrine and isoproterenol because of the possibility of increased additive effects and cardiotoxicity. When the action of one medication is considered complete (usually 4 hours), a different one may be administered.

Baseline assessments of the client's health status to be obtained are the same as for epinephrine.

■ **Nursing Diagnosis.** Because of the CNS effects of dizziness or light-headedness, nervousness or restlessness, trembling, and insomnia, the client should be evaluated for the nursing diagnoses of disturbed sleep pattern, anxiety, impaired oral mucous membrane (dry mouth), disturbed thought processes, and risk for injury (dizziness). There may also be impaired comfort because of the gastrointestinal, respiratory, and local effects of the drug. Evaluate for ineffective airway clearance related to the client's preexisting health status to determine the effectiveness of the drug. The potential complication of altered cardiac output may be evidenced by headache, hypertension, palpitations, tachycardia, and flushing of the face.

■ **Implementation**

■ ***Monitoring.*** Record the baseline blood pressure and pulse before starting IV administration of isoproterenol therapy. During infusion, document the blood pressure every 2 minutes until stabilized, then every 5 minutes during drug administration. Adjust the IV flow rate to maintain the desired rhythm or blood pressure—usually a systolic pressure of 80 to 100 mm Hg or, in clients with hypertension, 30 to 40 mm Hg below the preexisting blood pressure. Monitor ECG patterns and central venous pressure, as well as urine volume and blood gases for clients in shock. Pulmonary artery pressure and pulmonary capillary wedge pressure may also be monitored. Follow the prescriber's guidelines for titrating flow in relation to heart rate, central venous pressure, blood pressure, ECG changes, and volume of urine flow. IV isoproterenol often causes dysrhythmias in clients with heart disease. Monitor the client's respiratory pattern and lung sounds during administration. Discontinue the drug if precordial pain occurs. If the heart rate exceeds 110 beats/min, a slower infusion rate or a temporary discontinuance of the drug will be prescribed. Anticipate the development of ventricular dysrhythmias with doses that cause a heart rate of 130 beats/min.

Assess the effectiveness of the sublingual dosage forms carefully, because absorption of the drug may be erratic and unpredictable. If severe paradoxical airway resistance develops, discontinue the medication and institute alternative therapy.

Isoproterenol may increase blood glucose levels. Observe individuals with diabetes for a loss of diabetic control. The dosage of insulin or oral hypoglycemic agents may need to be increased. Evaluate the client's extremities for paresthesias, color changes, and coldness. The client receiving isoproterenol may also experience altered comfort related to mouth dryness.

■ ***Intervention.*** Read labels carefully; the solution for oral inhalation must not be administered intravenously.

Hypovolemia should be corrected if possible before beginning IV therapy. Plan nursing care so that the client is constantly attended while receiving the drug. Never leave the client unattended during the infusion. Use a two-bottle setup so that an IV infusion can be kept running if the isoproterenol is discontinued. Use an infusion pump for precise regulation of infusion rate. Have oxygen and other resuscitative equipment available. Barbiturates may be used for adjunct sedative therapy to manage the side effects of CNS stimulation.

■ ***Education.*** Instruct the client undergoing isoproterenol therapy to allow sublingual tablets to dissolve under the tongue and not to swallow saliva until the tablet is completely dissolved. Swallowing the drug with saliva causes epigastric pain. Instruct the client to rinse the mouth thoroughly with water between sublingual doses. Prolonged use can cause tooth decay. Instruct the client not to chew sustained-release tablets but to swallow them whole.

Instruct the client to use the oral inhalation correctly (see Box 38-2). The instructions for the metered powder nebulizer are the same as for the metered dose nebulizer except that deep inhalation is not necessary. The client should allow 1 to 5 minutes between the first and second inhalations. Advise the client to take no more than six inhalations in an hour in any 24-hour period. The prescriber should be contacted if the client needs more than three aerosol treatments within a 24-hour period. If the client has three to five treatments in a 6- to 12-hour period with minimal or no relief, additional medications need to be added to the therapeutic regimen.

Advise the client that isoproterenol may turn the sputum and saliva pink. Caution against overuse because tolerance can develop and sudden deaths have been reported. Instruct the client to notify the prescriber if prescribed doses are not producing desired relief or if there are adverse reactions.

Instruct the client to store the drug in a tight, light-resistant container. Instruct the client not to use the drug if a precipitate or discoloration is present (solutions become pink or brownish pink on exposure to light, air, heat, or on contact with metal or an alkali).

■ **Evaluation.** The expected outcome of isoproterenol therapy is that the client will demonstrate relief from respiratory distress, have vital signs within the normal range, and not experience any adverse reactions to the drug.

norepinephrine bitartrate [nor ep i nef′ rin] (Levophed)

Norepinephrine is a direct-acting sympathomimetic amine identical to the catecholamine synthesized in the postganglionic nerve endings of the sympathetic nervous system. This agent has a high affinity for the alpha receptors. The blood vessels of the skin and mucous membrane contain only alpha receptors, and therefore norepinephrine produces a powerful constriction in these tissues. In addition, the blood vessels (both arteriolar and venous beds) in the visceral organs, including the kidneys, contain predominantly alpha receptors. Consequently, norepinephrine causes vasoconstriction and a reduced blood flow through the kidneys and other visceral organs. This agent also activates $beta_1$ receptors in the heart and exerts an increase in the force of myocardial contraction, resulting in an increase in cardiac output.

The main therapeutic effect of norepinephrine results from peripheral arteriolar vasoconstriction in all vascular beds. Both systolic and diastolic pressures are elevated, causing an increase in mean arterial pressure. Of importance during shock is constriction of the venous capacitance vessels, which reduces splanchnic and renal blood flow. This is brought about by severe restriction of tissue perfusion in these regions. In cases of persistent hypotension after correction of blood volume deficit, norepinephrine helps to raise the blood pressure to an optimal level and establishes a more adequate circulation.

Norepinephrine is used selectively to restore blood pressure in certain acute hypotensive states such as sympathectomy, myocardial infarction, pheochromocytomectomy, and blood transfusion reaction. When used to treat hypotension associated with an acute myocardial infarction, an increase in cardiac output and oxygen demand plus the possibility of inducing dysrhythmias may offset the benefits of using the drug to increase blood pressure. These factors need to be carefully considered when selecting norepinephrine for use in such conditions.

Norepinephrine is also used as adjunct therapy for cardiac arrest and profound hypotension. The use of norepinephrine to treat shock has declined significantly since the advent of dopamine. It is usually prescribed for clients whose shock produces severe hypotension and vasodilation of the peripheral blood vessels.

Norepinephrine is administered only by IV infusion because oral norepinephrine is destroyed in the gastrointestinal tract and because subcutaneous norepinephrine is poorly absorbed. The onset of action by IV infusion is immediate or rapid, with distribution concentrating mainly in the sympathetic tissues. The duration of action is approximately 1 to 2 minutes after discontinuing the IV infusion. The drug is metabolized in the liver and other tissues and by reuptake into the sympathetic nerves; it is excreted by the kidneys.

The side effects/adverse reactions of norepinephrine include anxiety, dizziness, pallor, tremors, insomnia, headache, pounding heart rate, and perhaps swelling of the thyroid gland in the neck.

Stimulation of alpha receptors and $beta_1$ receptors with norepinephrine is dose related. At low dosages (<2 μg/min), $beta_1$ receptors are stimulated, thus producing an inotropic and chronotropic response. Dosages higher than 4 μg/min result in stimulation of the alpha receptors or increase total peripheral resistance.

When norepinephrine is used in the treatment of hypotension in adults, an IV infusion of 0.5 to 1 μg/min is administered; the dosage is adjusted as necessary to raise and maintain the desired pressure. The maintenance dosage ranges from 2 to 12 μg/min, with dosage adjustments made as necessary to raise and maintain the desired pressure.

BOX 22-1

Sulfite Sensitivity

Sulfite is contained in commercially available formulations of the following:
- inamrinone (Inocor)
- dobutamine (Dobutrex)
- dopamine (Intropin)
- epinephrine (Adrenalin)
- metaraminol (Aramine)
- methoxamine (Vasoxyl)
- norepinephrine (Levophed)
- phenylephrine (Neo-Synephrine)

These formulations should not be administered to individuals with a known sensitivity to sulfite agents (sulfur dioxide, potassium or sodium bisulfite, potassium or sodium metasulfite, sodium sulfite).

Symptoms of sulfite sensitivity include the following:
- Skin: clamminess, flushing, pruritus, urticaria, cyanosis
- Respiratory system: bronchospasm, shortness of breath, wheezing, laryngeal edema, respiratory arrest
- Cardiovascular system: hypotension, syncope
- CNS: severe dizziness, loss of consciousness
- Other: anaphylaxis, death

■ Nursing Management

Norepinephrine Therapy

■ **Assessment.** Review the client's health status for preexisting conditions that may preclude the use of norepinephrine or cause it to be used with particular caution, such as asymmetric septal hypertrophy or tachycardias. It is not to be used in clients who are in hypovolemic states except as an emergency measure to maintain cerebral and coronary artery blood flow. Hypovolemia should be corrected before administering norepinephrine.

Norepinephrine is contraindicated in pheochromocytoma because hypertension may be worsened. It may also increase the ischemia of myocardial infarction. Do not give to clients with mesenteric or peripheral vascular thrombosis because of the risk of increasing ischemia and extending the thrombosis. Because of its vasoconstricting effects, norepinephrine should be used with caution for clients with occlusive vascular diseases such as Buerger's disease or arteriosclerosis. It is also contraindicated in profound hypoxia or hypercapnia and during pregnancy. Determine whether the client is intolerant of sulfites, because the injection dosage form of norepinephrine contains sodium bisulfite as a preservative (Box 22-1).

Assess the client's current drug regimen for possible drug interactions. With the exception of the local-parenteral anesthetic interactions, the drug interactions with norepinephrine are similar to those listed under epinephrine. Be aware that norepinephrine solutions are incompatible with iron salts, alkalis (sodium bicarbonate), and oxidizing agents.

■ **Nursing Diagnosis.** The client receiving norepinephrine therapy should be assessed for the following selected nursing diagnoses/collaborative problems: risk for injury related to dizziness; impaired skin integrity related to extravasation (sloughing of skin); impaired comfort (headache); disturbed sleep pattern (insomnia); and the potential complications of sulfite allergy (rash, hives, swelling of the face, difficulty breathing) and altered cardiac output (dysrhythmias and hypertension).

■ **Implementation**

■ ***Monitoring.*** During the infusion of norepinephrine, adjust the dosage according to the prescriber's guidelines. This includes the client's response, with particular attention given to urinary output, respiration, blood pressure, pulse, central venous pressure, pulmonary wedge pressure, pulmonary capillary wedge pressure, and color and temperature of extremities (peripheral ischemia). These parameters must be accurately recorded to attain precise titration of the drug. It is advised that the blood pressure be measured every 2 to 3 minutes during norepinephrine administration until the desired blood pressure is reached, then every 5 minutes until the drug is discontinued. If the client was previously hypotensive, the desired systolic blood pressure range is 80 to 100 mm Hg; for clients who were previously hypertensive, blood pressure should be maintained at 30 to 40 mm Hg below their preexisting systolic values. Monitor the ECG; reduce or discontinue medication if cardiac dysrhythmia occurs.

Inspect the infusion site for extravasation every 10 to 15 minutes. Notify the prescriber immediately if extravasation occurs. Observe the client for blanching along the route of the infused vein and for cold, hard swelling around the injection site.

Observe the client for mentation (cerebral circulation), temperature of extremities, and color of earlobes, lips, and nail beds; also monitor for paresthesia.

Monitor intake and output. A decrease in urinary output after prolonged use of norepinephrine may indicate necrosis of the kidney.

■ ***Intervention.*** Be aware of the importance of maintaining adequate blood volume before administering norepinephrine. Blood should be administered separately. Maintaining adequate blood volume prevents tissue ischemia that can result from the vasoconstrictive effect of the drug. Administer norepinephrine only intravenously; its vasoconstrictor effect prohibits IM or SC administration.

Anticipate that the infusion will be administered through a plastic catheter deep into a large vein to minimize risk of extravasation. Leg veins are not recommended because of poor circulation, which can result in occlusive vascular disease.

If extravasation occurs, the area should be quickly infiltrated with 5 to 10 mg of phentolamine (Regitine) in 10 to 15 mL of sodium chloride to dilate blood vessels; a fine-gauge needle is used. Have phentolamine ready. To prevent sloughing of the skin secondary to extravasation, 5 to 10 mg of phentolamine may be added to every liter of norepinephrine solution.

Norepinephrine should be diluted with 5% dextrose in distilled water or 5% dextrose in sodium chloride solution because the dextrose prevents a significant loss of potency by oxidation. Anticipate the addition of heparin to the infusion solution to prevent thrombosis of the infused vein in clients experiencing severe hypotension after myocardial infarction.

Never leave the client unattended during infusion. An IV pump flow regulator should be used to ensure accuracy of the flow rate in drops per minute. Discontinue therapy gradually by slowing infusion rate, and continue to monitor the client and vital signs to ensure circulatory adequacy.

Store medication by protecting it from light. The solution deteriorates after 24 hours; discard it after that time. Do not use the solution if it is discolored or if precipitate is present.

■ ***Education.*** Alert the client to report immediately any breathing difficulties, discomfort at the infusion site, or headache.

■ **Evaluation.** The expected outcome of norepinephrine therapy is that the client will demonstrate an improvement of blood pressure and coronary artery blood flow with a blood pressure >90 to 100 mm Hg systolic and an absence of the clinical signs of shock (urinary output <30 mL/hr, weak and thready pulse, restlessness, confusion).

Drugs Used for Circulatory Shock

In any instance of shock, treatment must be directed to the cause. A main concern is the need to improve circulation so that enough oxygen is available for tissue perfusion. Hypoxia that denotes impaired tissue perfusion may result from inadequate pumping action of the heart, decreased blood volume, decreased peripheral resistance of arterial vessels, or an increased size of the venous bed.

During circulatory shock the autonomic nervous system plays an essential compensatory role in an attempt to restore normal circulation. Therefore many sympathomimetic drugs are used to manage this condition. Although there are other agents, the five drugs widely used for circulatory shock are dopamine, epinephrine, and norepinephrine (all of which are vasopressors), as well as dobutamine and isoproterenol (which possess cardiogenic activity). Inamrinone (Inocor), which has positive inotropic and vasodilator effects, can also be used for clients with congestive heart failure who are not responsive to standard therapy. Milrinone (Primacor), an analogue of inamrinone, is also available for short-term use in congestive heart failure (see Chapter 25).

Vasopressors have strong alpha activity, and dopamine produces less vasoconstriction than epinephrine and norepinephrine. Dobutamine and isoproterenol are important for improving cardiac output because of their capability to stimulate $beta_1$ receptors in the heart. Most of the agents are

TABLE 22-4 Vasopressor Effects in Shock

	Receptor Site Effects*			Organ Response†		
Drug	**β_1**	**β_2**	**α_1**	**Kidneys**	**Cardiac**	**Blood Pressure**
epinephrine	+++	+/++	+++	D	I	D
dobutamine	+++	+	0/+	0	I	—
dopamine	+++	0/+	++	I		0/I
isoproterenol	+++	+++	0	I/D	I	#
norepinephrine	++	0	+++	D	0/D	I

+, Minimal effect; ++, moderate effect; +++, greatest effect; 0, no effect; *I*, increased; *D*, decreased; #, usual doses maintain or increase systolic pressure.
*Receptor site effects: β_1, Inotropic effects; β_2, vasodilation; α_1, vasoconstriction.
†Organ response: *Kidneys*, renal perfusion; *cardiac*, cardiac output; *blood pressure*, blood pressure.

nonselective beta-acting drugs; norepinephrine lacks beta$_2$ activity. With the exception of isoproterenol and inamrinone, all of these agents stimulate alpha receptors (Table 22-4).

dobutamine hydrochloride [doe byoo′ ta meen] (Dobutrex)

Dobutamine is a synthetic catecholamine that acts directly on the heart muscle to increase the force of myocardial contraction. This response is attributed to the direct stimulation of the beta$_1$-adrenergic receptors of the heart. At the same time dobutamine produces comparatively little increase in heart rate or peripheral vascular resistance. By enhancing stroke volume, this agent is an effective positive inotropic drug.

Dobutamine is administered intravenously for the *short-term* management of clients requiring inotropic support, such as with congestive heart failure or after cardiac surgery. Because of its minimal influence on heart rate and blood pressure (both are major determinants of myocardial oxygen demand), it is valuable for use in strengthening a decompensated heart in individuals with low cardiac output syndrome. Its beneficial effects include a progressive increase in cardiac output and a decrease in pulmonary capillary wedge pressure, thereby improving ventricular contraction. Dobutamine is also used as an agent for stress echocardiography (Dhond et al., 1999).

The concomitant use of sodium nitroprusside and dobutamine is sometimes beneficial in clients with congestive heart failure or after an acute myocardial infarction. This combination results in a higher cardiac output and a lower pulmonary capillary wedge pressure than when either drug is used alone. Because of the vasodilating effect of nitroprusside, the decrease in peripheral resistance lessens the workload on the heart.

Dobutamine is administered by IV infusion and has an onset of action within 1 to 2 minutes; the plasma half-life is 2 minutes because it is rapidly metabolized by the liver and is excreted in the urine.

The side effects/adverse reactions of dobutamine include nausea, headache, angina, respiratory distress, palpitation, increased heart rate and blood pressure, and perhaps premature ventricular beats.

The adult dosage of dobutamine is by IV infusion, 2.5 to 15 μg/kg/min. For children, the dosage ranges between 5 and 20 μg/kg/min.

■ Nursing Management
Dobutamine Therapy

■ **Assessment.** Use dobutamine cautiously in clients with tachycardia and increased blood pressure, because the drug may intensify both of these conditions. The safe use of this drug after myocardial infarction has not been established. There is concern that a drug that increases the force of myocardial contraction and heart rate may intensify ischemia by increasing oxygen demand. Note that dobutamine is contraindicated in cases of idiopathic hypertrophic subaortic stenosis (obstruction may increase). Use dobutamine cautiously in individuals with occlusive vascular disease (e.g., Buerger's or Raynaud's disease, atherosclerosis, diabetic endarteritis, or arterial embolism) or with dysrhythmias (e.g., tachydysrhythmias, ventricular fibrillation). Note that dobutamine is contraindicated in pheochromocytoma. Hypovolemia should be corrected before beginning dobutamine therapy. Adequate fluid balance is required for the course of therapy. Clients with pheochromocytoma may experience severe hypertension.

Be aware of potential drug interactions, which are the same as those that occur with the administration of epinephrine.

■ **Nursing Diagnosis.** The client receiving dobutamine therapy should be monitored for the following nursing diagnoses/collaborative problems: impaired comfort (nausea, chest pain, palpitations, headache, nervousness); impaired tissue perfusion related to peripheral vasoconstriction (changes in color, tingling or numbness in fingers or toes); decreased cardiac output (hypotension, hypertension, tachycardia); and the potential complications of angina and dysrhythmia.

■ **Implementation**

■ ***Monitoring.*** The ECG and blood pressure should be continuously monitored during dobutamine therapy to ascertain any alteration in cardiac output. If possible, pulmonary capillary wedge pressure and cardiac output should be monitored to ensure safe infusion and precise titration of the drug. If the client responds with an increase in the heart rate (an increase of 30 beats/min or more) and an increase in systolic blood pressure (an increase of 50 mm Hg or greater), a reduction of dosage usually reverses these adverse reactions because the drug is rapidly metabolized. Monitor for peripheral ischemia by observing the client's extremities for color and temperature.

Monitor intake and output. Increased urinary output indicates improved cardiac output and urinary perfusion. NOTE: Clients with atrial fibrillation and rapid ventricular response should be treated with a digitalis preparation before undergoing dobutamine therapy.

If a significant decrease in pulse pressure (a disproportionate rise in diastolic pressure) is observed, decrease the infusion rate. Continue to observe the client for further evidence of vasoconstrictor activity. Decrease the medication or stop it temporarily and notify the prescriber if the following occurs: reduced urinary output without hypotension, increasing tachycardia, dysrhythmia, and marked decrease in pulse pressure. When appropriate, decrease the dosage gradually to prevent severe hypotension. Monitor for sulfite sensitivity (see Box 22-1).

Continue to observe the client carefully after discontinuing dobutamine therapy. The duration of action of this drug is brief, and the beneficial effects of the drug may terminate quickly.

■ ***Intervention.*** Administer dobutamine using an infusion pump or other device to control the rate of flow and avoid bolus dosing. As with norepinephrine and isoproterenol, adjust the dosage of dobutamine according to the clinical response of the client The concentration of solution for administration should not exceed 5 mg/mL of dobutamine. (See Nursing Management: Isoproterenol Therapy, p. 466, for information on the IV administration of isoproterenol.

For precautions and care regarding extravasation, see Nursing Management: Norepinephrine Therapy, p. 468. Have available a syringe with phentolamine mesylate (Regitine), 5 mg in 10 mL saline for use by the physician if extravasation occurs.

The IV solution of dobutamine remains stable for 24 hours. A color change during this period indicates some oxidation, but there is no loss of potency during the first 24 hours. Dobutamine is incompatible with alkaline solutions and should not be mixed with products such as 5% sodium bicarbonate injection. Check for drug incompatibilities when considering administration through an IV line with other drugs.

■ ***Education.*** Alert the client to report immediately any breathing difficulties, headache, or chest pain.

■ **Evaluation.** The expected outcome of dobutamine therapy is that the client will demonstrate an improvement in cardiovascular status, with vital signs within normal limits, improved hemodynamic monitor measurements (central venous pressure and pulmonary wedge pressures), urinary output >30 mL/hr, and an absence of adventitious lung sounds.

✓ dopamine hydrochloride [doe' pa meen] (Intropin)

Dopamine is a catecholamine that occurs as an immediate precursor of norepinephrine (see Figure 20-5). It acts both directly and indirectly by releasing norepinephrine. It stimulates dopaminergic receptors, $beta_1$ receptors and, in high doses, alpha receptors. Receptor activity is dose dependent; it depends on the amount of drug administered.

Unlike norepinephrine, dopamine is unique in low dosages (0.5 to 2 μg/kg/min) because it acts mainly on dopaminergic receptors to cause vasodilation of the renal and mesenteric arteries. Renal vasodilation increases renal blood flow with usually a greater amount of urine and sodium excretion. This prevents kidney failure secondary to shock.

In low to moderate dosages (usually 2 to 10 μg/kg/min), dopamine acts directly on the $beta_1$ receptors of the myocardium and indirectly by releasing norepinephrine from its neuronal storage sites in the sympathetic neuron. These actions increase myocardial contractility and stroke volume, thereby increasing cardiac output. Systolic blood pressure and pulse pressure may increase with either no effect on or a slight elevation in diastolic blood pressure. Total peripheral resistance usually remains unchanged. Coronary blood flow and myocardial oxygen consumption increase. Heart rate increases only slightly at low dosages.

With higher dosages of dopamine (10 μg/kg/min or more), alpha-adrenergic receptors are stimulated, which increases peripheral resistance. Blood pressure increases because of a rise in cardiac output. As a consequence, a high-dosage level may reduce urinary output, eliminating the benefit of vasodilation because the renal artery becomes constricted. From a therapeutic standpoint, it is important to note that dopamine in low to moderate dosages causes vasodilation in the renal, mesenteric, coronary, and cerebral blood vessels. These vasodilator properties suggest the presence of specific dopamine receptors.

Therefore, unlike norepinephrine, dopamine helps to alleviate inadequate tissue perfusion through the vital splanchnic organ systems. The combination of cardiac and circulatory effects has led to the successful use of dopamine in the treatment of circulatory shock and refractory heart failure. Dopamine is used to correct hemodynamic imbalances associated with shock syndrome caused by myocardial infarction, trauma, endotoxin septicemia, open heart surgery, renal failure, and chronic cardiac decompensation (as in congestive heart failure).

Dopamine must be administered by IV infusion. The drug has a rapid onset of action (2 to 5 minutes) and a short duration of action (5 to 10 minutes); it is widely distributed by the body but does not cross the blood-brain barrier. Dopamine is rapidly metabolized by the liver, kidney, and plasma to inactive substances. It is excreted in the urine.

The side effects/adverse reactions of dopamine include headaches, nausea, vomiting, angina, respiratory difficulties, decreased blood pressure or, less commonly, hypertension, irregular or ectopic heartbeats, tachycardia, and palpitations.

For vasopressor effects, the adult dosage ranges according to the effect desired (see the discussion earlier in this section). Pediatric IV infusion rates range between 5 and 20 μg/kg/min.

For the nursing management of dopamine therapy, see Nursing Management: Dobutamine Therapy, p. 470.

Indirect- and Dual-Acting Adrenergic Drugs

The direct-acting adrenergic (catecholamine) drugs act directly on alpha and beta receptors to stimulate an adrenergic response. The indirect-acting adrenergic drugs act indirectly on receptors by first triggering the release of the catecholamines norepinephrine and epinephrine from their storage sites; these neurotransmitters then activate the alpha and beta receptors. *Dual-acting* adrenergic drugs have both indirect and direct effects. Indirect- and dual-acting adrenergic drugs have many and varied uses in medicine.

ephedrine [e fed′ rin]

Ephedrine has both a direct and an indirect sympathomimetic action. It acts indirectly by stimulating the release of norepinephrine from presynaptic nerve terminals and also acts directly on both alpha and beta receptors. Like epinephrine and norepinephrine, ephedrine has positive inotropic and chronotropic activities, but it is a less effective vasoconstrictor. However, it does raise blood pressure and is used for this purpose during spinal anesthesia and in the treatment of orthostatic hypotension.

Parenteral ephedrine has been used in clients with hypotension who do not respond to fluid replacement, position changes, and specific antidotes in cases of drug overdose. However, the nurse should be aware that ephedrine may be ineffective and may actually worsen the situation if severe peripheral vasoconstriction is present (Table 22-5). Ephedrine is also used as a pressor agent in hypotensive states during spinal anesthesia or after sympathectomy.

Ephedrine has been used to produce bronchodilation in the treatment of milder forms of bronchial asthma but, in general, more beta_2-selective drugs are preferred (e.g., albuterol, metaproterenol, and terbutaline). It is also used to relieve nasal mucosal congestion.

Absorption of this drug is rapid after oral, IM, or SC administration. The onset of action for bronchodilation occurs within 15 to 60 minutes with the oral dosage form and within 10 to 20 minutes with the IM dosage form. The duration of action is 3 to 5 hours for the oral dosage form and 30 to 60 minutes for IM or SC injections of 25 to 50 mg. The pressor effects and cardiac responses usually occur within 60 minutes of the parenteral administration of ephedrine. This drug is metabolized in the liver and excreted by the kidneys.

The side effects/adverse reactions of ephedrine are similar to epinephrine, although coughing and local irritation are not reported because ephedrine is not available in aerosol form. Ephedrine may also cause mood changes and hallucinations.

For vasopressor effects, the adult dosage of ephedrine is 25 to 50 mg IM or SC, repeated if necessary. It may be administered intravenously if a faster effect is desired. For bronchodilator or decongestant effects, the dosage is 25 to 50 mg PO or 12.5 to 25 mg SC, IM, or slow IV every 3 or 4 hours as needed. For decongestion, several drops of a 0.5% to 1% ephedrine solution may be applied topically and repeated every 4 hours if necessary.

■ Nursing Management

Ephedrine Therapy

■ **Assessment.** The client's health status needs to be reviewed for conditions for which ephedrine may be contraindicated or used with additional caution. Use ephedrine with caution in clients with hypertension, hyperthyroidism, prostatic hypertrophy, and diabetes mellitus. Do not use in clients with severe hypertension, narrow-angle glaucoma, or a history of hypersensitivity to sympathomimetic drugs.

The significant interactions of ephedrine with anesthetics, antidepressants (tricyclic and MAO inhibitors), beta-blocking agents, cocaine, digitalis glycosides, ergoloid mesylates, and ergotamine are the same as those reported with epinephrine.

A baseline assessment of the client's cardiovascular and respiratory status is required.

■ **Nursing Diagnosis.** The client receiving ephedrine therapy should be assessed for the following selected nursing diagnoses: disturbed sleep pattern (insomnia); anxiety; impaired comfort (headache); and risk for injury related to drug sensitivity (rash, facial edema, wheezing). Impaired urinary elimination may occur as evidenced by sphincter spasm and retention as a result of the effects of ephedrine. There is the potential complication of altered cardiac output (tachycardia, dysrhythmias).

■ **Implementation**

■ ***Monitoring.*** During IV administration, closely monitor blood pressure repeatedly during the first 5 minutes, then check every 3 to 5 minutes until it is stable. Never leave the client unattended during IV administration.

If administered parenterally to maintain blood pressure in conjunction with spinal anesthesia during delivery, ephedrine may cause the fetal heart rate to accelerate. It should be discontinued when the maternal blood pressure reaches 130/80 mm Hg.

Monitor intake and output, and advise the client to report any difficulty in urinating (particularly older male clients).

■ ***Intervention.*** Administer ephedrine only if the solution is clear; discard any unused portion. If ephedrine is used as

TABLE 22-5 Indirect- and Dual-Acting Adrenergic Drug Effects

Receptors, Action Sites	Ephedrine	Phenylephrine	Mephentermine	Metaraminol	Methoxamine
Trade names	Ephedrine Sulfate	Neo-Synephrine	Wyamine	Aramine	Vasoxyl
Mode of action					
Alpha receptors	Stimulates	Stimulates	Stimulates	Stimulates	Stimulates
Beta receptors	Stimulates More prolonged but less intense action than epinephrine	NS	+	$Beta_1$ agonist	+
Effects					
Cardiovascular					
Myocardium	Variable	NS Bradycardia may occur reflexively	Increases contractility and rate May cause bradycardia	Some increase in contractility Bradycardia may occur	— Reflex bradycardia may occur
Pacemaker cells	NS	NS	NS	—	—
Coronary vessels	Dilates—increases blood flow	Dilates—increases blood flow	Dilates—increases blood flow	—	—
Blood pressure	Increases	Increases	Increases	Increases	Increases
Bronchi	Dilates	Dilates, but less than epinephrine	Dilates, but less than epinephrine	NS	—
Cerebral effects	Stimulating action	NS	NS	—	—
Blood vessels					
Skeletal muscle	NS	+	NS	NS	Decreases blood flow
Kidney	Constricts	Constricts	Constricts but less than ephedrine	Constricts—decreases blood flow	—
Gastrointestinal tract	Decreases peristalsis	Decreases motility	Relaxes smooth muscle—inhibits	Some inhibition	Inhibits
Metabolic	Increases metabolic rate	Some increase in metabolic rate	NS	NS	NS
Remarks	Serious dysrhythmias may occur if used with digitalis Can be given orally				Prolonged duration of action; cumulative effects may occur—give drug slowly May cause tissue sloughing—do not give subcutaneously
Uses	Vasopressor Allergic states Nasal decongestant Enuresis Myasthenia gravis	Nasal decongestant Vasopressor Paroxysmal atrial tachycardia Mydriatic	Vasopressor	Vasopressor	Vasopressor Paroxysmal atrial tachycardia

NS, Not significant.
+Effect is slight, nonexistent, or unknown in humans.

an ingredient within a cough and cold remedy, administer it a few hours before bedtime; avoid administering it at night to help prevent insomnia.

▪ ***Education.*** If ephedrine is self-administered for respiratory symptoms, advise the client not to take OTC drugs without consulting the prescriber. Caution the client not to overuse this drug because tolerance may develop. It may be necessary to withhold the medication for several days to restore effectiveness. Instruct the client to follow the correct dosage and to report any side effects or adverse reactions immediately to the prescriber. In addition, advise the client to prevent systemic effects by not swallowing nose drops.

▪ **Evaluation.** The expected outcome of ephedrine therapy is that the client will demonstrate an improvement in cardiovascular status with vital signs within normal limits, a urinary output >30 mL/hr, an absence of confusion and restlessness, and improved hemodynamic monitor measurements (central venous pressure and pulmonary wedge pressures). If administered for respiratory congestion, the client will demonstrate easier breathing without wheezing and rhinitis.

phenylephrine systemic [fen ill ef′ rin] (Neo-Synephrine injection)
phenylephrine nasal (Neo-Synephrine, Alconefrin)

Phenylephrine is a synthetic adrenergic drug chemically related to epinephrine, norepinephrine, and ephedrine. It is primarily a direct-acting agent; its main effects are stimulation of the alpha receptors, resulting in vasoconstriction and an increase in both diastolic and systolic blood pressures. The drug has little effect on the $beta_1$ receptors of the heart. Its vasoconstricting action is more prolonged than that of norepinephrine and therefore may be used for acute hypotension that occurs from spinal anesthesia. It is not effective in treating shock caused by a loss of blood volume. Phenylephrine is also contained in many combination cough-cold, antihistamine and decongestant, and ophthalmic preparations.

Phenylephrine exhibits fewer side effects than epinephrine and has longer-lasting therapeutic effects. It has little or no effect on the CNS.

When applied topically to mucous membranes, phenylephrine reduces swelling and congestion by constricting the small blood vessels. It is useful in the treatment of sinusitis, vasomotor rhinitis, and hay fever. It is sometimes combined with local anesthetics to slow their systemic absorption and to prolong their action.

Phenylephrine is used as a mydriatic for certain conditions in which pupil dilation is desired without cycloplegia paralysis of the ciliary muscle, and it may be applied intranasally for congestion caused by colds, hay fever, sinusitis, or allergies.

Administered intravenously, phenylephrine produces an immediate effect and has a duration of action of 5 to 20 minutes. The drug is metabolized partially in gastrointestinal tract tissues and in the liver by the enzyme monoamine oxidase. The route of excretion has not been identified.

The side effects/adverse reactions of phenylephrine are uncommon but include anxiety, restlessness, dizziness, tremors, difficulty breathing, pallor, increased weakness, angina and, with the preparations that contain sulfites, allergic reactions (see Box 22-1).

The adult dosage of phenylephrine for hypotension is 2 to 5 mg IM or SC of 1% solution, repeated if necessary. The IV injection dosage is 0.2 mg, repeated in 15 minutes if necessary; the IV infusion dosage is 100 to 180 μg/min until the blood pressure stabilizes, at which point it is reduced to 40 to 60 μg/min.

▪ Nursing Management

Phenylephrine Therapy

▪ **Assessment.** Before administering phenylephrine, the client should be assessed for any preexisting health problems for which the drug would be contraindicated or used only with extreme caution. The risk-benefit ratio should be considered if phenylephrine is used in clients with narrow-angle glaucoma (ophthalmic preparations), severe coronary disease, severe hypertension, or ventricular tachycardia. Use with caution in individuals with hyperthyroidism, hypertension, diabetes mellitus, ischemic cardiac disease, or cerebral arteriosclerosis.

Review the client's current medication regimen for the risk of significant drug interactions, such as those that may occur when phenylephrine is given concurrently with the following drugs:

Drug	Possible Effect and Management
Bold/color type indicates the most serious interactions.	
alpha-receptor blocking agents	May reduce or block the vasopressor effect of phenylephrine, resulting in hypotension.
anesthetics; inhalation of hydrocarbons such as chloroform, enflurane, halothane, and others; plus digitalis glycosides	**Increases the risk of inducing serious cardiac dysrhythmias. If necessary to use concurrently, monitor closely with ECG readings because therapeutic interventions may be necessary. Avoid concurrent use or a serious drug interaction may occur.**
beta-blocking agents	**The therapeutic effects of both drugs may be inhibited. This can occur with both oral and ophthalmic beta-adrenergic blocking drugs. Avoid concurrent use.**
cocaine, maprotiline (Ludiomil), or tricyclic antidepressants	**May potentiate the cardiovascular effects of phenylephrine (e.g., dysrhythmias, increased heart rate, and severe hypertension) and elevate body temperature. Avoid concurrent use or a serious drug interaction may occur.**
doxapram (Dopram)	The vasopressor effects of either or both drugs may increase. Monitor blood pressure closely because dosage adjustments may be necessary.

Drug	Possible Effect and Management
ergotamine and ergoloid mesylates	Increases vasoconstriction; severe hypertension and peripheral vascular ischemia and gangrene may occur. This combined use is not recommended. Avoid concurrent use or a serious drug interaction may occur.
MAO inhibitors	May cause increased release of accumulated neurotransmitters into the synapse area, causing severe headaches, dysrhythmias, vomiting, severe hypertension, and/or high fevers. Avoid concurrent use or a serious drug interaction may occur. Phenylephrine should not be given during or within 2 weeks of the administration of an MAO inhibitor.

Obtain a baseline assessment of the client's underlying condition for which the phenylephrine is being prescribed.

■ **Nursing Diagnosis.** The client's risk of impaired comfort is related to the cardiovascular (chest pain) and neurologic effects (restlessness, trembling) of phenylephrine and to the local effects of topical preparations (stinging). Altered cardiac output should be considered as a potential complication to the administration of phenylephrine related to its cardiovascular effects (hypertension, dysrhythmias).

■ **Implementation**

■ ***Monitoring.*** The blood pressure of clients with hypertension should be monitored carefully while they are receiving phenylephrine, even nasal or ophthalmic preparations. Any signs of angina should be reported to the prescriber immediately. Monitor the infusion site for extravasation. Monitor intake and output. Observe the client for rebound miosis (pupil constriction) after ophthalmic administration. Monitor for sulfite sensitivity (see Box 22-1). Children are more likely to be sensitive to the vasopressor effects of phenylephrine. Older adults may demonstrate confusion, sedation, hypotension, dryness of mouth, and urinary retention.

■ ***Intervention.*** After each use, wash nasal droppers with hot water to prevent contamination of the solution; eyedroppers should not touch the eye or any other surface. Solutions lose potency with exposure to air, strong light, or heat. Keep the container tightly sealed and away from light. Discard if the solution is dark brown or contains a precipitate.

If nasal or ophthalmic phenylephrine preparations are administered to clients with hypertension, they should not be administered at the end of the antihypertensive dosing period, when therapeutic levels of antihypertensive medications are low.

■ *Nasal Preparations.* Before administering a nasal preparation of phenylephrine, instruct the client to blow his or her nose to clear the nasal passages. Instill the nose drops by having the client tilt the head back and remain in position a few minutes to permit the medication to spread through the nose. When administering a spray, have the client hold the head upright; squeeze the bottle firmly and quickly to produce a spray into each nostril; after 3 to 5 minutes, have the client blow his or her nose and repeat.

■ *IV Administration.* See Nursing Management: Norepinephrine Therapy, p. 468, for the IV administration of phenylephrine. Have phentolamine (Regitine) available to treat extravasation ischemia.

■ *Ophthalmic Preparations.* Instruct the client to apply pressure to the lacrimal sac during the administration of phenylephrine eyedrops and for 1 or 2 minutes after instillation. Clients with contact lenses should consult the prescriber for specific instructions.

■ ***Education.*** For IV administration, alert the client to report discomfort at the infusion site, headache, or chest pain immediately. To prevent systemic effects, instruct the client not to swallow the nasal solutions. Instruct the client to swallow the extended-release capsules whole.

Emphasize to the client the importance of adhering to the drug regimen. Consult the prescriber about any modification—dosage, time interval, or others. Instruct the client to notify the prescriber if insomnia, dizziness, or tremors occur.

Caution the client about burning and stinging sensations after the instillation of eyedrops. Inform the client that the pupils will be dilated and may be sensitive to light after the instillation of drops. Notify the prescriber if sensitivity to light or blurred vision persists beyond 12 hours after discontinuing the drug. Instruct the client to wear sunglasses in bright light. Blurred vision will decrease with continued use.

If phenylephrine is used for nasal decongestion, contact the health care provider if symptoms are not relieved in 3 days; rebound nasal congestion may occur with nasal sprays and drops.

■ **Evaluation.** The expected outcome of phenylephrine therapy for hypotension is that the client will demonstrate a blood pressure >90 to 100 mm Hg systolic, a urinary output >30 mL/hr, and an absence of symptoms of shock (weak thready pulse, restlessness, confusion). For nasal congestion, the client will demonstrate easier breathing and report less nasal discharge and congestion. For pupillary dilation, the client will demonstrate dilated pupils and decreased intraocular pressure by tonometry.

mephentermine sulfate [me fen′ ter meen] (Wyamine)

The effects of mephentermine are similar to ephedrine, but mephentermine produces more cerebral stimulation. Mephentermine is a dual-acting (primarily) sympathomimetic. It releases catecholamines from storage sites in the heart and other tissues (indirect action). Therefore it tends to bring about both alpha- and beta-stimulating effects, including inotropic and chronotropic effects on the heart. Because mephentermine improves cardiac contraction and mobilizes blood from venous pools, thereby increasing cardiac output, it acts as a peripheral vasoconstrictor (see Table 22-5).

Mephentermine is used as a pressor agent in the treatment of hypotension secondary to spinal anesthesia and as adjunct therapy for hypotension secondary to hemorrhage, medications, and shock due to brain tumor or trauma.

The onset of action for IM administration occurs within 5 to 15 minutes, and the duration of action is 1 to 4 hours. Mephentermine is nearly immediate in action with IV administration, and the duration of action is 15 to 30 minutes. The drug is metabolized in the liver and excreted by the kidneys.

The side effects/adverse reactions of mephentermine include anxiety, nervousness, restlessness, and tachycardia.

The adult dosage of mephentermine for hypotension is 30 to 45 mg IV in a single injection, with doses of 30 mg repeated as needed to maintain blood pressure. The dosage for children has not been established.

■ Nursing Management
Mephentermine Therapy

■ **Assessment.** The client's health status should be evaluated to ensure that the client does not have a condition for which mephentermine would be contraindicated or require extreme caution. Use cautiously in chronically ill clients and in clients with arteriosclerosis, hypertension, cardiovascular disease, and hyperthyroidism. Hypoxia should be corrected before the administration of mephentermine, otherwise the response may be decreased or the risk of adverse reactions may be increased.

Mephentermine may cause uterine contraction, especially in the third trimester, and therefore should not be administered to pregnant women.

The client's current medication regimen should be reviewed to detect significant drug interactions. See the section on phenylephrine for potential drug interactions that may also occur with mephentermine.

Obtain a baseline assessment of the underlying condition for which the mephentermine is being prescribed.

■ **Nursing Diagnosis.** The client receiving mephentermine therapy is at risk for the following selected nursing diagnoses/collaborative problems: impaired comfort (restlessness, headache); anxiety; and the potential complication of altered cardiac output (dysrhythmias, hypertension).

■ **Implementation**

■ ***Monitoring.*** Monitor closely blood pressure, pulse, ECG, urinary output, central venous pressure, and other hemodynamic measures as appropriate. The blood pressure and pulse should be checked every 2 minutes until stabilized, then every 5 to 15 minutes during therapy. Blood pressure should be maintained at slightly less than the client's normal blood pressure. In clients with hypertension, blood pressure should be maintained at 30 to 40 mm Hg below the client's usual blood pressure.

Observe the client for possible development of tolerance if repeated injections are administered. Note that blood volume replacement must be instituted as soon as possible in the treatment of secondary shock.

■ ***Intervention.*** Administer mephentermine using an infusion device for precise regulation of dosage according to the response of the client. Mephentermine may also be administered intramuscularly. Do not use the solution if it is discolored or if a precipitate has formed.

■ ***Education.*** Alert the client to report headache and anxiety; these are early symptoms of overdose.

■ **Evaluation.** The expected outcome of mephentermine therapy is that the client will demonstrate a systolic blood pressure >90 to 100 mm Hg, a urinary output >30 mL/hr, and an absence of symptoms of shock (weak thready pulse, restlessness, confusion).

metaraminol [met a ram′ i nole] (Aramine)

Metaraminol is a vasopressor agent with both direct (primarily) and indirect effects on the sympathetic system. It acts indirectly by releasing norepinephrine from tissues and storage sites and directly on alpha receptors as a neurohormone.

Metaraminol has positive inotropic effects. Because it constricts blood vessels, increases peripheral resistance, elevates both systolic and diastolic blood pressure, and improves cardiac contractility and cerebral, coronary, and renal blood flow, it is used for the treatment of shock.

Because metaraminol exhibits beta- and alpha-adrenergic activity, it is often effective in raising blood pressure when alpha-adrenergic agents are ineffective. This may be because of its ability to bring about more effective venous flow. It does not appear to cause dysrhythmias. In general, it lacks CNS stimulatory effects, and its side effects are rare and often related to rapid drug administration. Although similar to norepinephrine in action, it is generally considered a less potent drug.

Metaraminol is used for acute hypotensive states occurring with spinal anesthesia. It is also administered for the prevention and treatment of acute hypotension associated with surgery, drug-induced reactions, and shock.

This drug is administered only parenterally. The onset of action is within 1 to 2 minutes with IV administration and within 10 minutes with SC or IM administration. The duration of action is between 20 to 60 minutes; it is metabolized in the liver and excreted in the bile and kidneys.

The adult dosage of metaraminol is 2 to 10 mg SC or IM to prevent acute hypotension. To avoid cumulative effects, 10 minutes should elapse before additional doses are administered. When metaraminol is given via IV infusion, 15 to 100 mg in 500 mL of sodium chloride injection (0.9%) or 5% dextrose in water is administered at a rate determined by the prescriber to maintain the desired blood pressure response. When given by direct IV injection for severe shock, 0.5 to 5 mg is administered followed by the IV infusion described above. The dosage for children has not been established.

■ Nursing Management
Metaraminol Therapy

■ **Assessment.** The client's health status should be reviewed for contraindications before the initiation of metaraminol therapy. This drug is to be used with caution in individuals with pheochromocytoma, hypertension, cardiac disorders, peripheral vascular disease, hyperthyroidism, or hypovolemia. Hypoxia should be corrected before or concurrently with the administration of metaraminol, otherwise its effectiveness may be reduced or the risk of adverse reactions may be increased. Do not use in individuals who are sensitive to metaraminol.

Review the client's current medication regimen for significant drug interactions. See the drug interactions for phenylephrine, because these may also occur with metaraminol.

Obtain a baseline assessment of the underlying condition for which the metaraminol is being prescribed.

■ **Nursing Diagnosis.** The client undergoing metaraminol therapy may experience the nursing diagnosis of impaired tissue integrity related to extravasation of IV fluid (sloughing at infusion site), as well as the potential complications of allergic reaction to sulfites (rash, facial edema, wheezing) and altered cardiac output (hypertension, dysrhythmias, hypotension when the drug is discontinued).

■ **Implementation**

■ ***Monitoring.*** Monitor blood pressure closely every 2 to 5 minutes during infusion (client must be constantly attended). Because metaraminol has a prolonged effect, adjust the flow rate carefully to avoid a cumulative response. Before terminating infusion, reduce the flow rate gradually to avoid abrupt withdrawal of the drug, which might result in severe hypotension. If possible, correct plasma volume before starting therapy. Continue to monitor blood pressure closely after the drug has been discontinued. The drug should be resumed quickly if severe hypotension occurs.

Monitor for cardiac dysrhythmias and for sulfite sensitivity (see Box 22-1). Monitor the infusion site frequently for extravasation because it will result in sloughing of the skin.

■ ***Intervention.*** IM and SC injection sites should be chosen carefully; areas with poor circulation may produce inadequate client response and increase the risk of tissue necrosis. Avoid extravasation during IV infusion; using larger veins may be helpful. Veins of the ankle and back of the hand should be avoided, particularly in clients with peripheral vascular disease. Phentolamine (decreases pressor effect) and atropine (for bradycardia) should be on hand. Metaraminol must be diluted before administration. Once diluted, it should be used within 24 hours. Because metaraminol is incompatible with many drugs, it should not be administered in a solution that contains other medications.

■ ***Education.*** Alert the client to report discomfort at the infusion site.

■ **Evaluation.** The expected outcome of metaraminol therapy is that the client will demonstrate a systolic blood pressure >90 to 100 mm Hg, a urinary output >30 mL/hr, and an absence of symptoms of shock (weak thready pulse, restlessness, confusion).

methoxamine hydrochloride [meth ox' a meen] (Vasoxyl)

Methoxamine is an alpha-adrenergic stimulator devoid of beta receptor activity, except in high doses. The direct-acting sympathomimetic agent is pharmacologically related to phenylephrine. Because it has no stimulating effect on the heart, the rise in blood pressure causes a reflex bradycardia. This effect makes it useful in treating paroxysmal supraventricular tachycardia and in restoring or maintaining blood pressure during anesthesia (see Table 22-5).

With IV administration the effects of methoxamine are immediate, and the duration of action as a vasopressor is 5 to 15 minutes. The effects are seen within 15 to 20 minutes following IM administration, with a duration of action between 60 and 90 minutes. Metabolism and excretion routes are unknown.

The side effects/adverse reactions of methoxamine are uncommon and include sweating, severe headaches, hypertension, vomiting, and urinary urgency with high doses.

The adult vasopressor dosage is 10 to 15 mg IM or 3 to 5 mg given slowly by direct IV injection. The dosage for children has not been established.

■ Nursing Management

Methoxamine Therapy

■ **Assessment.** Use methoxamine cautiously in clients with hyperthyroidism, pheochromocytoma, cardiovascular disease, or hypertension and also following the parenteral injection of ergot alkaloids. Hypoxia should be corrected before or concurrently with the administration of methoxamine, otherwise its effectiveness may be reduced or the risk of adverse reactions may be increased.

Review the client's current medications for significant drug interactions (see the drug interactions for phenylephrine).

Obtain a baseline assessment of the underlying condition for which the methoxamine is being prescribed.

■ **Nursing Diagnosis.** In addition to altered cardiac output, the client undergoing methoxamine therapy may also experience impaired comfort related to headache, increased perspiration, and the sensation of urinary urgency.

■ **Implementation**

■ ***Monitoring.*** Monitor the client's blood pressure and pulse continuously during therapy, and titrate the dose accordingly. Clients with hypertension are more apt to experience a greater reduction in blood pressure during spinal anesthesia than those with blood pressure in the normal range. Blood pressure should be maintained at slightly less than the client's normal blood pressure. In clients with hypertension, blood pressure should be maintained at 30 to 40 mm Hg below their usual blood pressure. Observe the ECG for cardiac dysrhythmias.

Monitor intake and output because output increases when normal blood pressure levels occur (if the client is not hypovolemic). Observe the client for sudden changes of blood pressure after the drug is terminated. Monitor for sulfite sensitivity (see Box 22-1).

■ ***Intervention.*** IM doses may need to be repeated. If so, allow sufficient time for the previous injection to take effect before considering administering another. Administer IV slowly if the systolic pressure falls below 60 mm Hg or if there is another emergency. Have atropine available if bradycardia occurs.

▪ **Evaluation.** The expected outcome of methoxamine therapy is that the client will demonstrate a systolic blood pressure >90 to 100 mm Hg, a urinary output >30 mL/hr, and an absence of symptoms of shock (weak thready pulse, restlessness, confusion).

▪ ▪ ▪

See Box 22-2 for information on the pro-drug midodrine (ProAmatine).

ADRENERGIC BLOCKING DRUGS

Alpha-Adrenergic Blocking Agents

Most **alpha-adrenergic blocking agents** are competitive blockers; they compete with the catecholamines at receptor sites and inhibit adrenergic sympathetic stimulation. They are more effective against the action of circulating catecholamines than against catecholamines released from storage sites in the neurons. These drugs may be obtained from natural sources, such as ergot and its derivatives, or they may be synthesized.

The alpha-adrenergic blocking agents fall into three categories:

1. *Noncompetitive, long-acting antagonists* (e.g., phenoxybenzamine [Dibenzyline]). The action persists for several days or weeks because a stable bond is formed between a specific component of the drug and the alpha receptor site.
2. *Competitive, short-acting antagonists* (e.g., phentolamine [Regitine], tolazoline [Priscoline]). The blocking action is reversible and competitive at the alpha receptor site, and the effects last only several hours.
3. *Ergot alkaloids.* Usually act as partial alpha-adrenergic antagonists. However, the drugs produce primarily a spasmogenic effect on the smooth muscle of blood vessels, thereby causing vasoconstriction.

BOX 22-2

Midodrine (ProAmatine)

Midodrine (ProAmatine) is indicated for the treatment of symptomatic orthostatic hypotension. It is a pro-drug that is converted to the active metabolite desglymidodrine, an alpha$_1$ agonist that activates arteriolar and venous receptors to increase blood pressure. It can raise systolic blood pressure by 15 to 30 mm Hg 1 hour after a 10-mg dose.

Pharmacokinetics

Midodrine metabolite peaks in 1 to 2 hours, and the half-life is 3 to 4 hours. Metabolism occurs in many tissues, including the liver. It is excreted by the kidneys.

Side effects/adverse reactions include paresthesia, pruritus, dysuria, and supine hypertension. The adult dosage is 10 mg PO three times daily during daytime hours (every 4 hours but not later than 6 PM). Because of the risk of supine hypertension, do not give midodrine after the evening meal or less than 4 hours before the client's bedtime.

Information from *Drug Facts and Comparisons.* (2000). St. Louis: Facts and Comparisons.

Noncompetitive, Long-Acting Antagonists

phenoxybenzamine [fen ox ee ben′ za meen] (Dibenzyline)

Phenoxybenzamine is a long-acting, irreversible alpha-adrenergic blocking agent that abolishes or decreases the receptiveness of alpha receptors to adrenergic stimuli. Because phenoxybenzamine competes with the catecholamines, it is also useful in decreasing the blood pressure of clients with pheochromocytoma. It does not block sympathetic impulses on the heart and therefore does not directly impair cardiac output.

All alpha$_1$ blockers are also used to relieve symptoms of benign prostatic hyperplasia; this indication is not included in the U.S. product labeling. By noncompetitively blocking alpha-adrenergic receptors of the bladder neck and proximal urethra, the internal sphincter is relaxed, which improves voiding efficiency in clients with functional outlet obstruction.

Phenoxybenzamine is used in the management of pheochromocytoma for preoperative preparation of the client for surgery, chronic treatment of individuals with malignant pheochromocytoma, and in individuals for whom pheochromocytoma surgery is contraindicated.

The oral absorption of phenoxybenzamine is variable. The onset of action occurs in 2 hours. This drug can persist for 3 or 4 days because it forms a stable bond with the receptor. The half-life is approximately 24 hours, with metabolism in the liver and excretion in the kidney and bile.

The side effects/adverse reactions of phenoxybenzamine include dizziness (postural hypotension), miosis, tachycardia, nasal congestion, confusion, dry mouth, fatigue, headache, and inhibition of ejaculation.

The initial adult dosage is 10 mg PO twice daily; the dosage may be increased by 10 mg every other day until the desired effect is noted. The maintenance dosage is 20 to 40 mg two or three times daily. The initial dosage for children is 0.2 mg/kg PO up to a maximum of 10 mg, administered once daily; this dosage may be increased every 4 days until the desired effect is noted. The maintenance dosage for children is 0.4 to 1.2 mg/kg body weight, given in 3 or 4 divided doses.

▪ Nursing Management

Phenoxybenzamine Therapy

▪ **Assessment.** Use phenoxybenzamine with caution in clients with renal insufficiency and upper respiratory infection (may aggravate nasal congestion). Consider the risk-benefit ratio in clients with compensated congestive failure or coronary artery disease (because this drug will cause angina and congestive heart failure), or in conditions when a decrease in blood pressure might be dangerous, such as cerebrovascular insufficiency. Sensitivity to the drug should be determined.

Review the client's current medication regimen for the risk of significant drug interactions. When phenoxybenzamine is given with other sympathomimetics, such as epinephrine, metaraminol, methoxamine, and phenylephrine, the results may be as follows:

- Blocking of the alpha-adrenergic receptor effects of epinephrine (Adrenalin), which may result in severe hypotension and tachycardia.
- Decrease in the vasopressor effect of metaraminol (Aramine).
- Blocking of the vasopressor effect of methoxamine (Vasoxyl), resulting in severe hypotension.
- Decrease in the vasopressor effect of phenylephrine (Neo-Synephrine). Avoid concurrent drug administration if at all possible.

Obtain a baseline assessment of the client's blood pressure and cardiovascular status.

■ **Nursing Diagnosis.** The client receiving phenoxybenzamine is at risk for the following nursing diagnoses: impaired comfort (headache, dry mouth); activity intolerance related to weakness and lethargy; sexual dysfunction related to alpha-adrenergic blockade (inability to ejaculate); and risk for injury related to miosis, postural hypotension, and confusion.

■ **Implementation**

■ ***Monitoring.*** Monitor blood pressure and pulse rate both in recumbent and standing positions during periods of dosage adjustment, particularly when dosage is increased. Observe the client for signs of hypotension and tachycardia. Inform the client that these signs usually disappear with continued therapy. However, these signs may recur with the vasodilation associated with exercise, drinking alcohol, or eating a large meal. Urinary catecholamine determinations during the initial treatment help in determining the appropriate dosage.

■ ***Intervention.*** Administer oral phenoxybenzamine with milk to reduce gastric irritation. The dosage should be adjusted according to the clinical response and level of urinary catecholamines. Dosage increases will be gradual from the lowest therapeutic dosage, but the increments should be no more frequent than every 4 days. Treat overdose with IV infusion of norepinephrine. Do not use epinephrine because it will cause a further drop in blood pressure.

■ ***Education.*** Advise the client to make position changes slowly (from recumbent to upright posture) to prevent orthostatic hypotension. Instruct the client to dangle the legs and exercise the feet for a few minutes at the bedside before standing. If faintness or weakness occurs, a head-low position should be assumed or the person must lie down immediately. Elastic support stockings help to prevent orthostatic hypotension. Because of the risk of injury related to orthostatic hypotension, instruct the client to not drink alcohol, not to stand for long periods, and not to exercise during hot weather because the possibility of increasing this effect. Advise the client to modify activities if dizziness and/or drowsiness occur because of the risk for injury.

Advise the client that regular dental checkups are required because phenoxybenzamine inhibits salivary flow and thus promotes the development of caries, periodontal disease, and buccal candidiasis. Dryness of the mouth can be relieved and the comfort of the client promoted with ice chips and sugarless gum. Warn the client against using any other drug, particularly OTC sympathomimetics (e.g., cough, cold, or allergy preparations) without consulting the prescriber.

Alert the client to notify other health care providers to phenoxybenzamine therapy if surgery, including dental surgery, or emergency treatment might be required.

An effect of this drug can be inhibition of ejaculation; this effect should be reported to the prescriber.

■ **Evaluation.** The expected outcome of phenoxybenzamine therapy is that the client with pheochromocytoma will note decreases in blood pressure, pulse, and sweating; these are signs of therapeutic effectiveness. The client's blood pressure will be within normal limits.

Competitive, Short-Acting Antagonists

phentolamine mesylate [fen tole' a meen]
(Regitine, Rogitine ♣)

Phentolamine is an alpha-adrenergic blocking agent that competitively blocks $alpha_2$ (presynaptic) and $alpha_1$ (postsynaptic) receptors. The action occurs at both arterial and venous vessels. This direct relaxation of vascular smooth muscle lowers total peripheral resistance. Phentolamine also decreases pulmonary vascular resistance.

Phentolamine is used to prevent or control hypertensive episodes in clients with pheochromocytoma. It is also used to reverse the vasoconstrictive action of an overdose or an excessive response to IV administration or extravasation of norepinephrine (Levophed) or dopamine. An SC injection of phentolamine (Regitine) following extravasation of IV norepinephrine or dopamine will prevent tissue necrosis if prompt action is taken.

Parenteral phentolamine is administered intravenously, and the half-life is approximately 19 minutes. Metabolism and excretion sources are unknown, because only 13% (approximately) of the drug is found in urine after parenteral administration.

The side effects/adverse reactions of phentolamine include diarrhea, dizziness (postural hypotension), nausea, vomiting, abdominal pain, and tachycardia.

When phentolamine is used preoperatively, 5 mg IV is administered 1 to 2 hours before surgery; this dose may be repeated if necessary during surgery. As an antiadrenergic preoperative in children, 1 mg IM or IV is administered 1 to 2 hours before surgery and repeated if necessary.

▪ Nursing Management
Phentolamine Therapy

▪ **Assessment.** Use phentolamine with caution in clients with coronary artery disease and myocardial infarction because reflex tachycardia as a result of the drug may precipitate congestive heart failure. Gastritis and peptic ulcers may be aggravated by phentolamine. Do not use in clients who have a hypersensitivity to phentolamine.

Significant drug interactions are the same as for phenoxybenzamine.

The client's blood pressure and cardiovascular status are essential for a baseline assessment.

▪ **Nursing Diagnosis.** Clients receiving phentolamine should be evaluated for the risk for injury related to the cardiovascular effects of the drug (orthostatic hypotension, reflex tachycardia). Diarrhea and impaired comfort (abdominal cramping, nasal stuffiness, facial flushing, nausea and vomiting) may also be an issue. If administered in a norepinephrine IV infusion or for extravasation, observe the client for impaired tissue integrity at the infusion site. With parenteral administration, the potential complications of cerebrovascular spasm (confusion, sudden loss of coordination or slurring of speech) and myocardial infarction (chest pain) may occur.

▪ **Implementation**

▪ ***Monitoring.*** If phentolamine is administered intravenously, monitor the client's blood pressure and pulse every 2 minutes until stabilized. Observe the extravasation site for tissue necrosis.

▪ ***Intervention.*** When administered intravenously as an antiadrenergic, the client should be in a supine position because the drug may cause severe and prolonged hypotension with fainting, tachycardia, and cardiac dysrhythmias.

When phentolamine is used to prevent sloughing of tissue with the administration of norepinephrine, 10 mg may be added to every liter of IV fluids containing norepinephrine without affecting its vasopressor effect. If extravasation has already occurred, 5 to 10 mg of phentolamine in 10 mL of 0.9% sodium chloride injection should be immediately infiltrated into the affected area. This treatment is ineffective if 12 or more hours have passed since the extravasation.

▪ ***Education.*** After therapy, advise the client to rise slowly from bed and remain in a sitting position for a few minutes before standing upright; this will prevent orthostatic hypotension.

▪ **Evaluation.** The expected outcome of phentolamine therapy is that the client's blood pressure will be within normal limits. There will be an absence of tissue necrosis at the IV infusion site.

tolazoline [toe laz' a leen] (Priscoline)

Like phentolamine, tolazoline produces a moderately effective, competitive alpha-adrenergic blocking action; however, tolazoline is considerably less potent. It acts as a vasodilator by having a direct relaxant effect on vascular smooth muscle. It usually reduces pulmonary arterial pressure and peripheral vascular resistance.

Tolazoline is used to treat persistent pulmonary hypertension in the newborn when systemic arterial levels of oxygen cannot be maintained by oxygen supplementation and/or mechanical ventilation machines.

When administered parenterally, the onset of action occurs within ½ hour of the initial dose. The half-life in neonates is 3 to 10 hours. Tolazoline is excreted mainly unchanged in the kidneys.

The side effects/adverse reactions of tolazoline include gastrointestinal bleeding, systemic alkalosis, hypotension, thrombocytopenia, and oliguria or acute renal failure.

The pediatric parenteral dosage is 1 to 2 mg/kg IV initially via a scalp vein over a 5- to 10-minute period. The maintenance dosage is 0.2 mg/kg by IV infusion for each 1 mg/kg loading dose. The drug may be gradually withdrawn when arterial blood gases appear to be remaining stable.

▪ Nursing Management
Tolazoline Therapy

▪ **Assessment.** Tolazoline should not be used when systemic hypotension (systolic blood pressure less than 40 mm Hg) exists. Caution must be used when administering tolazoline in the presence of acidosis (may increase pulmonary vasoconstriction) or mitral stenosis (may increase or decrease pulmonary artery pressure and total pulmonary resistance). Determine the client's sensitivity to tolazoline.

If epinephrine or norepinephrine is used to treat a tolazoline overdose, a paradoxical hypotensive effect followed by an exaggerated hypertensive response may occur. Avoid using epinephrine or norepinephrine with large amounts of tolazoline.

A baseline assessment should include the client's blood pressure, pulse, ECG, complete blood count (CBC), electrolytes, and blood gases. If long-term therapy is considered, renal function studies should be obtained.

▪ **Nursing Diagnosis.** Evaluate the client for the risk for injury related to the cardiovascular (systemic hypotension) and gastrointestinal (hemorrhage) effects of tolazoline. Impaired comfort may occur due to the adverse reactions of nausea and vomiting, goose bumps, and flushing of the skin. Diarrhea may occur. The potential complications of systemic alkalosis, acute renal failure, tachycardia, and thrombocytopenia may occur.

▪ **Implementation**

▪ ***Monitoring.*** Monitor the client's response to the drug through ECG, blood gases, blood pressure, and pulse rates. Also observe CBCs and serum electrolyte levels, particularly sodium and potassium levels. Renal function studies are to be performed periodically.

Perform a hematest of gastric aspirates to monitor for gastrointestinal bleeding. Monitor for pain in the upper abdominal area, increased pulse, and coffee-ground emesis.

▪ ***Intervention.*** Tolazoline is administered only in pediatric or neonatal intensive care units where respiratory support is immediately available. Use an infusion pump or microdrip regulator for administration to allow for precise flow regulation. Do not mix in a syringe or solution with other drugs. Pretreating the client with antacids may be necessary to prevent stress ulcers secondary to increased gastric secretion caused by the drug. Provide a warm environment for the infant to enhance the efficacy of the drug. Check the diluent carefully; diluents containing benzyl alcohol are not recommended for neonates and may lead to fatal toxic syndrome.

■ **Evaluation.** The expected outcome of tolazoline therapy is that the client's vital signs, arterial blood gases, acid-base balance, and electrolytes will be within the normal limits.

Ergot Alkaloids

Ergot is a fungus that grows on rye; when it is hydrolyzed, many of its derivatives dissociate to yield lysergic acid diethylamide (LSD). These alkaloids have diverse and somewhat contradictory effects. Ergot alkaloids are partial agonists or antagonists at alpha-adrenergic receptors. The primary effect of the ergot alkaloids used to treat or prevent migraine and other vascular headaches is alpha-adrenergic blockade. Only ergoloid mesylates is not used to treat headaches; it is indicated as adjunct therapy to treat dementia symptoms, but this therapy is controversial (*USP DI*, 1999). The following are examples of ergot preparations:

dihydroergotamine mesylate [dye hye droe er got' a meen] (D.H.E. 45)
ergoloid mesylates [er' goe loid mess' i lates] (Hydergine)
ergotamine tartrate [er got' a meen] (Ergomar ✤, Gynergen ✤)
ergotamine tartrate and caffeine (Cafergot)
ergotamine tartrate inhalation (Medihaler Ergotamine ✤)
ergotamine, belladonna alkaloids, and phenobarbital (Bellergal-S, Bellergal ✤)
methysergide maleate [meth i ser' jide] (Sansert)

The exact mechanism of action of ergoloid mesylates is unknown, but it may increase nerve cell metabolism, which can result in improved oxygen uptake and cerebral metabolism. Thus lowered neurotransmitter levels may increase to normal. Other ergot alkaloids stimulate smooth muscle, especially of the blood vessels and the uterus, so they decrease the cerebral blood supply.

The early phase of a migraine attack is associated with constriction of the cranial blood vessels. It is characterized by visual symptoms and malaise and appears as a warning or "aura" of an oncoming attack. This is followed by the painful phase of a migraine headache that results in cranial vasodilation. The increase in blood flow in the vessels produces pulsations that appear to be the source of the pain. The ergot alkaloids act as alpha-adrenergic blocking agents and depress the central vasomotor center. They cause direct vasoconstriction of cranial blood vessels during the vasodilation phase, thereby reducing the pulsation thought to be responsible for the headache.

Ergot alkaloids also possess antiserotonin activity. Abnormalities in serotonin metabolism may play a role in the migraine syndrome. Evidence exists that the drugs that act favorably in alleviating migraine have an influence on serotonin metabolism. Methysergide is a serotonin inhibitor and also acts as a potent vasoconstrictor (see Chapter 39 for information on serotonin). Ergotamine tartrate inhalation is used to abort or reduce a migraine attack, whereas ergotamine, belladonna alkaloids, and phenobarbital are used in combination to prevent vascular headaches. Some of these drugs are used for the treatment of vascular headaches (e.g., migraine and cluster headaches). Dihydroergotamine mesylate or ergotamine tartrate must be given early in the attack; neither drug prevents migraine attacks.

Dihydroergotamine is administered parenterally. Ergoloid mesylates and ergotamine tartrate (and its combinations without caffeine) are slowly and erratically absorbed from the gastrointestinal tract. Caffeine is said to aid oral absorption. The aerosol dosage form, such as methysergide, is well absorbed. Rectal suppositories of ergotamine tartrate (available in combination products) produce higher plasma concentrations than the oral dosage form and may be used if other routes are ineffective.

The onset of action for dihydroergotamine mesylate following IM, SC, or IV administration is fairly rapid—15 to 30 minutes after IM administration, and within minutes after IV administration. The half-life for an IV dose is 1.4 to 15 hours. The duration of action for an IM dose is 3 to 4 hours; for an IV or SC dose, the duration of action is 8 hours. Dihydroergotamine is mainly excreted in the bile.

Ergotamine tartrate and its combinations have onset of action within 1 to 2 hours and half-lives of approximately 2 hours. Methysergide maleate has an onset of action and a duration of 24 to 48 hours; the half-life of ergoloid mesylates is 3.5 hours.

All of the ergot alkaloids are metabolized in the liver and primarily excreted by the kidneys. Dihydroergotamine nasal is excreted primarily in the feces.

The side effects/adverse reactions of ergot alkaloids include dizziness, nausea, vomiting, headache, diarrhea, pruritus, edema of the lower extremities, and peripheral vasoconstriction or vasospasms (dose-related) that may result in cold hands or feet, leg weakness, pain in arms, legs, or lower back. Long-term use of methysergide may result in retroperitoneal fibrosis; therefore this product should not be routinely administered for longer than 6 months.

Dihydroergotamine mesylate, 1 mg IM, is administered at the start of an attack of migraine or cluster headaches. This dose is repeated in 1 hour if needed, up to a 3-mg maximum per day or a 6-mg maximum per week. The IV dose is 0.5 mg initially with an antiemetic, which is repeated once in 1 hour if necessary. The dosage for ergoloid mesylates is 1 to 2 mg PO three times daily. The ergotamine dose is 1 to 2 mg PO initially, repeated in ½ hour if needed; the maximum daily dose is 6 mg no more than twice weekly and at least 5 days apart. With ergotamine aerosol, one inhalation is administered at the beginning of the attack and repeated every 5 minutes if needed to a maximum of 6 sprays per day. Methysergide, 4 to 6 mg PO is administered in divided doses and taken with milk or after meals.

▪ Nursing Management

Ergot Alkaloid Therapy

▪ **Assessment.** Do not use ergot alkaloids with clients with severe hypertension (the condition may be aggravated) or with clients who have unstable angina or recent myocardial infarction (drug-induced vasospasm may precipitate a recurrence). Clients with a history of cerebrovascular accident (CVA) or transient ischemic attack (TIA) may be prone to a recurrence as a result of increased blood pressure caused by the use of ergot alkaloids. Caution should also be used if the client has undergone vascular surgery or has cardiovascular or peripheral vascular disease (may increase ischemia), sepsis (more sensitive to the effects of ergonovine), or hepatic (may result in ergot overdose) or renal disease. Older adults are also more at risk from the vasospastic and hypothermic effects of these drugs. Ergotamine is not recommended for use during pregnancy because of its oxytocic effects. It is contraindicated in clients who are breastfeeding because it inhibits lactation and may cause peripheral ischemia or nausea and vomiting in the infant.

When ergot alkaloids are given with other ergot alkaloids, vasopressors, or vasoconstrictors, the combination may result in increased vasoconstriction, ischemia, and possibly gangrene. Avoid this drug combination. A delay of 24 hours is recommended between the use of sumatriptan (Imitrex) and dihydroergotamine.

Obtain a baseline assessment of the client's headaches; their precipitating factors, aura, frequency, and severity; and past efforts and success of relief. A baseline assessment of blood pressure and ECG is essential. The examination of the extremities and palpation of peripheral pulses provides a baseline for older adults.

▪ **Nursing Diagnosis.** The client receiving ergot alkaloid therapy may experience the following selected nursing diagnoses/collaborative problems: impaired comfort related to underlying vascular headache because of ineffectiveness of the drug, a developing tolerance to the drug, dizziness, or nausea; risk for injury related to a decrease in peripheral sensation because of vasoconstriction (paleness, coolness, numbness, or tingling of fingers and toes); excess fluid volume (edema); and the potential complications of CNS toxicity, cardiovascular effects, rectal ulceration, and pleural or retroperitoneal fibrosis.

▪ **Implementation**

▪ ***Monitoring.*** Discuss with the client the frequency and severity of headaches. Examine the extremities and palpate the peripheral pulses at monthly intervals so that ischemia and edema can be detected as early as possible. Blood pressure and ECG monitoring are necessary with multiple dosing.

▪ ***Intervention.*** Nonpharmacologic interventions for pain relief of migraine should be used to supplement the medication, such as a quiet environment, relaxation therapy, and other measures specific to the client. Because nausea and vomiting may be increased by the administration of ergotamine before headache relief occurs, phenothiazine antiemetics may be required to promote the comfort of the client. Safety measures should be taken to prevent injury to the client's extremities, and they should be monitored for the ischemic effects of the drug.

▪ ***Education.*** Tell the client to take the initial dose of the ergot alkaloid during the early part of a migraine attack—during the "aura" (visual field defects, paresthesia, and nausea). The client should then lie down in a quiet, dark room for several hours. Assure the client that the quality of relief is related to the promptness with which the medication is started after the onset of symptoms.

Warn the client to take the drug exactly as prescribed. Prolonged use or overdose can cause circulatory impairment (ergot poisoning), which is evidenced by numbness, tingling sensations, weakness, intermittent claudication, cyanosis of the extremities, muscle pain, and coldness of the extremities. Report symptoms immediately to the prescriber. If this condition is not corrected, gangrene may develop. Warmth is to be applied, taking care to avoid excessive heat. Severe peripheral vasoconstriction may be treated by administering IV sodium nitroprusside. Discontinuing the drug for 2 to 3 days may relieve these symptoms.

Instruct the client to avoid alcohol ingestion because it aggravates the headache. Counseling should be provided for smoking cessation because nicotine increases the peripheral vasoconstrictive effects of the drug. For the same reason, the client should be instructed to avoid exposure to cold. Alert the client to the signs and symptoms of infection; caution the client to report these signs and symptoms to the prescriber because infection increases sensitivity to the drug.

Teach the client how to monitor for fluid volume excess by checking for edema, weighing daily, and maintaining a low salt intake. Inform the client of the possible occurrence of hypertension or hypotension. Position changes from recumbent to upright should be made slowly to avoid dizziness or fainting. Alert the client to the possible need to modify activities if dizziness and drowsiness occur as side effects. Warn female clients of childbearing age not to use ergot alkaloids because of potential oxytocic effects during pregnancy.

Clients with migraines may require assistance in identifying the physical and emotional stresses that cause migraine attack. Relaxation techniques, adequate rest, and avoidance of stressful situations may alleviate the severity or frequency of attacks.

Instruct the client in the proper method of taking sublingual tablets, including the avoidance of eating, drinking, and smoking until the tablet is completely dissolved. The correct use of an inhaler should be taught. If suppositories are to be used and only half a dose is required, instruct the client to cut them in half lengthwise after refrigeration.

▪ **Evaluation.** The expected outcome for ergot alkaloid therapy is that the client will experience diminished headaches or will not experience any headaches.

methysergide maleate [meth i ser′ jide] (Sansert)

Although methysergide is not as potent a vasoconstrictor as ergotamine, the nursing measures discussed under Nursing Management: Ergot Alkaloid Therapy, p. 482, should be observed. Administer an oral dose of methysergide with food to minimize gastrointestinal irritation.

Methysergide is not administered continuously for more than 6 months; a drug-free period of 3 to 4 weeks must occur before the drug is restarted. Advise the client to withdraw the drug gradually over a 2- to 3-week period to prevent "headache rebound" resulting from abrupt drug withdrawal. If the drug does not provide a therapeutic response after a 3-week trial period, it is unlikely that longer administration will be of benefit.

Because there is a potential for serious side effects with methysergide, the client should be advised to report dyspnea and chest or abdominal pain and to keep clinical appointments so that blood count, sedimentation rate, renal function, pulmonary function, and cardiac status may be assessed. Regular examination must be performed by the prescriber for the possible development of fibrotic (formation of tissue) and vascular complications. Retroperitoneal fibrosis, as well as cardiac fibrosis, has been noted in a small number of individuals. These conditions often regress when the drug is discontinued.

Beta-Adrenergic Blocking Agents

Beta-adrenergic blocking agents inhibit beta receptors by competing with the catecholamines at the receptor site. **Beta-adrenergic blocking agents** are differentiated into two subclasses: $beta_1$ and $beta_2$ blockers. Drugs that selectively inhibit only one type of receptor—$beta_1$ or $beta_2$—are called selective. $Beta_1$-selective blocking agents are often referred to as cardioselective blockers because these agents block the $beta_1$ receptors in the heart. Drugs that inhibit both types of receptors are referred to as nonselective beta-adrenergic blocking agents.

A further differentiation often identifies beta-adrenergic blocking agents that have intrinsic sympathomimetic activity (ISA). The ISA property was initially believed to be advantageous when compared with agents that possess only beta-blocking effects. It was projected that fewer serious side effects would occur with such agents, but the significance of this property has not been proven clinically. ISA causes partial stimulation of the beta receptor, but this effect is less than that of a pure agonist. For example, if the client has a slow heart rate at rest, the partial agonists may help to increase the heart rate by their partial agonist property. If the client has a rapid heart rate or tachycardia from exercise, these agents may help to slow down the heart rate secondary to the predominant beta-blocking effect. It is believed that the only role for the ISA property might be to treat clients who experience severe bradycardia from the non-ISA medications (Carter, Furmaga, & Murphy, 1995). Drugs with ISA properties should not be used to prevent myocardial infarction because of their partial agonist properties.

Examples of adrenergic-blocking drugs by classification include the following (Carter et al., 1995; *Drug Facts and Comparisons*, 2000):

$Beta_1$-antagonist effects

1. Selective $beta_1$-adrenergic blocking agents (cardioselective) include atenolol (Tenormin), betaxolol (Kerlone), bisoprolol (Zebeta), esmolol (Brevibloc), and metoprolol (Lopressor).
2. Selective $beta_1$-adrenergic blocking agents with ISA effects include acebutolol (Sectral).

$Beta_1$-and $beta_2$-antagonist effects

1. Nonselective beta-adrenergic blocking agents include labetalol* (Normodyne), nadolol (Corgard), propranolol (Inderal), sotalol (Betapace) and timolol (Blocadren).
2. Nonselective beta-adrenergic blocking agents with ISA effects include carteolol (Cartrol), carvedilol* (Coreg), penbutolol (Levatol), and pindolol (Visken).

The prototype beta-adrenergic blocking drug is propranolol.

Beta-adrenergic blocking agents compete with beta-adrenergic agonists (e.g., catecholamines) for available beta receptor sites located on the membrane of cardiac muscle, smooth muscle of bronchi, and smooth muscle of blood vessels. Cardiac muscle contains $beta_1$ receptors, whereas the smooth muscle sites contain primarily $beta_2$ receptors. Pharmacologically, the $beta_1$-adrenergic blocking action in the heart decreases heart rate, conduction velocity, myocardial contractility, and cardiac output.

The antianginal effects produced by the beta blockers are primarily caused by their ability to lower myocardial oxygen requirements. Their antihypertensive actions are not specifically identified, but these effects may result from a decrease in cardiac output, a diminished sympathetic outflow from the vasomotor center in the brain to the peripheral blood vessels, and an inhibition of renin release by the kidney. The result is a decrease in peripheral vascular resistance, which lowers blood pressure.

To prevent a recurrence of a myocardial infarction, beta blockers (without ISA properties) are used for their antidysrhythmic effect plus their ability to decrease the myocardial oxygen demands on the heart. The latter effect may reduce the progression of ischemia and its severity on the heart.

Various mechanisms may be involved in the prevention of vascular headaches, such as prevention of arterial vasodilation, inhibition of platelet aggregation, and increased oxygen release to tissues.

Indications. The beta-adrenergic blocking agents are used to treat chronic angina pectoris, hypertension, hypertrophic cardiomyopathy, tremors and anxiety; to prevent and/or treat cardiac dysrhythmias; to prevent a second myocardial infarction; and to prevent and/or treat vascular head-

*Labetalol and carvedilol are also $alpha_1$ antagonists.

aches; as an adjunct to thyrotoxicosis and pheochromocytoma therapy; and to treat mitral valve prolapse syndrome. Esmolol (Brevibloc) is a parenteral agent indicated for the treatment of supraventricular tachycardia and noncompensatory sinus tachycardia.

Pharmacokinetics. See Table 22-6 for the pharmacokinetics and usual adult dosage of the beta-adrenergic blocking agents. Propranolol, metoprolol, and penbutolol are highly lipid soluble and therefore have a larger volume of distribution in the body, a greater first-pass liver metabolism, and a wider range of effective doses (individual variability) than do the other agents. For example, the range for propranolol is 10 to 640 mg/day (see Table 22-6) as compared to a drug with a less lipophilic (more water-soluble) profile, such as atenolol (50 to 100 mg), betaxolol (10 to 20 mg), and others. The less lipophilic agents are not as affected by liver metabolism and are excreted unchanged by the kidneys to a greater extent; therefore dosage adjustments are required in persons with renal impairment (Carter et al., 1995).

Side Effects/Adverse Reactions. The side effects/adverse reactions of beta-adrenergic drugs include drowsiness, weakness, difficulty sleeping, anxiety, nasal congestion, abdominal distress, dizziness, bradycardia, nausea, vomiting, depression, cold hands and feet, and difficulty breathing (bronchospasm).

■ Nursing Management

Beta-Adrenergic Blocking Drug Therapy

■ **Assessment.** The client's health status should be reviewed for preexisting health problems that might contraindicate the use of beta-adrenergic blocking agents or indicate a need for special precautions with the client (see

TABLE 22-6 Beta-Adrenergic Blocking Agents: Pharmacokinetics and Adult Dosing

Drug	Time to Peak Effect (hours)	Half-life (hours)	Metabolism/ Excretion (%)*	Usual Adult Dosage (range)
acebutolol (Sectral)	2.5-3.5	3-8	Liver/renal (30-40) Bile/feces (50)	200 mg twice daily (600-1200 mg/day)
atenolol (Tenormin)	2-4	6-7	Renal (85-100)	50 mg daily (50-100 mg/day)
betaxolol (Kerlone)	3-4	14-22	Liver/renal (>80)	10 mg daily (10-20 mg/day)
bisoprolol (Zebeta)	N/A	9-12	Liver/renal (50)	5 mg daily (2.5-20 mg/day)
carteolol (Cartrol)	1-3	6	Liver/renal (60-70)	2.5 mg daily (2.5-10 mg/day)
carvedilol (Coreg)	N/A	7-10	Liver renal (2) Bile/feces	6.25 mg twice daily (6.25-50 mg/day)
labetalol (Normodyne)	PO: 2-4 IV: 5 minutes	6-8 5.5	Liver/renal (55-60)	PO: 100 mg twice daily (400-1200 mg/day) IV: 20 mg
metoprolol (Lopressor,  Toprol XL ◆)	PO: 1-2	3-7	Liver/renal (3-10)	100 mg daily (50-450 mg/day)
nadolol (Corgard)	4	20-24	Renal (70)	40 mg daily (40-240 mg/day)
penbutolol (Levatol)	1.5-3	5	Liver/renal (90)	20 mg daily (10-40 mg/day)
pindolol (Visken)	1-2	3-4	Liver/renal (40)	5 mg twice daily (5-45 mg/day in Canada; 60 mg/day in United States)
propranolol (Inderal)	1-1.5	3-5	Liver/renal (<1)	40 mg twice daily (10-640 mg/day)
sotalol (Betapace)	2-3	7-18	Liver/renal (75)	80 mg twice daily (80-320 mg/day)
timolol (Blocadren)	1-2	4	Liver/renal (20)	10 mg twice daily (10-60 mg/day)

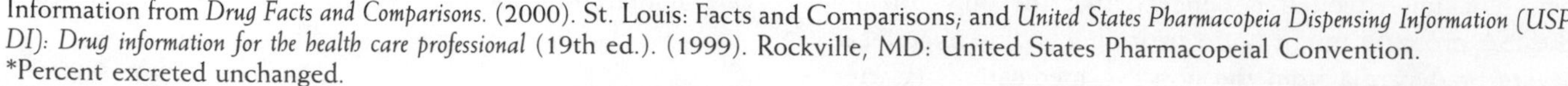
Information from *Drug Facts and Comparisons*. (2000). St. Louis: Facts and Comparisons; and *United States Pharmacopeia Dispensing Information (USP DI): Drug information for the health care professional* (19th ed.). (1999). Rockville, MD: United States Pharmacopeial Convention.

*Percent excreted unchanged.

the Pregnancy Safety box below). The risk of decreasing myocardial contraction, thus increasing the risk of heart failure, must be considered when selecting a beta-blocking agent. Such agents are contraindicated for clients with cardiac failure, cardiogenic shock, second- or third-degree heart block, and sinus bradycardia (<45 beats/min). Long-term use of beta-adrenergic blockers may aggravate congestive heart failure because of decreased cardiac output. If a beta-blocking agent is necessary for a client with stabilized congestive heart failure, labetalol or drugs with ISA activity (e.g., pindolol) at low dosages may be the agents of choice.

Blockade of the $beta_2$ receptors of the bronchial smooth muscle leads to bronchoconstriction. This effect is particularly hazardous for individuals with a history of allergy, asthma, bronchitis, and emphysema. There is less risk of inducing bronchospasm in these clients when a cardioselective beta blocker ($beta_1$ blocker) is used.

$Beta_2$-adrenergic blockade prevents the appearance of the warning signs and symptoms of acute hypoglycemia (sweating, increased heart rate, and anxiety). Therefore these agents should be used with caution in individuals with diabetes mellitus who take insulin or hypoglycemic drugs. In general, labetalol and other selective $beta_1$-adrenergic blockers do not potentiate insulin-induced hypoglycemia.

Because these drugs may mask the clinical signs of hyperthyroidism (e.g., tachycardia), they give a false impression of improvement of hyperthyroidism. Abrupt withdrawal of the drug will exacerbate symptoms of hyperthyroidism; therapy should be discontinued gradually.

Exacerbation of depression has been reported in clients with depression or with a history of depression; they should be closely monitored if taking a beta-blocking agent.

Review the client's current medication regimen for the risk of significant drug interactions, such as those that may occur when beta-adrenergic blocking agents are given concurrently with the following drugs:

Drug/Herb	Possible Effect and Management
Bold/color type indicates the most serious interactions.	
allergen immunotherapy or allergic extracts for skin testing	**The use of these agents places the client at risk for a serious systemic reaction; another drug should be substituted for the beta-adrenergic blocking agent. Avoid concurrent use or a potentially serious drug interaction may occur.**
antidiabetic agents, oral hypoglycemic agents or insulin	May cause hyperglycemia or hypoglycemia. Symptoms of hypoglycemia (e.g., increased heart rate and decreased blood pressure) may be blocked, thus making it difficult to monitor. Monitoring of blood glucose levels and dosage adjustments of the hypoglycemic agent may be necessary.
calcium channel blocking agents, clonidine (Catapres), or guanabenz (Wytensin)	May result in potentiated antihypertensive effects; monitor blood pressure closely. If therapy with a beta-adrenergic blocking agent, clonidine, or guanabenz is to be discontinued, taper the dosage of the beta blocker gradually over several days. When the beta blocker is discontinued, the clonidine or guanabenz should be tapered and discontinued over several days. Monitor blood pressure closely throughout this procedure. Use caution when high doses of calcium blocking agents are given concurrently with a beta-adrenergic blocking agent. In some instances nifedipine (Procardia, Adalat) may result in excessive hypotension in clients receiving concurrent therapy.
cocaine	May reduce or cancel the effects of the beta-adrenergic blocking agents. Although beta-blocking agents are used to treat the symptoms induced by cocaine (e.g., increased heart rate, cardiac dysrhythmias), an increased risk of inducing hypertension, severe bradycardia, and heart block can occur. If a beta blocker is necessary, labetalol may present less risk than the other beta-adrenergic blocking agents (because of its alpha-adrenergic blocking effect).
monoamine oxidase (MAO) inhibitors	**This combination is not to be used; severe hypertension may result, even up to 14 days after the MAO inhibitor is discontinued.**

Continued

Pregnancy Safety
Drugs Affecting the Sympathetic System

Category	Drug
B	acebutolol, pindolol
C	betaxolol, bisoprolol, carteolol, dopamine, ephedrine, epinephrine, inamrinone, isoproterenol, labetalol, mephentermine, metaraminol, metoprolol, nadolol, norepinephrine, penbutolol, phenoxybenzamine, phenylephrine, propranolol, timolol, tolazoline
X	ergotamine tartrate, methysergide
Unclassified	dihydroergotamine,* dobutamine, ergoloid mesylates, phentolamine

*Not recommended.

Drug/Herb	Possible Effect and Management
monoamine oxidase (MAO) inhibitors —cont'd	Avoid concurrent use or a potentially serious drug interaction may occur. Effects of both drugs may be reduced or blocked (sympathomimetics with beta activity). In sympathomimetics with both alpha and beta activity, beta blockade may result in increased alpha effects (i.e., hypertension, severe bradycardia, and possibly heart block). Avoid concurrent use or a potentially serious drug interaction may occur.
sympathomimetics	Labetalol may be used if combination therapy is necessary because it has alpha-blocking effects. In sympathomimetic drugs with beta-adrenergic activity, the beta-blocking agent may cancel the $beta_1$ cardiac activity of dopamine or dobutamine or the $beta_2$ bronchodilating effects of isoproterenol and metaproterenol.
xanthines (aminophylline or theophylline)	The therapeutic response of both drugs may be reduced or blocked. May also result in theophylline accumulation in the body. Monitor vital signs closely when this drug combination is prescribed.
yohimbine	Active ingredient in this herbal may increase blood pressure. Monitor.

Obtain a baseline assessment of the underlying condition for which the beta-adrenergic blocking agent is being prescribed. This may include pulse, blood pressure, ECG, and other cardiac functioning determinations.

▪ **Nursing Diagnosis.** The client receiving beta-adrenergic blocking agents may experience the following nursing diagnoses/collaborative problems: disturbed thought processes (confusion); sexual dysfunction (decreased sexual ability); risk for injury related to dizziness or orthostatic hypotension; ineffective airway clearance (bronchospasm); ineffective protection related to leukopenia or thrombocytopenia; disturbed sleep pattern (insomnia, drowsiness); activity intolerance related to lethargy and weakness; and the potential complications of mental depression, hepatotoxicity, and altered cardiac output (bradycardia, dysrhythmias, congestive heart failure).

▪ **Implementation**

▪ ***Monitoring.*** Always check the apical pulse rate before administering a beta-adrenergic blocking drug. If the pulse is slower than 60 beats/min or the rate is irregular, hold the drug and call the prescriber immediately. Also check and report significant variations in blood pressure. Low parameters indicate overdose.

Because of the potential for altered cardiac output and ineffective airway clearance related to the blockade of cardiac and bronchial beta-adrenergic receptors, monitor ECG, blood pressure, and pulmonary wedge pressure when these agents are administered intravenously. Have available atropine (for bradycardia), vasopressors (for hypotension), and bronchodilators (for bronchoconstriction). Institute oral therapy as soon as tolerated to reduce the risk of decreased cardiac output. Report to the prescriber a considerable slowing of the pulse rate regardless of how the drug is administered. Beta-blocking action can result in cardiac standstill.

Monitor closely individuals with hypertension who have congestive heart failure controlled by digitalis and diuretics. The effects of digitalis and beta blockers are additive in depressing AV conduction. Discontinue therapy if cardiac failure continues with digitalis administration. Cardiac failure may be precipitated because of drug-depressed myocardial contractility. Evaluate the effectiveness of drug therapy by assessing the frequency of anginal attacks and activity tolerance. When the drug is used as an antihypertensive, a reduction in blood pressure will indicate effectiveness.

To monitor for potential/actual fluid volume excess, measure intake and output, and weigh the client daily. Fluid retention may cause dyspnea, orthopnea, nocturnal cough, pulmonary rales, distended neck veins, and edema, all of which are signs of impending heart failure. Report weight gain and other such symptoms to the prescriber.

Observe the client for possible signs of thyrotoxicosis, because the drug may mask the clinical signs of hyperthyroidism. In individuals with renal and hepatic impairment, monitor for signs of excessive drug accumulation.

Monitor for adherence to the therapeutic regimen; noncompliance may be an issue related to sexual dysfunction, fatigue, and/or depression.

▪ ***Intervention.*** To minimize variations in absorption, be consistent in administering oral beta-blocking agents with regard to taking them with food or on an empty stomach. The bioavailability of labetalol, propranolol, and possibly metoprolol may be enhanced by food. Other oral beta-blocking agents may have delayed absorption with food but, with the exception of sotalol, bioavailability is not affected.

Notify the anesthetist if the client is scheduled for surgery and is receiving a beta blocker, because caution should be used if a hydrocarbon anesthetic (e.g., halothane) is to be administered. Note that beta-blocking drugs must be withdrawn slowly to prevent abrupt withdrawal syndrome with tremors, sweating, severe headache, malaise, palpitation, rebound hypertension, life-threatening dysrhythmias, myocardial infarction (in clients with cardiac problems and angina pectoris), and hyperthyroidism (in clients with thyrotoxicosis) (Box 22-3). If the drug is to be discontinued, reduce the dosage over a 1- to 2-week period. It may be recommended that the drug be withdrawn well before surgery. In individuals with pheochromocytoma, the drug is usually not discontinued before surgery.

For the administration of parenteral labetalol, the client should be in a supine position during injection and for 3 hours afterward. Increase the client's activity and move the client to an upright position gradually.

BOX 22-3

Withdrawal of a Beta-Adrenergic Blocking Agent

Withdraw beta-adrenergic blocking agents slowly by tapering or lowering the dose over approximately 14 days.

Advise the client to avoid vigorous physical exercises or activities during this time to decrease the risk of a reinfarction or cardiac dysrhythmia.

If withdrawal signs occur (angina or chest pain, sweating, tachycardia, respiratory distress), temporarily reinstitute the beta-blocking agent to stabilize the client; then lower the dose slowly with close supervision.

■ ***Education.*** Instruct the client to take his or her own pulse rate before each dose; withhold the medication and inform the prescriber if the pulse rate drops below 60 beats/min.

Counsel the client not to alter the drug regimen established by prescriber. Beta-blocking drugs control but do not cure hypertension; therefore lifetime compliance is necessary. The medication should be taken even if the client feels well, and the client should always have available an adequate supply of drug so that strict compliance is observed. Advise the client of the hazards of untreated hypertension. Emphasize the importance of keeping appointments for periodic laboratory tests.

Advise the client to carry medical identification to alert health care professionals during an emergency situation that a beta blocker is being taken.

Caution the client not to take OTC medications, especially decongestants and cough and cold medications, without consulting his or her health care provider.

To reduce the risk of myocardial infarction and/or dysrhythmias, advise the client to avoid physical exertion while the drug is being withdrawn. Instruct the client to restrict sodium intake to prevent unnecessary fluid retention. Caution the client to avoid cold temperatures because there is an increased sensitivity to cold. Painful, cold, and tender hands and feet are a sign of impaired circulation. Take peripheral pulses to monitor for a decrease in peripheral circulation.

Advise clients with hypertension to make position changes slowly to prevent light-headedness and dizziness. Alcohol ingestion, standing still for long periods, exercise, and hot weather enhance the orthostatic hypotensive effects of the drug. Notify the prescriber if the problem continues to exist. Because drowsiness and dizziness are common side effects, caution the client about operating a car or hazardous equipment.

When a beta-blocking agent is used to treat angina pectoris, exercise tolerance should increase and pain should be reduced. Caution the client to avoid overexertion because he or she has less pain. Instruct the client to inform the prescriber if adequate relief is not obtained from the drug.

Instruct the client to monitor weight and to report to the prescriber the possible signs of congestive heart failure: a weight gain of 3 to 4 pounds per day, dyspnea, cough, fatigue, rapid pulse, and anxiety. (A weight gain of 1 pound represents approximately 500 mL of retained fluid; 4 pounds of weight gain represent approximately one-half gallon of retained fluids.)

Alert clients with diabetes that beta-adrenergic blocking agents mask the signs and symptoms of hypoglycemia, may prolong hypoglycemia, or may cause increased levels of blood glucose.

■ **Evaluation.** The expected outcome of beta-adrenergic blocking drug therapy is that the client will experience an absence of signs and symptoms of the underlying condition without experiencing adverse reactions to the drug. If the drug is given for hypertension, the blood pressure will be within normal limits; if given for dysrhythmias, there will be a normal sinus rhythm on the ECG.

SEROTONERGIC DRUGS

sumatriptan [soo ma trip' tan] (Imitrex ◆)
naratriptan [nair' uh trip tan] (Amerge)
rizatriptan [rye zah trip' tan] (Maxalt)
zolmitriptan [zole mih trip' tan] (Zomig)

Sumatriptan, naratriptan, rizatriptan, and zolmitriptan are antimigraine products believed to produce their effects at selective serotonin receptor subtypes. Zolmitriptan, naratriptan, and rizatriptan have 5-HT_{1B} and 5-HT_{1D} selectivity; zolmitriptan has a much greater affinity for 1B receptors than 1D receptors. Sumatriptan is primarily selective for 5-HT_{1D} receptors. This selectivity results in the binding and stimulation of receptors located on cranial blood vessels (*Drug Facts and Comparisons,* 2000). The response of the receptors is constriction of the blood vessels and, perhaps, cerebral blood vessel constriction that results in the reduction of pulsation associated with pain from vascular headaches (*USP DI,* 1999). The serotonin agonists may also inhibit the release of the pro-inflammatory neuropeptides, which also helps in migraine relief.

Sumatriptan is available in oral, nasal, and parenteral dosage forms. It has an onset of action within 15 minutes (nasal), in ½ hour (oral), or in 10 minutes by SC injection (parenteral). The peak effect is reached in approximately 2 hours for an oral dosage (in up to 75% of clients) and within 1 hour for an SC injection (up to 70% of clients). It is metabolized in the liver (and by monoamine oxidase) and is excreted by the kidneys.

Naratriptan is available in an oral dosage form. It reaches peak serum levels in 2 to 3 hours, has a half-life of 6 hours, and is metabolized in the liver and excreted by the kidneys.

Rizatriptan is available in oral tablets and oral disintegrating tablets (Maxalt-MLT); the latter can be placed on the tongue, where it dissolves and is then swallowed (no water required). Rizatriptan has a half-life of 2 to 3 hours; it is metabolized in the liver and excreted by the kidneys.

Zolmitriptan is available in an oral dosage form; it reaches a peak serum level within 2 hours, is metabolized in the liver to an active (N-desmethyl) metabolite and inactive metabolites, and is excreted primarily in the urine (65%) and feces (30%) (Zolmitriptan, 1999).

The side effects/adverse reactions of sumatriptan and zolmitriptan include nausea, vomiting, weakness, tingling, and warm or hot sensations. Naratriptan, risatriptan, and zolmitriptan may also produce dizziness and drowsiness. Because many of these symptoms also occur during and/or after a migraine headache, it may be difficult to determine the contribution of the serotonin agonist to these effects.

Adverse reactions that require medical attention include chest pain or pain/pressure type sensations in the chest, neck, throat, or jaw. Dysrhythmias have also been reported. Several deaths have resulted 3 hours or more after the administration of sumatriptan (strokes, cerebral hemorrhage); it is not certain if these deaths were due to underlying disease or directly related to the sumatriptan. Individuals with migraines are at increased risk for CVAs or TIAs, and it has been postulated that perhaps a CVA rather than a migraine caused the symptoms that resulted in the administration of sumatriptan (*USP DI*, 1999).

The adult dosage of sumatriptan is 25 mg to 100 mg PO (maximum of 300 mg/day), 5 or 10 mg intranasally (1 or 2 sprays in each nostril), 20 mg intranasally (1 spray into one nostril), or 6 mg SC injected in the outer thigh or outer upper arm. If the client responds in 1 to 2 hours, an additional dose may be given if the headache pain returns or increases.

The adult dosage of naratriptan is 1 or 2.5 mg PO as a single dose, which may be repeated in 4 hours if necessary. The maximum dose is 5 mg in 24 hours or 2.5 mg in clients with mild to moderate liver or kidney impairment.

The adult dosage of rizatriptan is 5 or 10 mg PO, which is repeated in 2 hours if necessary. The maximum daily dose is 30 mg.

The adult dosage of zolmitriptan is 1.25 to 2.5 mg PO initially; additional doses may be administered in 2 hours if necessary. The maximum daily dose is 10 mg.

■ Nursing Management
Serotonergic Drug Therapy

■ **Assessment.** The client should be assessed for conditions for which serotonergic drugs would be contraindicated, such as sensitivity to the drug, ischemic heart disease, Prinzmetal's angina, history of myocardial infarction, uncontrolled hypertension (may worsen the condition), or sensitivity to sumatriptan. These drugs are used cautiously in clients with a history of or predisposition to coronary artery disease, CVA, or renal or hepatic function impairment. Safety has not been established for use during pregnancy, lactating clients, or children.

A baseline assessment should include a description of the aura, location, severity, duration, predisposing factors, and any associated symptoms (nausea and vomiting, photophobia) that the client experiences during a migraine episode.

■ **Nursing Diagnosis.** The client undergoing serotonergic therapy may experience the following nursing diagnoses/collaborative problems: pain related to migraine and the ineffectiveness of the drug; risk for injury related to dizziness and vertigo; fatigue; anxiety; impaired tissue integrity (site of injection); disturbed sensory perception (warm or cold sensations, tingling, burning, numbness of the jaw, mouth, throat, nasal cavity, or sinuses); and the potential complications of coronary vasospasm, angina, and myocardial infarction (chest pain/pressure).

■ **Implementation**

■ ***Monitoring.*** If the client is receiving a serotonergic drug for the first time, monitor blood pressure before and for 1 hour following the dose. If chest pain occurs, monitor with an ECG for ischemic changes.

■ ***Intervention.*** Administer the initial SC injection under observation in a health agency.

■ ***Education.*** Instruct the client not to take the drug if an atypical headache occurs but to contact the prescriber. Serotonergic drugs should be used only during a migraine episode; they do not prevent or reduce the number of migraines. The drug should be administered as soon as a migraine attack begins, but it may be used at any time during an attack. Caution against using additional doses if the first dose does not provide substantial relief.

If the client receives incomplete relief after the initial injection of sumatriptan, a second injection may be used after an hour, with no more than a total of two injections being used in a 24-hour period. However, if the client does not experience substantial relief within 1 to 2 hours of the initial injection, a second injection should not be used. Analgesics may be used if the migraine does not respond to the sumatriptan injection for that episode; the use of ergot alkaloids is not recommended because of the risk of additive or prolonged vasoconstriction. Instruct the client on SC administration of the drug. Advise the client that any redness or tenderness at the injection site usually lasts 1 hour.

Sumatriptan tablets have a special coating to disguise an unpleasant taste; they are to be swallowed whole, not broken, crushed, or chewed.

Advise the client that resting in a darkened room after taking the medication will also help to relieve the migraine. To prevent injury secondary to dizziness, caution the client against hazardous activities until the response to the drug has been determined. Advise female clients on contraception methods while they are undergoing sumatriptan therapy.

If the client experiences chest pain or tightness with the use of any serotonergic drug, notify the prescriber before using the drug again. If the pain is severe, notify the prescriber or other health care provider immediately. If the usual dose fails to relieve three consecutive headaches, notify the prescriber, and alternative therapy will be sought.

■ **Evaluation.** The expected outcome of serotonergic drug therapy is that the client will experience relief from the migraine attack.

SUMMARY

Being knowledgeable about drugs that affect the sympathetic nervous system is essential for all areas of nursing practice. Because of the ability of the sympathetic nervous system to produce generalized physiologic responses, drugs that act on this system may affect a wide range of body functions. These agents are described as either adrenergic (sympathomimetic) drugs—those that mimic the effects of sympathetic nerve stimulation—or adrenergic blocking (sympatholytic) drugs—those that compete with the catecholamines at receptor sites and inhibit adrenergic sympathetic stimulation. The adrenergic drugs may be direct-acting, indirect-acting, or dual-acting (direct and indirect) agents. Knowledge of these agents is essential, because many of them are used to rectify life-threatening situations in which the nurse must act quickly to provide the necessary pharmacologic intervention. Other drugs that act on the sympathetic nervous system are used quite commonly in practice for a wide range of clients.

The adrenergic direct-acting drugs, the catecholamines, interact with and stimulate adrenergic effector cells (alpha and beta receptors). Alpha-adrenergic activity includes vasoconstriction of arterioles in the skin and splanchnic area, which increases blood pressure, pupil dilation, and relaxation of the gut. Beta-adrenergic activity includes cardiac acceleration and increased contractility, vasodilation of the arterioles of the skeletal muscles, bronchial relaxation, and uterine relaxation. Beta receptors can be either $beta_1$ receptors, which are located mainly in the heart, or $beta_2$ receptors within the bronchioles and arterial smooth muscle. Understanding the placement of these receptor cells assists the nurse in conceptualizing the activities of the various drugs that affect the sympathetic nervous system.

Epinephrine is a direct-acting catecholamine that stimulates alpha, $beta_1$, and $beta_2$ receptors. It is considered to be the classic or standard drug of this classification because of its long history of use for symptomatic treatment of asthma, emergency treatment of anaphylactic shock and cardiac arrest, local homeostasis, and management of simple, open-angle glaucoma. Isoproterenol is a nonselective beta-adrenergic drug.

Norepinephrine, on the other hand, has a high affinity for alpha receptors. Dobutamine is valuable for individuals with low cardiac output because it directly stimulates the $beta_1$-adrenergic receptors of the heart. Dopamine acts mainly to cause vasodilation of the renal and mesenteric arteries. All of these drugs are used for the treatment of circulatory shock.

The indirect-acting adrenergic agents act indirectly on receptors by triggering the release of epinephrine and norepinephrine from their storage sites, which then stimulate alpha and beta receptors. Dual-acting adrenergic agents have both indirect and direct effects. Ephedrine has both a direct and an indirect sympathomimetic action and is used more commonly for bronchodilation for milder forms of asthma and as a nasal decongestant. Phenylephrine is also commonly found in many combination cough-cold, antihistamine and decongestant, and ophthalmic preparations. Mephentermine sulfate and metaraminol, as dual-acting adrenergic agents, are used primarily for their vasopressor effects with hypotensive clients.

The adrenergic blocking, or sympatholytic, drugs are also classified by alpha and beta receptors and by their ability to inhibit adrenergic sympathetic nervous stimulation at these sites. There are noncompetitive, long-acting antagonists such as phenoxybenzamine, which is used mainly for vasodilation and inhibition of vasospasm; competitive, short-acting antagonists such as phentolamine, which is used locally to reverse the action of an extravasation of vasoconstricting drugs; tolazoline, which is indicated for pulmonary hypertension in the newborn; and the ergot alkaloids, which are used for the management of vascular headaches. Sumatriptan is also an antimigraine agent but is believed to produce its effects at serotonin receptors.

The beta-adrenergic blocking agents are differentiated into selective $beta_1$-adrenergic blocking agents such as atenolol and metoprolol, which decrease heart rate, conduction velocity, myocardial contractility, and cardiac output; and the nonselective beta-adrenergic blocking agents such as carteolol, penbutolol, pindolol, propranolol, and timolol. The nonselective beta-adrenergic blocking agents affect cardiac muscle and smooth muscle of the bronchi and blood vessels but are used primarily to treat chronic angina, hypertension, and cardiac dysrhythmias and to prevent a second myocardial infarction, vascular headaches, and cardiac dysrhythmias.

Serotonergic drugs are antimigraine products that stimulate 5-HT receptors located on cranial blood vessels. This stimulation constricts the vessels and so reduces the pulsation associated with vascular headaches.

Critical Thinking Questions

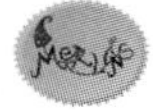

1. Sean Murphy is admitted to the emergency department with a massive myocardial infarction. His blood pressure has dropped to 80/40 mm Hg, his pulse has increased to 128 beats/min, and his skin is cool and moist. The physician indicates that Mr. Murphy is in cardiogenic shock and orders an infusion of dopamine, 10 μg/kg/min. How will this dose affect adrenergic receptors? What would you expect to occur as a result of Mr. Murphy receiving this infusion? As the nurse, what should you be monitoring? What action should you take if the infusion infiltrates?
2. Mrs. Melanie Freedman is 43 years old and has a history of migraine headaches. She has tried a number of therapies without success. Ergotamine tartrate

(Ergomar ✤) has now been prescribed for her. Mrs. Freedman calls the clinic and indicates that she vomits each time she takes the drug. As the nurse, how should you respond to Mrs. Freedman's comment?

3. Dr. Harry Lewis, a 56-year-old university professor, has been admitted to the hospital with atrial tachycardia. He has been started on propranolol (Inderal), 30 mg four times daily. Dr. Lewis also has diabetes mellitus. What nursing interventions will you take?

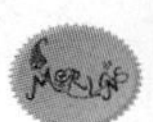

Collaborative Learning Activities

For Collaborative Learning Activities, go to mosby.com/MERLIN/McKenry/.

CASE STUDY

For a Case Study that will help ensure mastery of this chapter content, go to mosby.com/MERLIN/McKenry/.

BIBLIOGRAPHY

Ahrens, S.P., Farmer, M.V., Williams, D.L., Willoughby, E., Jiang, K., Block, G.A., & Visser, W.H. (1999). Efficacy and safety of rizatriptan wafer for the acute treatment of migraine. Rizatriptan Wafer Protocol 049 Study Group. *Cephalalgia*, 9(5), 525-530.

American Hospital Formulary Service. (1998). *AHFS drug information '98*. Bethesda, MD: American Society of Hospital Pharmacists.

American Medical Association. (1995). *Drug evaluations: Annual 1995*. Chicago: Author.

Anderson, K.N., Anderson, L.E., & Glanze, W.D. (Eds.). (1998). *Mosby's medical, nursing, & allied health dictionary* (5th ed.). St. Louis: Mosby.

Asmus, M.J., Sherman, J., & Hendeles, L. (1999). Bronchoconstrictor additives in bronchodilator solutions. *Journal of Allergy & Clinical Immunology, 104*(2 pt 2), S53-S60.

Carter, B.L., Furmaga, E.M., & Murphy, C.H. (1995). Essential hypertension. In L.Y. Young & M.A. Koda-Kimble (Eds.), *Applied therapeutics* (6th ed.). Vancouver, WA: Applied Therapeutics.

Dhond, M.R., Donnell, K., Singh, S., Garapati, S., Whitley, T.B., Nguyen, T., & Bommer, W. (1999). Value of negative dobutamine stress echocardiography in predicting long-term cardiac events. *Journal of American Society of Echocardiography*, 12(6), 471-475.

Drug Facts and Comparisons. (2000). St. Louis: Facts and Comparisons.

Dulli, D.A. (1999). Naratriptan: An alternative for migraine. *American Pharmacotherapy*, 33(6), 704-711.

Fitzgerald, M. (1995). Pharmacologic highlights: The beta-2 agonists. *Journal of the American Academy of Nurse Practitioners*, 7(6), 304-307.

Foster, S., Tyler V.E. (2000). *Tyler's honest herbal* (4th ed.). New York: Haworth Herbal Press.

Freemantle, N., Cleland, J., Young, P., Mason, J., & Harrison, J. (1999). Beta blockade after myocardial infarction: Systematic review and meta regression analysis. *British Medical Journal*, 318(7200), 1730-1737.

Grouhi, M., Alshri, M., Hummel, D., & Roifman, C.M. (1999). Anaphylaxis and epinephrine auto-injector training: Who will teach the teachers? *Journal of Allergy & Clinical Immunology*, 104(1), 190-193.

Hardman, J.G. & Limbird, L.E. (Eds.). (1996). *Goodman and Gilman's The pharmacological basis of therapeutics* (9th ed.). New York: McGraw-Hill.

Katzung, B.G. (1998). *Basic and clinical pharmacology* (7th ed.). Norwalk: Appleton & Lange.

Sterling, L.P. (1995). Beta adrenergic agonists. *AACN Clinical Issues in Advanced Practice Acute Critical Care* 6(2), 271-278.

United States Pharmacopeia Dispensing Information (USP DI): Drug information for the health care professional (19th ed.). (1999). Rockville, MD: United States Pharmacopeial Convention.

Zolmitriptan. (1999). *Canadian Family Physician, 45*, 1491-1494, 1497-1501.

23 Drugs for Specific Dysfunctions of the Central and Peripheral Nervous Systems

Chapter Focus

Dysfunctions of the central and peripheral nervous systems are often progressive and incapacitating. Therefore appropriate assessment, intervention, and evaluation are important measures for nursing. Parkinson's disease, myasthenia gravis, dementia, Alzheimer's disease, and skeletal muscle relaxants are discussed in this chapter.

Learning Objectives

1. Explain the neurotransmitter balance theory in Parkinson's disease.
2. Name the two neurotransmitters that centrally affect motor function and balance.
3. Discuss medications used to treat Parkinson's disease, myasthenia gravis, dementia, and Alzheimer's disease.
4. Describe the physiology of muscle movement and motor nerve response.
5. Compare the manifestations of the two primary types of muscle spasticity.
6. Compare the action of central-acting and direct-acting skeletal muscle relaxants.
7. Summarize the drug interactions associated with skeletal muscle relaxants.
8. Implement the nursing management of drug therapy prescribed for the treatment of Parkinson's disease, myasthenia gravis, dementia, Alzheimer's disease, and muscle spasm/spasticity.

Key Terms

akinesia, p. 493
Alzheimer's disease, p. 508
anticholinergic drug, p. 493
anticholinesterase agent, p. 505
dementia, p. 507
designer drugs, p. 492
dystonia, p. 511
myasthenia gravis, p. 504
on-off syndrome, p. 497
Parkinson's disease, p. 492
spasms, p. 511
spasticity, p. 511

Key Drugs [✔]

baclofen, p. 512
benztropine, p. 493
levodopa, p. 495
selegiline, p. 502
tacrine, p. 510

The personal tragedy of the progressive nature of Parkinson's disease, myasthenia gravis, dementia, and Alzheimer's disease, as well as the emotional distress of family members and the increasing cost of care to families and society, challenge health care providers to develop and mange rational pharmacologic treatments. Because there are currently no "cures," drug therapy attempts to minimize the symptoms of these conditions.

Skeletal muscle spasticity can also be debilitating, but these muscles are affected by many pharmacologic substances. Their effects may be at the neuromuscular junction or at different levels in the central nervous system (CNS), (i.e., at the brain or spinal cord). These agents are also discussed in this chapter.

PARKINSON'S DISEASE

Parkinson's disease is a progressively debilitating disorder of the CNS. This condition is characterized by resting tremor, bradykinesia (abnormal slowing of all voluntary movements and speech), forward flexion of the trunk, muscle rigidity, and weakness. It usually occurs between the ages of 50 to 80, and it affects both sexes equally. The prevalence for Parkinson's disease is 100 per 100,000 persons, although it affects several percent of those in the older-adult age-group (Van Den Nort, 1999).

Although the cause is unknown, genetic factors, viral influences, and environmental contaminants have been suspected. The correct balance of dopamine and acetylcholine is important in regulating posture, muscle tone, and voluntary movement (Figure 23-1). In Parkinson's disease, there is a disorder of the extrapyramidal system in the brain, especially the basal ganglia area. Degeneration of the dopamine-producing neurons in this area produces a dopamine/acetylcholine imbalance, a progressive loss of dopamine (inhibitory neurotransmitter), and an increase in acetylcholine (excitatory neurotransmitter). Other neurotransmitters (e.g., norepinephrine and serotonin) are also decreased in the brain of a person with Parkinson's disease. This condition can also be induced by the use of designer drugs (Box 23-1).

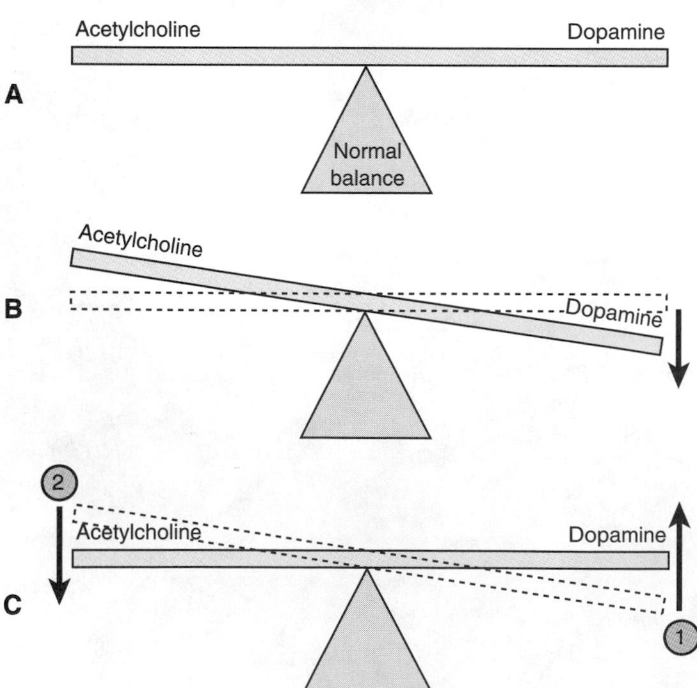

Figure 23-1 Central acetylcholine/dopamine balance. **A,** Normal "balance" of acetylcholine and dopamine. **B,** In Parkinson's disease, a decrease in dopamine results in an acetylcholine/dopamine imbalance. **C,** Drug therapy in Parkinson's disease aims at increasing the dopamine level, which restores the acetylcholine/dopamine balance toward normal by (*1*) increasing the supply of dopamine or (*2*) blocking or lowering acetylcholine levels.

The CNS has two major types of dopamine receptors, D_1 and D_2 receptors. The role of the D_1 receptor role is not currently known, but D_2 and especially D_{2A} receptors are involved with the effects of levodopa and the other dopamine agonists (Flaherty & Gidal, 1995). The use of drug therapy is aimed at correcting the dopamine/acetylcholine imbalance by increasing dopamine levels and blocking acetylcholine levels. Two classes of drugs are used in the treatment of Parkinson's disease: (1) drugs with central anticholinergic activity (anticholinergics and antihistamines), and (2) drugs that affect brain dopamine levels to enhance dopaminergic mechanisms.

For a Concept Map on Parkinson's disease, go to mosby.com/MERLIN/McKenry/.

Drugs with Central Anticholinergic Activity

Symptoms of Parkinson's disease caused by an excess of cholinergic activity are muscle rigidity and muscle tremor. The muscle rigidity or increased tone appears as "ratchet resistance," or "cogwheel rigidity," in which the affected

BOX 23-1

Parkinson's Disease Induced by Designer Drugs

Designer drugs, or chemical variations of illegal or controlled substances, are an ever-increasing problem in North America. Such products are usually not illegal but generally are produced to induce the psychoactive effects of selected illegal products. Often the user consumes an unknown substance that may or may not be the desired product. Reports indicate that MPTP, a chemical produced as an analog of meperidine in clandestine laboratories, has been sold on the streets as heroin, cocaine, or a contaminant of other products.

MPTP has reportedly induced a degenerative CNS disorder characterized by tremors and muscle paralysis similar to the symptoms of Parkinson's disease. In a number of cases the paralysis has been permanent.

muscle moves easily then meets resistance or remains fixed in the new position. The muscle tremors appear to have a "to-and-fro" movement caused by the sequence of contractions of the agonistic and antagonistic muscles involved. The tremors are usually worse at rest and are commonly manifested as a "pill-rolling" motion of the hands and a bobbing of the head. Anticholinergics are more useful early in the course of this disease because the side effects of dopamine depletion are not prominent at this stage.

Various drugs with central anticholinergic activity are used to treat Parkinson's disease and include benztropine (Cogentin), trihexyphenidyl (Artane), and diphenhydramine (Benadryl). These agents are used in the treatment of mild Parkinson's disease and as an adjunct to dopamine replacement.

Anticholinergic Agents

benztropine [benz troe' peen] (Cogentin, Apo-Benztropine ♣)
biperiden [bye per' i den] (Akineton)
procyclidine [proe sye' kli deen] (Kemadrin, Procyclid ♣)
trihexyphenidyl [trye hex ee fin' i dill] (Artane)

Drugs that inhibit or block the effects of acetylcholine are referred to as **anticholinergic drugs.** The belladonna alkaloids atropine and scopolamine were the first centrally active (i.e., crossing the blood-brain barrier) anticholinergic agents used to treat parkinsonism and for many years were the only drugs available for such treatment. These drugs have been supplanted by synthetic anticholinergics, which were developed in an effort to produce drugs as effective as the belladonna drugs but with fewer side effects. In this group, benztropine is the key drug.

Anticholinergic agents that readily cross the blood-brain barrier can produce some improvement in functional capacity. The usefulness of these drugs is limited because of their side effects and their tendency to be less effective with continued use. Some anticholinergics are also used to control extrapyramidal reactions, such as rigidity, **akinesia** (difficulty in or lack of ability to initiate muscle movement), tremor, and akathisia, which are caused by antipsychotic drugs such as the phenothiazines.

Anticholinergic agents block central cholinergic excitatory pathways, returning the dopamine/acetylcholine balance in the brain (especially in the basal ganglia) to normal. The effects of the anticholinergic agents include decreased salivation and relaxation of smooth muscle with a decrease in tremors. Decreased rigidity and akinesia (in nearly 50% of the clients) is also reported.

Anticholinergic agents are indicated for use as antidyskinetics, for treatment of Parkinson's disease, and for treatment of drug-induced extrapyramidal reactions.

These drugs are very well absorbed. The onset of action for specific drugs is as follows: benztropine oral, 1 to 2 hours; benztropine IM/IV, within minutes; biperiden IM, within 10 to 30 minutes; biperiden IV, within minutes; and trihexyphenidyl oral, 1 hour. (For the onset of action for diphenhydramine, see Antihistamines, Chapter 39.) The duration of effect for specific agents is as follows: benztropine (Cogentin) oral, IM, or IV, 24 hours; biperiden (Akineton) IV, 1 to 8 hours; procyclidine (Kemadrin, Procyclid) oral, 4 hours; and trihexyphenidyl (Artane) oral, 6 to 12 hours. The metabolism of the anticholinergics is undetermined. They are most likely excreted by the kidneys.

The side effects/adverse reactions of anticholinergic drugs include blurred vision, mydriasis, constipation, dry skin, anhidrosis, urinary hesitancy, pain on urination, nausea, vomiting, photophobia, drowsiness, xerostomia, and dysphagia.

The adult dosage of benztropine for Parkinson's disease is 1 to 2 mg PO, IM, or IV daily, adjusted as necessary; for drug-induced extrapyramidal reactions, the dosage is 1 to 4 mg PO, IM, or IV once or twice daily. The maximum dosage is 6 mg/day. The adult dosage of biperiden for Parkinson's disease is 2 mg PO three to four times daily, or 2 mg IM or slow IV. The adult dosage of procyclidine for Parkinson's disease or drug-induced extrapyramidal reactions is 2.5 mg PO three times daily after meals. The adult dosage of trihexyphenidyl is 1 to 2 mg initially, adjusted at three to five intervals as needed for Parkinson's disease; for drug-induced extrapyramidal reactions, the dosage of trihexyphenidyl is 1 mg PO initially, adjusted as necessary.

■ Nursing Management
Anticholinergic Therapy

■ **Assessment.** Clients who have a history of sensitivity to one belladonna alkaloid or derivative may experience a cross-sensitivity to other belladonna alkaloids or derivatives. Dyskinetics with anticholinergic activity may inhibit lactation and are therefore contraindicated in clients who are breastfeeding. Older adults are at risk for the development of health problems caused by the anticholinergic effects of these agents, such as dryness of the mouth, constipation, and urinary retention, particularly in males (see the Special Considerations for Older Adults box on p. 494). Although there is no information available on the age-specific effects of the antidyskinetics on children, children younger than 3 years are very susceptible to the toxic effects of anticholinergic agents (see the Special Considerations for Children box on p. 494).

Older adults may respond to the usual doses of anticholinergic agents with agitation, confusion, and altered thought processes (hallucinations and psychotic-like symptoms). The anticholinergics block the actions of acetylcholine, which supports many functions of the brain (including memory); as a result, older adults, particularly those with existing memory problems, may become more impaired with continued use of anticholinergics. Caution should be exercised when using anticholinergics in individuals over the age of 40 because of the possibility of precipitating undiagnosed glaucoma.

The anticholinergic activity that decreases the tone and motility of the gastrointestinal tract necessitates caution in

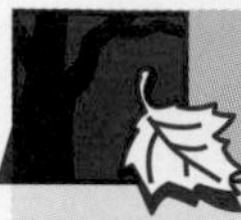

Special Considerations for Older Adults
Anticholinergic Agents

Older adults are highly susceptible to anticholinergic side effects, especially constipation, dry mouth, and urinary retention (usually in men).

Avoid using anticholinergic agents in clients with narrow-angle glaucoma or a history of urinary retention.

Memory impairment has been reported with continuous administration of these agents, especially in older clients.

When usual adult dosages are administered, some older adults may experience a paradoxical reaction: hyperexcitability, agitation, confusion, and sedation.

Chronic use decreases or inhibits the flow of saliva, which may contribute to oral discomfort, periodontal disease, and candidiasis.

Overheating resulting in heat stroke has been reported in persons receiving anticholinergic drugs during vigorous exercise or in periods of hot weather.

Blurred vision and/or increased sensitivity to light may occur.

Anticholinergic dosing in older adults should begin with the lowest dosage, with gradual increases until maximum improvement is noted or intolerable side effects occur.

the use of these drugs in clients with a history of or actual complete or partial intestinal obstruction. In addition, clients with or who have a predisposition to prostatic hypertrophy, urinary retention, or other obstructive uropathy may find the condition precipitated or exacerbated. The heart rate may be increased, and this should be carefully considered before administering drugs with anticholinergic properties to clients with preexisting tachycardia or other cardiac dysrhythmias, in whom such an increase would be undesirable. The mydriatic effect of these drugs increases intraocular pressure, which may precipitate an acute episode of angle-closure glaucoma or necessitate an adjustment in the therapy of clients with open-angle glaucoma.

Review the client's current medication regimen for the risk of significant drug interactions, such as those that may occur when anticholinergic agents are given concurrently with the following drugs:

Drug	Possible Effect and Management
alcohol and CNS depressants	May result in enhanced CNS depressant effects. Monitor closely for hypoventilation, sedation, confusion, and ataxia.
antacids	Concurrent administration may reduce the absorption and therapeutic effects of anticholinergic agents. Separate the administration of antacids and anticholinergics by at least 1 to 2 hours.
anticholinergic or other antimuscarinic* medications	May result in enhanced anticholinergic effects. Monitor for constipation because bowel impaction and/or paralytic ileus may be produced. Increased fluid intake, exercise, stool softeners, and/or laxatives may be necessary.

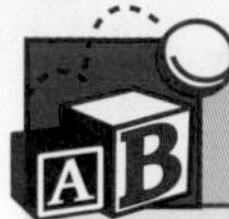

Special Considerations for Children
Anticholinergic Agents

Infants and young children are very susceptible to anticholinergic side effects/adverse reactions.

Closely monitor children with spastic paralysis or brain damage, because they usually have an increased reaction to anticholinergic agents and thus require a dosage reduction.

Anticholinergics, especially in high doses, may cause a paradoxical-type reaction of increased nervousness, confusion, and hyperexcitability.

Anticholinergic drugs suppress sweat gland activity. Therefore children receiving these agents in environments where hot weather prevails or temperatures are high have an increased risk of developing a rapid body temperature increase.

Dosage adjustments are often necessary for infants, clients with Down's syndrome, and clients with blonde hair because they usually have an increased response to this drug category. Flushing, increased temperature, irritability, increased pulse, and increased respiratory rate may occur.

Start with low dosages and increase gradually as needed and as tolerated.

A baseline assessment should include the client's mobility status and other symptoms related to the underlying disease for which the anticholinergic agent is being prescribed. Intraocular pressure should be measured for clients at risk for glaucoma.

■ **Nursing Diagnosis.** Once the client begins dyskinetic therapy with anticholinergic drugs, assessment should relate to the potential development of a number of nursing diagnoses/collaborative problems related to the drug. There may be disturbed sensory perception related to the effects of the drug on vision and somatosensory function, especially in older adults. Older adults are also more at risk for disturbed thought processes (confusion and hallucinations) and are at risk for injury related to the CNS effects of the drug. There may be anxiety, disturbed sleep pattern (extreme drowsiness or insomnia), constipation because of the gastrointestinal effects, and impaired urinary elimination that results primarily from urinary retention. There may be impaired comfort related to xerostomia, blurred vision, rash, and the gastrointestinal and genitourinary effects of the anticholinergics.

*Drugs that block cholinergic receptors at postganglionic parasympathetic synapses and a small number of postganglionic sympathetic synapses (atropine, scopolamine) (see Chapter 21).

Potential complications might be decreasedcardiac output (dysrhythmias), extrapyramidal symptoms, and increased intraocular pressure.

■ **Implementation**

■ ***Monitoring.*** The client's vital signs should be monitored, and changes in the cardiac status should be observed and reported. Dysrhythmias have been noted as a result of anticholinergic agents, but these effects are dose related.

Urinary retention may occur in clients with bladder neck obstruction. Male clients in particular should be monitored for difficulty in starting their urinary stream. Because of the decrease in peristalsis, gastrointestinal transit is prolonged and the absorption of other drugs may be impaired. Caution should be taken in clients with chronic pulmonary disease because the resultant decrease in bronchial secretions may lead to bronchial mucus plugs.

Older adults are more sensitive to anticholinergic agents and require dosages smaller than the usual adult dosage. Monitor closely for agitation, sleepiness, and altered thought processes.

Observe the client for xerostomia, a reduction in the volume of saliva. This symptom is important and should be reported, not only because extreme dryness of the mouth is usually a discomfort to the client but also because the severity of xerostomia limits the amount of drug that can be administered. From this symptom, the progression of adverse reaction is interference with visual accommodation and difficulty in urination.

■ ***Intervention.*** When therapy is initiated, the dosages are low and increase every 5 to 6 days until a therapeutic level can be obtained. The drug is withdrawn in the same manner—gradually. Sudden withdrawal may cause vomiting, lassitude, and excessive sweating and salivation. Tolerance may develop if the therapy is prolonged; this may require an increase in dosage. The dosage is titrated according to the client's symptoms. If another antiparkinson agent is to be substituted for the initial drug, the dosage of the first drug should be gradually decreased while the substitute is gradually increased.

Oral dosage forms of anticholinergic agents may be taken with or immediately after meals to minimize heartburn. With the parenteral administration of anticholinergics, the client may experience a temporary sensation of light-headedness; take precautions to meet the client's safety needs by having him or her rest in a sitting or, preferably, a prone position for approximately 20 minutes.

■ ***Education.*** Arrange for the client undergoing anticholinergic therapy to check with a pharmacist, physician, or other prescriber for drug interactions before taking any other drugs, including over-the-counter (OTC) drugs. The client should be instructed to avoid CNS depressants such as alcohol, barbiturates, and narcotics while taking anticholinergic agents.

The client should be cautioned that anticholinergic agents impair physical and mental functioning (i.e., they cause drowsiness and blurred vision) and that care should be taken when driving or operating machinery. Alert the client to the dangers of heat exhaustion and inform him or her to avoid exercising in warm weather because of the decreased ability to perspire. The client should also be instructed to change positions slowly if orthostatic hypotension is a problem.

Advise the client to use sugarless hard candy, gum, mouthwash, or ice chips to relieve dryness of the mouth.

The client should be counseled to have annual ophthalmic examinations. Intraocular pressure determinations are of particular importance because increased ocular tension may occur with the anticholinergic agents.

■ **Evaluation.** The expected outcome of anticholinergic therapy for parkinsonism is that the client will demonstrate improved mobility with a reduction in muscular rigidity and tremor and will not experience any adverse reactions to the drug.

Drugs Affecting Brain Dopamine

Three classifications of drugs affect brain dopamine: those that release dopamine, those that increase brain levels of dopamine, and dopaminergic agonists. The drugs of choice in the treatment of Parkinson's disease are those that increase brain levels of dopamine. The other two classifications are used as adjuncts or when the usual therapy is contraindicated.

The drugs that affect brain dopamine have their major effect on the akinesia seen in Parkinson's disease. Akinesia is difficulty or the lack of ability in initiating muscle movement; this condition is caused by decreased levels of brain dopamine in Parkinson's disease. The client with akinesia exhibits a masklike facial expression, impairment of postural reflexes, and eventually an inability for self-care. Drugs are used to increase the levels of dopamine in the brain, thus creating a balance between dopamine and acetylcholine in the brain, especially in the basal ganglia area.

Drugs That Increase Levels of Dopamine in the Brain

levodopa [lee voe doe′ pa] (L-Dopa, Dopar, Larodopa)

A small percentage of levodopa crosses the blood-brain barrier intact. It is decarboxylated to dopamine, stimulates dopamine receptors, and helps to balance the dopamine/acetylcholine concentrations. Levodopa is indicated for the treatment of Parkinson's disease (idiopathic, postencephalitic, symptomatic, or parkinsonism associated with cerebral atherosclerosis) (Jankovic, 1999, Simuni & Stern, 1999).

Levodopa is absorbed by active transport, with approximately 30% to 50% reaching the systemic circulation. It is distributed to most body tissues; the CNS receives less than 1% of the dose because of peripheral metabolism. The enzyme decarboxylase converts levodopa (95%) to dopamine in the stomach, intestines, and also the liver. Levodopa has a half-life of 1 to 3 hours.

Improvement is usually seen within 2 to 3 weeks, although some clients may require levodopa for up to 6 months to obtain a therapeutic effect. Peak concentration is achieved in 1 to 3 hours. The duration of action is up to 5 hours per dose. The drug is excreted by the kidneys.

The side effects/adverse reactions of levodopa include anxiety, nervousness, confusion (especially in older adults), constipation, nightmares, difficulty with urination, depression, orthostatic hypotension, mood changes, increased aggressiveness, irregular heart rate, severe nausea or vomiting, and choreiform and involuntary movements of the body (face, arms, hands, tongue, head, and upper body) (King, 1999).

For adults and children 12 years and older, the dosage of levodopa (Dopar, Larodopa) is 250 mg PO two to four times daily, increased by 100 to 750 mg/day at 3- to 7-day intervals until a therapeutic response is achieved. The maximum dosage is 8 g/day. Older adults and postencephalitic clients may require lower dosages because they are more sensitive to this medication. The dosage for children younger than 12 years has not been established.

▪ Nursing Management

Levodopa Therapy

▪ **Assessment.** The client's health status should be assessed for any preexisting conditions in which the administration of levodopa would place the client at higher risk for injury or would require a greater degree of caution. Levodopa is not recommended for children younger than 12 years of age, pregnant women, or clients with undiagnosed skin lesions or a history of melanoma (the lesions may be activated). (See the Pregnancy Safety box below for pregnancy safety ratings.) Levodopa may inhibit lactation in nursing mothers and is excreted into breast milk. Levodopa should be administered with great caution to clients with severe cardiovascular, renal, hepatic, or endocrine disease; peptic ulcer (increases risk of gastrointestinal bleeding); diabetes; or psychiatric disturbances (increases risk of depression and suicidal tendencies). Levodopa may increase dysrhythmias in predisposed clients. The respiratory effects of levodopa may aggravate pulmonary conditions, especially bronchial asthma and chronic obstructive pulmonary disease. Intraocular pressure may increase and precipitate an acute attack of glaucoma. The administration of levodopa may precipitate or aggravate urinary retention, particularly in male clients.

Pregnancy Safety
Drugs Affecting Brain Dopamine

Category	Drug
B	bromocriptine, pergolide
C	amantadine, biperiden, carbidopa-levodopa, edrophonium, entacapone, neostigmine, pramipexole, ropinirole, selegiline, tolcapone
Unclassified	ambenonium, benztropine, levodopa, procyclidine, pyridostigmine, trihexyphenidyl

Review the client's current medication regimen for the risk of significant drug interactions, such as those that may occur when levodopa is given concurrently with the following drugs:

Drug	Possible Effect and Management
Bold/color type indicates the most serious interactions.	
anesthetics, hydrocarbon inhalation	May result in dysrhythmias. Discontinue levodopa 6 to 8 hours before hydrocarbon anesthetics, especially halothane.
anticonvulsants, haloperidol (Haldol), or phenothiazines	May result in decreased levodopa effects because hydantoin anticonvulsants increase levodopa metabolism, whereas haloperidol and phenothiazines block dopamine receptors in the brain. Monitor closely when hydantoin and levodopa are given concurrently; increased dosages of levodopa may be necessary. If at all possible, avoid the combination of haloperidol or phenothiazines with levodopa.
cocaine	May result in an increased risk of dysrhythmias. If medically necessary to give both drugs concurrently, reduce dosages and monitor closely with electrocardiogram (ECG) monitoring.
monoamine oxidase (MAO) inhibitors	**This combination may result in a hypertensive crisis. Avoid concurrent use or a potentially serious drug interaction may occur. MAO inhibitors should be discontinued 2 to 4 weeks before starting levodopa therapy.**
pyridoxine (vitamin B_6)	Doses of 10 mg or more may reverse the antiparkinsonian effect of levodopa. Monitor closely.
selegiline (Eldepryl)	Although this combination may be used, it may result in increased levodopa-induced nausea, dyskinesia, confusion, hypotension, and hallucinations. If this combination is used, the dosage of levodopa should be reduced within several days of starting the selegiline.

Obtain a baseline assessment of the client's parkinsonian symptoms. This should include self-care deficits, the amount of assistance required for the client to accomplish activities of daily living, and the client's physical and emotional adaptation to the illness.

▪ **Nursing Diagnosis.** After beginning levodopa therapy, the client should be assessed for the following nursing diagnoses/collaborative problems: impaired physical mobility related to the underlying Parkinson's disease and dose-related side effects of choreiform movements (50% to 80% of clients); disturbed thought processes (anxiety, confusion, nervousness) related to adverse CNS reactions to the drug; disturbed sleep pattern (nightmares, insomnia); risk for injury related to orthostatic hypotension (30% of clients in early therapy); impaired urinary elimination (urinary retention); constipation; impaired comfort (headache, dry mouth, nausea and vomiting); and the potential complications of depression, hypertension, duodenal ulcer, hemolytic anemia, and dysrhythmias.

■ **Implementation**

■ ***Monitoring.*** The client's vital signs should be monitored during periods of dosage regulation for indications of hypotension and dysrhythmias. Monitor the client's progress by observing body movements for signs of improvement. Periodic evaluations need to be performed for hepatic, cardiovascular, and renal functioning, including hemoglobin determinations and a complete blood count. Ophthalmologic testing for glaucoma is especially important with the administration of levodopa. The client should also be observed for symptoms of nightmares and mood changes, such as agitation, anxiety, depression, and confusion.

■ ***Intervention.*** Levodopa should be administered before meals because food impedes its action. Nausea and vomiting occur in 80% of the clients early in levodopa therapy, but tolerance develops with continued use of the drug. For older adults and clients receiving other medications, the dosage of levodopa should be titrated to reach the client's therapeutic level with minimal side effects.

■ ***Education.*** The client undergoing levodopa therapy should be instructed to change to the upright position slowly if orthostatic hypotension is a problem. Hypotension can be minimized with the use of elastic stockings. In addition, older clients who respond to levodopa therapy, particularly those with osteoporosis, should be cautioned to resume higher activity levels gradually to minimize the risk of fractures. Because levodopa has mydriatic effects, clients should be encouraged to have their intraocular pressure checked periodically for the detection of glaucoma.

The client should be instructed to call the prescriber if symptoms of overdose develop (involuntary muscle twitching and involuntary winking). Caution the client receiving prolonged high-dose therapy that an "on-off" syndrome may occur (Box 23-2). The client should be advised that involuntary movement of the face, mouth, tongue, and head often develop with prolonged therapy and that the prescriber should be notified of these symptoms so that the dosage can be adjusted.

Clients need to be alerted that the response to levodopa may not occur until several weeks after treatment has begun. Urine and perspiration may be darker, but this is of no significance. Clients with diabetes need to be aware that levodopa may interfere with the control of blood glucose. Alert clients to the necessity for compliance, because full withdrawal of the drug may worsen parkinsonian symptoms, depression, and immobility and may also increase the risk of thromboembolic disease.

Dietary counseling should be provided regarding the ingestion of protein and pyridoxine (B_6). Proteins are metabolized into amino acids, which may compete with levodopa for transport to the brain and make the response to levodopa unpredictable. Rather than restrict the client's protein intake, it should be divided in equal parts to be taken over the entire day. Vitamin compounds and foods high in pyridoxine (e.g., pork, beef, liver, ham, egg yolks, avocado, beans, sweet potato, dry skim milk, and oatmeal) may decrease the effects of levodopa and should be avoided. Dietary teaching should include the necessity of a high fiber and fluid intake to minimize the side effect of constipation with the drug, along with gradual increases in activity and the establishment of an elimination routine. Other eating difficulties may arise if the client has full dentures; some clients experience difficulty retaining their dentures while undergoing levodopa therapy.

■ **Evaluation.** The expected outcome of levodopa therapy is that the client will demonstrate an improvement in mobility with a decrease in muscular rigidity and tremor without experiencing adverse reactions to the drug.

carbidopa-levodopa [kar bi doe' pa/lee voe doe' pa] (Sinemet, Sinemet CR)

Sinemet and Sinemet CR (control or extended release) are combinations of levodopa with carbidopa, a dopa decarboxylase inhibitor. Carbidopa competes for the enzyme dopa decarboxylase, thus slowing the peripheral break-

BOX 23-2

Levodopa On-Off Syndrome

On-off syndrome refers to a complication following prolonged levodopa therapy (2 years or more). During therapy, the client fluctuates from being symptom free ("on") to demonstrating full-blown Parkinson's symptoms ("off"). These effects may last from minutes to hours and may be due to a decrease in the delivery of dopamine centrally, an alteration in sensitivity of the dopamine receptors, a variation in the amount and rate of drug absorption, an interference with dopamine metabolites, or a combination of effects.

Treatment may require more frequent administration of levodopa or levodopa-carbidopa and perhaps the addition of bromocriptine, a direct-acting dopamine agonist. Some clients may demonstrate an improved response to the drug therapy following a drug holiday (drug withdrawal) of several days to a week. This may be because of the reestablishment of dopamine receptor sensitivity to levodopa, which is usually only temporary. Because many individuals worsen during the drug-free period, this approach should be instituted in a hospital setting (Flaherty & Gidal, 1995).

down of levodopa. Unlike levodopa, carbidopa does not cross the blood-brain barrier, and therefore it does not interfere with the intracerebral transformation of levodopa to dopamine. Because carbidopa prevents much of the peripheral conversion of levodopa to dopamine, the incidence of systemic side effects of levodopa, such as nausea, vomiting, and cardiac dysrhythmias, is decreased. The CNS effects of levodopa are a greater risk with this combination because more levodopa is reaching the brain to be converted to dopamine.

The addition of carbidopa to levodopa reduces the required dose of levodopa to approximately 20% to 25% of the original dose. The available carbidopa-levodopa combination dosage forms include 10/100 (10 mg of carbidopa and 100 mg of levodopa), 25/100 (25 mg of carbidopa and 100 mg levodopa), and 25/250 (25 mg of carbidopa and 250 mg of levodopa). To obtain the peripheral inhibitor effect of carbidopa, a minimum of 75 mg (range: 75 to 100 mg) per day is necessary. Saturating peripheral dopa decarboxylase requires between 75 and 100 mg/day of carbidopa (Flaherty & Gidal, 1995). Nausea and vomiting are reported in clients receiving dosages of carbidopa lower than 75 mg/day. Therefore three combination dosage forms are available to permit greater flexibility in prescribing sufficient amounts of both levodopa and carbidopa for the client. The manufacturer recommends that not more than 200 mg/day of carbidopa be prescribed. As with levodopa alone, the decarboxylation to dopamine replaces the missing brain dopamine and restores a balance to dopamine/acetylcholine concentrations.

Carbidopa-levodopa is indicated for the treatment of idiopathic, postencephalitic, and symptomatic Parkinson's disease. (See the previous section for the pharmacokinetics of levodopa.) Between 40% and 70% of an oral dose of carbidopa is absorbed. Carbidopa is distributed widely to many body tissues with the exception of the CNS. The metabolism of the drug is insignificant. It is excreted by the kidneys.

The side effects/adverse reactions of carbidopa-levodopa are similar to those for levodopa. Eyelid spasms or closing may be an early sign of drug overdose. Mental or mood changes may also occur earlier and may be dose related.

Drug interactions are the same as for levodopa, with the exception of the pyridoxine interaction. The interaction between levodopa and pyridoxine does not occur in the presence of carbidopa.

For clients not previously undergoing levodopa therapy, the oral dosage is initiated at 10/100 or 25/100 three times daily. Increase the dosage as needed every 1 or 2 days until the desired response is obtained. For clients previously undergoing levodopa therapy, discontinue levodopa at least 8 hours before instituting combination therapy. If the client has been receiving less than 1.5 g levodopa daily, the dosage is initiated with 10/100 or 25/100 of carbidopa-levodopa three or four times daily; it is increased at 1- or 2-day intervals until the desired response is obtained. If the client is receiving more than 1.5 g of levodopa daily, 25/250 carbidopa-levodopa PO is administered three or four times daily, increasing if necessary at 1- or 2-day intervals until the desired response is obtained.

The conversion from levodopa to a carbidopa-levodopa combination requires only 25% of the original dosage of levodopa, with a maximum of up to 200 mg carbidopa and 2 g levodopa daily. If additional levodopa is necessary, it is given as a single agent. (For more information, see the Case Study box on p. 499.)

Older adults and postencephalitic clients may require a lower dosage because they are more sensitive to this combination. The dosage for children under 18 years of age has not been established.

For the nursing management of carbidopa-levodopa, see Nursing Management: Levodopa Therapy, p. 496.

Dopamine-Releasing Drugs

amantadine [a man′ ta deen] (Symmetrel)

Amantadine is a synthetic antiviral compound. Although the exact mechanism of its action is not completely known, it is postulated that amantadine releases dopamine and other catecholamines from neuronal storage sites. It also blocks the uptake of dopamine into presynaptic neurons, thus permitting the peripheral and central accumulation of dopamine. Amantadine may also give the client a sense of well-being and elevate his or her mood. It is less effective than levodopa but produces more rapid clinical improvement and causes fewer untoward reactions.

Amantadine is indicated for use as an antidyskinetic (treatment of Parkinson's disease) and as an antiviral (systemic agent). Amantadine is well absorbed; it is not metabolized. It has a half-life of 11 to 15 hours. Peak serum levels are reached within 2 to 4 hours, with the onset of antidyskinetic action within 48 hours. A steady state is reached within 2 to 3 days with daily drug administration; the drug serum level is 0.2 to 0.9 μg/mL. Levels above 1 μg/mL are considered toxic. Amantadine is excreted by the kidneys.

The side effects/adverse reactions of amantadine include impaired concentration, dizziness, increased irritability, anorexia, nausea, nervousness, purple-red skin spots (livedo reticularis, usually seen with chronic therapy), confusion, hallucinations, mental or mood variations, orthostatic hypotension, and difficult urination. Symptoms of overdose include severe confusion, insomnia, nightmares, and seizures.

The adult dosage for antidyskinetic action is 100 mg PO once or twice daily. The maximum dosage is 400 mg/day. Older adults are given 100 mg daily to start, titrating to two or three times daily as necessary.

■ Nursing Management

Amantadine Therapy

■ **Assessment.** Before the initiation of amantadine therapy, the client should be assessed for preexisting peripheral edema, congestive heart failure, and epilepsy because the drug may exacerbate these conditions. Because amantadine is not metabolized and is excreted by the kidneys, clients who have renal function impairment are at risk for drug toxicity and require a reduced dosage. A baseline assessment

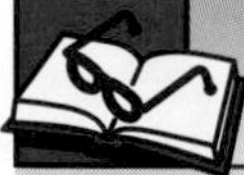

Case Study *Parkinson's Disease*

Mr. Edwards is 64 years of age and has been diagnosed with Parkinson's disease. He is to begin taking carbidopa-levodopa (Sinemet) 10/100 PO three times daily. After 3 days his dosage is increased by one tablet per day. His final dosage is now one tablet of Sinemet, 25/100 four times daily.

1. How does levodopa contribute to the improved function of the client with Parkinson's disease?
2. Explain the rationale for giving carbidopa with the levodopa.
3. What points should the nurse include in teaching Mr. Edwards about his drug therapy?

After 2 years of therapy, Mr. Edwards' symptoms have improved, with adverse reactions limited to occasional nausea, dry mouth, and anorexia. However, he experiences periodic increases in his disease symptoms even though he continues to take his medication. The prescriber has decided to add amantadine (Symmetrel) 100 mg PO daily to the drug treatment.

4. Why did Mr. Edwards experience an increase in his symptoms?
5. Amantadine is pharmacologically classified as an antiviral agent. Explain its role in the treatment of Parkinson's disease.

Six months later Mr. Edwards comes to the clinic reporting that he has started to have episodes of confusion, insomnia, nightmares, and hallucinations. He has waited several months to discuss these episodes and expresses concern that he is "losing his mind." In addition, the nurse notices that he has developed some involuntary movements of his tongue and face.

6. How should the nurse respond to Mr. Edwards' concerns?
7. What is the significance of the involuntary movements noted in the nurse's assessment of the client?

After reviewing Mr. Edwards' case, the prescriber decides to discontinue the amantadine. Within 6 weeks Mr. Edwards reports that the nightmares and insomnia have stopped. He no longer experiences the hallucinations, and the confusion is minimal. The involuntary movements have decreased significantly.

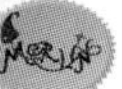

For answer guidelines, go to mosby.com/MERLIN/McKenry/.

of the client's vital signs and parkinsonian movements should be documented.

Review the client's current medication regimen for the risk of significant drug interactions, such as those that may occur with amantadine is given with the following drugs:

Drug	Possible Effect and Management
Bold/color type indicates the most serious interactions.	
alcohol	Increased CNS side effects such as confusion, light-headedness, orthostatic hypotension, and fainting spells are reported. Avoid concurrent use or a potentially serious drug interaction may occur.
anticholinergics	May enhance anticholinergic side effects, such as confusion, hallucinations, and frightening dreams. Dosage adjustments may be necessary. Also monitor for paralytic ileus.
CNS stimulants	Additive CNS stimulation is reported; side effects include increased nervousness, irritability, difficulty sleeping and, at times, seizures and cardiac dysrhythmias. Closely monitor clients who are receiving concurrent stimulant therapy.

■ **Nursing Diagnosis.** The client receiving amantadine should be assessed for the following nursing diagnoses/collaborative problems: disturbed thought processes (confusion, mental or mood variations); disturbed sleep pattern (insomnia); risk for injury related to blurred vision, dizziness, and orthostatic hypotension; imbalanced nutrition; impaired comfort related to rash, headache, xerostomia, anorexia, and nausea; impaired urinary elimination; constipation; and the potential complications of CNS toxicity (seizures, depression), congestive heart failure, corneal deposits (impaired vision), and livedo reticularis (red, blotchy spots on skin).

■ Implementation

■ ***Monitoring.*** The client's mobility status should be monitored for muscular rigidity, tremors, and the ability to accomplish activities of daily living. The side effects of nausea, dizziness, insomnia, nervousness, and impaired concentration are common with this drug. For clients receiving doses greater than 200 mg/day, there is a higher risk of CNS toxicity; these clients should be monitored carefully. Vital signs should be monitored four times daily when dosages are increased. Clients with epilepsy are at greater risk for seizures and should be monitored accordingly. In long-term therapy, monitor for congestive heart failure, which has symptoms such as increased edema of the feet and lower legs, difficulty in breathing, and rapid increase of body weight.

■ ***Intervention.*** Changing the client's medication schedule from a once-daily to a twice-daily schedule may decrease some of the unpleasant side effects such as light-headedness, insomnia, and nausea. However, be aware that increasing the number of doses of a drug increases the risk of ineffective management of the medication regimen by the client. Therapy should be discontinued gradually. Abrupt cessation of the drug may cause exacerbations of parkinsonian symptoms within 24 hours and an onset of parkinsonian crisis within 3 days.

■ ***Education.*** The client should be informed that it may require 2 weeks of amantadine therapy to reach a full effect and that a reduction in benefits occurs after 4 to 12 weeks of therapy. Increasing the dose or taking a brief holiday from the drug will restore its benefits. Compliance with a full course of therapy is necessary.

Instruct the client not to drink alcohol while taking this drug because doing so may result in dizziness, fainting, and confusion. (See also the general discussion under Nursing Management: Anticholinergic Therapy, p. 493.)

■ **Evaluation.** The expected outcome of amantadine therapy is that the client will demonstrate improved mobility with decreased muscular rigidity and tremor without experiencing adverse reactions to the drug.

Dopaminergic Agonists

bromocriptine [broe moe krip′ teen] (Parlodel)

Bromocriptine is an ergot alkaloid derivative marketed as the first agonist of dopamine receptor activity. It activates postsynaptic dopamine receptors, stimulating the production of dopamine and correcting dopamine/acetylcholine imbalances in the brain. This drug is indicated as an antidyskinetic, a growth hormone suppressant, an antihyperprolactinemic, and a prophylactic for lactation after a loss of pregnancy in the second or third trimester. Approximately 28% of a dose is absorbed, but only 6% reaches systemic circulation.

The half-life of bromocriptine is biphasic: alpha, 4 to 4½ hours; beta, 15 hours. The onset of activity from a single dose used for antiparkinsonism is 30 to 90 minutes, with a peak concentration reached in 2 hours. This drug is metabolized in the liver. Metabolites of bromocriptine are excreted primarily in bile.

The side effects/adverse reactions of bromocriptine include drowsiness, headache, nausea, hypotension and, less commonly, confusion, hallucinations, and uncontrolled movements of the body, face, tongue, arms, hands, and head.

The adult dosage for antidyskinetic effects is 1.25 to 2.5 mg PO daily, titrated as necessary. The maintenance dosage ranges from 2.5 to 40 mg daily in divided doses. The dosage for children younger than 15 years of age has not been established.

■ Nursing Management

Bromocriptine Therapy

■ **Assessment.** Bromocriptine should not be administered to mothers planning to breastfeed, because this drug inhibits lactation. In addition, bromocriptine is contraindicated for clients with a history of hypertension or pregnancy-induced hypertension because it may be aggravated. Use with caution in clients with hepatic dysfunction, because metabolism of the drug may be reduced. Clients with psychiatric disorders may experience a worsening of symptoms with the administration of bromocriptine.

Bromocriptine has an additive effect with other antiparkinson drugs. Clients with an intolerance of ergot derivatives may also be intolerant of bromocriptine. Review the client's current medication regimen for the risk of significant drug interactions, such as those that may occur when bromocriptine is given concurrently with the following drugs:

Drug	Possible Effect and Management
Bold/color type indicates the most serious interactions.	
alcohol	**Concurrent use may result in a disulfiram-like reaction (i.e., tachycardia, flushing, increased sweating, nausea, vomiting, severe headache, blurred vision, confusion, and chest pain). Avoid concurrent use or a potentially serious drug interaction may occur.**
erythromycin	A vast increase (over 200%) in the serum level of bromocriptine may occur. Monitor closely for bromocriptine toxicity. It has been proposed that this interaction may also occur with clarithromycin (Biaxin) and troleandomycin (TAO) (*United States Pharmacopeia Dispensing Information*, 1999).
risperidone (Risperdal)	May increase prolactin levels and also interfere with the effects of bromocriptine. Monitor closely because dosage adjustments may be needed.
ritonavir (Norvir)	Serum levels of bromocriptine may increase by 300% in combination with ritonavir. It is recommended that the dose of bromocriptine be decreased by 50% when this combination is used (*USP DI*, 1999).

A baseline assessment of the client's health status should include blood pressure determinations as well as a description of the client's motor status. If bromocriptine is being administered for hyperprolactinemia, a baseline serum prolactin should be obtained. To rule out a pituitary tumor as the cause of the hyperprolactinemia, a computed tomography (CT) scan or magnetic resonance imaging (MRI) of the sella turcica is recommended. Once menses resumes in clients being treated for amenorrhea, a pregnancy test is recommended whenever a period is missed.

■ **Nursing Diagnosis.** Clients receiving bromocriptine therapy have the potential for the following nursing diagnoses/collaborative problems: risk for injury related to hypotension and CNS effects (drowsiness, confusion, hallucinations); impaired comfort (nausea, dry mouth, stuffy nose, leg cramps); constipation; diarrhea; and the potential complications of dyskinesia, myocardial infarction (chest pain, shortness of breath, sweating, weakness), mental depression, seizure or stroke (headache, vision changes, sudden weakness), peptic ulcer (stomach pain, black tarry stools), Raynaud's phenomenon (tingling or pain of fingers and toes when exposed to cold), enlargement of pituitary tumor (severe nausea and vomiting, sudden headache, blurred vision), and retroperitoneal fibrosis (abdominal pain, anorexia, nausea, vomiting).

■ **Implementation**

■ ***Monitoring.*** Blood pressure should be monitored; 1% to 5% of the clients have symptomatic hypotension. Other common effects include constipation, nausea, nasal congestion, and tingling or pain in the fingers and toes when exposed to cold. These effects occur in 30% to 60% of the clients being treated with bromocriptine for Parkinson's disease. The most common side effects occur when the client first begins therapy; most of these effects are dose related and seldom occur with doses less than 20 mg daily.

If bromocriptine is administered for female infertility, periodic serum prolactin levels and ovulation evaluations are recommended. If used for the treatment of acromegaly, growth hormone serum levels aid in determining dosages.

■ ***Intervention.*** Administer bromocriptine with meals or milk to decrease the adverse reaction of nausea. Bedtime administration may minimize the effects of dizziness and nausea for the client. Give the first dose at bedtime or with the client lying down, because the hypotensive effects of the drug are more likely to occur after the initial dose. The dosage is initiated at a low level and gradually increased to the minimum effective dosage.

■ ***Education.*** Clients with infertility who are not taking bromocriptine for that indication should be cautioned to use a contraceptive measure, because this drug may result in a restoration of fertility. A mechanical barrier device, such as a diaphragm or condom, should be suggested rather than oral contraceptives, because oral estrogen contraceptives increase the risk of stimulating prolactin-secreting cells. In addition to these contraceptive measures, pregnancy tests should be performed every 4 weeks during therapy. A positive pregnancy test should be reported to the prescriber immediately.

Caution clients that bromocriptine may impair physical and mental functioning and that they should exercise caution when driving or operating machinery. The client should be instructed to limit alcohol consumption because it increases the CNS side effects. Taking this drug with alcohol may also result in a disulfiram-type reaction, tachycardia, pounding heart rate, facial flushing, sweating, nausea, vomiting, headache, blurred vision, chest pain, and lethargy.

The client should be taught to prevent or minimize constipation by increasing dietary fiber, increasing fluid intake to 3000 mL daily, performing moderate exercise daily, and establishing a regular time of day for bowel elimination. Advise the client to limit exposure to the cold or to wear protective clothing to prevent discomfort of the fingers and toes.

The client should be cautioned to get up slowly from a sitting or supine position because of the hypotensive effects of bromocriptine. Regular dental examinations are advised because bromocriptine inhibits salivation and thereby increases the client's risk of discomfort, caries, and periodontal disorders. See also the general discussion under Nursing Management: Anticholinergic Therapy, p. 493.

■ **Evaluation.** The expected outcome of bromocriptine therapy is that the client will demonstrate an increase in physical mobility and a decrease in muscular rigidity and tremor without experiencing any adverse reactions to the drug. If bromocriptine is administered for infertility, conception will occur.

pergolide [per′ go lide] (Permax)

Pergolide is a dopamine agonist, usually used in conjunction with levodopa or carbidopa-levodopa to treat the signs and symptoms of Parkinson's disease. It is more potent and longer acting than bromocriptine and directly stimulates both D_1 and D_2 receptors (Flaherty & Gidal, 1995). In combination therapy, the dose of levodopa or carbidopa-levodopa is often reduced. According to Flaherty and Gidal, up to 75% of clients who did not respond to levodopa did improve with the addition of pergolide. In addition, clinical fluctuations reported in clients receiving carbidopa-levodopa may be reduced; that is, the "on" period was prolonged, whereas the "off" period was decreased in most of the clients studied.

Pergolide stimulates dopamine receptors in the nigrostriatal area. However, unlike bromocriptine, its action is independent of dopamine synthesis or dopamine storage sites. It also inhibits prolactin secretion. Pergolide is indicated as an adjunct treatment for Parkinson's disease. It is well absorbed, and serum protein binding is high (approximately 90%). This drug is excreted by the kidneys.

The side effects/adverse reactions of pergolide include stomach distress/pain, constipation, light-headedness, sedation, hypotension, cold-type symptoms, nausea, lower back pain, confusion, dyskinesia (e.g., uncontrollable body movements), and hallucinations.

The recommended dosage of pergolide for adults and older adults is 0.05 mg PO daily for 2 days, increased by 0.1 to 0.15 mg every 3 days over the next 12 days. The dosage may then be increased by 0.25 mg every 3 days until the maximum therapeutic effect is reached. Doses should be divided and given three times daily. The maximum dosage is 5 mg/day. The dosage for children has not been established.

■ Nursing Management

Pergolide Therapy

■ **Assessment.** Pergolide should not be administered to clients who had a previous allergic experience with ergot alkaloids. Clients with altered thought processes such as confusion or hallucinations may experience a worsening of these symptoms. The increased risk of atrial premature contractions and sinus tachycardia should be considered before administering pergolide to clients with cardiac dysrhythmias. This drug inhibits lactation and therefore is contraindicated in mothers who anticipate breastfeeding.

No significant drug interactions are reported to date, but be aware that dopamine antagonists (e.g., the phenothiazines and haloperidol [Haldol]), may decrease the effects of pergolide. Medications that produce hypotension may have an additive hypotensive effect.

A baseline assessment of the client's mobility status, including previous "on-off" fluctuations and blood pressure determinations, is essential to monitoring the effectiveness of pergolide therapy.

■ **Nursing Diagnosis.** The client receiving pergolide therapy should be assessed for the following nursing diagnoses/collaborative problems: disturbed thought processes (confusion, hallucinations); risk for injury related to CNS toxicity (dyskinesia), urinary tract infection (burning on urination), and hypotension (dizziness); impaired comfort (dry mouth, rhinitis, nausea); disturbed sleep pattern (drowsiness); constipation; and the potential complications of myocardial infarction (chest pain, shortness of breath, tachycardia, weakness) and cerebrovascular hemorrhage (severe headache, vision changes, seizures, sudden weakness).

■ **Implementation**

■ ***Monitoring.*** The client's blood pressure should be monitored on a regular basis because changes in blood pressure occur. Hypotension is more common than hypertension. Fluctuations in blood pressure are more apt to occur during periods of dosage adjustment. Monitor the client's comfort level, mental status, mobility status, and bowel elimination pattern.

■ ***Intervention.*** The dosage of pergolide should be titrated so the client obtains the maximum therapeutic benefits and minimal side effects. Administer pergolide with meals to minimize nausea and vomiting; these effects usually subside with continued therapy. Nausea and dizziness are not uncommon with the first dose. These effects can be mitigated by administering the first dose at bedtime or while the client is lying down. Careful oral hygiene is required because of the reduced salivary flow.

■ ***Education.*** Encourage the client undergoing pergolide therapy to seek regular appointments with the prescriber so that the client's progress may be monitored. Alert the client that possible sleepiness or dizziness may make it unsafe to drive or perform other tasks that require alertness. The client should be taught to come to an upright position slowly from a sitting or prone position because of the hypotensive effects of the drug. Advise the client that sugarless candies or gum, ice chips, and saliva substitutes may be used to minimize the possible dryness of the mouth.

■ **Evaluation.** The expected outcome for pergolide therapy is that the client will demonstrate increased mobility with decreased muscular rigidity and tremor, as well as longer "on" periods and shorter "off" periods, without experiencing any adverse reactions to the drug.

Non-Ergot Dopamine Agonists

pramipexole [pra mi pex′ ol] (Mirapex)
ropinirole [roh pin′ a rohl] (Requip)

Pramipexole and ropinirole are non-ergot dopamine receptor agonists used in the treatment of Parkinson's disease. Although their exact mechanism of action is unknown, they are postulated to stimulate dopamine receptors in the striatum (Hobson, Pourcher, & Martin, 1999).

These agents are rapidly absorbed orally, reaching peak serum levels in 1 to 2 hours. The half-life of pramipexole is 8 hours (12 hours in older adults); the half-life of ropinirole is 6 hours. Ropinirole is extensively metabolized, with only 1% to 2% excreted unchanged by the kidneys. Pramipexole is not metabolized and is primarily excreted unchanged in the urine.

The side effects/adverse reactions of pramipexole and ropinirole include nausea, constipation, dizziness, sedation, dyskinesia, hallucinations, confusion, and dystonia. Ropinirole has a higher reported incidence of dizziness, sedation, nausea, vomiting, stomach pain, and dyspepsia (Korczyn et al., 1999).

The adult dosage of pramipexole ranges from 0.375 to 4.5 mg/day in divided doses. The adult dosage of ropinirole is 0.25 to 1 mg three times daily, with dosages adjusted weekly as necessary.

■ **Nursing Management**

Pramipexole and Ropinirole Therapy

Nursing management of the therapy for the non-ergot dopamine agonists is essentially the same as for the ergot dopamine agonists, with the exception of the drug interactions. Review the client's current medication regimen for the risk of significant drug interactions, such as those that may occur when pramipexole and ropinirole are given concurrently with the following drugs:

Drug	Possible Effect and Management
carbidopa-levodopa combination, levodopa	Both ropinirole and pramipexole increase serum levels of levodopa. This activity may potentiate the dopaminergic side effects of levodopa and require a dosage reduction of levodopa.
cimetidine (Tagamet)	Increases the serum level of pramipexole by up to 50% and also extends its half-life. Monitor closely because dosage adjustments may be necessary or, preferably, consider switching to a different histamine antagonist.
other renally excreted drugs, such as quinidine, ranitidine (Zantac), diltiazem (Cardizem), triamterene (Dyrenium), and verapamil (Calan)	Concurrent administration of drugs eliminated by the same system may result in a decrease in pramipexole elimination (by approximately 20%). Monitor closely (*USP DI*, 1999).

Monoamine Oxidase Inhibitors

✓ **selegiline** [se le′ jell een] or deprenyl (Eldepryl, SD-Deprenyl ♣)

Selegiline is used in combination with levodopa or carbidopa-levodopa to treat Parkinson's disease. There are two types of MAO in the body: MAO A is necessary to metabolize norepinephrine and serotonin, and MAO B metabolizes dopamine. Selegiline irreversibly inhibits MAO B, thus preventing the breakdown of dopamine. As a result, it enhances or prolongs the antiparkinson effect of levodopa, which may result in a lowering of the daily dose of levodopa.

Selegiline is well absorbed orally, reaches peak serum levels in ½ to 2 hours, and has three active metabolites (with half-lives of 2 to 20 hours). It readily crosses the blood-brain barrier and is excreted slowly via the kidneys.

The side effects/adverse reactions of selegiline include dry mouth, nausea, vomiting, insomnia, dizziness, stomach distress or pain, dyskinesia, and mood alterations.

The usual adult dosage of selegiline is 5 mg at breakfast and lunch.

▪ Nursing Management

Selegiline Therapy

The nursing management of the client undergoing selegiline therapy is essentially the same as for pergolide, except for its significant drug interactions.

Review the client's current medication regimen for the risk of significant drug interactions, such as those that may occur when selegiline is given concurrently with the following drugs:

Drug	Possible Effect and Management
Bold/color type indicates the most serious interactions.	
antidepressants (tricyclic)	Hypertension, syncope, asystole, changes in behavior and mental status, impaired consciousness, fever, seizures, and tremors have occurred with concurrent use. Such use is not recommended; 14 days should elapse between the discontinuance of one of these drugs and the initiation of the other.
fluoxetine (Prozac), fluvoxamine (Luvox), nefazodone (Serzone), paroxetine (Paxil), sertraline (Zoloft), venlafaxine (Effexor)	**Concurrent use may result in mania and a reaction similar to the serotonin syndrome (confusion, restlessness, hyperreflexia, sweating, shivering, tremors, diarrhea, ataxia, and fever). Avoid concurrent use or a potentially serious drug interaction may occur. These drugs should not be initiated until at least 2 weeks after selegiline is discontinued. Selegiline should not be initiated in persons taking fluoxetine until at least 5 weeks after fluoxetine has been discontinued or 7 days after venlafaxine has been discontinued.** (*USP DI*, 1999).
levodopa (Larodopa)	Although selegiline is indicated to be given concurrently with levodopa, be aware that this combination may increase levodopa-induced side effects, such as dyskinesias, nausea, hypotension, confusion, and hallucinations. To reduce this potential, the dosage for levodopa should be lowered within 2 to 3 days after initiating selegiline therapy.
meperidine (Demerol)	**Concurrent drug administration may result in severe adverse reactions, such as severe hypertension, respiratory depression, sweating, excitation, rigidity, seizures, hyperpyrexia, vascular collapse, coma, and death. Avoid concurrent use or a potentially serious drug interaction may occur. Avoid administration of meperidine for at least 2 to 3 weeks after the use of an MAO inhibitor. Although the use of other opioids, such as morphine, is not as likely to result in such a severe reaction, they should also be used very cautiously in lowered dosages in any person receiving an MAO inhibitor.**
tyramine	**The use of tyramine or foods and beverages that contain tyramine or high-pressor amines should be avoided or, if consumed in very small quantities, should be very carefully monitored. This combination may result in an immediate, severe hypertensive episode that requires medical attention. Avoid concurrent use or a potentially serious drug interaction may occur. It is recommended that dietary restrictions continue for at least 2 to 3 weeks after the discontinuing an MAO inhibitor.**

Antiparkinson Adjunct Medication

tolcapone [tol′ ca pone] (Tasmar)

Tolcapone is an adjunct treatment drug used in combination with levodopa and carbidopa for the symptoms of Parkinson's disease. Although its exact mechanism of action is unknown, tolcapone inhibits catechol-O-methyltransferase (COMT), which results in a more sustained serum level of levodopa. COMT is responsible for metabolizing catecholamines such as dopamine, norepinephrine, and epinephrine; its inhibition therefore causes levels of levodopa that may result in a more constant dopaminergic effect in the brain and may lead to an improvement in the symptoms of Parkinson's disease (Rivest, Barclay, & Suchowersky, 1999). The effects of tolcapone are selective and reversible.

Tolcapone is rapidly absorbed orally (administer on an empty stomach for best results) and is very highly protein bound (>99%). It reaches peak serum levels in approximately 2 hours, has a half-life of 2 to 3 hours, is metabolized in the liver, and is excreted by the kidneys (60%) and feces (40%).

The side effects of tolcapone include constipation, gastric distress, increase in dream time, sweating, and dry mouth. Adverse reactions that require medical attention may include orthostatic hypotension, diarrhea, dizziness, anorexia, dyskinesia, hallucinations, headache, insomnia, syncope, chest pain, confusion, dyspnea, hematuria, and upper respiratory infection.

The usual adult dosage for antiparkinson effects is 100 to 200 mg three times daily in conjunction with carbidopa-levodopa therapy. The maximum daily dose is 600 mg.

■ Nursing Management

Tolcapone Therapy

■ Assessment. The client's health status should be assessed for any preexisting conditions in which the administration of tolcapone would place the client at a higher risk of injury or would require a degree of caution, such as severe renal damage, moderate cirrhotic liver disease, or severe liver impairment of any etiology. The use of tolcapone is contraindicated if the client is hypersensitive to the drug or any of its ingredients.

The client's current drug regimen should be reviewed for significant drug interactions. Because MAO and COMT are the two major enzyme systems involved in the metabolism of catecholamines, the concurrent administration of tolcapone and a nonselective MAO inhibitor (e.g., phenelzine [Nardil] or tranylcypromine [Parnate]) may result in inhibition of the majority of the pathways responsible for normal catecholamine metabolism. This combination is contraindicated. However, tolcapone may be administered with a selective MAO-B inhibitor such as selegiline (Eldepryl). Because of the additive effects of tolcapone, monitor the client closely if any drug is administered in which orthostatic hypotension may be an issue. Monitor prothrombin times carefully when warfarin and tolcapone are administered concurrently.

Obtain a baseline assessment of the client's vital signs and parkinsonian symptoms.

■ Nursing Diagnosis. After beginning tolcapone therapy, the client should be assessed for the following nursing diagnoses/collaborative problems: constipation; diarrhea; impaired comfort (headache, dry mouth, anorexia, gastrointestinal disturbance); risk for injury related to orthostatic hypotension, dizziness, or syncope; disturbed sleep pattern (insomnia, increased dream time); disturbed thought processes (confusion, hallucinations); and the potential complications of dyskinesia, chest pain, hematuria, dyspnea, and upper respiratory infection.

■ Implementation

■ *Monitoring.* The client's vital signs need to be monitored during periods of dosage adjustment. Evaluate the client's progress by observing body movements for signs of improvement. It is recommended that hepatic transaminases be monitored monthly for the first 3 months and then every 6 weeks for the next 3 months. Treatment may be discontinued with increases of alanine aminotransferase (ALT).

■ *Intervention.* Tolcapone may be administered without regard to food, but the first dose of the day is usually administered with the first dose of the day of carbidopa-levodopa.

■ *Education.* To prevent orthostatic hypotension, the client undergoing tolcapone therapy should be instructed to sit or stand slowly and gradually. Advise the client not to drive or undertake other hazardous tasks that require alertness until he or she has sufficient experience with tolcapone to determine whether or not it affects mental or motor performance. Alert the client that nausea may occur when treatment is initiated but will abate in time. Encourage the client to report symptoms of chest pain, shortness of breath, and changes in motor function to the prescriber.

■ Evaluation. The expected outcome of tolcapone therapy is that the client will demonstrate an improvement in mobility with a decrease in rigidity and tremors and will not experience adverse reactions to the drug.

entacapone [en′ ta ca pone] (Comtan)

Entacapone is used as an adjunct drug to the levodopa-carbidopa (Sinemet) combination for the treatment of Parkinson's disease in individuals who have signs and symptoms of end-of-dosage or drug-wearing-off effects. It is a selective, reversible inhibitor of COMT and therefore alters the pharmacokinetics to increase levodopa serum levels.

Entacapone is rapidly absorbed and highly protein bound. With this drug, the elimination half-life of levodopa is extended from 1.3 hours to 2.4 hours. It is metabolized in the liver and excreted by the kidneys (10%) and in the feces (90%).

Significant side effects/adverse reactions of entacapone include nausea, diarrhea or, to a lesser degree, constipation, stomach pain, dyskinesia, hyperkinesia or hypokinesia, and dizziness.

The usual adult dosage is a 200-mg entacapone tablet administered with each levodopa-carbidopa dose, to a maximum of 8 doses daily (*Drug Facts and Comparisons*, 2000).

■ Nursing Management

Entacapone Therapy

In addition to the following discussion, see Nursing Management: Tolcapone Therapy, at left. Assess the client's current drug regimen, because there is a risk for dysrhythmias with concurrent administration of isoproterenol and epinephrine.

MYASTHENIA GRAVIS

Myasthenia gravis is a progressive, incurable disease characterized by the loss of or a decrease in acetylcholine receptors; it is caused by an autoimmune process and results in skeletal muscle weakness and fatigue. Because of its involvement with the production of antibodies, the thymus gland is believed to play a role in the development of myasthenia gravis. Nearly 15% of all clients with myasthenia gravis have a thymoma, or a tumor of the thymus gland.

Symptoms of myasthenia gravis usually become worse with exertion and are less noticeable with rest. Stress, infection, menses, surgery, and other factors may also increase the symptoms. The most common early reported symptoms are ptosis and diplopia. Dysarthria, dysphagia, and limb weakness, especially of the upper extremities, also occur in the advanced stages. The client may complain of hand weakness or of shoulder fatigue after shaving or combing the hair; the client may find it difficult to open doors or kitchen jars or to perform repetitive tasks, such as lawn work or playing the piano (Figure 23-2).

The most serious effects of myasthenia gravis are dysphagia and respiratory muscle weakness; these effects may result in aspiration pneumonia or respiratory failure. Treatment of this disease may include thymectomy, cholinesterase inhibitors, plasmapheresis and, at times, corticosteroids. The mainstay of therapy is cholinesterase-inhibitor drugs, such as anticholinesterase drugs.

Anticholinesterase Agents

The **anticholinesterase agents,** or antimyasthenics, are drugs that enhance cholinergic action by blocking the effect of cholinesterase. These drugs act by inactivating or inhibiting cholinesterase at the sites of acetylcholine transmission, thus permitting the accumulation of acetylcholine. Because of their ability to increase the amount of acetylcholine at the myoneural junction, the cholinesterase inhibitors are primarily used for the diagnosis and treatment of myasthenia gravis and for their local effects in the eye (see Chapter 43). These drugs are also used for urinary retention and paralytic ileus and as an antidote for the curariform effects of the nondepolarizing skeletal muscle relaxants, such as tubocurarine (Tubarine) and pancuronium (Pavulon).

In the oral form, all anticholinesterase agents are poorly absorbed from the gastrointestinal tract. The onset of action of these drugs is as follows: ambenonium (Mytelase), orally within 30 minutes; edrophonium (Tensilon), IM within 2 to 10 minutes and IV within 30 to 60 seconds; neostigmine (Prostigmin), orally within 45 to 75 minutes, IM within 30 minutes, and IV within 4 to 8 minutes; and pyridostigmine (Mestinon), oral tablet or syrup within 30 to 45 minutes, extended-release tablet within 30 to 60 minutes, IM within 15 minutes, and IV within 2 to 5 minutes.

The duration of effect of each is as follows: ambenonium, 3 to 8 hours; edrophonium, IM within 5 to 30 minutes and IV within approximately 10 minutes; neostigmine oral and IM, within 2 to 6 hours; and pyridostigmine, oral syrup or tablet within 3 to 6 hours, extended-release tablet within 6 to 12 hours, and parenteral within 2 to 4 hours. Neostigmine and pyridostigmine are metabolized mainly in the liver and are excreted in the kidneys; edrophonium is excreted primarily unchanged by the kidneys.

The side effects/adverse reactions of the anticholinesterase agents include nausea, vomiting, diarrhea, abdominal cramps, increased sweating, drooling, increased urge to urinate, pinpoint pupils, eye watering, and increased bronchial secretions. Overdose effects include blurred vision, severe diarrhea, increased salivation, increase in bronchial secre-

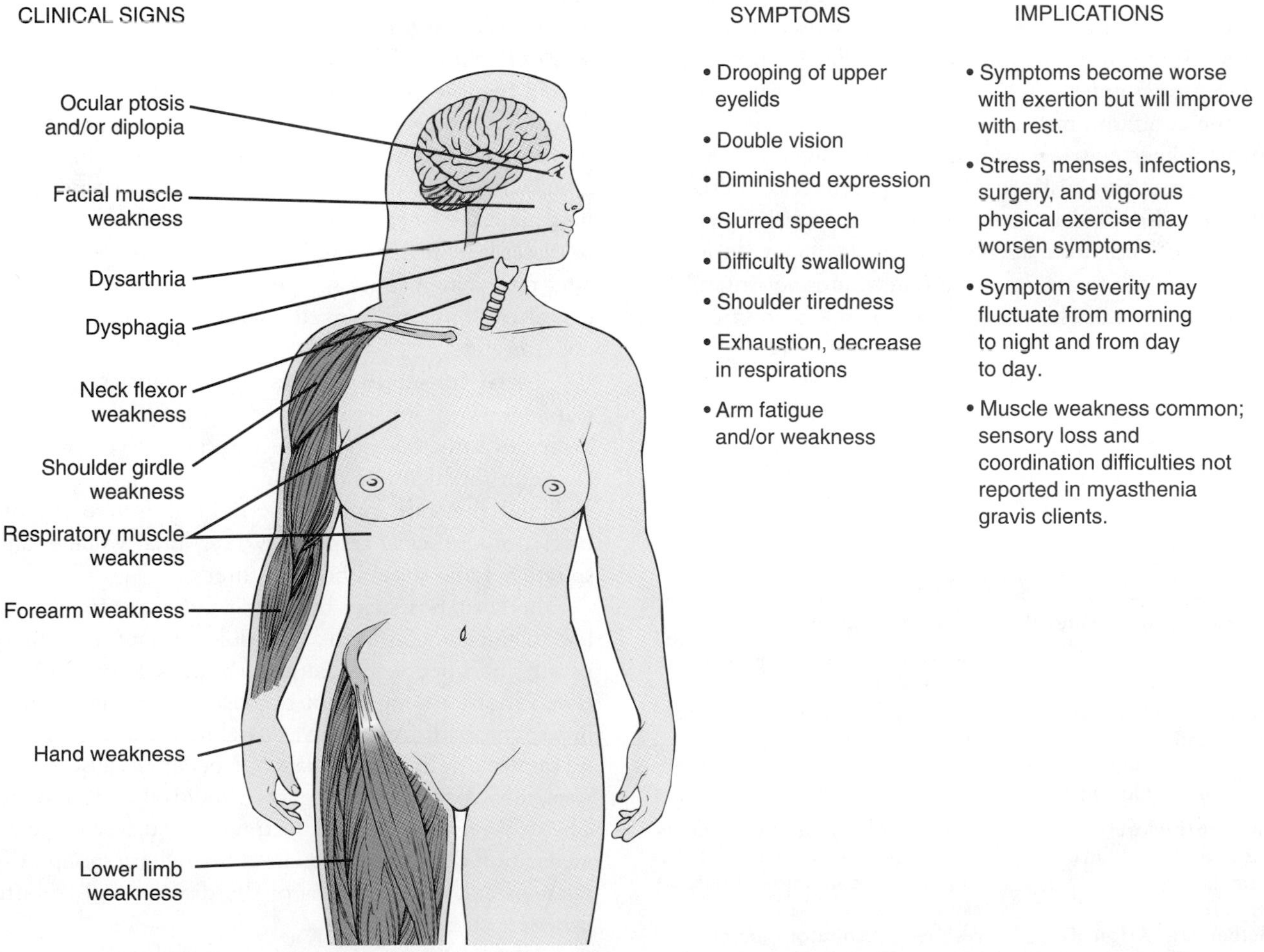

Figure 23-2 Signs, symptoms, and implications of myasthenia gravis.

tions, severe nausea or vomiting, respiratory difficulties, severe abdominal pain, bradycardia, increased weakness, ataxia, confusion, slurred speech, and muscle weakness.

Ambenonium (Mytelase) is a slowly reversible cholinesterase inhibitor; therefore it may accumulate at cholinergic synapses and produce increased, prolonged effects. Because of the narrow margin between the first appearance of side effects and serious toxicity, ambenonium is usually reserved for clients who have not responded adequately to neostigmine or pyridostigmine or for clients who are hypersensitive to the bromide component in both drugs. The usual adult dosage is 5 mg PO three to five times daily, as necessary. The dosage for children is 0.3 mg/kg in divided doses.

Edrophonium chloride injection (Tensilon) is used to diagnose myasthenia gravis. Because of its short duration of action, it is not indicated for the treatment of myasthenia gravis.

■ Nursing Management

Anticholinesterase Therapy

■ **Assessment.** Caution should be used in clients with asthma, pneumonia, or atelectasis. An increase in bronchial secretions may aggravate these conditions. Antimyasthenics may cause an increase in cardiac dysrhythmias. Clients who have a hypersensitivity to bromides, usually demonstrated by a rash, may also be sensitive to the bromide ion of neostigmine or pyridostigmine. Note that these drugs are contraindicated in clients with urinary tract infection or obstruction, because an increase in bladder muscle tone may aggravate symptoms. They should be avoided in clients with decreased gastrointestinal motility or bowel obstruction because the condition may be worsened.

Anticholinesterase agents need to be considered carefully before being administered during pregnancy. Muscular weakness has been demonstrated in some newborns whose mothers received these agents during pregnancy. In addition, anticholinesterase agents promote uterine irritability and may induce early labor in pregnant women who are near term.

Review the client's current medication regimen for the risk of significant drug interactions, such as those that may occur when cholinesterase inhibitors are given concurrently with the following drugs:

Drug	Possible Effect and Management
Bold/color type indicates the most serious interactions.	
other cholinesterase inhibitors, such as demecarium (Humorsol), ecothiophate (Phospholine), and isoflurophate (Floropryl)	**This combination of drugs is not recommended. Avoid concurrent use or a potentially serious drug interaction may occur.**
guanadrel (Hylorel), guanethidine (Ismelin), mecamylamine (Inversine), or trimethaphan (Arfonad)	**These ganglionic blocking agents may antagonize the action of the cholinesterase-inhibitor drugs, resulting in increased muscle weakness, respiratory muscle weakness, and difficulty in swallowing. Avoid concurrent use or a potentially serious drug interaction may occur.**
procainamide (Pronestyl) or quinidine	The neuromuscular blocking action and possibly antimuscarinic effect of procainamide may antagonize the action of the cholinesterase inhibitor drugs. Monitor client closely if these drugs are used concurrently.

Assess neuromuscular status (ptosis, diplopia, speed of movement, ability to swallow, respiratory function, extremity strength) before administering the drug. A baseline assessment should include the client's neuromuscular and respiratory status.

■ **Nursing Diagnosis.** Once the client begins antimyasthenic therapy, the nurse's assessment should focus on the potential development of nursing diagnoses/collaborative problems related to the effects of these drugs. There may be diarrhea related to the muscarinic effects; risk for injury related to the visual and CNS effects, especially in older adults; impaired comfort (increased watering of the mouth and eyes); and impaired urinary elimination, such as urinary frequency, urgency, and incontinence. The increase in bronchial secretions may result in ineffective airway clearance. The client's comfort may also be impaired because of rash, gastrointestinal effects, and muscle weakness.

■ **Implementation**

■ ***Monitoring.*** When treatment is initiated, the client should be observed closely for signs of toxic effects. Atropine sulfate and equipment for respiratory support should be on hand. Observation for cholinergic effects should be ongoing when these drugs are used. The time of onset of weakness indicates whether the weakness is caused by overdose or underdose. If the weakness begins approximately 1 hour after drug administration, overdose is a possibility. If it occurs after 3 or more hours, the weakness is usually caused by underdose.

Observe for subtle changes in the client's speech and facial expression. Ptosis increases and the ability to swallow decreases early, because more weakness occurs with an increase in the nicotinic effects.

Blood pressure, pulse, respirations, movement of the respiratory muscles, respiratory rate, tidal volume, and inspiratory force should be monitored.

Check vital capacity by asking the client to take a deep breath and count as high as possible without taking another breath; most people can count as high as 40 or 50. All these observations are important because symptoms usually seen in respiratory distress, such as nasal flaring and intercostal or suprasternal retractions, may not occur because of muscle weakness. Arterial blood gases should also be monitored. The dosage, route of administration, and frequency of the medication depend on the client's clinical response, the remissions and exacerbations of the disease, and the stresses experienced by the client.

CNS effects are evidenced by altered thought processes (confusion, irritability), increasing unsteadiness, slurred speech, dyspnea, and seizures. Blurred vision, bradycardia, increasing bronchial secretions and salivation, severe vomiting, and diarrhea result from the muscarinic effects.

■ ***Intervention.*** Anticholinesterase agents are initiated at a dosage less than that required to produce the client's maximum strength; the dosage is gradually increased at intervals of 48 hours or more according to the severity of the disease and the response of the client. Oral dosage forms may take several days to produce any change. If the last dosage increment does not produce a corresponding increase in the client's muscle strength, the dosage needs to be reduced to its previous level. Because it is essential that the smallest dosage for maximum result be used, it is crucial that the nurse assess and document the client's health status.

The drugs administered for myasthenia gravis are best given with food or milk to decrease adverse muscarinic effects, such as abdominal cramping, nausea, and vomiting. However, if dysphagia is a problem, the medication should be administered 30 to 45 minutes before meals, and a rest period from the time of medication until mealtime should be provided to allow for peak muscle strength for eating. Serving frequent, regular, soft foods and encouraging the client to take small bites of food with frequent rest intervals may enhance the client's ability to eat. The main meal should be served at the time of day when the client has the most strength.

Be prepared for crisis intervention with medications—edrophonium and neostigmine for a myasthenic crisis, and atropine for a cholinergic crisis. Basic resuscitative equipment should be available: suction catheters, Ambu bag, oxygen, and intubation tray.

The drugs should be administered on time because they are rapidly metabolized. A delay of 15 to 20 minutes in administration may begin to impair the muscles involved in swallowing and respiration. Around-the-clock therapy is often necessary.

Be especially alert to the route of administration because the oral dosage is 30 times greater than parenteral dosages.

It should be noted that atropine sulfate, 0.06 to 1.2 mg, may be administered before or concurrently with anticholinesterase agents to prevent adverse reactions such as excessive secretions or bradycardia.

When using these agents to counteract the neuromuscular blocking agents (e.g., tubocurarine), administer them along with artificial ventilation and oxygen therapy. They should be used only when some definite sign of voluntary respiration can be observed.

Administer IV pyridostigmine bromide (Mestinon) very slowly to prevent thrombophlebitis. The syrup dosage form of pyridostigmine may be more easily tolerated by clients with impaired swallowing or when the client's condition warrants frequent fractional doses (less than 60 mg). Although there is an extended-release form of pyridostigmine, it is usually not recommended because it increases the risk of cholinergic crisis, may need to be supplemented temporarily with other oral dosage forms to control symptoms, or may pass intact through the gastrointestinal tract if the client has increased intestinal activity or diarrhea.

A client who has had prolonged pyridostigmine therapy may become refractory to the drug. Responsiveness may be restored by decreasing the dosage or withdrawing the drug for a few days under medical supervision.

■ ***Education.*** The client with myasthenia gravis should be instructed to take the medication as ordered, using an alarm clock for precise timing of doses if necessary. An adequate supply of medications should be kept on hand. The family should also be instructed about the timing of doses.

The client and family should maintain a log of symptoms. This will help them to be aware of what events, such as emotional stress, menstruation, or infection, worsen the symptoms and how the client responds to medication. The client should be taught to observe for the therapeutic effects of the drug: a decrease or absence of ptosis; improved chewing, swallowing, and speech; increased skeletal muscle strength; and less fatigue. Activities should be planned to take advantage of the peak effectiveness of the drug.

When stabilized, the client can be taught to recognize the muscarinic effects (diaphoresis, salivation, slowed heart rate, and decreased blood pressure) and modify the medication dosage or take atropine if needed. The greater control the client has over the therapeutic regimen, the less the client's feeling of powerlessness in the face of a devastating and debilitating disease.

The client should be cautioned to avoid alcoholic beverages for 1 hour after medications because they hasten drug absorption. Tonic water should be avoided because it may contain quinine, which increases weakness.

■ **Evaluation.** The expected outcome of anticholinesterase therapy is that the client will demonstrate greater muscle strength and an increased ability to swallow, chew, and speak without experiencing adverse reactions to the drug.

DEMENTIA

Dementia, a progressive mental disorder characterized by chronic personality disintegration, confusion, and deterioration of intellectual capacity and impulse control, affects 3% to 16% of Americans over the age of 65. Alzheimer's disease accounts for approximately 50% to 60% of dementia cases; vascular dementia (including multiinfarct dementia, formerly known as cerebrovascular arteriosclerosis), Pick's disease, Parkinson's disease dementia, and other forms account for the balance (Williams, 1995). It has been estimated that irreversible dementias occur in approximately 90% of persons with dementia (Bravyak & Schechter, 1992).

Drugs, emotion, metabolic or endocrine alterations, nutrition, trauma, infection, alcoholism, and systemic illness may cause reversible dementias. The medications most associated with this type of dementia include anticholinergic agents, cardiac drugs, selected antihypertensives, and psychotropics. Box 23-3 lists selected, potentially reversible causes of dementia.

The syndrome of dementia usually develops slowly. Early signs include depression, loss of ability to concentrate, and increased anxiety, irritability, and agitation. Intellectual ability is usually the first to decline, then recent memory (e.g.,

BOX 23-3

Potentially Reversible Causes of Dementia

Drugs, Chemicals, or Toxins

Bromides
Mercury
Drugs such as butyrophenones, phenothiazines, diuretics, sedatives, alcohol

Emotional Problems

Depression
Chronic alcoholism

Metabolic Disorders

Hyperglycemia
Hypopituitarism
Hyperparathyroidism
Hypoparathyroidism
Hypothyroidism

Eye/Ear Deprivation

Blindness
Deafness

Nutritional Deficits

Vitamin B_{12} deficiency
Folic acid deficiency
Niacin deficiency

Acute Tumors/Trauma

Subdural hematoma
Brain metastasis
Brain tumors

Infections and/or Fever

Viral infections
Bacterial (tuberculosis)
Bacterial (endocarditis)
Syphilis

Arteriosclerotic Events

Vascular occlusion
Stroke

Information from Isselbacher, K.J., Braunwald, E., Wilson, J.D., Martin, J.B., Fauci, A.S., & Kasper, D.L. (Eds.). (1994). *Harrison's principles of internal medicine.* New York: McGraw-Hill.

names of acquaintances or recent events); this is followed by the loss of orientation to time, place, and person. Personal habits will change. The person may become loud or obscene, or some personality characteristics that were present might become magnified.

Helplessness, total dependency, and a loss of manual skills may occur next. In the final stages, the person may be bedridden and experience a loss of sphincter control. Eventually the person will die, usually as a result of bronchopneumonia.

The prescriber should first rule out all possible reversible causes of dementia. Treatment should be instituted to try to prevent or reduce the ongoing damage and to support the client and family in managing this disease process. Drug treatment is indicated only for symptom control, that is, the use of low-dose antipsychotic agents for treating severe agitation, delusions, and hallucinations, or the use of antidepressants for severe depression. Supportive care should include proper nutrition, moderate exercise if permitted, vitamins if indicated, and the use of environmental aids in a consistent fashion, such as night lights and daily calendar reminders. (See the Complementary and Alternative Therapies box on p. 509.)

ALZHEIMER'S DISEASE

Alzheimer's disease is a presenile dementia characterized by confusion, memory failure, disorientation, restlessness, speech disturbances, and hallucinosis; tragically, this condition is incurable. It affects approximately 4 million Americans, and approximately 250,000 new cases are diagnosed each year (Lamy, 1992). Alzheimer's disease has been estimated to be the major underlying reason for more than 50% of all nursing home admissions (Miller, 1995). It has been estimated that approximately 3% of Americans over the age of 65 have Alzheimer's disease; this rate increases with age to 19% in persons between 75 and 84 years of age and to 47% in persons 85 years of age and older (Miller, 1995).

Clinically, a progressive decline in intellectual functions is noted, such as memory loss, a loss of logical thinking or judgment, time and space disorientation, and an increased tendency to wander as a result of progressive disorientation. Profound memory loss, personality changes, hyperactivity, hostility, and paranoia may occur as the disease progresses. This middle phase in Alzheimer's disease is also characterized by the presence of aphasia (loss of speech or ability to express oneself), apraxia (loss of complex or intentional movements), and anomia (loss of ability to remember the names of persons and objects). In the terminal phase, nearly all higher mental functioning is lost, and the client needs assistance with activities of daily living; as a result, the client requires continuous nursing care.

In this final period clients may be unable to speak intelligibly, walk, sit up in bed, eat or groom themselves, smile, or recognize simple objects or familiar persons. Table 23-1 summarizes the stages of cognitive decline.

In the terminal or last phase of Alzheimer's disease, the client wants to touch or examine all objects with the mouth (hyperorality), exhibits a decrease or loss in emotions, may be bulimic, and may also have a compulsion to touch everything in sight. Insomnia, nighttime wandering, and restlessness have also been reported. The progressive deterioration of brain cells may lead to increased dependency for all needs, decreased mobility to the point of being bedridden and, eventually, death.

Researchers are still searching for the cause of Alzheimer's disease, and many theories have been proposed. The

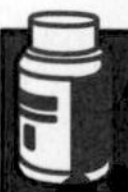

Complementary and Alternative Therapies
Ginkgo

The ginkgo tree is the world's oldest surviving tree species; fossils more than 200 million years old have been found. Various forms of the leaves and seeds of this tree have been used by humans for at least 5000 years. Recently, an extract of ginkgo leaves known as EGb 761 has shown promise for diminishing the symptoms of cerebrovascular insufficiency, such as memory loss, dizziness, difficulty concentrating, and mood disturbances. The results of one large study (Lebars et al., 1997) indicated positive findings for the use of EGb 761 for the treatment of dementia. Study subjects with mild to moderate dementia secondary to Alzheimer's disease or multiinfarct dementia experienced improved cognition and social functioning with the use of ginkgo.

Ginkgo extract affects cognitive impairment in two ways. It stimulates populations of functional nerve cells, and it protects nerve cells from pathologic influences. Ginkgo leaf extract increases cerebral blood flow and may improve cerebral metabolism and protect neural tissue from oxidative injury.

Standardized ginkgo extract taken orally is considered safe when used appropriately (except for people with sensitivity to ginkgo biloba). Side effects may be mild gastrointestinal complaints, headache, dizziness, palpitations, and allergic skin reactions. Large amounts of ginkgo may cause restlessness, nausea, vomiting, diarrhea, and weakness. Because there is insufficient information about the use of ginkgo extract in pregnancy and lactation, such use should be avoided. Bleeding is also cited as a side effect of ginkgo. Ginkgo can increase a client's risk of bleeding with the concurrent use of anticoagulant and antiplatelet drugs. It may also increase blood pressure when used concurrently with thiazide diuretics, and it may theoretically enhance the effects of MAO inhibitors and prevent cyclosporine-induced nephrotoxicity. Ginkgo extract may be used to reverse sexual dysfunction resulting from fluoxetine or sertraline therapy.

The typical oral dosage of ginkgo is 120 to 240 mg daily divided into 2 to 3 doses for dementia syndromes. Therapy should continue for a minimum of 8 weeks and should be reviewed for efficacy at the end of 3 months. Ginkgo leaf extract is used orally in a dosage of 120 to 160 mg daily divided into 2 or 3 doses for the treatment of peripheral vascular disease and vertigo or tinnitus. (See Chapter 12 for additional information.)

Information from Cirigliano, M.D. (1999). Ten most common herbs in clinical practice. In M.S. Micozzi (Ed.), *Current review of complementary medicine.* Philadelphia: Current Medicine; and Jellin, J.M., Batz, F., & Hitchens, K. (1999). *Pharmacist's letter/prescriber's letter natural medicines comprehensive database.* Stockton, CA: Therapeutic Research Faculty.

TABLE 23-1 Stages of Cognitive Decline

Stage	Clinical Phase	Symptoms
1	Normal	No change in cognition
2	Very mild	Forgets object location; some deficit in word finding
3	Mild (early confusion)	Early cognitive decline in one or more areas, memory loss, decreased ability to function in work situation, name-finding deficit, some decrease in social functioning, recall difficulties, anxiety
4	Moderate	Unable to perform complex tasks such as managing personal finances, planning a dinner party, concentrating, and knowing current events
5	Moderately severe (early dementia)	Usually needs assistance for survival, reminders to bathe, help in selecting clothes, and other daily functions; may be disoriented as to time and recent events, but this can fluctuate; may become tearful
6	Severe (dementia)	Needs assistance with dressing, bathing, and toilet functions (e.g., flushing); may forget names of spouse/family/caregivers and details of their personal life; may be generally unaware of their surroundings; incontinence of urine and feces may occur; CNS disturbances such as agitation, delusions, paranoia, obsessive anxiety, and the potential for violent behavior may increase.
7	Very severe (late dementia)	Unable to speak (speech limited to 5 words or less); may scream or make other sounds; unable to ambulate, sit up, smile, or feed self; unable to hold head erect; ultimately slips into stupor or coma

theories currently under study include the following: (1) a deficiency in acetylcholine, a major neurotransmitter, and perhaps other neurotransmitters in the brain; (2) a slow virus or infection that attacks selected brain cells; (3) genetic predisposition; (4) autoimmune theory—the theory that the body fails to recognize host tissue and attacks itself; and (5) beta-amyloid protein accumulation in the CNS (Williams, 1995). A primary hypothesis is that Alzheimer's results from loss of related cholinergic nerves in the CNS (Miller, 1995).

Current pharmacotherapy is directed toward improving cognitive functioning or limiting disease progression and symptom control (Richards & Hendrie, 1999). Unfortunately, no known current medication cures, slows, or prevents Alzheimer's disease. The ergoloid mesylates (Hydergine), tacrine (Cognex), and donepezil (Aricept) have been approved by the Food and Drug Administration (FDA) to treat memory deficits. The ergoloid mesylates have been used to treat early dementia, but their use is controversial in Alzheimer's disease. One study reported some *worsening* of cognitive ability and behaviors with its use (*USP DI*, 1999).

Symptom management includes small dosages of antipsychotic agents, such as haloperidol (Haldol) 0.5 to 5 mg/day for delusions and hallucinations. Two precautions exist: (1) start with a low dosage, increase it gradually only if necessary, and monitor the client closely for side effects; and (2) be aware that antipsychotic agents or any medications with a high anticholinergic potential could worsen cognitive function.

For depression, antidepressants with a low anticholinergic profile, such as desipramine (Norpramin) or trazodone (Desyrel, Trazon) have been used. The dosages should start at one-third to one-half the usual adult dosage for clients with Alzheimer's disease and increase slowly as necessary.

In general, the antianxiety agents, especially those with a short to intermediate half-life (e.g., lorazepam [Ativan], oxazepam [Serax], or alprazolam [Xanax]), are selected for clients who exhibit severe anxiety. However, if such agents are used to treat agitation in clients with dementia (or specifically, Alzheimer's disease), the potential for inducing a paradoxical reaction is present. Such clients may respond with an increase in activity, restlessness, and agitation. Therefore it is important for the prescriber to differentiate between agitation and anxiety. If the benzodiazepine antianxiety agents are used, they should be closely monitored because symptoms change with time. Short-term use or a reevaluation at least every 3 to 6 months is necessary.

tacrine [tack′ rin] (Cognex)

Tacrine (Cognex), a centrally acting cholinesterase inhibitor, has a longer duration of action than physostigmine. It appears to improve cognitive function in a limited number of persons with mild to moderate Alzheimer's disease.

Tacrine is rapidly absorbed orally, reaches peak serum levels in 0.5 to 3 hours, and has a half-life of 1.5 to 4 hours. It is metabolized in the liver, with one major metabolite having central cholinergic effects.

The side effects of tacrine include nausea, vomiting, loss of appetite, diarrhea, headache, ataxia, muscle aches, and hepatotoxicity. Refer to the current literature for a recommended schedule of routine testing of serum alanine aminotransferase for liver toxicity.

The oral adult dosage of tacrine is 10 mg four times daily, increased at 6-week intervals as necessary. The maximum daily dose is 160 mg.

Because the benefits from tacrine have been limited, many other drugs are under investigation. These agents include the nonsteroidal antiinflammatory agents (piracetam [Nootropil] and indomethacin [Indocin]); velnacrine maleate (Mentane), a centrally acting cholinesterase inhibitor; nimodipine (Nimotop), a calcium antagonist; and selegiline (Eldepryl), an MAO-B inhibitor that may have antioxidant effects and also increases concentrations of serotonin and norepinephrine (Eggert & Crismon, 1994; Bravyak & Schechter, 1992). It has also been reported that postmenopausal women treated with estrogen were less likely to get Alzheimer's disease than those left untreated (Williams, 1995). Serotonin antagonists and ACE inhibitors are also under investigation.

donepezil [don e′ pe zil] (Aricept)

Donepezil (Aricept) is the second drug released for the treatment of Alzheimer's disease. This drug inhibits the enzyme acetylcholinesterase, which permits an increased accumulation of acetylcholine in the brain.

Donepezil is well absorbed orally, reaches peak serum levels between 3 and 4 hours, and has an elimination half-life of 70 hours. It is metabolized in the liver to four major metabolites (two of which are active) and excreted primarily by the kidneys.

The side effects/adverse reactions of donepezil include muscle cramping, nausea, vomiting, diarrhea, and insomnia. The usual adult dosage for Alzheimer's dementia is 5 mg daily, taken in the evening.

rivastigmine [riv as tig′ mine] (Exelon)
galantamine [gah lan′ tah meen] (Reminyl)

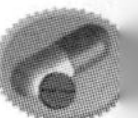

Rivastigmine and galantamine are acetylcholinesterase inhibitors for the treatment of Alzheimer's disease. Rivastigmine may cause significant gastrointestinal adverse effects, more so than the other cholinesterase inhibitors. It is therefore recommended that dose titration proceed slowly to reduce the possibility of inducing severe vomiting (Pharmacist's Letter, 2001). The initial dosage is 1.5 mg twice daily titrated every 2 weeks as necessary to a maximum of 6 mg twice daily. The medication should be administered with food (morning and evening) (*Drug Facts & Comparisons*, 2001). Galantamine is better tolerated than rivastigmine. The adult dosage starts at 4 mg twice daily for at least 1 month, then it may be increassed to 8 mg twice daily. This product should be taken with food (Pharmacist's Letter, 2001). For nursing management of anticholinesterase therapy, see pp. 506-507.

■ Nursing Management

Drug Therapy for Alzheimer's Disease

In the pharmacologic management of clients with Alzheimer's disease, care needs to be taken to provide for their safety and comfort. In older adults, most of the medications prescribed for the treatment of Alzheimer's disease are excreted and metabolized less efficiently. Smaller dosages are required to produce the desired effect. The nurse's assessment and documentation of subtle changes in the client's health status will allow prescribers to individualize medication dosages more closely. Drugs that compromise respiratory function or cause depression, confusion, or sleep alterations should be avoided.

In many ways Alzheimer's disease remains a perplexing illness. Besides providing appropriate care, keep abreast of medical and nursing research findings, be committed to conducting nursing studies on the care of clients with Alzheimer's disease, and share ideas about effective nursing interventions with colleagues.

SKELETAL MUSCLE RELAXANTS

Most muscle strains and spasms are self-limited and respond to rest, physical therapy, and short-term skeletal muscle relaxants. **Spasticity** (a form of muscular hypertonicity with increased resistance to stretch) as the result of stroke, closed head injuries, cerebral palsy, multiple sclerosis, spinal cord trauma, and other neurologic disorders requiring the long-term use of skeletal muscle relaxants will challenge the nurse's rehabilitative skills and knowledge. In both short- and long-term care, the nurse's role is not only to administer medications but also to provide comfort and rehabilitative measures in collaboration with physical therapists and other members of the health care team.

Neuromuscular Junction

Skeletal muscles are striated (striped) muscles attached to the skeleton. They are usually under voluntary control, and they produce body movements, maintain body position against the force of gravity, and counteract environmental stressors such as wind. A muscle is made of numerous muscle cells or muscle fibers. Each muscle cell is connected to only one motor nerve fiber, but each nerve fiber is connected to several muscle cells. Therefore stimulation of one nerve fiber causes stimulation and activation of a group of muscle cells. The region where a motor nerve fiber makes functional contact with a skeletal muscle fiber (synaptic contact) is known as the neuromuscular junction.

Skeletal Muscle Spasm and Spasticity

Skeletal muscle **spasms** result when there is an involuntary contraction of a muscle or group of muscles that is accompanied by pain or limited function. Most skeletal muscle spasms are caused by local injuries, but some may result from low calcium levels or epileptic myoclonic seizures. Each type of spasm is treated according to its cause.

Skeletal muscle injuries are usually self-limiting and can be treated with rest; physical therapy; immobility with the use of casts, neck collars, crutches, or arm slings; or whirlpool baths. Antiinflammatory drugs may be used for tissue damage and edema.

Central skeletal muscle relaxants are used mainly for conditions in which muscle spasms do not quickly respond to other forms of therapy. Such conditions include musculoskeletal strains and sprains, trauma, and cervical or lumbar radiculopathy as a result of degenerative osteoarthritis, herniated disk, spondylosis, or laminectomy. Unlike diazepam (Valium), the centrally acting drug baclofen (Lioresal)—which is used for skeletal muscle spasticity—has not been found to be useful in the treatment of muscle spasms.

Skeletal muscle spasticity is characterized by skeletal muscle hyperactivity and occurs when gamma motor neurons (which tonically control muscle spindle contractile activity) become hyperactive. There are two primary types of muscle spasticity: spinal and cerebral. Spinal spasticity can be identified by a marked loss of inhibitory influences with hyperactive tendon stretch reflexes, clonus (alternate contraction and relaxation of muscles), primitive flexion withdrawal reflexes, and a flexed posture. Varying degrees of spasticity of the bladder and bowel can also be seen. Cerebral spasticity has less reflex excitability, increased muscle tone, and no primitive flexion withdrawal reflexes or flexed posture. **Dystonia,** an impairment of muscle tone, may also be present in individuals with cerebral spasticity.

Muscle spasticity is most commonly seen in clients with CNS injuries and strokes. Moderate to severe spasticity can be seen in two thirds of clients with multiple sclerosis. Individuals with cerebral palsy and rare neurologic disorders can also have muscle spasticity, but it is seen less commonly in these instances.

Central-acting and direct-acting skeletal muscle relaxants are the drugs of choice in the treatment of muscle spasticity. These drugs include baclofen (Lioresal), diazepam (Valium), and dantrolene (Dantrium). They are more effective in the treatment of spinal spasticity than cerebral spasticity. Optimal therapy cannot be achieved in the treatment of either condition unless physical therapy is given concurrently.

Central-Acting Skeletal Muscle Relaxants

The exact mechanism of action of the central-acting skeletal muscle relaxants is not known. Action results from CNS depression in the brain (brainstem, thalamus, and basal ganglia) and spinal cord that results in the relaxation of striated muscle spasm. Removing the CNS depressant action from the central-acting skeletal muscle relaxants is not currently possible. As a result, these drugs create the side effects of drowsiness, blurred vision, light-headedness, headache, and feelings of weakness, lassitude, and lethargy; such effects make long-term use of these drugs undesirable. The drugs used primarily as antispastic agents are baclofen, diazepam, and dantrolene. Dantrolene, a direct-acting skeletal muscle relaxant (peripheral action), is discussed later in this chapter.

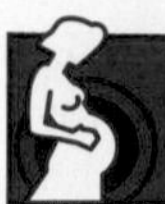

Pregnancy Safety
Central-Acting Skeletal Muscle Relaxants

Category	Drug
B	cyclobenzaprine, donepezil
C	tizanidine
Unclassified	baclofen, carisoprodol, chlorphenesin, chlorzoxazone, dantrolene, diazepam,* metaxalone, methocarbamol, orphenadrine

*To be avoided during pregnancy, especially during the first trimester.

■ Nursing Management
Central-Acting Skeletal Muscle Relaxant Therapy

■ **Assessment.** The client should be assessed for a history of allergic reaction to the specific agent. CNS depression may be exacerbated with the administration of central-acting muscle relaxants, so caution should be taken with these clients. The drugs should also be used cautiously in the presence of hepatic or renal dysfunction and in pregnant women. The FDA disapproves of prolonged administration of these drugs and discourages their use for periods longer than 3 weeks (see the Pregnancy Safety box above).

Obtain a baseline assessment of the client's spasticity: the frequency, location, severity, and factors that exacerbate and ameliorate the spasm.

■ **Nursing Diagnosis.** Once the client begins taking a central-acting skeletal muscle relaxant, the nurse's assessment should consider the potential development of a number of nursing diagnoses/collaborative problems related to the effects of the drug. Because of the CNS effects of the drug, the client may experience disturbed thought processes (confusion), activity intolerance related to weakness, and a risk for injury related to ataxia, drowsiness, dizziness, or syncope. Elimination patterns may be impaired, such as with constipation and dysuria. Impaired comfort may appear as muscle weakness, nausea, headache, stomach discomfort, hiccough, and rash. Disturbed sensory perception (visual and auditory hallucinations) may also occur. With overdose, the potential complications of seizures and respiratory depression exist.

■ **Implementation**

■ ***Monitoring.*** Document the progress of the client's muscle spasticity. Assess for the nursing diagnoses/collaborative problems discussed previously.

■ ***Intervention.*** For ease of administration, the tablets may be crushed and mixed with fluid, jelly, or other food. The drugs should be administered with meals or milk to prevent the side effects of nausea, vomiting, heartburn, and abdominal distress associated with large doses.

■ ***Education.*** Inform individuals undergoing central-acting skeletal muscle relaxant therapy to avoid activities that require mental alertness, judgment, and physical coordination (e.g., operating dangerous machinery or driving an automobile). Instruct the client that alcohol and other CNS depressants will increase the CNS effects of these drugs. Because many clients experience postural hypotension with these medications, clients should be cautioned about standing suddenly and instructed to rise slowly, in keeping with individual physical limitations.

■ **Evaluation.** The expected outcome of central-acting skeletal muscle relaxant therapy is that the client will demonstrate increased comfort, decreased involuntary movement and muscle tonicity, and an increased range of motion without experiencing adverse reactions to the drug.

baclofen [bak' loe fen] (Lioresal)

Baclofen, a gamma-aminobutyric acid (GABA) inhibitory neurotransmitter, inhibits the transmission of monosynaptic and polysynaptic reflexes. Although its exact mechanism of action is unknown, it is a spasmolytic agent at the spinal level, where it inhibits transmission. It is used in the treatment of spasticity resulting from multiple sclerosis or from injuries to the spinal cord. Baclofen may reduce pain in spastic clients by inhibiting the release of substance P in the spinal cord (Katzung, 1998).

Absorption is generally good but may vary with different individuals. The time to peak concentration is 2 to 3 hours. The onset of action is variable and may occur in hours or up to weeks. Baclofen has a half-life of 2.5 to 4 hours and a therapeutic serum level of 80 to 400 ng/mL. Baclofen is metabolized in the liver and excreted by the kidneys.

The side effects/adverse reactions of baclofen include transient drowsiness, vertigo, confusion, sleepiness, weakness, and nausea.

The adult dosage of baclofen is 5 mg PO three times daily, increased by 5 mg per dose every 3 days until the desired response is achieved; the dosage is not to exceed 80 mg/day. The dosage for children has not been determined.

■ Nursing Management
Baclofen Therapy

In addition to the information discussed under Nursing Management: Central-Acting Skeletal Muscle Relaxant Therapy (p. 511), baclofen requires the following management (see also the Case Study box on p. 513).

■ **Assessment.** The combination of baclofen and alcohol or other CNS depressants may result in enhanced CNS depressant effects and hypotension. Monitor closely because a reduction in dosage of one or both drugs may be necessary.

■ **Nursing Diagnosis.** Some clients receiving baclofen, particularly by intrathecal administration, may experience activity intolerance related to decreased extensor tone as an effect of the drug. The risk for injury related to ataxia, drowsiness, dizziness, or confusion is a significant nursing diagnosis with the administration of baclofen. Others to be considered are constipation, disturbed thought processes (paranoia), sexual dysfunction in males, impaired urinary elimination, and impaired comfort (dry mouth, nausea, nervousness).

■ **Implementation**

■ ***Monitoring.*** The administration of baclofen may increase the blood glucose levels of clients with diabetes, thus requiring an adjustment of the insulin dosage during therapy

Case Study *The Client Receiving Skeletal Muscle Relaxants*

Jimmy Culver is a 17-year-old male high school student who sustained a T3-T4 spinal cord injury a year ago in a car accident. He has been hospitalized for a recurrent urinary tract infection and right ischial decubitus ulcer. In addition, he has severe muscle spasms in his lower extremities. The prescriber has ordered baclofen (Lioresal) 10 mg PO twice daily and diazepam (Valium) 10 mg PO twice daily for his muscle spasms.

1. What should a baseline assessment of Jimmy include before beginning the administration of baclofen and diazepam?
2. Jimmy tells you that he is still having the muscle spasms even after taking baclofen for 1 week. What should you tell him?
3. What side effects of baclofen should Jimmy and his parents be looking for?
4. If for some reason Jimmy stops taking baclofen, he and his parents should be alert for what adverse reactions?
5. Jimmy tells you that sometimes he experiences severe nausea and abdominal distress after taking tablets between classes. How can you help to alleviate his discomfort?

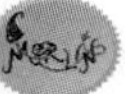

For answer guidelines, go to mosby.com/MERLIN/McKenry/.

and when baclofen therapy is stopped. Older adults are at risk for adverse CNS reactions and should be assessed for the development of altered thought processes (e.g., hallucinations, depression, confusion, and excessive sedation). Observe for increased seizure activity in clients with epilepsy because the seizure threshold may be lowered. Monitor the client's clinical state and electroencephalogram (EEG) results during therapy.

■ ***Intervention.*** The dosage of baclofen should be increased gradually to therapeutic levels to decrease the incidence of adverse reactions. A gradual reduction in dosage over a period of 2 weeks is recommended, because abrupt withdrawal may cause hallucinations, paranoia, nightmares, confusion, and rebound spasticity. If using an intrathecal pump, it may be programmed to give higher doses at night to decrease spasm and to give lower doses during the day, when the client may need some rigidity for walking.

■ ***Education.*** Inform the client undergoing baclofen therapy that the maximum benefit of the medication may not be reached for 1 to 2 months. Caution the client about driving and other activities that require alertness because of the CNS effects of the drug (dizziness, drowsiness, impaired mental or physical abilities, or visual disturbances).

If abrupt withdrawal is required, instruct the client that hallucinations and rebound spasticity may occur. Alert the client to possible side effects such as dermatitis, CNS effects, and syncope. If orthostatic hypotension is a concern, instruct the client to come to an upright position slowly and stay seated until the light-headedness dissipates.

■ **Evaluation.** The expected outcome of baclofen therapy is that the client will experience increased comfort, demonstrate decreased involuntary movement and muscle tonicity, and demonstrate an increased range of motion without experiencing adverse reactions to the drug.

diazepam [dye az′ e pam] (Valium, Apo-Diazepam ✤)

Although the mechanism of action for diazepam is unknown, it appears to act primarily by inhibiting afferent spinal polysynaptic (and possibly monosynaptic) pathways. It may also directly suppress muscle function at the neuromuscular synapse. Diazepam is used in the treatment of skeletal muscle spasm caused by reflex spasm or local pathologic conditions such as inflammation of muscle and joints or secondary to trauma. It is also used to treat spasticity caused by upper motor neuron disorders (cerebral palsy and paraplegia), athetosis, tetanus, and stiff-man syndrome (to overcome the widespread chronic muscular rigidity, pain, and skeletal muscle spasms). (See Chapter 16 for more information on diazepam.)

■ Nursing Management

Diazepam Therapy

In addition to the information discussed under Nursing Management: Central-Acting Skeletal Muscle Relaxant Therapy (p. 511), greater detail relating to diazepam may be found in Chapter 16. The unique nursing management of diazepam muscle relaxant therapy is discussed in the following sections.

■ **Assessment.** Baseline vital signs should be assessed before diazepam is given and then at frequent intervals after the injection.

■ **Implementation**

■ ***Monitoring.*** Observe clients, particularly older adults, for oversedation and impaired coordination. Clients undergoing long-term therapy can become physically dependent on the drug and show signs and symptoms of withdrawal when it is discontinued.

■ ***Intervention.*** Diazepam is insoluble in water, and therefore the parenteral form is prepared in a specific solvent. Do not mix or dilute parenteral doses with other fluids or add to IV fluids. Administer IM injections slowly and deeply into a large muscle to diminish local irritation.

Administer IV diazepam slowly, at least 1 minute for each 5 mg of the drug, to prevent apnea, hypotension, bradycardia, or cardiac arrest. After receiving a parenteral dose, the client should be observed and should stay in bed for at least 3 hours. Resuscitative equipment should be available. To avoid phlebitis and venous thrombosis, small veins on the back of the hand and wrist should not be used for IV administration. To minimize the occurrence of thrombophlebitis after IV administration of diazepam, flush the vein with 1 mL of saline per 1 mg of diazepam.

Continuous IV infusion is not recommended because diazepam may precipitate in the infusion bag and the medication may be adsorbed to the plastic of the infusion bags and tubing. Diazepam may be injected through the IV tubing if it cannot be administered by direct IV infusion, but the injection should be as close as possible to the insertion point.

■ ***Education.*** The client undergoing diazepam therapy should be alerted to the risk for injury related to the CNS effects of drowsiness, dizziness, and confusion.

■ **Evaluation.** The expected outcome of diazepam therapy is that the client will report feeling relaxed and will demonstrate decreased involuntary movement and muscle tonicity and increased range of motion without experiencing adverse reactions to the drug.

Other Central-Acting Skeletal Muscle Relaxants

carisoprodol [kar eye soe proe′ dole] (Soma)
chlorphenesin carbamate [klor fen′ e sin] (Maolate)
chlorzoxazone [klor zox′ a zone] (Paraflex)
cyclobenzaprine [sye kloe ben′ za preen] (Flexeril)
metaxalone [met ax′ ah lone] (Skelaxin)
methocarbamol [meth oh kar′ ba mole] (Robaxin, Marbaxin)
orphenadrine [or fen′ a dreen] (Disipal)
orphenadrine extended-release (Norflex)
tizanidine [ti zan′ i deen] (Zanaflex)

Muscle spasms are treated with central-acting skeletal muscle relaxants that are analogues to various antianxiety medications. The exact mechanism of action of these drugs has not been determined, but it is believed that the muscle relaxant effects of many of these drugs may be related to this CNS depressant activity. Carisoprodol interferes with nerve transmission in the descending reticular formation and spinal cord, whereas chlorzoxazone produces its effects in the spinal cord and subcortical brain areas. In addition to skeletal muscle relaxant effects, orphenadrine is also an analgesic.

These drugs are used in adjunct treatment for skeletal muscle spasms along with rest and physical therapy.

See Table 23-2 for information on the pharmacokinetics of these central-acting skeletal muscle relaxants.

The side effects/adverse reactions of these central-acting skeletal muscle relaxants include drowsiness, dizziness, dry mouth, and abdominal distress. Metaxalone (Skelaxin) may also cause nausea, vomiting, increased excitability, and restlessness; methocarbamol (Robaxin) and orphenadrine (Disipal) may also cause visual disturbances.

Enhanced CNS depressant effects may occur when a skeletal muscle relaxant is given with alcohol, CNS depressants, or opioid analgesics. Monitor closely because the dosage of one or both drugs should be reduced.

See Table 23-3 for the dosage and administration of the central-acting skeletal muscle relaxing agents.

■ Nursing Management

Other Central-Acting Skeletal Muscle Relaxants

For all of the following drugs, see also the general discussion of Nursing Management: Central-Acting Skeletal Muscle Relaxant Therapy, p. 511. See also the Pregnancy Safety box on p. 512.

■ **Carisoprodol (Soma).** Carisoprodol is found in the milk of lactating mothers at levels two to four times the concentration of the maternal plasma, causing sedation and gastrointestinal distress in the infant. The risk-benefit ratio should be considered before using this drug for a client who is pregnant or lactating. Carisoprodol is contraindicated in clients with acute intermittent porphyria. On occasion, an idiosyncratic reaction to carisoprodol has occurred within minutes or hours of the first dose. Symptoms may include disorientation, agitation, vision disturbances, impaired verbal communication, and extreme weakness. The symptoms are temporary, but supportive therapy may be needed and may require hospitalization. There have been rare reports of psychologic dependence and abuse. Drowsiness is more common with carisoprodol than with most other muscle relaxants.

■ **Chlorphenesin (Maolate).** Watch for sensitivity reactions. Hold the dose and notify the prescriber if unusual reactions occur. Observe for unusual bleeding and indications of blood dyscrasia. The safety of chlorphenesin when used for longer than 8 weeks has not been determined.

■ **Chlorzoxazone (Paraflex).** Chlorzoxazone is contraindicated in clients with hepatic disease. Liver function studies should be monitored closely during therapy because hepatotoxicity is a possible side effect. Tell the client that the drug may discolor the urine to an orange or a purple-red color. Drowsiness and/or dizziness are more common with chlorzoxazone than with most other muscle relaxants.

■ **Cyclobenzaprine (Flexeril).** Cyclobenzaprine is contraindicated in clients with dysrhythmias, conduction disturbances, congestive heart failure, or hyperthyroidism. Assess the client's medication regimen, because the concurrent use of other CNS depressants will enhance CNS depression, the effects of anticholinergics will be potentiated, and MAO inhibitors may cause a hypertensive crisis. This drug is intended for short-term (2 to 3 weeks) use only.

■ **Metaxalone (Skelaxin).** Metaxalone is contraindicated in individuals with renal and hepatic disease. Monitor liver function studies. Monitor the blood studies because hemolytic anemia may occur. Clinitest may give a false-positive reading in urine tests of clients taking metaxalone; Clinistix, Diastix, or Tes-Tape should be used instead. Caution the client to notify the prescriber if a skin rash or yellowish discoloration of skin or eyes occurs (signs of liver-related jaundice). Gastrointestinal irritation with nausea, vomiting, and abdominal cramps is more common with metaxalone than with other muscle relaxants.

TABLE 23-2 Other Central-Acting Skeletal Muscle Relaxants: Pharmacokinetics

Drug	Onset of Action	Time to Peak Concentration (hours)*	Peak Serum Concentration*	Duration of Action (hours)	Half-life (hours)	Metabolism/ Excretion
carisoprodol	30 minutes	4 (350 mg)	4-7 μg/mL	4-6	8	Liver/kidneys
chlorphenesin	N/A	1 to 3	3.8-17 μg/mL (800 mg)	N/A	2.5-5	Liver/kidneys
chlorzoxazone	Within 60 minutes	1 to 2	10-30 μg/mL (750 mg)	3-4	1-2	Liver/kidneys
cyclobenzaprine	Within 60 minutes	3 to 8	15-25 ng/mL (10 mg)	12-24	24-72	Gastrointestinal tract and liver/ kidneys
metaxalone	60 minutes	2 (800 mg)	295 μg/mL (800 mg)	N/A	2-3	Liver/kidneys
methocarbamol						
PO	Within 30 minutes	2 (2 g)	16 μg/mL (2 g)	N/A	0.9-2.2	May be liver/ kidneys and feces
IV	Immediate	Nearly immediate	19 μg/mL (1 g)	N/A		
orphenadrine						
Extended release	Within 60 minutes	6 to 8 (100 mg)	60-120 ng/mL (100 mg)	12	14†	Liver/kidneys and feces
IM	5 minutes	0.5 (60 mg)				
IV	Immediate	Immediate				
orphenadrine HCl	Within 60 minutes	3 (50 mg)	110-210 ng/mL (100 mg)	8	14†	Liver/kidneys and feces
tizanidine	N/A	1.5	N/A	3-6	2.5‡	Liver/kidneys

N/A, not available.
*Single dose.
†Parent drug half-life. The half-life of metabolites may range between 2 and 25 hours.
‡The half-life of metabolites ranges from 20 to 40 hours.

TABLE 23-3 Other Central-Acting Skeletal Muscle Relaxants: Dosage and Administration

Drug	Adults	Children
carisoprodol (Soma)	350 mg PO 4 times daily	Under 5 years: not recommended 5-12 years: 6.25 mg/kg 4 times daily
chlorphenesin (Maolate)	800 mg PO 3 times daily initially; later decreased to 400 mg 4 times daily	Not determined
chlorzoxazone (Paraflex)	250-750 mg PO 3-4 times daily, adjusted as necessary	20 mg/kg in 3 or 4 divided doses daily
cyclobenzaprine (Flexeril)	20-40 mg daily in divided doses	Not determined
metaxalone (Skelaxin)	800 mg PO 3-4 times daily	Not determined
methocarbamol (Robaxin)	1.5 g PO 4 times daily for 2-3 days, increased if necessary; parenteral dose: 1-3 g IM or IV daily for 3 days	Not determined
orphenadrine (Disipal, Norflex)	Extended-release dose: 50 mg PO 3 times daily or 100 mg twice daily; parenteral dose: 60 mg IM or IV q12h	Not determined
tizanidine (Zanaflex)	4 mg q6-8h as needed; adjust dosage if necessary.	Not determined

▪ **Methocarbamol (Robaxin, Marbaxin).** Be aware that methocarbamol is not recommended for individuals receiving anticholinesterase agents, for those who have epilepsy, or for those who are in renal failure (preexisting acidosis and urea retention may increase). Have epinephrine, injectable steroids, and/or injectable antihistamines available for IV injection to treat syncope should it occur. Anaphylactic reactions have occurred after IM and IV administration. Position the client in the recumbent position during IV infusion; have the client remain in this position 10 to 15 minutes after infusion to decrease the incidence of adverse reactions such as syncope, hypotension, and bradycardia.

Do not administer methocarbamol subcutaneously. Administer a deep (IM) injection to decrease local irritation. Avoid IV extravasation; thrombophlebitis, pain, and tissue sloughing may result. The IV infusion should not be refrigerated. In addition, its compatibility with other solutions is limited; see a specialized reference before mixing. It may be diluted in normal saline or 5% dextrose in water, but do not dilute to more than 10 mL (1 g) in 250 mL. If administering the undiluted solution intravenously, inject at a rate no greater than 3 mL/min. Note that tablets may be crushed and suspended in water or saline for administration via a nasogastric tube.

Advise the client to notify the prescriber if skin rash, itching, fever, or nasal congestion occurs. Tell the client that urine may darken to green, black, or brown if it is left standing.

▪ **Orphenadrine (Disipal).** Use orphenadrine with caution in individuals with cardiac decompensation, coronary insufficiency, cardiac dysrhythmias, or tachycardia. Note that orphenadrine is contraindicated in clients with glaucoma, prostatic hypertrophy, bladder neck obstruction, and myasthenia gravis. Periodic blood, urine, and liver function studies should be performed with prolonged therapy. Discuss the side effects with the client.

▪ **Tizanidine (Zanaflex).** The drug clearance of tizanidine is reduced in clients with renal impairment, older adults, and women who are taking oral contraceptives. Monitor closely for dry mouth, fatigue, orthostatic hypotension, and CNS depression. Dosage increments are made gradually in 2- to 4-mg steps based on decreasing spasm and muscle tone.

Direct-Acting Skeletal Muscle Relaxant

dantrolene [dan′ troe leen] (Dantrium)

Dantrolene is used for the prophylaxis and treatment of malignant hyperthermia (see Chapter 15) and spasticity, especially upper motor neuron disorders (e.g., multiple sclerosis, cerebral palsy, spinal cord insults, and cerebrovascular accident [CVA]). Dantrolene acts directly on the skeletal muscles to relax them by inhibiting the release of calcium from the sarcoplasmic reticulum to the myoplasm. This results in a decreased muscle response to the action potential and decreased muscle contraction. As an antispastic agent, the direct effect of dantrolene on skeletal muscle dissociates the excitation-contraction coupling. This effect is probably induced by the interference with calcium ion release from the sarcoplasmic reticulum. Dantrolene reduces both monosynaptic- and polysynaptic-induced muscle contractions.

Dantrolene is available orally and parenterally. The oral absorption of this drug is fair; when used to treat the spasticity of upper motor neurons, the onset of action is 1 week or more. The oral form of this drug has a half-life of 8.7 hours (100-mg dose); the IV half-life is 4 to 8 hours. The time to peak concentration is 5 hours (oral dose). It is metabolized in the liver and excreted by the kidneys.

The side effects/adverse reactions of dantrolene include diarrhea, dizziness, sleepiness, uncomfortable feelings, unusual fatigue, muscle weakness, nausea, vomiting, severe diarrhea, respiratory difficulty, and respiratory depression.

See Table 23-4 for the dosage and administration of dantrolene.

▪ Nursing Management

Dantrolene Therapy

▪ **Assessment.** Dantrolene should not be administered to clients with active hepatic disease because of the increased risk for hepatotoxicity. Use with caution in clients with impaired cardiac, hepatic, or pulmonary function. These precautions do not apply to the short-term IV use of dantrolene to treat malignant hyperthermia. Women over age 35 are also at higher risk for hepatotoxicity. Clients who are lactose intolerant may also react adversely to dantrolene capsules, which contain lactose. Determine if there is sensitivity to dantrolene. (See also the Pregnancy Safety box on p. 512.)

Careful assessment of the client is particularly important when dantrolene is prescribed for spasticity. Because there is no way of knowing if a client will benefit without a clinical trial, the observations of the relief of spasticity are critical. The decision for long-term use of dantrolene depends on the balance between the drug-induced weakness and the other adverse and beneficial effects of the drug. Clients with paraplegia may not consider the adverse reaction of weakness as detrimental as spasticity. Ambulatory clients who use spasticity to remain upright or for balance are not candidates for dantrolene therapy.

Review the client's current medication regimen for the risk of significant drug interactions, such as those that may occur when dantrolene is given concurrently with the following drugs:

Drug	Possible Effect and Management
Bold/color type indicates the most serious interactions.	
alcohol and other CNS depressants	Enhanced CNS depression may occur when dantrolene is given for short-term use (1 to 3 days) or chronic use. The dosage of one or both drugs may need to be decreased. Monitor closely.
calcium channel blockers	**If dantrolene is given intravenously for malignant hyperthermia, avoid the concurrent use of verapamil while attempting management of a**

TABLE 23-4 Dantrolene: Dosage and Administration

Adults	Children
Antispastic	
25 mg PO daily initially, increased by 25 mg as necessary every 4-7 days until an adequate response or 100 mg 4 times daily is reached.	0.5 mg/kg PO twice daily, increased by 0.5 mg/kg/day as necessary every 4-7 days until an adequate response or a dosage of 3 mg/kg 4 times daily is reached; do not exceed 400 mg/day
Prophylaxis for Malignant Hyperthermic Crisis	
4-8 mg/kg PO in 3 or 4 divided doses daily for 24-48 hours before surgery. Last dose is given 3-4 hours before surgery, with minimum water. IV infusion: 2.5 mg/kg over a 1-hour period before anesthesia.	Not available
Acute Malignant Hyperthermic Reaction	
IV push of minimum of 1 mg/kg; continue this dose until symptoms abate or a maximum cumulative dose of 10 mg/kg is reached. After IV therapy, 4-8 mg/kg PO in 4 divided doses daily is given for 1-3 days.	See adult dose

	malignant hyperthermic emergency. There is some evidence to suggest that these drugs may interact to produce cardiovascular collapse.
hepatotoxic drugs	For chronic use only, the risk of inducing liver toxicity increases. Women over 35 years of age taking estrogen products are at particular risk for this toxicity.

A baseline assessment of the client's involuntary movement, muscle tonicity, and range of motion should be determined. Because of the risk of hepatotoxicity, hepatic function studies should be performed before the start of chronic dantrolene therapy.

■ **Nursing Diagnosis.** The client receiving dantrolene therapy is at risk for the following selected nursing diagnoses/collaborative problems: impaired physical mobility related to muscle spasm because of ineffectiveness of the drug; impaired gas exchange related to respiratory depression; disturbed sleep pattern (drowsiness); fatigue; diarrhea; constipation; impaired urinary elimination (frequency); risk for injury related to dizziness or weakness; impaired comfort (headache, nausea); impaired skin integrity (acne-like rash); disturbed thought processes (confusion); and the potential complications of mental depression, pleural effusion with pericarditis, convulsions, hepatotoxicity, and thrombophlebitis.

■ **Implementation**

■ ***Monitoring.*** When dantrolene is administered to prevent malignant hyperthermia, carefully monitor the client postoperatively for possible delayed effects of the drug. The client receiving long-term therapy should be monitored for blood cell counts and hepatic and renal functioning. The risk of hepatotoxicity is greater in clients with previous liver disease, in clients taking 800 mg daily for short-term therapy or 200 mg daily for longer than 2 months, and in women over 35 concurrently receiving estrogen therapy. Hepatitis most commonly occurs between 3 and 12 months into therapy and is generally preceded by gastrointestinal symptoms such as anorexia, nausea, and vomiting. Starting with low dosages and increasing them gradually may minimize side effects. With short-term use, diarrhea may be a concern and may be severe enough to result in discontinuation of therapy. Constipation may occur with chronic use; health teaching should focus on its prevention.

The client's spasticity should be assessed periodically early in therapy, but the effects may not be seen for a week. If no improvement is noted after 45 days, therapy should be discontinued.

■ ***Intervention.*** The contents of the capsule may be mixed with fruit juice for oral administration to a client who is unable to swallow capsules. Administer immediately after mixing. When IV dantrolene is used to treat malignant hyperthermia, the use of all anesthetic agents is discontinued, oxygen is administered, metabolic acidosis and fluid and electrolyte imbalances are corrected, and the client is cooled. Reconstitute IV dantrolene with 60 mL of sterile water for injection without a bacteriostatic agent, and shake the mixture until it is clear; use this mixture within 6 hours of preparation. Dantrolene is incompatible with acidic solutions, including 5% dextrose injection and 0.9% sodium chloride injection. Oral dantrolene may be given after the IV dose to prevent a recurrence of symptoms. Avoid extravasation of IV dantrolene, which is painful and irritating to the tissue because of the high pH of the solution.

Dantrolene may be given orally or intravenously for malignant hyperthermic crisis prophylaxis. The IV solution is administered over a 1-hour period before anesthesia; the oral dosage form is administered 1 to 2 days before surgery, with the last dose administered 3 to 4 hours before scheduled surgery with a minimum of water.

▪ ***Education.*** Caution clients to avoid exposure to the sun, because photosensitivity is possible with dantrolene. Improvement should be seen within 45 days or the drug should be discontinued. Regular visits to the prescriber should be encouraged for assessment of progress and to monitor for side effects with blood studies. For other nursing considerations, see Nursing Management: Central-Acting Skeletal Muscle Relaxant Therapy, p. 511.

▪ **Evaluation.** The expected outcome of dantrolene therapy is that the client will demonstrate increased comfort, decreased involuntary movement and muscle tonicity, and increased range of motion without experiencing adverse reactions to the drug. If the drug is administered for malignant hyperthermia, the client will not demonstrate fever, cardiac dysrhythmias, or muscle rigidity.

SUMMARY

The major CNS-neuromuscular disorders discussed in this chapter—Parkinson's disease, myasthenia gravis, dementia, Alzheimer's disease, and muscle spasticity—are progressive and often incapacitating syndromes. Pharmacologic therapy is essential for symptom control, which allows the client to function as independently as possible for as long as possible.

Clients with Parkinson's disease require correction of the disorder's imbalance of dopamine and acetylcholine. For this reason, the client is treated with drugs that have central anticholinergic activity, anticholinergics and antihistamines, and drugs that affect dopamine levels to enhance dopaminergic mechanisms. Because the condition is debilitating and long term, clients and caregivers require support and education to maintain compliance with the medication regimen.

Myasthenia gravis is characterized by skeletal muscle weakness and fatigue and is also progressive and incurable. The anticholinesterase drugs are central to the treatment of this disorder.

Drug therapy is not as specific for dementia and Alzheimer's disease. Tacrine, donepezil, and low doses of antipsychotic drugs are used in both disorders to control severe agitation, delusions, and hallucinations.

Pharmacologic agents administered as skeletal muscle relaxants affect skeletal muscle at the neuromuscular junction or at different levels in the CNS, such as the spinal cord or the brain. The effects of the central-acting skeletal muscle relaxants result from CNS depression in the brain and spinal cord. Direct-acting skeletal muscle relaxants affect striated muscle to dissociate the excitation-contraction coupling and thus reduce monosynaptic- and polysynaptic-induced muscle contractions. Although most skeletal muscle spasm is the result of local injury, other instances may be of a more systemic nature; the treatment of each type of spasm is related to its cause.

An essential part of the nurse's role is to identify the subtle changes in the client's health status in any of the discussed conditions, which enables the prescriber to individualize the medication regimen and sustain the highest quality of life for the client.

Critical Thinking Questions

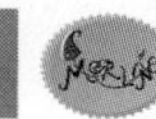

1. Mrs. Ross has been diagnosed with myasthenia gravis, for which she has been prescribed pyridostigmine syrup. Her most distressing symptom is a mild dysphagia. How could the nurse best manage Mrs. Ross's drug therapy?
2. Mrs. Kelly brings her 72-year-old husband to the clinic for a periodic assessment of his Alzheimer's disease and the effectiveness of his drug therapy. Formulate a line of inquiry to elicit information from Mrs. Kelly that will assist you in determining the effectiveness of her husband's drug therapy.
3. In evaluating the effectiveness of skeletal muscle relaxant therapy for a client with spasticity, what would constitute an appropriate assessment of the client's status?
4. What would be essential to include in a teaching plan for a client who will be self-administering muscle relaxant therapy?

Collaborative Learning Activities

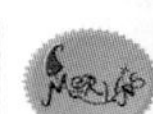

For Collaborative Learning Activities, go to mosby.com/MERLIN/McKenry/.

CASE STUDY

For a Case Study that will help ensure mastery of this chapter content, go to mosby.com/MERLIN/McKenry/.

BIBLIOGRAPHY

American Hospital Formulary Service. (1999). *AHFS drug information '99*. Bethesda, MD: American Society of Hospital Pharmacists.

Anderson, K.N., Anderson, L.E., & Glanze, W.D. (Eds.) (1998). *Mosby's medical, nursing, & allied health dictionary* (5th ed.). St. Louis: Mosby.

Bravyak, J.A.T. & Schechter, B.R. (1992). *Alzheimer's disease management*. Philadelphia: Philadelphia College of Pharmacy and Science.

Conley, S.C. & Kirchner, J.T. (1999). Medical and surgical treatment of Parkinson's disease: Strategies to slow symptom progression and improve quality of life. *Postgraduate Medicine, 106*(2):41-44, 49, 52.

Cutson, T.M., Laub, K.C., & Schenkman, M. (1995). Pharmacological and nonpharmacological interventions in the treatment of Parkinson's disease. *Physical Therapy, 75*(5), 363-373.

Drug Facts and Comparisons. (2000). St. Louis: Facts and Comparisons.

Drug Facts and Comparisons. (2001). St. Louis: Facts and Comparisons.

Eggert, A. & Crismon, M.L. (1994). Current concepts in understanding Alzheimer's disease. *Clinical Pharmacy Newswatch, 1*(1), 1-8.

Flaherty, J.F. & Gidal, B.E. (1995). Parkinson's disease. In L.Y. Young & M.A. Koda-Kimble (Eds.), *Applied therapeutics: The clinical use of drugs* (6th ed.). Vancouver, WA: Applied Therapeutics.

Grimes, D.A. & Lang, A.E. (1999). Treatment of early Parkinson's disease. *Canadian Journal of Neurological Science, 26* (suppl 2), S39-44.

Guttman, M. & Suchowersky, O. (1999). Parkinson's disease management: Toward a new paradigm. *Canadian Journal of Neurological Science, 26*(suppl 2), S53-57.

Hobson, D.E., Pourcher, E., & Martin, W.R. (1999). Ropinirole and pramipexole, the new agonists. *Canadian Journal of Neurological Science, 26*(suppl 2), S27-33.

Jankovic, J. (1999). New and emerging therapies for Parkinson's disease. *Archives of Neurology, 56*(7), 785-790.

Katzung, B.G. (1998). *Basic and clinical pharmacology* (7th ed.). Norwalk, CT: Appleton & Lange.

Kernich, C.A. & Kaminski, H.J. (1995). Myasthenia gravis: Pathophysiology, diagnosis and collaborative care. *Journal of Neuroscience Nursing,* 27(4), 207-218.

King, D.B. (1999). Parkinson's disease: Levodopa complications. *Canadian Journal of Neurological Science, 26*(suppl 2), S13-20.

Korczyn, A.D., Brunt, E.R., Larsen, J.P., Nagy, Z., Poewe, W.H., & Ruggieri, S. (1999). A 3-year randomized trial of ropinirole and bromocriptine in early Parkinson's disease: The 053 study group. *Neurology, 53*(2), 364-370.

Lamy, P.P. (1992). Alzheimer's disease: 1906-1991. *Elder Care News, 8*(4), 27-37.

Lebars, P.L., Katz, M.M., Berman, N., Itil, T.M., Freedman, A.M., & Schatzberg, A.F. (1997). A placebo-controlled, double-blind, randomized trial of an extract of ginkgo biloba extract for dementia, *Journal of the American Medical Association, 278,* 1327-1332.

Lopate, G. & Pestronk, A. (1993). Autoimmune myasthenia gravis. *Hospital Practice, 28*(1), 109.

Miller, S. (1995). Management strategies for the Alzheimer's disease patient. *Clinical Consultant, 14*(1), 1-9.

Pharmacist's Letter.(2001). Alzheimer's, 17(5):26.

Richards, S.S. & Hendrie, H.C. (1999). Diagnosis, management, and treatment of Alzheimer disease: A guide for the internist. *Archives of Internal Medicine, 159*(8), 789-798.

Rivest, J., Barclay, C.L., & Suchowersky, O. (1999). COMT inhibitors in Parkinson's disease. *Canadian Journal of Neurological Science, 26*(suppl 2), S34-38.

Ross, A.P. (1999). Neurological degenerative disorders. *Nursing Clinics of North America, 34*(3), 725-742.

Schneider, L.S. & Tariot, P.N. (1994). Emerging drugs for Alzheimer's disease: Mechanisms of action and prospects for cognitive enhancing medications. *Medical Clinics of North America, 78*(4), 911-934.

Segatore, M. & Miller, M. (1995). The pharmacotherapy of spinal spasticity: A decade of progress. II. Therapeutics. *Science of Nursing, 12*(1), 2-7.

Simuni, T. & Stern, M.B. (1999). Does levodopa accelerate Parkinson's disease. *Drugs Aging, 14*(6), 399-408.

United States Pharmacopeia Dispensing Information (USP DI): Drug information for the health care professional (19th ed.). (1999). Rockville, MD: United States Pharmacopeial Convention.

Van Den Nort, S. (1999). Parkinson's disease. In R.E. Rakel (Ed.), *Conn's current therapy* (51st ed.). Philadelphia: W.B. Saunders.

Williams, B.R. (1995). Geriatric dementias. In L.Y. Young & M.A. Koda-Kimble (Eds.), *Applied therapeutics: The clinical use of drugs* (6th ed.). Vancouver, WA: Applied Therapeutics.

mosby.com/MERLIN/McKenry/

24 Overview of the Cardiovascular System

Chapter Focus

Although progress has been made in increasing public awareness about the lifestyle changes necessary to promote good cardiovascular health, more than 75 million people in North America have some type of cardiovascular disorder. Cardiovascular disease is the leading cause of death in American women; one third of all deaths in females each year is a result of heart disease (Sifton, 1994). "Heart disease kills more women each year than cancer, accidents, and diabetes combined" (Sifton, 1994). As longevity increases, it can be expected that more people will be living with chronic cardiovascular conditions and coping with the results of acute ones. As a result, nurses will be not only providing care within acute facilities but also assisting clients to manage their therapeutic cardiovascular regimens effectively in a variety of community and home settings. A thorough knowledge of anatomy and physiology is essential for assessment of the client, interpretation of diagnostic examinations, provision of care, and client teaching.

Learning Objectives

1. Describe the anatomy and physiology of the heart.
2. Name the three major tissues of the heart.
3. Describe the role of electrical excitation in myocardial contraction.
4. Explain ion exchange during depolarization and repolarization of the myocardial cell.
5. Describe the events occurring in the cardiac cycles, systole, and diastole.
6. Describe the effect of the vagus nerve on the heart.
7. Describe the energy balance between expenditure and restoration maintained by the coronary blood vessels.

Key Terms

action potential, p. 523
atria, p. 521
automaticity, p. 525
AV junction, p. 525
cardiac output, p. 521
conduction system, p. 525
conductivity, p. 526
depolarization, p. 523
diastole, p. 525
electrocardiogram, p. 527
electrophysiologic properties, p. 525
myocardium, p. 521
refractoriness, p. 526
repolarization, p. 523
rhythmicity, p. 526
sarcomere, p. 521
stroke volume, p. 525
systole, p. 525
ventricles, p. 521

The rapid development of science and technology has resulted in new knowledge and a greater understanding of cardiac activity. The resulting anatomic, electrophysiologic, and pharmacologic information has permitted greater precision in diagnosing and treating cardiac disease, particularly the dysrhythmias. Along with these advances has come the increased use of electrocardiographic monitoring of acutely ill clients and those with known or suspected cardiovascular disorders. In addition, the nurse's clinical role has expanded and now includes the care of clients on many other types of monitoring equipment. This requires the nurse to recognize and understand abnormal electrocardiographic patterns and in some cases to begin therapy, including pharmacologic therapy, to prevent serious complications and unnecessary deaths. To keep their knowledge current and their nursing care therapeutically effective, nurses must understand the electrical and physiologic properties of the heart and the effects that drugs have on cardiac activity.

Microelectrode techniques have grown increasingly sophisticated and have helped to provide greater understanding of the electrical properties of cardiac fibers and the causes of various cardiac disorders. Fortunately, these advances have led to the discovery of new drugs that are useful in treating cardiac conditions.

Cardiac drugs largely affect three major tissues of the heart: cardiac muscle (**myocardium**), coronary vessels, and the conduction system. The normal function of these structures is discussed in this chapter. The physiologic properties of these structures and the drug groups used therapeutically are summarized in Table 24-1.

THE HEART

The heart is a hollow muscular organ that consists of two main pumping chambers: (1) the right ventricle, which is linked with the pulmonary circulation; and (2) the left ventricle, which is connected to the systemic circulation. The cardiac muscle, or myocardium, is the largest and most important structure of the heart. As a contractile muscle, it can adapt its performance under normal conditions by adjusting the cardiac output according to needs of the body. **Cardiac output** is the volume of blood expelled by the ventricles of the heart; it is equal to the amount of blood ejected at each beat multiplied by the number of beats in the time used in computation. When the heart cannot produce a variable output, the therapeutic use of digitalis or cardiac glycosides (i.e., the digitalis drugs) produces changes at the cellular level. The following description of myocardial ultrastructure and the contractile process facilitates an understanding of the basic mechanisms in the action of cardiac glycosides.

Cardiac Muscle

The pumping action of the heart depends on the ability of the cardiac muscle to contract. The myocardium is the thick, contractile, middle layer of the heart, and it is composed of many interconnected branching fibers or cells that form the walls of the two **atria** (the upper chambers of the heart) and the two **ventricles** (the lower chambers of the heart). Each individual myocardial fiber contains a nucleus in the middle and a plasma membrane (cell membrane) called the sarcolemma (Figures 24-1, *2*, *3*). The cells form a long fiber by joining end to end, with each cell separated from the other by a plasma membrane called an intercalated disk. This disk is believed to provide sites of low electrical resistance to permit the spread of electrical impulses throughout the cardiac muscle.

Each individual muscle fiber (cell) is part of a group of multiple parallel myofibrils; each myofibril is arranged end to end in a series of repeating units called the **sarcomere**—the basic unit of contraction in the heart (Figure 24-1, *4*). The tremendous energy requirements for cardiac muscle contraction may be seen by the great numbers of mitochondria lined up in long chains between the myofibrils (Figure 24-1, *3*). Under examination with a light microscope, the sarcomere reveals its most characteristic feature, alternating light A bands and dark I bands. These bands result from the crossing of multiple parallel myofibrils, which are aligned in register with one another (Figure 24-1, *3*). The darkness of the A bands results from the thicker myosin filaments,

TABLE 24-1 Effect of Cardiac Drug Groups on Cardiac Tissues

Cardiac Tissue	Physiologic Property	Drug Group	Pharmacologic Action
Cardiac muscle (myocardium)	Force of myocardial contraction (Frank-Starling law)	Cardiac glycosides	Positive inotropic effect—increases cardiac output
Sarcomere (functional unit)	Contractility and conductivity		
Cardiac conduction system	Automaticity (rhythm and rate) Conductivity	Antidysrhythmic drugs Calcium channel blockers	Converts to normal sinus rhythm or abolishes dysrhythmia
Coronary arteries	Nutritional blood flow to myocardium and other cardiac structures	Antianginal drug Calcium channel blockers	Coronary vasodilation or lessens work of the heart

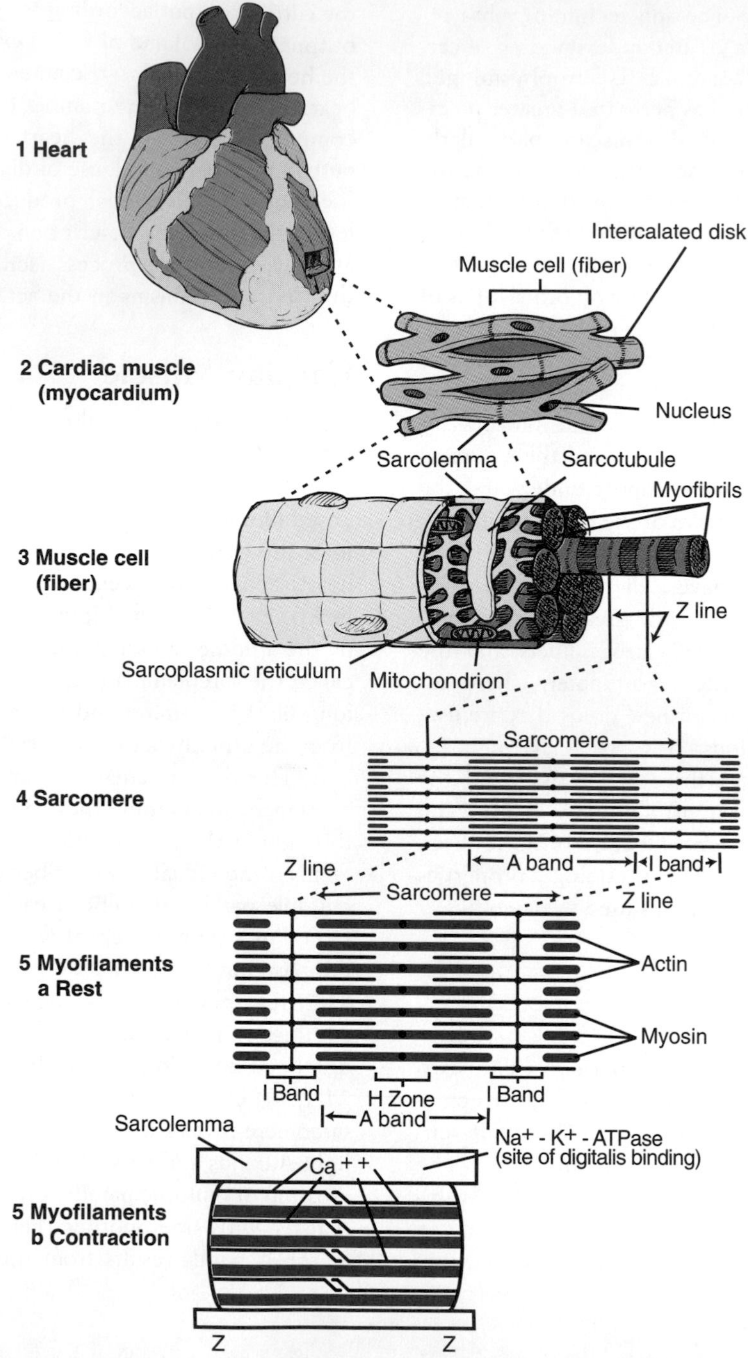

Figure 24-1 Structure of the heart and cardiac muscle cell fibers. The heart (*1*) is mainly a muscular organ. The enlargement of the square illustrates a portion of the cardiac muscle (myocardium) (*2*), which is composed of myocardial cells. Each cell contains a centrally located nucleus and a limiting plasma membrane (sarcolemma), which forms the intercalated disk at the termination of each cell. An individual muscle cell (fiber) (*3*) consists of multiple parallel myofibrils. Each myofibril is arranged longitudinally in a series of light and dark repeating units; the content of a unit is called a sarcomere. The sarcomere (*4*) is the unit of muscle contraction. It is composed of two types of bands, the A band and the I band. The latter is divided by the Z line. At the Z line, the sarcolemma invaginates to form the transverse sarcotubules, or T system. An extensive network, called the sarcoplasmic reticulum, encircles groups of myofibrils and makes contact with the sarcotubules. The sarcoplasmic reticulum contains a high concentration of calcium ions. The mitochondria appear in long chains between the myofibrils. Myofilaments of the sarcomere (*5*) include the thin filament (actin) and the thick filament (myosin). The dark appearance of the A band is caused by the myosin and the lighter appearance of the I band by the actin. Here, the sarcomere is at rest (*a*). On contraction (*b*), the sarcomere shortens so that the thick filaments approach the Z line and the width of the H zone narrows between the thin filaments. Calcium ions are needed for systolic contractions.

and the lightness of the I bands reflects the thinner actin filaments.

The sarcomere lies between two successive Z lines of the myofibril. The end unit of the myofibril is the myofilament. At the Z line, the sarcolemma of the muscle fiber interlocks (invaginates) at its end with the sarcomere to form the transverse sarcotubule, or T system, which penetrates deeply into the cell. Internal membranes form an extensive network called the sarcoplasmic reticulum. This structure encircles groups of myofibrils and makes contact with the sarcotubules.

Cross-bridges, which are small projections that extend from the sides of the myosin filament, appear along the entire length of the thick filament. The interaction between the cross-bridges of myosin and the active sites of actin produces contraction. In the sarcomere, the H zone represents the middle, less dense portion of the A band; the myosin filament runs the entire length of this band. On the other hand, the I band is divided by the Z line. The actin filament runs through the entire I band and terminates at the H zone. This arrangement is shown in Figure 24-1, *5*.

Myocardial Contraction

During the past decade there has been a tremendous increase in the understanding of the fundamental mechanisms governing contraction of cardiac muscle in both normal and pathologic states. However, some aspects of this complicated process remain unknown. Cardiac muscle contraction begins with a rapid change in the electrical charge of the cell membrane. This electrical current spreads to the interior of the cell, where it causes a release of calcium ions from the sarcoplasmic reticulum. The calcium ions then initiate the chemical events of contraction. The overall process for controlling cardiac muscle contraction, called excitation-contraction coupling, involves electrical excitation, mechanical activation, and contractile mechanisms.

Electrical Excitation. Cardiac muscle contraction begins with electrical excitation or stimulus of the myocardial fiber. The source of electricity in the heart is found in the charges of ion concentration—mainly sodium, potassium, and calcium ions—across the cardiac cell membrane of the sarcolemma. The difference in electrical charge, called the **action potential**, produces the rapid ion changes. These changes occur in the membrane of the myocardial cell and result in a self-propagating series of polarization and depolarization. The resting state of an inactive muscle cell in the ventricle is created by the difference in electrical charge across the sarcolemma. In this case the inside of the cell is negative with respect to the outside of the cell, which is positively charged. Because the sarcolemma separates these opposite charges, the membrane in effect is polarized. At rest, the extracellular environment is rich in sodium ions (Na^+) and the intracellular environment is rich in potassium ions (K^+); calcium ion (Ca^{++}) concentration is highest in the region of the sarcolemma and where it invaginates on the sarcotubule (Figure 24-2, *B*).

The cardiac action potential is divided into two stages: depolarization and repolarization. **Depolarization** is the stage in which an electrical impulse results in contraction of the ventricular muscle; it is represented by the QRS complex on the electrocardiogram (ECG). **Repolarization** is the recovery phase after muscle contraction; this stage is represented by the T wave on the ECG. These stages are subdivided into five phases of ionic changes. The resting potential of an inactive myocardial cell is called phase 4; in this phase the membrane is polarized with a charge of approximately −90 millivolts (mv). At this voltage the interior of the cell is negative with respect to the exterior, and the membrane cannot be penetrated by ions. Any stimulus that changes the resting membrane potential to a critical value (the threshold) can generate an action potential. (Follow Figure 24-2, *A*, for steps of the action potential.)

Threshold may be reached by normal pacemaker activity or by propagation of an electrical impulse from a nearby cell, which opens the sodium channels. The fast inward current of sodium ions (fast channel) results in a membrane that is positively charged to +20 mv. This difference in membrane potential results in depolarization and is designated as phase 0 of the action potential. Phase 0 in the ventricular muscle is the contraction phase and is represented by the QRS complex on the surface ECG. Soon after, the repolarization period occurs in three phases. The beginning of phase 1 is the overshoot, and it makes a brief change toward repolarization. Phase 2 is a slow period that forms a plateau with a slow inward current of calcium ions (slow channel) and an outward flow of potassium ions. Calcium ion entry into the cell is essential for the excitation-contraction coupling mechanism, which is explained later in this chapter.

Phase 3 is accomplished by the rapid efflux of potassium ions from the cell. After repolarization, phase 4 recovery (the resting period) begins. This phase is represented by the T wave, whereby the cell membrane actively transports sodium ions outside and potassium ions inside, returning the cell membrane to a state of rest or polarization. These cation exchanges require the energy-utilizing transport mechanism of the Na^+-K^+ pump, or Na^+-K^+-ATPase. Adenosine triphosphatase (ATPase) is powered by oxygen and is an enzyme located in the cell membrane or sarcolemma; it furnishes the energy needed for active transport to return sodium ions and potassium ions to their original resting positions at the membrane. Digitalis plays a key role at this site. By binding to the sarcolemma Na^+-K^+-ATPase, digitalis inhibits the return of sodium ions and potassium ions to their resting positions. Consequently, digitalis allows more sodium ions and calcium ions to enter the cell to strengthen myocardial contraction. It is also thought that digitalis toxicity may occur if an excessive amount of these ions appears intracellularly.

Mechanical Activation. As previously stated, the unit that contracts is the sarcomere. The sarcomere consists of two contractile proteins, actin and myosin. These two filaments combine to help produce cardiac contraction. Myosin, the thicker filament, contains the ATPase enzyme

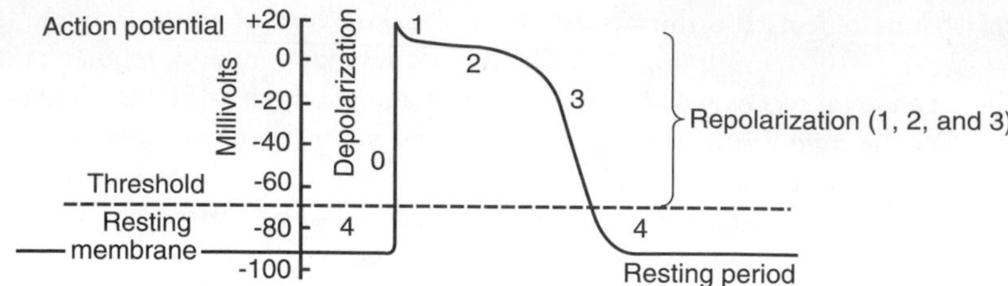

A

Depolarization

Phase 0—membrane becomes permeable to Na^+, which rapidly flows into the cell

Repolarization

Phase 1—membrane potential becomes slightly positive because of the rapid influx of Na^+

Phase 2—slow inward flow of Ca^{++} and outward flow of K^+

Phase 3—rapid outward flow of K^+

Resting period

Phase 4—cell membrane actively transports Na^+ outside and K^+ inside, returning cell membrane to state of polarization

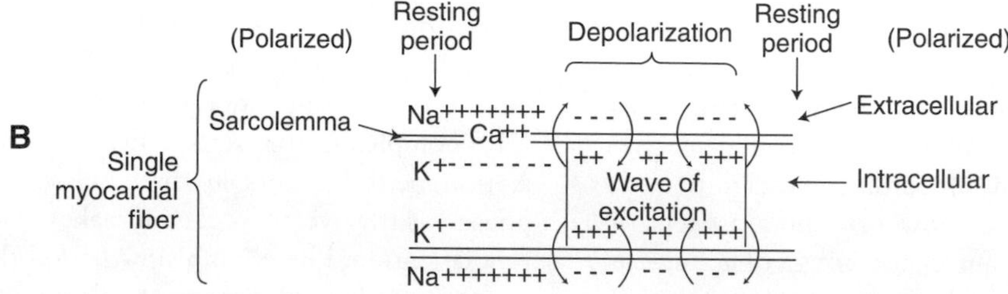

Figure 24-2 A, Action potential of a single myocardial fiber (cell). B, Ionic exchanges that occur across the cell membrane of a single myocardial fiber during an action potential.

system that is needed to hydrolyze ATP (adenosine triphosphate). Hydrolysis is required to provide the energy for contraction. ATP is synthesized in the mitochondria, which are normally abundant in cardiac muscle. Actin, the thin filament, is involved with calcium ion activity.

Contraction is initiated when the nerve impulse reaches the myocardial cell and travels along the sarcolemma of the muscle fiber. As the depolarization wave spreads along the sarcotubules, it arrives at the sarcoplasmic reticulum to cause the release of its large quantities of calcium ions. These ions then bind to special receptors on the actin filaments. The plateau, which is phase 2 of the action potential, is reached through the slow inward calcium current flow (slow channel). *Calcium ion movement is the chief component that links or couples electrical excitation of the sarcolemma with muscle activation of the myofilaments in the sarcomere. Mechanical activation* is finally accomplished when calcium ions bind to troponin, a regulator protein located on the actin filaments. This in turn mediates the interaction of actin and myosin.

Contractile Mechanism. As soon as the actin filaments are activated by the calcium ions, the myosin filaments become attracted to the active sites of the actin filament. This interaction pulls the actin along the immobile myosin filaments toward the center of the A band, thus shortening the sarcomere and producing muscle contraction. In this process the lengths of individual filaments remain unchanged. The I band narrows as the thick filaments approach the Z line, and the H zone narrows between the ends of the thin filaments when they meet at the center of the sarcomere (see Figure 24-1, *5a, 5b*). The greater the quantity of calcium ions delivered to troponin (a relaxing protein), the faster the rate and numbers of interactions between actin and myosin. As a result of this response, the development of tension and contractility is increased.

ATP is cleaved by myosin ATPase in the presence of magnesium. This reaction releases the energy needed to perform work. *The conversion of chemical energy to mechanical energy by ATP plays an essential role in energizing muscle shortening.* In other words, it provides energy so the actin-myosin filaments can move and produce muscle contraction. Although this is a somewhat simplified explanation of the contractile mechanism, it illustrates the events important to understanding cardiotonic drug action.

Muscle relaxation depends on removing calcium ions from the sarcomere. The calcium ATPase (located in the walls of the sarcoplasmic reticulum) actively returns calcium ions to the sarcoplasmic reticulum and the sarcolemma, thereby allowing the actin-myosin filaments of the sarcomere to return to their resting positions.

In the normal heart, the Frank-Starling relationship holds true. This relationship means that the longer the muscle fibers are at the end of **diastole** (period of heart relaxation), the more forceful the contraction during **systole** (the period of contraction). This mechanism applies only when the muscle fiber is lengthened within its physiologic limits. If a diseased heart is dilated and the fibers are stretched to a critical point beyond their limits of extensibility, the forces of contraction and cardiac output are both diminished and ineffective. Thus the functional significance of the Frank-Starling relationship is that effective cardiac output can be brought about only by adequate relaxation and refilling of cardiac chambers after each myocardial contraction.

Cardiac Conduction System

The effective pumping action of the heart depends on the regularity of events occurring in the cardiac cycle. Each cycle consists of a period of relaxation (diastole) followed by a period of contraction (systole). The rhythm and rate of the cardiac cycle are regulated by the **conduction system,** specialized tissue that has the ability to initiate and transmit the electrical impulses needed to stimulate contraction of the cardiac muscle.

The conduction system is made up of the following structures: (1) sinoatrial (SA) node, (2) internodal pathways, (3) atrioventricular (AV) node, (4) bundle of His, (5) right and left bundle branches, and (6) Purkinje fibers. The Purkinje fibers penetrate the endocardium and end in the myocardial cells. The AV node and the His area form the **AV junction,** which extends from the atrial fibers through the AV node to the bifurcation of the bundle of His. When referring to this region, the term *AV junction* is considered to be more accurate than *AV node* (Figure 24-3).

In the normal heart the SA node initiates the heartbeat. The impulses generated here are conducted through the internodal pathways to the "working" fibers of the atrial myocardium, producing atrial contraction. Electrical conduction is delayed when the impulses move through the AV junction. At the bundle of His, conduction speeds up and the impulses travel through the right bundle branch and the left bundle branch, then through the posteroinferior and anterosuperior fascicles of the left bundle branch. The transmission of impulses at the Purkinje fibers, which consist of tiny fibrils that spread around the ventricles and connect directly with the myocardial cells, is very rapid. The simultaneous depolarization of both ventricles produces ventricular contraction, resulting in **stroke volume,** the volume of blood propelled through the pulmonary artery and aorta by the ventricles.

Electrophysiologic Properties

The coordinated pumping action of the heart is initiated and regulated by specialized fibers of the conduction system. The individual fibers of this system possess three basic **electrophysiologic properties:** (1) automaticity, (2) conductivity, and (3) refractoriness.

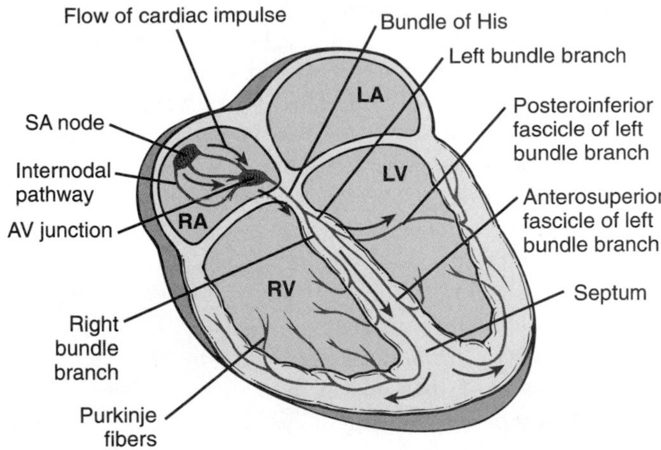

Figure 24-3 Conduction system of the heart. The cardiac impulse is initiated at the SA node and is transmitted through the internodal pathways to the two atria, resulting in atrial contraction. The electrical impulse is delayed at the AV node. Conduction speeds up at the bundle of His, with the impulse traveling through the right bundle branch and the left bundle branch and continuing through the posteroinferior fascicle and anterosuperior fascicle of the latter bundle branch. Finally, the arrival of impulses at the Purkinje fibers results in their distribution to all parts of both ventricles where, upon excitation, ventricular contraction is produced. *RA,* Right atrium; *RV,* right ventricle; *LA,* left atrium; *LV,* left ventricle.

Automaticity. The specialized fibers of the conduction system have the inherent ability to initiate a spontaneous electrical impulse without any external stimuli. This is the most fundamental mechanism of impulse formation. The cells that possess this property of **automaticity,** the ability to initiate an impulse, are called pacemaker cells. Automaticity is a property of fibers of the conduction system that normally controls heart rhythm; it is not a feature of "working" muscle—atria and ventricles.

Pacemaker cells are found in specialized conducting tissues such as the SA node, the AV junction, and the His-Purkinje system. Normally, the impulse of the heart is spontaneously and regularly initiated at the pacemaker cells of the SA node. During resting potential (phase 4), the membrane of the cell depolarizes itself—spontaneously and gradually—until it reaches threshold and an action potential occurs. The slow depolarization of the membrane in the resting state is called spontaneous diastolic depolarization, or phase 4 depolarization, and defines automaticity. Thus the membrane of pacemaker cells is never at rest; this property is attributed to the continuous influx of sodium ions into the interior of the cells, which readily drives the membrane to threshold. The resting potential of automatic pacemaker cells differs from that of the nonautomatic myocardial cells. After full repolarization, the membrane of nonautomatic myocardial cells maintains a steady resting potential until an external stimulus causes it to achieve threshold. However, under pathologic conditions, nonautomatic myocardial cells do have the potential to exhibit spontaneous depolarization.

The spontaneous excitation of pacemaker cells establishes the normal rhythm of the heart. The regularity of such pacemaking activity is termed **rhythmicity.** Under normal circumstances, only one functional pacemaker, the SA node, predominates because it has the highest frequency of depolarization. The normal rate of impulse formation is approximately 72 beats/min. If the SA node decreases its rate of impulse formation to a level below that of the AV junction (40 to 60 beats/min), then the AV junction becomes the primary pacemaker of the heart and will drive the heart at approximately 40 beats/min.

Conductivity. **Conductivity** refers to the ability to transmit an action potential or nerve impulse from cell to cell. The property of conductivity therefore exists not only in the cells of the conduction system but also in the cardiac musculature. The speed of impulse conduction varies as it passes from one tissue to another in the heart. It is slowest in the AV junction and fastest in the Purkinje fibers. The significant delay of conduction at the AV junction allows more time for ventricular filling. On the other hand, the rapid depolarization of Purkinje fibers creates an instantaneous spread of impulses from the terminals to the ventricular muscles. Simultaneous activation of the musculature is essential for producing powerful ventricular contraction.

The speed with which electrical activity is spread within the sinus node is quite slow, approximately 0.05 m/sec. The impulse then spreads out rapidly over the atrial musculature at a rate of approximately 1 m/sec. When the impulse reaches the AV node, a delay of approximately 0.05 m/sec occurs, and atrial systole takes place. The impulse then spreads rapidly, at 2 to 4 m/sec, along the right and left bundle branches and Purkinje fibers. Studies indicate that no more than 22 m/sec may elapse while the impulse is spreading. This rapid activation of contractile elements evokes a synchronous contraction of the ventricles.

The velocity of conduction is determined by the size of the resting potential of the cell membrane and the rate of rise of phase 0 of the action potential. This defines membrane responsiveness. Antidysrhythmic drugs may affect conduction by slowing the phase 0 depolarization rate, thereby decreasing membrane responsiveness.

Refractoriness. Cardiac tissue is nonresponsive to stimulation during the initial phase of systole (contraction). This nonresponsiveness is known as **refractoriness** and determines how closely together two action potentials can occur. Throughout most of repolarization, the cell cannot respond to a stimulus. The effective refractory period represents that period in the cardiac cycle during which a stimulus, no matter how strong, fails to produce an action potential. Antidysrhythmic drugs can lengthen or shorten the refractory period of cardiac tissues by influencing the level of responsiveness of the cell membrane. A relative refractory period occurs after the effective refractory period and as repolarization nears completion. During this time a propagated action potential can be elicited if the stimulus is stronger than normally required in diastole. When this happens, the fiber is stimulated to contract prematurely.

Autonomic Nervous System Control

Although the conduction system possesses the inherent ability for spontaneous, rhythmic initiation of the cardiac impulse, the autonomic nervous system has an important role in regulating the rate, rhythm, and force of myocardial contraction of the heart. The heart is innervated by both the parasympathetic and the sympathetic nerves. The vagal nerve fibers of the parasympathetic branch are found primarily in the SA node, atrial muscles, and AV junction, whereas the sympathetic fibers innervate the SA node, AV junction, and the atrial and ventricular muscles.

Vagal stimulation of the heart is mediated by the release of acetylcholine, a neurohormone that acts on the muscarinic receptors to decrease heart rate and is also believed to decrease ventricular contraction. The main effect of acetylcholine on the AV junction is to slow the rate of conduction and lengthen the refractory period. By contrast, sympathetic fiber stimulation is mediated by the release of norepinephrine, which acts specifically on the $beta_1$ receptors in the cardiac tissue. Circulating epinephrine from the adrenal medulla may also elicit cardiac responses. By acting on the beta-adrenergic receptors, norepinephrine and epinephrine increase both heart rate and the force of myocardial con-

BOX 24-1

Common Cardiac Dysrhythmias

Heart block Impaired impulse conduction through the heart; the impaired conduction usually occurs between the atria and the ventricles.

First-degree heart block Conduction time is prolonged, but all impulses are conducted from the atria to the ventricles.

Second-degree heart block Some but not all atrial impulses are conducted to the ventricles.

Third-degree heart block No atrial impulses are conducted to the ventricles.

Ectopic beats A contraction of the heart that originates at some place other than the SA node.

Extrasystole "premature beat" A premature contraction of the heart that arises independent of the normal rhythm.

Tachycardia Unusually rapid heart rate (usually over 100 beats/min in adult).

Bradycardia Unusually slow heart rate (usually less than 60 beats/min in adult).

Atrial flutter Extremely rapid rate of atrial contraction; may be 200 to 350 beats/min.

Atrial fibrillation Rapid and uncoordinated contraction of the atria.

Ventricular fibrillation Rapid and uncoordinated contraction of the ventricles; because of the incoordination of contractions, there is little or no effective pumping of blood; death will result if not immediately treated.

traction. They also increase conduction velocity and shorten the refractory period of the AV junction. Epinephrine has a very potent effect on the heart. In large doses its direct effect on the electrophysiologic properties of cardiac tissue can create cardiac dysrhythmias (Box 24-1). Normally the heartbeat is under the continuous influence of both parasympathetic and sympathetic control, with the resting heart rate the result of their opposing influences.

Electrocardiograms

Electrocardiograms (ECGs) are graphic representations of electrical currents produced by the heart. Nurses caring for clients on monitoring equipment should be able to detect and interpret changes in the cardiac rate or rhythm or in the conduction of the wave of electric activity or excitation. The ECG is a useful tool in determining the therapeutic effectiveness of certain drugs. Drugs used to treat cardiovascular disease may alter the electric activity of the heart. The ECG may provide the earliest objective evidence of the effectiveness or toxic manifestations of a drug. A knowledgeable and observant nurse can use the information obtained from the ECG to assess the effectiveness of drug therapy for cardiac dysrhythmias.

Electrical activity always precedes mechanical contraction. Immediately after a wave of electrical activity moves through atrial muscle, the muscle contracts and blood flows from the atria into the ventricles. Figure 24-4 illustrates a normal ECG. The P wave is produced by a wave of excitation through the atria (atrial depolarization). The onset of the P wave follows the firing of the SA node. After the P wave, a short pause or interval (PR interval) occurs while the electrical activity is transmitted to the AV junction, conduction tissue, and ventricles. Repolarization, or recovery, of the ventricles is indicated by the T wave. Atrial recovery or repolarization does not show on the ECG because it is hidden in the QRS complex.

Physiology of Fast and Slow Channels of Cardiovascular Fibers

A review of the normal physiology of the fast and slow channels that exist in the membrane of the cardiovascular fibers is necessary for understanding the clinical application of calcium channel blockers. The cell membrane is composed of two types of channels that are controlled by "gates." When opened, these gates allow the movement of an inward current of (1) sodium ions through the fast channels, and (2) calcium ions through the slow channels into the cell, depending on the type of fibers involved. These channels appear in the cell membrane of three types of cardiovascular fibers. The heart contains two types: (1) fast-channel fibers, which appear in the myocardial cells of the

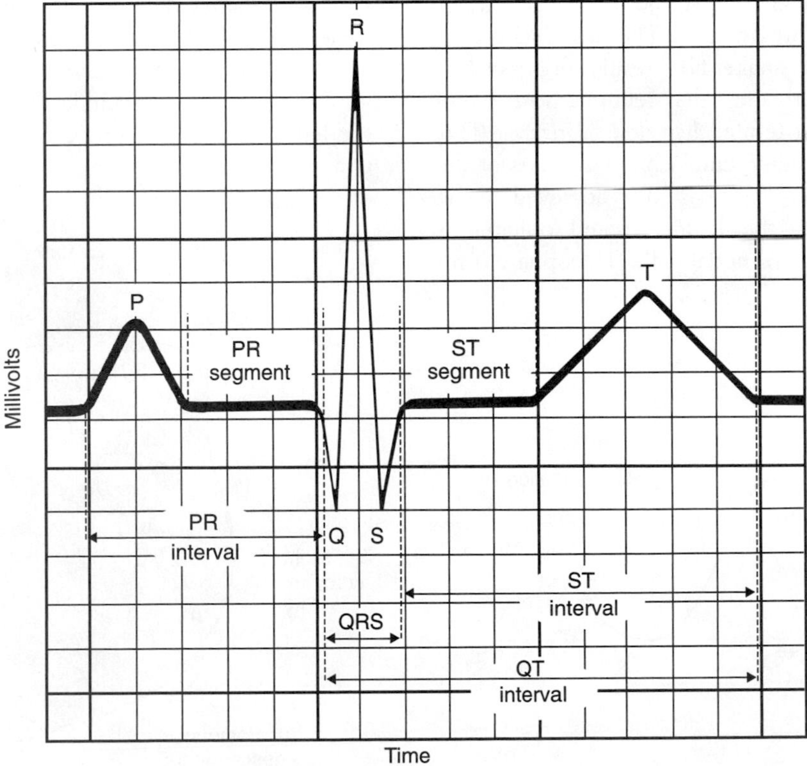

Figure 24-4 Graphic representation of the normal ECG. Vertical lines represent time, each square represents 0.04 second, and every five squares (set off by heavy black lines) represents 0.20 second. The normal PR interval is less than 0.20 second; the average is 0.16 second. The average P wave lasts 0.08 second, the QRS complex is 0.08 second, the ST segment is 0.12 second, the T wave is 0.16 second, and the QT interval is 0.32 to 0.40 second if the heart rate is 65 to 95 beats/min. Each horizontal line represents voltage; every five squares equals 0.5 millivolt.

atria and ventricles and the Purkinje fibers, and (2) slow-channel fibers, which occur in the SA node and the AV junction. The third type, slow fibers, are present in the smooth muscle of the coronary and peripheral arterial vessels.

In this mechanism, the role of calcium ions is essential in producing three physiologic processes:

1. Increasing the strength of myocardial contraction (fast fibers)
2. Enhancing automaticity and conduction speed (slow fibers)
3. Vasoconstriction of coronary arteries and peripheral arterioles (slow fibers)

As previously described, the action potential that generates excitation-contraction coupling in the fast fibers consists of five phases. Depolarization (phase 0) results from an electrical stimulus that produces a fast inward current of sodium ions (fast channel). This is followed by repolarization, which begins with a short phase 1; more important, phase 2 (the plateau phase) produces a slow inward current of calcium ions into the cell (slow channel). The influx of calcium ions is responsible for linking electrical excitation to myocardial contraction (excitation-contraction coupling), which is required to promote the sliding of actin and myosin filaments for myocardial contraction (positive inotropic effect). Rapid repolarization occurs during phase 3; finally, phase 4 reestablishes the resting state. (See the configuration of an action potential in Figure 24-2, *A.*)

In the slow fibers of the SA and AV nodes, the action potential consists of only three phases. The principal distinguishing feature of the pacemaker fiber resides in phase 4. A slow spontaneous depolarization that requires no external stimulus occurs here and is termed *diastolic depolarization.* This is responsible for automaticity. Unlike the fast fibers of the myocardium, depolarization (or phase 0) is achieved by the slower current carried by both calcium ions and sodium ions through the slow channels of nodal cells. Thus phase 0 results in a slower conduction velocity in nodal cells than in myocardial cells. Calcium channel blockers inhibit these slow channels. Repolarization is more gradual and involves only phase 3. The membrane then finally returns to phase 4 (Figure 24-5). The smooth muscle of blood vessels depends primarily on the presence of calcium ions to initiate and sustain contraction. The main source of calcium ions in cardiac muscle cells is the sarcoplasmic reticulum. In the action potential for smooth muscle, it is believed that the onset of depolarization (phase 0) is caused mainly by calcium ions rather than by sodium ions.

Calcium ions enter the smooth muscle cell through slow channels; the rise in free calcium ion concentration is considered to be the primary event in excitation-contraction coupling that is responsible for increasing muscle tone and vasoconstriction. In addition, the activation of smooth muscle can markedly reduce the caliber of small vessels, as is apparent from the "spasm" that may occur in coronary vessels. The calcium channel blockers (specifically verapamil, nifedipine, and diltiazem) are capable of blocking the slow calcium ion influx in the smooth muscle of blood vessels, thereby producing relaxation.

CORONARY VASCULAR SUPPLY

The entire blood supply to the myocardium is provided by the right and left coronary arteries, which arise from the base of the aorta (Figure 24-6). The right atrium and ventricle are supplied with blood from the right coronary artery. The left coronary artery divides into the anterior (descending) branch and the circumflex branch and supplies blood to the left atrium and ventricle. These main coronary vessels continue to divide, forming numerous branches. The result

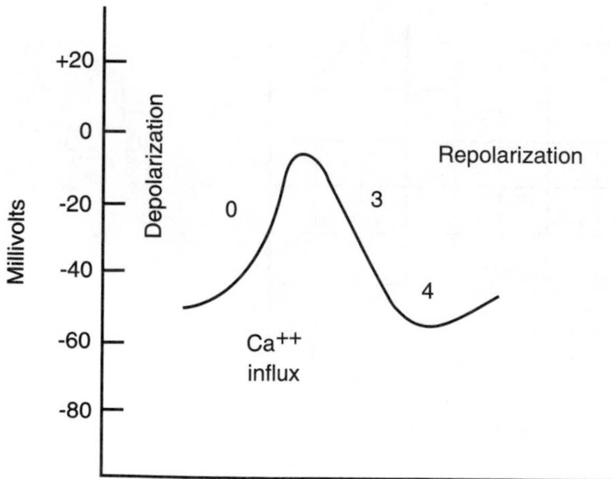

Figure 24-5 Action potential of a slow channel fiber, the SA node. It consists of three phases. Unlike the fast fibers of myocardial cells, depolarization (phase 0) is attributed primarily to Ca^{++} inflow through slow channels of the cell membrane. Repolarization involves only phase 3, which is followed by phase 4.

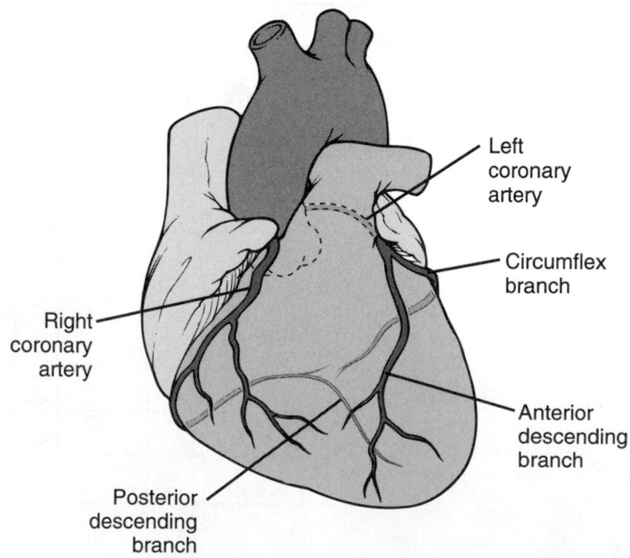

Figure 24-6 Coronary blood supply to the heart. Dark-shaded vessels are those located on the external surface of the ventricles; light-shaded vessels show the penetration of arterial branches toward the endocardial surface.

is a profuse network of coronary vessels. The major arterial vessels are located on the external surface of the ventricles. Arterial branches penetrate the myocardium toward the endocardial surface.

Increased oxygen delivery to the myocardium is supported almost exclusively by increased coronary blood flow. When the demand for oxygen and nutrients by body tissues increases, the heart must increase its output. At the same time, the heart muscle itself must be supplied with enough oxygen and nutrients to replace the energy expended. In other words, a balance must be maintained between energy expenditure and energy restoration. During systole the myocardial contraction compresses the coronary vascular bed. This restricts coronary inflow but increases coronary outflow. Coronary inflow in the left ventricle occurs primarily during diastole when the ventricles have relaxed and the coronary vessels are no longer compressed. Blood is driven through the coronary arteries by aortic pressure perfusing the myocardium.

A change in heart rate is accomplished by shortening or lengthening diastole. With tachycardia the increased number of systolic contractions per minute reduces the time available for diastole and coronary inflow. An increase also occurs in the metabolic needs of the rapidly beating heart. Coronary dilation normally occurs in an attempt to meet increased metabolic demand and to overcome restricted blood inflow. With bradycardia, the decreased number of systolic contractions per minute prolongs the diastolic period. Resistance to coronary flow and metabolic requirements of the myocardium are reduced.

Myocardial ischemia occurs whenever the delivery of oxygen to the myocardium is inadequate to meet the oxygen consumption needs of the heart. One of the major causes of ischemia is coronary artery disease, which is caused by atherosclerosis of the coronary arteries. Figure 24-7 gives an overview of heart, blood flow, and valves.

SUMMARY

It is essential for nurses to understand the electrical and physiologic properties of the heart and the effects of drugs on cardiac activity. The drugs used therapeutically affect the myocardium, the conduction system, and coronary vessels. The action of the myocardium to adjust cardiac output according to the needs of the body is based on electrical excitation, mechanical activation, and the contractile mechanism of myocardial fiber. Effective cardiac output can be achieved only with adequate relaxation and refilling of the cardiac chambers after each contraction. The cardiac conduction system initiates and transmits electrical impulses required for contraction of the myocardium. Automaticity, conductivity, and refractoriness are the essential properties of the fibers of the conduction system. The sequence of cardiac excitation is graphically represented by electrocardi-

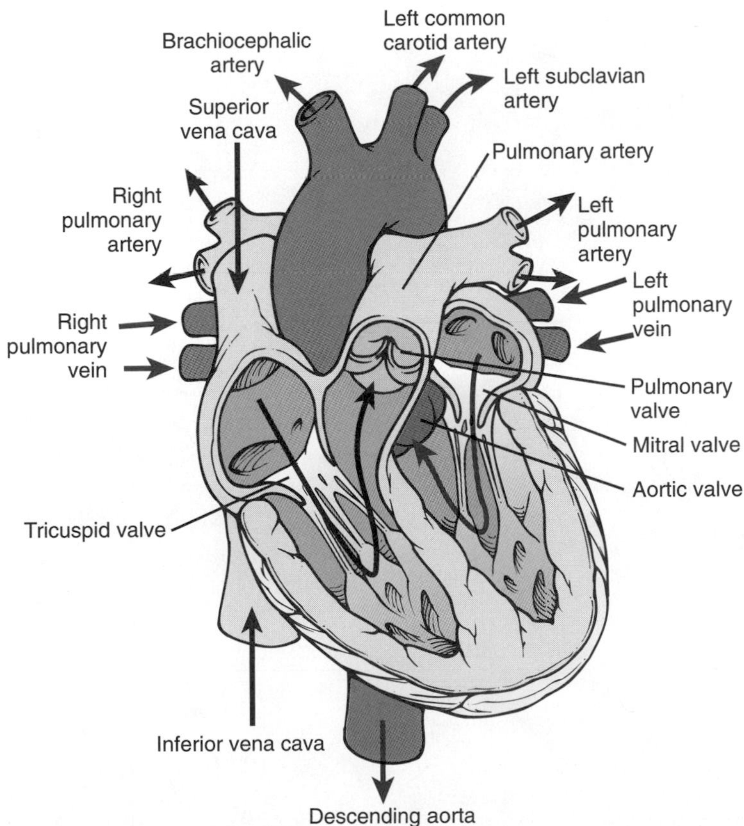

Figure 24-7 Overview of the heart, blood flow, and valves.

ography. The ECG is a useful tool for monitoring cardiac activity to assist nurses in evaluating the effectiveness of a number of drugs used to treat cardiovascular disease.

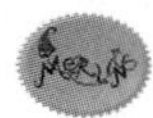

Critical Thinking Questions

1. What is the role of systole and diastole in the cardiac conduction system?
2. What are the effects of acetylcholine, norepinephrine, and epinephrine on vagal stimulation of the heart, sympathetic fiber stimulation, heart rate, myocardial contraction force, and conduction velocity?

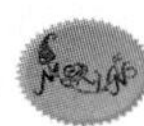

Collaborative Learning Activities

For Collaborative Learning Activities, go to mosby.com/MERLIN/McKenry/.

BIBLIOGRAPHY

Anderson, K.N., Anderson, L.E., & Glanze, W.D. (Eds.). (1998). *Mosby's medical, nursing, & allied health dictionary* (5th ed.). St. Louis: Mosby.

Hardman, J.G. & Limbird, L.E. (Eds.). (1996). *Goodman & Gilman's The pharmacological basis of therapeutics.* (9th ed.). New York: Macmillan.

Seeley, R.R., Stephens, T.D., & Tate, P. (1996). *Essentials of anatomy and physiology* (2nd ed.). St. Louis: Mosby.

Sifton, D.W. (1994). *The PDR family guide to women's health and prescription drugs.* Montvale, NJ: Medical Economics.

Thibodeau, G.A. & Patton, K.T. (1996). *Anatomy and physiology* (3rd ed.). St. Louis: Mosby.

Van Wynsberghe, D., Noback, C.R., & Carola, R. (1995). *Human anatomy and physiology* (3rd ed.). New York: McGraw-Hill.

25 Cardiac Glycosides

Chapter Focus

Cardiac glycosides have been used since the first century A.D. and are still commonly prescribed for the treatment of specific cardiac disorders. However, there is a very narrow therapeutic range, and toxicity is life threatening. Nurses must be knowledgeable about the administration of these drugs and be able to recognize the toxicities that commonly occur with them.

Learning Objectives

1. Describe right- and left-sided heart failure, including at least three major signs and symptoms.
2. Name the two primary mechanisms of action for digitalis glycosides.
3. Describe the first symptoms of digitalis toxicity and the different dysrhythmias usually seen in young children and in adults.
4. Name at least three drugs that interact with digitalis glycosides, and describe the possible effects and the management of any interaction.
5. Describe both the fast (rapid) and slow method of digitalization.
6. Discuss factors that predispose a client to digitalis toxicity.
7. Implement the nursing management for the care of clients who are receiving cardiac glycosides.

Key Terms

chronotropic, p. 532
congestive heart failure, p. 532
digitalization, p. 537
dromotropic, p. 532
inotropic, p. 532

Key Drugs [✔]

digoxin, p. 535

Various medications may change the force of myocardial contraction and the rate and rhythm of the heart. Pharmacologic terms that have specific meaning for the actions of drugs on the cardiovascular system include *inotropic, chronotropic,* and *dromotropic* effects.

Drugs with an **inotropic** (Gr. *inos,* fiber; *tropikos,* a turning or influence) effect influence myocardial contractility. Drugs with a positive inotropic effect strengthen or increase the force of myocardial contraction (e.g., digitalis, dobutamine, dopamine, epinephrine, and isoproterenol), whereas drugs with a negative inotropic effect weaken or decrease the force of myocardial contraction (e.g., lidocaine, quinidine, and propranolol).

Drugs with **chronotropic** (Gr. *chronos,* time) action affect heart rate. A positive chronotropic effect is produced if the drug accelerates the heart rate by increasing the rate of impulse formation in the sinoatrial (SA) node (e.g., norepinephrine). A negative chronotropic drug has the opposite effect and slows the heart rate by decreasing impulse formation (e.g., acetylcholine).

A **dromotropic** (Gr. *dromos,* a course) effect refers to drugs that affect conduction velocity through specialized conducting tissues. A drug having a positive dromotropic action speeds conduction (e.g., phenytoin), whereas a drug with a negative dromotropic action delays conduction (e.g., verapamil).

Drugs in the digitalis group are among the oldest drugs known as therapeutic agents for the treatment of heart failure. The effects of digitalis glycosides are twofold. They increase the strength of contraction (positive inotrope), and they alter the electrophysiologic properties of the heart by slowing the heart rate (negative chronotrope) and by slowing conduction velocity (negative dromotrope). Other agents may produce varying effects with the same objective of treating heart failure. To better understand the beneficial and toxic effects of the digitalis glycosides and other agents, the mechanisms of heart failure will first be described.

HEART FAILURE

Congestive heart failure (CHF) occurs in 2 to 4 million Americans annually, nearly twice as often in males as in females. After 50 years of age, the prevalence of CHF increases in every decade of life until approximately 9% of the population over age 80 is affected (Kradjan, 1995). CHF is primarily a disease of older adults, with 10% of the clients dying within 1 year; the 5-year mortality rate is 50% (Agency for Health Care Policy and Research, 1994; Hsu, 1996). Heart failure is the leading cause of hospitalization in adults older than 65 years, and it is currently the most costly cardiovascular disorder in the United States, with estimated annual expenditures in excess of $20 billion (Rich & Nease, 1999). Because CHF adversely affects quality of life and has a high mortality rate, an understanding of its etiology and the appropriate interventions is important.

CHF, or pump failure, is a pathologic state in which the weakened myocardium is unable to pump sufficient blood from the ventricles (i.e., cardiac output) to sustain the normal circulation required to meet the metabolic demands of the body organs. The etiologic factors of heart failure are listed in Box 25-1. Despite the etiologic factors, depressed myocardial contractility is primarily the underlying cause of heart failure. Therefore it is important to identify and remove the cause and correct the problem whenever possible and then to treat the heart failure state as follows:

1. Remove excess water and salt in the body. Sodium restrictions, reduction of physical activity, and initiation of diuretic and/or digitalis glycoside therapy are the usual measures.
2. Enhance myocardial contraction. The positive inotropic effect of digitalis glycosides has been related to excitation-contraction coupling. (See Chapter 24 for an explanation of this phenomenon.)

The nurse should be aware that some drugs may exacerbate or precipitate CHF (Box 25-2). Many drugs also contain sodium; avoiding their use must be considered with a salt-restricted diet (Table 25-1).

Pathogenesis. On a cellular level, heart failure may be associated with a defect in excitation-contraction coupling, and in some individuals dysfunction of *contractile proteins* may occur as an additional abnormality. Ineffective calcium pumping by the sarcoplasmic reticulum may alter the normal relaxation process. Furthermore, the mitochondria—*not* the sarcoplasmic reticulum—may act as the dominant calcium uptake storage site. If so, less calcium is available for release from the sarcoplasmic reticulum to activate contraction. Thus the amount of coupling is reduced, and depressed myocardial contractility ensues.

With regard to the dysfunction of contractile proteins in heart failure, attention has been focused on abnormal energy utilization. Some researchers have shown that the activity of myosin adenosine triphosphatase (ATPase) is decreased. When the activity of this enzyme is reduced in heart failure, the interaction between actin and myosin fila-

BOX 25-1

Etiology of Heart Failure

Organic Heart Disorders

Cardiac dysrhythmia
Hypertension
Infective endocarditis
Valvular disorders (e.g., mitral valve stenosis, regurgitation)
Myocardial infarction
Pulmonary embolism

Other Causes

Alcoholism
Anemia
Hyperthyroidism
Liver disease
Nutritional deficiency
Renal disease

ments is reduced in intensity, and thus the force of contractility is lowered.

An important consequence of inadequate performance of the myocardium is hemodynamic alterations. Compensatory mechanisms are activated, and incomplete emptying of the heart during ventricular systole eventually allows blood to accumulate inside the heart chambers. This accumulation causes dilation or enlargement of the heart and is referred to as low output, systolic dysfunction. During this process, blood backs up into the atria. This condition can lead to pulmonary congestion in the left atrium; systemic congestion, including ascites, may occur in the right atrium. During the interim, the heart attempts to pump the blood forward in the circulation, but instead the increased fluid in the left ventricle produces stretching of the myocardial fibers and dilation of the ventricles.

Athletes commonly have cardiac hypertrophy, which is an enlargement of cardiac muscle and the ventricular chambers. As a result, the overall effectiveness of the heart as a pump is increased. The Frank-Starling law states that an increase in the length of the muscle fibers of the heart results in increased contraction and cardiac output. This stretching of cardiac muscle results from increased preload, an increased amount of blood returning to the heart and entering the heart chambers. The more the cardiac muscles are stretched during diastole, the greater the contraction in systole.

BOX 25-2

Drugs That May Precipitate or Exacerbate Congestive Heart Failure

Drugs That Cause Sodium and Water Retention or Expand Intravascular Volume

Albumin
Androgens
Corticosteroids (e.g., cortisone, hydrocortisone, fludrocortisone [Florinef])
Diazoxide (Proglycem, Hyperstat)
Estrogens
Guanethidine (Ismelin)
Mannitol
Methyldopa (Aldomet)
Minoxidil (Loniten)
NSAIDs
Urea

Drugs That Inhibit Myocardial Contractility (Negative Inotropic or Cardiotoxic Agents)

Beta-blocking agents
Calcium channel blockers (especially verapamil)
Disopyramide (Norpace)
Doxorubicin (Adriamycin)
Quinidine

TABLE 25-1 Sodium Content of Selected Prescription and Over-the-Counter Medications

Medications	Sodium/Unit	Sodium/Maximum Daily Dose (Adult)
Antibiotics		
carbenicillin disodium (Geopen, Pyopen)	108-150 mg/g	4.5 to 6 g/40 g
ticarcillin injection (Ticar)	120-150 mg/g	2.9 to 3.6 g/24 g
ampicillin sodium (Polycillin-N, Omnipen-N, and others)	62-78 mg/g	1 to 1.2 g/16 g
cephalosporins		
cefamandole naftate (Mandol)	77 mg/g	0.9 g/12 g
ceftriaxone sodium (Rocephin)	83 mg/g	0.33 g/4 g
cephradine injection (Velosef)	136 mg/g	1 g/8 g
Over-the-Counter Medications		
Alka-Seltzer Effervescent Pain Reliever and Antacid Tablets	0.5 g/tablet	
Alka-Seltzer, Lemon-Lime	506 mg/tablet	
Alka-Seltzer, Original	567 mg/tablet	
Bellans	144 mg/tablet	
Bromo-Seltzer powder	0.76 g/capful	
Eno Powder	0.8 g/teaspoon	
Rolaids	53 mg/tablet	
Soda Mint Tablets	90 mg/tablet	
Food Supplements		
Ensure	844 mg/L	
Meritene	880-1078 mg/L	
Osmolite	549 mg/L	
Sustacal	924-940 mg/L	

CHF is a myocardial dysfunction resulting in a decreased cardiac output. Regardless of the primary cause, the result is that preload can increase until a massive overload results. The ventricles are unable to meet the needs for contraction or pumping. Mechanisms to compensate, involving sympathoadrenergic stimulation, may occur as the body attempts to maintain an adequate cardiac output. The increased heart rate and peripheral vascular resistance also elevate the heart's demand for oxygen, thus further contributing to myocardial dysfunction. The inability to obtain adequate cardiac output is referred to as myocardial insufficiency or cardiac decompensation. Chronic progressive ventricular failure generally leads to CHF, which means that the ability of the heart to contract decreases to the extent that the heart pumps out less blood than it receives. Subsequently, myocardial infarction produces circulatory failure.

A decrease in cardiac output means that less blood is in the blood vessels and that the various organs of the body are receiving less blood. The kidneys respond by retaining more water and electrolytes, producing fluid retention and electrolyte disturbances. This is called right-sided heart failure; the clinical signs include jugular vein distention, hepatomegaly, ascites, and peripheral edema. Left-sided heart failure leads to fluid accumulation in the lungs—pulmonary edema—which produces dyspnea and interferes with oxygen and carbon dioxide exchange. Failure of one side of the heart is usually followed by failure of the other side, which produces complete heart failure (Figure 25-1).

In summary, the failing heart may show increases in both preload (increased blood volume return to the heart chambers) and afterload (the increased pressure in the aorta that the ventricle muscles must overcome to open the aortic valve and push blood through). The decrease in renal perfusion just described may activate the renin-angiotensin-aldosterone (RAA) feedback mechanism. Sodium and water are then retained, and intravascular volume and blood flow back to the heart increase. In less serious situations this is usually enough to maintain arterial blood pressure, and the RAA system is turned off. Sodium and water are retained, and intravascular volume and blood flow back to the heart increases. However, in individuals who have conditions bordering on heart failure, this can produce a frank decompensation or acute heart failure. The increase in circulatory blood volume increases the demands on the heart, which may result in acute pulmonary edema.

General Treatment Goals. The overall treatment goals for CHF are multiple. It is necessary to treat any correctable underlying causes of the heart failure, such as hypertension or dysrhythmias. Following nonpharmacologic recommendations, such as dietary restrictions (sodium consumption restricted to 2 to 3 g/day, alcohol consumption limited to one drink per day, avoidance of excessive fluid intake) and activity (exercise, when appropriate during the treatment program), is essential. Counseling the client and family members on the signs and symptoms of heart failure and the need to adhere to the nonpharmacologic and pharmaco-

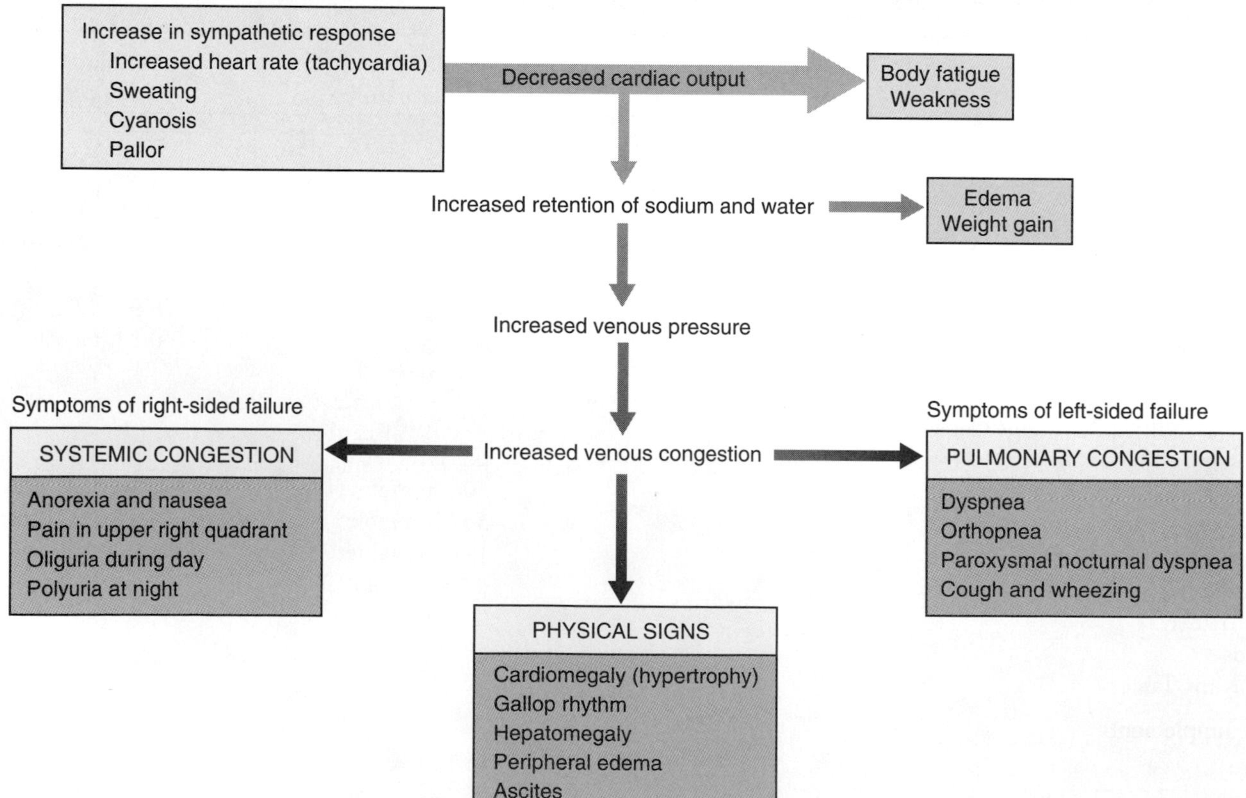

Figure 25-1 Signs and symptoms of heart failure.

logic treatments as prescribed are also fundamental to the management of CHF.

Drug therapy is also a combined approach. Diuretics are prescribed to reduce the increase in blood volume and edema. An angiotensin-converting enzyme (ACE) inhibitor (e.g., enalapril, captopril) is usually prescribed for left-ventricular systolic dysfunction. Vasodilators, such as nitrates that pool blood in the extremities and so reduce blood return or preload, as well as arterial vasodilators that decrease arterial resistance and reduce afterload, may also be part of the therapy. Dobutamine to increase myocardial contractility (see Chapter 22) and the cardiotonic drugs such as digitalis glycosides to increase cardiac contractility are also used.

ACE inhibitors decrease peripheral vascular resistance (afterload), pulmonary capillary wedge pressure (preload), pulmonary vascular resistance, and the secretion of aldosterone; thus these are important drugs in the treatment of heart failure. Although digoxin improves some symptoms, there is conflicting or no evidence that it alone improves client survival (AHCPR, 1994; Kienle, 1995). The ACE inhibitors are discussed in Chapter 27. This chapter focuses on digitalis glycosides, digoxin immune Fab (Digibind), inamrinone (Inocor), and milrinone lactate (Primacor).

DIGITALIS GLYCOSIDES

The story of the origin of digitalis is interesting in that it was an herbal remedy used for hundreds of years by common people (called "housewife's recipe"). Farmers and housewives prepared the remedy for dropsy (fluid accumulation). More than 400 years ago Dr. Leonhard Fuchs recommended that physicians use it "to scatter the dropsy, to relieve swelling of the liver, and even to bring on menstrual flow" (Silverman, 1942). Dr. Fuchs was a botanist-physician, and at that time the medical profession paid little attention to a "mere flower picker."

In the mid-1700s a female client shared an old family recipe for curing dropsy with Dr. William Withering. Dr. Withering used this recipe for his dropsy clients and, after spending 10 years studying digitalis, published his conclusions in *An Account of the Foxglove*. This remarkable publication stressed instructions that are still valid today—the necessity of individualizing dosage according to the client's response. Digitalis was finally admitted to the London Pharmacopeia in 1722.

The digitalis glycosides belong to many different botanical families. The action of each is fundamentally the same; with minor differences, the description for digitalis applies to all of them. The principal forms are discussed here.

digitoxin [di ji tox′ in] (Digitaline ✤)
100 **digoxin** [di jox′ in] (Lanoxin ◆, Lanoxicaps)

Digoxin is the most commonly used digitalis glycoside and is generally considered the prototype drug in this classification. Digoxin affects cardiac function through two important mechanisms: (1) positive inotropic action, and (2) negative chronotropic and negative dromotropic actions.

Digitoxin has been discontinued in the United States but may be available in other countries.

Positive Inotropic Action. The main function of digitalis is inotropic action. The increased myocardial contractility is associated with more efficient use of available energy. If the failing heart is enlarged, the positive inotropic action of digitalis can cause the myocardium to beat more forcefully, thereby increasing cardiac output and decreasing oxygen use. The improved pumping action of the heart in individuals with CHF may reach levels that approach normal because the net effect is not only reduced heart size but also decreased venous pressure to relieve edema.

Although the positive inotropic mechanism is not precisely known, one theory asserts that digitalis is bound to sites on the myocardial cell membrane (sarcolemma), where it inhibits the action of membrane-bound Na^+-K^+-ATPase enzyme. Normally this enzyme hydrolyzes ATP to provide the energy needed by the Na^+-K^+ pump to release Na^+ and transport K^+ into the cardiac cell during repolarization. By binding specifically to Na^+-K^+-ATPase, digitalis inhibits the active transport of Na^+ and K^+ (Figure 24-1, *5b*). Intracellular Na^+ accumulates, which stimulates the release of large quantities of free calcium ion from the sarcoplasmic reticulum. The free calcium ion is essential for linking the electrical excitation of the cell membrane to the mechanical contraction of the myocardial cell, a mechanism known as excitation-contraction coupling.

More free calcium ion produces a greater degree of coupling of actin and myosin to form actinomyosin, which results in more forceful myocardial contraction with a concomitant increase in cardiac output. Inhibition of Na^+-K^+-ATPase activity is projected to be the mechanism by which the digitalis glycosides increase myocardial contraction without causing increased oxygen consumption. (See Myocardial Contraction in the Cardiac Muscle, Chapter 24.)

Negative Chronotropic and Negative Dromotropic Actions. Digitalis has negative chronotropic effects (decreased heart rate) and negative dromotropic effects (slowed conduction velocity) because it can alter three electrophysiologic properties of cardiac tissues:

1. *Automaticity.* Cardiac tissue has the inherent ability to initiate and propagate an impulse without external stimulation. This property affects the rate and rhythm of the heart. Low to moderate doses of digitalis slow the heart rate because the SA node depolarizes less frequently. On the other hand, toxic concentrations of digitalis can directly increase automaticity. This increases the rate of both action potentials and spontaneous depolarization. This is one of the mechanisms responsible for digitalis-induced ectopic pacemakers. Toxic doses of digitalis may significantly increase impulse formation in latent or potential pacemaker tissue, causing dysrhythmia.

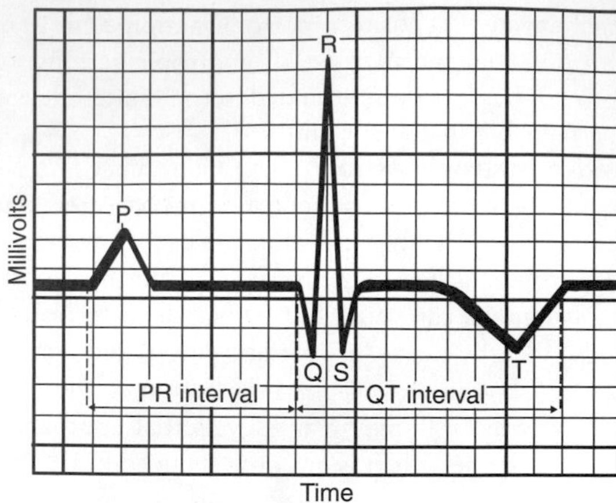

Figure 25-2 Representation of the typical effects of digitalization on the electric activity of the heart as shown on the ECG. Note the prolonged PR interval, the shortened QT interval, and the T-wave inversion.

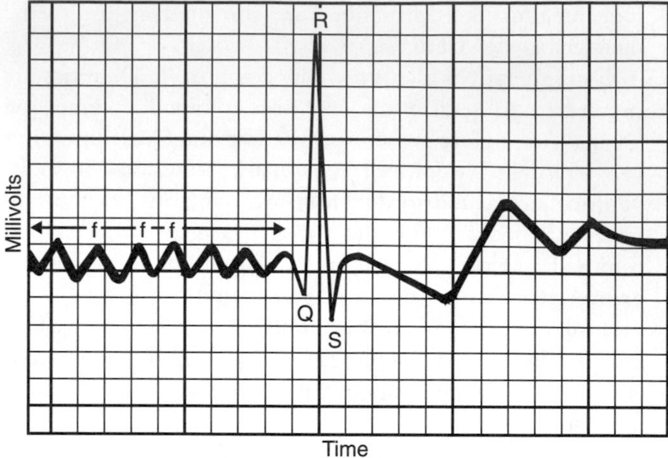

Figure 25-3 Graphic representation of atrial fibrillation as seen on the electrocardiographic monitor or tracing paper. No true P waves are noted, but f (fibrillation) waves consisting of rapid, small, and irregular waves are noted. The QRS complex is normal in configuration and duration but occurs irregularly.

2. *Conduction velocity.* All concentrations of digitalis decrease conduction velocity. Atrioventricular (AV) conduction velocity is slowed both by the direct action of digitalis and by increased vagal action. The ECG shows a prolonged PR interval, and in toxic doses the drug can lead to increased heart block (Figure 25-2).
3. The *refractory period* effects of digitalis vary in different parts of the heart. If the refractory period in the ventricles is reduced, nearly toxic amounts of digitalis are required. A prolonged refractory period occurs in the AV conduction system, which is very sensitive to digitalis action. This action is partly direct and partly caused by increased vagal tone. Toxic doses of digitalis may prolong the refractory period and depress conduction in the AV conduction system until complete heart block may occur.

Congestive Heart Failure. A heart in failure is no longer capable of supplying body tissue with adequate oxygen and nutrients or of removing metabolic waste products. The positive inotropic effect of digitalis that results in increased myocardial contractility benefits the client with a failing heart. The increased force of systolic contraction causes the ventricles to empty more completely. A slower heart rate permits more complete filling, which results in the following:

1. Venous pressure falls, and the pulmonary and systemic congestion and their accompanying signs and symptoms are either diminished or completely abolished.
2. Coronary circulation is enhanced, myocardial oxygen demand is reduced, and the supply of oxygen and nutrients to the myocardium is improved.
3. Heart size is often decreased toward normal.

Some cardiac glycosides have a true but mild diuretic effect. However, marked diuresis in a client with edema primarily results from improved heart action, improved circulation to all body tissues, and improved tissue and organ function, including renal function. When digitalis is effective, the client is noticeably improved and has an increased sense of well-being.

Atrial Fibrillation. During atrial fibrillation several hundred impulses originate from the atria, but only a fraction of them are transmitted through the AV junction. Figure 25-3 shows the electrocardiographic pattern of atrial fibrillation. Digitalis is ideal for slowing the ventricular rate because it increases the refractory period of the AV junction and also slows conduction at this site. It is important to know that the purpose of using digitalis in atrial fibrillation is to slow the ventricular rate to reduce the possibility of inducing ventricular tachycardia. It also may prevent or eliminate cardiac failure. Digitalis does not convert the fibrillating atria into normally contracting ones.

Indications. Digoxin and digitoxin are used in the treatment of CHF and in the treatment or prevention of cardiac dysrhythmias, especially atrial fibrillation, atrial flutter, and paroxysmal atrial tachycardia. These agents are more effective in low output heart failure (depressed ventricular function) than in high output failure (anemia, AV fistula, bronchopulmonary insufficiency).

Pharmacokinetics. The bioavailability of digoxin is approximately 60% to 80% with tablets, 70% to 85% with the elixir, and 90% to 100% with the capsule dosage form. Digitoxin is very lipophilic and therefore is almost completely absorbed orally. Digitalis glycosides can be categorized into two main groups: rapid-acting agents and long-acting agents. Table 25-2 lists specific pharmacokinetic information for digitalis glycosides.

Side Effects/Adverse Reactions. The side effects/adverse reactions of the digitalis glycosides include anorexia, nausea, bradycardia, stomach pain, and dysrhythmias. The dysrhythmias seen with digitalis toxicity are premature ven-

TABLE 25-2 Digitalis Glycosides: Pharmacokinetics

Drug	Route	Onset of Action	Peak Effect (hours)	Plasma Half-life	Duration of Action	Therapeutic Plasma Level (ng/mL)	Metabolism	Excretion
Rapid Acting								
digoxin (Lanoxin)	IV	5-30 minutes	1-4	36-48 hours	6 days	0.5-2	Liver	Kidney (50%-70% unchanged)
	Oral	½-2 hours	2-6	36-48 hours	6 days	0.5-2	Liver	Same as above
Long Acting								
digitoxin (Crystodigin)	Oral	1-4 hours	8-14	5-9 days	14 days	13-25	Liver	Kidney (metabolites)

tricular beats, paroxysmal atrial tachycardia with AV block, progressing AV blocks, and ventricular dysrhythmias such as ventricular tachycardia (*United States Pharmacopeia Dispensing Information,* 1999). A loss of appetite is usually the first sign of toxicity; nausea and vomiting and abdominal distress usually occur several days after the anorexia.

Although glycoside serum levels are of limited value in establishing therapeutic serum levels, they are sometimes helpful as an indicator of toxicity. For example, older adults may have age-related renal or hepatic impairment and a decreased volume of distribution for digitalis; thus lower dosages are necessary to avoid digitalis toxicity.

Dosage and Administration. See Table 25-3 for the dosage and administration of the digitalis glycosides. The maintenance dosage of digoxin for adults is usually 0.125 mg or 0.25 mg PO daily; the adult dosage of digitoxin is 0.05 to 0.3 mg PO daily. The pediatric dosage is usually one fifth to one third of the total digitalization daily dose. (See the Special Considerations for Children box on p. 540.)

The nurse should also be aware of the following issues related to the administration of the digitalis glycosides.

Bioavailability. Bioavailability (discussed in more detail in Chapter 3) refers to the amount of administered drug that is usable in the target tissue. Bioavailability must be considered when a client is transferred from one dosage form to another; a dosage adjustment may be required to compensate for the pharmacokinetic differences of the dosage form. A 100-μg (0.1-mg) dose of the injection or of the digoxin-solution capsule is bioequivalent to a 125-μg (0.125-mg) dose of the tablet or elixir. This difference in bioavailability must be kept in mind when switching clients from capsules to tablets or vice versa.

Digitalization. **Digitalization** is the saturation of body tissues with enough digitalis to cause the signs and symptoms of heart failure to disappear. Although nomograms and formula calculations are available to estimate digoxin dosage based on lean body weight and renal function, most prescribers still prescribe digoxin according to the client's body weight (see Table 25-3). However, digitalis glycosides have a very narrow therapeutic index; in other words, the therapeutic dose is very close to the toxic dose. Many clients experience digitalis toxicity, so it is vital for the nurse to monitor for, and to teach the client to watch for, signs and symptoms of improvement and of drug toxicity. Drug serum levels should also be monitored. There are essentially two methods of digitalization: the rapid (fast) method, which requires hospitalization of the client, and the slow method, which is usually prescribed in an ambulatory setting.

The rapid digitalization (loading) method is reserved for the client who is in acute distress from heart failure. If the client has not previously received any digitalis glycoside, IV digoxin is given in divided doses in a 24-hour period. The goal of treatment is to obtain the maximum therapeutic effect of the glycoside as rapidly as possible. With this method, the drug toxicities quickly become evident, while the client is in the controlled environment of the hospital unit. An advantage is that the toxicities can be easily correlated to a specific drug concentration. For example, the prescriber decides to administer a total IV dose of 1 mg digoxin. Digoxin may be prescribed as 0.5 mg IV now and 0.25 mg IV every 6 hours for two doses (for a total of 1 mg). The nurse is expected to observe the client for signs of improvement. If the client demonstrates digitalis toxicity after the 1-mg dose, the prescriber will know that this person is not able to tolerate a 1-mg total dose and in the future will avoid any dosage regimen that might reach this level.

In general, the slow method of digitalization is used in less acute situations in the ambulatory setting. The length of time before an individual reaches full digitalization is much longer than with the rapid method. A daily oral maintenance dose of digitalis may be prescribed, with the client not reaching full digitalization until approximately the fifth half-life of the drug. Digoxin, which has a 36-hour half-life, takes approximately 7 days for digitalization, whereas digi-

TABLE 25-3 Digitalis Glycosides: Dosage and Administration

Drug	Route	Dosage Range: Digitalizing (Loading)	Dosage Range: Maintenance
digitoxin (Crystodigin, Digitaline ♣)	Oral	Adults: RAPID: 0.6 mg initially, followed in 4-6 hours by 0.4 mg, then 0.2 mg q4-6h SLOW: 0.2 mg 2 times daily for 4 days Children: Not recommended	0.05-0.3 mg/day
digoxin (Lanoxicaps, Lanoxin)	IV	Adults: 0.4-0.6 mg initially, then 0.1-0.3 mg q6-8h as needed	0.125-0.5 mg daily as a single dose or in divided doses daily
	IV	Children: give in the following divided doses—½ dose at once, remainder in fractional doses at 4-8 hour intervals: Premature infant, rapid: 15-25 μg/kg	20%-30% of loading dose daily in divided doses
		Full-term infant, rapid: 20-30 μg/kg	20%-35% of loading dose daily in divided doses
		Infant (1-24 months), rapid: 30-50 μg/kg	25%-35% of loading dose daily in divided doses
	IV	Children: 2 to 5 years: 25-35 μg/kg 5 to 10 years: 15-30 μg/kg Over 10 years: 8-12 μg/kg	25%-35% of loading dose in divided doses 2 or 3 times daily
	Tablet	Adults: RAPID: 0.75-1.25 mg divided into 2 or more doses, each administered at 6-8 hour intervals SLOW: 0.125-0.5 mg once daily for 7 days	0.125-0.5 mg once daily
		Children: 2 to 10 years: 0.03-0.04 mg/kg in divided doses q6-8h	20%-30% of digitalizing dose daily
	Capsule	Adults: RAPID: 0.4-0.6 mg, followed by 0.1-0.3 mg q6-8h as necessary SLOW: 0.05-0.35 mg daily in 2 divided doses; repeat dose for 1-3 weeks to reach steady-state serum levels Children: See current literature, because dosages vary according to age	0.05-0.35 mg PO once or twice daily, as necessary

toxin (with a half-life of 7.5 days) requires more than a month.

The advantages of the slow method include the following: (1) the individual may be treated on an outpatient basis, (2) it is a safer method, (3) close monitoring is not required, and (4) the doses may be taken orally. The following are disadvantages of the slow method: (1) the extended length of time before the individual is digitalized, and (2) the difficulty in determining when digitalis toxicity occurs, because the onset of symptoms may be very gradual. According to the Clinical Practice Guidelines of the Agency for Health Care Policy and Research, loading doses of digoxin are usually unnecessary *(AHCPR,* 1994).

■ Nursing Management
Digitalis Glycoside Therapy

■ **Assessment.** The client's health status should be assessed for underlying conditions (e.g., ventricular fibrillation or a toxic effect from a previous administration of the drug) for which digitalis glycosides might be contraindicated. Digitalis glycosides are to be used cautiously when the following conditions are noted:

- *Dysrhythmias.* Dysrhythmias may be caused by underlying heart disease or reflect digitalis intoxication; the drug should be withheld if the latter occurs.
- *Progression of AV block.* Incomplete AV block may progress to advanced or complete heart block in digi-

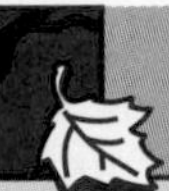

Special Considerations for Older Adults
Cardiac Glycosides

The administration of digoxin, one of the most commonly prescribed drugs in the world, must be closely monitored; the treatment dose is approximately 60% of the toxic dose (Long & Rybacki, 1995). Older adults often have a reduced tolerance for the cardiac glycosides; thus lower dosages may be necessary to reduce the potential for drug toxicity.

Early toxic signs often include anorexia, nausea, and vomiting; difficulty with reading, which may appear as visual alterations such as green and yellow vision, double vision, or seeing spots or halos; headaches; dizziness; fatigue; weakness; confusion; depression; increased nervousness; and diarrhea. Decreased libido and impotency have been reported in approximately 35% of males as a result of the estrogen-type effects of digoxin. Breast enlargement and breast tenderness have also been reported in males (Long & Rybacki, 1995).

Be aware that exercise reduces serum levels of digoxin because of increased uptake in skeletal muscles. The nurse must be cognizant of the physical activity of clients who are taking digoxin (Semla, Beizer, & Higbee, 1993).

Research indicates that bisacodyl (Dulcolax, Fleet Laxative) may reduce the absorption of digoxin (Lanoxin) (Graedon & Graedon, 1995). Do not administer these drugs concurrently.

talizing clients; this means that heart failure may need to be managed by other measures.

- *Older adults.* Because of their small body mass (i.e., lean body weight) and frequent renal impairments, older adults must be given digoxin cautiously. Digoxin has been identified as a cause of drug-induced cognitive impairment in older adults (Moore & O'Keefe, 1999). Digitoxin is less affected by renal function impairment (see the Special Considerations for Older Adults box above).
- *Clients with electronic cardiac pacemakers.* These clients require careful titration of their dosage because they may demonstrate symptoms of toxicity at dosages usually tolerated by other individuals.
- *Electrolyte imbalances.* Hypokalemia and hypomagnesemia increase the risk of digitalis toxicity. Exercise great caution in giving the drug to clients with hypercalcemia and hyperkalemia to avoid digitalis-induced dysrhythmia, principally heart block. Hypocalcemia may decrease the effectiveness of digitalis glycosides; calcium supplementation may be necessary.
- *Ventricular dysrhythmias.* Clients with premature ventricular contractions or ventricular tachycardia are at risk for exacerbation with the administration of digitalis glycosides.
- *Myocardial pathology.* Clients with acute myocarditis or myocardial infarction or ischemic heart disease are at higher risk for digitalis-induced dysrhythmias because of their increased sensitivity to the effects of the drug.
- *Conduction disorders.* The condition of clients with Wolff-Parkinson-White or sick sinus syndrome may worsen.
- *Renal dysfunction.* Clients with renal impairment (digoxin only) or acute glomerulonephritis may have reduced excretion and so a greater risk of toxicity.
- *Myxedema, severe pulmonary disease, or carotid sinus hypersensitivity.* These conditions may predispose the client to the toxic effect of digitalis glycosides.

Review the client's current medication regimen for the risk of significant drug interactions, such as those that may occur when digitalis glycosides are given concurrently with the following drugs:

Drug	Possible Effect and Management
Bold/color type indicates the most serious interactions.	
amiodarone (Cordarone)	May increase digoxin serum levels (and possibly other digitalis glycosides) to toxic levels. Reduce the dosage of digitalis preparation, and monitor serum digoxin levels closely.
antacids (especially aluminum and magnesium types)	May decrease digitalis absorption 25% to 35%. Space medications apart, preferably giving digitalis 1 to 2 hours before antacids.
antidiarrheal adsorbents (e.g., kaolin, pectin), cholestyramine (Questran), colestipol (Colestid), or large quantities of dietary fiber (bran)	May reduce the absorption of digitalis, resulting in a decreased therapeutic response. Administer digitalis products 1 to 2 hours before these agents, then monitor closely for the effectiveness of digitalis.
antidysrhythmic agents, injectable calcium salts, succinylcholine, or sympathomimetics	**Concurrent administration may enhance the risk of cardiac dysrhythmias. Avoid concurrent use or a potentially serious drug interaction may occur.**
calcium channel blocking agents (verapamil [Calan, Isoptin], diltiazem [Cardizem])	Concurrent use may require reduced digitalis dosages. Monitor closely for digitalis-related dysrhythmias.
indomethacin (Indocin)	Renal excretion of digitalis is reduced, leading to increased serum levels and possible toxicity. Reduce the dosage of digitalis by 50% when indomethacin is started. Monitor closely for both therapeutic and toxic effects, and make dosage adjustments accordingly.
magnesium sulfate injection	**Use with extreme caution in individuals receiving digitalis. Alterations in cardiac conduction and heart block may result. Avoid concurrent use or a potentially serious drug interaction may occur.**

Continued

Drug	Possible Effect and Management
potassium-depleting drugs, such as amphotericin B (parenteral), corticosteroids, or potassium-depleting diuretics	If used concurrently with digitalis preparations, the potential for inducing hypokalemia with these medications may increase the possibility of digitalis toxicity. Monitor potassium levels closely, and monitor the client for signs and symptoms of hypokalemia.
potassium salts	Although potassium salts are commonly prescribed to treat hypokalemia, especially when clients are also taking a digitalis glycoside, potassium salts are not indicated in clients with severe heart block who are receiving digitalis. Hyperkalemia may be very dangerous in such individuals.
propafenone (Rhythmol)	Concurrent use may increase digoxin levels by 25% to 85%, resulting in digitalis toxicity. Careful monitoring of serum digoxin levels and dosage adjustments may be necessary.
quinidine	May result in increased serum levels of digoxin and digitoxin. Monitor serum levels and the client's response closely; dosage reductions may be necessary.
spironolactone (Aldactone)	Concurrent administration may increase the half-life of digoxin. Monitor closely; a dosage reduction may be needed.
sucralfate (Carafate)	Concurrent use decreases the absorption of digoxin; space apart by at least 2 hours.

A baseline assessment of the client with CHF should include the following: weight; blood pressure, pulse pressure, and any postural change in blood pressure; apical pulse rate and rhythm; apical-radial pulse deficit; heart sounds; jugular vein distention; edema; lung sounds; capillary refill time; skin color and temperature; urinary output; determination of the presence of chest discomfort (pain or pressure), shortness of breath, syncope, fatigue, nausea, and perception of heart rate ("skipping beats"); level of consciousness and anxiety; cardiac enzymes; hepatic function studies, serum electrolyte levels, blood urea nitrogen (BUN), and creatinine levels; and ECG.

■ **Nursing Diagnosis.** The client receiving digitalis glycosides is at risk for the following selected nursing diagnoses/collaborative problems: impaired comfort (headache, nausea, vomiting); disturbed sensory perception (halos of green-yellow light around objects); diarrhea; disturbed thought processes (confusion); risk for injury (electrolyte imbalance, drowsiness, fainting); and the potential complications of allergic reaction, mental depression, decreased cardiac output, and dysrhythmias.

■ Implementation

■ ***Monitoring.*** Because altered cardiac output may occur in relation to the positive inotropic effects of the drug, measure the adult client's apical pulse for 1 minute before drug administration. Note the rate, rhythm, and quality of pulse. If the pulse is 60 beats/min or below or if a dysrhythmia that had not previously occurred is noted, withhold the drug and report immediately to the prescriber. In children, measure the apical pulse 1 minute before administering the drug. Consult with the prescriber to determine the apical rate at which the drug should be withheld in children. The baseline rate is usually higher in children than in adults (see the Special Considerations for Children box below).

Take the apical and radial pulse for 1 minute to monitor for atrial fibrillation before the administration of digitalis glycosides. In clients with atrial fibrillation, determine the pulse deficit (apical pulse minus radial pulse).

During digitalization, check the parameters as described in the following paragraphs. Observe the client for a positive response to digitalization. An increase in cardiac output reflects a more effective cardiac function, which includes improvement in the rate and rhythm of heartbeat and in respiration, diuresis, weight reduction (e.g., decrease in edema), and a feeling of well-being.

Know therapeutic digitalis serum levels and normal potassium, calcium, and magnesium ion serum levels. A fall in potassium serum levels enhances the effect of digitalis and the risk of digitalis toxicity. Clients taking digitalis often receive potassium-depleting diuretics, which promote renal

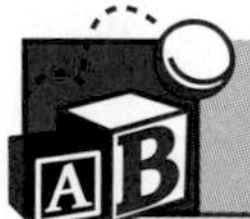

Special Considerations for Children
Cardiac Glycosides

A fall in serum potassium levels enhances the effect of digitalis and increases the risk of digitalis toxicity. Monitor serum potassium levels closely.

Early signs of CHF include tachycardia (especially during rest and minimum activity), increased fatigue and irritability, a sudden weight gain, respiratory distress, and profuse scalp sweating, especially in infants.

Individualize dosing with very close monitoring, especially in infants. Be extremely careful in calculating digitalis doses; a placement error of one decimal point can increase the dose tenfold. Double check all calculations with another health care professional (nurse, pharmacist, or physician).

Common signs of digoxin toxicity in children include nausea, vomiting, anorexia, bradycardia, and dysrhythmias.

Give digoxin on a regular time schedule, either 1 hour before or 2 hours after feedings.

Information from Wong, D.L., Hockenberry-Eaton, M., Wilson, D., Winkelstein, M.L., Ahmann, E., & DiVito-Thomas, P.A. (1999). *Whaley & Wong's nursing care of infants and children* (6th ed.). St. Louis: Mosby.

potassium excretion and lower serum potassium levels. Monitor serum potassium levels closely. Observe the client for symptoms of hypokalemia, such as drowsiness, hypoperistalsis, mental depression, paresthesia, muscle weakness, anorexia, depressed reflexes, orthostatic hypotension, and polyuria (Cooke, 1992). Provide the client who is taking potassium-depleting diuretics with foods that contain a high potassium content, such as bananas and orange juice if tolerated.

In addition, monitor serum BUN and creatinine levels as evidence of renal function, especially in older adults.

Observe the rhythm strip for digitalis-induced dysrhythmias if the client is on an ECG monitor. Dysrhythmias that might indicate digoxin toxicity are atrial tachycardia with AV block, progressing AV blocks, accelerated junctional rhythms, and ventricular dysrhythmias, including ventricular bigeminy and ventricular tachycardia (Kelso, 1992). Discontinue the drug if drug intoxication occurs. A serum level of digitalis is ordered by the prescriber if toxicity is suspected (Box 25-3). Be aware that the range of the therapeutic index of digitalis is extremely narrow. Note that digitoxin has the greatest potential for toxicity because its slow elimination can produce cumulative effects in the body, but it may be preferred if the prescriber wants to ensure that body stores will not be rapidly depleted if the client misses a dose. Digoxin may be preferred in individuals with impaired liver function because the drug does not require extensive hepatic metabolism. In contrast, digitoxin is slowly eliminated from the body by the liver, not the kidneys, which may make it the drug of choice for clients with renal disease.

Observe the client's food intake. Anorexia is almost always the first sign of toxicity; nausea and vomiting, sometimes with abdominal discomfort and increased salivation, usually occur 1 to 2 days after the anorexia.

Monitor intake and output. Delayed or diminished renal excretion of digitalis glycosides can lead to toxicity. Weigh the client daily, preferably before breakfast, to monitor for an alteration in fluid balance. A sudden weight gain is an early sign of fluid retention. Monitor the client for signs and symptoms of excess fluid volume, such as dependent edema (pedal or sacral), basilar crackles in the lungs, and jugular distention.

■ ***Intervention.*** Rapid-acting digoxin is the most commonly prescribed digitalis glycoside used in the coronary care unit (CCU). It may be given intravenously, intramuscularly, or orally. When given intravenously as an undiluted digoxin (0.25 mg/mL), administer it slowly at 0.25 mg/min. Rapid administration is avoided to prevent pulmonary edema. Digoxin may also be administered in diluted form. Administer IV digoxin with caution to clients with hypertension because it causes a temporary increase in blood pressure. Avoid IM injections of digoxin because it is painful and because the bioavailability of the IM injected drug is low and the absorption is unpredictable, especially in clients with severe heart failure, edema, and poor tissue perfusion (Marcus, 1991). However, if an IM injection of digoxin is ordered, administer it deep into the large muscle mass and follow with massage.

Maintenance doses of digoxin may be given orally if the client can tolerate food; otherwise IV injections are required. *Do not administer the oral preparation with meals that have a high fiber content.* Studies show that digoxin binds with the fiber, thereby reducing the amount of medication available for absorption from the gut. Advise the client to take the drug 1 hour before or 2 hours after meals.

Be aware that digitoxin, although infrequently used, can be given undiluted intravenously (slowly) or orally to avoid pulmonary edema. Oral administration is more consistently absorbed and is safer for individuals with renal disease because the metabolites excreted in the urine are inactive and do not affect the half-life of a digitalis glycoside.

■ ***Education.*** Instruct the client to take digitalis glycosides at the same time each day, precisely as prescribed. Doses should not be skipped, and they should not be doubled if missed. Inform the client that digoxin and Lanoxin are essentially the same drug, although there is a difference in bioavailability. Instruct the client not to change the brand of drug when a prescription is refilled because of this difference in bioavailability between the generic forms and Lanoxin. In some cases, clients were

BOX 25-3

Determining Serum Digoxin Concentration

The therapeutic serum digoxin concentration is 0.5 to 2 ng/mL. However, serum levels do not clearly distinguish between toxic clients and nontoxic clients. It has been reported that 38% of individuals with digoxin toxicity have a digoxin serum level below 2 μg/mL. Some clients with hypokalemia experience digoxin toxicity with serum levels of 1.5 ng/mL (Kradjan, 1995). Therefore serum levels should be used only as a guide; clinical impressions or evaluations are best in measuring therapeutic outcome.

The following are criteria for determining serum levels of digoxin:

1. Suspected toxicity
2. Questionable or unreliable client compliance
3. Client not responding appropriately to therapy
4. Presence of impaired renal function
5. Use of drugs with documented interference (e.g., quinidine, calcium channel blocking agents)
6. Confirming an unusual or seriously abnormal digoxin serum level

The time a blood sample is drawn for a digoxin serum level is critical. Serum levels are most reliable when obtained 6 to 8 hours after the last oral dose, 2 hours after an IV dose, or just before a dose is scheduled.

Case Study *The Client with Cardiovascular Disease*

Grace Markham is a 63-year-old widow who lives alone. She has a history of rheumatic heart disease, which is manifested by moderate mitral valve stenosis with slight mitral insufficiency. She has been maintained on digoxin, 0.125 mg PO daily for several years and has experienced few adverse effects. In general, her compliance with therapy has been excellent. She understands the drug therapy and her 2-g sodium diet.

She was admitted to the hospital complaining of dyspnea on exertion, ankle edema, mild chest pain on exertion, and fatigue. The ECG shows no signs of infarction but does show atrial fibrillation with a ventricular response of 124 beats/min. Her serum digoxin level was 0.9 ng/mL. A repeat cardiac catheterization shows no changes in the mitral valve but indicates some early coronary artery narrowing. The following medications are ordered for Mrs. Markham while she is in the hospital:

- digoxin, 0.25 mg PO daily
- Lasix, 20 mg PO twice daily
- K-Dur 20, 20 mEq PO daily
- verapamil SR, 240 mg PO daily
- Isordil, 10 mg PO three times daily

1. Describe the relationship between digoxin, Lasix, and K-Dur in the management of Mrs. Markham's symptoms.
2. What additional data should be included in the assessment of the client related to the use of these three medications?
3. What is the significance of a serum digoxin level of 0.9 ng/mL?
4. How will the use of digoxin affect Ms. Markham's atrial fibrillation?

Several weeks later Ms. Markham comes to the clinic complaining of nausea, vomiting, and diarrhea. She reports having had these symptoms for several days. She has continued to take her medications except for the K-Dur, which she found increased the nausea.

1. What additional assessment data (subjective, objective, laboratory) do you want to gather related to these new symptoms?
2. A serum digoxin level for Ms. Markham was 2.5 ng/mL. Explain the significance of this change in relationship to the symptoms she was having.

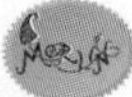

For answer guidelines, go to mosby.com/MERLIN/McKenry/.

prescribed digoxin and Lanoxin, each by a different prescriber, leading to an overdose. If using an elixir form of the drug, the dose should be determined using the special dropper that comes with the preparation. Caution the client not to take other medications without prior approval of the prescriber.

Instruct the client to restrict his or her sodium intake to 2 g daily. Advise clients who are not hospitalized to report a weight gain of 1 to 2 pounds a day. Caution clients to avoid licorice because it can induce sodium and water retention.

Advise the client to carry medical identification and to alert health care professionals unfamiliar with his or her drug regimen that the drug is being taken.

Teach the client how to take his or her own pulse, and recommend taking the pulse before each dose of medication. The dose should be withheld and the prescriber notified if the pulse is below 60 or above 110 beats/min and/or is erratic or if the client suffers from anorexia, diarrhea, nausea, vomiting, sudden weight gain, or apparent edema (see the Case Study box above). Visual disturbances, such as blurred vision or green or yellow halos around objects, should also be reported to the prescriber.

■ **Evaluation.** The expected outcome of digitalis glycoside therapy is that the client will demonstrate a normal sinus rhythm on the ECG and clinical improvement, such as an absence of S_3 and basilar crackles and dependent edema,improved activity tolerance, decreased cardiomegaly on x-ray studies, and an increased sense of well-being.

Antidote for Digitalis Glycosides

digoxin immune Fab (Ovine) (Digibind)

Digoxin immune Fab is an antidote for severe digitalis glycoside toxicity. It binds and makes complex molecules with digoxin or digitoxin in the serum. These molecules are then excreted by the kidneys. As more tissue digoxin is released into the serum to maintain an equilibrium, it is bound and removed by this product, which results in lower levels of digoxin in serum and body tissues.

This drug is indicated for the treatment of life-threatening digoxin or digitoxin overdose (Box 25-4).

The onset of action takes place in less than 1 minute, and the half-life is 15 to 20 hours. Initial signs of improvement in digitalis toxicity can be seen in 15 to 30 minutes after administration but can take up to several hours. Dysrhythmias and hyperkalemia are usually reversed first, whereas reversal of the inotropic effect may take several hours. This drug is excreted in the kidneys.

Close monitoring is necessary because the withdrawal of digitalis may result in a decrease in cardiac output, CHF, and hypokalemia. An increase in ventricular rate may be seen in persons with atrial fibrillation. No significant drug interactions have been reported.

The dosage of digoxin immune Fab in adults may be calculated on the amount of digoxin or digitoxin consumed, or it may be based on steady-state serum levels. Usually a 38-mg dose for injection will bind approximately 0.5 mg of

BOX 25-4

Digitalis Toxicity

Almost every type of dysrhythmia can be produced by digitalis toxicity. The type of dysrhythmia produced varies with the age of the client and other factors. Premature ventricular contractions and bigeminal rhythm (two beats and a pause) are common signs of digitalis toxicity in adults, whereas children tend to develop ectopic nodal or atrial beats. Digitalis-induced dysrhythmias are caused by depression of the SA and AV nodes of the heart. This results in various conduction disturbances (first- or second-degree heart block or complete heart block). Digitalis may also cause increased myocardial automaticity, producing extrasystoles or tachycardias.

Nurses must be aware of the predisposing factors to digitalis toxicity. The presence of any of the following factors in clients indicates the need for close observation for the signs and symptoms of digitalis intoxication:

1. *Potassium loss.* Hypokalemia (low potassium levels) can increase digitalis cardiotoxicity. Because potassium inhibits the excitability of the heart, a depletion of body or myocardial potassium increases cardiac excitability. Low extracellular potassium is synergistic with digitalis and enhances ectopic pacemaker activity (dysrhythmias). The following are causes of potassium loss:
   a. Hypokalemia occurs if large amounts of body fluids are lost as a result of vomiting, diarrhea, and gastric suctioning.
   b. The use of various diuretic agents (carbonic-anhydrase inhibitors, ammonium chloride, furosemide and thiazide preparations) induces potassium diuresis along with sodium and water diuresis.
   c. Poor dietary intake or severe dietary restrictions that decrease electrolyte intake can cause a loss of potassium.
   d. Adrenal steroids cause potassium loss and sodium retention.
   e. Surgical procedures associated with severe electrolyte disturbances (e.g., abdominoperineal resection, colostomy, ileostomy, colectomy, and ureterosigmoidostomy) can cause potassium loss.
   f. The use of potassium-free IV fluids can cause hypokalemia.
2. *Hypercalcemia.* Excess calcium in the presence of digitalis may cause sinus bradycardia, AV conduction block, and ectopic dysrhythmia.
3. *Pathologic conditions.* Kidney, liver, and severe heart disease are major factors in digitalis toxicity. Approximately 80% of digoxin is excreted by the kidneys, whereas approximately 90% of digitoxin is first metabolized by the liver. In a clinical setting, the prescriber may choose digitoxin as the drug of choice for a client in renal failure because of its mode of excretion (liver metabolism). For a client with liver impairment, the prescriber may select digoxin as the drug of choice, mainly because it does not rely on the liver for metabolism before excretion.

The long half-life of digitoxin is a disadvantage in treatment. If the client develops digitalis toxicity, the half-life of digoxin may increase from 36 hours to 120 hours, whereas the half-life of digitoxin increases from 120 to 210 hours.

digoxin or digitoxin. The formulas in Box 25-5 may be applied to determine the dose of the antidote.

MISCELLANEOUS AGENTS

inamrinone [in am′ rih none] (Inocor)

The mechanism of action of inamrinone has not been fully identified. Inamrinone increases the force and velocity of myocardial tissues, resulting in a positive inotropic effect. Experiments indicate that inamrinone inhibits phosphodiesterase activity, which in turn increases the concentration of cellular cAMP (cyclic adenosine monophosphate) and cardiac contractility. Inamrinone appears to produce a direct relaxant effect on the vascular smooth muscle (vasodilation) and to reduce preload and afterload. It is used to treat CHF in individuals who do not respond to standard therapies, such as digitalis glycosides, diuretics, and vasodilators.

Administered intravenously, the time to peak action of inamrinone is within 10 minutes. The duration of effect is dose related. If 0.75 mg/kg is administered, the duration of

BOX 25-5

Formulas for Digoxin Immune Fab (Ovine)

For digoxin tablets, oral solution, or IM injection:

$$\text{Dose (mg)} = \frac{\text{Dose ingested(mg)} \times 0.8}{0.5} \times 38$$

For digitoxin tablets, digoxin capsules, or IV digoxin:

$$\text{Dose (mg)} = \frac{\text{Dose ingested (mg)}}{0.5} \times 38$$

When the amount of digitalis ingestion is unknown and the steady-state serum level is unavailable, 760 mg of digoxin immune Fab (ovine) is usually administered because it is reportedly sufficient to treat most life-threatening ingestions.

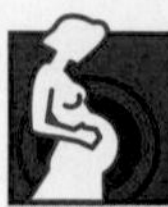

Pregnancy Safety
Cardiac Glycosides

Category	Drugs
C	digitoxin, digoxin, digoxin immune Fab (ovine), inamrinone, milrinone

action is approximately 30 minutes. If 3 mg/kg is administered, the duration of action is approximately 120 minutes. When administered for CHF, the half-life is between 5 and 8.3 hours. This drug is metabolized in the liver and excreted primarily via the kidneys.

The side effects/adverse reactions of inamrinone are infrequent and include nausea, vomiting, abdominal pain, fever, taste alterations, hypotension, dysrhythmias, chest pain, and thrombocytopenia. The inotropic effects of inamrinone are additive to those of digitalis.

The adult dosage of inamrinone is 0.75 mg/kg IV slowly over 2 to 3 minutes, repeated in 30 minutes if necessary. The maintenance dosage by IV infusion is 5 to 10 μg/kg/min, individualized according to response. The maximum dosage is 10 mg/kg/day; in several reports, dosages up to 18 mg/kg/day were given for short time periods.

For neonates and infants, the initial dosage is 3 to 4 mg/kg in divided doses; the maintenance dosage is 3 to 5 μg/kg/min for neonates and 10 μg/kg/min for infants. (See the Pregnancy Safety box above for pregnancy safety categories of the Food and Drug Administration [FDA]).

▪ Nursing Management
Inamrinone Therapy

▪ **Assessment.** Ascertain the status of the client's sensitivity to sulfites, because inamrinone lactate injection contains sodium metabisulfite; the client may be intolerant to this substance. Also ascertain the client's sensitivity to inamrinone. Inamrinone is not to be used for clients with severe aortic or pulmonic valvular disease. It is to be used with caution in clients with impaired hepatic or renal function; a dosage adjustment may be required because elimination of the drug will be impaired. Inamrinone may aggravate outflow tract obstruction in hypertrophic cardiomyopathy; use with caution.

▪ **Nursing Diagnosis.** The client receiving inamrinone is at risk for the following nursing diagnoses/collaborative problems: impaired comfort (burning at infusion site, chest pain, nausea, vomiting, abdominal pain); risk for injury related to hypotension (dizziness); hyperthermia; and the potential complications of decreased cardiac output, dysrhythmias, dose-dependent thrombocytopenia, hepatotoxicity, and hypersensitivity reactions.

▪ **Implementation**

▪ ***Monitoring.*** The client's blood pressure and pulse should be monitored to assess the hypotensive and dysrhythmic effects of the drug. The infusion rate should be slowed or stopped if the client becomes hypotensive. The appropriate range for blood pressure readings should be prescribed. In addition, assess the cardiac index and pulmonary wedge pressure if warranted. Assess electrolytes, central venous pressure, urine output, body weight, and the status of any orthopnea, dyspnea, and fatigue to evaluate the effectiveness of the drug and the client's progress.

Assess platelet counts before and frequently during therapy. Observe for unusual bleeding and bruising, which are clinical signs of thrombocytopenia. The drug may be discontinued if the platelet count falls below 150,000/mm^3.

Because of the possibility of hepatotoxicity, liver function studies are usually performed, and the client is monitored for clinical signs of jaundice. These signs include yellowish skin or sclera, dark urine, and pruritus. Report nausea and vomiting to the prescriber. It may be severe enough to require that the drug be discontinued.

Monitor for sulfite sensitivity (see Box 22-1). Also monitor for tachyphylaxis to the effects of inamrinone; this is common and usually occurs within the first 72 hours of therapy.

▪ ***Intervention.*** Examine the solution for color changes and/or precipitation. Inamrinone is incompatible with dextrose because it loses its potency. However, it may be diluted in saline and administered as a bolus through a line containing freely running D_5W. Do not mix with furosemide (Lasix) or inject it into the same tubing because it precipitates.

Inamrinone may be administered by direct IV injection over 2 to 3 minutes to minimize pain and burning at the injection site, or it may be diluted in 0.45% or 0.9% saline solution to a concentration of 1 to 3 mg/mL and given by continuous infusion. Use the prepared solution within 24 hours. Avoid extravasation. Change infusion sites every 48 hours, and administer with an infusion pump.

▪ ***Education.*** Instruct the client to move slowly from a sitting or lying position to a more upright position because of the hypotensive effects of the drug.

▪ **Evaluation.** The expected outcome of inamrinone therapy is that the client will demonstrate a normal sinus rhythm on the ECG and clinical improvement, such as an absence of S_3 and basilar crackles and dependent edema, improved activity tolerance, decreased cardiomegaly on x-ray studies, and an increased sense of well-being.

milrinone injection [mil reh' none] (Primacor IV)

Milrinone is indicated for the short-term treatment of CHF. It is a selective inhibitor of cAMP isozymes in cardiac and vascular muscle; thus it improves cardiac function, contractility, and vasodilation without increasing myocardial oxygen consumption and heart rate. It is a positive inotrope and vasodilator with very little chronotropic activity.

When administered intravenously, milrinone has a half-life of 2.5 hours and a duration of action between 3 and 6 hours. It is excreted by the kidneys.

Significant drug interactions have not been reported, but its administration with other hypotension-producing drugs may have an additive effect.

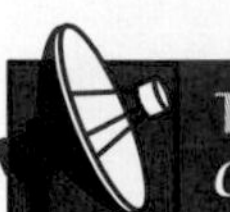

TechnologyLink
Cardiac Glycosides

Video Resources

Mosby's Medical-Surgical Nursing Videotape Series, Nursing Management of Congestive Heart Failure, ISBN 0-8151-6054-2 Mosby, Inc., 11830 Westline Industrial Drive, St. Louis, MO 63146; (800) 426-4545; www.mosby.com.

Web Resources

American Heart Association (www.americanheart.org/)
This site has information on heart disease, stroke, guidelines, and much more.

Cardiology Resources (www.medicalresourcesusa.com/cardiology.htm)
This site lists cardiology-related web links.

Mayo Clinic (www.mayoclinic.com)
This site contains information on heart disease, high blood cholesterol, coronary artery disease, stroke, congestive heart failure, and arrhythmias.

National Heart, Lung, and Blood Institute (www.nhlbi.nih.gov/index.htm)
This site has extensive information on health, clinical guidelines, and plans and programs relating to health matters.

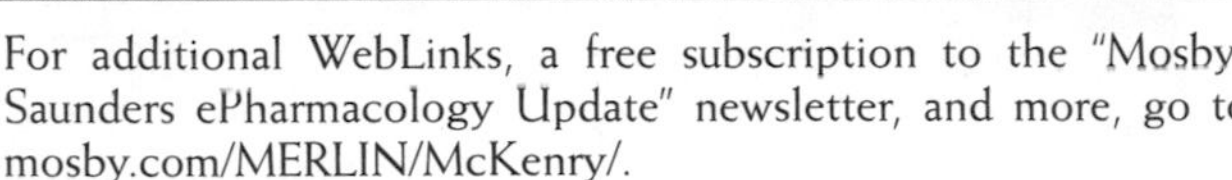

For additional WebLinks, a free subscription to the "Mosby/Saunders ePharmacology Update" newsletter, and more, go to mosby.com/MERLIN/McKenry/.

A chemical interaction (precipitate) has been reported when furosemide (Lasix) was administered via an IV line containing a milrinone infusion. This procedure should be avoided.

Significant side effects/adverse reactions of milrinone include headaches, hypotension, ventricular dysrhythmias and, rarely, angina and thrombocytopenia. Inotropic effects are additive to those of digitalis. See current guidelines for dosing recommendations.

The nursing management of milrinone is the same as for inamrinone except that the solution does not contain sulfites, which reduces the risk of hypersensitivity reactions. Milrinone may be prepared with dextrose solutions.

SUMMARY

Cardiac glycosides increase the strength of cardiac contraction and alter the electrophysiologic properties of the heart by slowing conduction velocity; this accounts for their therapeutic properties in the treatment of heart failure. Clients may be hospitalized for rapid digitalization—the saturation of the body tissues with enough digitalis to cause the signs and symptoms of heart failure to disappear—or may receive digitalization at a slower rate prescribed in an ambulatory setting. Because the therapeutic index of the drug is so narrow in either case, the nurse has the responsibility to monitor the client closely for signs of toxicity and also to teach the client about the therapeutic and nontherapeutic effects of the drug. The nurse must be aware of the predisposing factors to digitalis toxicity and assist the client in recognizing some of them. Potassium loss is the most common risk factor for digitalis toxicity. Digoxin immune Fab (ovine) for injection is used as an antidote for severe digitalis toxicity.

Inamrinone and milrinone are miscellaneous agents administered parenterally for their positive inotropic effects. They are used to treat CHF in individuals who do not respond to standard therapies.

The nurse has a major assessment and educational role with clients using cardiac glycosides, because many clients take these drugs on a long-term, if not a lifetime, basis. It is important that clients not only take their medications accurately but also be knowledgeable about them to minimize the risk for injury inherent in their administration.

Critical Thinking Questions

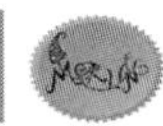

1. What electrolyte imbalances affect the development of digitalis toxicity? In what way?
2. Mrs. Stacy, a 74-year-old client with chronic CHF, is leaving the hospital with a medication regimen that includes digoxin, furosemide, and potassium supplements. What instructions would be essential to include in a teaching plan to enable Mrs. Stacy to self-administer her medications safely and accurately?

Collaborative Learning Activities

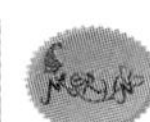

For Collaborative Learning Activities, go to mosby.com/MERLIN/McKenry/.

CASE STUDY

For a Case Study that will help ensure mastery of this chapter content, go to mosby.com/MERLIN/McKenry/.

BIBLIOGRAPHY

Agency for Health Care Policy and Research (AHCPR). (1994). *Heart failure: Evaluation and care of patients with left-ventricular systolic dysfunction.* Clinical Practice Guideline #11. Rockville, MD: Department of Health and Human Services.

American Hospital Formulary Service. (1999). *AHFS drug information '99.* Bethesda, MD: American Society of Hospital Pharmacists.

Anderson, K.N., Anderson, L.E., & Glanze, W.D. (Eds.). (1998). *Mosby's medical, nursing, & allied health dictionary* (5th ed.). St. Louis: Mosby.

Aronow, W.S. (1999). Management of the older person with atrial fibrillation. *Journal of the American Geriatric Society, 47*(6), 740-748.

Cawley, M. (1994). The role of digoxin in the treatment of atrial fibrillation. *Journal of Cardiopulmonary Rehabilitation, 14*(6), 373-375.

Cooke, D.M. (1992). Shielding your patient from digitalis toxicity. *Nursing, 22*(7), 44-47.

Drug Facts and Comparisons. (2000). St. Louis: Facts and Comparisons.

Graedon, J. & Graedon, T. (1995). *The people's guide to deadly drug interactions.* New York: St. Martin's Press.

Hsu, I. (1996). Optimal management of heart failure. *Journal of the American Pharmaceutical Association, NS36*(2), 92-106.

Kelso, L.A. (1992). Dysrhythmias associated with digoxin toxicity. *AACN Clinical Issues: Advanced Practice in Acute and Critical Care, 3*(1), 220-225.

Kienle, P.C. (1995). *Interventions to optimize management of congestive heart failure in long-term care: Application of the AHCPR guidelines—An inservice kit.* Philadelphia: Medical Education Systems.

Kradjan, W.A. (1995). Congestive heart failure. In L.Y. Young & M.A. Koda-Kimble (Eds.), *Applied therapeutics: The clinical use of drugs* (6th ed.). Vancouver, WA: Applied Therapeutics.

Long, J.W. & Rybacki, J.J. (1995). *The essential guide to prescription drugs.* New York: Harper Collins.

Marcus, F.I. (1991). Digitalis: How well are you using it? *Patient Care, 25*(17), 21.

Meisser, J.E. & Gever, L.N. (1993). Reducing the risks of digitalis toxicity. *Nursing, 23*(7), 47-51.

Moore, A.R. & O'Keefe, S.T. (1999). Drug-induced cognitive impairment in the elderly. *Drugs Aging, 15*(1), 15-28.

Rich, M.W. & Nease, R.F. (1999). Cost-effectiveness analysis in clinical practice: The case of heart failure. *Archives of Internal Medicine, 159*(15), 1690-1700.

Semla, T.P., Beizer, J.L., & Higbee, M.D. (1993). *Geriatric dosage handbook.* Hudson, OH: Lexi-Comp.

Silverman, M. (1942). *Magic in a bottle.* New York: Macmillan.

United States Pharmacopeia Dispensing Information (USP DI): Drug information for the health care professional (19th ed.). (1999). Rockville, MD: United States Pharmacopeial Convention.

Wong, D.L., Hockenberry-Eaton, M., Wilson, D., Winkelstein, M.L., Ahmann, E., & DiVito-Thomas, P.A. (1999). *Whaley & Wong's nursing care of infants and children* (6th ed.). St. Louis: Mosby.

Wright, J.M. (1995). Pharmacologic management of congestive heart failure. *Critical Care Nurse Quarterly, 18*(1), 32-44.

26 Antidysrhythmics

Chapter Focus

Although the use of antidysrhythmic drugs has increased tremendously during the last decade, the nurse should be aware that they can be as life threatening as they are lifesaving. An evaluation of the risk-benefit ratio is required with each client. The quality of client care is enhanced by the nurse's knowledge of antidysrhythmic therapy and role in client teaching.

Learning Objectives

1. Identify the medications most commonly used as antidysrhythmic agents.
2. Describe the primary electrophysiologic effects and electrocardiogram effects of the major antidysrhythmic agents.
3. Relate at least three nursing evaluation strategies for monitoring a client's response to antidysrhythmic therapy.
4. List the most common adverse reactions experienced by older adults receiving specific antidysrhythmic therapy.
5. Implement nursing management for the care of individual clients who require the administration of an antidysrhythmic agent.

Key Terms

Adams-Stokes syndrome, p. 557
automaticity, p. 548
conductivity, p. 548
dysrhythmia (arrhythmia), p. 548
sinus bradycardia, p. 548
sinus tachycardia, p. 548
Wolff-Parkinson-White syndrome, p. 557

Key Drugs [✔]

lidocaine, p. 556
procainamide, p. 555
quinidine, p. 550

A cardiac **dysrhythmia (arrhythmia)** may be defined as any deviation from the normal rhythm of the heartbeat. Dysrhythmia may be caused by a disorder that modifies the electrophysiologic properties of the cells of the conduction system or cardiac muscle. For a review of the electrophysiologic events of a normal action potential, see Chapter 24.

Antidysrhythmic drugs are used for the treatment and prevention of cardiac rhythm disorders. Dysrhythmias often develop in individuals approximately 4 to 72 hours after a myocardial infarction ("heart attack"). An abnormal rhythm may also occur in clients recovering from cardiac surgery, in clients with coronary artery disease, and in clients with extracardiac disorders such as pheochromocytoma, electrolyte imbalance, or thyroid disease. Cardiac pathology, such as the idiopathic long QT syndrome, may also be inherited (Vizgirda, 1999).

DISORDERS IN CARDIAC ELECTROPHYSIOLOGY

Disorders of cardiac rhythm arise as a result of (1) abnormality in the spontaneous initiation of an impulse, or **automaticity**; or (2) abnormality in impulse conduction, or **conductivity.** In some conditions, a combination of both processes may occur.

Abnormality in Automaticity. A disturbance in automaticity may alter the rate, rhythm, or origin of impulse formation in the heart. When the rate of pacemaker activity is affected, a decrease in automaticity of the sinoatrial (SA) node produces **sinus bradycardia** (an abnormal condition in which the myocardium contracts steadily but at a rate less than 60 beats/min); an increase in automaticity of the SA node results in **sinus tachycardia** (an abnormal condition in which the myocardium contracts regularly but at a rate greater than 100 beats/min). On the other hand, a shift in the origin of impulse formation can generate an abnormal pacemaker or an ectopic focus, resulting in activation of some part of the heart other than the SA node. This is called an ectopic pacemaker, and it may discharge at either a regular or an irregular rhythm. It occurs when the cardiac fibers depolarize more frequently than the SA node.

Abnormal automaticity may develop in cells that usually do not initiate impulses, such as atrial or ventricular cells. Clinical disorders such as hypoxia or ischemia can activate sympathetic receptors that in turn become centers to initiate impulses. In addition, ischemic sites can cause impulse disturbances in automaticity and also in conductivity; both manifestations are responsible for ectopic beats. The ectopic beats are classified as escape beats, premature beats or extrasystoles, and ectopic tachydysrhythmia.

Abnormality in Conductivity. Altered conduction of the cardiac impulse probably accounts for more dysrhythmias than a change in automaticity. A disturbance in conductivity may be caused by (1) a delay or block of impulse conduction or (2) the reentry phenomenon.

Delay or Block of Impulse Conduction. Normally, the SA node and atrioventricular (AV) junction are poor conductors of impulse transmission. Under abnormal circumstances, the conduction of an atrial impulse to the ventricles may be delayed or blocked in the AV junction or structures beyond this region in the conduction pathway. Impaired impulse transmission generally appears in the AV junction and occurs in varying degrees of block. In first-degree AV block, the impulses from the SA node pass through to the ventricles very slowly; this is noted by a prolonged PR interval on the electrocardiogram (ECG). In second-degree block, some atrial beats fail to pass into the ventricles through the AV junction. In third-degree block or complete heart block, no impulses reach the ventricle, in which case the Purkinje fibers initiate their own spontaneous depolarization at a very slow rate. This results in independent ventricular and atrial rhythms referred to as ventricular "escape."

Reentry Phenomenon. Reentry phenomenon is the mechanism responsible for initiating ectopic beats. A necessary condition for reentry is unidirectional block. When an impulse travels down the Purkinje fiber, it normally spreads along two branches; when the impulse enters the connecting branch, it is extinguished at the point of collision in the center (Figure 26-1, *A*). At the same time, other impulses that begin laterally from the Purkinje fibers activate ventricular muscle tissue. In an abnormal situation, the impulse descending from the central Purkinje fiber travels down the right branch normally but encounters a block in the left branch as a result of ischemia or injury (Figure 26-1, *B*). This is a unidirectional block, because the impulse is capable of passing in one direction but not in the other. In this left branch, where the impulse is blocked in the forward direction at the site of injury, a retrograde or reverse impulse from the ventricular tissue penetrates or reenters the depressed region from the other direction, provided that the pathway proximal to the block is no longer refractory. When the effective refractory period of the blocked area is over, reentry of the impulse from the ventricular muscle into this site causes the impulse to circulate or recycle repetitively through the loop, resulting in a circus-type movement that produces dysrhythmia.

As shown in Figure 26-1, *C*, reentry is abolished by certain drug groups, which are explained later in this chapter. *Drugs that decrease or slow conduction velocity can convert unidirectional block to a two-way or bidirectional block.* As the impulses traveling in the antegrade or forward direction and those appearing in a retrograde or reverse direction are blocked at the injured site, the reentry pathway is interrupted, thereby abolishing the ectopic beats. In Figure 26-1, *D*, the conditions required for preventing reentry by another mechanism are also illustrated. *The Group I-B drugs have no effect on conduction velocity, thus they eliminate reentry by stopping unidirectional block entirely.* Consequently, normal impulse conduction along the right and left branches of the Purkinje fibers is again restored.

■ ■ ■

In recent years an increasing number of antidysrhythmic drugs have required classification into categories based on their fundamental mode of action on cardiac muscle. Such a

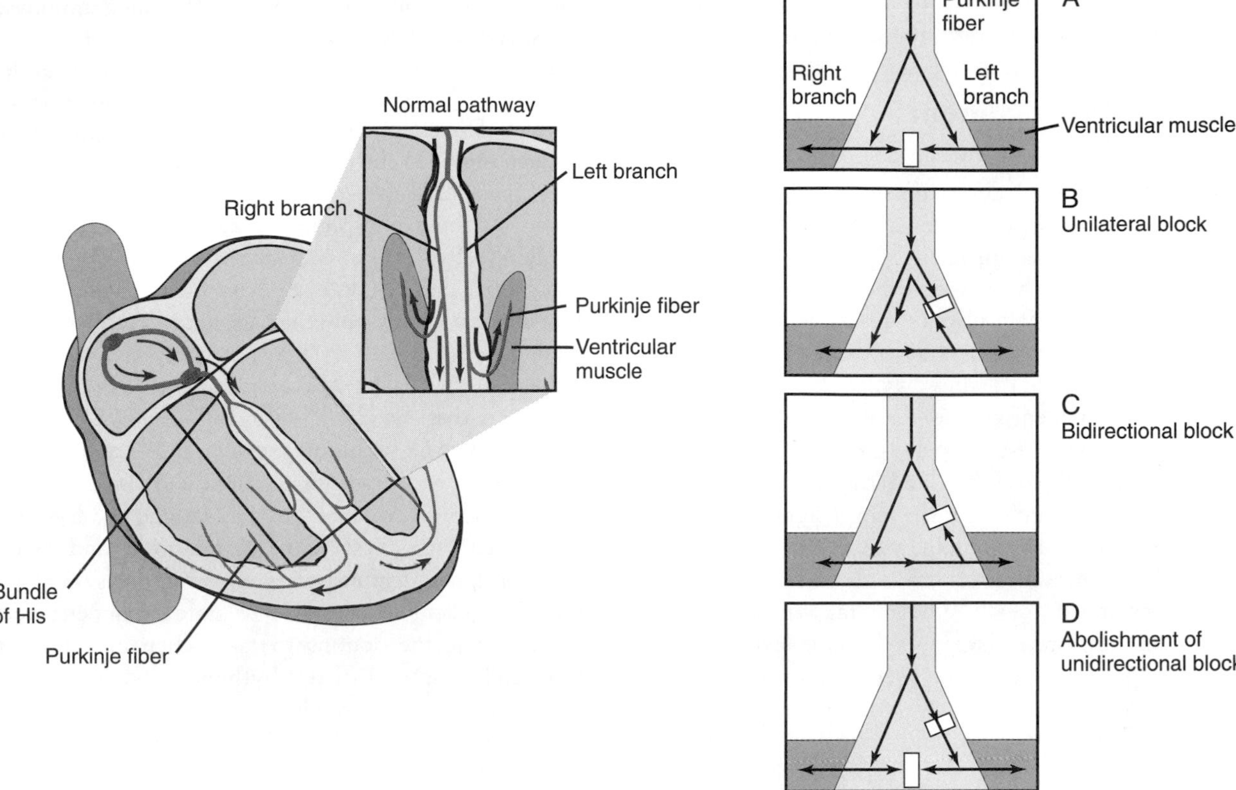

Figure 26-1 Reentry phenomenon. Illustration of a branched Purkinje fiber that activates ventricular muscle.

grouping of antidysrhythmic mechanisms should prove to be of value in predicting the therapeutic efficacy of the drug. All drugs belonging to a particular class do not necessarily possess totally identical actions. In some cases a given agent may have subsidiary properties (extracardiac effects) that alter the basic electrophysiologic actions on the cardiac muscle. The currently available antidysrhythmic drugs are classified into four categories according to their mechanisms of action (Box 26-1). All of these drugs have one major electrophysiologic property in common—the ability to suppress automaticity.

Group I compounds are subdivided into groups I-A, I-B, or I-C to reflect the similar electrophysiologic effects of each subgroup. The only exception to the subcategory division is moricizine. Moricizine (Ethmozine) is listed under Group I and has characteristics of all three subgroups (*Drug Facts and Comparisons,* 2000). Group I drugs bind to sodium channels and interfere with sodium influx during phase 0 of the action potential, thus depressing conduction velocity. Group I-A drugs include disopyramide (Norpace), procainamide (Pronestyl), and quinidine. Group I-B drugs are lidocaine, mexiletine (Mexitil), phenytoin (Dilantin), and tocainide (Tonocard). Group I-C includes flecainide (Tambocor) and propafenone (Rythmol). Because of their prodysrhythmic effects, Group I-C drugs should be carefully selected and closely monitored when prescribed.

Propranolol (Inderal), acebutolol (Sectral), and esmolol (Brevibloc) are considered Group II drugs because of their beta-adrenergic blocking action.

BOX 26-1

Antidysrhythmic Classifications

Group I drugs Fast sodium channel blockade in cardiac muscle, resulting in an increased refractory period; subclasses I-A, I-B, and I-C further define the differences between the drugs.

Group II drugs Beta-adrenergic blocking agents that reduce adrenergic stimulation on the heart.

Group III drugs In general, do not affect depolarization but work by prolonging cardiac repolarization.

Group IV drugs Block the slow calcium channel, resulting in the depression of myocardial and smooth muscle contraction, decreased automaticity and, perhaps, decreased conduction velocity.

Group III drugs include bretylium (Bretylol), amiodarone (Cordarone), ibutilide (Corvert), and sotalol (Betapace). The principal action of bretylium is antiadrenergic; it also has a positive inotropic action and prolongs repolarization. Contrary to the typical effects of bretylium, amiodarone increases the refractory period and increases the PR interval, QRS complex, and QT interval.

The last category, Group IV drugs, is characterized by a selective calcium antagonistic action. For this reason, verapamil is classified independently of other conventional compounds and is discussed in Chapter 28. Adenosine is listed under the unclassified antidysrhythmic agents.

Nursing Management

Antidysrhythmic Therapy

■ **Assessment.** Careful evaluation is necessary to determine the effect of a dysrhythmia on a specific client. The effect may range from benign to life threatening depending on the individual's health status and the degree of dysrhythmia. A thorough history, a physical assessment, and an interpretation of the dysrhythmia on the ECG are essential for formulating the possible nursing diagnoses.

A baseline assessment of the client with dysrhythmias should include blood pressure, pulse pressure, and any postural change; apical pulse rate and rhythm; apical-radial pulse deficit; heart sounds; jugular vein distention; edema; capillary refill time; urinary output; activity tolerance; determination of the presence of chest discomfort (pain or pressure), shortness of breath, syncope, fatigue, nausea, and perception of heart rate ("skipping beats"); level of consciousness, confusion, and anxiety; serum electrolyte levels; and ECG.

■ **Nursing Diagnosis.** Possible nursing diagnoses/collaborative problems that may be experienced by a client receiving an antidysrhythmic agent include, but are not limited to, the following: impaired comfort (nausea); risk for injury related to hypotension and dizziness; activity intolerance; deficient knowledge; anxiety related to altered heart action; and the potential complications of decreased cardiac output and altered cerebral and peripheral tissue perfusion. Consider these issues in the care and education of clients who are taking antidysrhythmic agents.

■ **Implementation**

■ ***Monitoring.*** To determine the effectiveness of antidysrhythmic therapy, continue to assess the indicators of the baseline assessment. The client should be questioned about episodes of light-headedness, dizziness, or confusion. Monitor lung sounds and heart rate and rhythm. The ECG is monitored for changes. Monitor laboratory data as ordered, especially potassium levels.

■ ***Intervention.*** Although some clients may require an artificial pacemaker to control their dysrhythmia, most are treated with antidysrhythmic agents some time during the course of their illness. Maintain a quiet environment for the client.

■ ***Education.*** If the client is in the hospital, provide a continuous explanation for the various diagnostic and/or monitoring devices. Instruction of the client receiving antidysrhythmic agents provides the opportunity for him or her to self-administer the medications safely and accurately. Much anxiety can be allayed through instruction regarding the dysrhythmia and its management. Such instruction is essential because medications may need to be taken for a lifetime. The client should be able to take and assess his or her pulse rate and rhythm accurately, counting for 1 full minute. He or she should be able to describe the medication regimen, including dosage scheduling, rationale, and the side effects/adverse reactions of the prescribed medications. Coffee, tea, and cola drinks may need to be limited because caffeine can cause an increase in abnormal heart rhythm. The client should be able to state signs and symptoms to report to the prescriber, including chest pain, dizziness, low blood pressure, gastrointestinal distress, blurred vision, a change in respiratory status or pulse rate or rhythm, swollen feet or ankles, or a sudden weight gain. He or she should be able to state the need for ongoing care and the importance of adhering to the prescribed treatment regimen.

■ **Evaluation.** The expected outcome of antidysrhythmic therapy is that the client will maintain normal cardiac output as evidenced by blood pressure, pulse, and capillary refill within normal limits. The client will also increase activity tolerance, as evidenced by less fatigue and less dyspnea; experience less chest pain, palpitations, and associated symptoms; and demonstrate no dysrhythmias on ECG tracings. The client will be able to state an understanding of dysrhythmia, the actions to take when experiencing the signs and symptoms of dysrhythmias, and administer antidysrhythmic therapy safely and accurately. The efficacy of the medications for a particular client is determined by the achievement of these goals. Modification of the nursing care plan may be necessary for the client to achieve the goals for management of the dysrhythmia.

GROUP I-A DRUGS

The pharmacologic effects of procainamide, quinidine, and disopyramide are similar: they bind to sodium channels and interfere with sodium influx during phase 0 of the action potential. The result is depression of conduction velocity. The ECG effects of these drugs include a widening of the QRS complex and a prolonged QT interval. Quinidine is the most widely used of these agents and serves as the key drug for this group.

quinidine gluconate [kwin′ i deen] (Quinaglute)
quinidine polygalacturonate (Cardioquin)
quinidine sulfate (Quinora)

Quinidine stabilizes the cell membrane by preventing the ready movement of sodium and potassium across this cellular barrier. This inhibition of cation exchange results in a decrease in the rate of diastolic depolarization from the resting potential during phase 4 and an increase in the threshold potential (the voltage shifts toward 0 mv). Therefore quinidine decreases impulse conduction and delays repolarization in the atria, ventricles, and Purkinje fibers. Quinidine suppresses or abolishes dysrhythmias by decreasing impulse generation at ectopic sites. Fortunately, abnormal or ectopic pacemaker tissue appears to be more sensitive to quinidine than normal pacemaker tissue (SA node), thus permitting the SA node to reestablish control over impulse formation in the heart.

Widening of the QRS complex indicates a decrease in intraventricular conduction, and lengthening of the PR interval represents slower conduction through the AV junction; these changes are observed on the ECG when quinidine is used. Thus caution must be used when quinidine is given to individuals with intraventricular conduction disorders.

Perhaps the most significant action of quinidine is its ability to prolong the effective refractory period of atrial and ventricular fibers. A delay in the completion of repolarization probably exerts an important antifibrillatory action. The tissue remains refractory for a period of time after full restoration of the resting membrane potential. This property is believed to influence the conversion of unidirectional block to bidirectional block, thereby abolishing the reentry type of dysrhythmia (see Figure 26-1, C).

The indirect anticholinergic effect of quinidine inhibits vagal action on the SA node and AV junction. This atropine-like effect permits the sinus node to accelerate and may often provoke a dangerous sinus tachycardia. Therefore digoxin, a beta blocking agent, or verapamil are usually administered before quinidine to prevent ventricular acceleration when attempting to convert atrial fibrillation to normal sinus rhythm. The chief noncardiac action of quinidine is peripheral vasodilation, which results from its alpha-adrenergic blocking effect on vascular smooth muscle. The combined effect of a decrease in peripheral vascular resistance and a reduced cardiac output caused by depressed myocardial contractility contributes to the development of hypotension, a condition that may reach serious proportions during quinidine therapy.

Quinidine is used in the management of ventricular and supraventricular dysrhythmias. Table 26-1 details the pharmacokinetics of this drug.

The side effects/adverse reactions of quinidine include anorexia, diarrhea, bitter taste, nausea, vomiting, abdominal distress, flushing, rash, tinnitus, confusion, and vision changes.

Quinidine salts contain different percentages of the active drug: quinidine gluconate, 62%; quinidine polygalacturonate, 80%; quinidine sulfate, 83%. Therefore these drugs are not interchangeable without an appropriate dosage adjustment. Quinidine sulfate 200 mg is considered equivalent to 275 mg of quinidine gluconate or quinidine polygalacturonate. The usual adult dosage of quinidine sulfate is 200 to 300 mg PO three to four times daily; the pediatric dosage is 6 mg/kg body weight in 5 divided doses.

■ Nursing Management

Quinidine Therapy

In addition to the following discussion, see Nursing Management: Antidysrhythmic Therapy, p. 550.

■ **Assessment.** The client's health status should be assessed to determine whether he or she has a medical condition for which the administration of quinidine might be contraindicated or incur some risk. Because of the additional cardiac depression produced by this drug, do not use in clients with complete AV block, digitalis toxicity with AV conduction disorder, or intraventricular conduction defects. With incomplete AV block and digitalis toxicity, the additive effects of quinidine will also increase conduction inhibition and result in more cardiac depression. If quinidine is administered to clients with myasthenia gravis, it may increase muscle weakness because of its weak curare-like action. Quinidine should be used with caution in clients with a history of thrombocytopenia. Clients with hepatic or renal function impairment may require decreased dosages to avoid accumulation of the drug. Clients sensitive to quinine may also be sensitive to quinidine.

Review the client's current medication regiment for the risk of significant drug interactions, such as those that may occur when quinidine is given concurrently with the following drugs:

Drug	Possible Effect and Management
anticoagulants, such as warfarin (Coumadin)	Monitor for signs of additional anticoagulant effects, such as excessive bruising, bleeding gums, black stools, hematuria, and hematemesis. It may be necessary to adjust the anticoagulant dosage both during therapy and after quinidine therapy is discontinued.
antidysrhythmic agents	May result in enhanced cardiac response. Monitor ECG tracings closely.
neuromuscular blocking agents	Monitor for increased or enhanced blocking effects, especially in the postsurgical client.
pimozide (Orap)	May potentiate cardiac dysrhythmias. Monitor closely, preferably with an ECG, because intervention may be necessary.
urinary alkalizers, such as carbonic anhydrase inhibitors, citrus fruit juices in large amounts, and antacids containing calcium and/or magnesium	May result in increased reabsorption of quinidine and elevated serum levels; dosage adjustments may be necessary.

■ **Nursing Diagnosis.** With the administration of quinidine, the client may experience the following nursing diagnoses/collaborative problems: impaired comfort (skin flushing, bitter taste, or abdominal cramping); risk for injury related to cinchonism (blurred vision, dizziness, headache, altered hearing), hypotension (syncope), and anemia (tiredness, weakness); imbalanced nutrition: less than body requirements related to gastrointestinal effects (anorexia, nausea, vomiting or diarrhea); disturbed thought processes (confusion); and the potential complications of allergic reaction (fever, rash, wheezing, dyspnea), thrombocytopenia (unusual bruising or bleeding), and further dysrhythmias.

■ **Implementation**

■ ***Monitoring.*** Use caution during the IV administration of quinidine because of possible vasodilation, depressed cardiac contraction, and cardiovascular collapse, which may lead to profound shock. NOTE: The IV route is seldom used.

TABLE 26-1 Selected Antidysrhythmics: Pharmacokinetics

Drug	Time to Peak Level or Effect (hours)	Duration of Action* (hours)	Therapeutic Serum Level† (μg/mL)
Group I-A Drugs			
disopyramide	0.5-3	1.5-8.5	3-6
procainamide	1-1.5	3	4-10
quinidine	1-4	6-8	3-6
Group I-B Drugs			
lidocaine	IV: 1 minute	10-20 minutes	1.5-5
tocainide	0.5-2	8	4-10
mexiletine	2-3	—	0.5-2
Group I-C Drugs			
flecainide	3	—	0.2-1 (trough)
propafenone	3.5	—	0.06-1 (trough)
Group I Drugs (A, B, C)			
moricizine	0.5-2 level 6-14 effect	10-24	—
Group II Drugs			
propranolol	1-1.5	3-5	0.05-0.1
Group III Drugs			
bretylium	IV: 5-10 minutes‡ IM: 1‡	6-8 —	0.5-1.5 0.5-2.5
amiodarone	3-7	Variable	1-2.5§
dofetilide (Tikosyn)	PO: SS 2-3 days	10	—
sotalol	2-3	7-18	—
Group IV Drugs			
Calcium antagonists (see Chapter 28)			

Information from *Drug Facts and Comparisons.* (2000). St. Louis: Facts and Comparisons; *United States Pharmacopeia Dispensing Information (USP DI): Drug information for the health care professional* (19th ed.). (1999). Rockville, MD: United States Pharmacopeial Convention; *Physicians' Desk Reference.* (1999). Montvale, NJ: Medical Economics Company; and Chow, M.S.S. & Kertland, H.R. (1995). Cardiac arrhythmias. In L.Y. Young & M.A. Koda-Kimble (Eds.), *Applied therapeutics: The clinical use of drugs* (6th ed.). Vancouver, WA: Applied Therapeutics.
SS, Steady state.
*Metabolism/excretion is primarily via the liver/kidneys, with the exception of amiodarone, mexiletine, and moricizine, which are mainly excreted via bile.
†Steady-state plasma level.
‡To treat ventricular fibrillation.
§Steady state following 2 months of drug therapy.

Continuously monitor both the ECG and the systemic arterial blood pressure during and immediately after parenteral administration. Quinidine is potentially cardiotoxic at doses that exceed 2.4 g daily. Toxic effects include widening of the QRS complex in excess of 25%, abolition of P waves, and ventricular extrasystoles. Notify the prescriber immediately when such effects occur.

Monitor blood pressure, ECG, intake and output, blood counts, serum electrolyte determinations, and kidney and liver function tests during prolonged therapy. The effect of quinidine is reduced if hypokalemia is present. Quinidine serum levels may also be monitored.

Use quinidine with caution in clients with atrial fibrillation or flutter. The vagal blocking effect of the drug may increase the number of atrial beats conducted across the AV junction, resulting in a sudden acceleration in ventricular rate. *Prior administration of digitalis slows AV conduction and reduces the hazard of ventricular tachycardia.* Monitor ECG and blood serum levels of quinidine and digitoxin to avoid toxicity. A reduction in the dosage of digoxin is suggested when quinidine is given simultaneously. Check plasma quinidine levels carefully. Be aware that concomitant administration with digitalis (digoxin) readily induces toxicity because it leads to an excessively high plasma concentration of digoxin (less digoxin is excreted by the kidney).

Be alert to premature ventricular contractions not noted before drug administration (appears as ectopic foci by reentry phenomenon), because they may lead to ventricular tachycardia or fibrillation and subsequently to cardiac standstill (asystole). Note that another form of ventricular disorder can cause "quinidine syncope." It produces ventricular tachycardia or fibrillation, causing a decrease in cardiac output and thereby diminishing blood flow to the brain. The symptoms are a feeling of faintness, loss of consciousness and, ultimately, sudden death.

■ ***Intervention.*** To determine if the client may have an idiosyncratic response or hypersensitivity to quinidine, give a test dose of 200 mg PO a few hours before initiating therapy. A parenteral dose of 200 mg is also administered before IM or IV therapy if time permits. Observe the client for fever, acute asthma, angioedema, and anaphylactic shock. Cinchonism may also be manifested as headache, dizziness, fever, tinnitus, nausea, tremor, and vision disturbances. Administer the oral preparation on an empty stomach 1 to 2 hours after meals with a full glass of water to promote absorption. Quinidine may be given with food to decrease gastric distress if it occurs.

■ ***Education.*** Instruct the client undergoing quinidine therapy to report any symptoms of rash, ringing in the ears, or visual disturbances. Caution the client to report feeling faint to the prescriber immediately. Examine the buccal mucosa for petechial hemorrhage. If bleeding occurs, report immediately; in this case quinidine is discontinued because of possible thrombocytopenic purpura.

Advise the client to have regular dental checkups and to practice good dental hygiene, because the antimuscarinic effects of the drug inhibit salivary flow and thus contribute to caries and gum disease, particularly in older adults. Recommend that the client carry medical identification. Caution the client to alert health care professionals, including dentists, that quinidine is being taken. Instruct the client to continue to take the drug, even if feeling well, and to check with the prescriber before discontinuing the medication.

■ **Evaluation.** The expected outcome of quinidine therapy is that the client's ECG will demonstrate an absence of atrial and ventricular ectopy.

disopyramide [dye soe peer′ a mide] (Norpace)

The effects of disopyramide are similar to those of quinidine with the exception that the anticholinergic effects of disopyramide are more prominent. This is the reason why a drug that slows AV conduction is administered with disopyramide for the treatment of atrial flutter or atrial fibrillation. Converting a unidirectional block into a bidirectional block (see Figure 26-1) abolishes reentrant dysrhythmias.

Disopyramide is indicated to treat ventricular dysrhythmias. See Table 26-1 for the pharmacokinetics of this drug.

The side effects/adverse reactions of disopyramide are similar to quinidine with exception of tinnitus, visual changes, and rash. In addition, disopyramide may cause dry mouth and throat, difficulty in urination, weight gain, and sexual impotency.

The dosage of disopyramide is individualized according to response and tolerance. The usual adult loading dose is 300 mg for clients weighing 50 kg or greater; the maintenance dosage is 150 mg every 6 hours. Older adults usually require a dosage reduction because they are more sensitive to the effects produced by the usual adult dosage. The dosage for children varies by age; the nurse should check a current reference for specific dosing recommendations.

■ Nursing Management

Disopyramide Therapy

In addition to the following discussion, see Nursing Management: Antidysrhythmic Therapy, p. 550.

■ **Assessment.** Despite the fact that little effect has been shown on the AV junction conduction time, do not use disopyramide in clients with greater than first-degree block. It should be discontinued if second- or third-degree block occurs during therapy; the PR interval will be prolonged. Do not use in clients with cardiogenic shock or known hypersensitivity to the drug.

Administering disopyramide to clients with cardiac conditions such as cardiac conduction abnormalities resulting in decreased conduction, congestive heart failure, and cardiomyopathies is not recommended because of its cardiac depressive effects. The client's serum potassium level must be within the normal range; if it is too high, serious dysrhythmias may occur; if it is too low, the drug may not be effective.

Disopyramide may cause hypoglycemia in clients with diabetes mellitus. Administer disopyramide phosphate cautiously in pregnant clients because it has been reported to produce uterine contractions in such clients.

The anticholinergic properties of disopyramide may cause urinary retention in clients with prostatic enlargement or bladder neck obstruction or a myasthenic crisis in clients with myasthenia gravis. The anticholinergic activity of this drug may also precipitate an acute condition in clients with a history of closed-angle glaucoma. If administered to clients with either renal or hepatic function impairment, an accumulation of disopyramide may result; dosage reductions may be required.

Review the client's current medication regimen for the risk of significant drug interactions, such as those that may occur when disopyramide is given concurrently with the following drugs:

Drug	Possible Effect and Management
Bold/color type indicates the most serious interactions.	
other antidysrhythmic agents, such as diltiazem (Cardizem), flecainide (Tambocor), lidocaine, procainamide (Pronestyl), beta-adrenergic blocking agents, quinidine, tocainide (Tonocard), or verapamil (Calan)	**Monitor closely for prolonged electrophysiologic conduction and decreased cardiac output. Beta-adrenergic blocking agents may exacerbate heart failure, especially in individuals with compromised ventricular function. Avoid concurrent use or a potentially serious drug interaction may occur. Do not administer disopyramide concurrently with, within 48 hours before, or 24 hours after verapamil, because fatalities have been reported.**
pimozide (Orap)	Concurrent therapy may prolong the QT interval, which may result in cardiac dysrhythmias. Monitor closely if used concurrently.

In addition to the assessment indicators discussed within the general nursing management of antidysrhythmic therapy, a baseline assessment of the client receiving disopyramide should include blood glucose determination, intraocular pressure, complete blood cell counts, and hepatic and renal function.

▪ **Nursing Diagnosis.** With the administration of disopyramide, the client has the potential to develop the following nursing diagnoses/collaborative problems: urinary retention related to the anticholinergic effects of the drug (10% to 20%); impaired comfort related to chest pain (1% to 10%) and dry mouth (40%); disturbed thought processes (confusion [1% to 10%], depression [<1%]); excess fluid volume (1% to 10%) (swelling of the feet and lower legs, rapid weight gain, shortness of breath); risk for injury related to dizziness, syncope, and weakness of hypotension (1% to 10%), blurred vision, and hypoglycemia (<1%); constipation related to the anticholinergic effects (1% to 10%); situational low self-esteem related to decreased sexual ability (1% to 10%); and the potential complications of decreased cardiac output (1% to 10%) and agranulocytosis (<1%) (sore throat and fever).

▪ **Implementation**

▪ ***Monitoring.*** Monitor blood pressure carefully; disopyramide should be discontinued if hypotension, bradycardia, or congestive heart failure becomes worse. The symptoms of congestive heart failure are difficulty in breathing, shortness of breath, weight gain, distended neck veins, and pulmonary rales.

Monitor ECG intervals carefully to avoid cardiac toxicity. The following signs are indications to collaborate with the prescriber in planning for drug withdrawal:

- The QRS complex widens more than 25%
- The QT interval is prolonged more than 25% (dose monitoring is required and discontinuing the drug is considered)

ECG monitoring is essential for clients with severe cardiac disease, hypertension, or renal or hepatic impairment. Monitor the serum level of potassium; it should be normal to achieve the optimal effect. Excessive potassium levels enhance toxic reactions. Measure intake and output, particularly in clients with impaired renal function or prostatic hypertrophy. Urinary retention may require stopping the use of disopyramide. Monitor blood glucose concentrations for those clients at risk for hypoglycemia.

▪ ***Intervention.*** Clients with preexisting closed-angle glaucoma should receive disopyramide only if cholinergic eye drops are also administered to control the ocular anticholinergic effects of the drug. If the client receives a loading dose of disopyramide, monitor for hypotension and congestive heart failure closely. Clients stabilized with other antidysrhythmic agents may be changed to disopyramide (6 to 12 hours after the last dose of quinidine sulfate, and 3 to 6 hours after the last dose of procainamide). Clients with atrial flutter and fibrillation should be digitalized before disopyramide therapy begins to ensure that the enhanced AV conduction does not increase the ventricular rate to inappropriate levels.

▪ ***Education.*** Instruct the client to make position changes slowly from the recumbent posture if hypotension should occur. Advise the client about the possibility of dry mouth, which can be relieved with sugarless hard candy, gum, or frequent clear water rinses. Recommend regular dental checkups for the prevention of caries and periodontal disease. In addition, instruct the client to avoid alcoholic beverages because of the potential hypotensive effects.

Emphasize the importance of not skipping doses or stopping the medication without consulting the prescriber; adverse cardiac effects may occur with sudden withdrawal. Instruct the client to swallow the extended-release forms whole and not to chew, crush, or break them.

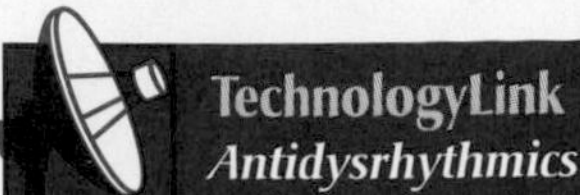

TechnologyLink
Antidysrhythmics

Audio Resources

Mosby Heart Sounds and Murmurs: A Practical Guide with Audiotape, 3rd ed., ISBN 0-8151-3146-1
Mosby, Inc. 11830 Westline Industrial Drive, St. Louis, MO 63146; (800) 426-4545; www.mosby.com.
Mosby Heart Sounds and Murmurs: A Practical Guide with Audio Compact Disk, ISBN 0-8151-3659-5

Video Resources

Mosby's Medical-Surgical Nursing Videotape Series, Nursing Management of Myocardial Infarction, ISBN 0-8151-6053-4

Web Resources

American Heart Association
Statistical Update on Heart and Stroke Disease: (www.americanheart.org/presenter.jhtml?identifier=1200026)
Official web site with guidelines, heart and stroke information, and more: www.americanheart.org

Cardiac Arrhythmias Research & Education Foundation, Inc. (www.longqt.org/)
This site provides articles, a newsletter, and other resources. Items can be translated from English to French, German, Italian, Portuguese, or Spanish.

Mayo Clinic Heart & Blood Vessels Center (www.mayoclinic.com)
This site provides the latest news and information on heart disease and cardiac-related problems.

National Heart, Lung, and Blood Institute (www.nhlbi.nih.gov/index.htm)
This site provides links to health information, scientific resources, guidelines, and other health information.

For additional WebLinks, a free subscription to the "Mosby/Saunders ePharmocology Update" newsletter, and more, go to mosby.com/MERLIN/McKenry/.

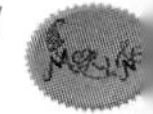

Instruct the client to weigh daily to monitor fluid retention. Report to the prescriber a weight gain of 2 or more pounds within a 24-hour period. Observe for edema.

Caution the client about driving or other hazardous activities, because blurred vision and dizziness may occur. Alert clients about the hypoglycemic effects of the drug, particularly clients with diabetes. Teach the signs and symptoms of hypoglycemia; instruct the client to take some form of sugar and notify the prescriber if they occur. Caution the client to avoid exertion and hot weather, because heat intolerance and reduced perspiration will occur. Constipation may result from the anticholinergic effects of the drug. Instruct clients about a high-fiber diet, increased fluid intake, moderate exercise, and regular bowel patterning.

■ **Evaluation.** The expected outcome of disopyramide therapy is that the client will have regular palpable pulses and demonstrate on the ECG the absence of or a decrease in ventricular ectopy.

procainamide [proe kane′ a mide] (Pronestyl)

The electrophysiologic effects of procainamide are similar to those of quinidine, with the following exceptions:

- Procainamide appears to be less effective in controlling abnormal ectopic pacemaker activity.
- Procainamide has fewer anticholinergic effects than quinidine.
- Procainamide has more potent negative inotropic effects than quinidine.

As a result, the direct depressant effect of procainamide on the SA node and AV junction may not be as effectively balanced by vagal blockade as it is with quinidine. Procainamide may also cause severe congestive heart failure in clients with a preexisting ventricular dysfunction.

The primary indications for procainamide for the treatment of atrial and ventricular dysrhythmias, such as premature ventricular contractions, ventricular tachycardia, atrial fibrillation, and paroxysmal atrial tachycardia. It is also used to treat cardiac dysrhythmias associated with anesthesia and surgery. See Table 26-1 for the pharmacokinetics of procainamide.

The side effects/adverse reactions of procainamide are similar to quinidine, with the exception of tinnitus and visual changes. In addition, a systemic lupus erythematosus (SLE)–type reaction may occur with fever, chills, painful joints, and rash.

The adult antidysrhythmic dosage of procainamide is 50 mg/kg PO or IM in 8 divided doses daily. The pediatric oral dosage is 12.5 mg/kg four times daily.

■ Nursing Management

Procainamide Therapy

In addition to the following discussion, see Nursing Management: Antidysrhythmic Therapy, p. 550.

■ **Assessment.** Because of its additive cardiac depressive effects, procainamide is contraindicated for use in second- or third-degree or complete AV block unless the client has an electric pacemaker. Clients with torsades de pointes (a type of ventricular tachycardia) may experience an aggravation of their condition. Use with caution in clients with atrial fibrillation or flutter; ventricular rate may increase suddenly because the atrial rate is slowed. Embolization may result from the dislodgment of mural thrombi as a result of forceful contraction of the atrium with conversion to sinus rhythm. There is a risk of increased cardiac depression with AV block, bundle branch block, or digitalis toxicity. Congestive heart failure and hepatic and renal impairment may cause drug accumulation, leading to toxicity. Procainamide may precipitate an active episode of SLE in clients with a history of this condition. This drug may also increase muscle weakness in clients with myasthenia gravis.

Review the client's current medication regimen for the risk of significant drug interactions, such as those that may occur when procainamide is given concurrently with the following drugs:

Drug	Possible Effect and Management
other antidysrhythmic agents	Monitor for enhanced or additive cardiac effects.
antihypertensives	Increased hypotension has been reported, especially when parenteral (IV) procainamide is given with antihypertensive agents. Monitor closely, because dosage adjustments may be necessary.
antimyasthenia agents	The effect of antimyasthenic agents on skeletal muscle may be blocked by the antimuscarinic effects of procainamide. Monitor closely, because dosage adjustments of the antimyasthenic agent may be required.
neuromuscular blocking agents	Concurrent use may result in enhanced neuromuscular blockade. Monitor closely because the reversal of blockade may be prolonged.
pimozide (Orap)	Prolonged QT intervals and cardiac dysrhythmias may be reported with concurrent use. Monitor closely, preferably with an ECG, because intervention may be necessary.

In addition to the indicators for the baseline assessment of clients receiving antidysrhythmic therapy, the baseline assessment for the administration of procainamide should include complete blood cell counts.

■ **Nursing Diagnosis.** With the administration of procainamide, the client may experience the following nursing diagnoses/collaborative problems: disturbed thought processes related to central nervous system (CNS) effects (confusion, hallucinations); risk for injury related to dizziness or light-headedness; risk for infection related to leukopenia and agranulocytosis (fever, sore mouth, gums, and throat); diarrhea; and the potential complications of allergic reaction, mental depression, SLE-like syndrome (30%) (fever, chills, skin rash, arthralgia), hemolytic anemia, and thrombocytopenia (unusual bleeding and bruising).

■ **Implementation**

■ ***Monitoring.*** Continue to monitor general cardiovascular status. Monitor IV administration constantly, and observe the following:

- *Infusion pump.* Maintain desired flow rate. Keep the client in the supine position. Avoid rapid administration to prevent "speed shock" (irregular pulse, tight feeling in chest, flushed face, headache, loss of consciousness, shock, cardiac arrest).
- *ECG monitoring.* Discontinue therapy if the QRS complex is widened greater than 50% and the PR interval is prolonged.
- *Arterial blood pressure.* Measure the client's blood pressure every 5 minutes during the loading dose; discontinue the infusion if the blood pressure drops more than 15 mm Hg. Have pressor solutions available, such as phenylephrine or norepinephrine to treat hypotension. Older adults are more apt to exhibit hypotension.

Monitor serum electrolytes, because hypokalemia predisposes the client to dysrhythmias. Blood pressure, ECG, and complete blood cell counts should be monitored with oral doses.

■ ***Intervention.*** To initiate IV therapy, the drug should be diluted in 5% dextrose to facilitate control of the dosage range; the dose should be administered at a rate not greater than 50 mg/min by direct IV administration or infusion. IV therapy is limited to use in hospitals, where monitoring facilities are available. Once prepared, the solution is stable for 24 hours at room temperature or 7 days if refrigerated. Procainamide is physically incompatible with many substances; check specific references when considering mixing with other drugs. The first oral dose should be administered at least 3 to 4 hours after the last IV dose.

■ ***Education.*** Urge the client undergoing long-term procainamide therapy to keep appointments for periodic laboratory work: antinuclear antibody (ANA) titers, blood counts, and plasma procainamide and *N*-acetylprocainamide (NAPA) determinations. This is particularly important in clients with congestive heart failure, in clients with hepatic or renal function impairment, or in clients who are changing from a regular oral to an extended-release preparation of the drug. Symptoms of SLE (polyarthralgia, cough, fever, and pleuritic pain) and steady increases in ANA titers should be reported to the prescriber so the drug can be discontinued.

Counsel clients to report to the prescriber symptoms such as unusual bleeding and/or bruising; sore mouth, gums, or throat; fever; rash; or symptoms of an upper respiratory tract infection. These symptoms are more apt to occur with the extended-release dosage form.

Some clients, particularly older adults, may be prone to dizziness. Alert them that driving and operating other mechanical equipment might be hazardous. Instruct the client to make positional changes gradually to avoid postural hypotension.

Advise the client to continue to take the medication even though he or she is feeling well. If a regular oral preparation dose is missed, instruct the client to take the dose if it is remembered within 2 hours (within 4 hours for the extended-release form). A missed dose remembered after this time *should not be taken.* Instruct the client not to double up on doses. Alert the client not to discontinue the medication without consulting the prescriber, because a gradual withdrawal may be necessary to prevent worsening the condition.

Recommend that the client carry medical identification. The client should be instructed to alert health care professionals, including dentists, that he or she is taking procainamide. The secondary anticholinergic effects of the drug decrease salivary flow and may contribute to caries and periodontal disease; recommend that the client maintain regular dental appointments. The oral forms of procainamide are hygroscopic (they will absorb moisture). Advise the client to keep these medications tightly closed in their original container and not to transfer them to less tightly sealed containers or leave them exposed to air.

Caution the client receiving the extended-release form of procainamide that the dose is contained in a wax matrix that may be detected in the stools. This has no effect on the absorption of the drug.

■ **Evaluation.** The expected outcome of procainamide therapy is that the client will demonstrate a regular palpable pulse and an absence of or decrease in atrial and ventricular ectopy on the ECG.

GROUP I-B DRUGS

The Group I-B drugs (e.g., lidocaine [Xylocaine], phenytoin [Dilantin], tocainide [Tonocard], and mexiletine [Mexitil]) differ from Group I-A drugs in that they either increase or have no effect on conduction velocity. Although not approved by the Food and Drug Administration (FDA), phenytoin is used in the therapy of digitalis-induced dysrhythmias. Lidocaine, tocainide, and mexiletine are related therapeutically and are particularly useful for acute ventricular dysrhythmias. The high incidence of side effects/adverse reactions with mexiletine has limited its use. Tocainide can cause the serious adverse reaction of agranulocytosis, and therefore it is usually reserved for clients who have not responded to other drug therapies.

lidocaine [lye' doe kane] (Xylocaine, Xylocard ♣)

Lidocaine, an agent used extensively as a local and topical anesthetic agent, is also an antidysrhythmic agent, especially for ventricular dysrhythmias seen after cardiac surgery or an acute myocardial infarction. Lidocaine appears to act primarily on the sodium channel, blocking both the activated and inactivated sodium channels; its greater effect is in depolarized or ischemic tissues. These effects are indicative of the efficacy of lidocaine for suppressing the dysrhythmias associated with depolarization (e.g., ischemia, digitalis-induced toxicity) and of its lack of effectiveness in dysrhythmias that occur in normal polarized tissues (atrial fibrillation, atrial flutter). Lidocaine has few electrophysiologic effects in normal cardiac tissue.

Unlike quinidine and procainamide, lidocaine has no vagolytic properties, nor does it influence cardiac output and arterial pressure. It does not depress myocardial contractility and thereby provides no potential for the development of congestive heart failure. Because lidocaine exerts a limited effect, if any, on the SA node and atrial myocardium, it has no use in the treatment of supraventricular tachycardias. Because electric activities are primarily limited to the ventricular cells, the major use of lidocaine is in abolishing ventricular dysrhythmias (see Figure 26-1, *D*).

See Table 26-1 for the pharmacokinetics of lidocaine.

The side effects/adverse reactions of lidocaine include dizziness, anorexia, nausea, vomiting, chest pain, and breathing difficulties. See Table 26-2 for the adverse effects of lidocaine as related to serum concentration.

The adult dosage of lidocaine is by IV bolus, 1 mg/kg at a rate of 25 to 50 mg/min; this may be repeated in 5 minutes if necessary (the maximum dose per hour is 300 mg). Children receive the same 1 mg/kg dose initially, but repeat doses in 5 minutes should not exceed a total of 3 mg/kg. With IV infusion, the dosage is usually 20 to 50 μg/kg given at a rate of 1 to 4 mg/min for both adults and children.

■ Nursing Management

Lidocaine Therapy

In addition to the following discussion, see Nursing Management: Antidysrhythmic Therapy, p. 550.

■ **Assessment.** Do not administer lidocaine to clients who have severe degrees of sinoatrial, atrioventricular, or intraventricular block or who have **Adams-Stokes syndrome** (sudden, recurring episodes of loss of consciousness, caused by the transient interruption of cardiac output by incomplete or complete heart block); the administration of lidocaine may worsen the heart block. The risk-benefit ratio should be considered with clients who have a known history of hypersensitivity to the amide type of local anesthetics. Use lidocaine with caution in individuals with hypovolemia, shock, all forms of heart block, sinus bradycardia, and **Wolff-Parkinson-White syndrome** (a supraventricular tachycardia), because these conditions may be aggravated. Use with caution and in lower dosages in older adults and in individuals with congestive heart failure or reduced cardiac output. To prevent toxicity in clients with impaired renal and hepatic function, exercise caution with prolonged use because lidocaine is metabolized mainly in the liver and excreted by the kidney.

TABLE 26-2 Adverse Reactions Related to Serum Concentrations of Lidocaine

Serum Concentration	Adverse Reactions
1.5-6 μg/mL	Anxiety, nervousness, drowsiness, dizziness, sensations of cold, heat, or numbness
6-8 μg/mL	Tremors, twitching, blurred or double vision, nausea, vomiting, tinnitus
>8 μg/mL	Dyspnea, severe dizziness, fainting, bradycardia, convulsions

The use of lidocaine during human pregnancy has not been established by adequate studies. Administer only when the potential benefits outweigh the potential hazards to the fetus, because lidocaine may constrict the arteries in the uterus, resulting in fetal hypoxia.

A significant drug interaction may occur when lidocaine is administered with phenytoin (hydantoin anticonvulsant); it may result in enhanced cardiac depressant effects. The anticonvulsant may reduce the serum concentration of lidocaine by increasing the liver metabolism of lidocaine.

A baseline assessment of the client should include the indicators described within the discussion of the general nursing management of antidysrhythmics.

■ **Nursing Diagnosis.** With the administration of lidocaine, the client should be assessed for the following selected nursing diagnoses/collaborative problems: impaired comfort related to prolonged IV use (pain at the site of injection) and specific serum levels of the drug (nervousness, dizziness, drowsiness, and feelings of numbness, cold, and heat); risk for injury related to drug toxicity (blurred vision, nausea, vomiting, tinnitus, tremors, dizziness, seizures, bradycardia); and the potential complications of allergic reaction (skin rash, urticaria, and dyspnea) and decreased cardiac output related to cardiac conduction disturbances (hypotension, dysrhythmias, heart block, and cardiac arrest).

■ **Implementation**

■ ***Monitoring.*** Constant ECG monitoring is essential for IV administration and is recommended during IM administration to observe for signs of toxicity. Monitor ECG and blood pressure to avoid potential overdose and toxicity. Stop the infusion immediately if excessive cardiac depression occurs, such as prolongation of the PR interval or QRS complex or aggravation of dysrhythmias. Serum electrolyte levels should be determined periodically during prolonged lidocaine infusions to correct imbalances. Observe the client for adverse reactions to lidocaine (see Table 26-2). Monitor serum lidocaine levels to minimize the chance of toxicity if high-dose infusions are used or if the client is receiving other drugs that might affect lidocaine clearance.

If the IV administration runs for more than 24 hours, observe for local thrombophlebitis and assess the client for the risk of accumulation.

■ ***Intervention.*** Recheck the drug label; administer only lidocaine hydrochloride *without preservatives or epinephrine.* The label will specifically read "IV use for cardiac dysrhythmias." Preparations intended for use as an anesthetic contain epinephrine and *should not* be used for treating dysrhythmias. IV infusions of lidocaine are usually prepared by adding 1 g of lidocaine to 1 L of 5% dextrose solution for a 1 mg/mL solution. The solution is stable for 24 hours. Do not add to blood transfusions. For IV administration, use a precision IV volume control set for continuous infusion.

A bolus dose is usually given to rapidly attain therapeutic serum concentrations. If the loading dose does not provide the desired therapeutic effect within 5 minutes, a second dose may be administered (one half to one third of the initial dose). However, administer no more than 200 to 300 mg in a 1-hour period. Monitor the prescribed IV rate of flow, usually at no more than 4 mg/min. Terminate the IV infusion as soon as the cardiac rhythm is stable or signs of toxicity develop. Have resuscitative equipment and drugs available to treat adverse reactions involving the cardiovascular system, respiratory system, and CNS.

Note that IV infusions are rarely continued beyond 24 hours. The client is then given an oral antidysrhythmic agent for maintenance therapy. After the initial use, discard partially used solutions of lidocaine that contain no preservatives.

In clients over age 65 or in those with congestive heart failure or renal or hepatic function impairment, the dose and rate of infusion is generally reduced by one half and adjusted in response to the client's condition.

▪ ***Education.*** Provide continuous explanation to the client about the monitoring equipment. Instruct the client to report any dizziness, chest pain, or shortness of breath.

▪ **Evaluation.** The expected outcome of lidocaine antidysrhythmic therapy is that the client will have regular palpable pulses and will experience an absence of or a decrease in ventricular ectopy on the ECG.

tocainide [toe kay′ nide] (Tonocard)
mexiletine [mex il′ e teen] (Mexitil)

Tocainide and mexiletine are chemically and therapeutically related to lidocaine. Because they resist first-pass liver metabolism, they may be administered orally. Dysrhythmias that respond to parenteral lidocaine are usually responsive to these drugs. They are indicated for the treatment and/or the prevention of ventricular dysrhythmias.

See Table 26-1 for the pharmacokinetics of tocainide and mexiletine.

The side effects/adverse reactions of tocainide and mexiletine are similar to lidocaine. In addition, paresthesia of the fingers and toes, rash, tremors and, usually with tocainide, pneumonitis and sweating are reported.

The adult dosage of mexiletine is usually 200 mg PO every 8 hours, titrated as necessary. The tocainide adult dosage is 400 mg PO every 8 hours. Older adults should receive smaller dosages because they may be more sensitive to these drugs. Pediatric dosages have not been established.

▪ Nursing Management

Tocainide Therapy

In addition to the following discussion, see Nursing Management: Antidysrhythmic Therapy, p. 550.

▪ **Assessment.** Determine that the client is not sensitive to tocainide or local amide-type anesthetics and has no preexisting second- or third-degree AV block unless he or she has an electric pacemaker. Note whether the client has renal or hepatic function impairment; in such cases tocainide must be used cautiously and with intensive monitoring because of the reduced elimination and biotransformation of the drug. Clients with congestive heart failure may have their condition worsen because of the small negative inotropic effect of tocainide. Caution should be used in clients with atrial flutter or fibrillation because acceleration of ventricular rate may infrequently occur. A baseline health assessment specific to this drug should include an ECG, a chest x-ray examination, and blood counts. No significant drug interactions are reported to date.

▪ **Nursing Diagnosis.** With the administration of tocainide, the client should be assessed for the development of the following nursing diagnoses/collaborative problems: impaired comfort related to CNS effects (dizziness, headache, blurred vision, trembling, numbness or tingling of the fingers and toes) and gastrointestinal effects (anorexia, nausea, vomiting); disturbed thought processes (confusion); risk for infection related to the development of leukopenia or agranulocytosis (fever, chills); impaired skin integrity related to skin reactions (peeling, scaling, and blisters of the skin); and the potential complications of thrombocytopenia (unusual bruising or bleeding), pneumonia, pulmonary fibrosis or edema (cough, dyspnea), and decreased cardiac output related to further cardiac dysrhythmias.

▪ **Implementation**

▪ ***Monitoring.*** Measure blood counts at periodic intervals to detect bone marrow suppression, and monitor ECG tracings for medication effectiveness. Chest x-ray examinations are required at the first sign of pulmonary complications, such as pneumonia, pulmonary edema, or pulmonary fibrosis. If the client shows evidence of tremor, it may be an indication that the highest tolerable dosage has been reached.

▪ ***Intervention.*** Administer tocainide with food or milk to reduce gastric distress. If the client has adverse reactions shortly after taking a dose, each individual dose may be decreased but administered with greater frequency. If the dysrhythmia returns before the next scheduled dose, a higher dosage or more frequent dosing should be considered.

▪ ***Education.*** Instruct the client to take the medication even if he or she is feeling better. Doses should not be missed and should be evenly spaced. A forgotten dose should be taken if remembered within 4 hours. If a longer interval has passed, the dose is not to be taken until the next scheduled time. Advise the client to maintain regular visits to the prescriber to monitor progress. Recommend that a medical identification card be carried or a bracelet worn.

Alert the client that dizziness may occur and that caution should be taken when driving or operating other mechanical equipment. Older adults have an increased risk of falling. Instruct the client to report signs and symptoms of leukopenia and thrombocytopenia (evidence of infection, delayed healing, fever, chills, sore throat, unusual bleeding, and bruising). If these symptoms occur, the client should postpone dental work and should be instructed to use toothbrushes, dental floss, and toothpicks cautiously.

▪ **Evaluation.** The expected outcome of tocainide therapy is that the client will have regular palpable pulses and will experience an absence of or a decrease in ventricular ectopy on the ECG.

■ Nursing Management

Mexiletine Therapy

The nursing management of the client receiving mexiletine is much the same as for tocainide, except that these clients may also experience constipation or diarrhea related to the gastrointestinal effects of the drug, and the risk for impaired skin integrity related to skin reactions is not quite so severe. (For more information, see Nursing Management: Tocainide Therapy, p. 558.)

GROUP I-C DRUGS

The Group I-C drugs include flecainide (Tambocor) and propafenone (Rythmol), which are used to treat and/or prevent supraventricular tachydysrhythmias. These agents can cause sinus arrest, AV block, and life-threatening ventricular dysrhythmias. This prodysrhythmic effect is of special concern, especially in clients with poor left ventricular function or sustained ventricular dysrhythmias. The Group I-C drugs can also aggravate congestive heart failure.

flecainide [fle kay′ nide] (Tambocor)

Flecainide is a sodium channel blocking agent used to treat ventricular dysrhythmias; it has minimal effects on repolarization and has no anticholinergic properties. It suppresses premature ventricular contractions and in high doses may exacerbate dysrhythmias in clients with a preexisting ventricular tachydysrhythmia or in clients with a previous myocardial infarction. It is indicated for the treatment of ventricular dysrhythmias and as prophylaxis of supraventricular dysrhythmias, such as AV junction reentrant tachycardia. See Table 26-1 for the pharmacokinetics of flecainide.

The side effects/adverse reactions of flecainide include blurred vision, dizziness, headaches, constipation, nausea, weakness, chest pain, irregular heartbeats, and dysrhythmias. Flecainide, if administered with other antidysrhythmic agents, may result in enhanced adverse cardiac effects. Irreversible ventricular tachycardia or ventricular fibrillation has been reported in persons with hypotensive ventricular tachycardia. Avoid concurrent use with other antidysrhythmic agents.

The adult dosage of flecainide is 50 to 100 mg PO every 12 hours, titrated every 4 days as necessary.

■ Nursing Management

Flecainide Therapy

In addition to the following discussion, see Nursing Management: Antidysrhythmic Therapy, p. 550. The nursing management of flecainide is essentially the same as for tocainide. However, pulmonary symptoms such as pneumonia and pulmonary fibrosis are not a concern with flecainide. Cigarette smoking induces the metabolism of flecainide with clinically significant results (Zevin & Benowitz, 1999). Dosage adjustments may be required.

propafenone [proe paff′ e nohn] (Rythmol)

Propafenone is similar to flecainide in its action and therapeutic uses. It also has some beta-blocking activity and weak calcium channel blocking activity. It prevents the passage of sodium ions into the fast sodium channels (phase 0), resulting in a decrease in depolarization rate. It also prolongs the refractory period in cardiac tissues. It is indicated for the treatment of life-threatening ventricular dysrhythmias.

See Table 26-1 for the pharmacokinetics of propafenone.

The side effects/adverse reactions of propafenone include dizziness, nausea, headaches, constipation, weakness, chest pain, irregular heartbeats, and dysrhythmias.

The usual adult dosage is 150 mg PO every 8 hours, with dosage adjustments at 3- to 4-day intervals as necessary. The pediatric dosage is unknown.

■ Nursing Management

Propafenone Therapy

In addition to the following discussion, see Nursing Management: Antidysrhythmic Therapy, p. 550.

■ Assessment. Because of the risk of complete heart block, propafenone is contraindicated in preexisting second- or third-degree AV block or right bundle branch block associated with left hemiblock without an electric pacemaker. Its use should be carefully considered in clients with congestive heart failure because of its negative inotropic effects and in clients with cardiogenic shock or sinus bradycardia because further myocardial depression may result. With sick sinus syndrome, sinus node recovery may be prolonged, resulting in sinus bradycardia, sinus pause, or sinus arrest. The effective dosage for older adults may be lower because of impaired hepatic or renal function in this age-group. As with the other antidysrhythmic agents, an ECG should be obtained before beginning therapy. Electrolyte imbalances should also be corrected because the effects of propafenone will be altered if imbalances are present. The client's sensitivity to propafenone should be ascertained.

A potentially significant drug interaction with digoxin has been reported; digoxin serum levels may increase from 35% to 85% depending on the dose of propafenone consumed, which increases the potential for digitalis toxicity. The digoxin dosage should be reduced when propafenone is started. Warfarin plasma concentrations also increase with concurrent administration, which may lead to an increase in prothrombin times (25% increase). Monitor closely, because warfarin dosage adjustments are usually necessary.

■ Nursing Diagnosis. Once propafenone has been administered, assess the client for the following nursing diagnoses/collaborative problems resulting from the effects of the drug: impaired comfort (chest pain, headache, dry mouth, taste disturbance, nausea and vomiting, rash, and dizziness); risk for injury related to hypotension; disturbed sensory perception related to CNS effects (trembling, shaking, blurred vision); diarrhea; constipation; risk for infection related to hematologic effects (agranulocytosis); fatigue; and the potential complication of decreased cardiac

Case Study *The Client Taking Antidysrhythmics*

James Cameron is a 62-year-old manager of a fast-food restaurant who had rheumatic heart disease as a child and who has a long family history of heart disease. He has been having chest pain for the past 3 months, and it is usually relieved by rest. He has come to the emergency department with pain that is more severe than usual and not relieved by rest. His ECG shows elevated ST segments. The chest pain persists, and his vital signs are as follows: blood pressure, 184/90 mm Hg; pulse, 114 beats/min and irregular; and respirations, 24. The physician finds that Mr. Cameron has developed ventricular dysrhythmias that are not only difficult to control with the usual medications—verapamil and lidocaine—but are also becoming life threatening. The physician prescribes propafenone hydrochloride (Rythmol); Mr. Cameron receives 150 mg PO every 8 hours.

1. What nursing diagnoses should be monitored with the administration of propafenone?
2. What side effects should the nurse be alert to?
3. What drug interactions are possible in the coadministration of propafenone?

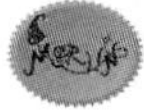

For answer guidelines, go to mosby.com/MERLIN/McKenry/.

output related to further dysrhythmias and the development of hypotension, angina, bradycardia, ventricular tachycardia, and/or congestive heart failure.

▪ **Implementation**

▪ ***Monitoring.*** Continuous ECG monitoring is recommended during the initiation of therapy. Periodic monitoring of the complete blood count (CBC) is recommended. If the client is also receiving digoxin, serum digoxin levels should be monitored. Prothrombin times should be monitored closely with concurrent administration of warfarin.

▪ ***Intervention.*** The therapeutic response to propafenone should be carefully recorded because the dosage is titrated by the prescriber on the basis of the client's response and tolerance (see the Case Study box above).

▪ **Evaluation.** The expected outcome of propafenone therapy is that the client's ventricular dysrhythmia will be suppressed or will diminish in severity.

GROUP I DRUGS (A, B, C)

moricizine [mor i′ si zeen] (Ethmozine)

Moricizine (Ethmozine) has the properties of all three classes (A, B, C) and therefore does not belong to one individual classification. It is a fairly potent sodium channel blocking agent that does not prolong the duration of the action potential. It has local anesthetic action and a membrane stabilizing effect; thus it decreases AV junction and His-Purkinje conduction. It is indicated for the treatment of life-threatening ventricular dysrhythmias.

See Table 26-1 for the pharmacokinetics of moricizine.

The side effects/adverse reactions of moricizine include light-headedness, dry mouth, blurred vision, nausea, vomiting, weakness, chest pain, heart failure, and ventricular tachydysrhythmias. The *United States Pharmacopeia Dispensing Information* (1999) does not list any significant drug interactions.

The adult dosage is 200 to 300 mg PO three times daily every 8 hours; the dosage is titrated as necessary at 3-day intervals. The maximum daily dose is 900 mg.

▪ Nursing Management

Moricizine Therapy

In addition to the discussion of Nursing Management: Antidysrhythmic Therapy, p. 550, the nursing management is essentially the same as for propafenone.

GROUP II DRUGS

propranolol [proe pran′ oh lole] (Inderal)
acebutolol [a se byoo′ toe lole] (Sectral)
esmolol [ess′ moe lol] (Brevibloc)

Propranolol, acebutolol, and esmolol are beta-adrenergic blocking agents used to control cardiac dysrhythmias caused by excessive sympathetic nerve activity. Dysrhythmias caused by an increased sympathetic discharge (hyperthyroidism) are effectively blocked by the beta-adrenergic blocking action of propranolol. Acebutolol is used to treat ventricular dysrhythmias, such as ventricular premature beats, whereas esmolol is indicated for the short-term treatment of supraventricular tachycardia induced by atrial fibrillation or atrial flutter (see the drug monographs in Chapter 22).

GROUP III DRUGS

The electrophysiologic properties of drugs in this group differ markedly from the drugs previously discussed. Drugs in this group prolong the effective refractory period by prolonging the action potential (delay repolarization).

bretylium tosylate [bre til′ ee um] (Bretylol, Bretylate 🍁)

Unlike the other antidysrhythmics, bretylium does not suppress automaticity and has no effect on conduction velocity. The direct electrophysiologic action on the heart appears to be prolongation of the action potential and lengthening of the effective refractory period. This mechanism is believed to help terminate dysrhythmias caused by the reentry phenomenon. Bretylium is also taken up and concentrated in the adrenergic nerve terminals where, after an initial release of norepinephrine, it prevents any further release. This sympatholytic action significantly increases the threshold, producing an antifibrillatory response in the ventricles. Bretylium produces a positive inotropic effect, increasing myocardial contractility. With long-term treatment, the drug shows increased responsiveness to circulating epinephrine and norepinephrine, which may account for the increased myocardial contractility. See Table 26-1 for the pharmacokinetics of bretylium.

The side effects/adverse reactions of bretylium include anorexia, headaches, nausea, vomiting, bitter taste, impotency, dizziness, cough, breathing difficulties, fever, paresthesia of the fingers or toes, hand tremors, and weakness.

The usual adult dosage for life-threatening ventricular fibrillation is 5 mg/kg IV of undiluted solution, followed by 10 mg/kg every 15 to 30 minutes as needed. Refer to a current reference for dosage recommendations for other ventricular dysrhythmias.

■ Nursing Management

Bretylium Therapy

In addition to the following discussion, see Nursing Management: Antidysrhythmic Therapy, p. 550.

■ **Assessment.** Bretylium should be administered with caution to clients with conditions that involve reduced cardiac output, such as aortic stenosis and pulmonary hypertension; in such cases severe hypotension may occur as a result of reduced peripheral resistance without an increase in cardiac output. Clients with renal function impairment require increased dosage intervals because elimination of the drug is reduced. Ascertain whether the client is sensitive to bretylium.

Do not administer digitalis glycosides to clients receiving bretylium. The initial release of norepinephrine produced by bretylium may increase digitalis toxicity.

■ **Nursing Diagnosis.** With the administration of bretylium, the client may be assessed for the following nursing diagnoses: impaired comfort related to rapid IV administration (nausea and vomiting); ineffective breathing pattern related to possible neuromuscular block (<0.1%) (dyspnea, respiratory depression); hyperthermia; risk for injury related to postural hypotension (dizziness, syncope); and the potential complications of angina (chest pain), decreased cardiac output, and renal function impairment.

■ **Implementation**

■ ***Monitoring.*** Continuously monitor ECG and blood pressure during bretylium administration.

■ ***Intervention.*** Administer bretylium to clients in an area that is adequately staffed by qualified personnel and equipped with appropriate facilities for constant ECG monitoring and the use of emergency equipment. Anticipate the possible development of transient hypertension and dysrhythmias during the early stage of therapy. This is caused by the initial release of norepinephrine from adrenergic nerve terminals.

Bretylium is always diluted for intermittent or continuous IV administration, unless it is a situation of life-threatening ventricular fibrillation. In this case, it is administered undiluted and as quickly as possible. In general, however, administer IV doses slowly to prevent nausea and vomiting.

Rotate the IM injection site, and do not administer more than 5 mL at one site. Necrosis, muscle atrophy, or fibrosis may occur if the injection is given repeatedly at the same site. Note that the IM injection is rarely used.

Bretylium is generally discontinued in 3 to 5 days, and an alternate antidysrhythmic agent may be substituted if indicated.

■ ***Education.*** Instruct the client to remain in a supine position during therapy until tolerance to the hypotensive effect of the drug occurs.

■ **Evaluation.** The expected outcome of bretylium therapy is that the client will have regular palpable pulses and will demonstrate an absence of ventricular tachycardia or fibrillation on the ECG.

amiodarone [a mee′ oh da rone] (Cordarone)

Amiodarone increases the refractory period in all cardiac tissues by having a direct effect on the tissues. It decreases automaticity, prolongs AV conduction, and decreases the automaticity of fibers in the Purkinje system. It may block potassium, sodium and calcium channels, and beta receptors. It has the potential to cause a variety of complex effects on the heart and has serious adverse effects. Therefore it is usually reserved for the prevention and treatment of life-threatening ventricular dysrhythmias in persons not responding to or tolerating other drug therapies (Aronow, 1999).

See Table 26-1 for the pharmacokinetics of amiodarone.

The side effects/adverse reactions of amiodarone include dizziness, bitter taste, headache, flushing, nausea, vomiting, constipation, ataxia, weight loss, tremors, numbness and tingling of the fingers and toes, photosensitivity, blue-gray skin discoloration, pulmonary fibrosis or pneumonitis, cough, dyspnea, fever, allergic reaction, and blurred vision.

The usual adult dosage for ventricular dysrhythmias is 800 mg to 1.6 g PO daily for 1 to 3 weeks until a therapeutic response is noted or side effects appear. The dosage is then reduced to 600 to 800 mg daily for 1 month, eventually decreasing to the lowest effective dosage. (See the Pregnancy Safety box on p. 562 for FDA pregnancy safety categories.)

The pediatric dosage is 10 mg/kg/day for 10 days or until a therapeutic response is noted or side effects appear. The dosage is then decreased and tapered to lowest effective dosage as outlined in the package insert.

■ Nursing Management

Amiodarone Therapy

In addition to the following discussion, see Nursing Management: Antidysrhythmic Therapy, p. 550.

■ **Assessment.** Determine that the client does not have either preexisting second- or third-degree AV block (be-

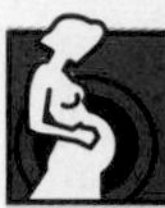

Pregnancy Safety
Antidysrhythmics

Category	Drug
B	lidocaine, moricizine
C	adenosine, bretylium, disopyramide, dofetilide, flecainide, ibutilide, mexiletine, procainamide, propafenone, quinidine, tocainide
D	amiodarone
Unclassified	sotalol

cause of the risk of complete heart block) or syncope as a result of severe bradycardia or sinus node function impairment (because of the risk of atropine-resistant sinus bradycardia) unless controlled by a pacemaker. Use caution if the client has congestive heart failure or impaired hepatic or thyroid function. Hypokalemia should be corrected before the initiation of amiodarone therapy to ensure the effectiveness of the drug. Hypersensitivity to amiodarone should be determined.

Review the client's current medication regimen for the risk of significant drug interactions, such as those that may occur when amiodarone is given concurrently with the following drugs:

Drug/Herb	Possible Effect and Management
anticoagulants, warfarin (Coumadin)	May increase the anticoagulant effect. The dosage of anticoagulant should be reduced by one third to one half when adding amiodarone to the client's drug regimen. Prothrombin times should also be closely monitored.
other antidysrhythmic agents	May increase cardiac effects and the risk of inducing tachydysrhythmias. Amiodarone also increases serum levels of quinidine, procainamide, flecainide, and phenytoin. If amiodarone must be given with Group I antidysrhythmic agents, reduce the dosage of the Group I antidysrhythmic drug by 30% to 50% several days after starting amiodarone, and gradually withdraw the Group I drug. If additional treatment with amiodarone is necessary, start therapy at half the usual recommended dosage.
chaparral	May cause hepatotoxicity. Monitor closely or, preferably, avoid concurrent use.
digitalis glycosides	May increase the serum level of digoxin and other digitalis glycosides, resulting in toxicity. Digitalis glycosides should be stopped or the dose reduced to 50% whenever amiodarone is given. Monitor serum levels closely. May also see the additive effects of both drugs on the SA node and AV junction.
phenytoin (Dilantin)	May result in increased serum levels of phenytoin, possibly resulting in toxicity. Monitor serum levels of phenytoin.

■ **Nursing Diagnosis.** With the administration of amiodarone, the client should be assessed for the development of the following nursing diagnoses/collaborative problems: impaired comfort (dizziness, bitter taste, headache, flushing, nausea, and vomiting); situational low self-esteem related to decreased libido and blue-gray coloring of the skin of the face, hands, and arms; constipation, 25%; imbalanced nutrition: less than body requirements related to anorexia, 25% (severe weight loss); and the potential complications of neurotoxicity, 20% to 40% (ataxia, tremors of the hands, numbness and tingling of fingers and toes, weakness of the arms and legs); photosensitivity; pulmonary fibrosis or pneumonitis, 10% to 15% (cough, dyspnea, fever); hyperthyroidism, 2% (weight loss, insomnia, nervousness, sensitivity to heat); hypothyroidism, 10% (weight gain, tiredness, sensitivity to cold, dry skin); ocular toxicity (blurred vision, corneal deposits [10%]); allergic reaction (rash); hepatitis (yellow skin and eyes); decreased cardiac output related to new dysrhythmias, sinus bradycardia, congestive heart failure (pulmonary edema, edema of feet and lower legs); and noninfectious epididymitis (pain and swelling of the scrotum).

■ **Implementation**

■ ***Monitoring.*** Perform ECG, thyroid function studies, liver function studies (ALT [SGPT], AST [SGOT], and serum alkaline phosphatase), chest x-ray examinations, and pulmonary studies before the initiation of therapy and periodically thereafter. Vital signs and fluid balance monitoring should occur with these clients. Ophthalmologic examinations should be performed initially and if eye symptoms occur. Pulmonary fibrosis may occur in 10% to 30% of clients receiving long-term amiodarone therapy. This is usually reversible if detected early enough, and thus chest x-ray examinations every 3 months are recommended. Thyroid function studies are to be performed at periodic intervals because of the risk for hyperthyroidism or hypothyroidism.

■ ***Intervention.*** Begin the loading dose phase at the beginning of amiodarone therapy in the hospital because of the difficulty in adjusting dosage and the potential for adverse reactions such as neurotoxicity and ocular, pulmonary, and thyroid toxicity. Because gastrointestinal disturbances occur in 25% of clients during loading, take care to minimize these as much as possible. Provide clients with a high-fiber diet and increased fluid intake, unless contraindicated, to prevent constipation. Administer with food or milk to decrease nausea. Make efforts to stimulate appetite to counteract anorexia.

With IV administration, a volumetric infusion pump should be used rather than a drop counter infusion set because amiodarone alters the surface tension of the solution and results in smaller drops. This phenomenon may result in underdosing of the client. It is recommended that a central venous catheter with an in-line filter be used for IV administration, with the initial rate not exceeding 30 mg/min.

■ ***Education.*** Instruct the client to continue the medication even if he or she is feeling well. If a dose is missed, the client should be advised not to take it at all to avoid doubling up on doses. If two or three doses are missed, instruct the client to contact the prescriber.

Instruct the client to maintain regular contact with the prescriber to monitor drug use. Advise the client to carry medical identification at all times. Instruct the client to alert health care professionals unfamiliar with the medication regimen to the amiodarone administration.

Photosensitivity is a potential adverse reaction with this drug. Caution the client to avoid exposure to the sun and to wear sun-protective clothing and dark glasses. Sunscreen agents are not effective because they do not block UVB light; therefore barrier sun blocks are needed (e.g., zinc or titanium oxide). In addition, a blue-gray coloration of the skin occurs with long-term use (more than 1 year) and affects sun-exposed parts of the body (e.g., face, neck, and arms) and those with fair skin.

Alert clients to report any of the following signs and symptoms to the prescriber: cough, dyspnea, fever (pulmonary toxicity); ataxia, numbness, tingling, weakness, or spasm of the extremities (neurotoxicity); blurred vision or increased sensitivity of the eyes to light (ocular toxicity); unusual weight gain or loss, increased sensitivity to heat or cold (thyroid toxicity); pain and swelling of the scrotum; jaundice (hepatic toxicity); or swelling of the lower limbs (congestive heart failure).

■ **Evaluation.** The expected outcome of amiodarone therapy is that the client will have regular palpable pulses and will demonstrate an absence of or decrease in atrial and ventricular ectopy on ECG.

dofetilide [doe fet' i lyde] (Tikosyn)

Dofetilide (Tikosyn), a class III agent, has been approved for the treatment and maintenance of atrial fibrillation and atrial flutter. This product is available only to hospitals. See Table 26-1 for pharmacokinetics. See Nursing Management: Antidysrhythmic Therapy, p.550.

ibutilide [eye byoo' ti lide] (Corvert)

Ibutilide has class III effects; it prolongs the action potential and increases the atrial and ventricular refractory period. It may produce its effect at the sodium channels by slowing the inward current or by blocking the potassium outward currents. It is indicated for the treatment of atrial fibrillation or atrial flutter.

Administered intravenously, ibutilide has an average 6-hour elimination half-life with excretion mainly in the urine. Significant side effects/adverse reactions include headache, nausea, cardiovascular alterations (e.g., AV block, bradycardia, ventricular extrasystoles), hypotension, and hypertension.

The adult dosage for clients weighing <60 kg is 0.01 mg/kg administered over 10 minutes. For clients weighing ≥60 kg, one vial (1 mg) is administered. If necessary, a second dose may be administered 10 minutes later or after the completion of the first infusion (*Drug Facts and Comparisons*, 2000).

■ Nursing Management

Ibutilide Therapy

In addition to the following discussion, see Nursing Management: Antidysrhythmic Therapy, p. 550.

■ **Assessment.** Ascertain that the client is not hypersensitive to ibutilide or any of the other product components. Ibutilide can induce or worsen ventricular dysrhythmias, particularly in clients with a history of congestive heart failure. Clients with chronic atrial fibrillation are at increased risk of recurrence of that state after conversion to sinus rhythm. Avoid its use in clients with prolongation of the QT interval. Hypokalemic and hypomagnesemic states also increase the risk of dysrhythmias.

Review the client's medication regimen to determine any significant drug interactions that might occur with the concurrent administration of ibutilide. Concomitant antidysrhythmics, such as the Class IA drugs (disopyramide, quinidine, and procainamide) and other Class III drugs (e.g., amiodarone and sotalol) should not be administered concurrently or within 4 hours after infusion because of their potential to prolong refractoriness. Avoid any other drugs that might prolong the QT interval, such as phenothiazines, tricyclic antidepressants, and some antihistamine agents (H_1 receptor antagonists). Ibutilide-induced supraventricular dysrhythmias may mask the cardiotoxicity associated with excessive digoxin levels.

■ **Nursing Diagnosis.** The client receiving ibutilide is at risk for the following nursing diagnoses/collaborative problems: impaired comfort (nausea, headache); risk for injury related to postural hypotension; and the potential complications of hypertension, ventricular dysrhythmias, and congestive heart failure.

■ **Implementation**

■ ***Monitoring.*** The client undergoing ibutilide therapy requires continuous ECG monitoring in an environment with personnel trained in the identification and management of acute ventricular dysrhythmias, including intracardiac pacing facilities, a cardioverter/defibrillator, and medication for the treatment of sustained ventricular tachycardia. Observe the ECG for at least 4 hours after the ibutilide infusion or until the QT interval has returned to baseline. The occurrence of any dysrhythmia requires longer monitoring.

■ ***Intervention.*** If the client has had atrial fibrillation of more than 2 to 3 days' duration, he or she should undergo anticoagulation at least 2 weeks before ibutilide therapy is initiated. If the dysrhythmia does not end within 10 minutes after the infusion, a second infusion of equal strength may be administered 10 minutes after the end of the first infusion. The infusion of ibutilide should be discontinued when the presenting dysrhythmia is terminated or if ventricular tachycardia occurs. The correction of any electrolyte imbalances is necessary before therapy is begun.

■ ***Education.*** Explain the procedure and equipment.

■ **Evaluation.** The expected outcome of ibutilide therapy is that the client will not experience atrial flutter/fibrillation or any adverse reactions to the drug.

sotalol [soe' ta lole] (Betapace)

Sotalol is a beta-adrenergic blocking agent that prolongs the duration of the action potential, increasing the effective refractory period in atrial, ventricular, and AV junction. It is indicated for life-threatening ventricular dysrhythmias. Sotalol is contraindicated in bronchial asthma, sinus bradycardia, AV block, cardiogenic shock, and heart failure and in persons who are hypersensitive to sotalol. (See Chapter 22 for additional information.)

▪ Nursing Management

Sotalol Therapy

In addition to the following discussion, see Nursing Management: Antidysrhythmic Therapy, p. 550, and Nursing Management: Beta-Adrenergic Agent Therapy, Chapter 22.

▪ Assessment. The client should be assessed for health conditions for which the use of sotalol is contraindicated, such as bronchial asthma, sinus bradycardia, second- and third-degree AV block, congenital or acquired long QT syndrome, cardiogenic shock, uncontrolled congestive heart failure, and hypersensitivity to sotalol. Determination should also be made of conditions for which there are precautions to sotalol use, such as reduced renal function and nonallergic bronchospasm. Sotalol may mask the signs of hypoglycemia in clients with diabetes mellitus and tachycardic symptoms of hyperthyroidism. Hypotension may occur in clients receiving anesthesia. Further dysrhythmias may be provoked in clients with conduction disturbances, prodysrhythmias, congestive heart failure, hypokalemia, acute myocardial infarction, and sick sinus syndrome (Dunnington, 1993).

As for other beta-adrenergic agents, an assessment should include the client's current medication regimen to detect significant drug interactions (see Chapter 22).

A baseline assessment is the same as for other antidysrhythmic agents.

▪ Nursing Diagnosis. The client receiving sotalol therapy is at risk for the following nursing diagnoses/collaborative problems: fatigue; ineffective sexuality patterns related to decreased libido and/or impotence; impaired comfort (headache); ineffective airway clearance related to bronchospasm; and the potential complications of mental depression, heart failure, hypoglycemia in clients with diabetes, and an exacerbation of peripheral vascular disease.

▪ Implementation

▪ *Monitoring.* Monitor the client's cardiovascular status as for other antidysrhythmic therapies.

▪ *Intervention.* The absorption of sotalol may be reduced by food, especially milk and milk products, due to an interaction with calcium; administer 1 hour before meal or 2 hours afterward.

▪ *Education.* Instruct the client on how to monitor his or her pulse and other pertinent indicators. Advise the client with ischemic heart disease not to discontinue the medication abruptly, because doing so may result in angina. Alert the client to consult with the prescriber before taking any other medications.

▪ Evaluation. The expected outcome of sotalol therapy is that the client will demonstrate an improvement in the underlying symptoms and a diminished dysrhythmia.

GROUP IV: MISCELLANEOUS DRUG GROUP

Calcium antagonists are selective antidysrhythmic agents and are reviewed in Chapter 28.

UNCLASSIFIED ANTIDYSRHYTHMIC DRUG

adenosine [a den' o seen] (Adenocard)

Adenosine, a natural constituent of muscle tissue, is used to slow AV node conduction and therefore is indicated for the conversion of paroxysmal supraventricular tachycardia (PSVT) to normal sinus rhythm. Administered by IV bolus, it is taken up almost immediately by red blood cells and vascular endothelial cells and metabolized to inosine and adenosine monophosphate (AMP) in the body.

The side effects/adverse reactions of adenosine include dyspnea, flushing, nausea, headache, dizziness, tingling in arms, new dysrhythmias such as premature ventricular contractions, sinus bradycardia, sinus tachycardia, skipped beats, and chest pain/pressure.

The usual dose is 6 mg administered rapidly by IV bolus over 1 to 2 seconds. If the dysrhythmia is still present 1 to 2 minutes after the injection, a 12-mg dose may be administered.

▪ Nursing Management

Adenosine Therapy

In addition to the following discussion, see Nursing Management: Antidysrhythmic Therapy, p. 550.

▪ Assessment. The client should be assessed to determine that there is no AV block or preexisting second- or third-degree block without a pacemaker; there is the risk of complete heart block if the drug is administered in such circumstances. The administration of adenosine in a client with sick sinus syndrome may result in prolonged sinus node recovery time, and sinus bradycardia or sinus arrest may occur. Hypersensitivity to the drug should be determined.

Review the client's medications, because the effects of adenosine are potentiated by the coadministration of carbamazepine (Tegretol) and dipyridamole (Persantine). Caffeine and theophylline reduce or antagonize the effects of adenosine. If possible, avoid concurrent drug administration.

A baseline assessment of blood pressure, pulse, and ECG should be obtained to confirm the efficacy of adenosine.

▪ Nursing Diagnosis. The client receiving adenosine may experience the following nursing diagnoses/collaborative problems: impaired comfort (flushing of the face, headache, nausea, or numbness or tingling in the arms); ineffective airway clearance related to transient bronchoconstriction; and the potential complications of new dysrhythmias and heart block.

▪ Implementation

▪ *Monitoring.* The client should be on a cardiac monitor, or the heart rate and blood pressure should be monitored every 15 to 30 seconds for several minutes.

■ ***Intervention.*** Adenosine is administered by IV rapidly, 6 mg over 1 to 2 seconds. It is given rapidly to achieve the desired negative dromotropic and chronotropic effect. Administer directly into the vein; if given by IV line, inject as proximal to the IV site as possible, and follow with a rapid saline flush. If the first dose is not effective within 1 to 2 minutes, a second one of 12 mg may be given in the same fashion and repeated if necessary. Do not repeat the dose if a high-level block occurs after the dose. Resuscitation equipment and drugs should be available during adenosine therapy. The solution may crystallize if refrigerated; warm it to room temperature. Ensure that the solution is clear before administering. Discard any unused solution, because it contains no preservatives.

■ ***Education.*** Alert the client that flushing of the face may occur and to report any symptoms of cough, dizziness, headache, nausea, or numbness or tingling of the arms.

■ **Evaluation.** The expected outcome of adenosine therapy is that the dysrhythmia for which the adenosine was administered will resolve without the client experiencing any adverse reactions to the drug.

SUMMARY

Antidysrhythmic agents are used for the treatment and prevention of cardiac rhythm disorders that result from some abnormality in the electrophysiologic properties of the cardiac conduction system cells or cardiac muscle cells. Although all drugs in this group have the ability to suppress automaticity, they are subdivided into groups I-A, I-B, and I-C to reflect the similar electrophysiologic properties of each subgroup. Group I-A includes disopyramide (Norpace), procainamide (Pronestyl), and quinidine, all of which decrease conduction velocity and prolong the action potential. Group I-B drugs—lidocaine, phenytoin (Dilantin), tocainide (Tonocard), and mexiletine (Mexitil)—either increase or have no effect on conduction velocity. Group I-C drugs—flecainide (Tambocor) and propafenone (Rythmol)—are used to treat or prevent supraventricular tachydysrhythmias; however, they have prodysrhythmic effects that are of concern and require careful monitoring of the client.

Group II drugs, such as propranolol (Inderal), acebutolol (Sectral), and esmolol (Brevibloc) have beta-adrenergic blocking action and are discussed mainly in Chapter 22. The Group III agents—bretylium (Bretylol), amiodarone (Cordarone), ibutilide (Corvert), and sotalol (Betapace)—are antiadrenergic. Group IV consists of the calcium channel blockers, such as verapamil; see the discussion in Chapter 28. Adenosine is an unclassified antidysrhythmic drug indicated for the conversion of paroxysmal supraventricular tachycardia.

The nursing management of cardiac dysrhythmias with the administration of antidysrhythmic agents should produce the following expected outcomes: the client will maintain cardiac output within normal limits, increase activity tolerance, experience less chest discomfort and associated symptoms, and demonstrate a decrease in or the absence of dysrhythmias on ECG tracings. Client education is focused on developing the client's knowledge of health status and medications, skill at pulse taking, and ability to recognize reportable changes in health status; this will enable the client to self-administer antidysrhythmic agents safely and accurately.

Critical Thinking Questions

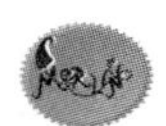

1. How would the differences in the groupings of antidysrhythmic agents affect nursing management of the client's care?
2. What concerns do you perceive a client might have if he or she is receiving antidysrhythmic therapy?

Collaborative Learning Activities

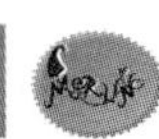

For Collaborative Learning Activities, go to mosby.com/MERLIN/McKenry/.

CASE STUDY

For a Case Study that will help ensure mastery of this chapter content, go to mosby.com/MERLIN/McKenry/.

BIBLIOGRAPHY

Abramowicz, M. (Ed.). (1994). Drugs for cardiac arrhythmias. *Medical Letter 36*(937):111-114.

American Hospital Formulary Service. (1999). *AHFS drug information '99.* Bethesda, MD: American Society of Hospital Pharmacists.

Anderson, K.N., Anderson, L.E., & Glanze, W.D. (Eds.). (1998). *Mosby's medical, nursing, & allied health dictionary* (5th ed.). St. Louis: Mosby.

Aronow, W.S. (1999). Management of the older person with ventricular arrhythmias. *Journal of the American Geriatric Society, 47*(7), 886-895.

Biffi, M., Boriani, G., Bronzetti, G., Capucci, A., Branzi, A., & Magnani, B. (1999). Electrophysiological effects of flecainide and propafenone on atrial fibrillation cycle and relation with arrhythmia termination. *Heart, 82*(2),176-182.

Chow, M.S.S. & Kertland, H.R. (1995). Cardiac arrhythmias. In L.Y. Young & M.A. Koda-Kimble (Eds.), *Applied therapeutics: The clinical use of drugs* (6th ed.). Vancouver, WA: Applied Therapeutics.

Drug Facts and Comparisons. (2000). St. Louis: Facts and Comparisons.

Dunnington, C.S. (1993). Sotalol hydrochloride (Betapace): A new antiarrhythmic drug. *American Journal of Critical Care, 2*(5), 397-406.

Kudenchuk, P.J., Cobb, L.A., Copass, M.K., Cummins, R.O., Doherty, A.M., Fahrenbruch, C.E., Hallstrom, A.P., Murray, W.A., Olsufka, M., & Walsh, T. (1999). Amiodarone for resuscitation after out-of-hospital cardiac arrest due to ventricular fibrillation. *New England Journal of Medicine, 341*(12), 871-878.

Paul, S.C. (1993). New pharmacologic agents for emergency management of supraventricular tachydysrhythmias. *Critical Care Nursing Quarterly, 16*(2), 35-45.

Physicians' Desk Reference. (1999). Montvale, NJ: Medical Economics Company.

Pinski, S.L. & Helguera, M.E. (1999). Antiarrhythmic drug initiation in patients with atrial fibrillation. *Progressive Cardiovascular Disease, 42*(1), 75-90.

Porterfield, L.M., Porterfield, J.G., & Collins, S.W. (1993). The cutting edge in arrhythmias. *Critical Care Nurse, 13*(3 suppl), 8-9.

Ramsay, J.G. (1999). Cardiac management in the ICU. *Chest, 115*(5 suppl), 138S-144S.

United States Pharmacopeia Dispensing Information (USP DI): Drug information for the health care professional (19th ed.). (1999). Rockville, MD: United States Pharmacopeial Convention.

Vizgirda, V.M. (1999). The genetic basis for cardiac dysrhythmias and the long QT syndrome. *Journal of Cardiovascular Nursing, 13*(4), 34-45.

Zevin, S. & Benowitz, N.L. (1999). Drug interactions with tobacco smoking. *Clinical Pharmacokinetics, 36*(6), 425-438.

27 Antihypertensives

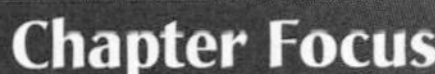

Chapter Focus

Hypertension (sustained, elevated blood pressure) is a chronic circulatory disease that affects millions of Americans. It has been estimated that approximately 50 million Americans have hypertension, or systolic and/or diastolic blood pressures higher than 140/90 mm Hg (Oates, 1996). Untreated hypertension or subtherapeutic treatment of hypertension increases the risk of stroke, cerebral hemorrhage, congestive heart failure, coronary heart disease, and renal failure. Risk factors for essential hypertension include family history, race (most common in African Americans), stress, obesity, a high dietary intake of saturated fats or sodium, the use of tobacco or oral contraceptives, sedentary lifestyle, and aging. The role of nursing is important not only in the direct care of clients with hypertension but even more so in the prevention and management of the condition through client education.

Learning Objectives

1. Describe the physiologic control of blood pressure.
2. Define hypertension on the basis of the criteria established by the Joint National Committee on Detection, Evaluation, and Treatment of High Blood Pressure.
3. Describe the stepped-care approach used in drug therapy for hypertension.
4. Discuss the special considerations for antihypertensive drug therapy: sexual dysfunction, concerns with children, older adults, pregnant clients, or surgical clients.
5. Define the six major categories of antihypertensive drugs: diuretics, adrenergic inhibitors, vasodilators, angiotensin-converting enzyme inhibitors, angiotensin II receptor antagonists, and calcium antagonists.
6. Identify the mechanism of action, pharmacokinetics, side effects/adverse reactions, interactions, and dosages in commonly used antihypertensive drugs.
7. Implement nursing management of the care of individual clients undergoing antihypertensive drug therapy.

Key Terms

adrenergic inhibitors, p. 575
angiotensin-converting enzyme inhibitors, p. 586
baroreceptor reflex, p. 569
calcium channel blocking agents, p. 589
diuretics, p. 575
hypertension, p. 568
potassium-sparing diuretic agents, p. 575
primary (idiopathic, essential) hypertension, p. 568
rebound hypertension, p. 574
renin-angiotensin-aldosterone mechanism, p. 571
secondary hypertension, p. 568
stepped treatment approach, p. 571
thiazides, p. 575
vasodilators, p. 589

Key Drugs [✔]

captopril, p. 586
clonidine, p. 576
losartan, p. 588
nitroprusside, p. 594
prazosin, p. 585

The number of persons with the silent killer hypertension is alarming. Although this condition seems relatively harmless, it severely damages major body organs. The American Heart Association has reported that, in the United States, 50% of individuals with hypertension are not receiving antihypertensive therapy. Of the individuals who are receiving treatment, only 21% are receiving adequate treatment (Portyansky, 1997). The need for improving medical care for clients with hypertension is apparent, because cardiovascular disease remains the number one cause of death in North America. (See the Nursing Research box at right.)

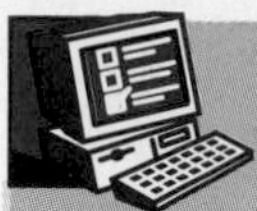

Nursing Research

Adherent and Nonadherent Medication Taking in Older Hypertensive Patients

Citation: Johnson, M.J., Williams, M., & Marshall, E.S. (1999). Adherent and nonadherent medication-taking in elderly hypertensive patients. *Clinical Nursing Research 8*(4): 318–335.

Abstract: Nonadherence to medications is a significant reason why clients fail to control their blood pressure. Little work has been attempted to conceptualize medication-taking behaviors from the client's perspective. This study examined factors that influence older hypertensive client's adherence or nonadherence to prescribed medications. Using a qualitative descriptive research design, 21 hypertensive older adults were interviewed. Two domains of adherence were identified: (1) purposeful use of medication for the control of client's blood pressure, and (2) establishing and maintaining patterns of medication taking. Two similar domains also emerged for nonadherence: purposeful and intentional. Adherence behaviors were dependent on the person's decision to take the hypertension medication, access to medications, and ability to initiate treatment and maintain a medication-taking pattern. The timing and location of pills were integral parts of establishing patterns of taking medications. Inadequate access to medications or interruption of a person's pattern were associated with the incidental missing of medications.

Critical Thinking Questions

- How would you assess a client's perspective in relation to medication taking?
- What nursing interventions would you incorporate in a plan of care for an older hypertensive client to enhance adherence to medication taking?
- What measurable health outomes would indicate that your client had been adherent in medication taking?

For answer guidelines for these *new Critical Thinking Questions,* go to mosby.com/MERLIN/McKenry/.

DEFINITION OF HYPERTENSION

Hypertension is defined as an elevated systolic blood pressure, diastolic blood pressure, or both. The classification for adult hypertension was defined by the Joint National Committee on Prevention, Detection, Evaluation, and Treatment of High Blood Pressure (JNC VI) (1997) as follows:

Hypertension	Systolic (mm Hg)	Diastolic (mm Hg)
Normal	<130	<85
High-normal	130-139	85-89
Stage 1	140-159	90-99
Stages 2 and 3	≥160	≥100

This classification has also stratified clients with hypertension on the basis of blood pressure levels, the presence of risk factors, and the degree of target organ damage secondary to hypertension. Table 27-1 presents the implications of risk stratification and antihypertensive treatment.

The major risk factors in clients with hypertension include smoking, diabetes mellitus, high blood cholesterol or lipids, being over 60 years of age, family history of heart disease (in females under 65 years of age and males under 55 years of age), and gender (males and postmenopausal women are at greater risk). The target organ damage or cardiovascular disease in clients with hypertension includes stroke or transient ischemic attacks (TIA), kidney disease, retinopathy, and various heart diseases such as angina, congestive heart failure, left ventricular hypertrophy, and prior myocardial infarction.

Clients in Stage 1 are instructed on lifestyle modifications such as weight loss if overweight; moderate alcohol intake; exercise; sodium restriction (Box 27-1); adequate consumption of dietary potassium, calcium, and magnesium; elimination of tobacco; and reduction of saturated fat intake. The client should be reevaluated in 6 to 12 months for the effectiveness of these nonpharmacologic measures. Clients in stage 2 and 3 require drug therapy.

Obtaining a careful and detailed drug history before diagnosis is also important, because many over-the-counter (OTC) and prescription medications may increase blood pressure or interfere with the effectiveness of an antihypertensive agent. Oral contraceptives (estrogen-containing agents), corticosteroids, nonsteroidal antiinflammatory drugs (NSAIDs), antidepressants, nasal decongestants, and appetite-suppressing agents are typical examples of interfering substances. Figure 27-1 illustrates the sites of drug effects that can induce or exacerbate hypertension.

CLASSIFICATION OF HYPERTENSION

In **primary (idiopathic or essential) hypertension,** the specific cause of the hypertension is unknown. This group accounts for approximately 90% of cases. **Secondary hypertension,** which represents approximately 10% of cases, may be a symptom of pheochromocytoma, toxemia of pregnancy, or renal artery disease; it may also result from the use of spe-

TABLE 27-1 Risk Stratification and Antihypertensive Treatment

	Treatment		
Blood Pressures	**High Normal (130-139/85-89 mm Hg)**	**Stage 1 (140-159/90-99 mm Hg)**	**Stages 2 and 3 (>160/>100 mm Hg)**
Rick Group A*	Lifestyle†	Lifestyle†	Drug therapy
Rick Group B‡	Lifestyle†	Drug therapy Lifestyle†	Drug therapy
Risk Group§	Drug therapy Lifestyle†	Drug therapy	Drug therapy

*Risk group A: client has no risk factors or target organ damage.
†Lifestyle changes are appropriate in all stages; these include weight loss if overweight, moderate alcohol intake, exercise, sodium restriction, adequate consumption of dietary potassium, smoking cessation, and reduction of saturated fat intake.
‡Risk group B: client has at least one risk factor (not diabetes) with no target organ damage.
§Risk group C: client has target organ damage and/or diabetes with or without other risk factors.

BOX 27-1

Fruits and Vegetables Low in Sodium and Calories and High in Potassium

artichokes	carrots	peaches
bananas	honeydew melon	potatoes
broccoli	orange juice	strawberries
brussels sprouts	oranges	tomatoes
cantaloupe		

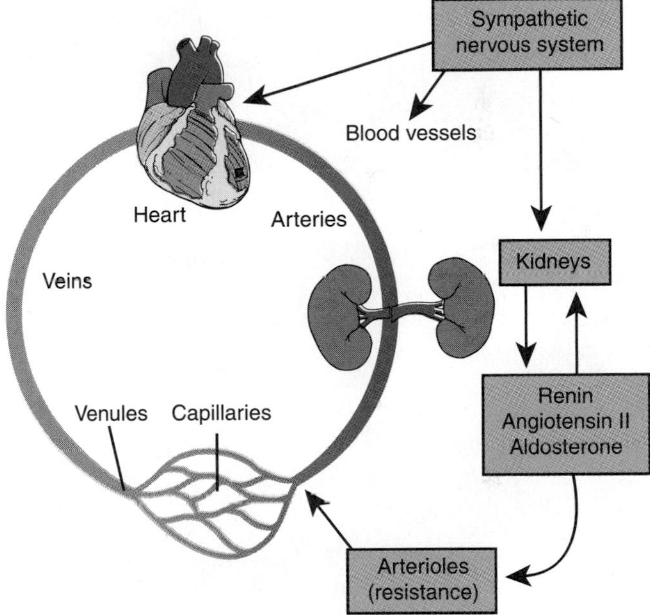

Figure 27-1 Sites of drug effects that can induce or exacerbate hypertension. Many drugs can do both. The sympathetic nervous system is affected by many drugs that can increase blood pressure by their action on the heart and blood vessels (i.e., sympathomimetics): cocaine, amphetamine, ergotamine, estrogen, MAO inhibitors, and NSAIDs. The kidneys are affected by NSAIDs, estrogens, corticosteroids, cocaine, and amphetamine. The renin-angiotensin II-aldosterone system is affected by estrogens, alcohol, and glycyrrhizic acid (licorice). Arterioles are affected by alcohol, sympathomimetics, cocaine, amphetamine, and ergotamine.

cific medications. If the cause of secondary hypertension is corrected, the blood pressure usually returns to normal.

PHYSIOLOGIC CONTROL OF BLOOD PRESSURE

Control of blood pressure involves a complex interaction between the nervous, hormonal, and renal systems; all play a part in regulating arterial blood pressure (Figure 27-2). The body has two primary mechanisms to control blood pressure:

1. Adrenergic nervous system or baroreceptor reflex—a rapid-acting system
2. Renin-angiotensin-aldosterone mechanism—a long-acting system

Adrenergic Nervous System

The adrenergic or sympathetic nervous system uses a reflex mechanism, the **baroreceptor reflex,** to maintain blood pressure. Baroreceptors are nerve endings located in the walls of the internal carotid arteries and the aortic arch. These sensory receptors rapidly respond to changes in blood pressure. Any elevation in pressure stretches the receptors, which causes an impulse to be transmitted along the afferent neuron (vagus nerve) to the vasomotor center in the brainstem. The vasomotor center responds to the impulse by causing two reactions: (1) a decrease in heart rate and force of myocardial contraction, which lowers cardiac output; and (2) vasodilation of peripheral vessels, which decreases total peripheral resistance. The subsequent reduc-

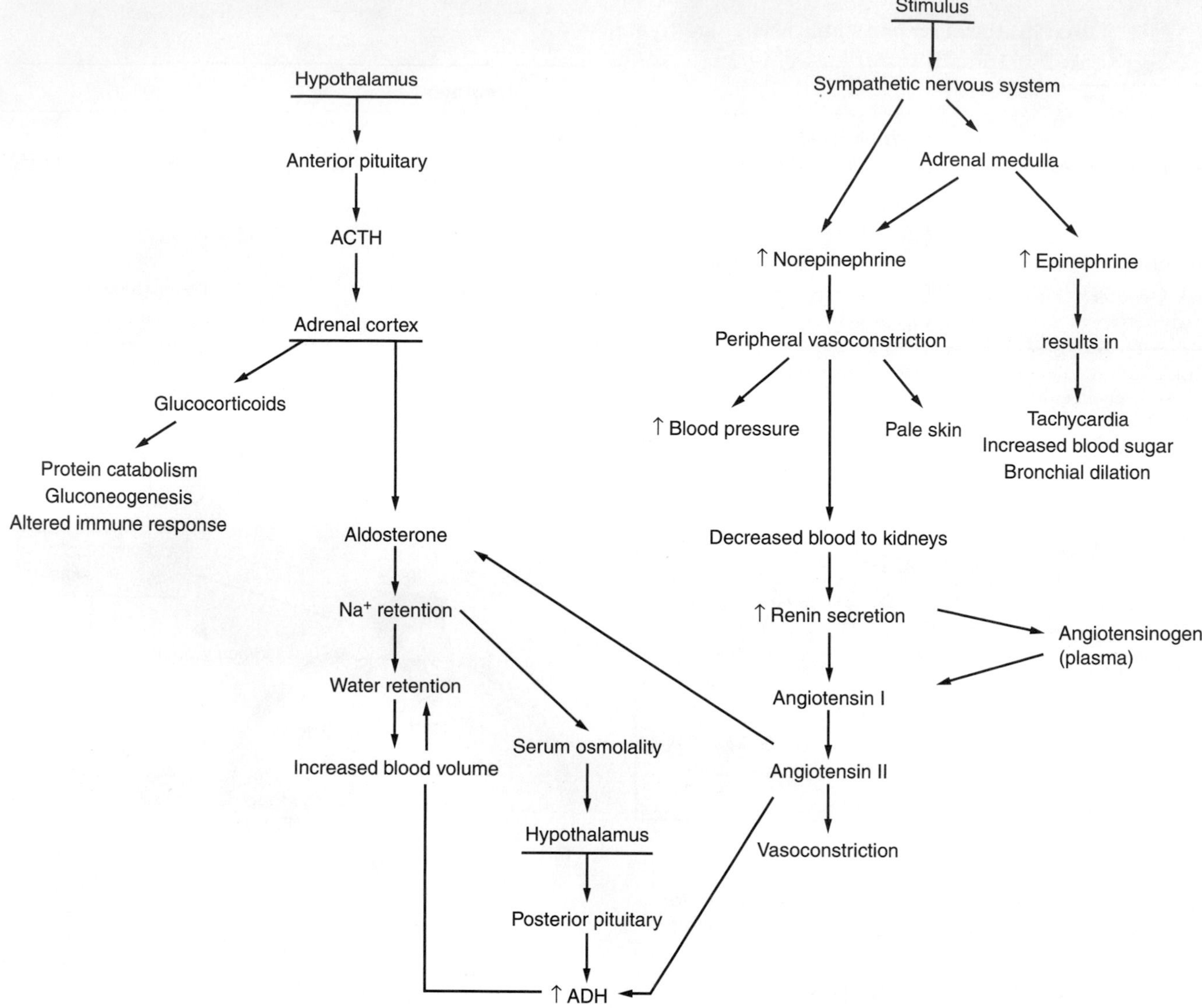

Figure 27-2 Physiologic control of blood pressure. Activation of the sympathetic nervous system results in an increased release of norepinephrine, resulting in peripheral vasoconstriction and increased blood pressure. An increased release of epinephrine increases heart rate and the force of myocardial contractions, which also results in an elevation of blood pressure. Vasoconstriction results in increased blood pressure plus decreased blood supply to the kidneys, which activates the angiotensin system. Ultimately, the release of angiotensin II (a potent vasoconstrictor) results in an increase in the release of aldosterone from the adrenal cortex, an increase in the release of ADH, and increased blood volume. (See the text for a description of mechanisms.)

tion in blood pressure is attributed to the reflex activity of the baroreceptor reflex.

When blood pressure is low, this information is projected to the vasomotor center, which then activates sympathetic nerves. Two hormones, norepinephrine and epinephrine, mediate the sympathetic nervous system. Norepinephrine acts mainly on alpha-adrenergic receptors (located in the arterioles), whereas epinephrine acts on both alpha- and beta-adrenergic receptors. The affinity of norepinephrine for these alpha receptors produces vasoconstriction, and blood pressure is increased. The $beta_1$-adrenergic receptors prevalent in the heart are also activated by norepinephrine. This response increases both the heart rate and the force of myocardial contraction, thereby indirectly elevating blood pressure.

Because it produces dilation of skeletal muscle blood vessels, epinephrine does not cause any increase in peripheral resistance. However, epinephrine does produce a considerable increase in heart rate and force of myocardial contraction; this elevation in cardiac output indirectly raises the blood pressure (Box 27-2).

The baroreceptor reflex functions as a rapidly acting system for short-term control of low and high blood pressure. It has been demonstrated that the rate of baroreceptor firing

BOX 27-2

Basic Blood Pressure Equations

Blood pressure (mean arterial pressure) = Cardiac output × Peripheral resistance
Cardiac output = Stroke volume × Heart rate

diminishes over a prolonged period, even if the blood pressure remains elevated. Therefore it has been speculated that in hypertension these receptors are "reset" to maintain a higher level of blood pressure.

Renin-Angiotensin-Aldosterone Mechanism

The **renin-angiotensin-aldosterone mechanism** regulates blood pressure by increasing or decreasing the blood volume through kidney function (Figure 27-3). The initiating factor is renin, an enzyme secreted from the juxtaglomerular cells located in the afferent arteriolar walls of the nephron. When blood flow through the kidneys is reduced, renal arterial pressure is reduced; this causes the release of renin into the circulation. Renin catalyzes the cleavage of a plasma protein to form angiotensin I, a weak vasoconstrictor. In the small vessels of the lung, angiotensin I is converted by angiotensin-converting enzyme (ACE) to angiotensin II.

Angiotensin II is one of the most potent vasoconstrictors known. It is particularly effective in constricting arterioles, which increases peripheral resistance and raises blood pressure. In addition, angiotensin II acts on the adrenal cortex to stimulate the secretion of aldosterone, a hormone that promotes sodium reabsorption by the kidneys. The increased sodium elevates the osmotic pressure in the plasma, causing a release of antidiuretic hormone from the posterior pituitary. Angiotensin II acts on the kidney tubules to promote reabsorption of water.

The renin-angiotensin-aldosterone system involves slow adjustments to changes in fluid volume. Excessive fluid retention is controlled by the negative-feedback mechanism operating within this system so that fluid balance is restored to a normal level. The kidneys are by far the most important organs in the body for long-term regulation of blood pressure. When the operation of the urinary system fails, increased peripheral resistance and retention of fluid volume produce a combination of hypertensive effects, which keep blood pressure constantly elevated.

Knowledge of the normal mechanisms for blood pressure control has led to the development of the pharmacologic agents. For example, beta-blocking agents suppress renin release, and ACE inhibitors prevent the conversion of angiotensin I to angiotensin II. The mechanism of action for the antihypertensive agents is reviewed in this chapter.

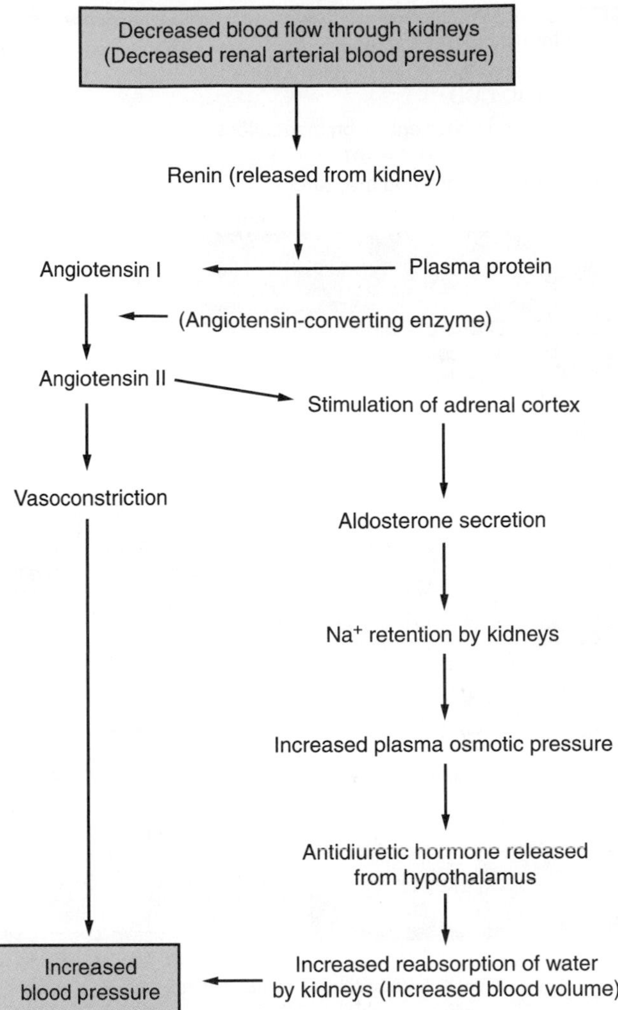

Figure 27-3 The renin-angiotensin-aldosterone system.

ANTIHYPERTENSIVE THERAPY

Client participation in antihypertensive therapy is essential for the control of blood pressure. The client needs to understand that hypertension is usually asymptomatic and that therapy does not cure but only controls hypertension. Long-term therapy is necessary to prevent the morbidity and mortality that result from primary hypertension. Compliance with an individualized antihypertensive regimen is associated with a good prognosis and a healthy lifestyle.

The careful use of antihypertensive drugs can effectively control blood pressure in a majority of clients with hypertension, with less risk of serious complications and intolerable side effects. The JNC VI (Kaplan, 1997) report proposes a new pharmacologic approach for hypertension based on the individual's risk factors and target organ damage. Figure 27-4 explains the **stepped treatment approach** for hypertension; this program is tailored to the individual and becomes more aggressive with each level of treatment.

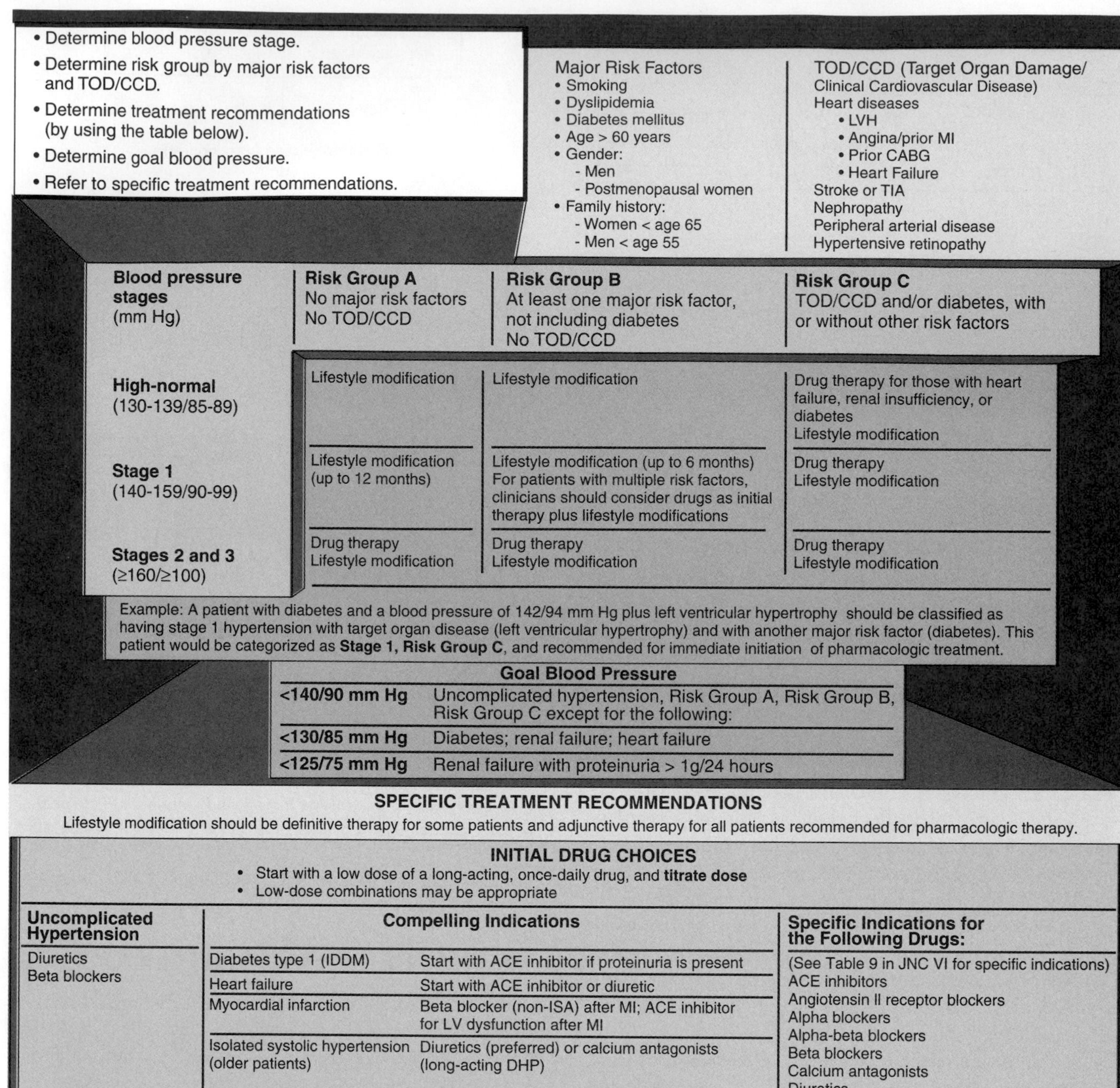

• Determine blood pressure stage.
• Determine risk group by major risk factors and TOD/CCD.
• Determine treatment recommendations (by using the table below).
• Determine goal blood pressure.
• Refer to specific treatment recommendations.
Major Risk Factors
• Smoking
• Dyslipidemia
• Diabetes mellitus
• Age > 60 years
• Gender:
- Men
- Postmenopausal women
• Family history:
- Women < age 65
- Men < age 55
TOD/CCD (Target Organ Damage/ Clinical Cardiovascular Disease)
Heart diseases
• LVH
• Angina/prior MI
• Prior CABG
• Heart Failure
Stroke or TIA
Nephropathy
Peripheral arterial disease
Hypertensive retinopathy
Blood pressure stages (mm Hg)
Risk Group A
No major risk factors
No TOD/CCD
Risk Group B
At least one major risk factor, not including diabetes
No TOD/CCD
Risk Group C
TOD/CCD and/or diabetes, with or without other risk factors
High-normal (130-139/85-89)
Lifestyle modification
Lifestyle modification
Drug therapy for those with heart failure, renal insufficiency, or diabetes
Lifestyle modification
Stage 1 (140-159/90-99)
Lifestyle modification (up to 12 months)
Lifestyle modification (up to 6 months)
For patients with multiple risk factors, clinicians should consider drugs as initial therapy plus lifestyle modifications
Drug therapy
Lifestyle modification
Stages 2 and 3 (≥160/≥100)
Drug therapy
Lifestyle modification
Drug therapy
Lifestyle modification
Drug therapy
Lifestyle modification
Example: A patient with diabetes and a blood pressure of 142/94 mm Hg plus left ventricular hypertrophy should be classified as having stage 1 hypertension with target organ disease (left ventricular hypertrophy) and with another major risk factor (diabetes). This patient would be categorized as **Stage 1, Risk Group C**, and recommended for immediate initiation of pharmacologic treatment.
Goal Blood Pressure
<140/90 mm Hg Uncomplicated hypertension, Risk Group A, Risk Group B, Risk Group C except for the following:
<130/85 mm Hg Diabetes; renal failure; heart failure
<125/75 mm Hg Renal failure with proteinuria > 1g/24 hours
SPECIFIC TREATMENT RECOMMENDATIONS
Lifestyle modification should be definitive therapy for some patients and adjunctive therapy for all patients recommended for pharmacologic therapy.
INITIAL DRUG CHOICES
• Start with a low dose of a long-acting, once-daily drug, and **titrate dose**
• Low-dose combinations may be appropriate
Uncomplicated Hypertension
Diuretics
Beta blockers
Compelling Indications
Diabetes type 1 (IDDM) Start with ACE inhibitor if proteinuria is present
Heart failure Start with ACE inhibitor or diuretic
Myocardial infarction Beta blocker (non-ISA) after MI; ACE inhibitor for LV dysfunction after MI
Isolated systolic hypertension (older patients) Diuretics (preferred) or calcium antagonists (long-acting DHP)
Specific Indications for the Following Drugs:
(See Table 9 in JNC VI for specific indications)
ACE inhibitors
Angiotensin II receptor blockers
Alpha blockers
Alpha-beta blockers
Beta blockers
Calcium antagonists
Diuretics

Figure 27-4 Stepped treatment approach for hypertension. (Redrawn from The *Sixth Report of the Joint National Committee on Prevention, Detection, Evaluation, and Treatment of High Blood Pressure.*(1997). *Arch Intern Med 157*, 2413-2446. Pub no 98-4080.)

Special Concerns in Antihypertensive Therapy

Demographics. African Americans generally respond better to diuretics and calcium antagonists than to ACE inhibitors or beta-blocking agents (Hall, 1999). (See the Cultural Considerations box on p. 573 for additional clinical responses to antihypertensive agents among different racial and ethnic groups.) Gender differences in response to antihypertensive agents have not been identified. Hypertension is reported to be two to three times more common in women who have used oral contraceptive agents for 5 years or longer as compared with those not taking any oral contraceptives. This risk increases with age, smoking, and higher doses of estrogen and progesterone. If hypertension occurs, the usual treatment is to discontinue the oral contraceptive; blood pressure usually normalizes in 3 to 6 months. If blood pressure does not return to normal, lifestyle modifications and antihypertensive drugs should be instituted according to Table 27-1 and Figure 27-4.

Age differences also affect blood pressure. Elevated systolic blood pressure, elevated diastolic blood pressure, or both, occurs in a significant proportion of persons over 65 years of age and increases their risk of cardiovascular mor-

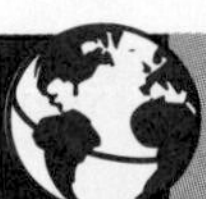

Cultural Considerations
Ethnic and Racial Differences in Response to Selected Antihypertensive Agents

Comparison Groups	Drug Class/Examples	Clinical Response
Blacks/whites	beta blockers, especially propranolol (also nadolol, pindolol, atenolol)	Blacks less responsive
Blacks/whites	diuretics (e.g., hydrochlorothiazide)	Blacks respond better to monotherapy
Blacks/whites	ACE inhibitors (e.g., captopril)	Monotherapy more effective in whites; no difference in diuretic
Chinese/whites	propranolol	Chinese twice as sensitive to effects of drug on blood pressure and heart rate

Information from Levy, R.A. (1993). *Ethnic and racial differences in response to medicines: Preserving individualized therapy in managed pharmaceutical programs.* Reston, VA: National Pharmaceutical Council.

bidity and mortality. Antihypertensive drugs should be started at smaller than usual doses, increased by smaller than usual amounts, and scheduled at less frequent intervals with older adults, because they are more sensitive to volume depletion and sympathetic inhibition than are younger clients. They commonly have impaired cardiovascular reflexes, which makes them more susceptible to hypotension.

In older adults with isolated systolic hypertension who are treated with antihypertensive drugs, the systolic pressure should be cautiously decreased to 140 to 160 mm Hg. Consideration should be given to further lowering the systolic value only if this medication level is tolerated without side effects. The response of older adults to both nonpharmacologic and pharmacologic therapies should be monitored closely.

The goal of therapy for children and adolescents with hypertension is to reduce blood pressure without producing adverse reactions that limit compliance or interfere with normal growth and development. The causative factors, the presence of complications, and the degree of hypertension will determine the type of intervention. Nonpharmacologic measures (weight control, reduction of dietary sodium, exercise, avoidance of smoking and alcohol, and reduction of saturated fat) are strongly recommended. Pharmacologic therapy should be considered if children do not respond to nonpharmacologic measures or if their blood pressures place them at risk for organ damage. (See the Special Considerations for Children box at right.)

Pharmacologic interventions for children also follow the stepped approach. Continued assessment of the child and family is necessary to ensure satisfactory blood pressure control and compliance with the pharmacologic or nonpharmacologic therapeutic program.

Concomitant Disease States. Persons with concurrent disease/illness may respond best or, in some instances, adversely to certain medications. For example, beta-blocking agents and calcium receptor antagonists are the preferred agents for hypertensive clients who also have angina or atrial tachycardia and fibrillation. In type 2 diabetes mellitus, diuretics in low doses are recommended. Beta-blocking agents are usually preferred with preoperative hypertension but should be avoided with asthma, heart block, depression, dyslipidemia, congestive heart failure (except carvedilol), and types 1 and 2 diabetes mellitus (Kaplan, 1997).

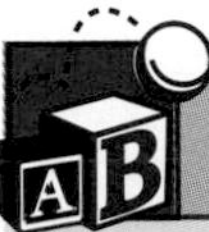

Special Considerations for Children
Hypertension

High blood pressure in children often occurs where there is a strong family history of hypertension. Close monitoring of these children is recommended.

Nonpharmacologic treatment or lifestyle modifications include weight loss (if obese), exercise, and dietary interventions. An increase in fresh fruits and vegetables and a reduction is salt intake are also recommended.

When drug therapy is necessary, it should be individualized according to the child's blood pressure, response to the drug therapy, and the potential side effects and adverse reactions of the medication. Diuretics, beta-blocking agents, and ACE inhibitors have been successfully used in this population.

Prescribers should avoid the use of ACE inhibitors and angiotensin II blocking agents in pregnant adolescents and in adolescent girls who are sexually active. These agents can cause fetal and neonatal injury and death (National Institutes of Health, 1996).

Pregnancy. Hypertension during pregnancy is a serious condition that requires early detection and treatment. The following are two major diagnostic categories and treatment:

1. *Chronic hypertension.* Hypertension is present before pregnancy or is diagnosed before the twentieth week of gestation. Diuretics, methyldopa (Aldomet), or other antihypertensive medications may be used. ACE inhibitors are to be avoided; serious neonatal problems, including renal failure and death, have been reported with their use. (For more information, see the Pregnancy Safety box on p. 574.)
2. *Preeclampsia-eclampsia.* This condition is a pregnancy-induced hypertension and is a primary factor in maternal and fetal morbidity and mortality. It has been

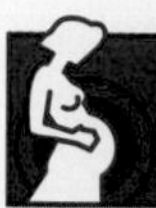

Pregnancy Safety
Antihypertensives

Category	Drug
B	guanadrel, guanfacine, methyldopa
C	clonidine, diazoxide, doxazosin, guanabenz, guanethidine, hydralazine, minoxidil, nitroprusside, prazosin, reserpine, terazosin; all ACE inhibitors in the first trimester; eprosartan, irbesartan, losartan, and valsartan in the first trimester
D	trimethaphan; all ACE inhibitors in the second and third trimesters; eprosartan, irbesartan, losartan, and valsartan in the second and third trimesters

estimated to occur in 10% of all pregnancies, mostly in teenagers or in primigravida women over 35 years of age (Sagraves, Letassy, & Barton, 1995).

The signs and symptoms of preeclampsia may range from mild to severe; the severe form may include diastolic blood pressure ≥110 mm Hg, systolic blood pressure ≥160 mm Hg, proteinuria, elevated serum creatinine, headache, visual disturbances, gastric pain, retinal damage (e.g., hemorrhage, exudate), pulmonary edema, decreased platelet count (<100,000/mm^3), and/or eclampsia or convulsions or seizures in a woman with preeclampsia.

Therapy includes bed rest, hospitalization (controversial today) and, if the fetus is mature, a timely delivery. The use of antihypertensive agents is based on maternal safety, with most clinicians initiating treatment when the diastolic blood pressure is ≥100 mm Hg. If delivery is not planned for within 24 hours, an oral agent such as methyldopa (Aldomet) is the drug of choice, although labetalol (Normodyne), magnesium sulfate, parenteral hydralazine, calcium blocking agents, and various beta-adrenergic agents have also been used. Published studies are suggesting the use of low-dose aspirin (60 mg) to prevent preeclampsia in high-risk clients. Aspirin reverses the imbalance between prostacyclin and thromboxane that may be responsible for preeclampsia. As mentioned previously, the ACE inhibitors are not recommended for use during pregnancy (Sagraves et al., 1995).

Women receiving continuous antihypertensive therapy should be advised not to breastfeed, because most of the agents are transferred to breast milk.

Sexual Dysfunction. Sexual dysfunction is a common complication of antihypertensive medications and may be manifested in males as decreased libido, impotence, impaired or retrograde ejaculation, and gynecomastia. In females it may be manifested as decreased libido, decreased vaginal lubrication, and inability to achieve orgasm. Such symptoms may lead to the client's poor compliance with the drug regimen. The nature of the disorder and a knowledge of the effects associated with different antihypertensive agents will assist in determining the cause of the symptoms. A dosage reduction or the substitution of another drug will often alleviate the problem.

BOX 27-3

Rebound Hypertension and Hypertensive Crisis

The abrupt withdrawal or discontinuation of antihypertensive medications may result in rebound hypertension and possibly a hypertensive crisis. In both instances, therapy is instituted to reduce blood pressure as soon as possible (Hawkins et al., 1993).

Rebound hypertension refers to the sudden increase of blood pressure to the pretreatment level or higher. Symptoms of rebound hypertension depend on the elevation of blood pressure. The symptoms usually involve sympathetic system hyperactivity (e.g., sweating, anxiety, tachycardia, insomnia, muscle cramps, chest pain, headache, and nausea).

A hypertensive crisis or hypertensive emergency is the elevation of diastolic blood pressure above 120 to 130 mm Hg (Hawkins et al., 1993). In a hypertensive emergency or crisis, the extremely elevated rise in blood pressure may cause target organ damage, such as to the eyes (retina), heart, kidneys, or neurologic system.

Surgical Clients. To prevent rebound hypertension, clients scheduled for elective surgery should receive their antihypertensive medications up to the time of surgery and as soon afterward as possible. Parenteral diuretics, adrenergic inhibitors, and vasodilators, plus sublingual nifedipine or transdermal clonidine, are available for clients who are unable to take oral medications. Clients taking an adrenergic inhibitor before surgery are more at risk for rebound hypertension (Box 27-3).

The client's electrolyte status should be carefully checked before surgery. If hypokalemia is detected, it should be corrected before the scheduled operation. The anesthetist should always be completely informed about the client's medication regimen; this is vital information that may alter the medications or the monitoring methods used.

▪ ▪ ▪

The antihypertensive drugs currently used to reduce blood pressure are classified into five major categories: diuretics, adrenergic inhibitors (central and peripheral), ACE inhibitors and antagonists, calcium antagonists, and vasodilators. The use of diuretics or the beta-blocking agents in hypertension have resulted in a reduction in morbidity and mortality.

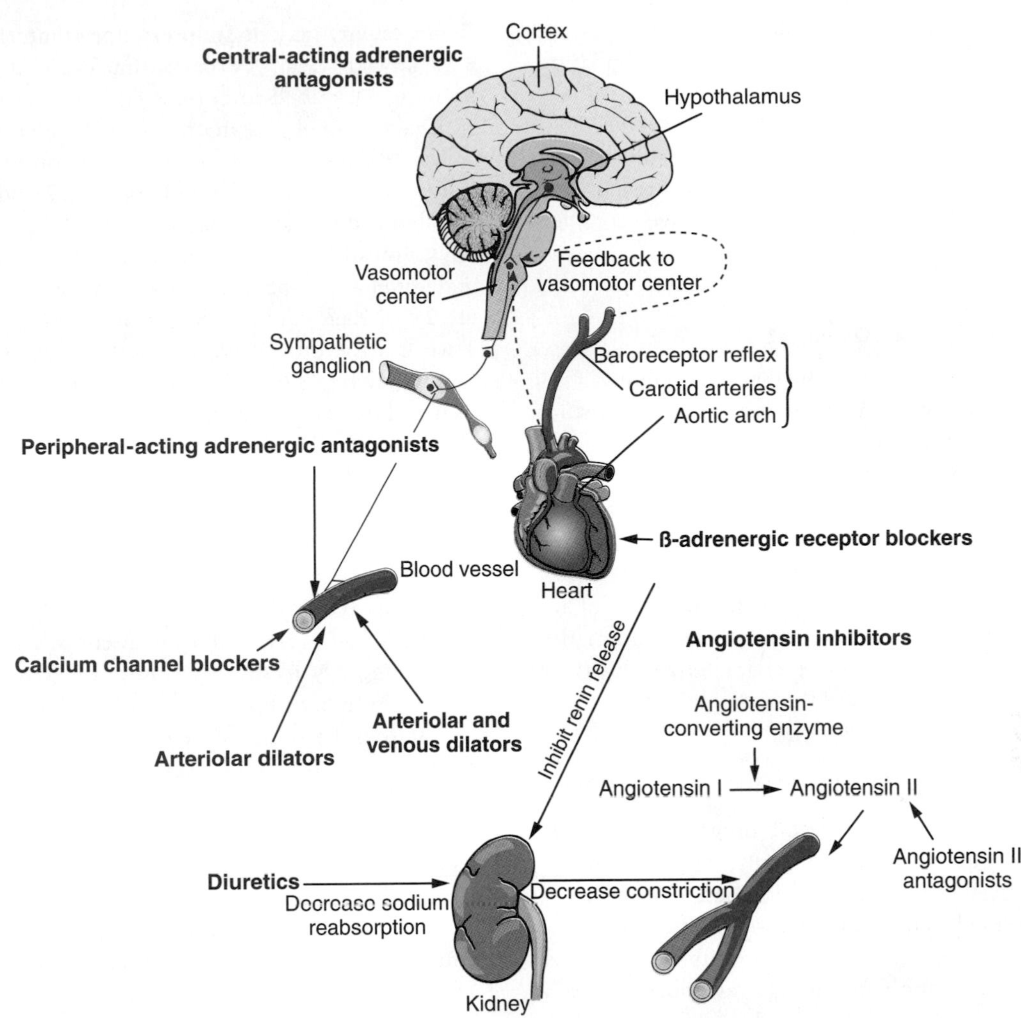

Figure 27-5 Site and method of action for various antihypertensive drugs, based on reported clinical and experimental evidence. (Modified from Lewis, S.M., Heitkemper, M.M., & Dirksen, S.R. (2000). *Medical-surgical nursing: Assessment and management of clinical problems* (5th ed.). St. Louis: Mosby.)

DIURETIC DRUGS

Diuretic drugs play a vital role in lowering blood pressure. The use of **diuretics**, agents that promote the formation and excretion of urine, results in a loss of excess salt and water from the body by renal excretion. The decrease in plasma and extracellular fluid volume subsequently depresses vascular reactivity to sympathetic stimulation. Thus volume depletion, plus the direct diuretic effect on the arterioles (which produces vasodilation), lowers the blood pressure. This response causes an initial decline in cardiac output followed by a decrease in peripheral resistance and a lowering of blood pressure (Figure 27-5).

When used in maximum therapeutic dosages, the **thiazides** and related sulfonamide diuretics (e.g., chlorthalidone and metolazone) are moderately effective in decreasing blood pressure. These mild diuretics can be used alone for individuals in the early stages of hypertension. In contrast, many of the other types of antihypertensive agents, when used alone on a long-term basis, cause a gradual retention of sodium and water and expansion of plasma fluid volume. Therefore a low-dose diuretic is often given in combination with ACE inhibitors, alpha-blocking agents, vasodilators, or adrenergic inhibitors to prevent fluid retention.

The **potassium-sparing diuretic agents,** such as spironolactone and triamterene, are useful in counteracting the potassium loss induced by other diuretics. They promote sodium and water loss without an accompanying loss of potassium. These drugs are indicated for the management of hyperaldosteronism and renal vascular hypertension when the client's condition is resistant to other diuretics. (See Chapter 34 for monographs on the diuretic drugs.)

ADRENERGIC INHIBITING (SYMPATHOLYTIC) AGENTS

Adrenergic inhibitors, the most effective antihypertensive drugs, are effective in reducing blood pressure and in preventing serious cardiovascular complications. These agents inhibit the activity of the sympathetic nervous system. The heart, blood vessels, and kidneys influence arterial pressure through various reflex mechanisms. Sympathetic stimulation increases heart rate and the force of myocardial contraction, constricts arterioles (resistance vessels) and venules (capacitance vessels), and releases renin from the kidneys. The sites at which these drugs modify sympathetic nervous system activity vary widely and usually involve complex mechanisms.

Beta-Adrenergic Blocking Agents

Beta-blocking agents decrease cardiac output and inhibit renin secretion, which results in a lowering of blood pressure. By competing with epinephrine for available beta receptor sites, they inhibit the typical organ or tissue response to beta stimulation. (See Chapter 22 for additional information about beta-blocking agents.)

The other adrenergic inhibitors are also effective in lowering blood pressure and generally have multiple sites of action or unknown mechanisms of action. For clarification, the drugs in the following sections are characterized by their primary proposed site of action.

Centrally Acting Adrenergic Inhibitors

Although thought of as antiadrenergic drugs, centrally acting adrenergic inhibitors are actually central alpha$_2$-adrenergic agonists. Central alpha$_2$-adrenergic stimulation results in a decreased sympathetic outflow to the heart, kidneys, and peripheral vasculature; this results in decreased heart rate, decreased peripheral vascular resistance and, as a result, decreased systolic and diastolic blood pressure. The centrally acting agents clonidine (Catapres), methyldopa (Aldomet), guanfacine (Tenex), and guanabenz (Wytensin) are effective antihypertensives, especially when combined with a diuretic. When given as a single agent, clonidine and methyldopa (and guanfacine and guanabenz to a lesser extent) usually produce sodium and water retention.

clonidine [klon′ i deen] (Catapres, Catapres-TTS)

Clonidine reduces systolic and diastolic blood pressure by stimulating central alpha$_2$ receptors, which decreases the sympathetic outflow of norepinephrine from the brain to the blood vessels and heart. Decreasing cardiac output, heart rate, and peripheral vascular resistance lowers blood pressure. The depressed cardiac output is the result of a reduction in both heart rate and stroke volume. Consequently, this action can cause bradycardia.

Although not approved indications in the United States, clonidine is also used in the diagnosis of pheochromocytoma; for prophylaxis of migraine or vascular headaches; for treatment of dysmenorrhea, menopause, and Tourette's syndrome; and for nicotine and opioid withdrawal (*United States Pharmacopeia Dispensing Information*, 1999).

Decreased sympathetic outflow to the kidneys reduces renal vascular resistance and thus preserves renal blood flow. Renin activity may be suppressed in some clients (Hoffman & Lefkowitz, 1996). With continued use of clonidine, a diuretic is prescribed to correct fluid retention.

Oral clonidine has an onset of action within ½ to 1 hour, a peak effect in 2 to 4 hours, a duration of action up to 8 hours, and a serum half-life between 12 and 16 hours. It is metabolized in the liver and excreted primarily by the kidneys. Transdermal clonidine is best absorbed from the chest and upper arm. The onset of action and time to peak effect are 2 to 3 days, and the duration of action is approximately 1 week if the drug is in continuous contact with the body (approximately 8 hours if removed from the body). Metabolism and excretion are the same as for oral clonidine.

The side effects/adverse reactions of clonidine include dry mouth, headaches, constipation, weakness, postural hypotension, impotency or decreased sexual drive, insomnia, anxiety, anorexia, nausea, vomiting, and pruritus.

The initial adult dosage is 0.1 mg twice daily; this is increased by 0.1 or 0.2 mg every 2 to 4 days as necessary to control blood pressure. For maintenance, the dosage is 0.2 to 0.6 mg daily in divided doses. The dosage for children has not been established.

Catapres-TTS (clonidine transdermal system). Clonidine transdermal is available in various strengths (0.1, 0.2, or 0.3 mg), which are programmed to deliver the specified strength daily for 1 week. The system is composed of four layers: a film that contains a drug reservoir of clonidine, a membrane that controls the rate of drug delivery, an adhesive layer that also contains clonidine to initially saturate the skin site, and a top backing or cover layer. This system was formulated for the drug to flow from a higher concentration to a lower concentration in the body; this is limited by the rate-controlling membrane layer. It takes approximately 2 to 3 days to reach a therapeutic serum level of clonidine on initial application; replacing the system weekly at a new body site will maintain the therapeutic serum level.

■ Nursing Management
Clonidine Therapy

■ **Assessment.** Use clonidine therapy cautiously with clients who have coronary insufficiency, recent myocardial infarction, or cerebrovascular disease, because the decrease in blood pressure may decrease tissue perfusion and increase ischemia. Chronic renal failure will decrease drug elimination and increase the risk of toxicity. Clients with thromboangiitis, Raynaud's disease, or a history of mental depression may experience a worsening of their condition. Clients with sinus or atrioventricular node dysfunction may experience further impairment. Older adults are also more sensitive to the hypotensive effects of clonidine and are at risk for injury related to orthostatic hypotension. Dosage adjustments may be necessitated by age-related renal function impairment.

If the transdermal dosage form of clonidine is to be applied, the client's skin should be assessed for any irritation or abrasion so that these areas can be avoided; absorption may be increased if the drug is applied to such areas. Areas of skin involvement with disorders such as systemic lupus erythematosus (SLE) or scleroderma might decrease drug absorption; these areas should also be avoided.

Review the client's current medication regimen for the risk of significant drug interactions, such as those that may occur when clonidine is given concurrently with the following drugs:

Drug/Herb	Possible Effect and Management
beta-adrenergic blocking agents	Concurrent administration with clonidine may lead to a loss of blood pressure control. Additive bradycardia effects may also occur. Monitor pulse rate closely. If the prescriber wants to discontinue both drugs, the beta-blocking agent should be stopped first. Discontinuing clonidine first may increase the risk of inducing a withdrawal hypertensive crisis (see Box 27-3).
tricyclic antidepressants	The antihypertensive effectiveness of clonidine may be reduced. This usually occurs in the first or second week of therapy. Monitor closely, because dosage adjustments and/or alternative hypotensive agents may need to be considered by the prescriber.
yohimbine	**Concurrent use may increase blood pressure. Monitor closely or, preferably, avoid concurrent use.**

A baseline assessment of the client's blood pressure, health status, and lifestyle should be performed before initiating clonidine therapy.

■ **Nursing Diagnosis.** The client receiving clonidine therapy has the potential for the following nursing diagnoses/collaborative problems: risk for injury related to orthostatic hypotension, rebound hypertension, or the ineffectiveness of clonidine therapy; impaired skin integrity related to an allergic reaction to the transdermal system (itching, redness of skin), 15% to 20%; excess fluid volume related to sodium and water retention (edema); constipation, 10%; disturbed sleep pattern (drowsiness), 33% with oral use; impaired oral mucous membrane (dry mouth), 40% with oral use; fatigue, 10%; sexual dysfunction (impotence, loss of libido), 1% to 5%; impaired comfort (anorexia, nausea, nervousness), 1% to 5%; disturbed thought processes (confusion); and the potential complications of mental depression and overdose (dyspnea, syncope, pinpoint pupils, bradycardia, fatigue). (See the Nursing Care Plan on p. 578 for other selected nursing diagnoses related to antihypertensive therapy.)

■ **Implementation**

■ ***Monitoring.*** Monitor blood pressure and pulse closely during initiation of therapy, and continue to observe these parameters until the dosage is properly titrated. Blood pressure should decrease within 30 to 60 minutes of oral administration, and the decrease may persist for 8 hours. Monitor blood pressure and pulse rate regularly on a long-term basis to determine the effectiveness of clonidine.

Observe the client for drug tolerance as evidenced by rising blood pressure levels. The prescriber may increase the dosage or add a diuretic to obtain the required antihypertensive response.

Weigh the client daily for 3 to 4 days after initiation of therapy; fluid volume excess may occur because of sodium retention and edema. Monitor intake and output, and check the client for dependent edema. If fluid retention exists, it may be necessary to add a diuretic to the regimen.

Monitor for the anticholinergic effects of dry mouth, constipation, and urine retention.

Closely monitor clients with a history of mental depression, because clonidine may intensify this condition. A self-concept disturbance related to impotence may also occur.

Older adults may experience impaired cognition, and younger clients may have diminished reaction times (Gray, Lai, & Larson, 1999; Jakala, Riekkinen, Sirvio, Koivisto, & Riekkinen, 1999).

■ ***Intervention.*** When applying the clonidine transdermal system, select a hairless, intact area of the client's upper arm or torso. Do not trim the patch; doing so will alter the dosage. Reapply a new patch to a different skin site once every 7 days. If the system loosens, cover it with an adhesive overlay from the drug package. The patch should remain in place during bathing or showering. Replace the patch if it falls off or becomes very loose. Discard used patches by folding them in half with the adhesive sides together. If local skin irritation occurs before the patch has been in place for 7 days, it may be removed and a new one applied to a different skin area. A change from transdermal therapy may be required if skin irritation persists.

Prescribed dosage reductions are performed over 2 to 4 days, or preferably longer (1- to 2-week period), to prevent rebound hypertension, a potentially serious adverse syndrome.

If a client cannot effectively manage the therapeutic regimen, consultation with the prescriber may result in a change from the oral dosage form to the transdermal therapeutic system or to another antihypertensive drug because of the risk of rebound hypertension. When a client is being switched from the oral to the transdermal dosage form, the oral dose needs to be reduced over 2 to 3 days; this is done to avoid a withdrawal response, because the onset of action for the transdermal dosage form is 2 to 3 days.

■ ***Education.*** Emphasize the importance of periodic follow-up visits so blood pressure can be closely monitored. Be explicit in instructions concerning the serious consequences of rebound hypertension caused by missing drug doses or abruptly discontinuing the drug (Leenen, 1999). Clients with serious side effects should immediately report the problem to the prescriber so that the dosage may be adjusted or the drug withdrawn gradually over a period of 2 to 4 days. Abrupt withdrawal, including the omission of sequential doses, can result in a hypertensive crisis within 8 to 24 hours. The symptoms of hypertensive crisis are anxiety, sweating, tachycardia, insomnia, salivation, abdominal and muscle cramps, headache, and chest pain. The client and caregivers should be taught to perform blood pressure monitoring at home, record the results, and report the results at regular visits to the health care provider.

As with all other antihypertensive agents, clonidine helps

Nursing Care Plan
Selected Nursing Diagnoses Related to Antihypertensive Therapy

Nursing Diagnosis	Outcome Criteria	Nursing Interventions
Deficient knowledge related to newly prescribed or altered antihypertensive drug therapy	Client will describe hypertension; how drug therapy relates to condition; how and when to take medications; common drug interactions, particularly with OTC drugs; safety precautions; common side effects and which are reportable; and storage requirements of drugs. Client will monitor effectiveness of drug therapy with sequential blood pressure readings.	Assess learning needs and learning readiness. Plan with client and family for achievement of realistic goals. Provide information to meet outcome criteria.
Ineffective therapeutic regimen management	Client will self-administer medications safely and accurately.	Check refill frequency to determine adherence to the medication regimen. Explore with the client the reasons for nonadherence, and take appropriate teaching/counseling interventions. Provide needed drug information concerning rationales for the specific client's hypertensive status. Emphasize that drug therapy controls but does not cure hypertension, and emphasize the possible need for lifelong therapy. Discuss the possibility of rebound hypertension with nonadherence to the medication regimen.
Sexual dysfunction related to antihypertensive drug therapy	Client will describe the nature of the dysfunction, consult with the prescriber for dosage reduction or drug substitution, and resume sexual activity.	Assess for causative factors. Encourage the client to share concerns. Provide health teaching and referrals when needed. Encourage a return to sexual activity.

to control but does not cure hypertension; therefore therapy may possibly be lifelong. It is important for the client to take the medication as prescribed, even if he or she is feeling well. Review the serious consequences of untreated hypertension.

Instruct the client to keep an adequate supply of the drug at all times, particularly during travel. Instruct the client to take the last dose before bedtime to ensure continuous blood pressure control during the night and to reduce daytime drowsiness, which occurs in approximately 33% of clients using oral dosage forms. Instruct the client to make position changes slowly. The client should move slowly from the recumbent to the upright position and dangle the feet from the edge of the bed to prevent dizziness and fainting. Because the potential for orthostatic hypotension is greatly increased, the client needs to be cautioned to avoid alcohol ingestion, prolonged standing and strenuous exercising, and exercising during hot weather.

Altered comfort related to dry mouth occurs in 40% of the clients using oral dosage forms. Encourage the client to use sugarless candy or gum or ice to obtain relief. A saliva substitute such as Salivart or Optimoist may also be used. If dry mouth persists longer than 2 weeks, the prescriber or dentist needs to be consulted because of the increased risk of caries and oral candidiasis.

Altered bowel function occurs as constipation in approximately 10% of clients. Instruction should be provided concerning adequate fluid and fiber intake, regular exercise, and establishing a regular bowel pattern to prevent or minimize constipation.

Advise the client undergoing long-term therapy to have a periodic eye examination (every 6 to 12 months) to identify possible retinal degeneration; this has occurred in rats who received clonidine. Instruct the client to carry a medical identification card or MedicAlert bracelet or pendant. Warn the client not to take an OTC medication without consulting the prescriber. Caution the client about the increased sedative effects of alcohol, barbiturates, and other central nervous system (CNS) depressants during clonidine therapy, particularly if the individual is operating a car or machinery.

Instruct the client on how to apply the transdermal patch and place it at a different site each week.

Advise the client in the nonpharmacologic management of hypertension, including sodium restriction, weight reduction, regular exercise, smoking cessation, moderate consumption of alcohol, reduction in dietary saturated fats, behavior modification to promote relaxation, and adequate dietary intake of potassium, calcium, and magnesium.

■ **Evaluation.** The expected outcome of clonidine therapy for hypertension is that the client's blood pressure will remain within normal limits. The client and family will state an understanding of effective self-management of the therapeutic clonidine regimen.

methyldopa [meth ill doe′ pa] (Aldomet)
methyldopate injection [meth ill doe′ payte] (Parenteral Aldomet)

Although the exact hypotensive mechanism is unknown, the theory is that a metabolite of methyldopa (alpha-methylnorepinephrine) stimulates the central $alpha_2$ receptors, which results in a reduction in norepinephrine (sympathetic) outflow to the heart, kidneys, and peripheral vasculature. It lowers blood pressure in a way that is similar to clonidine.

In the body, methyldopate is hydrolyzed to methyldopa, which then must undergo the previously described process to produce the hypotensive effect. The antihypertensive effect produced by the parenteral dosage form begins in approximately 4 to 6 hours and therefore should not be used as the primary single drug in a hypertensive emergency.

The peak effect for methyldopa occurs 4 to 6 hours after a single dose or in 48 to 72 hours with multiple dosing. The duration of action is 12 to 24 hours (after oral single dose), 1 to 2 days (after multiple oral doses), or 10 to 16 hours (after IV administration). Methyldopa is metabolized centrally to alpha-methylnorepinephrine. Excretion is primarily by the kidneys.

The side effects/adverse reactions include drowsiness, dry mouth, headaches, edema of feet and legs, postural hypotension, impotency, insomnia, depression, anxiety, and nightmares.

The initial adult oral dosage is 250 mg two to three times daily for 2 days, titrated as necessary. The maintenance dosage is 500 to 2000 mg/day, divided into 2 to 4 individual doses; the maximum daily dosage is 3 g/day. The initial pediatric dosage is 10 mg/kg PO in 2 to 4 divided doses, increased at 2-day intervals according to the child's response, up to 65 mg/kg or 3 g/day, whichever is less.

The parenteral adult dosage is 250 to 500 mg in dextrose 5% injection (100 mL) administered over ½ to 1 hour every 6 hours as needed. The maximum dosage is 1 g every 6 to 12 hours. The pediatric IV infusion dosage is 20 to 40 mg/kg in dextrose 5% injection over ½ to 1 hour every 6 hours as needed, up to 65 mg/kg or 3 g/day, whichever is less.

■ Nursing Management

Methyldopa Therapy

■ **Assessment.** Do not use methyldopa in clients with active hepatic disease (e.g., hepatitis or cirrhosis) or a hypersensitivity to methyldopa. Use with caution in clients with a history of autoimmune hemolytic anemia, pheochromocytoma (interference with catecholamines), or previous liver disease in association with the methyldopa administration. The risks-benefit ratio must be considered in childbearing and lactating women.

Review the client's current medication regimen for the risk of significant drug interactions, such as those that may occur when methyldopa is given concurrently with the following drugs:

Drug	Possible Effect and Management
Bold/color type indicates the most serious interactions.	
monoamine oxidase (MAO) inhibitors	**Hyperexcitability, hallucinations, headache, and hypertension have been reported with this combination. Avoid concurrent use or a serious drug interaction may occur.**
sympathomimetics (e.g., **cocaine, epinephrine, norepinephrine, phenylephrine**)	**A decrease in the antihypertensive effect of methyldopa is reported. Avoid concurrent use or a serious drug interaction may occur. If it is necessary to use sympathomimetics, the prescriber should prescribe very small doses of the sympathomimetic agent. Monitor closely.**

A baseline assessment of the client's blood pressure should be obtained, and a complete blood cell count (CBC) and a direct Coombs test should be performed.

■ **Nursing Diagnosis.** The client receiving methyldopa therapy has the potential for the following nursing diagnoses/collaborative problems: risk for injury related to orthostatic hypotension or the ineffectiveness of methyldopa therapy; ineffective protection related to leukopenia or thrombocytopenia; excess fluid volume related to sodium and water retention (edema); disturbed thought processes (nightmares, vivid dreams); anxiety; diarrhea; disturbed sleep pattern (drowsiness [>5%]); impaired oral mucous membrane (dry mouth [>5%]); impaired comfort (headache [>5%], nausea, stuffy nose); activity intolerance related to hemolytic anemia; sexual dysfunction (decreased libido, ejaculation failure); and the potential complications of mental depression, drug fever (fever within the first 3 months of therapy), myocarditis (fever, chills, tachycardia), pancreatitis (abdominal pain with nausea and vomiting), SLE–like syndrome (weakness, joint pain, rash), colitis (severe diarrhea, abdominal cramping), or cholestasis or hepatitis (dark urine, pale stools, jaundice).

■ **Implementation**

■ ***Monitoring.*** Take the client's blood pressure and pulse as prescribed during the initiation of therapy, and continue until the drug dosage is properly titrated. To determine the effectiveness of methyldopa, measure the blood pressure at regular intervals, with the client in the lying, sitting, and standing positions.

Observe the client for drug tolerance within the second or third month of therapy as evidenced by rising blood pressure levels. The prescriber may increase the dosage or add a diuretic to obtain the required antihypertensive response. Observe the client for drug-induced depression, and report any symptoms to the prescriber. Observe the client for side effects, especially unexplained fever or jaundice, and immediately report any to the prescriber.

If unexplained fever or rash occurs, obtain liver function studies (e.g., AST [SGOT], bilirubin), especially during the first 2 or 3 months of therapy. If jaundice is present, methyldopa is discontinued to avoid drug-induced hepatitis.

Monitor for fluid volume excess by measuring intake and output, weighing the client daily, and checking for dependent edema. Report fluid retention to the prescriber. If fluid retention occurs, it may be necessary to add a diuretic to the regimen.

Hemolytic anemia may occur with possible fatal complications. A CBC and a direct Coombs test should be performed periodically during treatment. A positive Coombs test may or may not indicate hemolytic anemia. With prolonged use of methyldopa, 10% to 20% of clients develop a positive direct Coombs test; this is not a contraindication to further use of the drug. However, if a positive Coombs test leads to a diagnosis of hemolytic anemia, the prescriber will discontinue therapy. A positive Coombs test produced by methyldopa therapy may interfere with the crossmatching of blood. If thrombocytopenia or reversible leukopenia occurs, drug therapy should be discontinued.

The refill frequency may be checked to determine the effectiveness of the client's management of the therapeutic regimen.

■ ***Intervention.*** Dosage increases should be initiated with the evening dose to minimize the effects of sedation.

IM or SC administration of methyldopa is not recommended because of unreliable absorption. Administer an IV infusion slowly over 30 to 60 minutes. When changing a client from the IV to the oral form once the blood pressure has stabilized, the same dosage is used.

■ ***Education.*** Emphasize to the client the importance of keeping clinical laboratory visits for blood cell counts and hepatic function studies. Methyldopa hepatotoxicity, which is reversible, may occasionally develop 2 to 4 weeks after initiation of therapy. The client should report any flu-like symptoms of chills, fever, headache, anorexia, fatigue, arthralgia, or pruritus. If the results of the liver function tests are positive, therapy will be discontinued. Instruct the client to follow the same precautions as for oral clonidine.

■ **Evaluation.** The expected outcome of methyldopa therapy is that the client's blood pressure will be within normal limits without the client experiencing any adverse reactions to the drug. The client and/or caregivers will manage the methyldopa regimen effectively.

guanabenz [gwahn′ a benz] (Wytensin)

The mechanism of action of guanabenz acetate is believed to be the same as for clonidine; it is a centrally acting alpha$_2$ agonist. Cardiac output remains unchanged, and the antihypertensive effect occurs without major changes in peripheral resistance. Peripheral resistance does eventually decrease with continued therapy.

Guanabenz has an onset of action within 1 hour (for a single dose); the peak effect occurs in 2 to 4 hours, and the duration of action is 12 hours. The serum half-life is 6 hours. This drug is metabolized in the liver, and excretion is via the kidneys and feces.

The side effects/adverse reactions of guanabenz include drowsiness, headaches, nausea, and impotency or decreased sexual drive.

The initial adult dosage is 4 mg PO twice daily, increased if necessary every 1 to 2 weeks by increments of 4 to 8 mg/day up to a maximum of 32 mg/day. The dosage for children is not established.

■ Nursing Management
Guanabenz Therapy

■ **Assessment.** Guanabenz is used during pregnancy only if the benefits outweigh the potential risk of adverse effects on the fetus. In animal studies an increase in skeletal abnormalities has been observed, as well as increased fetal loss and diminished body weight of the neonate. Always inquire whether a female client is pregnant or plans to become pregnant. Do not use guanabenz in clients who are hypersensitive to this substance. It should be used with caution in clients with cerebrovascular or cardiovascular disease or renal or hepatic impairment. A baseline assessment of the client's blood pressure should be obtained.

Giving guanabenz concurrently with a beta-adrenergic blocking agent or other hypotensive agents may result in additive hypotensive effects. Monitor blood pressure closely, because dosage adjustments may be necessary. When discontinuing both drugs in a client (for example, a beta-blocking drug and guanabenz), taper the beta blocker first to prevent a withdrawal hypertensive reaction.

■ **Nursing Diagnosis.** As with other antihypertensive agents, clients receiving guanabenz therapy might be at risk for the following nursing diagnoses/collaborative problems: risk for injury related to syncope or the ineffectiveness of guanabenz therapy (hypertension); impaired comfort (headache or nausea); impaired oral mucous membrane (dry mouth); fatigue; disturbed sleep pattern (drowsiness); sexual dysfunction; and the potential complications of sympathetic overactivity related to withdrawal (anxiety, chest pain, tachycardia, nausea, insomnia, headache, increased salivation and sweating).

■ **Implementation**

■ ***Monitoring.*** Monitor blood pressure and pulse closely during the initiation of therapy and until the dosage is properly titrated. Closely observe clients with severe hepatic or renal failure, severe coronary insufficiency, recent myocardial infarction, or cerebrovascular disease; also observe older adults closely, because they are particularly sensitive to the hypotensive effects of the drug. The client's blood pressure should be monitored on a long-term basis.

■ ***Intervention.*** The last dose of each day should be taken at bedtime to ensure overnight control of blood pressure and to reduce daytime drowsiness.

Although guanabenz is usually not discontinued before surgery, the anesthetist must be aware that the client is receiving the drug.

■ ***Education.*** Emphasize the importance of periodic follow-up visits so that the guanabenz dosage and blood pressure can be monitored. Some clients may be instructed to measure their own blood pressure and report the readings at regular visits to the prescriber.

Caution the client against abrupt withdrawal of the drug, even if he or she is experiencing unpleasant side effects. There is the possibility of withdrawal symptoms, although rebound hypertension does not generally occur. The prescriber should be consulted for recommendations as to how to proceed. Guanabenz needs to be taken even if the client is feeling well. The medication helps to control but not cure hypertension, and therapy may be lifelong.

Inform the client of the possible side effects, particularly dry mouth, and about the increased sedative effects if taken with alcohol, barbiturates, or other CNS depressants; caution in operating a car or other machinery is indicated. Caution the client not to take OTC medications without consulting the prescriber. Instruct the client to take the last dose before bedtime to ensure continuous blood pressure control during the night. Instruct the client to carry a medical identification card or a MedicAlert bracelet or pendant.

Instruct the client in the nonpharmacologic management of hypertension (see Figure 27-4).

■ **Evaluation.** The expected outcome of guanabenz therapy is that the client will maintain a blood pressure within normal limits without experiencing any adverse reactions to the drug.

guanfacine [gwahn′ fa seen] (Tenex)

Guanfacine (Tenex) is a centrally acting alpha$_2$-adrenergic agonist antihypertensive similar to clonidine. It is used to lower peripheral vascular resistance, heart rate, and blood pressure.

Guanfacine is well absorbed orally and has a peak effect in 8 to 12 hours (single dose) or 1 to 3 months (long-term dosing). The onset of action occurs within 7 days of chronic dosing. The duration of effect is 1 day (single dose). This drug is metabolized by the liver and excreted by the kidneys.

The side effects/adverse reactions of guanfacine include constipation, dry mouth, sedation, light-headedness, headache, nausea, vomiting, insomnia, impotency, dry or itching eyes, weakness, and depression.

The adult dosage is 1 mg PO daily at bedtime, increased if needed in 3 to 4 weeks (to 2 mg/day). If necessary, a third increase may be instituted in another 3 to 4 weeks. The pediatric dosage has not been determined.

■ Nursing Management

Guanfacine Therapy

Except for the precaution regarding the use of guanabenz during pregnancy, the nursing management for guanfacine is the same as for guanabenz. There is also the added concern that the client may experience depression with the use of guanfacine. The client and family/caregiver should report any symptoms of depression, including appetite disturbance (anorexia or overeating), significant weight gain or loss, sleep disturbance (insomnia or hypersomnia), fatigue, agitation, loss of interest or pleasure in activities, feelings of guilt or worthlessness, difficulty in concentration or decision making, or suicidal thoughts.

Peripheral Adrenergic Inhibitors

The peripherally active adrenergic inhibitors include guanethidine (Ismelin), guanadrel (Hylorel) and reserpine (Serpalan, Serpasil); the alpha-adrenergic blocking agents include doxazosin (Cardura), prazosin (Minipress), and terazosin (Hytrin).

guanethidine [gwahn eth′ i deen] (Ismelin)

Guanethidine sulfate is a powerful antihypertensive drug that acts as a postganglionic adrenergic neuron-blocking agent. It enters the storage vesicles of the adrenergic nerve terminal, where it gradually displaces the stored norepinephrine. The subsequent depletion of norepinephrine inhibits the transmission of nerve impulses at the neuroeffector junction. Although there is no significant change in peripheral resistance, this drug reduces blood pressure by decreasing vascular tone, primarily at the venous side and secondarily at the arterial side of the circulatory system.

A lower venous return reduces cardiac output, which consequently decreases cerebral, splanchnic, and renal blood flow. The venous pooling of blood is responsible for the severe orthostatic hypotension reported with this drug. This is a limiting factor for its use. The reduction in blood pressure is noticeably greater with the client in the standing position than in the recumbent position.

The adrenergic blocking action of guanethidine increases gastrointestinal motility, often causing diarrhea. This drug does not affect the catecholamines in the adrenal medulla. It is contraindicated for use in pheochromocytoma because it may cause the release of catecholamines, thus producing a hypertensive crisis.

Guanethidine has a variable absorption orally (3% to 30% absorbed) with long-term dosing. The peak effect occurs within 8 hours (single dose) or in 1 to 3 weeks (with long-term dosing). It has a biphasic half-life; that is, alpha is 1 to 2 days, and beta is between 4 and 8 days. When long-term dosing is discontinued, there is a gradual blood pressure increase to pretreatment levels within 1 to 3 weeks. Guanethidine is metabolized in the liver and excreted by the kidneys.

The side effects/adverse reactions of guanethidine include orthostatic hypotension, weakness, impaired ejaculation, diarrhea, bradycardia, stuffy nose, alopecia, blurred vision, ptosis of eyelids, nausea, vomiting, muscle pain or tremors, dry mouth, headache, edema, and chest pain (angina).

For adult ambulatory clients the dosage of guanethidine is 10 or 12.5 mg PO daily initially, increased by 10- or 12.5-mg increments at 5- to 7-day intervals as necessary. The maintenance dosage is 25 to 50 mg daily. For hospitalized clients, the initial dosage is 25 to 50 mg PO daily, increased by 25- to 50-mg increments at daily or every-other-day intervals as necessary. The pediatric dosage is 0.2 mg/kg PO daily, increased at 7- to 10-day intervals as necessary for blood pressure control.

■ Nursing Management
Guanethidine Therapy

■ **Assessment.** Do not use guanethidine in clients who are hypersensitive to this substance. The risk-benefit ratio should be considered carefully for clients with pheochromocytoma (the release of catecholamines may exacerbate symptoms) or congestive heart failure (the condition may be worsened by fluid retention).

Anticipate that hospitalized clients will receive a higher initial dosage than ambulatory clients because they can be monitored more carefully. A baseline measurement of the client's supine and standing blood pressure is necessary.

Review the client's current medication regimen for the risk of significant drug interactions, such as those that may occur when guanethidine is given concurrently with the following drugs:

Drug	Possible Effect and Management
Bold/color type indicates the most serious interactions.	
oral antidiabetic medications or insulin	May result in an increased hypoglycemic effect. Monitor blood glucose levels closely and communicate with the prescriber, because dosage adjustments may be necessary.
metaraminol (Aramine) and possibly other sympathomimetics	**The antihypertensive effectiveness of guanethidine may be reduced. Concurrent use of metaraminol and guanethidine may result in cardiac dysrhythmias, severe prolonged hypertension, or a hypertensive crisis. Avoid such use or a serious drug interaction may occur.**
minoxidil (Loniten) or hypotension-producing medications	**Concurrent use with guanethidine is not recommended, because antihypertensive effects may be potentiated.**
MAO inhibitors	**Severe hypertension may result. Avoid concurrent use or a serious drug interaction may occur. It is recommended that MAO inhibitors be discontinued for a minimum of 1 week before starting guanethidine.**
tricyclic antidepressants, loxapine (Loxitane), thioxanthenes, possibly other psychotropic medications, and trimeprazine (Temaril)	May reduce the antihypertensive effect of guanethidine by blocking its access to the adrenergic nerve site. Monitor closely, because dosage adjustments or alternate antidepressant medications on a trial basis may be ordered by the prescriber.

■ **Nursing Diagnosis.** With the administration of guanethidine, the client may experience the following nursing diagnoses/collaborative problems: ineffective tissue perfusion (renal, cerebral, and/or cardiopulmonary) related to ineffectiveness with the underlying condition or ischemic effects secondary to hypotension; excess fluid volume (dependent edema, pulmonary edema); sexual dysfunction as evidenced by ejaculation difficulties; impaired comfort related to headache or chest pain (angina); impaired oral mucous membrane (dry mouth, stuffy nose); diarrhea; fatigue; risk for injury related to the orthostatic hypotensive effects of the drug; and the potential complications of bradycardia.

■ **Implementation**

■ ***Monitoring.*** The most common problem with guanethidine is orthostatic hypotension. As a baseline for comparison, measure blood pressure before initiating drug therapy; during therapy, continue to keep a record of blood pressures while the client is supine and standing. The hypotensive effect of this drug is greater with the client in the standing position than in the supine position. Therefore the blood pressure is taken first while the client is in the supine position and then again after the client has been standing for 10 minutes or performing mild exercise. If there is no decrease from the previous blood pressure, an increase in dosage is indicated. The dosage should be reduced when the client has a normal supine blood pressure, an excessive fall in orthostatic pressure, or severe diarrhea.

Monitor intake and output, observing for reduced urine volume, particularly in clients with limited cardiac or renal function. Weigh the client daily, and watch for signs of edema or fluid retention. Report an increased weight (2 pounds or more in 24 hours) to the prescriber. Monitor the client's pulse rate carefully. Report occurrences of bradycardia to the prescriber. Closely monitor a client receiving long-term therapy, because the effects of guanethidine are cumulative.

Monitor the blood glucose levels of clients who are receiving antidiabetic medication, because guanethidine may produce additive hypoglycemic effects.

■ ***Intervention.*** Note that guanethidine has a long duration of action as well as a prolonged half-life. In addition, the full therapeutic benefits may not be noticed for 1 to 3 weeks. Therefore dosage increases, when needed, are made at intervals of 5 to 7 days.

■ ***Education.*** Forewarn the client that orthostatic hypotension (dizziness, light-headedness, or syncope) is common and is prominent when rising from sleep or making rapid position changes. Instruct the client to change positions gradually. Venous return to the heart can be increased by flexing the arms and legs slowly before sitting or standing. Recommend that the client don elastic stockings before getting out of bed.

During dosage adjustment, the hospitalized client should receive help when getting out of bed. Inform the client that orthostatic hypotension is aggravated by hot showers or baths, hot weather, prolonged standing, physical exercise, and alcohol ingestion. During an episode of orthostatic hypotension, caution the client to sit or lie down at the first sign of dizziness or weakness.

Instruct the client to report any signs of diarrhea. If it persists, the prescriber may order an anticholinergic agent (atropine), a paregoric, or a kaolin-pectin preparation. Guanethidine may be discontinued, or the dosage may be reduced. Note the state of hydration of the client, and check the level of electrolyte balance during this episode.

Alert the client to inform surgeons, anesthetists, and dentists that he or she is taking guanethidine before any invasive procedures are considered. Instruct the client to carry a medical identification card or a MedicAlert bracelet or pendant.

Emphasize the importance of drug compliance. Report side effects so the prescriber can modify the drug regimen without discontinuing the medication. Advise the client to avoid emotional encounters or any other form of stress; instruction on stress management techniques should be offered. Instruct the client not to take any other medication or OTC drugs, which may contain sympathomimetic agents, without consulting the prescriber. Stress the importance of keeping follow-up appointments with the prescriber.

As with guanabenz and other antihypertensive agents, instruct the client in the nonpharmacologic measures to take for blood pressure reduction.

■ **Evaluation.** The expected outcome of guanethidine therapy is that the client will maintain a blood pressure within normal limits without experiencing any adverse reactions to the drug.

guanadrel [gwahn′ a drel] (Hylorel)

The mechanism of action for guanadrel is the same as for guanethidine. Guanadrel has an onset of action within 2 hours and a peak effect between 4 and 6 hours (after a single dose). The half-life is variable but in general is approximately 10 hours. The duration of effect is approximately 9 hours. This drug is metabolized in the liver and excreted by the kidneys.

The side effects/adverse reactions of guanadrel include hypotension, weakness, impaired ejaculation, increased urination at night, muscle pain or tremors, dry mouth, headache, edema, and chest pain.

Metaraminol (Aramine) and other sympathomimetics, MAO inhibitors, tricyclic antidepressants, loxapine (Loxitane), thioxanthenes, and psychotropic agents (especially chlorpromazine [Thorazine]) may cause drug interactions; see the interactions for guanethidine, p. 582. In addition, trimeprazine (Temaril) may reduce the antihypertensive effect of guanadrel by displacement and by blocking guanadrel's access to the adrenergic neuron. Monitor blood pressures closely.

The initial adult dosage is 5 mg PO twice daily, which may be increased at daily, weekly, or monthly intervals as necessary for blood pressure control. The maintenance dosage is 20 to 75 mg/day in 2 to 4 divided doses. Pediatric dosages have not been established.

For the nursing management of guanadrel, see Nursing Management: Guanethidine Therapy, p. 582.

Rauwolfia Derivatives

reserpine [re ser′ peen] (Serpalan, Serpasil)

Rauwolfia derivatives are alkaloids obtained primarily from *Rauwolfia serpentina*, a shrub endemic to India and various tropical areas of the world. Reserpine, a rauwolfia alkaloid, lowers blood pressure by depleting the storage sites of norepinephrine in the peripheral postganglionic adrenergic neuron. Without adequate norepinephrine available for release, discharges of nerve impulses from the peripheral sympathetic neurons, which supply the smooth muscle of arterioles, produce little or no effect on these blood vessels. The resultant vascular relaxation decreases peripheral resistance, thereby reducing blood pressure. These compounds also decrease heart rate and thus lower cardiac output. Reserpine also depletes stores of serotonin.

Reserpine has an onset of antihypertensive action of days to 3 weeks with multiple dosing, and it has a peak antihypertensive effect within 3 to 6 weeks. The half-life is initially 4.5 hours, but with long-term dosing it is extended to be tween 45 and 168 hours. Reserpine is metabolized in the liver and excreted primarily in the feces.

The side effects/adverse reactions of reserpine include nausea, vomiting, anorexia, diarrhea, dizziness, dry mouth, stuffy nose, light-headedness, fluid retention, sexual dysfunction, chest pain, bradycardia, and bronchospasms.

The adult dosage is 0.1 to 0.25 mg PO daily.

■ Nursing Management
Reserpine Therapy

■ **Assessment.** Determine if the client has a history of mental depression, in which case the drug is used cautiously. Reserpine therapy is discontinued at the first sign of despondency; otherwise continued therapy could result in suicide. Use reserpine cautiously in clients with a history of gallstones to prevent biliary colic; also use cautiously in clients with a history of renal insufficiency (a diuretic is usually required) to avoid the decreased renal tissue perfusion that may result from lower blood pressure levels. Use cautiously in clients who are receiving electroconvulsive therapy or in clients with epilepsy, cardiac dysrhythmias, respiratory problems, parkinsonism, or pheochromocytoma. Clients with ulcerative colitis or acute peptic ulcer disease may experience increased gastrointestinal motility; use reserpine with caution in such cases. Do not use reserpine with clients who are hypersensitive to *Rauwolfia* derivatives.

Review the client's current medication regimen for the risk of significant drug interactions, such as those that may occur when reserpine is given concurrently with the following drugs:

Drug	Possible Effect and Management
Bold/color type indicates the most serious interactions.	
CNS depressants and/or alcohol	Enhanced CNS depressant effects. Monitor vital signs, level of consciousness, and mental status closely.
MAO inhibitors	**May result in hyperpyrexia and hypertension (moderate, severe, or even crisis level). Concurrent administration is not recommended. Clients receiving MAO inhibitors should be taken off this medication for at least 1 week before beginning administration of a rauwolfia alkaloid.**

A baseline assessment of the client's blood pressure should be obtained.

■ **Nursing Diagnosis.** With the administration of reserpine, the client may experience the following nursing diagnoses/collaborative problems: impaired tissue perfusion related to the client's underlying condition; risk for injury related to cardiovascular and CNS effects (light-headedness, dizziness, orthostatic hypotension); anxiety; disturbed thought processes (inability to concentrate); sexual dysfunction (impotence or decreased sexual interest); diarrhea; impaired oral mucous membrane (dry mouth, stuffy nose); disturbed sleep pattern (nightmares, early morning insomnia); ineffective protection (thrombocytopenia); impaired comfort (abdominal cramps, headache, chest pain); anxiety; and the potential complications related to gastrointestinal effects (tarry stools, hematemesis, peptic ulcer), mental depression, or dysrhythmias.

■ **Implementation**

■ ***Monitoring.*** Monitor the client's blood pressure and pulse rate frequently and compare with baseline readings, particularly before parenteral administration. A decrease in blood pressure may be a result of bradycardia. Weigh the client daily. Excessive weight gain indicates fluid retention, which should be reported to the prescriber.

■ ***Intervention.*** Administer the oral medication with meals or with milk or other food to minimize gastric irritation, because the drug increases gastric secretions.

Note that the *Rauwolfia* derivatives have a slow onset of action and a long duration of action; therefore therapeutic benefits may take approximately 2 weeks to develop. This means that dosage adjustments should be made no more frequently than every 7 to 14 days so that the full effect of the previous dosage can be evaluated. Action may persist for approximately 1 month after discontinuation of therapy. Reserpine no longer needs to be withdrawn if a client requires a general anesthetic, including for dental surgery; however, the anesthetist must be aware of the therapy. It is recommended that reserpine be withdrawn 2 weeks before electroconvulsive therapy is instituted.

■ ***Education.*** Although orthostatic hypotension does not usually occur, advise the client to make position changes slowly to avoid potential dizziness and fainting. Alert the client that the drug may cause drowsiness and to take precautions about driving and other hazardous activities until the CNS effects are known. Advise the client not to take alcohol or other CNS depressants, which will increase the sedative effects of reserpine.

Teach the client or caregiver the possible side effects that may occur and that should be reported to the prescriber, such as nightmares, weight gain, nasal stuffiness, or a significant change in blood pressure. Mental depression (anorexia, self-deprecation, detached attitude, and powerlessness) may lead to suicide. This usually occurs in clients who receive high dosages. Clients should report despondency, early-morning insomnia, anorexia, impotence, and feelings of low self-esteem.

If nasal stuffiness occurs, nasal decongestants or other OTC preparations containing sympathomimetics should not be used without first consulting the prescriber. A dry mouth may be relieved with warm water rinses, OTC saliva substitutes, sugarless gum, or sour hard candy.

Emphasize the importance of drug compliance even if the client is feeling well. Instruct the client not to discontinue the drug suddenly but to report unpleasant side effects to the prescriber. Also stress the need for medical follow-up visits. Instruct the client to carry a medical identification card or a MedicAlert bracelet or pendant.

As with other antihypertensive agents, instruct the client in nonpharmacologic measures for blood pressure reduction.

■ **Evaluation.** The expected outcome of reserpine therapy is that the client will maintain a blood pressure within normal limits without experiencing any adverse reactions to the drug.

Alpha-Adrenergic Blocking Drugs

The alpha-adrenergic blocking agents used in the management of hypertension include phenoxybenzamine (Dibenzyline), phentolamine (Regitine), doxazosin (Cardura), prazosin (Minipress), and terazosin (Hytrin). Phenoxybenzamine and phentolamine are relatively nonselective alpha blockers; they antagonize responses mediated by both $alpha_1$ and $alpha_2$ receptors. Hence, they lower blood pressure by preventing norepinephrine from activating $alpha_1$ receptors on vascular smooth muscle to produce vasoconstriction. (See Chapter 22 for monographs of phenoxybenzamine and phentolamine.) Doxazosin, prazosin, and terazosin are more selective in activity and are classed as $alpha_1$-adrenergic blocking agents.

doxazosin [dox ay′ zoe sin] (Cardura ◆)
prazosin [pra′ zoe sin] (Minipress)
terazosin [ter ay′ zoe sin] (Hytrin)

Doxazosin, prazosin, and terazosin are selective alpha$_1$-adrenergic blocking agents that dilate both arterioles and veins. This action results in decreased peripheral vascular resistance and lowered blood pressure. With prazosin and terazosin, the lowering of blood pressure is not associated with reflex tachycardia, whereas doxazosin may cause a small increase in heart rate. Prazosin has been used as adjunct therapy to digoxin and diuretics in the treatment of congestive heart failure. However, this combination has not resulted in improved survival (*USP DI,* 1999). Although all three drugs have been used for benign prostatic hyperplasia (BPH) to improve urinary flow and the symptoms of BPH, only doxazosin and terazosin have been approved by the Food and Drug Administration (FDA) for this indication (*USP DI,* 1999). Doxazosin and terazosin may be used in normotensive clients with BPH because they do not appear to significantly lower blood pressure. In individuals with both hypertension and BPH, they are effective in treating both conditions (Fawzy, Hendry, Cook, & Gonzales, 1999; Lowe, Olson, & Padley, 1999). Tamsulosin (Flomax) is an alpha$_1$-adrenergic blocking agent that is indicated only for the treatment of BPH.

The onset of action for doxazosin is 1 to 2 hours; the peak effect occurs in 5 to 6 hours, and the duration of action is 1 day. Prazosin has an onset of action within 0.5 to 1.5 hours, and it reaches a peak effect within 2 to 4 hours (within 1 hour for congestive heart failure). The duration of effect in clients with hypertension is 7 to 10 hours (single drug dose), whereas with congestive heart failure it is 6 hours. Terazosin is rapidly absorbed orally; it has an onset of action within 15 minutes, a peak effect in 2 to 3 hours, and a duration of action of approximately 1 day. All three drugs (active and inactive metabolites) are metabolized in the liver and are excreted primarily in the feces.

The side effects/adverse reactions of the alpha-adrenergic blocking drugs include weakness, nausea, vomiting, stuffy nose, orthostatic hypotension, angina, edema of the lower extremities, headaches, syncope, and shortness of breath. There are currently no known major drug interactions with these drugs (*USP DI,* 1999).

The initial adult dosage of doxazosin is 1 mg PO daily at bedtime, increased every 2 weeks if necessary. The maximum daily dose is 16 mg. A pediatric dosage has not been established. The adult dosage of prazosin is 0.5 mg PO two or three times daily for at least 3 days. If tolerated, the dosage may be increased if necessary according to individual response. The pediatric dosage is 0.05 to 0.4 mg/kg/day, administered in 2 or 3 divided doses. The adult dosage of terazosin is 1 mg PO daily at bedtime. The maintenance dosage is between 1 and 5 mg daily as needed to control blood pressure. The maximum daily dose is 20 mg. A pediatric dosage has not been established.

■ Nursing Management

Alpha-Adrenergic Blocking Agent Therapy

■ **Assessment.** Do not administer alpha-adrenergic blocking agents if the client has a sensitivity to these drugs. Clients with impaired renal function may require lower dosages. Older adults may be more sensitive to the effects of alpha-adrenergic blocking agents. Use prazosin with caution in clients who have angina pectoris or severe cardiac disease. Document a baseline blood pressure.

■ **Nursing Diagnosis.** The nursing diagnoses/collaborative problems to be considered with these agents include the following: risk for injury related to the cardiovascular and CNS effects (drowsiness, dizziness, and orthostatic hypotension); excess fluid volume (dependent edema, shortness of breath, and weight gain); fatigue; impaired oral mucous membrane (dry mouth); impaired comfort (nasal stuffiness, headache, chest pain, joint pain, nausea, and vomiting); altered cardiac output (tachycardia, palpitations); and the potential complication of "first-dose orthostatic hypotensive reaction." With prazosin, the client may also experience altered patterns of urinary elimination (urinary incontinence) and sexual dysfunction (priapism).

■ **Implementation**

■ ***Monitoring.*** Monitor the client's blood pressure and pulse rate frequently, and observe for tachycardia or any sudden drop in blood pressure.

■ ***Intervention.*** "First-dose hypotensive reaction," a syncope along with dizziness, light-headedness, or a sudden loss of consciousness, may occur, generally ½ to 2 hours after an initial dose or a rapid dosage increase. These symptoms may also appear when other antihypertensive agents are added to the regimen. Occasionally the syncopal episode is preceded by severe tachycardia (heart rate of 120 to 160 beats/min). To minimize this reaction, limit the initial dose of these drugs to 1 mg and then increase slowly. When adding a diuretic or other antihypertensive agent, reduce the dose to 1 or 2 mg and then increase as needed. It is recommended that the initial dose be administered at bedtime to minimize the "first-dose hypotensive reaction."

■ ***Education.*** Inform the client of "first-dose hypotensive reaction." Instruct the client to avoid rapid postural changes, particularly from recumbent to upright positions. The client should be instructed to lie down if dizziness occurs. Reassure the client that this effect tends to disappear with continued use of the drug or dosage reduction. Instruct the client not to drive or operate hazardous machinery during the early period of adjustment to drug therapy. Note that the full effect of the drug may not be achieved for 4 to 6 weeks.

Teach the client to weigh daily and to report any significant increase (over 1 kg per day) to the prescriber. Because these agents tend to increase fluid retention, instruct the client to minimize sodium intake.

Emphasize the importance of complying with the drug regimen and in keeping appointments with the prescriber. Ineffectiveness usually occurs within several months if tolerance develops, and the prescriber will need to alter the drug regimen. Instruct the client not to take any other drugs without first consulting the prescriber. This includes OTC medications that contain sympathomimetic agents used for a cold, cough, or allergic conditions.

As with other antihypertensive agents, instruct the client in nonpharmacologic measures to reduce hypertension (see Figure 27-4).

■ **Evaluation.** The expected outcome of alpha-adrenergic blocking therapy is that the client will maintain a blood pressure within normal limits and not experience any untoward effects of the drug.

ANGIOTENSIN-CONVERTING ENZYME INHIBITORS

Angiotensin-converting enzyme inhibitors competitively block the angiotensin I converting enzyme necessary for the conversion to angiotensin II. Angiotensin II is a powerful vasoconstrictor that raises blood pressure and also causes the release of aldosterone, resulting in sodium and water retention. Thus the inhibition of ACE has a number of results. First, there is a decrease in vascular tone, thereby directly lowering blood pressure. Second, the release of aldosterone is inhibited, which reduces sodium and water reabsorption. The resultant excretion of fluid is thought to cause only a secondary reduction in blood pressure (a decrease in aldosterone secretion does lead to a slight elevation in serum potassium). Third, there is an increase in plasma renin activity, which is caused by a loss of negative feedback on renin release. (See Figures 27-2 and 27-3 for physiologic blood pressure control and the renin-angiotensin-aldosterone system.) Captopril (Capoten) is the key or prototype drug for this category.

ACE inhibitors are used alone or in combination with thiazide diuretics to treat hypertension. Captopril, enalapril, and lisinopril are also used in combination with digoxin and diuretics for the treatment of congestive heart failure that does not respond to standard therapies. Captopril has also been used to treat diabetic nephropathy and left ventricular dysfunction after a myocardial infarction. It has been reported to increase survival and decrease the incidence of heart failure in such persons (*USP DI,* 1999).

It is apparent that a disturbance of the basic function of the renin-angiotensin-aldosterone system can cause increased vascular resistance or hypertension (Hawkins, Bussey, & Prisant, 1997). A damaged kidney that cannot regulate its renin release through normal feedback mechanisms may easily cause an elevation in blood pressure in certain individuals. This evidence has led to the development of the angiotensin II inhibitors. Benazepril (Lotensin), captopril (Capoten), enalapril (Vasotec) and its parenteral dosage form enalaprilat (Vasotec IV), fosinopril (Monopril), lisinopril (Prinivil, Zestril), moexipril (Univasc), perindopril (Aceon), quinapril (Accupril), ramipril (Altace), and trandolapril (Mavik) are ACE inhibitors. Enalapril and perindopril are pro-drugs that are converted to active metabolites (enalaprilat and perindoprilat) by the liver. Many of the other ACE inhibitors have active metabolites, which are listed in Table 27-2.

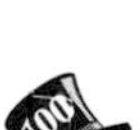

Combination drug therapies for hypertension are sometimes necessary to maintain blood pressure control (Messerli, 1999). Products that contain several active drugs in one tablet or capsule have been formulated to help improve compliance with prescribed therapy (Sheinfeld & Bakris, 1999). Examples of combination drugs include benazepril and amlodipine (Lotrel ◆), trandolapril and verapamil (Tarka), enalapril and diltiazem (Teczem), and hydrochlorothiazide and lisinopril (Zestoretic ◆).

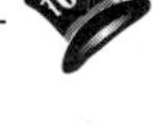

See Table 27-2 for the pharmacokinetics and adult dosage of the ACE inhibitors.

The side effects/adverse reactions of the ACE inhibitors include dry cough, headaches, diarrhea, loss of taste, weak-

TABLE 27-2 ACE Inhibitors: Pharmacokinetics and Dosing

Drug	Onset of Action (hours)	Duration of Effect (hours)	Active Metabolite	Usual Adult Dosage (mg/day)*
benazepril (Lotensin ◆)	Within 1	24	benazeprilat	5-40
captopril (Capoten)	0.25-1	6-12	—	25-300
enalapril (Vasotec ◆)	1	24	enalaprilat	5-40
fosinopril (Monopril ◆)	Within 1	24	fosinoprilat	10-40
lisinopril (Prinivil ◆, Zestril ◆)	1	24	—	10-40
moexipril (Univasc)	1	24	moexiprilat	7.5-30
perindopril (Aceon)	Pro-drug: 1 Metabolite: 3-7	24	perindoprilat	4 mg daily; titrate as necessary
quinapril (Accupril ◆)	Within 1	Up to 24	quinaprilat	10-80
ramipril (Altace)	1-2	24	ramiprilat	2.5-20
trandolapril (Mavik)	4	24	trandolaprilat	1-4

Information from *Drug Facts and Comparisons.* (2000). St. Louis: Facts and Comparisons; and *United States Pharmacopeia Dispensing Information (USP DI): Drug information for the health care professional* (19th ed.). (1999). Rockville, MD: United States Pharmacopeial Convention.
*Oral doses titrated as needed and as tolerated.

ness, nausea, dizziness, hypotension, rash, fever, and joint pain. The Management of Drug Overdose box below describes the treatment of ACE inhibitor overdose.

Nursing Management

ACE Inhibitor Therapy

■ **Assessment.** ACE inhibitors may cause fetal and neonatal morbidity and mortality when administered to pregnant women; discontinue them when pregnancy is suspected. Clients with a history of angioedema are at risk for ACE inhibitor–related angioedema. Because of the risk of hyperkalemia, clients with reduced renal function may require lower or less frequent doses of ACE inhibitors. The risk should be considered for clients who have hyperkalemia, hyponatremia, volume depletion, diabetes mellitus, or a sensitivity to the drug. Clients with cerebrovascular insufficiency or coronary insufficiency may have their ischemia aggravated by the reduced blood pressure, resulting in cerebrovascular accident or myocardial infarction.

Review the client's current medication regimen for the risk of significant drug interactions, such as those that may occur when ACE inhibitors are given concurrently with the following drugs:

Drug/Herb	Possible Effect and Management
Bold/color type indicates the most serious interactions.	
alcohol or diuretics	**Concurrent administration with an ACE inhibitor may result in a sudden, very severe hypotensive episode. Avoid such use or a potentially serious drug interaction may occur.** To reduce this reaction, either discontinue the diuretic for approximately 1 week before initiating ACE inhibitor therapy, increase the salt intake of the client for 1 week before, or start the ACE inhibitor at low dosages. In general, this reaction does not recur with continued dosing, and the diuretic may be given later if necessary.
potassium-sparing diuretics, low-salt milk, potassium supplements, or potassium-containing medications and salt substitutes (see also the Case Study box on p. 588)	Closely monitor serum electrolytes, especially potassium, because of the high risk for hyperkalemia.
yohimbine	**Concurrent use may increase blood pressure. Monitor closely or, preferably, avoid concurrent use.**

Before beginning therapy, a baseline assessment of the client's blood pressure, a complete white cell count, a proteinuria determination, and renal function studies are necessary.

■ **Nursing Diagnosis.** With the administration of ACE inhibitors, clients may experience the following nursing diagnoses/collaborative problems: imbalanced nutrition: less than body requirements related to taste impairment; risk for injury related to hypotension; ineffective protection related to neutropenia and agranulocytosis; impaired skin integrity (rash); impaired comfort (nausea, headache, dry cough, joint pain, or chest pain); diarrhea; fatigue; and the potential complications of anaphylaxis, pancreatitis, and hyperkalemia (confusion, weakness, cardiac dysrhythmias).

■ **Implementation**

■ ***Monitoring.*** Obtain white blood cell and differential counts every month for the first 3 to 6 months of therapy and periodically thereafter. Instruct the client to report any sign of infection (e.g., sore throat, fever), which indicates possible neutropenia.

Proteinuria associated with nephrotic syndrome may occur, particularly in clients with previous renal disease. Perform urinary protein determinations periodically on the client's first morning urine. If proteinuria is greater than 1 g/day, the drug regimen should be reevaluated. Instruct the client to report any edema or weight gain that may occur.

An elevation in potassium level may occur because of depressed aldosterone levels. Monitor the serum potassium and sodium levels.

Monitor blood pressure closely because a precipitous fall can occur in 1 to 3 hours, particularly in clients who have been receiving salt-restricted diets, diuretics, or dialysis. Vomiting, diarrhea, and dehydration can intensify hypotension. The client is to be instructed to discontinue the salt-restricted diet. The hypotensive effect is the same in both the standing and the supine positions. Monitor the pulse rate. If bradycardia occurs, document and report readings to the prescriber.

■ ***Intervention.*** Whenever possible, the current antihypertensive regimen should be discontinued for at least 1 week before initiating ACE inhibitor therapy. All other medications need prescriber approval. Captopril, moexipril, quinapril, and ramipril will have reduced absorption if given with meals. Administer captopril and moexipril to the client on an empty stomach 1 hour before meals. Absorption of the other ACE inhibitors is not affected by food (*Drug Facts and Comparisons*, 2000).

Clients with renal disease, particularly those with renal artery stenosis, may experience an increase in blood urea ni-

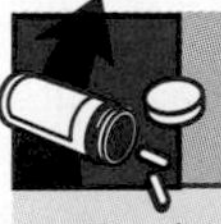

Management of Drug Overdose
ACE Inhibitors

- For hypotension, institute fluid volume expansion.
- An antihistamine may be useful if there is angioedema of the face or of the mucous membranes of the mouth, lips, and extremities. If angioedema affects the tongue, glottis, or larynx, withdraw the ACE inhibitor and hospitalize the client. SC epinephrine, IV diphenhydramine, and IV hydrocortisone may be necessary.
- Hemodialysis will remove captopril, enalaprilat, and lisinopril.

Case Study *The Client with Hypertension*

Ronald Sanford, age 37 years, is diagnosed with essential hypertension. His blood pressure has been ranging between 148 and 176 mm Hg (systolic) and 90 and 110 mm Hg (diastolic). His average blood pressure is 150/94 mm Hg. There is a strong family history of hypertension and stroke on both sides of the family. Mr. Sanford is married and has two school-aged children. He works full-time as a loading dock supervisor for a long-distance trucking company. His elevated blood pressure was detected during a routine physical examination. He reports no other manifestations. At this time there is no evidence of renal insufficiency or retinopathy.

Mr. Sanford is to begin taking atenolol, 50 mg daily, and hydrochlorothiazide, 50 mg daily.

1. Atenolol is a beta-adrenergic blocking agent. How will this drug contribute to the control of Mr. Sanford's blood pressure?
2. Describe the antihypertensive action of hydrochlorothiazide.
3. What will Mr. Sanford need to know about taking his medications and avoiding adverse reactions?
4. In addition to drug therapy, what nonpharmacologic measures will you teach Mr. Sanford to help lower his blood pressure?
5. After undergoing this drug therapy for 6 months, Mr. Sanford's blood pressure is maintained at 124 to 138 mm Hg (systolic) and 78 to 88 mm Hg (diastolic). However, he complains that he does not have the energy he used to have and is experiencing some decrease in sexual activity. What will you tell Mr. Sanford about these concerns and their relationship to the drug therapy?

Over the next 2 years, Mr. Sanford experiences a gradual increase in his blood pressure. Dosage adjustments in the atenolol and hydrochlorothiazide fail to lower his blood pressure effectively. Captopril, 25 mg three times a day, is added to his treatment program.

6. How does captopril lower blood pressure?
7. What does Mr. Sanford need to know about taking captopril in order to achieve the maximum therapeutic benefit?

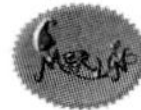

For answer guidelines, go to mosby.com/MERLIN/McKenry/.

trogen (BUN) and serum creatinine levels. Reduce the dosage of the ACE inhibitor or discontinue diuretic therapy if necessary.

A skin rash occurs in approximately 10% of clients during the first 4 weeks of therapy. A dosage reduction or cessation or the administration of an antihistamine usually causes the rash to disappear.

■ ***Education.*** Inform the client that the full therapeutic benefits of the drug will not be noticed until after several weeks of therapy. Therefore emphasize the importance of drug compliance. Report side effects so the prescriber can modify the drug regimen without discontinuing the medication. Advise the client against suddenly discontinuing the drug. Also advise the client to avoid emotional encounters or any forms of stress.

Advise the client that signs of infection (e.g., sore throat or fever) and easy bruising or bleeding (possible agranulocytosis) should be reported to the prescriber. If taste impairment (dysgeusia) occurs, it generally disappears in 2 or 3 months, but it may cause weight loss. Provide the client with nutritional guidance.

Instruct the client not to use potassium supplements or substances containing large amounts of potassium (i.e., salt substitutes or low-sodium milk, which may contain up to 60 mEq potassium/L) without prescriber approval. Caution clients with heart failure to increase their physical activity slowly in response to decreased chest pain.

As with other antihypertensive agents, instruct the client in nonpharmacologic measures to reduce hypertension (see Figure 27-4).

■ **Evaluation.** The expected outcome of ACE inhibitor therapy is that the client will maintain a blood pressure within the normal limits without experiencing adverse reactions to the drug.

ANGIOTENSIN II RECEPTOR ANTAGONISTS

A more recent discovery is the category of the angiotensin II receptor antagonists (AIIRAs), which includes candesartan cilexetil (Atacand), eprosartan (Teveten), irbesartan (Avapro), losartan potassium (Cozaar), telmisartan (Micardis), and valsartan (Diovan). These agents block the receptors for angiotensin II and thus block the vasoconstriction and increase of aldosterone release; however, they have very little effect on serum potassium (McConnaughey, McConnaughey, & Ingenito, 1999). Losartan is considered the key drug in this category.

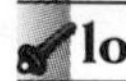

losartan potassium [lo zar′ tan] (Cozaar◆)

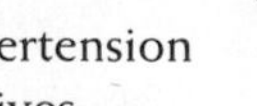

Losartan is indicated for the treatment of hypertension alone or in combination with other antihypertensives.

Losartan is administered orally and reaches a peak effect in 6 hours. It undergoes substantial first-pass metabolism in the liver and is converted to at least six metabolites; one active metabolite (carboxylic acid) is between 10 and 40 times more potent than the parent drug. The half-life of losartan is 2 hours; the half-life of the carboxylic acid metabolite is between 6 and 9 hours. The duration of action is at least 24 hours. Losartan is metabolized in the liver and excreted in the bile (approximately 60%) and kidneys (35%).

The side effects/adverse reactions of losartan include headache, tiredness, back or muscle pain, diarrhea, nasal congestion, dizziness, and upper respiratory infection. A dry cough and insomnia are considered rare effects.

The initial adult dosage is 50 mg PO daily; the maintenance dosage is 25 to 100 mg daily. The dosage for children has not been established.

■ Nursing Management

Losartan Therapy

In addition to the following discussion, see Antihypertensive Therapy, p. 571.

■ **Assessment.** The risk-benefit ratio of losartan administration should be considered if the initial evaluation of the client demonstrates sodium or volume depletion, an impairment in renal or hepatic function, or sensitivity to losartan.

■ **Nursing Diagnosis.** The client undergoing losartan therapy has the potential for the following nursing diagnoses/collaborative problems: risk for injury related to dizziness and hypotension; impaired comfort (headache, back or leg pain, muscle cramps, dry cough); disturbed sleep pattern (insomnia); fatigue; diarrhea; and the potential complications of sinusitis or other upper respiratory infections.

■ **Implementation**

■ ***Monitoring.*** Blood pressure should be measured and renal function studies performed periodically. Clients whose renal function is dependent on the renin-angiotensin-aldosterone system, particularly those with congestive heart failure, may be at risk for losartan-induced renal failure.

■ ***Intervention.*** A gradual dosage reduction is recommended to minimize the risk of rebound hypertension.

■ ***Education.*** As with other antihypertensive agents, the client should be cautioned to consult with the prescriber before taking other medications and to avoid using alcohol. The client should be cautioned about driving until his or her response to the medication is known. The client should also be instructed about the importance of maintaining regular visits to the prescriber for monitoring and of staying on the medication even if feeling well.

■ **Evaluation.** The expected outcome of losartan therapy is that the client's blood pressure will be within the normal range without the client experiencing any ill effects of the drug.

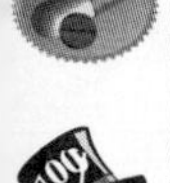

candesartan cilexetil [can de zar′ tan ci lex e til] (Atacand)
eprosartan (Teveten)
irbesartan [ir be zar′ tan] (Avapro)
telmisartan [tel mi zar′ tan] (Micardis)
valsartan [val zar′ tan] (Diovan ◆)

Additional angiotensin II receptor antagonists have been released in the United States. These drugs are approved for the treatment of hypertension, either alone or in combination with other antihypertensive agents.

Valsartan and irbesartan are metabolized in the liver to inactive metabolites. The time to peak serum level is 3 to 4 hours for candesartan, 1 to 2 hours for eprosartan, 1½ to 2 hours for irbesartan, ½ to 1 hour for telmisartan, and 2 to 4 hours for valsartan. The half-life (elimination) is 9 hours for candesartan, 5 to 9 hours for eprosartan, 11 to 15 hours for irbesartan, 24 hours for telmisartan, and 6 hours for valsartan. All of these drugs are primarily excreted in the feces.

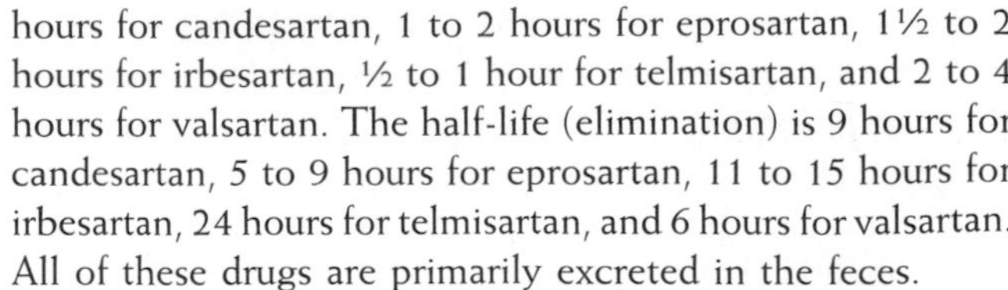

The side effects/adverse reactions of these agents are generally mild or are usually well tolerated (Mazzolai & Burnier, 1999). Candesartan may cause dizziness, musculoskeletal pain, upper respiratory tract infection and, to a lesser degree, headache, tiredness, diarrhea, nausea, vomiting, peripheral edema, and chest pain. Eprosartan may cause upper respiratory infection, urinary tract infection, hypotension, abdominal pain, arthralgia, and fatigue. Irbesartan can cause tiredness, diarrhea, gastric distress, upper respiratory tract infection, and cough. Less commonly reported are dizziness, headache, anxiety, nausea, vomiting, musculoskeletal pain, chest pain, edema, rash, urinary tract infection, and tachycardia. The more commonly reported effects of telmisartan include diarrhea, musculoskeletal pain, and upper respiratory tract infection; less commonly reported effects include dizziness, headache, tiredness, anxiety, gastrointestinal distress, chest pain, peripheral edema, and hypertension. The effects of valsartan are usually mild and infrequent, such as dizziness, headache, insomnia, fatigue, gastric distress, arthralgia, cough, upper respiratory tract infections, viral infection, and edema.

The usual adult dosage for candesartan is 16 mg daily (range: 8 to 32 mg), which can be given once or twice daily. The usual total daily dosage of eprosartan is 400 to 800 mg administered once or twice daily. The adult dosage for irbesartan is 150 mg PO daily, titrated as necessary to a maximum of 300 mg/day; The adult dosage for telmisartan is 40 mg daily (range: 20 to 80 mg). The adult dosage of valsartan is 80 mg daily, titrated as necessary to a maximum of 320 mg/day. The dosages for children have not been established.

The nursing management is the same as for losartan.

CALCIUM ANTAGONISTS

Calcium channel blocking agents are used for the treatment of hypertension, angina pectoris, supraventricular tachycardia, and vascular headaches. (See Chapter 28 for additional information.)

VASODILATORS

Vasodilators exhibit a direct action on the smooth muscle walls of the arterioles and veins, thereby lowering peripheral resistance and blood pressure. Although various theories have been proposed, the mechanism of action, at least in part, involves the direct relaxation of vascular smooth muscle by stimulation of the calcium-binding process. The drop in blood pressure stimulates the sympathetic nervous system and activates the baroreceptor reflexes, increasing heart rate and cardiac output. This also increases the release of renin. Therefore combined therapy is recommended. To inhibit sympathetic reflex response, the use of a beta-adrenergic blocker such as propranolol (Inderal) has been advocated along with a diuretic to alleviate the sodium and water retention that occurs during vasodilator therapy.

There are two types of vasodilators: (1) arteriolar dilators (e.g., diazoxide [Hyperstat IV], hydralazine [Apresoline], and minoxidil [Loniten]), which exert a selective effect on arterioles; and (2) arteriolar and venous dilators (e.g., sodium nitroprusside [Nipride, Nitropress]), which lower blood pressure by acting on both arteriolar resistance vessels and venous capacitance vessels.

Arteriolar Dilator Drugs

diazoxide [dye az ox′ ide] (Hyperstat IV)

The antihypertensive action of diazoxide results from the direct relaxation of smooth muscles in the peripheral arterioles, which causes a decrease in peripheral resistance. As blood pressure is reduced, a reflex increase in heart rate and cardiac output occurs, with a resultant maintenance of coronary and cerebral blood flow. This cardiovascular reflex mechanism also inhibits the development of orthostatic hypotension.

Diazoxide is a potent antihypertensive agent when administered intravenously. The oral form (Proglycem) produces only a slight decrease in blood pressure. The main action of diazoxide is to stimulate hyperglycemia and decrease plasma insulin levels by suppressing insulin release (see Chapter 50).

Diazoxide is administered intravenously to reduce blood pressure promptly in *hypertensive emergencies* such as malignant hypertension and hypertensive crisis. IV diazoxide is ineffective in reducing elevated blood pressure in clients with MAO-induced hypertension or pheochromocytoma. Because of its adverse effects, this drug is not used for the treatment of chronic hypertension.

Administered by IV push, the onset of action is 1 minute. The peak effect occurs within 2 to 5 minutes, the half-life is approximately 28 hours, and the duration of effect is 2 to 12 hours. Diazoxide is metabolized in the liver and excreted by the kidneys.

The side effects/adverse reactions of diazoxide include nausea, vomiting, tachycardia, anorexia, headache, constipation, abdominal cramps, changes in taste perception, and edema.

The adult dosage is up to 150 mg IV administered within 10 to 30 seconds, repeated in 5 to 15 minutes if necessary up to a maximum of 1.2 g/day. After the emergency period, diazoxide is administered for several days until an oral hypertensive agent is effective. The pediatric dosage is 1 to 3 mg/kg IV, repeated if necessary in 5 to 15 minutes.

■ Nursing Management

Diazoxide Therapy

■ Assessment. Clients who are unable to tolerate thiazide diuretics or sulfonamide-type medications may also show an intolerance to diazoxide. Do not use an IV injection of diazoxide in the treatment of compensatory hypertension, such as in aortic coarctation or arteriovenous shunt. Use with caution in clients with impaired cerebral or cardiac circulation, because an abrupt drop in blood pressure may seriously reduce blood flow to these organs. The risk-benefit ratio should be considered for clients with inadequate cardiac reserve, such as uncompensated congestive heart failure. Use diazoxide with caution in clients with hypokalemia, a history of gout, or hepatic or renal function impairment. Clients with diabetes may require a dosage adjustment of hypoglycemic agents due to the hyperglycemic effects of this drug.

A baseline assessment of the client should include blood pressure and blood glucose determinations.

Review the client's current medication regimen, because administering diazoxide concurrently with other antihypertensive medications or peripheral vasodilators may result in a severe hypotensive reaction. Smaller doses may be indicated if concurrent use is necessary. A concurrent use of hydantoin anticonvulsants and diazoxide may result in the diminished efficacy of both drugs. The client should be monitored closely for several hours for hypotension. The simultaneous use of anticoagulants with diazoxide may require reduction in the dosage of anticoagulants, because diazoxide potentiates their action.

■ Nursing Diagnosis. With the administration of diazoxide, the client may be assessed for the following nursing diagnoses/collaborative problems: risk for injury related to hypotension; ineffective protection related to thrombocytopenia; impaired tissue integrity related to extravasation of the IV preparation of diazoxide; impaired comfort (anorexia, nausea, vomiting, or abdominal distention); constipation; excess fluid volume related to sodium and water retention as evidenced by edema of the lower extremities and pulmonary edema; situational low self-esteem related to excessive hairiness with long-term use of the drug; and the potential complications of angina, myocardial infarction, extrapyramidal effects, hyperglycemia (drowsiness, fruity breath odor, polyuria), and allergic reaction.

■ Implementation

■ Monitoring. With IV administration, monitor blood pressure every 5 minutes until it is stable, then every hour during the duration of drug action. Before ending such frequent monitoring, measure blood pressure with the client standing. Take the pulse before and during therapy. If tachycardia occurs with IV administration, report it immediately to the prescriber. For oral administration, monitor blood pressure on a regular basis.

Because of sodium and water retention, weigh the client daily. Measure intake and output; report any weight gain to the prescriber because a diuretic may be indicated. After repeated injections, observe the client closely for signs of congestive heart failure (edema, dyspnea, cough, pulmonary rales, distended neck veins, and fatigue).

During treatment with IV diazoxide, monitor blood and urinary glucose levels, serum electrolytes, and CBCs. (Hypokalemia potentiates hyperglycemia.) An overdose of diazoxide requires that the client with hyperglycemia be observed up to 7 days until the blood sugar level is stabilized. Hyperglycemia occurs in most clients, especially when injections are repeated; closely monitor blood glucose levels, particularly in individuals with diabetes mellitus. Insulin may be indicated in some instances. Monitor the infusion site for extravasation; cellulitis may occur, but not usually necrosis.

■ ***Intervention.*** IV diazoxide should be administered only in a peripheral vein through an established IV line to avoid cardiac dysrhythmias. Avoid extravasation because the solution is alkaline and will cause pain and cellulitis of the tissue. Treat with cold packs if extravasation occurs.

Place the client in the recumbent position during therapy, and keep him or her in the same position for at least 30 minutes after injection. If a diuretic such as furosemide (Lasix) is administered, it is usually given ½ to 1 hour before diazoxide. Have the client remain in the supine position for 8 to 10 hours because of the additive hypotensive effect. The entire dose should be given by rapid IV injection (in less than 30 seconds). Slower administration may result in a reduced effect or a decreased duration of effect. Notify the prescriber if symptoms of abdominal distention, an absence of bowel sounds, or constipation occur.

■ ***Education.*** With the oral forms of diazoxide, instruct the client to monitor blood pressure, test urine ketones, and record his or her weight daily. The client should report any significant changes to the prescriber.

Alert the client not to take other medications without consulting the prescriber and to maintain regular appointments for surveillance. As with other antihypertensive medications, teach the client about nonpharmacologic therapies to reduce blood pressure (see Figure 27-4).

■ **Evaluation.** The expected outcome of diazoxide therapy is that the client will maintain a blood pressure within normal limits without experiencing any adverse reactions to the drug.

hydralazine [hye dral′ a zeen] (Apresoline)

Hydralazine is believed to produce its hypotensive effects by direct relaxation of vascular smooth muscle (particularly the arterioles) with little effect on the veins; this results in a reduction in peripheral resistance. Consequently, renal blood flow is increased, which provides an advantage to clients with renal failure. Hydralazine also maintains cerebral blood flow and produces sodium and water retention. However, the resultant hypotension is thought to stimulate the baroreceptor reflex, causing an increase in heart rate and cardiac output. Unfortunately, this response offsets the antihypertensive effects of the drug.

Tolerance to the antihypertensive action of hydralazine may be offset by the addition of a diuretic to the drug regimen. The diuretic enhances the antihypertensive effect and reduces the potential for increased cardiac output and fluid retention. Hydralazine decreases diastolic pressure more than systolic pressure. It also increases plasma renin activity.

The onset of action of hydralazine is 45 minutes for an oral dose or within 10 to 20 minutes for an IV dose. Its peak effect is within 1 hour (oral dose) or 15 to 30 minutes (IV dose). The half-life for both the oral and IV dosage forms is between 3 and 7 hours, and the duration of action is 3 to 8 hours. Hydralazine is metabolized in the liver and excreted by the kidneys.

The side effects/adverse reactions of hydralazine include diarrhea, nausea, vomiting, tachycardia, anorexia, headache, facial flushing, stuffy nose, edema, angina, rash peripheral neuritis, and SLE–like syndrome. The SLE-like syndrome may include myalgia, arthralgia, arthritis, weakness, fever, and skin changes.

The adult oral dosage is 40 mg daily PO for 2 to 4 days, then 100 mg daily in divided doses for the remainder of the first week. The maintenance dosage is 50 mg four times daily or the lowest effective dosage. Children receive 0.75 mg/kg divided into 2 to 4 doses, increased slowly over 1 to 4 weeks as necessary to a maximum of 7.5 mg/kg. For parenteral administration for hypertension, the adult dosage is 10 to 40 mg IM or IV; repeat if necessary. The parenteral pediatric dosage is 1.7 to 3.5 mg/kg divided into 4 to 6 daily doses.

■ Nursing Management

Hydralazine Therapy

■ **Assessment.** Hydralazine hydrochloride is administered with caution to clients with coronary artery disease (anginal attacks may be intensified); aortic aneurysm or acute aortic dissection (may be worsened); rheumatic mitral valvular disease (may increase pulmonary artery pressure and precipitate congestive heart failure); and hypersensitivity to hydralazine. Clients with cerebrovascular disease may be at risk for increased cerebral ischemia, and those with advanced renal disease may need lower dosages of hydralazine.

Before the initiation of hydralazine therapy, a baseline blood pressure is obtained.

If hydralazine and diazoxide or other hypotension-producing agents are used concurrently, a severe hypotension may result; monitor the client for at least several hours for this effect.

■ **Nursing Diagnosis.** With the administration of hydralazine, the client may experience the following nursing diagnoses/collaborative problems: risk for injury related to hypotension (dizziness, light-headedness); excess fluid volume related to sodium and water retention (swelling of feet or lower legs); impaired comfort (headache, nasal congestion, watery eyes, flushing of face, skin rash, anorexia, nausea, and vomiting); diarrhea; constipation; and the potential complications of SLE-like syndrome (malaise, sore throat, fever, arthralgia), angina (chest pain), blood dyscrasias (agranulocytosis, leukopenia, purpura), peripheral neuritis (tingling, numbness, and weakness in hands or feet), lymphadenopathy, and an allergic response.

■ **Implementation**

■ ***Monitoring.*** Check the blood pressure and pulse of clients receiving parenteral hydralazine every 5 minutes until stabilized; continue to check frequently (approximately every 10 to 15 minutes) during parenteral therapy. Monitor intake and output during parenteral therapy; output may be increased with improved renal blood flow. With the simultaneous use of parenteral diazoxide, observe the client for several hours to assess for profound hypotension. Monitor blood pressure periodically if oral hydralazine is used.

Weigh the client daily to check for fluid retention. Report to the prescriber any weight gain. Advise the client to reduce salt intake.

Observe the mental status of the client. Report to the prescriber any signs of anxiety or mental depression; this condition may indicate cerebral ischemia.

CBC, SLE cell preparation, and antinuclear antibody (ANA) titer tests are indicated if the client develops fever, sore throat, arthralgia, chest pain, and chronic malaise. Repeat these tests periodically if the client is receiving prolonged therapy. SLE-like syndrome may occur in clients receiving higher dosages (more than 200 mg/day), in slow acetylators, and in clients with renal impairment. Discontinue the drug if tests are positive.

■ ***Intervention.*** Administer the parenteral form of hydralazine as quickly as possible after opening the ampule. The drug may change color when added to infusion fluids. Most clients can be changed to oral dosage forms after 24 to 48 hours of parenteral therapy. Administer oral hydralazine with meals or food; this minimizes the first-pass metabolism of the drug in the intestinal wall, thereby enhancing bioavailability. The drug should be administered consistently in relation to food.

■ ***Education.*** Teach the client the importance of taking the medication at the same time each day and to take it exactly as prescribed, even when feeling well. Inform the client that the drug should not be discontinued even if side effects occur; instead, the prescriber should be contacted. This agent should be discontinued gradually; abrupt withdrawal will precipitate a sudden rise in blood pressure and heart failure.

Emphasize to the client the importance of keeping clinical appointments, including those involving laboratory studies. After long-term administration of hydralazine, drug tolerance may develop, which necessitates adjustment of the drug regimen.

Inform the client that palpitations and headache may occur during the early stages of oral administration, but these symptoms usually subside with continued therapy. A beta blocker such as propranolol is usually prescribed to prevent reflex tachycardia.

Instruct the client to report any signs of peripheral neuritis (numbness, tingling, and paresthesias) so that pyridoxine (vitamin B_6) may be prescribed to combat the antipyridoxine response of hydralazine.

Because orthostatic hypotension may occur, advise the client to make position changes slowly. Instruct the client to avoid standing still for long periods of time, taking hot baths or showers, or performing strenuous exercise. Warn the client against operating potentially hazardous machinery, because dizziness or faintness may occur. Instruct the client to carry a medical identification card or MedicAlert bracelet or pendant. As with other antihypertensive medications, teach the client about nonpharmacologic therapies to reduce blood pressure (see Figure 27-4).

■ **Evaluation.** The expected outcome of hydralazine therapy is that the client will maintain a blood pressure within normal limits and not experience any adverse reactions to the drug.

minoxidil [mi nox' i dill] (Loniten)

Minoxidil (Loniten) is an orally effective, direct-acting peripheral vasodilator. It reduces blood pressure by decreasing peripheral vascular resistance in the arteriolar vessels with little effect on veins. It does not cause orthostatic hypotension. It is a potent vasodilator and also causes a reflex increase in cardiac output, induces sodium retention, promotes the development of edema, and increases plasma renin activity.

Minoxidil is reserved for severe hypertension unresponsive to traditional agents (i.e., severe hypertension associated with chronic renal failure). Concomitant administration of a beta-adrenergic blocking agent such as propranolol (Inderal) is necessary to prevent severe reflex tachycardia. Administration of a diuretic agent is also essential to counteract sodium and water retention.

Minoxidil has an onset of action in 30 minutes and a peak effect in 2 to 3 hours (after a single dose). The half-life of this drug and its metabolites is 4.2 hours. Its duration of effect is between 1 and 2 days. It is metabolized in the liver and excreted mostly by the kidneys.

The side effects/adverse reactions of minoxidil include nausea; vomiting; tachycardia; anorexia; headaches; excessive hair growth (hypertrichosis), usually on the face, arms, and back; red flushing of the skin; angina; and pericarditis.

The dosage for adults and children 12 years and older is 5 mg PO daily, increased in 100% increments as necessary (e.g., to 10 mg, 20 mg, 40 mg). It is usually recommended that dosage increases be on a minimum 3-day schedule, but in certain cases increases can be made every 6 hours with close monitoring of the client. For children up to 12 years of age, the dosage is 0.2 mg/kg/day.

■ Nursing Management

Minoxidil Therapy

■ **Assessment.** Inquire if the client is pregnant or has plans for pregnancy, because studies about the risk to the fetus are inconclusive. Hypertrichosis has been reported in newborns following maternal therapy with minoxidil. Do not use in clients with pheochromocytoma, because minoxidil may stimulate catecholamine secretion from the tumor. Use minoxidil cautiously in clients with myocardial infarction, pericardial effusion, coronary insufficiency, or congestive heart failure not due to hypertension, because this drug may further limit blood flow to the myocardium. Clients with renal function impairment may require lower dosages.

Review the client's current medication regimen for the risk of significant drug interactions, such as those that may occur when minoxidil is given concurrently with the following drugs:

Drug	Possible Effect and Management
Bold/color type indicates the most serious interactions.	
diazoxide (Hyperstat IV), nitrates, nitroprusside (Nitropress)	**This combination may result in severe hypotensive reaction. Avoid concurrent use or a potentially serious drug interaction may occur. If administered, monitor the client closely for several hours.**
guanethidine (Ismelin)	**This combination is not recommended, because antihypertensive effects may be potentiated. Avoid concurrent or a potentially serious drug interaction may occur.**

A baseline assessment of the client should include blood pressure and weight determinations.

■ **Nursing Diagnosis.** With the administration of minoxidil, the client may experience the following nursing diagnoses/collaborative problems: excess fluid volume related to sodium and water retention (dependent edema, rapid weight gain); disturbed body image related to hypertrichosis; impaired comfort (rash, itching, paresthesia, and chest pain); and the potential complications of allergic reaction, angina, cardiac effusion, Stevens-Johnson syndrome, and reflex sympathetic activation (tachycardia, flushing of skin).

■ **Implementation**

■ ***Monitoring.*** When minoxidil is first administered, clients should be monitored in a hospital setting to prevent too rapid a decrease in blood pressure; this is especially important for clients who have been receiving guanethidine. Take blood pressure and pulse rate before administering minoxidil, and use these parameters as a guideline to determine progress. Monitor blood pressure and pulse rate regularly during therapy. Report to the prescriber any sharp drop in blood pressure, which can precipitate a cerebrovascular accident and myocardial infarction.

Monitor weight gain, intake and output, and the presence of edema. Inform the prescriber of an increase in weight (kg/day) so that fluid retention can be corrected. The client also should monitor his or her weight at home.

Monitor electrolyte balance, especially potassium levels if the client is receiving a diuretic, which may produce hypokalemia. Potassium replacement therapy should be prescribed. Watch for pericardial effusion with or without tamponade; this reaction may occur in approximately 3% of clients not receiving dialysis. This requires more vigorous diuretic therapy; if pericardiocentesis does not alleviate the condition, discontinuation of minoxidil is necessary.

Observe for anginal symptoms or tachycardia, which can be relieved by concomitant administration of a beta-adrenergic blocker.

■ ***Intervention.*** Closely monitor clients with renal failure or those receiving dialysis to prevent exacerbation of renal failure or precipitation of cardiac failure. Lower dosages of minoxidil are indicated for these clients. It is recommended that a 3-day interval occur between dosage adjustments. In an acute care setting, more rapid dosage changes may occur with careful monitoring of the blood pressure.

■ ***Education.*** Instruct the client to count the radial pulse rate for 1 minute before taking minoxidil and to report to the prescriber an increase of at least 20 beats/min above baseline. Advise the client receiving combination therapy to take each medication at the proper time and not to mix them. A diuretic is given to reduce salt and fluid retention, and a beta blocker is given to control reflex tachycardia. Combined therapy is indicated to increase the effectiveness of the drug and to minimize side effects by lowering the dosage of minoxidil. Advise the client to weigh daily and to report any sharp increase in weight to the prescriber.

Inform the client that a missed dose may be taken a few hours later. A missed dose should not be made up the next day; instead, the regular dosing schedule should be resumed. Consult the prescriber if there is any question.

Emphasize the importance of drug compliance despite uncomfortable side effects. Inform the client that minoxidil is a powerful drug for reducing blood pressure and that by relaxing small blood vessels, more blood flow protects vital organs (heart, kidney, and brain). Alert the client not to discontinue the drug without notifying the prescriber, because abrupt withdrawal will cause rebound hypertension.

Inform the client that hypertrichosis will likely occur (incidence is 80%) 3 to 6 weeks after starting therapy. This involves elongation, thickening, and increased pigmentation of fine body hair over the temples, eyebrows, sideburns, malar area, shoulders, back, legs, and forearms. This side effect is particularly troublesome to women. Advise the client that this condition is reversible within 2 to 6 months following discontinuation of therapy. No endocrine abnormalities have been found to account for this distressing effect. Hair remover (depilatory creams) or shaving may be effective in removing unwanted hair.

Instruct the client that minoxidil may be taken with or without food. Advise the client against increasing salt intake, and request that a dietitian provide information regarding appropriate dietary choices. Inform the client to notify the prescriber if difficulty in breathing occurs, especially when lying down, because this may indicate impending congestive heart failure.

Advise the client not to take other drugs, including OTC agents, without first consulting the prescriber. Instruct the client to carry a medical identification card or MedicAlert bracelet or pendant.

■ **Evaluation.** The expected outcome is that the client will maintain a blood pressure within normal limits and not experience any adverse reactions to minoxidil.

Arterial and Venous Dilator Drugs

nitroprusside [nye troe pruss' ide] (Nipride, Nitropress)

Nitroprusside is a potent and fast direct-acting vasodilator agent that greatly reduces arterial blood pressure. It relaxes both arterial and venous smooth muscles but is more active on veins. Therefore nitroprusside reduces cardiac load; that is, the decrease in systemic resistance results in a reduction in preload and afterload, which improves cardiac output in the client with congestive heart failure. It is indicated for rapid reduction of blood pressure in hypertensive emergencies, adjunct therapy in myocardial infarction and valvular regurgitation, and also as an antidote for ergot alkaloid toxicity.

Sodium nitroprusside has an almost immediate onset of action and peak effect (within minutes) after administration by IV infusion. The half-life of nitroprusside is 2 minutes; the half-life of thiocyanate, a possible toxic metabolite, is 3 days. The duration of effect is between 1 and 10 minutes after discontinuance of the infusion. It is metabolized by erythrocytes (to cyanide) and the liver (cyanide to thiocyanate), and it is excreted by the kidneys.

The side effects/adverse reactions of nitroprusside include dizziness, excessive sweating, headaches, anxiety, abdominal cramps, tachycardia, hypothyroidism, flushing, rash, and muscle twitching. If the client has thiocyanate toxicity, ataxia, blurred vision, headache, nausea, vomiting, tinnitus, shortness of breath, delirium, and unconsciousness may occur. Hypotension, metabolic acidosis, pink coloration, very shallow breathing pattern, decreased reflexes, coma, and widely dilated pupils may be observed in clients with cyanide toxicity.

For the adult and pediatric dosage, mix the contents of the vial in dextrose 5% injection only, and administer by IV infusion. The initial dosage is 0.3 μg/kg/min, which is slowly increased in increments of 0.3 μg according to client response. The usual dosage is 0.003 mg (3 μg)/kg/min.

▪ Nursing Management

Sodium Nitroprusside Therapy

▪ **Assessment.** Do not use the drug in clients with inadequate cerebral or coronary artery circulation because there is a reduced tolerance for hypotension. Sodium nitroprusside should be used cautiously in clients with renal or hepatic function impairment, Leber's hereditary optic atrophy, vitamin B_{12} deficiency, or tobacco amblyopia, because these conditions influence the metabolism and excretion of the drug. Clients with encephalopathy and other conditions in which they are at risk for increased intracranial pressure may experience pressure increases. A baseline blood pressure should be obtained.

If the client is also taking dobutamine, a higher cardiac output and lower pulmonary wedge pressure may result. Concurrent use of other antihypertensive agents is an indication for closer monitoring of the blood pressure, because there may be an additive effect.

▪ **Nursing Diagnosis.** With the administration of sodium nitroprusside, the client may experience the following nursing diagnoses/collaborative problems: risk for injury related to rebound hypertension with abrupt withdrawal of the drug or related to hypotension (dizziness, restlessness, tachycardia); impaired tissue integrity (pain at infusion site); impaired comfort (headache, abdominal cramping); and the potential complications of thiocyanate toxicity (ataxia, blurred vision, delirium, dizziness, nausea and vomiting, ringing of the ears) and cyanide toxicity (decreased consciousness progressing to coma).

▪ **Implementation**

▪ ***Monitoring.*** To prevent rapid hypotension, monitor the blood pressure every 30 seconds when the infusion is first started. Later, check it every 5 minutes. Facilities and personnel must be adequate for this purpose; intensive care facilities are recommended. Observe the client for any precipitous drop in blood pressure, which may occur if large doses are given. Do not allow the infusion rate to exceed 10 μg/kg/min. If an adequate reduction in blood pressure does not occur in 10 minutes, the drug is discontinued.

Monitor intake and output. Monitor the client for thiocyanate toxicity (tinnitus, blurred vision, and delirium). Because sodium nitroprusside is converted to thiocyanate, monitor the blood thiocyanate level when infusion is continued for more than 72 hours, especially in clients with renal dysfunction.

▪ ***Intervention.*** After preparing an IV solution of sodium nitroprusside, promptly wrap the container in the supplied opaque sleeve or aluminum foil or other opaque material to protect the drug from light. Use fresh solution, and do not keep it longer than 24 hours. Freshly prepared solution has a faint brown tinge; discard it if it is highly colored (e.g., blue, green, or dark red).

Administer the infusion using a volumetric infusion pump. These devices must be available to allow precise measurement of the prescribed flow rate. Do not add other drugs to the nitroprusside infusion. Avoid extravasation, because it results in tissue damage.

If the blood thiocyanate level exceeds 10 mg/dL, the infusion should be discontinued or decreased to prevent toxicity. A potential for cyanide intoxication exists with prolonged treatment and overdose. (Note that nitroprusside is metabolized first to cyanide, then to thiocyanate.) Discontinue nitroprusside in the event of cyanide toxicity (coma, dilated pupils, pink color, shallow respirations, imperceptible pulse rate, distant heart sounds, hypotension, and absent reflexes). Continue to observe the client for several hours to prevent the recurrence of signs of overdose. (See the Management of Drug Overdose box on p. 595.)

Be aware that the client's therapy will be changed to oral antihypertensive agents as soon as a response occurs. As oral therapy is instituted, the client will require lower doses of nitroprusside.

▪ ***Education.*** Keep the client advised about the care that is taking place.

▪ **Evaluation.** The expected outcome of sodium nitroprusside therapy is that the blood pressure will return to

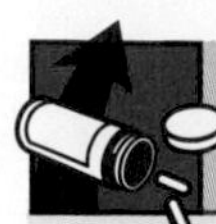

Management of Drug Overdose
Nitroprusside

- The structure of nitroprusside contains five cyanide groups. When the drug is administered intravenously, these groups split off to form free cyanide and nitric oxide, the active substance. Nitric oxide activates the enzyme guanylate cyclase to produce cyclic guanosine monophosphate (cGMP) and vasodilation. The free cyanide is converted to hydrogen cyanide (prussic acid), which is metabolized in the liver by rhodanase and a sulfur donor (such as thiosulfate) to thiosulfate, which is then excreted by the kidneys.
- When the amount of sulfur donors are limited or overwhelmed by high-dose nitroprusside therapy, hydrogen cyanide may accumulate in the body and cause toxicity. Some investigators report that the less toxic thiocyanate will be formed and excreted if sodium thiosulfate is mixed in the nitroprusside infusion at a 5:1 to 10:1 ratio during nitroprusside administration (e.g., 250 mg to 500 mg sodium thiosulfate to 50 mg nitroprusside). This method reduces the potential for cyanide accumulation and toxicity (Michocki, 1995; *USP DI,* 1999)
- Thiocyanate toxicity may occur in clients with chronic therapy and renal impairment. The half-life of nitroprusside in normal renal function is 2.7 days; in renal failure the half-life is 9 days. Therefore, depending on the amount of drug administered to the client, thiocyanate toxicity is usually more apt to occur than cyanide toxicity with chronic therapy (Michocki, 1995).
- For severe hypotension, slow or discontinue the infusion. Placing the client in the supine position with the legs elevated on pillows will maximize venous return.
- For cyanide toxicity, discontinue nitroprusside and administer sodium nitrite (3% solution) in a dose of 4 to 6 mg/kg IV over 2 to 4 minutes. Amyl nitrite inhalation should be used if IV sodium nitrite is not immediately available. Nitrites buffer the cyanide by converting approximately 10% of the client's hemoglobin to methemoglobin. After administering sodium nitrite, administer sodium thiosulfate (150 to 200 mg/kg) to convert the cyanide to thiocyanate. Thiocyanate is less toxic and is rarely a problem; use hemodialysis if thiocyanate toxicity occurs. Be aware, however, that hemodialysis does not remove cyanide. If necessary, this regimen (nitrite and thiosulfate) may be repeated after 2 hours in one-half the original dose.

normal parameters without the client experiencing any adverse reactions to the drug.

SUMMARY

Hypertension is the most common cardiovascular health problem and affects more than 30 million Americans. Ninety percent of such cases are considered to be essential, idiopathic, or primary hypertension—that is, the specific cause of the hypertension is not known. Because individuals with hypertension are at higher risk for cardiovascular injury, they are treated nonpharmacologically and/or pharmacologically to reduce their blood pressure and therefore reduce their risk of premature death or disability.

Nonpharmacologically, clients are encouraged to modify their lifestyles to include weight reduction, sodium restriction, elimination or limited consumption of alcohol and tobacco, reduction of dietary saturated fats, regular exercise, and behavior modification to promote relaxation.

Pharmacologically, a stepped-care approach is recommended by the Joint National Committee on the Detection, Evaluation, and Treatment of High Blood Pressure. This plan is a progressive approach that begins with the administration of a single drug, increases the dosage of that drug and then, in sequential order, gradually adds more potent agents as the need for more intensive therapy is indicated.

Diuretic drugs play an important role in the management of hypertension. Their administration results in the loss of excess salt and water from the body by renal excretion. This volume depletion, plus a direct effect on the arterioles to produce vasodilation, results in a decrease in blood pressure. Diuretic drugs are discussed primarily in Chapter 34.

Adrenergic inhibiting agents were discussed in Chapter 22. In terms of their modification of the effects of the sympathetic nervous system, they are the most effective antihypertensive drugs. The centrally acting drugs clonidine, methyldopa, guanabenz, and guanfacine are effective as stage 3 antihypertensives of the stepped-care regimen, especially when combined with a diuretic. The peripheral adrenergic inhibitors (guanethidine, guanadrel, and *Rauwolfia* derivatives) are also used as antihypertensives. Alpha-adrenergic blocking agents such as doxazosin, prazosin, and terazosin lower blood pressure by preventing norepinephrine from activating $alpha_1$ receptors on vascular smooth muscle to produce vasoconstriction. Beta-adrenergic blocking agents are also used successfully in the treatment of hypertension (see Chapter 22).

Vasodilators act on the smooth muscle walls of the arterioles and veins, lowering peripheral resistance and blood pressure. The arteriolar dilator agents commonly administered for hypertension are diazoxide, hydralazine, and minoxidil. Sodium nitroprusside is a direct-acting vasodilator that relaxes both arteriolar and venous smooth muscle, which greatly reduces arterial blood pressure. Captopril, enalapril, and doxazosin are angiotensin II antagonists that inhibit vasoconstriction and the action of the renin-angiotensin-aldosterone system, a disturbance of which may cause hypertension. Angiotensin II receptor antagonists, the newest class of antihypertensives, also inhibit vasoconstriction and the release of renin; they do this by blocking angiotensin II receptors.

Nurses have a major role in the administration of antihypertensive agents when involved in the direct care of the client. By far the greatest contribution of nursing is client education to sustain adherence to the accurate and safe self-administration of antihypertensive agents. This guidance will assist the client in changing his or her lifestyle to incorporate the modifications to promote a decrease in hypertension and thus a healthier life.

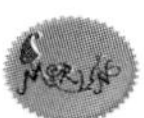

Critical Thinking Questions

1. Tim Rogers, age 46, has mild primary hypertension for which his health care provider has prescribed reserpine, 0.1 mg PO daily. What past medical conditions would the nurse specifically ask during the drug history, which is to be obtained before Mr. Rogers begins his reserpine therapy?
2. Stella Parr, age 52, expresses her relief now that her prescriber has placed her on a diuretic as part of her antihypertensive medications. She states, "Now I won't have to struggle with all that tasteless food without salt. If I get water retention, the diuretic will take care of it." How should the nurse respond? What other lifestyle issues need to be explored with Ms. Parr?

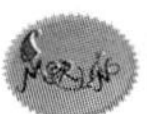

Collaborative Learning Activities

For Collaborative Learning Activities, go to mosby.com/MERLIN/McKenry/.

CASE STUDY

For a Case Study that will help ensure mastery of this chapter content, go to mosby.com/MERLIN/McKenry/.

BIBLIOGRAPHY

American Hospital Formulary Service. (1999). *AHFS drug information '99*. Bethesda, MD: American Society of Hospital Pharmacists.

Anderson, K.N., Anderson, L.E., & Glanze, W.D. (Eds.). (1998). *Mosby's medical, nursing, & allied health dictionary* (5th ed.). St. Louis: Mosby.

Carter, B.L., Furmaga, E.M., & Murphy, C.M. (1995). Essential hypertension. In L.Y. Young & M.A. Koda-Kimble (Eds.), *Applied therapeutics: The clinical use of drugs* (6th ed.). Vancouver, WA: Applied Therapeutics.

Chou, C.M. (1999). Evaluation and treatment of hypertension. *Rheumatic Disease Clinics of North America, 25*(3), 521-537.

Desmond S. et al. (1992). Perceptions of hypertension in black and white adolescents. *Health Values, 16*(2), 3-10.

Drug Facts and Comparisons. (2000). St. Louis: Facts and Comparisons.

Fawzy, A., Hendry, A., Cook, E., & Gonzales, F. (1999). Long-term (4-year) efficacy and tolerability of doxazosin for the treatment of concurrent benign prostatic hyperplasia and hypertension. *International Journal of Urology, 6*(7), 346-354.

Gray, S.L., Lai, K.V., & Larson, E.B. (1999). Drug-induced disorders in the elderly: Incidence, prevention and management. *Drug Safety, 21*(2), 101-122.

Hall, W.D. (1999). A rational approach to the treatment of hypertension in special populations. *American Family Physician, 60*(1), 156-162.

Hawkins, D.W., Bussey, H.I., & Prisant, L.M. (1997). Hypertension. In J.T. DiPiro, R.L. Talbert, G.C. Yee, G.R. Matzke, B.G. Wells, & L.M. Posey (Eds.), *Pharmacotherapy: A pathophysiological approach* (3rd ed.). Norwalk, CT: Appleton & Lange.

Hedner, T. (1999). Management of hypertension: The advent of a new angiotensin II receptor antagonist. *Journal of Hypertension, 17*(2), S21-S25.

Hoffman, B.B. & Lefkowitz, R.F. (1996). Catecholamines, sympathomimetic drugs, and adrenergic receptor antagonists. In J.G. Hardman & L.E. Limbird (Eds.), *Goodman & Gilman's The pharmacological basis for therapeutics* (9th ed.). New York: McGraw-Hill.

Jakala, P., Riekkinen, M., Sirvio, J., Koivisto, E., & Riekkinen, P. Jr. (1999). Clonidine, but not guanfacine, impairs choice reaction time in young healthy volunteers. *Neuropsychopharmacology, 21*(4), 495-502.

Johnson, M.J., Williams, M., & Marshall, E.S. (1999). Adherent and nonadherent medication-taking in elderly hypertensive patients. *Clinical Nursing Research 8*(4):318-355.

Kaplan, N.M. (1997). Perspectives on the new JNC VI guidelines for the treatment of hypertension. *Formulary, 32*(12), 1224-1231.

Kirkpatrick, M.K. (1992). *Review NAACOG's Women's Health Nursing Scan, 6*(5), 9.

Leenen, F.H. (1999). Intermittent blood pressure control: Potential consequences for outcome. *Canadian Journal of Cardiology, 15*(suppl C), 13C-18C.

Levy, R.A. (1993). *Ethnic and racial differences in response to medicines: Preserving individualized therapy in managed pharmaceutical programs.* Reston, VA: National Pharmaceutical Council.

Lowe, F.C., Olson, P.J., & Padley, R.J. (1999). Effects of terazosin therapy on blood pressure in men with benign prostatic hyperplasia concurrently treated with other antihypertensive medications. *Urology, 54*(1), 81-85.

Mabie, W.C. (1999). Management of acute severe hypertension and encephalopathy. *Clinical Obstetrics & Gynecology, 42*(3), 519-531.

Mazzolai, L. & Burnier, M. (1999). Comparative safety and tolerability of angiotensin II receptor antagonists. *Drug Safety, 21*(1), 23-33.

McConnaughey, M.M., McConnaughey, J.S., & Ingenito, A.J. (1999). Practical considerations of the pharmacology of angiotensin receptor blockers. *Journal of Clinical Pharmacology, 39*(6), 547-559.

Messerli, F.H. (1999). Combinations in the treatment of hypertension: ACE inhibitors and calcium antagonists. *American Journal of Hypertension, 12*(8 pt 2):86S-90S.

Michocki, R. (1995). Hypertensive emergencies. In L.Y. Young & M.A. Koda-Kimble (Eds.), *Applied therapeutics: The clinical use of drugs* (6th ed.). Vancouver, WA: Applied Therapeutics.

National Institutes of Health (1996). *Update on the Task Force Report (1987) on High Blood Pressure in Children and Adolescents: A Working Group Report from the National High Blood Pressure Education Program.* Bethesda, MD: Author. National Institutes of Health Pub. No. 96-3790.

Oates, J.A. (1996). Antihypertensive agents and the drug therapy of hypertension. In J.G. Hardman & L.E. Limbird (Eds.), *Goodman and Gilman's The pharmacological basis of therapeutics* (9th ed.). New York: McGraw-Hill.

Porsche, R. (1995). Hypertension: Diagnosis, acute antihypertension therapy, and long-term management. *AACN Clinical Issues: Advanced Practice Acute Critical Care, 6*(4), 515-525.

Portyansky, E. (1997). Hypertension: New treatment approaches target organ damage. *Drug Topics, 141*(21), 78-83, 87, 91.

Sagraves, R., Letassy, N.A., & Barton, T.L. (1995). Obstetrics. In L.Y. Young & M.A. Koda-Kimble (Eds.), *Applied therapeutics: The clinical use of drugs* (6th ed.). Vancouver, WA: Applied Therapeutics.

Sheinfeld, G.R. & Bakris, G.L. (1999). Benefits of combination angiotensin-converting enzyme inhibitor and calcium antagonist therapy for diabetic patients. *American Journal of Hypertension, 12*(8 pt 2), 80S-85S.

United States Pharmacopeia Dispensing Information (USP DI): Drug information for the health care professional (19th ed.). (1999). Rockville, MD: United States Pharmacopeial Convention.

28 Calcium Channel Blockers

Chapter Focus

Calcium channel blockers are indicated for a variety of cardiovascular conditions. They are used primarily for their antianginal, antidysrhythmic, and antihypertensive properties. Calcium channel blockers are being prescribed more often, and the nurse must be knowledgeable about them in order to administer them safely and provide guidance for clients to self-administer them.

Learning Objectives

1. State the mechanism of action of the calcium channel blockers on cardiac muscle, the cardiac conduction system, and the smooth muscle cells in the walls of blood vessels.
2. Compare and contrast the therapeutic effects of the calcium channel blockers: amlodipine, bepridil, diltiazem, felodipine, flunarizine, isradipine, nicardipine, nifedipine, nimodipine, nisoldipine, and verapamil.
3. Describe specific nursing interventions that may inhibit the side effects associated with calcium channel blockers.
4. Identify specific client education measures needed when calcium channel blockers are prescribed.
5. Implement the nursing management of the care of a client receiving calcium channel blocker therapy.

Key Terms

automaticity, p. 599
calcium channel blocker, p. 599
peripheral vascular resistance, p. 599

Key Drugs [✓]

verapamil, p. 599

OVERVIEW

The calcium channel blockers have diverse chemical structures, but all share a basic electrophysiologic property—they block the inward movement of calcium through the slow channels of the cell membranes of cardiac and smooth muscle cells. (See Chapter 24 for a discussion of the physiology of fast and slow channels of cardiovascular fibers.) The activity of the calcium channel blockers varies according to the specific type of cardiovascular cells involved. There are three types of tissues or cells:

1. Cardiac muscle or myocardium
2. Cardiac conduction system—sinoatrial (SA) node and atrioventricular (AV) junction
3. Vascular smooth muscle

Action on Cardiac Muscle. Calcium channel blockers decrease the force of myocardial contraction by blocking the inward flow of calcium ions through the slow channels of the cell membrane during phase 2 (the plateau phase) of the action potential (see Figure 24-2). The diminished entry of calcium ions into the cells fails to trigger the release of large amounts of calcium from the sarcoplasmic reticulum within the cell. This free calcium is needed for excitation-contraction coupling, an event that activates contraction by allowing cross-bridges to form between the actin and myosin filaments of muscle. The force of the contraction of the heart is determined by the number of actin and myosin cross-bridges formed within the sarcomere. Decreasing the amount of calcium ion released from the sarcoplasmic reticulum results in the formation of fewer actin and myosin cross-bridges; this decreases the force of contraction and results in a negative inotropic effect.

Action on the Cardiac Conduction System. In the cardiac conduction system, calcium channel blockers decrease automaticity in the SA node and decrease conduction in the AV junction. **Automaticity** means that a cell depolarizes spontaneously and initiates an action potential without an external stimulus. It is a normal characteristic of the SA nodal cells. Depolarization (phase 0) of the action potential is normally generated by the inward calcium ion current through the slow channels. Thus the agents that block the inward calcium ion current across the cell membrane of SA junction tissue decrease the rate of depolarization and depress automaticity. The result is a decrease in heart rate (negative chronotropic effect).

Similarly, an agent that decreases calcium ion influx across the cell membrane of the AV junction slows AV conduction (negative dromotropic effect) and prolongs AV refractory time. When AV conduction is prolonged, fewer atrial impulses reach the ventricles, and the rate of ventricular contractions is slowed. Diltiazem (Cardizem) depresses SA nodal automaticity, while verapamil (Calan, Isoptin) slows AV conduction; therefore verapamil is preferred to treat supraventricular tachycardia.

Action on Vascular Smooth Muscle. The smooth muscle of the coronary and peripheral vessels has a significant influence on the hemodynamics of circulation. Calcium channel blockers effectively inhibit calcium ion influx through the slow channels of the membrane of smooth muscle cells. The depressed interaction between actin and myosin results in a decreased force of smooth muscle contraction. As a result, coronary artery dilation occurs, which lowers coronary resistance and improves blood flow through collateral vessels, as well as oxygen delivery to ischemic areas of the heart. Hence drugs with these actions are useful in the treatment of angina pectoris.

Calcium channel blockers also inhibit the contraction of smooth muscle of the peripheral arterioles. This results in a widespread reduction in blood pressure and **peripheral vascular resistance** (resistance to blood flow through the body determined by the tone of the vascular musculature and the diameter of the blood vessels). The hemodynamic change reduces afterload, which also decreases the oxygen demands of the heart. This indirectly provides a beneficial effect in the management of angina.

■ ■ ■

The calcium channel blockers include amlodipine (Norvasc ◆), bepridil (Vascor), diltiazem (Cardizem, Cardizem CD ◆), felodipine (Plendil), flunarizine (Sibelium 🍁), isradipine (DynaCirc, DynaCirc CR), nicardipine (Cardene), nifedipine (Adalat, Adalat CC ◆, Procardia, Procardia XL ◆), nimodipine (Nimotop), nisoldipine (Sular), and verapamil (Calan, Isoptin). Flunarizine (Sibelium 🍁) is indicated for migraine prophylaxis and is marketed only in Canada. Verapamil was the first calcium channel blocker released and is the key drug for this category. It has direct effects on the heart and blood vessels, reducing AV conduction; it blocks the SA node (resulting in a decrease in heart rate), increases coronary perfusion (coronary vasodilation), and is considered a moderate peripheral vasodilator. Diltiazem has similar pharmacologic effects.

Calcium channel blockers dilate coronary arteries and arterioles, inhibit coronary artery spasm, dilate peripheral arterioles, and reduce total peripheral resistance (afterload), thus lowering arterial blood pressure at rest and during exercise. Table 28-1 compares the effects of calcium channel blockers.

Therapeutically, the calcium antagonists have been used to treat a variety of conditions. The following paragraphs list the indications approved by the Food and Drug Administration (FDA) along with the drugs approved to treat each condition (*United States Pharmacopeia Dispensing Information*, 1999; *Drug Facts and Comparisons*, 2000). Approved indications can be changed or expanded, and the nurse is encouraged to watch the current literature for any new changes. Current indications for calcium channel blockers include angina pectoris (bepridil, diltiazem, felodipine, mibefradil, nicardipine, nifedipine, verapamil), dysrhythmia (diltiazem parenteral, verapamil), hypertension (diltiazem, felodipine, isradipine, mibefradil, nicardipine, nifedipine extended-release tablets, verapamil), subarachnoid hemorrhage (nimodipine), and prophylaxis for vascular headaches (flunarizine). Some calcium channel blockers have also been prescribed for non–FDA approved indications, such as felodipine, isradipine,

TABLE 28-1 Calcium Channel Blockers: Comparison of Effects

Effects	amlodipine	bepridil	diltiazem	felodipine	nifedipine nicardipine isradipine	verapamil
Contractility	↑	↓	↓	↑	0/↓	↓↓
Vasodilation						
Coronary	↑	↑↑↑	↑↑↑	↑	↑↑↑	↑↑
Peripheral	↓↓↓	↓	↓	↓↓↓	↓↓↓	↓↓
Heart rate	+/−	↓	0/↓	↑	↑	↑↓
Cardiac output	↑	0	0/↑	↑	↑↑	↑↓

↑, Slight increase; ↓, slight decrease; ↑↑, intermediate increase; ↓↓, intermediate decrease; ↑↑↑, significant increase; ↓↓↓, significant decrease; +/−, minimal effect; ↑↓, slight effect; 0, no effect.

nicardipine, and nifedipine for Raynaud's phenomenon, and verapamil for vascular headache prophylaxis and hypertrophic cardiomyopathy. Because these agents differ in specificity and their individual effects on cardiac and peripheral tissues, they may have different indications, such as those discussed in the following paragraphs.

Bepridil is indicated only for chronic stable angina. Its potentially serious adverse effects, serious ventricular dysrhythmia and agranulocytosis, limit its use. The action of diltiazem is largely restricted to dilating the coronary and peripheral blood vessels; the long-acting tablet is indicated for hypertension, whereas the regular tablets are for angina and the parenteral dosage form is for dysrhythmias. Felodipine, nicardipine, and nifedipine are used to treat hypertension and angina, whereas isradipine is used to treat essential hypertension. Nicardipine is a very potent peripheral vasodilator that does not affect the SA node or AV junction. Because of its pronounced effect on the peripheral vascular bed, nifedipine causes the greatest hypotensive effect. However, it exerts minimal cardiac depressant action.

Nimodipine, which is highly lipophilic, crosses the blood-brain barrier and has a greater effect on the cerebral arteries than on other arteries in the body. It is indicated for the treatment of cerebral arterial spasm after subarachnoid hemorrhage. It also inhibits platelet aggregation. The adult dosage is 60 mg every 4 hours, starting within 96 hours after the subarachnoid hemorrhage and continuing for 3 weeks.

Pharmacokinetics. See Table 28-2 for the pharmacokinetics and usual adult dosage of the calcium channel blockers. Diltiazem is metabolized to a major metabolite, desacetyldiltiazem, which may be responsible for up to 50% of its coronary dilatation effect. The active metabolite of verapamil, norverapamil, accounts for approximately 20% of the antihypertensive effect of verapamil. Nifedipine has no known active metabolites. The other agents have metabolites that may or may not have significant therapeutic effects.

Side Effects/Adverse Reactions. The side effects/adverse reactions of the calcium channel blockers include headache, nausea, hypotension, dizziness, skin flushing or rash, edema of the ankles and feet, dry mouth, and tachycardia. (See the Management of Drug Overdose box on p. 601.)

Gingival hyperplasia is a rare side effect reported with amlodipine, diltiazem, felodipine, verapamil, and most often with nifedipine. This condition starts as an inflammation of the gums, usually within the first 9 months of therapy, and it usually improves within 1 to 4 weeks of discontinuing the drug. Good dental hygiene and professional teeth cleaning are necessary to reduce the potential for this adverse reaction.

■ Nursing Management
Calcium Channel Blocker Therapy

■ **Assessment.** The client's health status should be reviewed for conditions that contraindicate the use of calcium channel blockers or indicate the need for special caution with their administration. Do not administer these drugs to individuals who have severe hypotension (less than 90 mm Hg systolic). Bepridil, diltiazem, and verapamil are contraindicated for clients with heart block, sick sinus syndrome, and Wolff-Parkinson-White syndrome unless they have a functioning artificial ventricular pacemaker, because these drugs may cause severe bradycardia or dysrhythmias. Calcium channel blockers should be administered with caution to clients with severe aortic stenosis, bradycardia, heart failure, cardiogenic shock, acute myocardial infarction, and mild to moderate hypotension, because these conditions will be worsened.

Clients with renal or hepatic function impairment may have a reduced clearance of the drugs, which results in a prolonged half-life. Intolerance to the prescribed calcium channel blockers is also a contraindication. Ask female clients if they are pregnant or plan to become pregnant. Tests on laboratory animals have resulted in teratogenic effects on the fetus (FDA pregnancy category C).

Older adults may require more caution in the dosage of calcium channel blockers because of age-related renal impairment (see the Special Considerations for Older Adults box on p. 601). The half-life of diltiazem, nimodipine,

TABLE 28-2 Calcium Channel Blockers: Pharmacokinetics and Dosing

Drug	Onset of Action (minutes)	Time to Peak Concentration (hours)	Duration of Action (hours)	Metabolism/Excretion	Usual Adult Daily Dose
amlodipine (Norvasc)	2-5 (IV)	6-12	N/A	Liver/kidneys	PO: 5-10 mg Older adults: start at 2.5 mg
bepridil (Vascor)	60	2-3	24	Liver/kidneys	PO: 200-400 mg
diltiazem (Cardizem)	30	2-3	4-8	Liver/kidneys and bile	PO: 120-360 mg Parenteral: 15-25 mg
extended-release dosage form	30-60	6-11	12	Liver/kidneys and bile	PO: 60-360 mg
felodipine (Plendil)	120-300	2.5-5	24	Liver/kidneys	PO: 5-20 mg
isradipine (DynaCirc)	120	1.5	12	Liver/kidneys	PO: 2.5-20 mg
nicardipine (Cardene)	N/A	0.5-2	8	Liver/kidneys	PO: 60 mg
nifedipine (Procardia)	Oral: 20 (more rapid when given sublingually)	0.5-1	4-8	Liver/kidneys	PO: 30-120 mg
nimodipine (Nimotop)	N/A	1	Variable	Liver/bile and feces	PO: 60 mg q4h
nisoldipine (Sular)	N/A	N/A	24	Liver/kidneys	PO: 20-40 mg
verapamil (Calan, Isoptin)	Oral: 60-120 IV: 1-5	1-2	IV: 2 Oral (regular): 8-10 Oral (extended release): 24	Liver/kidneys and feces	PO: 240-480 mg Parenteral: 5-10 mg

N/A, Not available.

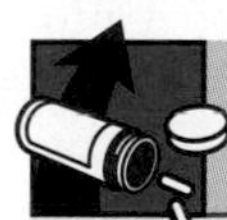

Management of Drug Overdose
Calcium Channel Blockers

- For symptomatic hypotension, administer IV fluids plus IV dopamine or dobutamine, metaraminol, isoproterenol, calcium chloride, or norepinephrine. Use Trendelenburg's position for parenteral verapamil-induced hypotension.
- Direct-current cardioversion, IV lidocaine, or IV procainamide is used for tachycardia, a rapid ventricular rate in clients with antegrade conduction, atrial flutter or fibrillation, and accessory pathway with Wolff-Parkinson-White syndrome.
- For bradycardia, use IV atropine, isoproterenol, norepinephrine, or calcium chloride. An electronic cardiac pacemaker may be necessary in some instances.

verapamil, and other calcium channel blockers may be increased because of decreased clearance; the half-life of nicardipine has shown no difference in young adults and in clients over age 65. In addition, the potential for adverse cognitive effects is greater in older adults (Maxwell, Hogan, & Ebly, 1999).

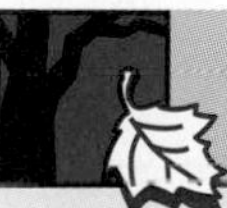

Special Considerations for Older Adults
Calcium Channel Blockers

Older adults are more susceptible to calcium channel blockers and the side effects of increased weakness, dizziness, fainting episodes, and falls.

Although nitroglycerin (or other nitrates) may be taken concurrently with these agents, the client should be advised to report any increase in frequency or intensity of angina attacks to his or her prescriber.

Nicotine may reduce the effectiveness of these agents; thus the reduction or avoidance of tobacco smoking is advisable (Long & Rybacki, 1995).

Alcohol consumption may result in hypotensive episodes in some clients. Whenever possible, the use of alcohol should be avoided.

The half-lives of diltiazem, nimodipine, and verapamil may increase because of accumulation from decreased elimination in older adults.

The risk of hypotension is increased with the use of nimodipine.

Calcium channel blockers should not be discontinued abruptly, because severe rebound angina attacks may result (gradual drug withdrawal is recommended).

Review the client's current medication regimen for the risk of significant drug interactions, such as those that may occur when calcium channel blockers are given concurrently with the following drugs:

Drug	Possible Effect and Management
Bold/color type indicates the most serious interactions.	
beta-adrenergic blocking agents, systemic and ophthalmic	Although advantageous in some clients, this combination should be closely monitored because adverse cardiac effects may occur (bradycardia, hypotension, and heart failure caused by prolonged AV conduction). Avoid concurrent use if possible in clients with impaired cardiac function.
carbamazepine (Tegretol), cyclosporine (Sandimmune), or quinidine	Diltiazem and verapamil may inhibit liver metabolism (cytochrome P-450 system), resulting in increased serum levels and toxicity of these drugs. Nifedipine with quinidine may result in reduced serum levels of quinidine. Monitor such combinations closely, because dosage adjustments may be necessary.
digitalis glycosides	Increased serum levels of digoxin are reported, especially when administered with verapamil (occur to a lesser degree with other calcium antagonists); monitor digoxin serum levels closely whenever a calcium channel blocker is started or discontinued or when the dosage is changed. Monitor for prolonged AV conduction, bradycardia, or AV blocks, especially during the initial week of therapy, because the dosage for digoxin may need to be changed.
disopyramide (Norpace)	**Do not administer disopyramide within 48 hours before or 24 hours after verapamil because the additive negative inotropic effects may result in serious reactions, including death. Use extreme caution when administering calcium antagonists with disopyramide. Avoid this combination if possible. Caution is also necessary when flecainide is given concurrently with calcium antagonists.**
grapefruit juice	Concurrent administration of 200 mL has been shown to increase felodipine serum levels more than twofold by inhibiting first-pass metabolism; a lesser effect has also been seen with nifedipine and nisoldipine.
hypokalemia-producing drugs, such as corticosteroids and potassium-depleting diuretics	**Increases the risk for bepridil-induced dysrhythmias.**
procainamide, quinidine, and any drugs that prolong the QT interval	**Both drug classifications have negative inotropic effects and may result in serious adverse reactions (e.g., hypotension, bradycardia, tachycardia, AV block, and pulmonary edema) when given concurrently. Avoid such combinations if possible.**

A baseline assessment should include pulse, blood pressure, lung sounds, and electrocardiogram (ECG) readings. Liver and renal function studies are recommended if long-term therapy is anticipated.

■ **Nursing Diagnosis.** The client undergoing calcium channel blocker therapy may be at risk for the following nursing diagnoses/collaborative problems: impaired oral mucous membrane (gingival hyperplasia); impaired comfort (dry mouth, flushing, dizziness, headache, chest pain, and nausea); excess fluid volume related to sodium and water retention as evidenced by swelling of the feet, ankles, and lower legs; risk for injury related to dizziness, drowsiness, and fainting; activity intolerance related to lethargy and weakness; disturbed sleep pattern (drowsiness); constipation; diarrhea; and the potential complications of allergic reaction (skin rash), depression, angina, congestive heart failure, and altered cardiac output related to hypotension, dysrhythmias, or tachycardia. With nifedipine, the client may experience the potential complications of arthritis or transient blindness at peak serum concentrations.

■ **Implementation**

■ ***Monitoring.*** Monitor blood pressure and pulse rate, particularly if the drug is coadministered with a beta-adrenergic blocking agent. Observe the ECG for a prolonged PR interval, which is caused by the slowing of AV conduction. Congestive heart failure may occasionally occur after the initiation of calcium channel blocker therapy, particularly in clients who are also receiving beta-blocking agents. Assess intake, output, and weight; also assess for edema. If beta blockers are withdrawn before initiating calcium channel blocker therapy, taper their dosage gradually. Abrupt withdrawal may provoke angina, especially when nifedipine is started. Hepatic and renal function studies may be required during long-term therapy with calcium channel blockers. Periodic potassium levels are recommended during bepridil therapy.

■ ***Intervention.*** Administer oral doses of calcium channel blockers on an empty stomach to promote rapid absorption. If nausea occurs with bepridil, administer it with meals or at bedtime. Take the client's pulse before each dose of a calcium channel blocker; if the pulse rate is 50 beats/min or below, withhold the dose and report to the prescriber.

For a verapamil injection, inspect the parenteral drug preparation, and discard it if cloudy. Administer the initial IV dose in a treatment center with appropriate facilities for monitoring and resuscitation. Administer the drug slowly as a direct injection over at least 2 minutes (over at least 3 minutes in older adults). Monitor with an ECG. Avoid repeated doses in clients with hepatic or renal failure, because an IV dose may prolong the duration of effects. If repeated injections are required, closely monitor blood pressure and the PR interval, and use smaller doses as prescribed. If bolus therapy is successful, the client may be placed on continuous IV administration; use a controlled infusion device for precise dosage. The maximum effects of verapamil occur in 15 to 30 minutes, and therefore adjustments in infusion rates are made at 30-minute intervals (Swavely, Molchany, & Jozefiak, 1993). Monitor the client carefully for a return of abnormal ECG readings for several hours after discontinuing the IV verapamil because the drug is excreted over 2 to 5 hours.

Clients receiving IV diltiazem should be monitored continuously on telemetry with frequent blood pressure measurements (Paul, 1993). Emergency equipment should be readily available. If the client becomes hypotensive, the infusion rate should be slowed or discontinued.

■ ***Education.*** Instruct the client to perform meticulous daily dental hygiene and to maintain regular dental examinations and cleaning; this may reduce the incidence or severity of gingivitis and gingival hyperplasia (a rare side effect).

Because calcium channel blockers may be coadministered with sublingual nitroglycerin and other nitrates, instruct the client to keep a record of nitroglycerin administration and anginal episodes and to report promptly if changes occur in the previous pattern (increased frequency, duration, and severity of anginal attacks). The symptoms may develop when starting calcium channel blockers or increasing dosages. (Nitroglycerin is used to abort acute angina attacks.)

Caution the client against smoking, because the effectiveness of calcium channel blockers is reduced in smokers (Jackson, 1993).

Instruct the client to move from a sitting or lying position to a standing position cautiously to avoid orthostatic hypotension. Advise the client to avoid alcohol to prevent dizziness and hypotension.

Teach the client to take his or her pulse and report a heart rate of less than 50 beats/min. Instruct the client to report headaches, rashes, nausea, and vomiting; in addition, instruct the client to report edema and weight gain (more than 1 kg/day), because these two symptoms may indicate congestive heart failure. If the client is taking a calcium channel blocker for hypertension, instruct the client how to measure blood pressure accurately (use the client's own equipment). Have the client keep a log of blood pressure values, pulses, and symptoms to share with the prescriber. Emphasize the importance of regular visits to a health care provider to monitor progress during therapy.

If the client is taking an extended-release form of the drug, caution against chewing, breaking, or crushing it. Alert the client if switching diltiazem brands, one preparation is for once-daily dosing and the other is for twice-daily dosing. Some calcium channel blockers may be taken without regard to food (bepridil); some are to be taken on an empty stomach (Adalat CC); others are to be taken with food (verapamil). Most calcium channel blockers are not to be taken with grapefruit juice, especially felodipine. It is recommended that flunarizine be taken in the evening. If a dose is missed, advise the client to take it as soon as it is remembered; however, if it is almost time for the next dose, the missed dose should be omitted.

If calcium channel blockers are being taken as antihypertensives, instruct the client to take the medication even if feeling well, because lifelong therapy may be required. Compliance may be ascertained by monitoring refill frequency. Advise the client regarding the hazards of untreated hypertension and the need for decreased sodium intake, smoking cessation, and weight control. Instruct the client in the procedure of periodic blood pressure determinations; have the client report results to the prescriber at follow-up visits. Caution the client to check with the prescriber before taking other medications, particularly OTC sympathomimetics, which are commonly found in cold remedies.

To reduce the hypotensive effects of calcium channel blockers, instruct the client to remain in the recumbent position for at least 1 hour following an IV bolus injection of verapamil.

■ **Evaluation.** The expected outcome of calcium channel blocker therapy is that the client will demonstrate a regular sinus rhythm on the ECG and have a blood pressure within the normal limits. If the drug is taken for angina, the client will report a decrease in the frequency and severity of angina, and the client's tolerance for activity will increase. The client will have a sufficient understanding of his or her condition and medications and will be able to self-administer medications safely and accurately.

SUMMARY

Calcium channel blockers are one of the newer groupings of cardiac drugs. They block the inward movement of calcium through the slow channels of the cell membranes of cardiac and smooth muscle cells. In cardiac muscle, this action decreases the force of myocardial contraction; in vascular smooth muscle, this action decreases the force of the smooth muscle contraction and in particular inhibits the contraction of the smooth muscle of the peripheral arterioles. Within the cardiac conduction system, calcium channel blockers decrease automaticity in the SA node and decrease conduction in the AV node.

At present a number of calcium channel blockers have been approved by the FDA for the treatment of angina pectoris and hypertension. Each of these drugs has distinct properties. Diltiazem is generally restricted to coronary blood vessel dilatation. Nicardipine and nifedipine are potent peripheral vasodilators but do not affect the cardiac conduction system; this makes them effective as antihypertensive agents and in the treatment of Raynaud's phenomenon. Flunarizine, nifedipine, and nimodipine have a greater effect than other calcium channel blockers on the cerebral arteries. Verapamil is also effective as an antidysrhythmic because it prolongs AV conduction time and depresses the contractility of cardiac muscle.

The goals for the administration of calcium channel blockers and client teaching include a decrease in the frequency and intensity of the angina attacks, blood pressure within the normal range, increased activity tolerance, and sufficient client understanding of his or her condition and medications to enable the safe and accurate self-administration of medications.

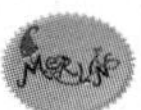

Critical Thinking Questions

1. John Samuels, age 56, developed a supraventricular tachycardia during a stress test and was transferred to the coronary care unit. He is prescribed verapamil (Isoptin), 5 mg IV push stat. Besides Mr. Samuels' ECG, what other assessments should the nurse be concerned with during the administration of the drug?
2. Alice Hooker, age 62, has angina. She has been prescribed nifedipine (Procardia), 10 mg PO three times daily. What laboratory values should the nurse monitor during the nifedipine therapy? Why?

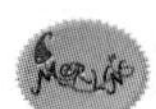

Collaborative Learning Activities

For Collaborative Learning Activities, go to mosby.com/MERLIN/McKenry/.

BIBLIOGRAPHY

American Hospital Formulary Service. (1999). *AHFS drug information '99.* Bethesda, MD: American Society of Hospital Pharmacists.

Anderson, K.N., Anderson, L.E., & Glanze, W.D. (Eds.). (1998). *Mosby's medical, nursing, & allied health dictionary* (5th ed.). St. Louis: Mosby.

Beattie, S. (1999). Management of chronic stable angina. *Nurse Practitioner, 24*(5), 44, 49, 53.

Brownley, K.A., Hurwitz, B.E., & Schneiderman, N. (1999). Ethnic variations in the pharmacological and nonpharmacological treatment of hypertension: Biopychosocial perspective. *Human Biology, 71*(4), 607-639.

Clem, J.R. (1995). Pharmacotherapy of ischemic heart disease. *AACN Clinical Issues in Advanced Critical Care, 6*(3), 404-417, 493-494.

Drug Facts and Comparisons. (2000). St. Louis: Facts and Comparisons.

Foley, J.J. (1994). Treatment of calcium-channel blocker overdose. *Journal of Emergency Nurse, 20,* 314-315.

Gillman, M.W., Ross-Degnan, D., McLaughlin, T.J., Gao, X., Spiegelman, D., Hertzmark, E., Goldman, L., & Soumerai, S.B. (1999). Effects of long-acting versus short-acting calcium channel blockers among older survivors of acute myocardial infarction. *American Journal of the Geriatric Society, 47*(5), 512-517.

Hall, W.D. (1999). A rational approach to the treatment of hypertension in special populations. *American Family Physician, 60*(1), 156-162.

Heidenreich, P.A., McDonald, K.M., Hastie, T., Fadel, B., Magan, V., Lee, B.K., & Hlatky, M.A. (1999). Meta-analysis of trials comparing beta-blockers, calcium antagonists, and nitrates for stable angina. *JAMA, 281*(20), 1927-1936.

Jackson, G. (1993). The management of stable angina. *Hospital Practice, 28*(1), 59.

Kayser, S.R. (1995). Pharmacology news. Calcium channel blockers—is vasoselectivity relevant? *Progress in Cardiovascular Nursing, 10*(1), 35-39.

Kelly, T. (1993). Medical management of calcium channel blocker overdoses. *Drug Newsletter, 12*(3), 18.

Long, J.W. & Rybacki, J.J. (1995). *The essential guide to prescription drugs.* New York: Harper Collins.

Maxwell, C.J., Hogan, D.B., & Ebly, E.M. (1999). Calcium-channel blockers and cognitive function in elderly people: Results from the Canadian Study of Health and Aging. *Canadian Medical Association Journal, 161*(5), 501-506.

Paul, S.C. (1993). New pharmacologic agents for emergency management of supraventricular tachydysrhythmias. *Critical Care Nursing Quarterly, 16*(2), 35-45.

Salerno, S.M. & Zugibe, F.T. Jr. (1994). Calcium channel antagonists: What do the second-generation agents have to offer? *Postgraduate Medicine, 95*(1), 181-188, 190, 201-202.

Sikes, P.J. & Nolan, S. (1993). Pharmacologic management of cerebral vasospasm. *Critical Care Nursing Quarterly, 154,* 78-87.

Swavely, D.A., Molchany, C.A., & Jozefiak, E. (1993). Continuous verapamil infusion: The nurse's role in monitoring patient outcomes. *Dimensions of Critical Care Nursing, 12*(4), 186-193.

Talbert, R.L. (1993). Ischemic heart disease. In J.T. DiPiro, R.L. Talbert, G.C. Yee, G.R. Matzke, B.G. Wells, & L.M. Posey (Eds.), *Pharmacotherapy: A pathophysiologic approach* (2nd ed.). Norwalk, CT: Appleton & Lange.

United States Pharmacopeia Dispensing Information (USP DI): Drug information for the health care professional (19th ed.). (1999). Rockville, MD: United States Pharmacopeial Convention.

29 Vasodilators and Antihemorrheologic Agents

Chapter Focus

Nitrates have been prescribed for more than 100 years to treat ischemic heart disease. Because these drugs have a short duration of action and poor bioavailability, manufacturers are continuously working on new forms to improve the therapeutic effect. The antihemorrheologics are relatively new therapeutic agents to improve microcirculatory flow.

Learning Objectives

1. Identify the three therapeutic objectives for the use of antianginal agents.
2. Compare the effects of nitrates, beta blockers, and calcium blocking agents on the heart.
3. Discuss the mechanism of action, side effects/adverse reactions, significant drug interactions, and dosages for nitrates.
4. Instruct a client in the self-management of a transdermal system for the administration of nitroglycerin.
5. Discuss isoxsuprine as an agent used in the treatment of peripheral vascular disease.
6. Implement nursing management for the care of a client receiving vasodilators.
7. Define the science of hemorrheology.
8. Implement nursing management for the care of a client receiving pentoxifylline.

Key Terms

angina pectoris, p. 606
hemorrheology, p. 612
ischemic, p. 606
nitrates, p. 606

Key Drugs [✓]

nitroglycerin, p. 607
pentoxifylline, p. 612

Vasodilators are used for the treatment of vascular disorders, including peripheral vascular conditions. These agents produce peripheral vasodilation by relaxing smooth muscle in the blood vessel walls. Some drugs act primarily on veins or arterioles, and others dilate both types of blood vessels.

The vasodilators used to treat hypertension are reviewed in Chapter 27. This chapter addresses the use of vasodilators for angina and peripheral occlusive arterial disease and the use of antihemorrheologic agents for the treatment of peripheral vascular disease. The antihemorrheologic drugs improve microcirculatory blood flow to **ischemic** tissues (tissues with a decreased oxygenated blood supply).

ANGINA

The term **angina pectoris** refers to a temporary interference with the flow of blood, oxygen, and nutrients to heart muscle, or intermittent myocardial ischemia. Angina is characterized by pain behind the sternum. The pain usually occurs with exercise or stress and is relieved by rest. Angina pectoris occurs when the workload on the heart is too great and oxygen delivery is inadequate. Coronary flow is very responsive to the oxygen requirements of the heart. Inadequate oxygenation of the heart implies that coronary blood flow is less than the amount actually needed.

Therefore angina pectoris is usually associated with myocardial ischemia. When coronary blood flow is inadequate, hypoxia causes an accumulation of pain-producing substances such as lactic acid (anaerobic metabolite) and other chemical irritants such as potassium ions, kinins, and prostaglandins. These products stimulate the cardiac sensory nerve endings, which transmit impulses to the central nervous system (CNS) to produce the typical anginal pain response.

Coronary atherosclerosis or vasomotor spasm of the coronary vessels may cause inadequate oxygenation. Other causes of anginal pain may be pulmonary hypertension and valvular heart disease. Individuals with severe anemia, even with minimal coronary artery disease, may suffer from anginal attacks because of inadequate oxygen supply. The presence of carbon monoxide hemoglobin (carboxyhemoglobin) in smokers, who have reduced amounts of available blood oxygen, is another factor in causing angina pectoris.

Drug therapy of angina pectoris is based on the belief that the relaxation of coronary smooth muscle will bring about coronary vasodilation, which in turn will improve blood flow to the heart. However, coronary arteries narrowed by disorders such as sclerosis and calcification cannot respond to any coronary vasodilator. Nitrates are the primary drugs prescribed for the treatment of angina.

VASODILATORS

The **nitrates** are very effective drugs for the treatment of angina pectoris because of their dilating effect on the veins and arteries. The pooling of blood in the veins (capacitance blood vessels) decreases the amount of blood returned to the heart (preload), which reduces left ventricular end-diastolic volume. This decrease in blood return may help to reduce the demand for myocardial oxygen. Chest pain induced by angina pectoris largely results from an inadequate supply of oxygen to the heart (Box 29-1).

The ideal antianginal drug would (1) establish a balance between coronary blood flow and the metabolic demands of the heart, (2) have a local rather than a systemic effect (would act directly on coronary vessels to promote coronary vasodilation with no effects on other organ systems), (3) promote oxygen extraction by the heart from arterial flow, (4) be effective when taken orally and have sustained action, and (5) have an absence of tolerance.

Currently, no drug meets these criteria. The drugs presently available provide only temporary relief. Evidence is increasing that the nitrates exert their effect not so much by coronary vasodilation but by lowering blood pressure and decreasing venous return and cardiac work. Table 29-1 compares the effects of nitrates, beta blockers, and calcium blocking agents.

BOX 29-1

Types of Angina Pectoris

Classic Angina (Stable or Effort)

This type of pain is usually associated with coronary arteriosclerosis. The attack can be precipitated by exertion or stress (e.g., cold, fear, and emotion) and by eating. The pain lasts approximately 15 minutes and disappears with rest or nitrates.

Unstable Angina (Crescendo or Preinfarction)

This is a progressive form of angina in which pain occurs more frequently and becomes more severe in time. The attack may appear during rest and may last longer, with less relief provided by antianginal drugs. Individuals with unstable angina eventually show signs and symptoms of impending myocardial infarction or coronary failure.

Variant Angina (Prinzmetal's or Vasospastic)

This type of pain may be associated with spasms of the coronary arteries, and it usually occurs in the presence of coronary stenosis. The pain often occurs during rest and without any cause. Its occurrence follows a regular pattern (e.g., it appears at the same time during the night). Dysrhythmias often accompany the attack, and the electrocardiogram shows an elevation in the ST segment during the anginal episode. Nitroglycerin acts to increase the oxygen supply by relaxing or preventing spasms in the coronary arteries.

TABLE 29-1 Comparison of Effects of Nitrates, Beta Blockers, and Calcium Blocking Agents

	Nitrates	Beta Blockers	Calcium Blocking Agents
Systolic blood pressure	(−)	(−)	(−)
Ventricular volume	(−)	(+)	(−) or (0)
Heart rate	(+)	(−)	(−),(+), or (0)
Myocardial contractility	(0)	(−)	(−)
Coronary blood flow	(+)	(+) or (0)	(+)
Coronary vessel resistance	(−)	(+) or (0)	(−)
Coronary spasms	(−)	(+) or (0)	(−)
Collateral flow of blood	(+)	(0)	(−)

(−), Decreased; (+), increased; (0), no change.

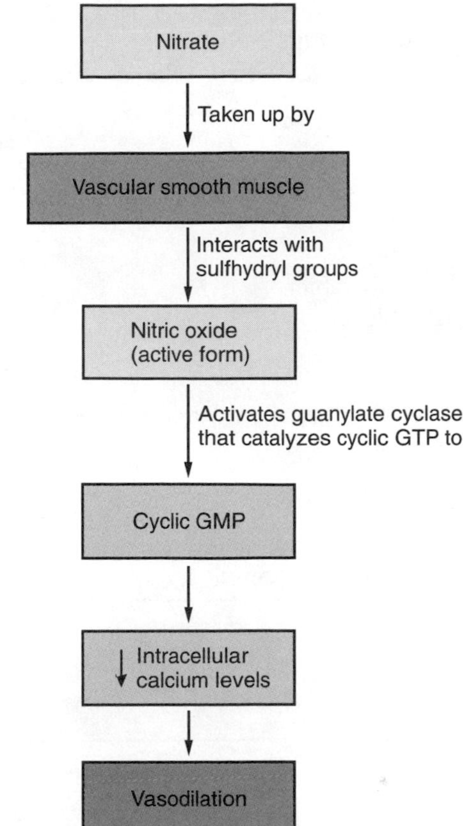

Figure 29-1 Biochemical steps on nitrates. (From Salerno, E. [1999]. *Pharmacology for health professionals*, St. Louis: Mosby.)

Nitrates

✓Nitroglycerin (NTG) is the key drug in the nitrate category. It is available as sublingual tablets (Nitrostat), extended-release buccal tablets (Nitrogard SR), lingual aerosols (Nitrolingual), extended-release capsules (Nitrocap), parenteral injections (Nitro-Bid, Nitrol), ointments (Nitro-Bid, Nitrostat), and transdermal topical systems (Nitrodisc, Transderm-Nitro, Nitro-Dur). The other drugs in the nitrate drug category include amyl nitrite inhalant and isosorbide dinitrate (Isordil, Sorbitrate).

Nitrates dilate venous capacitance and arterial resistance vessels, which results in reduced myocardial oxygen demand and a more efficient distribution of blood in the myocardium. The antihypertensive effect of nitrates is also a result of peripheral vasodilation. The biochemical steps for nitrates are illustrated in Figure 29-1.

Nitroglycerin and the other nitrates are used to reduce or prevent the pain of angina, to treat congestive heart failure associated or not associated with myocardial infarction, and to treat hypertension (nitroglycerin injection).

Amyl nitrite has been used to treat acute angina attacks, but the other, safer nitrate dosage forms have replaced it. Although not approved by Food and Drug Administration (FDA) labeling in the United States, amyl nitrite has been used as an antidote for cyanide poisoning and in cardiac function tests to assess reserve cardiac function. This product has also been abused and used as a sexual stimulant or euphoric agent, but such applications are extremely dangerous and should be avoided.

The pharmacokinetics of the nitrates are summarized in Table 29-2.

The side effects/adverse reactions include dizziness, headaches, nausea or vomiting, agitation, facial flushing, increased pulse rate, dry mouth, rash, prolonged headaches, and blurred vision.

Table 29-3 lists the dosage and administration of the nitrates. The FDA pregnancy safety classification is category C.

■ Nursing Management
Nitrate Therapy

■ **Assessment.** Although it is rare, clients who are intolerant of one nitrate may show an intolerance to other nitrates. A nitroglycerin injection is not considered appropriate for use in clients with cerebral hemorrhage or other head injury because of its tendency to increase cerebrospinal fluid pressure; it is also inappropriate for clients with pericardial tamponade or constrictive pericarditis. In addition, caution should be used in administering nitrates to clients with a recent myocardial infarction (the resultant hypotension may aggravate ischemia); glaucoma (may increase intraocular pressure); severe anemia; or hyperthyroidism. Any hypovolemia should be corrected before administering nitroglycerin by injection because it may precipitate severe hypotension and shock. Clients with hypotension evidenced by low systolic pressure may experience further hypotension with paradoxical bradycardia and increased angina pectoris.

TABLE 29-2 Nitrates: Pharmacokinetics

Drug	Onset of Action (minutes)	Duration of Action (hours)	Metabolism	Excretion
isosorbide dinitrate				
Oral tablet/capsule	15-40	4-6	Liver	Kidneys
Chewable tablet	2-5	1-2		
Extended-release tablet	30	12		
Sublingual tablet	2-5	1-2		
nitroglycerin				
Sublingual tablet	1-3	0.5-1	Liver	Kidneys
Extended-release (buccal) tablet/capsule	3	5		
Lingual aerosol	2-4	—		
IV infusion	Immediate	Several minutes		
Ointment	30	4-8		
Transdermal patch	30	8-24		
Extended-release tablet/capsule	—	8-12		

TABLE 29-3 Nitrates: Dosage and Administration

Drug	Usual Adult Dosage
isosorbide dinitrate	2.5-30 mg PO, SL or chewable q6h. Extended-release: 40-80 mg PO q8-12h.
nitroglycerin	0.15-0.6 mg SL or buccally, repeated at 5-minute intervals for up to 3 doses. If relief is not obtained, contact prescriber or transport individual to a hospital (maximum dosage is 10 mg/day). Lingual aerosol: 0.4-0.8 mg prn (maximum dosage is 1.2 mg/day). Oral tablets/capsules, extended-release: 2.5, 6.5, or 9 mg PO q12h. IV infusion: initial 5 μg/min increased in increments of 5 μg/min at 3- or 5-minute intervals as needed. Ointment: Apply 1-2 inches (15-30 mg) to skin q6-8h. Maximum is 5 inches (75 mg) per application. Transdermal topical system: Apply one patch q24h. To reduce the development of tolerance, it is recommended the patch be applied for 12 to 14 hours and removed for 10 to 12 hours.

SL, Sublingual.

The client's current medication regimen should be reviewed for significant drug interactions, such as with other vasodilators, because concurrent use may exaggerate the orthostatic hypotensive effects of the drugs; dosage adjustments may be necessary. The concurrent use of any drug with hypotensive effects such as alcohol, opioid analgesics, or antihypertensive agents should be avoided if at all possible for the same reasons. If it is not possible to avoid concurrent administration, monitor closely because dosage reductions may be necessary.

■ **Nursing Diagnosis.** With the administration of nitrates, the client may experience the following nursing diagnoses: impaired comfort related to dry mouth, flushing, headache, rash, dizziness, and nausea and vomiting; risk for injury related to orthostatic hypotension or blurred vision; and impaired skin integrity (erythema) related to the application of topical dosage forms.

■ Implementation

■ ***Monitoring.*** To determine effectiveness, assess the client's chest pain on a scale of 1 to 10 before administration and 5 minutes after administration of the sublingual dose. Monitor pulse and blood pressure before and after administration. Over the course of long-acting nitrate therapy used to prevent angina episodes, monitor for orthostatic hypotension and measure the client's blood pressure in both arms and in the sitting and standing positions.

For ointment administration, measure the baseline blood pressure and heart rate after the client has been at rest for 10 minutes; the client should be in a sitting position. Repeat the vital signs 1 hour after drug administration and report them to the prescriber. With the client in a resting position, an appropriate dosage produces a fall in blood pressure of 10 mm Hg or a rise in heart rate of 10 beats/min.

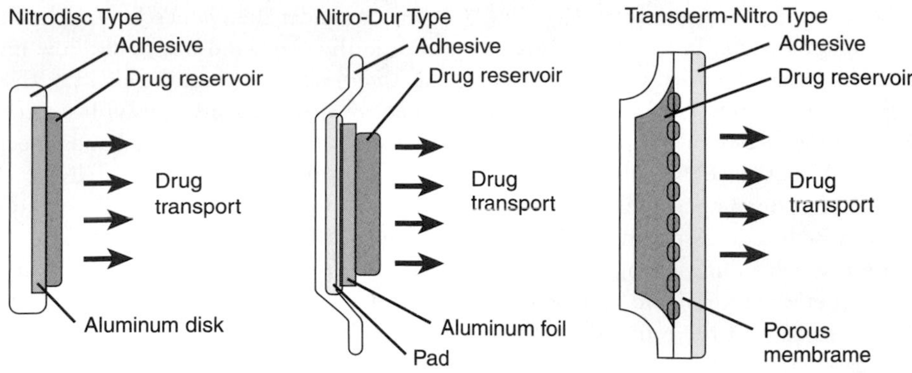

Figure 29-2 Transdermal system.

To titrate the IV dosage for desired hemodynamic function, monitor blood pressure, heart rate, and pulmonary capillary wedge pressure continuously until the correct dosage is obtained. Clients with normal or low capillary wedge pressure are likely to be sensitive to the hypotensive effects of IV nitroglycerin. The dosage after long-term or high-dose therapy should be reduced gradually to minimize withdrawal rebound angina.

Tolerance has been reported and is manifested by a lack of pain relief following the usual dose. Nitrates may be discontinued for several days until tolerance is lost; the drug is then reinstated. To help prevent tolerance, clients need to have an 8- to 12-hour "no nitrate" time. The paste and patches should be removed after 12 hours. If the client experiences pain during the day, the nitrate should be used during the day and removed at night; if the pain occurs at night, the nitrate should be removed during the day (Saunders, 1998).

■ ***Intervention.*** The dosage must be adjusted by the prescriber to the needs and tolerance of the individual client.

Store the stock supply of the drug in the original container; the container should be tightly closed with a metal screw cap. Federal regulation requires that the sublingual form of nitroglycerin be dispensed in the original unopened manufacturer's container. A supplementary stainless steel container has been approved for carrying small amounts of nitroglycerin. The pendant-like container may be worn on a chain around the neck to provide a convenient supply of the drug when it is needed.

■ *Intravenous Infusion.* Use special nitroglycerin disposable infusion sets provided by the manufacturer. They are made of non–polyvinyl chloride plastic to minimize the loss of nitroglycerin. Polyvinyl chloride (PVC) plastic may adsorb up to 40% to 80% of the nitroglycerin from a diluted solution of infusion; therefore use glass IV bottles or the administration set provided by the manufacturer.

Nitroglycerin is not to be used with a direct IV infusion. Dilute with 5% dextrose injection or 0.9% sodium chloride injection before infusion. Because the concentration and/or volume of the drug varies, carefully follow the dosage instructions of the manufacturer. Be aware that switching from a standard (PVC) set to a special (non-PVC) set is likely to affect the dosage—the PVC set requires a higher dosage, which would be excessive if switched to a non-PVC set. In addition, *do not mix nitroglycerin with other medications.*

■ *Ointment.* Squeeze the prescribed dose of nitroglycerin onto the specially designed dose-measuring applicator supplied with the package. Wash off the last application. *Avoid using the fingers* to spread the ointment. Apply a thin, uniform layer to a premarked, 6-square-inch surface (a clean, dry, nonhairy skin area of chest, abdomen, anterior aspect of thigh, or forearm). Rotate sites to prevent inflammation. Do not massage or rub in the ointment, because rapid absorption will interfere with the sustained action of the drug. Cover the area with a transparent wrap and secure it with tape. The ointment is usually applied every 8 hours during the day and at bedtime. If the client experiences breakthrough angina, the dose may be prescribed for application every 6 hours.

■ *Transdermal Application.* Rotate sites. Wash the skin when the patch is removed. Remove the patch for 8 to 12 hours every day. Patches with aluminum backings should be removed before defibrillation, because the electric current may cause it to burn (Figure 29-2).

■ ***Education.*** Instruct the client to avoid alcoholic beverages while taking nitrates because a shocklike syndrome (flushing, weakness, pallor, hypotension, and syncope) may occur. Inform the client about the importance of learning to identify stressful situations that precipitate anginal attacks. These include emotional stress, overeating, smoking, temperature extremes, and a sudden increase in physical activity. Explain the need to pace activities and to plan for rest periods. The client should receive support to modify behaviors that precipitate anginal attacks.

When the buccal, lingual, sublingual, and chewable oral dosage forms of nitrates are used to prevent angina, instruct the client to take the drug 5 to 10 minutes before the occurrence of the anticipated stressor.

Dizziness, light-headedness, and a slight headache may occur with the administration of nitrates. Have the client sit and rest until the symptoms pass. Advise changing positions slowly to avoid dizziness. Headache may be treated with a mild analgesic. Instruct the client to report to the prescriber if blurred vision, dry mouth, or severe headaches occur; these are signs of overdose and require immediate attention.

Inform the client about the inactivation of nitroglycerin by exposure to air, heat, and moisture. In general, it is recommended that unused tablets be discarded 6 months after the bottle is opened. The length of time of potency appears to vary with the manufacturer. Read the drug insert and check the expiration date. Do not leave the cotton or package insert in the container after opening; these articles may absorb some of the drug, which reduces potency.

Be sure the hands are dry if handling nitroglycerin, because moisture hastens its deterioration. Cold and heat affect nitroglycerin. Do not store it in the refrigerator or in the bathroom medicine cabinet.

Instruct the client not to change the dosage or medication without consulting the prescriber and to report regularly for cardiac function monitoring.

■ *Sublingual Tablets.* Instruct the client to sit or lie down and to take the medication on the first indication of an oncoming anginal attack. This position prevents postural hypotension. The signs and symptoms of postural hypertension include dizziness, syncope, and weakness.

Explain to the client that a sublingual tablet should be placed under the tongue or in the buccal pouch and allowed to dissolve; it is not to be swallowed. Avoid eating, drinking, or smoking while the drug dissolves. The potency of the drug is usually indicated by a burning or stinging sensation under the tongue. The newer, more stable preparations may not produce this effect.

Doses may be repeated at 5-minute intervals for three doses if necessary. The prescriber should be notified if pain is not relieved in 15 minutes. For a hospitalized individual, a specific number of tablets (approximately 25) may be prescribed to be placed at the bedside in an appropriate container and properly labeled for the client's use. Instruct the client to keep a record of the frequency of anginal attacks, the precipitating factors, the number of tablets used, and the occurrence of side effects. Warn the client of transient headaches, which usually last 5 to 20 minutes after the sublingual administration of nitroglycerin. The prescriber should be notified if the headache persists. Headaches may disappear within several days to weeks and may be relieved by aspirin, acetaminophen, or a temporary dosage reduction.

■ *Buccal Extended-Release Tablets.* Instruct the client to place the tablet between the upper lip and gum to dissolve or above the incisors if food or drink is to be taken within the 3 to 5 hours it takes to dissolve. Caution the client against using these tablets at bedtime, because aspiration is a risk. The tablet may be replaced if swallowed.

■ *Chewable Tablets.* Instruct the client to chew the tablet thoroughly and to hold it in the mouth for 2 minutes before swallowing.

■ *Oral Sustained-Release Tablets or Capsules.* Administer these tablets on an empty stomach (1 hour before or 2 hours after meals) with a full glass of water; instruct the client to swallow the medication whole. Alert the client to notify the prescriber if undigested tablets are found in stools.

■ *Lingual Aerosol.* Do not shake the can when administering a lingual aerosol. Hold the can vertically and spray it onto or under the client's tongue. Instruct the client not to inhale the spray and not to swallow immediately.

■ *Ointments.* Instruct the client in the application of ointment as described previously. Instruct the caregiver not to get ointment on his or her hands, because the medication may precipitate a headache. Tell the client to store nitroglycerin ointment in a cool place and in the original container with the tube tightly capped.

■ *Transdermal System.* Remove the old system and apply the new one at the same time each day. The system should be applied to clean, dry, and hairless skin areas of the chest, shoulder, or inside of the upper arm. Avoid skin folds, areas distal to the knee or elbow, and irritated or excessively scarred areas. Rotate application sites to prevent irritation. Apply a new system if the current one becomes loosened. Do not trim the units, because doing so will alter the dosage (Box 29-2). Alert the client to use caution near microwave ovens when wearing a transdermal system that has a metallic backing, because leaking radiation may heat the backing and cause a burn.

■ **Evaluation.** The expected outcome of nitrate therapy is that the client will report a decrease in the frequency and severity of angina attacks along with increased activity tolerance. If nitrates are administered for congestive heart failure, the client will demonstrate a clearing of peripheral edema and the lung fields, a urinary output of more than 30 mL/hr, and a blood pressure, pulmonary artery pressure, and pulmonary wedge pressure within normal limits.

MISCELLANEOUS AGENTS

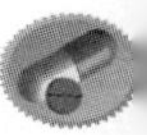

Epoprostenol (Flolan) directly dilates the pulmonary and systemic arteries and also inhibits platelet aggregation. It is administered via continuous injection through a central venous catheter. It is used for long-term treatment of pulmonary hypertension that has not responded to other therapies or for pulmonary hypertension associated with scleroderma. Epoprostenol should be reconstituted according to the manufacturer's instructions and not mixed with other parenteral solutions. In addition to the nursing care associated with an indwelling venous catheter to prevent sepsis and local infection, the client should be monitored for anxiety (21%), diarrhea (37%), dizziness (83%), flushing (42%), headache (83%), jaw pain (54%), tachycardia (35%), and thrombocytopenia. Epoprostenol therapy should not be discontinued abruptly.

PERIPHERAL VASCULAR DISEASE

Peripheral vascular disease results in coolness or numbness of the extremities, intermittent claudication, and leg ulcers; this condition is a common problem in older adults. The primary pathophysiologic factor is atherosclerosis or hyperlipidemia. In general, the use of various direct-acting vasodilators for peripheral occlusive arterial disease has been very disappointing. The FDA has classified cyclandelate (Cyclospasmol) as ineffective; it is not reviewed in this section. Papaverine (Pavabid) is an old drug that was exempted

BOX 29-2

Transdermal Nitroglycerin Systems

Transdermal nitroglycerin delivery systems are quite popular, and therefore the nurse should be familiar with several issues and concerns associated with these products. Three systems are currently available; the actual amount of nitroglycerin delivered by each system can vary depending on the system and the individual client's skin absorption of the nitroglycerin. Each system has a different mechanism of drug delivery:

1. Nitrodisc contains nitroglycerin mixed in a solid polymer similar to silicone. The drug is absorbed through the skin from this polymer, which also contains a co-solvent to enhance skin penetration.
2. Nitro-Dur contains a gel-like matrix surrounded by fluid. Nitroglycerin moves from the matrix to the fluid to the skin.
3. Transderm-Nitro contains a semipermeable membrane between the drug supply and the skin. The membrane is actually the controlling factor for the drug delivery (see Figure 29-2).

Drug absorption in all systems is by passive diffusion and is based on processes relating to heat transfer (or Fick's first law of diffusion).

These three systems are not interchangeable because patch size, nitroglycerin content, and the average amount of nitroglycerin delivered in 24 hours can differ. Although many individuals reportedly control their conditions with or have responded to this dosage form, other clients do not achieve adequate therapeutic blood levels or a clinically significant therapeutic response. Some researchers believe that maintaining stable nitroglycerin serum levels over 24 hours is not always desirable because this leads to drug tolerance and the need to increase dosages. The intermittent use of transdermal products (e.g., application for 12 to 16 hours and then removal for the night) results in prolonged clinical results without the development of significant drug tolerance.

Research and studies are ongoing in this area, and manufacturers are continuing their search for better methods for delivering their drug products.

from the FDA's review on drug effectiveness. After reviewing studies and open hearings, the Peripheral and Central from the FDA's review on drug effectiveness. After reviewing studies and open hearings, the Peripheral and Central Nervous System Drug Review Committee (the advisory committee of the FDA) concluded that papaverine has vasodilator effects but was not proven to be effective for its claimed indication, smooth muscle relaxation (*United States Pharmacopeia Dispensing Information,* 1999).

isoxsuprine [eye sox′ syoo preen] (Vasodilan)

The FDA requires substantial evidence of effectiveness in order to grade a drug "effective." Isoxsuprine lacks this information and is rated only "possibly effective" by the FDA for the treatment of symptoms of cerebrovascular insufficiency and peripheral vascular disease; it may relieve symptoms of Raynaud's disease, arteriosclerosis obliterans, and thromboangiitis obliterans (Buerger's disease). Isoxsuprine produces a direct relaxation effect on the smooth muscles of peripheral arterial walls located within skeletal muscle; it has little effect on cutaneous blood flow. It also causes an increase in heart rate, contractility and cardiac output, and uterine relaxation (*Drug Facts and Comparisons,* 2000).

Isoxsuprine has an onset of action of 10 minutes when given intravenously or 1 hour when administered orally. The half-life is 1.25 hours in adults. This drug is partially metabolized in the blood and excreted by the kidneys.

The side effects include nausea, vomiting or, rarely, chest pain, rash, and respiratory difficulties. No significant drug interactions are reported with isoxsuprine.

Isoxsuprine is administered in 10- to 20-mg tablets PO three or four times daily. The dosage to inhibit premature labor is 5 to 10 mg IM two to three times daily. Pregnancy safety has not been established, but in near-term neonates the drug has a half-life of 1.5 to 3 hours.

■ Nursing Management

Isoxsuprine Therapy

■ **Assessment.** Before the administration of isoxsuprine it should be ascertained that the client does not have severe cerebrovascular disease and has not recently had a myocardial infarction or severe coronary artery disease. Because it has a greater vasodilating effect on peripheral vessels than on vessels in coronary or cerebral areas, isoxsuprine may reduce blood flow and so increase ischemia in those areas. IV administration is not recommended for clients with hypotension or tachycardia; use caution if the drug is administered intramuscularly. If isoxsuprine is used for the management of premature labor, it should not be used immediately postpartum or if any of the following conditions exist: maternal cardiac disorders or hyperthyroidism (dysrhythmias may occur), intrauterine infection or fetal death or hemorrhage (immediate delivery is indicated), eclampsia, severe preeclampsia, or pulmonary hypertension.

■ **Nursing Diagnosis.** The client receiving isoxsuprine should be assessed for the following nursing diagnoses/collaborative problems: impaired comfort related to gastrointestinal effects such as nausea and vomiting (more common with parenteral dosing) and chest pain; ineffective tissue perfusion related to the client's underlying condition and ineffectiveness of the drug; risk for injury related to hypotension (dizziness, syncope); and the potential complications of pulmonary edema and allergic reaction.

■ **Implementation**

■ ***Monitoring.*** To detect hypotension, monitor the client's blood pressure with the client in the lying, sitting, and standing positions. Monitor peripheral pulses during drug administration to evaluate the effectiveness of this drug. For isoxsuprine use with clients with premature labor, monitor fetal and maternal heart rate, maternal blood pressure, and uterine activity. With prolonged IV administration for premature labor, assess blood glucose and fluid and electrolyte status.

■ ***Intervention.*** Administer isoxsuprine with milk, food, or antacids to prevent gastrointestinal distress.

■ ***Education.*** Instruct the client to move slowly to an upright from a sitting or lying position because of the hypotensive effects of the drug. Advise clients to avoid smoking, because the vasoconstrictive properties of nicotine are counterproductive to the use of isoxsuprine. Caution the client with premature labor to contact her health care provider if her water breaks or if her contractions begin again.

■ **Evaluation.** The expected outcome of isoxsuprine therapy is that the client with vascular insufficiency will experience an improvement in pulse volume, skin color, and temperature; report decreased extremity pain; report improved mental status; and demonstrate increased activity tolerance. For other clients, premature labor will cease.

HEMORRHEOLOGY

Hemorrheology is a science that deals with the deformation and flow properties of blood under physiologic and pathophysiologic conditions. Because arteriosclerosis reduces blood flow to tissues distal to the obstruction, blood viscosity is elevated; this further diminishes the flow of blood. In addition, impaired blood flow at the microcirculatory level affects the normal capacity of the red blood cells to flex as they enter the narrowed capillary lumen, which has a mean diameter smaller than the erythrocytes.

A major function of red blood cells is to transport the hemoglobin that carries oxygen, which during the metabolic process is converted to energy for muscle movement such as walking. The decreased flexibility of the red blood cells and the elevated blood viscosity are responsible for diminishing tissue oxygenation. Hence, during exercise the demand for an increase in blood flow and tissue oxygenation may result in claudication, thereby limiting the distance a person can walk.

Intermittent claudication is a syndrome that results from an insufficient supply of blood to the skeletal muscles in the legs. Reduced microcirculatory blood flow causes ischemia and pain. This syndrome is a common complication of atherosclerosis and is characteristic of Buerger's disease. While walking, affected individuals experience first pain and then cramps and weakness in the muscles.

Antihemorrheologic Agent

pentoxifylline [pen tox i′ fi lin] (Trental)

Pentoxifylline represents an important concept in the therapy for peripheral vascular disorders, because the ability of vasodilators to improve blood flow by the dilation of rigid, arteriosclerotic blood vessels is somewhat limited. Furthermore, capillary walls lack smooth muscle, and therefore dilation by this group of drugs is often unlikely to occur.

Pentoxifylline improves hemorrheologic disorders in microcirculation, which involves the flow of blood through the fine vessels (arterioles, capillaries, and venules). Although the mechanism of action of pentoxifylline is not completely understood, current evidence shows that it possesses several properties to improve microcirculatory blood flow to ischemic tissues:

1. It restores red blood cell flexibility, probably by its inhibition of phosphodiesterase, which results in an increase in cyclic adenosine monophosphate (cAMP) in red blood cells.
2. It lowers blood viscosity by decreasing fibrinogen concentrations and inhibiting the aggregation of red blood cells and platelets.

The result is increased microcirculatory blood flow and oxygenation of tissues.

Pentoxifylline is indicated as an adjunct to surgery for the treatment of intermittent claudication caused by occlusive arterial disease of the limbs. It is administered orally and on absorption binds to erythrocyte membranes. It has a half-life of 0.4 to 0.8 hours for the primary drug and 1 to 1.6 hours for the metabolites. Peak concentration in the blood occurs in 2 to 4 hours, and the onset of action with chronic dosing is between 2 and 4 weeks. It is metabolized by red blood cells and in the liver and is excreted primarily by the kidneys.

The side effects/adverse reactions of pentoxifylline include dizziness, headaches, abdominal distress, nausea, and vomiting. Rare adverse reactions are chest pain and an irregular heart rate. With an overdose the client experiences increased sedation, flushing of the skin, a feeling of faintness, increased excitability, or convulsions. No significant drug interactions have yet been reported with this drug.

The adult dosage is 400 mg PO three times daily with meals. If undesirable side effects occur, such as gastrointestinal upset or CNS disturbances, the dosage should be decreased to 400 mg twice daily. Pregnancy safety for pentoxifylline has been established as FDA category C.

■ Nursing Management

Pentoxifylline Therapy

■ **Assessment.** Because pentoxifylline is a xanthine derivative, do not administer it to clients who have an intolerance to other xanthine derivatives (e.g., caffeine, theophylline, or theobromine), because excessive CNS stimulation may result. Pentoxifylline should also be used with caution in clients with impaired hepatic and renal function; it may accumulate and dosages may need to be lowered. Because pentoxifylline enhances microcirculation, careful monitoring is required for any client at risk for bleeding, particularly a cerebral or retinal hemorrhage.

■ **Nursing Diagnosis.** With the administration of pentoxifylline, the client may be at risk for impaired comfort related to gastrointestinal effects (e.g., nausea, vomiting, and abdominal cramping) and the CNS effects (dizziness, drowsiness, and headache). The potential complications may be angina and dysrhythmias.

■ **Implementation**

■ ***Monitoring.*** Monitor blood pressure periodically in clients receiving concurrent antihypertensive therapy. Small decreases in blood pressure have been noted in clients receiving pentoxifylline alone, and a reduction of the hypotensive agent might be indicated. Monitor the client with peripheral vascular disease for an improvement in walking distance and duration. Monitor pulses, color, and temperature of the affected extremities.

■ ***Intervention.*** Administer pentoxifylline with food, milk, or antacids to decrease gastrointestinal distress. If gastrointestinal side effects persist, notify the prescriber to consider a reduction in the dosage.

■ ***Education.*** Instruct the client to swallow extended-release tablets whole without crushing or chewing them. Instruct the client that an improvement in clinical status may not occur before 8 weeks of therapy and that it is essential for the medication to be taken as prescribed until discontinued by the prescriber. Advise that the client quit smoking, because nicotine constricts the blood vessels and defeats the purpose of the medication. The client should receive support in smoking cessation through group or individual counseling.

■ **Evaluation.** The expected outcome of pentoxifylline therapy is that the client will experience an improvement in pulse volume and in skin color and temperature, report decreased pain, and demonstrate increased activity tolerance.

■ ■ ■

For information on horse chestnut and artichoke leaf, two complementary and alternative therapies that may be useful for clients with vascular disorders, see Appendix J.

SUMMARY

Both vasodilators and antihemorrheologics are used in the treatment of vascular disorders. Vasodilators produce vasodilation by relaxing smooth muscle in the blood vessel walls, whereas antihemorrheologic agents improve microcirculatory blood flow to ischemic tissues by lowering blood viscosity and increasing cAMP in the red blood cells. Vasodilators have been more effective in the treatment of angina and intermittent myocardial ischemia than they have been for peripheral vascular disease.

The goals of therapy with nitrates, the classic antianginal agents, are to decrease the duration and intensity of pain during an attack, decrease the frequency of attacks, and improve work capacity even though angina may occur. Nursing management of the client taking nitrates is to assist in determining the appropriate dosages for the client; this is accomplished through medication administration and evaluation and is based on symptom control. The nurse also prepares the client for the safe and accurate self-administration of nitrates.

Chronic occlusive arterial disease has been less successfully treated with vasodilating agents. The FDA has indicated that vasodilators are only effective in the treatment of peripheral vascular disease because the dilation of rigid, arteriosclerotic blood vessels is limited and because capillaries lack smooth muscle. The antihemorrheologic agent pentoxifylline increases microcirculatory blood flow and thereby oxygenation of the tissues. It is a valuable new adjunct treatment for occlusive arterial disease of the limbs, such as Buerger's disease.

Critical Thinking Questions

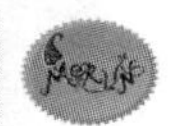

1. Mr. Scott has been taking sublingual nitroglycerin for years. He has now been prescribed a transdermal patch. How will Mr. Scott need to modify his therapeutic regimen?
2. In obtaining a drug history from Mr. Slattery, who is about to begin pentoxifylline therapy, you determine that he has an intolerance for milk and coffee and smokes a pack of cigarettes a day. What action would you take?

Collaborative Learning Activities

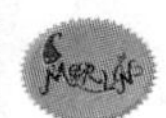

For Collaborative Learning Activities, go to mosby.com/MERLIN/McKenry/.

CASE STUDY

For a Case Study that will help ensure mastery of this chapter content, go to mosby.com/MERLIN/McKenry/.

BIBLIOGRAPHY

American Hospital Formulary Service. (1999). *AHFS drug information '99*. Bethesda, MD: American Society of Hospital Pharmacists.

Anderson, H.K., Anderson, L.F., & Glanze, W.D. (Eds.) (1998). *Mosby's medical, nursing, & allied health dictionary* (5th ed.). St. Louis: Mosby.

Beattie, S. (1999). Management of chronic stable angina. *Nurse Practitioner, 24*(5), 44, 49, 53.

Clem, J.R. (1995). Pharmacotherapy of ischemic heart disease. *AACN Clinical Issues: Advanced Practice in Acute and Critical Care, 6*(3), 404-417, 493-494.

Drug Facts and Comparisons. (2000). St. Louis: Facts and Comparisons.

Heidenreich, P.A. et al. (1999). Meta-analysis of trials comparing beta-blockers, calcium antagonists, and nitrates for stable angina. *JAMA, 281*(20), 1927-1936.

Katzung, B.G. & Chatterjee, K. (1998). Vasodilators and the treatment of angina pectoris. In B.G. Katzung (Ed.), *Basic and clinical pharmacology* (7th ed.). Norwalk, CT: Appleton & Lange.

Olson, H.G., & Aronow, W.S. (1996). Medical management of stable angina and unstable angina in the elderly with coronary artery disease. *Clinics in Geriatric Medicine, 12*(1), 121-140.

Saunders, C.S. (1998). Navigating the nitrate maze. *Patient Care, 32*(17), 23-24. 26, 31.

United States Pharmacopeia Dispensing Information (USP DI): Drug information for the health care professional (19th ed.). (1999). Rockville, MD: United States Pharmacopeial Convention.

30 Overview of the Blood

Chapter Focus

Because cells in the body are metabolically active, the blood plays an important role in maintaining homeostasis by providing constant nutrition and waste removal. Because the blood affects every other body system, it is a consideration in the assessment and care of most clients. Many drugs have adverse effects that cause disorders of the blood such as thrombocytopenia or agranulocytosis. The nurse therefore needs to be knowledgeable about hematology.

Learning Objectives

1. Describe the functions of the blood.
2. List the three types of blood cells and their functions.
3. Compare and contrast the five types of white blood cells.
4. Describe the role of platelets in blood clotting.
5. Name the three major blood proteins and their functions.

Key Terms

albumin, p. 616
anemia, p. 615
erythrocytes, p. 615
erythropoietin, p. 615
fibrinogen, p. 617
globulin, p. 617
hematocrit, p. 615
hemoglobin, p. 615
hemostasis, p. 617
leukocytes, p. 615
leukocytosis, p. 616
leukopenia, p. 616
phagocytosis, p. 616
plasma, p. 615
platelets, p. 615
thrombocytes, p. 616
thrombocytopenia, p. 616

Blood is the major transport system in the body. It is also vitally important for the proper functioning and regulation of the human body. Pumped by the heart, blood carries nutrients and oxygen from the digestive and respiratory systems to cells throughout the entire body. In addition, it picks up waste products from body cells and delivers them to the proper system for excretion, usually the liver, kidneys, and lungs. Hormones, enzymes, buffers, and many other biochemical substances are transported by the blood from one site in the body to the receptors or target cells. Blood also helps to regulate body heat by absorbing and transporting heat from the body core to where it can be more easily dispersed.

BLOOD VOLUME

Blood is composed of billions of cells and **plasma,** a fluid portion in which the cells are suspended. Although blood volume can vary from person to person, the average blood volume in a normal adult is approximately 5000 mL (5 L). Of this volume, 3000 mL is usually plasma; the remainder is primarily red blood cells. **Hematocrit** is the packed cell volume of the red blood cells expressed as a percentage of the total blood volume, or the blood viscosity. Hematocrit is measured by a laboratory test performed on a blood sample. The higher the hematocrit, the greater the blood viscosity. For example, persons with polycythemia may have a hematocrit of 60 or 70 because of an excessive number of red blood corpuscles. Increased blood viscosity can retard the flow of blood through blood vessels, resulting in headaches, fatigue, weakness, dyspnea, and perhaps an enlarged spleen and increased basal metabolism.

BLOOD COMPOSITION

Blood is composed of three types of blood cells: (1) red blood cells, or **erythrocytes,** which transport oxygen and carbon dioxide; (2) **leukocytes,** or white blood cells, which defend the body against bacteria and infections; and (3) **platelets,** or thrombocytes, which are necessary for blood coagulation. Proteins such as serum albumin, globulins, and fibrinogen are also present in the blood.

Plasma may contain thousands of other substances, such as glucose, electrolytes, vitamins, hormones, and waste products. The discussion in this chapter is limited to blood cells, blood proteins, and blood groups (or types).

Blood Cells

Red Blood Cells

Red blood cells (RBCs, erythrocytes) are small and disk shaped. They are the cells present in the largest quantities in the bloodstream, and they have a life span of approximately 120 days. The major function of the red blood cells is to carry hemoglobin. Each **hemoglobin** molecule contains four iron atoms; these four iron atoms combine with four oxygen molecules to transport oxygen from the lungs to the tissues. Hemoglobin can also combine with carbon dioxide and carry it from the cells to the lungs for excretion. It also serves as an acid-base buffering system in whole blood.

After birth, red blood cells are produced by the bone marrow. In early life most bones manufacture the red blood cells, but after 20 years of age most of them are produced in the bone marrow of the vertebrae, sternum, ribs, and ilia.

Males have more hemoglobin in their blood than do females. In general, most men have between 14 and 16 g/dL, whereas women have a range of 12 to 14 g/dL. A person with a hemoglobin count below 10 g/dL is usually diagnosed as having **anemia.** Anemias are classified according to both the size and the number of functional red blood cells in the blood.

Red blood cells are rapidly formed and destroyed in the body. It has been estimated that more than 100 million red blood cells are produced every minute during adulthood. The normal healthy adult has between 4.5 and 5.5 million cells/mm^3 of blood. The body balances the production versus the destruction of these cells to maintain a relatively constant level of red blood cells. The exact mechanism for this is unknown.

It is known that the rate of red blood cell production can be increased if a considerable decrease in red blood cells occurs or if tissue hypoxia develops. In such cases the kidneys are stimulated to increase the secretion of **erythropoietin,** a hormone that acts to stimulate the production of red blood cells by the bone marrow. With maximum bone marrow stimulation, red blood cell production can be increased to nearly seven times over normal.

To make new red blood cells, the bone marrow needs adequate supplies of vitamin B_{12}, iron, and other substances. A deficiency in the absorption of vitamin B_{12} from the gastric tract, which is caused by a lack of intrinsic factor (see Chapter 68), can lead to pernicious anemia.

Anemias can also be induced by increased red cell destruction, which can occur in infections or cancer, or from bone marrow suppression caused by radiation therapy and many cancer chemotherapeutic agents and other drugs (Box 30-1).

Leukocytes

There are five types of leukocytes, which are classified according to the presence or absence of granules in the cell cytoplasm. The granular leukocytes are neutrophils, eosinophils, and basophils; the nongranular leukocytes are lymphocytes and monocytes. The granular leukocytes have two or more nuclear lobes and are therefore referred to as polymorphonuclear leukocytes or "polys."

Under normal circumstances, blood contains between 5000 and 9000 leukocytes per cubic milliliter (Box 30-2). A differential count may be ordered by the physician or health care provider to aid in diagnosis. In acute appendicitis, for example, the percentage of neutrophils increases, as does the total leukocyte count.

Leukocytes are produced primarily in the bone marrow. However, lymphocytes are produced mainly in lymph tis-

BOX 30-1

Drugs That Cause Bone Marrow Depression

amphotericin B, systemic (Fungizone)
antithyroid medications
azathioprine (Imuran)
busulfan (Myleran)
carmustine (BCNU; BiCNU)
chlorambucil (Leukeran)
chloramphenicol (Chloromycetin)
cisplatin (Platinol-AQ)
colchicine
cyclophosphamide (Cytoxan, Procytox ♣)
cytarabine (Ara-C, Cytosar ♣)
dacarbazine (DTIC ♣, DTIC-Dome)
dactinomycin (Actinomycin-D, Cosmegen)
daunorubicin (Cerubidine)
doxorubicin (Adriamycin RDF)
etoposide (VePesid, VP-16)
floxuridine (FUDR)
flucytosine (Ancobon, 5-FC, Ancotil ♣)
fluorouracil, systemic (5-FU, Adrucil)
hydroxyurea (Hydrea)
interferon (Roferon-A, Intron-a)
lomustine (CCNU, CeeNU)
mechlorethamine, systemic (Mustargen, nitrogen mustard)
melphalan (Alkeran, L-PAM)
mercaptopurine (Purinethol)
methotrexate (Mexate)
mitomycin (Mutamycin)
pentamidine (Pentam)
plicamycin (Mithracin, mithramycin)
procarbazine (Matulane, Natulan ♣)
sodium iodide ^{131}I (Iodotope)
sodium phosphate P 32
streptozocin (Zanosar)
thioguanine (Lanvis ♣)
thiotepa (Thioplex)
uracil mustard
vinblastine (Velban, Velbe ♣)
vincristine (Oncovin)
zidovudine (Retrovir)

sues and organs (e.g., the spleen, thymus, tonsils) and in various other lymphoid tissue in the bone marrow, gastrointestinal tract, and elsewhere. Several terms are important to understand. **Leukopenia** refers to an abnormal decrease in the number of leukocytes to fewer than 5000/mm^3; **leukocytosis** refers to an abnormal increase in the number of leukocytes.

Neutrophils, monocytes, lymphocytes, and basophils are very mobile. They can leave the capillaries and migrate to organisms or foreign particles that have entered the body.

BOX 30-2

Differential Normal Leukocyte Count

Neutrophils (polymorphonuclear): 62%
Eosinophils (polymorphonuclear): 2.3%
Basophils (polymorphonuclear): 0.4%
Monocytes: 5.3%
Lymphocytes: 30%

Information from Guyton, A.C., & Hall, J.E. (2000.). *Textbook of medical physiology* (10th ed.). Philadelphia: W.B. Saunders.

Neutrophils and monocytes ingest and destroy the invaders in a process known as **phagocytosis.** Lymphocytes defend the body against bacteria, fungi, and viruses by forming B lymphocytes or T lymphocytes. (See Chapter 62 for an overview of the immune system.)

Eosinophils are considered weak phagocytes and have limited mobility. An increased level of eosinophils is usually seen with allergic reactions or a cell injury caused by parasites (e.g., hookworm).

The life span of granular leukocytes (granulocytes) is estimated to be 4 to 8 hours in the bloodstream and 3 to 5 days in body tissues. If involved in the ingestion of invading organisms, this life span can be reduced to only a few hours, because during this process they are also destroyed. Monocytes also have a short life span in blood, but they can live for months or even years in the body tissues if not destroyed by phagocytosis. Monocytes in the tissues often increase in size to become tissue macrophages, and in this way they often provide a first line of defense against tissue infections.

Platelets

Platelets, or **thrombocytes,** are small, round, or oval colorless cells produced by the bone marrow. They have a life span of 5 to 8 days. A normal platelet level in the blood is between 150,000 and 350,000/mm^3.

Platelets are key substances for blood clotting in the body. If a blood vessel is injured and blood is escaping, platelets quickly congregate at the site and clump together to form a plug and stop the bleeding. If the wound is large, platelets set off a series of chemical reactions within the body to form a clot and seal the injury (Figure 30-1).

Persons with **thrombocytopenia** have a low quantity of platelets. Such persons tend to bleed, and their skin usually displays small purple spots—hence the name thrombocytopenia purpura. Bleeding problems usually do not occur until the platelets decrease to levels below 50,000/mm^3. Thrombocytopenia is often induced by irradiation injury to the bone marrow or from aplasia of the bone marrow induced by specific drugs.

Blood Proteins

The blood contains three major proteins: albumin, globulins, and fibrinogen. **Albumin** is responsible for the osmotic

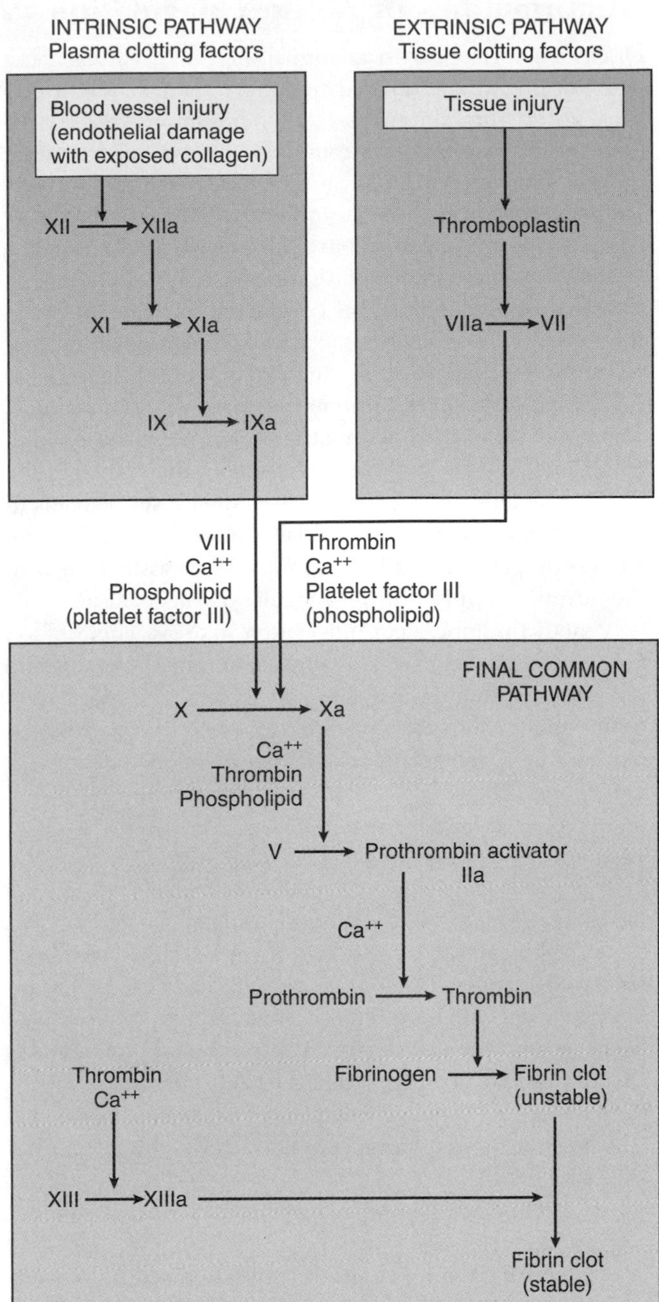

Figure 30-1 Coagulation mechanisms for intrinsic and extrinsic pathways for blood clotting. The final pathway (activation of factor X) is common to both the intrinsic and extrinsic coagulation systems.

pressure gradient produced at the capillary membrane. This prevents plasma fluid from leaving the capillaries to enter the interstitial spaces.

Globulins are divided into alpha, beta, and gamma globulins. Gamma globulin and perhaps beta globulin (to a lesser extent) help to protect the body against infections. Gamma globulin is involved with humoral immunity. Alpha and beta globulins are also believed to perform other functions, such as transporting certain substances in the blood by reversibly combining with them. They may also be a substrate to form other substances.

Fibrinogen, a plasma protein that is converted to fibrin by thrombin in the presence of calcium ions, is necessary for coagulation.

BLOOD COAGULATION

Hemostatic Mechanism

Hemostasis is a process that spontaneously stops the bleeding in damaged blood vessels. Blood is normally fluid while circulating in the vessels, but it rapidly clots at the site of vessel injury.

After any injury to a blood vessel, hemostasis is achieved by three sequential steps: (1) blood vessels constrict to slow blood flow from the injured area, (2) platelet plugs form to temporarily seal the leaking small arteries and veins, and (3) blood coagulates to plug openings within the damaged vessels and wounds to prevent further bleeding.

Blood Vessel Constriction. Vascular constriction occurs as a reflex response immediately after a blood vessel is injured. This response instantly slows the flow of blood from the ruptured vessel.

Platelet Plug Formation. When a blood vessel is injured, the interruption of the continuity of its endothelial lining exposes the collagen (a fibrous protein) in the underlying connective tissue. Platelets immediately adhere to this exposed collagen to form a dense aggregate in a process known as *platelet adhesion*. This attachment triggers the release of adenosine diphosphate (ADP), which causes the outer surface of the platelets to become extremely sticky so that other adjacent platelets adhere to one another at the damaged site. This process eventually forms the platelet plug. This plug is relatively unstable; it can stop bleeding quickly as long as the damage to the vessel is small. For long-term effectiveness the platelet plug must be reinforced with fibrin. This involves a chemical mechanism called blood coagulation.

Coagulation. Blood coagulation is the final stage of a complex series of events in hemostasis. This process ultimately results in the formation of a stable fibrin clot, which is composed of a meshwork of fibrin threads that entraps platelets, blood cells, and plasma. The physical formation of a blood clot or thrombus plays a key role in hemostasis by permanently closing the hole in the injured vessel to prevent further bleeding.

The chemical events in the blood coagulation mechanism involve two distinct pathways: the intrinsic pathway and the extrinsic pathway.

Intrinsic Pathway. Because all the chemical substances involved in coagulation are normally found in the circulating blood, this pathway is referred to as the *intrinsic system of coagulation*. In this pathway the activation of specific blood coagulation factors is initiated by injury to the endothelial lining of the blood vessel wall. When blood contacts the exposed underlying collagen, the Hageman factor (factor XII) is activated by enzymatically converting it to the active form (factor XIIa). The simultaneous damage of platelets also causes the release of platelet phospholipid (platelet factor 3), which is required later in the coagulation process. Factor XIIa then activates factor XI to XIa. The reaction of factor XIa with factor IX requires calcium ions for the formation of activated factor IX. In the presence of calcium ions and platelet phospholipids, factor IXa interacts with factor VIII and thrombin to form a complex. This combination speeds up the activation of factor X. Factor Xa combines with factor V, calcium ions, and platelet phospholipid to form a complex known as the *prothrombin activator (factor IIa)*. Factor IIa initiates the cleavage of prothrombin to form thrombin, which then enzymatically converts fibrinogen into fibrin, forming an unstable clot. The final step involves the action of factor XIII (a fibrin-stabilizing factor), thrombin, and calcium ions, which catalyze the formation of a stronger, stable fibrin clot. (See Figure 30-1 for a summary of the main events of the intrinsic pathway.)

Extrinsic Pathway. The extrinsic pathway is activated by trauma to the vascular wall or to the tissues outside the blood vessels. In this pathway, clotting occurs when products of tissue damage gain access to the blood. The tissue factor thromboplastin is released and becomes part of a complex with factor VII and calcium ions. This combination of components activates factor X, which is the step at which the extrinsic pathway converges with the intrinsic pathway; coagulation then continues through a common route with the resultant formation of a final stable clot. (See Figure 30-1 for the extrinsic pathway; Table 30-1 lists the blood coagulation factors.)

The final pathway, which is common to both the intrinsic and the extrinsic coagulation systems, begins with the activation of factor X and ends with the formation of fibrin. Both systems function simultaneously in the body. The lack of a normal factor in either system will usually result in a blood disorder.

TABLE 30-1 Blood Coagulation Factors and Synonyms

Factor	Name or Synonym
I	Fibrinogen
II	Prothrombin
III	Tissue thromboplastin
IV	Calcium
V	Proaccelerin (labile factor, accelerator globulin)
VII	Proconvertin (stable factor, serum prothrombin conversion accelerator [SPCA])
VIII	Antihemophilic factor (AHF)
IX	Plasma thromboplastin component, Christmas factor
X	Stuart-Prower factor
XI	Plasma thromboplastin antecedent (PTA)
XII	Hageman factor
XIII	Fibrin stabilizing factor

Abnormalities of Blood Coagulation

Diseases associated with abnormally clotting vessels cause many deaths. It is estimated that more than 1 million persons suffer from thrombosis or embolism in the United States each year. Diseases caused by intravascular clotting include some of the major causes of death from cardiovascular sources—coronary occlusion and cerebrovascular accidents. Drugs that inhibit clotting are therefore important.

Local trauma, vascular stasis, and systemic alterations in the coagulability of blood are considered the main factors in the initiation of thrombosis. Basically, coagulation mechanisms are responsible for forming two types of thrombi: arterial thrombi and venous thrombi. Arterial thrombi are most commonly associated with atherosclerotic plaques, high blood pressure, and turbulent blood flow that damages the endothelial lining of the blood vessel and causes platelets to stick and aggregate in the arterial system. Arterial thrombi are mostly platelets, and their formation is associated with the intrinsic pathway of the coagulation mechanism.

Venous thrombi occur most often in areas where blood flow is reduced or static. This appears to initiate clotting and produces a thrombus in the venous system. The formation of thrombi involves the extrinsic pathway of the coagulation mechanism. Current anticoagulants are more effective in preventing venous rather than arterial thrombi.

BLOOD TYPES

Blood type refers to the type of antigen located on red blood cell membranes. Although many antigens have been identified, antigens A, B, and Rh are the most important ones involved with blood transfusions and newborn survival. Every person belongs to one of the four blood groups and is also Rh positive or Rh negative. The ABO blood groups are as follows:

- Type A: A antigen on red blood cells (the plasma has antibody B)
- Type B: B antigen on red blood cells (the plasma has antibody A)
- Type AB: A antigen and B antigen on red blood cells (the plasma contains no antibodies)
- Type O: neither A nor B antigens on red blood cells (the plasma contains A and B antibodies)

Persons with type A blood can safely receive blood from type A and type O donors. Persons with type B blood can safely receive blood from type B and type O donors. People with AB blood are known as the universal recipients because their blood is compatible with types AB, A, B, and O. However, crossmatching of the blood is necessary before transfusion, because other agglutinins may be present. Type O persons can receive only type O blood; they are called universal donors because they can donate blood to anyone. (See Chapter 31 for additional information on blood transfusion.)

A person who is Rh-positive carries the Rh antigen on the red blood cells. A person who is Rh-negative does not have any Rh antigens on the red blood cells. Approximately 85% of the population is Rh-positive. Rh factor is particularly important when an Rh-negative woman is impregnated by an Rh-positive man. The mother may have antibodies against the Rh antigen, which can cross the placenta and attack the fetus should its blood be Rh-positive. If this occurs, the infant may develop jaundice or be dead on delivery.

An Rh-negative woman could acquire Rh antibodies via blood transfusions. It is also possible for her to develop them if fetal blood enters her bloodstream during childbirth or miscarriage. Regardless, the first pregnancy usually has less risk associated with it than subsequent pregnancies because there is less of a chance that the woman has Rh antibodies.

Prescribers can reduce this danger by administering an anti-Rh antibody (Gamulin Rh, RhoGAM, or HypRho-D) to Rh-negative women after each pregnancy. These drugs prevent their systems from making antibodies to Rh-positive blood. Rh-negative women who have a spontaneous or induced abortion or a termination of an ectopic pregnancy of up to and including 12 weeks' gestation are given a microdose of immune globulin (MICRhoGAM or Mini-Gamulin Rh) if the father is Rh-positive.

SUMMARY

The role of blood is to transport cellular requirements and products from one part of the body to another. The continuous exchange between the interstitial fluid and the blood serves to maintain a cellular environment that fluctuates only within narrow limits. An appreciation of the role of blood in maintaining homeostasis in the body is essential.

Critical Thinking Questions

1. Many medications have the adverse effect of depressing bone marrow production of various blood cells. What symptoms would you expect to see if a client had diminished production of platelets? Red blood cells? White blood cells?
2. Mrs. Chandler has type AB blood. At one time individuals with this blood type were considered to be universal recipients. Why was that so? Why might that term be misleading?

Collaborative Learning Activities

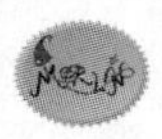

For Collaborative Learning Activities, go to mosby.com/MERLIN/McKenry/.

BIBLIOGRAPHY

Anderson, K.N., Anderson, L.E., & Glanze, W.D. (Eds.). (1998). *Mosby's medical, nursing, & allied health dictionary* (5th ed.). St. Louis: Mosby.

Drug Facts and Comparisons. (2000). St. Louis: Facts and Comparisons.

Guyton, A.C. & Hall, J. E. (2000). *Textbook of medical physiology* (10th ed.). Philadelphia: W.B. Saunders.

Guyton, A.C. & Hall, J. E. (1996.). *Human physiology and the mechanism of disease* (6th ed.). Philadelphia: W.B. Saunders.

Thibodeau, G. & Patton, K. (1998). *Anatomy and physiology* (4th ed.). St. Louis: Mosby.

United States Pharmacopeia Dispensing Information (USP DI): Drug information for the health care professional (19th ed.). (1999). Rockville, MD: United States Pharmacopeial Convention.

Van Wynsberghe, D., Noback, C.R., & Carola, R. (1995). *Human anatomy and physiology* (3rd ed.). New York: McGraw-Hill.

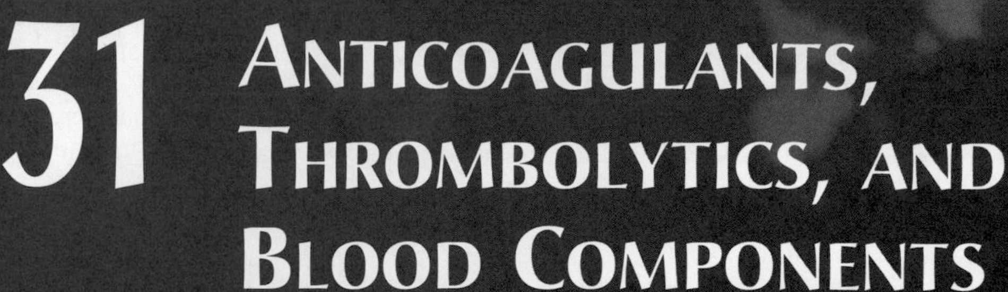

31 Anticoagulants, Thrombolytics, and Blood Components

Chapter Focus

Blood affects every body system because it transports gases, nutrients, metabolic wastes, blood cells, immune cells, and hormones throughout the body. The nurse must manage the client's therapeutic regimen for anticoagulants, thrombolytics, and blood components effectively to ensure the most positive outcome possible for clients with a wide variety of illnesses and injuries.

Learning Objectives

1. Identify the disease processes that require the administration of drugs to inhibit clotting.
2. Differentiate between the mechanisms of action of parenteral and oral anticoagulant agents.
3. Implement the nursing management of the care of a client with anticoagulant therapy.
4. Discuss the use of protamine sulfate and vitamin K as anticoagulant antagonists.
5. Differentiate between the actions of thrombolytic and anticoagulant drugs on blood clots.
6. Discuss drugs that may be successfully used in treating hemophilia.
7. Implement the nursing management of the care of a client receiving blood components.

Key Terms

embolus, p. 621
fibrinolytic activity, p. 633
hemophilia, p. 638
thrombolytic drugs, p. 633
thrombus, p. 621

Key Drugs [✓]

heparin, p. 622
streptokinase, p. 633
warfarin, p. 629

This chapter reviews the drugs and substances that affect hemostasis or blood clotting, preformed thrombi, and blood administration. Normal blood clotting is a defense mechanism constantly available for protection against excessive hemorrhage. However, the development of a thrombus in a blood vessel can obstruct blood flow and cause an infarction with resultant tissue necrosis. A **thrombus** is an aggregation of platelets, fibrin, clotting factors, and the cellular elements of the blood that becomes attached to the inner wall of a blood vessel—a blood clot. An **embolus**, a mass of undissolved matter that breaks off from the thrombus, can travel in the blood vessel and lodge in areas of the body; this can cause death. By contrast, a defect in the blood clotting mechanism may lead to excessive bleeding or hemorrhage, even after a minor injury. Both thrombotic and hemorrhagic disorders can be treated with drugs. The following discussion describes the rationale for the use of various groups of therapeutic agents.

Pregnancy Safety
Anticoagulants, Thrombolytics, and Blood Components

Category	Drug
B	aprotinin, clopidogrel, dalteparin, danaparoid, dipyridamole, enoxaparin, eptifibatide, lepirudin, ticlopidine, tranexamic acid, urokinase
C	abciximab, alteplase, aminocaproic acid, anagrelide, anistreplase, antiinhibitor coagulant complex, antithrombin III, ardeparin, cilostazol, factor IX, heparin, protamine, reteplase, streptokinase, tirofiban

Pregnancy safety has not been established for warfarin and anisindione, but they both cross the placenta and should not be used during pregnancy.

ANTICOAGULANT DRUGS

Anticoagulant drug therapy is primarily prophylactic because these agents act by preventing (1) fibrin deposits, (2) extension of a thrombus, and (3) thromboembolic complications. Although long-term anticoagulant therapy remains controversial, there is evidence that such therapy reduces the incidence of thrombosis and therefore prolongs life.

Anticoagulant therapy is directed toward preventing intravascular thrombosis by decreasing blood coagulability. This therapy has no direct effect on a blood clot that has already formed or on ischemic tissue injured by an inadequate blood supply because of the clot. The two main groups of anticoagulant drugs are (1) parenteral anticoagulant drugs, and (2) oral anticoagulant drugs. For effective anticoagulant therapy, the manner of use for both groups is important. They have been used to complement each other, and in some instances the administration of both a rapidly acting parenteral anticoagulant (heparin) and one of the synthetic oral anticoagulants is started simultaneously. Heparin is usually discontinued as soon as the prothrombin time has been sufficiently increased and the oral compound is producing a full therapeutic effect.

■ Nursing Management
Anticoagulant Therapy

The role of the nurse with the client receiving anticoagulant therapy is primarily one of assessing the client for altered protection related to the increased tendency for bleeding and educating the client for the safe and accurate self-administration of the particular anticoagulant agent.

■ **Assessment.** Before initiating anticoagulation therapy, the client should be assessed for any preexisting health conditions that would contraindicate anticoagulation or would indicate the need for caution in the use of anticoagulant therapy. Anticoagulation is contraindicated in instances in which bleeding would be imminently life threatening, such as threatened abortion, cerebral or aortic aneurysm, cerebrovascular hemorrhage, active hemorrhage, severe hypertension, hemophilia, thrombocytopenia, pericarditis, and recent or contemplated ophthalmic surgery or neurosurgery.

Caution is required if the client has any of the following conditions in which an increased risk of hemorrhage is present: recent childbirth; severe diabetes; severe renal function impairment; severe trauma, especially to the central nervous system (CNS); severe vasculitis; and active ulcers or lesions of the gastrointestinal, genitourinary, or respiratory tract.

Be concerned if the client has any condition that might increase the response to anticoagulant therapy, such as visceral carcinoma, severe hepatic impairment, and vitamin C or K deficiency; or if the client is to undergo a procedure that presents the risk of bleeding and a risk for injury, such as regional or lumbar block anesthesia or spinal puncture. (See the Pregnancy Safety box above for Food and Drug Administration [FDA] classifications of the various anticoagulant agents.)

The client's current medication regimen should be reviewed for significant drug interactions. In addition to the specific drug interactions listed within the discussion of heparin and the oral anticoagulants, consider that the risk of hemorrhage may be increased by the concurrent use of any medication that inhibits platelet aggregation or causes hypoprothrombinemia, thrombocytopenia, or gastrointestinal ulcers.

The appropriate laboratory tests to determine coagulation times, as well as a hematocrit and complete blood count (CBC), including platelets, should be performed before the initiation of anticoagulant therapy.

■ **Nursing Diagnosis.** The client receiving anticoagulant therapy is at risk for ineffective tissue perfusion (cardiopulmonary, cerebral, gastrointestinal, peripheral, renal) related to the client's underlying condition, and the potential complication of hemorrhage and excessive bruising related to the anticoagulant effect of the drugs.

▪ Implementation

▪ *Monitoring.* The nurse needs to remain vigilant to the early signs of bleeding in a client who is receiving anticoagulant therapy. The client should be assessed for signs of overdose, such as ecchymosis, petechiae, hematomas, nosebleeds, and unusual bleeding from gums, cuts, wounds, and tube insertion sites. Internal bleeding will reveal itself as abdominal pain or swelling, backache, bloody or black tarry stools, dizziness, headache, hematemesis, hematuria, hemoptysis, or joint pain. The client's urine and stool should be checked periodically for occult blood.

Laboratory values should be monitored before the drug is administered to ensure that the client's values are in the therapeutic, not the dangerous, range.

For heparin, the activated partial thromboplastin time (APTT) and/or the activated clotting time (ACT) is used to measure the effect of the drug on clotting; for the oral anticoagulants, prothrombin time (PT) or International Normalized Ratio (INR) determinations are used. These tests report the value in seconds along with the control value in seconds. The control value may vary somewhat from day to day because the reagents used may vary. Some laboratories report the values as ratios or percentages of normal activity, because the client's results are compared with the control. Normally the client's value is 85% to 100% without anticoagulation. In anticoagulant therapy the goal is to prevent thrombus formation, and therefore the therapeutic range desired is higher than the control, a prolonged coagulation time. For thromboembolic prevention, the therapeutic range for the APTT is 1.5 to 2.5 times the control value in seconds, for the ACT it is 2 to 3 times, and for the PT it is 1.3 to 1.5 times (INR 2.0 to 3.0).

▪ *Intervention.* The dosage of anticoagulants is individualized and adjusted according to the appropriate laboratory test.

▪ *Education.* Clients need to recognize and report the signs of bleeding: excessive bruising, bleeding gums, nosebleeds, cuts that do not stop bleeding, red or brown urine, and red or black bowel movements. Instruct the client to use a soft toothbrush for oral hygiene and an electric razor to shave and to avoid activities that have a potential for injury. Female clients who have a heavy menstrual flow should be cautioned, but treatment is not contraindicated unless the bleeding is excessive. Advise the client to alert any other health care providers, such as dentists, that an anticoagulant is being taken. A medical alert bracelet or card should be carried. The client should not take medications containing ibuprofen, aspirin, and other salicylates while receiving anticoagulant therapy. Instruct the client in how to read labels for over-the-counter (OTC) drugs that may contain these products.

In addition, nonpharmacologic measures should be reinforced with the client. The client should avoid wearing constrictive clothing, crossing legs at the knees, sitting or standing for long periods of time, or putting pressure on ischemic areas. Smoking cessation, regular exercise, and injury prevention should also be encouraged. The client should limit alcohol consumption to no more than an occasional drink or two. Encourage the client to have a normal, balanced diet and not to change dietary patterns radically or to take vitamins or dietary supplements without consulting the prescriber because of the possibility of altering the effect of anticoagulant therapy by changing the intake of vitamin K. Stress the importance of follow-up visits to the health care provider for laboratory testing and clinical monitoring.

▪ Evaluation. The expected outcome of anticoagulant therapy is that appropriate coagulation testing will show values in the therapeutic range. In addition, the client will not show any signs or symptoms of bleeding or thrombus formation.

Parenteral Anticoagulant Drugs

✔ heparin [hep′ a rin] (Hepalean ♣)

Heparin is formed in especially large amounts in the mast cells of the liver, lungs, and intestinal mucosa. The source of heparin for injection is bovine lung and the mucosal lining of pig intestines. It is a rapidly acting, injectable anticoagulant.

Heparin produces its anticoagulant effect by combining with antithrombin III (heparin cofactor), a naturally occurring anticlotting factor in the plasma. This compound is unrelated to factor III (tissue thromboplastin), a factor in the process of blood coagulation. The binding of heparin with antithrombin III forms a complex that acts at multiple sites in the normal coagulation system, inactivating factors IXa, Xa, XIa, and XIIa. Inactivation of factor Xa of the intrinsic and extrinsic pathways prevents the conversion of prothrombin to thrombin, thereby inhibiting the formation of fibrin from fibrinogen. Furthermore, by preventing the activation of factor XIII (fibrin stabilizing factor), heparin also prevents the formation of a stable fibrin clot. Because fibrin is associated with venous thrombi, heparin is useful in preventing venous thrombosis. Heparin does not have fibrinolytic activity; it will not dissolve existing clots but can prevent the extension of existing clots.

The normal function of antithrombin III is to maintain intravascular fluidity of the blood. Thromboembolism commonly occurs in individuals with acquired or congenital deficiency of this plasma protein. In the absence of antithrombin III, heparin is unable to perform its anticoagulating effect.

Heparin is used to prevent and treat all types of thromboses and emboli. It is used prophylactically to prevent blood clotting in surgery of the heart or blood vessels, during blood transfusion, in clients with disseminated intravascular coagulation (DIC), and in the hemodialysis process. It is considered the drug of choice for sudden arterial occlusion, because its action is immediate and can be readily reversed if surgery is necessary.

Heparin is superior to the coumarin drugs in preventing pulmonary complications in cases of thrombophlebitis. It is also preferred for the treatment of thrombophlebitis during pregnancy, because it does not cross the placental barrier and is not excreted in breast milk. When rapid anticoagulation is necessary, it is used before the oral anticoagulants (Table 31-1).

Heparin is administered via the parenteral route of administration because its large molecular size and polarity prevent any gastrointestinal absorption. The onset of action of the IV injection is immediate. An SC injection usually results in an onset of action within 20 to 60 minutes. The half-life is dose dependent but averages 1.5 hours (range: 1 to 6 hours). This drug is highly protein bound, metabolized in the liver, and excreted by the kidneys.

See Table 31-2 for the side effects/adverse reactions of heparin.

The dosage of heparin is expressed in USP heparin units/mL in the United States. In Canada, the dosage is expressed in USP units or in International Units (IU). USP heparin units are not equivalent to International Units. Because the potency may vary between USP and IU, the student should review the current package insert for dosage instructions whenever packages are labeled in International Units. The recommended dosages in the following paragraphs are given in USP units.

The adult dosage for heparin sodium is 10,000 to 20,000 USP units SC or 10,000 USP units IV initially, then 5,000 to 10,000 units IV every 4 to 6 hours. The pediatric dosage is usually 50 USP units/kg IV initially, followed by 50 to 100 units/kg IV every 4 hours.

The dosage of heparin is closely monitored with coagulation tests (e.g., APTT, ACT) or other tests as ordered. For consistency, it is recommended that a single laboratory be used to monitor a client undergoing heparin therapy.

TABLE 31-1 Anticoagulant Drugs: Comparison of Characteristics

	Heparin	Coumarins/ Indanediones
Onset of action	Immediate	Slow (24 to 48 hours)
Route of administration	Parenteral	Oral
Duration of action	Short (less than 4 hours)	Long (approximately 2 to 5 days)
Laboratory test for dosage control	APTT, ACT	Prothrombin time, INR
Antidote	Protamine sulfate	Vitamin K, whole blood, or plasma

TABLE 31-2 Anticoagulant Drugs: Side Effects/Adverse Reactions

Drug	Side Effects*	Adverse Reactions†
heparin		Less common or rare reactions: chest pain, chills, elevated temperature, respiratory difficulties, wheezing, rash, pruritus, hives, increase in nasal secretions (allergic reaction), anaphylaxis, paresthesia of the hands or feet, blue tinge on arms or legs, increased or persistent erections, thrombocytopenia Early signs of overdose: increased bruising; nosebleeds; excessive bleeding from minor cuts, wounds, brushing of teeth, or menstrual period Signs of internal bleeding: stomach pain or swelling; backaches; bloody urine; bloody or black stools; dizziness; severe, persistent headaches; swollen, stiff, or painful joints; vomiting or coughing up of blood Following 6 months or more of therapy: rib or back pain,* height decrease (osteoporosis), alopecia At site of injection: hematoma or blood accumulation under the skin, pain, local skin reaction such as irritation, peeling, or sloughing
anisindione		Although not yet reported with this drug, the following effects were reported with phenindione, another indanedione derivative, and may also be seen with this product: edema of the face or lower extremities, unexpected weight gain, leukopenia, agranulocytosis, liver toxicity, diarrhea, nausea, vomiting, severe abdominal distress
warfarin	Less frequent: alopecia	Less frequent or rare: leukopenia, nausea, vomiting, abdominal cramps or distress

*Inform the prescriber if side effects continue, increase, or disturb the client.
†Contact the prescriber if adverse reactions occur, because medical intervention may be necessary.

■ Nursing Management

Heparin Therapy

In addition to the following discussion, see Nursing Management: Anticoagulant Therapy, p. 621.

■ **Assessment.** The client should be assessed to determine that heparin is not contraindicated by preexisting conditions, such as those listed in the discussion of the nursing management of anticoagulant therapy. Caution must be used in administering heparin to clients who have any condition in which hemorrhage is possible. Clients over the age of 60, especially women, are more susceptible to the hemorrhagic effects of heparin. Heparin is the anticoagulant of choice for use during pregnancy because it does not cross the placenta and affect clotting mechanisms in the fetus. Because of the risk of maternal bleeding, it is used with caution only in the last trimester of pregnancy and during the postpartum period.

A baseline assessment should consist of an APTT, a platelet count, and a hematocrit evaluation. Anticipate that each dose of heparin will be individualized after the prescriber has evaluated the APTT or provided a sliding scale or protocol by which specific doses will be administered based on the laboratory values. Check to be sure that these tests are performed as ordered (before each IV or SC injection or daily) and that the results are reported promptly. If no dosage adjustments have been required for 2 weeks, further monitoring need not be as frequent. The exception is pregnant women, who need to be monitored throughout therapy because heparin requirements increase as the client's blood volume increases with the progression of pregnancy.

Review the client's current medication regimen for the risk of significant drug interactions, such as those that may occur when heparin is given concurrently with the following drugs:

Drug	Possible Effect and Management
Bold/color type indicates the most serious interactions.	
aspirin, sulfinpyrazone (Anturane), nonsteroidal antiinflammatory drugs (NSAIDs), or other platelet aggregation inhibitors	There is an increased risk of bleeding because of platelet inhibition by these drugs. Large doses of aspirin may also produce hypoprothrombinemia. All drugs increase the risk of toxicity because of their potential to produce gastrointestinal ulceration and bleeding. Avoid concurrent use or a potentially serious drug interaction may occur.
cefamandole (Mandol), cefoperazone (Cefobid), cefotetan (Cefotan), plicamycin (Mithramycin), or valproic acid (Depakene)	There is an increased risk of bleeding and hemorrhage possible with these drugs. These agents can cause hypoprothrombinemia. In addition, plicamycin and valproic acid inhibit platelet aggregation. Avoid concurrent use or a potentially serious drug interaction may occur.
methimazole (Tapazole), or propylthiouracil (PTU)	May produce a hypoprothrombinemic effect that can increase the anticoagulant effect of heparin. Avoid concurrent use or a potentially serious drug interaction may occur. If necessary to give concurrently, monitor closely for bleeding.
probenecid (Benemid)	May prolong and enhance the anticoagulant effects of heparin. Avoid concurrent use or a potentially serious drug interaction may occur. If necessary to give concurrently, monitor coagulation tests closely.
thrombolytics, such as alteplase, anistreplase, streptokinase, or urokinase	There is an increased risk of bleeding and hemorrhage possible with this combination. Avoid concurrent use or a potentially serious drug interaction may occur. Some studies indicate that heparin may be given with low doses of thrombolytic agents via the intracoronary route of administration. Heparin may be also be administered before or after thrombolytic therapy.

■ **Nursing Diagnosis.** With the administration of heparin, clients are at risk for the following nursing diagnoses/collaborative problems: ineffective tissue perfusion related to the underlying condition and ineffectiveness of the drug; risk for injury related to increased bleeding tendencies; impaired comfort such as irritation, pain, or redness at the injection site related to parenteral administration; disturbed body image related to unusual hair loss (long-term therapy); and the potential complications of allergic reaction, thrombocytopenia, and osteoporosis with long-term therapy. The Nursing Care Plan on p. 625 lists other selected nursing diagnoses for clients receiving anticoagulant therapy.

■ Implementation

■ ***Monitoring.*** Adjust the dosage of heparin to maintain the APTT between 1.5 and 2.5 times normal control level and the ACT between 2 and 3 times the control value, while observing that the client remains free of signs of hemorrhage as discussed in the section on the nursing management of anticoagulant therapy. Any value under or over this range should be reported to the prescriber immediately.

Test stools and urine for occult blood daily to determine hidden bleeding. Monitor the platelet count for any possible thrombocytopenia, which may be associated with arterial thrombosis or "white clot" syndrome. Perform hematocrit tests at frequent intervals.

There is the possibility of "heparin resistance" in conditions associated with infection, thrombophlebitis, fever, pleurisy, cancer, myocardial infarction, and extensive surgery. In addition, be aware that the abrupt withdrawal of heparin may precipitate an increase in coagulability; a full dose of heparin is usually followed by oral anticoagulants for

Nursing Care Plan
Selected Nursing Diagnoses for Clients Receiving Anticoagulant Therapy

Nursing Diagnosis	Outcome Criteria	Nursing Interventions
Ineffective tissue perfusion: reduced blood flow (prevention and treatment of thromboembolic disorders)	Clotting studies are maintained within therapeutic range; APTT is prolonged to 1.5-2.5 times the control (heparin). PT is prolonged to 1.5-2.5 times the control (warfarin) (INR 2.0-3.0). Extension of the thrombus or embolization of thrombi does not occur.	Monitor clotting studies as ordered. Administer anticoagulant therapy and assess effectiveness. Monitor vital signs and blood pressure every 4 hours. Report immediately any change in vital signs or a decrease in blood pressure. Ausculate breath sounds every 4 hours. Report the development of rales. In addition, assess for other developments of pulmonary emboli, such as dyspnea, cough, or hemoptysis. Apply antiembolism stockings as ordered. Measure calf dimension bilaterally; compare and record every 8 hours.
Risk for injury: hemorrhage	No signs of hemorrhage occur.	Administer SC heparin rather than IM heparin to prevent hematoma formation. Inject into lower abdomen using a small-gauge needle (25-27); do not massage injection sites. Rotate sites. All personnel should be alerted that the client is receiving anticoagulant therapy. Venipunctures and injections should be kept to a minimum and pressure applied to prevent bleeding when they are performed. Observe the client for excessive bruising; bleeding gums; nosebleed; blood in urine, feces, and/or secretions; report any findings.
Deficient knowledge related to medication regimen	Client will describe the underlying condition, how the drug relates to the condition, how and when to take the medication, common drug interactions, safety precautions, common side effects, and which side effects warrant reporting. Client will self-administer warfarin safely and accurately.	Assess learning needs and learning readiness. Plan with the client for the achievement of realistic goals. Provide information to meet outcome criteria. Caution the client to use a soft toothbrush and an electric razor. Recommended to the client that all health care personnel be informed of anticoagulant therapy before treatment. Advise the client on the importance of having blood studies performed as ordered. Instruct the client on the need to report any signs of bleeding.

prophylaxis. Thus there generally is an overlap of both drugs for 3 to 5 days while the heparin is being tapered off.

■ ***Intervention.*** Heparin comes in many concentrations: carefully check the vial and the prescriber's order. Errors have been known to occur between the vials of 1000 USP units/mL and 10,000 USP units/mL, as well as between the vials of 2500 USP units/mL and 25,000 USP units/mL; watch the decimal points. Be alert, too, that the heparin-lock flush solution maintains the patency of the indwelling venipuncture unit and that the solution is not used for systemic anticoagulation. The nurse working with premature neonates should be aware that some heparin sodium injections contain benzyl alcohol as a preservative; these preparations should not be administered to these infants. Clients with a history of allergies or asthma should receive a test dose of 1000 USP units of heparin before treatment is initiated, because heparin is derived from animal tissue.

For SC administration, use the smallest gauge (25 to 27) ⅜- to ⅝-inch needle to prevent hematoma at the injection site. Use a "bunching" technique (pull the fatty layer away from the underlying tissue). Inject the heparin deep into the fatty tissue above the iliac crest or into the abdominal fat layer. Avoid the umbilical veins by avoiding a 2-inch radius around the umbilicus. This distance should also be maintained from scars and lesions. Do not aspirate, and *do not massage the injection site.* Hold the needle in place for 10 seconds after administration, and withdraw it gently to minimize bruising. Apply direct pressure for 1 to 2 minutes if needed. Rotate sites to prevent the formation of hematomas.

Document the location of injection sites graphically. IM administration is not recommended because it causes hematomas, irritation, and pain at the injection site and causes erratic absorption.

With IV administration, a loading dose usually precedes a continuous infusion, or heparin may be administered intermittently via a heparin lock. This IV dose may be given undiluted over at least 1 minute. Many clinicians prefer continuous IV infusions for the administration of heparin because it provides a more constant blood level of the drug and because the risk for bleeding complications is decreased. For continuous IV infusion of heparin, use an infusion pump or a volume control unit so the flow rate and fluid volume of the drug can be controlled precisely. Check the system frequently to prevent overdose or underdose. Never add other drugs to the heparin infusion or piggyback other drugs into an IV line containing heparin, because many other drugs inactivate heparin.

For clients receiving intermittent doses of heparin—either subcutaneously or by heparin lock—the blood samples for the APTT should be drawn 30 minutes before each dose to avoid a falsely high APTT. This false reading can also be avoided for the client with a continuous heparin infusion by drawing the sample from the arm opposite the infusion site.

Although controversy exists in clinical practice regarding whether normal saline or diluted heparin solutions (10 to 100 units of heparin sodium/mL) should be used to irrigate and maintain patency of an indwelling venipuncture device, be aware that the purpose of the device is to maintain an open IV line so that intermittent bolus doses of drugs, IV solutions, or both may be administered through this line. The Nursing Research box below discusses research comparing heparinized vs. nonheparinized IV lines. Obtain information within each clinical practice setting about the ac-

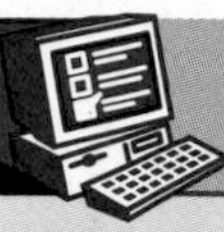

Nursing Research

Heparinized vs. Nonheparinized Intravascular Lines

Throughout the country in recent years, controversy has developed regarding the use of heparinized saline as opposed to normal saline as a flush solution in intermittent IV sets in acute-care settings. The question centers around whether heparin mixed in variable dilutions in saline is necessary to maintain the patency of an IV site used for intermittent infusions (McMullen et al., 1993). Peterson and Kirshhoff (1991) performed an analysis of the research about heparinized vs. nonheparinized intravascular lines and concluded that there is no significant difference in the duration of patency between intravascular catheters flushed with saline solution and those flushed with a heparinized solution. Many hospitals have decided to change their practice given the cost savings of discontinuing the use of heparin, as well as client well-being in the prevention of heparin-related complications (McAllister et al., 1993). However, the Intravenous Nursing Standards of Practice established by the Intravenous Nurses' Society supports the use of heparinized saline as the accepted solution for the maintenance of intermittent IV locks (Fry, 1992).

A large-scale multicenter trial has found that heparin does make a difference in keeping arterial pressure monitoring lines open, although other factors are also important (American Association of Critical Care Nurses, 1990). In the 3-year "Thunder Project" conducted by the American Association of Critical Care Nurses, clinicians at 198 institutions randomly assigned 5139 individuals on arterial pressure monitoring lines to flush solutions with or without heparin. Lines stayed clear more often when heparin was used—94% vs. 88% of nonheparinized lines—and were more likely to remain clear over time. Several other variables figured into whether lines stayed patent. Lines were more likely to stay clear among clients receiving other anticoagulants or thrombolytics than among clients receiving no anticoagulants. Catheters greater than 2 inches in length also enhanced the probability of patency. The researchers also found greater patency in femoral catheters than in other sites. In addition, whether heparinized or not, the lines were slightly more likely to remain open in men.

Interestingly enough, the issue of heparinized vs. nonheparinized (normal saline) flush solutions for maintaining the patency of peripheral intermittant infusion devices (PIIDs) has been reviewed again for neonates and children, and the results have been mixed. In the four double blind studies, two found no significant difference in the effectiveness of heparinized and nonheparinized flush solutions (Heilskov et al., 1998; Kotter, 1996), one found the heparin flush solution to be more effective (Mudge, Forcier & Slattery, 1998), and one found significantly longer catheter longevity with saline (Golberg et al., 1999). Further research appears to be necessary within the pediatric setting.

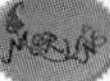

Critical Thinking Questions

- If you were assigned a client with an intermittent IV lock, what would be your preferred flush solution? Why?
- If you were assigned a client with an arterial pressure monitoring line who was intolerant of heparin, what recommendations would you make to maximize its patency?
- If you were assigned a neonatal client with a PIID, what would be your preferred flush solution? Why?

cepted protocol concerning the solution to be used and how often the device should be flushed if not in frequent use; then closely monitor the unit for patency.

If a heparin solution is being used to maintain the patency of an indwelling peripheral venipuncture device, 1 mL of a heparin-lock flush solution is usually effective for 4 to 8 hours. If the device is being used to administer a drug that is incompatible with heparin, it should be flushed with sterile water or 0.9% sodium chloride for injection before and after the drug is administered. Inject the heparin-lock flush solution after the second flush. If the device is being used to obtain blood samples for laboratory analysis and heparin might alter the results of the test, the heparin solution should be cleared from the device by aspirating and discarding 1 mL of solution before the blood sample is taken. After the blood sample is drawn, the device is again filled with 1 mL of heparin-lock flush solution.

Heparin is to be stopped immediately if the client complains of chills, low back pain (a sign of abdominal bleeding), or spontaneous bleeding. Notify the prescriber, and have protamine sulfate on hand. In some cases it may be necessary to administer whole blood or plasma.

Alert other staff members that the client is receiving heparin (i.e., place a sign over the client's bed). Pressure should be applied to venipuncture and injection sites to minimize bruising. These invasive procedures should be avoided if at all possible. Consult the prescriber regarding a change from the IM administration of other drugs to other routes of administration while the client is receiving heparin (see the Case Study box below).

■ ***Education.*** In addition to the client education information discussed in Nursing Management: Anticoagulant Therapy (p. 621), inform the client of the potential for diuresis beginning 36 to 48 hours after the initial dose of heparin and lasting 36 to 48 hours after the termination of therapy.

Advise the client that alopecia may occur several months after the initiation of heparin therapy and that the condition is reversible when the drug is discontinued.

■ **Evaluation.** The expected outcome of heparin therapy is that the client's APTT will show values 1.5 to 2.5 times the control value in seconds or ACT values 2 to 3 times the control value in seconds. In addition, the client will not show evidence of any signs or symptoms of bleeding or thrombus formation.

Low-Molecular-Weight Heparins

The low-molecular-weight (LMW) heparins are new antithrombins that have the potential to be more effective than heparin. They have longer half-lives, require less laboratory monitoring, and are safe and effective for the management of thromboembolic disease (Turpie, 1995). Four LMW heparins are currently on the market: ardeparin, dalteparin, enoxaparin, and tinzaparin.

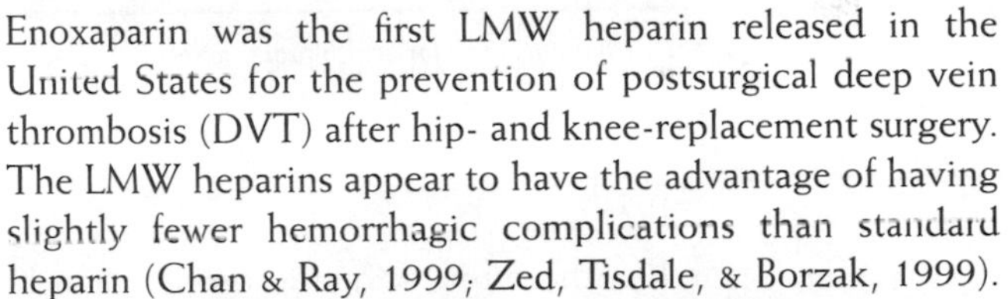

ardeparin [ar de′ pear in] (Normiflo)
dalteparin [dahl′ ta pear in] (Fragmin)
enoxaparin [ee nox′ uh pear in] (Lovenox)
tinzaparin [tinz′ ay pear in] (Innohep)

Enoxaparin was the first LMW heparin released in the United States for the prevention of postsurgical deep vein thrombosis (DVT) after hip- and knee-replacement surgery. The LMW heparins appear to have the advantage of having slightly fewer hemorrhagic complications than standard heparin (Chan & Ray, 1999; Zed, Tisdale, & Borzak, 1999).

LMW heparins are made by chemically processing regular heparin into fragments based on molecular weight. These LMW heparins have a mean molecular weight between 4000 and 6000 daltons, whereas the mean molecular weight of heparin ranges between 12,000 and 15,000 daltons. This difference in molecular weight produces an anticoagulant with considerably different properties than heparin. Both types of heparin can inactivate factor Xa, but

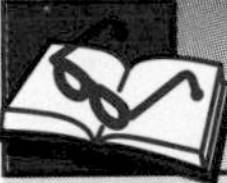

Case Study *The Client with Deep Vein Thrombosis*

John Tucker is a 53-year-old construction worker who has been admitted to the hospital with a diagnosis of DVT of the right leg. Mr. Tucker has experienced increasing pain and swelling of the right lower leg over several days. He has received an IV bolus of 5000 units of heparin followed by a continuous infusion of heparin (25,000 units in 1000 mL of 0.9% sodium chloride).

1. What measures should the nurse implement to ensure accurate administration of the continuous heparin infusion?
2. What data are used by the nurse to evaluate the client's response to the heparin therapy?
3. In preparation for discharge in 4 days, Mr. Tucker is started on warfarin sodium (Coumadin) at the same time he is started on the IV heparin. What is the reason for administering two anticoagulants?
4. The nurse carefully questions Mr. Tucker about his use of OTC medications. He admits to using aspirin for headaches and assorted muscle aches from his job. He also takes a multiple vitamin daily. How should the nurse respond to this information?
5. What additional information does the client need for safe self-administration during anticoagulant therapy?

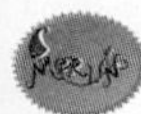

For answer guidelines, go to mosby.com/MERLIN/McKenry/.

TABLE 31-3 Comparison of Regular Heparin and Low-Molecular-Weight Heparin

Properties	Regular Heparin	LMW Heparin
Molecular weight range	3000-30,000	1000-10,000
Mean molecular weight	12,000-15,000	4000-6000
Mechanism of action	Inactivates factor Xa and IIa (thrombin)	Inactivates factor Xa
APTT monitoring required	Yes	No
Inhibits platelet function	++++ (high)	++(medium)
Route of administration	IV, SC	SC only
Protein binding	++++ (high)	+ (low)
Vascular permeability increased	Yes	No
Treatment of drug overdose	Protamine	Protamine

From Salerno E. (1999). *Pharmacology for health professionals*. St. Louis, Mosby.

inactivating factor IIa (thrombin) requires the larger molecular weight heparin. See Table 31-3 for a comparison of heparin and LMW heparins.

The LMW heparins are administered subcutaneously and have a very low protein-binding ratio, therefore their anticoagulant effect is more predictable. Peak serum levels are reached in 2 to 4 hours with ardeparin, 4 hours with dalteparin, and 3 to 5 hours with enoxaparin and tinzaparin. The elimination half-life is 1.2 to 3.3 hours for ardeparin, 3 to 5 hours for dalteparin and tinzaparin, and 3 to 6 hours for enoxaparin. These agents are primarily excreted by the kidneys.

The side effects/adverse reactions of the LMW heparins include local irritation effects such as erythema, hematomas, urticaria, and pain at injection sites. Thrombocytopenia and bleeding episodes may occur less frequently.

The usual adult dosage of ardeparin is 50 anti-factor Xa units/kg SC every 12 hours for up to 2 weeks or until the client is mobile. The usual adult dosage of dalteparin is 25,000 IU SC 1 to 2 hours before abdominal surgery; this is repeated daily for 5 to 10 days afterward until the client is mobile. For hip surgery, the dosage of dalteparin is 5000 IU SC the night before surgery; this is repeated each evening for 5 to 10 days or until the client is mobile. The usual adult dosage of enoxaparin is 30 mg SC twice daily for 7 to 14 days postsurgically, with the first dose administered within 24 hours after surgery. Treatment is continued throughout the postoperative period until the risk for DVT declines. The dosage of tinzaparin for DVT is 175 anti-Xa IU/kg body weight SC once daily for ≥6 days.

The nursing management for the LMW heparin therapy is as for heparin therapy, except that no special monitoring of coagulation times is required.

Miscellaneous Antithrombins

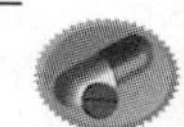

argatroban [are ga troe′ ban] (Acova)
bivalirudin [bye val i rue′ din] (Angiomax)
danaparoid [dan ah′ pa roid] (Orgaran)
lepirudin [le pir′ u din] (Refludan)

This is a miscellaneous group of antithrombin agents that directly inhibit thrombin. For example, argatroban binds to active thrombin sites to inhibit any thrombin-induced processes, such as the formation of fibrin, platelet aggregation, and activation of the coagulation factors (V, VIII, and XIII). Danaparoid is an LMW nonheparin glycosaminoglycan that is derived from porcine intestinal mucosa. This agent inhibits coagulation factor Xa and thrombin, with little effect on blood clotting tests. It is not equivalent in action to heparin or the LMW heparins.

The anticoagulants argatroban and lepirudin are indicated for the treatment and prophylaxis of thrombosis in clients with heparin-induced thrombocytopenia. Bivalirudin is used in individuals with unstable angina undergoing percutaneous transluminal coronary angioplasty (PTCA). Danaparoid is indicated for the prevention of postoperative DVT and pulmonary thromboembolism, especially in individuals undergoing hip replacement surgery.

Side effects/adverse reactions include bleeding events such as hematuria, a decrease in hemoglobin, and hemoptysis, as well as nonbleeding episodes of dyspnea, hypotension, elevated temperature, nausea, vomiting, diarrhea, and cardiac irregularities.

The dosage and administration for this drug group is very specific and detailed. Refer to current literature for instructions.

The nursing management of the miscellaneous antithrombin agents is the same as for the nursing management of LMW heparins.

Parenteral Anticoagulant Antagonist

protamine sulfate [proe′ ta meen] (Heparin Antidote)

Protamine sulfate, a proteinlike substance derived from the sperm and mature testes of salmon and other fish, is an antidote for a heparin overdose. Protamine is a very weak anticoagulant alone; however, when it is given in conjunction with heparin a combination is formed that dissociates the heparin–antithrombin III complex, thus reducing the anticoagulant action of heparin. Because protamine is a basic protein (has many free amino groups), it is able to combine with and inactivate the sulfuric acids of heparin.

Protamine is indicated for the treatment of a severe heparin overdose that has resulted in hemorrhaging. Blood transfusions may be necessary. Protamine is also used to neutralize the effects of heparin administered during dialysis or cardiac or arterial surgery.

When administered intravenously, protamine has an onset of action within 30 to 60 seconds, with a duration of effect of usually 2 hours.

When protamine is administered too rapidly, respiratory difficulties, bradycardia, and a sudden hypotensive effect may result. Less often reported are bleeding (caused by protamine overdose or a rebound of heparin activity), hypertension, anaphylaxis, back pain, a feeling of warmth and/or tiredness, flushing, nausea, or vomiting. Coughing spells, facial edema, or rash also occur and should be reported to the prescriber immediately.

Protamine is administered by slow IV injection at a rate of 1 mg/min. One milligram of protamine is necessary to neutralize approximately 100 USP units of heparin. It is recommended that not more than 50 mg of protamine be given in any 10-minute period and that no more than 100 mg be administered over a 2-hour period. Close monitoring with blood coagulation tests is required.

■ **Nursing Management**

Protamine Sulfate Therapy

■ **Assessment.** Protamine is used as an antidote to severe heparin overdose (including the LMW heparins) as evidenced by frank hemorrhaging or abnormally high values on the APTT or ACT. It is not used in instances of minor heparin overdose, which can be treated by withholding the doses of heparin. Ascertain that the client has not had a previous allergic reaction to protamine.

■ **Nursing Diagnosis.** The client receiving protamine sulfate is at risk for the following nursing diagnoses/collaborative problems: ineffective tissue perfusion and deficient fluid volume related to the underlying hemorrhage; impaired comfort (back pain, feelings of warmth and flushing, and nausea or vomiting); and the potential complications of cardiovascular collapse related to too rapid administration, anaphylaxis, bleeding related to protamine overdose or rebound heparin activity, and pulmonary edema.

■ **Implementation**

■ ***Monitoring.*** Frequent assessment of the client's vital signs, as well as some estimation of blood loss, is essential. An ACT, APTT, or thrombin time (TT) should be performed 5 to 15 minutes after the initial administration of protamine as an antidote for heparin and repeated as needed. APTT and TT may not be useful in monitoring protamine therapy after the administration of enoxaparin, because it does not alter the results of these tests in therapeutic doses. Observe the client for spontaneous bleeding or heparin "rebound" (the effects of heparin last longer than the effects of protamine) after procedures involving extracorporeal circulation such as cardiac or arterial surgery or dialysis. This may occur as long as 18 hours after the initial neutralization of the heparin.

■ ***Intervention.*** Protamine sulfate should be administered by a physician. It should be administered slowly intravenously—over 1 to 3 minutes—not more than 50 mg in any 10-minute period. Too rapid administration may cause injury, dyspnea, and shock. Emergency equipment should be available.

■ **Evaluation.** The expected outcome of protamine sulfate therapy is that the client will not evidence bleeding, the hemoglobin and hematocrit will stabilize, and the APTT or ACT will be within normal, or therapeutic, limits.

Oral Anticoagulant Drugs

There are two major types of oral anticoagulant drugs: coumarins and indanediones.

Coumarins

warfarin [war' far in] (Coumadin ◆)

Indanediones

anisindione [an iss in dye' one] (Miradon)

Both the coumarin and the indanedione derivatives interfere with liver synthesis of the vitamin K–dependent clotting factors. Thus they depress the synthesis of factors X, IX, VII, and II (prothrombin). Factor VII is depleted quickly; the sequential depletion of factors IX, X, and II follows. These agents do not affect established clots but do prevent further extension of formed clots, thereby diminishing the potential for secondary thromboembolic complications.

The oral anticoagulant drugs are used for the prophylaxis and treatment of DVT and pulmonary thromboembolism. They are also used for the prophylaxis of thromboembolism associated with chronic atrial fibrillation or myocardial infarction. The major advantages of these drugs are that they are effective orally and need to be given only once daily after the maintenance dosage has been established.

All the oral anticoagulants are absorbed well from the gastrointestinal tract. Oral anticoagulants are highly protein bound (99%), metabolized in the liver, and excreted by the kidneys. Table 31-4 provides additional information on the pharmacokinetics of these drugs.

The side effects/adverse reactions of the oral anticoagulant drugs include alopecia, anorexia, abdominal cramps or distress, leukopenia, nausea, vomiting, diarrhea, purple toes syndrome (rare), and kidney damage (rare). Fetal abnormalities and facial anomalies of newborns have been reported following use of the drug during pregnancy. If an anticoagulant is necessary during pregnancy, LMW heparins are the drugs of choice (Chan & Ray, 1999).

TABLE 31-4 Oral Anticoagulants: Pharmacokinetics and Dosage and Administration

Generic/Trade Name	Onset of Action (days)	Duration of Action (days)	Half-life (days)	Dosage and Administration
Coumarins				
warfarin (Coumadin)	0.5-3	2-5	1.5-2.5	Adult: 10-15 mg PO for 2-4 days; then 2-10 mg daily as indicated by PT or INR tests Injectable dosage form: same dosage as oral
Indanediones				
anisindione (Miradon)	2-3	1-3	3-5	Adult: 25-250 mg PO daily as indicated by PT

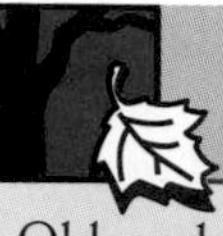

Special Considerations for Older Adults
Anticoagulants

Older adults may be more susceptible to the effects of anticoagulants, such as warfarin (Coumadin); thus a lower maintenance dosage is usually recommended for older adults along with very close supervision and monitoring.

The primary adverse effects of excessive drug use are prolonged bleeding from the gums when brushing the teeth or from small shaving cuts, excessive or easy skin bruising, blood in the urine or stools, and unexplained nosebleeds. These may be early signs of overdose that indicate the need for medical intervention.

Caution clients to carry an identification card indicating the use of an anticoagulant. Remind the client to always consult his or her prescriber before starting any new drug (including OTC medications and vitamins), when changing a medication dose, or when discontinuing any drug product. Many medications can change the effects of an anticoagulant in the body.

Be aware that the administration of concurrent drug therapy that may induce gastric irritation increases the risk for gastrointestinal bleeding. Drugs such as the NSAIDs (e.g., ibuprofen or indomethacin) that are commonly prescribed for older adults often cause gastrointestinal effects.

Alcohol consumption can alter the effect of anticoagulants in the body. Clients should be instructed to avoid alcohol or at the least limit their daily alcohol intake to one drink per day. Alcohol may cause liver damage, which increases the individual's sensitivity to anticoagulants (*USP DI,* 1999.)

The nurse should be aware that diet can interfere with the effects of anticoagulants. In a previously stabilized person, vitamin C deficiency, chronic malnutrition, diarrhea, or other illnesses may result in an increased anticoagulant effect. In contrast, an increased intake of green leafy vegetables (e.g., broccoli, cabbage, collard greens, lettuce, spinach) or the consumption of a nutritional supplement or multiple vitamin containing vitamin K can result in decreased effectiveness of the anticoagulant.

See Table 31-4 for the dosage and administration of the oral anticoagulant drugs.

■ Nursing Management

Oral Anticoagulant Therapy

In addition to the following discussion, see Nursing Management: Anticoagulant Therapy, p. 621.

■ **Assessment.** The client should be assessed for health conditions for which oral anticoagulant therapy is contraindicated or for which the client might be at risk for adverse reactions. (Review the assessment content within the discussion of the nursing management of anticoagulant therapy.) Before initiating therapy, inquire if client is pregnant, and inform her of the potential risk of congenital malformations. The Special Considerations for Older Adults box above discusses the issues involved in oral anticoagulant therapy with older adults.

The client's current medication regimen should be reviewed for significant drug interactions. Although all interactions between the coumarins, the indanediones, and the other medications have not been identified, a listing of the medications known to cause interactions is found in Box 31-1.

A baseline assessment should consist of a PT or INR determination, a platelet count, and a hematocrit evaluation. Anticipate that the dosage of these drugs will be individualized after the prescriber has evaluated the client's PT or INR.

■ **Nursing Diagnosis.** With the administration of oral anticoagulant therapy, clients are at risk for the following nursing diagnoses/collaborative problems: ineffective tissue perfusion related to the underlying condition; risk for injury related to increased bleeding tendencies; ineffective protec-

BOX 31-1
Significant Drug/Herb Interactions of Oral Anticoagulants

The oral anticoagulants have a great potential for causing drug interactions; therefore clients must be cautioned against taking any drug and/or making significant dietary changes without prior consultation with their prescriber. Check a current *USP DI* for major drug interactions.

Agents that may increase the anticoagulant effect, often necessitating a dosage reduction

allopurinol	cimetidine	ginkgo	plicamycin
amiodarone	clofibrate	ginseng	propylthiouracil
anabolic steroids	danazol	indomethacin	quinidine
androgens	dextran	mefenamic acid	salicylates
aspirin	dextrothyroxine	meperidine	stroptokinase
azlocillin	diflunisal	methimazole	sulfinpyrazone
carbenicillin (parenteral)	dipyridamole†	metronidazole	sulfonamides
cefamandole	disulfiram	mezlocillin	sulindac
cefoperazone	erythromycins	nalidixic acid	thyroid hormone
chloral hydrate*	fenoprofen	phenytoin‡	ticarcillin
chloramphenicol	gemfibrozil	piperacillin	urokinase

Agents that may decrease the anticoagulant effect, often necessitating an increase in anticoagulant dosage

oral antidiabetic agents§	colestipol	ethchlorvynol	rifampin
barbiturates	contraceptives, oral	griseifulvin	vitamin K
carbamazepine	estramustine	primidone	
cholestyramine	estrogens		

*Usually occurs during the first 2 weeks of therapy. With chronic concurrent therapy, the anticoagulant effect may return to normal or be decreased.

†With doses of dipyridamole more than 400 mg/day.

‡Increased anticoagulant effect occurs initially. Decreased activity may occur with chronic concurrent therapy. May also see a decrease in the metabolism of phenytoin, possibly leading to increased serum levels and toxicity.

§May initially increase anticoagulant effects, but such effects may decrease with long-term concurrent therapy. The decrease in metabolism of the antidiabetic agent may increase serum levels and cause a prolonged half-life, hypoglycemia, and toxicity.

tion related to agranulocytosis or leukopenia (chills, fever, sore throat, excessive fatigue); impaired skin integrity related to allergic dermatitis; impaired comfort (bloated stomach or gas); diarrhea related to gastrointestinal effects; disturbed body image related to unusual hair loss (long-term therapy); and the potential complications of acute adrenal insufficiency (diarrhea, nausea with or without vomiting, abdominal cramps) and hepatotoxicity (dark urine, yellow sclera and skin).

■ **Implementation**

■ ***Monitoring.*** Anticipate that the dosage is based on the PT or INR. Check to be sure that one of these tests is performed as ordered, and report the results to the prescriber immediately. The therapeutic aim for clients undergoing anticoagulant therapy is to prolong the PT to within 1.3 to 1.5 times (INR 2.0 to 3.0) the control value. If the client is at higher risk for thrombus, then a prolongation of the PT to within 1.5 to 2 times (INR 3.5 to 4.0) the control value is the therapeutic level sought. Once the maintenance dosage has been determined, further monitoring need not be as frequent. (Review client monitoring within the discussion of the nursing management for anticoagulant therapy.) In addition to the observations related to hemorrhage, clients receiving anisindione need to be observed for nephrotoxicity, hepatotoxicity, and blood dyscrasias.

■ ***Intervention.*** Be aware that the onset of action of the oral anticoagulants is slow; therefore heparin sodium is usually given during the first few days of treatment. Blood for PT or INR should be drawn just before or 5 hours after the administration of IV heparin.

Oral anticoagulant therapy is usually terminated gradually over a 3- or 4-week period to prevent rebound thromboembolic complications.

■ ***Education.*** In addition to the points discussed in Nursing Management: Anticoagulant Therapy (p. 621), instruct the client to carry an identification card that lists the client's and prescriber's names and phone numbers and the name and dosage of the oral anticoagulant drug. Because so many drugs interact with anticoagulant agents, emphasize the importance of not taking any other medication, especially ibuprofen, aspirin, or other salicylates, without checking with the prescriber. Clients with alcoholism should be closely monitored because of the risk for ineffective management of the therapeutic drug regimen.

Once maintenance therapy is established, stress the importance of adhering to the schedule of laboratory procedures and prescriber's appointments. PT or INR should be performed at intervals of 1 to 4 weeks, depending on dosage. Periodic urinalysis, blood counts, stool guaiac, and liver function tests should also be performed. Ensure that the client is aware of different dosage tablets, because the prescriber may vary the dosage by phone on the basis of the PT or INR.

Vitamin K_1 (phytonadione) should be readily accessible if bleeding occurs. Statistics show that bleeding occurs in approximately 10% of all clients undergoing long-term anticoagulant therapy; however, fatalities are rare.

▪ **Evaluation.** The expected outcome of oral anticoagulant therapy is that the client's PT will show values 1.3 to 1.5 (INR 2.0 to 3.0) times the control value, or 1.5 to 2 (INR 3.0 to 4.5) times the control value in clients at higher risk for thrombus. In addition, the client will not show evidence of any signs or symptoms of bleeding or thrombus formation.

Oral Anticoagulant Antagonists

Vitamin K

menadiol sodium diphosphate [men a dye′ ole] (Synkayvite)
phytonadione [fye toe na dye′ one] (Mephyton, AquaMephyton)

Vitamin K is essential to the hepatic synthesis of prothrombin (factor II) and factors VII, IX, and X. It contributes to the activation of an enzyme necessary to the formation of prothrombin. A deficiency of vitamin K leads to hypoprothrombinemia and hemorrhage.

Vitamin K is used to prevent and treat hypoprothrombinemia. A prothrombin deficiency may occur because of inadequate absorption of vitamin K from the intestine (usually caused by biliary disease, in which bile fails to enter the intestine) or because of the destruction of intestinal organisms, which may occur with antibiotic therapy. It is also seen in the newborn, in which case it is probably caused by the fact that the intestinal organisms have not yet become established. It may result from therapy with certain medications, such as salicylates, sulfonamides, quinine, quinidine, or broad-spectrum antibiotics.

Vitamin K is useful only in conditions in which the prolonged bleeding time is caused by a low concentration of prothrombin in the blood and not by damaged liver cells. Vitamin K is routinely administered to newborns to help prevent hemorrhage. Although prothrombin levels may be normal at birth, they decline until about the sixth to the eighth day, when the liver is able to form prothrombin. Phytonadione is usually the preferred agent.

Vitamin K is also indicated in the preoperative preparation of individuals with deficient prothrombin, particularly those with obstructive jaundice. In addition, it is given as an antidote for an overdose of oral anticoagulants.

It is important to measure the prothrombin activity of the blood frequently when the client is receiving a preparation of vitamin K. Parenteral preparations should be administered if intestinal absorption is impaired. Natural vitamin K is normally synthesized by the intestinal flora. When synthetic forms of vitamin K are administered, the absorption is good, but phytonadione requires the presence of bile salts.

The onset of action for the menadiol sodium diphosphate injection is 8 to 24 hours; for oral phytonadione it is 6 to 12 hours, and for the injectable form it is 1 to 2 hours. Vitamin K is metabolized in the liver and excreted by the kidneys and in the bile.

The side effects/adverse reactions include facial flushing, taste alterations, and redness or pain at the injection site.

The dosage of menadiol (vitamin K) as a nutritional supplement for hypoprothrombinemia is 5 mg/day PO or 5 to 15 mg IM or SC once or twice daily. As an antidote for drug-induced hypoprothrombinemia, the oral dosage is 5 to 10 mg daily; the IM or SC dosage is 5 to 15 mg PO or IM daily.

▪ Nursing Management
Vitamin K Therapy

▪ **Assessment.** The client should be assessed for preexisting conditions in which vitamin K therapy would entail some risk, such as hepatic function impairment (large doses of vitamin K might increase the impairment), or glucose-6-phosphate dehydrogenase (G6PD) deficiency (menadiol might induce erythrocyte hemolysis).

Drug interactions with vitamin K in the client's current medication regimen need to be identified. When vitamin K is given concurrently with the oral anticoagulants, a decrease in anticoagulation effect is reported. If other hemolytics are used concurrently with vitamin K, especially menadiol, the potential for toxic side effects may increase.

▪ **Nursing Diagnosis.** The administration of vitamin K may place the client at risk for impaired comfort (facial flushing, unusual taste, and discomfort and redness at the injection site) and the potential complications of hemolytic anemia or a rare hypersensitivity-like reaction.

▪ **Implementation**

▪ ***Monitoring.*** Monitor PT as a baseline measurement and throughout vitamin K therapy to evaluate the client's response. During IV infusion, observe for signs of side effects such as flushing, weakness, and hypotension, and report them to the prescriber.

▪ ***Intervention.*** Because vitamin K has a delayed onset, the administration of plasma or fresh whole blood may be necessary with severe bleeding. IV administration is not recommended because of the risk of hypersensitivity reactions; if IV administration is necessary, administer the drug by slow IV infusion over 2 to 3 hours, and protect the infusion container from light by wrapping it in aluminum foil. AquaMephyton, a parenteral solution, contains benzyl alcohol, which may cause a toxic fatal syndrome in neonates; avoid using this solution with infants.

▪ ***Education.*** In general, dietary supplements of vitamin K are not necessary because a normal diet and intestinal bacterial synthesis supply sufficient amounts. Green leafy vegetables, meats, and dairy products are the best sources of vitamin K, with little nutritional loss of the vitamin during ordinary cooking. The client's intake of dietary vitamin K should be considered when determining therapeutic dosages for long-term use.

■ **Evaluation.** The expected outcome of vitamin K therapy is that the client's PT will be within 2 seconds of the control time, and the client will not show evidence of bleeding.

THROMBOLYTIC DRUGS

Thrombolytic (fibrinolytic) drugs are used to treat acute thromboembolic disorders. Unlike anticoagulants, they dissolve clots and are used in a hospital setting only by health care providers who are experienced in the management of diseases caused by thrombosis. These agents alter the hemostatic capability of the client more profoundly than does anticoagulant therapy. Consequently, when bleeding occurs, it is more severe and very difficult to control.

alteplase [al ti plase′] (Activase)
anistreplase [a ni′ strep lase] (Eminase)
reteplase [re′ te plase] (Retavase)
✓ **streptokinase** [strep toe kye′ nase] (Streptase)
tenecteplase [te nek′ te plase] (TNKase)
urokinase [yoor oh kin′ ase] (Abbokinase)

Thrombolytic drugs dissolve clots via the endogenous fibrinolytic system. All six drugs have similar biochemical mechanisms of action on the fibrinolytic system—converting plasminogen in the blood to plasmin. Plasmin, an enzyme with **fibrinolytic activity,** digests or dissolves fibrin clots wherever they exist and wherever they can be reached by plasmin. Streptokinase is a key drug because it was the first thrombolytic agent released. Alteplase, streptokinase, and urokinase are indicated for the treatment of acute pulmonary thromboembolism; anistreplase and streptokinase are indicated for the treatment of an acute DVT (*USP DI*, 1999). All of these drugs can be used to treat an acute coronary arterial thrombosis associated with an acute myocardial infarction. Alteplase is also indicated for the treatment of acute ischemic stroke (Hock, 1998; *USP DI*, 1999).

These agents are administered intravenously and/or intraarterially. Alteplase has an elimination half-life of 35 minutes; the half-lives for streptokinase and urokinase are 23 minutes and up to 20 minutes, respectively. Anistreplase, which is an acylated complex of streptokinase and human plasminogen, has a long half-life of approximately 90 minutes; the peak effect after IV injection is from 20 minutes to 2 hours. The duration of the thrombolytic effect is approximately 4 hours for alteplase, streptokinase, and urokinase; it is 6 hours for anistreplase. Tenecteplase has a long-life and may cause fewer bleeding complications.

Reteplase has an elimination half-life of 13 to 16 minutes and reaches a peak effect (fibrinogen levels decreased to under 100 mg/dL) within 2 hours; mean fibrinogen levels return to previous levels within 48 hours; it is metabolized in the liver and excreted by the kidneys.

In an acute coronary artery thrombosis that evolves into a transmural myocardial infarction, thrombolytic therapy is most effective when started within 3 to 4 hours after the onset of symptoms. Alteplase is usually given at 1.25 mg/kg IV in divided doses over 3 hours for clients weighing less than 65 kg, or 100 mg IV is given to clients 65 kg or over in divided doses over 3 hours. See the current literature for recommended dosages over each of the 3 hours.

For reteplase, the usual adult dosage is 10 units IV over 2 minutes, repeated in 30 minutes. The dosage of anistreplase is 30 units in solution administered by IV injection over 2 to 5 minutes. For streptokinase, the dosage is 1,500,000 IU IV administered within an hour of onset. Smaller doses of 20,000 IU initially followed by an additional 2000 IU/min are used for intraarterial administration. Urokinase 6000 IU/min is administered intraarterially until the artery is opened. For other indications, refer to a current package insert or *USP DI* for dosing information.

antithrombin III, human [an′ tee throm bin] (ATnativ, Thrombate III)

Antithrombin III is prepared from pooled human plasma of healthy donors. It is indicated for the treatment or prevention of thromboembolism associated with a hereditary antithrombin III deficiency. Heparin and antithrombin III will enhance each other's effects and therefore have been administered concurrently depending on the situation. ATnativ is an orphan drug, and Thrombate III is marketed by Bayer (*Drug Facts and Comparisons*, 2000).

The side effects/adverse reactions of antithrombin III include diuresis, hypotension, chest pain, fever, hives, nausea, hematoma, and shortness of breath in some persons. The dosage is determined by antithrombin III levels before therapy; if the levels are subnormal, a formula is used to determine the number of units required. (See the current literature of *Drug Facts and Comparisons* for the formula and administration information.)

■ Nursing Management
Thrombolytic Therapy

■ **Assessment.** Note that thrombolytic therapy is contraindicated for clients in whom there is the risk of uncontrollable bleeding because of preexisting conditions such as aneurysm or arteriovenous malformation, active bleeding, brain tumor, cerebrovascular accident, intracranial or intraspinal surgery within the last 2 months, recent thoracic surgery, or recent CNS trauma. Such therapy is also contraindicated for severe uncontrolled hypertension (>200 mm Hg systolic and/or >120 mm Hg diastolic) because of the risk of cerebral hemorrhage. Alteplase therapy for acute ischemic stroke is initiated only after the exclusion of intracranial hemorrhage by a cranial computed tomographic scan or other diagnostic imaging method. Use with caution in high-risk clients who have experienced major surgery, childbirth, serious gastrointestinal bleeding, organ biopsy, previous puncture of noncompressible blood vessels, or severe trauma other than CNS trauma within the past 10 days. Use with caution for any condition in which the risk of bleeding is present or would be difficult to control because of its location. In addition to those already listed are coagulation defects secondary to severe hepatic and renal disease, neurosurgical procedures within the last 2 months, suspected left heart thrombus involving mitral stenosis with atrial fibrillation, subacute bacterial endocarditis, and diabetic hemorrhagic retinopathy. If the client has been treated previously with anistreplase or streptokinase, the formation of antibodies to the drug may cause either a resistance to the therapeutic effects of the drug or a severe allergic reaction.

Before thrombolytic therapy, coagulation tests such as TT, APTT, PT, fibrin/fibrinogen degradation product (FDP/fdp) titer, and fibrinogen concentration must be performed; however, therapy for acute coronary arterial occlusion must not be delayed until the test results are available. In addition, an electrocardiogram (ECG) and hematocrit, hemoglobin, and platelet counts are needed.

Review the client's current medication regimen for the risk of significant drug interactions, such as those that may occur when thrombolytic agents are given concurrently with the following drugs:

Drug	Possible Effect and Management
Bold/color type indicates the	**most serious interactions.**
aminocaproic acid or other antifibrinolytic drugs	May inhibit the effectiveness of thrombolytic agents. Reserve such drugs to treat severe bleeding induced by the thrombolytic agents.
anticoagulants, oral or heparin	Increased risk of bleeding and hemorrhage. Heparin has been administered with thrombolytic agents to treat an acute coronary arterial occlusion. Monitor closely when concurrent therapy is prescribed.
antiinflammatory agents, nonsteroidal, aspirin,* other platelet aggregation inhibitors, especially sulfinpyrazone and ticlopidine	**Inhibition of platelet aggregation may increase the potential for gastrointestinal ulceration and bleeding. Avoid concurrent use or a potentially serious drug interaction may occur.**
carbenicillin, dextran, dipyridamole, divalproex, ticarcillin	**These drugs inhibit platelet aggregation; they may increase the risk of severe bleeding and hemorrhage if used concurrently with the thrombolytic agents. Avoid concurrent use or a potentially serious drug interaction may occur.**
cefamandole, cefoperazone, cefotetan, plicamycin, or valproic acid	**May cause hypoprothrombinemia and inhibit platelet aggregation. The use of these drugs is not recommended because of the increased risk of hemorrhage. Avoid concurrent use or a potentially serious drug interaction may occur.**

*Low doses of aspirin have been given concurrently with thrombolytic therapy, especially with streptokinase. This combination is reported to decrease the risk of reocclusion, stroke, and death more significantly than streptokinase alone (USP DI, 1999).

■ **Nursing Diagnosis.** With the administration of thrombolytic agents, the client is at risk for the following nursing diagnoses: risk for injury related to increased bleeding tendencies; impaired comfort (chest pain); ineffective tissue perfusion related to cardiac dysrhythmias; hyperthermia; and the potential complication of stroke (hemorrhagic or thromboembolic). In addition, the client is at risk for the complication of an allergic reaction with the use of anistreplase, streptokinase, and urokinase.

■ **Implementation**

■ ***Monitoring.*** During the early phase of therapy, observe the client carefully for allergic reactions. With urokinase, relatively mild reactions (e.g., bronchospasm, skin rash) are reported. Anistreplase and streptokinase may produce more serious reactions, and possibly anaphylaxis. If allergic manifestations occur, discontinue the infusion and treat with epinephrine, antihistamines, and corticosteroids. Fever should be treated symptomatically with acetaminophen. Alteplase is not antigenic and does not cause antibody formation; this allows for a second course of the drug if reocclusion occurs without fear of anaphylaxis.

Monitor vital signs frequently (i.e., pulse rate, temperature, respiratory rate, and blood pressure), at least every 4 hours. To avoid possible dislodgement of deep vein thrombi, do not take blood pressure in the lower extremities. Monitor the client carefully for bleeding: every 15 minutes for the first hour, every 30 minutes for the next 8 hours, and every 4 hours until therapy is discontinued. The prescriber should be notified immediately if bleeding occurs. Therapy should be discontinued if bleeding occurs that is not controlled by local pressure. In addition to observing for overt bleeding, observe the client for internal bleeding—bloody sputum, hematuria, hematemesis, dark stools (i.e., guaiac positive), flank and abdominal pain, and neurologic and mental status changes (intracranial bleeding). For uncontrollable bleeding, stop treatment and be ready to administer whole blood (fresh blood if available), packed red cells, cryoprecipitate or fresh-frozen plasma, and aminocaproic acid.

Observe the extremities and palpate the pulses of the affected extremities every hour. The prescriber should be notified immediately if there are signs of circulatory impairment. Observe the client carefully for dysrhythmias during and after intracoronary infusion of streptokinase. Rapid lysis of coronary thrombi has caused atrial and ventricular dysrhythmias. ECG monitoring is recommended.

Continue to observe the client for bleeding during and after treatment. Coagulation tests such as APTT, PT, and TT are used to assess fibrinolytic activity. Because the thrombolytic effects of the drug last for several hours, the sites of invasive devices are common areas for hematoma formation.

After therapy, monitor fibrinogen levels—which are decreased by thrombolytic agents—until they return to normal.

■ ***Intervention.*** Thrombolytic therapy is administered only by personnel who are experienced in the management of thrombotic diseases and only where skilled personnel and laboratory resources are available. Typed and crossmatched whole blood and packed red cells should be available in case of hemorrhage. Follow the manufacturer's instructions when reconstituting and diluting the drug to minimize the formation of fibrin:

- *Alteplase.* Reconstitute using the diluent supplied with the drug (sterile water for injection); do not use bacteriostatic water for injection. It may be used as is or diluted further. If it is diluted further, use only 0.9% sodium chloride solutions or 5% dextrose injection without preservatives. Mix gently to prevent foaming. Leave the solution undisturbed for a few minutes; any bubbles created will dissipate. Treatment with alteplase for acute ischemic stroke should be instituted within 3 hours of the onset of stroke symptoms.
- *Anistreplase.* Slowly add 5 mL of sterile water for injection to the vial using a large-bore (18-gauge) needle, aiming the stream of diluent at the side of the vial. The vial should be rolled, not shaken, to dissolve the drug. The reconstituted solution should be used within 30 minutes. Unused solution needs to be discarded because it contains no preservative.
- *Streptokinase.* Slowly add diluent according to the manufacturer's directions, depending on the purpose of drug therapy. Direct the stream toward the side of the vial rather than into the powder. Do not shake the vial, but gently roll it and tilt it for reconstitution. Note that shaking may cause foaming and increase flocculation (small, thin fibers). The solution may be used if there is slight flocculation but should be discarded if it is extensive. If reconstituting for arteriovenous cannula obstruction clearance, use 2 mL of sodium chloride injection or 5% dextrose injection for each 250,000 IU of streptokinase. If the solution is not used soon after reconstitution, store it at 2° to 4° C, and use it within 24 hours.

  Note that a client with a recent streptococcal infection may require a higher loading dose because of higher resistance levels. Have equipment and drugs for treating anaphylaxis available in the immediate environment. A glucocorticoid and/or antihistamine may be administered before streptokinase administration to reduce the risk of adverse reactions, such as hypersensitivity and fever. However, the effectiveness of these interventions has not been proven. Streptokinase therapy may continue for up to 72 hours.
- *Urokinase.* For intracoronary arterial administration, add 5 mL of sterile water without preservatives (not bacteriostatic water) for injection to each of three 250,000 IU vials immediately before use. Roll and tilt, but do not shake for reconstitution. Further dilute by adding the contents of the three vials to 500 mL of 5% dextrose solution to make a solution of 1500 IU/mL. For IV infusion, see the manufacturer's instructions. For IV catheter clearance (for the 250,000 IU size only), add 5 mL of sterile water (without preservatives) to the vial. Add 1 mL of the reconstituted solution to 9 mL of sterile water for injection to make a solution of 5000 IU/mL. Discard the unused portion of the reconstituted material.

Do not add any other medication to the container of alteplase, anistreplase, streptokinase, or urokinase solution or administer other medications through the same IV line. Do not administer by IM injection because of the danger of hematoma. Use venipuncture sites as seldom as possible (use a 23-gauge or smaller needle), and perform this procedure with care. Maintain pressure dressings at the site for at least 30 minutes, and check frequently for bleeding.

Start thrombolytic therapy as soon as possible after the thrombotic event. With coronary thrombosis, the therapy still has benefit up to 6 to 12 hours after the onset of symptoms; arterial thrombus, 3 days; DVT, 3 to 4 days; and pulmonary embolus, 5 to 7 days. Administer using a constant infusion pump.

For arteriovenous cannula occlusion, administer heparinized saline solution to clear the cannula. If adequate flow is not reestablished, use streptokinase.

To prevent bruising during therapy, avoid unnecessary handling of the client. The client should be prescribed bed rest, and the side rails of the client's bed should be padded.

After the completion of thrombolytic therapy, begin continuous IV infusion of heparin (without a loading dose) when TT has decreased to less than twice the normal control value (usually within 2 hours after completion of the infusion). Use an infusion pump for heparin. Later the client will probably receive oral anticoagulant therapy, a procedure that prevents the recurrence of thrombosis.

■ **Evaluation.** When thrombolytic therapy is used for the emergency treatment of coronary artery thrombosis, the expected outcome is that the client will experience a cessation of chest pain, improved ECG values, and the absence of coronary occlusion with cardiac catheterization. When thrombolytic therapy is administered for the treatment of venous thrombosis, pulmonary embolism, and arterial thrombosis and embolism, the client will demonstrate increased tissue perfusion as evidenced by the absence of ischemic pain, a return of normal peripheral pulses, and good capillary refill. When administered for pulmonary embolus, the client will demonstrate normal blood gases and a normal lung scan. The expected outcome of alteplase therapy for acute ischemic stroke is that the client's symptoms of stroke will resolve and the client will not experience intracranial hemorrhage.

ANTIPLATELET AGENTS

The antiplatelet drugs, or drugs that inhibit platelet aggregation, include aspirin, anagrelide (Agrylin), cilostazol (Pletal), clopidogrel (Plavix), dipyridamole (Persantine), ticlopidine (Ticlid), and glycoprotein IIb/IIIa inhibitors (abciximab [ReoPro], eptifibatide [Integrilin], and tirofiban [Aggrastat]). Aspirin inhibits cyclooxygenase, an enzyme necessary for the synthesis of thromboxane A_2. As mentioned previously, thromboxane A_2 promotes platelet aggregation and vasoconstriction, and thus aspirin suppresses these actions (see Chapter 11). The other drugs are discussed in the following paragraphs.

The composition of arterial thrombi is primarily platelet aggregates; venous thrombi are usually composed of fibrin and red blood cells. Therefore the anticoagulant drugs are used to reduce the risks or complications of venous thrombi, whereas the antiplatelet agents are used for arterial thrombi.

anagrelide [a na' gre lyde] (Agrylin)

The antiplatelet effect of anagrelide is unknown, but studies indicate that it decreases megakaryocyte hypermaturation, inhibits cyclic adenosine monophosphate (cAMP) phosphodiesterase and adenosine diphosphate (ADP), and inhibits collagen-related platelet aggregation. It is indicated for the treatment of essential thrombocythemia.

The side effects/adverse reactions of anagrelide include stomach pain, tachycardia, edema, diarrhea, and headaches. Adverse reactions may include congestive heart failure, cardiomyopathy, heart block, atrial fibrillation, pulmonary hypertension, and seizures.

The initial adult dosage is 1 mg twice daily for 1 week; the dosage is then adjusted to the lowest effective dose that maintains a platelet count <600,000/mcL. The dosage may be increased by 0.5 mg/day weekly.

cilostazol [sil oe' sta zol] (Pletal)

Cilostazol and several of its metabolites are inhibitors of cAMP phosphodiesterase III, which results in an increase in cAMP levels, vasodilation, and the inhibition of platelet aggregation. The antiplatelet effects of this drug may also be induced by a variety of other mechanisms. Cilostazol is indicated for intermittent claudication.

The side effects of cilostazol include headache, pharyngitis, diarrhea, nausea, and peripheral edema. Adverse reactions include tachycardia, congestive heart failure, cerebral ischemia, atrial fibrillation, and atrial flutter.

The adult dosage is 100 mg twice daily administered ½ hour before or 2 hours after the morning and evening meals. If the client is taking ketoconazole, itraconazole, erythromycin, or diltiazem (CYP3A4 inhibitors) or omeprazole (CYP2C19 inhibitor), the adult dosage is 50 mg twice daily. Clients should avoid the consumption of grapefruit juice because it is associated with CYP3A4 inhibition.

clopidogrel [kloe pi'doe grel] (Plavix ◆)

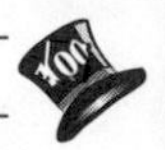

Clopidogrel is an antithrombotic and inhibitor of platelet aggregation and therefore is indicated for the prophylaxis of myocardial infarction, thromboembolic stroke, and vascular death. It inhibits ADP binding to platelet receptors, thus interfering with the ADP activation of a glycoprotein complex; this results in the inhibition of platelet aggregation.

Administered orally, clopidogrel is biotransformed in the liver to an active metabolite that produces approximately 85% of its effects. It has an onset of action in 2 hours after a single dose and reaches peak serum levels in 1 hour and peak effects with repeated dosing between day 3 and day 7. It is excreted by the kidneys (50%) and in the feces (approximately 46%).

The side effects/adverse reactions of clopidogrel include gastrointestinal distress, arthralgia, back pain, headache, dizziness, anxiety, weakness, constipation, cough, diarrhea, hypoesthesia or paresthesia, insomnia, pruritus, nausea, leg cramps, depression, vomiting, and rash. Adverse reactions include chest pain, purpura, upper respiratory infection, dysrhythmias, bronchitis, dyspnea, edema, gastrointestinal hemorrhage, hypertension, urinary tract infection, and syncope.

The usual adult dosage of clopidogrel is 75 mg PO daily.

dipyridamole [dye peer id' a mole] (Persantine)

The mechanism of action for dipyridamole has been postulated to be inhibition of the following:

1. Thromboxane A_2 formation, a potent platelet activator
2. Phosphodiesterase, which results in an increase in cyclic-3', 5' monophosphate in the platelets
3. Red blood cell uptake of adenosine, a platelet aggregation inhibitor

Dipyridamole is used in combination with coumarin anticoagulants for the prevention of postsurgical thromboembolic complications after cardiac valve replacement.

After an oral dose, dipyridamole reaches peak serum levels in approximately 75 minutes. This drug is highly protein bound, metabolized in the liver, and excreted in bile.

The side effects/adverse reactions include headache, dizziness, abdominal upset, and rash.

The usual adult (adjunctive) dosage is 75 to 100 mg PO four times daily.

ticlopidine [tye kloe' pih deen] (Ticlid)

Ticlopidine is believed to produce an irreversible, ADP-induced inhibition of platelet-fibrinogen binding. It is indicated to decrease the risk of stroke for clients who have had warning of a thrombotic stroke or for those who have had a thrombotic stroke.

Administered orally, this drug reaches peak serum levels in approximately 2 hours and a peak effect with repeated dosing in 8 to 11 days. It is metabolized by the liver and excreted by the kidneys.

The side effects/adverse reactions of ticlopidine include nausea, stomach cramps, bloating or gas, dizziness, skin rash, diarrhea, tinnitus, bleeding, pruritus, neutropenia, agranulocytosis, thrombocytopenia, and purpura.

The recommended adult dosage is 250 mg twice daily with food.

Glycoprotein IIb/IIIa Inhibitors

abciximab [ab six′ i mab] (ReoPro)

Abciximab, a monoclonal antibody fragment, inhibits platelet aggregation by binding or blocking the glycoprotein (GP) IIb/IIIa receptor involved in the pathway for platelet aggregation. It is indicated as adjunct therapy (to aspirin and heparin) for the prevention of acute cardiac vessel ischemic complications in clients undergoing percutaneous transluminal coronary angioplasty or atherectomy (PTCA).

The side effects/adverse reactions of abciximab include major bleeding episodes and hypotension.

The recommended adult dosage is 0.25 mg/kg administered 10 to 60 minutes before the procedure. The maintenance dosage by IV infusion is 0.01 mg/min up to 12 hours.

eptifibatide [ep ti fib′ a tide] (Integrilin)
tirofiban [tir oe fib′ an] (Aggrastat)

Eptifibatide and tirofiban are platelet glycoprotein IIb/IIIa receptor antagonists. They prevent fibrinogen, von Willebrand's factor, and other potential adhesion substances from binding to this receptor site, thus inhibiting platelet aggregation. These drugs are indicated for the treatment of acute coronary syndrome (unstable angina or non–Q wave myocardial infarction).

The most common adverse reaction is bleeding, which can range from minor bleeding to intracranial (stroke) and retroperitoneal bleeding. Thus close monitoring of platelet counts, hemoglobin, and other laboratory tests are necessary before treatment and at regular intervals (at least daily if not more often) during treatment. Other adverse reactions include bradycardia, edema, and leg pain.

The adult dosage of eptifibatide for acute coronary syndrome is an initial IV bolus of 180 μg/kg. This is followed by an IV infusion of 2 μg/kg/min until hospital discharge or until a coronary artery bypass graft (CABG) surgery is initiated, which is usually up to 3 days. Refer to a current package insert or reference for additional dosing parameters and monitoring guidelines.

Tirofiban is administered in combination with heparin for acute coronary syndrome. Most clients receive an initial IV dose of 0.4 μg/kg/min for 30 minutes, followed by 0.1 μg/kg/min.

■ Nursing Management

Antiplatelet Agent Therapy

■ **Assessment.** Antiplatelet therapy is contraindicated for clients with hematopoietic disorders such as neutropenia and thrombocytopenia. Because these drugs prolong bleeding times, they are also contraindicated for clients with a hemostatic disorder, a history of bleeding within the last 6 weeks, active bleeding (e.g., a peptic ulcer or intracranial bleeding), or hepatic dysfunction (may be prone to bleeding). Use with caution in clients who are at risk for trauma, surgery, or lesions that might bleed (e.g., intracranial aneurysm, arteriovenous malformation, or neoplasm), as well as in clients with severe uncontrolled hypertension, recent major surgery (within 6 weeks), or a cardiovascular accident in the last 2 years.

With abciximab, clients are at an increased risk for bleeding if they are over 65 years of age, have a history of gastrointestinal disease, weigh more than 75 kg, or have a failed PTCA, a PTCA lasting more than 70 minutes, or a PTCA within 12 hours of the onset of symptoms for acute myocardial infarction. Because of the positive ionotropic effects and cardiac side effects of anagrelide, it should be used with extreme caution in clients with known or suspected cardiac disease. With dipyridamole, clients with unstable angina will experience an increased risk of myocardial ischemia, which may lead to hypotension, ventricular dysrhythmias, and cardiac arrest. Clients with hypotension and asthma may experience an aggravation of their condition. Hypersensitivity to the particular antiplatelet agent is also an issue for assessment.

The client's current medication regimen should be reviewed for significant drug interactions. With the antiplatelet agents, the concomitant use of anticoagulants, platelet aggregation inhibitors (e.g., aspirin and other NSAIDs), thrombolytic agents, and other antiplatelet agents would result in additive bleeding effects.

The concurrent use or subsequent use of dextran and abciximab will increase bleeding tendencies.

A baseline assessment of the client receiving antiplatelet therapy should include a CBC, including a white cell differential and platelet count, and coagulation studies (ACT, APTT, and PT). A baseline cardiovascular examination is required for clients receiving anagrelide and dipyridamole.

■ **Nursing Diagnosis.** The client receiving antiplatelet therapy may be at risk for the following nursing diagnoses/collaborative problems: impaired comfort (headache [12.2% with IV dipyridamole], flushing, nausea, dyspepsia, and gastrointestinal cramping); ineffective airway clearance related to bronchospasm (shortness of breath, dyspnea, wheezing); risk for injury related to dizziness (13.6%

with dipyridamole); impaired skin integrity (rash [5.1% with ticlopidine], pruritus, or purpura); diarrhea (>10% with anagrelide, 12.5% with ticlopidine); ineffective protection related to neutropenia and thrombocytopenia; and the potential complications of angina pectoris or its exacerbation (>19% with dipyridamole), pulmonary infiltrates or fibrosis (>10% with anagrelide), bleeding, ECG changes, and dysrhythmias.

■ **Implementation**

■ ***Monitoring.*** All platelet aggregate inhibitor therapy should be discontinued if the platelet count is less than 80,000 cells/mm^3. Monitor the client for bleeding—epistaxis, hematuria, conjunctival hemorrhage, gastrointestinal bleeding, excessive bruising, catheter insertion sites, arterial and venous puncture sites, cutdown sites, and needle puncture sites. Coagulation studies should also be performed.

With abciximab, platelet counts are recommended 2 to 4 hours after the initial IV injection and at 24 hours or at discharge, whichever comes first. In addition, monitor for hypersensitivity reactions.

With anagrelide and dipyridamole, monitor ECG tracings and vital signs, particularly the blood pressure.

With ticlopidine, monitor the CBC every 2 weeks until the third month of therapy; monitor more frequently if the neutrophil count is declining or is 30% less than the baseline count. After the third month, obtain a CBC only if the client has signs and symptoms of an infection.

■ ***Intervention.*** Administer ticlopidine with food to minimize gastrointestinal distress. With abciximab, administration is with a continuous infusion pump with an in-line filter. Be aware that hypersensitivity or anaphylaxis may occur at any time during the administration of abciximab. Minimize the use of invasive procedures to reduce the risk of bleeding.

■ ***Education.*** Instruct the client to apply direct pressure to the site if bleeding does occur and to seek medical attention for any unusual bleeding. Encourage the client to wear medical identification that indicates this medication and alert other health care providers that antiplatelet therapy is being taken. Other medications should not be taken without consultation with the prescriber.

Advise the client undergoing antiplatelet therapy to report any symptoms of chest pain, palpitations, or edema to the prescriber.

With ticlopidine, advise the client on the importance of routine blood testing and of any symptoms of infection that may indicate neutropenia (e.g., fever, chills, and sore throat), which should be reported to the prescriber. Symptoms of hepatic dysfunction, such as yellowing skin and sclera and darker urine and lighter stools, should also be reported.

■ **Evaluation.** The expected outcome of antiplatelet therapy is that the client will not experience any thrombotic episodes, such as stroke, and will not experience adverse reactions to the drug.

ANTIHEMOPHILIC DRUGS

Hemophilia is a hereditary disorder caused by a deficiency of one or more plasma protein clotting factors. This condition usually leads to persistent and uncontrollable hemorrhage after even a minor injury. Symptoms include excessive bleeding from wounds and hemorrhage into joints, the urinary tract, and on occasion the CNS. There are two types of hemophilia: (1) hemophilia A, the classic type, in which factor VIII activity is deficient; and (2) hemophilia B, or Christmas disease, in which factor IX complex activity is deficient. In recent years a correct diagnosis of the coagulation disorder has led to specific factor replacement therapy; this medical advance has resulted in effective management of the client at home.

factor VIII (Koate-HP, Recombinate)

Factor VIII, or the antihemophilic factor (AHF), is a glycoprotein necessary for hemostasis and blood clotting. In the intrinsic pathway of the coagulation mechanism, AHF is required for the transformation of prothrombin to thrombin. In the treatment or prevention of hemophilia A, factor VIII administration is based on replacing the missing plasma clotting factor to control and prevent bleeding.

When administered intravenously, factor VIII has a distribution half-life of 2.4 to 8 hours and an elimination half-life of 8.4 to 19.3 hours. The time to peak effect is between 1 and 2 hours after IV administration.

Mild to severe allergic reactions have been reported, such as bronchospasm, elevated temperature, chills, or rash. Other side effects/adverse reactions, which may be related to the rate of infusion, include headache, increased heart rate, tingling of fingers, fainting, lethargy, sedation, hypotension, back pain, nausea or vomiting, visual disturbances, and chest constriction. No significant drug interactions are reported with factor VIII.

The dosage of factor VIII must be individualized according to the client's weight, severity of the deficiency, and the amount of blood loss. During hemorrhage the dosage is adjusted so that a level of 25% of normal levels of factor VIII can produce hemostasis. Clients who develop inhibitors to factor VIII may not respond to factor VIII therapy. After careful evaluation of the client, the administration of antiinhibitor coagulant complex, which reduces factor VIII inhibitors, may be indicated to correct this condition.

Two recombinant DNA-derived factor VIII preparations (Recombinate and Kogenate) were marketed in 1993. Before these products, concentrates were prepared from donor plasma pools; some concentrates have been the source of transmission of various viruses, such as hepatitis, human immunodeficiency virus (HIV), and others. The recombinant products are essentially free of viruses because they are prepared by genetic engineering in a controlled laboratory setting. They appear to be as effective as the plasma source concentrates, although presently they are much more expensive than the other products (Abramowicz, 1993).

■ Nursing Management

Factor VIII Therapy

■ **Assessment.** Obtain baseline values of factor VIII antibody determinations and vital signs before administering AHF. If the pulse increases significantly, reduce the rate of administration or discontinue the drug.

■ **Nursing Diagnosis.** The client undergoing factor VIII therapy may experience fatigue, impaired comfort (headache, dermatitis, chills, fever, back pain, nausea and vomiting) related to mild allergic reaction, and ineffective airway clearance (bronchospasm) related to allergic response.

■ **Implementation**

■ ***Monitoring.*** Monitor the client's vital signs over the course of administration. Adverse reactions are related to the rate of administration. Slow the rate of flow or stop the infusion until the symptoms of flushing, headache, and alterations of blood pressure and pulse disappear. Periodic plasma factor VIII determinations will determine that adequate concentrations have been achieved for the client. Periodic determinations of factor VIII antibodies will help to predict the client's ability to respond to AHF therapy.

■ ***Intervention.*** Refrigerate the concentrate until ready for use, but do not freeze it. Do not refrigerate after reconstitution, because the active ingredient may precipitate. Warm the concentrate and diluent to room temperature before reconstitution. Gently rotate (do not shake) the vial containing the concentrate and diluent until it is completely dissolved. This may take as long as 5 to 10 minutes. Because the AHF is filtered before administration, the active components will be filtered out if it is not fully dissolved. Although AHF remains stable for 24 hours at room temperature after reconstitution, it should be used within 3 hours. Do not mix it with other medications.

AHF is for IV infusion only. Use only plastic syringes to prepare for administration, because the solution adheres to the ground surfaces of glass syringes.

■ ***Education.*** Instruct the client to wear a MedicAlert bracelet to alert medical personnel in an emergency situation that factor VIII may be required. Encourage clients with newly diagnosed hemophilia to be vaccinated for hepatitis A and B.

■ **Evaluation.** The expected outcome of factor VIII therapy is that the client's plasma factor VIII levels will be adequate and the client will not experience any abnormal bleeding.

antiinhibitor coagulant complex (Autoplex, Feiba VH Immuno)

Antiinhibitor coagulant complex is made from pooled human plasma. It contains variable quantities of clotting factors and kinin system factors and has been standardized to help correct clotting time in factor VIII–deficient individuals or to treat factor VIII–deficient individuals who have plasma-containing inhibitors to factor VIII.

Antiinhibitor coagulant complex is indicated for clients with factor VIII inhibitors who are bleeding or are being prepared for surgery. Approximately 10% of factor VIII–deficient individuals have inhibitors to factor VIII. Clients with factor VIII inhibitor levels greater than 10 Bethesda units are usually treated with this product.

Allergic reactions and hypersensitivity reactions (fever, chills, rash, hypotension) have been reported with the use of antiinhibitor coagulant complex. If antiinhibitor coagulant complex is administered too rapidly, the recipient may experience flushing, headache, and changes in blood pressure and heart rate. These are indications to slow the rate of flow or to stop the infusion until the symptoms disappear.

Concurrent administration with epsilon-aminocaproic acid or tranexamic acid is not recommended. Antiinhibitor coagulant complex is administered only by IV infusion. The recommended dosage varies from 25 to 100 units/kg depending on the site and severity of the hemorrhage. Check the current package insert or *USP DI* for specific recommendations.

In addition to the nursing management for factor VIII, weigh the benefits of the antiinhibitor complex against the risk of hepatitis associated with its administration. The client is also at risk for the potential complications of thrombotic complications such as DIC, myocardial infarction, and DVT.

Because this complex is prepared from human plasma, the risk of transmitting hepatitis, HIV, and other viral diseases exists.

factor IX complex (Mononine, Proplex T)

Factor IX complex is a purified plasma fraction prepared from pooled units of plasma. It contains factors II, VII, IX, and X, which are known as the vitamin K coagulation factors. This agent is used for therapy during hemorrhage or before surgery in individuals with a deficiency of these factors. It is also indicated for hemophilia B in which factor IX (Christmas disease) is deficient. Factor IX complex is used to prevent or control bleeding in individuals with factor IX deficiency. It is also used to treat clients with bleeding problems who have inhibitors to factor VIII and will reverse the hemorrhage induced by coumarin anticoagulants.

Factor IX has an elimination half-life of 18 to 32 hours; the time to peak effect after IV administration is 10 to 30 minutes.

The side effects/adverse reactions of factor IX include chills and fever, especially when large doses are given. If the IV infusion is given too rapidly, headache, flushing, rash, nausea, vomiting, sedation, lethargy, elevated temperature, and tingling have been reported. The infusion should be stopped; in most clients it can be resumed at a much slower rate.

Thrombosis and DIC have occurred as a result of the administration of factor IX. Myocardial infarction, pulmonary embolism, and anaphylaxis have also been reported. Factor

IX should not be used in individuals undergoing elective surgery, because they are at a greater risk for thrombosis. No significant drug interactions have been reported to date.

Factor IX should be administered slowly by IV injection or IV infusion. The dosage is individualized according to the client's coagulation assay, which is performed before treatment. Check current references for specific dosing recommendations.

■ Nursing Management
Factor IX Therapy

The considerations for factor IX therapy are the same as for factor VIII; only the instructions for preparation differ. Factor IX is administered intravenously or by IV infusion only at a rate not to exceed 3 mL/min. Warm the diluent to room temperature before reconstitution. Gently rotate the mixture in the vial until it is completely dissolved, or the active components will be filtered out when it is administered through the filter needle. Although stable for 12 hours at room temperature, it should be used within 3 hours of reconstitution. Do not refrigerate the reconstituted preparation, because the active ingredients may precipitate.

Factor IX is derived from pooled plasma. Therefore the risk of hepatitis, HIV, and other viral diseases exists as for antiinhibitor coagulant complex.

HEMOSTATIC DRUGS

Hemostatic agents are compounds used to hasten clot formation to reduce bleeding. The purpose of these agents is to control the rapid loss of blood.

Systemic Hemostatics

aminocaproic acid [a mee noe ka proe′ ik] (Amicar)

Aminocaproic acid is a synthetic compound that inhibits fibrinolysis when excessive bleeding occurs. This drug acts as a competitive antagonist of plasminogen, therefore reducing the conversion of plasminogen to plasmin or fibrinolysin. To a lesser degree, it directly inhibits plasmin (fibrinolysin) by noncompetitive mechanisms.

Aminiocaproic acid is used in the treatment of hyperfibrinolysis-induced hemorrhage such as fibrinolytic bleeding after heart surgery, prostatectomy, nephrectomy, and for hematologic disorders such as aplastic anemia, hepatic cirrhosis, and neoplastic disease states. Although not an approved indication, it has also been used as a specific antidote for an overdose of thrombolytic drugs.

Aminocaproic acid is absorbed orally and reaches a peak concentration within 2 hours. The therapeutic serum concentration is 130 μg/mL to inhibit systemic hyperfibrinolysis or 150 to 300 μg/mL to prevent recurrent subarachnoid hemorrhage. It is excreted mainly by the kidneys.

The side effects/adverse reactions include nausea; diarrhea; menstrual difficulties; increased weakness; severe muscle pain; a decrease in urination; edema of the face, feet, or lower legs; unusual weight gain; slow or irregular heart rate; abdominal pain; rash; stuffy nose; tinnitus; bloodshot eyes; and thrombosis.

The recommended adult dosage of aminocaproic acid is 5 g PO or parenterally (IV infusion) initially, followed by 1 g/hr for up to 8 hours or until the desired response is achieved. The maximum dosage is 30 g/24 hr. The pediatric dosage (oral or parenteral) is 100 mg/kg body weight the first hour followed by 33.3 mg/kg/hr up to 18 g/m^2/24 hr.

■ Nursing Management
Aminocaproic Acid Therapy

■ **Assessment.** Aminocaproic acid is contraindicated for use in clients with active intravascular clotting because of the risk of serious thrombus formation. It is used cautiously in individuals with a predisposition to thrombosis or in those with cardiac disease (may cause hypotension and bradycardia), hepatic disease (may make diagnosing the cause of bleeding more difficult), or renal disease (may accumulate). Assess the female client's current drug regimen for estrogen or estrogen-containing contraceptives, because they will increase the risk for thrombus formation if administered concurrently with aminocaproic acid.

Assess baseline vital signs and coagulation studies initially and periodically during administration.

■ **Nursing Diagnosis.** With the administration of aminocaproic acid, the client is at risk for development of the following nursing diagnoses/collaborative problems: impaired comfort (headache, myopathy, tinnitus, stuffy nose, rash, nausea, abdominal cramping, or unusual menstrual cramping); diarrhea; impaired urinary elimination related to bladder obstruction caused by blood clot formation; fatigue; sexual dysfunction (dry ejaculation); risk for injury related to hypotension; and the potential complications of renal failure (sudden decrease in urinary output, edema) or thromboembolism (sudden headache; pains in chest, groin, or legs; sudden shortness of breath; slurred speech; vision changes; or weakness of arm or leg).

■ **Implementation**

■ ***Monitoring.*** Monitor the client for signs of thromboembolic complications such as thrombophlebitis, pulmonary embolus, myocardial infarction, and cerebrovascular accident. Monitor for the signs and symptoms of the previously listed nursing diagnoses. Aminocaproic acid therapy is usually discontinued when bleeding stops or when laboratory values of fibrinolysis indicate that the drug is no longer necessary.

■ ***Intervention.*** Dilute before administering intravenously. Dilution with sterile water for injection is not recommended for clients with subarachnoid hemorrhage. Administer slowly; an infusion that is too rapid may result in hypotension or bradycardia. Take care with insertion and positioning of the infusion needle to minimize thrombophlebitis. The syrup form of the drug may be used as an oral rinse to prevent bleeding during dental and oral surgery in clients with hemophilia.

■ ***Education.*** Inform the client of the purpose of the medication and subjective symptoms to report, such as headache, dizziness, tinnitus, and abdominal cramping.

■ **Evaluation.** The expected outcome of aminocaproic acid therapy is that the client's laboratory values for fibrinolysis will be within normal limits and that the client will have no signs of bleeding.

tranexamic acid [tran ex am′ ik] (Cyklokapron)

Tranexamic acid is a competitive inhibitor of plasminogen activation; at high doses, it is a noncompetitive inhibitor of plasmin. Its effects are similar to aminocaproic acid, but it is approximately 5 to 10 times more potent in vitro. It is used after dental surgery in clients with hemophilia to reduce or prevent bleeding episodes.

Peak plasma levels are reached 3 hours after oral administration; the peak plasma level is 8 μg/mL after a 1-g dose. The duration of action in serum is 7 to 8 hours, and excretion is by the kidneys.

The side effects/adverse reactions of tranexamic acid include nausea, vomiting, and diarrhea. Visual disturbance, thrombosis, and menstrual discomfort have been infrequently reported. No significant drug interactions have been reported.

The dosage before dental surgery for adolescents and adults with hemophilia is 25 mg/kg PO three or four times daily, starting 1 day before the planned dental procedure. Clotting factors VIII or IX should also be given before surgery. Postsurgically, the dosage is 25 mg/kg PO three or four times daily for 2 to 8 days. The parenteral postsurgical dose is usually reserved for persons who are unable to take the oral product. By injection, the dosage is 10 mg/kg IV before surgery and 10 mg/kg IV postsurgically three or four times daily for 2 to 8 days.

■ Nursing Management

Tranexamic Acid Therapy

In addition to the following discussion, see Nursing Management: Aminocaproic Acid Therapy, p. 640. Tranexamic acid places the client at risk for visual disturbances. For this reason ophthalmologic examinations (visual acuity, color vision, eye grounds, and visual fields) are suggested before and periodically during therapy. It is recommended that administration of the drug be discontinued if visual changes occur or if thromboembolic complications occur.

Tranexamic acid, as an IV medication, should not be mixed with blood or added to any solution containing penicillin.

aprotinin [a pro ti′ nin] (Trasylol)

Aprotinin is a proteinase inhibitor obtained from bovine lung that directly prevents fibrinolysis by inhibiting plasmin and kallikrein, an enzyme of the renal cortex. It is used in cardiopulmonary bypass surgery to reduce blood loss and the need for blood transfusions.

Aprotinin is administered intravenously and is rapidly distributed in the extracellular space with a terminal half-life between 5 and 10 hours. It is slowly metabolized by lysosomes in the kidneys and excreted primarily in the urine.

Side effects/adverse reactions are rare but include allergic-type reactions (skin rash, respiratory difficulties, nausea, tachycardia, hypotension, bronchospasm) and anaphylaxis. The recommended adult dosage is 10,000 KIU (1 mL) as a test IV dose first, administered at least 10 minutes before the loading dose. If no allergic-type reaction occurs, all other dosages should be administered via a central venous line, and no medications should be given in this line. See the current *USP DI* or the package insert for dosing recommendations.

■ Nursing Management

Aprotinin Therapy

■ **Assessment.** Determine if the client is allergic to aprotinin by obtaining a history and/or administering a test dose. All clients should receive a test dose (1 mL) IV at least 10 minutes before a loading dose. There is an increased risk of allergic reactions with reexposure to the drug. Assess the client's pulse, blood pressure, respirations, breath sounds, and skin for color, temperature, and other indicators of peripheral perfusion. A baseline ECG and renal and hepatic function studies should be performed.

Review the client's current medication profile to determine drug-drug interactions, such as thrombolytic agents that will increase the risk for hemorrhage.

■ **Nursing Diagnosis.** The client receiving aprotinin has the potential for the following nursing diagnoses/collaborative problems: risk for injury related to hypotension; ineffective airway clearance related to asthma; and the potential complication of anaphylaxis.

■ **Implementation**

■ ***Monitoring.*** Continue to monitor the client by the indicators in the baseline assessment and ACT and partial prothrombin time (PTT).

■ ***Intervention.*** After a loading dose over 20 to 30 minutes, a continuous infusion of 50 mL/hr is used. All IV doses are to be administered through a central venous line, and no other medication should be administered through the same line.

■ ***Education.*** Inform the client of the purpose of aprotinin and any subjective symptoms that should be reported, such as palpitations and beginning dyspnea.

■ **Evaluation.** The expected outcome of aprotinin therapy is that the client will show no evidence of blood loss or anaphylaxis, and the pulse, blood pressure, and ECG will remain within normal limits.

Topical Hemostatics

absorbable gelatin sponge (Gelfoam)

Absorbable gelatin sponge is a specially prepared, nonantigenic gelatin capable of holding many times its weight in whole blood. It is used in thin strips to control capillary bleeding and may be left in place in a surgical wound because it is completely absorbed in 4 to 6 weeks. It should be well moistened with isotonic saline solution or thrombin solution before being applied to a bleeding surface. Its presence does not induce excessive scar formation. Sterile technique must be used to avoid infection.

When inserted into cavities or tissue spaces, the gelatin sponge reduces bleeding by acting as a tampon. The contact with the sponge damages platelets, liberating the thromboplastin needed for clot formation. This product completely dissolves within 2 to 5 days when applied to bleeding areas on the skin or in the nose, rectum, or vagina.

An absorbable gelatin sponge is indicated in surgical procedures as an adjunct to hemostasis when bleeding is not controlled by ligature or when such methods are impractical. It is also used by dentists to aid in hemostasis.

Insertion of the gelatin sponge in the prostatic cavity promotes hemostasis in open prostatic surgery. The gelatin sponge may provide a site for infection. Monitor the surgical incision and implantation site closely for redness, swelling, or discomfort, as well as for signs of recurrent bleeding.

No significant drug interactions have been reported. This product is available in different sizes and diameters. Application instructions and size depend on the area to be treated.

absorbable gelatin film (Gelfilm)

A sterile absorbable gelatin film (Gelfilm) is also available for specific indications, such as neurosurgery or thoracic or ocular surgery. When it is implanted in tissues, the rate of absorption can range from 2 to 5 months depending on the site of implantation and the size of the film implanted. This product is useful as a dural substitute (neurosurgery) or to repair pleural defects during thoracic surgery.

absorbable gelatin powder (Gelfoam)

A sterile absorbable gelatin powder (Gelfoam) is also available to promote hemostasis. This powder can be made into a paste to control bleeding from bone areas when standard procedures such as ligatures are ineffective or impractical. It is also used to treat chronic leg ulcers and decubitus ulcers.

oxidized cellulose (Oxycel, Surgicel)

Oxidized cellulose is a specially treated form of surgical gauze or cotton that exerts a hemostatic effect but is absorbable when buried in the tissues. The hemostatic action is caused by the formation of an artificial clot by cellulosic acid. Absorption of oxidized cellulose occurs between the second and the seventh days following implantation, although the absorption of large amounts of blood-soaked material may take 6 weeks or longer. Oxidized cellulose is valuable in controlling bleeding during surgery that involves organs such as the liver, pancreas, spleen, kidney, thyroid, and prostate. Its hemostatic action is not increased by the addition of other hemostatic agents. It should not be used as a surface dressing except for the control of bleeding, because cellulosic acid inhibits the growth of epithelial tissue. It also interferes with bone regeneration and therefore should not be implanted in fractures.

No significant drug interactions are reported. Do not moisten the oxidized cellulose, and use sterile technique when applying or inserting it. Serious adverse reactions are related to the site of application, the amount used, and the pressure applied to a blood vessel or specific area. Careful application and monitoring are necessary to reduce complications such as obstruction, necrosis, and stenosis. A burning sensation has been reported when used after nasal polyp removal or hemorrhoidectomy. Headache, stinging, and sneezing may also occur.

microfibrillar collagen hemostat (Avitene)

Microfibrillar collagen hemostat is an absorbable topical hemostatic substance that will attract platelets and platelet aggregation in the area when placed on a bleeding surface, forming thrombi. It is used as an adjunct to hemostasis during surgery when ligature or standard procedures are ineffective or impractical.

Adhesions, allergic or foreign body reactions, hematomas, or infections such as abscesses may occur. Monitor the client closely, because these conditions may cause serious problems. No significant drug interactions have been reported.

In general, microfibrillar collagen hemostat is applied directly on the source of bleeding in a dry form. Do not moisten or wet this substance, and do not resterilize it. Apply pressure over the area with a dry sponge for a minute or more. Use dry forceps to handle it because it will adhere to wet gloves or instruments. Do not use gloved fingers to apply the necessary pressure.

thrombin (Thrombinar, Thrombostat)

Thrombin is a hemostatic agent prepared as a sterile powder; it is obtained from bovine prothrombin that has been treated with thromboplastin in the presence of calcium. Thrombin catalyzes the conversion of fibrinogen to fibrin. It has several additional mechanisms, which may include stimulating the release, reaction, and aggregation of platelets. It is used topically to treat capillary bleeding. It has also been used during various surgeries with absorbable gelatin sponge for hemostasis.

Febrile and allergic-type reactions have been reported when thrombin is used for epistaxis. No significant drug interactions are reported.

Thrombin may be applied topically as a powder or solution. Concentration of the preparation varies with its use (see the package insert).

■ Nursing Management

Thrombin Therapy

■ **Assessment.** Ascertain whether or not the client is sensitive to bovine products.

■ **Nursing Diagnosis.** The client undergoing thrombin therapy may be at risk for infection and the potential complications of an allergic reaction and bleeding related to the ineffectiveness of the therapy.

■ **Implementation**

■ ***Monitoring.*** Monitor the client for recurrent bleeding, infection, and allergic reaction.

■ ***Intervention.*** Do not inject thrombin into large blood vessels, because extensive intravascular clotting and even death may result. Sponge—do not wipe—all blood from the recipient surface before applying the thrombin as a powder or a solution. If applied as a powder, thrombin may need to be pulverized with a sterile instrument before use. To avoid disturbing the clotting, do not sponge once the thrombin is applied. Thrombin may be used in association with an absorbable gelatin foam. In this case the saturated sponge is applied to the bleeding area for 10 to 15 seconds to promote hemostasis. Use the solution within a few hours of reconstitution, or freeze it and use within 48 hours.

■ **Evaluation.** The expected outcome of thrombin therapy is that the client's bleeding will diminish and eventually cease.

BLOOD AND BLOOD COMPONENTS

The bloodstream is the main mode of transport and distribution in the body. As such, it functions to deliver vital nutrients, water, and oxygen from the digestive and respiratory systems to all body parts. Wastes are retrieved for excretion by the bloodstream. In the kidneys, the bloodstream provides the hydrostatic pressure necessary to create urine as an excretory vehicle for those waste products. It conveys hormones from endocrine glands and enzymes, vitamins, buffers, and other biochemical substances to target areas. The bloodstream buffers and regulates the body's heat exchange processes by absorbing and transferring core body heat to the surface for dissipation, and it buffers the body's acid-base balance. The bloodstream also carries components such as platelets, blood cells, and antibodies to sites where a sudden need for these exists, such as in hemorrhage, inflammation, or infection.

The bloodstream creates oncotic or colloid osmotic pressure to regulate the volume of interstitial fluids. It also transports therapeutic additives such as medications, fluids, electrolytes, and nutrients to their respective sites of action.

Abnormal States of Blood Components

Normally, a thrifty bodily balance is maintained between the production and loss, attrition, or excretion of all components that comprise the bloodstream. Pathologic conditions result from a disturbance in production or an excessive loss or excretion of one or more components. Hemorrhage results in a generally impoverished bloodstream and may significantly alter many body functions. Impaired production or the increased destruction of any one component may impinge on one or more functions. All this is a matter of degree. If the impairment is minor or is detected early, correction of the cause and replenishment by natural or therapeutic means may restore functioning.

Naturally harmful or foreign substances may build up in the bloodstream when excretory systems fail (e.g., renal failure) or when metabolizing capabilities fail (e.g., liver failure). Some examples of abnormal states of blood components follow.

Depending on the individual's size and preexisting blood integrity, an acute whole blood loss of more than 500 mL is manifested by signs of anemia. Chronic, gradual, and unnoticed blood loss from gastrointestinal tract malignancy, ulcers, or hemorrhoids may be compensated for naturally, or iron deficiency anemia may develop. Signs of anemia usually reflect the true importance of red blood cell loss. Deficiencies in intake or in the functioning of certain essential nutritional elements may result in iron deficiency anemia or one of the megaloblastic anemias, which usually are caused by deficiencies in vitamin B_{12} or folic acid. A pathologic overabundance of erythrocytes can be compensation for long-standing hypoxia from pulmonary or cardiac disease, certain tumors, or polycythemia vera. Delayed or disordered production of erythrocytes (aplastic anemia) may result from disorders of the reticuloendothelial system, primarily the bone marrow, which is responsible for their systematic production. The bone marrow is particularly vulnerable to certain drugs, poisons, and antineoplastic agents. On the other hand, too-rapid destruction of erythrocytes can lead to hemolytic anemia.

Leukocytes also are lost in hemorrhage, but reductions in their numbers most often are associated with certain specific conditions. Each of the five types of white blood cells—neutrophils, eosinophils, basophils, lymphocytes, and monocytes—is associated with different disorders. For example, abnormally low neutrophil counts are associated with certain aplastic diseases, as well as with acute reactions to drugs such as sulfonamides, propylthiouracil, and chloramphenicol. Excessively high neutrophil counts are found primarily with bacterial infections, as well as with some inflammatory disorders, leukemia, and hyperplastic disorders.

Thrombocytes may be present in inadequate numbers because of their rapid destruction, typically caused by idiopathic thrombocytopenia purpura. Conversely, excessive platelet counts are associated most often with hyperplastic disorders, iron deficiency anemia, splenectomy, and chronic inflammatory conditions such as tuberculosis. Other factors crucial to the clotting process may be absent in hemophilia and similar disorders.

Losses of the liquid portion of the blood can create dehydration problems, impede metabolic processes that function only through the use of hydrogen or oxygen molecules, or subvert hydrodynamic and hydraulic processes.

In addition to hemorrhage, plasma proteins may be lost through burn wounds or wound drainage or may be insufficient because of a lack of adequate available substrates such as amino acids. The results vary depending on the type of plasma protein and may include deficiencies in immune sta-

TABLE 31-5 Indications for Common Blood Component Therapies

Component	Indications
Whole blood	Hemorrhage, hypovolemic shock
Fresh whole blood	Multiple transfusions, exchange transfusions; priming agent for hemodialysis machines (normal saline may also be used)
Packed red blood cells	Transfused when whole blood could result in circulatory overload
Deglycerolized or washed red cells	Transfused when hypersensitivity reactions are likely, as in immunosuppressed clients and those with a history of reactions or extreme hypersensitivity
Fresh-frozen plasma (FFP)	Clotting deficiencies, especially factors V and VII; blood volume expansion in burns, shock, or protein deficiencies (believed to be overused for these deficiencies)
Plasma exchange (plasmapheresis): blood drawn off, cleansed, and components returned	Immune-related disorders: multiple myeloma, glomerulonephritis, systemic lupus erythematosus, rheumatoid arthritis, myasthenia gravis
Plasma expanders (Dextran—large polysaccharide polymer)	Temporary volume expansion in hemorrhagic shock states (sole use for Dextran 70 or 75); not a substitute for blood or plasma
Granulocytes	Granulocyte counts below $500/mm^3$
Platelets	Platelet counts at or below $20{,}000/mm^3$
Cryoprecipitate (fresh-frozen plasma precipitate; contains factors I and VIII)	Hemophilia, fibrinogen deficiency, von Willebrand's disease
Antihemophilic factor concentrate	Treatment of hemophilia; preferred over fresh-frozen plasma
Factor VIIa	
Factor IX complex	Hemophilia B; deficiencies of clotting factors II, VII, X; coumarin overdose
Plasma protein fraction (PPF)	Hypovolemic shock, protein replacement, burns, adult respiratory distress syndrome, dehydration, and hypoalbuminemia; as an additive to complement packed cells when necessary
Fibrinogen	When fibrinogen levels are insufficient for adequate control of bleeding
Albumin	Blood volume expansion by oncotic pressure; prevention and treatment of cerebral edema
Gamma globulins	Exposure to hepatitis; to prevent complications of mumps

tus, blood viscosity, or colloid osmotic pressure (oncotic pressure).

Replacement Therapies

Therapy to replace all or certain components of the bloodstream is a common practice in most health facilities. Because blood is considered a tissue, transfusions are technically tissue transplants. The usual treatment of choice is replacement of the blood component that is deficient rather than whole blood, because the body is better able to replace intravascular fluids than formed elements of the blood. Transfusing only the depleted blood fraction serves two other purposes: (1) it prevents fluid overload in high-risk individuals such as older adults and those with cardiovascular or renal disease, and (2) it more efficiently uses the remaining blood fractions for other clients' needs. Table 31-5 outlines the indications for this therapy. When a client is to receive blood, the nurse is largely responsible for its safe administration.

■ Nursing Management
Blood and Blood Component Replacement Therapies

■ **Assessment.** Obtain the client history regarding previous transfusions and the client's response to them. Report any history of an adverse reaction to the prescriber and the blood bank. Assess the client for adequacy of venous access. Gather baseline data about the client's blood studies and vital signs before administration, and observe the general appearance and demeanor of the client.

■ **Nursing Diagnosis.** The client is at risk for injury related to a hemolytic or allergic reaction (anaphylactic shock), volume overload (pulmonary congestion, circulatory overload), or a response to aged blood (hyperkalemia).

■ **Implementation**

■ ***Monitoring.*** As administration begins, observe the client closely for reactions for 15 minutes or more while the flow rate is kept at 20 to 30 drops/min. Assess and record vital signs several times during the first 15 minutes. If reactions occur, stop the transfusion and administer the prescribed corrective measures. Observe the client for the development of the following:

- Apprehension; restlessness; flushed skin; increased pulse and respiratory rates; burning sensations; fever; chills; dyspnea; chest, head, or back pain; shock—hemolysis (possible blood type incompatibility)
- Rash; swellings of the skin, face, or throat; pruritus; shock—allergic reaction
- Fever and chills starting 1 hour after administration and lasting up to 10 hours—febrile reaction
- Nausea, weakness, jaundice considerably later—possible viral hepatitis
- Fever and chills, hypotension, vomiting, abdominal pain, bloody diarrhea—bacterial contamination
- Dyspnea, tight chest, cough with basilar rales, pulmonary edema—circulatory overload
- Cyanosis, dyspnea, abrupt onset of localized pain, shock—air embolism

Frequent assessment of the needle insertion site is essential because the absorption of infiltrated blood is very slow. If no symptoms of reactions appear after the first 15 minutes, the flow rate may be calculated and set so that therapy is concluded in ½ to 2 hours (volumes are usually between 250 and 500 mL). Continue monitoring vital signs and observing for symptoms throughout administration.

■ ***Intervention.*** Administer blood components promptly to ensure that the transfused product is fresh, uncoagulated, and without toxic breakdown products. Before administration, the product should remain out of the blood bank's refrigerator and untransfused for no longer than 30 minutes. Refrigeration in the standard hospital units or home refrigerator will not prevent deterioration. Blood and blood components must not lie unused at the nursing station but must be returned to the blood bank refrigerator if administration has not started within ½ hour. A unit of whole blood or packed red blood cells cannot be returned to a blood bank if it has been out of a monitored environment (1° to 6° C) for more than 30 minutes. Once the infusion has started, whole blood or packed red blood cells should be transfused within 2 hours, 4 hours at the most.

Because incompatibility is a possibility, especially after multiple doses of these products, take precautions such as scrupulously comparing the product ordered with the label on the product before administration. The worst adverse reactions to blood transfusions often result from misidentification of the blood or the client. Although the procedures of various institutions vary, at least two persons (often two registered nurses) must verify the identification of blood product and client. This will vary with the administration of blood products in the home (see the Community and Home Health Considerations box at right). Client identification must match, as well as the prescriber's name, the blood type, the Rh factor, and the unit number. Note the Venereal Disease Research Laboratories' (VDRL) information and expiration date. Compare the client's identifying armband or tag with the label on the container.

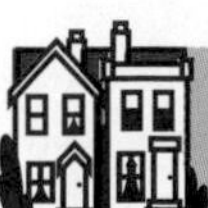

Community and Home Health Considerations
Blood Component Administration

It is becoming increasingly common for whole blood, blood components, or expanders to be administered in the home setting. The administration of these substances allows for the restoration of blood volume or the replacement of serum, plasma, RBCs, platelets, or albumin in a more cost-effective and comfortable environment for the client.

The client and caregiver(s) need to understand the purpose of the blood administration. Ask them if they understand the procedure and why it is being performed. Assess the client's allergy history, and ascertain any previous reactions to blood products.

Make the client comfortable in bed or in a reclining chair. Have the client void before the procedure begins. Check the blood bag information against the client identification with at least one other person. Check the bag for leaks. Select an appropriate site and perform the venipuncture using aseptic technique (see the discussion of nursing management for infusion techniques discussed in this chapter). Determine the drip rate per minute and the time for blood completion. Administer the blood slowly for the first 15 minutes, and monitor the client and vital signs carefully during this time. Monitor the vital signs every hour while the blood is infusing; check the drip rate every 15 minutes. Assess the infusion site for infiltration. Assess the client for symptoms of transfusion reaction as discussed in the text. Change the blood tubing and filter if more than one unit is to be administered. Remove the IV needle or cannula after transfusion and ensure that it is intact. Document the procedure as described in the text.

If the client experiences any untoward symptoms, stop the transfusion and transfuse normal saline. Follow the health care agency protocols for emergency action. Stay with the client until the situation is resolved.

Nurses should be aware of transfusion hazards in certain blood-type combinations. Careful typing and crossmatching help to prevent serious complications. ABO antigen-antibody reactions result from the following and must be avoided:

Recipient's Blood Type	Should Not Receive
A	Type B or AB
B	Type A or AB
O	Any type except type O

Recipient's Blood Type	Reactions with Multiple Transfusions
A	Type O
B	Type O
AB	Type A, B, or O

Immediately report to the blood bank any discrepancies between the information on the compatibility tag, the unit of blood, and the prescriber's order on the clinical record; blood that is past its expiration date; or any signs of contamination.

Hypersensitivity is also common, because most of these products are essentially foreign proteins. Exceptions include autologous transfusions collected previously from the client's own blood or transfusions of inert, synthetic products. Diphenhydramine (Benadryl) 25 mg, taken orally or injected into blood transfusion tubing before the transfusion, is recommended to prevent mild allergic reactions.

Return the product to the blood bank or laboratory if the contents appear unusual because of discoloration, gas bubbles, or an overly full (gaseous) appearance. Mix the contents by gently upending the container once or twice; take care not to bruise or damage blood cells or other fragile components by squeezing or agitating the bag carelessly. Note that many of these agents require the concomitant use of a 170-μg filter incorporated into the transfusion tubing to remove the debris and tiny clots found in the blood. Check the filter often to ensure that it is not clogged and slowing the transfusion. If the rate of transfusion is too slow, it may be necessary to use a filter with a larger surface area. This may also be necessary when administering packed RBCs because of the viscosity of the product. Access to the vein should be provided by fresh tubing and a needle no smaller than 19 gauge. However, a 22- or 23-gauge needle is recommended for adults with small veins and for children.

A normal saline solution should be hung in tandem with the blood product using a Y-set multiple lead tubing. Use the saline solution to flush the tubing before connecting it to the insertion site. Using straight tubing limits the possibility of stopping the transfusion while keeping the vein open if the client has an untoward response to the blood. Piggybacking on an established IV line increases the risk of

BOX 31-2

Legal Implications: Consent for Transfusion

The law is clear that ordinarily a physician has the sole and exclusive right to obtain his or her client's informed consent to surgery. However, who bears the responsibility to obtain the client's informed consent to a blood transfusion? Whose duty is it to apprise the client of all of the risks attendant to the transfusion of donated blood? Must the client be informed that there are several options, including donations from "anonymous" sources, direct donations (usually from family or friends), or an autologous donation (in which the client donates blood before surgery) for use during surgery?

Informed consent was at issue in Jones *v.* Philadelphia Coll. of Osteo. Med. (813 F. Supp. 1125-PA [1993]). On October 6, 1986, J. Jones was admitted to the hospital by his primary treating physician for a lumbar myelogram to diagnose the cause of his severe low back pain. Following this examination, his physician recommended surgery to alleviate his condition. During surgery Mr. Jones lost blood and received 9 units of packed cells and 2 units of fresh-frozen plasma. One of the units of fresh-frozen plasma came from an "anonymous" donor who was infected with the HIV virus. Before his transfusion, Mr. Jones was never advised by the physicians or the hospital of the potential risk of contracting AIDS as a result of the use of contaminated blood products. He brought suit against the hospital and physicians involved in the surgery, alleging that he received HIV-contaminated blood during the surgery.

The United States District Court for the Eastern District of Pennsylvania held that informed consent was necessary for blood transfusions. The law of Pennsylvania states that consent is valid only if the individual grants it after being fully apprised of important matters such as the nature of the therapy, the seriousness of the situation, the disease and organs involved, and the potential results of the treatment. In determining whether a client's consent was "informed," the standard is whether the physician disclosed all the facts, risks, and alternatives that a reasonable person in the situation would deem significant. In Pennsylvania the doctrine of informed consent is limited to cases involving surgery or operative procedures. However, the Court held that a physician cannot inform a client of all of the risks of a surgical procedure without also informing him or her of the risks associated with blood transfusion when transfusion is a potential part of the procedure.

Although the Court held that only the primary treating physician could be held liable for failure to obtain informed consent, there was also a basis for liability on the part of the hospital. Because the hospital was bound by FDA regulations requiring it to obtain informed consent and because the hospital could also be held liable for battery (lack of informed consent) by intending that the client come in contact with a foreign substance as a part of a planned procedure, the hospital had Mr. Jones sign two documents for informed consent for transfusion. In doing so the hospital "gratuitously undertook an obligation to obtain informed consent." Because of this the Court concluded that Mr. Jones may indeed have a valid claim against the hospital as well as against the physician.

How would this knowledge of informed consent influence your nursing practice in relation to clients receiving a blood transfusion?

Information from Tammelleo A.D. (Ed.). (1993). Must hospitals obtain "consent" for transfusions? *Reagan Report,* 33(12), 1.

contamination, especially with the administration of multiple units of blood. Change the filter and administration set at least every 4 hours; do not transfuse more than 2 units per administration set.

Infuse approximately 60 mL of saline through the tubing before and after the transfusion. Do not use dextrose and other solutions with red blood cell products, because they may react with the product in the tubing to clump cells and cause hemolysis. When inserting the spike of the administration set into the port of the blood bag, guide it straight into the container to avoid puncturing the side of the bag. Note that infusion pumps intended specifically for maintaining transfusion rates are safe and reliable when used with the appropriate tubing and filters. Raising the height of the container or applying a pressure sleeve to the bag (at pressures up to 300 mm Hg) is also useful to maintain transfusion flows at prescribed rates. Higher pressures may burst the bag.

To maintain the prescribed infusion rate, agitate the blood by inverting the bag frequently during administration. A blood-warming device (up to 37° C [98.6° F]) is necessary if a rapid transfusion is to be made through a central venous catheter line. Do not administer any medications through the same tubing while any blood products are being infused.

Documentation should include the client's baseline vital signs before the transfusion was started; the signatures of the two persons who identified the client and the blood product; the blood product administered; the time the transfusion was started and completed; the total volume of fluid transfused, listing the starter solution separately; the client's response to the transfusion; and any nursing interventions taken in response to an adverse reaction to the blood.

Be aware that the risks of nursing personnel contracting diseases such as hepatitis when accidentally injected with pooled blood, especially repeatedly, are not entirely known. Therefore take care when manipulating these products and their equipment. Use universal precautions.

If the client experiences any of the untoward symptoms previously discussed, stop the transfusion and infuse normal saline. Notify the prescriber. Continue to monitor vital signs, monitor intake and output, observe the client, and follow the health agency's emergency measures. Obtain a blood sample and the first voided urine specimen after the reaction.

■ ***Education.*** Explain the transfusion procedure to the client, especially the reason why it has been ordered. Many older adults associate a blood transfusion with being critically ill and may be upset about the need for the transfusion. Ensure that a consent form for the procedure has been signed (Box 31-2).

Instruct the client to report any symptoms of an adverse reaction, such as nausea, chills, burning sensations, or headache.

■ **Evaluation.** The client will experience increased hemoglobin and hematocrit levels. One unit of whole blood typically raises the average adult's hemoglobin level by 1 to 1.5 g/dL and the hematocrit by 2% to 3%.

SUMMARY

This chapter reviewed substances that concern anticoagulant therapy, thrombolytic therapy, antiplatelet agents, hemostatic agents, and blood and blood component administration. Anticoagulant therapy is primarily prophylactic; it acts to prevent fibrin deposits, thrombus extension, and thromboembolic complications by decreasing blood coagulability. Anticoagulants may be administered parenterally or orally. Administered parenterally, heparins act almost immediately but have a short duration of action (less than 4 hours). Coumarin and the indanedione derivatives are administered orally; the onset of action is slow (24 to 48 hours) and the duration is long (2 to 5 days). This allows heparin and coumarin to be used in a complementary fashion. They may be started simultaneously; heparin is used when an immediate anticoagulant effect is needed, and its dosage is tapered off as the oral agent produces its full therapeutic effect. In the administration of both types of anticoagulants, the client has the potential for injury related to increased bleeding tendencies; nursing care focuses on the observation, protection, and education of the client to prevent injury. There are specific antidotes for both parenteral and oral anticoagulants: protamine sulfate is the antidote for heparin, and vitamin K is the antidote for the oral anticoagulants.

Whereas anticoagulants are used prophylactically, thrombolytic agents are used to dissolve clots in the treatment of acute thromboembolic disorders. Thrombolytic enzyme therapy with streptokinase, urokinase, alteplase, or anistreplase alters the hemostatic capability of the client to a greater extent than anticoagulant therapy; therefore when bleeding does occur, it is more severe and more difficult to control. Antiplatelet drugs are used for the treatment and prevention of ischemic events.

Hemostatic agents are compounds used to hasten clot formation to reduce bleeding and therefore control rapid blood loss. Aminocaproic acid, a hemostatic agent, has been used as an antidote for the thrombolytic agents, but this use is not approved.

The antihemophilic agents are specific factors within the clotting process that can be used in replacement therapy for clients who have hemophilia, a deficiency of one or more plasma protein clotting factors. With accurate diagnosis of the specific missing factor, this replacement therapy has allowed for the successful management of these clients at home.

Blood and blood components may need to be replaced as the result of impaired production, excessive loss, or increased destruction of any of the components. Because blood is considered a tissue, transfusions are essentially tissue transplants. The preferred therapy is replacement of the sole blood component that is deficient rather than whole blood. However, the nurse needs to be alert to the many responses that clients may have to such transfusions. Careful typing and crossmatching helps to prevent many serious complications, but careful observation of the client is essential during the transfusion of blood and blood components.

Critical Thinking Questions

1. Mary Brickland, age 58, is admitted to a general medical unit for the treatment of acute thrombophlebitis in her right calf. Strict bed rest and heparin 5000 U by IV bolus followed by 1000 U/hr are prescribed. Why would heparin be the anticoagulant of choice? How would you best monitor the effectiveness of the heparin therapy?
   In preparation for discharge, the prescriber adds coumadin to Ms. Brickland's medication regimen. How will this affect her response to the heparin therapy?
2. George Thomas, age 45, has been admitted to the emergency department with an acute myocardial infarction. In the brief medical history that was obtained, it was determined that Mr. Thomas was seeing his primary care physician for an active peptic ulcer for which he was taking antacids and cimetidine. The emergency physician decides to administer streptokinase IV. What will be of major concern for the client's safety? What assessments are required to monitor Mr. Thomas' condition?
3. What is the informed consent policy for the transfusion of blood products within your practice setting? What part do you play in this policy as a nursing student? What will your role be as a registered nurse?

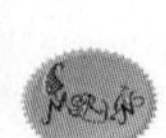

Collaborative Learning Activities

For Collaborative Learning Activities, go to mosby.com/MERLIN/McKenry/.

CASE STUDY

For a Case Study that will help ensure mastery of this chapter content, go to mosby.com/MERLIN/McKenry/.

BIBLIOGRAPHY

Abramowicz, M. (Ed.). (1993). Recombinant antihemophilic factor. *Medical Letter 35*(898), 51.

American Association of Critical Care Nurses. (1990). Nationwide practice survey results announced. *AACN News*, August, 3.

American Hospital Formulary Service. (1999). *AFHS drug information '99*. Bethesda, MD: American Society of Hospital Pharmacists.

Anderson, K.N., Anderson, L.E., & Glanze, W.D. (Eds.) (1998). *Mosby's medical, nursing, & allied health dictionary* (5th ed.). St. Louis: Mosby.

Bick, R.L. & Strauss, J. (1995). Thrombolytic therapy and its uses. *Laboratory Medicine, 26*(5), 330-337.

Boysen, G. (1999). Bleeding complications in secondary stroke prevention by antiplatelet therapy: A benefit-risk analysis. *Journal of Internal Medicine, 246*(3), 239-245.

Chan, W.S. & Ray, J.G. (1999). Low molecular weight heparin use during pregnancy: Issues of safety and practicality. *Obsterical & Gynecological Survey, 54*(10), 649-654.

Craig, V. & Bower, J.O. (1997). Perioperative pharmacology: Blood administration in perioperative settings. *AORN Journal, 66*(1), 133-136.

Dreger, V. & Tremback, T. (1998). Blood and blood product use in perioperative care. *AORN Journal, 67*(1), 153-154, 156, 158.

Drug Facts and Comparisons. (2000). St. Louis: Facts and Comparisons.

Friedman, M.M. (1997). Risk management strategies for home transfusion therapy. *Journal of Intravenous Therapy, 20*(4), 179-187.

Fry, B. (1992). Intermittent heparin flushing protocols: A standardization issue. *Journal of Intravenous Nursing, 15*(3), 160.

Golberg, M., Sankaran, R., Givelichian, L., & Sankaran, K. (1999). Maintaining patency of peripheral intermittent infusion devices with heparinized saline and saline: A randomized double blind controlled trial in neonatal intensive care and a review of literature. *Neonatal Intensive Care, 12*(1), 18-22.

Hardman, J.G. & Limbird, L.E. (Eds.).(1996). *Goodman and Gilman's The pharmacological basis of therapeutics* (9th ed.). New York: McGraw-Hill.

Heilskov, J., Kleiber, C., Johnson, K., Miller, J. (1998). A randomized trial of heparin and saline for maintaining intravenous locks in neonates. *J Soc Pediatr Nurs, 3*(3), 111-116.

Hock, N. (1998). Neuroprotective and thrombolytic agents: Advances in stroke therapy. *Journal of Neuroscience Nursing, 30*(3), 175-184.

Jaffee, M.S. & Skidmore-Roth, L. (1988). *Home health nursing care plans*. St. Louis: Mosby.

Kotter, R.W. (1996). Heparin vs saline for intermittent intravenous device maintenance in neonates. *Neonatal Network, 15*(6), 43-47.

Majerus, P., Broze, Jr., G.J., Miletich, J.P., & Tollefsen, D.M. (1996). Anticoagulant, thrombolytic, and antiplatelet drugs. In J.G. Hardman & L.E. Limbird (Eds.), *Goodman and Gilman's The pharmacological basis of therapeutics* (9th ed.). New York: McGraw-Hill.

Mazur, W., Kaluza, G., & Kleiman, N.S. (1999). Antiplatelet therapy for treatment of acute coronary syndromes. *Cardiology Clinics, 17*(2), 345-357.

McAllister, C.C., Lenaghan, P.A., & Tosone, N.C. (1993). Changing from heparin to saline flush solutions: A research utilization model for implementation. *Journal of Emergency Nursing, 19*(4), 306-312.

McCloskey, J.C. & Bulechek, G.M. (Eds.) (1996). *Nursing interventions classification (NIC)*. St. Louis: Mosby.

McMullen, A. et al. (1993). Heparinized saline or normal saline as a flush solution in intermittent intravenous lines in infants and children. *MCN, 18*(2), 78.

Mudge, B., Forcier, D., Slatterly, M.J. (1998). Patency of 24-gauge peripheral intermittent infusion devices: A comparison of heparin and saline flush solutions. *Pediatric Nursing, 24*(2), 142-149.

Pagana, K.D. & Pagana, T.J. (1997). *Mosby's diagnostic and laboratory test reference* (3rd ed.). St. Louis: Mosby.

Peterson, F.Y. & Kirshoff, K.T. (1991). Analysis of the research about heparinized versus nonheparinized intravascular lines. *Heart & Lung, 20*(6), 631.

Tootill, D.M. (1995). Thrombolytic therapy: Nursing strategies for successful outcomes. *Progress in Cardiovascular Nursing, 10*(1), 3-12.

Turpie, A.G.G. (1995). Management of deep vein thrombosis: Prevention and treatment. *P & T Journal, 20*(6S), 7S-15S.

United States Pharmacopeia Dispensing Information (USP DI): Drug information for the health care professional (19th ed.). (1999). Rockville, MD: United States Pharmacopeial Convention.

Willerson, J.T. & Zoldhelyi, P. (1999). Future directions in thrombolysis. *Clinical Cardiology, 22*(8 suppl), IV44-53.

Wittkowsky, A.K. (1995). Thrombosis. In L.Y. Young & M.A. Koda-Kimble (Eds.), *Applied therapeutics: The clinical use of drugs* (6th ed.). Vancouver, WA: Applied Therapeutics.

Zed, P.J., Tisdale, J.E., & Borzak, S. (1999). Low-molecular-weight heparins in the management of acute coronary syndromes. *Archives of Internal Medicine, 159*(16), 1849-1857.

Zusman, R.M., Chesebro, J.H., Comerota, A., Hartmann, J.R., Massin, E.K., Raps, E., & Wolf, P.A. (1999). Antiplatelet therapy in the prevention of ischemic vascular events: Literature review and evidence-based guidelines for drug selection. *Clinical Cardiology, 22*(9), 559-573.

32 Antihyperlipidemic Drugs

Chapter Focus

A strong link exists between coronary artery disease and elevated plasma lipoprotein concentrations. These elevated lipids, or hyperlipidemia, may develop as the result of high dietary fat intake, systemic disease, or genetic factors. The nurse needs to be knowledgeable about drugs that lower serum lipids, as well as factors that increase lipid levels, in order to provide appropriate information to clients to prevent the coronary artery disease that might result from hyperlipidemia.

Learning Objectives

1. Define hyperlipidemia and describe the pathophysiology of this condition.
2. Identify the four types of lipoprotein and differentiate them according to their lipid content.
3. Discuss the importance of combining dietary modifications with drug therapy to treat hyperlipidemia.
4. Implement nursing management for the care of clients receiving antihyperlipidemic agents.

Key Terms

atherosclerosis, p. 650
chylomicrons, p. 650
high-density lipoproteins, p. 650
hyperlipidemia, p. 650
lipoprotein, p. 650
low-density lipoproteins, p. 650
very low-density lipoproteins, p. 650

Key Drugs [✓]

cholestyramine, p. 653
lovastatin, p. 660

Hyperlipidemia is a metabolic disorder characterized by increased concentrations of cholesterol and triglycerides, two of the major serum lipids in the body. Antihyperlipidemic or antilipemic drugs are used along with dietary modifications to treat hyperlipidemia. Clinical and experimental studies offer evidence that an important relationship exists between atherosclerosis and high levels of circulating triglycerides and cholesterol. **Atherosclerosis** is a disorder characterized by lipid deposits in the lining of large- and medium-sized arteries, which eventually produces degenerative changes and obstructs blood flow.

Atherosclerosis is a causative factor in coronary heart disease (CHD), which may result in angina, heart failure, myocardial infarction, cerebral arterial disease that results in senility or cerebrovascular accidents, peripheral arterial occlusive disease (which may cause gangrene and loss of limb), and renal arterial insufficiency. It is also a factor in hypertension. Intensive research is being conducted to develop more effective and safer antihyperlipidemic drugs. If serum lipid or blood lipid levels can be controlled within normal limits, the development and progression of atherosclerosis might be inhibited or prevented.

HYPERLIPIDEMIC DISORDERS

Lipid compounds do not circulate freely in the bloodstream but are bound to plasma proteins (albumin, globulin), which act as carriers. These complexes are called lipoproteins. A **lipoprotein** has a protein shell and an interior composed of a core lipid (cholesterol, triglycerides) (Table 32-1). Hyperlipoproteinemia is always associated with an increased concentration of one or more lipoproteins, particularly cholesterol.

Classification of Lipoproteins. Lipoprotein complexes are classified according to their densities and electrophoretic mobilities. The three primary lipoproteins found in the blood of fasting individuals are very low-density lipoproteins (VLDLs), low-density lipoproteins (LDLs), and high-density lipoproteins (HDLs).

The **very low-density lipoproteins** contain a large amount of triglycerides (50% to 65%) and 20% to 30% cholesterol. VLDLs are formed in the liver from endogenous fat sources and contain 15% to 20% of the total blood cholesterol and most of the triglycerides found in the body (McKenney, 1995). Because these particles are quite large, they are not believed to be involved in atherosclerosis.

After secretion from the liver, the VLDL particles will in time become smaller particles as the triglyceride content is removed. Two enzymes, lipoprotein lipase and hepatic lipase, are involved with triglyceride removal. Medications that increase the action of lipoprotein lipase will lower triglyceride levels. Triglyceride-depleted lipoprotein is smaller and contains a higher quantity of cholesterol. VLDL is eventually broken down into intermediate-density lipoprotein (IDL), which contains 50% each of cholesterol and triglycerides. Approximately 50% of this substance is converted to the cholesterol-rich lipoprotein, or LDL. These smaller remnant VLDL particles include VLDL, IDL, and LDL. These lipoproteins can now be involved in the development of atherosclerosis.

The **low-density lipoproteins** contain the major portion of cholesterol in the blood and are considered to be the most harmful. They carry 60% to 70% of total blood cholesterol. Elevated LDL levels suggest that an individual has a greater potential for developing atherosclerosis.

The **high-density lipoproteins** are the smallest and most dense lipoproteins. Their function is to transport cholesterol from peripheral cells to the liver, where it is metabolized and excreted. This transport mechanism prevents the accumulation of lipids in the arterial walls, thereby providing protection against the development of CHD. Thus high levels of HDL are considered beneficial. The higher the HDL levels, the lower the potential risk for developing cardiovascular disease.

Chylomicrons are large particles that transport cholesterol and fatty acids from the diet and/or the gastrointestinal tract to the liver. This is known as the *exogenous* system of transport. The lipoproteins transporting cholesterol from the liver to peripheral cells are part of the *endogenous* system. Chylomicrons consist mainly of triglycerides (85% to 95%). Normally they are produced in the small intestine during absorption of a fatty meal and are cleared from the bloodstream by lipoprotein lipase after 12 to 14 hours. A deficiency of this enzyme is rare and results in increased levels of chylomicrons, causing a disease called *exogenous hyperlipoproteinemia*. This condition is usually found in children but may also be induced by alcoholism. Therapy is aimed at keeping the diet low in fat.

Apolipoproteins. Lipoproteins contain proteins on their surface called apolipoproteins. These proteins have a number of functions, including helping the lipoprotein bind with cell receptors, activating the enzyme system, and providing structure for the lipoprotein. An increased risk of

TABLE 32-1 Lipoproteins: Core Lipids and Transport/Function

Lipoproteins	Core Lipid	Transport/Function
Chylomicrons	Dietary triglycerides	Dietary triglycerides
Chylomicron remnants	Dietary cholesterol	Dietary cholesterol
VLDL	Endogenous cholesterol	Endogenous triglycerides
IDL	Endogenous cholesterol and triglycerides	Endogenous cholesterol
LDL	Endogenous cholesterol	Endogenous cholesterol
HDL	Endogenous cholesterol	Removes cholesterol

atherosclerosis exists if the metabolism of apolipoproteins is impaired. Therefore blood levels of apolipoproteins are important in evaluating lipid disorders. The clinically important apolipoproteins are A-I, A-II, B-100, C-II, and E. A deficiency of the C-II apolipoprotein in VLDL particles results in impaired triglyceride metabolism and hypertriglyceridemia. The quantity of apolipoprotein B present is used to determine the number of VLDL and LDL substances in circulation. High levels of apolipoprotein A-I in HDL correlates more closely with a lower incidence of CHD than do HDL particles that have both A-I and A-II (McKenney, 1995).

Figure 32-1 reviews the normal lipid transport system. Dietary fats and cholesterol are orally consumed and transported into the system by bile acids; in the endogenous transport system, the liver converts excess calories from carbohydrates and fatty acids into triglycerides. The liver ultimately produces both HDL and LDL. The function of HDL is to carry approximately 25% of blood cholesterol to the liver, where it is processed into bile acids. Because the cholesterol carried by HDL is for ultimate excretion, HDL is known as "good cholesterol." LDL carries more than 50% of the total blood cholesterol, and this LDL-cholesterol combination can penetrate arterial walls, resulting in atherosclerotic plaques; thus in excess, this combination is referred to as "bad" cholesterol.

Plasma lipoproteins are usually in a state of dynamic equilibrium because the LDL needed to transport fats such

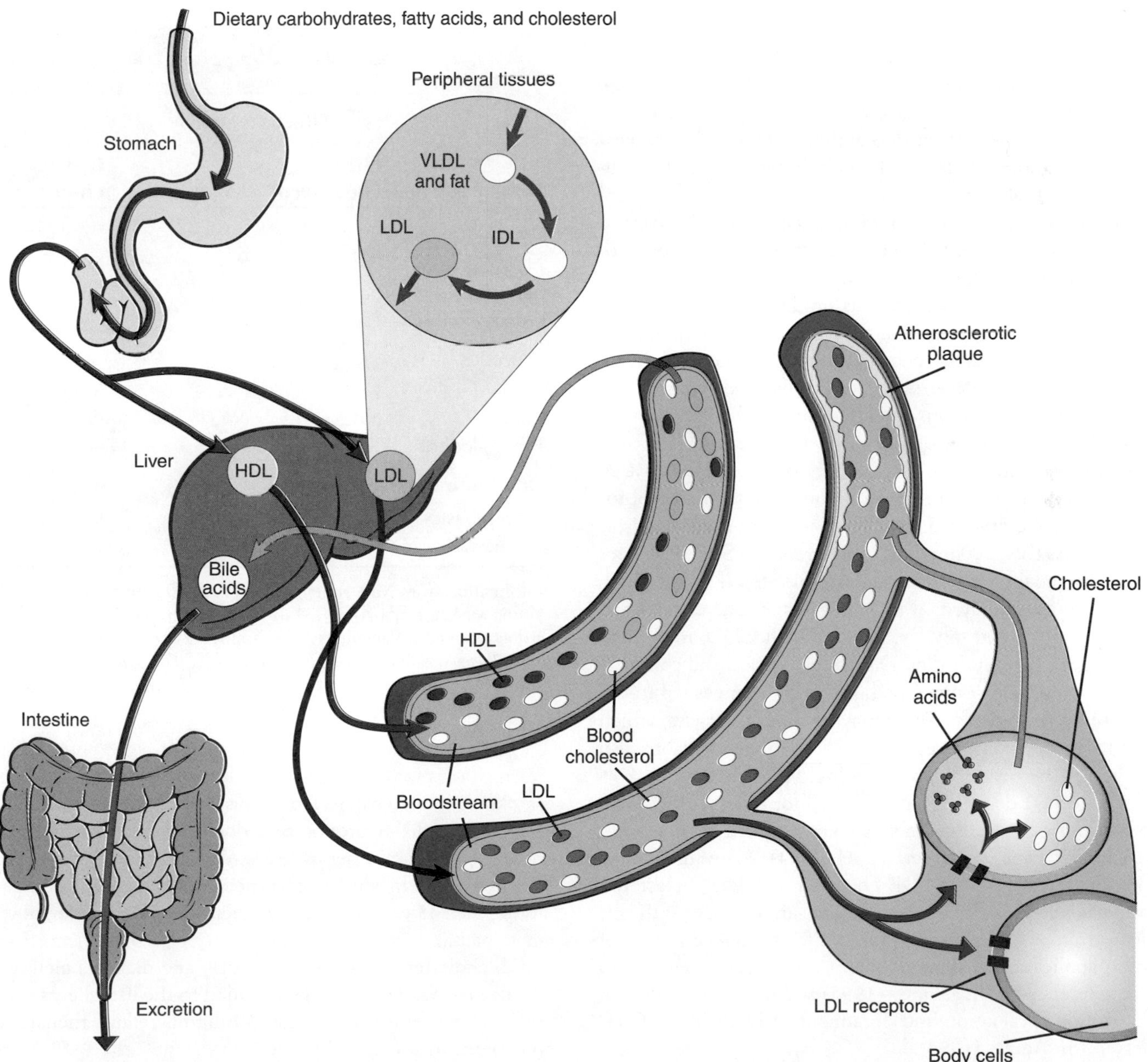

Figure 32-1 Dietary carbohydrates, fatty acids, and cholesterol: conversion sites and processes.

TABLE 32-2 Pharmacologic Treatment for Lipid Disorders

Lipid Disorder	Test Results	Drug Therapy Recommendations
Hypercholesterolemia	↑LDL, TG <200 mg/dL	Bile acid sequestering agent, niacin, or reductase inhibitor
Hypertriglyceridemia		Niacin, reductase inhibitor, or gemfibrozil
Combined hyperlipidemia	↑LDL, TG 200-400 mg/dL	Niacin, reductase inhibitor, or gemfibrozil
Low HDL (<35 mg/dL)	↑LDL	Niacin, reductase inhibitor, or gemfibrozil
	↑TG	Niacin, gemfibrozil, or reductase inhibitor
	Alone, with CHD	Niacin, reductase inhibitor

From Expert Panel on Detection, Evaluation, and Treatment of High Blood Cholesterol in Adults, National Cholesterol Education Program. (1994). Second report of the Expert Panel (Adult Treatment Panel II). *Circulation, 89,* 1329-1445.
TG, Triglycerides.

as fatty acids and cholesterol is located throughout the body. When cells outside the liver need cholesterol, they produce LDL receptors on their surfaces (see Figure 32-1). These receptors are necessary for LDL to enter the cell, where it is broken down into amino acids and free cholesterol. When the cellular need for cholesterol is met, the production of LDL receptors stops, and the excess cholesterol is discarded into the plasma. LDL receptors are also located in the liver, where they function to monitor plasma levels of LDL; when the appropriate level of LDL is present in the plasma, the liver will suppress its production. This is essentially a feedback system that functions like a thermostat in the home; it maintains adequate plasma levels of LDL in order to provide cholesterol to body cells on demand.

Dietary modifications are important in the treatment of high levels of LDL cholesterol. Dietary management consists of a two-step plan. Step I limits saturated fat to 8% to 10% of total calories, permits that no more than 30% of total calories be obtained from fat, and limits cholesterol intake to less than 300 mg/day. If adherence to Step I does not meet the goal of lowering cholesterol, Step II is instituted. Step II limits saturated fat to 7% or less of total calories and cholesterol to 200 mg/day. Persons with CHD are usually started on the Step II diet. Dietary evaluation and consultation are highly recommended. If dietary changes fail to decrease hyperlipidemia, there may be a genetic cause, which usually requires drug treatment; dietary noncompliance also indicates the need for pharmacologic intervention.

Table 32-2 describes the approach for the pharmacologic treatment of lipid disorders as recommended by the Adult Treatment Panel II (Expert Panel, 1994). Many drugs may affect serum levels of LDL cholesterol, HDL cholesterol, and triglycerides; Table 32-3 presents an overview of the effect of drugs on lipids. In addition, for a detailed review of drug application and management the reader is referred to the reference by McKenney (1995) and the Expert Panel on Detection, Evaluation and Treatment of High Blood Cholesterol in Adults (1994).

TABLE 32-3 Effects of Drugs on Serum Lipids

	Effect on Lipids		
Drug	LDL Cholesterol	Triglycerides	HDL Cholesterol
Beta Blockers			
Nonselective	N/C	I	D
Selective	N/C	I	D
Corticosteroids	I	I	—
Diuretics			
Thiazides	I	I	I
Loop	N/C	N/C	D
Ethyl alcohol	N/C	I	—
Oral Contraceptives			
Monophasics	I	I	I/D
Triphasics	I	I	I

Information from McKenney, J.M. (1995). Dyslipidemias. In L.Y. Young & M.A. Koda-Kimble (Eds.), *Applied therapeutics: The clinical use of drugs* (6th ed.). Vancouver, WA: Applied Therapeutics; and *United States Pharmacopeia Dispensing Information (USP DI): Drug information for the health care professional* (19th ed.). (1999). Rockville, MD: United States Pharmacopeial Convention.
I, Increased; *D,* decreased; *N/C,* no change; —, unknown.

Treatment Guidelines. Treatment recommendations are based on the client's cholesterol level and the presence of CHD or two other risk factors, such as current cigarette smoking, hypertension, family history of premature CHD (i.e., myocardial infarction or sudden death before 55 years of age in father or other male first-degree relatives, or before the age of 65 in mother or other female first-degree relatives), men 45 years or older, women 55 years or older, postmenopausal woman without estrogen replacement, low HDL cholesterol level (<35 mg/dL), and diabetes mellitus. A negative risk factor has been added to the list: clients with HDL cholesterol greater than 60 mg/dL reduce their total number of risk factors by one.

Total serum cholesterol and HDL cholesterol should be evaluated in a nonfasting state at least every 5 years in adults 20 years and older. As noted in Table 32-4, an LDL choles-

TABLE 32-4 Guidelines for Cholesterol Levels

Risk	Total Cholesterol (mg/dL)	LDL Cholesterol (mg/dL)
Desirable	<200	<130
Borderline/high risk	200-239	130-159
High risk	≥240	≥160

Information from Expert Panel on Detection, Evaluation, and Treatment of High Blood Cholesterol in Adults, National Cholesterol Education Program. (1994). Second report of the Expert Panel (Adult Treatment Panel II). *Circulation, 89,* 1329-1445.

terol level of 130 to 159 mg/dL is classified as borderline/high risk, and 160 mg/dL and over is considered high risk. Assessment by a prescriber includes a clinical evaluation to determine if high levels of LDL cholesterol are secondary to other risk factors or causes and to evaluate for familial disorders.

The primary goals of treatment are as follows:

- Clients without CHD and who have fewer than two risk factors but LDL cholesterol levels >160 mg/dL should receive dietary instructions and be reevaluated in 1 year. Drug therapy should be initiated if the client has an LDL cholesterol level >190 mg/dL.
- Clients without CHD but with two or more risk factors and an LDL cholesterol level >130 mg/dL should receive a complete clinical evaluation plus dietary instructions. Further treatment is based on evaluation findings. If the LDL cholesterol is >160 mg/dL, drug therapy is indicated.
- Clients with CHD and an LDL cholesterol level of >100 mg/dL should receive dietary instructions; if LDL cholesterol is 130 mg/dL or greater, drug therapy should be instituted.
- If a negative response to dietary alterations is noted, drug therapy may be indicated.

Hormone replacement therapy with estrogen to reduce menopause symptoms and osteoporosis in postmenopausal women may have the additional benefit of reducing the risk for CHD by up to 50%. Doses of estrogen (e.g., 0.625 mg conjugated estrogen or 2 mg micronized estradiol per day) may reduce LDL cholesterol by 25% and increase HDL cholesterol by approximately 15%. Clinical studies have not been performed to evaluate the risk-benefit ratio of estrogen. If it is used for its primary indications of treatment for menopausal symptoms or the prevention of osteoporosis in women with hypercholesterolemia, lipoprotein cholesterol levels should also be monitored to evaluate the potential additional effect of estrogen (McKenney, 1995).

Antihyperlipidemic agents offer the client a pharmacologic method for reducing serum lipid levels and ideally reducing the risk of atherosclerosis with its many complications. The use of antihyperlipidemic agents is reserved for clients specifically identified to be at significantly increased

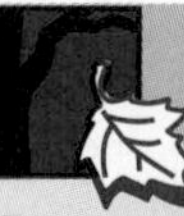

Special Considerations for Older Adults
Antihyperlipidemic Drugs

Dietary modifications and recommendations are vital to a successful lipid reduction program. Drug therapy should be considered when goals are not obtainable by diet alone.

Older adults often take multiple medications for their illnesses in addition to antihyperlipidemia medications. Therefore obtain a thorough drug history to determine if the client is taking medications that can increase lipid levels. For example, thiazides can increase triglycerides by 30% to 50%, nonselective beta blockers by 20% to 50%, ethanol by up to 50%, and so on (McKenney, 1995).

Constipation, a common and sometimes severe side effect, has been reported in older adults who are taking cholestyramine and colestipol. Encourage the client to increase daily fluid intake to 2500 mL help reduce the constipating effects of this drug.

Be aware that long-term use of cholestyramine or colestipol may lead to deficiencies in folic acid, calcium, and vitamins A, D, E, and K. Additional nutritional supplementation may be necessary (Long, 1990).

Administer antihyperlipidemic drugs before or with meals (follow manufacturer's instructions), because these drugs are generally ineffective if not administered with food. Because the highest rate of cholesterol production occurs from midnight to 5 AM, lovastatin is often given with dinner to obtain its maximum beneficial effects (Long, 1990).

risk and unable to lower their serum lipid levels satisfactorily through exercise, diet, and other nondrug methods. Drug therapy for these clients augments the therapy aimed at lowering serum lipids and cardiovascular risk. (See the Special Considerations for Older Adults box above.)

BILE ACID SEQUESTERING AGENTS

cholestyramine [koe less tir′ a meen] (Questran)
colesevelam [coal see vel′ am] (Welchol)
colestipol [koe les′ ti pole] (Colestid)

These agents are nonabsorbable anion-exchange resins that are also called bile acid sequestrants. These drugs are used for their cholesterol-lowering effects. Cholesterol is the major precursor of bile acids that are normally secreted from the gallbladder and liver into the small intestine. Here the bile acids perform two functions: (1) they emulsify the fat present in food to facilitate chemical digestion, and (2) they are required for the absorption of lipids (including fat-soluble vitamins A, D, E, and K). After their physiologic performance, the major portion of the bile acids is returned to the liver.

The anion-exchange resins bind bile acids in the intestine, thus preventing their absorption and producing an insoluble complex that is excreted in the feces. To compensate for the loss of bile acids removed by the drugs, the liver increases the rate of oxidation of cholesterol by converting more cholesterol to bile acids. Subsequently, the long-term fecal loss of bile acids causes a reduction of serum cholesterol levels and LDL cholesterol.

All three drugs are used in the treatment of hyperlipidemia of primary hypercholesterolemia. Cholestyramine is also used to treat the pruritus induced by bile acid deposits in dermal tissues (from partial biliary obstruction). Cholestyramine is also used as an antidiarrheal agent for diarrhea caused by bile acids (not for common diarrhea) and as an antidote for negatively charged drugs and other medications (e.g., digoxin, oral penicillin, tetracyclines, and thyroid medication); these are not approved indications.

Pharmacokinetics. Plasma cholesterol levels usually decrease 1 to 2 weeks after the initiation of therapy. With cholestyramine, plasma cholesterol levels may continue to fall for up to 1 year. After the initial decrease, plasma cholesterol levels may increase to previous levels in some individuals or even exceed these levels with continued therapy. Close monitoring for effectiveness is necessary. Diarrhea induced by increased bile acids will respond to cholestyramine within 24 hours, but it usually takes 1 to 3 weeks of therapy before a response is noted in cases of pruritus caused by cholestasis. Colesevelam is water soluble; maximum effect is achieved within 2 weeks.

Pharmacokinetics. The peak effect of colestipol is noted within 1 month. After the initial decrease in cholesterol, some clients may exhibit an increased cholesterol level that equals or surpasses the previous level. Plasma cholesterol levels increase approximately 2 to 4 weeks after the withdrawal of colestipol and cholestyramine. If used to treat pruritus, pruritus often returns within 1 to 2 weeks.

Side Effects/Adverse Reactions. The side effects/adverse reactions of the bile acid sequestering agents include constipation, indigestion, abdominal pain, nausea and vomiting, abdominal pain, gas, dizziness, headache, and, rarely, gallstones, pancreatitis, bleeding ulcers, and malabsorption syndrome.

Dosage and Administration. Cholestyramine is available as Questran and Questran Light (sugar free) powders for oral suspension. The adult dosage of cholestyramine is 4 g once or twice daily before meals; the maintenance dosage is 8 to 24 g/day in 2 to 6 divided doses as necessary. The pediatric dosage is 4 g/day in 2 divided doses initially, then 8 to 24 g in 2 or more divided doses as necessary.

The adult dosage of colestipol is 15 to 30 g PO before meals in 2 to 4 divided doses. The pediatric dosage has not been established. The adult dosage of colesevelam is three 625-mg tablets twice daily with meals.

■ Nursing Management

Cholestyramine and Colestipol Therapy

■ **Assessment.** Ascertain whether the client has a preexisting condition for which the drug would be used with great caution or contraindicated. The risk of cholestyramine and colestipol therapy should be considered in clients with constipation because it may induce fecal impaction. Because of its tendency to enhance constipation, this therapy should be used with caution in clients with medical conditions that could be aggravated by severe constipation, such as hemorrhoids or CHD. It should also be used with caution in older adults and in clients with peptic ulcer, gallstones, steatorrhea, bleeding disorders, and impaired renal function. Clients with complete biliary obstruction or complete atresia will have no bile acids in the gastrointestinal tract to bind with cholestyramine and colestipol. These drugs are contraindicated for use in clients who have an allergy to bile acid sequestrants. Clients with phenylketonuria will be sensitive to the phenylalanine in aspartame in the sugar-free preparation of cholestyramine. Colestipol is contraindicated in clients with primary biliary cirrhosis because it may further increase concentrations of serum cholesterol.

The safety of these drugs for use by pregnant women and lactating mothers has not been established (see the Pregnancy Safety box below for FDA pregnancy safety classifications). However, because the drugs are almost totally unabsorbed after ingestion, there is a risk for impaired maternal absorption of vitamins and other nutrients.

Review the client's current medication regimen for the risk of significant drug interactions, such as those that may occur when cholestyramine or colestipol are given concurrently with the following drugs:

Drug	Possible Effect and Management
oral anticoagulants, warfarin, or indanediones	Concurrent use significantly decreases the absorption of oral anticoagulants and vitamin K; thus the anticoagulant effect may be increased or decreased. It is suggested that oral anticoagulants be given 6 hours before cholestyramine or colestipol. Monitor prothrombin times closely, because dosage adjustments may be necessary.
digitalis glycosides, especially digitoxin	The half-life of digitalis glycosides, as well as gastrointestinal absorption, may be reduced. It is recommended that cholestyramine or colestipol be administered at least 8 hours after digoxin to reduce the potential for

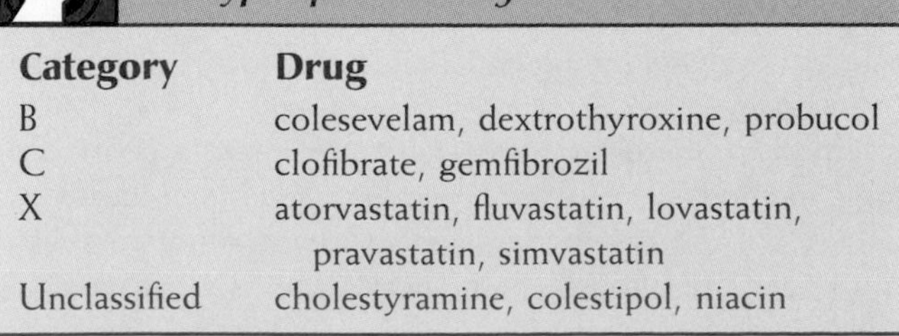

Pregnancy Safety
Anithyperlipidemic Drugs

Category	Drug
B	colesevelam, dextrothyroxine, probucol
C	clofibrate, gemfibrozil
X	atorvastatin, fluvastatin, lovastatin, pravastatin, simvastatin
Unclassified	cholestyramine, colestipol, niacin

	interactions. If cholestyramine or colestipol is discontinued in a client who is also taking a digitalis product, monitor the client closely for digitalis toxicity.
thiazide diuretics (oral), oral propranolol, oral penicillin G, oral tetracyclines, or oral vancomycin	Decreased absorption of these medications been reported. Administer such medications several hours before or after cholestyramine or colestipol. Whenever possible, administer these medications before cholestyramine or colestipol.
thyroid hormones	Decreased absorption of thyroid products is reported. Administer thyroid first on the medication administration schedule, then administer cholestyramine or colestipol several hours later.

Before beginning cholestyramine and colestipol therapy, the client should undergo serum cholesterol and triglyceride concentration determinations to provide a baseline by which to evaluate therapy.

■ **Nursing Diagnosis.** Clients receiving cholestyramine and colestipol are at risk for the following nursing diagnoses/collaborative problems: constipation in approximately 10% of clients (mild to severe) and possible fecal impaction; impaired comfort (headache, belching, bloating, heartburn, nausea or vomiting, and abdominal discomfort); and the potential complications of gallstones or pancreatitis (severe stomach pain with nausea and vomiting), gastrointestinal bleeding or peptic ulcer (black, tarry stools), or steatorrhea or malabsorption syndrome (sudden loss of weight).

■ **Implementation**

■ ***Monitoring.*** Continue to monitor serum cholesterol and triglyceride levels in relation to baseline periodically and at regular intervals. (Table 32-5 compares the antilipemic effects of these drugs.) In addition, it is recommended that prothrombin time (PT) values be monitored, because a vitamin K deficiency may occur with the chronic use of both drugs, which would put the client at risk for increased bleeding tendencies. With the chronic use of cholestyramine, serum calcium concentrations should be monitored because of decreased calcium absorption.

Monitor digitalis glycoside levels in clients who are receiving digitalis glycoside and a bile sequestering agent simultaneously. To avoid toxicity, adjust the dosage of the digitalis glycoside before discontinuing the anion-exchange resin.

The client should be placed on a fluid balance record to monitor hydration and bowel status in relation to the side effect of constipation.

■ ***Intervention.*** Administer cholestyramine and colestipol before meals. To increase the palatability of the drug, sprinkle the powder on the surface of 2 ounces of a preferred liquid or semiliquid, such as cold beverages, hot cereals, thin

TABLE 32-5 Antihyperlipidemic Effects of Various Drugs

	Effect on Lipids		Effect on Lipoproteins			
Drug	**Cholesterol**	**Triglycerides**	**VLDL**	**LDL**	**HDL**	**Typical Response**
Bile Acid Sequestering Agents						
cholestyramine	↓	0 or slight ↑	0 or↑	↓	0 or ↑	Decreases cholesterol 20%-40%
colestipol	↓	0 or slight ↑	↑	↓	0 or ↑	Decreases cholesterol 20%-40%
Other Antihyperlipidemic Agents						
clofibrate	↓	↓ (greatest effect)	↓	0 or ↓	0 or ↑	Lowers triglycerides; only slight decrease in cholesterol
dextrothyroxine	↓	0	0 or ↓	↓	0	—
gemfibrozil	↓	↓	↓	0 or ↓	↑	Decreases triglycerides; only slight decrease in cholesterol; increases HDL
niacin	↓	↓	↓	↓	↑	Decreases triglycerides and cholesterol 10%-20%
probucol	↓	0 or ↑	↑ or ↓	↓	↓	Decreases cholesterol 12%-25%; also decreases HDL
Reductase Inhibitor						
lovastatin	↓	↓	↓	↓	↑	LDL cholesterol levels reduced 19%-39%; total cholesterol levels reduced 18%-34%

↑, Increased; ↓, decreased; 0, no change. Typical response was approximated with individual taking drug while concurrently on a specified diet.

soups (tomato, chicken noodle), or pulpy fruit (fruit cocktail, pears, peaches, or pineapple). Allow the drug to sit on the surface of the liquid for 1 to 2 minutes before stirring vigorously to prevent lumpiness. Add an additional 2 to 4 ounces of diluent, and shake vigorously again. Be sure the drug is thoroughly mixed, because it does not dissolve. Incomplete mixing of the dry form may result in mucosal irritation and esophageal impaction, or it may be accidentally inhaled. Rinse the glass or cup with a small amount of liquid, and have the client drink it to ensure that the complete dose is taken.

Concurrent administration of a laxative or stool softener may help to prevent constipation. The client should also increase fluid intake to 2500 mL if not contraindicated.

Because resins interfere with the absorption of other drugs when taken concurrently, administer other drugs 1 hour before or 4 to 6 hours after cholestyramine or colestipol.

■ ***Education.*** Instruct the client in the preparation of the medication for administration as discussed previously. Warn the client that the sudden withdrawal of resins could lead to uninhibited absorption of other drugs taken concomitantly, resulting in overdose or toxicity.

Supplemental parenteral or water-soluble vitamins A, D, E, and K, as well as folic acid, are prescribed to prevent vitamin deficiencies in clients receiving long-term therapy. Instruct the client to report early symptoms of bleeding immediately: petechiae, ecchymoses, bleeding from mucous membranes of gums or nose, or tarry stools (which indicate hypoprothrombinemia). The administration of vitamin K_1 (parenteral) and vitamin K_2 (oral) may be necessary.

Encourage the client to observe bowel elimination patterns and to adhere to a high-fiber diet (e.g., grains, fruits, raw vegetables) and an increased fluid intake as an adjunct therapy to the drug. If constipation occurs, the dosage may be lowered to prevent fecal impaction, or a stool softener or laxative may be prescribed. Instruct the client to report gastrointestinal symptoms to the prescriber: gastric distress, nausea and vomiting (pancreatitis), and unusual weight loss (steatorrhea).

■ **Evaluation.** The expected outcome of bile acid sequestering agent therapy is that the client's serum cholesterol and LDL levels will decrease to within normal range. The drug is usually withdrawn if the response is unsatisfactory after 3 months of therapy.

ADDITIONAL ANTIHYPERLIPIDEMIC AGENTS

clofibrate [kloe fye' brate] (Atromid-S, Claripex ♣)

The results of several large studies raise specific warnings concerning the use of clofibrate. First, the use of this product may possibly increase the risk of inducing malignancy and cholelithiasis in humans. Individuals taking clofibrate had twice the risk of nonusers for cholelithiasis and cholecystitis that required surgery. Second, there is no evidence of reduced cardiovascular mortality with its use. In fact, studies reported an increase in cardiac dysrhythmias, angina, and thromboembolic episodes (*Drug Facts and Comparisons,* 2000). As a result, the clinical use of clofibrate has declined tremendously.

Clofibrate is more effective in reducing VLDLs rich in triglycerides than in lowering LDLs high in cholesterol. The exact mode of action of the drug is unknown, but VLDL breakdown may contribute to its effect.

Clofibrate is indicated for the treatment of hyperlipidemia. It is slowly but completely absorbed from the intestines, is highly protein bound (96%), and reaches peak plasma levels 2 to 6 hours after a dose. The peak effect with continued therapy is seen in approximately 3 weeks. A reduction in plasma concentrations of VLDL is seen within 2 to 5 days. The half-life of this drug ranges from 6 to 25 hours for a single dose or 54 hours at a steady state in normal healthy individuals. It is metabolized in the liver and gastrointestinal tract and is excreted by the kidneys.

The side effects/adverse reactions of clofibrate therapy include diarrhea, nausea, muscle pain or cramps, fatigue, headache, weight gain, abdominal pain, gas, nausea, vomiting, flu-like syndrome and, rarely, anemia, leukopenia, angina, gallstones, pancreatitis, cardiac dysrhythmias, and kidney disease.

The adult dosage is 1.5 to 2 g PO daily in 2 to 4 divided doses. A pediatric dosage has not been established.

■ Nursing Management
Clofibrate Therapy

■ **Assessment.** A complete health assessment should be obtained to ensure that the client does not have a preexisting condition for which the administration of clofibrate would be contraindicated or entail risk. The presence of primary biliary cirrhosis precludes the use of clofibrate because the drug may further raise serum cholesterol levels. Hepatic dysfunction may require a reduced dosage of clofibrate because the protein binding of the drug is reduced but the half-life remains unchanged, which leads to increased side effects/adverse reactions. With renal dysfunction the reduced protein binding and clearance of the drug also leads to an increased incidence of side effects, especially myopathy. Hypothyroidism may also predispose the client to drug-induced myopathy. Reactivation of peptic ulcers has been reported as well as an increased risk of biliary complications in the presence of gallstones with clofibrate.

Obtain a family health history; because of the genetic tendency of the disease, children and other family members should be screened for abnormal lipid levels.

As a baseline assessment, a complete blood count, liver function tests, and serum cholesterol and triglyceride levels should be determined.

Inquire if the client is pregnant. Strict birth control measures must be observed to prevent pregnancy and thus fetal damage. The drug must be withdrawn at least 2 months before conception.

Review the client's medication regimen to detect significant drug interactions. An increased anticoagulant effect is reported when clofibrate is given with oral anticoagulants (coumarin- or indanedione-type). Monitor prothrombin times closely because the anticoagulant dosage may need to be decreased significantly.

■ **Nursing Diagnosis.** Clients undergoing clofibrate therapy are at risk for developing the following nursing diagnoses/collaborative problems: impaired comfort (nausea, vomiting, flu-like syndrome, headache, heartburn, and abdominal discomfort); diarrhea; impaired oral mucous membrane (stomatitis); sexual dysfunction (decreased sexual ability); and the potential complications of myopathy (muscle aches or cramps), angina (chest pain, shortness of breath), cardiac dysrhythmias, anemia or leukopenia (abnormal blood counts and signs of infection—fever or chills, cough, painful urination), pancreatitis or gallstones (severe stomach pain with nausea and vomiting), and renal toxicity (blood in urine, decreased urinary output, pedal edema).

■ **Implementation**

■ ***Monitoring.*** In addition to clinically monitoring the client for signs and symptoms of side effects/adverse reactions, monitor complete blood counts for signs of anemia or leukopenia, and monitor serum cholesterol and triglyceride levels for the effectiveness of the drug. Clofibrate may increase the risk of biliary diseases such as cholelithiasis and cholecystitis; the appropriate diagnostic tests should be performed if signs and symptoms of biliary disease occur. This drug may produce hyperglycemia and glycosuria in clients with diabetes, and therefore serum glucose levels should be monitored. Consult with the prescriber to withdraw the drug if any of the test results are abnormal.

■ ***Intervention.*** Administer clofibrate with meals to prevent gastric distress.

■ ***Education.*** Before initiating clofibrate therapy, advise the client to adhere to the diet recommended by prescriber. The diet is usually low in fats, cholesterol, and/or sugars. Encourage weight reduction and physical exercise.

A decrease in serum lipid levels during the first and second months of therapy indicates a therapeutic response. Warn the client that a paradoxical rise in levels may occur in 2 or 3 months, but afterward a further decrease is customary.

Instruct the client to keep clinical appointments for laboratory studies and reevaluation by the prescriber. If serum cholesterol and triglyceride levels are not lowered within 3 months, drug therapy is usually discontinued.

Advise the client to report any flu-like symptoms (muscular aching, soreness, cramping). This condition may be remedied by a dosage reduction. Instruct the individual to check with the prescriber about alcohol intake, because alcohol may be restricted to prevent hypertriglyceridemia.

The client should be aware that there is no substantial evidence that the drug reduces the incidence of CHD or fatal myocardial infarction. Increased incidences of cardiac dysrhythmias, thromboembolism, intermittent claudication, and angina have been reported in clients treated with clofibrate.

■ **Evaluation.** The client undergoing clofibrate therapy will experience a reduction in serum lipid levels to within normal limits.

gemfibrozil [jem fi′ broe zil] (Lopid)

Gemfibrozil is an agent that primarily decreases the serum triglycerides found in VLDL and increases HDL. The mechanism of this action has not been established but may involve an inhibition of peripheral lipolysis and a decrease in the hepatic extraction of free fatty acids, which result in a reduction of triglyceride production. In addition, the drug may accelerate the turnover and removal of cholesterol from the liver, which is ultimately excreted in the feces.

Gemfirozil is indicated for the treatment of hyperlipidemia. It may be used in conjunction with HMG-CoA reductase inhibitors for the treatment of mixed lipid disorders (Murdock et al., 1999; Rader & Haffner, 1999). Oral gemfibrozil is well absorbed from the gastrointestinal tract and reaches peak levels in 1 to 2 hours. The onset of action in reducing serum VLDL levels is within 2 to 5 days, and the peak effect is seen in 4 weeks. It is metabolized in the liver and excreted by the kidneys and in the feces.

The side effects/adverse reactions of gemfibrozil include muscle aches and cramps, nausea, vomiting, rash, diarrhea, gas, and abdominal distress. An increased anticoagulant effect is reported when gemfibrozil is given with oral anticoagulants (coumarin or indanedione-type). Monitor PTs closely because the anticoagulant dosage may need to be decreased significantly. If administered with lovastatin, an increased risk of rhabdomyolysis and myoglobinuria may result in acute renal failure. This has been reported after 3 weeks to several months of combined drug therapy. If possible, avoid concurrent drug administration.

The adult dosage is 1.2 g daily in 2 divided doses, preferably before breakfast and dinner. Pediatric dosages have not been established.

Gemfibrozil has chemical, pharmacologic, and clinical effects that are similar to those of clofibrate. For the nursing management of gemfibrozil, see Nursing Management: Clofibrate Therapy on p. 656.

fenofibrate [fen oh fee′ brate] (Tricor)

Fenofibrate is similar to clofibrate and gemfibrozil. Although its exact mechanism of action is unknown, the active metabolite fenofibric acid is believed to lower triglyceride levels by inhibiting triglyceride synthesis and stimulating the breakdown of triglyceride-rich lipoproteins (VLDL). It is indicated as an adjunct to diet for the treatment of very high plasma levels of triglycerides (types IV and V hyperlipidemia) in adults who have not responded to diet alone or in persons who are at risk for pancreatitis.

Fenofibrate reaches peak levels in 6 to 8 hours, is highly protein bound (99%), and has a half-life of 20 hours. It is metabolized in the liver and excreted primarily by the kidneys.

The side effects/adverse reactions of fenofibrate therapy include constipation, gastrointestinal distress, eye irritation, decreased libido, skin photosensitivity or rash, dizziness, flu-like syndrome, infections, and pruritus.

The usual adult dosage is 67 mg PO initially; the dosage is then adjusted according to the client's response. The maximum daily dose is 201 mg.

For the nursing management of fenofibrate, see Nursing Management: Clofibrate Therapy on p. 656.

dextrothyroxine [dex tro thy rox′ seen] (Choloxin)

The mechanism of action of dextrothyroxine as an antihyperlipidemic agent is not fully understood. Dextrothyroxine appears to act in the liver to increase the formation of LDL and, to a greater extent, to increase the breakdown of LDL. The result is an increased excretion of cholesterol and bile acids via bile into the feces, which results in a decrease in serum cholesterol and LDL.

A definite relationship exists between thyroid function and serum cholesterol levels. Hypothyroidism is associated with high serum cholesterol levels, and the administration of thyroid hormones lowers serum cholesterol. Dextrothyroxine apparently stimulates the liver to increase the rate of oxidation of cholesterol, and it promotes the biliary excretion of cholesterol and its byproducts.

Dextrothyroxine is used as an adjunct to diet and other measures to reduce elevated LDL cholesterol levels in clients with no evidence of heart disease. Other antihyperlipidemic agents have replaced this drug because significant cardiac side effects are associated with its use. Dextrothyroxine is approximately 25% absorbed from the gastrointestinal tract, is highly protein bound, has a half-life of 18 hours, and reaches its peak effect as an antihyperlipidemic agent in 1 to 2 months. The duration of action after the drug is withdrawn is 6 weeks to 3 months. It is metabolized in the liver and excreted by the kidneys and in the feces.

The side effects/adverse reactions of dextrothyroxine are rare and include nausea, vomiting, chest pain, abdominal pain, irregular heart rate, skin rash, and gallstones.

The adult dosage of dextrothyroxine for an antihyperlipidemic effect is 1 to 2 mg/day PO, increased monthly if necessary to achieve the desired effect. The maximum recommended dosage is 8 mg/day. For children 2 years and older, the dosage is 0.05 mg/kg/day, titrated monthly as necessary to achieve the desired effect; the maximum recommended dosage is 4 mg/day.

■ Nursing Management

Dextrothyroxine Therapy

■ **Assessment.** Because of the risks associated with increased metabolic demands caused by thyroid hormone administration, do not administer dextrothyroxine to clients with cardiovascular disease, such as angina pectoris, CHD, a history of myocardial infarction, cardiac dysrhythmias, congestive heart failure, or rheumatic heart disease. Dextrothyroxine should be used with caution in clients with liver or kidney disease, diabetes mellitus (may increase the need for an antidiabetic agent), or a history of iodism. Use this medication with caution in older adults, who may be more sensitive to thyroid hormones. Monitor therapy closely.

When dextrothyroxine is given with oral anticoagulants (coumarin or indanediones), the anticoagulant effects may be increased or decreased depending on the thyroid status of the client. Monitor prothrombin times closely because the oral anticoagulant dosage may need to be adjusted. If given concurrently with cholestyramine or colestipol, the absorption of dextrothyroxine is reduced unless the dextrothyroxine is taken approximately 4 to 5 hours before or after these drugs.

■ **Nursing Diagnosis.** Clients receiving dextrothyroxine should be monitored for the following nursing diagnoses/collaborative problems: impaired comfort (headache, rash, itching, sweating, flushing) and the potential complications of myocardial infarction and angina (chest pain, shortness of breath), gallstones (severe stomach pain with nausea and vomiting), and hyperthyroidism (irritability, nervousness, insomnia, sweating, increased sensitivity to heat, weight loss, tremors).

■ **Implementation**

■ ***Monitoring.*** Baseline serum cholesterol and triglyceride levels are determined and monitored every 2 months to determine the effectiveness of therapy. Laboratory values will show that a decrease in cholesterol levels may not occur until 2 to 4 weeks after the initiation of drug therapy; a maximum decrease occurs approximately 2 or 3 months later. If the response is inadequate after 3 months of therapy, discontinue the drug. Vital signs and weight loss should be monitored at clinical visits to determine if hyperthyroidism is a problem.

Bone age, growth, and psychomotor development should be measured periodically in children receiving long-term therapy.

■ ***Intervention.*** Dextrothyroxine should be discontinued at least 2 weeks before surgery to reduce the potential for precipitating cardiac dysrhythmias during the procedure. In clients receiving digitalis, do not administer more than 4 mg/day of dextrothyroxine to prevent the danger of increasing the myocardial oxygen requirement. In addition, closely monitor the effects of both drugs.

Diabetes mellitus should be controlled if present. The drug may increase blood sugar levels, and therefore an increase in antidiabetic drugs or a decrease in dextrothyroxine may be required. A loss of diabetic control is noted by the symptoms of glycosuria, polydipsia, and polyuria.

■ ***Education.*** Before initiating dextrothyroxine therapy, advise the client to adhere to the diet recommended by the prescriber. The diet is usually low in fats, cholesterol, and/or sugars. Encourage weight reduction and physical exercise.

Instruct the client to keep clinical appointments so the prescriber can check progress.

Advise the client to report the following side effects immediately: chest pain, palpitation, headache, sweating, diarrhea, nocturnal coughing, and dyspnea. In addition, report promptly any signs of iodism: stomatitis, bronchitis, laryngitis, rhinitis, brassy taste, conjunctivitis, acneiform rash, and pruritus. Side effects may not occur for 6 weeks.

■ **Evaluation.** The client taking dextrothyroxine will evidence serum lipid levels within normal limits.

niacin [nye' a sin] (nicotinic acid, Nicobid)

Niacin (vitamin B_3) is a water-soluble vitamin that can lower total cholesterol and triglyceride levels by inhibiting VLDL synthesis and can also increase HDL cholesterol levels. It is used as an adjunct to other therapies because its vasodilating effects and other side effects limit its usefulness. Because nicotinic acid inhibits lipolysis in adipose tissue, it lowers the plasma concentration of free fatty acids, which usually is the main source of triglyceride synthesis in the liver. Niacin is used as adjunctive therapy in the treatment of both hypertriglyceridemia and hypercholesterolemia (Hunninghake, 1999). It is also used to prevent and treat niacin (vitamin B_3) deficiency.

Niacin is well absorbed orally and has a half-life of approximately 45 minutes. It reduces cholesterol levels several days after initiating therapy; a reduction in triglyceride levels occurs within several hours of taking an oral dose. Niacin is metabolized in the liver and excreted by the kidneys.

The side effects/adverse reactions of niacin include increased feelings of warmth, flushing or red skin on the face and neck, headache, pruritus, skin rash and, rarely, anaphylactic reactions. Dysrhythmias, dry skin or eyes, hyperglycemia, dizziness, diarrhea, hyperuricemia, myalgia, pruritus, and aggravation of peptic ulcers have been reported with high dosages. Liver toxicity has been reported with chronic use of the extended-release niacin. No significant drug interactions have been reported to date.

The adult dosage of niacin for an antihyperlipidemic effect is 1 g PO three times daily. The dosage may be increased to 500 mg/day every 2 to 4 weeks as necessary. The maximum dosage is 6 g/day.

■ Nursing Management
Niacin Therapy

■ **Assessment.** Niacin should be used cautiously in clients with allergies or peptic ulcers, because nicotinic acid causes a release of histamine and stimulates the secretion of hydrochloric acid. Niacin should be used with caution in individuals with arterial bleeding and hypotension (the vasodilating effects of the drug may worsen these conditions), hepatic dysfunction (may cause hepatic damage), glaucoma (may worsen the condition), diabetes mellitus (may impair glucose tolerance), and gout (may cause hyperuricemia).

■ **Nursing Diagnosis.** With the administration of niacin, the client may experience the following nursing diagnoses/collaborative problems: impaired comfort (flushing of the skin of the head and neck, headaches, dizziness, nausea, and vomiting); diarrhea; impaired skin integrity (pruritus); and the potential complications of peptic ulcer (stomach pain), hyperglycemia (frequent urination, unusual thirst), hyperuricemia (joint pain, flank pain), or myalgia (fever, muscle aches, or cramping).

■ **Implementation**

■ ***Monitoring.*** Serum cholesterol levels should be monitored periodically to evaluate the effectiveness of drug therapy; blood glucose, uric acid, and hepatic function studies should be performed to determine adverse reactions. Monitor for orthostatic hypotension, especially if the client is also taking antihypertensive agents. Prolonged treatment with niacin has resulted in hepatic disease.

■ ***Intervention.*** Giving the drug with meals or with antacids may reduce the incidence and severity of gastric distress.

■ ***Education.*** Instruct the client to swallow the extended-release form whole, without chewing or crushing. The powder within the capsule may be mixed with jam or applesauce for ease of administration. Advise the client to adhere to the dietary regimen—low cholesterol and low saturated fats. Instruct the client to maintain clinical appointments so that serum cholesterol and triglycerides may be monitored on a periodic basis.

Alert the client that numerous and often disagreeable side effects may occur from nicotinic acid. Common side effects include severe gastrointestinal upset, flushing, pruritus, nervousness, and urticaria. Although tolerance to the flushing, pruritus, and gastrointestinal effects usually occurs within 2 weeks, these effects may be minimized by starting the client's therapy with a low dosage and increasing it slowly. If flushing continues to be a discomfort for the client, 300 mg of aspirin may be taken 30 minutes before each dose of niacin.

■ **Evaluation.** The client undergoing niacin therapy will have serum lipid levels within the normal limits. If used for niacin deficiency, the client will experience a decrease or absence in the symptoms of pellagra, such as dermatitis, dementia, and diarrhea.

probucol [proe' byoo kole] (Lorelco)

Probucol is an antihyperlipidemic agent for persons with primary hypercholesterolemia who have not responded to other measures. It lowers levels of both LDL cholesterol and the desired HDL cholesterol, which limits the usefulness of this product. In addition to lowering cholesterol levels, probucol induces the regression of xanthomas in persons with homozygous familial hypercholesterolemia and inhibits atherosclerosis as result of its antioxidant properties (Witztum, 1996).

Probucol is administered orally and has a variable absorption pattern. It tends to accumulate in fatty tissues with chronic therapy. Peak serum levels increase slowly and reach a steady state after 3 or 4 months of treatment; the peak effect usually occurs in 20 to 50 days after initiation of the drug. The half-life ranges from 12 to 500 hours. Probucol is excreted as bile in the feces.

The side effects/adverse reactions of probucol include gas, diarrhea, nausea, vomiting, abdominal distress, ventricular dysrhythmias and, rarely, anemia, angioneurotic edema, and thrombocytopenia. It has no reported significant drug interactions.

The adult dosage is 500 mg PO twice daily with breakfast and dinner. A pediatric dosage has not been established.

■ Nursing Management
Probucol Therapy

■ **Assessment.** Probucol is usually administered to individuals who do not respond adequately to dietary management and weight reduction. Do not give probucol to clients with primary biliary cirrhosis because it may further raise cholesterol levels, and do not give to clients with QT interval prolongation because the risk of additive QT interval may increase the risk of ventricular tachycardia. If there is evidence of myocardial damage and unresponsive congestive heart failure, the drug should be used with caution and only with electrocardiogram (ECG) monitoring, because these conditions may be exacerbated.

A baseline assessment should include serum cholesterol and serum triglycerides.

▪ **Nursing Diagnosis.** With the administration of probucol, the client may experience the following nursing diagnoses/collaborative problems: impaired comfort related to gastrointestinal irritation (bloating, nausea, vomiting, abdominal discomfort), dizziness, headache, and tingling of the fingers and toes; and potential complications that include eosinophilia, anemia, thrombocytopenia, QT interval prolongation, and ventricular dysrhythmias.

▪ **Implementation**

▪ ***Monitoring.*** Serum cholesterol and triglyceride levels should be obtained periodically during therapy to determine the efficacy of treatment. A baseline and periodic ECG readings should be monitored, especially for QT prolongation. Observe for syncope and pulse irregularities.

▪ ***Intervention.*** If syncope occurs, probucol should be discontinued and the client monitored with an ECG. Probucol is usually discontinued if the client's response is not adequate after 4 months of therapy. When the drug is discontinued, continue to monitor serum lipids because serum cholesterol levels may rise up to or above the original base.

▪ ***Education.*** If medication is given, adherence to a low-cholesterol, low-fat diet and physical exercise should continue. Instruct the individual to take the drug with food to minimize gastric irritation.

▪ **Evaluation.** The client will show evidence of serum lipid concentrations that are within normal limits.

REDUCTASE INHIBITORS

atorvastatin [a tor va′ sta tin] (Lipitor ◆)
fluvastatin [floo vah stat′ in] (Lescol ◆)
100 ✓**lovastatin** [loe vah stat′ in] (Mevacor)
pravastatin [pra vah stat′ in] (Pravachol ◆)
simvastatin [sim vah stat′ in] (Zocor ◆)

The reductase inhibitors are the most effective drugs to lower LDL cholesterol levels. They are competitive inhibitors of HMG-CoA reductase, an enzyme necessary for cholesterol biosynthesis. The decrease in cholesterol production in the liver leads to an increase in the synthesis of cholesterol and also stimulates hepatocytes to produce more LDL receptors. The result is that more LDL cholesterol is removed from the blood. In summary, these drugs convert HMG-CoA reductase to mevalonate, which results in an increase in HDL cholesterol and a decrease in LDL cholesterol, VLDL cholesterol, and plasma triglycerides.

Indications. These agents are indicated as adjuncts for the treatment of primary hypercholesterolemia caused by an elevated LDL cholesterol level not controlled by diet or other treatment measures.

Pharmacokinetics. On absorption, the reductase inhibitors have extensive first-pass hepatic extraction; all but pravastatin are highly protein bound. Peak serum levels are reached in 1 to 2 hours for atorvastatin, 0.5 to 0.7 hours for fluvastatin, 2 to 4 hours for lovastatin, 1 hour for pravastatin, and 1.3 to 2.4 hours for simvastatin.

Lovastatin and simvastatin are converted by the liver to several active metabolites. The initial response is seen within 1 to 2 weeks, with the maximum therapeutic response occurring within 4 to 6 weeks of chronic drug administration. Excretion is primarily fecal.

Side Effects/Adverse Reactions. The side effects/adverse reactions of the reductase inhibitors include gas, stomach cramps or pain, rash, constipation or diarrhea, nausea, headaches, myalgia, myositis, rhabdomyolysis and, rarely, impotency and insomnia. A significant drug interaction may occur if the drugs are administered with cyclosporine (Neoral, Sandimmune), gemfibrozil (Lopid), or niacin (vitamin B_3). An increased risk of rhabdomyolysis (necrosis of skeletal muscle with the release of myoglobulin, which may result in myopathy and acute renal failure) may occur. Monitor closely if concurrent administration is necessary.

Dosage and Administration. The recommended adult dosage for atorvastatin is 10 mg daily, titrated monthly as needed (range is 10 to 80 mg/day); and for fluvastatin, 20 mg PO daily at bedtime, titrated monthly as necessary. The adult dosage of lovastatin is 20 mg daily with the evening meal, increased monthly as necessary according to the client's response to therapy, up to a maximum of 80 mg/day. The adult dosage of pravastatin is 10 to 20 mg at bedtime, with dosage adjustments at monthly intervals as needed. The adult dosage of simvastatin is 5 to 10 mg in the evening, titrated monthly as necessary and tolerated; the maximum dosage is 40 mg/day.

▪ Nursing Management

Reductase Inhibitor Therapy

▪ **Assessment.** Do not administer reductase inhibitors to clients with active liver disease or unexplained persistent elevations of serum transaminase. Use with caution in clients with organ transplant and immunosuppressant therapy because of the increased risk of rhabdomyolysis and renal failure. Administer with caution in those conditions in which there is increased risk of secondary renal failure if rhabdomyolysis occurs, such as hypotension, severe infection, uncontrolled seizures, major surgery, trauma, and severe metabolic, endocrine, or electrolyte disorders. A baseline assessment should include serum cholesterol, serum creatine kinase (CK), and liver function studies.

▪ **Nursing Diagnosis.** Clients receiving reductase inhibitor therapy are at risk for the following nursing

BOX 32-1

Summary of Drug Treatment Goals and Selected Drug Therapies

Drug Treatment Goals

Primary goal: reduce risk of coronary heart disease

Approaches: lower LDL cholesterol and triglyceride serum levels; increase HDL cholesterol serum level

Selected Drug Therapies

Bile acid sequestering agents to lower high LDL cholesterol levels

Niacin to lower total and LDL cholesterol levels and increase HDL cholesterol level

Reductase inhibitors, which are very potent drugs that lower LDL cholesterol and triglyceride levels and increase HDL serum levels

Gemfibrozil to lower triglycerides

diagnoses: impaired comfort related to myalgia or myositis (fever, muscle aches), headache, and nausea; risk for injury related to blurred vision and dizziness; disturbed sleep pattern (insomnia—lovastatin only); sexual dysfunction (impotence—lovastatin only); and impaired skin integrity (rash).

■ **Implementation**

■ ***Monitoring.*** Liver function studies should be performed periodically, because reductase inhibitors may elevate transaminase levels and serum creatine concentrations. Serum CK levels should be determined if the client develops muscular tenderness. Serum cholesterol levels will determine the efficacy of treatment.

■ ***Intervention.*** Discontinue reductase inhibitor therapy if serum transaminase concentrations increase to three times the upper limit of normal, if CK concentrations markedly increase, or if myositis occurs.

■ ***Education.*** As with other antihyperlipidemic medications, an appropriate diet, exercise, and weight reduction in obese clients should be instituted along with drug therapy. Alert clients to notify the prescriber if grapefruit juice is a regular part of their diet, because it greatly increases the bioavailability of atorvastatin, lovastatin, and simvastatin (but not pravastatin) (Lilja, Kivisto, & Neuvonen, 1999).

■ **Evaluation.** The client's serum lipid concentrations will be within the normal limits.

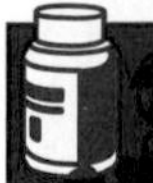

Complementary and Alternative Therapies
Garlic

Garlic is widely used for flavoring in foods and beverages. Medicinally, it is used to reduce blood pressure, prevent age-related vascular changes, decrease LDLs and VLDLs, increase HDLs, and reduce blood clotting (antiplatelet effect). The lipid-lowering effects of garlic are attributed to its inactivation of the enzymes involved in lipid synthesis through an interaction with enzyme thiol groups. It is considered to be effective for lowering blood pressure and reducing serum cholesterol, LDLs, and triglycerides when taken orally as fresh garlic. Some controversy exists about the particular garlic supplements used in some studies. In general, data suggest that in addition to its lipid-lowering abilities, garlic has demonstrated antihypertensive, antithrombotic, and hypoglycemic activity.

Garlic ingestion in the amounts commonly found in foods is considered safe unless the person has a sensitivity to garlic. It is possibly safe in larger amounts, but it may be contraindicated in clients with bleeding disorders, gastrointestinal infection, or inflammation. Close monitoring is required for all clients with diabetes (because of garlic's hypoglycemic effects) and for clients taking anticoagulants (because additive effects may increase bleeding tendencies). The dose-related effects of garlic are breath odor, oral and gastrointestinal burning or irritation, nausea, vomiting, flatulence, and diarrhea. Large amounts of garlic are contraindicated in children and in women who are pregnant or lactating. Garlic enhances the effects of warfarin as measured by the International Normalized Ratio (INR). Theoretically, it may also increase the effects of other anticoagulant drugs, antiplatelet drugs, and hypoglycemic drugs. Monitor more carefully clients with diabetes who are taking larger amounts of garlic, because the control of diabetes may be affected by the garlic.

Although larger doses are taken to obtain the cholesterol-lowering and antihypertensive effects of garlic, the usual dosage is 1 clove of fresh garlic daily. Garlic is also available in various over-the-counter preparations. (For further information, see Chapter 12.)

Information from Cirigliano, M.D. (1998). Ten most common herbs in clinical practice. In M.S. Micozzi (Ed.), *Current review of complementary medicine.* Philadelphia: Current Medicine; and Jellin, J.M., Batz, F., & Hitchens, K. (1999). *Pharmacist's letter/prescriber's letter natural medicines comprehensive database.* Stockton, CA: Therapeutic Research Faculty.

SUMMARY

Along with dietary modifications, antihyperlipidemic agents are used to treat hyperlipidemia, a metabolic disorder characterized by increased serum concentrations of cholesterol and triglycerides. High levels of these serum lipids have been associated with atherosclerosis, in which lipids are deposited in the linings of medium- and large-sized arteries. Box 32-1 summarizes the drug treatment goals and selected drug therapies. (See also the Complementary and Alternative Therapies box above.)

Atherosclerosis is a causative factor in hypertension, CHD, cerebral artery disease, peripheral artery occlusive disease, and renal arterial insufficiency. Although atherosclerosis has many causes, such as dietary saturated fats, faulty fat metabolism, genetic influences, and others, some clinicians believe that the progression of atherosclerosis can be controlled if serum lipid levels can also be controlled. At the present time, however, the available antihyperlipidemic agents remain controversial.

The bile acid sequestering agents, cholestyramine, colesevelam, and colestipol hydrochloride, combine with bile acids in the intestine to prevent their absorption and promote their loss from the body in feces. To compensate for their loss, the liver increases its rate of oxidation of cholesterol to replace the bile acids, which causes a reduction of serum cholesterol levels. Clofibrate is more effective in lowering serum triglyceride levels; it appears to block the synthesis of triglycerides in the liver. Dextrothyroxine and probucol enhance the excretion of cholesterol. Gemfibrozil and niacin lower both triglyceride and cholesterol levels. As enzyme inhibitors, atorvastatin, fluvastatin, lovastatin, pravastatin, and simvastatin inhibit the synthesis of cholesterol in the liver and are effective for clients with primary hypercholesterolemia. Each agent is indicated for specific instances of hyperlipidemia (see Table 32-2).

Nursing management focuses on client education for compliance with lifestyle changes, particularly adherence to a low-fat dietary regimen as a long-term commitment and, in the short term for most clients, adherence to the prescribed medication regimen until the hyperlipidemia is resolved.

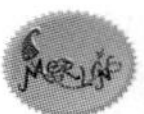

Critical Thinking Questions

1. Mr. Clark has been taking cholestyramine for 6 months. During this office visit he indicates that he has been experiencing nosebleeds more frequently. What might be happening?
2. How would the nurse counter the common belief of clients that drug therapy replaces dietary restrictions in the management of hyperlipidemia?

Collaborative Learning Activities

For Collaborative Learning Activities, go to mosby.com/MERLIN/McKenry/.

CASE STUDY

For a Case Study that will help ensure mastery of this chapter content, go to mosby.com/MERLIN/McKenry/.

BIBLIOGRAPHY

American Hospital Formulary Service. (1999). *AHFS drug information '99*. Bethesda, MD: American Society of Hospital Pharmacists.

Anderson, K.N., Anderson, L.E., & Glanze, W.D. (Eds.) (1998). *Mosby's medical, nursing, & allied health dictionary* (5th ed.). St. Louis: Mosby.

Clark, J. (1995). Lipid-lowering drugs in heart disease prevention. *Community Nurse, 1*(2 Nurse Prescriber), 3-4.

Drug Facts and Comparisons. (2000). St. Louis: Facts and Comparisons.

Expert Panel on Detection, Evaluation, and Treatment of High Blood Cholesterol in Adults, National Cholesterol Education Program. (1994). Second report of the Expert Panel (Adult Treatment Panel II). *Circulation, 89*, 1329-1445.

Haffner, S.M. (1999). Diabetes, hyperlipidemia, and coronary artery disease. *American Journal of Cardiology, 83*(9B), 17F-21F.

Hardman, J.C. & Limbird, L.E. (Eds.) (1996). *Goodman & Gilman's The pharmacological basis of therapeutics* (9th ed.). New York: Macmillan.

Hunninghake, D.B. (1999). Pharmacologic management of triglycerides. *Clinical Cardiology,, 22*(6 suppl), II44-48.

Knopp, R.H. (1999). Drug treatment of lipid disorders. *New England Journal of Medicine, 341*(7), 498-511.

Lilja, J.J., Kivisto, K.T., & Neuvonen, P.J. (1999). Grapefruit juice increases serum concentrations of atorvastatin and has no effect on pravastatin. *Clinical Pharmacology & Therapeutics, 66*(2), 118-127.

Long, J.W. (1990). *The essential guide to prescription drugs.* New York: Harper Collins.

McKenney, J.M. (1995). Dyslipidemias. In L.Y. Young & M.A. Koda-Kimble (Eds.), *Applied therapeutics: The clinical use of drugs* (6th ed.). Vancouver, WA: Applied Therapeutics.

Murdock, D.K., Murdock, A.K., Murdock, R.W., Olson, K.J., Frane, A.M., Kersten, M.E., Joyce, D.M., & Gantner, S.E. (1999). Long-term safety and efficacy of combination gemfibrozil and HMG-CoA reductase inhibitors for the treatment of mixed lipid disorders. *American Heart Journal, 138*(1 Pt 1), 151-155.

Rader, D.J. & Haffner, S.M. (1999). Role of fibrates in the management of hypertriglyceridemia. *American Journal of Cardiology, 83*(9B), 30F-35F.

Ross, S.D., Allen, I.E., Connelly, J.E., Korenblat, B.M., Smith, M.E., Bishop, D., & Luo, D. (1999). Clinical outcomes in statin treatment trials: A meta-analysis. *Archives of Internal Medicine, 159*(15), 1793-1802.

United States Pharmacopeia Dispensing Information (USP DI): Drug information for the health care professional (19th ed.). (1999). Rockville, MD: United States Pharmacopeial Convention.

Wilson, B.A. (1994). Understanding management of hyperlipidemia. *MEDSURG Nursing, 3*(4), 319-321.

Witztum, J.L. (1996). Drugs used in the treatment of hyperlipoproteinemias. In J.G. Hardman & L.E. Limbird (Eds.), *Goodman & Gilman's The pharmacological basis of therapeutics* (9th ed.). New York: McGraw-Hill.

33 Overview of the Urinary System

Chapter Focus

The urinary system functions with other organs to regulate the volume and composition of fluid within the body, retaining essential materials and excreting waste. Because of this function, the urinary system affects other body systems and the client's general health. Many pharmacologic effects are diminished or enhanced by the activity of the urinary system, and therefore the nurse must be knowledgeable about its anatomy and physiology.

Learning Objectives

1. Describe the anatomy and physiology of the urinary system
2. Identify the functions of the various segments of the nephron.
3. Describe the major functions of the kidneys.
4. Describe the sites of action and primary effects of antidiuretic hormone, vasopressin, and aldosterone on the nephrons.

Key Terms

electromagnetic gradient, p. 665
glomerular filtration, p. 664
glomerulus, p. 664
hypertonic, p. 665
hypotonic, p. 665
osmotic gradient, p. 665
threshold concentration, p. 665
tubular reabsorption, p. 665
tubular secretion, p. 665
tubular transport maximum, p. 665

The urinary system is composed of organs that manufacture and excrete urine from the body: two kidneys, two ureters, the bladder, and the urethra (Figure 33-1). Urine formed in the kidneys flows through the ureters to the bladder, where it is stored. When approximately 250 mL of urine is collected, bladder expansion results in a feeling of distention and a desire to void. The urine flows from the bladder into the urethra to be expelled from the body.

In males the urethra is surrounded by the prostate gland; it then passes through fibrous tissue connected to the pubic bones and terminates at the urinary meatus, or tip of the penis (Figure 33-2). The male urethra serves a dual purpose—elimination of urine from the body and the transport of semen. In females the urethra is the final vehicle for urination (Figure 33-3).

The kidneys regulate homeostasis in the body; they are responsible for the maintenance of body fluids, electrolytes, and acid-base balance as well as the elimination of body waste, urea, and urine. The primary focus of this chapter is the kidneys.

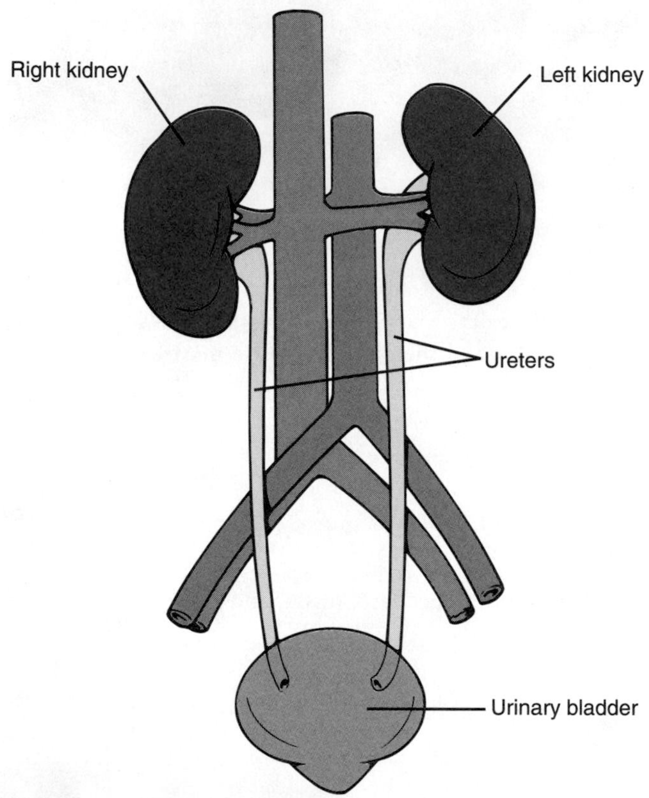

Figure 33-1 Urinary system.

ANATOMY AND PHYSIOLOGY OF THE KIDNEY

The kidney is composed of millions of individual units called nephrons. Each nephron consists of a glomerulus and a tubular system. The volume and composition of urine as a result of concentration and dilution depend on three major processes in the kidney: glomerular filtration, tubular reabsorption, and tubular secretion.

Glomerular Filtration. **Glomerular filtration** occurs as a result of plasma flowing across a cluster of capillary blood vessels and into the urinary space of the Bowman's capsule. This capillary cluster is enveloped within a thin wall, branching into uriniferous tubules; it is called the **glomerulus.** The heart works to create pressure in the blood vessels, which in turn provides the force necessary to accomplish glomerular filtration. Blood flow to the kidney occurs at a rate of 1200 mL/min, which is 20% to 25% of cardiac output. The blood pressure within the glomerular capillaries is approximately 60% of arterial pressure. Systemic blood pressure must be significantly reduced before glomerular filtration is greatly altered. Usually some degree of filtration exists if the mean blood pressure remains above 50 mm Hg. Maintenance of glomerular hydrostatic pressure is aided by the ability of the afferent and efferent arterioles to alter vessel resistance effectively.

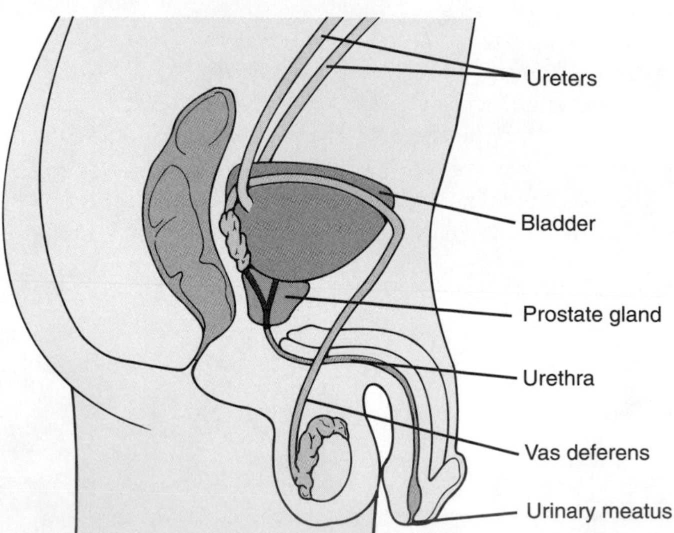

Figure 33-2 Sagittal section of male pelvis.

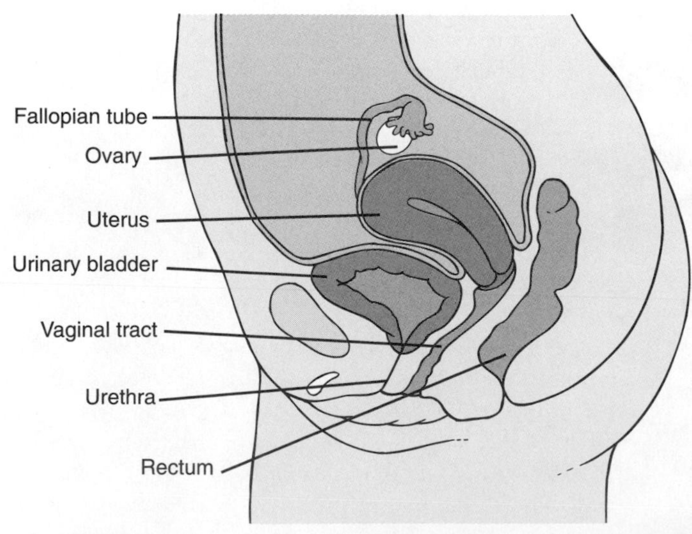

Figure 33-3 Sagittal section of female pelvis.

In the absence of disease, the glomerular membrane does not filter plasma proteins greater than 100 angstroms in diameter (e.g., hemoglobin and albumin and the small amount of protein-bound substances). Otherwise the glomerular filtrate is almost identical to plasma. The rate of filtration in an average adult is approximately 125 mL/min; 99% of this tubular filtrate is ultimately reabsorbed throughout the tubule.

Tubular Reabsorption. **Tubular reabsorption** involves both active and passive transport of substances into the tubular epithelial cell and into the extracellular fluid compartment. Passive transport, or diffusion, through the tubular membrane occurs because of a difference in particle concentration (**osmotic gradient**) or electrical charge (**electromagnetic gradient**).

In the proximal tubule, sodium is *actively* transported across the tubular cell membrane from the tubule filtrate. Chloride follows passively because of an electromagnetic gradient. Water in turn follows passively in response to an osmotic gradient established by sodium chloride solute. Then diffusion of 60% of urea content occurs to maintain a chemical gradient. Weak acids and weak bases may be reabsorbed by diffusion depending on the amount of a drug in ionized or nonionized form and the pH of the tubular fluid.

For almost every substance that is actively transported across the membrane, there is a maximum rate at which the transport mechanism can function; above this maximum, the excess substance will not be reabsorbed and the substance will appear in the urine. This is called the **tubular transport maximum**. For example, the tubular transport maximum for glucose averages 320 mg/min for most adults. If the tubular load becomes greater than 320 mg/min, the excess will not be reabsorbed and will appear in the urine. Every substance that has a tubular transport maximum also has a **threshold concentration**, the plasma concentration below which none of the substance appears in the urine and above which progressively larger quantities appear.

Tubular Secretion. **Tubular secretion** affects the composition of urine by allowing compounds such as penicillin, histamine, probenecid, methotrexate, and thiazides to enter into tubular fluid from peritubular or interstitial capillaries. This is accomplished via specific transport mechanisms for the secretion of organic compounds. Other very important examples of tubular secretion include that of the hydrogen ions, ammonia, and potassium ions.

Proximal Tubule. Most of the glomerular filtrate is reabsorbed in the proximal tubule and returned to the bloodstream. Approximately 70% of salt and water is reabsorbed rapidly, maintaining nearly the same osmolality between tubular fluid and interstitial fluid at the end of the proximal tubule (isotonic). The general mechanism for sodium, chloride, water, and urea reabsorption is tubular reabsorption with respect to gradient transport. There are no dilutional or concentration changes of these ions in the proximal tubule.

Other substances reabsorbed in the proximal tubule include glucose, amino acids, phosphate, uric acid, and a major portion of potassium. Nearly 90% of bicarbonate in tubular filtrate is reabsorbed as carbon dioxide if hydrogen ions are secreted in the tubular lumen. Plasma carbon dioxide is hydrolyzed in the tubular cell to form carbonic acid, which dissociates to give bicarbonate and hydrogen ion. This reversible reaction is catalyzed by carbonic anhydrase. The hydrogen ion secreted into the lumen combines with the bicarbonate of the glomerular filtrate to form carbonic acid in the lumen. This again dissociates to give water and carbon dioxide, which are reabsorbed. This reaction is catalyzed at both steps by carbonic anhydrase. Proximal tubule reabsorption is usually constant in spite of moderate changes in the glomerular filtration rate.

Descending Loop of Henle. This portion of the nephron is permeable to water; water is passively taken up to equilibrate medullary interstitial osmolality. This produces a **hypertonic** (more concentrated) filtrate at the tip of the loop of Henle, the papilla. There is very low sodium and urea permeability in this segment.

Ascending Loop of Henle. Water permeability is almost nil in the ascending limb of the loop of Henle, whereas sodium and chloride permeability is high. Approximately 20% to 25% of sodium load in glomerular filtrate is reabsorbed, and chloride follows passively. As a result, two very important situations occur. The concentration of tubular filtrates becomes very dilute, or **hypotonic**; this is often termed "free water production." Meanwhile, the medullary interstitium becomes hypertonic, which is necessary to the concentration capacity of the countercurrent multiplier. The concentration gradient established across the tubular epithelium becomes multiplied in a longitudinal direction, resulting in a large osmotic gradient between the isosmotic renal cortex and the hyperosmotic medulla and papilla. Unlike other segments, the ascending limb of the loop of Henle is not responsive to any hormones.

Distal Convoluted Tubule. Between 5% and 10% of sodium reabsorption actively occurs in the distal tubule. This uptake is largely determined by the presence of a hormone called aldosterone. When the extracellular fluid volume is decreased, the renin-angiotensin system becomes involved and stimulates the release of aldosterone. Increased levels of aldosterone act to increase the active reabsorption of sodium. Although an increase in potassium secretion is seen, a simple sodium-potassium exchange pump is no longer recognized.

Collecting Duct. The hypotonic fluid entering the collecting duct may be altered in the medullary portion by the presence of antidiuretic hormone (ADH), or vasopressin. The released ADH acts at the distal tubule and collecting duct to reabsorb water to increase plasma volume, thus lowering plasma osmolality. Urinary output is more concentrated, or fluid is lost because of the osmotic gradient set up by hypertonic medullary interstitium. Thus the collecting duct is responsible for urine concentration.

PHYSIOLOGIC REGULATION BY THE KIDNEY

The kidneys excrete metabolic byproducts of the body, especially nitrogenous-type substances such as urea. They maintain electrolyte homeostasis (e.g., sodium, potassium, chloride) and body fluids. Sodium is actively reabsorbed in the proximal tubules (approximately 65%) and ascending loop of Henle (27%). Approximately 8% of sodium reaches the distal tubules; the rate of reabsorption in the distal tubules depends on the presence of aldosterone. If large quantities of aldosterone are present, sodium is reabsorbed. A lack of aldosterone will result in the elimination of sodium in the urine. In general, healthy kidneys excrete the daily sodium intake. Potassium is reabsorbed from the proximal tubules and loop of Henle in percentages equivalent to sodium. Thus approximately 8% of the filtered potassium reaches the distal tubules. Aldosterone controls potassium secretion; in its presence, sodium is reabsorbed and potassium is secreted in the distal tubules. The daily potassium intake is generally excreted daily in the kidneys. Figure 33-4 and Table 33-1 explain nephron functions.

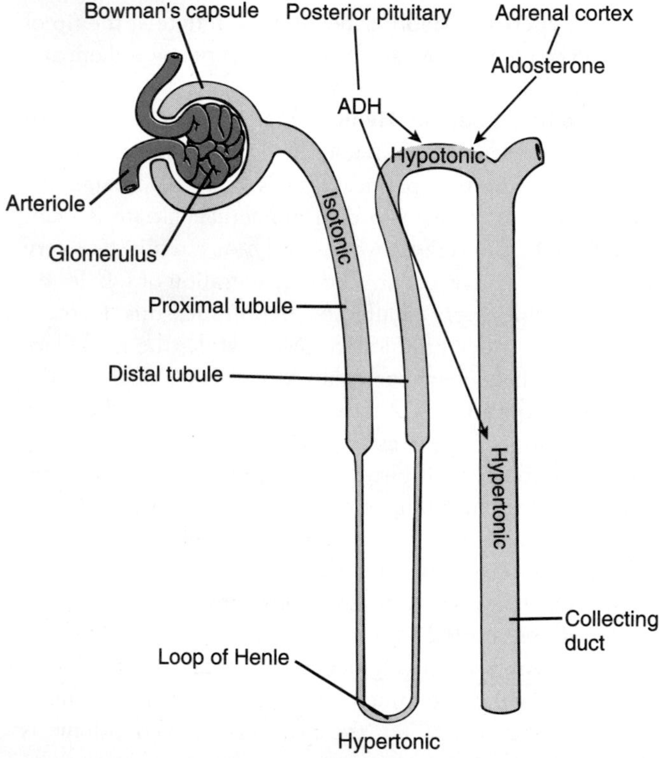

Figure 33-4 Components of a nephron.

ADH is a water-conserving hormone synthesized in the hypothalamus and stored in the posterior pituitary gland. When plasma osmolarity increases as a result of dehydration or water deprivation, osmoreceptors in the supraoptic area of the hypothalamus stimulate the release of ADH. The released ADH acts at the distal tubule and collecting duct to reabsorb water to increase plasma volume, thus lowering plasma osmolality. Urine output is decreased, and the urine is more concentrated.

Acid-base balance is partially controlled in the kidneys. The kidneys are one of three pH control mechanisms in the body; the others are blood buffering and the respiratory adjustment mechanism. As the blood pH becomes more acidic, the kidneys respond by increasing the renal tubule excretion of hydrogen and ammonia, which results in an increase in blood bicarbonate and an increase in pH (toward normal). This is an effective method of adjusting hydrogen ions within the system.

The hormone erythropoietin is synthesized in the kidneys. A decrease in red blood cells below normal, or tissue hypoxia, stimulates an increased release of erythropoietin from the kidneys. The increased serum concentration of erythropoietin stimulates the bone marrow to increase its production of red blood cells so that the red blood cell average is restored to normal.

SUMMARY

The kidneys as part of the urinary system participate with other body organs to regulate the volume and composition of interstitial fluid within a narrow range of values. They remove waste products from the blood and are important in controlling blood volume, the concentration of ions in the

TABLE 33-1 Nephron Functions

Site	Major Functions
Glomerulus	Filtration
Proximal tubule	Reabsorption of glucose, potassium, sodium, amino acids, water, and nutrients; remaining fluid isotonic.
Loop of Henle	Sodium and chloride reabsorbed in ascending loop. Countercurrent mechanism produces decrease in osmolality of filtrate in ascending loop of Henle (i.e., sodium chloride but not water is transported into the body). Filtrate leaves loop of Henle as hypotonic urine.
Distal tubule	Sodium and bicarbonate are reabsorbed. Potassium, hydrogen, and ammonia may be secreted. ADH is necessary to reabsorb water at this site. Filtrate leaves the distal tubule as hypotonic urine.
Collecting duct	ADH, if present, will reabsorb water at this site. Urine may be hypertonic. If ADH is unavailable or not functioning, dilute urine (hypotonic) may be excreted.

blood, and the pH of the blood. The kidneys also function in the control of red blood cell production. As the major excretory organs in the body, the kidneys are essential in maintaining a normal environment for the body cells.

Critical Thinking Questions

1. Sally Bownes has eaten a large box of salty pretzels. What effect will this have on her urine concentration and volume? Why?
2. Mr. Smith has had a course of acyclovir for a week at the high level of the dosage range and needs continued encouragement to drink fluids. Knowing that a potential complication of this drug is renal toxicity, what laboratory values would you be monitoring? How would you expect them to change if Mr. Smith began to develop toxicity and why?

Collaborative Learning Activities

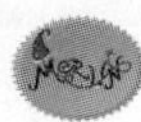

For Collaborative Learning Activities, go to mosby.com/MERLIN/McKenry/.

BIBLIOGRAPHY

Anderson, K.N., Anderson, L.E., & Glanze, W.D. (Eds.) (1998). *Mosby's medical, nursing, & allied health dictionary* (5th ed.). St. Louis: Mosby.

Seeley, R.R., Stephens, T.D., & Tate, P. (1996). *Anatomy & physiology* (3rd ed.). St. Louis: Mosby.

Thibodeau, G.A. & Patton, K. (1999). *Anatomy and physiology* (4th ed.). St. Louis: Mosby.

Van Wynsberghe, D., Noback, C.R., & Carola, R. (1995). *Human anatomy and physiology* (3rd ed.). New York: McGraw-Hill.

34 Diuretics

Chapter Focus

Diuretics play a leading role in many therapies, including congestive heart failure and hypertension. Although diuretics can be beneficial, they may also result in many side effects and drug interactions. With the appropriate nursing assessment and intervention, diuretic therapy can have positive effects in the treatment of hypertension and edema with a minimum of adverse effects.

Learning Objectives

1. Compare and contrast the five classifications of diuretics.
2. Identify the most common agents within the five classifications of diuretics, as well as the site within the nephron where the action of each classification occurs.
3. Identify the signs and symptoms of fluid and electrolyte imbalance associated with diuretic therapy.
4. Explain the nursing care and client education required for clients receiving potassium-depleting diuretics and those receiving potassium-sparing diuretics.
5. Implement the nursing management of the care of a client receiving diuretic therapy.

Key Terms

diuretic, p. 669
loop diuretics, p. 676
osmotic diuretics, p. 679
potassium-sparing diuretics, p. 678
proximal tubule diuretics, p. 669
thiazide-type diuretics, p. 671

Key Drugs [✓]

furosemide, p. 676
hydrochlorothiazide, p. 671
spironolactone, p. 678

Diuretics modify renal function to induce diuresis, or the loss of body water by urination. In addition to water, diuretics increase the excretion of electrolytes, primarily sodium chloride. Understanding their action requires knowledge of the events that take place along each of the tubular segments (see Chapter 33). Diuretics are among the most commonly used medications. They represent the mainstay in the treatment of hypertension (see also Chapter 27) and are an integral part of drug therapies in edematous conditions such as cirrhosis, nephrotic syndrome, chronic renal failure, and acute and chronic congestive heart failure.

Therapeutically, drug selection is best understood if each diuretic is presented according to its major site of action. This approach does not preclude the drug's effect at other sites in the nephron. Figure 34-1 shows the various sites of action of diuretic drug groups by means of water and electrolyte transport system in a kidney nephron.

PROXIMAL TUBULE DIURETICS: CARBONIC ANHYDRASE INHIBITORS

acetazolamide [a set a zole′ a mide] (Diamox, Acetazolam ♣)

Acetazolamide, a sulfonamide, is the prototype of the **proximal tubule diuretics,** which act primarily to reduce the volume of sequestered fluids, especially of the aqueous humor. It inhibits the action of the enzyme carbonic anhydrase, which in turn prevents the reabsorption of bicarbonate ions from the proximal tubules. These bicarbonate ions then act to increase tubular osmotic pressure, causing osmotic diuresis. With long-term use, however, the diuretic effect of these drugs is lost.

Acetazolamide is widely used as an antiglaucoma agent because it lowers intraocular pressure by decreasing the production of aqueous humor by more than 50% (see Chapter 43 for further discussion).

Acetazolamide is indicated for the treatment of open-angle glaucoma and is also used as adjunct treatment with

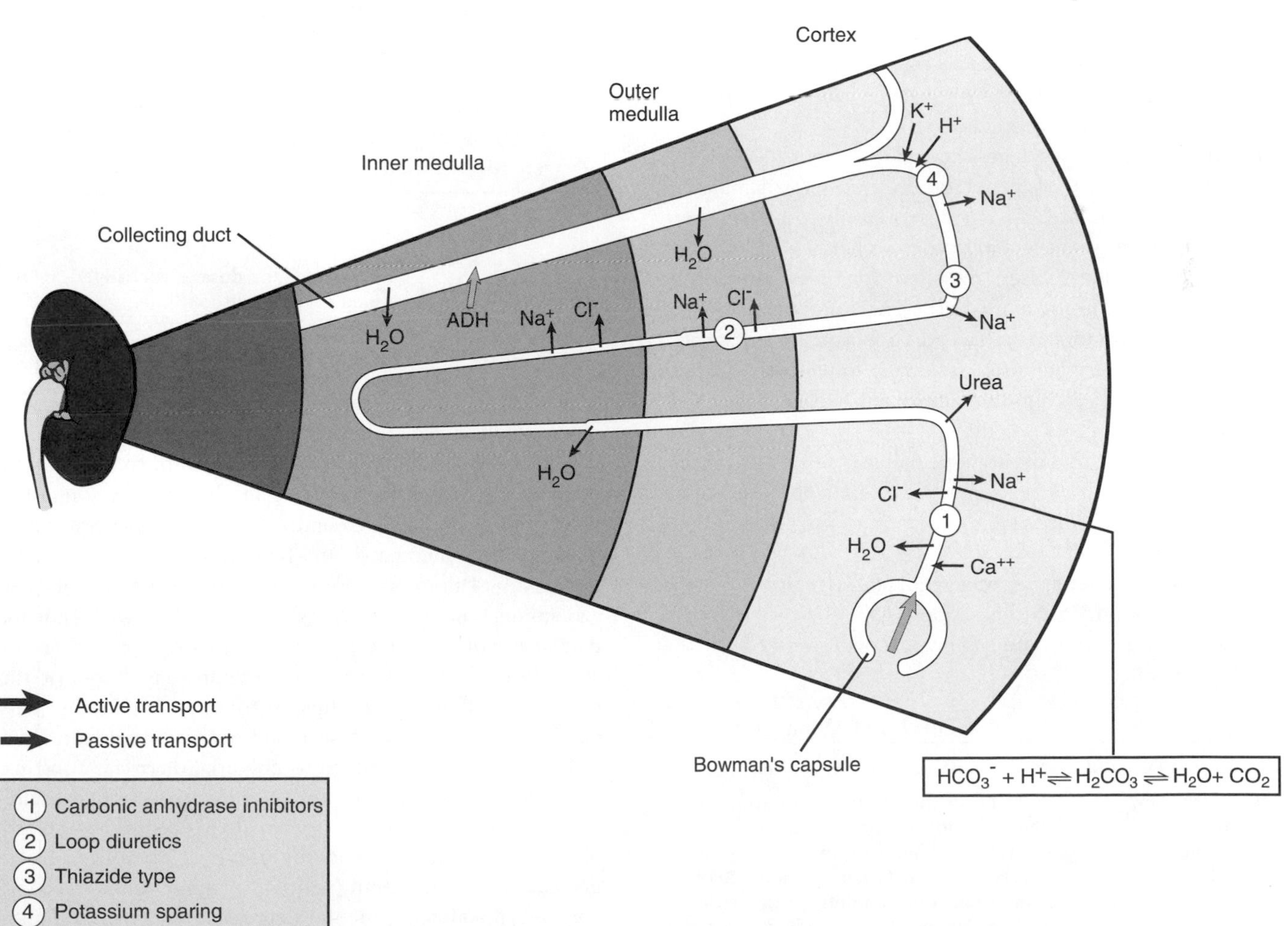

Figure 34-1 Site of action of diuretics by means of water and electrolyte transport.

anticonvulsants to manage absence seizures (petit mal), generalized tonic-clonic seizures (grand mal), mixed seizure patterns, and myoclonic seizures. It has been found especially useful for women who experience an increase in seizures during their menstrual periods. It has also been found to decrease the incidence and severity of symptoms of altitude sickness in mountain climbers when taken orally. In addition, acetazolamide produces an alkaline urine, which may help to increase the excretion of weakly acidic drugs in cases of drug overdose. It is also used to reverse metabolic alkalosis (Mazur et al., 1999).

Acetazolamide is well absorbed orally. It reaches a peak level in 2 to 4 hours after a 500-mg dose or in 8 to 12 hours after a 500-mg extended-release capsule. Its half-life is 10 to 15 hours, and excretion is mainly by the kidneys.

The side effects/adverse reactions of acetazolamide therapy include headaches, increased nervousness, anorexia, nausea, vomiting, depression, tremors, rash, alopecia, ataxia, and chest, groin, or leg pain.

The adult dosage for glaucoma is 250 mg PO one to four times daily. The anticonvulsant dosage is 4 to 30 mg/kg PO divided into 4 doses per day. For altitude sickness the dosage is 250 mg PO two to four times daily. The pediatric dosage for glaucoma is 8 to 30 mg/kg PO daily in divided doses. Acetazolamide is also available as a parenteral injection for IV or IM use. Refer to the current package insert for dosing instructions.

■ Nursing Management

Acetazolamide Therapy

■ Assessment. Ascertain whether the client has diabetes or a familial history of diabetes, because acetazolamide has caused elevations of blood glucose and glycosuria in these clients. Do not give acetazolamide to clients who are allergic to sulfonamides. Assess the client for preexisting health conditions that might increase the risk for exacerbation of electrolyte imbalances, such as adrenocortical insufficiency, renal or respiratory acidosis, or hepatic impairment. Clients with a history of calcium-containing renal stones may experience a recurrence of calculi.

Note that older adults are especially susceptible to excessive diuresis and may be unable to tolerate the usual adult dosages (see the Special Considerations for Older Adults box at right).

Review the client's current medication regimen for the risk of significant drug interactions, such as those that may occur when acetazolamide is given concurrently with the following drugs:

Bold/color type indicates the most serious interactions.

Drug	Possible Effect and Management
amphetamines, mecamylamine (Inversine), or quinidine	**Because of the alkalinization of urine, the excretion of these drugs is decreased. Therefore increased serum levels and toxicity may be seen. Avoid concurrent drug administration with mecamylamine. Dosage adjustments may be necessary with the other two drugs whenever a carbonic anhydrase inhibitor is started, the dosage is changed, or the medication is discontinued.**
methenamine mandelate (Mandelamine)	**Alkaline urine will reduce the effectiveness of methenamine. Avoid concurrent use.**

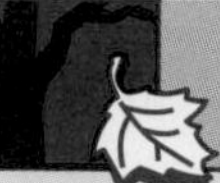

Special Considerations for Older Adults
Diuretics

Older adults may be more sensitive to diuretic-induced hypotension and electrolyte disturbances than the average adult.

Pharmacologically, older adults are started with the lowest dosage possible, generally one-half the recommended adult dosage, which is titrated slowly to effect (Menscer, 1992).

Advise clients to drink sufficient fluids. Because diuretics are often referred to as "water pills," many persons believe fluid intake is restricted with this drug category. This erroneous belief should be discussed with the client.

Avoid concurrent administration of a potassium supplement or a potassium chloride salt substitute with clients receiving a potassium-sparing diuretic, or use *extreme* caution and close monitoring. Hyperkalemia and fatality have been reported with this combination.

Be aware that all diuretics will increase urinary incontinence.

Report any signs and symptoms of diuretic toxicity to the prescriber, such as anorexia, nausea, vomiting, confusion, increased weakness, and paresthesia of the extremities.

When a diuretic is to be discontinued, reduce the drug gradually to avoid the possible development of fluid retention and edema.

A baseline assessment of the client's underlying condition should be obtained; the neurologic status of the client with seizures, the presence of edema in clients with congestive heart failure, and the eye comfort and intraocular pressure of clients with glaucoma should be determined.

■ Nursing Diagnosis. With the administration of acetazolamide, clients are at risk for the following nursing diagnoses/collaborative problems: impaired comfort (headache, bitter taste, nausea, vomiting, and numbness or tingling of the fingers, toes, lips, or tongue); impaired urinary elimination with an increase and frequency of urination; disturbed sleep pattern related to polyuria; diarrhea; constipation; fatigue; imbalanced nutrition: less than body requirements related to anorexia (weight loss); disturbed thought processes (confusion); and the potential complications of decreased cardiac output (ventricular dysrhythmias secondary to hypokalemia), mental depression, electrolyte imbalance such as hypokalemia (dry mouth, increased thirst, irregular heartbeats, muscle cramps, fatigue), renal calculi or nephrotoxicity (hematuria, lower back pain, burning on urination), and blood dyscrasias (fever, sore throat, unusual bleeding or bruising).

■ **Implementation**

■ ***Monitoring.*** Observe the client for signs of allergic reaction and photosensitivity. Weigh the client daily. A rapid loss of body water (which may cause hypotension) will be reflected in a rapid weight loss. Monitor blood pressure for indications of hypotension. Monitor intake and output and electrolytes, especially serum potassium levels. Perform complete blood cell counts periodically to monitor for blood dyscrasias. Monitor blood glucose levels for clients with diabetes or those at risk for diabetes.

■ ***Intervention.*** Reconstituting acetazolamide with at least 5 mL sterile water is necessary before parenteral use. Discard it after 24 hours of reconstitution, because it contains no preservatives.

Administer the oral forms of acetazolamide with meals or with antacids to decrease gastrointestinal distress. For clients who are unable to tolerate tablets for oral administration, crush acetazolamide tablets and mix them with a flavored syrup such as chocolate or cherry. Although up to 500 mg may be prepared in 5 mL syrup, it is more palatable if only 250 mg/5 mL is used. Refrigeration also increases the palatability but not the stability of the preparation; use within a week of preparation. Mixing the drug with fruit juices and elixirs is not as satisfactory.

Planning a high fluid intake for the client with gout or hypercalciuria (excessive calcium in the urine) is necessary because of the risk of renal calculi. Establish dosing schedules that minimize the inconvenience of diuresis that results from altered urinary elimination patterns. When acetazolamide is used in diuretic therapy, consult the prescriber and the dietitian to provide a high-potassium diet.

Acetazolamide is used to prevent or minimize high-altitude sickness, but it is not a substitute for rapid descent if the climber manifests signs of pulmonary or cerebral edema.

■ ***Education.*** The oral and IV routes of administration are preferred. If acetazolamide is to be given intramuscularly, alert the client that the injection will be painful because of the alkalinity of the drug.

Alert the client that constipation is common with diuretic therapy and may be prevented or minimized by increased fluid intake, a high-fiber diet, and moderate exercise if these are not contraindicated by the client's health status. A high fluid intake, 2500 to 3000 mL/day, is necessary to reduce the risk of renal calculi.

Instruct the client to move gradually from a sitting or lying position to a more upright position to prevent the lightheadedness caused by orthostatic hypotension. Caution the client that the ability to accomplish tasks requiring mental alertness or physical coordination may be impaired.

Advise the client that dryness of the mouth may occur but that its discomfort may be minimized by the use of sugarless hard candies and frequent mouth rinses. Advise the client to get regular dental checkups to monitor the development of caries and gum disease, which may occur as the result of xerostomia.

Although the sensation of "not feeling well" is common with the use of acetazolamide, malaise should be reported to the prescriber so that monitoring for acidosis, blood dyscrasias, or hypokalemia may be done. Advise the client to notify the prescriber if paresthesias (numbness, tingling, or burning) of the mouth, fingers, or toes occur.

Instruct the client and the family member who shops for and prepares the food about a high-potassium diet in keeping with the client's usual dietary patterns.

Advise the client to consult the prescriber before switching brands or using a generic formulation of acetazolamide, because bioequivalence problems have been noted.

■ **Evaluation.** The expected outcome for the client receiving acetazolamide therapy for glaucoma is a reduction of intraocular pressure readings to within the normal limits when measured with a tonometer. If the drug is administered for the prevention of seizures, the client will be free of seizures. If taken for altitude illness, the client will not evidence signs of an attack, such as shortness of breath, headache, or syncope.

DILUTING SEGMENT DIURETICS: THIAZIDE AND THIAZIDE-TYPE DRUGS

bendroflumethiazide [ben droe floo me thye′ a zide] (Naturetin)
benzthiazide [benz thye′ a zide] (Exna, Hydrex)
chlorothiazide [klor oh thye′ a zide] (Diuril)
chlorthalidone [klor thal′ i done] (Hygroton)
cyclothiazide [sye kloe thye′ a zide] (Anhydron)
✓**hydrochlorothiazide** [hye droe klor oh thye′ a zide] (HydroDiuril, Esidrix)
hydroflumethiazide [hye droe flu me thye′ a zide] (Diucardin, Saluron)
indapamide [in dap′ a mide] (Lozol)
methyclothiazide [meth ee cloe thye′ a zide] (Enduron)
metolazone [me toe′ la zone] (Zaroxolyn)
polythiazide [pol ee thye′ a zide] (Renese)
quinethazone [kwin eth′ a zone] (Hydromox)
trichlormethiazide [try klor me thye′ a zide] (Metahydrin, Naqua)

Thiazide diuretics are the major diuretics active in the diluting segments of the kidney. They are synthetic drugs that are chemically related to the sulfonamides. Hydrochlorothiazide is one of the most commonly used thiazides. Because these agents are similar, all the diluting segment diuretics will be described collectively as the **thiazide-type diuretics**; important differences will be mentioned later. Table 34-1 presents an overview of the pharmacokinetics and dosages of selected thiazide-type and other diuretics.

TABLE 34-1 Selected Diuretics: Pharmacokinetics and Dosages*

Category/Generic (Trade Name)	Onset of Action (hours)	Peak Effect (hours)	Duration of Action (hours)	Initial Dosage: Adults	Initial Dosage: Children
Thiazide Diuretics					
chlorothiazide (Diuril)	PO: 2	4	6-12	250 mg q6-12h	6 months and older: 10-20 mg/kg/day
chlorthalidone (Hygroton)	PO: 2	2	48-72	25-100 mg/day	2 mg/kg/day
hydrochlorothiazide (Esidrix)	PO: 2	4	6-12	25-100 mg/day	1-2 mg/kg/day
metolazone (Zaroxolyn)	PO: 1	2	12-24	5-20 mg/day	Not established
Loop Diuretics					
bumetanide (Bumex)	PO: 0.5-1	1-2	4-6	0.5-2 mg/day	Not established
	IV: minutes	0.25-0.5	3.5-4		
ethacrynic acid (Edecrin)	PO: 0.5	2	6-8	50-100 mg/day	25 mg/day
	IV: within 5 minutes	0.25-0.5	2	50 mg; repeat in 2-4 hours if needed	1 mg/kg
furosemide (Lasix)	PO: ⅓-1	1-2	6-8	20-80 mg/day, then adjust as necessary q6-8h	2 mg/kg/day
	IV: within 5 minutes	0.5	2	20-40 mg IM or IV	1 mg/kg IM or IV
torsemide (Demadex)	PO: 0.5-1	1-2	6-8	10-20 mg/day	Not established
	IV: within 10 minutes	0.5-1	6-8		
Potassium-Sparing Diuretics					
amiloride (Midamor)	PO: 1-2	6-10	24	5-10 mg/day	Not established
spironolactone (Aldactone)	PO: 24-48	48-72	48-72	25-200 mg/day	1-3 mg/kg/day
triamterene (Dyrenium)	PO: 2-4	24-72	7-9	25-100 mg/day	2-4 mg/kg/day
Osmotic Diuretics					
glycerin (Osmoglyn)	PO: 20 minutes	1	5	1-1.5 g/kg initially, then 0.5 g q6h	Same initial dose; may repeat in 4-8 hours
isosorbide	PO: N/A	1-1.5	5-6	1.5 g/kg 2-4 times/day	Not established
mannitol (Osmitrol)	IV Diuresis: 1-3 Lowering intraocular pressure: 0.25	0.5-1	6-8	50-100 g as 5%-25% IV infusion	0.25-2 g/kg as 15%-20% IV infusion
urea (Ureaphil)	IV: 10 minutes	1-2	3-10	0.5-1.5 g/kg as 30% IV infusion	2 years and older: see adult dosage

Information from *Drug Facts and Comparisons.* (2000). St. Louis: Facts and Comparisons; and *United States Pharmacopeia Dispensing Information (USP DI): Drug information for the health care professional* (19th ed.). (1999). Rockville, MD: United States Pharmacopeial Convention.

*Dosages are titrated as needed and tolerated.

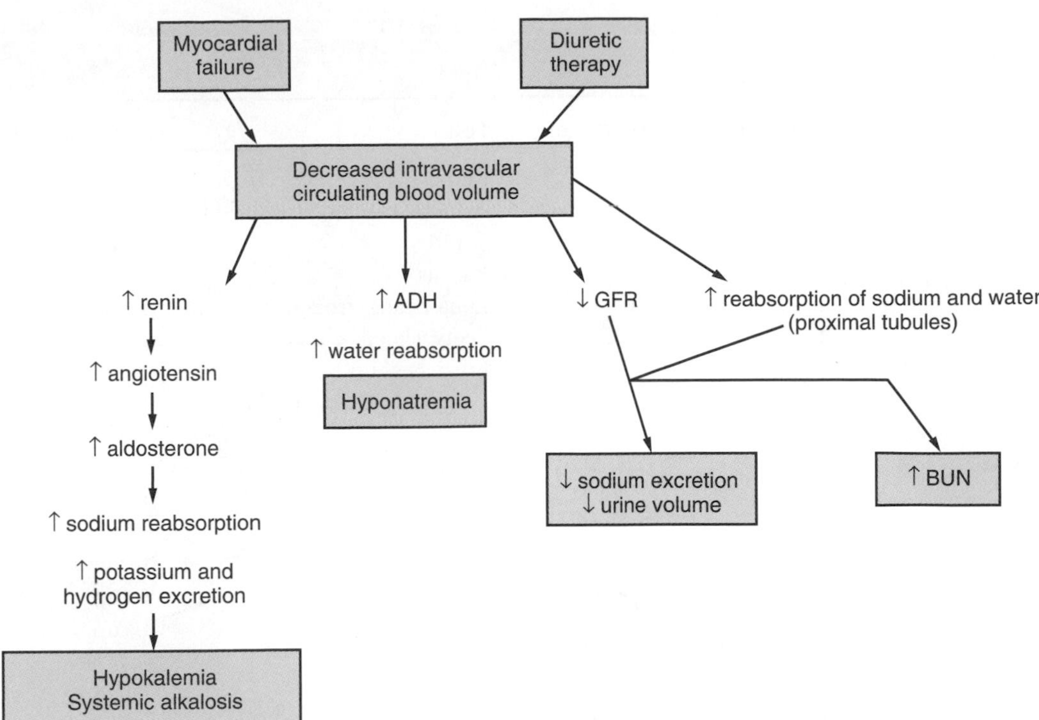

Figure 34-2 Body adaptation to extracellular volume depletion.

The primary action and site of action appear to be inhibition of sodium reabsorption in the early distal tubules in the nephron, the cortical diluting segment. These drugs are less potent than the loop diuretics, because the maximum portion of the sodium load they can affect at the distal tubule is less than 10% of the glomerular filtrate. Therefore the thiazide-type diuretics primarily promote the renal excretion of water, sodium, chloride, potassium, and magnesium; they also may increase serum levels of calcium, glucose, and uric acid.

An especially important feature of thiazide-type diuretics is their ability to impair free water clearance with no effect on concentration ability. The initial natriuretic effect lasts for approximately 1 week and then resets at a lower level. This diuretic tolerance occurs because of increased aldosterone levels and a decreased sodium load at the distal tubule. The mechanisms of antihypertensive action are believed to be initially due to the reduction in plasma and extracellular fluid volume, which results in a decrease in cardiac output. In time, the cardiac output returns to normal. Thiazide-type diuretics also decrease peripheral resistance by a direct action on the peripheral blood vessels.

When an increased sodium load is presented to the distal tubule, there is a corresponding increase in potassium secretion. In addition, plasma renin activity and aldosterone levels increase as extracellular fluid volume decreases, with a resulting potassium loss (Figure 34-2). Potassium is one of the most common electrolytes lost, with a loss occurring in 14% to 60% of ambulatory clients with hypertension. This loss is dose related, occurring early in treatment (first month) and more commonly with larger diuretic doses or with the long-acting type of diuretics (e.g., chlorthalidone) and in individuals with a high sodium intake (Tang & Lau, 1995). However, in many cases the loss is intermittent and neither harmful nor clinically observable. Potassium loss may be a serious threat in clients who are taking digitalis preparations, because it can precipitate serious dysrhythmias as a result of digitalis toxicity. Hypokalemia may predispose the client with cirrhosis to hepatic encephalopathy and coma. Health care providers should caution clients with prescribed thiazide therapy to increase their dietary intake of potassium (Table 34-2).

If hypokalemia occurs, the prescriber may order oral potassium preparations; if urgent replacement is necessary, IV potassium chloride administration may be performed. Potassium loss may also be reversed by the addition of a potassium-sparing diuretic that acts to inhibit potassium loss at the distal tubule. However, potassium replacement is usually not necessary in 80% to 90% of clients taking thiazide-type diuretics, particularly for the treatment of nonedematous states. Potassium replacement may be dangerous in older adults, in renal dysfunction, or when used in combination with potassium-sparing diuretics, because dangerously high serum potassium levels may occur.

Clients receiving the thiazide-type diuretics may experience an increase in serum uric acid. The 1 to 2 mg/dL increase in serum uric acid level is persistent and probably results from the inhibition of the tubular secretion of uric acid. This effect is reversible when the drugs are discontinued. In the absence of gout or genetic predisposition, hyperuricemia is usually asymptomatic and requires no treatment. In clients with a history of gout, the use of allopurinol (Zy-

TABLE 34-2 Foods Rich in Potassium

Food	Amount	Potassium (mg)	Food	Amount	Potassium (mg)
Apricots			Prunes		
Fresh	1	105	Juice, canned or bottled	1 cup	706
Canned in water	1 cup	409	Dried	1 cup	1200
Dried, uncooked	1 cup	1791	Raisins	1 cup	1089
Avocado	1	1097	Lima beans, frozen, cooked	1 cup	694
Banana	1	451	Beets, sliced, cooked	1 cup	532
Figs			Brussels sprouts, cooked	1 cup	494
Fresh	1	116	Peanuts roasted in oil	1 ounce	200
Canned in heavy syrup	1 cup	258	Potato		
Dried, uncooked	1 cup	1418	Baked	1	610
Grapefruit			Boiled	1	515
Canned in water	1 cup	322	Spinach		
Fresh	½	312	Cooked, fresh	1 cup	838
Juice, canned, unsweetened	1 cup	378	Canned	1 cup	709
Melon, fresh cantaloupe	1 cup	494	From frozen	1 cup	566
Orange			Squash		
Fresh	1	237	Acorn, baked	1 cup	896
Juice, frozen, diluted	1 cup	474	Hubbard, mashed	1 cup	504
Peaches			Winter, mashed	1 cup	895
Fresh	1	171	Zucchini, canned	1 cup	622
Canned in water	1 cup	241	Sweet potato, baked	1	397
Dried	1 cup	1594	Tomato	1	297
Pears			Tomato juice, canned	1 cup	535
Fresh	1	208			
Canned in juice	1 cup	238			
Dried	1 cup	959			

Information from Wardlaw, G.M., Insel, M., & Paul, M. (1995). *Perspectives in nutrition* (3rd ed.). St. Louis: Mosby.

loprim) or probenecid (Benemid) is suggested to counteract any elevation of serum uric acid.

Hyperglycemia or impaired glucose tolerance has also been reported with the thiazide-type and loop diuretics. This effect is reported most often in older adults. The thiazides can precipitate diabetes in individuals with overt or subclinical disease patterns. Thiazide-type diuretics are not contraindicated for use in clients with diabetes, because if hyperglycemia is noted it can usually be controlled by diet alterations or by increasing the dosage of insulin. When hyperglycemia does occur in a nondiabetic client, many prescribers may try another type of diuretic (e.g., furosemide) to see if the problem can be reduced or alleviated.

The thiazide-type diuretics and perhaps furosemide have been associated with increasing serum levels of cholesterol and triglycerides. Because elevated serum lipid levels are associated with an increase in coronary heart disease, it is important that serum lipids be monitored and perhaps a specific dietary approach or weight loss program implemented if necessary.

Indications for thiazide-type diuretics include treating hypertension, edema associated with congestive heart failure, hepatic cirrhosis with ascites, and some types of renal impairment, such as nephrotic syndrome, acute glomerulonephritis, and chronic renal failure. These agents are well absorbed orally and are usually excreted unchanged by the kidneys. See Table 34-1 for the pharmacokinetics and dosages of these drugs.

■ Nursing Management

Thiazide and Thiazide-Type Diuretic Therapy

■ **Assessment.** Thiazide-type diuretics are given with caution to clients with severe renal impairment (may be ineffective or precipitate azotemia), hepatic impairment (may precipitate hepatic coma), diabetes mellitus (the dosages of hypoglycemic agents may need to be altered), or electrolyte imbalances (may be exacerbated). They are contraindicated or given carefully to pregnant women, because they cross the placental barrier (see the Pregnancy Safety box on p. 675). Check the creatinine clearance of older adults to ensure adequate renal function before administering thiazide-type diuretics. Approximately 60% of all adverse drug reactions in older adults are the result of diuretics.

Review the client's current medication regimen for the risk of significant drug interactions, such as those that may

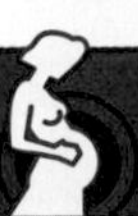

Pregnancy Safety
Diuretics

Category	Drug
B	amiloride, chlorothiazide, chlorthalidone, ethacrynic acid, hydrochlorothiazide, indapamide, isosorbide, mannitol, methyclothiazide, metolazone, torsemide, triamterene
C	acetazolamide, bendroflumethiazide, benzthiazide, bumetanide, cyclothiazide, furosemide, glycerin, hydroflumethiazide, trichlormethiazide, urea
Not established	quinethazone, spironolactone

occur when thiazide or thiazide-type diuretics are given concurrently with the following drugs:

Drug	Possible Effect and Management
Bold/color type indicates the most serious interactions.	
cholestyramine (Questran) or colestipol (Colestid)	Concurrent administration may reduce the gastrointestinal absorption of thiazide-type diuretics. Schedule the administration of diuretics 1 hour before or 4 hours after the administration of these drugs.
digitalis glycosides	There is an increased risk of digitalis toxicity in the presence of hypokalemia. Monitor the pulse and electrocardiogram (ECG) closely.
lithium	**Not recommended. An increased risk of lithium toxicity is possible because of decreased lithium excretion. Lithium also has the potential for nephrotoxic side effects. Avoid this combination.**

A baseline assessment of the client's underlying condition should be obtained: the blood pressure in hypertension and the extent and severity of edema in clients with congestive heart failure and other edematous conditions. A baseline blood chemistry for glucose, electrolytes, blood urea nitrogen (BUN), serum uric acid, and serum creatinine is recommended before diuretic therapy is begun.

■ **Nursing Diagnosis.** Clients receiving thiazide or thiazide-type diuretics are at risk for the following nursing diagnoses/collaborative problems: impaired comfort (nausea); impaired urinary elimination (frequency and amount); diarrhea; constipation); risk for injury related to orthostatic hypotension; and the potential complications of electrolyte imbalances (hypokalemia, hyponatremia, and hypochloremic alkalosis), allergic reaction, agranulocytosis (fever, low back pain, dysuria), gout, hepatotoxicity, and thrombocytopenia (unusual bleeding and bruising, petechiae, and blood in the urine or stools).

BOX 34-1

Signs and Symptoms of Fluid and Electrolyte Imbalances Associated with Diuretic Therapy

Hypovolemia: hypotension, weak pulse, tachycardia, clammy skin, rapid respirations, and reduced urinary output

Hyponatremia: low serum sodium levels (normal range 135 to 145 mEq/L), lethargy, disorientation, muscle tenseness, seizures, and coma

Hypokalemia: low serum potassium levels (normal range 3.5 to 5.0 mEq/L), weakness, abnormal ECG, postural hypotension, and flaccid paralysis

Hypocalcemia: low serum calcium levels (normal range 8.4 to 10.2 mg/dL), irritability, vomiting, diarrhea, twitching, hyperactive reflexes, cardiac dysrhythmias, tetany, and seizures

Hypochloremia: low blood chloride levels (normal range 100 to 110 mEq/L)

Hypomagnesemia: low serum magnesium levels (normal range 1.3 to 2.1 mEq/L), nausea and vomiting, lethargy, muscle weakness, tremors, and tetany

With potassium-sparing diuretics, be alert for the following:

Hyperkalemia: above-normal values for potassium serum levels, nausea, diarrhea, muscle weakness, postural hypotension, and ECG changes

■ **Implementation**

■ ***Monitoring.*** Take the client's blood pressure before administering the diuretic to ensure that the client is not hypotensive. Obtaining a daily weight and monitoring fluid balance will assist in determining the progress of the diuretic therapy. Because electrolyte imbalances are possible, monitor laboratory reports, particularly serum potassium levels. Monitoring is particularly important when digitalis compounds are part of the regimen, because hypokalemia primes clients taking digitalis preparations for the toxic cardiac effects of the digitalis (e.g., bradycardia or ventricular irritability). Latent diabetes or gout may occasionally occur; laboratory reports should be monitored for hyperglycemia or hyperuricemia. Observe the client for the signs and symptoms of fluid and electrolyte imbalances: hypovolemia, hyponatremia, hypokalemia, hypocalcemia, hypochloremia, or hypomagnesemia (Box 34-1).

■ ***Intervention.*** Although potassium loss is usually not significant enough to require potassium supplementation, add potassium-rich foods to the diet to help prevent hypokalemia. Discontinue thiazide-type diuretics before performing parathyroid function tests, because they may alter serum calcium concentrations.

As with other diuretics, plan dosing schedules to minimize the inconvenience of diuresis for the client.

■ ***Education.*** Teach clients that thiazide-type diuretics may make them feel unusually tired. Because of the potential for digitalis toxicity when these drugs are taken in combination with digitalis glycosides, clients also need to know how to take their pulse rate before taking digitalis medications. If the pulse rate is less than 60 beats/min or is irregular, digitalis medications should be discontinued and the prescriber notified. Anorexia, nausea, and vomiting are even earlier signs of digitalis toxicity that nurses and clients should recognize.

Clients should understand that diuretic drugs prescribed for a chronic condition need to be taken as an integral part of their lifestyle.

As with acetazolamide, the client should receive instruction related to the prevention and minimization of the effects of dry mouth, constipation, and orthostatic hypotension. The signs and symptoms of electrolyte imbalances and blood dyscrasias should be taught, with proper referral to the prescriber.

Instruct clients to eat foods rich in potassium if a supplement is not prescribed.

■ **Evaluation.** Because thiazide-type diuretics are indicated for hypertension, an expected outcome is that the client's blood pressure will decrease or be within normal limits. If the thiazides are used for fluid volume excess, the client will experience an increased urinary output, a decrease in pedal edema, weight loss, and an absence of rales and edema.

LOOP DIURETICS

bumetanide [byoo met′ a nide] (Bumex)
ethacrynic acid [eth a krin′ ik] (Edecrin)
furosemide [fur os′ e myde] (Lasix, Furoside ♣)
torsemide [tore′ seh mide] (Demadex)

The **loop diuretics** are so called because they inhibit the reabsorption of sodium and water in the ascending loop of Henle. Agents that work here at the Na^+-K^+-$2Cl^-$ cotransport (or carrier transfer site) in the ascending limb are most effective because the diuretic effect is greater than that reported with the other diuretic sites (Jackson, 1996). For the most part, these drugs are very similar to the thiazide-type diuretics pharmacologically and in the side effects they produce. Hyperglycemia, hyperuricemia, increases in low-density lipoprotein (LDL) cholesterol and triglycerides, and a decrease in high-density lipoprotein (HDL) cholesterol plasma levels are reported. The loop diuretics also increase the excretion of magnesium and calcium, which may result in hypomagnesemia and hypocalcemia; thus they are administered with a normal saline infusion to treat hypercalcemia (Jackson, 1996).

Bumetanide inhibits sodium reabsorption in the ascending limb of the loop of Henle, as shown by the marked reduction of free-water clearance during hydration and tubular free-water reabsorption during dehydration. The reabsorption of chloride in the ascending loop is also blocked by bumetanide, which may have an additional action in the proximal tubule. Because phosphate reabsorption takes place largely in the proximal tubule, phosphaturia during bumetanide-induced diuresis indicates this additional reaction. Bumetanide does not appear to have a noticeable action on the distal tubule.

The indications for the loop diuretics include the treatment of edema associated with congestive heart failure, cirrhosis, or renal disease. Furosemide is also used to treat hypertension. These agents are also used as adjunct therapy in clients with acute pulmonary edema and in clients who are refractory to the other diuretics. The loop diuretics have fair-to-good absorption orally, are highly protein bound, are metabolized in the liver, and are excreted by the kidneys and in bile.

See Table 34-1 for the pharmacokinetics and dosage information for the loop diuretics.

The side effects/adverse reactions of the loop diuretics include postural hypotension, blurred vision, headaches, abdominal distress, diarrhea, anorexia, anxiety, confusion, and ototoxicity. Photosensitivity has been reported with furosemide.

■ Nursing Management
Loop Diuretic Therapy

■ **Assessment.** The use of loop diuretics is not recommended in the presence of anuria or severe renal impairment because of decreased effectiveness. If they are used, the reduced clearance with renal function impairment may require higher doses but at more prolonged dosing intervals to reduce accumulation and the resultant risk of ototoxicity. The use of loop diuretics with liver dysfunction increases the risk of dehydration and electrolyte imbalance.

Review the client's current medication regimen for the risk of significant drug interactions, such as those that may occur when loop diuretics are given concurrently with the following drugs:

Drug/Herb	Possible Effect and Management
Bold/color type indicates the most serious interactions.	
amphotericin B injectable	Increases the risk for ototoxicity, nephrotoxicity, and electrolyte imbalance (especially hypokalemia). Avoid concurrent use or a potentially serious drug interaction may occur.
anticoagulants; coumarin-type (Coumadin), indanedione-type, or heparin	Anticoagulant effects may be decreased with concurrent therapy. The anticoagulant effects may be enhanced with ethacrynic acid because of displacement of the anticoagulant from its protein binding sites. Gastrointestinal ulcers or bleeding is a possible adverse reaction to ethacrynic acid, which may increase the risk for hemorrhage. When possible, avoid giving ethacrynic acid to clients receiving anticoagulants. If loop diuretics are given concurrently, monitor clients closely for increased or decreased effectiveness of the anticoagulant.

Drug/Herb	Possible Effect and Management
ginseng/germanium combination	May induce diuretic resistance. Avoid concurrent use.
gossypol	May decrease potassium levels. Monitor closely if given concurrently.
hypokalemia-causing drugs	There is an increased risk of hypokalemia when loop diuretics are administered concurrently. Monitor serum potassium levels and ECGs carefully; potassium supplements may be required.
lithium	There is an increased risk of lithium toxicity due to reduced renal clearance. Monitor closely.
nephrotoxic medications or other ototoxic medications	There is an increased risk of ototoxicity and nephrotoxicity, especially in clients with renal impairment. Avoid concurrent use or a potentially serious interaction may occur.

A baseline assessment of the client's underlying condition should be obtained: the blood pressure in clients with hypertension and the extent and severity of edema in clients with congestive heart failure, cirrhosis, and renal disease. Blood chemistries will be monitored for electrolyte concentrations, BUN, carbon dioxide, glucose, and uric acid.

■ **Nursing Diagnosis.** Clients receiving loop diuretics should be assessed for the development of the following nursing diagnoses/collaborative problems: impaired comfort related to headache, local irritation at the site of injection, and abdominal cramping; impaired urinary elimination (frequency and amount); diarrhea; constipation; disturbed sensory perception (visual: blurred vision); risk for injury related to orthostatic hypotension (most common adverse reaction) and increased skin sensitivity on exposure to sunlight; and the potential complications of allergic reaction (rash), ototoxicity as evidenced by tinnitus (deafness), gout (joint pain, back pain), hepatotoxicity (yellow eyes or skin), pancreatitis (severe abdominal pain with nausea and vomiting), thrombocytopenia (unusual bleeding or bruising, black stools, hematuria, petechiae), and agranulocytosis or leukopenia (fever, chills, cough, dysuria).

■ **Implementation**

■ ***Monitoring.*** Weigh the client at the initiation of therapy and periodically thereafter to monitor fluid loss. When these diuretics are administered for acute excess fluid volume, it may be necessary to weigh the client daily. For the most accurate readings, weigh the client at the same time each day, preferably before breakfast, in similar clothing, and on the same scale. Weight loss and a reduction in the extent of the edema indicate effectiveness of the drug. Monitor blood pressure periodically; a reduction in blood pressure to values within normal limits is also sought. Monitor clients closely, especially older adults, for the following: extreme blood pressure changes; postural hypotension; dehydration (e.g., weight loss of more than 2 pounds per day); allergic reactions (rashes); constipation, nausea, vomiting, and diarrhea; ototoxicity (tinnitus, hearing loss); and serum potassium deficiency.

Monitor carefully clients who may be experiencing potassium loss through other causes (e.g., vomiting, diarrhea, diaphoresis, gastrointestinal drainage, or paracentesis) for signs and symptoms of hypokalemia.

Be aware that hyperuricemia may occur. A reversible elevation of BUN and creatinine levels may occur, especially in association with dehydration and particularly in clients with renal insufficiency.

Check reports of serum electrolytes, uric acid, blood and urine glucose tests, and BUN levels for abnormalities. Excessive doses or too-frequent administration can lead to prolonged water loss, electrolyte depletion, dehydration, blood volume reduction, and circulatory collapse, with possible vascular thrombosis and embolism, especially in older adults.

Be aware that hypokalemia can occur. The prevention of hypokalemia requires giving particular attention to the following conditions: individuals receiving digitalis glycosides and diuretics for congestive heart failure, hepatic cirrhosis, or ascites; states of aldosterone excess with normal renal function; potassium-losing nephropathy; and certain diarrheal states. Monitor serum potassium levels periodically; potassium supplements or potassium-sparing diuretics may be necessary. Periodic determinations of other electrolytes is advised in clients who are taking high dosages for prolonged periods, particularly in clients on low-salt diets.

Determine blood sugar periodically, particularly in clients with diabetes or suspected latent diabetes.

■ ***Intervention.*** Liquid potassium for oral use, although unpleasant tasting, may be disguised in cold juices and taken with food. Regular tomato juice is not recommended for this purpose because its sodium content is high; low-sodium juices do well to disguise the taste of potassium. Enteric-coated potassium tablets should be avoided because they have been implicated in ulcerations of the gastrointestinal tract lining.

If loop diuretics are added to the medication regimen of hypertensive clients, expect that the medications will be adjusted to minimize the potential for orthostatic hypotension.

The use of the IM route can produce temporary pain at the site; therefore oral or IV routes are preferable. Administer these drugs so that the onset and peak of action coincides with access to toilet facilities. Administer with food if gastrointestinal upset occurs with oral forms. When administering oral solutions, use the calibrated dropper provided by the manufacturer for accurate dosages.

Administer IV injections of bumetanide and furosemide slowly over 2 minutes. Administer ethacrynic acid intravenously at a controlled rate over 30 minutes; if a second dose is required, use a different injection site to prevent thrombophlebitis.

Because many glass ampules must be broken to prepare large doses of furosemide IV infusions, there is the possibility that glass fragments will appear in the solution. Use a filter to remove these particles while drawing the drug into the syringe and also during IV administration.

■ ***Education.*** Caution the client to move carefully from a sitting or lying position to an upright position because of positional hypotension. Alcohol ingestion, hot weather, and standing or lying for long periods also increases the risk of orthostatic hypotension. Instruct the client in the symptoms of electrolyte imbalances (see Box 34-1), particularly hypokalemia. Provide dietary counseling so the client will know which foods are rich in potassium.

Checking refills of the medication prescription provides a basis for client counseling for compliance with the regimen, as well as the opportunity for appropriate feedback.

Photosensitivity is a problem for some clients taking furosemide; caution them to avoid prolonged exposure to the sun or to sunlamps. Encourage clients to use sun-blocking lotions and to cover skin areas with protective clothing.

▪ **Evaluation.** The expected outcome of loop diuretic therapy is that the client will experience diuresis and an absence of rales and edema. In addition, the client's blood pressure, central venous pressure (CVP), and pulmonary artery pressure (PAP) will be within normal limits.

DISTAL TUBULE DIURETICS/ POTASSIUM-SPARING DIURETICS

amiloride [a mill′ oh ride] (Midamor)
✓**spironolactone** [speer on oh lak′ tone] (Aldactone)
triamterene [trye am′ ter een] (Dyrenium)

The **potassium-sparing diuretics** are similar in action to other diuretics and are generally considered to be weak diuretics that act at the distal renal tubules. They block sodium reabsorption in the distal tubule, thus increasing sodium and water excretion; at the same time, they conserve potassium so generally that they are primarily considered useful when combined with other potassium-losing diuretics. In 1999, spironolactone (Aldactone) was discovered to be beneficial for heart failure. When compared with other therapies for severe heart failure, the addition of spironolactone reduced the risk of death and hospitalization by 30%. The combination of spironolactone with an angiotensin-converting enzyme (ACE) inhibitor provides an additive blockade on aldosterone (i.e., the ACE inhibitor lowers the synthesis of aldosterone), whereas spironolactone blocks the aldosterone receptors. Therefore the addition of spironolactone protects the heart from too much aldosterone, which can reduce the capability of the heart to pump (Pharmacist Letter, 1999; Pitt et al., 1999).

Amiloride and triamterene directly inhibit the reabsorption of sodium and water, whereas spironolactone is an aldosterone antagonist. Any of the three agents may be used when it is necessary to restore or preserve the normal serum potassium level if other concurrent diuretic therapy challenges it and when potassium supplementation by medication or diet is inappropriate. These agents are highly effective for this purpose. If prescribed singly, however, their efficacy may actually result in an undesirable and rapidly developing hyperkalemia.

Spironolactone, a synthetic steroidal compound, antagonizes the effect of aldosterone by binding competitively to the protein that permits potassium secretion at the distal tubule. This response is directly related to the amount of circulating aldosterone in the serum. Spironolactone produces a very mild diuresis of sodium and water at the distal tubule by means of this mechanism. It does not interfere with the renal tubule transport of sodium and chloride and does not inhibit carbonic anhydrase. Triamterene directly depresses the renal tubular transport of sodium in the distal tubule independent of the presence of aldosterone.

The potassium-sparing diuretics are indicated for the prevention and treatment of hypokalemia. They are also used as adjunct therapy in the treatment of edema and hypertension, and spironolactone is indicated in the diagnosis and treatment of primary hyperaldosteronism.

These agents have low (amiloride), moderate (triamterene), or good (spironolactone) absorption from the gastrointestinal tract. Spironolactone and triamterene are metabolized in the liver. Amiloride and spironolactone are excreted mainly by the kidneys, and triamterene is excreted primarily in bile. Amiloride is excreted unchanged (not metabolized). See Table 34-1 for the pharmacokinetics and dosages of these potassium-sparing diuretics.

The side effects/adverse reactions of the potassium-sparing diuretics include abdominal cramps, diarrhea, nausea, vomiting, dry mouth, sedation, and hyperkalemia. Photosensitivity is reported with triamterene.

▪ Nursing Management

Distal Tubule/Potassium-Sparing Diuretic Therapy

▪ **Assessment.** Before administering these compounds, ascertain that the client has no related drug history of allergy or hyperkalemia, because the potassium-sparing diuretics may further increase serum potassium levels. Greater caution is required in the administration of these diuretics to clients who are at risk for developing hyperkalemia because of preexisting conditions (e.g., impaired renal or hepatic function or diabetes mellitus), to severely ill clients, and to clients with decreased urine volumes, which might aggravate electrolyte imbalances.

Review the client's current medication regimen for the risk of significant drug interactions, such as those that may occur when distal tubule/potassium-sparing diuretics are given concurrently with the following drugs:

Drug/Herb	Possible Effect and Management
anticoagulants	Anticoagulant effects may be decreased when used concurrently with potassium-sparing diuretics as a result of plasma volume reduction, which concentrates procoagulant factors in the blood. Dosage adjustments of anticoagulants may be necessary.
blood from bank, ACE inhibitors, cyclosporine (Sandimmune), other potassium-sparing diuretics, low-salt milk, potassium-containing medications, or potassium supplements	May increase potassium levels and result in hyperkalemia. Monitor serum electrolytes closely.

Drug/Herb	Possible Effect and Management
digoxin	With spironolactone only, the half-life of digoxin may be increased. Dosage reductions of digoxin may be required by either reducing the dose or the frequency of dosing. Monitor serum digoxin levels carefully.
licorice	**Chronic intake of large doses of licorice may offset spironolactone effects. Avoid concurrent usage.**
lithium	Concurrent use increases the risk of lithium toxicity by reducing renal clearance.

In addition to an assessment of the underlying condition for which the diuretic was prescribed, a baseline health assessment should include blood pressure, serum electrolyte concentrations (especially potassium), and BUN and/or serum creatinine levels; for triamterene, a platelet and white blood cell count should be performed.

■ **Nursing Diagnosis.** With the administration of distal tubule/potassium-sparing diuretics, the client should be assessed for the following nursing diagnoses/collaborative problems: impaired comfort related to muscle cramps, headache, dizziness, and gastrointestinal effects (nausea, vomiting, and abdominal cramping); constipation; diarrhea; disturbed body image related to decreased libido, gynecomastia in males, and hirsutism in females secondary to the antiandrogenic effects of the drug; and the potential complications of hyperkalemia (confusion, dysrhythmias, paresthesia, fatigue), allergic reactions (shortness of breath, rash), nephrolithiasis (flank pain), agranulocytosis (fever, chills, dysuria), and thrombocytopenia (unusual bleeding or bruising, black stools, hematuria, petechiae).

■ **Implementation**

■ ***Monitoring.*** Monitor blood pressure, weight loss, and fluid balance to evaluate the effectiveness of the diuretic. Evaluate client compliance at frequent intervals. Especially at first, be alert to an irregular heartbeat (often the first clinical sign of hyperkalemia) or peaked T waves on the ECG. Other warning signs of hyperkalemia are confusion, tingling in the extremities, breathing difficulties, unexplained anxiety, fatigue, and physical weakness. Serum electrolyte determinations and an ECG are probably indicated if these occur.

Check laboratory reports closely, especially if the client is taking other similar drugs or potassium-rich foods. Rapidly increased serum potassium levels may occur. Act immediately to reverse hyperkalemia if the serum potassium level exceeds 6 to 6.5 mEq/L, and anticipate treatment with sodium bicarbonate, glucose and regular insulin preparations, or other therapy. Hyponatremia may occur as evidenced by fatigue, drowsiness, increased thirst, and dry mouth.

If the client is receiving spironolactone, remain sensitive to cues that he or she may be concerned about body image changes that may threaten sexual identity.

Note that when triamterene is being given, a complete blood count is probably indicated if the client has an unexplained sore throat, mouth ulcerations, or fever; all of these symptoms are indications of a possible blood dyscrasia.

■ ***Intervention.*** Administering distal tubule/potassium-sparing diuretics with food or milk may allay some gastrointestinal symptoms and possibly enhance bioavailability. Deal with unpleasant side effects such as dry mouth, thirst, or drowsiness if they arise.

Plan nursing measures common to diuretic agents, such as measuring fluid intake and output, monitoring daily weight changes, monitoring vital signs and heart rhythm, and assessing postural hypotension, weakness, or confusion. Monitor closely for hyperkalemia when transfusing blood. Whole blood may contain up to 30 mEq of potassium per liter; this amount may double if blood has been stored for more than 10 days.

■ ***Education.*** The client should be counseled to avoid excessively stringent low-salt diets and relatively concentrated potassium intake in the form of citrus juices, cola beverages, low-sodium milk, some salt substitutes, and other potassium supplements.

■ **Evaluation.** The expected outcome of distal tubule and potassium-sparing diuretic therapy is that the client will experience diuresis and an absence of rales and edema; blood pressure and serum potassium values will be within normal limits.

OSMOTIC DIURETICS

glycerin [gli′ ser in] (Osmoglyn)
isosorbide [eye sew sore′ bide] (Ismotic)
mannitol [man′ i tole] (Osmitrol)
urea [yoor ee′ a] (Ureaphil)

Osmotic diuretics include the parenteral agents (mannitol and urea) and the oral agents (glycerin and isosorbide). The two parenteral agents cause diuresis by adding to the solutes already present in the tubular fluid; they are particularly effective in increasing osmotic pressure because they are not reabsorbed by the tubules. Thus more water is pulled into tubular fluid, and the kidneys reabsorb less sodium, chloride, and water in an effort to equalize the higher solute content. These excesses are then excreted in the urine. The oral agents are primarily used to reduce intraocular pressure before and after intraocular surgery and to interrupt an acute attack of glaucoma.

The parenteral agents (mannitol and urea) are used to treat cerebral edema and secondary glaucoma when other methods have been unsuccessful. Mannitol has also been used to increase the urinary excretion of toxic substances (salicylates, barbiturates, lithium, bromides), as an irrigating preparation to prevent hemolysis and hemoglobin accumulation during transurethral prostatic resection, and as an adjunct to other therapies in the treatment of edema in acute renal failure.

Very little if any mannitol is metabolized in the liver. Urea is partially metabolized in the gastrointestinal tract to ammonia and carbon dioxide, which may be resynthesized into urea. Both mannitol and urea are excreted by the kidneys. Glycerin is metabolized in the liver and excreted by the kidneys. See Table 34-1 for the pharmacokinetics and dosages of the osmotic diuretics.

The side effects/adverse reactions of the parenteral agents (mannitol and urea) include nausea, vomiting, dry mouth, headache, increased urination, and weakness. Mannitol may also cause visual disturbances, dizziness, and rash. The oral agents (glycerin and isosorbide) may induce nausea, vomiting, headache, increased thirst, dry mouth, diarrhea, and confusion.

■ Nursing Management

Osmotic Diuretic Therapy

■ **Assessment.** Ascertain that the client does not have preexisting severe dehydration, anuria, or severe pulmonary congestion; osmotic diuretics are contraindicated for these conditions. Intracranial bleeding, except during craniotomy, would negate the use of mannitol and urea. Caution should be used in administering osmotic diuretics to clients with significant renal dysfunction or severe cardiopulmonary impairment, because the sudden increase in extracellular fluid might lead to circulatory overload and congestive heart failure. The concurrent use of osmotic diuretics with digitalis glycosides may increase the risk of digitalis toxicity associated with hypokalemia. The risk-benefit ratio should be considered in administering invert sugar IV preparations of urea to clients with hereditary fructose intolerance (aldolase deficiency).

Recommend baseline serum electrolyte and renal function determinations if they have not already been performed, and monitor the results.

Note that mannitol is different from the drug mannitol hexanitrate; do not confuse them.

■ **Nursing Diagnosis.** Clients receiving osmotic diuretics should be assessed for the following nursing diagnoses/collaborative problems: impaired comfort (dry mouth, nausea, vomiting, headache, dizziness, rash); hyperthermia; impaired urinary elimination (frequency and amount); and the potential complications of electrolyte imbalance, blurred vision, chest pain, pulmonary congestion, and thrombophlebitis.

■ **Implementation**

■ ***Monitoring.*** Because these are potent osmotic drugs, it is essential to be alert to rapidly changing client conditions; assess urinary output and vital signs at frequent intervals for changing intravascular volume, pulmonary edema, or hemoconcentration. Monitor fluid and electrolyte balance, particularly serum and urine potassium and sodium levels. When urea is administered, BUN determinations should be performed before and frequently during IV administration. If the BUN exceeds 75 mg/dL or if there is no diuresis within 1 to 2 hours, slow or stop the infusion and have the client reevaluated. If the osmotic diuretics are administered for a reduction of intraocular pressure, monitor the pressure determinations closely.

■ ***Intervention.*** If the adequacy of renal function is suspect before the administration of mannitol, a test dose is usually prescribed and is given as an IV infusion over 3 to 5 minutes. Urine flow should increase to at least 30 to 50 mL/hr for 2 to 3 hours after this or a second test dose. If it does not, mannitol should be withheld and the client reevaluated.

Infuse mannitol and urea separately from other drugs and blood. Crystallization in solution is common; it may be countered by warming the solution until the crystals are invisible and by inserting a filter in the line whenever this drug is infused. Avoid the extravasation of urea and mannitol; observe the IV site periodically for tissue inflammation, irritation, and necrosis. Electrolyte-free mannitol should not be administered concurrently with blood, because pseudoagglutination may occur. If concurrent administration is necessary, at least 20 mEq of sodium chloride should be added to each liter of mannitol to minimize this effect.

Infuse urea into large veins. For both urea and mannitol, avoid using lower extremity IV sites because phlebitis and thrombosis may occur, particularly in older adults. Do not infuse urea more rapidly than 4 mL/min, because hemolysis and cerebral vasomotor symptoms may occur.

To assist in the prevention and relief of headache caused by cerebral dehydration, have the client lie down during and after the administration of these parenteral drugs.

Use an indwelling catheter with comatose clients to ensure urinary drainage. The use of a urometer that allows for precise measurement of output is important because the therapy is based on the accurate evaluation of intake and output.

When osmotic diuretics are administered preoperatively, the dosing schedule should be as follows: glycerin, isosorbide, and mannitol, ½ to 1 hour before surgery; urea, 1 hour before surgery if administered for the reduction of intraocular pressure or at the time of scalp incision during intracranial surgery.

To increase palatability, isosorbide comes in a vanilla-mint–flavored syrup that may be iced, and glycerin may be mixed with iced, unsweetened fruit juice; sip through a straw. With repeated doses of these drugs, maintain adequate fluid and electrolyte balance.

■ ***Education.*** Prepare the client for the diuresis that will occur with these drugs. Provide for the convenience, comfort, and privacy of the client.

Advise the client to visit the physician regularly for intraocular pressure monitoring if taking glycerin and isosorbide for the reduction of intraocular pressure.

■ **Evaluation.** If osmotic diuretics are administered for increased intracranial pressure, the expected outcome is that the client will have an intracranial pressure value within an acceptable range. If the indication for the drugs is increased intraocular pressure, the client will demonstrate a reduced intraocular pressure value with tonometer measurement. If these drugs are being given for acute renal failure, the client will experience diuresis and an improvement in BUN and serum creatinine values.

TABLE 34-3 Examples of Fixed-Dose Diuretic Combinations

Trade Name	Contents
Aldactazide 25/25	spironolactone, 25 mg; hctz,* 25 mg
Aldactazide 50/50	spironolactone, 50 mg; hctz, 50 mg
Capozide 50/15, 25/25, & 50/25	captopril, 25 or 50 mg; hctz, 15 or 25 mg
Dyazide	triamterene, 37.5 mg; hctz, 25 mg
Hydropres-50	reserpine 0.125 mg; hctz, 50 mg
Hyzaar ◆	losartan, 50 mg; hctz, 12.5 mg
Inderide LA 80/50, 120/50, or 160/50	propranolol, 80, 120, or 160 mg; hctz, 50 mg
Lopressor HCT 50/25, 100/25, or 100/50	metoprolol, 50 or 100 mg; hctz, 25 or 50 mg
Maxzide	triamterene, 75 mg; hctz, 50 mg
Timolide 10/25	timolol, 10 mg; hctz, 25 mg
Ziac ◆ 2.5, 5, or 10	bisoprolol fumarate, 2.5, 5, or 10 mg; hctz, 6.25 mg

*_hctz,_ Hydrochlorothiazide.

DIURETIC COMBINATIONS

As mentioned previously, a thiazide diuretic may be combined with a potassium-sparing diuretic. Fixed-dose combinations, which are commercially available, may provide additional diuretic activity and decrease the potassium depletion characteristic of the thiazide diuretics. In addition, diuretics are combined with antihypertensive agents to simplify medication regimens for clients whose hypertensive status has somewhat stabilized (Table 34-3).

SUMMARY

Diuretics are valuable assets in the therapeutic regimen for the treatment of hypertension and other conditions in which fluid volume excess is an issue, such as congestive heart failure, cirrhosis, and nephrotic syndrome. These drugs act on the tubular function of the kidneys and inhibit solute reabsorption; water reabsorption is affected because water diffuses passively across the tubular membrane when sodium transport occurs. In general, diuretics are grouped by the major site of their action along the tubule: proximal tubule diuretics, diluting segment diuretics, loop diuretics, and distal tubule diuretics. Osmotic diuretics act by adding to the solutes already present in tubular fluid; because they are not reabsorbed, more water is pulled into tubular fluid and less sodium, chloride, and water are reabsorbed by the kidneys in an effort to equalize the higher solute volume that is excreted in the urine. Combinations of diuretic agents are used for clients with stabilized conditions.

Nursing management focuses on the education of the client for the safe and accurate self-administration of diuretics, particularly in the early recognition of adverse reactions. Hypokalemia is common except in clients taking potassium-sparing diuretics; clients should understand the importance of including potassium-rich foods in their diet if a potassium supplement has not been prescribed. An evaluation of the effectiveness of the therapeutic regimen through accurate measurement of the client's blood pressure, fluid balance, and weight is essential.

Critical Thinking Questions

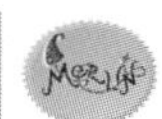

1. What conditions place clients receiving loop diuretics at higher risk for hypokalemia? What observations by the nurse are particularly important for these clients?
2. What conditions place clients receiving distal tubule and potassium-sparing diuretics at higher risk for hyperkalemia? What observations by the nurse are particularly important for these clients?
3. Mrs. Williams, an 82-year-old woman, lives alone in substandard urban housing. Although she has hypertension and chronic congestive heart failure, she maintains her independence with the assistance of members of her church, who shop for her, bring her meals occasionally, and take her for visits to her doctor. Her current medication regimen is as follows: digoxin, 0.25 mg PO daily; furosemide, 20 mg PO two times daily; K-Dur 20, one tablet PO daily; verapamil SR, 240 mg PO daily; and isosorbide dinitrate, 10 mg PO four times daily. For what nursing diagnoses/collaborative problems is Mrs. Williams at risk? Why? As her home health care nurse, what will be your plan of care?

Collaborative Learning Activities

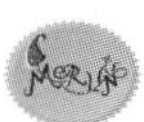

For Collaborative Learning Activities, go to mosby.com/MERLIN/McKenry/.

CASE STUDY

For a Case Study that will help ensure mastery of this chapter content, go to mosby.com/MERLIN/McKenry/.

BIBLIOGRAPHY

American Hospital Formulary Service. (1999). *AHFS drug information '99.* Bethesda, MD: American Society of Hospital Pharmacists.

Anderson, K.N., Anderson, L.E., Glanze, W.D. (Eds.) (1998). *Mosby's medical, nursing, & allied health dictionary* (5th ed.). St. Louis: Mosby.

Drug Facts and Comparisons. (2000). St. Louis: Facts and Comparisons.

Hewa, Z.A., Gradman, A.H. (1998). Combination therapy in elderly hypertension patients. *Clinical Geriatrics, 6*(10), 65-74.

Jackson, E.K. (1996). Diuretics. In J.G. Hardman, & L.E. Limbird (Eds.), *Goodman & Gilman's The pharmacological basis of therapeutics* (9th ed.). New York: McGraw-Hill.

Larsen, G.Y. & Goldstein, B. (1999). Consultation with the specialist: Increased intracranial pressure. *Pediatric Review, 20*(7), 234-239.

Mazur, J.E., Devlin, J.W., Peters, M.J., Jankowski, M.A., Iannuzzi, M.C., & Zarowitz, B.J. (1999). Single versus multiple doses of acetazolamide for metabolic alkalosis in critically ill medical patients: A randomized, double-blind study. *Critical Care Medicine, 27*(7), 1257-1261.

Menscer, D. (1992). Hypertension. In R.J. Ham, & P.D. Sloane (Eds.), *Primary care geriatrics: A case-based approach* (2nd ed.). St. Louis: Mosby.

Mickley, T.F. (1998) A patient-focused approach to managing diuretic therapy. *Critical Care Nursing Clinics of North America 10*(4), 421-431.

Paradiso, C. (1999). *Fluids and electrolytes* (2nd ed.). Philadelphia, J.B. Lippincott.

Pharmacist Letter. (1999). Spironolactone (Aldactone) is beneficial for heart failure. *Pharmacist's Letter, 15*(8), 43.

Pitt, B., Zannad, F., Remme, W.J., Cody, R., Castaigne, A., Perez, A., Palensky, J., & Wittes, J. (1999). The effect of spironolactone on morbidity and mortality in patients with severe heart failure: Randomized Aldactone Evaluation Study Investigators. *New England Journal of Medicine, 341*(10), 709-717.

Tang, I. & Lau, A.H. (1995). Fluid and electrolyte disorders. In L.Y. Young, & M.A. Koda-Kimble (Eds.), *Applied therapeutics: The clinical use of drugs* (6th ed.). Vancouver, WA: Applied Therapeutics.

United States Pharmacopeia Dispensing Information (USP DI): Drug information for the health care professional (19th ed.). (1999). Rockville, MD: United States Pharmacopeial Convention.

Williams, S.R. (1997). *Nutrition and diet therapy* (8th ed.). St. Louis: Mosby.

35 Uricosuric Drugs

Chapter Focus

Gout, a disorder of uric acid metabolism in the body, affects nearly half a million Americans. Although it can affect both males and females, nearly all of the cases affect men; fewer than 5% of diagnosed cases involve postmenopausal women, probably because estrogen promotes the excretion of uric acid (McCance & Huether, 1998). The nurse manages care during the acute episodes but primarily provides teaching and counseling for clients to self-manage the therapeutic regimen to prevent the painful attacks of gout.

Learning Objectives

1. Recall the process of the production of uric acid in the body.
2. Describe the classic symptoms of gout and the objectives for the treatment of gout.
3. Identify other diseases in which a secondary hyperuricemia may occur and the common drugs that may increase or decrease a client's uric acid level.
4. List the common side effects/adverse reactions and the significant drug interactions for uricosuric drugs.
5. Implement the nursing management for the care of a client receiving a uricosuric drug.

Key Terms

gout, p. 684
hyperuricemia, p. 684
urate nephropathy, p. 686

Key Drugs [✔]

allopurinol, p. 686
colchicine, p. 684

Hyperuricemia and gout occur in persons with an abnormality in uric acid production and/or excretion. Risk factors for gout include obesity, hypertension, alcohol consumption, and lead exposure (Brooks, 1997). Recurrent gouty arthritis is painful and can cause crystal deposits throughout the body, which results in an inflammatory response and, in some instances, kidney stones.

GOUT

Gout is a disease associated with an inborn error of uric acid metabolism that increases the production or inhibits the excretion of uric acid. The hallmark of gout is **hyperuricemia,** or high levels of uric acid in the blood.

Gout is characterized by a defective purine metabolism and manifests itself by attacks of acute pain, swelling, and tenderness of joints, such as those of the big toe, ankle, instep, knee, and elbow. The amount of uric acid in the blood becomes elevated, and tophi, which are deposits of uric acid or urates, form in the cartilage of various parts of the body. These deposits tend to increase in size and are seen most often along the edge of the ear. Chronic arthritis, nephritis, and premature sclerosis of the blood vessels may develop if gout is uncontrolled.

The goals of treatment for gout are to (1) end the acute gouty attack as soon as possible, (2) prevent a recurrence of acute gouty arthritis, (3) prevent the formation of uric acid stones in the kidneys, and (4) reduce or prevent disease complications that result from sodium urate deposits in the joints and kidneys.

The drugs used to treat an acute attack of gout include colchicine, nonsteroidal antiinflammatory drugs (NSAIDs), and corticosteroids. The NSAIDs are primarily used to treat the acute inflammation and have no effect on the underlying metabolic problem; they are often prescribed to relieve an acute gout attack. Colchicine is reserved for persons who do not respond to or cannot tolerate these agents (*United States Pharmacopeia Dispensing Information,* 1999). The NSAIDs are reviewed in Chapter 14. Colchicine is used specifically to treat gout and is reviewed in this chapter. Allopurinol, probenecid, sulfinpyrazone, and salicylates have also been used to treat chronic gouty arthritis or to prevent gout attacks. Salicylates require very high daily dosages, such as 4 to 6 g/day. Because few individuals can tolerate such high dosages on a long-term basis, they are not commonly prescribed for gout.

The nurse should be aware that low dosages of aspirin can interfere with the excretion of uric acid, resulting in an exacerbation of gout, and that a secondary hyperuricemia may occur from neoplastic diseases, cancer, psoriasis, Paget's disease, and other common and rare disease states. Many drugs have also been reported to increase or decrease levels of uric acid (Box 35-1).

It is preferable for the prescriber to identify the cause of the hyperuricemia and then decide whether or not to treat it. Asymptomatic hyperuricemia in an older adult may or may not be drug induced and often is not treated by the prescriber because of the potential adverse drug reactions and the cost of the medications (Figure 35-1). However, specific treatments are indicated if symptoms are present or a treatable disease state is identified.

BOX 35-1

Medications Affecting Serum Uric Acid Levels

Increase Levels

alcohol
aminoglycosides
cancer chemotherapeutic agents
diuretics (thiazides, furosemide)
ethambutol
levodopa
methyldopa
pancrelipase
salicylates (less than 2 g/day)

Decrease Levels

acetohexamide
adrenocorticotropic hormone
allopurinol
chloramphenicol
probenecid
radiopaque dyes
salicylates (more than 3 g/day)
streptomycin
tetracycline (outdated)

Information from Pagana, K.D. & Pagana, T.J. (1997). *Mosby's diagnostic and laboratory test reference* (3rd ed.). St. Louis: Mosby; *United States Pharmacopeia Dispensing Information (USP DI): Drug information for the health care professional* (19th ed.). (1999). Rockville, MD: United States Pharmacopeial Convention; and Young, L.Y. & Campagna, K.D. (1995). Gout and hyperuricemia. In L.Y. Young & M.A. Koda-Kimble. *Applied therapeutics: The clinical use of drugs* (6th ed.). Vancouver, WA: Applied Therapeutics.

colchicine [kol' chi seen]

The mechanism of action of colchicine for the treatment of gout is unknown but is reported to have antiinflammatory effects in gout. It also decreases phagocytosis, leukocyte motility, lactic acid production, and the release of a glycoprotein produced during urate crystal phagocytosis. These effects result in a decrease in urate deposits and inflammation even though the drug does not affect levels of uric acid in the circulatory system.

Colchicine is used in the treatment and prophylaxis of acute gouty arthritis and in the treatment of chronic gouty arthritis. In acute gouty arthritis, colchicine has an onset of action within 12 hours after oral administration and IV injection. The peak effect for relief of pain and inflammation is reached in 1 to 2 days, but the reduction of swelling may

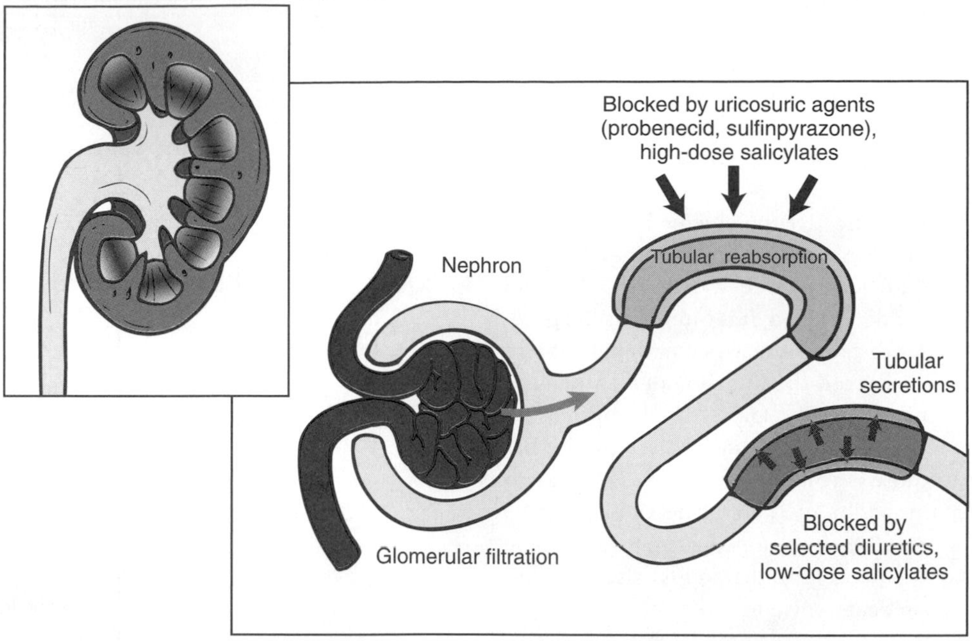

Figure 35-1 Drug effects on uric acid excretion in the kidney.

require 3 days or more. Colchicine is metabolized in the liver and excreted mainly in bile.

The side effects/adverse reactions with the oral administration of colchicine include diarrhea, nausea, vomiting, abdominal pain, anorexia and, with chronic therapy, alopecia. Colchicine-induced toxicity depends on the total dose given over time, as well as the amount of single doses, especially IV doses.

The adult dosage for gout prophylaxis is 0.5 to 0.6 mg PO daily, increased if necessary to twice daily. The dosage for acute gouty attacks is 0.5 to 1.2 mg (1 to 2 tablets) initially, followed by 1 tablet every 1 to 2 hours until pain is relieved; until the side effects of nausea, vomiting, or diarrhea occur; or until the maximum dose of 6 mg has been reached. The parenteral adult dosage for prophylaxis is 0.5 to 1 mg IV once or twice daily. For use in acute gouty attacks, the dosage is 2 mg IV initially followed by 0.5 mg every 6 to 12 hours until the desired effect is achieved. Pediatric dosages have not been established.

■ Nursing Management

Colchicine Therapy

■ **Assessment.** Caution should be used when this drug is given to older adults, because they have diminished renal function and are more likely to experience cumulative toxicity, as are those with cardiac, renal, or hepatic disease. Colchicine may cause additional injury to gastrointestinal tissues in clients with gastrointestinal disorders. Sensitivity to colchicine should also be assessed. The risk of inducing bone marrow depression or other serious, toxic, hematologic effects may be increased when colchicine is given concurrently with radiation therapy or drugs that induce blood dyscrasia or bone marrow depression (e.g., chloramphenicol [Chloromycetin], antineoplastics). (See the Pregnancy Safety box above.)

Pregnancy Safety
Uricosuric Drugs

Category	Drug
C	allopurinol
D	colchicine
Unclassified	probenecid, sulfinpyrazone

Before initiating therapy, obtain a baseline assessment of the client's general health status, uric acid levels, complete blood count (CBC), frequency and severity of gout symptoms, and current joint pain and stiffness.

■ **Nursing Diagnosis.** The assessment of the client receiving colchicine should include consideration of the following selected nursing diagnoses/collaborative problems: diarrhea (up to 80% with oral doses); impaired comfort related to pain at the injection site (thrombophlebitis), rash, stomach pain, anorexia, nausea, and vomiting; hyperthermia; ineffective protection related to agranulocytosis; disturbed thought processes related to mood and mental changes; disturbed body image related to hair loss; and the potential complications of thrombocytopenia (increased tendency to bleed), aplastic anemia, hypersensitivity, myopathy (muscle weakness), pulmonary edema, and peripheral neuritis (numbness and tingling of the hands and feet).

■ **Implementation**

■ ***Monitoring.*** Monitor the client's affected joints for range of motion, pain, and swelling. Because of the risk of bone marrow depression, the client's CBC should be monitored. Serum uric acid levels should also be monitored. Monitor fluid intake and output to assess the adequacy of urinary output. The drug should be discontinued as soon as the pain of the acute gout episode is relieved, the maximum dose is reached, or diarrhea, nausea, vomiting, or stomach pain occur.

▪ ***Intervention.*** To be effective, colchicine must be given properly at the first indication of an oncoming attack, and the dosage must be adequate. Once the dosage that will cause diarrhea has been determined, it is often possible to reduce subsequent doses to prevent diarrhea and still achieve satisfactory pain relief. Record the total amount of the drug taken before the occurrence of gastrointestinal symptoms, so that in subsequent attacks treatment may be discontinued before this cumulative dose is reached. To avoid the toxic effects of accumulation, additional colchicine should not be administered for at least 3 days after a course of oral therapy or for at least 7 days (21 days for older adults) after a course of IV treatment for an acute episode.

Oral colchicine may be administered with food to prevent gastrointestinal distress. Oral administration is preferred for prophylaxis. However, IV administration is preferable for clients who are alcoholic because they are more susceptible to gastrointestinal toxicity, which is more likely to occur with oral administration.

Colchicine cannot be given subcutaneously or intramuscularly because it is highly irritating and will cause tissue necrosis. Extravasation must be avoided when colchicine is given intravenously. Colchicine is incompatible with IV tubing containing 5% dextrose solution, solutions containing a bacteriostatic agent, or any solution that would change the pH of the colchicine solution; it will precipitate if mixed with or injected into these substances. To dilute colchicine, use 0.9% sodium chloride injection or sterile water for injection. Change the needle before administration. Administer the IV injection over a period of 2 to 5 minutes.

Fluid intake needs to be encouraged to ensure a urinary output of at least 2000 mL daily.

▪ ***Education.*** Alert the client to start the medication at the earliest sign of an attack but to discontinue it when the pain is relieved, when the maximum dose is reached, or at the first sign of diarrhea, nausea, vomiting, or stomach pain. The course of therapy should not be repeated for at least 3 days unless otherwise instructed by the prescriber. Because colchicine has such a narrow margin of safety, alert the client to report to the prescriber as soon as possible any signs of nausea, vomiting, diarrhea, sore throat, unusual bleeding or bruising, or unusual tiredness. Advise the client to visit the health care provider regularly so that progress can be monitored.

Alert the client undergoing prophylactic colchicine therapy not to increase the drug dosage if an attack occurs but to contact the prescriber for other drug therapy (i.e., NSAID or corticosteroid therapy).

Caution the client not to drink alcoholic beverages while taking colchicine, because alcohol increases the risk of gastrointestinal toxicity and decreases the effectiveness of the medication by increasing levels of uric acid.

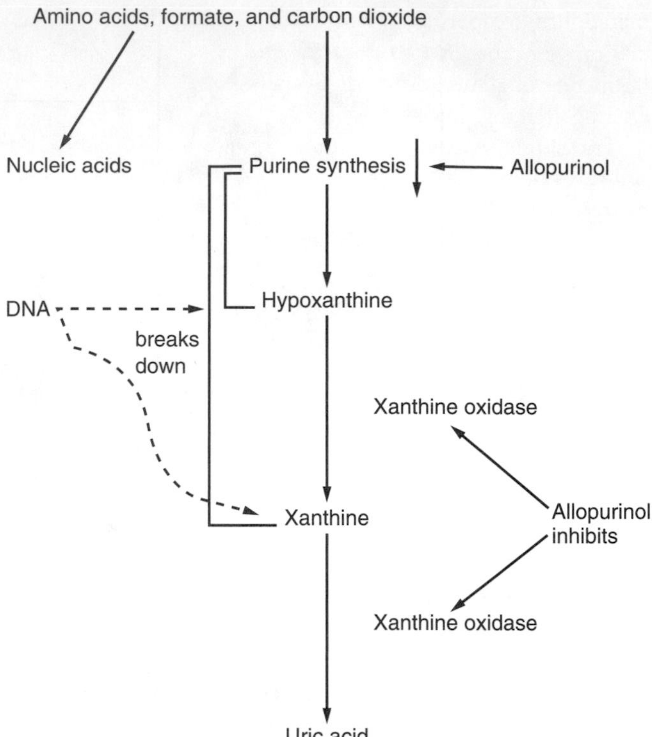

Figure 35-2 Uric acid production and allopurinol effects in the body.

Instruct the client to inform other health care providers that colchicine is being taken before any surgical or dental procedures are performed.

▪ **Evaluation.** The expected outcome of colchicine therapy is that the client will experience pain relief associated with the gout attack or will not experience an acute episode of gout.

allopurinol [al oh pure' i nole] (Zyloprim, Purinol ♣)

Allopurinol decreases the production of uric acid by inhibiting xanthine oxidase, the enzyme necessary to convert hypoxanthine to xanthine and xanthine to uric acid (Figure 35-2). It also increases the reutilization of both hypoxanthine and xanthine for nucleic acid synthesis, thus resulting in a feedback inhibition of purine synthesis. The result is a decrease of uric acid in both the serum and in the urine.

This decrease of uric acid will prevent or decrease urate deposits, thus preventing or reducing both gouty arthritis and urate nephropathy. The reduction in urinary urate levels prevents **urate nephropathy**, the formation of uric acid or calcium oxalate calculi in the kidneys.

Allopurinol is indicated for the treatment of chronic gouty arthritis and for the prophylaxis and treatment of hyperuricemia, urate nephropathy, and renal calculi (Jones & Ball, 1999). This drug is well absorbed orally; the onset of action in reducing serum uric acid is 2 to 3 days. Approximately 70% of a dose is metabolized in the liver to an active metabolite, oxypurinol. The reduction of uric acid to a normal range occurs in 1 to 3 weeks, whereas a decrease in the frequency of acute gout attacks may require several months of drug therapy. Excretion is via the kidneys.

The side effects/adverse reactions of allopurinol include pruritus, allergic reaction, rash, hives, diarrhea, abdominal distress, nausea, vomiting, alopecia, dermatitis and, rarely, bone marrow depression, liver toxicity, hypersensitivity reaction, peripheral neuritis, renal failure, and nosebleeds.

The adult antihyperuricemic dosage is 100 mg PO daily initially, increased by 100 mg/day at 7-day intervals if necessary. The maximum daily dosage should not exceed 800 mg. The maintenance dosage is 100 to 200 mg PO two to three times daily or 300 mg once daily. For the treatment of hyperuricemia (from antineoplastic therapy), initially administer 600 to 800 mg PO daily, beginning 2 to 3 days before chemotherapy or radiation therapy. For maintenance therapy, adjust the dosage according to serum uric acid levels, which are analyzed approximately 2 days after the initiation of allopurinol and periodically thereafter. Discontinue allopurinol during the period of tumor regression.

To treat uric acid calculi, the dosage is 100 to 200 mg PO one to four times daily or 300 mg daily as a single dose. For the pediatric dosage as an antihyperuricemic agent in antineoplastic therapy, refer to a current package insert or the *USP DI.*

■ Nursing Management

Allopurinol Therapy

■ **Assessment.** Monitoring of renal function and a reduction in dosage may be necessary if the client has impaired renal function or any illness that may predispose him or her to a change in renal function (e.g., diabetes mellitus or hypertension), because allopurinol may accumulate and increase the risk of allergic reactions and other adverse effects. The client's sensitivity to allopurinol should be ascertained.

Review the client's medication regimen for the risk of significant drug interactions, such as those that may occur when allopurinol is given concurrently with the following drugs:

Drug	Possible Effect and Management
anticoagulants, oral (coumarin or indanedione)	Allopurinol may inhibit the metabolism of the oral anticoagulant, resulting in an increase in serum levels, activity, and perhaps toxicity. Monitor prothrombin levels closely, because a dosage adjustment may be necessary.
azathioprine (Imuran) or mercaptopurine (Purinethol)	The effect of allopurinol in inhibiting xanthine oxidase may result in a decreased metabolism of these medications, leading to an increased potential for therapeutic and/or toxic effects (especially bone marrow depression). Monitor closely, because interventions or dosage adjustments may be necessary.

A baseline assessment of the client should include serum uric acid levels, CBC, hepatic and renal function determinations, and assessments of joint stiffness and pain.

■ **Nursing Diagnosis.** An assessment of the client receiving allopurinol should include consideration of the following nursing diagnoses/collaborative problems: impaired comfort (headache, stomach pain, anorexia, nausea, and vomiting); impaired skin integrity (exfoliative dermatitis); diarrhea; disturbed body image related to hair loss; and the potential complications of peripheral neuritis (numbness and tingling of the hands and feet), allergic dermatitis (rash, hives, itching), hepatitis, bone marrow suppression (thrombocytopenia [increased tendency to bleed], anemia [fatigue], agranulocytosis [fever, mouth ulcers, sore throat]), erythema multiforme (chills, fever, sores in mouth, skin rash), Stevens-Johnson syndrome, or toxic epidermal necrolysis (chills, fever, muscle ache, skin peeling).

■ **Implementation**

■ ***Monitoring.*** For proper dosing, serum uric acid levels should be monitored. CBCs and renal and hepatic function studies are recommended at periodic intervals during therapy, particularly during the first few months. Monitor the client's intake to ensure an adequate fluid intake. Observe the client's pain level and the mobility status of the affected joints.

■ ***Intervention.*** Administer allopurinol with food to minimize gastrointestinal distress. For ease of administration to clients who have difficulty swallowing, the tablets may be crushed and mixed with a small amount of applesauce or jelly.

A high fluid intake (80 to 96 ounces daily to produce 2 L of urine) and alkalinization of the urine are necessary to lessen the risk of stone formation and sludging of the tubules with urates.

A single dose of allopurinol should not exceed 300 mg; it may be given in divided doses.

■ ***Education.*** Encourage the client to comply with the medication regimen. The client should be advised that allopurinol helps to prevent, but does not relieve, acute episodes of gout.

Caution the client not to drink alcoholic beverages, because alcohol increases concentrations of uric acid. Alert the client that drowsiness may occur and that hazardous activities requiring mental alertness, such as driving, need to be avoided until the response to the medication has been determined. Stress the importance of a large amount of fluid intake to ensure the adequacy of fluid output.

To minimize the formation of calcium oxalate stones, the client should maintain a diet that enhances the alkalinity of the urine. This diet includes milk, fruits (except plums, prunes, and cranberries), carbonated beverages, vegetables (except corn and lentils), molasses, and baking soda and baking powder. Aspirin and large doses of vitamin C should be avoided.

The client should be advised to report to the prescriber immediately any signs of a skin rash or other adverse reactions. A skin rash usually precedes severe hypersensitivity reactions. Regular visits to the prescriber are necessary to monitor progress through periodic blood testing and the assessment for side effects/adverse reactions. Contact the prescriber if an acute attack of gout occurs while undergoing prophylaxis therapy; additional drug therapy with NSAIDs or corticosteroids may be prescribed.

■ **Evaluation.** The expected outcome of allopurinol therapy is that the client will experience fewer or no acute attacks of gout.

probenecid [proe ben′ e sid] (Benemid, Benuryl ♣)

Probenecid is indicated for the treatment of hyperuricemia and chronic gouty arthritis and as an adjunct to antibiotic therapy. It lowers serum levels of uric acid by competitively inhibiting the reabsorption of urate at the proximal renal tubule, thus increasing the urinary excretion of uric acid. It has no antiinflammatory action or analgesic effects.

As an adjunct to antibiotic therapy, probenecid competitively inhibits the secretion of weak organic acids, such as penicillin and some of the cephalosporins, at both the proximal and distal renal tubules in the kidneys. The result is an increase in blood concentrations and the duration of action of these antibiotics. This combination is used to treat sexually transmitted diseases (e.g., gonorrhea, acute pelvic inflammatory disease [PID], and neurosyphilis).

Probenecid is well absorbed orally and is highly bound to plasma proteins, especially to albumin. The therapeutic serum level is 100 to 200 μg/mL for uricosuric effects and 40 to 60 μg/mL for the suppression of penicillin excretion. The peak uricosuric effect is reached within 30 minutes, whereas the peak suppression of penicillin excretion is noted in 2 hours and lasts nearly 8 hours. Probenecid is metabolized in the liver and excreted by the kidneys.

The side effects/adverse reactions of probenecid include headaches, anorexia, mild nausea or vomiting, sore gums, pain and/or blood on urination, and lower back pain.

The adult dosage is 250 mg twice daily for 7 days, then increased to 500 mg twice daily. As an adjunct to penicillin/cephalosporin drug therapy, the dosage is 500 mg four times daily. The pediatric dosage as an antihyperuricemic agent has not been established. As an antibiotic adjunct, check a current drug reference for recommended dosing schedules.

■ Nursing Management

Probenecid Therapy

■ **Assessment.** Probenecid is well tolerated by most clients. However, probenecid is contraindicated for clients in whom there is an increased risk of uric acid renal calculi formation or urate nephropathy, such as clients undergoing cancer chemotherapy or radiation therapy or clients with moderate to severe renal function impairment. Its use should be carefully considered in clients with blood dyscrasias, a history of uric acid kidney stones, or mild renal function impairment, because these conditions may be exacerbated. Allergies to probenecid should be assessed.

Review the client's drug history for the risk of significant drug interactions, such as those that may occur when probenecid is given concurrently with following drugs:

Drug	Possible Effect and Management
Bold/color type indicates the most serious interactions.	
antineoplastic cytolytic drugs	**Increases the potential toxicity of uric acid nephropathy. In addition, the rapidly acting antineoplastic drugs may increase plasma levels of uric acid and interfere with any control of the previous hyperuricemia and gout. Avoid concurrent use or a potentially serious drug interaction may occur.**
aspirin or salicylates	**Not recommended because salicylates in moderate to high doses given chronically will inhibit the effectiveness of probenecid. In addition, if high doses of salicylates are being given for their uricosuric effects, probenecid may lower the excretion of salicylates, which may result in elevated serum salicylate levels and toxicity. Avoid concurrent use or a potentially serious drug interaction may occur.**
cephalosporins, penicillins	Probenecid decreases the renal tubular secretion of penicillin and selected cephalosporins, which may result in an increased serum level and a prolonged duration of action of the antibiotic. An increased risk of toxicity may also be present. Monitor serum levels closely if given concurrently. Cephalosporins not affected by probenecid include cefoperazone (Cefobid), ceforanide (Precef), ceftazidime (Fortaz), ceftriaxone (Rocephin).
heparin	**The anticoagulant effects of heparin may be enhanced and prolonged. Avoid concurrent use or a potentially serious drug interaction may occur.**
indomethacin (Indocin), ketoprofen (Orudis), and other NSAIDs	**Probenecid decreases the renal excretion of ketoprofen by 66%, decreases protein binding by 28%, and decreases the formation and renal clearance of ketoprofen conjugates. This leads to an increase in ketoprofen serum levels and possibly toxicity. Avoid concurrent use or a potentially serious drug interaction may occur.** **Probenecid may also decrease the excretion of indomethacin and possibly other NSAIDs from the body, thus leading to increased serum levels, an extended half-life, and an increased potential for NSAID toxicity. Monitor closely because the prescriber may need to lower the daily dose of NSAID if adverse reactions are reported.**
methotrexate (Folex, Mexate)	Probenecid may decrease the renal excretion of methotrexate, which may increase the risk of serious toxicity with methotrexate. If used concurrently, administer a lower dosage of methotrexate and monitor closely for toxicity, or monitor serum levels of methotrexate.

Drug	Possible Effect and Management
nitrofurantoin (Microdantin)	Probenecid may decrease the renal tubular secretion of nitrofurantoin, resulting in an increase in serum levels and possibly toxicity. This may reduce the urinary levels and effectiveness of nitrofurantoin. A reduction in the dosage of probenecid may be necessary before using nitrofurantoin for urinary tract infections. Monitor effectiveness closely.
zidovudine (AZT)	Concurrent drug administration may lead to an inhibition of zidovudine metabolism and secretion, resulting in elevated serum levels and an increased risk of zidovudine toxicity. The administration of probenecid may permit a reduced daily dose schedule for zidovudine. In one trial, a high incidence of skin rash was reported.

A baseline assessment of the client should include serum uric acid determinations, acid-base balance determinations, and an assessment of the frequency and severity of acute episodes of gout.

■ **Nursing Diagnosis.** An assessment of clients receiving probenecid should include consideration of the following selected nursing diagnoses/collaborative problems: impaired comfort (headache, stomach pain, anorexia, nausea, and vomiting); hyperthermia; disturbed body image related to hair loss; and the potential complications of allergic dermatitis, uric acid renal calculi (low back pain), thrombocytopenia (increased tendency to bleed), or anemia.

■ **Implementation**

■ ***Monitoring.*** Monitor the client's involved joints for range of motion, pain, and swelling during the course of medication, as well as serum uric acid levels and CBCs and, if urinary alkalizers are used, acid-base balance values. Fluid intake and output is monitored to ensure adequacy of urinary output (2000 to 3000 mL daily) to minimize urate stone formation.

■ ***Intervention.*** Probenecid may be administered with an antacid or food to minimize gastrointestinal distress. A high fluid intake (2500 to 3000 mL of water daily) to produce copious volumes of urine is recommended to minimize the formation of uric acid stones and the occurrence of renal colic and hematuria.

Alkalinization of the urine may be required to minimize the formation of kidney stones. Sodium bicarbonate, potassium citrate, and acetazolamide are agents recommended for the alkalinization of urine. As with allopurinol therapy, diet therapy is recommended with probenecid.

■ ***Education.*** Encourage the client to comply with the medication regimen. Variations in the dosage may precipitate an acute episode of gout. It is important for the client to understand that probenecid helps to prevent attacks but does not relieve acute episodes of gout. Regular visits to the prescriber are necessary to monitor progress. If an acute attack of gout occurs, contact the prescriber for additional medication (i.e., NSAIDs or colchicine).

Stress the importance of maintaining adequate fluid intake. Caution the client not to drink alcohol, because doing so increases uric acid levels.

Aspirin and other salicylates should be avoided because they decrease the effectiveness of probenecid and may precipitate a gout attack. Advise the client to read the labels of over-the-counter (OTC) medications carefully because aspirin and other salicylates are common ingredients of OTC medications for cold and flu-like symptoms.

The client should be cautioned to report to the prescriber any symptoms of hypersensitivity (skin rash), renal stones (hematuria, dysuria, low back pain), or blood dyscrasias (sore throat, fever, unusual bleeding or bruising, unusual fatigue).

■ **Evaluation.** The expected outcome of probenecid therapy is that the client will not experience attacks of gout, or the attacks will be diminished in frequency and severity.

sulfinpyrazone [sul fin peer′ a zone] (Anturane)

The mechanism of action of sulfinpyrazone is similar to probenecid; it inhibits the reabsorption of urate at the proximal renal tubule, thus increasing the excretion of uric acid in the urine. It is indicated for the treatment of chronic gouty arthritis and hyperuricemia.

Sulfinpyrazone is well absorbed orally and is highly bound to plasma proteins. It is metabolized in the liver into four active metabolites; the p-hydroxy-sulfinpyrazone metabolite contributes between 33% and 50% of the uricosuric effect of sulfinpyrazone. The duration of the uricosuric effect is usually 4 to 6 hours. Sulfinpyrazone is excreted by the kidneys.

The side effects/adverse reactions of sulfinpyrazone include nausea, vomiting, abdominal pain, and a rash or allergic reaction.

The adult antigout dosage is 100 to 200 mg PO twice daily initially, increased gradually at 2-day intervals if necessary until it is sufficient to control the elevated serum uric acid levels (usually 400 to 800 mg/day). The maintenance dosage is 200 to 400 mg daily. The pediatric dosage has not been established.

■ Nursing Management

Sulfinpyrazone Therapy

■ **Assessment.** Sulfinpyrazone is contraindicated for clients in whom there is an increased risk of uric acid renal calculi formation or urate nephropathy, such as clients undergoing cancer chemotherapy or radiation therapy or clients with moderate to severe renal function impairment. Its use should be carefully considered in clients with blood dyscrasias, active peptic ulcer disease, or mild renal function impairment, because the condition may be exacerbated. Allergies to sulfinpyrazone should be assessed.

Review the client's current medication regimen for the risk of significant drug interactions, such as those that may

occur when sulfinpyrazone is given concurrently with the following drugs:

Drug	Possible Effect and Management
Bold/color type indicates the most serious interactions.	
alprostadil (Prostin VR), anagrelide, aspirin, dextran, carbenicillin (parenteral), dipyridamole (Persantine), divalproex (Depakote), NSAIDs, plicamycin (Mithramycin), ticarcillin (Ticar), ticlopidine (Ticlid), or valproic acid (Depakene)	These drugs inhibit platelet aggregation; therefore concurrent drug administration may increase the potential of bleeding episodes. Monitor closely for early signs of bleeding.
anticoagulants (coumarin or indanedione, heparin) or thrombolytics (streptokinase or urokinase)	**Sulfinpyrazone may increase the anticoagulant effect by displacing coumarin or indanedione from their protein-binding sites and by inhibiting their metabolism. Monitor prothrombin time closely, because dosage adjustments may be necessary. An increase in bleeding episodes or hemorrhage may result from the concurrent administraion of sulfinpyrazone and anticoagulant or thrombolytic therapy. The potential for this reaction is caused by the inhibitory effect of sulfinpyrazone on platelet aggregation and its possibility of causing gastrointestinal ulceration or hemorrhage. Avoid concurrent use or a potentially serious drug interaction may occur.**
antineoplastic agents, rapidly cytolytic	An increased risk of inducing uric acid nephropathy or losing control of uric acid serum levels (preexisting levels) and gout is possible. Avoid concurrent use or a potentially serious drug interaction may occur.
aspirin or salicylates	**When salicylates are given long term in moderate to high doses, the uricosuric effect of sulfinpyrazone may be inhibited (see comments about probenecid). Avoid concurrent use or a potentially serious drug interaction may occur.**
cefotetan (Cefotan), cefoperazone (Cefobid), or plicamycin (Mithramycin)	These drugs can cause platelet function inhibition and hypoprothrombinemia. Monitor closely for bleeding tendencies. Avoid concurrent use or a potentially serious drug interaction may occur.
nitrofurantoin (Macrodantin)	**Sulfinpyrazone may decrease kidney excretion of nitrofurantoin, which may increase the risk of nitrofurantoin toxicity and reduce the effectiveness of nitrofurantoin as a urinary tract antiinfective agent. Avoid concurrent use or a potentially serious drug interaction may occur.**

A baseline assessment of the client should include serum uric acid determinations, blood counts, renal function determinations, and an assessment of the frequency and severity of acute gout episodes.

■ **Nursing Diagnosis.** An assessment of the client receiving sulfinpyrazone should include consideration of the following selected nursing diagnoses/collaborative problems: impaired comfort (stomach pain, anorexia, nausea, and vomiting); hyperthermia (allergic reaction); activity intolerance related to anemia; diarrhea; and the potential complications of thrombocytopenia (increased tendency to bleed), allergic dermatitis, renal failure, and uric acid renal calculi (low back pain).

■ **Implementation**

■ ***Monitoring.*** CBCs, uric acid determinations, and renal function studies should be performed at periodic intervals during therapy. Monitor fluid intake and output to ensure that intake is adequate for sufficient urinary output (2 to 3 L/day) to help prevent urinary stones. Monitor the client's frequency and severity of gouty episodes.

■ ***Intervention.*** Sulfinpyrazone may be administered with an antacid or food to minimize gastrointestinal distress. Clients should maintain adequate fluid intake (8 ounces 10 to 12 times daily) and urinary alkalinization by the administration of sodium bicarbonate, potassium citrate, or acetazolamide if necessary, because sulfinpyrazone is a potent uricosuric agent that may cause urolithiasis and renal colic, especially in the initial stages of therapy.

■ ***Education.*** Encourage the client to comply with therapy. This is essential because optimal effectiveness of the drug may not be reached for several months. Advise the client that sulfinpyrazone helps prevent gout attacks but does not relieve acute episodes. Regular visits to the health care provider should be maintained to monitor progress. Stress the importance of adequate fluid intake in the prevention of stone formation.

Caution the client not to use alcohol because it increases levels of uric acid. Aspirin and other salicylates should be avoided because they decrease the effectiveness of sulfinpyrazone and may precipitate a gout attack.

■ **Evaluation.** The expected outcome of sulfinpyrazone therapy is that the client will experience diminished attacks of gout or none at all.

■ ■ ■

The NSAIDs naproxen (Naprosyn) and sulindac (Clinoril) are also used in the treatment of acute gouty arthritis. See Chapter 14 for information on these drugs.

SUMMARY

Gout is a metabolic disorder characterized by hyperuricemia. The aims of therapy for gout are to end the acute attack quickly, prevent a recurrence, prevent uric acid renal calculi, and prevent or minimize the complications of sodium urate deposits in the joints. Agents used for these purposes are colchicine, allopurinol, probenecid, and sulfinpyrazone.

Critical Thinking Questions

1. Mr. Stevens, 56 years of age, comes to the clinic with a red, swollen big toe on his left foot. He is accompanied by his wife. He indicates that he has had pain, redness, and swelling for approximately 1 week, and it has been unrelieved by aspirin. For what risk factors of gout will you assess Mr. Stevens? How will his medical diagnosis be confirmed? Given what Mr. Stevens has already said, what health teaching does the client and family require?
2. Why is a diet that enhances alkalinity of the urine recommended for clients with gout? What should be included in such a diet? What dietary limitations are prescribed for these clients?

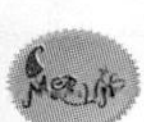

Collaborative Learning Activities

For Collaborative Learning Activities, go to mosby.com/MERLIN/McKenry/.

CASE STUDY

For a Case Study that will help ensure mastery of this chapter content, go to mosby.com/MERLIN/McKenry/.

BIBLIOGRAPHY

American Hospital Formulary Service. (1999). *AHFS drug information '98.* Bethesda, MD: American Society of Hospital Pharmacists.

Anderson, K.N., Anderson, L.E., & Glanze, W.D. (Eds.). (1998). *Mosby's medical, nursing, & allied health dictionary* (5th ed.). St. Louis: Mosby.

Brooks, P.M. (1997). Rheumatic disorders. In T.M. Speight & N.H.G. Holford (Eds.), *Avery's drug treatment* (4th ed.). Auckland, New Zealand: Adis International.

Drug Facts and Comparisons. (2000). St. Louis: Facts and Comparisons.

Jones, R.E. & Ball, E.V. (1999). Gout: Beyond the stereotype, *Hospital Practice, 34*(6), 95-102.

McCance, K.L. & Huether, S.E. (1998). *Pathophysiology: The biologic basis for disease in adults and children* (3rd ed.). St. Louis: Mosby.

Pagana, K.D. & Pagana, T.J. (1997). *Mosby's diagnostic and laboratory test reference* (3rd ed.). St. Louis: Mosby.

Physicians' Desk Reference. (1999). Montvale, NJ: Medical Economics.

Seeley, R.S. & Tate, P. (1995). *Anatomy and physiology* (3rd ed.). St. Louis: Mosby.

Thibodeau, G.A. & Patton, K.T. (1999). *Anatomy and physiology* (4th ed.). St. Louis: Mosby.

United States Pharmacopeia Dispensing Information (USP DI): Drug information for the health care professional (19th ed.). (1999). Rockville, MD: United States Pharmacopeial Convention.

Young, L.Y. & Campagna, K.D. (1995). Gout and hyperuricemia. In L.Y. Young & M.A. Koda-Kimble. *Applied therapeutics: The clinical use of drugs* (6th ed.). Vancouver, WA: Applied Therapeutics.

36 Drug Therapy for Renal System Dysfunction

Chapter Focus

Renal dysfunction can alter the bioavailability, distribution, and protein binding of drugs by modifying systemic pH, altering the configuration and amount of albumin, and altering body hydration and renal excretion. Even with drugs that are not excreted renally, renal dysfunction may cause toxic metabolites to accumulate. Drug-induced nephrotoxicity may also occur. The nurse needs to be acutely aware of the effects of renal system dysfunction on drug therapy and vice versa.

Learning Objectives

1. Differentiate between acute renal failure and chronic renal failure.
2. Describe two laboratory tests used to evaluate renal impairment.
3. Explain why dietary protein, fluid intake, potassium, magnesium, and phosphorus are restricted in chronic renal failure.
4. Describe the differences between the drug dosage reduction method and the interval extension method of treatment, and describe the advantages of each.
5. Implement the nursing management of drug therapy for the client with renal system dysfunction.

Key Terms

acute renal failure, p. 693
azotemic, p. 693
chronic renal failure, p. 693
end-stage renal disease, p. 693
hemodialysis, p. 693
peritoneal dialysis, p. 693

Because many potentially toxic drugs are excreted by the kidneys, people with impaired renal function who receive standard drug dosages on a regular schedule may experience drug accumulation and toxicity. It is important for the health care provider to monitor and evaluate clients with impaired renal function, because drug dosages or time intervals often need to be adjusted.

ACUTE VS. CHRONIC RENAL FAILURE

Acute renal failure, a condition characterized by oliguria, a rapid accumulation of nitrogenous wastes in the blood, and a rapid decline in renal function, occurs in 2% to 5% of all hospitalized individuals and in up to 1% of hospital admissions from the community (Bailie, 1995). Primary causes include trauma, pregnancy, and renal ischemia as a result of surgery, severe hemorrhage, severe volume depletion, and shock. In some instances, nephrotoxic agents such as heavy metals and aminoglycosides may also induce acute renal failure. If recognized early and treated promptly, acute renal failure may be reversed before acute tubular necrosis or permanent damage occurs.

Chronic renal failure (CRF) is a progressive disease usually caused by an irreversible kidney injury that results in the permanent loss of nephrons or renal mass. It is a major health concern in North America. In 1991, nearly 215,000 persons in the U.S. Medicare program had end-stage renal disease (Ateshkadi & Johnson, 1995). The most common causes of CRF are glomerulonephritis, diabetes mellitus, hypertension, polycystic kidney disease, and other diseases that may lead to the destruction or impaired functioning of the kidneys. Initially, individuals with CRF may be treated conservatively, but in **end-stage renal disease (ESRD)** the kidney is so severely damaged or scarred that hemodialysis or organ transplantation may be necessary for survival. **Hemodialysis** is a procedure in which impurities or wastes are removed from the blood; the blood is shunted from the body through a machine for diffusion and ultrafiltration and then returned to the client's circulation. **Peritoneal dialysis** is another form of dialysis but one in which the peritoneum is used as the diffusible membrane. A solution known as dialysate is placed into the peritoneal cavity via a catheter and retained for a specified time; osmosis, diffusion, and filtration pass needed electrolytes into the bloodstream and remove wastes into the dialysate, which is then drained by gravity from the abdominal cavity.

Because the focus of this text is pharmacology, this chapter concentrates on the therapeutic regimen and recommendations for drug dosage adjustments in clients with impaired renal function.

SIGNS AND SYMPTOMS OF RENAL FAILURE OR INSUFFICIENCY

One of the more common signs of acute renal failure is a marked alteration in expected urine output, usually a significant reduction (<400 mL/day). Thus the first phase is the oliguric phase. Phase two is the diuretic phase; in this phase the individual experiences an increase in urine volume for a few days but remains **azotemic,** retaining excessive amounts of nitrogenous compounds (blood urea nitrogen [BUN] and creatinine) in the blood. Phase three is considered the recovery phase as azotemia decreases and renal function is recovering. The recovery phase may occur over weeks to months, depending on the damage caused by the original insult to the kidneys (Bailie, 1995). Signs of acute renal failure in the presence of reduced urine production are usually the result of fluid overload: edema, weight gain, weakness, hypertension, and tachycardia.

The most common complaints with CRF are increasing weakness, fatigue, and lethargy. Gastrointestinal signs include anorexia, gastrointestinal distress, nausea, vomiting, thirst, and weight loss. Paresthesias, peripheral neuropathy, convulsions, and neuromuscular irritability may also occur. On examination, the client may appear pale and dehydrated and have an increased respiratory rate and uremic breath. Hypertension with retinopathy, cardiac hypertrophy, pulmonary edema, or pericarditis may often be present.

A detailed client history, thorough physical examination, urinalysis, and blood chemistry levels are important for the assessment, diagnosis, and determination of an appropriate treatment plan. The degree of renal impairment is usually estimated by reviewing the levels of serum creatinine and BUN. Elevated levels indicate a decrease in renal clearance, which predisposes the individual to drug toxicity.

MEASUREMENT OF RENAL FUNCTION

Many formulas and nomograms are available to determine the client's approximate creatinine clearance and the drug dosage adjustment necessary to minimize the possibility of toxicity. Normal values may vary from laboratory to laboratory, but in general a normal BUN ranges between 5 and 20 mg/dL; the range of serum creatinine, which varies with age, is usually between 0.5 and 1.2 mg/dL. The most reliable test is the creatinine clearance test. Because it is difficult to obtain an accurate collection of all urine excreted for a 24-hour period, many clinicians use a formula to estimate creatinine clearance; others may prefer to use a nomogram. The formulas most commonly used are noted in Box 36-1. The mean endogenous creatinine clearance in an adult is usually between 90 and 130 mL/min/1.73 m^2 body surface/24 hr. Reductions in this quantity signify an impairment of renal function (Table 36-1).

Another important factor in evaluating serum levels of drugs in clients with renal failure or renal impairment is an assessment of serum albumin and total protein. Serum protein is decreased in individuals with renal insufficiency; this can alter the interpretation of serum levels of drugs that are protein bound (90% or more) in persons with normal renal function. Individuals with a lower albumin or protein value may have a drug concentration in the low range that appears

BOX 36-1

Formulas for Estimating Creatinine Clearance

Adult male

$$= \frac{(140 - \text{Age}) \times (\text{Ideal body weight in kg})}{72 \times \text{Serum creatinine (mg/dL)}}$$

Adult female

$$= \frac{(140 - \text{Age}) \times (\text{Ideal body weight in kg})}{72 \times \text{Serum creatinine (mg/dL)} \times 0.85}$$

Ideal Body Weight (IBW) Calculations

IBW (males) = 52 kg + (1.9 kg × Inches over 5 feet)
IBW (females) = 49 kg + (1.7 kg × Inches over 5 feet)

Information from Katzung, B.G. (Ed.). (1998). *Basic and clinical pharmacology* (7th ed.). Stamford, CT: Appleton & Lange.

TABLE 36-1 Typical Grading of Renal Impairment Using Creatinine Clearance

Degree of Renal Failure	Creatinine Clearance
Normal	Men: 90-139 mL/min Women: 80-125 mL/min
Mild impairment	50-80 mL/min
Moderate impairment	10-50 mL/min
Severe impairment	<10 mL/min

Information from Bennett, W.M., Aronoff, G.R., Morrison, G., Golper, T.A., Pulliam, J., Wolfson, M., & Singer, I. (1983). Drug prescribing in renal failure: Dosing guidelines for adults. *American Journal of Kidney Disease,* 3(3), 155.

to be therapeutic. This is possible if the laboratory does not differentiate between the bound and unbound drug in the testing. Lower protein levels may lead to a higher unbound concentration of the drug (the active form), thus producing an adequate therapeutic response.

SPECIAL NEEDS OF THE CLIENT WITH RENAL FAILURE

Clients with CRF have special dietary, electrolyte, and fluid requirements. In general, dietary protein is usually restricted to 0.5 to 1 g/kg of lean body weight daily. This limitation will reduce the incidence of azotemia, hyperkalemia, and acidosis. Fluid intake is based on daily losses and metabolic needs.

Dietary sodium is restricted to approximately 2 g or 90 mEq/day. Potassium, magnesium, and phosphorus are also restricted. An aluminum hydroxide gel is often prescribed to decrease phosphate absorption from the gastrointestinal tract. The reduced excretion of phosphates, magnesium, and potassium from the kidneys in CRF can lead to elevated serum levels or hypermagnesemia, hyperkalemia, and hyperphosphatemia, which in turn lead to hypocalcemia and osteodystrophy.

Thus dietary restrictions are absolutely necessary. Calcium supplements and vitamin D are often prescribed for these clients to reduce or prevent hyperparathyroidism and bone disease. Magnesium levels are kept somewhat in check if the client avoids magnesium-containing antacids and laxatives.

Decreased production of red blood cells (erythropoiesis) in CRF leads to anemia, weakness, and fatigue. Iron therapy may be prescribed for clients with iron deficiency anemia resulting from chronic blood loss; folic acid, vitamin C, and soluble B-complex vitamins are often given to replace the substances usually lost during dialysis. It is not unusual to care for CRF clients who have many dietary and fluid restrictions, as well as prescriptions for vitamins, calcium, specific antacids, and additional drugs as necessary. Epoetin is used specifically to stimulate erythropoiesis in CRF (Barrett et al., 1999).

epoetin [eh poe′ ee tin] (Epogen)

Epoetin is a glycoprotein chemically identical to human erythropoietin. It is produced by recombinant DNA technology that contains the same 165 amino acids in the same sequence as human erythropoietin. Epoetin stimulates bone marrow erythropoiesis and also induces the release of reticulocytes from the marrow so they can mature into erythrocytes. Human erythropoietin is produced mainly in the kidneys.

Because endogenous erythropoietin is manufactured mainly in the kidneys, the anemia resulting from CRF is caused by an inadequate production of the hormone. With the use of epoetin, an initial increase in reticulocytes is seen within 7 to 10 days; an increase in red cell count, hematocrit, and hemoglobin occurs within 2 to 6 weeks. Epoetin reaches a peak serum level within 15 minutes of IV administration and within 5 to 24 hours of an SC dose. The half-life is between 4 and 13 hours after IV or SC administration. When therapy is discontinued, the hematocrit decreases in approximately 2 weeks (duration of action).

The side effects/adverse reactions of epoetin include arthralgias or bone pain, asthenia (severe muscle weakness), nausea and vomiting, weakness, diarrhea, chest pain, edema of the extremities or face, weight gain, tachycardia, headache, hypertension, clotting of the arteriovenous (AV) shunt and/or dialyzer, and polycythemia. No significant drug interactions have been reported.

The initial adult dosage is 50 to 100 units/kg IV or SC three times weekly. Dosage increments of 25 units/kg may be instituted if the hematocrit has not increased after 2 months of therapy by at least 5 to 6 points and the client is still below the desired range of 30% to 33%. For maintenance, decrease the dosage gradually by 25 units/kg monthly to the lowest dosage that maintains the hematocrit at the desired level. The dosage has not been determined for children below 12 years of age. Pregnancy safety has been established by the Food and Drug Administration (FDA) as category C.

■ Nursing Management

Epoetin Therapy

■ **Assessment.** The client with hypertension is at risk with the administration of epoetin because the resultant increase in hematocrit increases blood viscosity and peripheral vascular resistance, leading to a rise in blood pressure.

Clients with poorly controlled hypertension should delay undergoing epoetin therapy until the hypertension is controlled. Even then, the blood pressure of the hypertensive client (and the previously normotensive client) should be monitored closely because of the increased risk of hypertension, which may lead to hypertensive encephalopathy. The drug should not be used if the client is hypersensitive to human albumin or to products derived from mammalian cells, such as beef and pork insulin.

■ **Nursing Diagnosis.** Clients receiving epoetin may be at risk for the following selected nursing diagnoses/collaborative problems: impaired comfort related to arthralgias (11%), headache (16%), chest pain (7%), nausea (10.5%), vomiting (8%), and flu-like syndrome for 1 to 12 hours after IV administration; fatigue (9%); excess fluid volume (weight gain, swelling of the face, fingers, feet, and ankles [9%]); impaired skin integrity (skin reaction at administration site [7%]); diarrhea (8.5%); and the potential complications of polycythemia (increased clotting tendency [6.8%]), severe muscle weakness (7%), seizures (1.1%), and increased blood pressure (24%).

■ **Implementation**

■ ***Monitoring.*** As mentioned, the client's blood pressure should be monitored. A complete blood count (CBC), as ordered by the prescriber, should be assessed for change. Hematocrit values are particularly important, with baseline and twice-weekly frequencies recommended as a guide for dosage and efficacy. A rise in the hematocrit of more than 4 points in a 2-week period or a value over 36%, which is considered the safety limit for the prevention of adverse reactions, should be brought to the prescriber's attention.

It is recommended that the status of the client's iron stores be monitored to determine the need and the amount of iron supplementation for the client. Because iron is incorporated into hemoglobin as a result of the effectiveness of the drug, the client's iron stores may be depleted, causing a decrease in the efficacy of epoetin.

Neurologic assessments for premonitory signs for the risk of seizures should be performed periodically, particularly during the first 90 days of therapy and at times when the hematocrit rises rapidly. Renal function studies (BUN, serum creatinine, serum phosphorus, serum potassium, serum sodium, and serum uric acid) should be monitored, because the need to begin or increase dialysis may occur with the administration of epoetin. The client should be weighed daily, and the fluid balance should be monitored by intake and output measurements.

■ ***Intervention.*** Each vial of epoetin should be used to administer one dose only because the injection contains no preservative. Discard any unused portion of the drug. Do not shake the vial; shaking may denature the substance and render it biologically inactive. Do not mix epoetin with other medications.

■ ***Education.*** Alert the client to avoid activities that may be hazardous if seizures would occur, especially during the first 90 days of therapy. The client should be instructed about dietary sources of iron, folic acid, and B_{12} as an adjunct to iron and other vitamin supplementation. Dietary restrictions as part of the antihypertensive regimen and those pertinent to clients with chronic renal failure should be reviewed with the client. The correction of anemia may result in an increased appetite, making it more difficult for the client to maintain compliance with the required dietary restrictions. The client should be encouraged to keep prescriber and dialysis appointments.

If epoetin is prescribed for the client to self-administer, ensure that the client knows the proper injection technique.

■ **Evaluation.** The expected outcome of epoetin therapy is that a clinically significant increase in the red cell count, hematocrit, and hemoglobin should be seen in 2 to 6 weeks of the initiation of therapy. The hematocrit should stabilize in the 30% to 33% range. With correction of the client's anemia, the client will demonstrate an improved activity tolerance, decreased fatigue, and an improved appetite, sleep pattern, cognitive function, and sense of well-being.

SELECTED DRUG MODIFICATIONS IN RENAL FAILURE

As previously mentioned, BUN and serum creatinine are waste products to be excreted by the kidneys. Serum levels of these substances are used to measure renal function. Unfortunately, neither test is useful in discovering early renal impairment because abnormal levels do not appear until 50% or more of renal function is impaired. Fortunately, human kidneys are functional even if 90% of the glomerular filtration rate is lost. However, the continuing progressive loss may result in ESRD, or renal loss that necessitates hemodialysis, peritoneal dialysis, kidney transplantation, and other interventions discussed in this chapter.

In individuals with renal insufficiency or impairment, the drug dose may be decreased (dosage reduction method) while maintaining the usual dosage interval; if the dose remains the same, the interval between doses is lengthened (interval extension method). Usually the dosage reduction method is preferred for drugs that require a constant therapeutic level in the blood. For most clients receiving a loading dose, the dose is similar to the dose given to a client without renal impairment. This permits a therapeutically desirable blood level that is then maintained by either the dosage reduction method or the interval extension method. Table 36-2 gives typical dosing recommendations for selected medications along with a list of drugs that may or may not be removed by hemodialysis or peritoneal dialysis.

TABLE 36-2 Selected Medication Dosing for Adults with Renal Insufficiency

	Creatinine Clearance (mL/min)*			
	Normal Dosage	Renal Failure		
Medication	**>50**	**10-50**	**<10**	**Half-life (hours)**
acyclovir (Zovirax)	5 mg/kg q8h (IV infusion)	5 mg/kg q12-24h	2.5 mg/kg q24h	N: 2.5 A: 20
ampicillin (Omnipen-N)	1-2 g q4-6h	1-1.5 g q6h	1 g q8-12h	N: 0.8-1.5 A: 20
cefazolin (Ancef)	0.5-1 g q8h	250-500 mg q12h	250-500 mg q24h	N:1.8-2.6 A: 12-40
ciprofloxacin (Cipro)	250-750 mg PO q12h	250-500 mg q12h	250-500 mg q24h	N: 4 A: 8.5
fluconazole (Diflucan)	100-200 mg q24h	50-100 mg q24h	50-100 mg q24h	N: 20-50 A: 98
gentamicin (Garamycin)	1 mg/kg q8h	0.15-0.5 mg/kg q8h	0.1 mg/kg q8h	N: 1.5-3 A: 20-54
meperidine (Demerol)	50-100 mg IV/IM q3-4h	75%-100% of dose q6h	50% of dose q6-8h	N: 3-7 A: ?
vancomycin (Vancocin)	500 mg q6h	1 g every 3-7 days	1 g every 1-2 weeks	N: 4-9 A: 129-190

Information from Aweeka, F.T. (1995). Dosing of drugs in renal failure. In L.Y. Young & M.A. Koda-Kimble (Eds.), *Applied therapeutics: The clinical use of drugs* (6th ed.). Vancouver, WA: Applied Therapeutics; *United States Pharmacopeia Dispensing Information (USP DI): Drug information for the health care professional* (19th ed.). (1999). Rockville, MD: United States Pharmacopeial Convention; *Physicians' Desk Reference.* (1998). Montvale, NJ: Medical Economics; *Mosby's GenRx* (1999). St. Louis: Mosby.
N, Normal; *A*, anuric.
*Creatinine clearance or glomerular filtration rate.

The reader is referred to the current package inserts or renal failure dosing guides for specific data.

■ Nursing Management
Pharmacologic Therapies for Clients with Renal System Dysfunction

■ **Assessment.** The initial assessment should include a history of recent weight changes, edema, malaise, increasing irritability or mental changes, metallic taste in the mouth, polyuria and nocturia (caused by reduced ability to concentrate urine), headache, dizziness, gastrointestinal disturbances, and hypertension.

Because other body systems may be affected by renal dysfunction, a thorough multisystem assessment should be conducted. A baseline assessment of the client's laboratory values should include BUN, serum creatinine, serum electrolytes, CBC, and urinalysis. The client's current drug regimen requires a review to determine the risk for drug toxicities related to drug accumulation. If the client is receiving medications with significant toxicities, the appropriate serum drug levels should be carefully monitored to help prevent overdosing the client. Table 36-3 lists the medications most commonly associated with inducing renal dysfunction.

■ **Nursing Diagnosis.** The client undergoing pharmacologic therapy for renal system dysfunction is at risk for the following selected nursing diagnoses/collaborative problems: excess fluid volume related to an inability to adequately excrete fluids and electrolytes and/or an excessive fluid intake during periods of decreased renal function; ineffective breathing pattern related to circulatory volume overload and/or metabolic acidosis leading to hyperventilation; imbalanced nutrition: less than body requirements related to anorexia, nausea, and vomiting; fatigue secondary to anemia and uremia; risk for infection related to a debilitated state and the use of indwelling catheters and other invasive procedures; and the potential complications of dysrhythmias related to renal failure, anemia related to bone marrow suppression and increased hemolysis and bleeding tendencies, and altered levels of consciousness related to electrolyte imbalances, the accumulation of waste products in the blood, and hypoxia.

■ **Implementation**

■ ***Monitoring.*** The client should be weighed at the same time each day, with the same amount of clothing, and with the same scale. The client at home may be better able to establish a routine by weighing first thing in the morning after the first voiding and before dressing or eating. The daily weight can be evaluated in light of the 24-hour intake and output balance for determining fluid volume excess or fluid volume deficit.

The fluid intake and output of the client should be recorded accurately on a 24-hour basis. The 24-hour balance should be calculated by subtracting the output from the in-

TABLE 36-3 Medications Associated with Renal Toxicity or Dysfunction

Medications	Possible Toxicity or Dysfunction
kanamycin, colistin, amikacin (rare), tobramycin (rare), gentamicin, cephaloridine, lithium, amphotericin B, cisplatin, rifampin, bacitracin, tetracycline, nitrofurantoin, kanamycin, neomycin, polymyxin B, streptozocin, cyclosporine	Renal tubule damage and/or necrosis
penicillins, methoxyflurane, cephalothin, sulfonamides, nonsteroidal antiinflammatory drugs, allopurinol	Acute interstitial nephritis
trimethadione, paramethadione, gold, probenecid, lithium, heroin	Glomerular damage
Injectable antihypertensive drugs given to older adults, excessive dosages of low-molecular-weight dextran, diuretics, opioid medications	May induce acute ischemic renal failure

From Douglas, S. (1992). Acute tubular necrosis: Diagnosis, treatment, and nursing implications. *AACN Clinical Issues,* 3(3),688-697. Reprinted with permission, Nursecom, Inc.

take. The balance, whether positive or negative, should relate to a weight loss or gain of approximately 500 mL to a pound of body weight. BUN and serum creatinine levels should be monitored to ascertain the client's degree of ESRD and to anticipate the clinical signs and symptoms of physiologic injury that require nursing intervention and client education.

Serum potassium levels should be monitored daily. Cardiovascular monitoring should become more intense when the level exceeds 6 mEq/L. In addition to blood pressure and apical heart rate determinations, assessment by cardiac monitor is required. Serum levels of calcium and phosphate should be monitored every 3 to 4 days, and the client should be clinically assessed for hypocalcemia and hyperphosphatemia as evidenced by irritability, muscular twitching, and tetany.

The client's arterial blood gases should be monitored. Clinically, the client should be observed for increased respiratory rate and depth and changes in mental status that would indicate impending metabolic acidosis. CBCs should be performed periodically, and the client should be assessed for signs and symptoms of anemia that might necessitate interventions such as iron supplements and anabolic steroids or, in the extreme, the transfusion of packed or frozen red blood cells.

■ ***Intervention.*** Fluid intake may be restricted. If so, fluid allotments should be planned with the client regarding the types of fluids and time of intake to enhance the client's acceptance of the regimen and to maintain the client's feeling of control. Dietary sodium is usually restricted, and intake will need to be planned with the client based on the degree of restriction. Drug therapy is based on each client's particular form of dysfunction and its cause. Many body systems are affected by renal dysfunction, and therefore several medications may be used. The more common agents are diuretics to control fluid balance, edema, and hypertension and antibiotics to treat infection. Because altered renal function also alters the pharmacokinetics of many drugs, dosages and dose intervals are adjusted based on the drug and degree of renal system dysfunction.

■ ***Education.*** As with any condition, particularly those with multisystem consequences, knowledge deficit is likely. The client should be instructed in the purpose of the medications, such as antihypertensives, diuretics, calcium supplements, vitamin D, and phosphate binders. In addition, the client should be told of the side effects/adverse reactions, because with increasing renal insufficiency the margin of safety with any medication is diminished. Multiple drug therapy increases the chance of a drug interaction. The stressors placed on the client with increasing renal insufficiency are multiple. Changes in lifestyle and body image, as well as the impact of the disease on the client, require the nurse to exercise skill in supporting and educating the client and family to minimize the potential for ineffective coping.

■ **Evaluation.** The expected outcome of pharmacologic therapy for renal system dysfunction is that the client will adhere to the prescribed fluid restrictions and will be normovolemic as evidenced by stable weight, normal breath sounds, an absence of edema, and a blood pressure and pulse within the client's normal range. In addition, the client will verbalize orientation to person, place, and time; will experience a decrease in fatigue; and will increase participation in activities. The client will be free of infection, as evidenced by normothermia, a white blood cell count (WBC) within normal limits, clear urine, normal breath sounds, and an absence of drainage at catheter sites.

SUMMARY

Renal system dysfunction may be a source of tremendous stress for the client and family, and it also presents a challenge for the nurse. Therapy is complicated by multiple drug therapy and altered pharmacokinetics. Drug interactions or adverse reactions may appear at any time, and therefore it is essential that the nurse monitor closely the client's renal function and the effects of the drug. Additional areas for nursing intervention include nondrug therapy (e.g., diet modification and fluid restriction) and the involvement of other body systems.

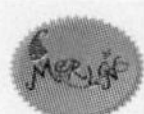

Critical Thinking Questions

1. Mrs. Defrees, a 54-year-old female client, has been admitted to your unit for congestive heart failure. She has a height of 5 feet, 3 inches, and she weighs 175 pounds. She has been prescribed digoxin, 0.25 mg daily for her condition. She indicates a history of renal failure, and you are concerned about the level of her renal function with the administration of digoxin. You are aware that a creatinine clearance is the best indicator of renal function, but it is a 24-hour test. The laboratory has just called to the unit with her serum creatinine value of 3.2 mg/dL. Estimate her creatinine clearance to determine the severity of her renal impairment. What action would you take on the basis of your findings?
2. Two commonly used tests of renal impairment determination are the BUN and the serum creatinine. Which test is considered to be the most sensitive of renal function and why?

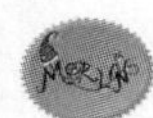

Collaborative Learning Activities

For Collaborative Learning Activities, go to mosby.com/MERLIN/McKenry/.

CASE STUDY

For a Case Study that will help ensure mastery of this chapter content, go to mosby.com/MERLIN/McKenry/.

BIBLIOGRAPHY

Anderson, K.N., Anderson, L.E., & Glanze, W.D. (Eds.). (1998). *Mosby's medical, nursing, & allied health dictionary* (5th ed.) St. Louis: Mosby.

Ateshkadi, A. & Johnson, C.A. (1995). Chronic renal failure. In L.Y. Young & M.A. Koda-Kimble (Eds.), *Applied therapeutics: The clinical use of drugs* (6th ed.). Vancouver, WA: Applied Therapeutics.

Aweeka, F.T. (1995). Dosing of drugs in renal failure. In L.Y. Young & M.A. Koda-Kimble (Eds.), *Applied therapeutics: The clinical use of drugs* (6th ed.). Vancouver, WA: Applied Therapeutics.

Bailie, G.R. (1995). Acute renal failure. In L.Y. Young & M.A. Koda-Kimble (Eds.), *Applied therapeutics: The clinical use of drugs* (6th ed.). Vancouver, WA: Applied Therapeutics.

Barrett, B.J., Fenton, S.S., Ferguson, B., Halligon, P., Langlois, S., McCready, W.G., Muirhead, N., & Weir, R.V. (1999). Clinical practice guidelines for the management of anemia coexistent with chronic renal failure. Canadian Society of Nephrology. *Journal of the American Society of Nephrology, 10*(suppl 13), S292-S296.

Briglia, A. & Paganini, E.P. (1999). Acute renal failure in the intensive care unit: Therapy overview, patient risk stratification, complications of renal replacement, and special circumstances. *Clinical Chest Medicine, 20*(2), 347-366.

Brundage, D.J. (1992). *Renal disorders.* St. Louis: Mosby.

Chambers, J.K. (1993). Renal insufficiency: Implications for care of the medical-surgical patient. *MEDSURG Nursing, 2*(1), 33.

Mosby's GenRx (1999). St. Louis: Mosby.

Pagana, K.D. & Pagana, T.J. (1997). *Mosby's diagnostic and laboratory test reference* (3rd ed.). St. Louis: Mosby.

Physicians' Desk Reference. (1998). Montvale, NJ: Medical Economics.

Thibodeau, G.A. & Patton, K.T. (1999). *Anatomy and physiology* (4th ed.). St. Louis: Mosby.

United States Pharmacopeia Dispensing Information (USP DI): Drug information for the health care professional (19th ed.). (1999).Rockville, MD: United States Pharmacopeial Convention.

37 Overview of the Respiratory System

Chapter Focus

The respiratory system functions to maintain the exchange of oxygen and carbon dioxide in the lungs and cells and to regulate the pH of body fluids; therefore a change within this system affects other body systems. The reverse is also true—disorders of other body systems may increase the body's need for oxygen, such as with fever, and therefore increase the work of respiration. Many respiratory problems require direct nursing care and education of the client and caregivers for effective management of the therapeutic regimen at home. This chapter provides a review of anatomy and physiology as a background for understanding the drugs affecting the respiratory system.

Learning Objectives

1. Explain the three interrelated processes of respiration.
2. Name the two sources of respiratory secretions.
3. Describe the $beta_2$ receptor theory of bronchodilation.
4. Describe the parasympathetic effect on the respiratory system.
5. Discuss the central and peripheral control of respiration.

Key Terms

bronchial glands, p. 700
bronchoconstriction, p. 701
bronchodilation, p. 701
cellular respiration, p. 700
gas transport, p. 700
goblet cells, p. 700
mucokinesis, p. 700
pulmonary ventilation, p. 700

The respiratory system includes all structures involved in the exchange of oxygen and carbon dioxide, such as the airway passages, lungs, nasal cavities, pharynx, larynx, trachea, bronchi, bronchioles, pulmonary lobules with their alveoli, the diaphragm, and all muscles concerned with respiration itself.

The most urgent and critical need for maintaining life is a continued, uninterrupted supply of oxygen. Oxygen is supplied to the body through the process of respiration. The term *respiration* is loosely used to describe three distinct but interrelated processes:

- **Pulmonary ventilation,** which involves the movement of air into and out of the lungs
- **Gas transport,** which involves the exchange of gases between the air in the lungs, the blood, and the cell
- **Cellular respiration,** which involves the use of oxygen in the catabolism of energy-yielding substances for the production of energy

Respiration, one of the body's regulating systems, helps to maintain physiologic dynamic equilibrium. It also compensates for rapid adjustment to changes in metabolic states.

The air passages permit air to flow from the external environment to pulmonary blood, and they modify the air taken in by warming it, moistening it, and removing noxious substances. Airway efficiency is determined by the following factors:

- Shape and size of each portion of the respiratory tract (nasal cavity, pharynx, larynx, trachea, bronchi, bronchioles, alveolar sacs)
- Presence of a ciliated, mucus-secreting, epithelial lining throughout most of the respiratory tract
- Character and thickness of respiratory tract secretions
- Compliance of the cartilaginous and bony supports
- Pressure gradients
- Traction on airway walls
- Absence of foreign substances in the lumen of the respiratory tract

An alteration of any of these factors will affect the ease with which air flows through the air passages, or effective airway clearance. Congenital anomalies, injuries, allergies, or disease will cause airflow resistance if these factors are abnormally affected. For example, resistance occurs if there is stenosis or narrowing of any portion of the respiratory tract, a loss of the cilia that ordinarily sweep out foreign substances, any thick or tenacious secretions, a loss of elasticity, or the presence of foreign objects.

RESPIRATORY TRACT SECRETIONS

The tracheobronchial tree is made up of repeated branching tubes. It is a tubular airway that serves as a conduit for the passage of air from the external environment to the alveolar-capillary exchange unit (Figure 37-1). The inner surface of the tracheobronchial tree is lined with ciliated columnar epithelium interspersed with goblet cells (see Figure 37-1, *B*). The gelatinous mucus (gel layer) produced by **goblet cells** is normally discharged into the tubular lumen. In some obstructive pulmonary diseases, mucus secretion is greatly increased, making it difficult for the cilia to transport secretions along the airway.

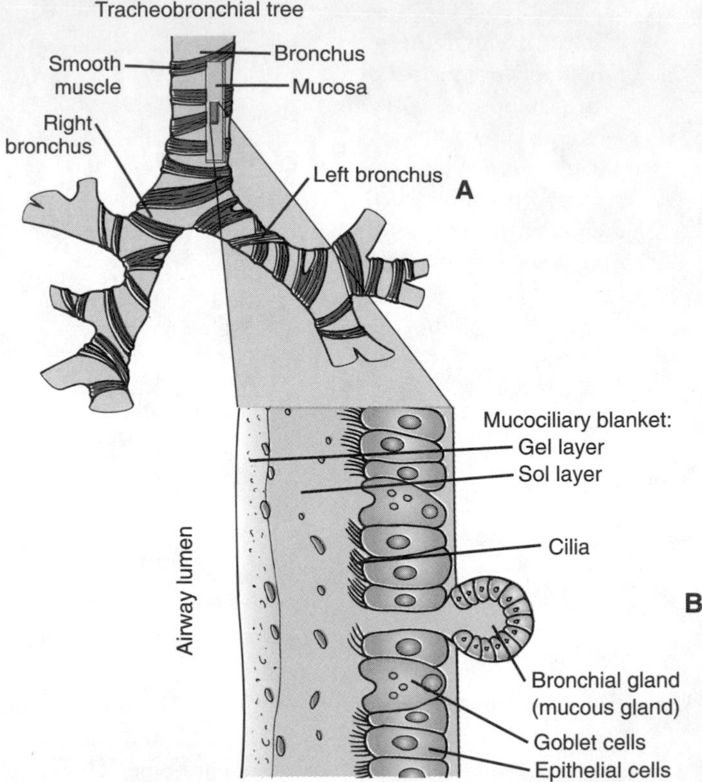

Figure 37-1 Tracheobronchial tree and bronchial smooth muscle. **A,** Diagram of the tracheobronchial tree. **B,** Cut-out section of inner lining of the bronchus.

The **bronchial glands,** which are located in the submucosa of the tracheobronchial tree, secrete a relatively watery fluid (sol layer) through ducts leading to the surface of the ciliated epithelium (see Figure 37-1, *B*). Under vagal (parasympathetic) control, the bronchial glands can be stimulated by irritant agents or aerosol drugs to release their contents into the lumen of the airway.

The products of the goblet cells and bronchial glands form the sol-gel film that makes up the mucociliary blanket. This protective blanket of fluid bathes the ciliated epithelium of the tracheobronchial tree. In addition, the cilia continuously propel the sol-gel film up toward the larynx along the respiratory tree. The normal adult produces approximately 100 mL of respiratory secretions per day and swallows this material without being aware of it. The process of moving mucus along the tracheobronchial tree is called **mucokinesis.** The mucociliary blanket is a basic concern in most chronic obstructive pulmonary disease. The cilia must sustain appropriate function; a dry atmosphere causes the respiratory secretions to become thick and tenacious, which tends to interfere with ciliary movements. Thus adequate humidity should be maintained to prevent a change in the normal consistency of the respiratory secretions.

BRONCHIAL SMOOTH MUSCLE

Smooth Muscle Arrangement. An important structure of the tracheobronchial tree is the smooth muscle. The mass of muscle fibers along the bronchi progressively increases as it extends down toward the distal bronchioles. Isolated muscle fibers may be found as far down as the alveolar ducts. The smooth muscle fibers are arranged along the length of the tubular tree in a double helical or spiral pattern, and this formation profoundly influences the diameter or the lumen of the airways. Because of this structural feature, the effect of muscle contraction reduces both the diameter and the length of the bronchus (see Figure 38-1, C).

Nerve Supply. The airway or tracheobronchial tree is innervated by the autonomic nervous system. The balance maintained between parasympathetic and sympathetic stimuli during rest influences the tone of the bronchial smooth muscle. Activation of the parasympathetic fiber (vagus nerve) releases acetylcholine, which results in **bronchoconstriction,** a narrowing of the lumen of the bronchial airway. By contrast, stimulation of the sympathetic fiber and the sympathoadrenal system releases epinephrine and norepinephrine from the adrenal medulla into the circulation. Their action on the $beta_2$ receptor sites in the bronchial smooth muscle produces **bronchodilation** by means of smooth muscle relaxation, which improves ventilation to the lungs.

Receptors. Several types of receptors are found along the bronchial airway. The release of acetylcholine activates muscarinic receptors during stimulation of the parasympathetic system, whereas the sympathetic system affects adrenergic receptors. Most of the adrenergic receptors present in the bronchial smooth muscle are $beta_2$ receptors that are stimulated mainly by epinephrine released from the adrenal medulla. $Beta_1$ receptors are also found, although the ratio of $beta_2$ to $beta_1$ receptors is approximately 3:1. Thus bronchial smooth muscle is supplied primarily by $beta_2$ receptors. The sympathomimetic drugs used principally as bronchodilators stimulate the $beta_2$ receptors. Because many of these agents are not purely selective in their pharmacologic effect, they also stimulate the $beta_1$ receptors in the heart, as well as alpha receptors in the lungs and peripheral arterioles. The side effects on the heart are increased cardiac output, tachycardia, and dysrhythmia. The presence of alpha receptors on the bronchial smooth muscle is relatively scarce, and their stimulation results in only mild bronchoconstriction.

Bronchodilation. The $beta_2$ adrenergic receptors mediate bronchodilation. Presumably this mechanism is initiated by epinephrine released from the adrenal medulla and norepinephrine released from the peripheral sympathetic nerves. Also located in the cell membrane is an enzyme system known as adenyl cyclase. In the presence of magnesium ions, adenyl cyclase catalyzes the action of adenosine triphosphate (ATP) in the cytoplasm of the cell to produce cyclic 3′5′ adenosine monophosphate (cyclic 3′5′ AMP). Cyclic 3′5′ AMP then performs its important function—inducing the relaxation of bronchial smooth muscle, or bronchodilation. The hormone epinephrine is designated as the "first messenger"; cyclic 3′5′ AMP is designated as the "second messenger." As a final action, cyclic 3′5′ AMP is inactivated by an enzyme, phosphodiesterase, which catalyzes it to the inactive 5′ AMP. This results in a fall in the cyclic 3′5′ AMP level. A xanthine drug such as theophylline may inhibit the action of phosphodiesterase. As a consequence, the cyclic 3′5′ AMP level remains elevated, thereby affecting smooth muscle dilation (see Figure 38-4).

Circulating catecholamines can exert their effects on $beta_1$, $beta_2$, and alpha receptors. Clients with asthma may have a normal reaction to both alpha and beta stimulation through a reduced cyclic AMP response, by an abnormally sensitive response to alpha stimulation, and by an exaggerated response to the muscarinic agonists via the vagal pathways. This exaggerated bronchoconstrictive airway response may result from the effects of a decrease in cyclic AMP, histamine effects on smooth muscle, the vagal reflex pathway, an increase in cyclic guanylic acid secondary to calcium influx, and a histamine-induced release of the contents of mast cells. Bronchodilation is induced by circulating catecholamines or the administration of a sympathomimetic agent.

Circulating catecholamines reach the lung via the circulation and interact with the $beta_2$-adrenergic receptors in the cell membrane of the bronchial smooth muscle cell.

Bronchoconstriction. The bronchial smooth muscle is innervated by the parasympathetic fibers from the vagus nerve. Acetylcholine released from the terminal interacts with the muscarinic receptors on the membrane of the cell. Stimulation of the muscarinic receptor increases the activity of the enzyme guanylate cyclase in the membrane, thereby promoting the rate of formation of cyclic 3′5′ guanosine monophosphate (cyclic 3′5′ GMP) from guanosine triphosphate (GTP) (see Figure 38-4). The cyclic 3′5′ GMP level affects the bronchial muscle by producing bronchoconstriction. Alpha receptors found on the bronchial smooth muscle have a similar involvement with this mechanism. On activation, the alpha receptors also increase the level of cyclic GMP. Furthermore, cyclic 3′5′ GMP stimulates the release of chemical mediators from the mast cell during an asthmatic attack, and these mediators are responsible for causing bronchoconstriction.

CONTROL OF RESPIRATION

Central Control. The basic rhythm for respiration is initiated and maintained in the medullary rhythmicity area, which is located beneath the lower part of the floor of the fourth ventricle in the medial half of the medulla. Neurons that control inspiration and expiration intermingle and discharge or fire impulses alternately. Signals from the spinal cord, the cerebral cortex and midbrain, the apneustic area of the pons, and the pneumotaxic area of the upper pons can enter the medullary rhythmicity area, modify the rhythm of respiration, and contribute to the normal pattern of respiration.

Normally, the human organism is unaware of the respiratory process. However, voluntary influence and control of breathing are possible. This is important when a client must learn to voluntarily control breathing patterns.

Peripheral Control. The medullary rhythmicity area is also influenced by various sensory and peripheral stimuli, the vasomotor center, reflex mechanisms (e.g., the Hering-Breuer reflex), the chemoreceptors in the carotid and aortic bodies, and the baroreceptors in the carotid sinus and aortic arch. Fear, pain, stress, blood pressure, body temperature, and blood levels of oxygen and carbon dioxide can all modify the activity of the respiratory centers.

The humoral regulation of respiration is achieved primarily through changes in the concentrations of oxygen, carbon dioxide, or hydrogen ions in body fluids. In a healthy individual, carbon dioxide is the chief respiratory stimulant. An increase in the carbon dioxide tension of the blood directly stimulates the inspiratory and expiratory centers, which increases both the rate and the depth of breathing. This results in a blowing off of carbon dioxide to keep the carbon dioxide tension of the blood constant. The pH of the blood is determined by the ratio of bicarbonate ion (HCO_3) to carbon dioxide. When the carbon dioxide content of the blood is increased, there is a subsequent increase in the formation of carbonic acid in the blood. This alters the bicarbonate/carbonic acid ratio from the normal value of 20:1 and results in acidosis. Conversely, a decrease in the carbon dioxide content of the blood results in alkalosis. Therefore respiration is important for regulating the pH of the blood by controlling the carbon dioxide tension of the blood.

Basically, changes in arterial oxygen concentration have little, if any, direct effect on the respiratory center. However, if the arterial oxygen concentration falls below normal, the chemoreceptors in the carotid and aortic bodies are stimulated and in turn stimulate the respiratory center to increase alveolar ventilation. This mechanism operates primarily under abnormal conditions such as chronic obstructive pulmonary disease.

SUMMARY

The highest priority for the survival of the human organism is an adequate, uninterrupted supply of oxygen. Oxygen is supplied to the various body tissues by the processes of pulmonary ventilation, gas transport, and cellular respiration. Although it is possible to influence and control the respiratory pattern voluntarily, the rhythm and depth of pulmonary ventilation are generally initiated and maintained centrally in the medulla and influenced peripherally by reflex mechanisms, chemoreceptors, and baroreceptors.

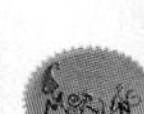

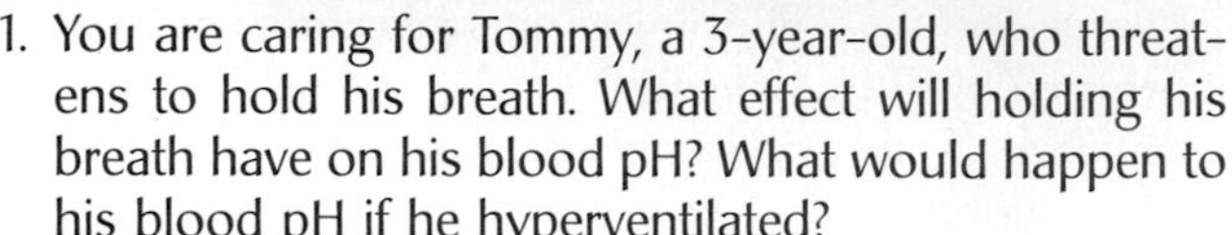

Critical Thinking Questions

1. You are caring for Tommy, a 3-year-old, who threatens to hold his breath. What effect will holding his breath have on his blood pH? What would happen to his blood pH if he hyperventilated?
2. It is known that smoking decreases the number of cilia in the respiratory airway. What will occur as the result of this change?

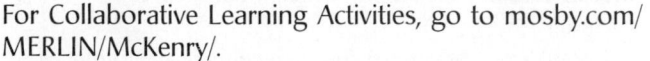

Collaborative Learning Activities

For Collaborative Learning Activities, go to mosby.com/MERLIN/McKenry/.

BIBLIOGRAPHY

Anderson, K.N., Anderson, L.E., & Glanze, W.D. (Eds.). (1998). *Mosby's medical, nursing, & allied health dictionary* (5th ed.). St. Louis: Mosby.

Guyton, A.C. & Hall, J. E. (2000). *Textbook of medical physiology* (10th ed.). Philadelphia: W.B. Saunders.

McCance, K.L. & Huether, S.E. (1998). *Pathophysiology: The biological basis for disease in adults and children* (3rd ed.). St. Louis: Mosby.

Seeley, R.R., Stephens, T.D., & Tate, P. (1995). *Anatomy and physiology* (3rd ed.). St. Louis: Mosby.

Thibodeau, G.A. & Patton, K. (1999). *Anatomy and physiology* (4th ed.). St. Louis: Mosby.

Van Wynsberghe, D., Noback, C.R., & Carola, R. (1995). *Human anatomy and physiology* (3rd ed.). New York: McGraw-Hill.

38 Mucokinetic, Bronchodilator, and Antiasthmatic Drugs

Chapter Focus

Clients using mucokinetic and bronchodilator drugs may have ineffective breathing patterns, ineffective airway clearance, or impaired gas exchange. Nurses involved in caring for clients with these nursing diagnoses use a variety of technologies with which they must be knowledgeable. These agents are used with clients who have respiratory disorders and with clients who have respiratory problems caused by nonrespiratory disorders.

Learning Objectives

1. Describe effective aerosol therapy, including the number and size of droplets, side effects, and expected outcomes for client respiratory status.
2. Compare the advantages and disadvantages of water and saline as diluents.
3. Identify the therapeutic goals of mucolytic and bronchodilator drugs.
4. Compare and contrast the sympathomimetic bronchodilator drugs.
5. Identify drugs and beverages in the xanthine group.
6. Discuss the use of cromolyn and nedocromil, sympathetic agonists, ipratropium, leukotriene antagonists, xanthine derivatives, and corticosteroid drugs in the treatment of asthma.
7. Implement the nursing management of the care of clients receiving mucokinetic and bronchodilator drug therapy.

Key Terms

aerosol therapy, p. 705
expectorants, p. 706
mucokinetic agents, p. 704
mucolytics, p. 706
mucus, p. 704
nebulizer, p. 705
sputum, p. 704
xanthine derivative, p. 709

Key Drugs [✓]

albuterol, p. 716
cromolyn, p. 724
ipratropium, p. 718
theophylline, p. 720
zafirlukast, p. 719

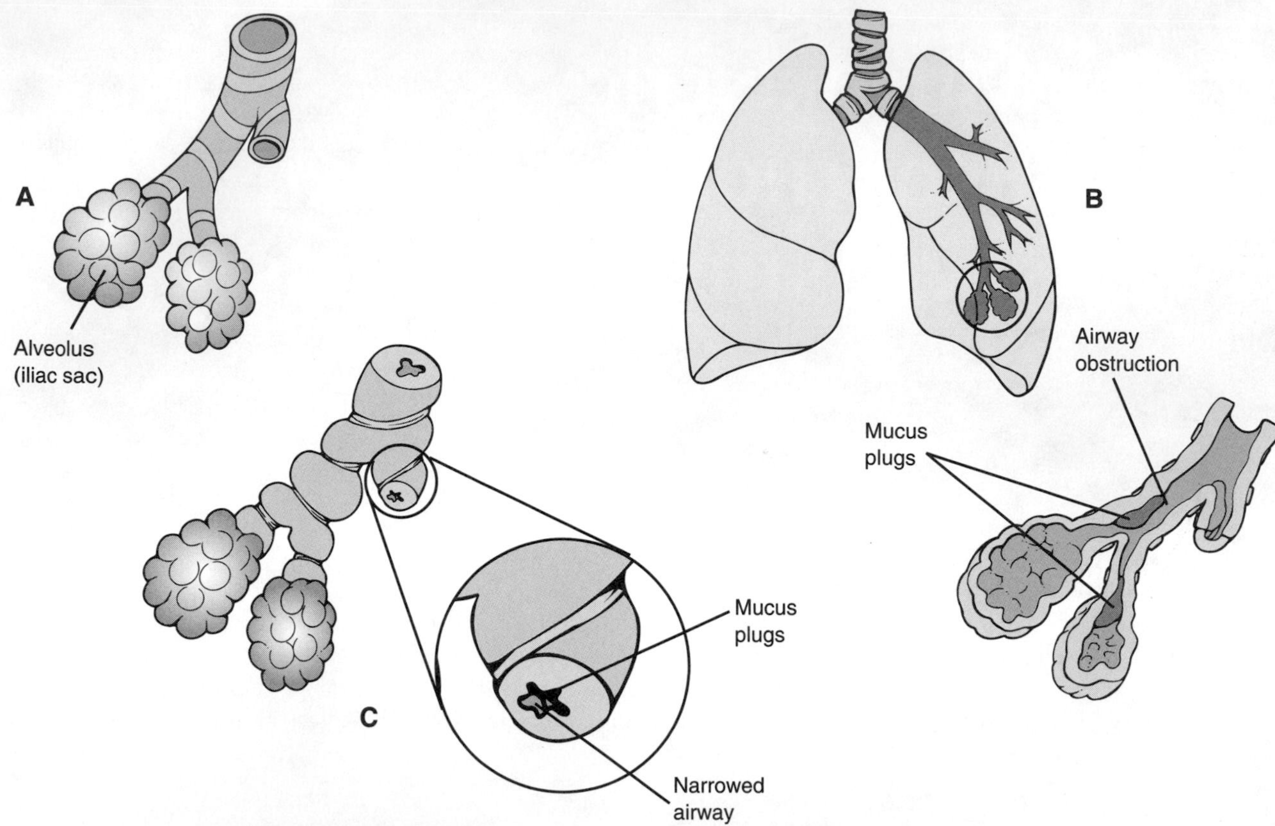

Figure 38-1 Bronchiole in normal state (A) and during an asthma attack (B). An asthmatic attack is illustrated by bronchial muscle spasms, inflammation, and excessive mucus, resulting in mucus plugs, edema, and trapped air in the air sacs (alveoli); this causes airway obstruction. C, Total amount of air inhaled and exhaled is decreased because of air trapped in the lungs after expiration.

Mucokinetic and bronchodilator drugs help to maintain the patency of the respiratory tract. They are the two main groups of drugs discussed in this chapter.

Mucokinetic Drugs

Mucokinetic agents promote the removal of abnormal or excessive respiratory tract secretions by thinning hyperviscous mucus, which allows for a more effective ciliary action. These agents prevent sputum retention, which may result from abnormal ciliary activity, defects in airflow, or a modification in cough effectiveness. **Sputum** (or phlegm) may be defined as an abnormal, viscous secretion that is an excretory production of the lower respiratory tree. It consists mainly of **mucus**, a proteinaceous material that has a mucopolysaccharide as its major component. In addition, sputum contains deoxyribonucleic acid (DNA) molecules, which are derived from the breakdown of mucosal cells, leukocytes, and bacteria. These products are responsible for the characteristic heavy quality and yellow color of the sputum. The terms *sputum* and *mucus* should not be used interchangeably. Sputum is an abnormal secretion originating in the lower respiratory tract, whereas mucus is a normal secretion produced by the surface cells in the mucous membrane.

Individuals with respiratory disorders such as chronic bronchitis develop disturbances of the mucociliary blanket, resulting in a significant impairment of the process of mucus clearance (Figure 38-1).

Mucus plugging and the pathogenic colonization of microorganisms occur in the lower respiratory tract. These changes lead to an overproduction of thick, tenacious sputum. The advantage provided by the mucokinetic drugs is that they alter the consistency of the sputum, thereby promoting the eventual expectoration, or expulsion, of these secretions.

DILUENTS

Water

The most commonly used agent to dilute respiratory secretions is water. Persons with chronic obstructive pulmonary disease (COPD) often suffer from dehydration; thus respiratory secretions are retained. These secretions become highly viscous in consistency and lead to widespread plug formation in the respiratory tree. Water may be administered by ultrasonic **nebulizer,** a device for producing a fine spray. Small amounts of water deposited on the gel layer of the respiratory tree appear to reduce the adhesive characteristics and general viscosity of the gelatinous substances found in this layer. Care is needed with clients receiving restricted fluid intake, because water can be absorbed through the inhalation route. If fluid intake is being measured, water added to the nebulizer and absorbed through the inhalation route must be added to the client's intake record. If a client's fluid intake is not restricted, large amounts of water are usually encouraged to liquefy the respiratory secretions.

Saline Solutions

Normal saline (0.9% sodium chloride) is a physiologic (isotonic) salt solution that exerts the same osmotic pressure as plasma fluids. Therapy by nebulization is well tolerated, resulting in the hydration of respiratory secretions. A hypotonic solution (0.45% sodium chloride) is thought to provide deeper penetration into the more distal airways or into the alveoli via the inhalation route, whereas inhalation of a hypertonic solution (1.8% sodium chloride) stimulates a productive cough because the particles deposited on the respiratory mucosa are irritating. A hypertonic solution osmotically attracts fluid out of the mucosa and into the respiratory secretions, thereby promoting their excretion.

AEROSOL THERAPY

Aerosol therapy is a form of inhaled, topical pulmonary treatment. An aerosol is a suspension of fine liquid or solid particles dispersed in a gas or in a solution that is deposited in the respiratory tract. Dry powder inhalers are also available. Liquid or solid particles range in size from approximately 0.005 to 50 μm in diameter. Nebulizers are designed to deliver a maximum number of particles of a desired size. Thus aerosol therapy is delivered through nebulization. The terms *aerosol therapy* and *nebulization therapy* are often used interchangeably. Aerosol therapy promotes the following:

- Bronchodilation and pulmonary decongestion
- Loosening of secretions
- Topical application of corticosteroids and other drugs
- Moistening, cooling, or heating of inspired air

The effectiveness of nebulization therapy depends on the number of droplets that can be suspended in an inhaled aerosol. This number is directly related to the size of the droplets, with smaller droplets suspended in greater numbers than large droplets. Small droplets (approximately 2 to 4 μm in diameter) are more likely to reach the periphery of the lungs—the alveolar ducts and sacs. Small droplets are more effective for the absorption of bronchodilators. Larger droplets (8 to 15 μm in diameter) are deposited primarily in the bronchioles and bronchi. Droplets of more than 40 μm in diameter are deposited primarily in the upper airway (mouth, pharynx, trachea, and main bronchi).

The rate and depth of breathing are other factors that determine the effectiveness of nebulization therapy. Rapid or shallow breathing decreases the number, as well as the retention, of droplets that reach the periphery of the lungs. Rapid breathing permits significant amounts of fine droplets to escape during expirations; few droplets will escape if the breath is held long enough after deep inspiration to permit droplet deposit in the lung periphery.

Almost all large droplets are retained somewhere in the larger air passages. Large droplets are used for keeping large airways (nose, trachea) moist and for loosening secretions. Slow and deep breathing is required for proper lung aeration and penetration of the mist into peripheral lung areas. The breath should be held for a few seconds after a full inspiration.

Droplet size can be controlled by the amount of pressure used to force oxygen or room air through the solution to produce a mist. The nebulizer tubing diameter, its length, and its number of bends affect turbulent flow and mist temperature. With most nebulizers the maximum density of the inhaled mist is achieved by making the flow of mist as smooth and direct as possible. Nebulizers commonly used in hospitals produce similar mists. A *note of precaution:* drug reconcentration can occur with both jet and ultrasonic nebulizers if a humidity deficit occurs.

The evaporation of water molecules causes a gradual increase in drug concentration in the droplets, thus increasing the risk of drug toxicity. Controlling temperature and humidity can prevent this toxicity.

The main groups of drugs conventionally administered by aerosol include bronchodilators, cromolyn (Intal), nedocromil (Tilade), and steroid preparations. It is important to remember that the lung is an absorptive organ and is therefore a route of access for drugs to enter the systemic circulation. For example, after entering the blood, inhalation anesthetic agents exert their main effect on the central nervous system (CNS). When used as a method of administering drugs, aerosol therapy is supposed to minimize systemic absorption and side effects. Certain bronchodilator aerosols produce cardiovascular effects simply because the drug may possess a property that adversely influences cardiac action after absorption into the bloodstream.

When combination inhalation aerosols are prescribed for a client without specific instructions for the sequence of administration, the nurse should be aware of the proper recommendations for drug administration. For example, if corticosteroids (Beclovent, Vanceril) or cromolyn (Intal) or nedocromil (Tilade) are prescribed to be administered with ipratropium (Atrovent), the ipratropium should be administered 5 minutes before either of the other drugs to promote bronchodilation. Whenever a beta agonist (Alupent, Proventil) is prescribed with ipratropium (Atrovent), the beta agonist is always administered first, with a 5-minute wait before administration of the second drug. Do not administer both aerosols in rapid sequence, because there is the possibility of inducing fluorocarbon toxicity; such rapid adminis-

BOX 38-1

Therapeutic Tips

Selective $beta_2$ drugs such as albuterol, salmeterol, and others provide the most rapid relief of acute asthmatic symptoms. An SC injection is not more effective than inhalation therapy and often causes more side effects/adverse reactions; therefore its use is usually reserved for persons with very severe dyspnea that prevents them from responding to inhalation therapy. These products are used in combination with inhaled corticosteroids or other antiinflammatory drugs.

Oral selective $beta_2$ drugs are considered less effective than the same agents administered by inhalation. They also have a longer onset of action time and often cause more tremors than inhaled preparations.

Corticosteroid inhalation products are less toxic than oral preparations and are preferred for long-term use. Corticosteroids are very potent agents and effective antiinflammatory agents (Gross & Ponte, 1998). Oral candidiasis can occur with use if proper preventive measures are not followed, such as rinsing and/or gargling with water after each use. Other adverse reactions may occur with continuous, long-term use; check a current drug reference for information.

Theophylline is considered a less potent bronchodilator than inhaled adrenergic drugs; thus it has limited usefulness in acute, intermittent asthma. Theophylline is more useful in chronic asthma.

Cromolyn and nedocromil are drugs used to inhibit bronchospasm (the response of a client with asthma to allergens and exercise). These drugs are used to decrease airway hyperreactivity in mild to moderate bronchial asthma (Gross & Ponte, 1998). They do not have bronchodilator effects and thus should not be used for the treatment of acute asthma.

Clients need to be taught the proper techniques for use of a metered dose inhaler and other inhaling devices as ordered. Spacer units are often suggested for young children; at times, other clients with coordination difficulties may also benefit from their use. Home use of peak flow meters (PFMs*) and documentation of the results are also often recommended for clients with moderate to severe asthma. With proper use, this device may help in the early detection of airflow obstruction, which allows for a more timely intervention (National Asthma Education and Prevention Program, 1998).

*PFM readings provide an objective measurement of peak expiratory flow rate and daily variability determinations before and after the use of medications, especially bronchodilators.

tration also decreases the effectiveness of the drug. Combivent contains ipratropium and albuterol combined in an aerosol container. It is indicated for bronchospasm in clients with COPD. Box 38-1 lists additional therapeutic tips.

MUCOLYTIC DRUGS

Mucolytics are drugs that exert a disintegrating effect on mucus. These agents, also called **expectorants,** promote coughing or spitting and thereby the removal of mucus or other exudates from the lung, bronchi, or trachea. One of the more commonly used mucolytics is acetylcysteine.

acetylcysteine [a se teel sis′ tay een] (Mucomyst, Airbron ♣)

Acetylcysteine reduces the thickness and stickiness of purulent and nonpurulent pulmonary secretions by decreasing the viscosity of the respiratory mucoprotein molecules into smaller, more soluble, and less viscous strands. It also effects similar changes in the DNA molecule and cellular debris. This decrease in the viscosity of bronchial secretions aids their removal by coughing, postural drainage, or suctioning.

Acetylcysteine is indicated as an adjunct treatment for thick or abnormal mucus in bronchopulmonary disease, cystic fibrosis, or atelectasis caused by a mucus obstruction. It is also used as a diagnostic aid in a variety of bronchial studies, such as bronchospirometry and bronchograms.

When administered systemically, acetylcysteine is a specific antidote for an acetaminophen overdose; it reduces the extent of liver injury by altering hepatic metabolism, and it maintains or restores concentrations of glutathione. Glutathione is necessary for the inactivation of an intermediate metabolite of acetaminophen, which is believed to be hepatotoxic on accumulation.

With inhalation therapy, some acetylcysteine is absorbed from the pulmonary epithelium, although its primary effects are local on the mucus in the lungs. It produces an effect within 1 minute when inhaled; direct instillation via an intratracheal catheter produces an immediate effect. The peak response from inhalation occurs within 5 to 10 minutes. Acetylcysteine is metabolized in the liver.

The side effects/adverse reactions of acetylcysteine include fever, nausea, vomiting, runny nose, throat or lung irritation, unpleasant odor during drug administration, clammy skin, sore mouth, stomatitis, hemoptysis, rash, and respiratory difficulties. No significant drug interactions have been reported with acetylcysteine when administered by inhalation.

The usual dosage for adults and children by nebulization using a face mask, mouthpiece, or tracheostomy is 3 to 5 mL of a 20% solution or 6 to 10 mL of a 10% solution inhaled three or four times daily. To treat an acetaminophen overdose, acetylcysteine is administered orally in a dose of 140 mg/kg initially, then 70 mg/kg every 4 hours for an additional 17 doses.

■ Nursing Management

Acetylcysteine Therapy

■ **Assessment.** Use acetylcysteine with caution in older adults, in debilitated clients, and in clients with asthma or severe respiratory insufficiency. This drug may increase airway obstruction, and bronchospasm may occur in susceptible clients. Determine the client's sensitivity to acetylcysteine.

■ **Nursing Diagnosis.** With the administration of acetylcysteine, the client is at risk for the following nursing diagnoses/collaborative problems: impaired comfort related to the unpleasant odor of the drug during administration, facial stickiness after nebulization by face mask, nausea or vomiting, and throat irritation; impaired oral mucous membrane (stomatitis); ineffective airway clearance related to increased amounts of sputum; and the potential complications of allergic dermatitis, bronchospastic allergic reaction, and hemoptysis.

■ **Implementation**

■ ***Monitoring.*** The frequency of the client's cough and its character should be monitored and documented. The character and quantity of expectorated material should be observed. Percussion and auscultation of the chest should be accomplished on a periodic basis.

■ ***Intervention.*** Ultrasonic nebulizers are recommended for administration of the drug. Hand nebulizers are discouraged because the output is too small and the fluid particles too large. The prescriber may order the administration of a bronchodilator before acetylcysteine therapy. The nebulized drug may be inhaled either directly or by the use of a plastic face mask, face tent, mouthpiece, or oxygen tent. The nebulizer may be used with an intermittent positive pressure breathing (IPPB) apparatus. An IPPB apparatus is a ventilator that assists or controls respiration by delivering compressed gas under positive pressure into a person's airways until a preset pressure is reached. Passive exhalation is allowed through a valve, and the cycle begins again as the flow of gas is triggered by inhalation. When the drug is nebulized using a dry gas, the drug may become concentrated because of evaporation of the solution. The last remaining quarter of the drug can be diluted with an equal part of sterile water for injection to continue nebulization so the client is ensured of receiving the appropriate dosage.

After nebulization, the face should be washed with water to remove the sticky coating left by the drug. The equipment should be cleaned immediately after use to prevent blockage of the fine parts and corrosion of the metal ones. In many health care agencies, respiratory therapists administer these treatments, but nurses are responsible for evaluating the effectiveness of treatments, and they may be responsible for administering them at night and with the client in the home.

Some clients may develop nausea and vomiting; this may result from the disagreeable odor of the nebulized drug and quantity of respiratory secretions eliminated. With the aid of these agents and postural drainage, most individuals can expectorate pulmonary secretions without further assistance; however, suctioning may be indicated for older adults or debilitated clients. Provide mouth care after inhalation treatment to minimize nausea and vomiting.

Because of the release of hydrogen sulfide, solutions of acetylcysteine will harden rubber and become discolored on contact with certain metals. Acetylcysteine solutions should be used with equipment made of glass, plastic, or stainless steel. If the vacuum seal has been broken on the bottle, the solution should be refrigerated to slow oxidation and used within 48 hours.

When acetylcysteine is administered orally, it is tolerated better if it is well chilled (over ice), diluted in soft drinks or citrus juices, and sipped with a straw from a covered container. The diluted solution should be used within the hour.

■ ***Education.*** Alert the client to the disagreeable odor of the drug and the expected result of increased expectoration. The client should clear the airway by coughing before the drug is administered by aerosol. Instructions should be provided on the correct use of the nebulizer.

■ **Evaluation.** The expected outcome of acetylcysteine mucolytic therapy is that the client will experience increased sputum production and expectoration and a decrease or absence of adventitious breath sounds.

■ **Antidotal Use.** When acetylcysteine is administered as an antidote for acetaminophen overdose, it is most beneficial when started within 10 hours of the overdose, but it is still beneficial if started within the first 24 hours (Zed & Krenzelok, 1999). The client should be supported through gastric lavage or induced emesis, the administration of activated charcoal, and other appropriate therapies. The greatest risk of acetaminophen overdose is hepatotoxicity. The potential for hepatotoxicity can be assessed from plasma acetaminophen concentrations; monitoring these concentrations and liver function studies is essential. Liver function studies should be performed every 24 hours for at least 96 hours after the ingestion of the overdose. Monitor fluid and electrolyte balances, renal function, and cardiac function. Nursing care is provided for the client with a knowledge deficit or a high risk for self-harm.

The expected outcome of acetylcysteine as an antidote for acetaminophen toxicity is that the client's liver function studies will be within normal limits and that the underlying issue, knowledge deficit or high risk for self-harm, will be resolved.

Other Expectorants

Over the years many other products have been used as expectorants in both prescription and over-the-counter (OTC) medications. Guaifenesin is the only expectorant listed by the Food and Drug Administration (FDA) in Category I (safe and effective); it is reviewed in Chapter 11. A prescribed respiratory inhalant product is recombinant human DNase or dornase alfa (Pulmozyme). This product is used to increase expectoration in cystic fibrosis.

dornase alfa (Pulmozyme)

Cystic fibrosis is a respiratory disease associated with thick secretions caused by an accumulation of DNA from degenerating neutrophils and inflammation. Dornase alfa is an enzyme that digests extracellular DNA, thus improving pulmonary function and reducing the risk for the respiratory tract infections common with cystic fibrosis (Johnson, Butler, Konstan, Breen, & Morgan, 1999). The use of this product has resulted in a decrease in respiratory infections, hospitalizations, and medical costs (Franz & Cohn, 1994).

A significant improvement in pulmonary function is seen within 3 to 7 days, and a decrease in respiratory infections is seen within weeks to several months. The side effects/adverse reactions of dornase alfa include chest pain, sore throat, laryngitis, skin rash, conjunctivitis, hoarseness, upset stomach, dyspnea, fever, and rhinitis.

The usual dosage for adults and children 5 years and older is 2.5 mg daily inhaled via nebulization.

▪ Nursing Management

Dornase Alfa Therapy

▪ **Assessment.** It should be determined that the client does not have a sensitivity to dornase alfa, Chinese hamster ovary cell products, or any other component of the product. Although drug interactions have not been studied with dornase alfa, it has been administered safely with other medications commonly taken by clients with cystic fibrosis (e.g., bronchodilators, antibiotics, corticosteroids, enzymes, vitamins, and analgesics). Establish a baseline assessment of the client's respiratory status.

▪ **Nursing Diagnosis.** The client receiving dornase alfa has the potential for the following nursing diagnoses: impaired comfort (chest pain, sore throat, conjunctivitis); impaired skin integrity (rash); and disturbed body image (hoarseness, voice changes).

▪ **Implementation**

▪ ***Monitoring.*** The client's respiratory status should be carefully monitored for cough, breath sounds, sputum, forced expiratory volume, vital capacity, and tidal volume.

▪ ***Intervention.*** Dornase alfa is administered via a nebulizer. Refer to the package literature for recommended devices. Wash hands thoroughly before assembling the nebulizer and mouthpiece. Do not mix or dilute dornase alfa with other agents. It should be administered every day; a decrease in pulmonary function occurs within 48 hours after therapy is stopped.

▪ ***Education.*** Instruct the client on the appropriate nebulizer and ensure its correct use with dornase alfa. Advise the client not to use a face mask but only a mouthpiece. Do not use the medication if it is cloudy or discolored. Advise the client that the treatment should be administered at the same time each day and that compliance is essential. Although some improvement may be seen a week after therapy starts, it may require weeks or months for the full benefits to be experienced.

▪ **Evaluation.** The expected outcome of dornase alfa therapy is that the client's airway is patent, the breathing pattern is effective without fatigue or dyspnea, and the breath sounds are clear.

DRUGS THAT ANTAGONIZE BRONCHIAL SECRETIONS

Anticholinergic agents decrease secretions and also make them hard to expectorate. Although not generally used for this purpose, atropine may be given cautiously to decrease secretions and excessive expectoration in certain forms of bronchitis. Many remedies used to treat colds contain atropine, an anticholinergic. Ipratropium, which is described in the following section, is an anticholinergic agent more commonly used for respiratory conditions but primarily for its bronchodilating effects.

BRONCHODILATOR DRUGS

Bronchodilator drugs are primarily used to treat chronic pulmonary diseases such as asthma, chronic bronchitis, and emphysema. The major causes of ineffective airway clearance include (1) bronchial smooth muscle contraction (asthma), (2) mucus hypersecretion (chronic bronchitis), and (3) mucosal edema or inflammation (chronic bronchitis). Bronchial asthma may appear with some or all of these symptoms (see Figure 38-1).

In the past asthma was classified on the basis of the stimuli that induce the attack, such as intrinsic asthma caused by emotional factors or exercise and extrinsic asthma caused by pollens, molds, dust, or animal hair. Because many asthmatics have a combination-type asthma, this type of classification is not considered useful. The National Institutes of Health (NIH) defines asthma as a lung disease with reversible airway obstruction, airway inflammation, and increased airway sensitivity to stimuli (Self & Kelly, 1995). Clients are classified according to the frequency and severity of their asthma attacks (mild, moderate, or severe); this information is the most useful when considering pharmacologic interventions:

- *Mild.* Intermittent attacks occur less than 1 to 2 times weekly, or nocturnal asthma symptoms occur less than 1 to 2 times monthly. Peak expiratory flow (PEF) is >80% and is normal after bronchodilator use; PEF variability is <20%.
- *Moderate.* Attacks occur more than 1 to 2 times weekly, or nocturnal asthma symptoms occur more than twice a month. A beta-agonist inhaler is used almost daily. PEF is 60% to 80% and is normal after bronchodilator use; PEF variability is 20% to 30%.
- *Severe.* Asthmatic symptoms are frequent and continuous (including nocturnal asthma), plus the client has been hospitalized for asthma in the previous year.

The major drugs used in the treatment of asthma include sympathomimetic drugs, theophylline, cromolyn, nedocromil, and the corticosteroids. Figure 38-2 gives an overview of the effects of the antiasthmatic medications, and Figure 38-3 illustrates their primary sites of action. The

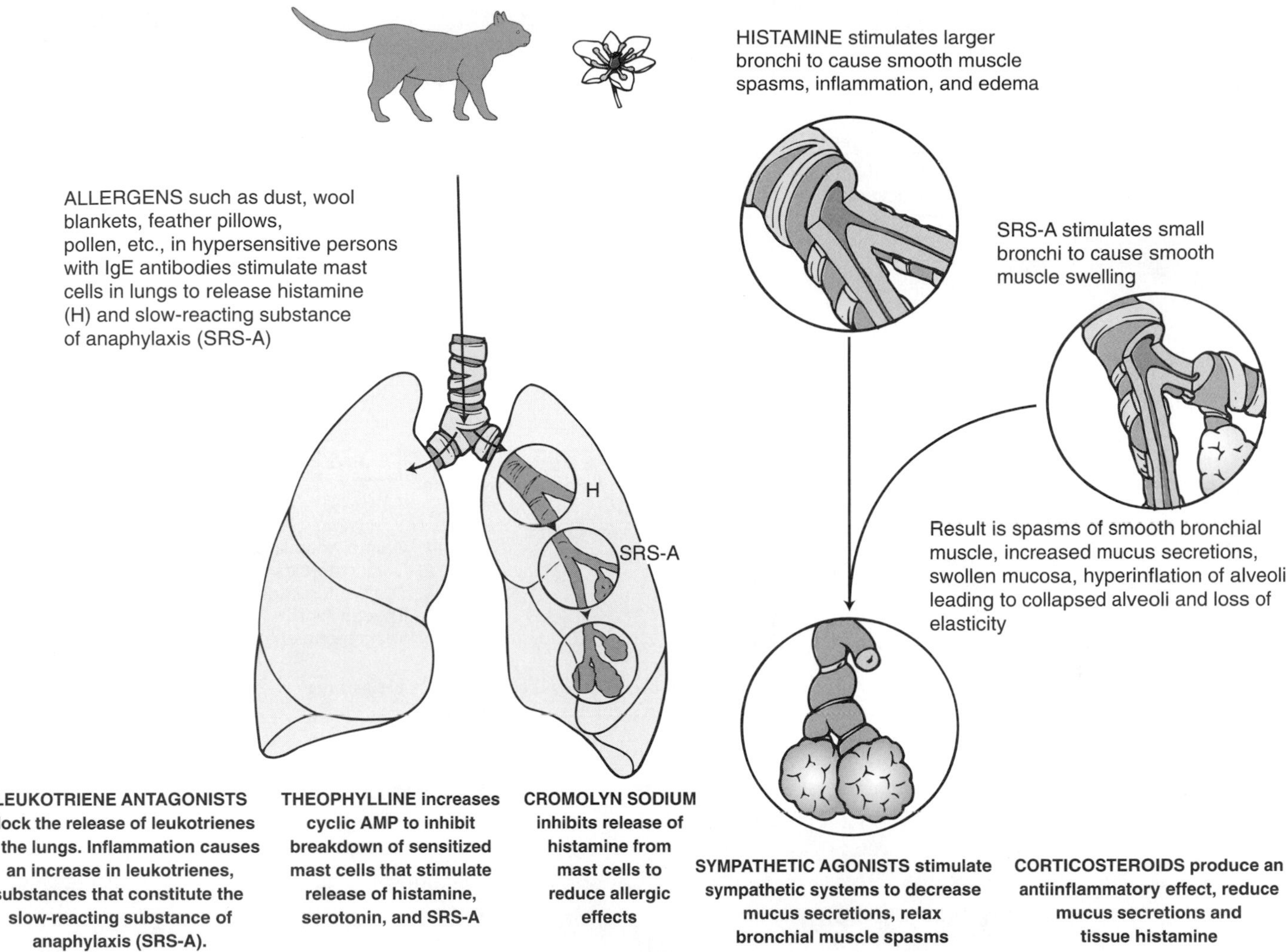
HISTAMINE stimulates larger bronchi to cause smooth muscle spasms, inflammation, and edema
ALLERGENS such as dust, wool blankets, feather pillows, pollen, etc., in hypersensitive persons with IgE antibodies stimulate mast cells in lungs to release histamine (H) and slow-reacting substance of anaphylaxis (SRS-A)
SRS-A stimulates small bronchi to cause smooth muscle swelling
H
SRS-A
Result is spasms of smooth bronchial muscle, increased mucus secretions, swollen mucosa, hyperinflation of alveoli leading to collapsed alveoli and loss of elasticity
LEUKOTRIENE ANTAGONISTS block the release of leukotrienes in the lungs. Inflammation causes an increase in leukotrienes, substances that constitute the slow-reacting substance of anaphylaxis (SRS-A).
THEOPHYLLINE increases cyclic AMP to inhibit breakdown of sensitized mast cells that stimulate release of histamine, serotonin, and SRS-A
CROMOLYN SODIUM inhibits release of histamine from mast cells to reduce allergic effects
SYMPATHETIC AGONISTS stimulate sympathetic systems to decrease mucus secretions, relax bronchial muscle spasms
CORTICOSTEROIDS produce an antiinflammatory effect, reduce mucus secretions and tissue histamine

Figure 38-2 Overview of the effects of various antiasthmatic medications.

principal agents used in the treatment of airway obstruction include sympathomimetic drugs and **xanthine derivatives.** A xanthine derivative is any one of the closely related alkaloids (caffeine, theobromine, and theophylline) and has properties to stimulate the CNS, produce diuresis, and relax smooth muscle. Prophylactic antiasthmatic agents also prevent airway obstruction in individuals with certain types of asthma. Most of these drugs enhance the production of cyclic 3′5′ adenosine monophosphate (AMP) in bronchial smooth muscle cells to cause bronchodilation (Figure 38-4).

For a Concept Map on asthma, go to mosby.com/MERLIN/McKenry/.

■ Nursing Management

Bronchodilator Drug Therapy

■ **Assessment.** Bronchodilators are primarily indicated for the treatment of chronic pulmonary conditions such as asthma, chronic bronchitis, and emphysema. A baseline assessment should include a description of the client's respiratory status—respiratory rate and effort, the use of accessory muscles, nasal flaring or lip pursing, breath sounds per auscultation, circumoral pallor or cyanosis, the presence of cough and/or sputum, activity intolerance, PEF readings, and signs of impaired gas exchange (e.g., anxiety, confusion, and irritability). In addition, the following diagnostic tests are usually performed: arterial blood gas (ABG) values, chest x-ray examination, sputum culture, complete blood count (CBC), pulmonary function studies, and electrocardiogram (ECG).

■ **Nursing Diagnosis.** Because these diseases interfere with the basic human need for air, expect the client to exhibit anxiety, not only during acute episodes but also in anticipation of them. Ineffective airway clearance, ineffective breathing pattern, impaired gas exchange, and activity intolerance are nursing diagnoses common to clients receiving bronchodilator therapy. (See the Nursing Care Plan on p. 711 for other selected nursing diagnoses.)

■ **Implementation**

■ ***Monitoring.*** The client's respiratory status should be monitored on an ongoing basis to evaluate the drug's effectiveness using indicators from the baseline assessment. Monitor for side effects of bronchodilators, including tachycardia and dysrhythmias. Depending on the specific drug, serum levels may be monitored.

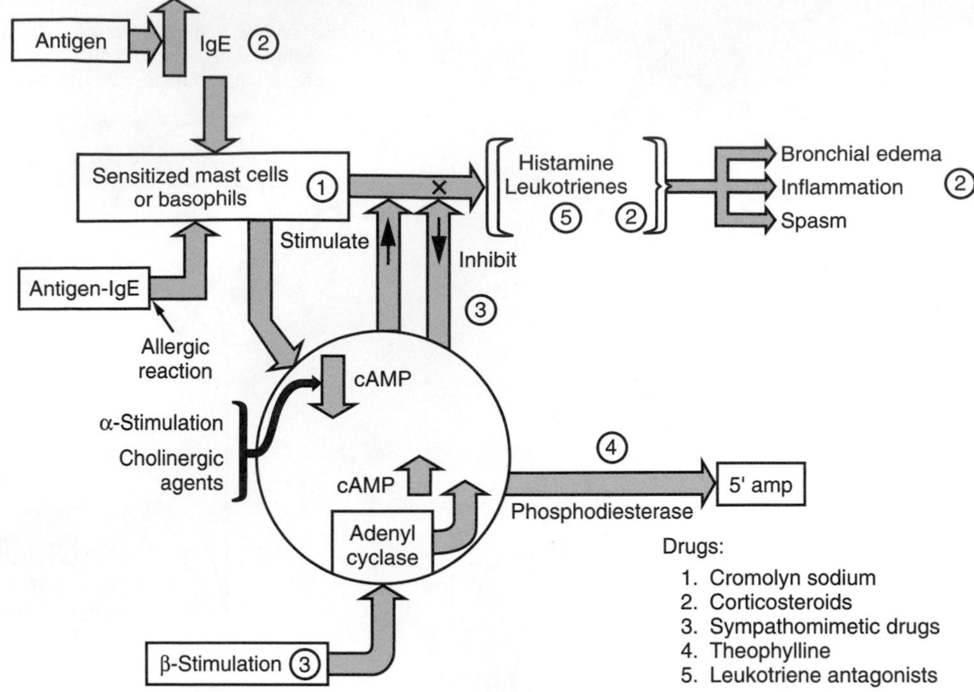

Figure 38-3 Major sites of action of drugs used to treat asthma.

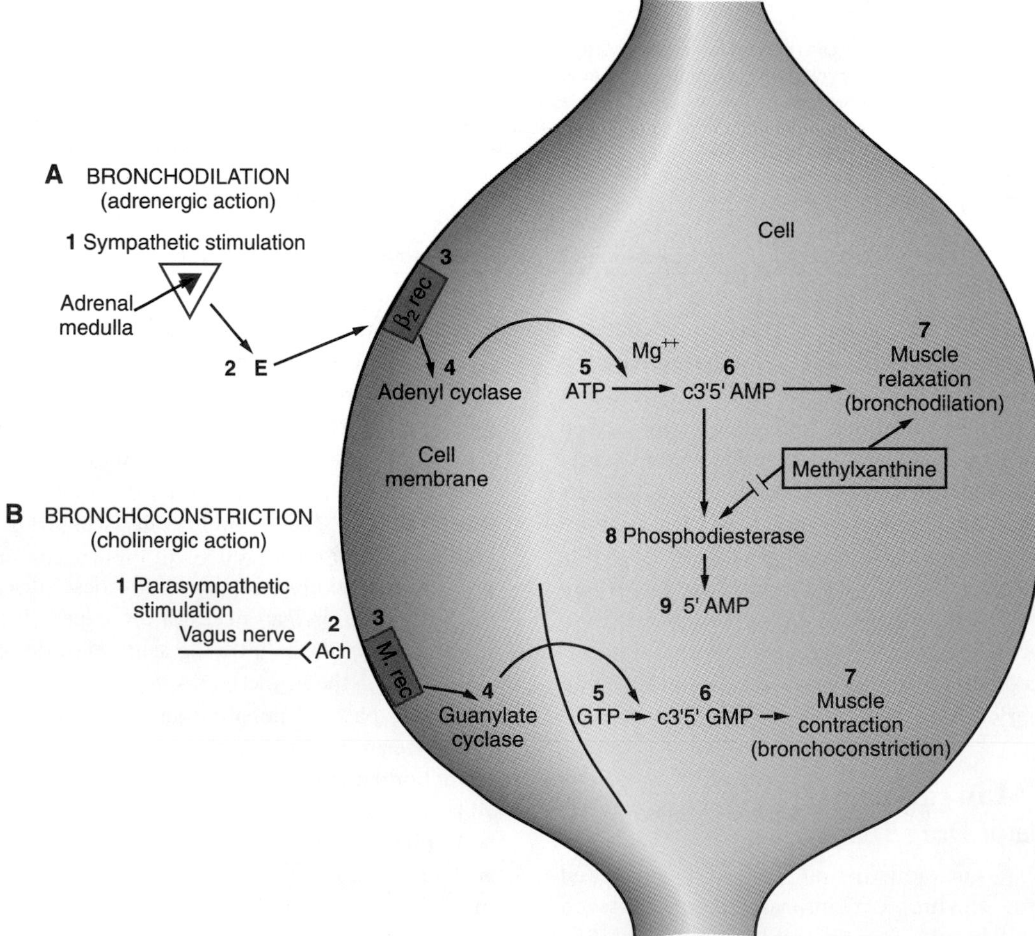

Figure 38-4 Mechanism of bronchial smooth muscle action. **A,** Bronchodilation pathway. **B,** Bronchoconstriction pathway. (*E,* Epinephrine; *Ach,* acetylcholine; β_2 *rec,* β_2 receptor; *M. rec,* muscarinic receptor.)

Nursing Care Plan
Selected Nursing Diagnoses Related to Bronchodilators

Nursing Diagnosis	Outcome Criteria	Nursing Interventions
Ineffective airway clearance related to reversible airway obstruction	Coughs effectively and expectorates sputum Absence of abnormal breath sounds Absence of sputum production Fluid intake of at least 3000 mL/24 hr unless contraindicated	Assess respiratory status every 4 hours. Assist client to turn, cough, and deep breathe as necessary. Provide adequate humidification as ordered. Monitor characteristics of sputum every 8 hours and record. Encourage fluids to at least 3000 mL daily.
Activity intolerance related to reversible airway obstruction	Increasing level of activity Pulse, respiration, and blood pressure remain within acceptable limits during activity	Plan with client for increasing levels of activity, including activities that have priority for the client. Identify and limit the factors that decrease the client's tolerance for activity. Monitor pulse rate, respiration, and blood pressure while increasing the level of activity.
Deficient knowledge related to medication regimen	Client will describe underlying condition and how the drug relates to the condition, how and when to take the medication, common drug interactions, safety precautions, common side effects/adverse reactions, and which of those warrant reporting Client will self-administer medication safely and accurately	Administer oral forms with food to minimize gastrointestinal distress. Emphasize the need for the drug to be taken as prescribed around-the-clock. Caution the client not to self-administer any OTC drugs without prescriber consultation. Advise the client to notify the prescriber if the usual dosage fails to be therapeutic or if the condition worsens after treatment. Instruct the client to minimize the ingestion of foods and beverages containing xanthine (coffee, chocolate, colas). Emphasize the need for ongoing contact with the prescriber for serum levels and evaluation.

■ ***Intervention.*** Provide supportive nursing care with oxygen and fluid replacement to bring respirations within the normal range for rate, depth, and effort during acute episodes.

Nebulized bronchodilator solutions are available as both nonsterile and sterile-filled products. Nonsterile products contain additives (e.g., sulfites, benzalkonium chloride, or chlorobutanol) to prevent bacterial growth. These additives are capable of inducing bronchospasm in a concentration-dependent manner that diminishes the bronchodilator effects of the drug for some clients. For hourly or continuous nebulization of bronchodilator drugs, use only additive-free solutions (Asmus, Sherman, & Hendeles, 1999).

■ ***Education.*** An important aspect of nursing management is to provide clients with information that enables them to maintain some measure of control over what is happening to them and thus decrease their anxiety. Education for clients receiving bronchodilators should be an integral part of their care and include instruction on factors that tend to precipitate an acute episode. They should also be instructed to maintain a diary of symptoms and the time and dose of medications during attacks, to explain their medication program, to demonstrate how to take inhaled medications (see the Nursing Research box on p. 712) and care for the inhaler, to describe the measures to take during an attack, and to identify the signs and symptoms to report to the health care provider. Advise the client against floating the metered dose inhaler in water to estimate the amount of drug remaining in the canister; instead, the client should keep a record of the number of inhalations for accuracy.

■ **Evaluation.** The expected outcome of bronchodilator therapy is that the client will have an adequate respiratory status as evidenced by the absence of adventitious breath sounds, PEF readings in the satisfactory range, a normal arterial blood oxygen saturation of 95% or more, ABGs within normal limits (PaO_2 >60 mm Hg, $PaCO_2$ 35 to 45 mm Hg), pH 7.35 to 7.45, and respirations that are unlabored and within the normal limits for age.

SYMPATHOMIMETIC DRUGS

Based on their receptor action, three types of sympathomimetic drugs are recognized: (1) nonselective adrenergic drugs that have alpha, $beta_1$ (cardiac), and $beta_2$ (respirato-

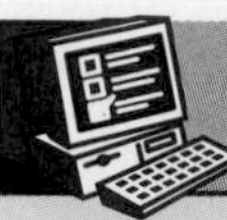

Nursing Research
Teaching the Use of Metered Dose Inhalers

Citation: Interiano, B. & Guntupalli, K.K. (1993). Metered-dose inhalers: Do health care providers know what to teach? *Archives of Internal Medicine, 153*(1), 81-85.

Abstract: Many clients do not know how to use a metered dose inhaler and depend on their health care providers to instruct them. Nurses and physicians may need more skill themselves.

Interiano and Guntupalli, investigators from Baylor College of Medicine, reached this conclusion after surveying 100 asthmatic clients and 170 health care professionals and evaluated their ability to complete the 6 steps that should be followed when using the device. They found that 65% of the clients, 82% of the nurses, and 39% of the house medical staff received a "poor" rating. This rating means they were unable to perform more than 2 steps correctly. Respiratory therapists performed the best—85% of them knew at least 5 of the 6 steps.

The investigators concluded that better training is essential for both clients and health care providers, so that everyone is familiar with the following procedure:

1. Remove the inhaler cap and shake.
2. Exhale normally.
3. Administer the medication at the beginning of the next inhalation.
4. Slowly inhale.
5. Hold your breath for up to 10 seconds.
6. Wait at least 30 seconds before inhaling a second puff.

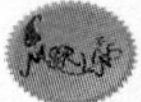

Critical Thinking Questions

- Why is it essential for clients to use an inhaler correctly?
- How could you effectively evaluate the client's/nurse's ability to use an inhaler correctly?

ry) activities (e.g., epinephrine); (2) nonselective beta-adrenergic drugs with $beta_1$ and $beta_2$ effects (e.g., isoproterenol); and (3) selective $beta_2$ agents (e.g., albuterol [Proventil], bitolterol [Tornalate], formoterol (Foradil), isoetharine [Bronkosol], metaproterenol [Alupent], pirbuterol [Maxair], salmeterol [Serevent], terbutaline [Brethine]), which act primarily on $beta_2$ receptors with minor activity at $beta_1$ receptors in the lungs (bronchial smooth muscle). Two additional bronchodilator drugs are available in Canada: fenoterol (Berotec) and procaterol (Pro-Air).

Nonselective Adrenergic Drugs

Nonselective adrenergic drugs such as epinephrine, ephedrine, and others possess both alpha- and beta-receptor stimulating properties. Alpha stimulation appears to mediate vasoconstriction to reduce mucosal edema, whereas $beta_2$ stimulation produces bronchodilation and vasodilation. In contrast, $beta_1$ receptor action causes unwanted cardiac side effects such as increases in heart rate and the force of myocardial contraction.

Undesirable effects on $beta_2$ receptors include skeletal muscle tremors, tachycardia, palpitations, increased CNS stimulation, hypokalemia (after large doses are administered), glycogenolysis (the breakdown of glycogen to glucose), and gluconeogenesis (the formation of glycogen from fatty acids and proteins rather than from carbohydrates).

epinephrine [ep i nef′ rin] (Adrenalin)

Epinephrine induces the relaxation of bronchial smooth muscle by stimulating $beta_2$ receptors in the lungs, thus relieving bronchospasm, increasing vital capacity, and reducing airway resistance. It also inhibits the bronchoconstriction induced by the release of histamine and substances released during anaphylaxis.

Epinephrine is indicated for the treatment of bronchial asthma, bronchitis, and other pulmonary disease states and for the prevention of bronchospasm and bronchial asthma. Only slight absorption occurs with inhalation, but systemic absorption increases if large doses of epinephrine are administered. Systemic absorption is rapid with IM or SC administration.

The onset of action is within 3 to 5 minutes with inhalation, 6 to 15 minutes with SC injection, and variable by IM injection. The duration of action is between 1 and 3 hours with inhalation or between 1 and 4 hours by the parenteral routes. It is metabolized at sympathetic nerve endings and other tissues with a small amount of excretion by the kidneys.

The side effects/adverse reactions of epinephrine include nervousness, insomnia, dizziness, headaches, hypotension, anorexia, nausea, a pounding tachycardia, sweating, vomiting, cold and pale skin, trembling, increased anxiety, blurred vision, mental alterations, severe muscle cramps, increased blood pressure, hallucinations, chills, fever, and difficulty in urination.

Many drug interactions have been reported with epinephrine. For example, fluorocarbon toxicity may result when epinephrine is given concurrently with a corticosteroid (or other) inhaler that also contains a fluorocarbon propellant. Teach the client to allow at least a 5-minute interval between the use of such inhalants. Alpha-adrenergic blocking agents (e.g., prazosin, tolazoline), other medications with alpha-blocking properties (e.g., phenothiazines, haloperidol), or the fast-acting vasodilators (nitrates) may block the alpha-stimulating effects of epinephrine; this may result in severe hypotension and tachycardia. Monitor closely because medical interventions may be necessary. The vasodilator effects of nitrites may also be decreased with concurrent drug administration.

The concurrent use of epinephrine with anesthetics such as chloroform, cyclopropane, and halothane may increase the risk for severe dysrhythmias. Tricyclic antidepressants or cocaine and epinephrine may increase the risk of cardiac dysrhythmias, tachycardia, hypertension, and hyperpyrexia. Such combinations should be avoided.

Beta-adrenergic blocking agents (oral, parenteral, and ophthalmic) may reduce the therapeutic effects of both agents. In addition, adverse cardiovascular side effects (e.g., hypertension, bradycardia, and heart block) may be enhanced. Avoid concurrent administration whenever possible. With the digitalis glycosides (digoxin, digitoxin), an increase in the risk for cardiac dysrhythmias may occur. If concurrent therapy is necessary, monitor with an ECG.

Ergotamine and the ergoloid mesylates may result in peripheral vascular ischemia, gangrene or, with ergotamine, severe hypertension. These drug combinations should be avoided.

Various forms of epinephrine are available, such as epinephrine (Bronkaid Mist, Primatene Mist), epinephrine bitartrate (AsthmaHaler, Medihaler-Epi), and racepinephrine (AsthmaNefrin, Vaponefrin). By inhalation, the adult dosage is usually 10 drops of a 1% solution or a diluted racepinephrine solution (2.25%) in a nebulizer. In general, one inhalation of the 1% solution or 2 or 3 inhalations of the diluted racepinephrine solution are administered. Doses may be repeated at sufficient intervals as stated in the current package inserts or the *United States Pharmacopeia Dispensing Information (USP DI)*. With the aerosol preparations, one inhalation is administered, which may be repeated in 1 minute if needed. Subsequent doses are usually administered in 3 to 4 hours. Pediatric dosages are individualized by the prescriber according to the response.

Many other adrenergic bronchodilators are available. In choosing a beta-receptor agonist, the $beta_2$ selectivity, potency, and duration of action of the drug are considered. The high incidence of undesirable cardiotoxic effects caused by the $beta_1$ property of sympathomimetic agents (nonselective agents) led to the search for a more specific $beta_2$ receptor agonist, such as isoetharine and the noncatecholamine $beta_2$ receptor agonists (albuterol, metaproterenol, and terbutaline).

■ Nursing Management

Epinephrine Therapy

The nursing management of clients receiving epinephrine is discussed in detail in Chapter 22 (p. 463). This selection should be consulted because the drug has far-reaching systemic effects. In addition, see Nursing Management: Bronchodilator Drug Therapy, p. 709. However, some nursing management relates specifically to the administration of epinephrine by inhalation.

Epinephrine and other beta-adrenergic agents may be used interchangeably during inhalation therapy. Do not administer them concurrently; allow 4 hours between doses when changing from one to another.

Instruct the client in the use of the metered dose inhaler. Teach the client to take his or her pulse rate before inhalation therapy. One inhalation may be repeated after 1 minute if necessary. Do not administer more frequently than every 3 hours as required to relieve symptoms, because excessive use may cause paradoxical bronchospasm. Symptoms should be relieved within 20 minutes. The prescriber should be notified if symptoms are not relieved with the usual dosage, because this may indicate a worsening of bronchospasm, which requires a reassessment of therapy. Advise the client to rinse his or her mouth with water to prevent the mucosal absorption of the drug. In case of emergency, the client should be taught to self-inject epinephrine subcutaneously.

Nonselective Beta-Adrenergic Drugs

Nonselective beta-adrenergic drugs exhibit both $beta_1$- and $beta_2$-agonist activity. Their main action is on the bronchial smooth muscle and on the heart. Isoproterenol is the prototype example for this drug category.

isoproterenol solution [eye soe proe ter′ e nole] (Vapo-Iso, Isuprel)

Isoproterenol is indicated for the treatment of bronchial asthma, bronchitis, and other pulmonary disease states. The onset of action by inhalation is within 2 to 5 minutes; sublingually, within 15 to 30 minutes; and by IV injection, immediately. Its duration of action is 0.5 to 2 hours by inhalation, 1 to 2 hours sublingually, and less than 1 hour by IV injection. It is metabolized in the liver, lungs, and other body tissues and excreted by the kidneys.

The side effects/adverse reactions of isoproterenol include restlessness, anxiety, insomnia, pink- or red-colored saliva, and a dry mouth or throat after inhalation. Dizziness, flushing of the skin, headache, tremors, palpitations, sweating, tachycardia, weakness, vomiting, and hypertension or hypotension have also been reported. Significant drug interactions are similar to those of epinephrine, except for the interactions noted with parenteral local anesthetics, alpha-blocking agents, and the ergoloid mesylates or ergotamine. These exceptions are due to the fact that isoproterenol does not have alpha effects.

The usual dosage with a metered dose inhaler is 1 to 2 inhalations. The client should start with 1 inhalation; a second inhalation may be taken if no relief is experienced after 2 to 5 minutes. For daily maintenance, 1 to 2 inhalations are used four to six times daily. Do not use more than 2 inhalations at a time or 6 inhalations in an hour. Using a hand bulb nebulizer in an acute asthmatic attack, 5 to 15 deep inhalations of a 0.5% nebulized solution or 3 to 7 inhalations of a 1% nebulized solution are administered. The sequence is repeated once if needed after waiting 5 to 10 minutes. Up to 5 subsequent doses per day may be administered, if necessary. For bronchospasm in COPD, a nebulizer of IPPB drug administration may be used. Pediatric dosage recommendations are similar to those for an adult, but a 0.25% to 0.5% solution is used (*Drug Facts and Comparisons*, 2000).

An isoproterenol IV injection is used as a bronchodilator for bronchospasm during anesthesia at a dose of 10 to 20 μg. The dose may be repeated if necessary.

▪ Nursing Management
Isoproterenol Therapy

The nursing management of clients receiving isoproterenol is discussed in detail in Chapter 22 (p. 466); see also Nursing Management: Bronchodilator Drug Therapy, p. 709. These selections should be consulted because the drug has both bronchodilating and cardiotonic effects. However, some interventions relate specifically to its administration by inhalation.

Instruct the client to use the nebulizer correctly. If using a metered dose inhaler, the client should allow 2 to 5 minutes between the first and second inhalations. Advise the client of the number of doses permitted in a 24-hour period, based on the literature for the particular form or delivery device of the drug. The prescriber should be notified if this limit is reached within a 24-hour period. Treatment of this frequency may indicate that other medications may need to be added to the therapeutic regimen.

Available evidence indicates that high-dose preparations of isoproterenol are associated with increased mortality, probably as the result of both long-term effects with regular use leading to worsening asthma control and acute effects resulting from their overuse in a life-threatening attack of asthma (Beasley, Pearce, Crane, & Burgess, 1999). Advise the client that sputum and saliva may turn pink with the use of the drug. Isoproterenol needs to be stored in a tight, light-resistant container and is not to be used if a precipitate or discoloration occurs. Some preparations of isoproterenol contain enough sulfites as preservatives to produce bronchospasm in clients with asthma (Asmus et al., 1999).

Selective Beta$_2$ Receptor Drugs

Catecholamine Beta$_2$ Agents

isoetharine inhalation [eye soe eth′ a reen]
(Bronkosol)

Isoetharine is a direct-acting sympathomimetic catecholamine that selectively stimulates beta$_2$ receptors to relax bronchial smooth muscle. Because it possesses a weak beta$_1$ response, there is less risk of cardiotonic side effects than with epinephrine and isoproterenol. The beta$_2$-adrenergic receptor activity of isoetharine relieves bronchospasm, increasing vital capacity and decreasing the resistance of bronchial airways. It may also inhibit the antigen-induced release of histamine by stimulating the production of cyclic 3′5′ AMP, which stabilizes the mast cell.

Isoetharine has the same indications as epinephrine. It has an onset of action of 1 to 6 minutes and a peak effect between 15 and 60 minutes. Its duration of action is 1 to 4 hours. It is metabolized in the liver, lungs, gastrointestinal tract, and other body tissues and is excreted by the kidneys.

The side effects/adverse reactions of isoetharine include dizziness, headaches, dry mouth, and a foul taste in the mouth or throat after use of the inhalation product. Nausea, anxiety, palpitations, tremors, insomnia, tachycardia, weakness, and vomiting have also been reported. Significant drug interactions are the same as for isoproterenol.

The adult bronchodilator dosage with a hand nebulizer is 4 inhalations of an undiluted 0.5% or 1% solution, usually administered every 4 hours. For IPPB or oxygen aerosolization dosage, refer to a current package insert or *USP DI*. The dosage for children has not been established.

▪ Nursing Management
Isoetharine Therapy

▪ **Assessment.** Determine initially if the client has a preexisting condition that would indicate cautious use of the drug: cardiovascular disease (e.g., hypertension, coronary artery disease, or limited cardiac reserve), hyperthyroidism, pheochromocytoma, or sensitivity to sympathomimetics. Baseline assessments are the same as those discussed in the nursing management of bronchodilator drugs. Some preparations of isoetharine contain enough sulfites to produce bronchospasm in most clients with asthma, even in those with no prior history of sulfite sensitivity (Asmus et al., 1999).

▪ **Nursing Diagnosis.** With the administration of isoetharine, the following nursing diagnoses/collaborative problems should be considered for the client: impaired comfort (dryness of the mouth and throat, headache, nausea, nervousness, trembling, and palpitations); disturbed sleep pattern (insomnia); anxiety; activity intolerance (weakness) related to overdose; ineffective airway clearance related to paradoxical bronchospasm (increase in wheezing and difficulty breathing); and the potential complication of tachycardia.

▪ **Implementation**

▪ ***Monitoring.*** The client's respiratory status should be monitored on an ongoing basis to evaluate the effectiveness of the drug. Monitor for the side effects of isoetharine, including tachycardia and dysrhythmias.

▪ ***Intervention.*** Isoetharine may be administered by metered dose inhaler or by nebulizer, IPPB, and oxygen aerosolization. The use of IPPB is currently limited as a method of aerosol deposition; the amount of drug lost in the room air and the apparatus is approximately 40% to 65%, and the amount of drug deposited in the lower airways is only about 5% to 15%. However, IPPB is a convenient procedure for helping clients with airway obstruction to breathe deeply. IPPB is generally administered by the respiratory therapist.

▪ ***Education.*** Instruct the client in the use of the inhaler (Box 38-2). Warn the client to avoid getting the spray in the eyes and to rinse his or her mouth after therapy to prevent dryness and throat irritation. Advise the client to use inhalation therapy as prescribed, because rapid relief encourages overuse. Thus tolerance to a bronchodilator agent may occur, with a potential for causing cumulative drug toxicity (e.g., palpitations, tachycardia, headache, dizziness, and nausea).

Repeated use of the inhaler may cause paradoxical airway resistance, which produces sudden dyspnea. To relieve possible bronchospasm, the prescriber may discontinue therapy and use another drug. Instruct the client to take no more

BOX 38-2

Client Education: Using an Inhaler

It is important that the client be instructed in the correct use of a metered dose inhaler before it is needed to relieve an asthma attack. The prescriber will indicate whether the closed-mouth or open-mouth technique is to be used. If the client has a choice, encourage him or her to use the open-mouth technique, because it provides better inhalation of the drug. If used incorrectly, the dose may be dispersed into the air or even swallowed. Because only 10% of an inhaled dose reaches the lungs under the best of conditions, the ability to use the metered dose inhaler appropriately is essential for the client.

A placebo inhaler should be used for the demonstration. This will enable the client to repeat the demonstration a number of times until the inhaler can be used easily and correctly.

Closed-Mouth Technique

1. Shake the container for 2 to 5 seconds.
2. Hold the inhaler with the drug container upside down.
3. Place the mouthpiece in the mouth, closing the lips tightly around it.
4. Exhale steadily and completely through the nose.
5. Inhale slowly and deeply while pressing the container down on the mouthpiece.
6. Hold your breath for as long as possible before exhaling, and then remove the mouthpiece from your mouth.
7. Wait 15 seconds.
8. Repeat steps 1 through 6.
9. Contact the prescriber if no relief is achieved after 5 minutes and the condition worsens.

Open-Mouth Technique

1. Shake the container for 2 to 5 seconds.
2. Hold the inhaler with the drug container upside down.
3. Hold the mouthpiece two finger widths (approximately 1.5 inches) in front of your widely opened mouth. Hold the container upright.
4. Exhale deeply, then inhale slowly through your mouth while pressing down firmly on the container. Continue to breathe deeply.
5. Hold your breath for a few seconds, then exhale slowly. Wait approximately 15 seconds, and then repeat steps 3 to 5 for a second inhalation. (Keep your eyes closed; a temporary blurring of vision may occur if the aerosol is sprayed into the eyes.)

Many practitioners are now advising the use of a spacer, a small tube that fits into the inhaler mouthpiece and goes into the client's mouth, to enhance the delivery of the nebulized agent to the bronchioles.

• • •

Advise the client that rinsing the mouth after using the inhaler prevents systemic absorption and minimizes dryness of the mouth. The mouthpiece should be rinsed at least once daily to avoid clogging. Stress the importance of keeping the equipment clean to prevent infection. If using a refillable inhaler, do not place more than a day's supply of drug in the inhaler. Change the solution daily.

Clients with asthma benefit greatly from the use of sympathomimetic inhalers, but they should be discouraged from using OTC inhalers because of the nonselective beta-agonist effect of the epinephrine base. The nurse needs to recognize the possibility of misuse and the consequences of abuse in order to successfully help the client with inhalant drug therapy.

Cleaning

1. Clean the inhaler and cap once a day by rinsing it in warm running water. Let it dry before using it again. Have another inhaler to use while it is drying.
2. Wash the plastic mouthpiece twice a week with mild dishwashing soap and warm water. Rinse and dry it well before putting it back.

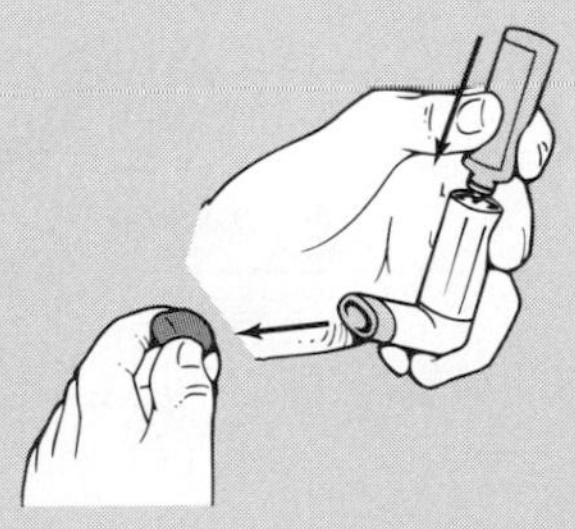

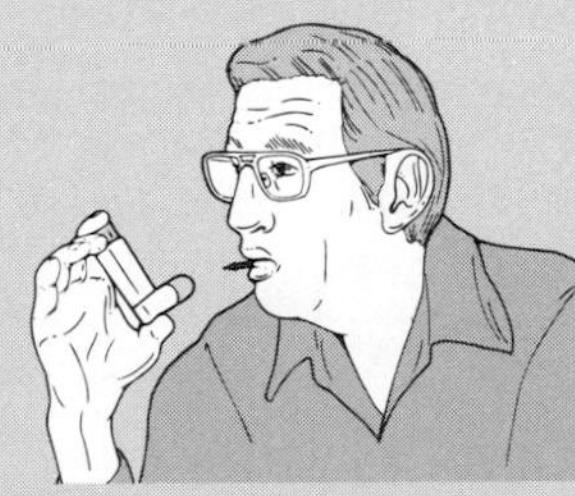

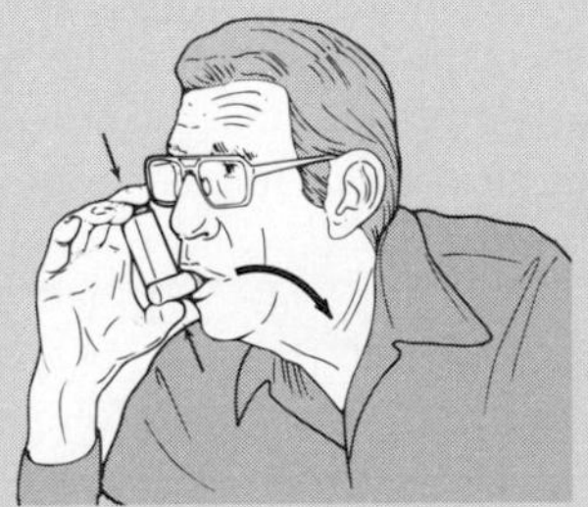

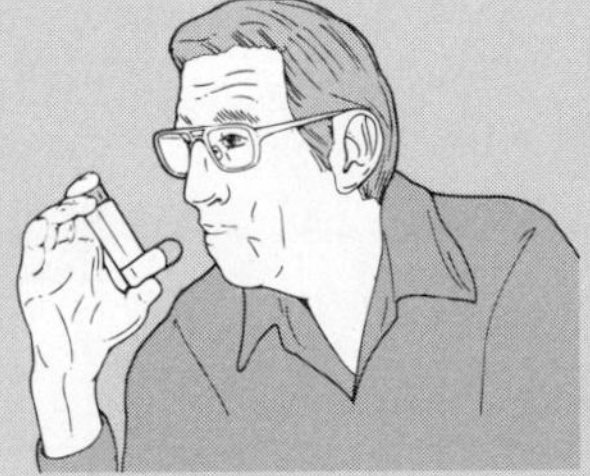

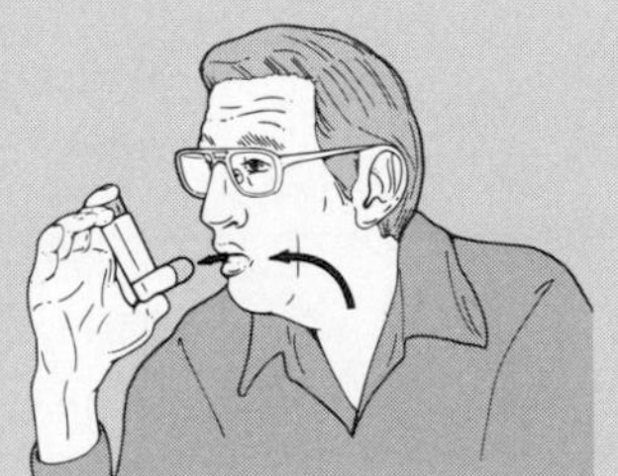

than 2 inhalations at a time and to allow 1 to 2 minutes between inhalations.

Encourage an increase in fluid intake to adequately hydrate the client, which will also aid in liquefying bronchial secretions. Inform the client that sputum may be rust-colored because of oxidation of the medication.

▪ **Evaluation.** The expected outcome of isoetharine therapy is that the client will have an adequate respiratory status as evidenced by the absence of adventitious breath sounds. The client will also have satisfactory PEF readings, a normal arterial blood oxygenation above 95%, ABGs within normal limits (PaO_2 >60 mm Hg, $PaCO_2$ 35 to 45 mm Hg), pH 7.35 to 7.45, and unlabored respirations of 12 to 20 breaths/min or within the client's normal baseline.

Noncatecholamine Beta$_2$ Receptor Drugs

Noncatecholamine drugs have two advantages over the catecholamine type agents: they are longer acting and produce fewer cardiovascular side effects. Albuterol, formoteral, and metaproterenol represent this category, although salmeterol (Serevent) is the first long-acting bronchodilator inhaler approved for twice-daily dosing.

albuterol [al byoo′ ter ole] (Proventil, Ventolin)

Albuterol, a sympathomimetic bronchodilator, possesses a relatively selective specificity for beta$_2$-adrenergic receptors in the lungs and therefore is less likely to cause unwanted cardiovascular effects. Its interaction with the beta$_2$ receptor in the cell membrane of the bronchial smooth muscle stimulates the enzyme adenyl cyclase to produce cyclic 3′5′ AMP, which results in relaxation of the smooth muscle of the bronchi (see Figure 38-4), thus relieving bronchospasm and decreasing airway resistance. In addition, this mechanism causes relaxation of the smooth muscle of the uterus and the blood vessels of skeletal muscle. However, it has been reported that high IV doses of the drug would be required to inhibit uterine contractions to delay premature labor (see the Pregnancy Safety box below).

An R-isomer of racemic albuterol, levalbuterol (Xopenex), is also available as a nebulized solution to prevent and treat bronchospasm in clients at least 12 years of age (Abramowicz, 1999). The characteristics of this drug are the same as for albuterol; it is yet to be determined whether it is more effective than albuterol (Abramowicz, 1999; Costello, 1999; Nelson, 1999) (Box 38-3).

Albuterol has the same indications as epinephrine. By inhalation, albuterol has an onset of action between 5 and 15 minutes, a peak effect in 1 to 1½ hours after two inhalations, and a duration of action of 3 to 6 hours. Orally, its onset of action is between 15 and 30 minutes, its peak effect is in 2 to 3 hours, and its duration of action is 8 hours or more (12 hours for the sustained-release dosage form). This drug is metabolized in the liver and excreted by the kidneys and in the feces.

The side effects/adverse reactions of albuterol include nausea, increased anxiety, palpitations, tremors, tachycardia, sedation, hypokalemia, difficulty in urination, dizziness, headaches, heartburn, muscle cramping, insomnia, increased sweating, vomiting, increased weakness, hypotension or hypertension, and an unusual taste in the mouth.

The adult bronchodilator dosage for inhalation is 200 to 400 μg every 4 to 6 hours. The oral dosage is 2 to 6 mg three or four times daily. This dose may be increased to a maximum of 8 mg four times daily if necessary. Extended-release tablets are administered 4 or 8 mg PO every 12 hours. Refer to the package insert for the pediatric dosage schedule.

▪ Nursing Management

Albuterol Therapy

▪ **Assessment.** Initially clients should be assessed for a previous intolerance to other sympathomimetic agents, because this may indicate an intolerance to albuterol. Albuterol should be used with caution in clients with cardiac dysrhythmias, coronary insufficiency, hypertension, or pheochromocytoma. Clients with diabetes mellitus may need an increased dosage of insulin when receiving albuterol because of drug-induced hyperglycemia. Clients with hyperthyroidism may have an exaggerated response to albuterol. Older adults are more susceptible to the effects of the drug and usually require lower dosages.

Pregnancy Safety
Mucokinetic, Bronchodilator, and Antiasthmatic Drugs

Category	Drug
B	acetylcysteine, cromolyn, dornase alfa, ipratropium, montelukast, nedocromil, terbutaline, zafirlukast
C	albuterol, aminophylline, beclomethasone, flunisolide, formoterol, isoetharine, isoproterenol, levalbuterol, metaproterenol, oxtriphylline, salmeterol, theophylline, zileuton
D	triamcinolone

BOX 38-3

Levalbuterol (Xopenex)

Levalbuterol (Xopenex) is a new sympathomimetic released in 1999 for the treatment of bronchospasm in adolescents (12 years and older) and adults with reversible obstructive airway disease. The usual dosage is 0.63 mg by nebulization three times daily (every 6 to 8 hours). For nonresponsive clients, the dose may be doubled (1.25 mg) and administered three times daily. This product must be protected from light (store in a protective foil pouch) and excessive heat; once opened, the vial is good for up to 2 weeks. The solution should be colorless; if it develops a color, discard it (*Drugs Facts and Comparisons*, 2000).

Determine interactions with the client's medication regimen. Significant drug interactions are similar to those of epinephrine, with the exception of the interactions noted with alpha-adrenergic blocking agents, ergoloid mesylate, and ergotamine. Albuterol also has a significant drug interaction with monoamine oxidase (MAO) inhibitors; the effects of albuterol on the vascular system may be enhanced.

A baseline assessment is the same as that discussed for the nursing management of the client undergoing bronchodilator therapy.

▪ **Nursing Diagnosis.** With the administration of albuterol, the client should be assessed for the following nursing diagnoses/collaborative problems: impaired comfort (dryness of the mouth and throat, unusual taste, coughing, flushing of the face, increased sweating, nausea and vomiting, heartburn, headache, weakness, muscle cramps, nervousness, trembling, palpitations, and chest pain); anxiety; disturbed sleep pattern (drowsiness or insomnia); and the potential complications of paradoxical bronchospasm (increase in dyspnea and wheezing), hypertension, and tachycardia.

▪ **Implementation**

▪ ***Monitoring.*** Monitor as discussed for other bronchodilating drugs.

▪ ***Intervention.*** A mouthpiece or a face mask may be used to administer the inhalation solution through a nebulizer. The nebulizer may be used with compressed air or oxygen, 6 to 10 L/min. A treatment lasts about 10 minutes.

▪ ***Education.*** The client should be taught the correct use of the inhaler. Inform the client that the drug may have a shorter duration of action (1 to 2 hours) after long-term use. The client should report to the prescriber a failure to respond to the usual dosage, which may mean the development of drug tolerance or worsening of the disease state. The development of tolerance may stimulate adverse reactions such as cardiac arrest if the dosage continues to be increased. Advise the client to rinse his or her mouth after inhalation therapy to prevent dryness, throat irritation, and systemic absorption. Any foul taste that occurs as a result of treatment will gradually disappear with repeated use.

Warn the client that the excessive use of aerosol may be harmful and cause paradoxical (rebound) bronchospasm, meaning that the effects of the drug are no longer therapeutic. Stress the importance of not changing the dosage or frequency of albuterol without consulting the prescriber. Chest pain, extreme dizziness and light-headedness, severe headache, palpitations, continuing tachycardia, dysrhythmias, and hypertensive episodes should be reported to the prescriber.

▪ **Evaluation.** The expected outcome of albuterol therapy is that signs of the client's anxiety should decrease as breathing becomes more effective. Wheezing, if present, should also decrease. Signs of respiratory distress such as an increased effort to breathe, increased use of accessory muscles, contraction of the abdominal muscles on expiration, and diaphoresis will decrease as the medication becomes effective. The client will respond subjectively if relief from the respiratory distress is felt.

formoterol [for mo′ ter ole] (Foradil)

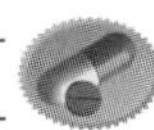

Formoterol (Foradil) is a long-acting beta-2 agonist used PRN to prevent exercise-induced bronchospasm in adults and children 12 years and older. It is administered by inhalation and has side effects similar to the other selective beta-2 agonists.

metaproterenol [met a proe ter′ e nole] (Alupent, Metaprel)

The mechanism of action for metaproterenol is the same as for albuterol; its indications are the same as epinephrine. The inhalation form of metaproterenol has an onset of action within 1 minute, a peak effect in 1 hour, and a duration of action of 1 to 5 hours after a single dose. The oral form has an onset of action within 15 to 30 minutes, a peak effect in 1 hour, and a duration of action of up to 4 hours. It is metabolized in the liver and excreted by the kidneys.

The side effects/adverse reactions of metaproterenol include anxiety, restlessness, dizziness, headaches, hypertension, muscle cramps, nausea, vomiting, palpitations, tremors, sweating, tachycardia, and weakness. Respiratory difficulties are a rare adverse reaction. The significant drug interactions are similar to those for albuterol.

The adult dosage for the bronchodilator inhalation form is 1.3 to 2.25 mg (2 or 3 inhalations) every 3 to 4 hours, not to exceed 9 mg (12 inhalations) in 24 hours. The oral dosage is 20 mg three or four times daily. A dosage has not been established for children under 6 years of age. For children 6 to 9 years old who weigh up to 27 kg, the oral dosage is 10 mg three or four times daily. Apply the adult dosage scale for children over 9 years of age who weigh at least 27 kg.

For the nursing management of metaproterenol, see the Nursing Management: Albuterol Therapy, p. 716.

salmeterol [sal met′ er ole] (Serevent ◆)

The mechanism of action of salmeterol is the same as for albuterol. Its indications are for the maintenance therapy of asthma and for the prevention of bronchospasm in clients over 12 years of age with reversible airway disease. Because of its long onset of action, it is not used for acute asthmatic attacks or for clients who can be managed with the occasional use of short-acting bronchodilator inhalers (Rosenthal et al., 1999). It may be used with clients who experience nocturnal asthma (Wiegand et al., 1999).

The inhalation form of salmeterol has an onset of action within 20 minutes, a peak effect in 3 to 4 hours, and a duration of action of 12 hours. It is metabolized in the liver and excreted by the kidneys.

Side effects/adverse reactions of salmeterol include anxiety, insomnia, dizziness, headaches, nausea, vomiting, palpitations, tremors, sweating, tachycardia, and weakness. Respiratory difficulties are a rare adverse reaction. Significant drug interactions are similar to those for albuterol.

The bronchodilator inhalation dosage for adults and children over 12 years of age is 2 inhalations (42 μg) twice daily, morning and evening, approximately 12 hours apart.

For the nursing management of salmeterol, see Nursing Management: Albuterol Therapy, p. 716.

terbutaline aerosol [ter byoo′ ta leen] (Brethaire)
terbutaline tablets and injection (Brethine, Bricanyl)

The mechanism of action of terbutaline is similar to albuterol, and the indications are the same as for epinephrine. The onset of action of terbutaline by inhalation is 5 to 30 minutes; it has a peak effect within 1 to 2 hours and a duration of action of 3 to 6 hours. Orally its onset of action is within 1 to 2 hours, with a peak effect in 2 to 3 hours and a duration of action of 4 to 8 hours. Parenterally, its onset of action is within 15 minutes, with a peak effect in ½ to 1 hour and a duration of action of 1.5 to 4 hours. It is metabolized in the liver and excreted by the kidneys.

The side effects/adverse reactions of terbutaline include tremors, increased anxiety, restlessness, dizziness, sedation, headaches, hypertension, muscle cramps, nausea, vomiting, palpitations, insomnia, sweating, tachycardia, weakness, dry mouth or throat, and an unusual taste in the mouth. Rare adverse reactions include chest pain and an increase in respiratory difficulties.

The adult bronchodilator dosage is 1 to 2 inhalations (200 to 500 μg); the second inhalation is given at least 1 minute after the first, then every 4 to 6 hours. For oral administration, a 2.5- to 5-mg tablet three times daily every 6 hours is recommended. For children 12 to 15 years of age, the dosage is 2.5 mg PO three times daily. Parenterally, the dosage is 250 μg SC, which may be repeated in 15 to 30 minutes. A total dose of 500 μg is the maximum in a 4-hour period.

For nursing management regarding terbutaline, see Nursing Management: Albuterol Therapy, p. 716.

ANTICHOLINERGIC BRONCHODILATOR AGENT

ipratropium [i pra troe′ pee um] (Atrovent)

Ipratropium is an anticholinergic drug that produces a local bronchodilation after inhalation. It is indicated for maintenance therapy (not for acute episodes) in clients with COPD (chronic bronchitis or emphysema). Although not an FDA-approved use, it is commonly used as an adjunct bronchodilator inhaler with other therapies for asthma. After administration, the onset of action is between 5 and 15 minutes, with a peak effect in 1 to 2 hours and a duration of action of 3 to 6 hours.

The side effects/adverse reactions of ipratropium include dry mouth or throat, coughing, headache, anxiety, gastrointestinal distress and, rarely, eye pain, blurred vision, tremors, tachycardia, bronchospasms, glaucoma, hives, skin rash, or stomatitis.

The usual adolescent or adult dosage is 1 or 2 inhalations three or four times daily, administered every 4 hours. Shake the unit well before using.

Combivent aerosol ◆ is a combination of ipratropium and albuterol for the treatment of bronchospasm in COPD.

▪ Nursing Management

Ipratropium Therapy

▪ **Assessment.** Because ipratropium has primarily a local, site-specific effect, the risk of side effects in proportion to its bronchodilatory benefits is minimal. However, this anticholinergic drug may precipitate or exacerbate urinary retention and angle-closure glaucoma. Concurrent use with other anticholinergic drugs might produce an additive effect. Determine any sensitivity to ipratropium or belladonna alkaloids. If a client is using the metered dose inhaler, determine if he or she is allergic to soya lecithin, soybean proteins, or other legumes such as peanuts. An accurate baseline status of the client's respiratory status should be documented.

▪ **Nursing Diagnosis.** The client receiving ipratropium therapy may be at risk for the following nursing diagnoses/collaborative problems: impaired mucous membrane (stomatitis); impaired comfort (rash, cough/dryness of mouth or throat, headache, metallic taste, nausea, sweating, trem-

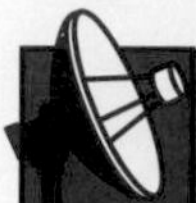

TechnologyLink
Mucokinetic, Bronchodilator, and Antiasthmatic Drugs

Video Resources

Mosby's Medical-Surgical Nursing Videotape Series, Nursing Management of COPD, ISBN 0-8151-6052-6
Mosby, Inc., 11830 Westline Industrial Drive, St. Louis, MO 63146; (800) 426-4545; www.mosby.com.

Web Resources

JAMA Asthma Information Center (www.ama-assn.org/special/asthma/asthma.htm)
This site is a resource for the health care professional. It provides an asthma newsline for current articles and reports, a treatment center with clinical guidelines for asthma management, educational resources, information on support groups, and more.

American Lung Association (www.lungusa.org/)
This site provides information on asthma, tobacco use, and related lung diseases. There is also a section on school programs and occupational health.

Asthma Information Center (www.mdnet.de/)
This site has numerous links for clients and physicians. It also lists available research grants.

alt.support.asthma (www.radix.net/~mwg/asthma-gen.html)
This site is a discussion forum approach on asthma, symptoms, causes, and treatment. It offers an interesting lay approach to the topic.

For additional WebLinks, a free subscription to the "Mosby/Saunders ePharmacology Update" newsletter, and more, go to mosby.com/MERLIN/McKenry/.

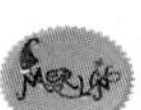

bling); impaired urinary elimination (urinary retention); ineffective airway clearance; risk for injury related to blurred vision or dizziness; and the potential complications of paralytic ileus (especially in clients with cystic fibrosis), palpitations, angle-closure glaucoma (acute eye pain), or increased bronchospasm, which may be due to other agents in the preparation (e.g., benzalkonium chloride).

■ **Implementation**

■ ***Monitoring.*** Continuing assessment of the client should include lung sounds, respirations, pulse, and blood pressure before and after each inhalation therapy until the client's response has stabilized. Monitor for the occurrence of the nursing diagnoses mentioned previously.

■ ***Intervention.*** A gas flow of 6 to 10 L/min of oxygen or compressed air is necessary for nebulization of ipratropium. A face mask or mouthpiece may be used, but the mouthpiece is preferable to reduce the risk of getting the drug into the eyes. If more than one inhalation is necessary, allow 1 minute between inhalations for the most effective results. Consult with the prescriber immediately if the client's symptoms do not improve within 30 minutes. If the client also uses a beta-agonist inhalation aerosol, it should be used 5 minutes before the ipratropium. For clients also using a corticosteroid or cromolyn inhalation aerosol, the ipratropium should be used 5 minutes before the corticosteroid or cromolyn aerosol. Do not mix ipratropium and cromolyn in a nebulizer, because they will form a precipitate.

■ ***Education.*** Caution the client to avoid contact with the eyes because temporary irritation will occur and because precipitation or worsening of narrow-angle glaucoma has been reported. As an anticholinergic, the drug may cause dryness of the mouth and throat; tell the client about the use of sugarless candies and gum or ice chips for relief. Instruct the client to inspect the oral cavity for candidiasis and to seek regular dental attention for the detection of caries.

Alert the client to contact the prescriber immediately if symptoms do not improve within 30 minutes of using ipratropium or if the client's condition becomes worse; this may indicate a worsening airway clearance or the development of another illness requiring medical care.

Advise the client against floating the metered dose inhaler in water to estimate the amount of drug remaining in the canister; the client should instead keep a record of the number of inhalations for accuracy.

■ **Evaluation.** The expected outcome of ipratropium inhalation therapy is that the client will experience and maintain a decrease or absence in respiratory distress; the respiratory rate and effort will be within the normal limits for the client.

LEUKOTRIENE ANTAGONISTS

montelukast [mon te loo′ cast] (Singulair ◆)
zafirlukast [za feer′ loo cast] (Accolate)
zileuton [zye loo′ tahn] (Zyflo)

Zafirlukast blocks the leukotriene receptors D_4 and E_4, which are components of the slow-reacting substance of anaphylaxis. Zileuton blocks the synthesis of leukotriene. Zileuton is the first lipoxygenase inhibitor approved in the United States. By blocking lipoxygenase, it interferes with the formation of substances that cause mucus plugs and constrict bronchial airways. Therefore these drugs can reduce the inflammation, mucus secretion, and bronchoconstriction associated with asthma. Montelukast is a selective leukotriene receptor inhibitor; it inhibits cysteinyl leukotriene receptors. Cysteinyl leukotrienes, by-products of arachidonic acid metabolism, bind to leukotriene receptors and are associated with the pathophysiology of asthma (airway edema, smooth muscle contraction and inflammation) (Devillier, Baccard, & Advenier, 1999a). Therefore montelukast is a more selective leukotriene antagonist. All three agents are indicated for the treatment and/or prophylaxis of chronic asthma (Devillier et al., 1999b; Nicosia, 1999).

When administered orally, all three drugs are rapidly absorbed and bound to plasma proteins (mainly albumen). Zafirlukast and montelukast are 99% bound; zileuton is 93% bound. The onset of action for zileuton is 2 hours; with zafirlukast, it is about 1 week before an improvement in asthma symptoms is noted. With montelukast, the onset of action occurs after the first dose, and peak levels are reached in 3 to 4 hours; the duration of action of montelukast is 24 hours. These drugs are metabolized in the liver, with montelukast and zafirlukast excreted primarily in feces.

The side effects/adverse reactions of the leukotriene antagonists include headache, nausea, an increased incidence of infection (especially in clients over 55 years of age), abdominal upset or pain, weakness, liver function impairment with zileuton (flu-like symptoms, fatigue, lethargy, pruritus, upper right abdominal pain, jaundice), and perhaps Churg-Strauss syndrome with zafirlukast when corticosteroid therapy is reduced or discontinued. Churg-Strauss syndrome is an allergic disorder that presents with a flu-like syndrome, fever, muscle pain, weight loss, eosinophilia, vasculitic rash, cardiac problems, neuropathy and, if left untreated, damage to major organs. The side effects/adverse reactions of montelukast include headache, gastrointestinal distress, weakness, cough, dental pain, fever, nasal congestion, and rash.

The adult and adolescent dosage of zileuton is 600 mg PO four times daily; for zafirlukast, it is 20 mg PO twice daily, 1 hour before or 2 hours after a meal; and for montelukast, it is 10 mg PO in the evening.

■ Nursing Management
Leukotriene Antagonist Therapy

■ **Assessment.** The use of leukotriene antagonists is not recommended during breastfeeding. Clients over 55 years of age may experience a greater incidence of mild or moderate infections, particularly respiratory infections. Because there have been incidences of hepatitis with the administration of zileuton and elevated hepatic enzymes with all of these drugs, clients with a history of alcoholism or hepatic impairment should not take these drugs or should take them only with great caution. Sensitivity to the leukotriene antagonists should be determined. Because leukotriene antagonists are known to inhibit cytochrome P-450 3A4 in vitro, concurrent use of medications known to be metabolized by that cytochrome should be monitored carefully (e.g., astemizole [Hismanal], cisapride [Propulsid], cyclosporine [Sandimmune], felodipine [Plendil], isradipine [DynaCirc], nicardipine [Cardene], nifedipine [Procardia], or nimodipine [Nimotop]). The same holds true with montelukast and zafirlukast and drugs metabolized by cytochrome P-450 2CP, such as carbamazepine (Tegretol), phenytoin (Dilantin), or tolbutamide (Orinase). Both zafirlukast and zileuton significantly increase prothrombin times when administered concurrently with warfarin. Monitor the prothrombin times and International Normalization Ratios (INRs) closely, and monitor the client for bleeding tendencies; warfarin dosages may need to be decreased. Zileuton increases the serum levels of beta-blocking agents and theophylline (Theo-Dur). Dosage adjustments and close monitoring are necessary with the concurrent use of zileuton with either beta blockers or theophylline.

A baseline assessment of the client should include a description of the respiratory status—respiratory rate and effort, the use of accessory muscles, nasal flaring or lip pursing, breath sounds per auscultation, circumoral pallor or cyanosis, the presence of cough and/or sputum, activity intolerance, PEF readings, and signs of impaired gas exchange (e.g., anxiety, confusion, and irritability). In addition, the following diagnostic tests are usually performed: ABG values, chest x-ray examination, sputum culture, CBC, pulmonary function studies, hepatic function studies, and ECG.

■ **Nursing Diagnosis.** With the administration of leukotriene antagonist therapy, the client should be assessed for the following nursing diagnoses/collaborative problems: impaired comfort (headache, dental pain, nausea, nasal congestion, rash); hyperthermia; risk for infection; ineffective airway clearance; and the potential complications of liver function impairment and Churg-Strauss syndrome.

■ **Implementation**

■ ***Monitoring.*** In addition to monitoring the client's respiratory status as described in previous nursing management sections, hepatic enzyme determinations should be monitored for increases that would indicate impaired liver function. For clients who are taking zafirlukast and being weaned from corticosteroid asthma medications, monitor for Churg-Strauss syndrome, which is a systemic eosinophilic vasculitis characterized by flu-like symptoms (fever, muscle aches, weight loss), rash, increasing respiratory symptoms, or neuropathy.

■ ***Intervention.*** Administer zafirlukast on an empty stomach, at least 1 hour before or 2 hours after meals.

■ ***Education.*** Advise the client on the importance of using leukotriene antagonist therapy every day at regularly scheduled times, even if symptom-free. Although these drugs are not to be used to treat acute episodes of asthma, they should continue to be used through any acute episodes. Alert the client not to discontinue or reduce the dosage of any drugs without consulting with the prescriber. In addition, advise the client to contact the prescriber if more inhaled, short-acting drugs are needed to relieve an acute episode or if more than the prescribed maximum number of bronchodilator inhalations in 24 hours are required for asthma control. Encourage regular visits to the prescriber for monitoring with liver enzyme tests.

■ **Evaluation.** The expected outcome of leukotriene antagonist therapy is that the client will experience fewer, less severe, or no acute episodes of asthma without any adverse reactions to the drug.

XANTHINE DERIVATIVES

The xanthine group of drugs includes caffeine, theophylline, and theobromine. Beverages from the extracts of plants containing these alkaloids have been used by humans since ancient times. Xanthine derivatives relax smooth muscle (particularly bronchial muscle), stimulate cardiac muscle and the CNS, and also produce diuresis, probably through a combined action of increased renal perfusion and increased sodium and chloride ion excretion.

The drugs in this category are methylated forms of xanthines or methylxanthines. The effectiveness of these preparations as bronchodilators depends on their conversion to theophylline, which is the active constituent. Therefore, with the exception of dyphylline, the action of xanthine depends on the content of theophylline. Xanthines inhibit mast cell degranulation and the release of histamine and other mediators that are responsible for bronchoconstriction. Because the methylxanthines impede enzymatic action, they are also called phosphodiesterase inhibitors (see Figures 38-3 and 38-4).

Slow-release theophylline products can vary in their rate of absorption and therapeutic effects, even if they have the same strength and active ingredient. It has been recommended that pharmacists not substitute for these drugs if the new product does not have proven bioequivalence (*United States Pharmacopeia Dispensing Information,* 1999). Some states do not permit generic substitution for theophylline slow-release products.

The upper therapeutic level is 20 μg/mL, although theophylline toxicity may occur in some persons at 15 μg/mL. Dosage adjustments with theophylline are also necessary under certain conditions, especially when concurrent factors affecting therapeutic effects are present. Box 38-4 lists factors that affect the therapeutic effects of theophylline.

aminophylline [am in off′ i lin] (Aminophylline, Palaron ✦)
oxtriphylline [ox trye′ fi lin] (Choledyl, Apo-Oxtriphylline ✦)
✓ **theophylline** [thee off′ i lin] (Bronkodyl, Elixophyllin)

Theophylline is the prototype of the xanthine derivatives. It competitively inhibits the action of phosphodiesterase (the enzyme that degrades cyclic 3′5′ AMP); this inhibition results in bronchodilation, as illustrated previously (see Figure 38-4). These drugs are used for the prevention and treatment of bronchial asthma and for the treatment of bronchitis, pulmonary emphysema, and COPD.

BOX 38-4

Factors Affecting the Therapeutic Effects of Theophylline

May Increase Therapeutic Effects

Age: older adults and newborns
Drugs: erythromycin, cimetidine, ciprofloxacin
Disease states: cirrhosis, pulmonary edema, congestive heart failure, and severe COPD
Diet: high carbohydrate

May Decrease Therapeutic Effects

Age: adolescence
Drugs: phenobarbital, phenytoin
Substances: tobacco, marijuana
Diet: high protein

Oral liquids and uncoated tablets of aminophylline, oxtriphylline, and theophylline are rapidly absorbed, whereas enteric-coated tablets have a delayed and, at times, an unreliable pattern of absorption. The extended-release dosage forms are slowly absorbed and sometimes unreliable. The retention enema is rapidly absorbed, whereas rectal suppositories are slow and unreliable. Dyphylline has good oral absorption. Peak levels of theophylline are reached in 1 to 2 hours with the oral solution, immediate-release capsules, or tablets; in approximately 4 hours with delayed-release tablets; and in 4 to 13 hours with extended-release products.

The half-life of theophylline varies by age and with concurrent illness. For example, with premature newborns, the half-life is approximately 30 hours during the first 15 days of life; for children 1 to 4 years of age, it is 3.4 hours; for adult nonsmokers with uncomplicated asthma, 8.2 hours; and for older adults, nearly 10 hours. In clients with acute hepatitis, the half-life is 19 hours; for cirrhosis, 32 hours; and for hyperthyroidism, 4.5 hours (*USP DI*, 1999). The half-life of theophylline in an adult smoker is only 3 to 4 hours (Self & Kelly, 1995).

Aminophylline, oxtriphylline, and theophylline salts release free theophylline in vivo. Theophylline is metabolized by the liver to caffeine. Caffeine concentrations may average approximately 30% of the theophylline concentration in adults, but in neonates it may be much more. Caffeine does not accumulate in adults.

The therapeutic serum levels for bronchodilator effects with theophylline are usually between 10 and 20 μg/mL. Some studies have indicated that a therapeutic response may be seen with serum levels of 5 to 15 μg/mL; however, some clients have minimal gain at this level, and others experience toxicity at levels of 15 to 20 μg/mL (Kelly & Kamada, 1997). Therefore it is necessary to provide close supervision with dosage adjustments according to client's therapeutic response or the presence of toxic effects. As a respiratory stimulant, serum levels of theophylline are between 5 and 10 μg/mL. Theophylline is metabolized in the liver and excreted by the kidneys.

The side effects/adverse reactions of theophylline preparations include nausea, increased anxiety, restlessness, gastric upset, vomiting, gastroesophageal reflux, headache, increased urination, insomnia, trembling, increased nervousness, tachycardia and, with aminophylline, dermatitis.

The dosage of theophylline preparations must be tailored to the medical circumstances in each case. The usual efficacy of a theophylline preparation depends on the attainment of a serum concentration of 10 to 20 μg/mL (see previous comments on serum levels). The rapid IV administration of theophylline and its derivatives has caused severe and even fatal acute circulatory failure; therefore the drug should be administered slowly, over 20 to 30 minutes. Because theophylline has a low therapeutic index, it is essential to use caution when determining the dosage. The various xanthine preparations contain the following:

Drug	Percentage of Anhydrous Theophylline Present
aminophylline anhydrous	86
aminophylline dihydrate	79
oxtriphylline	64
theophylline monohydrate	91

Nursing Management

Xanthine Derivative Therapy

■ **Assessment.** Use with caution in individuals with active gastritis, active peptic ulcers, or a history of peptic ulcers; theophylline products may cause local gastric irritation or act centrally to stimulate the secretion of gastric acid. This condition can be aggravated when the serum level of theophylline exceeds 20 μg/mL. Use cautiously with clients who have congestive heart failure (CHF), because circulatory impairment may cause very slow clearance of serum xanthines, and xanthines are potentially cardiotoxic. Aminophylline, oxtriphylline, and theophylline should be used with caution in clients with acute pulmonary edema, sepsis, hypothyroidism, seizure disorders, and hepatic disease. Xanthines are contraindicated in clients who are hypersensitive to any of its components. In addition, use xanthine derivatives cautiously in young children and older adults. (See the Management of Drug Overdose box on p. 722).

Theophylline crosses the placenta; dangerous levels of caffeine concentration may occur in the neonate because of the newborn's inability to metabolize this compound. The xanthines are excreted in breast milk and can produce toxicity in the neonate. Symptoms of theophylline toxicity include tachycardia, jitteriness, irritability, gagging, and vomiting.

Smoking one to two packs of cigarettes every day decreases the serum half-life of theophylline (Zevin & Benowitz, 1999). Consequently, smokers require larger dosages of xanthines than nonsmokers. This effect may persist for months to years, even after the person has stopped smoking (see the Case Study box on p. 723).

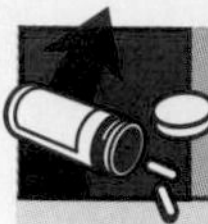

Management of Drug Overdose
Theophylline (Xanthine)

- Treatment is supportive and symptomatic because there is no known specific antidote.
- To decrease drug absorption, administer an activated charcoal preparation orally or via a nasogastric tube. Charcoal should be premixed with sorbitol, or a single dose of sorbitol should follow the charcoal dose. Sorbitol is considered to be more effective than magnesium-containing laxatives.
- A gastric lavage (if instituted early—within 1 hour of ingestion) or a whole bowel irrigation with a polyethylene glycol and electrolyte solution are useful for very large overdoses of theophylline.
- If the client has seizures, establish an airway and administer oxygen. Diazepam or phenobarbital IV may be administered to control the seizures.
- Charcoal hemoperfusion may be necessary when the serum concentration of theophylline is very high (greater than 40 μg/mL in chronic overdose) or if other risk factors are present, such as older age or concurrent illnesses. Hemodialysis is less effective and peritoneal dialysis is ineffective for theophylline toxicity (*USP DI*, 1999).
- Monitor vital signs; give supportive care as needed.

Review the client's current drug regimen for the risk of significant drug interactions, such as those that may occur when xanthine products are given concurrently with the following drugs:

Drug/Herb	Possible Effect and Management
beta-adrenergic blocking agents, systemic or ophthalmic	The therapeutic effects of both drugs may be inhibited. Concurrent use may also decrease theophylline excretion. Monitor closely, because dosage adjustments may be necessary.
black pepper	May increase theophylline levels. Monitor closely.
cimetidine (Tagamet), macrolide antibiotics (clarithromycin [Biaxin], erythromycin [Erythrocin], or troleandomycin [TAO]), fluvoxamine (Luvox), recombinant interferon alfa, mexiletine (Mexitil), pentoxifylline (Trental), tacrine (Cognex), thiabendazole (Mintezol), ticlopidine (Ticlid)	May decrease theophylline clearance, resulting in elevated serum levels of theophylline and possible toxicity. Monitor closely, because dosage adjustments may be necessary.
ciprofloxacin (Cipro), enoxacin (Penetrex)	Concurrent drug administration may reduce theophylline excretion, resulting in an increase in the half-life, serum level, and potential toxicity of theophylline. Monitor serum levels closely, because a dosage adjustment may be indicated.
moricizine (Ethmozine), rifampin (Rifadin)	Increase clearance and lower serum levels of theophylline. Monitor theophylline when the drugs are used concurrently or when theophylline is added or discontinued.
phenytoin (Dilantin), ketamine (Ketalar)	Increased metabolism of xanthines occurs. Increased clearance of phenytoin, leading to low serum levels, may be seen with concurrent administration. May lower seizure threshold. Serum levels of both drugs should be closely monitored, because dosage adjustments may be necessary.
St. John's wort	**May increase theophylline metabolism. Avoid concurrent use if possible.**
tobacco or marijuana	Aromatic hydrocarbons in smoke may result in increased metabolism and increased clearance of xanthines (except dyphylline); this may result in low serum levels of theophylline. Dosage adjustments of 50% to 100% greater have been required in smokers.

A baseline assessment of the client's respiratory status should be accomplished as discussed in Nursing Management: Bronchodilator Drug Therapy, p. 709.

■ **Nursing Diagnosis.** With the administration of the xanthine derivatives, the client should be assessed for the following nursing diagnoses/collaborative problems: risk for aspiration related to the ability of the drug to induce gastroesophageal reflux in clients who may have impaired gag reflex, infants under 2 years of age, older adults, or clients who are debilitated or stuporous; impaired comfort (flushing of the face, headache, nausea, nervousness, and palpitations); impaired oral mucous membrane (rectal irritation with rectal dosage forms of the drug); and the potential complications of allergic reaction and drug toxicity.

■ **Implementation**

■ ***Monitoring.*** Anticipate adverse reactions if the serum level of theophylline exceeds the normal serum therapeutic range of 10 to 20 μg/mL. Because of the variation in the metabolism of xanthines, monitoring serum theophylline concentration and client response is necessary to prevent toxicity. In clients with low serum albumin, total theophylline levels may be in the therapeutic range, but unbound serum theophylline concentrations may be a better indicator for setting dosages and predicting toxicity. Serum levels obtained immediately before the next dose (trough concentrations) tend to be more consistent than peak serum levels.

Be sure that IV administration is given slowly with an infusion pump. Monitor vital signs and observe the client for signs of toxicity such as hypotension, tachycardia, ventricular dysrhythmias, or convulsions. Earlier, less severe signs of toxicity may not occur. Have oxygen, respirator, and IV diazepam (for convulsions) available during the initiation of therapy. Maintain airway, hydration, and normal temperature with tepid water sponges or a hypothermic blanket for hyperpyrexia (Potter & Perry, 1997).

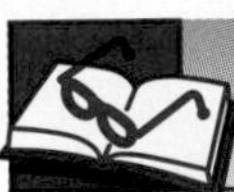

Case Study *The Client with Asthma*

Christine Newman is a 32-year-old woman with a long history of bronchial asthma. She is currently being maintained on theophylline (Theo-Dur), 200 mg twice daily. When respiratory wheezing increases, she uses an albuterol (Proventil) inhaler, 2 puffs every 4 hours until her breathing improves. In spite of her history of asthma, Christine continues to smoke at least half a pack of cigarettes daily. She is making an effort to quit smoking but finds it hard to stop.

1. What is the pharmacologic effect of the Theo-Dur in the management of the client with asthma?
2. Explain the effect the Proventil inhaler has on the client's wheezing.
3. Why is it especially important to support Ms. Newman's effort to stop smoking, in light of her drug therapy and her asthmatic condition?

One evening Ms. Newman is brought to the emergency department by her family. She is having an acute asthma attack and has difficulty talking because of respiratory distress. Her breathing is extremely labored, with accessory muscle use. She has audible wheezing. Her family tells the nurse that Ms. Newman's breathing became more difficult 2 days ago. She began using the Proventil inhaler, but it did not provide any relief.

After a brief examination she is given metaproterenol (Alupent) by nebulization. She experiences some decrease in respiratory distress, but the wheezing continues. A continuous IV infusion of aminophylline is started. Ms. Newman is admitted to the hospital. The Alupent inhaler treatments continue at 4-hour intervals.

4. What will you include in your assessment (subjective, objective, and laboratory data) of Ms. Newman while she is receiving aminophylline intravenously?
5. Compare the actions of Alupent and Proventil in the treatment of asthma.

Christine is to be discharged with the following medications: Theo-Dur, 200 mg twice daily; Proventil inhaler, 2 puffs every 6 hours; and beclomethasone (Vanceril) inhaler, 2 puffs every 6 hours.

6. Ms. Newman asks why she needs a second inhaler. How will you respond to her need for this information about the use of the Vanceril inhaler?
7. What does Ms. Newman need to be taught about the combined use of the Vanceril and Proventil inhalers?

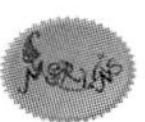

For answer guidelines, go to mosby.com/MERLIN/McKenry/.

Pulmonary studies are performed to assess the client's progress while taking the drug. Intake and output should also be monitored.

Observe children closely because they are more susceptible than adults to the CNS effects of the drug (nervousness, restlessness, insomnia, hyperactive reflexes, twitching, and convulsions).

Monitor the client when changing from one route of administration to another until the dosage is regulated. Wait 4 to 6 hours after changing from IV to oral therapy and 12 hours when changing from rectal administration, because its absorption tends to be less consistent.

If a client with status asthmaticus does not respond quickly to bronchodilating agents, additional medications (e.g., corticosteroids) will be required. Note positive responses to the medication, such as an increased ease of respiration, decreased wheezing, and a decrease in the client's anxiety regarding the dyspnea.

▪ ***Intervention.*** A loading dose may be used to reach therapeutic levels as soon as possible for all ages, including neonates. Although IV administration has the most rapid effect, immediate-release oral liquids, tablets, or capsules may be used. Before the loading dose is given, a determination should be made of the last dose of any of the xanthine derivatives, including time, amount, dosage form, and route of administration. Once a therapeutic level is reached, it is maintained with an oral or IV form of the drug. Clients should be switched from IV to oral forms as soon as an oral form is tolerated. For chronic therapy, transient and caffeine-like side effects may be minimized by starting with a low dosage and increasing it by 25% every 3 days until the best therapeutic response is achieved with the least side effects. Whenever a client experiences nausea, vomiting, or signs of CNS stimulation, hold the next dose of theophylline and ensure that serum theophylline levels are determined, even if another reason is suspected (e.g., the flu).

When administering theophylline by "piggyback," turn off the other IV solution already in place or start another IV line, because theophylline will need to be titrated according to the client's response. For IV administration, monitoring theophylline serum concentrations and the client's response is essential to prevent toxicity.

Administer oral doses on an empty stomach to promote faster absorption; to lessen local gastrointestinal irritation, the drug may be given with food. Whether or not the dose is administered with food, it is important that it be given consistently with or without food and at approximately the same time each day. The client should chew the chewable tablet forms before swallowing but should swallow enteric-coated or extended-release tablet forms whole without crushing, breaking, or chewing. For clients with difficulty in swallowing, some extended-release capsules may be opened and the contents mixed with 1 teaspoon of jelly, jam, or applesauce. The elixir dosage forms have a high alcohol content (20%); the alcohol-free liquid forms are generally preferred. Some of the liquid forms contain sorbitol, which may cause diarrhea and hyperglycemia.

Rectal suppositories are not recommended because they are irritating to tissues, and absorption is unreliable. If they are administered, schedule the administration when the rectum is free of feces to enhance absorption. Have the client remain in the recumbent position for 15 to 20 minutes after inserting the drug. Administer before meals to enhance retention. Suppositories are contraindicated if irritation or infection of the rectum or lower colon is present.

■ ***Education.*** Caution the client not to take OTC remedies that contain ephedrine or other sympathomimetics for the treatment of asthma or cough. Instruct the client to limit his or her intake of xanthine-containing beverages (e.g., coffee, tea, chocolate, cocoa, and cola beverages), because these may increase the CNS stimulant effects of the xanthine derivatives. Advise the client to avoid radical and sustained changes in diet: high-carbohydrate, low-protein diets decrease theophylline elimination; and low-carbohydrate, high-protein diets and charcoal-broiled foods increase theophylline metabolism and excretion, resulting in decreased serum concentrations of the drug.

Warn older adults of possible dizziness during therapy, and have them take necessary precautions for safety.

If the client is taking the extended-release form of the drug, advise against changing brands unless prescribed to do so, because the various brands may not be bioequivalent.

The client should notify the prescriber of any fever, flu-like symptoms, or diarrhea, because the prescribed dosage may need to be changed. Advise the client to keep medical and laboratory appointments to check the progress of therapy.

■ **Evaluation.** The expected outcome of therapy with xanthine derivatives is that the client will have an adequate respiratory status as evidenced by ease of respiration at rest, the absence of adventitious breath sounds, PEF readings in the client's best range, ABGs within normal limits (PaO_2 >60 mm Hg, $PaCO_2$ 35 to 45 mm Hg), pH 7.35 to 7.45, and a respiratory rate of 12 to 20 breaths/min or a return to the baseline rate.

PROPHYLACTIC ANTIASTHMATIC DRUGS

cromolyn [kroe' moe lin] (Intal, Novo-Cromolyn ♣)
nedocromil [ned o kroe' mill] (Tilade)

Cromolyn and nedocromil are antiinflammatory agents that inhibit the release of histamine, leukotrienes, and other mediators of inflammation from mast cells, macrophages, and other cells associated with asthma. Neither drug has any bronchodilator effect, nor do they have any effect on inflammatory mediators already released in the body. Nedocromil appears to be more effective than cromolyn (Serafin, 1996) and in some persons is therapeutically effective with twice-daily dosing (*USP DI*, 1999).

Both drugs are indicated for the prevention of bronchospasms and bronchial asthmatic attacks. Administered by oral inhalation, cromolyn has approximately 8% to 10% absorption in the lungs; it has an onset of action within 4 weeks and is excreted in the kidneys and bile. Nedocromil has a systemic absorption of 7% to 9%, a half-life of 1.5 to 3.3 hours, and an onset of action as maintenance therapy between 2 and 4 weeks; it is excreted by the kidneys. Nedocromil can also prevent bronchospasm if given up to ½ hour before exposure to allergens or exercise.

The side effects/adverse reactions of cromolyn and nedocromil include cough, hoarseness, dry mouth or throat, nasal congestion, sneezing, diarrhea, myalgia, difficulty sleeping, stomach pain, rash, sneezing, bronchospasm, and a bad taste in the mouth after use of the inhaler.

The dosage of cromolyn for adults and children (5 years and older) to prevent bronchial asthma is 2 oral inhalations (1.6 or 2 mg) four times daily at 4- or 6-hour intervals. To prevent exercise-induced or allergen-induced bronchospasms, the dosage is 2 oral inhalations approximately 10 to 15 minutes before exercise or exposure. A dosage has not been established for children under 5 years of age.

The initial dosage of nedocromil for adults and adolescents is usually 2 oral inhalations four times daily. A reduction of the dosage to three and then two times daily may be attempted in persons whose symptoms are under good control.

■ Nursing Management

Prophylactic Antiasthmatic Drug Therapy

■ **Assessment.** During the initial assessment, determine that the client does not have a sensitivity to cromolyn or nedocromil. Documentation of a baseline history of the client's frequency and severity of asthma episodes will help with the evaluation of drug therapy.

■ **Nursing Diagnosis.** With the administration of cromolyn and nedocromil, the client has the potential for impaired comfort (unpleasant taste). Cromolyn administration has the risk of impaired comfort (throat irritation) and the potential complication of anaphylactic reaction. Clients receiving nedocromil may experience ineffective airway clearance related to increased bronchospasm secondary to nedocromil or its propellants, impaired comfort (headache, rhinitis, throat irritation, nausea and vomiting), and the potential complications of arthritis and neutropenia or leukopenia.

■ **Implementation**

■ ***Monitoring.*** The client should be monitored for the frequency and intensity of asthma attacks or other symptoms of allergy.

■ ***Intervention.*** Cromolyn and nedocromil help to prevent but do not relieve asthma or bronchospasm attacks. They may be continued during an attack unless the client becomes intolerant to the use of inhaled drugs. If the client is also using a bronchodilator inhaler, it should be used 15 minutes before the cromolyn or nedocromil inhalation. Cromolyn solution should be administered from a power-operated nebulizer because hand-squeezed bulb nebulizers do not provide sufficient force.

■ ***Education.*** A client using the aerosol, capsule, or solution dosage form for inhalation should be aware that instructions come with each preparation. Make sure the client can administer the drug correctly. Demonstration kits are available for the inhalation capsule dosage form of cromolyn. Caution clients using the aerosol form to avoid getting the medication in the eyes. Inhalation capsules are to be used with a special inhaler; they are not effective if swallowed. Instruct the client not to float the canister to test fullness but to keep a record of sprays.

The client should be taught to rinse the mouth and gargle after an inhalation treatment to relieve dryness of the mouth and throat and the unpleasant aftertaste.

The client should be advised that it may be as long as 4 weeks before the drug is fully beneficial. Compliance with the regimen is necessary to achieve these results. With the use of these prophylactic agents it may be possible to lower the dosages of other antiasthmatic medications. However, alert the client that it is important to maintain any concurrent therapies, such as adrenocorticoids, until modified or discontinued by the prescriber. The prescriber should be notified if the client's condition does not improve or worsens.

Advise the client using a nedocromil inhaler to prime it with 3 sprays into the air before using it the first time or if it has not been used in more than 7 days.

■ **Evaluation.** An expected outcome of cromolyn or nedocromil therapy is a reduction in the number of attacks, reduced cough, decreased sputum production, and/or a decreased need for other antiasthma drugs in 4 weeks of therapy. Some clients show improvement in pulmonary function. Only clients showing improvement should continue to receive cromolyn and nedocromil.

CORTICOSTEROIDS

Corticosteroid drugs are used in chronic asthma to decrease airway obstruction. As antiinflammatory agents, they stabilize the membranes of lysosomes, thus preventing the release of hydrolytic enzymes that produce the inflammatory process in the tissues. The exact mechanism in asthma is still poorly understood but involves the suppression of antibody formation that is responsible for provoking the asthmatic attack. In addition, corticosteroids inhibit the synthesis of leukotriene, thus reducing bronchoconstriction and mucus secretion.

Daily administration of systemic corticosteroid therapy provides great therapeutic benefits, but the high incidence of side effects has led to the use of the alternate-day schedule of treatment. This regimen provides the best risk-benefit ratio for prolonged therapy because it minimizes the likelihood of unwanted side effects. The corticosteroids generally used have an intermediate-acting duration of action. These corticosteroids include prednisone, fluticasone (Flovent ◆), prednisolone, and methylprednisolone (see Chapter 49 for details).

Chronic use of the steroid aerosols has resulted in a decrease in bronchial hyperreactivity and respiratory symptoms. Inhaled corticosteroids are the most important therapeutic agents for the pharmacologic control of pulmonary inflammation in asthma (Weltman, 1999). Topical corticosteroid therapy offers the possibility of limiting action at the site of application and thereby avoiding the systemic effects of the oral agents. By chemically modifying the structural arrangement of the steroid molecule, compounds were developed to diminish systemic absorption from the respiratory tract. The products available are beclomethasone (Vanceril, Beclovent), budesonide (Pulmicort), flunisolide (AeroBid), fluticasone nasal (Flonase ◆), mometasone intranasal (Nasonex ◆), and triamcinolone (Azmacort).

These products offer the advantage of producing few systemic adverse reactions, including that of limited or no adrenal suppression. This category also includes dexamethasone (Decadron), but it is used less often today because it has a higher incidence of side effects than the other agents. (Table 38-1 explains the step approach to the therapeutic management of asthma for the current recommendations for corticosteroids.) The aerosols are rapidly absorbed from the pulmonary tissues with limited gastrointestinal absorption. The maximum improvement in pulmonary function may take 1 to 4 weeks.

The side effects/adverse reactions of the corticosteroid drugs include abdominal distress, anorexia, cough without infection, dizziness, headache, unpleasant taste in the mouth, and oral fungal infection or candidiasis.

The adult dosage of beclomethasone (Vanceril, Beclovent) is 2 oral inhalations three or four times daily. For severe asthma, 12 to 16 sprays daily are used initially, with the dosage decreased according to client response. The dosage has not been established for children under 6 years of age; for children 6 to 12 years of age, administer 1 or 2 metered sprays three or four times daily.

In severe asthma, the initial adult dosage for the inhalation powder of budesonide (Pulmicort) is 0.2 to 2.4 mg daily, divided in 2 to 4 doses. The maintenance dosage is 0.2 to 0.4 mg twice daily, with the dosage adjusted according to the client's response. The dosage for children 6 to 12 years of age with severe asthma is 0.1 to 0.2 mg twice daily; this product is not recommended for children under 6 years of age.

The dosage of flunisolide (AeroBid) for adults and children 4 years and older is 2 oral inhalations twice daily, morning and night. Fluticasone (Advair Diskus) is used for long-term, twice-daily maintenance treatment of asthma in clients 12 years and older.

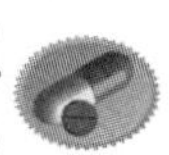

The adult dosage of triamcinolone (Azmacort) is 2 inhalations three or four times daily. In very severe asthma, 12 to 16 inhalations per day may be used. For children 6 to 12 years of age, 1 or 2 inhalations three or four times daily are recommended. The dosage for children should not exceed 12 inhalations per day. (See Special Considerations for Children.)

TABLE 38-1 Step Approach for the Therapeutic Management of Asthma

Step 4: Severe	For long-term prophylaxis control, a high-dose corticosteroid inhaler *plus* a long-acting beta_2-agonist tablet, or an inhaler or a long-acting theophylline *plus* an oral corticosteroid (2 mg/kg/day, not exceeding 60 mg/day) daily should be used. A short-acting beta_2-agonist inhaler is available for symptom control.
Step 3: Moderate	Intermediate-dose corticosteroid inhaler *plus* a long-acting beta_2-agonist inhaler, tablets, or long-acting theophylline daily. A short-acting beta_2-agonist inhaler is available for symptom control.
Step 2: Mild (persistent)	Low-dose corticosteroid inhaler or nedocromil daily. Children may start with cromolyn or nedocromil. Zafirlukast, zileuton, or a long-acting theophylline product are alternatives for clients 12 years of age or older. A short-acting beta_2-agonist inhaler is available for symptom control.
Step 1: Mild (intermittent)	A short-acting beta_2-agonist inhaler is available for symptom control. If the inhaler is used more than twice weekly, consider step 2 therapy.

Information from National Heart, Lung, and Blood Institute (1997). *Expert Panel Report II: Guidelines for the diagnosis and management of asthma.* National Asthma Education and Prevention Program, NHLBI Information Center. Bethesda, MD: Author.

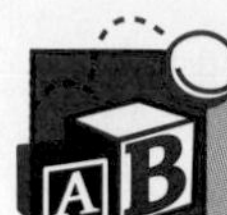

Special Considerations for Children
Asthma

More than 17 million Americans have asthma, with the prevalence of asthma increasing by 75% from 1980 to 1994 (Centers for Disease Control and Prevention, 1998).

Asthma affects nearly 5 million children in the United States. It is more prevalent in black children and accounts for approximately 3 million prescriber office visits yearly (Fast Facts, 1999).

The prevalence rate of asthma from 1982 and 1994 increased approximately 42% in males and 81% in females (American Lung Association, 1998).

Infants and preschool children with two or more asthma symptoms per week should receive an inhaled antiinflammatory medication, such as a corticosteroid, cromolyn (Intal), or nedocromil (Tilade). Such medications may be administered via a metered dose inhaler with a spacer/holding chamber and face mask.

School-age children and adolescents generally follow the same treatment regimen as recommended for adults (Practical Guide, 1998).

■ Nursing Management

Inhalation Corticosteroid Therapy

■ **Assessment.** Tuberculosis may be reactivated with long-term corticosteroid inhalation therapy; asthmatic clients with a positive Mantoux test should be monitored carefully. Osteoporosis may be exacerbated in postmenopausal women who take high dosages over a long period of time. Significant systemic absorption of inhaled corticosteroids as the result of high dosages over an extended period has been reported to cause growth inhibition in children related to hypothalamic-pituitary-adrenal (HPA) axis suppression; glaucoma and cataracts may also result. With the use of properly administered doses of inhalation corticosteroid, systemic adverse reactions do not often occur unless the client has bronchitis or is taking systemic corticosteroid drugs; in such cases, all concerns related to systemic corticosteroids may occur (see Chapter 49).

A baseline assessment of the client's respiratory status should be completed (see the assessment within Nursing Management: Bronchodilator Drug Therapy, p. 709). Drug interactions are unlikely to occur with the usual dosages of inhalation corticosteroids.

■ **Nursing Diagnosis.** With the administration of corticosteroids by inhalation, the client is at risk for the following nursing diagnoses/collaborative problems: impaired comfort (unpleasant taste, dry/irritated mouth and throat, and cough and hoarseness without signs of infection, headache, nausea); and the potential complications of oral candidiasis (creamy, white patches within the mouth), monilial esophagitis (difficulty in swallowing), upper respiratory tract infection, bronchospasm, and allergic reaction. Psychologic changes (nervousness, restlessness, depression) have been reported with budesonide only.

■ **Implementation**

■ ***Monitoring.*** The client's respiratory status should be monitored on an ongoing basis to evaluate the effectiveness of the drug. Monitor for side effects of corticosteroid therapy. Check the client's proper use of the inhaler at periodic intervals.

■ ***Intervention.*** If the client also uses a bronchodilator, it should be used 15 minutes before the corticosteroid inhalation. If the client's response to the corticosteroid begins to diminish, the prescriber should be notified so the dosage can be adjusted. Box 38-5 reviews the inhalants used for the treatment of asthma.

The use of a spacer greatly decreases the occurrence of candidiasis and hoarseness.

■ ***Education.*** Stress the importance of self-management. Assess the client's ability to hold and manipulate a metered dose inhaler. Provide instructions on inhaler use. After inhaling, the client should hold the inhaled drug for a few

BOX 38-5

Nursing Review: Inhalants for Asthma Treatment

With the wide variety of medications that may be used concurrently for the treatment of asthma, the nurse should be aware of the following:

- For prophylactic use, the antiinflammatory inhalation drugs cromolyn (Intal) or nedocromil (Tilade) are recommended. These drugs have no role in the treatment of acute asthmatic attacks.
- Corticosteroid inhalers such as beclomethasone (Beclovent, Vanceril) and flunisolide (AeroBid) are for preventive use only, and they may cause localized fungal infections in the mouth and pharynx. Advise the client to rinse the mouth with water or mouthwash after each use and to thoroughly rinse and dry the inhaler tip after each use. This will help reduce the incidence of a dry and sore throat and oropharyngeal candidiasis.
- Beta$_2$-agonist inhalers have no antiinflammatory effects but are considered the most effective drugs for the treatment of acute bronchospasm and asthma. An SC injection of beta agonists has not been found to be more effective than inhalation, and it has been reported to cause more systemic adverse reactions (Abramowicz, 1999). Examples include albuterol (Proventil, Ventolin), bitolterol (Tornalate), pirbuterol (Maxair), terbutaline (Brethaire), and salmeterol (Serevent), a drug that acts twice as long as albuterol (Dyer, 1993).

Clients with asthma often have multiple inhalers prescribed, such as ipratropium (Atrovent), an anticholinergic; beclomethasone (Vanceril), a corticosteroid; and albuterol (Ventolin), a beta$_2$ agonist.

What instructions would you offer the client with asthma?

If the prescriber has not given specific dosing instructions, the order of administration to obtain optimal drug effects is generally as follows:

1. The beta agonist is used first to open the airways.
2. The anticholinergic agent is administered.
3. The corticosteroid is administered.

Instruct the client to wait approximately 5 minutes between each medication and to rinse his or her mouth thoroughly (without swallowing the rinse) after the corticosteroid dose.

seconds before exhaling and allow a minute to elapse between each inhalation to increase its effectiveness. Written instructions should be provided in addition to verbal discussion. Ensure that the client is able to use the inhaler.

Encourage the client to use a diary to record the administration of as-needed (prn) medications and his or her response. The diary should be reviewed routinely by a health care provider to monitor for continued beneficial effects or the presence of side effects/adverse reactions and early treatment failures. This information may provide the first warning of the incorrect use of the medication or failure to take early preventive measures, or it may indicate the need for a change in dosage, a change in medication, or additional medication.

BOX 38-6

Control of Known Risk Factors for Asthma

Although some allergens may be impossible to avoid, many occupational or environmental allergens may be reduced or eliminated. For example, smoking is an irritant to many asthmatics, especially children; asthmatic attacks may be precipitated or aggravated by dust, dust mites, cat or dog hair, hairspray, perfumes, temperature changes, and physical exertion. Whenever possible, changes that can reduce or eliminate the irritants should be attempted, such as keeping the house as dust free as possible and avoiding shag carpeting, heavy draperies, dust on silk flower arrangements, the use of perfumed soap and products, and smokers or smoke-contaminated areas.

The client should be told that fungal infections of the mouth may occur with the inhalation of corticosteroids. The mouth should be thoroughly examined daily for the presence of infection. In addition, tell the client that rinsing the mouth after each treatment and washing and drying the inhaler thoroughly after use will help to prevent infection.

Instruct the client in ways to control known risk factors whenever possible to support the treatment plan and help to prevent recurrences (Box 38-6).

■ **Evaluation.** The expected outcome of corticosteroid therapy for the client with asthma is that there will be fewer asthmatic episodes of lesser severity without adverse reactions to the drug. If the inhalation therapy has been for rhinitis, the client will have decreased nasal secretions and sneezing.

SUMMARY

In clients with ineffective airway clearance, nursing interventions and mucokinetic and bronchodilator drugs are used together to prevent or minimize the client's condition. Mucokinetic agents promote the removal of abnormal or excessive respiratory tract secretions by thinning hyperviscous secretions, thereby enhancing the ciliary action of the respiratory tract. Bronchodilators diminish airway obstruction by bronchial smooth muscle relaxation. Mucokinetic agents are either diluents of respiratory secretion or mucolytics by dissolving the linkages of mucoprotein molecules of the respiratory secretions. Bronchodilators may be sympathomimetic drugs—either nonselective adrenergic, nonselective beta-adrenergic, or selective $beta_2$ agents. Use of the nonselective adrenergic drugs (e.g., epinephrine) not only results in bronchodilation and vasodilation but also in unwanted side effects such as increased heart rate, muscle tremors, CNS stimulation, glycogenolysis, and gluconeogenesis. The nonselective beta-adrenergic agents (e.g., isoproterenol) act on bronchial smooth muscle and on the heart, whereas the selective $beta_2$-receptor agents (e.g., isoetharine and albuterol) have less cardiotonic effect and act primarily to relieve bronchospasm. Xanthine derivatives and ipratropium, an anticholinergic agent, are also used as bronchodilators. Cromolyn and nedocromil are used as prophylactic asthmatic agents, as are the leukotriene antagonists. Leukotriene antagonists reduce inflammation, mucus secretion, and bronchoconstriction associated with asthma. Corticosteroids are also used in chronic asthma to prevent or minimize inflammation.

Nursing management of the care of the client receiving mucokinetic and bronchodilator drugs is focused on the client experiencing increased ease of respiration, decreased wheezing, and a decrease in medication use. The nurse should stress the need for responsible self-management of the therapeutic medication regimen. The nurse can play a crucial role in reducing the morbidity and mortality of asthma by keeping current on the guidelines and treatment of asthma and by taking an active role in applying the clinical skills of assessment, intervention, client education, and evaluation.

Critical Thinking Questions

1. John Holt, age 62, was admitted to the hospital with the symptoms of fatigue, weakness, dyspnea, malaise, and a persistent, nonproductive cough. He was diagnosed as having a viral upper respiratory tract infection. Would a mucolytic drug be appropriate for this client? Why or why not?
2. What nursing interventions would be considered appropriate to the nursing management of a client receiving either a mucolytic or bronchodilating drug?
3. Stanley Myers, age 22, a college student with a history of asthma, has come to the clinic for a regularly scheduled visit. In reviewing his inhalant therapy, he indicates that he takes the medications in any order "just to get it over with." What should be the response of the nurse?

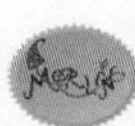

Collaborative Learning Activities

For Collaborative Learning Activities, go to mosby.com/MERLIN/McKenry/.

CASE STUDY

For a Case Study that will help ensure mastery of this chapter content, go to mosby.com/MERLIN/McKenry/.

BIBLIOGRAPHY

Abramowicz, M. (Ed.). (1999). Levalbuterol for asthma. *The Medical Letter, 41*(1054), 51-53.

American Hospital Formulary Service. (1999). *AHFS drug information '99.* Bethesda, MD: American Society of Hospital Pharmacists.

American Lung Association (1998). Epidemiology and Statistics Unit. *Trends in asthma morbidity and mortality.* Washington, D.C.: Author.

Anderson, K.N., Anderson, L.E., & Glanze, W.D. (Eds.). (1998). *Mosby's medical, nursing, & allied health dictionary* (5th ed.). St. Louis: Mosby.

Asmus, M.J., Sherman, J., & Hendeles, L. (1999). Bronchoconstrictor additives in bronchodilator solutions. *Journal of Allergy & Clinical Immunology, 104*(2 pt 2), S53-S60.

Beasley, R., Pearce, N., Crane, J., & Burgess, C. (1999). Beta-agonists: What is the evidence that their use increases the risk of asthma morbidity and mortality? *Journal of Allergy & Clinical Immunology, 104*(2 pt 2):S18-S30.

Centers for Disease Control and Prevention (CDC), US Department of Health and Human Services. (1992). Asthma—United States, 1980-1990. *Journal of the American Medical Association, 268*(15), 1995.

Centers for Disease Control and Prevention (1998). Forecasted state-specific estimates of self-reported asthma prevalence—1998. *Morbidity and Mortality, 47,* 1022-1025.

Costello, J. (1999). Prospects for improved therapy in chronic obstructive pulmonary disease by the use of levalbuterol. *Journal of Allergy & Clinical Immunology, 104*(2 pt 2), S61-S68.

Devillier, P., Baccard, N., & Advenier, C. (1999a). Leukotrienes, leukotriene receptor antagonists and leukotriene synthesis inhibitors in asthma: An update. Part I: Synthesis, receptors and role of leukotrienes in asthma. *Pharmacology Research, 40*(1), 3-13.

Devillier, P., Baccard, N., & Advenier, C. (1999b). Leukotrienes, leukotriene receptor antagonists and leukotriene synthesis inhibitors in asthma: An update. Part II: Clinical studies with leukotriene receptor antagonists and leukotriene synthesis inhibitors in asthma. *Pharmacology Research, 40*(1), 15-29.

Drug Facts and Comparisons. (2000). St. Louis: Facts and Comparisons.

Dyer, J. (1993). Drug watch: New long-lived bronchodilator knocks out albuterol. *American Journal of Nursing, 93*(5), 53.

Fast Facts (1999). *Statistics on asthma and allergic diseases.* Updated October, 1999. Patient Public Resource Center (www.aaaai.org/public/fastfacts/statistics.stm [2/3/2000]).

Franz, M.N. & Cohn, R.C. (1994). Management of children and adults with cystic fibrosis: One center's approach. *Hospital Formulary, 29*(9), 364-378.

Gross K.M. & Ponte C.D. (1998). New strategies in the medical management of asthma. *American Family Physician,* 58(1), 89-109.

Interiano, B. & Guntupalli, K.K. (1993). Metered-dose inhalers: Do health care providers know what to teach? *Archives of Internal Medicine, 153*(1), 81.

Johnson, C.A., Butler, S.M., Konstan, M.W., Breen, T.J., & Morgan, W.J. (1999). Estimating effectiveness in an observational study: A case study of dornase alfa in cystic fibrosis. The Investigators and Coordinators of the Epidemiologic Study of Cystic Fibrosis. *Journal of Pediatrics, 134*(6), 734-739.

Kelly, H.W. (1997). The 1997 Expert Panel Report II: Guidelines for the diagnosis and management of asthma. *Pharmacist's Letter,* Document #130417.

Kelly, H.W. & Kamada, A.K. (1997). Asthma. In J.T. DiPiro, R.L. Talbert, G.C. Yee, G.R. Matzke, B.G. Wells, & L.M. Posey (Eds.), *Pharmacotherapy: A pathophysiologic approach* (3rd ed.). Norwalk, CT: Appleton & Lange.

Kuschner, W.G. (1999). Ten asthma pearls every primary care physician should know. *Postgraduate Medicine, 106*(3), 99-104.

National Asthma Education and Prevention Program (1998). Considerations for the diagnosing and managing of asthma in the elderly. National Institutes of Health. (www.nhlbi.nih.gov/nhlbi/lung/asthma/prof/as_elder.txt [6/16/98]).

Nelson, H.S. (1999). Clinical experience with levalbuterol. *Journal of Allergy & Clinical Immunology, 104*(2 pt 2), S77-S84.

Nicosia, S. (1999). Pharmacodynamic properties of leukotriene receptor antagonists. *Monaldi Archives of Chest Disease, 54*(3), 242-246.

Potter, P.A. & Perry, A.G. (1997). *Fundamentals of nursing: Concepts, process, and practice* (4th ed.). St. Louis: Mosby.

Practical Guide (1998). Practical guide for the diagnosis and management of asthma. National Heart, Lung, and Blood Institute 97(4053). (www.medscape.com/govmt/NHLBI/1998/guidelines/nih4053-01.html. [2/3/2000]).

Public Health Service, U.S. Department of Health and Human Services. (1991). *Executive summary: Guidelines for the diagnosis and management of asthma.* National Institutes of Health Pub. No. 91-3042A.

Rosenthal, R.R., Busse, W.W., Kemp, J.P., Baker, J.W., Kalberg, C., Emmett, A., & Rickard, K.A. (1999). Effect of long-term salmeterol therapy compared with as-needed albuterol use on airway hyperresponsiveness. *Chest, 116*(3), 595-602.

Self, T.H. & Kelly, H.W. (1995). Asthma. In L.Y. Young & M.A. Koda-Kimble (Eds.), *Applied therapeutics: The clinical use of drugs* (6th ed.). Vancouver, WA: Applied Therapeutics.

Serafin, W.E. (1996). Drugs used in the treatment of asthma. In J.G. Hardman & L.E. Limbird (Eds.), *Goodman & Gilman's The pharmacological basis of therapeutics* (9th ed.). New York: McGraw-Hill.

Weltman, J.K. (1999). The use of inhaled corticosteroids in asthma. *Allergy Asthma Proceedings, 20*(4), 255-260.

Wiegand, L., Mende, C.N., Zaidel, G., Zwillich, C.W., Petrocella, V.J., Yancey, S.W., & Rickard, K.A. (1999). Salmeterol vs. theophylline: Sleep and efficacy outcomes in patients with nocturnal asthma. *Chest, 115*(6), 1525-1532.

United States Pharmacopeia Dispensing Information (USP DI): Drug information for the health care professional (1999). (19th ed.). Rockville, MD: United States Pharmacopeial Convention.

Zed, P.J. & Krenzelok, E.P. (1999). Treatment of acetaminophen overdose. *American Journal of Health System Pharmacy, 56*(11), 1081-1091.

Zevin, S. & Benowitz, N.L. (1999). Drug interactions with tobacco smoking: An update. *Clinical Pharmacokinetics, 36*(6):425-438

39 Oxygen and Miscellaneous Respiratory Agents

Chapter Focus

An understanding of oxygen therapy and other associated therapies is essential to the delivery of effective respiratory care. Clients with different types of respiratory conditions may require varied treatment modalities and respiratory agents. Assessment and management of the client with altered respiratory function is more efficacious when the approach is multidisciplinary and collaborative.

Learning Objectives

1. Describe how the body uses oxygen and the result of oxygen deprivation.
2. Implement the nursing interventions applicable to each of the various methods of oxygen administration.
3. Discuss the effects of carbon dioxide.
4. Implement nursing management for the care of clients receiving respiratory stimulants and depressants.
5. Discuss antitussive agents and the proper method of administration.
6. Explain the three actions of histamine in the body.
7. Implement nursing management for the care of clients receiving antihistamine therapy.
8. Discuss the pharmacokinetics and pharmacologic effects of serotonin and its relationship to drugs and several disease states.

Key Terms

analeptics, p. 736
hypercapnia, p. 733
hypoxemia, p. 731
hypoxia, p. 731
pulse oximetry, p. 734

Key Drugs [✓]

cyproheptadine, p. 745
diphenhydramine, p. 738

DRUGS THAT AFFECT THE RESPIRATORY CENTER

Therapeutic Gases

Oxygen

Oxygen—a gas that is essential for life—is colorless, odorless, and tasteless. It is not flammable, but it supports combustion much more vigorously than does air. Inspired air normally contains 20.9% oxygen which, at an atmospheric pressure of 760 mm Hg, exerts a partial pressure (PO_2) or tension of 159 mm Hg. As oxygen passes through the bronchial airway, the inspired air becomes saturated with water vapor, which reduces the PO_2 in the alveoli to approximately 100 mm Hg. Finally, the oxygen appears in dissolved form in the arterial blood. The PO_2 of arterial blood is normally above 80 mm Hg.

Oxygen must be continuously supplied to tissue cells; no fiber or cell can survive very long without oxygen. The adult human brain consumes from 40 to 50 mL of oxygen per minute. The cortex consumes more than the centers in the medulla or spinal cord. Cerebral oxygen consumption proceeds without pausing, and the replenishment of oxygen by the blood must be maintained continuously. Whenever any circulatory stress exists, cerebral blood flow tends to be preserved at the expense of other, less vital organs. Of all the tissues affected by **hypoxia** (inadequate cellular oxygen), the brain is most susceptible to disruption of normal function and irreversible damage. An acute reduction of the PO_2 to 50 mm Hg decreases mental functioning, emotional stability, and finer muscular coordination. Further reduction of the PO_2 to 40 mm Hg produces impaired judgment, decreased pain perception, and impairment of muscular coordination. When the PO_2 is reduced to 32 mm Hg or less, unconsciousness and a progressive, descending depression of the central nervous system (CNS) ensue.

The kidneys are vital organs in which there must be considerable constancy of blood flow and oxygen supply. Oxygen consumption is greater in the renal cortex; renal medullary tissue has an oxygen consumption that is 15% less than that of the renal cortex. This difference is related to the variation in pressure gradient and to the fact that cortical flow is rapid whereas the medullary flow is slower. The renal cortex is highly dependent on oxygen, whereas the renal medulla can function relatively independently of the oxygen supply.

The rate of oxygen consumption by the kidneys is approximately 0.06 mL/g/min, more than most other tissues. For each 100 mL of blood entering the kidney, 1.4 mL of oxygen is consumed. The oxygen consumed by the kidneys is primarily used for sodium reabsorption.

Renal vasoconstriction occurs when the renal arterial content falls to less than 55% of normal. This response is believed to be mediated by chemoreceptors, which stimulate the vasomotor center to produce renal vasoconstriction. Renal vasoconstriction also occurs as a result of the action of ether, barbiturates, and other anesthetics. Renal blood flow is also decreased during periods of exercise. It is important to note that autoregulation of renal perfusion does occur.

In the skeletal muscles, oxygen consumption is related to blood flow. Oxygen consumption and blood flow are decreased when the muscle is at rest and significantly increased during exercise.

Some investigators regard the reduction of oxygen supply to the intestinal tract as a key factor for inadequate splanchnic vasoconstriction during hypotension. An inadequate oxygen supply impairs myocardial metabolism and function.

When used alone, arterial blood pressure determinations are unreliable indicators of the adequacy of tissue perfusion. Arterial blood gas determinations should be obtained, because these results provide a more accurate and reliable indication of the shifts in the partial pressures of oxygen and carbon dioxide. Severe hypoxia may produce changes in the ST segment and T wave of the electrocardiogram (ECG), dysrhythmias, ectopic beats, and myocardial infarction.

Indications. Oxygen is used chiefly to treat hypoxia and **hypoxemia** (diminished oxygen tension in the blood). Basically, there are four types of hypoxia:

1. Hypoxemic hypoxia: decreased oxygen level in the blood, resulting in decreased oxygen diffusion into the tissues
2. Ischemic hypoxia: inadequate blood flow to an organ or tissue in the presence of a normal PO_2 and hemoglobin content
3. Anemic hypoxia: inadequate hemoglobin to carry oxygen in the presence of a normal PO_2
4. Histotoxic hypoxia: adequate PO_2 and hemoglobin but an inability of the tissues to use the delivered oxygen because of a toxic agent

Clinically, hypoxemic hypoxia is the most common form of hypoxia. A variety of pathologic conditions result in hypoxemic hypoxia and necessitate the use of oxygen treatment. These conditions include hypoventilation, increased airway resistance, pneumothorax, respiratory center depression, abnormal ventilation-perfusion ratio, congenital cyanotic heart disease, decreased pulmonary compliance, and breathing oxygen-poor air. The use of oxygen is also indicated in cardiac failure or decompensation and coronary occlusion, as well as anesthesia administration (to increase the safety of general anesthesia).

Administration. Oxygen is administered by inhalation. Various methods are used, and each method has its advantages and disadvantages (Figure 39-1).

A *nasal catheter* is made of soft plastic. When used, it should be lubricated with water-soluble K-Y Jelly and passed through the nose until the tip is just above the epiglottis. This distance is usually the same as the distance from an individual's external nares to the tragus of the ear, minus 1 cm. The catheter should not be inserted so far that the client swallows oxygen, because this will cause stomach distention and abdominal discomfort. The catheter is fastened with tape to the forehead and/or nose. The flow rate varies according to individual need, but 4 to 8 L/min of a 25% to 40% concentration of oxygen is commonly used. This form of therapy is very drying to the mucous membrane, and

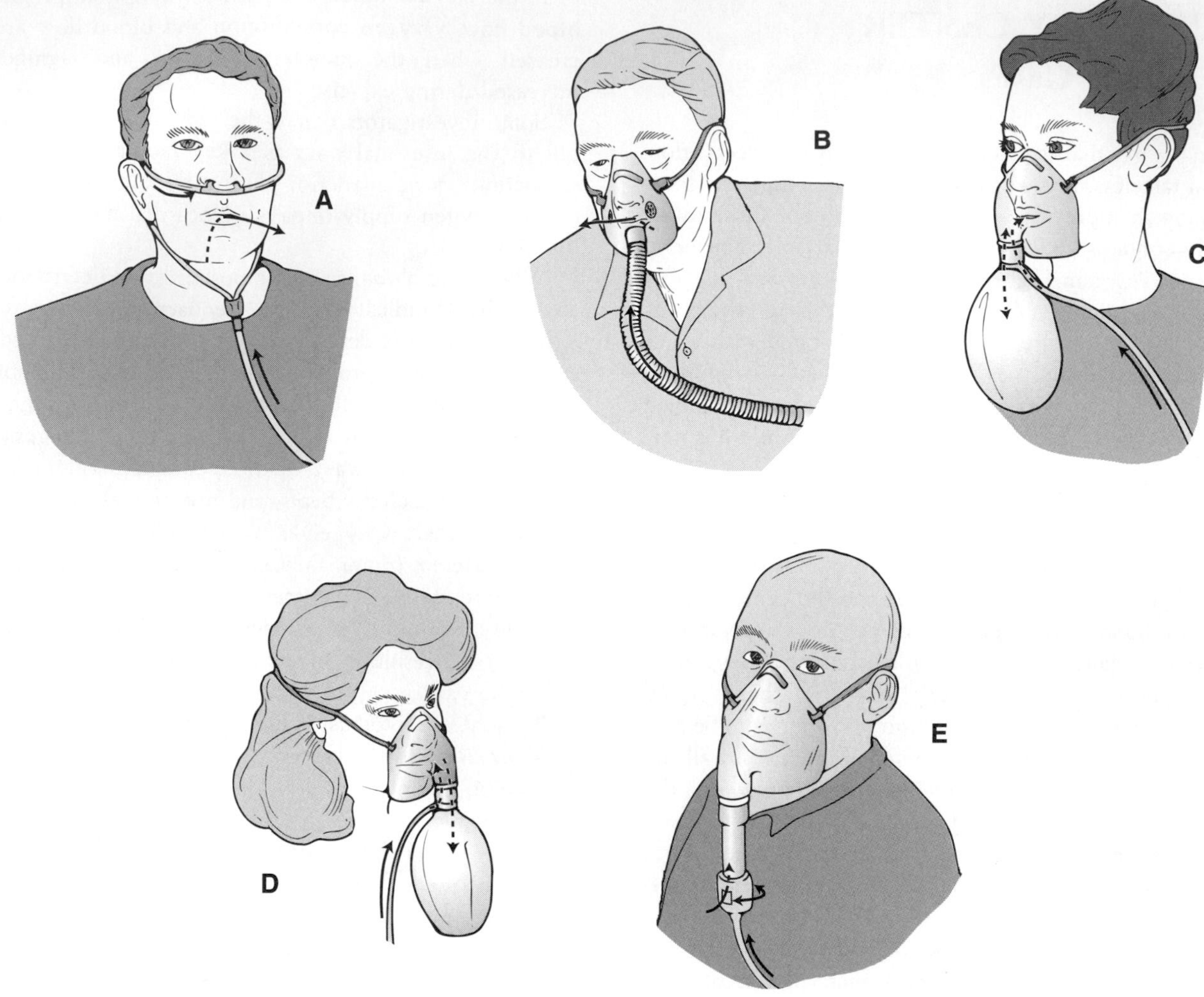

Figure 39-1 Various oxygen delivery systems. **A**, Nasal cannula. **B**, Simple face mask. **C**, Partial rebreathing mask. **D**, Nonrebreathing mask. **E**, Venturi mask.

therefore the oxygen should be humidified. In addition, nasal and oral hygiene are important to maintain cleanliness and an intact mucous membrane and to prevent infection and discomfort. Most clients receiving oxygen therapy are mouth breathers, and frequent mouth care is required to prevent alteration of the mucous membranes. Nasal catheters become obstructed with encrusted secretions and must be removed and cleaned or replaced several times a day.

A *nasal cannula* is much more comfortable for the client than is a catheter. Cannulas have either single or double, short prongs that are inserted into the lower part of the nostrils. Cannulas are less likely to become obstructed with secretions. Nasal and oral mucosa still require frequent attention. A flow of 1 to 6 L/min of a 23% to 42% concentration of oxygen is adequate for many clients.

An *oxygen mask* is the most effective means of delivering needed oxygen. Oxygen concentrations up to 100% can be administered by mask. To be effective, the mask must fit well over the nose and mouth; to some extent, high flow rates can compensate for a poor fit. Masks are better tolerated when used intermittently or when disposable plastic masks are used. Only absolutely clean and uncontaminated rubber masks should be used, because they can be a source of nosocomial infection. There are two main types of oxygen masks: those that deliver low concentrations of oxygen and those that deliver high concentrations of oxygen.

A *simple face mask,* which is lightweight and disposable, is useful for short-term oxygen administration, such as in the early postoperative period or when intermittent oxygen therapy is required. The flow rate is only 6 to 8 L/min at a low-oxygen concentration of 40% to 60%. Because the mask is loose fitting and can leak, simple face masks are suitable for individuals with carbon dioxide retention. They are also indicated for clients who cannot use a nasal cannula, such as those who have a nasal obstruction.

A *partial rebreathing* mask is a disposable, lightweight plastic face mask that consists of a reservoir bag and a partial rebreathing valve. It is commonly used by individuals who require oxygen. On expiration, only a portion of the exhaled air enters the reservoir bag; it conserves roughly one third of the client's exhaled air. Because this air comes from the trachea and bronchi and does not participate in gas exchange in the lungs, it is rich in oxygen. To prevent the rebreathing of carbon dioxide, the reservoir bag should deflate only slightly on inhalation. By this method, a concentration of 50% to 75% oxygen can be delivered at a flow rate of 8 to 11 L/min.

A *nonrebreathing mask* is designed to fit tightly over the face and is usually made of rubber with a reservoir bag and a nonrebreathing valve. On inhalation, oxygen flows into the bag and mask, and the one-way valve prevents exhaled air from flowing back into the bag. The expired air instead escapes through the one-way flap valve in the mask. The concentration of oxygen is 80% to 100%, and the flow is adjusted to keep the reservoir bag fully inflated. This type of mask is used for short-term therapy, such as counteracting smoke inhalation. The rubber can become hot and sticky; prolonged use can cause discomfort.

An *oxygen tent* is of limited value, particularly when it is necessary to open the canopy for monitoring vital signs and administering care to the client. The rate of flow is 20 L/min at an oxygen concentration of 60%. Obviously, the oxygen concentration falls each time the tent is opened, which makes the flow difficult to control. Oxygen tents are now used less frequently, except for children beyond early infancy.

Plastic hoods may be used to deliver oxygen to infants. The clear plastic head hood allows low and high concentrations of oxygen to be maintained without hampering most nursing care. A rate of 4 to 5 L/min is needed to maintain oxygen concentrations and remove the exhaled carbon dioxide.

The *Ventimask (Mix-O-Mask)* is a development originating from the Venturi mask. It is used for clients with chronic alveolar hypoventilation and carbon dioxide retention. Exact low-flow concentrations of oxygen are delivered to the individual. The Ventimask provides an air-oxygen mixture with the desired oxygen concentration. The size of the orifice to the mask determines the concentration of oxygen—24% or 28%, 31%, 35%, and 40% with flow rates of 4, 6, 8, and 10 L/min, respectively. A thin elastic band holds the Ventimask in position and tends to press into the skin behind the ears. A gauze padding under each side of the elastic band will alleviate this discomfort. The device must be removed when the client eats and may give the client a feeling of being smothered.

Most of the oxygen administered in hospitals for therapy is provided from a central source where it is stored as a gas or as liquid oxygen. The gas is piped into a client's room at a standard pressure of 50 pounds per square inch (psi) at the gauge. Compressed oxygen is marketed in steel cylinders that are fitted with reducing valves for delivery of the gas. The cylinders are usually color-coded; green is used in the United States. Because the gas is under considerable pressure, the tanks must be handled carefully to prevent falling or jarring.

The effectiveness of oxygen administration depends on the carbon dioxide content of the blood. Individuals with chronic obstructive pulmonary disease (COPD) have difficulty with carbon dioxide and oxygen exchange and are subject to **hypercapnia** (high carbon dioxide content in the blood). Because of chronic hypercapnia, the medullary center of these individuals is relatively insensitive to stimulation with carbon dioxide; rather, a low PaO_2 serves as a stimulant to respiration. Therefore oxygen flow rates are kept low (1 to 2 L/min) for clients with COPD. Nursing care should be used to prevent a greater accumulation of carbon dioxide by encouraging the improvement of gas exchange. This involves having the client turn, deep breathe, and use pursed lip breathing periodically. Toxic carbon dioxide levels may result in further depression of respiration and respiratory acidosis. The nurse should be alert to neurologic symptoms that indicate an accumulation of carbon dioxide, including drowsiness, mental confusion, paresthesias, and visual disturbances. The occurrence of carbon dioxide narcosis may be prevented by gradually increasing the concentration of oxygen administered.

Oxygen Administration in the Premature Infant. Nurses caring for premature infants in incubators must be constantly aware of the danger of retrolental fibroplasia (retinopathy of prematurity). This is a vascular proliferative disease of the retina that occurs in some premature infants who have received high concentrations of oxygen at birth.* Although there has been a considerable reduction in the incidence and severity of this condition, infants less than 28 weeks' gestational age or with birth weights less than 1000 g are still at considerable risk (Hussain, Clive, & Bhandari, 1999). Oxygen concentration should be kept between 30% and 40%. Higher concentrations can be administered to cyanotic infants without increasing the danger of retrolental fibroplasia because it is PaO_2, not inspired PO_2, that is implicated in this disease. Therefore careful monitoring of arterial blood gases is essential. Some incubators are equipped with a safety valve that automatically releases any excess oxygen outside the chamber. When orders for an infant include oxygen prn, the nurse must make certain that it is administered only as needed and at low concentrations rather than continuously. Often the removal of a very small plug of mucus can clear the airway and enable the infant to breathe oxygen without assistance.

Hyperbaric Oxygen. In recent years hyperbaric oxygen has been used in the treatment of various conditions. The intermittent use of hyperbaric oxygen is controversial in the treatment of infections caused by *Clostridium perfringens, C. septicum,* or *C. histolyticum*—anaerobic bacilli that produce gas gangrene. It is believed that increased oxygen pressure in the tissue may exert an inhibitory effect on the enzyme systems of these bacteria. This same inhibitory effect may be implicated in the use of hyperbaric oxygen on other anaerobic microorganisms.

Hyperbaric oxygen has also been used in certain circulatory disturbances, such as air or gas embolism, decompres-

*Excessive oxygen constricts the developing retinal vessels of the eye. Consequently, normal vascularization is suppressed; because the endothelial cells become disorganized, they cause destruction of the immature retina. The result is blindness.

sion sickness, carbon monoxide and cyanide poisoning, and exceptional blood loss. It has also been used in certain local circulatory disturbances such as necrotizing soft-tissue infections; acute traumatic ischemia, crush injury, and compartment syndrome; compromised (ischemic) grafts and flaps; radiation necrosis; refractory osteomyelitis; and enhancement of healing in selected problem wounds (Weaver, 1992).

Helium-Oxygen Mixtures. Helium-oxygen mixtures have been used to treat obstructive types of dyspnea. Helium is an inert gas and so light that a mixture of 80% helium and 20% oxygen is only one third as heavy as air. Helium is only slightly soluble in body fluids and has a high rate of diffusion. Because of its low specific gravity, mixtures of this gas with oxygen can be breathed with less effort than either oxygen or air alone when air passages are obstructed. These mixtures are recommended for individuals with status asthmaticus, bronchiectasis, and emphysema, as well as during anesthesia induction for clients with respiratory tract obstruction.

Oxygen Toxicity. Exposure to 100% oxygen for a period of 6 hours causes an inflammatory response with subsequent destruction of the alveolocapillary membrane of the respiratory tract and the development of pulmonary edema that is not cardiac in origin. Toxicity is often difficult to recognize, but the most common symptoms are substernal distress (ache or burning sensation behind the sternum), an increase in respiratory distress, fatigue, nausea, vomiting, restlessness, tremors, twitching, paresthesias, and convulsions.

■ Nursing Management

Oxygen Therapy

■ **Assessment.** Dyspnea or an increased respiratory rate may indicate the need for oxygen therapy. The best means of gauging the need for oxygen or the effectiveness of oxygen therapy is via arterial blood gas evaluations or pulse oximetry before and during therapy (Box 39-1). In addition, document the client's blood pressure and pulse, level of consciousness, and respiratory status, including respiratory rate, effort, adventitious breath sounds, cyanosis, and activity intolerance.

It is important to know normal blood gas values and be able to recognize deviations (Box 39-2). The goal of oxygen therapy is to return the arterial oxygen pressure to the client's normal baseline, a range between 60 and 90 mm Hg, or an oxygen saturation greater than 90%.

In chronic carbon dioxide retention, the PaO_2 may range from 55 to 60 mm Hg. An arterial blood gas analysis is required 30 minutes after the oxygen dosage is changed unless the oxygen saturation is being monitored.

Oxygen should be given with extreme caution to some clients. In clients with chronic hypoxemia, the central chemoreceptors no longer act as the primary stimulus for breathing. In such cases respiratory drive is maintained by peripheral chemoreceptors that are sensitive to changes in PaO_2. If oxygen therapy causes PaO_2 to exceed 60 mm Hg, the stimulus to breathe is lost, and apnea results. Low-flow oxygen is administered to these clients, and arterial blood gas evaluations should be checked frequently.

■ **Nursing Diagnosis.** The client receiving oxygen therapy may experience ineffective airway clearance, ineffective breathing pattern, and impaired gas exchange. In addition, oxygen therapy places the client at risk for the following nursing diagnoses/collaborative problems: impaired skin integrity of the face related to the mask; infection related to contamination of the oxygen equipment; risk for injury related to the combustibility of oxygen; impaired oral mucous membrane related to the drying effects of oxygen; and the potential complications of oxygen toxicity and, for infants, retrolental fibroplasia.

BOX 39-1

Pulse Oximetry

An advance in monitoring for tissue hypoxia is the development of **pulse oximetry.** Pulse oximetry has been called one of the most significant technologic advances ever made in monitoring the respiratory function of clients. Simply explained, pulse oximetry works by passing light of differing wavelengths through living tissue and analyzing the differences in absorption. Oxygenated hemoglobin absorbs light differently, and these variations in absorption serve as the basis for calculations that determine the presence and amount of oxygenated hemoglobin compared with nonoxygenated hemoglobin. This provides a continuous reading of oxygen saturation in arterial blood. A saturation of 90% or greater is desired; this correlates with a PaO_2 of 60 mm Hg.

Current pulse oximeters work with a small probe (light source and detector) that may be placed on a client's ear, finger, toe, bridge of the nose, nasal septum, or temple. Pulse oximetry monitors are relatively inexpensive, noninvasive, safe, and extremely accurate. They require no calibration and provide almost instantaneous results. Although initially used with clients during anesthesia, recovery, and critical care, pulse oximetry is now commonly used as an immediate and safe method of determining tissue oxygenation in any client experiencing respiratory difficulties.

BOX 39-2

Normal Values for Arterial Blood Gases

pH: 7.36-7.44
$PaCO_2$: 36-44 mm Hg
PaO_2: 80-100 mm Hg
O_2 saturation: 95% or above
HCO_3: 22-26 mEq/L

■ **Implementation**

■ ***Monitoring.*** Monitor the client's vital signs—pulse rate, blood pressure, and respiratory rate and pattern. Also observe level of consciousness, skin temperature, and color. Report any abnormal findings to the prescriber. Examine the client and the equipment frequently to see that the skin and mucous membranes in contact with the equipment are intact and without irritation; the equipment is patent, without leaks, and properly positioned; the flow rate is at the prescribed level; the humidifier contains solution; and, if an oxygen cylinder is being used, that it is stabilized and contains enough oxygen. Pulse oximetry, as well as blood gases, may be required periodically. If high concentrations of oxygen are used, positive end-expiratory pressure (PEEP) or continuous positive airway pressure (CPAP) values are used to determine the best oxygenation without hemodynamic compromise and thereby prevent oxygen toxicity.

■ ***Intervention.*** To prevent dryness of the nose and throat and respiratory complications, add sterile, distilled water to the humidifying device, and administer oxygen concentration and liter flow as prescribed. Because oxygen is a dry gas, adequate humidification is essential to the client and must be monitored frequently.

Oxygen supports combustion, and combustible materials (linens, wooden furniture, plastic articles) burn with greater ease and intensity in the presence of oxygen. Therefore smoking, matches, woolen blankets, clothing, or electric equipment (radios, electric razors, hair dryers) that may cause sparks are strictly forbidden in rooms where oxygen is being administered. "No smoking" signs are also posted within the home environment. In some health agencies, these signs are posted on the individual's door and above the bed, even though smoking is not permitted within the agency.

Because oxygen therapy is often administered to debilitated clients, take special care to avoid contamination of the equipment; this will help to prevent a nosocomial infection. Nasal cannulas, Ventimasks, other masks, tubing, nebulizers, and other equipment exposed to moisture need to be changed daily. Nasal catheters should be changed every 8 to 12 hours. If the client's condition permits, remove the oxygen mask periodically to dry, powder, and massage the skin around the mask.

■ ***Education.*** The equipment for oxygen administration should be shown to the client and family. Explain the procedure and the benefits of oxygen therapy. Explain to the client and visitors the importance of not lighting candles or smoking in the client's room. (Because oxygen supports combustion, the possibility of fire always exists.) Prepare the client and caregivers for oxygen use in the home (see the Community and Home Health Considerations box on p. 736).

■ **Evaluation.** The expected outcome of oxygen therapy is that the client will have adequate gas exchange as evidenced by a respiratory rate of 12 to 20 breaths/min or a rate in keeping with the client's baseline and blood gas values: PaO_2 >60 mm Hg, $PaCO_2$ 35 to 45 mm Hg, and pH 7.35 to 7.45.

Carbon Dioxide

Carbon dioxide is a colorless, odorless gas that is heavier than air. Carbon dioxide used as a pharmacologic agent affects respiration, circulation, and the CNS. Inhaling carbon dioxide for a short time increases both the rate and the depth of respiration unless the respiratory center is depressed by narcotics or disease.

Carbon dioxide stimulates the cells of the sympathetic nervous system, respiratory center, and peripheral chemoreceptors. It depresses the cerebral cortex, myocardium, and smooth muscle of the peripheral blood vessels. Carbon dioxide may also interfere with nerve conduction and transmission. When carbon dioxide increases the rate and force of respiration, venous return to the heart is usually enhanced as a result of decreased peripheral resistance; the rate and force of myocardial contraction improves, and there is less likelihood of myocardial irritability and dysrhythmias.

Although the use of carbon dioxide has been suggested for many commonly encountered clinical situations, other therapies are usually more effective and have fewer disadvantages. Too much carbon dioxide has a depressant effect and results in acidosis and unresponsiveness of the respiratory center to the gas. Therefore it is important that carbon dioxide be administered with caution.

Indications. The following sections explain indications for the use of carbon dioxide.

General Anesthesia. Most general anesthetics cause a reduction in the body's response to carbon dioxide, which is reflected in CNS depression. The degree of depression is directly related to the depth of anesthesia. The more deeply the individual is anesthetized, the greater the CNS depression. Carbon dioxide initially speeds up anesthesia by increasing pulmonary ventilation. By lessening the sense of asphyxiation, it reduces struggling. In the postanesthesia period, it hastens the elimination of many anesthetics. Inhalation of 5% to 7% carbon dioxide increases cerebral blood flow by approximately 75%, primarily by dilation of the cerebral vessels.

Respiratory Depression. The use of carbon dioxide as a respiratory stimulant in the presence of depressed respiration is limited. When used, close monitoring of pulse oximetry and PaO_2 is important; carbon dioxide should be discontinued if the desired results are not obtained. Mechanical assistance in respiration and oxygen administration is the usual treatment in cases of respiratory depression.

Postoperative Use. Occasionally, carbon dioxide is used postoperatively to increase ventilation and prevent atelectasis. However, most investigators believe better results are obtained with the use of deep breathing exercises, coughing, frequent turning, tracheal suction, and intermittent positive pressure breathing.

Carbon dioxide administration has also been used in the treatment of postoperative hiccups. Relief from hiccups is apparently accomplished by stimulating the respiratory center; this causes large excursions of the diaphragm that suppress spasmodic contractions of that muscle, thereby promoting regular contractions.

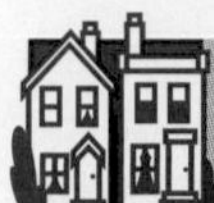

Community and Home Health Considerations
Home Management of Oxygen Therapy

For the home use of oxygen, the client and family must understand how the system works, how to determine that the system is not functioning, how to "troubleshoot" the system, how to contact the supplier, and what to do in an emergency. There are essentially three methods of delivery for home oxygen systems:

1. *The liquid oxygen system.* Liquid oxygen is provided in large reservoir canisters with smaller portable units that can be transfilled from the larger reservoir canister by the client. This system has the advantage of delivering 100% oxygen on all flow rates so that higher liter flow is achievable. The disadvantages are that the stationary unit must be refilled periodically (a small amount evaporates), and it may be the most costly method.
2. *The oxygen concentrator system.* This system, which extracts oxygen from ambient air, is inexpensive and convenient. However, the main unit is not portable, so the client also needs a portable unit. It is heavy and the client must have a backup system in case of power failure.
3. *Compressed oxygen tanks.* These tanks deliver 100% oxygen on all flow rates so a higher liter flow is achievable. However, they are heavy and unsightly, pose a safety hazard if not stored properly, and must be replaced by periodic delivery.

Whatever the system, it should be checked by the client or caregiver daily. The assessment should include proper functioning of the equipment, prescribed flow rates, remaining liquid or compressed gas content, and backup supply to meet the client's needs. The supplier's name and phone number need to be in a handy place for reordering or in case of emergency. Fire hazards should be prevented by instructing the client and family not to smoke or use an open flame in the room where the oxygen is on. Electrical appliances, such as razors and electric blankets, should not be used in the vicinity of the oxygen. No oil (Vaseline, hair oils, body oils), wool blankets, or flammable liquids (alcohol) should be used in the area. "No smoking" signs should be posted as reminders. The local fire department should be alerted to the presence of oxygen tanks in the house.

A respiratory care practitioner or nurse should visit at least monthly to provide a clinical assessment of the client, to reinforce appropriate practices and performance by the client and caregivers, and to ensure that the equipment is being maintained in accordance with the manufacturer's recommendations (American Association of Respiratory Care Clinical Practice Guideline, 1992).

To ensure consistent quality of care and to maximize the client's financial reimbursement, the physician's order for oxygen therapy needs to include the disorder for which the oxygen is required, the amount of oxygen flow, and the conditions for its use (i.e., continuous, prn, or nighttime only).

Administration. Carbon dioxide is kept in metal cylinders and vaporizes as it is delivered from the cylinder. It is administered in combination with oxygen when used for medical purposes. A 5% to 10% concentration of carbon dioxide delivered through a tight-fitting face mask is inhaled by the client until the depth of respiration is definitely increased, which usually occurs within 3 minutes. For postoperative clients, the procedure is repeated every hour or two for the first 48 hours and then several times a day for several days.

Another way of administering carbon dioxide is to allow the client to hyperventilate with a paper bag held over the face. Reinhaling expired air causes the carbon dioxide content to be continually increased.

Signs of carbon dioxide overdose are dyspnea, breath holding, markedly increased chest and abdominal movements, nausea, and increased systolic blood pressure. Administration of the gas should be discontinued when these symptoms appear. The administration of 5% carbon dioxide may produce severe mental depression if given over an hour; a 10% concentration can lead to a loss of consciousness within 10 minutes. The administration should be stopped as soon as the desired effects on the client's respiration have been obtained.

Direct Respiratory Stimulants

Direct respiratory stimulants come under a broader classification of CNS stimulants and are often referred to as **analeptics** (see Chapter 18). These drugs act directly on the medullary center to increase respiratory rate and tidal exchange. Although these drugs are available for stimulating the depth and rate of respiration, airway management and ventilation support are more effective in the treatment of respiratory depression. The mechanical support of ventilation is often superior to the use of drugs, because respiratory stimulants in large doses can cause convulsions.

In the past, respiratory stimulants (analeptics) have been advocated in the treatment of drug-induced respiratory depression. However, these drugs are not specific antagonists to sedatives or narcotics, and thus their use in drug-induced respiratory depression is now considered obsolete. Indeed, repeated doses of an analeptic may potentiate the depressant effects of CNS depressants. See Chapter 18 for information on the direct respiratory stimulant doxapram.

Reflex Respiratory Stimulants

An aromatic ammonia spirit is given by inhalation for its action as a reflex respiratory stimulant. In cases of fainting, it is administered by inhaling the vapor. Reflex stimulation of the medullary center occurs through peripheral irritation of sensory nerve receptors in the pharynx, esophagus, and stomach. The rate and depth of respiration are then increased through afferent messages to the respiratory control centers. Reflex stimulation of the vasomotor center results in a rise in blood pressure.

Respiratory Depressants

The most important respiratory depressants are barbiturates and opium and its derivatives. These agents depress the respiratory center, thereby making breathing slower and more shallow and lessening the irritability of the respiratory center. Respiratory depression is seldom desirable or necessary, but it is sometimes unavoidable. It is a side effect/adverse reaction of otherwise very useful drugs.

Occasionally an opiate such as codeine is administered to inhibit the rate and depth of respiration for a painful or harmful cough. Concentrations of carbon dioxide that are too high in inhalation mixtures may act paradoxically to depress respiration.

COUGH SUPPRESSANTS

The over-the-counter (OTC) cough suppressants are reviewed in Chapter 11; prescription-requiring cough suppressants are discussed in this chapter. Prescription cough suppressants are usually reserved for a nonproductive cough that is inadequately controlled by or nonresponsive to OTC medications.

Treatment of the cough is secondary to treatment of the underlying disorder; that is, the therapeutic objective is to decrease the intensity and frequency of the cough yet permit adequate elimination of tracheobronchial secretions and exudates.

Opioid Antitussive Drugs

Opioids such as morphine and hydromorphone are potent suppressants of the cough reflex, but their clinical usefulness is limited by their side effects. They inhibit the ciliary activity of the respiratory mucous membrane, depress respiration, and may cause bronchial constriction in clients with allergies or asthma. In addition, they can cause drug dependence. Codeine and hydrocodone are widely used; they exhibit fewer pronounced antitussive effects but have fewer side effects. (See Chapter 14 for information on opioid agents.)

Nonopioid Antitussive Drugs

The nonnarcotic, nonopioid antitussive drugs produce fewer gastrointestinal side effects than do codeine and the related compounds.

benzonatate [ben zoe′ na tate] (Tessalon Perles, Tessalon ♣)

Benzonatate is chemically related to the local anesthetic tetracaine. Benzonatate relieves coughing by peripherally anesthetizing the stretch or cough receptors in the lungs and respiratory passages, and it may also have a central effect on the cough reflex.

Benzonatate is indicated for the symptomatic treatment of a nonproductive cough. The onset of action is within 15 to 20 minutes after oral administration, with a duration of action of up to 8 hours.

Side effects include drowsiness, headache, dizziness, tightness or numbness in chest, nausea, constipation, abdominal upset, skin eruptions, nasal congestion, and a vague sensation of chill.

The dosage for adults and children over 10 years of age is 100 mg three times daily. The maximum daily dose is 600 mg.

■ Nursing Management
Benzonatate Therapy

■ **Assessment.** Assess from the client's history that there is no known hypersensitivity to benzonatate or related compounds (local anesthetics). Determine the cause of the cough, because the cough could indicate congestive heart failure or other disease. Benzonatate is contraindicated for a productive cough because secretions are retained if the cough is suppressed. No significant drug interactions have been reported with this drug. A baseline assessment of the client's respiratory status and cough should be obtained.

■ **Nursing Diagnosis.** With the administration of benzonatate, the client should be assessed for the following nursing diagnoses/collaborative problems: ineffective airway clearance; impaired comfort related to gastrointestinal effects (nausea, heartburn) and nasal congestion; constipation; impaired skin integrity related to the occurrence of rash; risk for injury related to CNS effects (sedation, dizziness); and the potential complications of allergic reaction, or bronchospasm or laryngospasm related to local anesthesia secondary to chewing or sucking the perle.

■ **Implementation**

■ ***Monitoring.*** Clients should be observed for drowsiness and dizziness, nausea, gastrointestinal distress, constipation, and rash. Assess the client's cough to determine if it is productive or nonproductive. Chest pain associated with the cough should be noted.

■ ***Intervention.*** Nursing actions supportive of antitussives are deep-breathing exercises, frequent changes of position, limitation or cessation of smoking, maintenance of adequate humidity in the environment, and adequate hydration. Attempt to pinpoint the cause of the cough and then direct nursing measures toward the cause. Infections should be treated with pulmonary hygiene (e.g., cough, deep breathing). If a specific stimulus for the cough can be identified (e.g., dust, smoking, or pollen), attempts should be made to minimize exposure to these substances.

■ ***Education.*** The capsule should be swallowed whole. Temporary local anesthesia of the oral mucosa results if it is chewed or dissolved in the mouth. Caution the client about operating a car or other machinery, because the drug may cause drowsiness or dizziness. Advise the client to report a cough that persists longer than a week.

■ **Evaluation.** The expected outcome of benzonatate therapy is that the client will experience a decrease in the intensity and frequency of coughing.

diphenhydramine [dye fen hye' dra meen] (Benylin, Benadryl, and others)

Diphenhydramine, available OTC and by prescription, depresses the cough center in the medulla of the brain (antitussive effect). It is reviewed in the antihistamine section of Chapter 11.

The adult dosage for an antitussive effect is 25 mg PO (syrup) every 4 to 6 hours; for an antihistamine effect, the dosage is 25 to 50 mg PO every 4 to 6 hours when necessary; and as a sedative-hypnotic, the dosage is 50 mg given 20 to 30 minutes before bedtime. The dosage for antidyskinetic or antiparkinson effects is 50 to 150 mg PO daily in divided doses. For antiemetic or antivertigo effects, the dosage is 25 to 50 mg PO 30 minutes before traveling and before each meal as necessary. Older adults may be more sensitive to the effects of this drug; lower adult dosages should be prescribed, with close monitoring for any adverse reactions. The maximum recommended daily dose is 300 mg in divided doses.

The antihistamine dosage for children is 1.25 mg/kg PO every 4 to 6 hours. The maximum daily dose is 300 mg. Do not use diphenhydramine in premature or full-term neonates.

The adult dosage of diphenhydramine injection for antihistamine or antidyskinetic effects is 10 to 50 mg IM or IV every 2 to 3 hours. For antiemetic or antivertigo effects, the initial dosage is 10 mg IM or IV, which may be increased to 20 to 50 mg every 2 or 3 hours. In children the parenteral dosage for antihistamine or antidyskinetic effects is 1.25 mg/kg IM four times daily. Do not use in premature or full-term neonates.

For a discussion of the nursing management of diphenhydramine, see Nursing Management: Antihistamine Therapy, p. 741.

■ ■ ■

See Chapter 11 for information on dextromethorphan, another nonopioid antitussive drug.

HISTAMINE

Distribution

Histamine is a chemical mediator that occurs naturally in almost all body tissues. It is present in highest concentration in the skin, lung, and gastrointestinal tract. These structures are often exposed to environmental assaults and require protection against damage. When liberated from its cells, the free form of histamine plays an early transient role in the inflammatory process that defends the exposed tissues against injury.

In many tissues the chief site of production and storage of histamine occurs in the cytoplasmic granules of the mast cell or, in the case of blood, the basophil (which closely resembles the mast cell in function). The mast cells are small, ovoid structures widely distributed in the loose connective tissue. They are especially abundant along small blood vessels and along the bronchial smooth muscle cell, which appears to have the highest concentration of mast cells of any organ in the body. Both the mast cells and basophils make up the mast-cell histamine pool.

A second major site of histamine production is known as the nonmast pool, where the amine is stored in the cells of the epidermis, gastrointestinal mucosa, and the CNS. Although histamine is present in various foods and is synthesized by intestinal flora, the amount absorbed does not contribute to the body's stores of this amine.

Pharmacologic Actions

The reactions mediated by histamine are attributed to receptor activity, which involves two distinct populations of receptors: H_1 and H_2. The principal actions of histamine are summarized in Table 39-1.

Vascular Effects. In the microcirculatory component of the cardiovascular system (arterioles, capillaries, venules), the liberation of histamine has been shown to involve both H_1 and H_2 receptors. Stimulation of these receptors dilates the capillaries and venules, producing an increased localized blood flow, increased capillary permeability, erythema, and edema. By activating the H_1 and H_2 receptors on the smooth muscles of the arterioles, histamine is also capable of eliciting a systemic response (vasodilation of the arterioles), which can result in a profound fall in blood pressure.

Smooth Muscle Effects. Although histamine exerts a powerful relaxing effect on the smooth muscle of the arterioles, it produces a contractile action on the smooth muscles of many nonvascular organs, such as the bronchi and gastrointestinal tract. In sensitized individuals, activation of the H_1 receptors of the lungs can cause marked bronchial muscle contraction that often progresses to dyspnea and airway obstruction.

Exocrine Glandular Effects. Histamine stimulates the gastric, salivary, pancreatic, and lacrimal glands, with the main effect seen in the gastric glands. Stimulation of H_2 receptors in the exocrine glands of the stomach increases the

TABLE 39-1 Histamine: Principal Actions

Structure	Histamine Receptors	Pharmacologic Effects
Vascular system		
Capillary (microcirculation)	H_1 and H_2	Dilation; increased permeability
Arteriole (smooth muscle)	H_1 and H_2	Dilation
Smooth muscle		
Bronchial, bronchiolar	H_1	Contraction
Gastrointestinal	H_1	Contraction
Exocrine glands		
Gastric	H_2	Gastric acid secretion (HCl)
Epidermis	H_1	Triple response (flush, flare, wheal)
Adrenal medulla	—	Epinephrine and norepinephrine release
Central nervous system	H_1	Motion sickness

production of gastric acid secretions. The high concentration of hydrochloric acid in the stomach is attributed to the activity of the parietal cells and is implicated in the development of peptic ulcers.

Central Nervous System Effects. Histamine is also known to be present throughout the tissues of the brain. Its effects seem to involve both H_1 and H_2 receptor mediation. The activation of H_1 receptors of the semicircular canals is associated with motion sickness.

Pathologic Effects

Histamine as a chemical mediator is implicated in many pathologic disorders. Conditions for which drugs are used to counteract this compound are concerned with the hypersensitivity response known as the allergic reaction. There are four different types of hypersensitivity responses to immunologic injury; the type I anaphylactic reaction is associated with the disorders caused by histamine release.

Individuals with type I–mediated hypersensitivity develop allergies as a result of sensitization to a foreign agent that may be ingested, inhaled, or injected. An incalculable number of these agents act as antigens. They vary widely—seasonal exposure to pollens, grasses, and weeds, or nonseasonal exposure to agents such as house dust, feathers, molds, and other similar substances can produce different forms of allergic reactivity.

Hypersensitivity to a variety of foods such as shellfish or strawberries requires ingestion of the antigen. Insects such as bees or wasps and even drugs, particularly penicillin, also possess allergic properties that may induce a severe response in hypersensitive individuals.

Thus type I anaphylactic hypersensitivity accounts for a substantial number of allergic disorders, and it involves a complex series of anomalies that range from mild urticaria to anaphylactic shock. The mechanism of type I anaphylactic reaction involves the attachment of an antigen (Ag) to an antibody (Ab), specifically immunoglobulin E (IgE); this complex becomes fixed to the mast cell. The pathologic manifestations of an Ag-IgE interaction are caused by mast cell degranulation, which results in the release of histamine and other mediators responsible for producing the allergic symptoms. The type I anaphylactic reaction is responsible for various disorders, such as urticaria, atopy (allergic rhinitis, hay fever), food allergies, bronchial asthma, and systemic anaphylaxis.

Urticaria. Urticaria is a vascular reaction of the skin; it is characterized by immediate formation of a wheal and flare and is accompanied by severe itching. Contact with an external irritant such as drugs or foods produces the Ag-IgE–mediated response with the resultant release of histamine from the mast cell into the skin. The local vasodilation produces the red flare, and the increased permeability of the capillaries leads to tissue swelling. These swellings are called "hives"; giant hives are known as angioneurotic edema. Antihistaminic drugs administered before exposure to the antigen will prevent this response.

Atopy. Atopy occurs in genetically susceptible individuals and is usually caused by seasonal pollen. This condition is manifested as an upper respiratory tract disorder known as allergic rhinitis (hay fever) (Table 39-2). (See Chapter 11 for additional information.) After the interaction of the Ag-IgE complex on the surface of the bronchial mast cells, histamine is released, producing local vascular dilation and increased capillary permeability. This change produces a rapid leakage of fluid into the tissues of the nose, which results in swelling of the nasal linings. Antihistaminic therapy can prevent the edematous reaction in certain individuals if the drug is administered before antigenic exposure.

Food Allergies. Food allergies involve the interaction of the Ab-IgE complex and mast cells in the intestine; this occurs when antigens are ingested. If the upper gastrointestinal tract is affected, vomiting results; if the lower gastrointestinal tract is invaded, cramps and diarrhea occur. The ingestion of a large amount of antigen has also been known to produce systemic anaphylaxis.

Bronchial Asthma. When the inhaled antigen combines with the IgE antibody, stimulation of the mast cells triggers the release of mediators in the lower respiratory tract, usually in the bronchi and bronchioles. Histamine plays a minor role in this response because the slow-reacting substance of anaphylaxis (SRS-A) is a more potent mediator, causing long-term contraction of the bronchiolar smooth muscle. The difficulty in breathing may be relieved by a bronchodilator such as epinephrine. Because more potent chemical mediators than histamine are responsible for caus-

TABLE 39-2 Colds, Allergic Rhinitis, and Influenza: Signs or Symptoms

Signs or Symptoms	Common Cold	Allergic Rhinitis	Influenza
Fever	Rare	Absent	Common: sudden onset, may range from 102° to 104° F
Aches and pains	Slight	Absent	May be severe
Sneezing	Usual	Common	Infrequent
Pruritus	Absent or rare	Common	Absent
Cough	Mild-moderate	Uncommon	Common
Headaches	Rare	Can occur	Prominent
Causative	Usually viruses	Usually allergens	Usually viruses
Occurrence	Anytime	Usually seasonal	Anytime
Complications	Sinus congestion, earache	Uncommon	Bronchitis, pneumonia

ing the reaction, the administration of antihistaminic drugs actually has no value in relieving this condition.

Systemic Anaphylaxis. Systemic anaphylaxis is a generalized reaction manifested as a life-threatening systemic condition. The Ag-IgE mediator response involves the basophils of the blood and the mast cells in the connective tissue. The most common precipitating causes of this response are drugs (particularly penicillin), insect stings (wasps and bees), and occasionally certain foods. The release of massive amounts of histamine into the circulation causes widespread vasodilation, resulting in a profound fall in blood pressure. The excessive dilation also allows plasma to leave the capillaries, and a loss of circulatory volume ensues. When the reaction is fatal, death is usually caused not only by shock but also by laryngeal edema. The symptoms of the latter condition include smooth muscle contraction of the bronchi and pharyngeal edema, which usually leads to asphyxiation. Because the mediator SRS-A is also released from the cells, the resulting spasm of the smooth muscle of the bronchioles elicits the asthma-like attack.

Antihistaminic drugs are less effective against systemic anaphylaxis because these agents do not antagonize the SRS-A mediator that causes the severe bronchoconstriction. Accordingly, a drug such as epinephrine, a bronchodilator, is indicated for this life-threatening situation. The relief produced by this drug results from the $beta_2$ receptor action that relaxes the bronchial smooth muscles.

Drug allergies often develop in susceptible individuals who show no adverse reactions after the first dose of drug administration. However, a second or subsequent reexposure to even an extremely small amount of this same antigen may elicit an exaggerated local or systemic IgE response. Individuals who exhibit such reactions are said to be allergic to the drug. The IgE-mediated response, particularly with penicillin, may occur either in the skin, producing severe urticaria, or in the respiratory tract, causing bronchial asthma.

In certain sensitized individuals, even limited contact can produce a fatal systemic anaphylaxis. Some of the drugs that elicit an allergic response include penicillin, chloramphenicol, streptomycin, sulfonamides, aspirin, and phenacetin. Allergic reactions to penicillin account for nearly 100 deaths per year in the United States. Therefore even the mildest sign of an allergic response, such as a slight skin rash, should be reported immediately to the prescriber. In all probability the drug will be discontinued to avoid the possibility of an exaggerated type I hypersensitivity reaction.

Histamine Testing: Gastric Function

Histamine is used to test for gastric acid secretory functions. If achlorhydria is the response to histamine, the client may have pernicious anemia, gastric polyps, gastric carcinoma, or atrophic gastritis. If hypersecretion of gastric acid occurs after the histamine, a duodenal ulcer of Zollinger-Ellison syndrome may be the problem.

Histamine testing of gastric function is contraindicated in clients who have a history of hypersensitivity to the drug, bronchial asthma, vasomotor instability, urticaria, or severe cardiac, pulmonary, or renal disease. Histamine should be used cautiously in clients with pheochromocytoma. Histamine H_2 receptor antagonists, such as cimetidine and ranitidine, are not to be administered for 24 hours before the test because they will antagonize the effects of the histamine. Antacids and anticholinergics are also withheld before the examination. The procedure and any anticipated effects of the histamine test should be explained to the client.

The client should fast for a minimum of 12 hours and be at rest under basal conditions. Use a nasogastric tube to empty the stomach contents before the examination and to obtain specimens during the examination. A baseline or basal acid output is obtained by obtaining four samples of aspirant 15 minutes apart; the nasogastric tube is clamped between samples. The histamine dose of 0.01 mg/kg (equal to histamine phosphate 0.0275 mg/kg) is administered subcutaneously. Epinephrine or ephedrine may be administered if the side effects of flushing, headache, nasal stuffiness, dizziness, faintness, and nausea become too severe. Epinephrine and ephedrine antagonize the effects of histamine (except the effects of gastric secretion).

Monitor the client's pulse rate and blood pressure closely. Prevent the client from swallowing saliva, because its alkalinity may interfere with test results. Obtain four samples for volume and acidity of gastric contents, 15 minutes apart for analysis. The maximal acid output is determined by adding the total milliequivalent of all samples collected after the injection of the gastric acid stimulant. The maximal acid output should be 1.5 to 3 times the baseline acid output. The maximum effect from the histamine is usually seen in approximately 30 minutes. *This test should be performed by or under the direction of a physician.*

Pentagastrin (Peptavlon) is another drug used to induce gastric secretion. It is a useful test for achlorhydria and is helpful in diagnosing pernicious anemia, atrophic gastritis, and gastric carcinoma. It is as effective as histamine and produces much fewer side effects and less severe adverse reactions (American Hospital Formulary Service, 1999).

ANTIHISTAMINES

Antihistamines are drugs that compete with histamine for its receptor sites. With the discovery of two histamine receptors (H_1 and H_2), the antihistamines are divided into the H_1 receptor antagonists and the H_2 receptor antagonists. The H_2 receptor blocking agents, which include cimetidine (Tagamet), ranitidine (Zantac), and others, are discussed in Chapter 41; the OTC antihistamines are reviewed in Chapter 11. The following section reviews the prescription antihistamines.

H_1 Receptor Antagonists

Antihistamines prevent the physiologic action of histamine by preventing it from reaching its site of action; thus the H_1 antihistamines have the greatest therapeutic effect on nasal allergies. They do not inhibit histamine already attached to receptors; therefore these drugs are more effective if administered before histamine is released. They relieve symptoms better at the beginning of the hay fever season than during its height, but they fail to relieve the asthma that often accompanies hay fever. These preparations are palliative and do not immunize the individual or protect him or her over time against allergic reactions.

Antihistamines do not replace other remedies such as epinephrine, ephedrine, and others. In acute asthmatic reactions the antihistamine drugs serve only as supplements to these remedies, and relief of various symptoms is obtained only while the drug is being taken. Dozens of antihistamine drugs are available and generally differ from each other by potency, duration of action, and incidence of side effects, particularly sedation. It is often necessary to try different types of antihistamines to determine the appropriate one for a client.

Antihistamines are indicated for the treatment of allergies, vertigo, motion sickness; for antitussive effects (diphenhydramine [Benadryl]); and for sedative and local anesthetic effects in dentistry. In general, their oral absorption pattern is good, with most of them having an onset of action within 15 to 60 minutes. With astemizole (Hismanal), the onset of action is 2 to 3 days. Rectal administration of dimenhydrinate (Dramamine) has an onset of action within 30 to 45 minutes. The time to peak effect can vary with each individual preparation. For example, the peak effect of astemizole occurs within 9 to 12 days, whereas the peak effect for triprolidine (Myidil) occurs within 2 to 3 hours. The duration of action is also variable: for dimenhydrinate, it is between 3 and 6 hours; for azatadine (Optimine), 12 hours; and for loratadine (Claritin), at least 24 hours. These agents are primarily metabolized in the liver and excreted by the kidneys, with the exception of astemizole, which is mainly excreted in the feces.

For the side effects/adverse reactions of the antihistamines, see the discussion of diphenhydramine on p. 738.

The dosage of antihistamine varies with the chemical classification and pharmacokinetic profile of each drug. The newer agents are generally longer-acting drugs with fewer sedative side effects, such as loratadine (Claritin) and cetirizine (Zyrtec), which are taken once a day and have few, if any, sedative and anticholinergic side effects (Kay & Harris, 1999).

The older agents that usually exhibit these side effects carry warnings about drug use in older adults; older adults are usually more sensitive to the effects of these drugs and may require a reduced dosage. The adult and pediatric dosages of the antihistamines are noted in Table 39-3.

Fexofenadine (Allegra), an antihistamine approved in 1996, is a metabolite of terfenadine (Seldane) that was chemically altered to eliminate the serious and potentially fatal cardiovascular drug interactions associated with terfenadine. Fexofenadine is indicated for the treatment of seasonal allergic rhinitis (Mason, Reynolds, & Rao, 1999).

Many prescription antihistamine-decongestant formulations are also available, such as acrivastine-pseudoephedrine (Semprex-D), brompheniramine and pseudoephedrine (Bromfed), fexofenadine and pseudoephedrine (Allegra-D), and others. The trend is for more antihistamines and antihistamine combinations to be allowed OTC marketing status in the future. See Chapter 11 for a discussion of antihistamine combinations.

■ Nursing Management

Antihistamine Therapy

■ **Assessment.** Use antihistamines with caution in clients with the following: asthma, because the drying effect may thicken secretions and diminish expectoration; bladder neck obstruction, prostatic hypertrophy, or a predisposition to urinary retention, because urinary retention may be aggravated; or a predisposition to angle-closure glaucoma, because the drug may precipitate an acute episode. Astemizole or terfenadine may induce dysrhythmias in clients with a history of QT interval prolongation or in clients with hepatic impairment, because increased plasma concentrations will occur. Hypokalemia should be corrected before astemizole and terfenadine therapy because of the risk of ventricular dysrhythmias.

TABLE 39-3 Antihistamines: Recommended Dosages

Antihistamine	Adult Dosage	Children's Dosage
astemizole (Hismanal)	10 mg daily	6-12 years: 5 mg/day
azatadine (Optimine)	1-2 mg q8-12h	12 years and older: 0.5-1 mg twice daily
brompheniramine (Dimetane)	4 mg q4-6h (maximum of 24 mg/day)	0.5 mg/kg in 3 or 4 divided doses
	Parenteral IM, IV, or SC: 10 mg q8-12h	12 years and under: 0.125 mg/kg 3 or 4 times daily
cetirizine (Zyrtec ◆, Reactine ♣)	5-10 mg daily	2-6 years: 5 mg daily 6-11 years: 10 mg daily
chlorpheniramine (Chlor-Trimeton)	4 mg q4-6h	6-12 years: 2 mg 3 or 4 times daily
	Parenteral IM, IV, SC: 5-40 mg as a single dose	SC: 87.5 μg/kg q6h
clemastine (Tavist)	1.34 mg twice daily or 2.68 mg 1 to 3 times daily	6-12 years: 670 μg to 1.34 mg twice daily
cyproheptadine (Periactin)	4 mg q8h, increase as necessary (range 4-20 mg/day)	0.125 mg/kg q8-12h
dexchlorpheniramine (Polaramine)	2 mg q4-6h	150 μg/kg in 4 divided doses
	Extended release: 4 or 6 mg q8-12h	Not recommended
dimenhydrinate (Dramamine)	50-100 mg q4h	5 mg/kg in 4 divided doses
	Parenteral, IM, IV: 50 mg IM or 50 mg in 10 mL normal saline for IV q4h (administer IV slowly)	1.25 mg/kg IM or IV q6h (maximum 300 mg/day)
diphenhydramine (Benadryl)	25-50 mg q4-6h	6-12 years: 12.5-25 mg q4-6h
doxylamine (Unisom)	12.5-25 mg q4-6h	6-12 years: 6.25-12.5 mg q4-6h
fexofenadine (Allegra ◆, Allegra-D ◆)	60 mg PO twice daily	Not available
loratadine (Claritin ◆, ClaritinD ◆)	10 mg daily, before eating	2-9 years: 5 mg daily before eating 10 years and older: see adult dosage
phenindamine (Nolahist)	25 mg q4-6h	6-12 years: 12.5 mg q4-6h
tripelennamine (Pyribenzamine)	25-50 mg q4-6h	1.25 mg/kg q6h (maximum 300 mg/day)
	Extended-release: 100 mg q8-12h	Not recommended
triprolidine (Myidil)	2.5 mg q4-6h	4 to 24 months: 312 μg q6-8h 2-4 years: 625 μg q6-8h 4 to 6 years: 937 μg q6-8h 6 to 12 years: 1.25 mg q6-8h

Review the client's health history to determine if there is a previous intolerance to antihistamines. In addition, review the client's current medication regimen for the risk of significant drug interactions, such as those that may occur when antihistamines are given with the following drugs:

Drug	Possible Effect and Management
Bold/color type indicates the most serious interactions.	
alcohol, CNS depressants	Concurrent use may enhance the CNS depressant effects. If the CNS depressant also has anticholinergic side effects, enhanced anticholinergic effects may be seen. Monitor closely, because interventions may be necessary.
anticholinergic medications, psychotropics, and others	Enhanced CNS depressant and anticholinergic side effects may be noted. Monitor closely, because intervention may be necessary.
clarithromycin (Biaxin), erythromycin (Erythrocin), troleandomycin (TAO)	**An increased risk of cardiotoxic effects has been reported with concurrent use of astemizole (Hismanal). Such use is contraindicated pending further investigation.**
grapefruit juice	Concurrent use inhibits the metabolism of astemizole; this leads to increased serum concentrations, which may prolong QT intervals with resultant dysrhythmias.
itraconazole (Sporanox) ketoconazole (Nizoral), mibefradil (Posicor)	**If administered concurrently with astemizole or loratadine, increased levels of antihistamines may result, which increases the potential for cardiotoxicity. Avoid concurrent use or a potentially serious drug interaction may occur.**
monoamine oxidase (MAO) inhibitors	**Prolonged anticholinergic and CNS depression effects may result. Avoid concurrent use or a potentially serious drug interaction may occur.**
quinine	**Concurrent use is contraindicated with astemizole (Hismanal), because a serious dysrhythmia may occur.**
zileuton	Concurrent use increases serum concentrations of astemizole (Hismanal). Although dysrhythmias have not been reported, concurrent use is not recommended pending further investigations.

A baseline assessment of the condition for which the antihistamine is being administered should be obtained.

■ **Nursing Diagnosis.** With the administration of antihistamines, the client should be assessed for the following nursing diagnoses/collaborative problems: impaired comfort related to dryness of the mouth and throat, rash, and/or tinnitus; risk for injury related to blurred vision, drowsiness, and hypotension (fainting); ineffective airway clearance related to thickened mucus; disturbed thought processes (confusion); impaired urinary elimination (difficult or painful urination); and the potential complications of blood dyscrasias (unusual bleeding or bruising, sore throat, fever), cardiac dysrhythmias, photosensitivity, and paradoxical reaction (excitement, restlessness, nightmares).

Pregnancy Safety
Antihistamines

Category	Drug
B	azatadine, brompheniramine, chlorpheniramine, clemastine, cyproheptadine, dexchlorpheniramine, dimenhydrinate, diphenhydramine, loratadine, triprolidine
C	astemizole, benzonatate
Unclassified	doxylamine, hydroxyzine, tripelennamine

■ **Implementation**

■ ***Monitoring.*** With IV administration, monitor the client's blood pressure before and after dosing. Observe the client for drowsiness that might be hazardous. Clients undergoing long-term antihistamine therapy should have periodic blood counts to monitor for the development of blood dyscrasias. Tolerance to some antihistamines may occur. If a tolerance develops, another antihistamine may be prescribed.

A paradoxical response to the drug may occur in an older child, with the child exhibiting hyperexcitability rather than the drowsiness that is usually seen. With older adults, sedation and hypotension are more likely to occur, as well as the antimuscarinic effects of the drug, resulting in dryness of the mouth or urinary retention, particularly in men.

Closely monitor clients with hypertension or cardiac or renal disease who are taking antihistamines. (See the Pregnancy Safety box above for ratings of the Food and Drug Administration [FDA]).

■ ***Intervention.*** Administer the oral dosage form with food, water, or milk to minimize gastric irritation. Do not break, crush, or chew sustained-release capsules or long-acting tablets.

■ ***Education.*** Advise the client who will be using antihistamines on a long-term basis to maintain dental hygiene by brushing and flossing, because the diminished salivary flow resulting from antihistamines will contribute to caries and gum disease. Regular dental checkups should also be advised. Ice, sugarless gum, or hard candy may minimize the discomfort of mouth dryness.

Drowsiness is a common effect of antihistamines. Caution the client about driving or using other hazardous equipment until the response to the drug has been ascertained. The client may modify his or her lifestyle accordingly when the effect of the drug is known. If the drowsiness is severe, another antihistamine may be prescribed.

Advise the client about using sun-protection lotions, wearing hats and long sleeves, and avoiding the sun from 10

AM to 3 PM to avoid the sunburn secondary to the photosensitivity effect of these drugs.

Alert the client to the symptoms of blood dyscrasias, such as sore throat, fever, unusual bruising and bleeding, and tiredness; these symptoms should be reported to the prescriber. Caution the client about ingesting alcohol or CNS depressants, because the effects of the drugs will be potentiated.

If the client is taking antihistamines as prophylaxis for motion sickness, the dose should be taken 30 minutes to 1 to 2 hours before its effect is needed. The client taking antihistamines should alert the allergist if scheduled for allergy skin tests, because these drugs interfere with the results.

▪ **Evaluation.** If antihistamines are taken for an antitussive effect, the expected outcome is that the client will report a decrease in coughing. If taken for symptoms of allergy, the client will demonstrate relief from itching, sneezing, and nasal secretions. If taken for the prevention of motion sickness, the client will report an absence or a decreased frequency or intensity of nausea episodes. If taken for sleep, the client will report having slept well.

Inhibitor of Histamine Release

Cromolyn sodium provides a local protective effect in the mucosal airways by inhibiting the granulation of pulmonary mast cells and thereby preventing the release of histamine and SRS-A. (See the section on cromolyn sodium in Chapter 38.)

SEROTONIN

As with histamine, serotonin (5-hydroxytryptamine or 5-HT) has no therapeutic application; however, its importance is related to the action of other drugs and several disease states. Serotonin is widely distributed in nature, occurring in both plants (pineapples, bananas, strawberries, tomatoes, nuts) and animals. In human beings, serotonin occurs in various body tissues but primarily in three tissue types:

1. The largest fraction (90%) is synthesized and stored in the enterochromaffin cells of the gastrointestinal tract mucosa, particularly in the pylorus of the stomach and in the upper region of the small intestine.
2. A much smaller fraction is stored but not synthesized in platelets; on disintegration this fraction is released in serum and in the spleen.
3. In the CNS the greatest concentration of serotonin occurs in the hypothalamus, midbrain, reticular formation, raphe (midline) regions of the medulla and pons, and pineal gland. A neuron that releases serotonin is termed a *serotoninergic* or *tryptaminergic fiber.*

Only a very low concentration of serotonin appears in cells.

Pharmacologic Actions

Serotonin appears to possess multiple pharmacologic actions; this variability has caused much controversy because of discrepant experimental findings. Despite the need for additional experimental analysis, it is now known that the primary function of serotonin is exerted on various smooth muscles and nerves. As previously stated, serotonin is not a therapeutic agent, but its more prominent effects are associated with its influence on other drugs and some disease states.

Gastrointestinal Tract. Serotonin is secreted from specialized cells of the stomach and intestine that are responsible for contraction of the gastrointestinal smooth muscle, thereby producing the peristaltic response.

Carcinoid syndrome is a condition elicited from carcinoid tumors; these tumors cause an overproduction of serotonin, and bradykinin and histamine may also be released. Serotonin is responsible for causing this syndrome, which is characterized by paroxysmal flushing, hyperperistalsis, diarrhea, bronchoconstriction, and cardiac valvular lesions. The diagnosis of carcinoid syndrome is confirmed by the presence of excess serotonin, which eventually is excreted in the urine.

Blood Platelets. Serotonin is released from platelets during their breakdown within the circulation. This compound activates receptors on the surface of other blood platelets, thereby promoting platelet aggregation. It has been suggested that through this mechanism the discharge of serotonin from platelets may contribute to the formation of pulmonary embolism.

Central Nervous System. Serotonin is manufactured and stored in the neurons of the brain. The central action of the neuronal system appears to elicit primarily an inhibitory response from the specific nuclei of the brain. Researchers now postulate that the altered function of serotoninergic pathways is a factor in various CNS dysfunctions.

Sleep. Serotonin-synthesizing cells are required for the induction of non–rapid eye movement (NREM) sleep (quiet brain, potentially excitable muscles) and the onset of REM sleep (active brain, rapid eye movements, dreams, atonic muscles). Normal sleep depends on serotonin along with the combined functions of the norepinephrine and cholinergic systems. The basic sleep pattern consists of four to six cycles that alternate between NREM and REM sleep. Destruction of the raphe nuclei results in insomnia. Other disorders of sleep are quite common; for example, narcolepsy is characterized by a sudden change from wakefulness directly to REM sleep.

Sleep hypnotics such as barbiturates tend to decrease REM sleep, which is an essential component of restful sleep. The drug *p*-chlorophenylalanine inhibits the formation of serotonin; this depletion can cause prolonged wakefulness when administered to animals.

Pain Perception. The serotoninergic neurons located in the raphe nuclei of the brainstem have axons that project to the spinal cord and forebrain. One important system related to the brain involves a substance called beta-endorphin, which is associated with neurons that interconnect various nuclei in the hypothalamus, limbic system, and thalamus. The beta-endorphin neurons mediate euphoric and emotional behavior. The thalamic nuclei mediate poorly

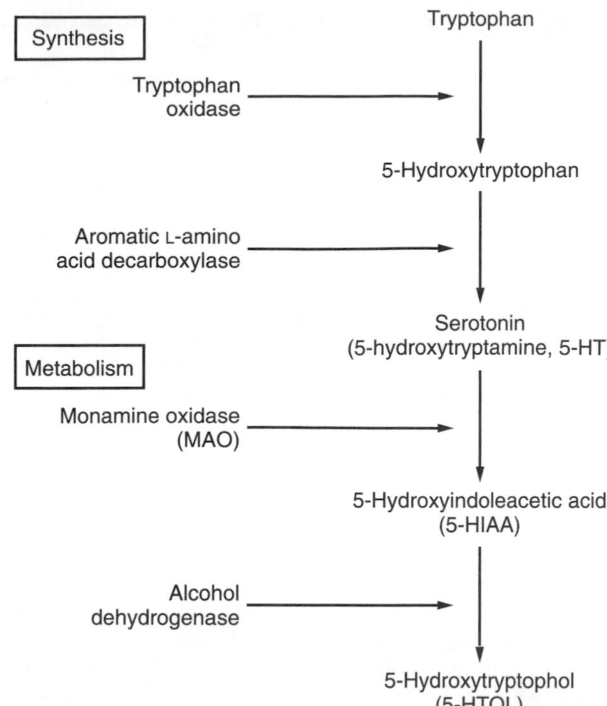

Figure 39-2 Synthesis and metabolism of serotonin.

localized deep pain, which is best influenced by opiates. The density of opiate receptors in the brain appears to be much greater in the medial and lateral thalamus. The extent of opiate addiction and withdrawal is influenced by the quantity of opiate receptors involved.

Serotonin is also implicated in the action of morphine. Studies suggest that the synthesis but not the accumulation of serotonin doubles with the development of tolerance to morphine. In addition, a decrease in serotonin levels in the brain increases a person's sensitivity to painful stimuli, thus decreasing the analgesic effect of morphine.

Mental Illness. CNS depression correlates with low levels of serotonin in the brain. The enzyme MAO metabolizes serotonin, resulting in a lower level of the transmitter (Figure 39-2). Accordingly, an MAO inhibitor blocks the degradation of serotonin and thereby increases its level of concentration in the brain. (The antidepressant effects of the MAO inhibitors are discussed in Chapter 19.) The tricyclic compounds also act as antidepressants, blocking the reuptake of serotonin and norepinephrine at the membrane of the neuron and thereby potentiating the action of the synapse. Selective serotonin reuptake inhibitors (SSRIs), a newer class of antidepressants, act by inhibiting the reuptake and destruction of serotonin from the synaptic cleft, thereby prolonging the action of the neurotransmitter.

ANTISEROTONINS

Antiserotonins, or serotonin antagonists, are considered complex compounds because they possess varying degrees of specificity; their exact mechanism of action is unknown. In addition to performing serotonin-blocking activity, many other pharmacologic actions are involved in inhibiting responses to serotonin.

cyproheptadine [si proe hep′ ta deen] (Periactin)

Cyproheptadine blocks serotonin activity in the smooth muscle of blood vessels and the intestine and also has antihistaminic and possibly anticholinergic properties. It may produce weight gain by blocking serotonin activity in the appetite center in the hypothalamus; in other words, cyproheptadine stimulates appetite. Although not approved by the FDA, it has also been used to treat vascular headaches. It is administered primarily for allergic disorders. (See Antihistamines, p. 741.)

lysergic acid diethylamide (LSD)

The basic mechanism underlying the hallucinogenic properties of LSD is not known. However, experts agree that its profound effects on behavior are mediated through the central neurotransmitter, serotonin. Studies performed in the 1970s suggested that the more powerful hallucinogenic drugs exert a dual function in the brain: (1) inhibiting the action of serotonin, and (2) stimulating the norepinephrine system. (See Chapter 9 for a discussion of LSD as a drug of abuse.)

methysergide maleate [meth i ser′ jide] (Sansert)

Although its mechanism of action in preventing vascular headaches is unknown, methysergide is both a potent antiserotonin and a vasoconstrictor agent. These properties apparently help to relieve migraine and other vascular headaches (see Chapter 22).

SURFACTANTS

For information on beractant (Survanta), calfactant (Infasurf), and colfosceril (Exosurf Neonatal), three new drugs in this classification, see Appendix E.

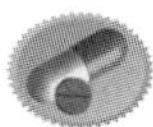

SUMMARY

The drugs discussed in this chapter cover a wide range of therapeutic effects on the respiratory system. Oxygen, a therapeutic gas, is essential to sustain life, and its administration is required for many clients. Although most acute care facilities have a respiratory therapy department, the nurse is responsible for evaluating the client's response to oxygen and, in some circumstances, initiating oxygen therapy.

In general, cough suppressants are used for nonproductive coughs in which prolonged coughing is annoying, exhausting, and painful. (Opioid antitussive drugs are discussed in Chapter 14.) Nonnarcotic antitussive drugs may be effective and produce fewer gastrointestinal side effects.

Histamine is a chemical mediator that occurs naturally in most body tissues and has been implicated in a number of pathologic conditions, such as urticaria, atopy, food allergies, bronchial asthma, and systemic anaphylaxis. This makes antihistamines, which compete with histamines at receptor sites to prevent their physiologic actions, invaluable as medications. Antihistamines are contained in numerous antitussive preparations, cold-cough products, OTC sleeping compounds, and oral analgesic products.

Serotonin is a naturally occurring substance with no therapeutic application. However, it is related to the action of other drugs, such as the opiates. CNS depression also correlates with low levels of serotonin in the brain. The antiserotonins (cyproheptadine and methysergide maleate) may be used to relieve vascular headaches, but cyproheptadine is used primarily for allergic disorders.

Critical Thinking Questions

1. Mr. Hodges, a 72-year-old with COPD, has been receiving low-flow oxygen therapy at 2 L/min per nasal cannula. When you check the flowmeter, you discover it is set at 6 L/min. What assessment do you need to make of Mr. Hodges immediately? Why?
2. You are preparing Mr. Hodges and his wife for his return home, where he will be continuing his oxygen therapy. Although Mr. Hodges has given up smoking since he became so ill, you have noticed that both his wife and his son, with whom he lives, smoke. What action will you take?

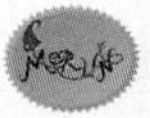

Collaborative Learning Activities

For Collaborative Learning Activities, go to mosby.com/MERLIN/McKenry/.

CASE STUDY

For a Case Study that will help ensure mastery of this chapter content, go to mosby.com/MERLIN/McKenry/.

BIBLIOGRAPHY

American Association of Respiratory Care Clinical Practice Guideline. (1992). Oxygen therapy in the home or extended care facility. *Respiratory Care, 37*(3), 918-922.

American Hospital Formulary Service. (1999). *AHFS drug information '99*. American Society of Hospital Pharmacists.

Anderson, K.N., Anderson, L.E., & Glanze, W.D. (Eds.) (1998). *Mosby's medical, nursing, & allied health dictionary* (5th ed.). St. Louis: Mosby.

Branson, R.D. (1993). The nuts and bolts of increasing arterial oxygenation: Devices and techniques. *Respiratory Care, 38*(6), 672-683.

Drug Facts and Comparisons. (2000). St. Louis: Facts and Comparisons.

Hussain, N., Clive, J., & Bhandari, V. (1999). Current incidence of retinopathy of prematurity: 1989-1997. *Pediatrics, 104*(3), e26.

Kay, G.G. & Harris, A.G. (1999). Loratadine: a non-sedating antihistamine: Review of its effects on cognition, psychomotor performance, mood and sedation. *Clinical and Experimental Allergy, 29*(suppl 3), 147-150.

Mason, J., Reynolds, R., & Rao, N. (1999). The systemic safety of fexofenadine. *Clinical and Experimental Allergy, 29*(suppl 3), 163-170.

Routledge, P.A., Lindquist, M., & Edwards, I.R. (1999). Spontaneous reporting of suspected adverse reactions to antihistamines: A national and international perspective. *Clinical and Experimental Allergy, 29*(suppl 3), 240-246.

Somerson, S.J. & Sicilia, M.R. (1992). Emergency oxygen administration and airway management. *Critical Care Nurse, 12*(4), 23-29.

United States Pharmacopeia Dispensing Information (USP DI): Drug information for the health care professional (19th ed.). (1999). Rockville, MD: United States Pharmacopeial Convention.

Weaver, L.K. (1992). Hyperbaric treatment of respiratory emergencies. *Respiratory Care, 37*(7), 720-730.

Wilson, S.F. & Thompson, J.M. (1990). *Respiratory disorders*. St. Louis: Mosby.

40 Overview of the Gastrointestinal Tract

Chapter Focus

The gastrointestinal (GI) system is responsible for the digestive processes of the body and for supplying nutrients to fuel the body. This function contributes to the client's wellness by influencing overall health. The nurse should assess every client's nutritional-metabolic need. This assessment requires a thorough knowledge of the anatomy and physiology of the GI system and provides the background for the nurse to plan for and deliver appropriate care to clients with GI disorders. This chapter provides a review of that anatomy and physiology.

Learning Objectives

1. Identify the major parts of the GI tract.
2. Describe the functions of individual components of the GI tract.
3. List the effects of parasympathetic and sympathetic innervation on the GI tract.
4. Describe common disorders affecting the GI tract.

Key Terms

acute gastritis, p. 749
cholecystitis, p. 750
cholelithiasis, p. 750
chronic gastritis, p. 749
digestion, p. 748
peptic ulcer disease, p. 749
peristalsis, p. 748

Disorders of the gastrointestinal (GI) tract such as indigestion, gastritis, constipation, and peptic ulcers are very common problems reported by large numbers of the population. Because the cause of many GI diseases remains unclear, pharmacologic management is often directed at relieving symptoms rather than at control or cure. In this chapter the anatomy and functions of the GI tract are reviewed.

The GI system is made up of the alimentary canal (or digestive tract), the biliary system, and the pancreas (Figure 40-1). The alimentary canal extends from the mouth to the anus. Food substances entering the canal undergo mechanical and chemical changes called **digestion.** These changes permit nutrients to be absorbed and indigestible materials to be excreted by the body. Absorbed nutrients may be used as an energy source or stored (as glycogen for glucose or as fat for carbohydrates). **Peristalsis** is the movement of the smooth muscle fibers surrounding the canal that (1) mixes the contents by segmental contractions and (2) moves the mass through the tract by peristalsis.

The secretory and muscular activities of the GI system are regulated by neural mechanisms. An interconnecting network of neurons is located in the smooth muscle and secretory cells. This system is self-regulating; it is capable of controlling exocrine gland secretions and muscular contractions without any external influence.

By contrast, the external innervation of the GI system is supplied by the divisions of the autonomic nervous system. Their major function is to correlate activities between different regions of the GI system and also between this system and other parts of the body. The influence of the parasympathetic division is mediated by two branches of the vagus nerve and exerts an excitatory action, which increases digestive secretions and muscular activity. In contrast, the splanchnic nerves of the sympathetic division are primarily inhibitory, depressing digestive secretions and muscular activity. Under normal conditions, the two divisions of the autonomic nervous system maintain a delicate balance of control of functions.

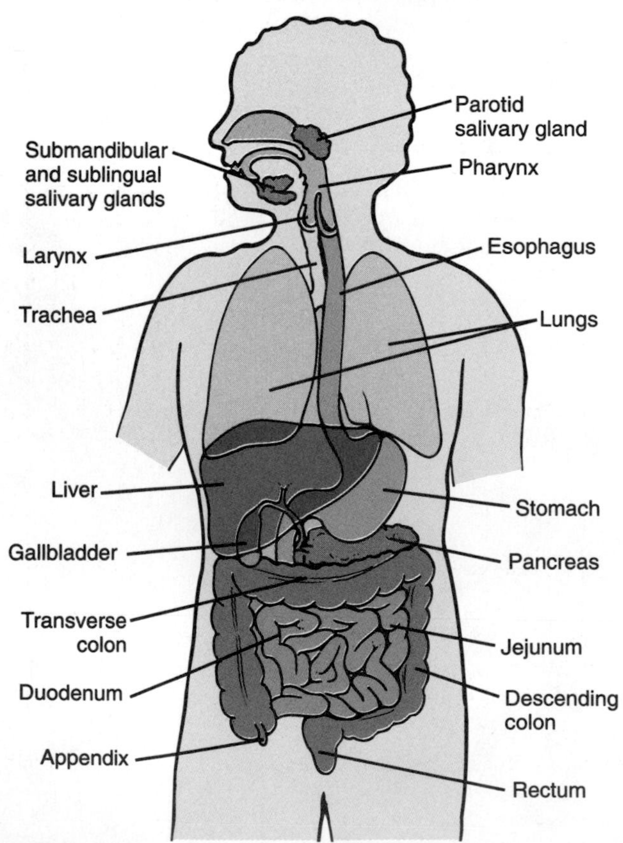

Figure 40-1 Gastrointestinal and respiratory systems.

Drugs affecting the GI tract exert their action mainly on muscular and glandular tissues. The action may be directly on the smooth muscle and gland cells or indirectly on the autonomic nervous system. Drugs may also increase or decrease function, tone, emptying time, or peristaltic action of the stomach or bowel. In addition, they may be used to relieve enzyme deficiency, to counteract excess acidity or gas formation, to produce or prevent vomiting, or to aid with diagnosis.

MOUTH (ORAL CAVITY)

The mouth, or oral cavity, functions as the starting point of the digestive process. Food is taken in, chewed, and mixed with saliva, which contains the enzyme amylase (ptyalin) and begins the process of chemical digestion.

Three pairs of salivary glands secrete saliva into the ducts that empty into the mouth. The sublingual and submandibular salivary glands are located beneath the tongue; the largest pair, the parotid glands, are found in front of and slightly below the ears. When the food bolus has been chewed and reduced in the mouth, it is swallowed. Swallowing (deglutition) is a complex process that begins as a voluntary movement but continues as an involuntary muscular reflex as the food is propelled through the GI tract.

Disorders Affecting the Mouth. Systemic diseases, nutritional deficiencies, and mechanical trauma can cause irritation or inflammation of the buccal structures. Dental disorders (e.g., caries, gingivitis, and pyorrhea) and bacterial, viral, or fungal infections (e.g., candidiasis or herpes simplex) can affect the structures of the oral cavity, causing symptoms such as mouth blistering or other lesions, swelling, pain, and inflammation.

Agents acting on the oral cavity are discussed in Chapter 41.

PHARYNX

The pharynx (throat), a tubelike passageway connecting the mouth and the esophagus, is important in swallowing. Food and fluid pass through the pharynx into the esophagus. During this passage the trachea is closed to prevent aspiration into the lungs.

Disorders Affecting the Pharynx. Like the mouth, various systemic diseases can affect the pharynx. It can become irritated and inflamed (e.g., from sinusitis or the "common cold") and treated symptomatically with an antiinflammatory agent. It can also become a locus of infection (e.g., strep throat), which requires systemic antibiotic therapy.

ESOPHAGUS

The esophagus is a pliable muscular structure approximately 25 cm long that extends from the pharynx to the cardiac end of the stomach. It extends through the diaphragm as it drops from the thoracic cavity into the abdominal cavity.

The esophagus is considered the beginning of the digestive system proper; the rest of the organs of the GI tract function only in digestion and/or excretion. The esophagus continues the process of swallowing and begins the peristaltic process, or the squeezing of the food bolus down the GI tract by band contraction. The peristaltic band wave stimulates the lower esophageal sphincter, which closes to prevent gastroesophageal reflux and then returns the esophagus to its normal resting state.

Disorders Affecting the Esophagus. Esophageal disorders are characterized by retrosternal pain (heartburn) and difficulty in swallowing (dysphagia). The sources of pain are numerous; potential causes include diffuse esophageal spasm, achalasia, pyloric or duodenal ulcers, scleroderma, postural changes (bending forward), excessive alcohol ingestion, and nonspecific dysmotility.

Heartburn commonly results from reflux esophagitis, in which the incompetent lower esophageal sphincter permits gastric contents to flow back into the esophagus; or from hiatal hernia, in which a part of the stomach protrudes into the diaphragm. One type of hiatal hernia, paraesophageal hernia, may be associated with esophageal obstruction and strangulation. Difficulty in swallowing can be a symptom of esophageal obstruction, mechanical interference with or paralysis of the muscles of deglutition, neuromuscular incoordination, achalasia, carcinoma of the esophagus, anxiety states, hysteria, or schizophrenic hallucinations.

Inflammation of the esophagus can have many causes: reflux esophagitis associated with hiatal hernia, irritant ingestion, infection, peptic ulceration, prolonged gastric intubation, and uremia.

STOMACH

The stomach, a pouchlike structure lying below the diaphragm, has three divisions: the fundus, the body, and the pylorus. Two sphincter muscles—the cardiac sphincter and the pyloric sphincter—regulate the stomach opening. Gastric glands secrete mucus and gastric juice composed of enzymes and hydrochloric acid. They also produce intrinsic factor, a protein essential for the absorption of vitamin B_{12}. Vitamin B_{12} is needed for erythropoiesis (red blood cell formation).

The stomach functions as a temporary storage site for food as it is being digested. It also manufactures gastrin, a hormone that regulates enzyme production to facilitate digestion. The stomachs of males and females differ both in storage capacity and in size; females have smaller and more slender stomachs. The stomach is capable of holding 1500 to 2000 mL. It distends after eating and gradually collapses as the food bolus moves into the small intestine. Its churning action further breaks down the food bolus and mixes it with gastric juice to continue chemical digestion. A limited amount of nutrient and drug absorption takes place in the stomach.

The time required for digestion in the stomach depends on the amount of food eaten. Normal emptying time is 2 to 6 hours. However, gastric emptying time may be affected by drug administration, physical activity of the individual, and body position during digestion. Gastric emptying time is a factor to consider in the timing of drug administration, because the presence of food may block the absorption of some drugs.

Disorders Affecting the Stomach. **Acute gastritis** is an inflammatory response of the stomach lining to the ingestion of irritants, such as ethanol or nonsteroidal antiinflammatory agents, including aspirin. Symptoms include epigastric discomfort, nausea, abdominal tenderness, and GI hemorrhage. Treatment consists of lifestyle modifications and drugs such as antacids, antiemetic agents, anticholinergics, and antihistamines (see Chapter 41).

Chronic gastritis is a long-term inflammation of the stomach lining, generally with degeneration of the gastric mucosa; its causes are not well established. It is more common in women, and the incidence increases with age, excessive smoking, and ethanol use. Symptoms are nonspecific but may include flatulence, epigastric fullness after meals, diarrhea, and bleeding. Iron deficiency anemia and pernicious anemia may result from chronic gastritis. Treatment is the same as for acute gastritis. The usual therapeutic regimen involves treatment of symptoms with antacids, anticholinergics, and sedatives (and vitamin B_{12} if pernicious anemia is present), as well as the elimination of possible causative or aggravating factors (e.g., aspirin use).

Peptic ulcer disease is a broad term encompassing both gastric and duodenal ulcers. Although both types of ulcers produce a "break" in the gastric mucosa, the causes differ. With gastric ulcers the ability of the gastric mucosa to protect and repair itself seems to be defective; with duodenal ulcers the hypersecretion of gastric acid is responsible for the erosion of the gastric mucosa. Gastric colonization with *Helicobacter pylori*, a gram-negative bacillus, has been identified as a causative agent in clients with peptic ulcer disease not caused by nonsteroidal antiinflammatory drugs. Treatment with various antibacterial combinations has resulted in healing and a low recurrence rate (Abramowicz, 1994). *H. pylori* has been identified in nearly all persons with duodenal ulcers and in nearly 75% of persons with gastric ulcers (Berardi & Dunn-Kucharski, 1993).

Duodenal ulcers are more common than gastric ulcers; they account for nearly 80% of all peptic ulcers. Duodenal ulcers usually occur more often in younger persons. Overall, the reported incidence of peptic ulcers is much lower in females. In addition to antibacterial combination therapies, pharmacologic treatment of peptic ulcer disease may include the use of antacids, H_2 receptor antagonists, and sucralfate. Nondrug treatment (diet and lifestyle modifications) is equally important (see Chapter 41). Hereditary factors, the use of some drugs (e.g., aspirin and corticosteroids), psychologic factors, stress, and diet have been implicated in the development of peptic ulcer disease.

LIVER

Immediately under the diaphragm and above the stomach is the liver, the largest gland in the body. It weighs approximately 1.5 kg and is an extremely active and important organ that performs more than 100 different functions.

The liver consists of two lobes, which are composed of multitudes of lobules that function to remove toxins from the bloodstream, store nutrients such as iron and some vitamins, and secrete bile. Bile is transported via the hepatic ducts to the gallbladder for storage. In the intestine, bile aids in the digestion, emulsification, and absorption of fat. Because it is normally alkaline, bile also functions to neutralize gastric acid in the duodenum.

Venous blood goes directly to the liver from the intestinal tract; nutrients and absorbed drugs pass through the liver before reaching the systemic circulation. Thus the liver plays an active role in absorbing and metabolizing fats, carbohydrates, and proteins. It also stores iron and vitamins A, B_{12}, and D. Some drugs are taken up by the liver, released into the bile, and excreted in the feces. Other drugs move from the bile into the small intestine, where they are reabsorbed and recirculated. Still other drugs are transformed by the liver and excreted in the urine. In all of these cases the liver metabolizes the drug to make it more water soluble. This biotransformation changes the parent compound to a metabolite that may have greater, lesser, or equal activity; cytochrome P-450 in the liver is responsible for biotransformation. There are also drugs that pass through the body and are excreted unchanged in the urine.

Disorders Affecting the Liver. Viral hepatitis, Laënnec's cirrhosis, postnecrotic cirrhosis, carcinoma, and chronic alcoholism cause liver damage and liver cell dysfunction.

GALLBLADDER

Lying on the undersurface of the liver is the gallbladder, a pear-shaped organ 7 to 10 cm long and 2.5 to 3.5 cm wide. The gallbladder can hold 30 to 50 mL of bile. It concentrates the bile and stores it until it is needed for digestion in the stomach and small intestine.

Disorders Affecting the Gallbladder. Cholecystitis, inflammation of the gallbladder, is often associated with the presence of gallstones (**cholelithiasis**). The stones lodge in the ducts or neck of the gallbladder, causing congestion and edema as bile builds up. This condition may be acute or chronic. Treatment of cholecystitis and cholelithiasis includes the administration of analgesics, antispasmodics, and chenodeoxycholic acid. Malignant tumors of the gallbladder are uncommon.

PANCREAS

The pancreas is a gland that is approximately 15 to 20 cm long and 5 cm wide, and it weighs approximately 75 g. The gland has three major segments: the head (found in the curve of the duodenum), the body, and the tail (which touches or nearly touches the spleen). The role of the pancreas is twofold: the exocrine cells secrete the digestive enzymes found in pancreatic juice, and the endocrine cells help to control the metabolism of carbohydrates by producing glucagon and insulin.

Disorders Affecting the Pancreas. With the exception of diabetes mellitus, many pancreatic diseases have symptoms that are not readily diagnosed. Inflammation of the pancreas may be acute or chronic. Among the many causes are blockage of the pancreatic ducts, trauma to the pancreas, alcohol consumption, drug use, tumors, cysts, or abscesses. Symptoms are nonspecific but ultimately include severe pain. Carcinoma of the pancreas is as difficult to diagnose as other pancreatic disorders.

SMALL INTESTINE

The small intestine is a coiled tube approximately 21 feet long. It consists of the duodenum, jejunum, and ileum. Within the small intestine the food bolus is thoroughly mixed with the digestive juices to complete the "breakdown" process. The intestinal mucosa then absorbs nutrients and drugs, which are filtered through the liver before entering the circulatory and lymphatic systems.

Disorders Affecting the Small Intestine. Diarrhea and constipation are two disorders that affect the entire lower GI tract. These disorders are discussed in Chapters 11 and 41 along with the drugs used in their treatment.

Other disorders affecting the small intestine include obstruction, malabsorption syndrome, and blind loop syndrome. Symptomatic treatment is customary while the underlying causative factors are investigated.

LARGE INTESTINE

The cecum, colon, and rectum make up the large intestine. The distal 2.5 cm of the rectum is known as the anal canal. The large intestine is approximately 5 feet long and completes the digestive and absorptive processes. The large intestine is involved mainly with water absorption (from 1800 to 3000 mL/day) and synthesis of vitamin K. The lining of the large intestine secretes mucus to coat the undigested residue and protect the bowel lining. The indigestible residue is expelled through the reflex action known as defecation.

Disorders Affecting the Large Intestine. Diarrhea and constipation, which are discussed in Chapters 11 and 41, also affect the large intestine. Other disorders include diverticular disease, which has no specific therapy; ulcerative colitis, which is treated with lifestyle modifications, antidiarrheals, and steroids; carcinoma; and irritable bowel syndrome. Hemorrhoids (varicosities of the external or internal hemorrhoidal veins) are common.

SUMMARY

Food sustains life and determines nutritional status, which contributes to an individual's state of health, levels of achievement, and resistance to and ability to handle disease. The primary function of the GI tract is to provide the body cells with nutrients, electrolytes, and water through the processes of ingestion, digestion, and absorption of food and fluid and the elimination of waste products and residue. Drugs affect the GI tract by acting primarily on muscular and glandular tissue. Although some drugs are prescribed primarily for their effect on the GI tract, the nurse needs to be aware that most drugs prescribed for other reasons also produce GI side effects/adverse reactions.

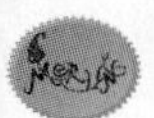

Critical Thinking Questions

1. Imagine being a bolus of food progressing through the GI tract; describe what the journey would be like.
2. Patty Smith has been diagnosed as having achlorhydria, a condition in which the stomach stops producing hydrochloric acid. What effect will this have on her digestion? On her red blood cell count?

Collaborative Learning Activities

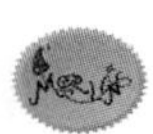

For Collaborative Learning Activities, go to mosby.com/MERLIN/McKenry/.

BIBLIOGRAPHY

Abramowicz, M. (Ed.). (1994). Drugs for the treatment of peptic ulcers. *The Medical Letter, 36*(927), 65-67.

Anderson, K.N., Anderson, L.E., & Glanze, W.D. (Eds.). (1998). *Mosby's medical, nursing, & allied health dictionary* (5th ed.). St. Louis: Mosby.

Berardi, R.R. & Dunn-Kucharski, V.A. (1993). Peptic ulcer disease: An update. *American Pharmacy, NS33*(6), 26-34.

McCance, K.L. & Huether, S.E. (1998). *Pathophysiology: The biological basis for disease in adults and children* (3rd ed.). St. Louis: Mosby.

Melmon, K.L., Morrelli, H.F., Hoffman, B.B., & Nierberg, D.W. (1992). *Clinical pharmacology: Basic principles in therapeutics* (3rd ed.). New York: McGraw-Hill.

Thibodeau, G.A. & Patton, K.T. (1999). *Anatomy and physiology* (4th ed.). St. Louis: Mosby.

Van Wynsberghe, D., Noback, C.R., & Carola, R. (1995). *Human anatomy and physiology* (3rd ed.). New York: McGraw-Hill.

41 Drugs Affecting the Gastrointestinal Tract

Chapter Focus

The gastrointestinal (GI) tract affects the overall health of the individual because it has the essential task of supplying necessary nutrients to fuel the physiologic processes of other vital organs (brain, lungs, and heart) and of eliminating the body's wastes. Many GI disorders are manifested as pain, nausea, constipation, and diarrhea, which negatively affect the client's quality of life. To assist clients toward self-management and optimal health, the nurse needs to be knowledgeable and skillful in the management of the pharmacologic therapeutic regimen related to the GI tract.

Learning Objectives

1. Discuss the use and side effects of antacids.
2. List four drugs administered to promote digestion.
3. Differentiate the five classes of antiemetic medications and their sites of action.
4. Describe the emetic agents and their use.
5. Discuss the effect of proton pump inhibitors and H_2 receptor antagonists on gastric acid secretion.
6. Discuss the use of mesalamine, olsalazine, sulfasalazine, and infliximab in the treatment of inflammatory and ulcerative bowel disease.
7. Differentiate between the various types of laxatives and their mechanisms of action, and state the best indication for each type.
8. Implement nursing management for the care of clients receiving agents that affect the GI tract.

Key Terms

adsorbents, p. 785
antiemetics, p. 759
chemoreceptor trigger zone, p. 759
constipation, p. 778
diarrhea, p. 756
emetic center, p. 759
laxatives, p. 779

Key Drugs [✓]

cimetidine, p. 772
mesalamine, p. 776
metoclopramide, p. 760
misoprostol, p. 769
omeprazole, p. 770
ondansetron, p. 764

Drugs That Affect the Upper Gastrointestinal Tract

DRUGS THAT AFFECT THE MOUTH

In general, medications have little effect on the mouth. Good oral hygiene, which includes brushing properly after meals and at bedtime, flossing, and stimulating the gums, has more influence on the tissues of the mouth than most medicines. Many mouth and throat preparations are available with steroids, anesthetics, and antiseptics for various disorders of the oral cavity, including chapped lips, sun and fever blisters, inflammatory lesions, ulcerative lesions secondary to trauma, gingival lesions, teething pain, toothache, irritation caused by orthodontic appliances or dentures, and abrasions of the oral cavity. Most agents that affect the mouth may be purchased over-the-counter (OTC).

Mouthwashes and Gargles

Mouthwashes and gargles are dilute aromatic solutions that contain a sweetener and an artificial coloring agent. They may also contain an antiseptic (e.g., alcohol, cetylpyridinium chloride, phenol), anesthetic (eugenol, clove oil), astringent (zinc chloride), or anticaries agent (sodium fluoride). Mouthwashes with a high alcohol content may be problematic for certain populations (Box 41-1).

Although several products claim to contain ingredients that reduce plaque formation, clinical trials have demonstrated some success with volatile oils and cetylpyridinium chloride alone or in combination with domiphen bromide. Commercial products that contain at least one of these active ingredients include Cepacol (cetylpyridinium chloride), Listerine (volatile oils), and Scope (cetylpyridinium chloride and domiphen bromide). A detergent-type product to lessen plaque (Plax) is also available on the market. The client should be informed that these products do not replace good oral hygiene but instead are recommended as an adjunct to proper brushing and flossing of the teeth (Flynn, 1996).

Mouthwashes are often used for halitosis, or "bad breath," or as gargles to treat colds or sore throats. In general, they are not considered effective for such problems. Mouthwashes may improve mouth odor briefly; however, if such a problem persists, the underlying cause needs to be identified and treated (e.g., poor dental hygiene, various gum diseases, and many other potential causes).

Sore throats are usually caused by infection, most often viral rather than bacterial. Gargling cannot reach the site of infection, which is usually deep in the throat tissues. Sodium chloride solution (½ teaspoon of salt to an 8-ounce glass of warm water) has been recommended for use as a gargle and mouthwash and is probably as effective as some of the remedies sold today.

BOX 41-1

Warnings for Mouthwashes with High Alcohol Content

Pediatric Alert

The leading mouthwashes usually contain between 14% and 27% alcohol. Because safety closures may not be used with mouthwashes, parents of young children should be cautioned to store these products in a safe area, preferably a locked cabinet. The use of mouthwashes in young children is not recommended, because children often swallow the mouthwash rather than expectorate it (Covington, 1996).

Alcohol Abuse

Alcoholics may substitute alcohol-containing products such as mouthwashes and cough-cold preparations when beverage alcohol is not readily available. The health care professional should be alert for the ingestion of alcohol-containing products in persons with a history of alcohol abuse (Katzung, 1992; Ruskosky, 1996).

Oxygen-Releasing Agents

Hydrogen peroxide is a weak antibacterial agent used to clean topical and oral wounds. The antibacterial effect depends on the liberation of oxygen, which occurs when the peroxide comes in contact with the tissue enzyme catalase. The resulting effervescence (bubbling action) loosens pus and tissue debris, which helps to reduce bacterial content. Hydrogen peroxide is usually used in a 1.5% to 3% solution for cleaning wounds or as a mouthwash. As a gargle, the 3% solution should be diluted with an equal amount of water before use.

A number of other oxygen-releasing products are commercially available. Perimax Perio Rinse (hydrogen peroxide) is used for the treatment of canker sores, denture irritation, and irritation following orthodontic intervention. The solution is expectorated. Hydrogen peroxide gel (Peroxyl) is also available for minor mouth irritation and is applied and expectorated after use.

Fluoridated Mouthwashes

A number of fluoride-containing preparations, including mouthwash (Fluorigard), toothpaste, tablets, and solutions are available for use as anticaries agents. Although the exact mechanism of action of fluoride in preventing caries is not fully understood, fluoride ions appear to exchange for hydroxyl or citrate (anion) ions and then settle in the anionic space on the surface of the enamel (Marcus, 1996). This results in a harder outer layer of tooth enamel (a fluoridated hydroxyapatite) that is more resistant to demineralization. Fluoridated mouthwashes have been used in communities with both limited fluoridated and unfluoridated water supplies, and their use has been associated with a significant decrease in tooth decay (between 17% and 47%) (Flynn, 1996).

Fluoridated mouthwashes are generally used once a day (rinsed for a minute and expectorated), preferably after brushing and flossing. The client should be taught to avoid taking anything by mouth for approximately 30 minutes after use. See Box 41-2 for information regarding fluoride toxicity.

Antiseptic Mouthwashes

Phenol penetrates plaque and is a local anesthetic and antimicrobial agent. Chloraseptic mouthwash contains phenol and sodium phenolate. Preparations that provide temporary relief of sore gums caused by teething often contain phenol or benzocaine. Phenol or phenol-type compounds are also present in several OTC lozenges, liquids, and sprays for the treatment of sore throat. The liquid is diluted with equal parts of water or may be sprayed full strength.

Dentifrices

A dentifrice is a substance used to aid in cleaning the teeth. An ordinary dentifrice contains one or more mild abrasives, a foaming agent, and flavoring materials made into a powder or paste (toothpaste) to aid in the mechanical cleansing of accessible parts of the teeth. Fluoride dentifrices are effective anticaries agents. These products carry a seal of the American Dental Association Council on Dental Therapeutics to indicate its endorsement.

Dentifrices are also available for the treatment of hypersensitive teeth, which usually occur from exposed root areas at the cement-enamel junction. The exposed area allows pain stimuli access to the nerve fibers in the pulp area. Dentists often suggest desensitizing dentifrices that contain potassium nitrate, such as Promise, Mint Sensodyne, or Denquel.

BOX 41-2

Fluoride Toxicity

Fluoride is capable of producing an acute toxic reaction that may be fatal if not treated promptly. A chronic toxic state resulting in mottling or discoloration of the tooth enamel and possible osteosclerosis has been reported. This effect may occur when excessive fluoride is consumed during childhood. In severe cases, the teeth have brown- to black-stained corroded areas.

Fluoridated water supplies usually contain 1 ppm (part per million) of fluoride, which is accepted as a safe and effective level in reducing the incidence of caries in permanent teeth. Health care professionals, particularly in primary health care settings, need to be aware of the amount of fluoride in their water supplies and to recommend and/or closely supervise the use of additional fluoride products by their clients. Fluoride supplements are recommended when community drinking water contains less than 0.7 ppm of fluoride (*United States Pharmacopeia Dispensing Information*, 1999).

Oral Antifungal Agents

clotrimazole [kloe trim′ a zole] (Mycelex)
nystatin [nye stat′ in] (Mycostatin, Nilstat)

Clotrimazole and nystatin inhibit the synthesis of sterols in the fungal wall; this increases the permeability of the fungal cell membrane, which results in the loss of important cellular contents. Clotrimazole also inhibits oxidative enzyme activity, which may increase intracellular hydrogen peroxide to toxic levels and thus contribute to the destruction of the fungal cells and their contents. In addition, they inhibit fungal synthesis of triglycerides and phospholipids. Clotrimazole and nystatin are indicated for the oral-local treatment of candidiasis or fungal infections caused by *Candida* species. Fluconazole (Diflucan), ketoconazole (Nizoral), and itraconazole (Sporanox) are more potent systemic drugs used to treat severe candidal infections. These antifungal agents are reviewed in Chapter 60.

The usual dosage of clotrimazole for adults and children (5 years of age and over) is one lozenge (10 mg) dissolved slowly in the mouth, five times daily for 2 weeks. The dosage of nystatin for adults and children (over 5 years of age) is 400,000 to 600,000 units of oral suspension, four times daily (one half of the dose in each side of mouth, retaining the drug as long as possible before swallowing), or 200,000-400,000 units of troches, four to five times daily.

■ Nursing Management

Oral Antifungal Agent Therapy

See also Chapter 60 for information related to the systemic use of antifungal agents.

■ **Assessment.** Inspect the oropharynx using a tongue depressor and a flashlight. Ask the client to remove any partial or complete dentures. Poorly fitting dentures can be a source of inflammation. Clients who have acquired immunodeficiency syndrome (AIDS) or are taking antineoplastic or immunosuppressive drugs (e.g., steroids) are particularly at risk for oral candidiasis. The normal mucosa is pink, although dark-skinned clients may have bluish or patch-type pigmented mucosa. Candidiasis presents as cream-colored or bluish white patches of exudate on the tongue, mouth, or pharynx that reveal bloody engorgement when scraped. A culture of the fungus may be obtained before initiating antifungal therapy. Ascertain that the client is not allergic to clotrimazole or nystatin.

■ **Nursing Diagnosis.** Clients receiving oral antifungal agents for candidiasis may experience the following nursing diagnoses: impaired oral mucous membrane related to the underlying condition and the ineffectiveness of the oral antifungal drug; or impaired comfort related to the GI effects of the drug as evidenced by nausea or vomiting, diarrhea and, perhaps, abdominal cramping.

■ **Implementation**

■ ***Monitoring.*** Using a tongue blade and flashlight, inspect and document the size and condition of the affected areas of the mouth on a daily basis.

■ ***Intervention.*** Brush the client's teeth (or have the client brush his or her teeth) and cleanse the area carefully before each dose is administered. For infants and dependent clients, gently swab nystatin on the oral mucosa. Clients with full or partial dentures need to soak them nightly in an oral suspension of nystatin to eliminate the fungus.

When administering the oral suspension, shake it well to ensure consistency in dosing. When preparing the oral suspension from powder, shake it well and use it immediately, because it contains no preservatives.

To improve retention within the mouth, nystatin can be administered in the form of flavored frozen water on a stick.

■ ***Education.*** Instruct the client in good oral hygiene techniques. Inform the client that an annual dental examination is recommended.

When using the oral suspension forms of nystatin, instruct the client to swish the medication around in the mouth and maintain contact with the mucosa as long as possible before swallowing. The client may also gargle the solution. If the client is using the troche form, provide a careful explanation that the troche is to be dissolved slowly in the mouth (15 to 30 minutes). It is not to be chewed or swallowed whole. The client is to swallow the saliva. The troche may be cut in half to facilitate administration. Avoid the use of troches with children under 5 years of age, because they may be unable to safely manage that form of the medication.

Instruct the client to continue taking the medicine for the full time of prescription and to report to the prescriber if symptoms persist. Inform the client that therapy is continued for 48 hours after symptoms have disappeared to prevent relapse.

Before an initial course of antineoplastic chemotherapy, instruct the client to consult a dentist to complete any care needed to help prevent oral complications, such as candidiasis.

■ **Evaluation.** The expected outcome of antifungal therapy for the prevention and/or treatment of altered oral mucous membranes is that the client will experience normal-colored, intact oropharyngeal mucous membranes.

Saliva Substitutes

Saliva substitutes (Orex, Xero-Lube, Moi-Stir, Salivart) are used for the relief of dry mouth and throat in xerostomia. They are available as solutions in squirt bottles and as pump or aerosol sprays. They contain electrolytes (potassium phosphate, magnesium chloride, potassium chloride, calcium, and sodium), sodium fluoride, sorbitol, and carboxymethylcellulose as the base.

Drugs Used to Treat Mouth Blistering

Acute and chronic diseases contribute to mouth blistering and erosions. Acute viral diseases such as herpes simplex, herpes zoster, and varicella have previously been treated only symptomatically. Acyclovir (Zovirax), an antiviral agent, is effective against herpes simplex virus and varicella zoster virus, the viruses associated with skin manifestations. It acts to reduce viral shedding, time to crusting, duration of local pain, and severity of symptoms (American Hospital Formulary Service, 1999). Acyclovir is available in topical, oral, and parenteral dosage forms. It and other antivirals are covered in Chapter 60.

Local irritation, medications, radiation, dental manipulations, or systemic disease may cause mouth lesions or blistering (acute or chronic). To treat this condition properly, the causative factor must first be identified and the appropriate treatment instituted.

DRUGS THAT AFFECT THE STOMACH

Conditions of the stomach that require drug therapy include hyperacidity, hypoacidity, ulcer disease, nausea, vomiting, and hypermotility. Some of the drugs used for these conditions are not unique in their treatment of gastric dysfunction but are members of other major groups of drugs, such as anticholinergic preparations, antihistamines, and antidepressants.

Drugs Used to Treat Gastric Hyperacidity: Antacids

Antacids are chemical compounds that buffer or neutralize hydrochloric acid in the stomach and thereby increase gastric pH. The major ingredients in antacids include aluminum salts, calcium carbonate, magnesium salts, and sodium bicarbonate, alone or in combination. Most antacids may be purchased as OTC preparations.

Traditionally, the antacids have been classified as nonsystemic or systemic. The term *nonsystemic* indicates that an almost negligible amount of drug is absorbed into the circulation; activity occurs only locally within the GI tract. The nonsystemic metal ion is absorbed to some degree. The aluminum ion is absorbed the most and magnesium the least; calcium is absorbed slightly more than magnesium. Long-term, chronic use of antacids or their use in the presence of impaired renal function may result in increased adverse reactions from the absorption of metal ions, especially calcium carbonate or magnesium hydroxide.

Antacids are indicated for the relief of symptoms associated with the hyperacidity related to peptic ulcer, gastritis, gastric esophageal reflux disease (GERD), gastric hyperacidity, heartburn, or hiatal hernia. In general, antacids have a rapid onset of action. The antacid effect lasts from 20 to 40 minutes when administered in a fasting state. If administered 1 hour after meals, the effects may be extended for up to 3 hours. A small amount of absorbable antacid is absorbed (15% to 30%), with the remainder broken down via the digestive process and excreted in the feces.

See Table 11-2 for the side effects/adverse reactions of the antacids. See Chapter 11 for the dosage and administration of antacids.

Altered Drug Solubility, Stability, and Absorption. Many drugs are either weak acids or weak bases, and the pH of the stomach is an important factor in their absorption. Changes in pH modify drug solubility and stability, which also affects absorption. Therefore antacids affect the absorption of most drugs to some degree (Humphries & Merritt, 1999). Drugs that are weak acids are nonionized in the acidic environment of the stomach, are lipid soluble, and are absorbed by simple diffusion across the gastric mucosal cells. The administration of an antacid either with a weak acidic drug or shortly before or after its administration will raise the pH of the stomach contents; as a result, a more ionized drug is formed and is not absorbed to the degree to which the nonionized, lipid-soluble form was absorbed. A weakly basic drug is absorbed in a more alkaline medium.

Drugs that are weak bases include morphine sulfate, quinine, pseudoephedrine, antihistamines, amphetamines, theophylline, tricyclic antidepressants, and quinidine. Examples of weak acids are isoniazid, barbiturates, nalidixic acid, nonsteroidal antiinflammatory drugs, sulfonamides, salicylates, nitrofurantoin, and coumarins.

Additional Drug Interactions. Antacids have been reported to reduce the absorption of many drugs, such as quinolone antibiotics, tetracyclines, ketoconazole, sucralfate, and digoxin. Therefore the nurse should carefully schedule the majority of medications hours apart from the administration time for an antacid. Close monitoring for both therapeutic response and possible side effects is also recommended.

■ Nursing Management

Antacid Therapy

Although antacids are considered to be OTC preparations (and are therefore discussed in Chapter 11), these medications are commonly administered by nurses in a variety of health care settings. In addition, the nurse is ideally placed within the health care delivery system to offer clients instruction on the safe use of antacids as OTC medications.

■ Assessment. A baseline assessment of the client receiving antacids should include the client's discomfort or pain and nutritional status. Sensitivity to medications containing aluminum, calcium, magnesium, simethicone, or sodium bicarbonate should be determined.

All antacids should be carefully considered in clients with renal function impairment. Clients who have renal failure and are receiving magnesium-containing antacids are particularly at risk for hypermagnesemia. If such antacids are given to clients with renal dysfunction, low dosages (50 mEq magnesium/day) should be administered under close monitoring by a health care provider. Antacids that contain magnesium may also cause **diarrhea**, the frequent passage of loose, watery stools; caution should be used in clients with an ostomy or any condition that might be worsened by diarrhea, such as hemorrhoids, ulcerative colitis, or diverticulitis.

On the other hand, aluminum- and calcium-containing antacids tend to be constipating and should be administered with caution to clients with constipation or hemorrhoids, which might be aggravated. Clients with hypercalcemia or hypoparathyroidism should not receive calcium-containing antacids. The cautious use of antacids is recommended if the client has symptoms of appendicitis, undiagnosed GI bleeding, and intestinal obstruction, because the laxative or constipating effects may worsen the condition. Aluminum-containing antacids may exacerbate Alzheimer's disease, and calcium-containing antacids may affect hypothyroidism and sarcoidosis. Consult with the prescriber about low-sodium antacids for clients with sodium restrictions.

Review the client's current medication regimen, keeping in mind that antacids have an effect on most oral forms of drugs. In particular, consider the following significant drug interactions, which may occur when antacids are given concurrently with the following drugs:

Drug	Possible Effect and Management
Bold/color type indicates the most serious interactions.	
cellulose sodium phosphate	Concurrent use with calcium-based antacids may prevent the hypercalcemic effects of this agent. Magnesium binding may occur with magnesium-based antacids; avoid administering within 1 hour of each other.
fluoroquinolones	Aluminum- and magnesium-containing antacids may reduce the absorption of these drugs; advise taking norfloxacin (Chibroxin, Noroxin) and ofloxacin (Floxin) at least 2 hours before or 2 hours after an antacid; ciprofloxacin (Cipro) and lomefloxacin (Maxaquin), 6 hours after an antacid; and enoxacin (Penetrex), 8 hours after an antacid.
ion-exchange resin (e.g., sodium polystyrene sulfonate)	**The neutralization of gastric acid may be impaired when calcium- or magnesium-containing antacids are given concurrently with this agent. The binding of the calcium and magnesium may result in anion absorption and systemic alkalosis. Avoid concurrent oral administration of this combination.**
isoniazid (INH)	Aluminum antacids interfere with the absorption of isoniazid. Separate the administration of these drugs by at least 1 hour, or administer a non–aluminum containing antacid to prevent this interaction.
ketoconazole (Nizoral)	Increased gastric pH may decrease the absorption of ketoconazole. Advise clients to take antacids at least 3 hours after ketoconazole.
mecamylamine (Inversine)	**The effects of mecamylamine may be prolonged because an alkaline urine decreases its excretion. Concurrent administration should be avoided.**

Drug	Possible Effect and Management
methenamine (Mandelamine, Hiprex)	An alkaline urine may decrease the effectiveness of methenamine by prohibiting its conversion to formaldehyde. Concurrent administration is not recommended. Because urine alkalinization may occur with antacids, monitor the client for an increased risk of crystalluria and nephrotoxicity.
tetracyclines, oral	Antacids may combine with tetracyclines, decreasing their absorption in the GI tract. Advise clients to take antacids at least 3 to 4 hours before or after tetracycline.

■ **Nursing Diagnosis.** With the administration of antacids, the client may experience pain related to the underlying condition and the ineffectiveness of the antacid or noncompliance related to its chalky taste. Other concerns for the client are related to the type of antacid administered. With aluminum- or calcium-containing antacids, constipation may result from an alteration of bowel function, whereas diarrhea may result from magnesium-containing antacids. Excessive use of calcium- and sodium bicarbonate–containing antacids may place the client at risk for the potential complication of metabolic alkalosis (mood/mental changes, muscle twitching, decreased respiratory rate, unpleasant taste, fatigue). With the long-term use of aluminum- and sodium bicarbonate–containing antacids, hypercalcemia associated with milk-alkali syndrome (headache, urinary frequency, anorexia, nausea/vomiting, fatigue) and osteomalacia/osteoporosis caused by phosphate depletion (bone pain, wrist or ankle joint swelling) may occur. Clients with renal impairment may experience neurotoxicity (mood swings, mental changes) with the chronic use of aluminum-containing antacids, or hypermagnesemia (fatigue, dizziness) with the chronic use of magnesium-containing antacids.

■ **Implementation**

■ ***Monitoring.*** Assess epigastric discomfort at the time of each dose, and record the client's progress. An evaluation of antacid therapy is important. The client's subjective response to antacid therapy and the nurse's objective observations (e.g., frequency with which the client takes the antacid) can help determine the effectiveness of therapy.

Note the frequency and consistency of stools. If diarrhea occurs, it may be advantageous to change to another antacid, such as magnesium hydroxide with magnesium trisilicate or aluminum hydroxide. If constipation occurs, a magnesium hydroxide antacid or an increase in the intake of bran and roughage in the diet may be instituted.

Monitor clients undergoing long-term aluminum antacid therapy regularly for serum phosphate levels, because phosphate depletion may result in osteoporosis; monitor serum calcium levels for milk-alkali syndrome.

■ ***Intervention.*** The dosing schedule of antacid therapy is important. Antacids given immediately after meals will delay gastric emptying and the buffering effect. When given at 1 and 3 hours after meals and at bedtime, the gastric pH remains at approximately 3 throughout the day. Because of their ability to interact with numerous medications, scheduling in relation to other medications should be considered. Administer antacids 1 hour before or 2 hours after digoxin, tetracyclines, phenothiazines, and all enteric-coated medications. Antacids combined with ibuprofen, indomethacin, phenylbutazone, potassium chloride supplements, reserpine, sulindac, and tolmetin can help to reduce the gastric distress associated with these drugs.

Shake liquid preparations of antacids vigorously before administration to achieve a uniform suspension. When administering antacids via a nasogastric tube, assess the placement and patency of the tube before giving the medication, and follow the dose with sufficient water to clear the tube. Refrigerate antacids to make them more palatable, but do not freeze them.

Do not administer calcium carbonate antacids with milk, milk products, or other foods or vitamin supplements high in vitamin D, because milk-alkali syndrome may occur.

■ ***Education.*** Discuss with the client the sodium content and side effects of various antacids (see Table 11-2 for the side effects/adverse reactions of antacids). Inform clients that antacids vary in their sodium content, which can be significant for clients who are on low-sodium diets or who take antihypertensive drugs or diuretics. Instruct clients with hypertensive, cardiac, or renal disease to avoid antacids containing sodium, particularly if antacids are used frequently.

Inform clients that liquid antacids have superior neutralizing properties compared with tablets. However, clients who must take liquid antacids at frequent intervals may lose their desire for food or drink. For this reason chewable tablets may be advised. Instruct clients taking chewable antacid tablets to chew or pulverize the tablets thoroughly. The tablets may not mix well with water. A full glass of water will facilitate the action of the antacid tablets.

Stress adherence to antacid therapy schedules. Allow clients to take their own antacids while hospitalized to encourage effective management of the therapeutic regimen. Caution clients about side effects, and instruct them to consult their prescriber if these occur. Alert clients to check the expiration dates of the antacids, because the effectiveness of antacids decreases with age. Alert clients to check the name carefully when purchasing OTC antacids. Names may be similar (Mylanta vs. Mylanta II), but dosage requirements differ. Advise clients to seek medical care if they are self-medicating with antacids for recurring GI symptoms, because they are treating the symptoms rather than the cause of the problem. Because antacids are OTC drugs and there is no medically supervised restriction, clients may abuse or misuse antacids.

Help clients to identify sources of gastric discomfort, such as overeating, smoking, tension, anxiety, or other emotional stress; this may teach them to avoid the causes of discomfort and eliminate the need for antacid therapy.

■ **Evaluation.** The expected outcome of antacid therapy is that the client will experience decreased discomfort or an absence of pain without adverse reactions (i.e., constipation or diarrhea).

For a Concept Map on gastroesophageal reflux, go to mosby.com/MERLIN/McKenry/.

Digestants

Digestants are drugs that promote the process of digestion in the GI tract. Problems with digestion may be caused by a deficiency of hydrochloric acid, digestive substances, enzymes, or bile salts; organic disease states (stomach cancer, pernicious anemia, cholecystectomy); or, possibly, a reaction to emotional situations or stress.

Digestive enzymes secreted by the mouth, stomach, small intestine, pancreas, and liver are necessary for the digestion of food. Pepsin is the stomach enzyme that reduces protein to smaller particles. It can be given alone or in combination with a hydrochloric acid source in clients with hypochlorhydria or achlorhydria.

Hydrochloric acid keeps the gastric pH level below 4 and protects the proteolytic activity of pepsin. A pH level of 1.5 to 2.5 is usually the optimal range. Pepsin is not considered a critical enzyme because proteolytic enzymes released from the pancreas and intestine cause the same effects.

pancreatin [pan′ kree a tin] (Entozyme, Donnazyme)
pancrelipase [pan kre li′ pase] (Pancrease, Viokase)

The pancreas releases digestive enzymes and bicarbonate into the duodenum to help in the digestion of fats, carbohydrates, and proteins. Bicarbonate neutralizes acid and thus helps to protect the enzymes from both acid and pepsin. When acid chyme enters the duodenum, vagal stimulation regulates pancreatic secretion; therefore enzyme replacement therapy may be necessary for clients who have had their vagal fibers surgically severed or have undergone surgical procedures that cause food to bypass the duodenum.

Both pancreatin and pancrelipase aid in the digestion and absorption of fats, carbohydrates, and triglycerides. Replacement therapy is usually necessary in cases of exocrine pancreatic enzyme deficiency states, chronic pancreatitis, cystic fibrosis, pancreatic tumors, pancreatic obstruction, and pancreatectomy.

Both pancreatin and pancrelipase contain the enzymes amylase, trypsin, and lipase, but pancrelipase has greater enzyme activity in the neutral or alkaline media of the GI tract. It has approximately 12 times the lipolytic and 4 times the proteolytic and amylolytic activities of pancreatin. These agents are not interchangeable because they are not bioequivalent.

Both products are available in enteric-coated capsules to avoid destruction in the stomach. The enteric-coated microsphere formulation resists gastric inactivation, so enzymes reach the duodenum to hydrolyze fats into glycerol and fatty acids, proteins into proteases, and starch into dextrins and sugars.

The side effects/adverse reactions of pancreatin and pancrelipase include nausea, abdominal cramps, hyperuricemia, intestinal obstruction, allergic reaction, and loose stool.

The usual adult dosage for pancreatin is 1 to 2 tablets with meals or snacks; the adult dosage for pancrelipase is 1 to 3 capsules or tablets or 1 or 2 packets before or with meals or snacks. The dosage should be adjusted as necessary. With extreme deficiency, the dosage interval may be changed to hourly if no nausea or diarrhea develops.

▪ Nursing Management

Digestant Therapy

▪ **Assessment.** A baseline assessment should include the client's discomfort levels associated with eating, as well as bowel status and serum and urine uric acid levels. Treatment with pancrelipase is contraindicated if the client has acute pancreatitis or a sensitivity to pork protein, pancrelipase, or pancreatin. Consideration should be given to clients whose religious beliefs prohibit the use of pork products.

Review the client's medications for drug interactions. The most significant drug interaction occurs when calcium and magnesium antacids negate the action of the enzyme pancrelipase. A serum iron response to oral iron therapy is decreased by pancreatic extracts.

▪ **Nursing Diagnosis.** The client receiving digestant therapy may experience the following nursing diagnoses/collaborative problems: impaired comfort (nausea and abdominal cramps); impaired oral mucous membrane related to the enzymatic digestion of mucous membranes when the tablet is held in the mouth; diarrhea; and potential complications related to an allergic reaction (rash), sensitization induced by inadvertent inhalation of the powder dosage form (dyspnea, nasal congestion, wheezing), hyperuricemia, or hyperuricuria.

▪ **Implementation**

▪ ***Monitoring.*** Monitor for discomfort associated with eating, diarrhea, irritated mouth, respiratory status, and elevated serum and urine levels of uric acid.

▪ ***Intervention.*** Pancreatin is inactivated by gastric pepsin and acid pH; therefore cimetidine or antacids (except for those containing calcium and magnesium) may be prescribed to be taken with it. For children or adults who cannot swallow the capsules, sprinkle the powdered form or the powder from the opened capsule on food. Avoid the inhalation of capsule contents.

▪ ***Education.*** Instruct the client to take pancrelipase and pancreatin before or with meals for the greatest effectiveness. Instruct the client to swallow enteric-coated tablets whole; do not crush them or allow them to be chewed, because irritation of the mouth may occur. Instruct the client on the rationale for taking the pancreatic enzyme preparations, and instruct the client not to stop taking the medication without prescriber approval. Urge the client to adhere to the prescribed diet, because the dosage for pancrelipase is individualized and determined by the client's indigestion and malabsorption and the fat content of the diet.

If capsules need to be opened to be administered, advise the client to be careful not to inhale the contents or spill them on the hands; the contents are very irritating to the nasal membranes, respiratory tract, and skin. If the capsules contain enteric-coated spheres, they should be taken with liquids or small amounts of foods that do not need chewing. Tablet forms should be followed with 1 or 2 mouthfuls of food to decrease the risk of esophageal irritation, particularly in clients in a recumbent position. Instruct the client to contact the prescriber if side effects such as nausea, abdominal cramping, and diarrhea occur. Consult with the prescriber before changing brands.

■ **Evaluation.** The expected outcome of digestant therapy is that the client will experience normal digestion and manage the digestant therapy effectively without experiencing any side effects/adverse reactions.

Antiemetics

The vomiting or **emetic center**, which is located in the medulla oblongata, may be stimulated by smells, strong emotion, severe pain, increased intracranial pressure, labyrinthine disturbances (motion sickness), endocrine disturbances, toxic reactions to drugs, GI disease, radiation treatments, and chemotherapy (Figure 41-1). The stimuli may involve neurotransmitters and vagal and/or sympathetic afferent nerve transmission.

The **chemoreceptor trigger zone (CTZ)** is an area of sensory nerve cells; this area is activated by chemical stimuli and relays messages to the emetic center. It has various receptors (serotonin, dopamine, opiate) that detect irritating drugs or toxins in the blood to stimulate or mediate emesis. The CTZ itself is not able to induce vomiting. Because the CTZ is located close to the respiratory center in the brain, it is difficult to completely control vomiting initiated from this site without affecting respiration.

The cerebral cortex is involved in anticipatory nausea and vomiting, a conditioned response caused by a stimulus connected with a previous unpleasant experience. For example, a client who vomited after receiving cancer chemotherapy might vomit at the sight of the hospital, doctor, or nurse, even before treatment is given (Koda-Kimble & Young, 1995). (See Chapter 56.)

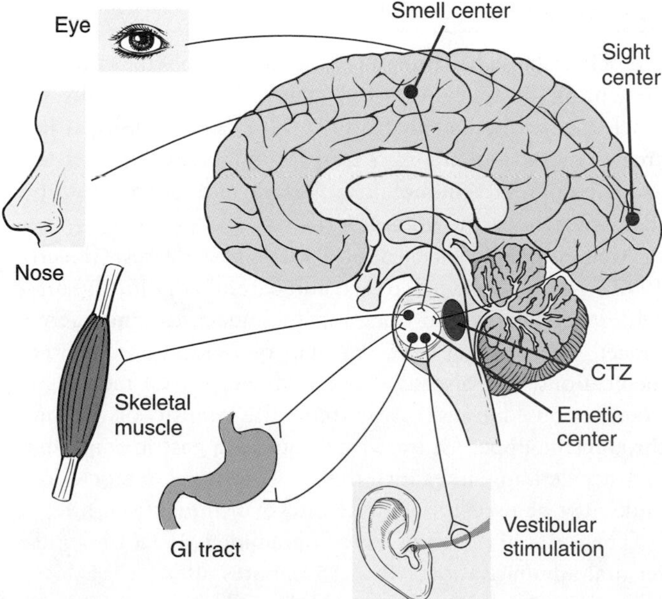

Figure 41-1 CTZ and other sites that activate the emetic center.

If the emetic center is activated by stimuli, it sends impulses (via the efferent nerves) to the diaphragm, stomach muscles, esophagus, and salivary glands, resulting in vomiting.

Antiemetics are drugs given to prevent or relieve nausea and vomiting. Control of vomiting is important and at times may be difficult. Numerous preparations have been used, but effective treatment usually depends on treating the cause. The primary pathways for the vomiting reflex are as follows:

1. Higher central nervous system or cerebral cortex stimulation
   a. Emotional or anticipatory vomiting
2. Peripheral or central nerve transmission secondary to body tissue or organ alterations
   a. Irritation of GI tract
   b. Increased intracranial pressure
   c. Vestibular stimulation
3. Stimulation from the CTZ
   a. Toxins circulating in blood

Antiemetics may exert their effects on the vomiting center, the cerebral cortex, the CTZ, or the vestibular apparatus (Table 41-1).

The neurotransmitters and pharmacologic agents used to control and/or prevent nausea and vomiting include the following:

1. *Neurotransmitter:* dopamine (D_2) receptors located in the GI tract and CTZ

TABLE 41-1 Proposed Sites of Action for Antiemetic Drugs

Proposed Sites	Drugs
Emetic center	anticholinergics
	antihistamines
	thiethylperazine maleate*
Chemoreceptor trigger zone	benzquinamide hydrochloride
	butyrophenones
	metoclopramide*
	phenothiazine
	thiethylperazine maleate*
	trimethobenzamide HCl
Cerebral cortex	cannabinoids (THC, nabilone, dronabinol)
	diazepam
	lorazepam
	scopolamine*
	antihistamines
Peripheral	metoclopramide*
	scopolamine*
Unknown	corticosteroids

*Dual action.

Pharmacologic agents: Phenothiazines, such as chlorpromazine (Thorazine), promethazine (Phenergan), and metoclopramide (Reglan) are dopamine antagonists. They act on the CTZ, GI tract, and other dopamine neurotransmitter areas. These are the most effective antiemetics and are often the drugs of choice.

2. *Neurotransmitter:* acetylcholine (ACh) receptors in the vestibular and vomiting center; overstimulation of the labyrinth (inner ear) results in the nausea and vomiting of motion sickness

   Pharmacologic agents: Anticholinergics, such as scopolamine, reduce the excitability of labyrinth receptors, depress conduction in the vestibular cerebellar pathways, or prevent impulses from stimulating the CTZ.
3. *Neurotransmitter:* histamine (H_1) receptors in the vestibular and vomiting centers

   Pharmacologic agents: H_1 antihistamines affect neural labyrinth pathways; examples include cyclizine (Marezine), dimenhydrinate (Dramamine), and diphenhydramine (Benadryl). Many antihistamines have anticholinergic side effects (see point 2).
4. *Neurotransmitter:* serotonin ($5\text{-}HT_3$) receptors in the GI tract, CTZ, and vomiting centers (Lichter, 1993)

   Pharmacologic agents: Ondansetron (Zofran), granisetron (Kytril) and dolasetron (Anzemet) are selective serotonin receptor antagonists approved for the prevention of nausea and vomiting induced by cancer chemotherapy.
5. *Miscellaneous agents:* Antacids relieve gastric irritation, and benzquinamide (Emete-Con) acts on the CTZ to reduce nausea and vomiting. Steroids (dexamethasone, methylprednisolone) and cannabinoids (nabilone, tetrahydrocannabinol [THC]) are also used.

Vomiting as a result of cancer chemotherapy can be serious enough to limit the dosages of chemotherapeutic agents given to a client. Because antiemetics are usually more effective in preventing vomiting than they are in treating it, they should be administered prophylactically before chemotherapy administration. The effective treatment of chemotherapy-induced vomiting may require several antiemetic agents with different sites of action—for example, metoclopramide (Reglan) and lorazepam (Ativan), metoclopramide and dexamethasone, or prochlorperazine (Compazine) and dexamethasone. A number of clients respond well to the serotonin receptor antagonists alone if properly scheduled according to the manufacturer's recommendations (see the Nursing Research box on p. 761).

▪ Nursing Management

Antiemetic Therapy

▪ **Assessment.** A baseline assessment should include an allergy history in relation to the antiemetic, fluid balance data, the degree of nausea reported by the client, and the frequency of vomiting. Do not give antiemetics until the underlying cause of nausea has been established. For example, a drug overdose or increased intracranial pressure may cause nausea.

▪ **Nursing Diagnosis.** With the administration of antiemetic therapy, the client may experience the following nursing diagnoses: impaired comfort (nausea) related to the underlying health condition, chemotherapy, and/or ineffectiveness of the antiemetic agent; deficient fluid volume or imbalanced nutrition: less than body requirements related to vomiting secondary to the underlying condition or chemotherapy and ineffectiveness of the antiemetic drug; or disturbed sleep pattern (drowsiness).

▪ **Implementation**

▪ ***Monitoring.*** Monitor for nausea and vomiting, a general sense of well-being, and fluid balance.

▪ ***Intervention.*** Give antiemetics before the administering chemotherapeutic agents. The time of administration of the antiemetic agent will depend on the chemotherapeutic regimen prescribed. To support the administration of antiemetics (or if antiemetic therapy is unavailable or cannot be given), provide a quiet environment, make the client comfortable, and give ice chips, a carbonated beverage or, if allowed, hot tea to drink.

▪ ***Education.*** Instruct the client that any hypersensitivity necessitates that the effects be reported to the prescriber and the drug discontinued.

Most antiemetics cause drowsiness as a side effect. Caution clients against performing hazardous tasks until the effects of the drug have subsided. Caution clients against combining antiemetics with alcohol or any central nervous system (CNS) depressants. The CNS depressant effects of the drug can be potentiated when these drugs are combined.

Vomiting during pregnancy or as the result of cancer chemotherapy can cause serious electrolyte imbalance and a nutritional deficit. Instruct the pregnant client to eat small frequent meals or small nutritional snacks between meals.

▪ **Evaluation.** The expected outcome of antiemetic therapy is that the client will experience the absence of or diminished nausea and vomiting.

metoclopramide [met oh kloe′ pra mide] (Reglan, Maxeran 🍁)

Metoclopramide has both a central and peripheral action in preventing or relieving nausea and emesis. Centrally, it blocks dopamine receptors in the CTZ; peripherally, it increases motility of the upper GI tract, increases peristalsis, and overcomes the immobility, dilation, and reverse motility that occurs with the vomiting reflex.

Metoclopramide is used for diabetic gastroparesis (Koch, 1999), gastroesophageal reflux, and parenterally for the prevention of nausea and vomiting secondary to emetogenic cancer chemotherapeutic agents, radiation, and opioid medications. It is also used as an adjunct for GI radiologic examinations because it hastens the transit of barium through the upper GI tract by stimulating gastric emptying and accelerating intestinal transit. Parenteral metoclopramide may be used to facilitate intestinal intubation.

The onset of action of metoclopramide is ½ to 1 hour after oral administration, 10 to 15 minutes after an IM dose, and within 3 minutes after an IV dose. The duration of action is 1 to 2 hours, and the half-life is 4 to 6 hours. It is metabolized by the liver and excreted by the kidneys.

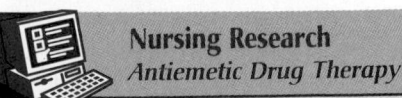

Nursing Research
Antiemetic Drug Therapy

Citations: Marchioro, G., et al. (2000). Hypnosis in the treatment of anticipatory nausea and vomiting in patients receiving cancer chemotherapy, *Oncology 59*(2):100-104; Mayer, D.J. (2000). Acupuncture: An evidence-based review of the clinical literature, *Annual Review of Medicine 51*:49-63; Plezia, P.M., et al. (1990). Randomized crossover comparison of high-dose intravenous metoclopramide versus a five-drug antiemetic regimen. *Journal of Pain Symptom Management, 5*(2), 101.

Abstract: Despite recent advances, antineoplastic drug–induced nausea and vomiting remain a serious problem for clients with cancer. Not only can these effects be physically harmful, but they may also directly contribute to client noncompliance. It has been suggested that up to 50% of clients with potentially curable cancers refuse treatment and/or are noncompliant in some treatment programs.

New antiemetic agents are being evaluated with the hope of decreasing the incidence of nausea and vomiting associated with cancer chemotherapy on a continuing basis. In a randomized open crossover study, Plezia et al. (1990) demonstrated the antiemetic efficacy of a five-drug antiemetic regimen consisting of metoclopramide, dexamethasone, diazepam, diphenhydramine, and thiethylperazine compared to a regimen of high-dose metoclopramide.

The study was terminated before the accrual of the planned number of individuals because of the statistically significant difference in efficacy between treatments found at interim analysis. In general, both regimens were well tolerated; however, when given the choice of continuing antiemetic therapies, 92% of the clients preferred the five-drug antiemetic combination.

Because drug administration always carries inherent risk, other methodologies are being sought to deal with the nausea and vomiting associated with chemotherapy. Marchioro and others (2000) recorded major positive responses to hypnosis in the management of anticipatory nausea and vomiting. Mayer (2000) concludes that acupuncture is effective for the treatment of postoperative and chemotherapy-induced nausea and vomiting.

Critical Thinking Questions

- How could a combination of drugs be expected to function more effectively than a single agent? Although the client is receiving a greater number of drugs, why might combination therapy be safer for the client?
- What ethical considerations might have contributed to the termination of this study before the accrual of the planned number of participants?
- What would be the advantages and/or disadvantages of having chemotherapy-induced nausea and vomiting managed by complementary/alternative therapies, such as hypnosis or acupuncture?

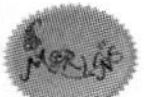

For answer guidelines for these *new Critical Thinking Questions*, go to mosby.com/MERLIN/McKenry/.

Most common side effects of metoclopramide include diarrhea, sleepiness, restlessness, increased weakness and, rarely, extrapyramidal (parkinsonian) effects, hypotension, hypertension, tachycardia, and agranulocytosis.

To treat diabetic gastroparesis or gastroesophageal reflux in an adult, the oral dosage of metoclopramide is 10 mg 30 minutes before each meal and at bedtime (up to four times daily). Check the package insert for further instructions. The IV dosage is 10 mg as a single dose. The antiemetic adult dosage (for chemotherapy-induced emesis) is 2 mg/kg by IV infusion 30 minutes before chemotherapy; the dose may be repeated every 2 to 3 hours as necessary.

The oral pediatric dosage of metoclopramide is 0.1 to 0.2 mg/kg 30 minutes before meals and at bedtime to increase peristalsis in delayed gastrointestinal emptying. Refer to current drug references for additional dosing recommendations.

■ Nursing Management
Metoclopramide Therapy

In addition to the following discussion, see Nursing Management: Antiemetic Therapy, p. 760.

■ Assessment. Do not give metoclopramide to clients with epilepsy (isolated seizures have been reported) or to those in whom stimulation of GI motility is hazardous (e.g., those with GI hemorrhage, perforation, or mechanical obstruction); these conditions may be aggravated by increased bowel motility. Clients with liver or renal dysfunction may experience decreased clearance of these agents. Extrapyramidal effects may be increased if metoclopramide is administered to clients with chronic renal failure. With metoclopramide, clients with pheochromocytoma are at risk for a hypertensive crisis. Assess for sensitivity to both agents. Clients with intolerance to procaine and procainamide may experience a cross-sensitivity to metoclopramide.

Review the client's medication regimen for the risk of significant drug interactions, such as those that may occur when metoclopramide is given concurrently with the following drugs:

Drug	Possible Effect and Management
Bold/color type indicates the most serious interactions.	
alcohol and CNS depressants	**Concurrent administration may increase the CNS depressant effects of either or both drugs. It may also result in an increased rate of alcohol absorption from the small intestine. Avoid concurrent use or a potentially serious drug interaction may occur.**
anticholinergic agents and opioid analgesics	Concurrent administration of these agents may antagonize the motility effects of metoclopramide and increase the sedative effects of all the agents.

Obtain a baseline assessment of blood pressure, mental status, and underlying nausea and vomiting.

■ **Nursing Diagnosis.** With the administration of metoclopramide, the client may be at risk for the following nursing diagnoses/collaborative problems: disturbed sleep pattern (drowsiness); impaired comfort (headache, dryness of the mouth, breast tenderness and swelling, and dizziness); disturbed thought processes (confusion, agitation, restlessness, depression); fatigue; ineffective protection related to agranulocytosis (chills, fever, sore throat, fatigue); risk for injury related to postural hypotension; constipation; diarrhea; and the potential complications of parkinsonian extrapyramidal effects, tardive dyskinesia, and altered cardiac output related to tachycardia and hypertension.

■ **Implementation**

■ ***Monitoring.*** For metoclopramide, monitor the client's complete blood count (CBC), blood pressure, mental status, and bowel status; also monitor for the presence of extrapyramidal effects and tardive dyskinesia and the incidence of nausea and vomiting. Be aware that extrapyramidal side effects may be seen with therapeutic dosages of metoclopramide and are more likely to occur in children and young adults.

■ ***Intervention.*** For metoclopramide, administer oral preparations 30 minutes before meals and at bedtime.

Administer IV injections of metoclopramide slowly over 1 to 2 minutes; a more rapid administration will produce a brief episode of anxiety and restlessness followed by drowsiness. For an IV infusion, dilute in 50 mL of the appropriate IV solution and infuse for a period of time (not less than 15 minutes). Solutions of parenteral metoclopramide may be kept for 48 hours after dilution if protected from light; if solutions are not protected from light, discard unused portions after 24 hours.

■ ***Education.*** Because metoclopramide can cause drowsiness, caution the client against operating any potentially hazardous equipment. Caution the client against using alcohol or other CNS depressants. Instruct the client on symptoms to report to the prescriber. Instruct the client to obtain medical attention if fainting, dizziness, irregular heartbeat, or any other unusual symptoms occur.

■ **Evaluation.** The expected outcome of metoclopramide is that the client will report relief from nausea without experiencing any side effects/adverse reactions or vomiting episodes.

dexpanthenol [deks pan′ thah nol] (Ilopan, Ilopan-Choline)

Dexpanthenol (Ilopan, parenteral) and dexpanthenol with choline bitartrate (Ilopan-Choline tablets) are also gastrointestinal stimulants. The parenteral dosage form (dexpanthenol) is prescribed after abdominal surgery to reduce the potential of paralytic ileum and intestinal atony. It is an alcohol analogue of D-pantothenic acid, which is a precursor of coenzyme A—a necessary substance for reactions that involve the transfer of acetyl groups in the body. This transfer is the final step necessary for the synthesis of acetylcholine. A reduction in acetylcholine with result in a decrease in peristalsis and possibly an adynamic ileus. Side effects include pruritus, respiratory difficulties, rash, colic, vomiting, and diarrhea. The usual adult dosage is 250 to 500 mg IM, which may be repeated in 2 hours, then every 6 hours as necessary. The usual dosage of the oral tablets (50 mg dexpanthenol and 25 mg choline bitartrate per tablet) is 2 to 3 tablets three times daily. The oral dosage form is also available in a liquid suspension (*Drug Facts and Comparisons*, 2000).

thiethylperazine maleate [thye eth il per′ a zeen] (Torecan)

Thiethylperazine is a phenothiazine derivative with antiemetic effects, probably through an inhibiting action on the CTZ and vomiting center. It is used to prevent nausea and vomiting caused by toxins, surgery, chemotherapy, and radiation therapy.

For the pharmacokinetics of thiethylperazine, see the discussion of phenothiazines in Chapter 19.

The reported side effects of thiethylperazine include sleepiness, dizziness, dry mouth, skin rash, fever, ringing of the ears, and headache. Adverse reactions are less common or rare and are mainly related to the phenothiazine structure, extrapyramidal effects (parkinsonism in older adults and dystonia in younger persons), and agranulocytosis and cholestatic jaundice. Confusion, seizures, and peripheral edema have also been noted.

The adult dosage is 10 mg PO, IM, or rectally one to three times daily. Thiethylperazine is not recommended for children.

■ Nursing Management

Thiethylperazine Therapy

In addition to the following discussion, see Nursing Management: Antiemetic Therapy, p. 760.

■ **Assessment.** Clients with preexisting severe cardiovascular disease or CNS depression or comatose states may experience a worsening of their condition with the administration of thiethylperazine. Hepatic dysfunction may decrease the metabolism of the drug and enhance its CNS effects. Clients with active alcoholism increase their risk of hypotension and CNS depression with administration of this drug. Because of the anticholinergic effects of thiethylperazine, clients with a predisposition to angle-closure glaucoma may experience an acute episode.

Review the client's medication regimen for the risk of significant drug interactions, such those that may occur when thiethylperazine is given concurrently with the following drugs:

Drug	Possible Effect and Management
Bold/color type indicates the most serious interactions.	
alcohol and CNS depressants	Concurrent use may result in increased CNS and respiratory depression. Dosage reductions of either drug may be necessary.

Drug	Possible Effect and Management
epinephrine (Adrenalin)	**Avoid the use of epinephrine to treat severe hypotension induced by thiethylperazine. Avoid concurrent use or a potentially serious drug interaction may occur. Norepinephrine and phenylephrine are drugs of choice for this purpose.**
levodopa (Larodopa)	**Concurrent administration may cancel the therapeutic antiparkinson effect of levodopa. Avoid concurrent drug administration.**
metrizamide, intrathecal (Amipaque)	**Concurrent drug administration may result in an increased risk of seizures, because thiethylperazine lowers the seizure threshold; a potentially serious drug interaction may occur. Thiethylperazine should be discontinued at least 48 hours before metrizamide is administered.**
phenothiazines, other medications that cause extrapyramidal effects	Monitor for an increased potential for and severity of extrapyramidal reactions.
quinidine	**An increase in adverse cardiac effects may result with this combination. Avoid concurrent use or a potentially serious drug interaction may occur.**

■ **Nursing Diagnosis.** With the administration of thiethylperazine, the client is at risk for the following nursing diagnoses/collaborative problems: disturbed sleep pattern (drowsiness—more frequent); constipation related to the anticholinergic effects of the drug; impaired comfort (headache, decreased sweating, nasopharyngeal dryness); risk for injury related to postural hypotension and dizziness; disturbed sensory perception (ringing in ears); ineffective protection (agranulocytosis); and the potential complications of paradoxical reaction, cholestatic jaundice (fever and chills, fatigue, abdominal discomfort, nausea, yellow skin or eyes), convulsions, and extrapyramidal effects.

■ **Implementation**

■ ***Monitoring.*** Blood pressure and CBC should be monitored. Depending on the client's preexisting health condition, an assessment of cardiovascular status and hepatic function, neurologic tests, or ophthalmologic examinations may be required.

■ ***Intervention.*** Thiethylperazine may be taken with food or milk to decrease gastric irritation. After long-term therapy, a gradual dosage reduction is recommended to prevent withdrawal symptoms. (See Chapter 19 for additional nursing management for phenothiazine drugs.)

■ ***Education.*** Dryness of the mouth may be relieved with ice chips, sugarless gum, or candy. Instruct the client to avoid alcohol and other CNS depressants and to use caution when driving until the effects of the drug are known. Caution the client about sitting or standing abruptly because of the hypotensive effects of thiethylperazine.

■ **Evaluation.** The expected outcome of thiethylperazine therapy is that the client will experience a reduction in nausea and vomiting without experiencing any side effects/adverse reactions to the drug.

trimethobenzamide [trye meth oh ben′ za mide] (Tigan)

Trimethobenzamide may depress the CTZ in the medulla rather than the vomiting center directly. As an antiemetic, it is not as effective as metoclopramide (Brunton, 1996).

Trimethobenzamide is metabolized in the liver and excreted in the urine.

The reported side effects include sleepiness, blurred vision, diarrhea, dizziness, headache, muscle cramps and, rarely, allergic reactions, seizures, blood dyscrasias, impaired liver function, tremors, Reye's syndrome, and depression (*USP DI*, 1999).

The adult oral dosage of trimethobenzamide is 250 mg three or four times daily. For rectal or IM administration, 200 mg is given three or four times daily. With children, the dosage is 15 mg/kg PO daily, divided into 3 or 4 doses. Refer to a current drug reference for additional recommendations.

■ Nursing Management

Trimethobenzamide Therapy

In addition to the following discussion, see Nursing Management: Antiemetic Therapy, p. 760.

■ **Assessment.** Trimethobenzamide is not recommended for use in children with viral illness, because it may contribute to the development of Reye's syndrome, an acute encephalopathy. Administer with caution to clients with dehydration, electrolyte imbalance, high fever, gastroenteritis, or encephalitis because of the increased risk for adverse CNS reactions such as convulsions, coma, and extrapyramidal symptoms. Suppositories contain 2% benzocaine; use with caution in clients who are allergic to this substance. Determine the client's sensitivity to trimethobenzamide. The concurrent use of trimethobenzamide with other CNS depressants may potentiate the CNS effects of both drugs; avoid such use.

A baseline assessment should include determining the etiology of the underlying nausea and vomiting, as well as monitoring the client's blood pressure and neurologic status.

■ **Nursing Diagnosis.** The client receiving trimethobenzamide is at risk for the following nursing diagnoses/collaborative problems: disturbed sleep pattern (drowsiness); impaired comfort (headache, muscle cramps); diarrhea; disturbed sensory perception (blurred vision, dizziness); ineffective protection related to blood dyscrasias; and the potential complications of allergic reactions (rash), convulsions, mental depression, hepatic function impairment, Parkinson-like syndrome, or Reye's syndrome.

■ **Implementation**

■ ***Monitoring.*** Monitor closely if trimethobenzamide is given concurrently with CNS depressants, because these effects may be potentiated. Hypotension can occur in the surgical client when trimethobenzamide is administered parenterally. Assess blood pressure before administering the medication and at frequent intervals after its administration.

Trimethobenzamide may mask symptoms of appendicitis or signs of ototoxicity (tinnitus, dizziness) secondary to large doses of ototoxic drugs, such as salicylates.

▪ ***Intervention.*** To minimize injection site irritation, inject trimethobenzamide deeply into the upper outer quadrant of the gluteal area.

▪ ***Education.*** Caution the client against using alcohol or other CNS depressants with this drug. Use caution when driving or performing other activities that require alertness, because this drug may cause dizziness and drowsiness.

▪ **Evaluation.** The expected outcome of trimethobenzamide therapy is that the client will experience relief from nausea and vomiting without experiencing side effects/adverse reactions to the drug.

scopolamine transdermal [skoe pol′ a meen] (Transderm-Scop)

Scopolamine is an anticholinergic agent used to prevent motion-induced nausea and vomiting by depressing conduction in the labyrinth of the inner ear. Overstimulation in this area is responsible for the nausea and vomiting of motion sickness. Scopolamine is metabolized in the liver and excreted by the kidneys.

The side effects/adverse reactions of scopolamine are related to its anticholinergic effects: decreased sweating, sleepiness, dry mouth, nose, throat, or skin. Impaired memory and insomnia (paradoxical reaction) have been reported in older adults.

Scopolamine transdermal is recommended for use in adults only. In the United States, the product is a four-layered film that releases 0.5 mg of scopolamine over a 3-day period. It is applied on the skin behind the ear, usually 4 hours before the antiemetic effect is desired. In Canada, it is formulated to release 1 mg of scopolamine over a 3-day period, and it should be applied 12 hours before the antiemetic effect is desired.

▪ Nursing Management

Scopolamine Transdermal Therapy

In addition to the following discussion, see Nursing Management: Antiemetic Therapy, p. 760.

▪ **Assessment.** Take precautions when clients have asthma, narrow-angle glaucoma, pyloric or intestinal obstruction, urinary tract obstruction, or diminished renal or hepatic function. Older adults are more susceptible to the effects of scopolamine. Do not use with children because of adverse reactions. Use cautiously, if at all, in women who are pregnant or breastfeeding.

The effects of anticholinergic/antimuscarinic drugs or CNS depressants may be potentiated when used concurrently with scopolamine.

▪ **Nursing Diagnosis.** The client using a scopolamine transdermal patch is at risk for the following nursing diagnoses: disturbed sleep pattern (drowsiness); impaired comfort (headache, nasal congestion, dry mouth); constipation; impaired urinary elimination (urinary hesitancy and retention); and risk for injury related to blurred vision.

▪ **Implementation**

▪ ***Monitoring.*** The client may have a dilated pupil on the side that the patch is worn. Be aware that clients can develop tolerance to the drug after prolonged use.

▪ ***Intervention.*** Depending on the type of patch, apply the system at least 4 hours or 12 hours before the antiemetic effect is desired. Wash and dry the hands thoroughly before and after applying the system. Apply it to intact skin in the hairless area behind the ear.

▪ ***Education.*** Warn the client that operating machinery or driving a motorized vehicle is hazardous because of drowsiness, disorientation, confusion, and blurred vision.

▪ **Evaluation.** The expected outcome of scopolamine transdermal therapy is that the client will not experience motion sickness, nausea, and vomiting or any side effects/adverse reactions to the drug.

ondansetron hydrochloride [on dan′ si tron] (Zofran)
granisetron [gran iz′ e tron] (Kytril)
dolasetron [doe laz′ e tron] (Anzemet)

Ondansetron was the first of a new class of serotonin receptor (5-HT_3) antagonists approved by the Food and Drug Administration (FDA) for the prevention of nausea and vomiting associated with the use of antineoplastic agents. Granisetron and dolasetron are also selective serotonin antagonists. Serotonin (5-HT_3) receptors are located peripherally on the vagus nerve terminal and centrally in the CTZ. It is believed that antineoplastics cause the release of stored serotonin from the enterochromaffin cells of the GI tract (*USP DI*, 1999). Serotonin stimulates serotonin receptors in the vagus nerve in the GI tract, which then stimulates serotonin receptors in the CTZ, inducing vomiting. When ondansetron or granisetron are administered before antineoplastic therapy, they block serotonin receptors in the brainstem and GI tract. As a result, serotonin released in response to the administration of antineoplastic agents cannot bind with the serotonin receptors, and vomiting is prevented. Ondansetron is also effective for postoperative nausea and vomiting (Domino, Anderson, Polissar, & Posner, 1999).

Ondansetron peaks in 1 to 2 hours when administered orally; the elimination half-life is 3 to 4 hours, and it is metabolized in the liver and excreted primarily by the kidneys. Pharmacokinetic information on granisetron is limited; the elimination half-life may be 9 to 12 hours for IV doses and 6.23 hours for oral doses. Granisetron is metabolized in the liver and excreted in the urine and feces. Dolasetron peaks in 1 hour when administered orally and in 0.6 hour when given intravenously. The elimination half-life of dolasetron is 8.1 hours; it is metabolized by the liver and excreted in the urine and feces.

The side effects/adverse reactions of granisetron include stomach pain, diarrhea or constipation, headache, increased weakness and, rarely, cardiac dysrhythmias, fainting, and hypersensitivity or allergic-type reactions. The side effects/adverse reactions of ondansetron include fever, headache, constipation, diarrhea and, rarely, anaphylaxis, chest pain, and bronchospasm. The side effects/adverse reactions of dolasetron include diarrhea, headache, stomach pain, dizziness, fatigue, hypertension or hypotension and, rarely, anaphylaxis, bradycardia, tachycardia, edema, urinary retention, and pancreatitis.

The parenteral dosage for ondansetron to prevent cancer chemotherapy–induced nausea and vomiting in adults and children 4 to 18 years of age is 0.15 mg/kg IV infused over 15 minutes beginning ½ hour before chemotherapy, followed by 0.15 mg/kg 4 and 8 hours after the first dose of ondansetron. The oral adult dosage is 8 mg ½ hour before cancer chemotherapy, then 8 mg at 8 hours after the first dose, followed by 8 mg every 12 hours for several days. The oral dosage for children is 4 mg in the same schedule as for adults.

The parenteral dosage for granisetron to prevent cancer chemotherapy–induced nausea and vomiting in adults and children 2 years of age and older is 10 μg/kg IV over 5 minutes (30 minutes before the chemotherapy or radiation therapy). The oral dosage for adults is 1 mg twice daily, with the first dose administered 1 hour before chemotherapy and the second dose 12 hours after the first dose (*USP DI*, 1999; *Drug Facts and Comparisons*, 2000).

The adult dosage of dolasetron for the prophylaxis of cancer chemotherapy–induced nausea and vomiting is 100 mg PO (1 hour before therapy) or IV (½ hour before therapy). The oral dosage for children 2 to 16 years of age is 1.8 mg/kg, up to a maximum of 100 mg, administered 1 hour before chemotherapy (Coppes et al., 1999). The IV dosage for children is the same and should be administered approximately ½ hour before chemotherapy.

■ Nursing Management

Ondansetron, Granisetron, and Dolasetron Therapy

In addition to the following discussion, see Nursing Management: Antiemetic Therapy, p. 760.

■ **Assessment.** The use of these drugs is contraindicated in clients with a sensitivity to them. Ondansetron may increase hepatic enzymes and therefore is contraindicated at its standard dosage and schedule for clients with hepatic impairment. Use granisetron with caution in children under 2 years of age. Dolasetron is used with caution when the client has an underlying condition that may increase the risk for developing prolonged cardiac conduction intervals, especially the QT interval (e.g., antidysrhythmic drug therapy or potassium-wasting diuretics).

A baseline assessment should include a description of the client's previous experience with antiemetic therapy, nutritional status, bowel status, serum electrolytes, ECG determinations, and respiratory status.

■ **Nursing Diagnosis.** The client receiving ondansetron, granisetron, and dolasetron therapy is at risk for the following nursing diagnoses: impaired comfort (headache, abdominal cramping, dry mouth, rash); fatigue; disturbed sleep pattern (drowsiness); diarrhea; and constipation. The client is also at risk for the following potential complications: with ondansetron, bronchospasm; with granisetron, weakness; and with dolasetron, cardiac dysrhythmias.

■ **Implementation**

■ ***Monitoring.*** Monitor the client's fluid and electrolytes, and monitor the bowel status for diarrhea or constipation. Monitor the client's vital signs, nausea, vomiting, and comfort status.

■ ***Intervention.*** With ondansetron, dilute the IV injection in 50 mL of 5% dextrose or 0.9% sodium chloride solution before administering; infuse over 15 minutes. This dose may be repeated twice at 4-hour intervals. Ondansetron sometimes precipitates in the vial; shake the vial vigorously to restabilize it.

Dilute granisetron with 5% dextrose or 0.9% sodium chloride injection to a total volume of 20 to 50 mL; infuse over 5 minutes ½ hour before the administration of cancer chemotherapy. Doses of granisetron are often described in micrograms, but the vial concentration is identified by mg/mL. Granisetron injection also contains benzyl alcohol as a preservative; this should not be administered to newborns and immature infants.

Dolasetron is to be administered before chemotherapy; 1 hour before with oral doses and 30 minutes before for IV doses. The injection solution may be mixed in apple juice or grape juice for oral administration to children. The IV injection preparation of dolasetron is not to be mixed with other medications, and the IV infusion line should be flushed before and after administration.

■ ***Education.*** Alert the client that headache may occur; this can be relieved by an analgesic.

■ **Evaluation.** The expected outcome of ondansetron, granisetron, or dolasetron therapy is that the client will not experience postoperative or antineoplastic drug–induced nausea and vomiting or any adverse reactions to the drug.

Cannabinoids

dronabinol [droe nab' i nol] (Marinol)

Dronabinol is the synthetic derivative of THC (delta-9-tetrahydrocannabinol), which is indicated for the treatment of nausea and vomiting related to cancer chemotherapy. Dronabinol is indicated as a second-line agent to prevent the nausea and vomiting associated with chemotherapy when other antiemetics are ineffective. It is also used as an appetite stimulant to treat anorexia and weight loss in persons with AIDS.

Dronabinol reaches peak serum levels in 2 to 4 hours; the duration of action is 4 to 6 hours for psychologic effects and 1 day or longer for appetite-stimulating effects. It is metabolized in the liver and excreted mainly in the feces.

The side effects/adverse reactions of dronabinol include ataxia, light-headedness, nausea, vomiting, blurred vision, dry mouth, restlessness, weakness, drowsiness, tachycardia or bradycardia, and CNS side effects such as confusion, delusions, hallucinations, depression, mood alterations, restlessness, and anxiety. Older adults are particularly prone to the adverse reactions in the CNS.

The oral dosage for adults is 5 mg/m^2 of body surface 1 to 3 hours before chemotherapy, then every 2 to 4 hours afterward (4 to 6 doses daily). If the initial dose is ineffective, it may be increased in increments of 2.5 mg/m^2 (the maximum dose is 15 mg/m^2 per dose). The dosage for appetite stimulation is 2.5 mg twice daily before lunch and supper, which may be increased if necessary up to a maximum of 20 mg/day. The pediatric dosage is similar to the adult dosage.

nabilone [na' bi lone] (Cesamet ♣)

Nabilone is a synthetic derivative of cannabinoid (not THC); it is approved for selected persons receiving emetogenic chemotherapy who are nonresponsive to other first-line antiemetic agents.

Nabilone has an onset of action within ½ to 1 hour and has a peak effect in 2 hours. It is metabolized in the liver and excreted primarily in the feces.

The side effects include ataxia, sedation, dry mouth, euphoria, headache, and difficulty concentrating.

The adult dosage is 1 or 2 mg twice daily. The pediatric dosage has not been established.

■ Nursing Management

Cannabinoid Therapy

In addition to the following discussion, see Nursing Management: Antiemetic Therapy, p. 760.

■ **Assessment.** Sensitivity to dronabinol, nabilone, other marijuana products and, with dronabinol, sesame oil may preclude the use of cannabinoids. These agents should be used with caution in clients with cardiac disorders and hypertension, because dysrhythmias and hypertension may occur with an increase in sympathomimetic activity. Clients with mental disorders such as manic, depressive, and schizophrenic states may have increased symptoms. Clients with a history of substance abuse may tend to abuse these agents. The concurrent use of cannabinoids with alcohol and other CNS depressants may potentiate the effects of the CNS depressants. Assess the client's cardiac and mental status before therapy.

■ **Nursing Diagnosis.** The client receiving cannabinoid therapy is at risk for the following nursing diagnoses/collaborative problems: disturbed sleep pattern (drowsiness); disturbed thought processes as a result of the psychotomimetic effects of the drug (mood swings, confusion, inability to think, anxiety, hallucinations); impaired oral mucous membrane (dry mouth); risk for injury related to blurred vision, orthostatic hypotension, and light-headedness; and the potential complications of mental depression and altered cardiac output (tachycardia, hypertension).

■ **Implementation**

■ ***Monitoring.*** Monitor the client's vital signs and mental status. Some clients report feelings of well-being and euphoria; others have transient psychoses characterized by hallucinations and depersonalization.

■ ***Intervention.*** The cannabinoids should be administered while the client is being supervised. They are administered 1 to 3 hours before chemotherapy. The amount dispensed should be limited to that necessary to accompany a single cycle of chemotherapy. Clients may experience withdrawal (irritability, insomnia, restlessness, diarrhea, sweating, anorexia) when the drugs are abruptly discontinued after 12 to 16 days of therapy; to prevent this, clients should be weaned gradually from the drug.

■ ***Education.*** Alert the client to make position changes slowly, particularly from the recumbent to upright position, to prevent the dizziness and fainting of orthostatic hypotension. Caution the client to avoid ingesting alcoholic beverages and other CNS depressants while taking cannabinoids. Alert the client to use caution when driving or performing other activities that require alertness.

■ **Evaluation.** The expected outcome of cannabinoid therapy is that the client will not experience nausea and vomiting or any adverse reactions to dronabinol or nabilone.

Corticosteroids

Corticosteroids have been reported to be effective for chemotherapy-induced nausea and vomiting alone or when used in combination with other antiemetics (Koda-Kimble & Young, 1995). The mechanism of action is unknown, but it has been proposed that these drugs may inhibit the synthesis of prostaglandins, which may be involved in chemotherapy-induced vomiting. Research has indicated that certain prostaglandins (especially the PGE series) can induce nausea and vomiting.

Many studies with corticosteroids have involved the use of dexamethasone and methylprednisolone, but corticotropin and hydrocortisone may also be used. Their effectiveness as antiemetics was a serendipitous discovery—clients receiving various chemotherapeutic regimens experienced less nausea and vomiting when prednisone was one of the agents administered. Thus the corticosteroids are used as antiemetics in cancer chemotherapy, especially in clients who are not responsive to other drug therapies. See Chapter 49 for a discussion related to corticosteroids, and see the Complementary and Alternative Therapies box on p. 767.

Emetic Agents

Emetic drugs exert their effects on the same centers as antiemetic drugs but have the opposite effect. They are used to induce vomiting as part of the treatment for certain drug overdoses and poisonings.

ipecac syrup [ip' e kak]

Ipecac syrup is an OTC drug for home emergency treatment; it is the emetic of choice. Its major alkaloids are emetine and cephaeline, which stimulate the CTZ and irritate the gastric mucosa to induce vomiting.

Approximately 80% to 90% of clients vomit within ½ hour of oral drug administration; the average time for vomiting is 20 minutes. Although this product is generally given in the home, a poison control center or health care provider should be called for advice before administration. If medical

Complementary and Alternative Therapies
Ginger

Ginger is an herbal remedy that has been used throughout the world to flavor foods as well to aid digestion, relieve nausea, and treat motion sickness. The active components of ginger are thought to include the volatile oils composed of shogaol and gingerols. Both of these components have cardiotonic activity, but gingerols also have analgesic and sedative effects and effects on GI motility. Studies have found ginger to have possible effectiveness in preventing motion sickness, morning sickness related to pregnancy, and nausea.

The ingestion of ginger in the amounts commonly found in foods is considered safe unless the person has a sensitivity to ginger. A ginger sensitivity usually results in dermatitis. Ginger is considered safe when taken as an oral medication in the recommended dosage amounts. Overdoses can cause CNS depression and cardiac dysrhythmias. Theoretically, ginger may be harmful to clients with bleeding conditions, diabetes, cardiac conditions, and high or low blood pressure. This is related to its ability to increase the risk of bleeding, interfere with blood glucose control, interfere with therapy for heart conditions, and interfere with blood pressure control. It may increase the effects of inotropic drugs, hypoglycemic drugs, anticoagulant and antiplatelet drugs, and barbiturates; it may also decrease the effects of acid-inhibiting drugs. Ginger is considered safe in pregnancy and lactation when used in food amounts; however, greater amounts are contraindicated in pregnancy because of ginger's abortifacient (abortion-inducing) activity.

Oral preparations of ginger are in the form of dried root, teas, and tinctures. The typical dosage is 0.25 g of dried root three times daily. The tea is prepared by steeping 0.5 to 1 g of dried root in 150 mL of boiling water for 5 to 10 minutes and straining the preparation before administration. There are weak and strong tincture preparations of ginger. Read the label carefully, because the dosage will vary according to the concentration of ginger in the tincture. Ginger 250 mg four times daily is used to reduce morning sickness. The maximum dosage of ginger is 4 g of the root daily. (See Chapter 12 for more information.)

Information from Cirigliano, M.D. (1998). Ten most common herbs in clinical practice. In M.S. Micozzi (Ed.), *Current review of complementary medicine.* Philadelphia: Current Medicine; and Jellin, J.M., Batz, F., & Hitchens, K. (1999). *Pharmacist's letter/prescriber's letter natural medicines comprehensive database.* Stockton, CA: Therapeutic Research Faculty.

help is not available, this product can still be used. Up to 78% of the gastric contents can be recovered by this method (the mean is 28%). Therefore clients need further monitoring and/or treatment, because not all the toxic substances are recovered from the GI tract.

Ipecac syrup has the advantage of oral administration. The active alkaloid emetine is a cardiotoxic substance. Although the administration of a single dose does not usually lead to major problems, the chronic use of this product by persons with eating disorders such as anorexia or bulimia has led to serious complications, including fatalities. Emetine is excreted very slowly; it accumulates in the body with repeated doses. It may produce systemic effects for months, even after the drug is discontinued.

Myopathy or muscle aching and weakness (especially in the muscles of the neck and extremities), hyporeflexia, slurred speech, and dysphagia have been reported with the use of ipecac syrup. Cardiotoxicity has caused some fatalities. The cardiac and muscle effects are due to emetine toxicity and are usually symptoms associated with misuse or overdose of this drug.

The dose for adults and children over 12 years of age is 15 to 30 mL PO. Children 1 to 12 years of age are given 15 mL PO. For adults, follow each dose of ipecac syrup with 8 ounces (240 mL) of water; 4 to 8 ounces of water is given to children. A second dose may be given if vomiting does not occur in 20 to 30 minutes. If vomiting still does not occur, gastric lavage should be implemented.

■ Nursing Management
Ipecac Syrup Therapy

See Chapter 73 for a detailed discussion of the nursing management of the client with poisoning.

■ **Assessment.** Assess the client's vital signs and level of consciousness, and determine the substance ingested. Call the poison control center or emergency department before administering ipecac syrup. CAUTION: Vomiting should never be induced in a client who is unconscious, has swallowed corrosive substances or petroleum distillates, or has depressed gag or cough reflexes. Vomiting may result in the aspiration of gastric contents into the lungs, which may be fatal. The use of ipecac syrup for strychnine poisoning may precipitate seizures.

■ **Nursing Diagnosis.** The client receiving ipecac syrup therapy is at risk for the potential complication of cardiotoxicity if vomiting does not occur within 20 minutes of the second dose.

■ **Implementation**

■ ***Monitoring.*** Monitor the client for vomiting, and document the amount and character of the vomitus. Monitor the client's vital signs and ECG before and after administering the drug. If the client does not vomit, monitor for drug toxicity (abdominal pain, hypotension, dyspnea, cardiac disturbances, shock, seizures, coma). Daily bowel activity and consistency should be noted. Monitor fluid balance and for signs of dehydration (dry mucous membranes, poor skin turgor).

▪ ***Intervention.*** Follow the administration of ipecac syrup with water as previously described. Giving the water before the medication is sometimes more helpful in young or frightened children. Dilute, clear juice (apple) may be substituted if a child will not drink water. Do not give milk, because it will delay the emetic effect of the drug.

Drug-induced vomiting is usually preferable to gastric lavage for conscious clients, particularly children, because the aspiration of vomitus is less likely to occur. Nurses should undertake the necessary measures to reduce the likelihood of aspiration (e.g., proper positioning of client).

If activated charcoal is also to be administered, do so only after vomiting has been induced and completed.

▪ ***Education.*** Parents should be encouraged to keep ipecac syrup in their home first aid kit and be aware of its proper use. Advise the family to post the poison control center phone number near the phone or on the ipecac syrup bottle.

▪ **Evaluation.** The expected outcome of ipecac syrup therapy is that the client will vomit the noxious agent without aspiration or cardiotoxicity.

Drugs Used to Treat Peptic Ulcers

The treatment of peptic ulcer disease may involve a variety of drugs—antimicrobials, antacids, anticholinergics, antidepressants, anxiolytics, H_2 receptor antagonists, and cytoprotective agents (substances that protect cells from damage) such as sucralfate. This section is limited to the more specific agents: the cytoprotective agents and the H_2 receptor antagonists. (See the Special Considerations for Older Adults box at right.)

Helicobacter pylori bacteria have been found in persons with gastritis and gastric and duodenal peptic ulcers. It has been reported that persons who have a colony of *H. pylori* in the stomach are more prone to gastritis and gastric and duodenal ulcers (Fedotin, 1993). It has been recommended that all persons with a non–drug-induced peptic ulcer be treated with a combination of antibacterials to eradicate *H. pylori* (Laheij, Rossum, Jansen, Straatman, & Verbeek, 1999). Controlling or eradicating these bacteria vastly improves the chances that the ulcer will not recur. The drug regimen usually includes a bismuth preparation (Pepto-Bismol), tetracycline, metronidazole (Flagyl), and an H_2 blocking agent. Some resistance to metronidazole has been reported, and side effects have been reported with all three drugs; this has led to the use of other combinations, such as bismuth and amoxicillin or amoxicillin and omeprazole (Abramowicz, 1994; Graham, 1993; Smith, 1995).

Combination medications include ranitidine bismuth citrate (Tritec), which is used in combination with clarithromycin; a bismuth subsalicylate, metronidazole, and tetracycline combination (Helidac) may be used for active duodenal ulcers associated with *H. pylori* infection (*Drug Facts and Comparisons,* 2000). Combining individual agents in a single product helps simplify a complicated drug schedule.

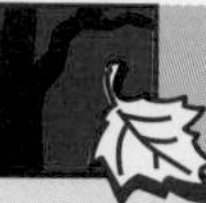

Special Considerations for Older Adults
Antiulcer Therapies

GI symptoms are very common in older adults. Every symptom should be properly evaluated before instituting drug therapy.

Acid secretion reaches its peak during sleep—between 10 PM and the early morning hours (Covington, 1996). Therefore H_2 receptor antagonists prescribed as a daily dose should be administered at bedtime.

Cigarette smoking, which increases the amount of acid produced in the stomach, may decrease the effect of H_2 blockers.

Clients should be advised to stop smoking if possible, or at least not to smoke after taking the last daily dose of medication (*USP DI,* 1999).

With the routine administration of H_2 blockers, confusion and dizziness are more commonly reported by older adults than by younger adults (*USP DI,* 1999). Mental status changes have been reported with cimetidine, famotidine, and ranitidine, especially in older adults who have impaired liver or renal function or are severely ill. Acute mental changes in older adults may indicate the need for lowering the drug dose or discontinuing the medication.

Antacids effectively neutralize gastric acid; food also serves as a buffer for gastric acid. Thus antacids are most beneficial if administered between meals and at bedtime.

When H_2 receptor antagonists are prescribed with antacids, schedule medications at least 1 hour apart, and administer the antacid first.

Cytoprotective Agents

sucralfate [soo kral′ fate] (Carafate, Sulcrate ♣)

Sucralfate is a local topical agent composed of sulfated sucrose and aluminum hydroxide; in the presence of albumin and fibrinogen, this substance forms a protective, acid-resistant shield in the ulcer crater. This barrier hastens the healing of the peptic ulcer by protecting the mucosa for up to 6 hours.

This drug is indicated for short-term treatment of a duodenal ulcer (up to 8 weeks) (see the Case Study box on p. 769).

Sucralfate is administered orally, and there is minimal systemic absorption (up to 5%). Excretion is primarily in the feces.

The side effects of sucralfate are minimal; the most common one reported is constipation. Other possible effects include diarrhea, nausea, gastric discomfort, dry mouth, dizziness, drowsiness, back pain, rash, and itching.

The adult dosage for the treatment of a duodenal ulcer is 1 g four times daily, 1 hour before each meal and at bedtime.

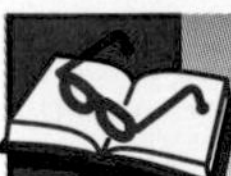

Case Study *The Client with a Duodenal Ulcer*

Annette Jones, a 24-year-old white female, has been diagnosed with duodenal ulcer disease. She was prescribed antacids after her initial attack. However, recurrent symptoms have caused her family physician to hospitalize her. You are told that Annette is an exceptionally bright young woman but is "very sensitive and childish." She entered law school last year at the insistence of her father, Arthur Jones, a prominent trial attorney. Annette is an only child and lives with her parents, who are very demanding of her and do not appear to tolerate mistakes. She is treated medically and her symptoms again resolve.

When she is discharged this time, the prescriber puts her on sucralfate (Carafate) 1 g PO four times daily.

1. How does sucralfate work differently from other agents used in the treatment of duodenal ulcer?
2. You are teaching Annette the most common side effects of sucralfate, of which constipation is the most common. What other side effects should she be told about?
3. What other important information will Annette need to know about sucralfate?
4. Considering Annette's health history, what other drug issues should be included in her health instruction?
5. If Annette experiences a recurrence of her ulcer, what other drug regimens are available for her treatment?

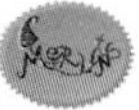

For answer guidelines, go to mosby.com/MERLIN/McKenry/.

The dosage for the prophylaxis of duodenal ulcer is 1 g twice daily on an empty stomach.

■ Nursing Management

Sucralfate Therapy

■ **Assessment.** A baseline assessment should include the client's underlying condition, sensitivity to sucralfate, and renal status. Obtain a serum aluminum level in clients with renal failure. Sucralfate should be used with caution in clients with renal failure because the absorption of the aluminum in the drug may cause aluminum toxicity, especially with long-term use.

Review the client's current medication regimen for the risk of significant drug interactions, such as those that may occur when sucralfate is given concurrently with the following drugs:

Drug	Possible Effect and Management
antacids	Concurrent use may interfere with sucralfate binding, thus reducing its effect. Administer antacids either 30 minutes before or 1 hour after the administration of sucralfate.
ciprofloxacin (Cipro), norfloxacin (Noroxin), or ofloxacin (Floxin)	Sucralfate is reported to decrease the absorption and serum levels of these antibiotics. Advise clients to take antibiotics 2 to 3 hours before sucralfate.
digoxin (Lanoxin) or theophylline (Elixophyllin)	Sucralfate interferes with the absorption of digoxin and theophylline. Advise clients to take digoxin or theophylline 2 hours before or after sucralfate.
phenytoin (Dilantin)	Concurrent administration with sucralfate may decrease serum levels of phenytoin, resulting in a loss of seizure control. Advise clients not to take sucralfate within 2 hours of phenytoin administration.

■ **Nursing Diagnosis.** The client receiving sucralfate is at risk for the following nursing diagnoses: constipation; diarrhea; disturbed sleep pattern (drowsiness); impaired oral mucous membrane (dry mouth); and impaired comfort (nausea, itching, indigestion, dizziness, backache).

■ **Implementation**

■ ***Monitoring.*** Monitor the client's bowel elimination for constipation or diarrhea. The ulcer will be monitored by x-ray or endoscopic examination.

■ ***Intervention.*** Administer sucralfate with water to the client 1 hour before meals and at bedtime; sucralfate is taken on an empty stomach. If the client's regimen also includes antacids, they may be administered ½ hour before or 1 hour after the sucralfate. The use of sucralfate via a nasogastric tube has resulted in the formation of bezoar as a result of the protein-binding properties of the drug.

■ ***Education.*** Instruct the client not to chew the tablet. An oral suspension is available for clients who are unable to swallow tablets. Encourage compliance with the regimen for at least 4 to 8 weeks, until healing has been documented by x-ray or endoscopic examination. Sucralfate therapy is not recommended for longer than 8 weeks.

■ **Evaluation.** The expected outcome of sucralfate therapy is that the client's duodenal ulcer will heal within 8 weeks as evidenced by x-ray or endoscopic examination.

misoprostol [mye soe prost' ole] (Cytotec)

Misoprostol, a gastric mucosa–protecting agent, is indicated for the prevention of gastric ulcers associated with the use of nonsteroidal antiinflammatory drugs (NSAIDs), especially in persons at increased risk for developing complications from gastric ulcers (La Corte, Caselli, Castellino, Bajocchi, & Trotta, 1999; Raskin, 1999). Prostaglandins normally protect the stomach by decreasing gastric acid secretion and increasing gastric cytoprotective mucus and bicarbonate. NSAIDs inhibit prostaglandin synthesis, which reduces the protective mechanisms and may result in gastric ulcers. Misoprostol, a synthetic prostaglandin E_1 analogue, suppresses gastric acid secretion and thus helps to heal gastric ulcers (Brunton, 1996).

Misoprostol is rapidly absorbed orally; it reaches a peak serum level in approximately 15 minutes and has a duration of action of 3 to 6 hours. It is metabolized to an active metabolite that is later metabolized to inactive metabolites in various tissues. It is excreted primarily by the kidneys.

The most common side effects associated with misoprostol are stomach distress and diarrhea, which are dose related. Less common side effects include constipation, gas, headache, nausea, or vomiting. At the present time, no significant drug interactions have been noted with misoprostol.

The adult dosage is 0.2 mg PO four times daily after meals and at bedtime, or 0.4 mg PO twice daily, with the last dose at bedtime. A pediatric dosage has not been established.

▪ Nursing Management

Misoprostol Therapy

▪ **Assessment.** Determine if the client is sensitive to other prostaglandins or prostaglandin analogues, because there may be cross-sensitivity. Use misoprostol with caution in clients with cerebrovascular or coronary artery disease; although it has not been reported with this drug, prostaglandins can cause hypotension, which would worsen these conditions. Use this drug cautiously in clients with epilepsy; prostaglandins administered by routes other than the oral route have been reported to cause seizures, although this effect has not been reported with misoprostol itself. It should be determined if the client is pregnant, because this drug increases the frequency and intensity of uterine contractions and may cause miscarriages (Scheepers, van Erp, & van den Bergh, 1999; Surbek, Fehr, Hosli, & Holzgreve, 1999).

▪ **Nursing Diagnosis.** The client receiving misoprostol is at risk for the following nursing diagnoses/collaborative problems: diarrhea (13% to 40%); constipation (1.1%); impaired comfort (mild abdominal pain, flatulence, 2.9%; headache, 2.4%); deficient fluid volume related to nausea and vomiting; and the potential complications of uterine stimulation and vaginal bleeding.

▪ **Implementation**

▪ ***Monitoring.*** Monitor for GI distress and discomfort and the stools for type, amount, color, and guaiac determinations.

▪ ***Intervention.*** Administer misoprostol with or after meals. Start the course of therapy at the same time as the NSAIDs. Misoprostol may be administered with antacids; magnesium-containing antacids are not recommended because they may aggravate misoprostol-induced diarrhea.

Therapy should continue for 4 weeks unless healing has been documented by endoscopic examination.

▪ ***Education.*** Alert the client to report to the prescriber any episode of diarrhea that lasts more than 1 week. Misoprostol is not to be taken for longer than 4 weeks unless otherwise prescribed, and then only for another 4 weeks if necessary. Instruct the client not to give the drug to any other person. Misoprostol has an expiration date of 18 months after its manufacture.

▪ **Evaluation.** The expected outcome of misoprostol therapy is that the client will remain ulcer free as evidenced by endoscopic examination and will not experience any side effects/adverse reactions to misoprostol.

Proton Pump Inhibitors

Proton pump inhibitors suppress gastric acid secretion by inhibiting the hydrogen/potassium adenosine triphosphatase (ATPase) enzyme system at the secretory surface of the gastric parietal cells. Therefore they block the final step of acid production, inhibiting both basal and stimulated gastric acid secretion. Omeprazole binds irreversibly at this site, whereas the effects of lansoprazole are dose related.

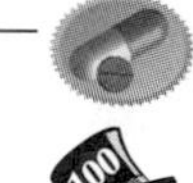

esomeprazole [e soe meh′ pray zole] (Nexium)
lansoprazole [lan′ soe pray zole] (Prevacid ◆)
omeprazole [oh meh′ pray zole] (Prilosec ◆)
pantoprazole [pan toe′ pray zole] (Protonix)
rabeprazole [ra beh′ pray zole] (Aciphex)

Omeprazole (the prototype drug) and the other drugs in this category are indicated for the treatment of severe erosive esophagitis that occurs with gastroesophageal reflux, for the treatment of duodenal ulcer, and for the long-term treatment of hypersecretory gastric conditions (Bardhan et al., 1999; Kromer, Horbach & Luhmann, 1999).

Administered orally, the onset of action for omeprazole is within 1 hour, the peak effect is in 2 hours, and the duration of action is 3 to 4 days (the time needed for production of new enzyme). It is metabolized in the liver and excreted by the kidneys. The onset of action of lansoprazole, esomeprazole, and pantoprazole is within 1 to 3 hours (depending on dose), and these agents have a duration of action of 24 hours. They are metabolized in the liver and excreted primarily in the bile and feces. Plasma concentrations of rabeprazole peak in approximately 2 to 5 hours; it is metabolized in the liver and excreted in the urine.

The side effects/adverse reactions include stomach colic or pain for omeprazole and diarrhea for lansoprazole. Other potential side effects of the proton pump inhibitors include abdominal distress, increased weakness, muscle aches, dizziness, headache, sedation, chest pain, heartburn, constipation or diarrhea, gas, nausea, vomiting, or skin rash. Rare adverse reactions reported with omeprazole include anemia, neutropenia, pancytopenia, thrombocytopenia, and urinary tract infections. The adult dosage of esomeprazole is 20 to 40 mg PO daily.

The adult dosage of omeprazole for gastroesophageal reflux is 20 mg PO (delayed-release capsule) daily for 1 to 2 months. For gastric hypersecretory conditions, the dosage is 60 mg PO daily, with dosage adjustments as necessary. For older adults the dosage should not exceed 20 mg/day. The pediatric dosage has not been established.

The adult dosage of lansoprazole for duodenal ulcer is 15 mg PO before breakfast for up to 1 month; for erosive esophagitis, 30 mg PO daily before breakfast for up to 2 months; for hypersecretory conditions, 60 mg PO daily before breakfast. The pediatric dosage has not been established.

The adult dosage of pantoprazole is 40 mg PO daily for up to 8 weeks for GERD and gastric ulcer, and up to 4 weeks for duodenal ulcer.

For healing and maintenance rabeprazole therapy, the daily dose is 20 mg PO. For chronic hypersecretory conditions, including Zollinger-Ellison syndrome, the dosage is 60 mg PO once daily.

■ Nursing Management

Proton Pump Inhibitor Therapy

■ **Assessment.** It should be determined if the client has a sensitivity to the drug or a history of or current chronic hepatic disease that would require a reduced dosage (hepatic dysfunction increases the half-life). Review the concurrent medications of the client, because proton pump inhibitors increase gastric pH and have the potential to affect the bioavailability of medications that depend on pH for absorption. Omeprazole may interact and cause an inhibition of the liver-metabolizing enzyme system (P-450), thus decreasing the metabolism of coumarin and indanedione anticoagulants, diazepam, and phenytoin. Serum levels of these agents can rise, resulting in toxicity. The absorption of lansoprazole is delayed and its bioavailability decreased by the concurrent administration of sucralfate; administer lansoprazole at least 30 minutes before sucralfate.

■ **Nursing Diagnosis.** The client receiving proton pump inhibitor therapy is at risk for the following nursing diagnoses: impaired comfort (heartburn, flatulence, abdominal pain, itching of skin, headache, chest pain); anxiety; ineffective protection related to blood dyscrasias (thrombocytopenia, eosinopenia, leukocytosis, anemia); fatigue; diarrhea; constipation; and risk for injury related to CNS disturbance (dizziness). With lansoprazole, the potential complications of mental depression and urinary tract infection (frequency, urgency, and burning on urination; hematuria; proteinuria) may occur.

■ **Implementation**

■ ***Monitoring.*** Monitor the client for decreased GI reflux or heartburn. Record the frequency, character, and color of stools. Monitor CBCs, urinalysis, and hepatic function studies. Monitor concurrent therapy closely.

■ ***Intervention.*** Therapy for the healing of ulcers should continue for at least 4 to 6 weeks but rarely beyond 8 weeks. Maintenance therapy for ulcer prophylaxis or hypersecretory gastric conditions may be long-term. Administer immediately before meals, preferably in the morning. Omeprazole may be taken with antacids to minimize gastric discomfort.

■ ***Education.*** Instruct the client in administration times and about swallowing the capsule whole; it is not to be crushed or chewed. If the client has difficulty swallowing, the lansoprazole capsule may be opened and the intact granules sprinkled on a tablespoon of applesauce and swallowed immediately. For clients with a nasogastric tube, the intact granules of the lansoprazole capsule may be mixed in 1½ ounces of apple juice and placed in the tube; flush the tube with additional apple juice to clear it.

■ **Evaluation.** The expected outcome of proton pump inhibitor therapy is that the client's hyperacidity is alleviated without producing side effects/adverse reactions to omeprazole, lansoprazole, or rabeprazole.

H_2 Receptor Antagonists

Histamine is found in the mucosal cells of the GI tract; this substance activates H_2 receptors to increase gastric acid secretion. The major components of gastric secretion include hydrochloric acid (HCl) and intrinsic factor (IF), both of which are produced by the parietal (acid-forming) cells; pepsinogen, which is synthesized by the chief cells; and mucus. The principal function of mucus is to protect the epithelial cells of the GI tract from an attack by pepsin and irritation by the HCl secreted by the stomach. Pepsinogen, an enzyme, is the precursor of pepsin; HCl catalyzes the cleavage of pepsinogen to active pepsin by providing a low pH environment in which pepsin can initiate the digestion of proteins.

Gastric secretion is regulated by a neural mechanism (parasympathetic [vagus] fibers) and a hormonal mechanism (gastrin). Activation of the vagus nerve causes the secretion of vast quantities of pepsinogen and HCl. The hormonal mechanism involves the actual presence of food, which distends the stomach and stimulates the antral mucosa to release gastrin. This hormone is then absorbed into the blood and carried to the parietal cells and chief cells, which secrete HCl and pepsinogen, respectively. It is believed that histamine activates the gastric mucosa much the same as gastrin does. In addition, caffeine and alcohol are potent stimuli for gastrin release. When the acidity of the gastric juice is increased to a pH of 2, a negative feedback mechanism helps to block gastric secretion from the parietal and chief cells. Thus the inhibition of gastric gland secretion plays an essential role in protecting the stomach against excessively acidic secretions, which are responsible for causing peptic ulcerations.

Normally the mucosal surface of the stomach and upper duodenum is protected from the irritation of gastric acid by a layer of mucus. If a circumscribed area of the mucosal surface is damaged and fails to repair rapidly, it may become eroded, forming an ulcer at one of these sites. When gastric acid comes in contact with this inflamed region, pain may result. Moreover, clinical studies have suggested that esophageal, gastric, and duodenal ulcers (peptic ulcers) are associated with the excessive production of gastric acid. Infection with *H. pylori* is also a major cause of gastric and duodenal ulcers. H_2 receptor antagonists are used as a part of the combination therapies for the eradication of *H. pylori*.

Clinical evidence has shown that histamine released by severe injuries, particularly burns, may lead to the formation of peptic ulcers.

The H_2 receptor blockers include cimetidine (Tagamet), ranitidine (Zantac), famotidine (Pepcid), and nizatidine (Axid). They act to prevent histamine from stimulating the H_2 receptors on the gastric parietal cells, thus reducing the volume of gastric acid secretion (from stimuli such as food, pentagastrin, histamine, caffeine, and insulin) and the concentration (acid content) of these secretions. All four drugs are presently considered to be equally potent and effective, but the pharmacokinetics, side effects/adverse reactions, and drug interactions may differ.

TABLE 41-2 H_2 Receptor Antagonists: Pharmacokinetics

Drug	Absorption	Time to Peak Plasma Levels	Plasma Half-life (hours)	Duration of Action (hours)	Metabolism/Excretion
cimetidine (Tagamet)	Very good orally, 60%-70%	45-90 minutes after oral dose	2	Basal: 4-5 Nocturnal: 6-8	Liver/kidneys
famotidine (Pepcid)	Fair orally, 40%-45%	1-3 hours after oral dose	2.5-3.5	Basal and nocturnal: 10-12	Liver/kidneys
nizatidine (Axid)	Very good orally, 90%	0.5-3 hours after oral dose	1-2	Basal: up to 8 Nocturnal: up to 12	Liver (has active metabolite)/kidneys
ranitidine (Zantac)	Good orally, 50%	2-3 hours after oral dose	2-2.5	Basal: up to 4 Nocturnal: up to 13	Liver/kidneys

Case Study *The Client with Peptic Ulcer Disease*

Henry Blake is a 47-year-old electrical engineer who has had a gastric ulcer for 3 years. The prescriber is seeing him because his symptoms have worsened. The nursing history reveals that Mr. Blake is experiencing increased gastric pain after he eats; the pain is relieved by antacids. He smokes a pack of cigarettes daily and has an occasional glass of wine before dinner. He has been taking two aspirin three to four times daily to treat the elbow pain he experiences when playing racquetball. His prescriber is placing him on cimetidine (Tagamet) 300 mg PO four times daily.

1. What is the mechanism of action for histamine H_2-blocking agents?
2. What side effects of cimetidine should Mr. Blake be aware of?
3. What is important to teach Mr. Blake regarding his smoking habit? Considering his health history, what other issues should be included in his health instruction?

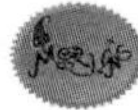

For answer guidelines, go to mosby.com/MERLIN/McKenry/.

cimetidine [sye met′ i deen] (Tagamet)
ranitidine [ra nit′ te deen] (Zantac)
famotidine [fa moe′ ti deen] (Pepcid ◆)
nizatidine [ni za′ ti deen] (Axid)

These agents are used to treat and prevent duodenal ulcers and to treat gastric ulcers, gastroesophageal reflux, and hypersecretory gastric states. See Table 41-2 for the pharmacokinetics of these agents.

The side effects of H_2 receptor blockers include diarrhea, constipation, headache, stomach cramps or pain, dizziness, and rash. Breast swelling or pain in males and females has been reported. Famotidine may also cause dry mouth or skin, anorexia, and tinnitus. Less common and rare adverse reactions include confusion, neutropenia, bradycardia, tachycardia, and agranulocytosis.

For the treatment of duodenal and benign active gastric ulcers, the adult dosage is as follows:

- cimetidine: 300 mg PO four times daily with meals and at bedtime, 600 mg twice daily, or 800 mg at bedtime; the adult dosage by IM, IV, or IV infusion is 300 mg every 6 to 8 hours
- famotidine: 40 mg at bedtime; the parenteral adult dosage is 20 mg IV injection or IV infusion every 12 hours
- nizatidine: 300 mg PO at bedtime
- ranitidine: 150 mg PO twice daily or 300 mg PO at bedtime; the parenteral dosage is 50 mg IM, IV, or IV infusion every 6 to 8 hours

Refer to a current reference for additional dosing recommendations. In addition, see the Case Study box above.

■ Nursing Management

H_2 Receptor Antagonist Therapy

■ **Assessment.** Determine the client's sensitivity to H_2 receptor blockers. Note that clients with impaired renal function may require a dosage reduction for cimetidine, famotidine, ranitidine, or nizatidine because of delayed excretion and the risk for increased side effects, particularly CNS effects. A further reduction in dosage may be necessary in clients with impaired liver function. (See also the Pregnancy Safety box on p. 773.)

Assess the underlying condition. These drugs are not to be used for minor digestive complaints. Before administering, the potential existence of a malignant GI neoplasm should be ruled out. Assess the client's smoking history.

A baseline assessment of the client's GI pain should be obtained along with a CBC and a stool guaiac for occult blood.

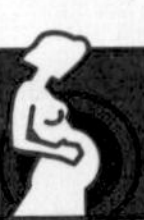

Pregnancy Safety
Drugs Affecting the Gastrointestinal Tract

Category	Drug
B	cimetidine, dolasetron, esomeprazole, famotidine, granisetron, lansoprazole, mesalamine, metoclopramide, ondansetron, pantoprazole, ranitidine, sucralfate, sulfasalazine, ursodiol
C	cisapride, difenoxin and atropine, diphenoxylate and atropine, dronabinol, ipecac syrup, infliximab, monoctanoin, nizatidine, olsalazine, omeprazole, pancreatin, pancrelipase, scopolamine
X	chenodiol, misoprostol
Not established	rabeprazole, trimethobenzamide; thiethylperazine is not recommended for use during pregnancy

Review the client's current medication regimen for the risk of significant drug interactions, such as those that may occur when the H_2 receptor antagonists are given concurrently with the drugs in the following table. Unlike the other H_2 receptor antagonists, cimetidine inhibits drug metabolism in the liver; therefore the major drug interactions noted in the following table occur with cimetidine. However, all of the H_2 receptor antagonists may exhibit a similar effect with the use of itraconazole, ketoconazole, and antacids.

Drug	Possible Effect and Management
antacids	Concurrent use is often prescribed, but the absorption of any of the H_2 receptor antagonists may be decreased if given concurrently with an antacid. Antacids should not be administered within 1 hour of administration of the H_2 receptor antagonist.
anticoagulants (coumarins, indanediones), tricyclic antidepressants, metoprolol (Lopressor), phenytoin (Dilantin), propranolol (Inderal), or the xanthines (exception: dyphylline)	A decrease in the metabolism and excretion of these medications may occur when administered with cimetidine. Because dosage adjustments may be necessary, monitoring of serum concentrations for phenytoin and xanthines, prothrombin time (for anticoagulants), and blood pressure (for metoprolol and propranolol) are indicated.
itraconazole (Sporanox), ketoconazole (Nizoral)	An increase in GI pH induced by the H_2 receptor antagonist (any of the four agents) may result in a reduced absorption of itraconazole and ketoconazole. Advise clients to take the H_2 receptor antagonist at least 2 hours after these antifungals.

■ **Nursing Diagnosis.** With the administration of H_2 receptor antagonists, the client is at risk for the following nursing diagnoses/collaborative problems: impaired comfort (headache, breast tenderness, muscle ache, anorexia, nausea or vomiting, rash, and dizziness); sexual dysfunction (decreased sexual ability); constipation; diarrhea; disturbed sleep pattern (drowsiness); disturbed thought processes (confusion); hyperthermia; ineffective protection related to blood dyscrasias; and the potential complications of allergic reaction, bradycardia or tachycardia, and bronchospasm.

■ **Implementation**

■ ***Monitoring.*** Assess the client regularly for GI pain. A periodic evaluation of blood counts is required during therapy.

Be aware that mild bilateral gynecomastia in males and galactorrhea in females have been observed in some clients after long-term treatment with cimetidine (1 month or more). This drug also may cause a reversible decline in sperm count or impotence. No such problems have been reported with ranitidine.

■ ***Intervention.*** Administer H_2 receptor antagonists with meals, because the maximum therapeutic effect occurs when the stomach is protected by the buffering effect of food. A bedtime dose protects the stomach from the nocturnal hypersecretion of gastric acid. To prevent drug interactions, administer antacids to relieve acute ulcer pain 1 hour before or 1 hour after the administration of an H_2 antagonist. Although the symptoms of duodenal ulcers may diminish in a week or two, therapy should be continued for 4 to 6 weeks (rarely beyond 8 weeks).

Note that the parenteral form of the drug is stable for 48 hours at room temperature. Cimetidine, ranitidine, and famotidine are compatible for dilution with IV solutions of 0.9% sodium chloride and dextrose 5%. Rapid IV bolus administration (less than 2 minutes) may result in cardiac dysrhythmias and hypotension.

■ ***Education.*** Warn the client that IM administration may be painful. Instruct the client to keep clinical and laboratory appointments as scheduled.

Encourage the client with peptic ulcer disease to discontinue smoking altogether or at least after the last dose of the day. The effectiveness of H_2 receptor antagonists in inhibiting nocturnal gastric acid secretions is diminished by smoking.

■ **Evaluation.** The expected outcome of H_2 antagonist therapy is that the client will report diminished pain or an absence of pain and demonstrate healing or an absence of ulceration by endoscopic or x-ray examination.

Drugs That Affect the Gallbladder

chenodiol [kee noe dye′ ole] (Chenix)

Chenodiol (chenodeoxycholic acid) is a normal bile acid synthesized in the liver. Bile acids and lecithin break down cholesterol; when the amount of cholesterol exceeds the capacity of bile acids and lecithin to perform this effect, crystallization and gallstones may result. Chenodiol blocks the synthesis of cholesterol in the liver; this reduces biliary cholesterol levels, which leads to a gradual dissolving of floating, radiolucent cholesterol gallstones.

Chenodiol is indicated for the client with radiolucent stones who has a well-opacified, functioning gallbladder but who is at increased risk with elective surgery because of systemic disease, age, or cardiovascular, renal, or respiratory disease. A number of warnings about the use of this drug have been used and include the following: (1) this drug may cause hepatotoxicity, (2) poor response rates have been reported by some subgroups of chenodiol-treated clients, and (3) other treated subgroups required cholecystectomy after treatment. Laparoscopic surgery for cholelithiasis may be more appropriate given the length of treatment time with chenodiol. For these reasons, chenodiol should be reserved only for select clients; if used, liver function tests should be closely monitored. The nurse should review the most current drug information (package insert) available before using this drug (Chenodiol, 2000). (See the Complementary and Alternative Therapies box at right.)

monoctanoin [mon oe ock′ ta noyn] (Moctanin)

Monoctanoin is a solubilizing agent (dissolves cholesterol stones) indicated for the treatment of cholesterol gallstones in the bile duct or after an unsuccessful cholecystectomy. It is more effective for a single radiolucent stone than for multiple gallstones. Monoctanoin is administered directly into the common bile duct.

Monoctanoin is absorbed by the portal vein and metabolized by pancreatic lipases to fatty acids and glycerol.

The most commonly reported side effects are abdominal irritation and pain. Less commonly reported side effects include diarrhea, anorexia, nausea, or vomiting.

The adult dosage via a catheter (continuous perfusion) is 3 to 5 mL/hr administered at a pressure of 10 cm of water for 1 to 3 weeks. This drug is not to be given by IM or IV administration.

■ Nursing Management
Monoctanoin Therapy

■ **Assessment.** It should be determined that the client does not have a condition for which the administration of monoctanoin is contraindicated, such as severe biliary tract infection, obstructive jaundice, recent duodenal ulcer, or pancreatitis, which might be aggravated. Hepatic dysfunction might interfere with the metabolism of the fatty acids generated from monoctanoin and result in adverse reactions. It might also increase the risk of ulceration and hemorrhage in jejunitis or duodenal ulcer. Monoctanoin should be used with caution in clients who are sensitive to this substance or to vegetable oils and in clients who have biliary duct obstruction.

A baseline assessment of pulse, blood pressure, and temperature; hepatic function studies; and a cholangiogram is obtained.

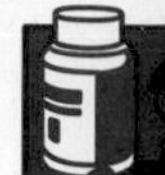

Complementary and Alternative Therapies
Milk Thistle

The above-ground parts of milk thistle, as well as its fruit and seed, have been used for thousands of years for treating dysfunction of the gallbladder and liver and other dyspeptic disorders. In Europe, the edible peeled stalk of the plant has been used as a vegetable, and the leaves have been used as salad greens. The above-ground parts of the plant are likely to be safe when consumed in this form and in amounts commonly used in food.

The fruit and seed of milk thistle are thought to have therapeutic use and are taken orally for the treatment of hepatic cirrhosis and acute and chronic hepatitis related to drugs, alcohol, toxins, and viral conditions. Silymarin, a milk thistle fruit and seed extract, seems to be therapeutic in two ways. The first is a protective mechanism that alters the outer hepatic cell membrane to prevent the penetration of toxins. The second is the stimulation of ribosomal RNA polymerase, which increases hepatocyte protein synthesis and the formation of new hepatocytes. Recent studies (Buzzelli et al., 1993; Pares et al., 1998) indicate that the use of milk thistle has been beneficial in clients with alcohol-related cirrhosis and chronic active hepatitis.

Milk thistle is considered safe when taken in recommended doses, but it may have a laxative effect with some people. People sensitive to ragweed, marigolds, daisies, and other members of the Asteraceae/Compositae family may experience mild allergic reactions with use. Clients with diabetes who are using milk thistle should monitor their blood sugar levels carefully, because this substance may lower blood sugar levels.

Typical dosages of milk thistle involve 140-mg capsules, standardized to 70% silymarin extract, two to three times daily. For the dried fruit or seed, the typical dosage is 12 to 15 g daily prepared as tea and taken as one cup three to four times daily 30 minutes before meals. Each cup of tea is prepared by steeping 3 to 5 g of the crushed fruit or seed in 150 mL of boiling water for 10 to 15 minutes and then straining it before consuming.

Information from Cirigliano, M.D. (1998). Ten most common herbs in clinical practice. In M.S. Micozzi (Ed.), *Current review of complementary medicine.* Philadelphia: Current Medicine; and Jellin, J.M., Batz, F., & Hitchens, K. (1999). *Pharmacist's letter/prescriber's letter natural medicines comprehensive database.* Stockton, CA: Therapeutic Research Faculty.

■ **Nursing Diagnosis.** The client receiving monoctanoin is at risk for the following nursing diagnoses/collaborative problems: impaired comfort (abdominal pain, backache, flushing of the face, metallic taste); diarrhea; deficient fluid volume related to nausea and vomiting; and the potential complication of cholangitis, gallbladder perforation, and biliary peritonitis.

■ **Implementation**

■ ***Monitoring.*** Monitor the client's blood pressure, pulse, temperature, and comfort status every 4 to 6 hours during the perfusion. An elevated temperature with increasing upper abdominal pain might be indicative of ascending cholangitis. Monitor the white cell count (WBC) for leukopenia. Hepatic function studies are suggested.

After placing a percutaneous T-tube or nasobiliary tube directly into the common bile duct by endoscopy, an infusion pump with an overflow manometer is used to regulate the continuous perfusion of monoctanoin into the duct. Monitor perfusion flow pressure to prevent exceeding the prescribed pressure level. Adjust if necessary; GI side effects, such as nausea and diarrhea, are more likely to occur if the infusion pump rate is too fast.

A cholangiogram is recommended every 3 days to monitor stone dissolution. Therapy is discontinued if endoscopy or an x-ray examination does not show a significant decrease in stone size after 10 days. Complete stone dissolution is variable from 7 to 21 days.

■ ***Intervention.*** The perfusion may be interrupted for 1 to 2 hours at mealtime to reduce GI effects. Hourly aspiration of bile will reduce pressure and distention in the biliary tract and may decrease abdominal and back discomfort.

■ ***Education.*** Instruct the client to alert the nurse to any nausea, diarrhea, or discomfort that may occur. Provide counseling related to low-fat, high-fiber dietary changes if required.

■ **Evaluation.** The expected outcome of monoctanoin therapy is that the client's gallstones will be dissolved without any adverse drug reactions.

ursodiol [ur soh' dee ole] (Actigall)

Ursodiol, an analog of chenodiol, is an oral product used to dissolve cholesterol gallstones in clients with uncomplicated gallstone disease. It is more effective against small, floatable stones and is not indicated for the treatment of calcified cholesterol stones, radiopaque (calcium-containing) stones, or radiolucent bile pigment–type stones or when surgery is clearly necessary.

Although its exact mechanism of action is unknown, ursodiol inhibits the intestinal absorption of cholesterol and also decreases cholesterol synthesis and secretion in the liver. It concentrates in the bile. A decrease in cholesterol saturation allows for the gradual dissolution of cholesterol from the gallstones. Ursodiol also increases the flow of bile in the body. However, 6 to 24 months of oral therapy may be necessary for gallstone dissolution depending on the composition and size of the stone. Therapy is monitored by performing ultrasonograms at 6-month intervals during the first year. If partial effectiveness is not recorded after 1 year of treatment, ursodiol is usually determined to be ineffective and drug therapy is discontinued. If therapy is successful, ursodiol is recommended for at least 3 months after complete dissolution of the stones to ensure the removal of small particles that are not visible with the ultrasonogram.

When administered orally, ursodiol is absorbed from the small intestine, reaches a peak concentration in 1 to 3 hours, and is metabolized by the liver to taurine and glycine conjugates that are secreted in bile. Excretion is mainly in the feces.

An uncommon side effect reported with ursodiol is diarrhea. Ursodiol may cause hepatotoxicity, but liver injuries have not been reported to date.

The oral dosage for adults is 8 to 10 mg/kg daily, divided into 2 or 3 doses taken with meals. A pediatric dosage has not been established.

■ Nursing Management

Ursodiol Therapy

■ **Assessment.** Although ursodiol is indicated for the dissolution of cholesterol gallstones, it is administered with caution if the client's health status is further compromised with bile duct abnormalities, complications of gallstones such as cholecystitis or pancreatitis, or chronically impaired hepatic function. The client will usually undergo ultrasonogram and/or hepatic function studies to determine if these conditions exist before beginning a regimen of ursodiol. Hepatic function studies are performed to rule out preexisting liver disease. No significant drug interactions have been reported with ursodiol, but keep in mind that antacids (containing aluminum), cholestyramine, or colestipol may decrease the absorption and effectiveness of ursodiol when administered concurrently. A nursing baseline assessment includes ursodiol sensitivity, pain status, and bowel status.

■ **Nursing Diagnosis.** During the course of ursodiol therapy the client may experience diarrhea as an adverse reaction to the drug.

■ **Implementation**

■ ***Monitoring.*** Ultrasonograms, cholecystograms, and/or hepatic function studies are usually performed periodically over the course of drug therapy to determine the dissolution of gallstones and the development of hepatotoxicity. Monitor the client's bowel elimination for the frequency and character of stools.

■ ***Intervention.*** Administer ursodiol with meals, but pace antacids and the bile sequestering agents at least 2 hours apart from ursodiol. If partial dissolution has not occurred after 6 to 12 months of therapy, the drug is considered ineffective and is discontinued.

■ ***Education.*** The client should be instructed to take ursodiol with meals because it dissolves more rapidly when bile and pancreatic enzymes are present. Compliance is encouraged and the client is cautioned to be patient, because gallstone dissolution may take 6 months to 2 years depending on the size and number of stones.

■ **Evaluation.** If ursodiol therapy is successful, the client's gallstones should diminish in size and number as demonstrated by the ultrasonogram, and the client will not experience any adverse reactions to the drug.

Drugs Used to Treat Inflammatory Bowel Disease

The miscellaneous GI medications include mesalamine or 5-aminosalicylic acid (Asacol, Pentasa, Rowasa), olsalazine (Dipentum), sulfasalazine (Azulfidine) and infliximab (Remicade). Mesalamine is used to treat chronic inflammatory bowel disease, sulfasalazine is indicated for the treatment of ulcerative colitis, and olsalazine is used to maintain the remission of ulcerative colitis in persons who cannot tolerate sulfasalazine. Infliximab, a monoclonal antibody, is the first drug approved to treat fistulizing Crohn's disease; it may also be prescribed to treat moderate to severe, active Crohn's disease.

Mechanism of Action. Although the exact mechanism of action of mesalamine is unknown, it appears to decrease inflammation by inhibiting cyclooxygenase and lipoxygenase, which results in a decrease in the production of prostaglandin and leukotriene. Bacteria in the colon splits sulfasalazine into sulfapyridine and mesalamine, and it is theorized that mesalamine is the active ingredient for the treatment of ulcerative colitis. Olsalazine is a salicylate compound that is converted in the colon by bacteria to mesalamine. Therefore the active ingredient in these three products is mesalamine. Infliximab is a monoclonal antibody that binds and neutralizes the tumor necrosis factor alpha, which is a primary cytokine that is believed to activate the inflammatory response in clients with Crohn's disease (McCusker, 1998).

Pharmacokinetics. Mesalamine is available in extended-release capsules and tablets (Pentasa), delayed-release tablets (Asacol) and rectal suppositories and rectal suspensions (Rowasa). The nurse should be aware that there is a difference between the extended-release and delayed-release preparations; therefore one product should not be substituted for the other.

The absorption of oral mesalamine is 20% to 30%. Asacol has a coating (acrylic-based resin) that delays dissolution until the tablet is at a pH of 7 or more; therefore it is released in the distal ileum and colon. Pentasa contains cellulose-coated granules, which permits the continuous release of mesalamine in the small and large intestine, independent of pH. The half-life of mesalamine from Asacol is 3 hours; the half-life of Pentasa cannot be determined because of the continuous release of the product. A peak serum level occurs in 4 to 12 hours for Asacol and in 3 hours for Pentasa. Excretion of the unchanged drug is primarily in the feces for Asacol (80%) and Pentasa (13%). The absorbed mesalamine is excreted renally as the metabolite (*N*-acetyl-5-aminosalicylic acid [Ac-5-ASA]).

Sulfasalazine is poorly absorbed orally (20%); the remaining dose is converted by bacteria in the colon to sulfapyridine and mesalamine. Most of the sulfapyridine (60% to 80%) and approximately 25% of the mesalamine is absorbed in the colon. The half-life of sulfapyridine is 6 to 14 hours; for mesalamine it is 0.6 to 1.4 hours. The peak serum level is between 1.5 and 6 hours for sulfasalazine (oral suspension and tablets) and between 9 and 24 hours for sulfapyridine. Enteric-coated tablets take longer to peak—between 3 and 12 hours for sulfasalazine and between 12 and 24 hours for sulfapyridine. Excretion is primarily by the kidneys for sulfasalazine and sulfapyridine, whereas it is mainly fecal for mesalamine.

Olsalazine remains primarily unabsorbed until it reaches the colon, where it is converted to mesalamine by colonic bacteria. Mesalamine is absorbed slowly, which results in a high local concentration of mesalamine in the colon. The time to peak serum levels for mesalamine is 4 to 8 hours. The excretion of mesalamine occurs in the feces (80%); the absorbed portion is excreted by the kidneys as the metabolite (Ac-5-ASA).

Infliximab is administered by IV infusion and has a prolonged half-life; a single infusion of 5 mg/kg has a half-life of approximately 9.5 days.

Side Effects/Adverse Reactions. The side effects/adverse reactions of mesalamine include stomach cramps or pain, diarrhea, headache, nausea, vomiting, weakness, rhinitis and, infrequently or rarely, acne, alopecia, loss of appetite, back pain, indigestion, hepatitis, pancreatitis, or pericarditis. The side effects/adverse reactions of olsalazine include similar GI side effects; infrequent or rare effects include acne, joint and muscle pain, mood alterations, sedation, headache, insomnia, exacerbation of ulcerative colitis, hepatitis, and pancreatitis. For sulfasalazine, the side effects/adverse reactions include similar GI side effects, continuous headache, allergic reaction, photosensitivity; infrequent or rare effects include blood dyscrasias, hepatitis, Stevens-Johnson syndrome, systemic lupus erythematosus–like syndrome, and exacerbation of colitis. Undesirable infliximab effects include headache, nausea, upper respiratory infections, stomach pain, weakness, fever, vomiting, pharyngitis and, infrequently, hypotension, hypertension, tachycardia, acne, alopecia, and other skin disorders, constipation, gas, intestinal obstruction, and urinary tract infection (*Drug Facts and Comparisons*, 2000).

Dosage and Administration. The adult dosage of mesalamine is 1 g four times daily, up to 2 months for the extended-release preparations; or 800 mg three times daily for 6 weeks for the delayed-release tablet (Asacol). The adult dosage of olsalazine is 500 mg twice daily. The adult dosage of sulfasalazine is 1 g every 6 to 8 hours initially, which is reduced to 500 mg every 6 hours for maintenance dosing. The adult dosage of infliximab for moderate to severe cases of Crohn's disease is 5 mg/kg by a single dose (IV infusion). Fistulizing Crohn's disease may require additional doses 2 and 6 weeks after the first dose.

■ Nursing Management

Drug Therapy for Inflammatory Bowel Disease

■ **Assessment.** Determine if the client has a sensitivity to mesalamine, olsalazine, sulfasalazine, infliximab, or salicylates. Before administering sulfasalazine, determine if the client is sensitive to a wider range of agents: sulfonamides, furosemide, thiazide diuretics, sulfonylureas, or carbonic anhydrase inhibitors. Concern for renal function impairment exists with all of these agents, but the use of sulfasalazine is contraindicated in clients with intestinal or urinary obstruction. Clients with severe allergies or asthma risk developing an increasing hypersensitivity to sulfasalazine. Clients with blood dyscrasias, a deficiency of glucose-6-phosphate dehydrogenase (G6PD), and porphyria may develop more symptomatic conditions. Sulfonamides are metabolized in the liver and may cause hepatitis in clients with a preexisting hepatic impairment.

Review the client's concurrent medication regimen for the risk of significant drug interactions, such as those that may occur when these drugs are given concurrently with the following drugs:

Drug	Possible Effect and Management
anticoagulants (coumarin or indanedione derivatives), anticonvulsants (hydantoins), oral antidiabetic agents, methotrexate (Folex)	Sulfasalazine may displace these drugs from protein-binding sites and/or inhibit their metabolism, resulting in a prolonged effect or toxicity. Dosage adjustments may be necessary during and after sulfonamide therapy.
other hemolytics, such as methyldopa (Aldomet), nitrofurans, quinidine (Quinaglute)	Increases the potential for toxic hematologic side effects. Monitor CBCs carefully.
other hepatotoxic drugs, such as alcohol, angiotensin-converting enzyme (ACE) inhibitors, NSAIDs, isoniazid, valproic acid (Depakene), zidovudine (Retrovir), and others	Increases the risk of hepatotoxicity, especially in clients with a history of liver disease. Monitor hepatic function studies carefully.

A baseline assessment of the client's health status should include weight, dietary patterns, bowel status, CBCs, liver function studies, and proctoscopy and sigmoidoscopy determinations.

■ **Nursing Diagnosis.** The client undergoing mesalamine therapy is at risk for the following nursing diagnoses/collaborative problems: impaired comfort (heartburn, abdominal cramping, flatulence, headache, anorexia, nausea or vomiting, rhinitis); fatigue; and the potential complications of acute intolerance syndrome (severe abdominal cramping, fever, skin rash, severe headache), hepatitis (jaundice, right upper abdominal quadrant tenderness), pancreatitis (severe back or stomach pain, fever, nausea and vomiting), and pericarditis (anxiety, chest pain, chills, shortness of breath, tiredness). Olsalazine may lead to diarrhea; impaired comfort (headache, abdominal cramping, anorexia, nausea or vomiting); disturbed sleep pattern (drowsiness or insomnia); anxiety; and the potential complications of mental depression, pancreatitis, hepatitis, or exacerbation of the client's ulcerative colitis. Sulfasalazine therapy may result in impaired comfort (headache, abdominal cramping, anorexia, nausea or vomiting); diarrhea; and the potential complications of blood dyscrasias (agranulocytosis, neutropenia, aplastic anemia, thrombocytopenia), hepatitis, Stevens-Johnson syndrome (aching of joints, peeling of skin, fatigue), systemic lupus erythematosus–like syndrome (skin rash or blisters, general feeling of illness), or hypersensitivity reaction.

■ **Implementation**

■ ***Monitoring.*** CBCs and renal and hepatic function studies are performed periodically. Client progress is monitored by proctoscopy and sigmoidoscopy. The client's comfort, weight, diet, bowel status, and general health should also be monitored. Serum sulfapyridine levels may be useful, because concentrations greater than 50 μg/mL seem to result in a higher incidence of adverse reactions in clients receiving sulfasalazine.

■ ***Intervention.*** Mesalamine is to be administered before meals and at bedtime with a full glass of water. Olsalazine and sulfasalazine should be administered with food. The client may be placed on maintenance doses when improvement is demonstrated by endoscopy.

■ ***Education.*** Stress the importance of adherence to the full course of therapy, consulting with the prescriber on a regular basis to check progress, and not switching brands of medications without checking with the prescriber. Instruct the client to swallow mesalamine tablets whole and not to chew, crush, or break them; the empty tablet may be seen in the stool after the medication has been absorbed. Olsalazine and sulfasalazine should be taken in evenly divided doses throughout the day.

Advise clients on the instructions discussed in the intervention section. With sulfasalazine, maintain a fluid intake of 1200 to 1500 mL/daily. Alert the client taking sulfasalazine about the following sun precautions to protect against photosensitivity effects: avoid sun exposure between 10 AM and 3 PM, apply sunscreen lotion with at least a 15 SPF to sun-exposed body parts, and wear sunglasses, long sleeves, pants, and a hat when outside during the day. The client taking sulfasalazine may experience an orange-yellow discoloration of the urine and skin, but this coloration is clinically insignificant.

■ **Evaluation.** The expected outcome for inflammatory bowel disease drug therapy is that the client's underlying condition will improve as evidenced by an absence of abdominal cramping and diarrhea, a weight gain to a normal weight for height, and an improved sense of well-being.

Drugs That Affect the Lower Gastrointestinal Tract

Bowel elimination is often a major concern of clients, particularly constipation in the older client and diarrhea in children and immunosuppressed clients. Most of the agents that affect the lower GI tract may be purchased over-the-counter and are discussed in Chapter 11. Clients admitted to various health care agencies for short stays in acute care institutions or for extended stays in long-term care facilities often experience constipation or diarrhea.

BOX 41-3

NANDA Nursing Diagnoses Related to Altered Bowel Elimination

Colonic constipation is a state in which an individual's pattern of elimination is characterized by hard/dry stool that results from a delay in the passage of food residue. Its major defining characteristics are decreased frequency, hard/dry stool, painful defecation, abdominal distention, and a palpable mass. Minor characteristics are rectal pressure, headache, appetite impairment, and abdominal pain. Related factors are less than adequate fiber, less than adequate dietary intake, immobility, lack of privacy, emotional disturbance, chronic use of medications and enemas, stress, a change in daily routine, and metabolic problems such as hypothyroidism, hypocalcemia, and hypokalemia (accepted by the Eighth National Conference on the Classification of Nursing Diagnoses, 1988).

Perceived constipation is a state in which an individual makes a self-diagnosis of constipation and ensures a daily bowel movement through the use of laxatives, enemas, and suppositories. The defining characteristic is an expectation of a daily bowel movement; it may be expected at the same time every day. This results in the overuse of laxatives, enemas, and suppositories. Related factors are cultural and family health beliefs, faulty appraisal, and impaired thought processes (accepted by the Eighth National Conference on the Classification of Nursing Diagnoses, 1988).

Rectal constipation is a state in which an individual's pattern of elimination is characterized by stool retention, normal stool consistency, and delayed elimination that results from biopsychosocial disruptions. There is also abdominal discomfort, rectal fullness, and a change in flatus. Related factors are weak pelvic floor muscles, painful anorectal lesions, self-care deficits, environmental constraints, altered mobility, low or no social support, impaired communication, altered awareness, and emotional disturbances (accepted by the Eighth National Conference on the Classification of Nursing Diagnoses, 1988).

Diarrhea is the frequent passage of loose, watery stools, generally as the result of increased motility in the colon. The cause of the condition includes stress and anxiety, dietary intake, the side effects of medications, inflammation, toxins, contaminants, or radiation. The defining characteristics include abdominal pain, cramping, increased frequency of elimination, increased frequency of bowel sounds, loose or liquid stools, urgency of defecation, and a change in the color of the feces (accepted by the Fourth National Conference on the Classification of Nursing Diagnoses, 1975).

Information from Carpenito, L.J. (2000). *Nursing diagnosis: Application to clinical practice* (8th ed.). Philadelphia: J.B. Lipppincott; and Anderson, K.N., Anderson, L.E., & Glanze, W.D. (Eds.).(1998). *Mosby's medical, nursing, & allied health dictionary* (5th ed.). St. Louis: Mosby.

Constipation is defined as difficult fecal evacuation as a result of degree of hardness and perhaps infrequent movements. Regular bowel movements may range from three per day to three per week. The Eighth National Conference on the Classification of Nursing Diagnoses has further classified the condition into colonic and rectal constipation (Box 41-3). A subjective aspect of constipation is the individual's feeling or attitude of dissatisfaction regarding bowel function, pattern of elimination, or perceived constipation. Chronic constipation is sometimes caused by organic disease (e.g., tumors); bowel obstruction; megacolon; metabolic abnormalities (e.g., diabetes mellitus or hypercalcemia); rectal disorders; diseases of the liver, gallbladder, or muscles; neurologic abnormalities (e.g., multiple sclerosis and Parkinson's disease); and pregnancy. Persons who suffer from disorders of the GI tract often complain of constipation. On the other hand, many persons complain of constipation when no organic disease or lesion can be found.

When not a result of organic factors, constipation is generally attributable to faulty eating habits, a failure to respond to defecation impulses, insufficient fluid intake or exercise, or being hospitalized, off the usual routine, and in a strange place. For example, a diet that provides inadequate bulk and residue will contribute to the development of constipation. The GI tract should function normally if fluids and residue are supplied in sufficient quantities to keep the stool formed but soft.

Another common cause of constipation is a failure to respond to the normal defecation impulses and insufficient time to permit the bowel to produce an evacuation. Sedentary habits and insufficient exercise may be factors. Clients with impaired physical mobility may be constipated because of inactivity or an unnatural position for defecation, such as using a bedpan.

Another causative factor is the effect of drugs. The use of antacids, diuretics, morphine, tricyclic antidepressants, codeine, aluminum hydroxide, and anticholinergics often leads to constipation as a side effect. Constipation can also be a symptom of both functional and organic disorders, such as febrile states, psychosomatic disorders, anemias, and tension headaches. A less common cause of constipation may be atonic and hypotonic conditions of the musculature of the colon. These conditions may result from habitual use of cathartics, substances that produce a liquid or fluid evacuation of the bowel.

BOX 41-4

Selected Types of Laxatives

Saline laxatives retain and increase the water content of feces by virtue of their osmotic qualities.

Stimulant laxatives increase peristalsis in the colon by irritating intramural sensory nerve plexi endings in the mucosa.

Bulk laxatives absorb water and increase the volume, bulk, and moisture of nonabsorbable intestinal contents, thereby distending the bowel and initiating reflex bowel activity.

Intestinal lubricants mechanically lubricate the feces to facilitate defecation.

Emollients, or fecal softening agents act as dispersing wetting agents, facilitating the mixture of water and fatty substances within the fecal mass. The feces become soft when a homogeneous mixture is produced.

Hyperosmotic agents increase intraluminal osmotic pressure in the bowel. Because these agents are not absorbed, they draw water into the intestine, resulting in an increased volume that stimulates peristalsis.

LAXATIVES

Laxatives are drugs given to induce defecation. Laxatives may be classified according to their source, site of action, degree of action, or mechanism of action (see Chapter 11). Box 41-4 summarizes the types of laxatives discussed in Chapter 11. The monographs for the prescription laxatives (Lactulose and GoLYTELY), as well as the nursing management of laxative therapy in general, are discussed in this chapter (Table 41-3).

lactulose [lak′ tyoo lose] (Chronulac, Duphalac)

Lactulose is composed of galactose, fructose, and other sugars; in the GI tract, the normal colonic bacteria (*Lactobacillus, Bacteroides, Escherichia coli,* and *Streptococcus faecalis*) metabolize lactulose syrup to organic acids, primarily lactic, acetic, and formic acids. These acids produce an osmotic effect, with an increase in fluid accumulation, distention, peristalsis, and bowel movements within 24 to 72 hours. Lactulose is also used to decrease serum levels of ammonia in persons with hepatic encephalopathy secondary to chronic liver disease.

The absorption of lactulose is minimal after oral administration, and it is excreted by the kidneys. Lactulose syrup is used in clients who have a history of chronic constipation that generally does not respond sufficiently to the bulk laxatives. It increases the number of daily bowel movements and the number of days on which bowel movements occur. Dose-related flatulence and intestinal cramps, gas, and belching are reported. Excessive doses may produce some

TABLE 41-3 Overview of Prescription Laxatives

	Lactulose Syrup or PEG 3350*
Disadvantages with repeated frequent (long-term) administration?	Early, transient flatulence and cramps; nausea reported
Increases rate of transit in small bowel?	Possibly
Causes net secretion of water and electrolytes in small bowel?	No
Inhibits absorption in small bowel?	Not reported
Increases mucosal permeability in small bowel?	No
Causes mucosal damage in small bowel?	No
Acts only in colon (not small bowel)?	Yes
Indicated for long-term treatment?	Yes: lactulose No: PEG
Examples of types	Chronulac (lactulose) CoLyte GoLYTELY
Physical or chemical property responsible for action	Colon-specific increase in stool water content and stool softening by increasing osmotic pressure (hyperosmotic) and colon acidification

*PEG 3350, Polyethylene glycol electrolyte solution.

diarrhea (hypokalemic) and nausea (caused by the sweet taste).

The effectiveness of lactulose may be reduced if it is used concomitantly with an antibiotic that destroys the normal colonic bacteria. A nonabsorbed antibiotic such as neomycin destroys enough luminal colonic bacteria to interfere with lactulose. Most systemic, highly absorbable antibiotics do not affect the colonic bacteria in the lumen.

The adult dosage is 1 to 2 tablespoons (15 to 30 mL) daily after breakfast, which is increased in 5- and 10-mL increments to 60 mL daily after breakfast.

polyethylene glycol (PEG) and electrolytes (GoLYTELY)

This powder consists of a mixture of polyethylene glycol (nonabsorbable osmotic substance) with sodium salts (sulfate, bicarbonate, and chloride) and potassium chloride; this mixture is isotonic with body fluids. Because it is isotonic, fluids and electrolytes are neither absorbed nor secreted in the GI tract; thus it can be used in clients who are dehydrated or have renal impairment or cardiac disease. The drug acts as an osmotic agent.

GoLYTELY is used for bowel cleansing before colonoscopy and before the administration of a barium enema for radiologic examination. There is a low incidence of nausea, vomiting, bloating, cramps, and abdominal fullness with GoLYTELY.

Nursing Management

Laxative Therapy

■ **Assessment.** Determine the client's bowel status by careful assessment. The occurrence of the last bowel movement, the quality of bowel sounds, defecation habits, dietary patterns, fluid intake, level of daily activity, and the use of laxatives are important components of the nurse's assessment (Wilson, 1999). Ensure that the client does not have intestinal obstruction, paralytic ileus, perforated bowel, or toxic bowel; laxatives are contraindicated for these conditions. Review the client's medical history for causative factors. Assess the client's current medication regimen for drugs that might contribute to the constipation or produce significant drug interactions. These include the following:

- High-fiber and bulk-forming laxatives may decrease the effects of tetracycline, anticoagulants, digitalis glycosides, or salicylates by binding with the drug or delaying its absorption. Separate the administration of these substances by at least 2 hours.
- Saline or osmotic laxatives that contain calcium may interact with the same drugs as the magnesium-containing antacids. Calcium or magnesium salts may interact with tetracycline, forming a nonabsorbable complex when administered within 1 to 2 hours of tetracycline. The diarrhea produced by these drugs may interfere with absorption.
- Stimulant/contact/irritant laxatives such as bisacodyl oral tablets, which contain an enteric coating, will be prematurely released in the stomach when administered with antacids or proton pump inhibitors, producing severe cramping in the stomach and duodenum.
- Lubricant/emollient laxatives such as mineral oil may interfere with the absorption of antibiotics, anticoagulants, oral contraceptives, digitalis glycosides, and fat-soluble vitamins when concurrently administered; this reduces their therapeutic effectiveness.
- Mineral oil is not recommended for children under the age of 6 years or for bedridden older adults because they are more at risk for aspirating the droplets coating the pharynx; this may result in lipid pneumonia. Do not give mineral oil routinely to pregnant women; it decreases vitamin K availability to the fetus, resulting in hypoprothrombinemia and hemorrhagic disease. The chronic use of mineral oil in any client may decrease vitamin K absorption and lead to an increased potential for bleeding. In addition, clients may experience anal leakage of the oil with long-term use.
- Stool softener/surfactant or wetting agent laxatives may increase the absorption of mineral oil if administered together. Granuloma formation or tumor-like deposits in tissues are also reported.
- The use of lactulose during pregnancy has not been evaluated. Lactulose use in clients with diabetes may cause elevations in blood glucose levels; therefore another type of laxative without galactose or lactose may be better. Older adults and debilitated clients receiving lactulose for 6 months or more should undergo periodic evaluations of serum electrolytes (potassium, chloride, and carbon dioxide). Lactulose contains galactose (less than 2.2 g/15 mL) and is therefore contraindicated in low-galactose diets.
- Other oral medications given within an hour of administration of a PEG-electrolyte solution may be expelled from the GI tract without absorption.
- Do not use laxatives when an emergency surgical condition in the abdomen might be suspected, such as appendicitis, bowel obstruction, hemorrhage, or intussusception.

■ **Nursing Diagnosis.** Clients receiving laxatives are at risk for the following nursing diagnoses/collaborative problems: constipation related to ineffectiveness of the laxative or to intestinal obstruction (bulk laxatives); diarrhea related to the misuse of laxatives; impaired comfort (abdominal cramping, flatulence, nausea); and the potential complications of allergic reaction or electrolyte imbalance (weakness, muscle cramping, confusion).

■ **Implementation**

■ ***Monitoring.*** Observe the client's stools for frequency, consistency, and color. Determine the client's comfort during defecation.

■ ***Intervention.*** Encourage nonpharmacologic interventions to relieve constipation. Depending on the client's health assessment, measures to relieve constipation include adding fresh fruits, vegetables, and whole grains to increase bulk to the diet; allowing for a calm, adequate, and routine time for defecation; ensuring a daily fluid intake of eight to ten glasses of water for adequate hydration; and increasing the amount of daily exercise. When laxatives are indicated, use the mildest laxative necessary.

■ *Lactulose.* Mix lactulose in water, juice, or milk to make it more palatable. Results may occur 24 to 36 hours after administration. The solution may darken on exposure to high temperature, but this does not change its therapeutic effect. Freezing does not alter the therapeutic effect.

■ *GoLYTELY.* GoLYTELY is given orally, 4 L at a rate of 240 mL every 10 minutes (rapidly swallowed). Fasting 3 to 4 hours before use is necessary. In general, a midmorning examination permits 3 hours for consumption followed by a 1-hour period for bowel movement. Less stool is retained after its use, but the water or electrolyte balance does not change. Only clear liquids are permitted after its administration and before examination.

After reconstitution of the powder, refrigerating the solution improves palatability. The reconstituted solution must be used within 48 hours.

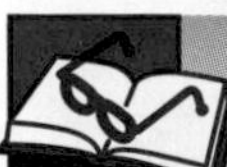

Case Study *Drug Therapy for Bowel Elimination*

Margaret Gordon, a 73-year-old widow, is recovering at home from an internal fixation of a fractured left hip. Mrs. Gordon is recovering well from the surgery. She continues with physical therapy, but she does not go out much and spends most of the day sitting in a chair watching television. Her primary meal of the day is delivered to her home by a voluntary agency. The remainder of her food intake includes snack foods and occasionally soup and crackers.

Mrs. Gordon takes the following medications:

- Colace, 100 mg PO at bedtime as needed
- Milk of Magnesia, 1 tablespoon at bedtime as needed
- Metamucil, 2 teaspoons daily
- Kaopectate, 2 tablespoons after each loose stool

A review of the client's history by the community health nurse reveals that Mrs. Gordon takes the Colace daily. When questioned, she reports that this is the same way it was given to her in the hospital. Her physician routinely orders Colace for all clients who have orthopedic surgery. If she goes more than one day without a bowel movement, she takes the Milk of Magnesia. She has been taking Metamucil daily for several years. She began using the Metamucil again when she returned home from the hospital. Several weeks later she developed diarrhea. She began taking the Kaopectate without consulting her physician.

Mrs. Gordon readily admits that she believes "normal" bowel habits are essential to her health. She believes that one well-formed stool daily is her normal pattern. She believes that any deviation from this pattern is diarrhea or constipation; she promptly treats the problem with any or all of the above medications, which she purchases over-the-counter. The physician's office renews the prescription for Colace at her request.

1. What factors during Mrs. Gordon's postoperative recovery may have contributed to the present situation?
2. What effect does each medication have on Mrs. Gordon's bowel elimination?

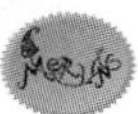

For answer guidelines, go to mosby.com/MERLIN/McKenry/.

■ *Castor Oil.* Castor oil may be unpleasant and nauseating. This effect may be overcome by disguising the taste of the oil. To do this, emulsify it in a blender or mix it with cold orange juice or other fruit juices, and have the client drink the mixture immediately. Neoloid is a preemulsified preparation. Castor oil is contraindicated in pregnancy. Its administration often results in engorgement of the pelvic area, which may reflexively stimulate the gravid uterus.

■ *Bulk-Forming Laxative (Metamucil and Others).* Because there is a possibility of impaction or obstruction if fluid intake is not substantial, avoid the use of bulk-forming laxatives in clients with stenosis, adhesions, or dysphagia. Administer these laxatives with a full glass of liquid (240 mL) plus additional liquid every day to prevent intestinal impaction. Some preparations contain sugar and sodium and may not be used with clients for whom these substances are restricted.

■ ***Education.*** Instruct clients on measures to prevent constipation appropriate to the lifestyle information obtained in your assessment.

Encourage clients to avoid the habitual use of laxatives. Inform them that misuse or overuse may result in a dependence on laxatives for routine bowel function. Instruct clients not to take laxatives unnecessarily. For example, some individuals believe that laxatives are to be taken to "clean out" the system, as a tonic, in the case of colds, or at the change of seasons (see the Case Study box above).

■ *Bisacodyl (Dulcolax).* Because bisacodyl tablets are enteric coated, instruct clients not to chew them or ingest them when they are chipped. Instruct clients to swallow bisacodyl tablets whole no sooner than 1 hour before or after the ingestion of dairy products or antacids. (Milk or antacids can break down the enteric coating, which can lead to gastric irritation, cramping, and vomiting.) See Chapter 11 for additional information on bisacodyl.

■ *Calcium Polycarbophil (Mitrolan).* Instruct the client with constipation to follow each dose of calcium polycarbophil with at least 8 ounces of water or other liquid. If this drug is being used to treat diarrhea, administer less fluid with each dose. Instruct the client to chew polycarbophil tablets thoroughly before swallowing.

Caution clients to forbid children free access to laxative preparations that are in a candylike form, chewing gum, or mint. Children are likely to regard these substances as ordinary candy or gum and take an overdose of the drug. Deaths have been reported from such accidents.

■ **Evaluation.** The expected outcome of laxative therapy is that the client reports bowel movements of soft stool without straining or pain. If the drug was administered for bowel cleansing before a colonoscopy or barium enema, there will be an absence of stool in the colon.

ANTIDIARRHEALS

This section focuses on the prescription drugs that have a direct pharmacologic effect on the GI tract. Although many antidiarrheal preparations may be purchased over-the-counter (as discussed in Chapter 11), the nurse may administer these same preparations within a health agency setting.

■ Nursing Management

Antidiarrheal Therapy

■ **Assessment.** The objectives of treatment of the client with diarrhea are to replenish fluid and electrolyte loss;

Nursing Care Plan
Selected Nursing Diagnoses/Potential Complications: Antidiarrheal Medication Administration

Nursing Diagnosis	Outcome Criteria	Nursing Interventions
Diarrhea	Decrease in number of stools to less than three per day Formed stools	Record the frequency, number, and consistency of stools. Encourage a bland diet and liquids. Administer antidiarrheal agents as prescribed.
Risk for impaired comfort related to abdominal cramping and diarrhea	The client will: Verbalize comfort or pain relief Maintain activities of daily living without disruption because of discomfort	Assess the comfort status of the client. Instruct the client in an appropriate diet to minimize intestinal cramping. Provide suggestions for nondrug pain management (positioning, activities, distraction). Administer antidiarrheal medications as prescribed. Consult prescriber if additional pain relief is needed.
Potential complications: hypovolemia and electrolyte imbalance	The client will: Maintain electrolytes within normal limits Maintain normal fluid balance Experience less diarrhea Maintain a normal body weight	Monitor client's intake and output. Monitor bowel movements, recording diarrhea as output. Weigh client daily. Administer antidiarrheal agents as prescribed. Assess the client for signs of dehydration and hypokalemia. Encourage a high fluid intake. Monitor serum electrolyte determinations.

ascertain, if possible, the cause or causes of diarrhea; and treat the underlying cause or causes. Reducing the frequency of evacuation may be contraindicated if the diarrhea is infectious and self-limiting. It is important to determine the cause of the diarrhea through careful evaluation of the individual client. Evaluative questions for discovering the cause or causes may be used in assessing the following criteria:

- Age of the client
- Occupation
- Duration of diarrhea (precipitating factors tantamount to onset)
- Stool description (frequency of evacuation, rectal bleeding or black stool appearance, foul odor, light color, or greasy consistency)
- Medication profile (prescribed and self-administered OTC drugs)
- Presence or absence of anorexia, weight reduction (involuntary), fever, abdominal tenderness, dehydration
- Ingestion of foods, toxic substances, milk, alcohol
- Travel outside the United States or Canada
- Symptom description (location)
- Relief obtained, if any, and treatment modality
- Chronic diseases, the presence of acute or concurrent illness, emotional or behavioral problems

■ **Nursing Diagnosis.** The client undergoing antidiarrheal therapy is at risk for the following nursing diagnoses/collaborative problems: diarrhea related to the underlying cause and ineffectiveness of the antidiarrheal agent; impaired comfort related to abdominal cramping; and the potential complications of hypovolemia and electrolyte imbalances.

■ **Implementation**

■ ***Monitoring.*** Fluid and electrolyte loss may cause tachycardia, postural hypotension, elevated hematocrit or blood urea nitrogen, and poor skin turgor. The stool specimen may reveal occult blood (GI bleeding), fecal leukocytes, parasites, or fat.

■ ***Intervention.*** Nonspecific measures are directed at treating stool frequency, which burdens daily lifestyle; alleviating abdominal cramps; preventing dehydration and metabolic acidosis from fluid and electrolyte loss; and minimizing weight loss and nutritional deficits resulting from malabsorption. Specific treatment is directed at the cause or condition creating the diarrhea, as demonstrated by the Nursing Care Plan above.

Hospitalization is needed for dehydration that would compromise a client with congestive heart failure or chronic renal disease; these conditions complicate fluid replacement efforts. If a child or infant is unable to consume oral replacement fluids, hospitalization is needed to replace fluids and maintain urine flow. Bed rest alone may reduce stool frequency. Children, infants, older adults with a poor medical history, clients with chronic illness (heart disease, asthma), and pregnant women are at risk from acute or chronic diarrhea.

Maintaining fluid and electrolyte balance is the most important goal of supportive therapy in acute diarrhea. If left untreated, a loss of anions (bicarbonate, organic anions as short-chain fatty acids) will create a gain of hydrogen ions, resulting in metabolic acidosis. This gain will be exacerbated by the (often) concomitant ketoacidosis of starvation and the acidosis of prerenal azotemia. As volume increases in diarrhea, a rise in sodium and chloride develops with a decrease in potassium concentration. The decreased contact time of the luminal contents with the mucosal surface decreases the passive secretion of potassium. The electrolyte composition of stool water is then close to that of plasma. The electrolyte loss of sodium, potassium, chloride, and bicarbonate is the basis of therapy.

It is recommended that clear liquids (noncarbonated soft drinks, fruit juice, diluted and flavored gelatin, and apple juice) and a bland diet be continued for 1 to 2 days. According to the cause of the diarrhea, several different medications can be given along with bed rest. Such medications include activated charcoal, absorbents, anticholinergic drugs, and many other drug products.

OTC antidiarrheals may contain the following ingredients: limited amounts of opiates; adsorbents such as bismuth salts, aluminum salts, attapulgite, kaolin, pectin, activated charcoal, and belladonna alkaloids (hyoscyamine, hyoscine, scopolamine, atropine); and calcium salts. Inactive ingredients vary, but the nurse should be aware of the variation in alcohol content (1.5% to 18%).

Antidiarrheal products have a warning stating that they are not to be used for longer than 2 days, not to be used if a fever is present, and not to be used in infants or children under 3 years of age. The prescriber may modify these instructions.

Intractable diarrhea of infancy is traditionally treated with clear liquids and a gradual reintroduction of milk or formula, with the addition of oral elemental diets or total parenteral nutrition. The infant syndrome is described as loose stools that result in dehydration and a failure to thrive. Because a newborn's total body weight is usually 75% water, a 10% or greater weight loss may occur with severe diarrhea. If an infant has eight to ten bowel movements in a 24-hour period, the fluid loss may cause circulatory collapse and renal impairment. Diarrhea in infants should be considered serious enough to warrant referring the client to a prescriber for evaluation.

Persistent diarrhea in older adults can result in fluid and electrolyte loss, dehydration, and perhaps more serious medical complications. Such clients should be referred to a prescriber.

■ ***Education.*** Explain the effects of diarrhea on hydration and electrolytes. Instruct the client on interventions to prevent future episodes.

■ **Evaluation.** The expected outcome of antidiarrheal drug therapy is that the client will experience a decrease in the number, frequency, and fluidity of stools.

Prescription Antidiarrheal Agents

Opioids

The opioids (codeine and paregoric—DEA Class III) act by virtue of their constipating and sedative action. They lower the propulsive motility of the bowel, reduce pain, and relieve tenesmus (rectal spasms). The delay in transit time of food permits intestinal contact time with the absorptive surface of the bowel; this increases the reabsorption of water and electrolytes and reduces stool frequency and net volume.

The anticholinergics and opium derivatives decrease bowel motility. They should not be used when the cause of diarrhea is an invading organism (e.g., toxigenic bacteria or pseudomembranous enterocolitis), because these drugs decrease intestinal motility and subsequently lower the excretion of the organisms and their toxins, resulting in epithelial penetration and multiplication of the organisms.

Codeine and paregoric cause depression and sedation. Because of the additive effects, this factor must be considered if the client is taking other CNS depressant drugs. The opiates are short acting; frequent administration (4 to 6 hour intervals) is needed to control the function of smooth muscle in the GI tract. The opiates are discussed in greater detail in Chapter 14.

opium tincture, deodorized

Tincture of opium, a hydroalcoholic (19% alcohol) solution, contains 10% opium. The average dosage is 0.6 mL four times daily. This substance is a class II prescription under the Controlled Substances Act.

paregoric

Paregoric (camphorated opium tincture, although camphor is no longer required in this formulation in the United States) requires a prescription. It is a class III drug that is equivalent to 2 mg of morphine/5 mL. It is important that the nurse not confuse deodorized opium tincture (10 mg morphine equivalent/1 mL), and camphorated opium tincture (0.4 mg morphine equivalent/1 mL); deodorized opium tincture has 25 times more morphine equivalent than camphorated opium tincture. Addiction liability has been reported with these preparations. Paregoric becomes a class V product when combined with another drug if the combination contains no more than 100 mg of opium or 25 mL of paregoric/100 mL of the mixture.

The adult antidiarrheal dosage is 5 to 10 mL one to four times daily. The pediatric dosage is 0.25 to 0.5 mL/kg one to four times daily.

Synthetic Opioids

The synthetic opioids used to treat diarrhea include diphenoxylate and difenoxin.

diphenoxylate and atropine [dye fen ox′ i late] (Lomotil)

Diphenoxylate, a controlled substance in the United States (class V), inhibits intestinal propulsive motility by acting directly on intestinal smooth muscles to decrease transit time. It is indicated as an adjunct to fluid and electrolyte replacement for the treatment of acute and chronic diarrhea in adults. It is not recommended for use in children.

The onset of action for diphenoxylate is between 45 to 60 minutes; the half-life is 2.5 hours, and the duration of action is 3 to 4 hours. It is metabolized in the liver and excreted primarily by the kidneys.

The side effects of diphenoxylate include drowsiness, dizziness, tachycardia, dry mouth, hyperthermia, abdominal distress, rash, and agitation.

For adults and children 12 years of age and older, the dosage is 1 to 2 tablets PO three or four times daily.

▪ Nursing Management

Diphenoxylate Therapy

▪ **Assessment.** The client's health status should be assessed for conditions for which diphenoxylate therapy would be contraindicated or would indicate risk. For example, it should not be used with clients with pseudomembranous colitis (*Clostridium difficile* toxin) secondary to broad-spectrum antibiotic therapy; in this case, slowing peristalsis would inhibit the evacuation of toxins from the bowel and thereby worsen the client's diarrhea. The risk associated with the use of diphenoxylate for dehydration, particularly in children, requires caution because it may predispose the client to delayed diphenoxylate intoxication. Antidiarrheal agents (e.g., diphenoxylate, loperamide, or narcotics) should be carefully considered in instances of acute diarrhea or traveler's diarrhea caused by bacteria (enterotoxin-producing strains of *E. coli*, *Campylobacter jejuni*, *Salmonella*, or *Shigella*), parasites (*Giardia lamblia*), and viruses (parvovirus or rotavirus); these organisms penetrate the intestinal wall if retained in the intestine and therefore must be eliminated in the feces. The cautious use of antidiarrheals is also true of diarrhea that is caused by poisoning until the toxic materials have been eliminated from the GI tract.

Diphenoxylate may precipitate a hepatic coma in clients with impaired hepatic function. Children and older adults are more susceptible to the respiratory depressant effects of diphenoxylate. Toxic megacolon may develop as the result of inhibition of intestinal motility in clients with acute ulcerative colitis. The client's current drug regimen should be reviewed for significant drug interactions, which include the following:

- The CNS depressant effects are potentiated by alcohol and other CNS depressant drugs.
- Concurrent use with monoamine oxidase (MAO) inhibitors may precipitate a hypertensive crisis because of the chemical similarity to meperidine.
- Additive effects are seen with drugs that have anticholinergic/antimuscarinic effects because of the atropine present.
- The administration of naltrexone will block the therapeutic effects of diphenoxylate and will precipitate withdrawal symptoms if the client is physically dependent on diphenoxylate.

A baseline assessment of the client's bowel disorder should be obtained and should include GI status and the frequency of diarrhea.

▪ **Nursing Diagnosis.** The client undergoing diphenoxylate therapy is at risk for the following nursing diagnoses/collaborative problems: diarrhea related to ineffectiveness of the drug regimen; constipation related to the side effects; ineffective breathing pattern related to the effect of the drug on respiratory depression; disturbed thought processes related to the CNS effects of drug (confusion); urinary retention related to the anticholinergic effects of the drug; impaired comfort (blurred vision, dry mouth, flushing of skin, dizziness) related to the anticholinergic effects of the drug; and the potential complications of paralytic ileus (nausea, vomiting, constipation, severe abdominal pain), mental depression, or withdrawal symptoms.

▪ **Implementation**

▪ ***Monitoring.*** Monitor hepatic function in the client receiving long-term therapy. Dehydration in clients may cause variability in the response to diphenoxylate. Clients can have a delayed toxic response; observe for bloating, constipation, abdominal pain, and diminished bowel sounds indicative of paralytic ileus or toxic megacolon. Discontinue the drug if abdominal distention occurs. Electrolytes must be monitored and dehydration corrected in hospitalized clients. If the client is not hospitalized, fluid intake should be increased to prevent dehydration. Until diarrhea is controlled, weigh the client daily to monitor fluid loss. Monitor the client's intake and output.

The frequency and character of stools should be carefully monitored to observe for constipation (a potential side effect) or to see if diarrhea is diminishing, which indicates the efficacy of therapy.

▪ ***Intervention.*** Modify the client's diet to support hydration and help control diarrhea. Provide good skin care to the perianal area.

▪ ***Education.*** Caution clients about taking alcohol and CNS depressants with diphenoxylate. Instruct about its habit-forming potential. Because dizziness and drowsiness are common side effects, caution the client regarding tasks that involve alertness. Refer the client to the prescriber if diarrhea increases or fever develops.

▪ **Evaluation.** The expected outcome of diphenoxylate therapy is that the client will experience a decrease in or an absence of diarrhea without experiencing side effects/adverse reactions to the drug.

difenoxin [dye fen ox' in] (Motofen)

A second product in the synthetic opioid category is difenoxin with atropine (Motofen). Difenoxin is the active metabolite derived from diphenoxylate; therefore it is effective at one-fifth the dose of diphenoxylate. It is indicated for the treatment of acute nonspecific diarrhea and acute exacerbations of chronic diarrhea.

Peak serum levels of difenoxin are reached between 40 and 60 minutes. It is metabolized in the liver and excreted primarily by the kidneys and in the feces.

The adult oral dosage is 2 tablets initially, then 1 tablet after each loose stool or 1 tablet every 3 to 4 hours as needed. The maximum daily dose is 8 tablets.

The nursing management of difenoxin is the same as for diphenoxylate.

Complementary and Alternative Therapies
Peppermint Oil

Peppermint oil is a common flavoring agent in foods and beverages. When taken orally, peppermint oil is used for nausea and vomiting, colds, cough, inflammation of the mouth and pharynx, liver and gallbladder complaints, dyspepsia, and as an antiflatulent. Topically, peppermint oil is used for headache, neuralgias, toothaches, mucosal inflammation, and pruritus. When used for relief of irritable bowel syndrome (IBS), it is considered to be possibly effective. There is some evidence (Pittler & Ernest, 1998) that peppermint oil can reduce abdominal pain, distention, flatulence, and bowel movements in clients with IBS. Although there may be some burning and ulceration of the mouth in clients with contact sensitivity, enteric-coated capsules may reduce the incidence of these symptoms and heartburn. The usual dose of peppermint oil for irritable bowel syndrome is 0.2 to 0.4 mL three times daily in enteric-coated capsules.

Information from Pittler, M.H., Ernst, T. (1998). Peppermint for irritable bowel syndrome: A critical review and meta analysis. *American Journal of Gastroenterology* 93(7):1131-1135.

Adsorbents

Adsorbents are substances that take up or attach to (adsorb) another substance. They act by coating the wall of the GI tract, absorbing the bacteria or toxins causing the diarrhea, and passing them out with the stools. Examples of drugs in this class that require a prescription are the anion-exchange resins colestipol and cholestyramine.

cholestyramine [koe less tir′ a meen] (Questran)

Cholestyramine has a direct adsorbent affinity for acidic materials (e.g., bile acids). It is indicated as an adjunct therapy to diet in the treatment of hypercholesterolemia. Although not an FDA-approved indication, cholestyramine has also been used to treat diarrhea. (See Chapter 32 for the nursing management of cholestyramine.)

SUMMARY

Drugs and agents that affect the mouth are usually used for the provision of good oral hygiene. Dentifrices are helpful as mechanical aids for brushing teeth. Clotrimazole and nystatin are specific agents for the treatment of oral candidiasis.

Drugs that affect the stomach are classified as antacids, antiflatulents, digestants, antiemetics, emetics, and those used in the treatment of peptic ulcer. Antacids are used to neutralize hydrochloric acid in the stomach and may be composed of aluminum salts, calcium carbonate, magnesium salts, or sodium bicarbonate (alone or in combination). Digestants are administered to promote the process of digestion when there is a deficiency of some substance essential to that process. Antiemetics are given for the relief of nausea and vomiting; it is essential to determine the cause of the gastric distress, because these drugs may mask the symptoms of more serious illnesses. Emetics are administered to induce vomiting, usually as a part of drug overdoses or poisonings. Drugs used in the treatment of peptic ulcer are cytoprotective agents, which act locally to promote healing; H_2 receptor antagonists, which prevent histamine from stimulating the H_2 receptor; and proton pump inhibitors, which block acid production and so increase the pH of the stomach.

Chenodiol and ursodiol, which affect the gallbladder, are administered to dissolve radiolucent cholesterol gallstones in clients who may be surgical risks because of preexisting conditions.

Miscellaneous agents, such as mesalamine, olsalazine, sulfasalazine, and infliximab, are used for the treatment of Crohn's disease and other inflammatory bowel diseases.

Drugs affecting the lower GI tract are either laxatives or antidiarrheal agents. Laxatives are given to relieve or prevent constipation, to expel parasites or poisonous substances, to obtain a specimen, or to cleanse the bowel for diagnostic examination. They are usually classified by their mechanism of action: saline, stimulant, bulk-forming, emollient, lubricant laxatives, or bowel evacuants. The goal is to return the client to a normal, adequate bowel pattern.

Antidiarrheals are administered to reduce the frequency of evacuations. This is only part of a treatment plan that should also include replenishment of fluid and electrolyte loss, diagnosis and treatment of the underlying cause, and restoration of the intestinal flora. Again, the goal of treatment is to return the client to a normal, adequate bowel pattern.

Critical Thinking Questions

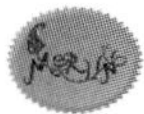

1. Given the efficacy of the products, why is advertising money spent for mouthwashes and gargles?
2. Why is it important to establish the underlying cause of vomiting before administering any antiemetic?
3. How would you use ipecac syrup for a 2-year-old who has ingested half a bottle of baby aspirin?
4. What lifestyle teaching would be important in supporting H_2 receptor antagonist therapy?
5. What would be the laxative of choice for Mr. Preston, a 56-year-old client, 3 days after his myocardial infarction? For Jimmy Tyrone, 7 years old, whose last bowel movement was 4 days ago? For Mrs. White, a 42-year-old client being prepared for a colonoscopy? Why would it be the drug of choice, and what disadvantages are involved in its use?
6. Alice Reagan, a 27-year-old teacher, has just returned from a week's vacation in Mexico with severe diarrhea of 3 days' duration. What criteria should be considered in the selection of an antidiarrheal agent?

Collaborative Learning Activities

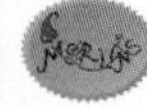

For Collaborative Learning Activities, go to mosby.com/MERLIN/McKenry/.

CASE STUDY

For a Case Study that will help ensure mastery of this chapter content, go to mosby.com/MERLIN/McKenry/.

BIBLIOGRAPHY

Abramowicz, M. (1994). Drugs for treatment of peptic ulcers. *Medical Letter, 36*(927), 65-67.

Abramowicz, M. (1999). Rabeprazole. *Medical Letter, 41*(1066), 110-112.

American Hospital Formulary Service. (1999). *AHFS drug information '99*. Bethesda, MD: American Society of Pharmacists.

Anderson, K.N., Anderson, L.E., & Glanze, W.D. (Eds.).(1998). *Mosby's medical, nursing, & allied health dictionary* (5th ed.). St. Louis: Mosby.

Bardhan K.D., Crowe J., Thompson R.P., Trewby P.N., Keeling P.N., Weir D., Crouch S.L. (1999). Lansoprazole is superior to ranitidine as maintenance treatment for the prevention of duodenal ulcer relapse. *Alimentary Pharmacologic Therapy, 13*(6), 827-832.

Brunton, L.L. (1996). Agents affecting gastrointestinal water flux and motility; emesis and antiemetics; bile acids and pancreatic enzymes. In J.G. Hardman & L.E Limbird (Eds.), *Goodman & Gilman's The pharmacological basis of therapeutics* (9th ed.). New York: McGraw-Hill.

Buzzelli, G., Moscarella, S., Giusti, A., Duchini, A., Marena, C., & Lampertico, M. (1993). A pilot study on the liver protective effect of silybin-phosphatidylchlorine complex [IdB 1016] in chronic active hepatitis. *International Journal of Clinical Pharmacology, Therapy & Toxicology, 31*(9), 450-460.

Carpenito, L.J. (1989-90). *Nursing diagnosis: Application to clinical practice.* (3rd ed.). Philadelphia: J.B. Lippincott.

Carpenito, L.J. (2000). *Nursing diagnosis: Application to clinical practice* (8th ed.). Philadelphia: J.B. Lippincott.

Chenodiol (2000). MD Consult—Drug text; home.mdconsult.com/das/drug/body/12878930/1/712.html (4/16/00).

Coppes, M.J. et al. (1999). Safety, tolerability, antiemetic efficacy, and pharmacokinetics of oral dolasetron mesylate in pediatric patients receiving moderately to highly emetogenic chemotherapy. *Journal of Pediatric Hematology & Oncology, 21*(4), 274-283.

Covington, T.R. (Ed.). (1996). *Handbook of nonprescription drugs: Product updates* (11th ed.). Washington D.C.: The American Pharmaceutical Association.

Domino. K.B., Anderson, E.A., Polissar, N.L., & Posner, K.L. (1999). Comparative efficacy and safety of ondansetron, droperidol, and metoclopramide for preventing postoperative nausea and vomiting: A meta-analysis. *Anesthesia Analogue, 88*(6), 1370-1379.

Drug Facts and Comparisons. (2000). St. Louis: Facts and Comparisons.

Fedotin, M.S. (1993). *Helicobacter pylori*-associated ulcer disease: Current treatment options. *Hospital Formulary, 28*(7), 632-634, 636, 639-640.

Flynn, A.A. (1996). Oral health products. In T.R. Covington (Ed.). *Handbook of nonprescription drugs* (11th ed.). Washington, D.C.: American Pharmaceutical Association.

Graham, D.Y. (1993). Treatment of peptic ulcers caused by *Helicobacter pylori. New England Journal of Medicine, 328*(5), 349-350.

Hall, G.R. et al. (1995). Managing constipation using a research-based protocol. *MedSurg Nursing, 44*(1), 11-20.

Humphries, T.J. & Merritt, G.J. (1999). Review article: Drug interactions with agents used to treat acid-related diseases. *Alimentary Pharmacologic Therapy, 13*(suppl 13), 18-26.

Katzung, B.G. (1992). *Basic and clinical pharmacology* (5th ed.). Norwalk, CT: Appleton & Lange.

Koch, K.L. (1999). Diabetic gastropathy. Gastric neuromuscular dysfunction in diabetes mellitus: A review of symptoms, pathophysiology, and treatment. *Digestive Disease Science, 44*(6), 1061-1075.

Koda-Kimble, M.A. & Young, L.Y. (1995). Nausea and vomiting. In L.Y. Young & M.A. Koda-Kimble (Eds.), *Applied therapeutics: The clinical use of drugs* (6th ed.). Vancouver, WA: Applied Therapeutics.

Kromer, W., Horbach, S., & Luhmann, R. (1999). Relative efficacies of gastric proton pump inhibitors: Their clinical and pharmacological basis. *Pharmacology, 59*(2), 57-77.

LaCorte, R., Caselli, M., Castellino, G., Bajocchi, G., & Trotta, F. (1999). Prophylaxis and treatment of NSAID-induced gastroduodenal disorders. *Drug Safety, 20*(6), 527-543.

Laheij, R.J., Rossum, L.G., Jansen, J.B., Straatman, H., & Verbeek, A.L. (1999). Evaluation of treatment regimens to cure *Helicobacter pylori* infection: A meta-analysis. *Alimentary Pharmacologic Therapy, 13*(7), 857-864.

Lichter, I. (1993). Forum: Which antiemetic? *Journal of Palliative Care, 9*(1), 42.

Marcus, R. (1996). Agents affecting calcification and bone turnover. In L.Y. Young, & M.A. Koda-Kimble (Eds.), *Applied therapeutics: The clinical use of drugs* (6th ed.). Vancouver, WA: Applied Therapeutics.

Marchioro, G., et al. (2000). Hypnosis in the treatment of anticipatory nausea and vomiting in patients receiving cancer chemotherapy, *Oncology 59*(2):100-104.

Mayer, D.J. (2000). Acupuncture: An evidence-based review of the clinical literature, *Annual Review of Medicine 51*:49-63.

McCusker, C. (1998). Monoclonal antibody approved for the treatment of Crohn's disease. *Pharmacy Today, 4*(10), 1, 7.

Mera, R., Realpe, J.L., Bravo, L.E., DeLany, J.P., & Correa, P. (1999). Eradication of *Helicobacter pylori* infection with proton pump-based triple therapy in patients in whom bismuth-based therapy failed. *Journal of Clinical Gastroenterology, 29*(1), 51-55.

Pares A., Planas R., Torres M., Caballeria J., Viver J.M., Acero D., Panes J., Rigau J., Santos J., Rodes J. (1998). Effects of silymarin in alcoholic cirrhosis of the liver: Results of a controlled, double-blind, randomized, and multicenter trial. *Journal of Hepatology, 28*(1), 615-621.

Pittler, M.H., Ernst, T. (1998). Peppermint for irritable bowel syndrome: A critical review and meta analysis. *American Journal of Gastroenterology 93*(7):1131-1135.

Plezia, P.M. et al. (1990). Randomized crossover comparison of high-dose intravenous metoclopramide versus a five-drug antiemetic regimen. *Journal of Pain Symptom Management, 5*(2), 101.

Raskin, J.B. (1999). Gastrointestinal effects of nonsteroidal anti-inflammatory therapy. *American Journal of Medicine, 106*(5B), 3S-12S.

Ruskosky, D.R. (1996). Alcohol and alcohol substitutes: An overview. *Florida Pharmacy Today, 60*(3), 22, 25.

Scheepers, H.C., van Erp, E.J., & van den Bergh, A.S. (1999). Use of misoprostol in first and second trimester abortion: A review. *Obstetrics & Gynecology Survey, 54*(9), 592-600.

Smith, C. (1995). Upper gastrointestinal disorders. In L.Y. Young & M.A. Koda-Kimble (Eds.), *Applied therapeutics: The clinical use of drugs* (6th ed.). Vancouver, WA: Applied Therapeutics.

Surbeck, D.V., Fehr, P.M., Hosli, I., & Holzgreve, W. (1999). Oral misoprostol for third stage of labor: A randomized placebo-controlled trial. *Obstetrics & Gynecology Survey, 54*(2), 255-258.

United States Pharmacopeia Dispensing Information (USP DI): Drug information for the health care professional (19th ed.). (1999). Rockville, MD: United States Pharmacopeial Convention.

Wilson, J.A. (1999). Constipation in the elderly. *Clinical Geriatric Medicine, 15*(3), 499-510.

42 Overview of the Eye

Chapter Focus

Approximately 70% of all sensory information is perceived through the eyes. Visual impairment, which often accompanies ophthalmic disorders, affects the client's ability to function independently and diminishes his or her perception of the environment. Disorders of the eye are becoming increasingly common as the population ages. To appropriately assess and care for clients with ophthalmic problems, the nurse needs to have a thorough understanding of the anatomy and physiology of the eye.

Learning Objectives

1. Describe the anatomy and physiology of the eye.
2. Identify the muscles involved with miosis and mydriasis, and explain their functions.
3. Define accommodation and cycloplegia.
4. Name four protective mechanisms associated with the eye.

Key Terms

accommodation, p. 788
cataract, p. 788
cornea, p. 788
cycloplegia, p. 789
miosis, p. 788
mydriasis, p. 788

The eye is the receptor organ for one of the most delicate and valuable senses—vision. Figure 42-1 shows the parts of the eye. The eyeball has three layers or coats: the protective external layer (cornea and sclera), the middle layer (which contains the choroid, iris, and ciliary body), and the light-sensitive retina.

The eyeball is protected in a deep depression of the skull called the orbit. It is moved in the orbit by six small extraocular muscles.

The anterior covering of the eye is the **cornea.** The cornea is normally transparent and allows light to enter the eye. It has no blood vessels and receives its nutrition from the aqueous humor and its oxygen supply by diffusion from the air and surrounding structures. The corneal surface consists of a thin layer of epithelial cells that are quite resistant to infection. An abraded cornea, however, is very susceptible to infection. The cornea is also supplied with 60 to 80 sensory fibers that elicit pain whenever the corneal epithelium is damaged. Seriously injured corneal tissue is replaced by scar tissue, which is usually not transparent. Increased intraocular pressure also results in a loss of transparency.

The sclera, which is continuous with the cornea, is nontransparent; it is the white fibrous envelope of the eye. The conjunctiva is the mucous membrane that lines the anterior part of the sclera and the inner surfaces of each eyelid.

The iris gives the eye its brown, blue, gray, green, or hazel color. It surrounds the pupil; the size of the pupil is altered by the sphincter and dilator muscles in the iris. The sphincter muscle, which encircles the pupil, is parasympathetically innervated; the dilator muscle, which runs radially from the pupil to the periphery of the iris, is sympathetically innervated. Contraction of the sphincter muscle, either alone or with relaxation of the dilator muscle, causes constriction of the pupil, or **miosis.** Contraction of the dilator muscle and relaxation of the sphincter muscle causes dilation of the pupil, or **mydriasis** (Figure 42-2). Drugs producing miosis (miotics) act by (1) interfering with cholinesterase activity or (2) acting like acetylcholine at receptor sites in the sphincter muscle. Drugs producing mydriasis (mydriatics) act by (1) interfering with the action of acetylcholine or (2) stimulating sympathetic or adrenergic receptors. Pupil constriction normally occurs in bright light or when the eye is focusing on nearby objects. Pupil dilation normally occurs in dim light or when the eye is focusing on distant objects.

The lens is situated behind the iris. It is a transparent mass of uniformly arranged fibers encased in a thin elastic capsule. Its protein concentration is higher than that of any other tissue of the body. The function of the lens is to ensure that the image on the retina remains in sharp focus. The lens does this by changing shape (**accommodation**) to adjust to variations in distance. This occurs readily in young persons, but the lens becomes more rigid with age. The ability to focus on close objects is then lost, and the near point (the closest point that can be seen clearly) recedes.

With age the lens may also lose its transparency and become opaque; this is known as a **cataract.** Blindness can occur unless the cataract can be treated or removed surgically. Vision is not compromised if the opaque (cataract) portion is located peripherally in the lens.

The lens has suspensory ligaments called zonular fibers around its edge. These fibers connect with the ciliary body, and their tension helps to change the shape of the lens. In the unaccommodated eye the ciliary muscle is relaxed and the zonular fibers are taut. When zonular fibers contract, the pupil dilates; this results in sharp distant vision and blurred

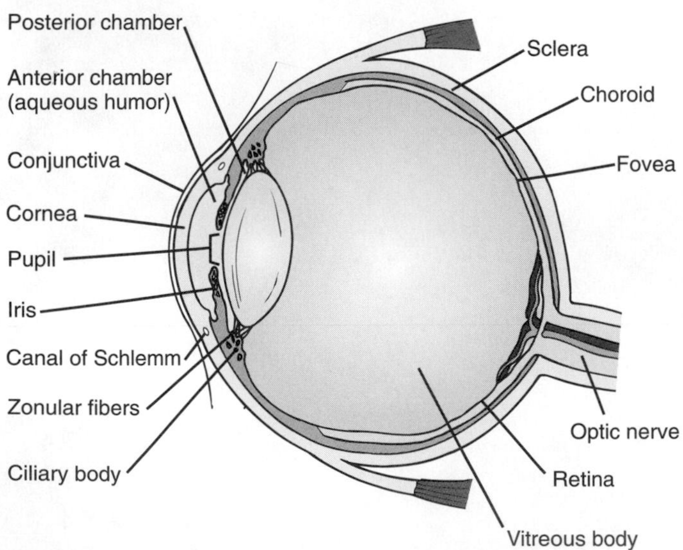

Figure 42-1 Parts of the eye.

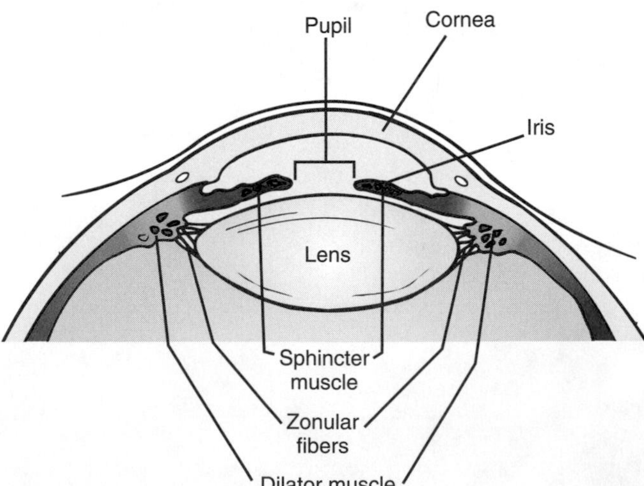

Figure 42-2 Accommodation and pupillary alterations. When zonular fibers contract, the pupil dilates, resulting in sharp distant vision and blurred near vision (unaccommodated eye). Parasympathetic stimulation accommodates the eye for near vision; the pupil constricts in response to contraction of the sphincter muscle, and the zonular fibers are relaxed. *Pupillary diameter:* Constriction (miosis) involves contraction of the sphincter muscle (parasympathetic stimulation) alone or with relaxation of the dilator muscle. Dilation (mydriasis) involves contraction of the dilator muscle (sympathetic stimulation) alone or with relaxation of the sphincter muscle.

near vision (unaccommodated eye). Parasympathetic stimulation accommodates the eye for near vision; the pupil constricts in response to contraction of the sphincter muscle, and the zonular fibers are relaxed.

Accommodation depends on two factors: (1) ciliary muscle contraction and (2) the ability of the lens to assume a more biconvex shape when tension on the ligaments is relaxed. The ciliary muscle is innervated by parasympathetic fibers. Paralysis of the ciliary muscle is termed **cycloplegia.**

Aqueous humor is formed by the ciliary body. It bathes and feeds the lens, iris, and posterior surface of the cornea. After it is formed, it flows forward between the lens and the iris into the anterior chamber. It drains out of the eye through drainage channels located near the junction of the cornea and sclera. A trabecular meshwork called the canals of Schlemm drains the aqueous humor into the venous system of the eye (see Figure 43-2).

The retina contains nerve endings plus the rods and cones that function as visual sensory receptors. It is connected to the brain by the optic nerve, which leaves the orbit through a bony canal in the posterior wall.

Eyelashes, eyelids, blinking, and tears serve to protect the eye. Each eye has approximately 200 eyelashes. A blink reflex occurs whenever a foreign body touches the eyelashes. The lids close quickly to prevent the foreign substance from entering the eye. Blinking, which is bilateral, occurs every few seconds during the waking hours. This process keeps the corneal surface free of mucus and spreads the lacrimal fluid evenly over the cornea. Tears are secreted by the lacrimal glands and contain lysozyme, a mucolytic enzyme with bactericidal action. Tears provide lubrication for lid movements, and they wash away noxious agents. By forming a thin film over the cornea, tears provide a good optical surface. Tear fluid is lost by evaporation and by draining into two small ducts (the lacrimal canaliculi) at the inner corners of the upper and lower eyelids.

SUMMARY

The eyes provide much of the information of the world around us. These delicate structures are protected from direct sunlight, damaging particles, and dryness of the environment by accessory structures such as eyelids, eye muscles, and tear glands.

Critical Thinking Questions

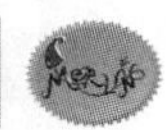

1. Mrs. B. has come to have her eyes examined. During the examination her pupils will be dilated. As part of your postexamination instructions, you tell her she will be unable to drive home. Why?
2. One of your classmates cannot see the whiteboard during class and moves to the front row, but still gets headaches. What do you think is happening, and what causes this?

Collaborative Learning Activities

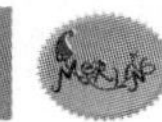

For Collaborative Learning Activities, go to mosby.com/MERLIN/McKenry/.

BIBLIOGRAPHY

Anderson, K.N., Anderson, L.E., & Glanze, W.D. (Eds.). (1998). *Mosby's medical, nursing, & allied health dictionary* (5th ed.). St. Louis: Mosby.

Thibodeau, G.A. & Patton, K. (1999). *Anatomy and physiology* (4th ed.). St. Louis: Mosby.

Van Wynsberghe, D., Noback, C.R., & Carola, R. (1995). *Human anatomy and physiology* (3rd ed.). New York: McGraw-Hill.

43 Ophthalmic Drugs

Chapter Focus

Eye disorders and the sensory-perceptual alterations that occur can cause varying degrees of disability. The early detection and treatment of eye disorders can minimize limitations of vision. Ophthalmic drugs make a significant contribution to the treatment of eye disorders and the preservation of vision.

Learning Objectives

1. Discuss the nursing management of ophthalmic drug administration.
2. Compare and contrast the antiglaucoma agents.
3. Discuss the systemic effects of ophthalmic drugs.
4. List antiinfective and antiinflammatory ophthalmic agents.
5. Implement the nursing management for the care of clients receiving ophthalmic agents.

Key Terms

glaucoma, p. 794
miotics, p. 796
mydriasis, p. 800

Drugs used to treat eye disorders can be divided into three major groups: the antiglaucoma agents, the mydriatics and cycloplegics, and the antiinfective/antiinflammatory agents. Many eye preparations are available, including ophthalmic diagnostic products, enzymes, irrigating solutions, eyewashes, and hyperosmolar preparations. This chapter discusses the major groups and selected other eye preparations, along with their major dosage and administration considerations and nursing management.

■ Nursing Management

Drugs Affecting the Eye

■ **Assessment.** Determine if the client wears glasses or contact lenses or has a history of glaucoma, cataracts, vision loss, or retinitis. Determine if the client is taking any medications; some drugs may cause visual disturbances. For example, digoxin causes the client to see yellow halos around bright lights. Assess the pregnancy safety of female clients of childbearing age (see the Pregnancy Safety box below). Assess the eyes for redness, swelling, tearing, discharge, a decrease in visual acuity, and pain. Check the pupils for size, equality, reactivity, light reaction, and accommodation. In the case of glaucoma, tonometry will indicate increased intraocular pressure (IOP).

■ **Nursing Diagnosis.** Once a client has begun a course of therapy with ophthalmic preparations, he or she should be evaluated for the following possible nursing diagnoses/collaborative problems: deficient knowledge related to self-administration of the medication and the condition for which it is administered; risk for injury related to blurred vision as the result of the instillation of drops or ointment into the eye; risk for infection related to contaminated eye drops or ointment; and the potential complications of hypersensitivity, superinfections, and systemic effects of the drug. The Nursing Care Plan on p. 792 provides other selected nursing diagnoses to consider for clients who are receiving ophthalmic conditions.

■ **Implementation**

■ ***Monitoring.*** Monitor the affected eye(s) on a daily basis for improvement of the condition for which the medication was prescribed. Assess for redness, itching, swelling, and a burning sensation that was not present before therapy started; such reactions might indicate hypersensitivity. Systemic absorption may occur with eyedrops and cause adverse systemic reactions (Table 43-1). Assess the client for ocular side effects/adverse reactions related to the administration of systemic medications (Table 43-2).

■ ***Intervention.*** In addition to developing a working knowledge of the available ophthalmic agents, be especially aware of the special considerations in administering these drugs. Ocular drugs are administered by topical application of a solution or ointment (Box 43-1). Ocular solutions are sterile and easily administered and usually do not interfere with vision. Their main disadvantage is that the drug is in contact with the eye for only a short time. Ocular ointments have the advantages of being quite comfortable on instillation and staying in longer contact with the eye for more prolonged effects. However, ointments form a film or haze over the eye that interferes with vision, and they have a higher incidence of contact dermatitis than do solutions. In addition, most ointments are not sterile.

Packs may also be used to apply drugs to the eye. Packs are cotton pledgets that are saturated with an ophthalmic solution and inserted into the inferior or superior cul-de-sac. Ocular drugs may also be physician-administered by iontophoresis, subconjunctival (sub-Tenon's) injection, retrobulbar injection, or injection directly into the vitreous or anterior chamber of the eye.

Ocular gel formulations and Ocuserts (an elliptical unit that is placed in the cul-de-sac of the eye to provide continuous drug release) provide delivery systems for pilocarpine and perhaps other medications. The newer systems were developed to overcome some of the problems with conventional eye drops or ointments. Their longer duration of action improves client management of the therapeutic regimen and avoids the peak-and-valley response associated with previous solutions and ointments. A steady release or range of pilocarpine should reduce drug-induced adverse reactions and improve treatment outcome.

■ ***Education.*** Instruct the client and/or home caregiver in the proper administration of eye medications (see Box 43-1). Caution the client to always check the bottle label for correct medication and concentration, such as 0.1% or 1%. Checking labels is increasingly important because many beauty aids and home products (glues) are now packaged in similar containers (Box 43-2). Discard ophthalmic solutions that have darkened or become cloudy.

Pregnancy Safety
Ophthalmic Drugs

Category	Drug
B	cromolyn, dipivefrin, erythromycin, lodoxamide, tobramycin
C	acetazolamide, atropine, betaxolol, carbachol, carteolol, cyclopentolate, dichlorphenamide, dorzolamide, echothiophate, epinephrine, homatropine, idoxuridine, latanoprost, levobunolol, levocabastine, methazolamide, metipranolol, naphazoline, natamycin, norfloxacin, phenylephrine, pilocarpine, polymyxin B, proparacaine, sulfonamides, tetracaine, timolol, trifluridine, vidarabine
X	demecarium, isoflurophate
Unclassified	chymotrypsin, gentamicin, hydroxyamphetamine, oxymetazoline, scopolamine, tetrahydrozoline, tropicamide

Nursing Care Plan
Selected Nursing Diagnoses Related to Ophthalmic Drugs

Nursing Diagnosis	Outcome Criteria	Interventions
Deficient knowledge related to new ophthalmic drug regimen	Client will: Express understanding of purpose, function, side effects/adverse reactions Demonstrate proper handling and administration Discuss possible drug interactions	Assess client's level of understanding. Determine the educational needs of the client. Instruct client in the following: Purpose and function of medicine Side effects/adverse reactions that may occur, and the appropriate response Proper storage and handling Correct method of administration Systemic reactions that may occur with topically applied eye preparations Provide client with a list of possible drug interactions.
Anxiety related to possible decrease in or loss of vision	Client will: Verbalize fears and concerns	Assess client for perceptions and fears related to the eye disorder. Encourage open communication about fears. Provide emotional support. Provide information related to the effectiveness of drug therapy. Allay unwarranted fears.
Impaired comfort related to ophthalmic disorder	Client will: Express a decrease in discomfort	Closely assess the client's symptoms and level of comfort. Provide rest and limiting of eye activity (e.g., reading). Provide emotional support and encouragement.
Risk for injury related to impaired vision	Client will: Maintain activity appropriate for level of vision without injury Discuss necessary lifestyle adjustments	Assess level of vision impairment. Provide safety measures as needed. Encourage client to adjust activities in accordance with client's level of vision.

TABLE 43-1 Ophthalmic Drugs: Adverse Systemic Reactions

Ophthalmic Drug	Reported Adverse Reaction
Antimicrobial Agents	
chloramphenicol eyedrops	Aplastic anemia
sulfacetamide eyedrops	Stevens-Johnson syndrome, systemic lupus erythematosus
Anticholinergic Drugs	
atropine eyedrops	Tachycardia, elevated temperature, fever, delirium
cyclopentolate	Convulsions, hallucinations
scopolamine eyedrops	Acute psychosis
Antiglaucoma Medications	
beta-blocking agents (timolol)	Bradycardia, syncope, low blood pressure, asthmatic attack, congestive heart failure, hallucinations, loss of appetite, headaches, nausea, weakness, depression
anticholinesterase (echothiophate)	Asthmatic attack, systemic cholinergic effects
parasympathomimetic (pilocarpine)	Nausea, stomach pain, increased sweating, salivation, tremors, bradycardia, lightheadedness
Adrenergic Medications	
phenylephrine (10%)	Severe hypertension, cerebral hemorrhage, dysrhythmias, myocardial infarction
epinephrine eyedrops	Tremors, increased sweating, headaches, hypertension

TABLE 43-2 Ocular Side Effects Induced by Systemic Medications

Drug	Possible Ocular Side Effect	Drug	Possible Ocular Side Effect
allopurinol	Retinal hemorrhage, exudative lesions	hydralazine	Lacrimation, blurred vision
aspirin	Allergic dermatitis, including keratitis and conjunctivitis	ibuprofen	Altered color vision, blurred vision
barbiturates	Nystagmus	indomethacin	Mydriasis, retinopathy
busulfan	Cataracts	isoniazid	Optic neuritis
cannabis, marijuana	Nystagmus, conjunctivitis, double vision	lithium carbonate	Exophthalmos
chloral hydrate	Eyelid edema, conjunctivitis, miosis	nitroglycerin	Transient elevation in IOP
chloroquine	Lenticular and corneal opacity, retinopathy	opiates	Miosis, nystagmus
clomiphene citrate	Blurred vision, light flashes	phenothiazines	Corneal and conjunctival deposits, cataracts, retinopathy, oculogyric crisis
clonidine	Miosis	phenytoin	Nystagmus
corticosteroids	Cataracts, increased IOP, papilledema	quinine	Blurring of vision, optic neuritis, blindness (reversible)
diazoxide	Oculogyric crisis	thiazide diuretics	Acute transient myopia, yellow coloring of vision
digitalis glycosides	Scotomas, optic neuritis	vincristine	Ptosis, paresis of extraocular muscles
ethyl alcohol	Nystagmus	vitamin A overdose or toxicity	Papilledema, increased IOP
guanethidine	Miosis, ptosis, blurred vision	vitamin D toxicity	Calcium deposits in cornea

BOX 43-1

Guidelines for the Instillation of Eyedrops and Ophthalmic Ointments

Instillation of Eyedrops

Wash your hands and put on gloves if necessary.

Gently cleanse exudate from the eye if necessary.

Ask the client to tilt the head toward the side of the affected eye.

Gently pull the lower eyelid down and ask the client to look up.

Instill the correct number of drops in the sac formed by the lower eyelid.

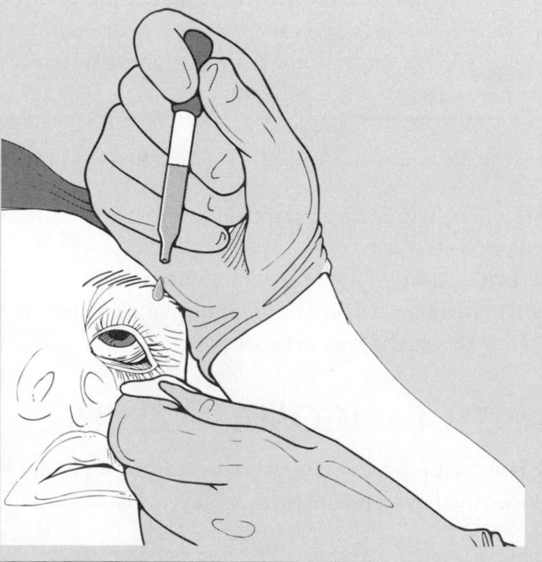

Take care not to touch the dropper to the eye or eyelashes.

Gently apply pressure for 30 seconds to 1 minute over the inner canthus next to the nose to prevent absorption through the tear duct and premature drainage of the medication away from the eye.

Ask the client to close the eye gently, which distributes the solution. Warn against squeezing the eye tightly, which forces out the medication.

Wipe away any excess medication.

If both eyes are to be medicated, do the second instillation quickly before the client begins to blink and tear as a reaction to the burning sensation occurring in the first eye.

Instillation of Eye Ointment

The procedure is the same except that the ointment is expressed directly into the exposed conjunctival sac from the inner to outer canthus with a small individual tube.

Have the client close his or her eye; gently massage the eye to distribute the medication.

BOX 43-2

Eyedrops and Look-Alikes

Containers that look like eyedrop containers are the culprits behind many ophthalmic emergencies. Thinking they are instilling eyedrops, adults and children have instead dropped in Superglue, contact lens cleaners, ear drops, and perfumes. These products are often sold in bottles that are similar in shape, size, and color. Older adults, who may have poor eyesight, are particularly at risk for mistaking one product for another.

In most cases the injured eye responds to copious flushing to dilute and wash out the offending agent. This is followed by topical antibiotics, lubricants or cycloplegics, and patching if needed. If the client has instilled glue in the eye and has no significant pain, irrigation and a sterile eye patch soaked in tap water and left overnight are sufficient. The solvents that dissolve glue are too toxic for the eye; therefore if the conservative approach does not work, the client may need to be referred to an ophthalmologist, who may cut the eyelids apart to prevent corneal abrasion.

Advise all clients to keep their eyedrops in one particular place and away from other chemicals. Recommend that they check the labels on the container while still wearing their glasses or contact lenses to ensure they have the right medicine before administering their eyedrops.

Critical Thinking Questions

- In what other ways could visually impaired clients prevent instilling inappropriate solutions into their eyes?
- Should there be regulation of packaging to prevent such accidents? What would be the social and economic effects of such regulation?

Information from O'Boyle, J.E. & Enzenaur, R.W. (1992). "Super glue" in the eye. *Emergency Medicine, 24*(6), 59-60, 62.

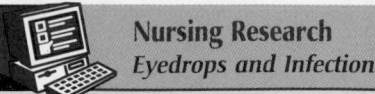

Nursing Research
Eyedrops and Infection

Citation: Schein, O.D., Hibberd, P.L.., Stark, T., Baker, A.S., & Kenyon, K.R. (1992). Microbial contamination of in-use ocular medications. *Archives of Ophthalmology, 110*(1):82-85.

Abstract: A study was performed at the Massachusetts Eye and Ear Infirmary to examine the incidence of contamination of eyedrops and ointments in use by clients. Schein et al. (1992) cultured 220 eye medications in use by 101 clients with nonmicrobial ocular surface disease at the Infirmary. Conjunctival cultures were taken from the study clients and from 50 age-matched controls with no eye surface disease or infection. Potentially pathogenic organisms were cultured from 64 medications (29%) and from 34 study clients (34%), compared with only 5 control clients. The most common contaminants were gram-negative organisms. Coagulase-negative staphylococci and diphtheroids—the usual conjunctival flora—were also commonly found in the eyedrops and ointments, as were small numbers of gram-positive organisms and fungi.

Medication caps had the highest rate of bacterial colonization. The contents also became colonized by contamination from the dropper or ointment drip. Contamination of the dropper or medication itself is clinically important because it guarantees delivery of the organism to the ocular surface.

Clients should be advised to discard old bottles of eye medications. They should be carefully instructed in the administration of eye medications so that the tip of the dropper or ointment tube does not come in contact with the skin, eye, or eyelashes. They should cap the medication promptly after each use.

Critical Thinking Questions

- How would this research influence your assessment of a client using eye medications? How would it influence your health teaching?
- Try administering eyedrops or an eye ointment while wearing garden gloves to simulate impaired mobility of the hands, which might occur with aging. How might this limitation affect contamination of the medication?

Store medications as directed on the label; some may need refrigeration. Once opened, most medications have a limited life (3 months or the end of the current illness). If stored longer, the medication is more likely to become contaminated and lead to an infection of the eye (see the Nursing Research box above). To avoid such contamination from the outset, the sterility of the preparation and/or dropper must be maintained. Do not allow the tube tip or dropper to touch anything, including the skin. Hold the dropper with the tip down. Never allow medication to flow into the bulb of the dropper. Keep the container closed when not in use. If two or more family members are using eye medications, each should have a separate vial to prevent cross-contamination.

Inform the client of the signs of side effects/adverse reactions of the medication, as well as signs of progress. Advise the client when to contact or return to the prescriber for assessment.

■ **Evaluation.** The expected outcome is that the client will experience a decrease in or absence of the symptoms for which the agent was prescribed.

ANTIGLAUCOMA AGENTS

Glaucoma is an eye disease characterized chiefly by an abnormally elevated IOP, which may result from the excessive

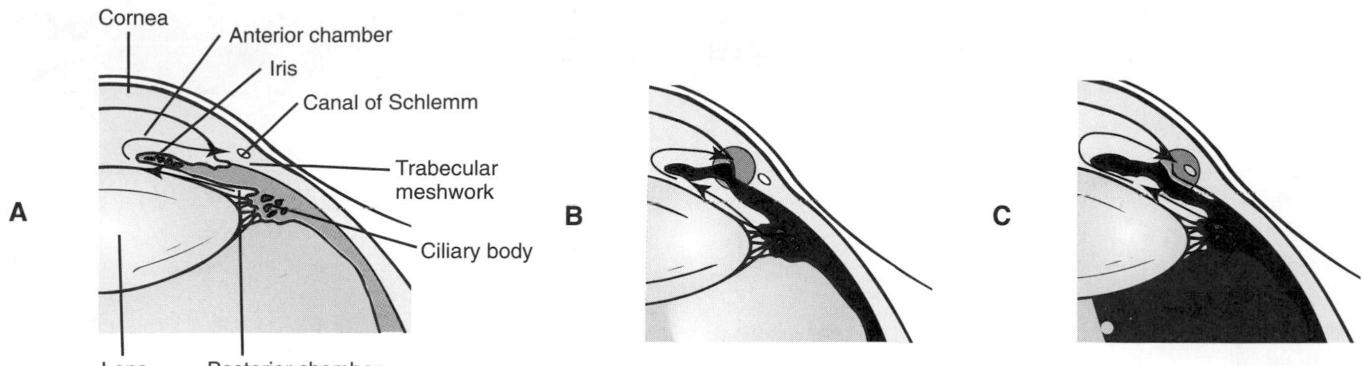

Figure 43-1 Main structures of the eye and enlargement of the canal of Schlemm showing aqueous flow in normal (A), angle-closure (B), and open-angle glaucoma (C).

production of aqueous humor or diminished ocular fluid outflow. Increased pressure, if sufficiently high and persistent, may lead to irreversible blindness. Although glaucoma is primarily a disease of middle age—occurring in approximately 2% of all persons 40 years and older—it has also been diagnosed in younger adults and children. There are three major types of glaucoma: primary, secondary, and congenital.

Primary glaucoma includes angle-closure (acute congestive) glaucoma and open-angle (chronic simple) glaucoma (Figure 43-1). Persons with angle-closure glaucoma have closure of the angle of the anterior chamber, possibly because of a physiologic or anatomic predisposition. Drugs are needed to control the acute attack associated with angle-closure glaucoma; this is usually followed by surgery, such as iridectomy or laser surgery. Open- or wide-angle glaucoma is more common, occurring in approximately 90% of individuals with primary glaucoma. The increased IOP is secondary to an increased production of aqueous humor or a decreased outflow caused by degenerative changes in the outflow system. It has a gradual insidious onset, and its control depends on drug therapy or perhaps a peripheral iridectomy. Secondary glaucoma may result from previous eye disease or may follow cataract extraction (Abel, 1995). Therapy for secondary glaucoma usually involves drug therapy, whereas congenital glaucoma requires surgical treatment.

Primary medications used to treat glaucoma include beta-adrenergic blocking agents, cholinergics, and sympathomimetics. The selection of a particular drug is determined largely by the requirements and individual response of the client.

Beta-Adrenergic Blocking Agents

The beta-adrenergic blocking agents include betaxolol (Betoptic), carteolol (Ocupress), levobunolol (Betagen C Cap), metipranolol (OptiPranolol), and timolol (Timoptic). Betaxolol is a cardioselective ($beta_1$) blocking agent, whereas all the other beta blockers are noncardioselective and block both $beta_1$- and $beta_2$-adrenergic receptors. These agents work alone or in combination with other drugs to decrease the production of aqueous humor, thus reducing IOP in open-angle glaucoma. However, the exact mechanism of action for these agents is unknown.

Timolol is also used to treat selected cases of secondary glaucoma. Betaxolol is indicated for the treatment of open-angle glaucoma and ocular hypertension and may be a drug of choice for clients with pulmonary disease because of its selective $beta_1$-blocking effects; the nurse should still monitor for respiratory difficulties.

The side effects/adverse reactions of the beta-adrenergic blocking ophthalmic agents are primarily local reactions, such as burning, stinging, or eye irritation. Rare effects include eye inflammation, visual disturbance, pruritus, or allergic reaction. These agents can be systemically absorbed to cause bradycardia or tachycardia, confusion, insomnia, weakness, wheezing, respiratory difficulties, depression, ataxia, edema of the lower extremities, nausea, and vomiting. Hallucinations have been reported with timolol only.

Table 43-3 lists the pharmacokinetics and dosing information for beta-adrenergic blocking agents.

■ Nursing Management

Beta-Adrenergic Blocking Ophthalmic Agent Therapy

In addition to the following discussion, see Nursing Management: Beta-Adrenergic Blocking Drug Therapy, Chapter 22.

■ **Assessment.** Use caution when administering beta-adrenergic blocking agents to clients with bronchial asthma, severe chronic obstructive pulmonary disease, sinus bradycardia or greater than first-degree heart block, cardiogenic shock, or overt cardiac failure. Determine the client's history of allergy to the solution. There is sufficient absorption from the conjunctiva and nasopharynx to produce systemic nonselective beta-adrenergic ($beta_1$ and $beta_2$) effects such as cardiopulmonary complications, exacerbation of asthma, and hypotension (Hayreh, Podhajsky, & Zimmerman, 1999). Symptoms of hypoglycemia may be masked if these agents are used for clients with diabetes mellitus. These agents may mask symptoms of hyperthyroidism and precipitate a thyroid storm if suddenly discontinued.

TABLE 43-3 Beta-Adrenergic Blocking Agents: Pharmacokinetics and Dosing

Drug	Onset of Action (hours)	Peak Effect (hours)	Duration of Action (hours)	Usual Adult Dosage
betaxolol (Betoptic)	0.5	2	12	0.25%, 0.5%: instill 1 drop twice daily
carteolol (Ocupress)	N/A	2	6-8	1%: instill 1 drop twice daily
levobunolol (Betagan)	1	2-6	Up to 24	0.25%: instill 1 drop 1-2 times daily 0.5%: instill 1 drop daily
metipranolol (OptiPranolol)	0.5	2	24	0.3%: instill 1 drop twice daily
timolol (Timoptic)	0.5	1-2	Up to 24	0.25%, 0.5%: instill one drop 1-2 times daily

Information from *United States Pharmacopeia Dispensing Information (USP DI): Drug information for the health care professional* (20th ed.). (2000). Rockville, MD: United States Pharmacopeial Convention.
N/A, not available.

Because the drug may be absorbed systemically, review the client's current medication regimen for drug interactions, such as those listed for systemic beta-adrenergic blocking agents in Chapter 22.

Obtain baseline assessments of the client's vision, IOP, and vital signs.

▪ **Nursing Diagnosis.** The client undergoing therapy with beta-adrenergic blocking agents is at risk for the following selected nursing diagnoses/collaborative problems: disturbed sensory perception (visual) related to the client's underlying condition or the development of ocular irritation; risk for injury related to decreased night vision; impaired comfort related to eye pain, dryness, increased sensitivity to light, crusting, itching, stinging, burning, or watering of eye; and the potential complications of decreased cardiac output and other symptoms related to systemic absorption of the drug.

▪ **Implementation**

▪ ***Monitoring.*** Assess the client's vision and IOP periodically. Monitor the eye for inflammation; although these agents are usually well tolerated, occasional signs of mild ocular irritation may occur. Local hypersensitivity (rash) occurs rarely. Monitor the client's vital signs because a slight reduction of resting heart rate may occur, and acute bronchospasm in clients with bronchospastic disease has been reported.

▪ ***Intervention.*** Use a nasolacrimal occlusion to minimize systemic absorption.

▪ ***Education.*** Instruct the client in the proper administration technique. Alert clients with diabetes that symptoms of hypoglycemia may be masked, such as tachycardia and trembling. Advise clients to wear sunglasses and avoid bright light. Instruct the client to alert health practitioners to the drug if surgery is considered; some prescribers recommend that these agents be gradually withdrawn 48 hours before surgery. Encourage regular consultation with the prescriber to check IOP.

▪ **Evaluation.** The expected outcome of beta-adrenergic blocking ophthalmic agent therapy is that the client will experience a therapeutic reduction in IOP without experiencing clinically significant, systemic beta-adrenergic blocking effects.

Cholinergic Agents

Cholinergic medications or **miotics,** so called because they cause pupillary constriction, are topically applied agents useful in treating open-angle and angle-closure glaucoma. Cholinergic miotics (direct acting) are chemically related to acetylcholine, the neurotransmitter that mediates nerve impulse transmission at all cholinergic or parasympathetic nerve sites. When applied topically to the eye, cholinergic drugs cause contraction of the sphincter muscle of the iris. This results in pupil constriction (miosis) and contraction of the ciliary muscle attached to the trabecular meshwork, thus opening the spaces in the meshwork and increasing the outflow of aqueous humor. The contracted ciliary muscle leaves the eye in accommodation of near vision.

Cholinergic miotics (direct-acting) drugs include carbachol (Carboptic) and pilocarpine (Isopto Carpine). Anticholinesterase drugs inhibit the enzymatic destruction of acetylcholine by activating cholinesterase. This action permits acetylcholine to act on the iris sphincter and ciliary muscles, producing pupil constriction (miosis) and ciliary muscle contraction (accommodation).

The irreversible anticholinesterase drugs (echothiophate [Phospholine Iodide] and isoflurophate [Floropryl]) form stable complexes with cholinesterase and thus irreversibly

TABLE 43-4 Cholinergic Agents: Pharmacokinetics and Dosing

Drug	Onset of Action (hours)	Peak Effect (hours)	Duration of Action (hours)	Usual Adult Dosage
Miotics–Direct Acting				
carbachol (Carboptic)	0.25	Miosis: 2-5 minutes IOP: within 4 hours	24	0.75%-3%: 1 drop topically 3 times daily
pilocarpine (Isopto Carpine)	Up to 0.5	1-1.25	4-8	0.25%-4%: 1 drop topically up to 4 times daily
Miotics–Cholinesterase Inhibitors				
demecarium (Humorsol)	Miosis: <1 IOP: 4	Miosis: 2 IOP: within 24	24-48	0.125%-0.25%: 1 drop topically once or twice daily
echothiophate (Phospholine Iodide)	Same as demecarium			0.03%-0.25%: 1 drop topically once or twice daily
isoflurophate (Floropryl)	Same as demecarium			0.025% ointment: thin strip topically once every 3 days to 3 times daily

Information from *Drug Facts and Comparisons*. (2000). St. Louis: Facts and Comparisons; and *United States Pharmacopeia Dispensing Information (USP DI): Drug information for the health care professional* (20th ed.). (2000). Rockville, MD: United States Pharmacopeial Convention.

impair the destructive function of the enzyme. The destruction of acetylcholine then depends on the synthesis of new enzymes. Demecarium (Humorsol) is more toxic than the other agents in this category and therefore is not as commonly used. Although it is a reversible inhibitor, its prolonged action has results similar to the irreversible inhibitors.

The cholinesterase inhibitors are usually reserved for clients who respond inadequately to the first-line agents, such as beta blockers, cholinergics (pilocarpine), and sympathomimetics (epinephrine).

The side effects/adverse reactions of the cholinergic agents include visual blurring, irritation, myopia, ciliary spasm, brow pain, and headache resulting from the stimulation of accommodative ancillary muscles. Miosis also makes it difficult to adjust quickly to changes in illumination. This may be serious in older adults, because their light adaptation and visual acuity are often reduced. Nighttime is particularly hazardous for these individuals.

Cysts of the iris, synechiae, retinal detachments, obstruction of tear drainage, and even cataracts may develop with prolonged use of cholinergic agents, especially with the long-acting anticholinesterases. In general, side effects caused by direct-acting cholinergic agents are less severe and occur less often than those caused by anticholinesterase agents. Systemic side effects include salivation, nausea, vomiting, diarrhea, precipitation of asthmatic attack, decrease in blood pressure, and other symptoms of parasympathetic stimulation.

Table 43-4 lists the pharmacokinetics and dosing information for cholinergic agents.

The nursing management is much the same as for the beta-adrenergic blocking ophthalmic agents, except there is not the concern for cardiac function. In addition, the cholinergic agents are contraindicated for clients with acute iritis or other conditions in which pupillary constriction is not desired.

Sympathomimetic Agents

The primary sympathomimetic agents are dipivefrin (Propine), which is converted to epinephrine by enzyme hydrolysis in the eye, and epinephrine, a direct-acting sympathomimetic agent. The chemical modification of dipivefrin results in a more lipophilic compound that facilitates absorption and penetration through the cornea into the anterior chamber of the eye. The penetration and absorption of dipivefrin is greater than that of epinephrine. The mechanism of action of the sympathomimetic agents is unknown, but it appears that they lower IOP by decreasing aqueous humor production and increasing its outflow. These agents are indicated for the treatment of open-angle glaucoma.

The side effects/adverse reactions of the sympathomimetic ophthalmic agents are rarely troublesome; they include burning, stinging or eye irritation, headache, brow pain, and watering eyes. The signs and symptoms of systemic absorption include tachycardia, palpitations, hypertension, increased sweating, tremors, and light-headedness.

Epinephrine has an onset of action within 1 hour, a peak effect in 4 to 8 hours, and a duration of action of up to 24 hours. It is available in 0.1% to 2% strengths.

The usual adult dosage is 1 drop topically once or twice daily. Dipivefrin has an onset of action within 30 minutes and reaches a peak effect in 1 hour. The pediatric and adult dosage is 1 drop (0.1%) topically every 12 hours.

■ Nursing Management

Sympathomimetic Ophthalmic Therapy

■ **Assessment.** Sympathomimetic ophthalmic agents are contraindicated in clients with narrow-angle glaucoma or a predisposition to it, because pupil dilation may aggravate the condition. Dipivefrin or epinephrine may cause macular edema in clients with aphakia (the absence of a crystalline lens). Ophthalmic epinephrine should be administered with caution to clients with hypertension or other cardiovascular disease, hyperthyroidism, parkinsonism, asthma, or diabetes mellitus. Determine the client's sensitivity to sulfites or the drug being used.

The client's drug history should be reviewed to determine the risk for drug interactions. Epinephrine may be absorbed systemically to interact with ophthalmic beta blockers, digitalis glycosides, or monoamine oxidase (MAO) inhibitors.

A baseline assessment of the client should include ocular pressure, pupil size, vision status, and vital signs.

■ **Nursing Diagnosis.** Clients receiving these sympathomimetic ophthalmic solutions may be at risk for impaired comfort related to possible photophobia and burning, stinging, or other eye irritations. If the agent is absorbed systemically, the client may experience the potential complication of altered cardiac output (tachycardia, hypertension).

■ **Implementation**

■ ***Monitoring.*** To ensure the effectiveness of therapy, the prescriber should evaluate the client's condition at periodic intervals throughout therapy with fundus and IOP examinations. Assess for decreased visual acuity and ocular discomfort. Obtain periodic pulse and blood pressure determinations to assess for systemic effects such as tachycardia and elevated blood pressure.

■ ***Intervention.*** Review the client's regimen carefully if dipivefrin is being administered with other antiglaucoma ophthalmic solutions. When dipivefrin is replacing epinephrine, the epinephrine should be discontinued when the dipivefrin is started. If the antiglaucoma agent to be replaced is something other than epinephrine, that agent should be discontinued on the second day of dipivefrin administration. If administered in addition to other antiglaucoma agents, dipivefrin is given at the usual adult dosage.

To minimize systemic absorption, pressure should be maintained on the lacrimal sac during and for 1 to 2 minutes after instillation of the drug. Discoloration or precipitation of epinephrine indicates oxidation to inactive products, and the solution should be discarded.

■ ***Education.*** Review with the client the safe and accurate techniques for the self-administration of ophthalmic agents. (See Nursing Management: Drugs Affecting the Eye, p. 791.)

Alert the client that pigment deposits in the conjunctiva may occur after the prolonged use of epinephrine. The client should seek medical advice regarding the use of contact lenses during therapy. Instruct the client about which symptoms to report to the prescriber.

■ **Evaluation.** The expected outcome of sympathomimetic ophthalmic agent therapy is that the client will experience therapeutic mydriasis and a reduction in IOP without adverse systemic effects.

Carbonic Anhydrase Inhibitor Agents

The oral carbonic anhydrase inhibitors include acetazolamide (Diamox), dichlorphenamide (Daranide), and methazolamide (Neptazane). Acetazolamide, the most widely used drug of this class, is the focus of this discussion. The carbonic anhydrase inhibitors are sulfonamides (nonbacteriostatic) with an undetermined mechanism of action, but they appear to lower IOP by decreasing the aqueous production to approximately one-half its baseline measurement.

The topical sulfonamide dorzolamide, a carbonic anhydrase inhibitor, is systemically absorbed to produce its antiglaucoma effects. The 2% eyedrop solution applied three times daily is approximately equivalent in effect to a 2-mg oral dose given twice daily.

The oral drugs are used for the treatment of open-angle, secondary, and angle-closure glaucoma, whereas eyedrops are indicated for open-angle glaucoma and ocular hypertension. Side effects with the oral carbonic anhydrase inhibitor agents include diarrhea, discomfort, diuresis, anorexia, metallic taste in mouth, nausea, vomiting, weight loss, and tingling or numbness (paresthesia) of the fingers, hands, and toes. Prescriber intervention is necessary if the client has the signs and symptoms of acidosis, blood dyscrasias, or hypokalemia. The side effects of the eyedrops include a topical allergic reaction of the eye, a bitter taste in the mouth, photosensitivity, and superficial punctate keratitis. Table 43-5 lists the pharmacokinetics and dosing information for the antiglaucoma agents.

■ Nursing Management

Carbonic Anhydrase Inhibitor Ophthalmic Therapy

■ **Assessment.** The client's health status should be assessed for conditions that might indicate that carbonic anhydrase inhibitors should be administered cautiously, such as clients with adrenocortical insufficiency who would be more inclined to electrolyte imbalances. Reactions to sulfonamide agents (thiazide diuretic, oral sulfonylureas) raise suspicion for cross-sensitivity and hypersensitivity. Contraindications include clients with decreased sodium/potassium serum levels or other electrolyte imbalances, or hepatic or renal dysfunction (potential for renal calculi formation).

Review the client's current medication regimen for the risk of significant drug interactions, such as those that may

TABLE 43-5 Antiglaucoma Agents: Pharmacokinetics and Dosing

Drug	Onset of Action (hours)	Peak Effect (hours)	Duration of Action (hours)	Usual Adult Dosage
Carbonic Anhydrase Inhibitors				
Oral				
acetazolamide (Diamox)				
capsules	2	8-12	18-24	500 mg PO twice daily, morning and evening
tablets	1-1.5	2-4	8-12	250 mg PO 1 to 4 times daily
IV	2 minutes	15 minutes	4-5	500 mg IV
dichlorphenamide (Daranide)	0.5-1	2-4	6-12	100-200 mg initially, then 100 mg q12h; maintenance dosage 25-50 mg 1 to 3 times daily
methazolamide (Neptazane)	2-4	6-8	10-18	50-100 mg 2 or 3 times daily
Eyedrops				
dorzolamide (Trusopt)	N/A	N/A	N/A	2% solution: 1 drop 3 times daily
Prostaglandin Agonist				
latanoprost (Xalatan ◆)	N/A	2	N/A	1 drop in affected eye(s) in the evening

Information from *United States Pharmacopeia Dispensing Information (USP DI): Drug information for the health care professional* (20th ed.). (2000). Rockville, MD: United States Pharmacopeial Convention.
N/A, not available.

occur when carbonic anhydrase inhibitors are given concurrently with the following drugs:

Drug	Possible Effect and Management
Bold/color type indicates the most serious interactions.	
amphetamines, quinidine, mecamylamine (Inversine)	**Carbonic anhydrase inhibitors decrease the excretion of these drugs because of alkalinization of the urine, which may result in a prolonged duration of drug action and possibly increased side effects. Avoid the concurrent use of mecamylamine. Monitor other agents closely, because dosage adjustments are usually necessary.**
methenamine (Mandelamine)	**Alkalinization of the urine prevents the conversion of methenamine to formaldehyde, thus reducing the effectiveness of methenamine. Concurrent drug administration is not recommended.**

Obtain a baseline assessment of the client's vision, IOP, ocular pain, vital signs, urinalysis, complete blood cell count (CBC), platelet count, and serum electrolytes.

■ **Nursing Diagnosis.** The client is at risk for impaired comfort in a variety of ways, including metallic taste, anorexia, nausea and vomiting, feelings of malaise, and numbness or tingling of the fingers, toes, mouth, and tongue. In addition, the client may experience fatigue, diarrhea, constipation, and impaired urinary elimination (polyuria). A deficient fluid volume may occur. The client's feelings of malaise should be carefully assessed, because he or she may also be at risk for collaborative problems related to the development of mental depression, crystalluria, sulfonamide-like nephrotoxicity, hypokalemia, blood dyscrasias, and acidosis.

■ **Implementation**

■ ***Monitoring.*** Carbonic anhydrase inhibitors cause some decrease in renal blood flow and glomerular filtration rate, which produces an increased excretion of sodium, potassium, bicarbonate, and water alkaline diuresis. Monitor appropriate serum concentrations for electrolyte imbalances. To monitor for fluid volume depletion, maintain an accurate record of intake and output and daily weights, and assess skin turgor and mucous membranes. Monitor the affected eye(s) on a daily basis for improvement.

■ ***Intervention.*** Administer these medications with meals to minimize gastrointestinal distress. Schedule doses early in the day to minimize nocturia. If potassium supplements are required, assess serum chloride levels; a potassium preparation that does not contain chloride is required if sodium chloride levels are elevated.

■ ***Education.*** Instruct the client in a high-potassium, low-sodium diet. Advise a fluid intake of 2 L daily to reduce the risk of renal calculi. Encourage the client to monitor his or her weight daily, and instruct him or her about the signs and symptoms of fluid and electrolyte imbalances.

Alert the client to report fever, rash, changes in urine color, or lumbar or abdominal pain to the prescriber.

Case Study *The Client with Glaucoma*

James Gibson, a 70-year-old male, has been having difficulty with his peripheral vision and has been diagnosed with closed-angle glaucoma. The provider prescribes pilocarpine (Isopto Carpine), 1 drop three times daily and acetazolamide (Diamox), 250 mg PO four times daily. The nurse's major responsibility becomes client teaching.

1. What are important issues in teaching Mr. Gibson how to instill his eyedrops?
2. How does pilocarpine affect glaucoma?
3. Why should the provider place Mr. Gibson on a carbonic anhydrase inhibitor (Diamox) in addition to the eyedrops?
4. Mr. Gibson has been taking furosemide (Lasix) 40 mg PO daily for another health condition. What side effects does he need to watch for while he is taking the Diamox?

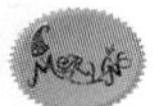

For answer guidelines, go to mosby.com/MERLIN/McKenry/.

■ **Evaluation.** The expected outcome of carbonic anhydrase inhibitor therapy is that the client will experience a decrease in IOP without any adverse reactions to the drug (see the Case Study box above).

Prostaglandin Agonist

Latanoprost (Xalatan) is the first prostaglandin agonist approved to treat open-angle glaucoma and ocular hypertension. It reduces IOP by increasing aqueous humor outflow.

The side effects/adverse reactions of latanoprost include blurred vision, burning and stinging, itching, photophobia, and conjunctival hyperemia. Clients should be informed that this drug may cause an increase in iris pigmentation (brown).

■ Nursing Management

Latanoprost Therapy

In addition to the following discussion, see Nursing Management: Drugs Affecting the Eye, p. 791.

■ **Assessment.** Determine if the client has a sensitivity to latanoprost or to benzalkonium chloride within the ophthalmic solution.

■ **Nursing Diagnosis.** The client receiving latanoprost may experience the following nursing diagnoses/collaborative problems: risk for injury related to blurred vision; impaired comfort (burning, itching or stinging of the eye, photophobia); and the potential complication of increased pigmentation of the iris, eyelashes, and periorbital tissue.

■ **Implementation.** Advise the client to remove contact lenses before administering the drug and to wait at least 15 minutes before reinserting the lenses. Latanoprost should be administered 5 minutes apart other antiglaucoma ophthalmic medications; pilocarpine should be administered 1 hour after the bedtime dose of latanoprost (Kent, Vroman, Thomas, Hebert, & Crosson, 1999). The once-a-day dosing of latanoprost should not be exceeded. Alert the client that the eyelashes may become longer, thicker, and darker, and the iris and skin around the eye may also become darker. This hyperpigmentation may be reason to discontinue the drug.

■ **Evaluation.** The expected outcome of latanoprost therapy is that the client's ophthalmic tonometry determinations will be within the normal range without significant hyperpigmentation of the iris and periorbital tissue.

Osmotic Agents

Osmotic agents are given intravenously or orally to reduce IOP. In general, these agents do not cross the blood aqueous barrier into the anterior chamber of the eye and are rarely found in the ocular humor. (See Chapter 34 for a discussion of the osmotic agents.)

MYDRIATIC AND CYCLOPLEGIC AGENTS

Adrenergic agonists cause pupil dilation (**mydriasis**), and cycloplegic agents paralyze ciliary muscle (accommodation). These agents are used primarily for the diagnosis of ophthalmic disorders. The effects of these agents depend on the client's age, race, and color of iris. For example, mydriatic agents evoke less of a response in persons with heavily pigmented (dark) irides than in those with lighter pigmented (blue) irides. Thus blacks tend to respond less to the agents than whites. Anticholinergic agents produce both mydriasis and cycloplegia via the blockade of muscarinic receptors. Contraction of the iris sphincter leads to relaxation and a possible increase in IOP. This discussion focuses on anticholinergic agents and adrenergic agonists.

Anticholinergic Agents

Anticholinergic agents are indicated for the treatment of inflammations such as uveitis and keratitis; they relieve ocular pain by relaxing inflamed intraocular muscles. They are also used for the relaxation of ciliary muscle to allow accurate measurement of refractive errors (which permits proper lens determination for eyeglasses) and for preoperative and postoperative use in intraocular surgery.

Local side effects/adverse reactions that are reported with the use of anticholinergic ophthalmic agents include stinging or an increase in IOP. Allergic lid reactions, red eye, and various eye irritation injuries may be induced with chronic use. Systemic absorption of these agents may result in mild to serious adverse reactions, such as dryness of the mouth, inhibition of sweating, flushing, tachycardia, ataxia, hallucinations, psychiatric and behavioral problems, fever, delirium, convul-

TABLE 43-6 Anticholinergic Agents: Pharmacokinetics and Dosing

Drug	Time to Maximal Mydriasis (minutes)	Recovery (days)	Time to Maximal Cycloplegia (minutes)	Recovery (days)	Usual Adult Dosage
atropine	30-40	7-10	60-180	6-12	1%: 1 drop
cyclopentolate	30-60	1	25-75	6-24 hours	0.5%-2%: 1 drop
homatropine	40-60	1-3	30-60	1-3	2%-5%: 1 drop
scopolamine	20-130	3-7	30-60	3-7	0.25%: 1 drop
tropicamide	20-40	6 hours	30	6 hours	1%: 1 drop

	Indication	Usual Adult Dosage
Combination Eyedrops		
cyclopentolate and phenylephrine (Cyclomydril)	Mydriasis	1 drop in each eye every 5-10 minutes as necessary; do not exceed 3 doses
scopolamine and phenylephrine (Murocoll-2)	Mydriasis, cycloplegia, and posterior synechiae in iritis	Mydriasis: 1-2 drops in eye, repeated in 5 minutes if necessary
tropicamide and hydroxyamphetamine (Paremyd)	Mydriasis with partial cycloplegia	1-2 drops into conjunctival sac

Information from Moroi, S.E. & Lichter, P.R. (1996). Ocular pharmacology. In J.G. Hardman & L.E. Limbird (Eds.), *Goodman & Gilman's The pharmacological basis of therapeutics* (9th ed.). New York: McGraw-Hill; *Drug Facts and Comparisons.* (2000). St. Louis: Facts and Comparisons; *United States Pharmacopeia Dispensing Information (USP DI): Drug information for the health care professional* (20th ed.). (2000). Rockville, MD: United States Pharmacopeial Convention.

sions, respiratory depression, andcoma. Deaths have been recorded in children after systemic absorption.

Pupillary dilation from either local or systemic administration can precipitate acute glaucoma in persons with a predisposition to this condition. Blindness can result if this condition is left unrecognized or untreated. Table 43-6 lists the pharmacokinetics and dosing information for the anticholinergic agents.

Combination eyedrops include Cyclomydril, Murocoll-2, and Paremyd. These agents in combination produce a greater mydriasis than either drug alone. Table 43-6 summarizes the indications for and dosages of these combinations.

■ Nursing Management

Anticholinergic Ophthalmic Therapy

■ Assessment. Anticholinergic therapy with atropine is contraindicated for clients with a history of severe systemic reaction to atropine. It is used with caution in clients with primary glaucoma or a predisposition to angle-closure glaucoma. Dilation of the pupil causes a narrowing of the iridocorneal angle where the canal of Schlemm is located. This restricts the drainage of intraocular fluids, although secretion continues and IOP rises. This may precipitate an attack of acute glaucoma.

Obtain a baseline assessment of the client's vision status and IOP.

■ Nursing Diagnosis. The client receiving anticholinergic ophthalmic therapy is at risk for the following nursing diagnoses: disturbed sensory perception related to blurred vision and increased sensitivity of the eyes to light; impaired tissue integrity related to eye irritation not present before therapy and swelling of the eyelids; and risk for injury related to systemic absorption (confusion, dizziness, dryness of skin, fever, slurred speech, tachycardia, drowsiness, dryness of the mouth).

■ Implementation

■ *Monitoring.* The client's IOP and vision should be monitored periodically over the course of therapy. The potential for systemic side effects is more pronounced in infants, young children, children with blond hair or blue eyes, clients with Down's syndrome, children with brain damage, and older adults. Monitor these clients for a fast, irregular pulse, skin dryness, confusion, slurred speech, dry mouth, fever, and unusual drowsiness or weakness.

■ *Intervention.* If the ointment form is to be used for refraction, it should be applied several hours before the vision examination to minimize any impairment of corneal transparency.

Although 2 drops are the recommended dosage by some manufacturers, the conjunctival sac will usually hold only 1 drop. To minimize systemic absorption, the lacrimal duct should be compressed during administration of the drops and for 2 to 3 minutes after administration.

■ *Education.* Instruct clients that the next instillation should be omitted if side effects (dryness of mouth, tachycardia) are present. Alert the client that he or she may be unable to focus on nearby objects during therapy (blurred vision) and will be unusually sensitive to light. Dark glasses should be worn to decrease the photophobia. The eye will be accommodated for distant vision. Because atropine is highly toxic, it should be stored in a safe place out of the reach of children.

■ Evaluation. The expected outcome of anticholinergic ophthalmic therapy is that the client will experience

TABLE 43-7 Adrenergic Ophthalmic Agents

Drug	Duration of Action (hours)	Market Availability	Usual Adult Dosage
epinephrine (Epifrin, Glaucon)	Vasoconstriction: <1 IOP: 12-24	Rx	0.5%-2%: 1 drop once or twice daily
hydroxyamphetamine (Paredrine)	1-3	Rx	1%: 1 or 2 drops for dilation of pupil
naphazoline			
(Allerest, VasoClear)	3-4	OTC	0.012%-0.03%: 1 drop up to 4 times daily
(Albalon, Vasocon)	3-4	Rx	0.1%: 1 drop q3-4h as necessary
oxymetazoline (OcuClear)	4-6	OTC	0.025%: 1 drop q6h as necessary
phenylephrine			
(Ak-Nefrin, Prefin)	0.5-1.5	OTC	0.12%: 1 or 2 drops up to 4 times daily as necessary
(Neo-Synephrine)	1-7	Rx	2.5%, 10%: 1 drop as necessary
tetrahydrozoline (Murine Plus, Visine)	1-4	OTC	0.05%: 1 or 2 drops up to 4 times daily

Information from *Drug Facts and Comparisons.* (2000). St. Louis: Facts and Comparisons; *United States Pharmacopeia Dispensing Information (USP DI): Drug information for the health care professional* (20th ed.). (2000). Rockville, MD: United States Pharmacopeial Convention.
IOP, Reduction in intraocular pressure; Rx, prescription.

cycloplegia. If administered for uveitis, the condition will be alleviated as evidenced by a lack of discomfort, redness, and drainage from the eye.

Adrenergic Agonist Agents

Topical adrenergic agents mimic (direct acting) or potentiate (indirect acting) the action of epinephrine on the dilator muscle of the iris; this results in mydriasis and decreased congestion of the conjunctival blood vessels. The primary adrenergic drugs used in ophthalmology include epinephrine (Epifrin, Glaucon), phenylephrine (Ak-Nefrin, Prefin, Neo-Synephrine), oxymetazoline (OcuClear), hydroxyamphetamine (Paredrine), naphazoline (Allerest, VasoClear), and tetrahydrozoline (Murine Plus, Visine).

Adrenergic drugs applied topically to the eye elicit the following sympathetic responses: vasoconstriction, pupil dilation, an increase in the outflow of aqueous humor, a decrease in aqueous humor formation, and relaxation of the ciliary muscle. Exactly how these effects are produced remains uncertain, but there is some evidence that alpha-adrenergic receptors are present in the outflow mechanism of the eye. When stimulated, they increase outflow of aqueous humor. It has also been shown experimentally that vasoconstriction decreases the rate of aqueous humor formation (Abel, 1995).

Adrenergic drugs are used to treat wide-angle glaucoma and glaucoma secondary to uveitis, to produce mydriasis for ocular examination, and to relieve congestion and hyperemia. Adrenergic drugs are contraindicated in the treatment of narrow-angle glaucoma or abraded cornea because dilation of the pupil will further restrict ocular fluid outflow, which may cause an acute attack of glaucoma. (See Chapter 22 for a discussion of pharmacokinetics of adrenergic agents.)

Serious systemic side effects are unusual; typical side effect include local pain and brow ache. Systemic absorption is a concern, especially in clients with cardiovascular disease, because tachycardia and elevated blood pressure can occur with these agents. Sweating, tremors, and confusion may also occur. As with other ophthalmic drugs, the potential for systemic drug interactions exists if significant absorption occurs.

Apraclonidine (Iopidine) reduces IOP in glaucoma and also in clients after laser trabeculoplasty or iridotomy. This drug is a selective alpha agonist that does not produce any local anesthetic action. The onset of action is usually within 60 minutes, with maximum IOP reduction occurring within 3 to 5 hours. After topical application, apraclonidine is absorbed and may induce systemic side effects/adverse reactions such as stomach pain, diarrhea, vomiting, and dry mouth; ophthalmic side effects include burning, pruritus, dryness, blurred vision, conjunctival blanching, and mydriasis.

Table 43-7 lists adrenergic ophthalmic drugs and their duration of action, market availability, and usual adult dosage.

ANTIINFECTIVE/ ANTIINFLAMMATORY AGENTS

To treat ocular infections, the drug of choice and the required dosage should be determined by laboratory isolation of the offending organism. The initial culture from the infected area is obtained before any ophthalmic agent is applied. However, treatment is not withheld if the time required to make these determinations may cause increased severity of infection and if the type of infection (e.g., most cases of conjunctivitis, which tend to be self-limiting) does not warrant the expense of laboratory analysis.

In general, the prophylactic use of antiinfective/antiinflammatory agents is useless, wasteful, and potentially dangerous because a large proportion of ophthalmic inflammatory diseases are caused by viruses or other agents that are not susceptible to any currently available antiinfective agents (Liesegang, 1999). Systemic medications that can induce ocular side effects need to be considered before an antiinfective or antiinflammatory agent is introduced. See Table 43-2 for drugs that induce ocular side effects.

Most antiinfective agents do not readily penetrate the eye when applied. Some drugs do penetrate the inflamed eye when the blood-aqueous barrier is decreased by injury or inflammation. Topically applied antiinfective agents can cause sensitivity reactions (stinging, itching, angioneurotic edema, urticaria, dermatitis). Clients who are sensitive to one drug may show cross-reactions to chemically related drugs. The topical application of antiinfective agents may also interfere with the normal flora of the eye, which may encourage the growth of other organisms.

Eye infections require prompt treatment to help prevent the spread of infection; severe infections may damage the eye and impair vision. Solutions are preferred for the treatment of eye infections, because ointment bases often tend to interfere with healing.

Antibacterial Agents

Antibiotics

To avoid possible sensitization to systemic antiinfective drugs and to discourage the development of resistant strains of offending organisms, the antibiotic of choice is not given systemically. Instead these agents are administered topically, subconjunctivally, or intrauveally. The selection of an antibiotic for ocular infection is based on (1) clinical experience, (2) the nature and sensitivity of the organisms most commonly causing the condition, (3) the disease itself, (4) the sensitivity and response of the client, and (5) laboratory results. Unfortunately, antibiotic resistance by pathogenic ophthalmic microorganisms is emerging (Garg, Sharma, & Rao, 1999; Goldstein, Kowalski, & Gordon, 1999; Sechi et al., 1999).

Some of the common ocular infections treated with antibiotics include the following:

- *Conjunctivitis:* An acute inflammation of the conjunctiva resulting from a bacterial invasion or viral infection. It is a common sign in severe colds. "Pink eye" is the acute contagious epidemic form of conjunctivitis usually caused by *Haemophilus* organisms. Symptoms include redness and burning of the eye, lacrimation, itching, and at times photophobia. Conjunctivitis is usually self-limiting. The eye should be protected from light.
- *Hordeolum (sty):* An acute localized infection of the eyelash follicles and the glands of the anterior lid margin, which results in the formation of a small abscess or cyst.
- *Chalazion:* Infection of the meibomian (sebaceous) glands of the eyelids. A hard cyst may form from blockage of the ducts.
- *Blepharitis:* Inflammation of the margins of the eyelid resulting from bacterial infection or allergy. Symptoms are crusting, irritation of the eye, and red and edematous lid margins.
- *Keratitis:* Corneal inflammation caused by bacterial infection; herpes simplex keratitis is caused by a viral infection.
- *Uveitis:* Infection of the uveal tract or the vascular layer of the eye, which includes the iris, ciliary body, and choroid.
- *Endophthalmitis:* Inflammation of the inner eye structure caused by bacteria.

Antibiotic ophthalmic preparations include bacitracin, chloramphenicol, ciprofloxacin, erythromycin, gentamicin, norfloxacin, ofloxacin, polymyxin B, and tobramycin. Combination preparations usually contain various combinations of these ingredients and/or neomycin, gramicidin, oxytetracycline, or trimethoprim. Selected antibiotic ophthalmic products are discussed in the following sections.

triple antibiotic ophthalmic ointment (neomycin, polymyxin B sulfate, and bacitracin ophthalmic ointment) [nee oh mye′ sin, pol ee mix′ in, bass i tray′ sin] (Mycitracin, Neosporin)

Bacitracin is rarely used systemically because of its nephrotoxic effects. It is particularly useful in treating surface superficial infections caused by gram-positive bacteria (it inhibits protein synthesis). Bacitracin does penetrate the conjunctiva or the cornea slightly, but in therapeutic amounts it is nonirritating to the eye, is excreted in the nasolacrimal system, and produces no systemic effects.

A broader spectrum of antimicrobial activity is produced when bacitracin is used in combination with other antibiotics than when used alone. Although all three of these agents have been or are available as single ophthalmic drugs, reports of sensitization to the individual drug somewhat limit their usefulness. The combination dosage form provides a bactericidal effect against many gram-positive and gram-negative organisms. It is indicated for the treatment of superficial ocular infections caused by susceptible organisms. A small amount (1 cm) of ointment is usually applied into the conjunctival sac every 3 to 4 hours.

■ Nursing Management

Triple Antibiotic Ophthalmic Therapy

■ **Assessment.** The use of a triple antibiotic is contraindicated if the client has had a previous allergic reaction to the drug. A baseline assessment of the ocular infection is required. A specimen for culture and sensitivity should be obtained before therapy is initiated.

▪ **Nursing Diagnosis.** The client should be assessed for the following nursing diagnosis/collaborative problem: risk for injury related to the ineffectiveness of the drug; and the potential complication of a hypersensitivity response (burning, itching, redness, and swelling not present before therapy).

▪ **Implementation**

▪ ***Monitoring.*** The status of the infected eye(s) should be monitored regarding pain, redness, swelling, and drainage.

▪ ***Intervention.*** The presence of exudate interferes with the effectiveness of the medication; it should be removed before the medication is applied. A thin strip (approximately 1 cm) of ointment is placed into the conjunctival sac. Be careful not to touch the tip of the tube to the surface of the eye. Keep ophthalmic ointments exclusive for each client.

▪ ***Education.*** Instruct the client and caregiver in the application of the ointment. Alert them to symptoms of hypersensitivity that need to be reported to the prescriber.

▪ **Evaluation.** The expected outcome is that the client's ocular infection will be resolved as evidenced by the absence of pain, redness, swelling, and drainage.

chloramphenicol [klor am fen′ i kole] (Chloroptic)

Chloramphenicol is a bacteriostatic that prevents peptide bond formation and protein synthesis in a wide variety of gram-positive and gram-negative organisms. Thus it is an extremely useful drug for superficial intraocular infections.

Side effects are usually rare. Burning and stinging on instillation have been reported. Irreversible aplastic anemia has not been reported with this form of chloramphenicol, although it would be prudent to monitor for blood dyscrasias.

In treating adults, a thin strip of ointment (1% solution) is applied into the conjunctival sac every 3 hours (more often if necessary). The adult dosage of the solution is 1 drop into the conjunctival sac every 3 hours.

The nursing management is the same as for triple antibiotic ophthalmic therapy. In addition, avoid prolonged (more than 3 days) or frequent use. Chloramphenicol has been implicated in the development of aplastic anemia after prolonged use; monitor CBCs. Monitor the client for pallor, sore throat and fever, unusual bleeding or bruising, and unusual tiredness, which may indicate irreversible bone marrow depression associated with aplastic anemia. See Table 43-1 for the systemic effects of a variety of ophthalmic agents.

erythromycin [er ith roe mye′ sin] (Ilotycin)

Erythromycin ophthalmic ointment is a bacteriostatic agent, but it may be bactericidal in high concentrations against very susceptible organisms. It is indicated for the treatment of neonatal conjunctivitis caused by *Chlamydia trachomatis* and for the prevention of ophthalmia neonatorum (against *Neisseria gonorrhoeae* or *C. trachomatis*) and other ocular infections caused by susceptible organisms.

Eye irritation not present before therapy is rarely reported with this drug. For adults and children with ocular infections, a thin ointment strip is applied into the conjunctival sac daily, or more often (up to 6 times daily) if necessary. To prevent ophthalmia neonatorum, the ointment should not be flushed from the eye.

Nursing management is the same as for triple antibiotic ophthalmic therapy. However, when used for the prevention of neonatal conjunctivitis, instillation of the ointment is delayed until an hour or so after birth so that eye contact and parent bonding are enhanced.

Aminoglycosides

gentamicin [jen ta mye′ sin] (Garamycin, Genoptic)

Gentamicin is effective against a wide variety of gram-negative and gram-positive organisms. It is particularly useful against *Pseudomonas, Proteus,* and *Klebsiella* organisms and *Escherichia coli,* as well as staphylococci and streptococci that have developed a resistance to other antibiotics. It is applied as an ointment two or three times daily; with the solution, 1 drop is applied every 4 hours.

The nursing management is the same as for triple antibiotic ophthalmic therapy.

tobramycin [toe bra mye′ sin] (Tobrex)

This water-soluble aminoglycoside is used topically on a wide variety of gram-positive and gram-negative external ophthalmic pathogens and is particularly valuable for treating gentamicin-resistant infections.

Adverse reactions include ocular toxicity and hypersensitivity, including lid itching, swelling, and conjunctival erythema. When topical aminoglycosides are used concurrently with systemic aminoglycosides, total serum concentration is affected and should be monitored. Systemic toxicity from absorption may occur from excessive use.

The dosage for mild to moderate infection is 1 drop in the affected eye every 4 hours.

The nursing management is the same as for triple antibiotic ophthalmic therapy.

Sulfonamides

sulfacetamide [sul fa see′ ta mide] (Bleph-10, Sulamyd)
sulfisoxazole [sul fi sox′ a zole] (Gantrisin)

Ophthalmic bacteriostatic antiinfective agents block the synthesis of folic acid in susceptible bacterial organisms. The action of sulfonamides is reduced by the presence of paraaminobenzoic acid (PABA) or its derivatives, procaine and tetracaine, and also by the presence of purulent drainage or exudate (purulent matter contains PABA). Therefore lid exudate should be removed before the drugs are instilled.

Because the activity of sulfacetamide may be inhibited by the concurrent administration of ophthalmic anesthetics, such drugs are applied 30 to 60 minutes apart. Sulfonamides are physically incompatible with thimerosal and silver preparations.

Before administration, the client should check to see that the solution has not darkened in color; if so, it is discarded. Solutions are instilled at a rate of 1 drop every 1 to 3 hours during the day, with increased time intervals during the night. Instillation of the drops may cause some mild pain and discomfort.

The nursing management is the same as for triple antibiotic ophthalmic therapy.

Antifungal Agents

natamycin [na ta mye′ sin] (Natacyn)

Natamycin ophthalmic suspension is used to treat fungal blepharitis, conjunctivitis, and keratitis. It produces altered membrane permeability by binding to steroids in the cell membrane of the fungus; this causes a loss of the cellular constituents. Because natamycin is retained mainly in the conjunctival area, significant drug levels in the ocular fluids are not achieved. It is not systemically absorbed. Natamycin may cause irritation of the eye.

For fungal keratitis, 1 drop of the 5% solution is instilled into the conjunctival sac at 1- to 2-hour intervals initially for 3 or 4 days, after which the solution is instilled 6 to 8 times daily. For fungal blepharitis and conjunctivitis, 1 drop 4 to 6 times daily is usually adequate.

The nursing management is the same as for triple antibiotic ophthalmic therapy.

Antiviral Agents

Antiviral ophthalmic preparations include idoxuridine, trifluridine, and vidarabine.

idoxuridine [eye dox yoor′ i deen] (Stoxil, Herplex)

Idoxuridine resembles thymidine, a substance necessary for viral DNA; thus idoxuridine replaces thymidine and inhibits the replication of viral DNA. It is indicated for the treatment of herpes simplex virus keratitis.

Less common side effects/adverse reactions include hypersensitivity (eye redness, pruritus, irritation), visual disturbance, and photosensitivity not present before therapy.

The adult dosage of the idoxuridine solution for the treatment of herpes simplex virus keratitis is 1 drop hourly during the waking hours and every 2 hours during the night. With the ointment, apply a thin strip every 4 hours (five times daily) during the waking hours.

Nursing management is the same as for triple antibiotic ophthalmic therapy. Burning of the eye after application or failure to respond may indicate the need for a fresh solution. Store in a cool place or refrigerate.

trifluridine [trye flure′ i deen] (Viroptic)

The mechanism of action of and indications for trifluridine are the same as those for idoxuridine. Trifluridine is also used to treat herpes simplex virus keratoconjunctivitis.

A commonly reported side effect is burning or stinging on application. Rare side effects/adverse reactions include increased IOP, blurred vision, and hypersensitivity reaction as evidenced by redness, swelling, or eye irritation not present before therapy.

The usual adult dosage is 1 drop (1% solution) into the conjunctival sac every 2 hours during the waking hours. The maximum daily dose is 9 drops. Therapy is continued until the cornea has recovered; the dosage is then reduced to 1 drop every 4 hours during the waking hours (minimum of 5 drops per day) for 1 week.

Nursing management is the same as for triple antibiotic ophthalmic therapy. In addition, the ophthalmic solution is refrigerated.

vidarabine [vye dare′ a been] (Vira-A)

The antiviral mechanism of action is due to the conversion of vidarabine to intracellular substances that inhibit viral DNA polymerase or other enzymes specific to virus DNA. It is indicated for the treatment of herpes simplex virus keratitis and keratoconjunctivitis. Systemic absorption is not expected after ocular administration.

The side effects/adverse reactions of vidarabine include increased tear flow and a sensation that something is in the eye. The prescriber should be contacted if there is an occurrence of photosensitivity, redness, eye swelling, or increased eye irritation not present before treatment.

The usual adult dosage is a thin strip of ointment applied into the conjunctival sac every 3 hours five times daily. Therapy is continued until the cornea is completely reepithelialized; the dosage is then decreased to twice daily for 7 to 10 days.

Nursing management is the same as for triple antibiotic ophthalmic therapy.

Antiseptics

Many antiseptics that were used to treat surface infections of the eye before the advent of antibiotics are now obsolete. Inorganic mercuric salts such as yellow mercuric oxide ophthalmic ointment (1% to 2%), thimerosal (Merthiolate), and ammoniated mercury formerly served as bacteriostatic agents. They are seldom used today because they do not completely sterilize, spores are resistant to them, and they are irritating to the eye.

silver nitrate

Silver nitrate is no longer commonly used to prevent neonatal conjunctivitis because it does not protect against chlamydial infection and can cause chemical conjunctivitis. Canadian hospitals have not recommended its use since 1985. When used, 2 drops of a solution of 1% silver nitrate are instilled into each eye immediately after birth as prophylaxis against gonorrheal ophthalmia neonatorum. Gonococci are particularly susceptible to silver salts. Liberated silver ions precipitate bacterial proteins.

Silver nitrate ophthalmic solution is available in collapsible capsules that contain approximately 5 drops of a 1% solution. The solution should be in contact with the conjunctival sac for not less than 30 seconds to produce a mild chemical conjunctivitis. The American Academy of Pediatrics does not recommend irrigation of the eyes following the instillation of silver nitrate.

Corticosteroids

Many corticosteroids are available as topical solutions, suspensions, or ointments for ophthalmic use. These include betamethasone (Betnesol), dexamethasone (Maxidex, Decadron), fluorometholone (FML S.O.P., FML), hydrocortisone (Cortamed ♣), medrysone (HMS Liquifilm]) and prednisolone (Pred-Forte, Predair-A). These drugs are available in varying strengths and in combination with various antibiotics or mydriatics. They are indicated for the treatment of allergic and inflammatory ophthalmic disorders of the conjunctiva, cornea, and anterior segment of the eye.

Rare side effects/adverse reactions include burning or lacrimation. Blurred vision or visual disturbances, eye pain, headaches, ptosis, or enlarged pupils should be reported to the prescriber. For dosage and administration, refer to the *United States Pharmacopeia Dispensing Information (USP DI)* or to current package inserts.

▪ Nursing Management

Ophthalmic Corticosteroid Therapy

▪ **Assessment.** Ophthalmic corticosteroid therapy is not used for pyogenic (pus-producing) inflammations of the eye because corticosteroids decrease defense mechanisms and reduce resistance to pathogenic organisms. Corticosteroid therapy is not recommended for minor corneal abrasions. Steroids may actually increase ocular susceptibility to fungal, viral, or tuberculosis infection. Cataracts and chronic open-angle glaucoma may be worsened. When steroids are used for various eye conditions, they should be used for a limited time only, and the eye should be checked for increased IOP. Corticosteroids may diminish the resistance to infection and may also mask the allergic reactions or hypersensitivity reactions to other drugs. A baseline assessment of the client's ocular inflammation and vision should be noted.

▪ **Nursing Diagnosis.** The client should be assessed for the following nursing diagnoses/collaborative problems: risk for injury related to ineffectiveness of the drug; impaired comfort (burning, stinging, or watering of the eyes); and the potential complications of hypersensitivity and the long-term effects of the drug (open-end glaucoma, optic nerve damage, cataracts, defects in vision).

▪ **Implementation**

▪ ***Monitoring.*** Periodic tonometry and slit-lamp examinations should be performed to monitor client progress. The eye should be assessed for infection at periodic intervals; infections are reported to the prescriber.

▪ ***Intervention.*** The glucocorticoids used in ophthalmology may be applied topically, injected into the conjunctiva, or given systemically to diminish leukocyte infiltration where inflammation exists.

▪ ***Education.*** Alert the client that temporary stinging may occur after application. For adequate dispersion of the active ingredients, instruct the client to shake the ophthalmic suspensions well before use. Contact lenses should not be used during and for some time after corticosteroid therapy because of the risk of infection. Caution the client not to stop taking the medication without consulting the prescriber. The return of inflammation secondary to the abrupt cessation of ophthalmic steroid administration may be overcome by using dose-frequency reduction (from every 3 hours, to every 6 hours, to 3 times daily, to twice daily, to once daily, and to every other day) or by decreasing the percentage strengths and using the dose-frequency reduction schedule.

▪ **Evaluation.** The expected outcome of ophthalmic corticosteroid therapy is that the client's inflammation will be resolved without the occurrence of infection.

TOPICAL ANESTHETIC AGENTS

Local anesthetics stabilize neuronal membranes so they become less permeable to ions; this prevents the initiation and transmission of nerve impulses. It is theorized that sodium ion permeability is limited by these agents.

Local anesthetics are used to prevent pain during surgical procedures (removal of sutures and foreign bodies) and tonometry examinations. The local anesthetics have a rapid onset (within 20 seconds) and last for 15 to 20 minutes.

proparacaine [proe par′ a kane] (Ophthaine, Ophthetic)

Proparacaine is similar to tetracaine. A 0.5% solution is administered by topical instillation. Anesthesia is produced within 20 seconds and lasts for 15 minutes. It is relatively free from the burning and discomfort of other anesthetics, but it is highly toxic if it enters the systemic circulation.

Side effects/adverse reactions include allergic contact dermatitis, softening and erosion of the corneal epithelium, pupillary dilation, cycloplegia, conjunctival congestion and hemorrhage, stromal edema, and delayed corneal healing after photorefractive keratectomy.

tetracaine [tet′ ra kane] (Pontocaine)

Tetracaine is a widely used anesthetic used topically for rapid, brief, superficial anesthesia. One to two drops of a 0.5% solution will produce anesthesia within 30 seconds;

the client may feel a burning or stinging sensation. The anesthetic effect lasts for 10 to 15 minutes. Tetracaine can cause epithelial damage and systemic toxicity and therefore is not recommended for prolonged home use by clients. It is physically incompatible with the mercury or silver salts often found in ophthalmic products.

■ Nursing Management
Topical Anesthetic Agents

■ Assessment. Question the client about past experiences with anesthetics to determine if a hypersensitivity reaction has occurred. Note the condition of the eye and vision status as a baseline assessment.

■ Nursing Diagnosis. The client receiving topical anesthetic agents should be assessed for the following nursing diagnoses/collaborative problems: impaired comfort related to ineffectiveness of the drug; and the potential complications of hypersensitivity, loss of sensation in the eye (delayed wound healing, perforation of the cornea, accidental trauma), and long-term effects of the drugs (permanent corneal opacification).

■ Implementation

■ *Monitoring.* Clients receiving local anesthetics that produce systemic toxicity should be monitored for central nervous system (CNS) excitation (blurred vision, dizziness, trembling, nervousness, restlessness) followed by CNS depression (drowsiness, dyspnea) and cardiovascular depression (dysrhythmias). The appearance of the eye and the status of vision should also be monitored.

■ *Intervention.* The practice of repeatedly applying a topical anesthetic agent to the eye after removing a foreign body is to be condemned. Besides delaying wound healing, this action can produce sensitivity, permanent corneal opacification, vision loss, or perforation of the cornea.

Patching the anesthetized eye is prudent because the blink reflex is lost, and the cornea needs to be protected from debris and irritants.

■ *Education.* To prevent damage to the eye, the client should be instructed not to touch or rub the eye until the anesthesia has worn off.

■ Evaluation. The expected outcome of topical ophthalmic anesthetic agent therapy is that the client will experience no discomfort and experience no adverse reactions or injuries.

OTHER OPHTHALMIC PREPARATIONS

Artificial Tear Solutions and Lubricants

Lubricants or artificial tears are used to provide moisture and lubrication for diseases in which tear production is deficient, to lubricate artificial eyes and moisten contact lenses, to remove debris, and to protect the cornea during procedures on the eye. These agents are also incorporated into ophthalmic preparations to prolong the contact time of topically applied drugs.

These products have a balanced salt solution (equivalent to 0.9% sodium chloride), buffers to adjust pH, highly viscous agents (methylcellulose, propylene glycol, and others) to extend contact time with the eye, and preservatives to maintain sterility. These products are usually administered three or four times daily.

An artificial tear insert (Lacrisert) was devised to extend the effect of this preparation. It is usually inserted daily or at most twice daily for selected clients.

Ointment preparations are also used as ocular lubricants. They help to protect the eye, such as during and after eye surgery, and to lubricate the eye. They are particularly valuable for clients who have an impaired blink reflex and for nighttime use. Examples include Lacri-Lube, Duratears, and Hypo Tears.

Antiallergic Agents

Antiallergic ophthalmic agents available include cromolyn, ketotifen fumarate, levocabastine, and lodoxamide tromethamine.

cromolyn sodium [kroe′ moe lin] (Opticrom)

Cromolyn sodium inhibits the degranulation of sensitized mast cells that occurs after exposure to a specific antigen. This inhibition of mast cell release prevents the mediators of inflammation (histamine and slow-releasing substance of anaphylaxis) from producing their characteristic effects. This drug is used for allergic eye disorders (vernal and allergic keratoconjunctivitis, papillary conjunctivitis, keratitis) that have symptoms of itching, tearing, redness, and discharge.

The side effects/adverse reactions of cromolyn sodium include a stinging and burning sensation in the eyes. Concomitant corticosteroids may be necessary. In adults and children over 4 years of age, instill 1 drop in each affected eye four to six times daily at regular intervals.

■ Nursing Management
Cromolyn Sodium Therapy

■ Assessment. Assess the client for itching, tearing, redness, and discharge from the eyes. Determine the client's sensitivity to the drug.

■ Nursing Diagnosis. The client receiving cromolyn sodium should be assessed for the following nursing diagnoses/collaborative problems: risk for injury related to the ineffectiveness of the drug; impaired comfort (burning, stinging, sensation of foreign body); and the potential complications of hypersensitivity or chemosis (severe swelling of the conjunctiva).

■ Implementation

■ *Monitoring.* Note that the signs and symptoms of relief will appear within days but that treatment may be required at regular intervals for as long as 6 weeks.

■ *Intervention.* Refrigerate this drug, keep it out of direct sunlight, and discard any unused portion after 4 weeks.

■ *Education.* Although manufacturers recommend not wearing soft contact lenses while using cromolyn ophthalmic solution, medical experts believe this precaution is unnecessary in most instances (*USP DI*, 2000). Have the client check with the prescriber about contact lens use before using the drug.

■ **Evaluation.** The expected outcome of cromolyn sodium is that client's eye will not evidence an allergic reaction; itching, tearing, redness, and discharge will not be present.

ketotifen fumarate [kee toe ti′ fen] (Zaditor)

Ketotifen fumarate (Zaditor) is a histamine antagonist and mast cell stabilizer used to treat allergic conjunctivitis. The usual adult dosage is 1 drop in the affected eye(s) every 8 to 12 hours.

levocabastine [lev oe ka bas′ teen] (Livostin)

Levocabastine is a topical antihistamine indicated for allergic conjunctivitis. The side effects are mild and consist of burning, stinging, visual alterations, eye pain, red eyes, and headaches. The usual adult dosage is 1 drop in the eyes four times daily.

The nursing management is the same as for cromolyn sodium. In addition, shake the medication well before using.

lodoxamide [loe dox′ a myde] (Alomide)

Lodoxamide ophthalmic, an antiallergic and mast cell stabilizer, is used for the treatment of vernal conjunctivitis, vernal keratitis, and several other eye disorders. Lodoxamide inhibits Type I immediate hypersensitivity reactions by interfering with histamine release, and it inhibits the release of SRS-A and eosinophil chemotaxis.

The side effects/adverse reactions of lodoxamide include a transient burning of the eye. Less commonly reported effects are blurred vision, pruritus of the eye, tearing, or eye irritation.

The usual dosage for adults and children 2 years and older is 1 drop in each affected eye four times daily for up to 3 months (*Drug Facts and Comparisons*, 2000).

The nursing management is the same as for cromolyn sodium therapy.

Diagnostic Aids

fluorescein [flure′ e seen] (Fluorescite, Fluor-I-Strip)

Fluorescein is a nontoxic, water-soluble dye that is used as a diagnostic aid. When applied to the cornea, corneal lesions or ulcers are stained a bright green, and foreign bodies appear to be surrounded by a green ring. These effects permit the location of foreign bodies and corneal epithelial defects caused by injury or infection.

Fluorescein dye is also used in fitting hard contact lenses. Areas that lack fluorescein-stained tears will appear black under ultraviolet light, indicating that the contact lens is touching the cornea at those areas. Fluorescein is used in retinal photography to determine retinal vascular status and to identify defects in the retinal pigment epithelium. In addition, it may be used to test the patency of the lacrimal apparatus; if the dye appears in the nasal secretions after being instilled into the eye, the nasolacrimal drainage system is open.

A fluorescein injection is used in ophthalmic angiography to examine the fundus, vasculature of the iris, and aqueous flow; to make a differential diagnosis of cancerous and noncancerous tumors; and to determine the time for circulation in the eye. Side effects/adverse reactions after injection include nausea, headache, abdominal distress, vomiting, hypotension, hypersensitivity reactions, and anaphylaxis.

If a topical solution is being used to detect foreign bodies and corneal abrasions, instill 1 or 2 drops of the 2% solution. Check a current drug reference for instructions regarding strip application and injection.

Enzyme Preparation

chymotrypsin [kye moe trip′ sin] (Catarase)

Chymotrypsin, a proteolytic enzyme, is used in selected cases to facilitate cataract extraction. It is injected behind the iris and into the posterior chamber to dissolve the filaments or zonules that hold the lens; this facilitates intracapsular lens extraction. This effect is usually obtained in 5 to 15 minutes, with total lysis of the entire zonular membrane reported within 30 minutes. Side effects/adverse reactions include a transient postoperative glaucoma that lasts approximately 1 week; this effect can be relieved by the use of pilocarpine.

Hyperosmolar Preparation

sodium chloride (ointment: Muro-128, solution: Adsorbonac)

The 5% ointment and 2% or 5% solution of sodium chloride are used to reduce the corneal edema that occurs in certain corneal dystrophies and after cataract extraction. The dosage is 1 to 2 drops or a small amount of the ointment in the affected eye(s) every 3 to 4 hours as directed.

Nonsteroidal Antiinflammatory Agents

Flurbiprofen, suprofen, diclofenac, and ketorolac tromethamine are available topically for ophthalmic use. These agents are nonsteroidal antiinflammatory drugs (NSAIDs). They have the following indications:

- flurbiprofen [flure bi′ proe fen] (Ocufen) and suprofen [sue′ proe fen] (Profenal) are used to inhibit intraoperative miosis.
- diclofenac [dye kloe′ fen ak] (Voltaren) is used to treat postoperative inflammation after a cataract extraction.

- ketorolac [kee toe' role ak] (Acular) is used to treat conjunctivitis and seasonal allergic ophthalmic pruritus.

These agents may produce a systemic effect if absorbed. Because they have the potential to cause increased bleeding, monitor their use closely in clients who are known to have bleeding tendencies.

The most commonly reported side effect is transient burning or stinging on application. Other minor symptoms of ocular irritation have also been reported, such as itching, redness, discomfort, allergic reaction. For dosing recommendations, refer to a current package insert or drug reference.

For the nursing management of nonsteroidal antiinflammatory agents, see Nursing Management: Drugs Affecting the Eye, p. 791. In addition, it should be determined if the client has a sensitivity to aspirin, phenylacetic acid derivatives, such as diclofenac, or other ophthalmic or systemic NSAIDs.

Irrigating Solutions

Sterile isotonic external irrigating solutions are used in tonometry, fluorescein procedures, and the removal of foreign material. They are also used to cleanse and soothe the eyes of clients who wear hard contact lenses. These external products do not require a prescription and are available as drops, irrigations, and eyewashes. Examples of irrigating solutions include Blinx, Dacriose, Eye Stream, and Eye Wash.

SUMMARY

Although there are a myriad of ophthalmic preparations, the drugs used to treat eye disorders can be divided into three major groups: the antiglaucoma agents, the mydriatics and cycloplegics, and the antiinfective/antiinflammatory agents. Antiglaucoma agents may be miotics. These cause pupillary constriction either by (1) direct action (cholinergic) to minimize the effects of acetylcholine at autonomic synapses or the neuroeffector junction of the parasympathetic nervous system, or (2) indirect action (anticholinesterase), inactivating the enzyme cholinesterase by preventing hydrolysis of acetylcholine. Antiglaucoma drugs may also be sympathomimetic agents that decrease the production of aqueous humor (beta-adrenergic effect) and increase its outflow (alpha-adrenergic effect). Beta-adrenergic blocking agents, carbonic anhydrase inhibitor agents, and osmotic agents are also used in the treatment of glaucoma.

Mydriatic and cycloplegic agents used for ophthalmic disorders are topically applied autonomic drugs that cause dilation of the pupils (mydriasis) and paralysis of accommodation (cycloplegia). In addition to being used for the specific treatment of ophthalmic disorders, they are also used during eye examinations and in preparation of the client for intraocular surgery.

Antiinfective/antiinflammatory agents used in the treatment of ocular infections may be antibacterial agents, antifungal agents, or antiviral agents, antiallergics, corticosteroids, and NSAIDs.

The role of the nurse in the clinical management of the client receiving ophthalmic drugs focuses on safe administration and the preparation of the client for the self-administration of these drugs.

Critical Thinking Questions

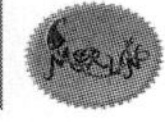

1. How would the teaching plan for the self-administration of ophthalmic agents vary between antiglaucoma agents, antiinfective agents, and corticosteroids?
2. Steve Cameron has had his ophthalmic medication changed from an optic solution to an optic ointment. What instruction will you provide Mr. Cameron to prepare him for safe self-administration of the new form of medication?

Collaborative Learning Activities

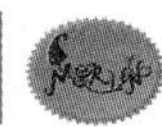

For Collaborative Learning Activities, go to mosby.com/MERLIN/McKenry/.

CASE STUDY

For a Case Study that will help ensure mastery of this chapter content, go to mosby.com/MERLIN/McKenry/.

BIBLIOGRAPHY

Abel, S.R. (1995). Eye disorders. In L.Y Young & M.A. Koda-Kimble (Eds.), *Applied therapeutics: The clinical use of drugs* (6th ed.). Vancouver, WA: Applied Therapeutics.

American Hospital Formulary Service. (1999). *AHFS drug information '99*. Bethesda, MD: American Society of Hospital Pharmacists.

Anderson, K.N., Anderson, L.E., & Glanze, W.D. (Eds.) (1998). *Mosby's medical, nursing, & allied health dictionary* (5th ed.). St. Louis: Mosby.

DiPiro, J.T., Talbert, R.L., Yee, G.C., Matzke, G.R., Wells, B.G., & Posey, L.M. (1997). *Pharmacotherapy: A pathophysiologic approach* (3rd ed.). Norwalk, CT: Appleton & Lange.

Drug Facts and Comparisons. (2000). St. Louis: Facts and Comparisons.

Eye drops and infection: The solution may be the problem. (1992). *Emergency Medicine, 24*(4):142.

Garg, P., Sharma, S., & Rao, G.N. (1999). Ciprofloxacin-resistant *Pseudomonas* keratitis. *Ophthalmology, 106*(7):1319-1323.

Goldstein, M.H., Kowalski, R.P., & Gordon, Y.J. (1999). Emerging fluoroquinolone resistance in bacterial keratitis: A 5-year review. *Ophthalmology, 106*(7):1313-1318.

Hayreh, S.S., Podhajsky, P., & Zimmerman, M.B. (1999). Beta-blocker eyedrops and nocturnal arterial hypotension. *American Journal of Ophthalmology, 128*(3):301-309.

Kent, A.R., Vroman, D.T., Thomas, T.J., Hebert, R.L., & Crosson, C.E. (1999). Interaction of pilocarpine with latanoprost in patients with glaucoma and ocular hypertension. *Journal of Glaucoma,* 8(4):257-262.

Liesegang, T.J. (1999). Perioperative antibiotic prophylaxis in cataract surgery. *Cornea* 18(4), 383-402.

Lowdermilk, D.L., Perry, S.E., & Bobak, I.M. (2000). *Maternity and women's health care* (7th ed.). St. Louis: Mosby.

Moreira L.B., Kasetsuwan N., Sanchez D., Shah S.S., LaBree L., & McDonnell P.J. (1999). Toxicity of topical anesthetic agents to human keratocytes in vivo. *Journal of Cataract Refractive Surgery,* 25(7), 975-980.

Moroi, S.E. & Lichter, P.R. (1996). Ocular pharmacology. In J.G. Hardman & L.E. Limbird (Eds.), *Goodman & Gilman's The pharmacological basis of therapeutics* (9th ed.). New York: McGraw-Hill.

O'Boyle, J.E. & Enzenaur, R.W. (1992). "Super glue" in the eye. *Emergency Medicine,* 24(6), 59-60, 62.

Schein, O.D., Hibberd, P.L., Stark, T., Baker, A.S., & Kenyon, K.R. (1992). Microbial contamination of in-use ocular medications. *Archives of Opthalmology,* 110(1), 82-85.

Sechi L.A., Pinna A., Pusceddu C., Fadda G., Carta F., & Zanetti S. (1999). Molecular characterization and antibiotic susceptibilities of ocular isolates of *Staphylococcus epidermis. Journal of Clinical Microbiology,* 37(9), 3031-3033.

United States Pharmacopeia Dispensing Information (USP DI): Drug information for the health care professional (20th ed.). (2000). Rockville, MD: United States Pharmacopeial Convention.

44 Overview of the Ear

Chapter Focus

Disorders of the ear can be painful and impair the client's ability to hear and maintain balance. Pharmacologic interventions for the ear are somewhat limited. However, many systemic drugs have ototoxic effects. To appropriately assess and care for clients with ear disorders, the nurse needs to have a thorough understanding of the anatomy and physiology of the ear.

Learning Objectives

1. Differentiate between the external, middle, and inner ear.
2. Name the three bones of the inner ear.
3. Describe the function of the eustachian tube.
4. List common ear disorders.

Key Terms

auditory ossicles, p. 812
cochlea, p. 812
eustachian tube, p. 812
external ear, p. 812
inner ear, p. 812
middle ear, p. 812
otitis media, p. 812
tympanic membrane, p. 812

ANATOMY AND PHYSIOLOGY

The ear consists of three sections or parts: external ear, middle ear, and inner ear (Figure 44-1). The **external ear** has two divisions, the outer ear (or pinna) and the external auditory canal. The external auditory canal leads to the eardrum (or **tympanic membrane**), which is a thin, transparent partition of tissue between the auditory canal and the middle ear. The function of the external ear is to receive and transmit auditory sounds to the eardrum. The tympanic membrane protects the middle ear from foreign substances and transmits sound to the bones of the middle ear.

The **middle ear** is an air-filled cavity in the temporal bone that contains three small bones called the **auditory ossicles.** The auditory ossicles consist of the malleus (hammer), incus (anvil), and stapes (stirrup). The tip of the malleus is attached to the surface of the tympanic membrane. Its head is attached to the incus, which in turn is attached to the stapes. The ossicles amplify and transmit sound waves to the inner ear.

The middle ear is also directly connected to the nasopharynx by the eustachian (auditory) tube. The **eustachian tube** is usually collapsed except during swallowing, chewing, yawning, or jaw movements. This tube joins the nasopharynx and the tympanic cavity, which allows for the equalization of air pressure in the inner ear with atmospheric pressure to prevent the tympanic membrane from rupturing. Pressure changes on airline flights are relieved by the action of the eustachian tube when the individual chews gum, yawns, or deliberately swallows.

The **inner ear** is the complex structure of the ear that communicates directly with the acoustic nerve, which transmits sound vibrations from the middle ear. The inner ear, also referred to as the labyrinth because of its series of canals, has two main divisions: the bony labyrinth and the membranous labyrinth. The bony labyrinth consists of the vestibule, cochlea, and semicircular canals, and the membranous labyrinth consists of a series of sacs and tubes within the bony labyrinth. The **cochlea** is the primary organ of hearing; fibers of the cochlear division of the acoustic nerve pass through this organ. The vestibular apparatus is necessary for maintaining equilibrium and balance (see Figure 44-1).

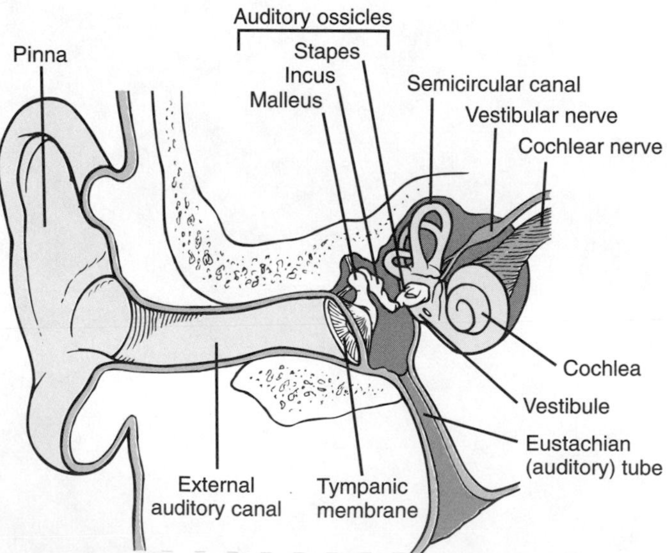

Figure 44-1 Anatomy of the ear.

COMMON EAR DISORDERS

The most common ear disorders include infections of the ear (bacterial or fungal), earwax accumulation, and various other painful or distressing conditions. Many ear disorders are minor and are easily treated or self-limiting. Persistent pain or ear problems should be professionally evaluated, because some untreated disorders can lead to hearing loss.

External ear disorders usually include trauma, such as lacerations or scrapes to the skin. These conditions are often minor and heal with time. If the injury results in bleeding and perhaps a hematoma, a referral to a primary health care provider is necessary. Localized infections of the hair follicles may result in boils. Clients with recurring boils and small boils that do not respond to good hygiene and topical compresses should be referred to a provider for evaluation and possible treatment with systemic antibiotics.

Dermatitis of the ear, itching, local redness, weeping, or drainage are also reported. Such conditions must be individually evaluated, because the causes can vary from inflammation induced by seborrhea, psoriasis, or contact dermatitis to head trauma that produces ear discharge. Self-medication should be discouraged when infection is suspected, when there are known injuries to the ear, or whenever drainage, pain, and dizziness are present.

Middle ear disorders are not to be treated with over-the-counter medications. The most commonly reported problem is middle ear inflammation, or **otitis media.** This condition occurs most often in children, but chronic otitis media may be caused in adults by a nasopharyngeal tumor. Pain, fever, malaise, pressure, a sensation of fullness in the ear, and hearing loss are common symptoms. Clients with such conditions should be treated promptly by a prescriber. Acute tympanic membrane perforation from foreign objects or from water sports (e.g., diving or water skiing) will result in a multitude of symptoms if left untreated. Pain at the time of injury that subsides, diminished hearing acuity, tinnitus, nausea, vertigo, and otitis media or mastoiditis may be noted. An examination by a physician is vital when a perforated tympanic membrane is suspected.

Loss of hearing, especially a unilateral hearing loss, may result from a viral infection of the inner ear. Genetic diseases or slowly progressive diseases such as otosclerosis or Meniere's disease may cause hearing deficits. Untreated external and middle ear infections may also affect hearing and the functioning of the inner ear.

The nurse also needs to be aware of drugs that include ototoxicity as an adverse reaction; this reaction results in impaired hearing for the client (see Chapter 45).

SUMMARY

Pharmacologic interventions for the ear are limited. To appropriately assess and care for clients receiving otic agents, the nurse needs to have a thorough understanding of the anatomy and physiology of the ear.

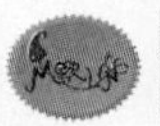

Critical Thinking Questions

1. It is not uncommon to hear infants begin to cry when airplanes begin their descent and cabin pressure changes. Why does this occur, and what action would you recommend to caregivers to minimize this response?
2. Mr. Jones worked with heavy equipment at construction sites for a number of years before regulations of the Occupational Safety and Health Administration required ear protection. He admits to having difficulty hearing. Why do you think this has happened?
3. Mrs. Harris, 84 years of age, has come to the emergency department with a broken arm from a fall in her home. She states having increasing problems maintaining her balance. Why might this be so?

Collaborative Learning Activities

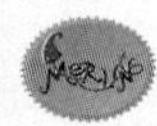

For Collaborative Learning Activities, go to mosby.com/MERLIN/McKenry/.

BIBLIOGRAPHY

Anderson, K.N., Anderson, L.E., & Glanze, W.D. (Eds.). (1998). *Mosby's medical, nursing, & allied health dictionary* (5th ed.). St. Louis: Mosby.

McCance, K.L. & Huether, S.E. (1998). *Pathophysiology: The biologic basis for disease in adults and children.* (3rd ed.). St. Louis: Mosby.

Thibodeau, G.A. & Patton, K.T. (1999). *Anatomy and physiology* (4th ed.). St. Louis: Mosby.

45 Drugs Affecting the Ear

Chapter Focus

Persons with ear disorders may experience impaired communication related to hearing loss, or they may experience difficulty with balance and vertigo. Otic drugs may be prescribed for ear disorders; however, systemic drugs prescribed for a variety of diagnoses may result in ototoxicity, causing a loss of both hearing and balance. The nurse needs to be concerned about the client's comfort, auditory perception, and risk of injury related to vestibular dysfunction; the nurse also needs to be knowledgeable about drugs that affect the ear in order to provide client instruction for effective self-management of the therapeutic drug regimen.

Learning Objectives

1. List the drugs commonly used to treat ear infections.
2. Discuss the various preparations used to treat ear ailments.
3. List five drugs reported to cause ototoxicity.
4. Implement the nursing management of the client receiving drugs that affect the ear.

Key Terms

cerumen, p. 815
ototoxicity, p. 816
tinnitus, p. 816
vertigo, p. 816

Disorders and infections of the external ear canal are treated with antibiotic solutions, corticosteroids, and miscellaneous preparations such as wax emulsifiers, antibacterials, antifungals, local anesthetics, antiinflammatory agents, and local analgesic–type preparations. The potent systemic medications that may adversely affect the client's hearing and/or balance are also reviewed in this chapter.

ANTIBIOTIC EAR PREPARATIONS

Antibiotic ear preparations are used as topical agents to treat infections of the external auditory canal surface. Systemic antibiotics are indicated for serious inner ear infections.

chloramphenicol [klor am fen′ a kole] (Chloromycetin Otic)

Chloramphenicol is a broad-spectrum antibiotic (bacteriostatic) solution used to treat external ear infections caused by *Staphylococcus aureus, Escherichia coli, Pseudomonas aeruginosa, Enterobacter aerogenes, Haemophilus influenzae,* and other susceptible organisms.

The possible side effects produced by chloramphenicol are burning, redness, rash, swelling, or other signs of topical irritation that were not present before the start of therapy. This medication should be discontinued if the hypersensitivity reaction occurs.

The usual dosage for adults and children is 2 or 3 drops inserted in the ear canal every 6 to 8 hours.

gentamicin sulfate otic solution [jen ta mye′ sin] (Garamycin)

Gentamicin is a bactericidal antibiotic. It has not been approved by the Food and Drug Administration for use as an otic preparation in the United States, but it is available in Canada. However, prescribers sometimes use the ophthalmic preparation, which is available in the United States, for otic infections.

The side effects of gentamicin are similar to those of chloramphenicol. The dosage is 3 or 4 drops inserted in the ear canal three times daily.

CORTICOSTEROID EAR PREPARATIONS

Corticosteroid otic solutions include betamethasone, hydrocortisone (Betnesol ♣ and Cortamed ♣), and dexamethasone (Decadron). Hydrocortisone combinations with acetic acid (VoSol HC, Acetasol HC), with alcohol (EarSol-HC), or with acetic acid and benzethonium (AA-HC Otic) are also available. Acetic acid, boric acid, benzalkonium chloride, benzethonium, and aluminum acetate (Burow's solution) are used for their antibacterial or antifungal effects. Hydrocortisone is included for its antiinflammatory, antipruritic, and antiallergic effects (*United States Pharmacopeia Dispensing Information,* 1999).

Corticosteroids may be combined with the antibiotics neomycin and polymyxin B to treat infections in the external ear canal or mastoid cavity. Many such products are available that may also include other ingredients, such as those included in over-the-counter (OTC) otic preparations. These are prescription otic solutions such as AK-Spore HC, Cort-Biotic, Cortisporin, and Cortomycin (*USP DI,* 1999).

OTHER OTIC PREPARATIONS

OTC otic preparations often contain acidified (acetic acid) solutions of alcohol, glycerin, or propylene glycol to help restore normal acid pH to the ear canal, especially after the client swims or bathes. Glycerin, mineral oil, and olive oil (sweet oil) are used as emollients to help relieve itching and burning in the ear, whereas propylene glycol enhances the antibacterial effect and acidity of acetic acid. Carbamide peroxide (urea hydrogen peroxide) is an antibacterial agent that releases oxygen to help remove accumulations of **cerumen** (earwax). Thus combinations of these ingredients are often included in OTC otic solutions (Covington, 1995).

A wide variety of both single and combination products is used to treat impacted cerumen, inflammation, bacterial or fungal infections, ear pain, and other minor or superficial problems associated primarily with the external ear canal. To prevent complications, a health care provider's thorough evaluation and intervention is required for more serious problems such as an earache secondary to an upper respiratory tract infection, ear discharge or drainage, persistent or recurrent otitis, or ear pain caused by recent injury or head trauma. Systemic medications with or without ear preparations are usually necessary in such cases.

Although most OTC otic preparations are considered safe and effective, clients should be advised to see a provider if symptoms do not improve within several days of using these preparations or if an adverse reaction occurs. Table 45-1 lists selected examples of OTC otic solutions.

■ Nursing Management

Drugs That Affect the Ear

■ **Assessment.** Before initiating therapy, assess the client's hearing and the extent of symptoms (earache, pain, erythema, vertigo, drainage, and others) that may be present. Before instilling the eardrops, assess that the ear canal is clear and not impacted with cerumen and that the tympanic membrane is intact.

To identify areas for education, assess the client for improper hygiene or health practices that may contribute to the development of infections, such as cleaning the ear canal with a cotton swab.

■ **Nursing Diagnosis.** The client is at risk for the following nursing diagnoses/collaborative problems: impaired verbal communication related to hearing loss; impaired comfort; risk for injury related to vertigo secondary to vestibular dysfunction; risk for infection related to the underlying condition; and the potential complication of deafness.

TABLE 45-1 Selected Examples of Over-the-Counter Otic Solutions

Ingredients (Trade Names)	Use/Indications
carbamide peroxide (Auro Ear Drops)	Earwax accumulation
isopropyl alcohol (Auro-Dri Ear Drops)	Swimmer's ear
boric acid and isopropyl alcohol (Aurocaine 2)	Swimmer's ear
isopropyl alcohol in glycerin (Swim-Ear Drops)	Swimmer's ear
carbamide peroxide and glycerin (Dent's Ear Wax Drops, E.R.O. Ear Drops, Ear Wax Removal System)	Earwax accumulation
hydrocortisone, propylene glycol, alcohol, benzyl benzoate (Earsol-HC Drops)	Antiinflammatory, antipruritic

Information from Otic Products. (1997). *Nonprescription products: Formulations and features '97-'98*. Washington, D.C.: American Pharmaceutical Association.

■ **Implementation**

■ ***Monitoring.*** Monitor the client's affected ear(s) for improvement of the condition for which the eardrops are being administered. Monitor for possible hypersensitivity to the eardrops as evidenced by burning, redness, and swelling that was not present when the medication was started. If hypersensitivity occurs, discontinue the drops and notify the prescriber. Monitor the client's level of comfort, ear drainage, hearing, and temperature at periodic intervals.

■ ***Intervention.*** Eardrops are more comfortably tolerated if they are warmed (if not contraindicated) before instillation. This can be achieved by running warm water over the bottle (on the side without the label) or by immersing the bottle in warm water in a medicine cup. Even simply carrying the bottle in a pocket for half an hour or so will take the chill off the drops.

Assist the client to a comfortable position before attempting to administer eardrops. To prepare for the instillation of eardrops, cleanse any drainage from the ear and position the client so that the ear to be medicated is facing upward.

The instillation of eardrops requires knowledge of anatomic structure across the life span; the shape of the auditory canal of a young child is different from that of an adult. To instill eardrops in children 3 years of age or younger, gently pull the pinna of the ear slightly down and back. In older children and adults, hold the pinna up and back. Gently massaging the area immediately anterior to the ear will facilitate the entry of the drops into the ear canal (see Figure 7-4).

■ ***Education.*** Instruct the client to remain on his or her side for 5 minutes after instillation. A small cotton pledget may be gently inserted into the ear canal if desired. Alert the client to the hazard of impaired hearing related to the eardrops, the cotton pledget, or the ear ailment itself. Instruct the client and/or family member in the appropriate method of eardrop instillation according to the client's age.

■ **Evaluation.** The expected outcome of otic drug therapy is that the client will show no clinical signs of infection (fever, pain, redness, heat, odor, drainage) or hearing loss and will have a normal white cell count (WBC). Cultures of the ear canal will be negative for pathogenic growth.

DRUG-INDUCED OTOTOXICITY

Many medications have reportedly caused **ototoxicity** in humans. This condition may affect hearing (auditory or cochlear function), balance (vestibular function), or both. The most common symptom reported is **tinnitus,** a ringing or buzzing sound in the ears.

Cochlear ototoxicity causes a progressive or continuing hearing loss. High-pitched tinnitus or a loss of the highest tones occurs first and then progresses to affect the lowest tones. Because of this slow progression, most clients are not aware that it is occurring. Vestibular toxicity may start with a severe headache of 1 to 2 days' duration; this is followed by nausea, vomiting, dizziness, ataxia, and difficulty with equilibrium. The client may feel as though the room is in motion (**vertigo**). Ototoxicity is usually bilateral and may be reversible, but it can become irreversible if not recognized early enough to stop the offending medications. Most drug-induced ototoxicity is associated with the use of aminoglycosides, such as streptomycin, gentamicin, tobramycin, and others. Table 45-2 lists selected drugs reported to induce ototoxicity.

■ Nursing Management

Drugs That Induce Ototoxicity

■ **Assessment.** Assess the client's hearing before starting therapy with an ototoxic drug. Concurrent administration of more than one ototoxic drug may increase the potential for hearing loss. Use caution when administering ototoxic drugs to clients who have any condition that may increase their risk of having an adverse reaction. One such condition is renal failure, which alters the elimination of aminoglycosides and may result in ototoxic serum levels.

Obtain a thorough drug history, particularly with a client who is experiencing tinnitus or a sudden hearing loss. Aspirin is the most widely used drug that causes tinnitus, but also keep in mind nonsteroidal antiinflammatory drugs, aminoglycosides, quinine and its synthetic substitutes, diuretics, and antineoplastics (see Table 45-2).

TABLE 45-2 Selected Drugs Reported to Cause Ototoxicity

Drug	Comments
Analgesics	
aspirin and NSAIDs	Salicylates, especially in high dosages, can cause tinnitus, vertigo, and hearing loss. This reaction is generally reversible if the drug is reduced or discontinued, but some cases of irreversible hearing loss are documented. Hearing disturbances and losses have been reported with NSAIDs.
Antibiotics	
aminoglycosides	The incidence of ototoxicity is 1% to 5% and may be irreversible.
clarithromycin	Hearing loss is reported (usually reversible); it occurs more often in older women.
erythromycin	Reversible hearing loss has been reported in persons with liver and/or kidney impairment. IV erythromycin has resulted in irreversible ototoxicity in persons 50 years of age and older and in individuals who received high dosages (>4 g/day).
vancomycin	Hearing loss is reported, especially in persons who have kidney impairment or are receiving another ototoxic medication concurrently.
Antineoplastic Agents	
cisplatin	Ototoxicity with tinnitus, hearing loss, and possible deafness has been reported. This effect is especially severe in children younger than 12 years of age. This effect is cumulative; therefore audiometric testing is recommended.
mechlorethamine	Tinnitus and, less commonly, hearing loss are reported.
Loop Diuretics	
bumetanide, ethacrynic acid, furosemide	Reversible and irreversible hearing loss have been reported, usually in association with too-rapid IV injection, high diuretic dosages, concurrent use with other ototoxic medications, and renal impairment.

Information from *Drug Facts and Comparisons* (2000). St. Louis: Facts and Comparisons.

■ **Nursing Diagnosis.** The client who is taking drugs that cause ototoxicity is at risk for the following nursing diagnoses/collaborative problems: disturbed sensory perception related to ototoxicity (auditory deficit, tinnitus); risk for injury related to vestibular dysfunction (ataxia, dizziness); and the potential complication of deafness.

■ **Implementation**

■ ***Monitoring.*** The serum levels of some drugs may be monitored to help detect the development of dangerously high blood levels. Monitor the client's ability to hear by observing for cues that indicate increasing hearing loss (inappropriate responses to the conversation of others, speaking loudly, moving closer to others when they speak) and by noting any comments by the client regarding an inability to hear or understand what others are saying. Report indications of increased hearing loss to the prescriber.

■ ***Intervention.*** When given intravenously, aminoglycosides should be administered over 30 to 60 minutes to avoid high peak levels.

■ ***Education.*** Instruct clients to report tinnitus or any other hearing impairment immediately. Auditory damage is usually reversible if the causative drug is discontinued early.

■ **Evaluation.** The expected outcome of therapy with drugs that induce ototoxicity is that the client will not experience tinnitus or deafness, will be able to understand others, and will express satisfaction with sensory input.

SUMMARY

Drugs that affect the ear may relate to the treatment of inflammation, excess cerumen, bacterial or fungal infection, or ear discomfort, or they may cause ototoxicity as an adverse reaction when administered for some other condition. In both instances the nurse needs to be concerned about the client's comfort and auditory perception and the risk for injury as a result of adverse reactions to the drugs or an extension of the client's symptoms.

Critical Thinking Questions

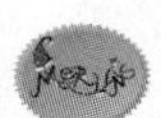

1. Joan Stevens is a 10-month-old infant who is brought to the clinic by her mother because of irritability, tugging at her ear, and a fever of 101° F. What would the nurse consider to be essential in her assessment of Joan?
2. What clients are particularly at risk for drug-related ototoxicity and why?

Collaborative Learning Activities

For Collaborative Learning Activities, go to mosby.com/MERLIN/McKenry/.

BIBLIOGRAPHY

Anderson, K.N., Anderson, L.E., & Glanze, W.D. (Eds.). (1998). *Mosby's medical, nursing, & allied health dictionary* (5th ed.). St. Louis: Mosby.

Covington, T.R. (1995). *Product update: Handbook of nonprescription drugs* (10th ed.). Washington, D.C.: American Pharmaceutical Association.

Drug Facts and Comparisons. (2000). St. Louis: Facts and Comparisons.

Semla, T.P., Beizer, J.L., & Higbee, M.D. (1998). *Geriatric dosage handbook: American Pharmaceutical Association.* Hudson, OH: Lexi-Comp.

United States Pharmacopeia Dispensing Information (USP DI): Drug information for the health care professional (19th ed.). (1999). Rockville, MD: United States Pharmacopeial Convention.

Zivic, R.C. & King, S. (1993). Cerumen-impaction management for clients of all ages. *Nurse Practitioner, 18*(3), 29.

46 Overview of the Endocrine System

Chapter Focus

The endocrine and nervous systems serve as the communication system of the body. The endocrine glands respond to signals from the internal and external environment by synthesizing and releasing hormones into the circulation. To provide care to clients with disorders of the endocrine system, it is essential that the nurse be knowledgeable about the anatomy and physiology of this complex system.

Learning Objectives

1. Define hormones and explain their functions.
2. List the primary hormones released from the anterior and posterior pituitary glands.
3. Describe the effects of the thyroid hormones on the body.
4. Discuss the functioning of the parathyroid glands in relationship to calcium and vitamin D.
5. Describe the functions of the three hormones released from the adrenal glands.
6. Compare the effects of insulin and glucagon on blood sugar levels.

Key Terms

HORMONES

Hormones are active, natural chemical substances secreted into the bloodstream from the endocrine glands. These substances initiate or regulate the activity of an organ or group of cells in another part of the body. They also have specific, well-defined physiologic effects on metabolism. The list of major hormones includes the secretions from the anterior and posterior pituitary glands, the thyroid hormones, parathyroid hormone, pancreatic insulin and glucagon, epinephrine and norepinephrine from the adrenal medulla, several potent steroids from the adrenal cortex, and the gonadal hormones of both sexes (Figure 46-1).

The major types of hormones are the steroid hormones and the hormones derived from amino acids. Steroid hormones are secreted by the adrenal gland and the sex glands. They transport proteins in the plasma; their physiologic effect begins when the steroid enters the cell, with subsequent binding to the specific cytosol or nuclear protein receptor.

Hormones from the various endocrine glands work together to regulate vital processes, including the following:

- Secretory and motor activities of the digestive tract
- Energy production
- Composition and volume of extracellular fluid
- Adaptation, such as acclimatization and immunity
- Growth and development
- Reproduction and lactation

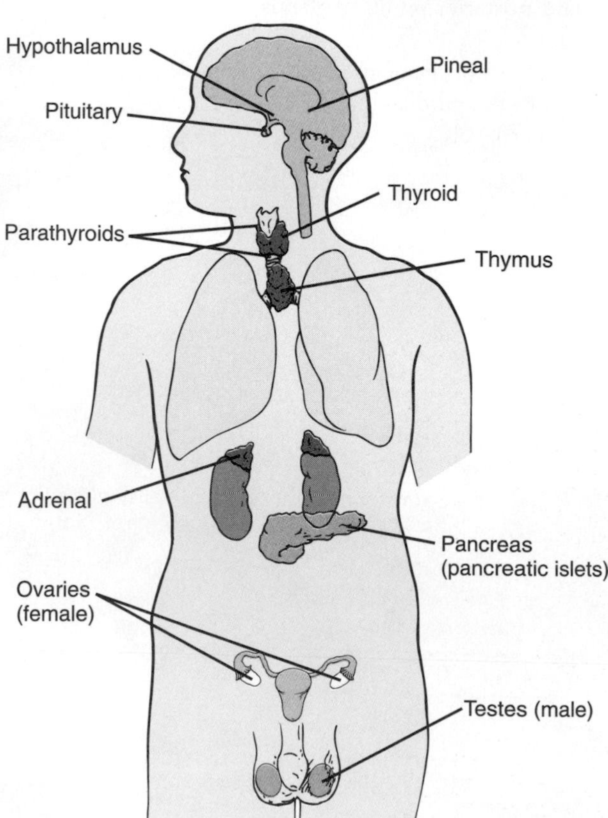

Figure 46-1 Locations of the major endocrine glands.

Hormones may exert their effects by controlling the formation or destruction of an intracellular regulator (cyclic 3′5′ adenosine monophosphate [cAMP]), controlling protein synthesis, or controlling membrane permeability and the movement of ions and other substances. The effect of a hormone depends on its interaction with a receptor and is determined by the level of the circulating active hormone.

To maintain the internal environment, hormone secretion must be controlled. This is achieved by a self-regulating series of events known as **negative feedback,** in which a hormone produces a physiologic effect that, when strong enough, inhibits further secretion of that hormone, thereby inhibiting the physiologic effect. Increased hormonal secretions may be evoked in response to stimuli from the external environment; the cessation of the external stimuli ends the internal secretion response (Figure 46-2).

Hormones are not "used up" in exerting their physiologic effects; they must be inactivated or excreted if the internal environment is to remain stable. Inactivation occurs enzymatically in the blood or intercellular spaces, in the liver or kidney, or in the target tissues. The excretion of hormones is primarily via the urine and, to a lesser extent, the bile.

The wide range in the onset and duration of hormonal activity contributes to the flexibility of the endocrine system. Most hormones are destroyed rapidly, with a half-life of 10 to 30 minutes in blood. Some hormones (e.g., catecholamines) have a half-life of seconds, and thyroid hormones have a half-life measured in days. Some hormones exert their physiologic effects immediately, whereas others require minutes or hours before their effects occur. Some effects end immediately when the hormone disappears from

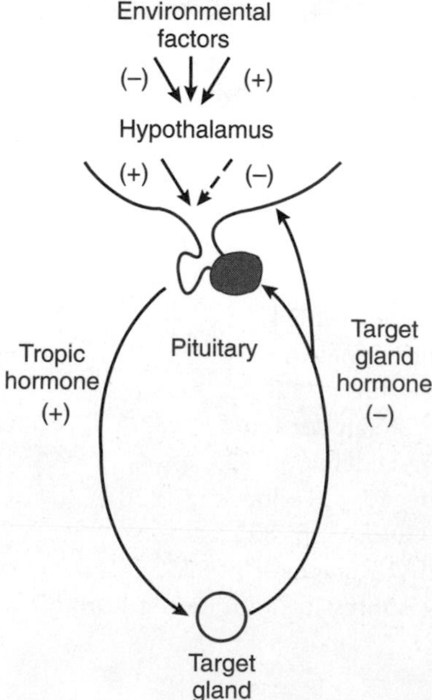

Figure 46-2 Various internal and external factors may inhibit or stimulate the hypothalamus to secrete inhibitory (−) or releasing (+) factors to control the output of hormones from the anterior pituitary and ultimate hormone release from the target glands.

the circulation; other responses may persist for hours after hormone concentrations have returned to basal levels. The exposure of a tissue to an active hormone is also controlled by that hormone's pathway for metabolism, including molecular alterations, consumption at the site of action, and hepatorenal excretion.

One of the major developments of this century in biology and medicine has been the recognition, isolation, purification, and chemical and cellular understanding of most known hormones. Duplicating hormones by chemical synthesis becomes theoretically possible once their chemical structure is known. This has been accomplished for some but not all hormones.

In medicine, hormones generally are used in three ways: (1) for replacement therapy, as exemplified by the use of insulin in diabetes or of adrenal steroids in Addison's disease; (2) for pharmacologic effects beyond replacement, as in the use of larger-than-endogenous doses of adrenal steroids for their antiinflammatory effects; and (3) for endocrine diagnostic testing.

Research in endocrinology has advanced the concept of specific receptors within or on the surface of cells. This has led to knowledge of hormone specificity and the essential cellular mechanisms involved in the hormone-receptor complex. The recognition and activation properties found in the hormone-receptor complex come from different receptor molecular sites. Only specific receptor material binds a hormone and begins its activity; the hormone has no effect on tissues that do not carry specific receptors.

Alterations in either hormone secretion or hormone receptor responses may culminate in endocrine disease states. Certain cell surface receptors may become antigenic and develop antibodies that accelerate receptor destruction, block receptor function, or mimic the action of the target tissue. Among the receptor-like disorders, which are referred to as antireceptor autoimmune diseases, are myasthenia gravis, Graves' disease, insulin-resistant diabetes mellitus, and bronchial asthma.

PITUITARY GLAND

The hormones of the pituitary gland exert an important effect in regulating the secretion of other hormones. The pituitary body is approximately the size of a pea and occupies a niche in the sella turcica of the sphenoid bone. It consists of an anterior lobe (adenohypophysis), a posterior lobe (neurohypophysis), and a smaller pars intermedia composed of secreting cells. The anterior lobe is particularly important in sustaining life. The function of the pars intermedia is not well understood. Figure 46-3 shows the major pituitary hormones and their principal target organs.

Regulation of Anterior Pituitary Function

The pituitary and target glands have a negative feedback relationship. A trophic hormone from the pituitary stimulates the target gland to secrete a hormone that inhibits further secretion of the trophic hormone by the pituitary. When the serum concentration of the target gland hormone falls below a certain level, the pituitary again secretes the trophic hormone until the target gland produces enough hormone to inhibit the pituitary secretion. However, the negative feedback concept alone is not enough to account for changes in the serum levels of target gland hormones, especially those caused by changes in the external environment. The central nervous system is believed to play a decisive role in regulating pituitary function to meet environmental demands.

The discovery of various hypothalamic-releasing factors is of great interest in research. These factors cause the release of inhibition of the various hormones from the anterior pituitary. Among these releasing factors are thyroid-stimulating hormone releasing factor, corticotropin-releasing factor, growth hormone releasing hormone, growth hormone pituitary hormone (somatostatin), luteinizing hormone releasing hormone, and prolactin inhibitory factor.

Anterior Pituitary Hormones

The number of hormones secreted by the anterior pituitary gland is unknown. However, at least seven relatively pure extracts have been prepared, and these have definite specific action:

1. A growth factor influences the development of the body and promotes skeletal, visceral, and general growth. Acromegaly, gigantism, and dwarfism are associated with pathologic conditions of the anterior lobe of the pituitary gland.

   Growth hormone (GH) (somatotropin, somatropin, somatotropic hormone [STH]) has been obtained as a small crystalline protein but currently has no established place in medicine, except in documented clinical and laboratory evidence of growth hormone deficiency, especially that associated with chronic renal insufficiency (*Drug Facts and Comparisons*, 2000). Its use in various clinical conditions is largely experimental. (See Chapter 47 for further discussion on growth hormone.)
2. Follicle-stimulating hormone (FSH) stimulates the growth and maturation of the ovarian follicle, which in turn brings on the characteristic changes of estrus (menstruation in women). This hormone also stimulates spermatogenesis in men. FSH appears to be a protein or associated with a protein, but this human pituitary gonadotropin has not yet been obtained in a highly purified form.
3. Luteinizing hormone (LH), also known as the interstitial cell–stimulating hormone (ICSH), together with FSH (Pergonal) causes maturation of the graafian follicles, ovulation, and the secretion of estrogen in females. It causes spermatogenesis, androgen formation, and the growth of interstitial tissue in males. LH also promotes the formation of the corpus luteum in females.

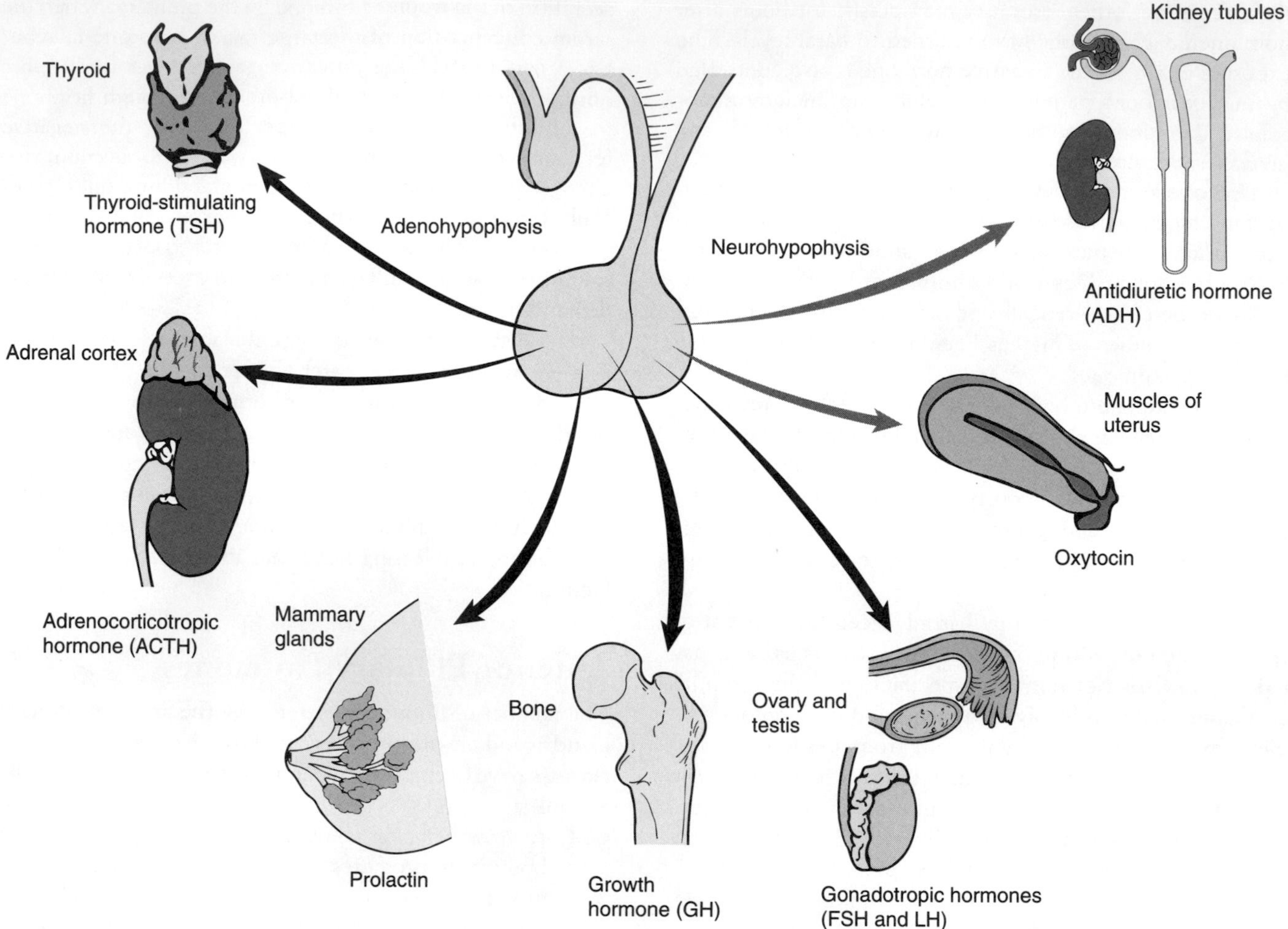

Figure 46-3 Pituitary hormones. Some of the major hormones of the adenohypophysis and neurohypophysis and their principal target organs.

4. Thyroid-stimulating hormone (TSH, thyrotropic hormone, thyrotropin) is necessary for the normal development and function of the thyroid gland. If too much is present, it produces hyperthyroidism and increases the size of the gland in laboratory animals.
5. A lactogenic factor (prolactin or mammotropin) plays a part in the proliferation and secretion of the mammary glands of mammals. This may be identical to the hormone responsible for the development of the corpus luteum. In its absence the corpus luteum fails to produce progesterone.
6. Adrenocorticotropic hormone (corticotropin or ACTH) stimulates the cortex of the adrenal gland.
7. Melanocyte-stimulating hormone (intermedin or MSH) is probably produced in the intermediate lobe. Its physiologic role is unknown, but it darkens the skin when injected into human beings.

The hormones produced by the anterior lobe of the pituitary gland are important physiologically, and purified preparations have become available, at least for clinical study; such preparations are both expensive and limited in supply. They may become useful in combating certain disorders in the future as chemically defined preparations become available.

Posterior Pituitary Hormones

Two hormones obtained from the posterior lobe of the pituitary gland have been identified and chemically analyzed. These compounds, **oxytocin** (a hormone that stimulates the smooth muscle of the uterus to contract) and **vasopressin** (the **antidiuretic hormone**), are both peptides; each contains eight amino acids. It has proved possible to synthesize them chemically. The availability of these hormones in pure form has clarified their mechanism of action and has allowed better control of their therapeutic use. A certain overlap of pharmacologic action exists even in the pure preparation; pure oxytocin has some vasopressor activity, and vice versa. The antidiuretic potency of vasopressin is much greater than its pressor potency.

Although vasopressin is available in a natural state, synthetic formulations (e.g., lypressin and desmopressin) have been developed, and they act primarily as antidiuretic hormone. They have very little, if any, pressor or oxytocic activity. Oxytocin is discussed in Chapter 53.

THYROID GLAND

The thyroid gland, one of the most richly vascularized tissues of the body, secretes three hormones essential for the proper regulation of metabolism: thyroxine (T_4), triiodothyronine (T_3), and calcitonin. Because of its role in calcium metabolism, calcitonin is discussed in greater detail in the section on parathyroid gland hormones (see Chapter 48).

The thyroid gland is composed of at least two types of cells: follicular, which produce T_3 and T_4; and parafollicular, the source of calcitonin.

Thyroid Hormones

The large amount of iodine in thyroid hormones and the availability of radioactive iodine have led to detailed knowledge about the physiology of the thyroid gland and its role in metabolism. Iodine is essential for the synthesis of thyroid hormone. Approximately 1 mg of iodine is required per week, most of which is ingested in food, water, and iodized table salt. Approximately two thirds of this iodine is reduced in the gastrointestinal tract, enters the circulation as iodide, and is excreted into the urine. The remaining third is taken up by the thyroid gland for hormone synthesis. This process is aided by the "iodide pump," which takes up the iodide from the extracellular fluid, traps it, and concentrates it to many times that found in plasma. The ratio of iodide in the thyroid gland to that in the serum is expressed as the T/S ratio; normally this ratio is 20:1. In hypoactivity the ratio may be 10:1; in hyperactivity it may be as great as 250:1.

Thyroglobulin is synthesized first. It contains tyrosine, an amino acid that reacts with iodine to form thyroid hormones. The thyroglobulin–thyroid hormone complex is stored in the follicles of the thyroid gland and is called "colloid." Approximately 30% of the thyroid mass is stored thyroglobulin, which contains enough thyroid hormone to meet normal requirements for 2 to 3 months without any further synthesis.

Normally thyroglobulin is not released into the circulation but undergoes proteolytic digestion (a coupling reaction), which releases the active thyroid hormones T_3 and T_4. Hormone synthesis—iodine trapping, iodination and proteolysis of thyroglobulin, and hormone release—is controlled by the thyroid-stimulating hormone (thyrotropin, TSH) from the beta cells of the anterior pituitary gland. Thyroid secretion is maintained by this TSH secretion. Decreased serum levels of T_3 and T_4 stimulate thyrotropin-releasing hormone (TRH) from the hypothalamus, which stimulates the pituitary gland to secrete TSH; this in turn stimulates release of thyroxin from thyroglobulin.

TSH secretion is negatively regulated by T_3 and T_4, which directly inhibit the thyrotropic cells of the pituitary gland. An increase in free, unbound thyroid hormone causes a decrease in TSH secretion and inhibits TRH production; a decrease in the free unbound hormone causes an increase in TSH secretion and stimulates TRH production—a negative feedback mechanism.

Overall Physiologic Effects. The precise physiologic role of the thyroid hormones is not yet known, but several hormonal actions have been identified and studied. Three generalizations can be made about thyroid hormones:

1. They have a diffuse effect and do not seem to have any specific target organ effect; no special cells or tissues appear to be particularly affected by the thyroid hormones.
2. Their long delay in onset of action and their prolonged action rule them out as minute-to-minute regulators of physiologic function. Instead, their role is more likely to be that of establishing and maintaining long-term functions such as growth, maturation, and adaptation.
3. They are not necessary for survival, although reduced levels can affect quality of life.

Thyroxine and triiodothyronine appear to have the same physiologic actions, but T_3 is far more potent than T_4.

Effects on Growth and Maturation. A normal, functioning thyroid is essential for normal growth. Thyroid hormones stimulate the production of messenger ribonucleic acid (RNA) molecules, which are involved in the synthesis of various proteins; this facilitates growth and development. The hormones must be present in the right amounts if growth is to occur at the normal rate. The growth rate is slowed in children with hypothyroidism; this may lead to shortness of stature. Conversely, children with hyperthyroidism may have excessive skeletal growth and become taller than they otherwise would. However, stunting of growth results if there is premature closing of the epiphyses because of accelerated bone maturation. In the adult, excess thyroid hormone causes increased bone demineralization and an increased loss of calcium and phosphate.

Calcitonin is produced by cells in the interstitial tissue between the follicles of the thyroid gland; the effect of this hormone is to reduce the concentration of calcium ions in the blood—the exact opposite effect of parathyroid hormone. Calcitonin is essential for bone formation in children because it promotes the deposition of calcium. Calcitonin has a very weak effect on plasma concentration in adults because the absorption and deposition of calcium are slow in the adult and because the effects of calcitonin are rapidly overridden by parathyroid hormone.

Effects on the Central Nervous System. From the time of birth through the first year of life, thyroid hormone must be present for normal cerebral development; irreversible mental retardation occurs if the hormone is not present. In the adult, hypothyroidism causes listlessness, a general dulling of mental capacity, decreased sensory capacity, slow speech, impaired memory, and somnolence. Hyperthyroidism in the adult results in hyperexcitability, irritability, restlessness, exaggerated responses to environmental stimuli, and emotional instability. Psychosis can occur in either hypothyroidism or hyperthyroidism.

Effects on Basal Metabolic Rate. Thyroid hormones increase oxygen consumption in most cells of the body; the lungs, spleen, gastric smooth muscle, gonads, and accessory sex organs are not affected. The basal metabolic rate is subnormal with hypothyroidism; it may be 40% to 60% above normal with hyperthyroidism.

Effects on Carbohydrate and Lipid Metabolism. Thyroid hormones accelerate glucose catabolism, increase cholesterol synthesis, and enhance the ability of the liver to excrete cholesterol in the bile. Because the effect on cholesterol excretion is greater than that on cholesterol synthesis, the result is a decrease in plasma cholesterol level. The hormones also stimulate the mobilization of fatty acids from adipose tissue. Individuals with hypothyroidism have an elevated serum cholesterol level and increased blood levels of phospholipids and triglycerides.

Effects on Protein Metabolism. Thyroid hormones are essential for the development of protein mass. In hypothyroidism both the synthesis and the breakdown of protein are diminished, but the effect on protein synthesis is more profound. The deposition of mucoproteins occurs in subcutaneous spaces, which osmotically attract water, causing "puffiness." Increased catabolism of protein, or the breakdown of muscle mass, and increased nitrogen excretion occur with hyperthyroidism.

Effects on Gastrointestinal Function. Thyroid hormones increase gastrointestinal motility, the absorption of food, and the secretion of digestive juices. Hypothyroidism decreases both intestinal absorption and the secretion of pancreatic enzymes. Constipation may also occur.

Effects on Water and Electrolyte Balance. Water and electrolytes accumulate in subcutaneous spaces when thyroid hormone is deficient. Administering thyroid hormone results in diuresis and a loss of fluid and electrolytes from the subcutaneous spaces.

Effects on Cardiovascular Function. Because the thyroid hormones increase metabolism, the tissues have an increased need for oxygen and nutrients; this in turn demands increased blood flow. In hyperthyroidism these effects cause increased cardiac output, increased pulse pressure, and tachycardia. If these effects are prolonged, cardiac hypertrophy and even high-output myocardial failure may occur. The opposite effects occur in hypothyroidism.

Effects on Muscle Function. Moderate increases in thyroid hormone make muscles react with vigor; large increases result in muscle weakness because of excess protein catabolism. A characteristic sign of hyperthyroidism is a fine muscle tremor. Hypothyroidism causes the muscles to be sluggish.

Effects on Temperature Regulation. Thyroid hormones must be present for an increase in heat production or a decrease in heat loss to occur. Although the hormones do not initiate the physiologic response to cold, they appear to magnify the body's response to catecholamine effects, which innervate the sympathetic system during exposure to cold. Hypothyroidism causes decreased tolerance to cold.

Effects on Lactation. Thyroid hormone is necessary for normal milk production; without thyroid hormone, the fat content of milk and total milk production are greatly reduced.

Effects on Reproduction. Thyroid hormone is required for normal rhythmicity in the reproductive cycle.

Thyroid Gland Disorders

Goiter

The synthesis of the thyroid hormones and their maintenance in the blood in adequate amounts depend largely on an adequate intake of iodine. Iodine ingested through food or water is changed into iodide and is stored in the thyroid gland before reaching the circulation. Prolonged iodine deficiency in the diet results in enlargement of the thyroid gland, known as a simple **goiter.** When thyroid hormones fail to be synthesized because of a lack of iodine, the anterior lobe of the pituitary is stimulated to increase the secretion of thyrotropic hormone, which in turn causes hypertrophy and hyperplasia of the gland. The enlarged thyroid then removes residual traces of iodine from the blood. Providing an adequate supply of iodine for young persons can prevent this type of goiter (simple or nontoxic). Iodine is not abundant in most foods except fish and seafood; iodized salt is often the primary source of iodine in areas where seafood is expensive or not readily available.

Hypothyroidism

Clients with primary hypothyroidism have decreased T_3 and T_4 levels and an elevated TSH level. Those with pituitary (secondary) hypothyroidism and hypothalamic (tertiary) hypothyroidism have decreased levels of T_3, T_4, and TSH.

The TSH test, the most sensitive index of hypothyroidism, is elevated in primary hypothyroidism and depressed in secondary hypothyroidism. The free thyroxine index is depressed in clients with both primary and secondary hypothyroidism but elevated in clients with hyperthyroidism. The T_3 resin uptake (RT_3U) is depressed in pregnancy and in clients with primary and secondary hypothyroidism but is elevated in clients with hyperthyroidism. The serum T_3 level is depressed in both secondary and primary hypothyroidism but elevated in hyperthyroid states and T_3 thyrotoxicosis. The total T_4 is elevated in pregnancy and hyperthyroidism but depressed in both primary and secondary hypothyroidism. The free T_4 (unbound) is depressed in both primary and secondary hypothyroid states but is elevated in hyperthyroid states.

Hypothyroidism in the young child is known as **cretinism** and is characterized by the cessation of physical and mental development, which leads to dwarfism and mental retardation. Clients with cretinism usually have thick, coarse skin; a thick tongue; a gaping mouth; a protruding abdomen; thick, short legs; poorly developed hands and feet; and weak musculature. This condition may result from faulty development or atrophy of the thyroid gland during fetal development. Failure of the gland to develop may be caused by a lack of iodine in the mother.

In children, normal skeletal growth is evidence of adequate therapy; an increase in serum alkaline phosphatase indicates that growth will occur. In cases of cretinism, thyroid hormone levels equal to or above those required for the adult must be established immediately after birth to prevent permanent mental and physical retardation. If cretinism is not treated until a later time, treatment will not reverse the mental retardation that has already occurred. Clients with hypothyroidism need to be informed of their lifelong need for replacement therapy.

Severe hypothyroidism in an adult is called **myxedema** (acid mucopolysaccharide accumulation). When it is the last stage of a long-standing, inadequately treated, or untreated hypothyroidism, coma sets in and is accompanied by hypotension, hypoventilation, hypothermia, bradycardia, hyponatremia, and hypoglycemia. The development of myxedema is usually insidious and causes gradual slowing of physical and mental functions. There is gradual infiltration of the skin and a loss of facial lines and facial expression, which results in a puffy, expressionless face. The formation of subcutaneous connective tissue causes the hands and face to appear puffy and swollen. The basal metabolic rate becomes subnormal, the skin is cold and dry, the hair becomes scant and coarse, movements become sluggish, cardiac output is reduced, and the client becomes hypersensitive to cold.

Hyperthyroidism (Thyrotoxicosis)

Excessive formation of the thyroid hormones and their escape into the circulation result in a toxic state called **thyrotoxicosis.** This occurs with diffuse toxic goiter, exophthalmic goiter (Graves disease), thyroid cancer, and in some forms of adenomatous goiters.

Primary hyperthyroidism is characterized by elevated levels of T_3 and T_4 and decreased levels of TSH. T_3, T_4, and TSH levels increase with pituitary (secondary) hyperthyroidism. Hyperthyroidism leads to symptoms quite different from those seen in myxedema. The metabolic rate is increased, sometimes as much as 60% or more. The body temperature is often above normal, the pulse rate is fast, and the client complains of feeling too warm. Other symptoms include restlessness, anxiety, emotional instability, muscle tremor and weakness, sweating, and exophthalmos. The increased thyroxine levels may cause cardiomegaly, tachycardia, congestive heart failure, hepatic alterations (necrosis, dysfunction, fatty changes), lymphoid hyperplasia, osteoporosis, pretibial myxedema, and neurologic irritability. In thyroid storm, elevated thyroxine levels cause a sudden onset of hyperthyroid symptoms, especially those affecting the nervous and cardiovascular systems.

Before the advent of antithyroid drugs, treatment was limited to a subtotal resection of the hyperactive gland. Propylthiouracil is the most commonly used antithyroid medication. However, antithyroid drugs provide less rapid control of hyperthyroidism than do surgical measures. Radioactive therapy is used primarily in treatment of middle-aged clients and older adults.

PARATHYROID GLANDS

Lying just above and behind the thyroid gland are bean-shaped glands known as the parathyroids. Humans have two pairs of these glands. The adult glands consist of encapsulated masses of cells, between which are abundant adipocytes and vascular channels. The primary function of the parathyroids is to maintain adequate levels of calcium in the extracellular fluid. Parathyroid hormone has multiple effects, ultimately culminating in the mobilization of calcium from bone. It also reduces the concentration of phosphate, which permits more calcium to be mobilized.

Parathyroid Hormones

Parathyroid hormone (PTH) is a polypeptide. The active component has a half-life of 30 minutes, and the inactive component has a half-life of 7 to 10 days. PTH circulates in elevated concentrations in clients with hyperplastic parathyroid glands as a result of diminished calcium levels; this condition occurs in persons with impaired renal function or intestinal malabsorption. Elevated PTH levels may cause metabolic bone disease, including osteoporosis and osteomalacia.

The mechanism of action of PTH in the bone or kidney is not completely understood. Some researchers suggest that PTH receptor binding and adenylate cyclase activity are coupled events that are subject to down regulation of the receptors. Clients with hyperparathyroidism may be resistant to PTH action in the kidney and bone. The decreased number of these receptors, not their altered affinity, produces a reduction in PTH-stimulated adenylate cyclase activity.

Cholesterol-derived provitamin D is converted to vitamin D_3 by the action of sunlight on the skin. The vitamin is also present as a milk additive. Along with PTH, vitamin D_3 is converted to its active form in the kidney. It is involved in the metabolism of calcium, phosphate, and magnesium in the bone and gastrointestinal tract. Primary hyperparathyroidism is the most common parathyroid disorder. In general, it is caused by adenomas, chief cell hyperplasia, or hypertrophy. PTH elevations alter the function of renal tubular cells, bone cells, and gastrointestinal tract mucosa. Elevated levels of calcium and increased bone resorption with the development of renal calculi generally occur in hyperparathyroidism. In secondary hyperparathyroidism, an overactive parathyroid gland causes increased calcium excretion and possibly kidney stones, but serum calcium levels generally remain stable because of an effective feedback mechanism.

Hypoparathyroidism leads to manifestations of hypocalcemia and tetany, the symptoms of which include muscle spasms, convulsions, gradual paralysis with dyspnea, and death from exhaustion. Gastrointestinal hemorrhages and hematemesis commonly occur before death. At death the intestinal mucosa is congested, and the calcium content of the heart, kidney, and other tissues is increased.

Symptoms of tetany are relieved by administration of calcium salts. Large doses of vitamin D also help to relieve tetany and to restore the normal calcium level in the blood. The client is hospitalized because frequent assessment of blood calcium and phosphate levels is essential.

ADRENAL GLANDS

The adrenal glands are located just above the kidneys. They consist of two parts: the inner medulla and the outer cortex. The adrenal cortex synthesizes three important classes of hormones: the **glucocorticoids** (cortisol), **mineralocorticoids** (primarily aldosterone), and **androgens** (primarily dehydroepiandrosterone). The glucocorticoids—adrenocortical steroid hormones that increase glyconeogenesis, exert an antiinflammatory effect, and influence many body functions—are synthesized primarily in the zona fasciculata and are under the control of ACTH from the pituitary gland.

The basal production rate averages 30 mg every 24 hours; under stressful conditions (trauma, major surgery, infection), there is a reserve capacity production of up to 300 mg daily. Increases in glucocorticoid production may be related to proportional increases in the release of ACTH by the pituitary. (See the discussion of steroid abuse in Chapter 9.)

The mineralocorticoids are synthesized specifically in the zona glomerulosa of the adrenal cortex. Production is primarily under the control of both the renin-angiotensin axis system (discussed later in this chapter) and the blood potassium level. The production of **aldosterone,** the primary mineralocorticoid, is stimulated by salt depletion and causes sodium retention in the kidney at the distal convoluted tubule to preserve extracellular fluid volume. Mineralocorticoids also increase the urinary excretion of potassium and hydrogen ions and maintain normal blood volume.

The androgens are synthesized in the zona fasciculata and the zona reticularis and essentially enhance male characteristics and control the growth of hair follicles in the skin.

A reaction to serious stress normally causes a prompt and noticeable increase in the production of cortisol and aldosterone; these hormones operate together to maintain the cardiovascular tone essential for survival. A client under stress who has impaired ability to produce these hormones incurs the risk of developing an acute adrenal crisis. The production of cortisol is under the control of a continuous feedback mechanism involving the pituitary and ACTH production, which in turn is inhibited by the circulating cortisol levels. Stress is a stimulus that overrides this inhibition and initiates the secretion of corticotropin-releasing factor; this culminates in the release of ACTH and activation of the adrenal cortex, which leads to an increased production of cortisol.

Mineralocorticoids: Aldosterone

Aldosterone is the primary mineralocorticoid to regulate the balance of sodium and potassium in the blood. It is synthesized in the adrenal zona glomerulosa, which is the outer edge of the adrenocortical tissue below the adrenal capsule. The production of aldosterone is maintained primarily by the renin-angiotensin system and the concentration of circulating serum potassium. A drop in the circulating arterial volume stimulates volume receptors in the juxtaglomerular apparatus. As a result, renin (a proteolytic enzyme) is produced and acts on angiotensinogen, which is synthesized by the liver to form angiotensin I. When the angiotensin I passes through the pulmonary circulation, two amino acids are cleared from it to form angiotensin II. Angiotensin II stimulates the adrenal zona glomerulosa to produce aldosterone. Aldosterone promotes sodium reabsorption in the kidney at the distal convoluted tubule to preserve extracellular fluid volume. Aldosterone secretion is normally stimulated by a decrease in circulating volume (e.g., loss of blood, excessive diuresis, low salt intake) and increased potassium levels. Aldosterone secretion is suppressed by an elevation of sodium levels in the blood (e.g., by excessive dietary salt intake). It restricts the loss of sodium and its accompanying anions, chloride and bicarbonate, and thereby helps to maintain extracellular fluid volume. It also maintains acid-base and potassium balance.

In adrenal insufficiency, aldosterone deficit occurs, sodium reabsorption is inhibited, and potassium excretion decreases. Hyperkalemia and mild acidosis occur. In adrenalectomy the loss of aldosterone leads to an overall reduction of sodium reabsorption and a powerful and uncontrolled loss of extracellular fluid. Plasma volume drops, and a state of hypovolemic shock may ensue. This may cause death unless a mineralocorticoid, salt, and water are administered. Excessive doses of aldosterone increase potassium excretion; hypokalemia results unless dietary intake compensates for the loss. Acidification of the urine then occurs, which leads to metabolic alkalosis.

Aldosterone is much more potent in its electrolyte effects than desoxycorticosterone, but it has not yet established a therapeutic status comparable to that of desoxycorticosterone. Its use has been limited because of its cost and relative unavailability and because it must be administered intramuscularly.

The amount of aldosterone secreted by the adrenal cortex apparently is affected by the concentration of sodium in the body fluids rather than by stimulation of the adrenal cortex by ACTH.

PANCREAS

The pancreas is a gland that lies transversely across the posterior wall of the abdomen. It secretes a limpid, colorless fluid that digests proteins, fats, and carbohydrates. It also produces internal secretions—insulin and glucagon—that affect blood sugar levels.

Insulin is a hormone secreted by the beta cells of the islets of Langerhans in the pancreas in response to increased levels of glucose in the blood. On hydrolysis, this hormone yields several amino acids. In its crystalline state it appears to be chemically linked with certain metals (zinc, nickel, cadmium, or cobalt). Normal pancreatic tissue is rich in zinc, which may be significant to the natural storage of the hormone. Insulin consists of two polypeptide chains and contains 48 amino acids, the exact sequence of which is known. Insulin is stored in the beta cells as a larger protein known as proinsulin. Because relatively small amounts of insulin are necessary in the body tissues, it is thought that insulin acts as a catalyst in cellular metabolism.

Carbohydrate metabolism is controlled by a finely balanced interaction of several endocrine factors (adrenal, anterior pituitary, thyroid, insulin), but the particular phase of carbohydrate metabolism that is affected by insulin is not entirely known. An SC injection of insulin produces a rapid lowering of blood sugar in both diabetic and nondiabetic persons. Moderate amounts of insulin in diabetic animals promote the storage of carbohydrate in the liver and also in the muscle cells, particularly after the ingestion of carbohydrate. The deposit of muscle glycogen also increases in the nondiabetic animal, but apparently the level of liver glycogen does not. In both diabetic and nondiabetic persons the oxygen consumption increases and the respiratory quotient rises.

Glucagon, like insulin, is a pancreatic extract and is thought to oppose the action of insulin. Glucagon is a product of the alpha cells of the islets of Langerhans. Glucagon acts primarily by mobilizing hepatic glycogen and converting it to glucose, which produces an elevation in the concentration of glucose in the blood.

Diabetes Mellitus

Diabetes mellitus is a heterogenous complex disorder of carbohydrate, fat, and protein metabolism that is primarily a result of a relative or complete lack of insulin or defects of the insulin receptors. Insulin is ineffective at the tissue site, or not enough insulin is available. Obesity, certain drugs, viruses, autoimmune phenomena, genetic predisposition, and age may have roles in its development. The blood sugar becomes elevated, and when it exceeds a certain amount, the excess is secreted by the kidney (glycosuria). Symptoms include increased appetite (polyphagia), thirst (polydipsia), weight loss, increased urine output (polyuria), weakness (fatigue), and itching (e.g., pruritus vulvae).

In diabetes mellitus, glycogen fails to store in the liver, although the conversion of glycogen back to glucose or the formation of glucose from other substances (**gluconeogenesis**) is not necessarily impaired. As a result, the level of blood sugar rapidly rises. This derangement of carbohydrate metabolism results in an abnormally high metabolism of proteins and fats. The ketone bodies, which result from the oxidation of fatty acids, accumulate faster than the muscle cells can oxidize them, resulting in ketosis and acidosis.

The course of untreated diabetes mellitus is progressive. The symptoms of diabetic coma and acidosis are directly or indirectly the result of the accumulation of acetone, beta-hydroxybutyric acid, and diacetic acid. Unless treatment is started promptly, respirations become rapid and deep, the breath has an odor of acetone, the blood sugar is elevated, the client becomes dehydrated, and stupor and coma develop.

The long-term complications of diabetes mellitus can lead to an increase in morbidity and mortality. Some of the most commonly associated problems are peripheral atherosclerosis, which may result in coronary artery disease, infections, gangrene, or strokes; and diabetic retinopathy, which can include vitreal hemorrhage, retinal detachment, and blindness. Renal disease, peripheral sensory neuropathy, and cardiomyopathy leading to heart failure are also reported.

Diabetes mellitus is usually treated with exogenous insulin, diet, and exercise. Glucose and insulin promote the formation and retention of glycogen in the liver, and the oxidation of fat in the liver is arrested. Therefore the rate of formation of acetone bodies is slowed and the acidosis is checked. Other supportive measures, such as restoring the fluid and electrolyte balance of the body, are very important in treatment.

Recent advances in diabetic therapy include (1) the synthesis of human insulin by bacteria genetically altered by recombinant DNA technology, (2) islet cell and/or pancreas transplantation, and (3) external and implanted continuous insulin infusion pumps.

SUMMARY

The endocrine system carries out integrative and regulatory functions within the body through the actions of hormones. Hormones regulate mechanisms that allow the body to meet its needs. The endocrine system consists of specialized glands and their hormones, which act on specific target cells and stimulate various responses. The overproduction or underproduction of hormones results in pathologic conditions. Hormonal replacement therapy is the major concern in the underproduction of hormones by the endocrine system.

Critical Thinking Questions

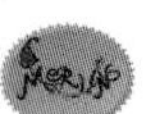

1. Given that the hospital laboratory has the ability to determine blood levels of TSH, T_3, and T_4, create a protocol for determining whether hyperthyroidism is the result of a pituitary abnormality or the production of a nonpituitary thyroid-stimulating substance.
2. A client is admitted to the emergency department with polydipsia (thirst), polyuria (excess urine production), and urine with low specific gravity. The prescriber wants to reverse these symptoms. Which of the following substances will he or she ask you to administer: insulin, glucagon, antidiuretic hormone, or aldosterone? Explain why.
3. A client arrives at the emergency department. He is unconscious, and his MedicAlert bracelet indicates that he has diabetes. The client may be in diabetic coma or insulin shock. How do you distinguish between these two conditions, and what treatment would you recommend for each condition (Seeley, Stephens, & Tate, 1995)?

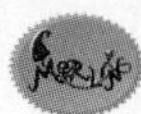

Collaborative Learning Activities

For Collaborative Learning Activities, go to mosby.com/MERLIN/McKenry/.

BIBLIOGRAPHY

Anderson, K.N., Anderson, L.E., & Glanze, W.D. (Eds.) (1998). *Mosby's medical, nursing, & allied health dictionary* (5th ed.). St. Louis: Mosby.

Drug Facts and Comparisons. (2000). St. Louis: Facts and Comparisons.

Melmon, K.L., Morrelli, H.F., Hoffman, B.B., & Nierenberg, D.W. (1992). *Melmon & Morrelli's clinical pharmacology: Basic principles in therapeutics* (3rd ed.). New York: McGraw-Hill.

Seeley, R.R., Stephens, T.D., & Tate, P. (1995). *Anatomy and physiology* (3rd ed.). St. Louis: Mosby.

Thibodeau, G.A. & Patton, K.T. (1999). *Anatomy and physiology* (4th ed.). St Louis: Mosby.

Toto, K.H. (1994). Endocrine physiology: A comprehensive review. *Critical Care Nursing Clinics of North America, 6*(4), 637-653, 655-659.

47 Drugs Affecting the Pituitary

Chapter Focus

Although the pituitary secretes numerous hormones, this chapter discusses only the growth hormones and the antidiuretic hormone vasopressin. Other hormones are discussed in chapters more directly related to the endocrine glands they affect. Although disorders involving these two hormones are not common, the nurse is expected to appropriately assess and care for clients with pituitary dysfunction.

Learning Objectives

1. Describe the primary functions of the anterior and posterior pituitary hormones.
2. Describe the effects of somatrem, somatropin, and octreotide.
3. List the effects of vasopressin.
4. Implement the nursing management for the care of the client receiving drugs affecting the pituitary.

Key Terms

diabetes insipidus, p. 832
dwarfism, p. 830
gigantism, p. 830
growth hormone-inhibiting hormone (somatostatin), p. 830
growth hormone-releasing hormone, p. 830

Key Drugs [✓]

somatrem, p. 830
vasopressin, p. 832

The variety of available preparations that affect the pituitary gland are generally used as replacement therapy for hormone deficiency, as drug therapy for specific disorders to produce a therapeutic hormonal response, and as diagnostic aids to determine hypofunctional or hyperfunctional hormone states.

A number of hormones have been identified, and many have been synthesized, including the following: growth hormone-releasing hormone (GH-RH), growth hormone–inhibiting hormone (somatostatin), thyrotropin-releasing hormone (TRH), corticotropin-releasing hormone (CRH), gonadotropin-releasing hormone (Gn-RH), and prolactin-inhibiting hormone (PIH or dopamine). Six anterior pituitary hormones and two posterior pituitary hormones have also been identified. The anterior pituitary hormones include growth hormone (GH), thyrotropin (thyroid-stimulating hormone [TSH]), adrenocorticotropin (ACTH), follicle-stimulating hormone (FSH), luteinizing hormone (LH), and prolactin. The posterior pituitary hormones are vasopressin and oxytocin. This chapter covers specific agents that affect the pituitary.

Gonadotropin-releasing hormone (gonadorelin) is discussed in Chapter 52; thyrotropin-releasing hormone and corticotropin-releasing hormone are discussed in Chapters 48 and 49, respectively. Although a true hormone with prolactin-inhibiting effects has not been identified, the substance is believed to be dopamine. Bromocriptine, a drug with dopamine-agonist properties, is reviewed in Chapters 23 and 53.

Of the remaining two substances, **growth hormone-releasing hormone** has been identified in vivo but is still under investigation. This substance has been found to stimulate the release of growth hormone after intranasal application. It is currently listed as an orphan drug and is manufactured by ICN Pharmaceuticals* (*Drug Facts and Comparisons*, 2000).

At one time the **growth hormone-inhibiting hormone (somatostatin)** was obtained from human cadaver pituitaries, but its distribution in the United States was stopped in 1985. Creutzfeldt-Jakob disease (a neurotropic virus), which is very rare in young people, was diagnosed in some clients and resulted in the death of several persons 5 to 7 years after receiving this product. Several biosynthetic hormones grown through recombinant DNA technology are available in the United States.

Growth hormone preparations include somatrem and somatropin; octreotide is used to inhibit the release of growth hormone.

ANTERIOR PITUITARY HORMONES

✔ **somatrem** [soe′ ma trem] (Protropin)

Somatrem contains the identical sequence of the pituitary-derived human growth hormone plus one additional amino acid, methionine. In tests it has been demonstrated to be therapeutically equivalent to somatropin, the pituitary human growth hormone.

The anabolic effects of somatrem result from the indirect effect of other hormones known as somatomedin-C or insulin-like growth factors (IGF-1) (Ascoli & Segaloff, 1996). IGF-1 is directly responsible for the growth of skeletal and soft tissue, and it increases the number of cells in the body rather than cell size. Therefore a major pharmacologic consequence of the use of somatrem is an increase in longitudinal growth; a deficiency in growth hormone usually results in **dwarfism.**

Somatrem also has metabolic effects. It decreases insulin sensitivity and may also affect glucose transport. It also increases lipolysis; promotes cellular growth by retaining phosphorus, sodium, and potassium; and enhances protein synthesis by increasing the retention of nitrogen.

Somatrem is indicated for the treatment of growth failure in children as a result of a deficiency in pituitary growth hormone. It is sometimes abused by athletes seeking increased size and strength (Box 47-1).

Although the half-life of parenteral (IV) somatrem is 20 to 30 minutes (3 to 5 hours for IM and SC forms), the duration of action for IV, IM, and SC preparations is 12 to 48 hours. This drug is metabolized in the liver and excreted by the kidneys.

Antibodies to somatrem have been reported in 30% to 40% of treated clients during the first 3 to 6 months of therapy, but only 5% of the clients develop neutralizing antibodies. It is rare that a client does not respond to therapy. However, pain and edema have been reported at the site of injection; an allergic-type reaction (rash, itching) is rare. Excessive doses may produce **gigantism** in children, an abnormal condition characterized by excessive size and stature. Therefore growth failure must be carefully documented before the drug is used, and dosages and individual responses must be closely monitored. Hypothyroidism is rarely reported.

The growth response effects of somatrem may be impaired when given concurrently with adrenocorticoids, glucocorticoids, or corticotropin (ACTH). ACTH should not be given concurrently; if it is necessary to treat with an adrenocorticoid agent, the daily doses should be limited. For example, the total daily dose per square meter of body area should not be greater than the following: cortisone (12.5 to 18.8 mg), hydrocortisone (10 to 15 mg), methylprednisolone (2 to 3 mg), prednisone or prednisolone (2.5 to 3.75 mg), betamethasone (300 to 450 μg), and dexamethasone (250 to 500 μg).

With children, the dosage and administration of somatrem for injection (Protropin) is up to 0.1 mg/kg IM or SC (preferred) three times weekly. The growth rate response is monitored in 3 to 6 months to determine if a dosage adjustment is necessary. Therapy is usually continued until epiphyseal closure occurs or there is no further response. If therapy is unsuccessful (<2 cm per year), treatment should be discontinued and the child reevaluated (*Drug Facts and Comparisons*, 2000; *United States Pharmacopeia Dispensing Information*, 1999).

*Information on orphan drug availability may be obtained from the Office of Orphan Products Development (HF-35), 5600 Fishers Lane, Rockville, MD 20857.

BOX 47-1

Growth Hormone Abuse

Some athletes use growth hormone either to increase their size and strength or to increase their ultimate height; the use depends on the age of the user. Although the effects of short-term usage are difficult to predict, there is a risk for adverse reactions to the drug, such as acromegalic syndrome, with symptoms such as increased size of facial bones, thickened hands and fingers, osteoporosis, long-term cardiac failure, diabetes, impotence, and amenorrhea. Because the drug is injectable, there is also the risk of contracting hepatitis and AIDS as the result of shared needles and syringes.

Under an amendment to the Food, Drug, and Cosmetic Act, "whoever knowingly distributes, or possesses, human growth hormone for any use in humans other than the treatment of disease or other recognized medical condition, or such use as has been authorized by the Secretary of Health and Human Services under Section 505 and pursuant to the order of a physician, is guilty of an offense punishable by not more than 5 years in prison, such fines as are authorized by Title 18, United States Code, or both." This legislation clearly defines the distribution of growth hormone as a serious federal offense, and federal authorities are authorized to investigate these practices.

Fortunately, the abuse of growth hormone is limited by its the cost and the fact that anabolic steroids are simply more enticing to the athlete. However, many athletes are unfamiliar with the adverse effects. Education of the potential consequences of growth hormone excess is important in counseling athletes who are considering its use.

Information from Haupt, H.A. (1993). Anabolic steroids and growth hormone. *American Journal of Sports Medicine, 21*(3), 468.

■ Nursing Management

Somatrem Therapy

■ **Assessment.** It should be ascertained that the client does not have a malignancy, especially an intracranial tumor. Somatrem is also contraindicated in clients with closed epiphyses or in those with a known sensitivity to benzyl alcohol, such as neonates. Use with caution in clients with untreated hypothyroidism, because the growth response will be adversely affected.

Review the client's current medication regimen to ensure the client is not receiving adrenocorticoids, glucocorticoid, or corticotropin, which inhibit the growth response to somatrem.

■ **Nursing Diagnosis.** The client receiving somatrem therapy is at risk for the following nursing diagnoses/collaborative problems: delayed growth and development related to an underlying lack of endogenous growth hormone secretion and an ineffective response to the drug; impaired tissue integrity (pain and swelling at the injection site); and the potential complications of allergic reaction (rash), slipped capital femoral epiphysis (limp, pain in hip or knee), and hypothyroidism.

■ **Implementation**

■ ***Monitoring.*** Obtain baseline data from bone age determinations, thyroid function studies, and anti–growth hormone antibodies. Monitor these data periodically during therapy. If the growth rate does not exceed the pretreatment rate by 2 cm per year, the client should be monitored for noncompliance or other factors such as antibody formation, hypothyroidism, or malnutrition. Antibodies to somatrem may form in some clients after several months of therapy, but these rarely reduce the response to therapy. Ineffectiveness to therapy is more a function of the binding capacity of antibodies rather than the antibody titer.

Observe the injection site; pain and swelling can occur at the site of injection.

Monitor for signs of hypothyroidism such as lethargy, intolerance to cold, weight gain, constipation, dry skin, and brittle, lackluster hair, which have been reported in clients with hypopituitarism who are receiving somatrem therapy.

■ ***Intervention.*** Prepare the drug for parenteral use by diluting it with 1 to 5 mL of Bacteriostatic Water for Injection USP (benzyl alcohol preserved only). Do not shake the vial; rotate it gently between the palms of the hands until the solution is clear. A cloudy solution should not be used. Store the solution in the refrigerator. If reconstituted with Water for Injection without a preservative, such as for neonates, use the vial for one dose only and discard the unused portion.

■ ***Education.*** Advise the client of the importance of regular visits to the pediatric endocrinologist for the monitoring of blood and urine studies, thyroid function studies, and growth rate and bone age determinations.

■ **Evaluation.** The expected outcome of somatrem therapy is that the client will experience an increase in the growth pattern at a minimum of 2 cm per year. Therapy is usually continued as long as the client is responsive and until a mature adult stature is reached or the client's epiphyses close.

somatropin, recombinant [soe ma troe' pin] (Humatrope)

Somatropin is a DNA recombinant product that is identical to the amino acid sequence of human growth hormone. It is used to stimulate linear growth in clients who lack sufficient endogenous growth hormone; this stimulation results in increased skeletal growth (an increased length of the epiphyseal plates of long bones is reported). The number and size of muscle cells, organs, and red cell mass are also increased. An increase in cellular protein synthesis and lipid mobilization resulting in a decrease in body fat stores is also reported.

The mechanism of action, indications, and other properties of somatropin are similar to somatrem. The recommended dosage is individualized—up to 0.06 mg/kg SC or IM three times weekly (*Drug Facts and Comparisons,* 2000).

The nursing management is the same as for somatrem.

octreotide [ok tree′ oh tide] (Sandostatin)

Octreotide is a long-acting agent with an effect similar to somatostatin, the growth hormone-inhibiting hormone; however, octreotide is a more potent inhibitor of growth hormone, glucagon, and insulin (*Drug Facts and Comparisons,* 2000). It is indicated to lower blood levels of growth hormone and IGF-1 to normal in persons with acromegaly who have not responded to other therapies, such as surgery, radiation, and bromocriptine. It is also used to treat the symptoms associated with carcinoid tumors, such as flushing and severe diarrhea. It also has many unapproved uses, including the treatment of diarrhea associated with acquired immunodeficiency syndrome (AIDS). Refer to a current reference for additional approved and unapproved indications.

Octreotide is rapidly absorbed after SC injection and reaches a peak serum concentration in approximately 25 minutes; the half-life is 1.7 hours. Its duration of action is variable but can be up to 12 hours depending on the tumor. The IV and SC dosages are considered equivalent in effect.

The side effects/adverse reactions of octreotide include pain, swelling, and pruritus at the injection site; sinus bradycardia; diarrhea and stomach distress (30% to 58% in clients with acromegaly, and only 5% to 10% in clients with other disorders); headache, dysrhythmias, and cold-like symptoms. Hyperglycemia, hypoglycemia, and hypothyroidism are also reported primarily in clients with acromegaly. Refer to a current reference for a list of other potential side effects/adverse reactions.

The dosage for the treatment of acromegaly is 50 μg SC or IV three times daily; the dosage is adjusted according to the client's response and the presence of side effects/adverse reactions.

■ Nursing Management

Octreotide Therapy

■ **Assessment.** It should be determined that the client does not have active gallbladder disease or gallstones or a history of these conditions; there is an increased risk of cholelithiasis because of decreased gallbladder motility and the alteration of fat absorption with the administration of octreotide. A baseline and periodic ultrasonograms may be necessary to assess for the presence of gallstones.

Review the client's current medication regimen for oral antidiabetic agents, insulin, glucagon, or growth hormone; the use of these medications in combination with octreotide may result in hypoglycemia or hyperglycemia. A baseline determination of blood glucose concentrations is recommended.

A detailed assessment of the condition for which the octreotide is administered should be recorded before initiating therapy. The client's sensitivity to octreotide should also be determined.

■ **Nursing Diagnosis.** The client receiving octreotide is at risk for the following nursing diagnoses/collaborative problems: impaired comfort (abdominal cramping, headache, flushing of the face, nausea and vomiting); impaired tissue integrity (pain and redness at the injection site); diarrhea; fatigue; and the potential complications of hypoglycemia or hyperglycemia.

■ **Implementation**

■ ***Monitoring.*** Monitor blood glucose determinations, particularly during dosage changes in the medication regimen. Observe the client for hypoglycemia (anxiety, cool/pale skin, headache, hunger, nausea, difficulty concentrating, nervousness, shakiness, weakness, unconsciousness) and hyperglycemia (drowsiness, red/dry skin, anorexia, acetone-like breath, thirst, nausea and vomiting, rapid weight loss, lethargy, unconsciousness). Urinary 5-hydroxyindoleacetic acid (5-HIAA) determinations are recommended periodically during therapy for clients with carcinoid tumors.

■ ***Intervention.*** Octreotide is administered subcutaneously, with the hip, thigh, and abdomen being the preferred sites. Administer octreotide slowly at room temperature, and rotate injection sites to prevent tissue irritation. Administer between meals and at bedtime to minimize the gastrointestinal symptoms of octreotide.

■ ***Education.*** Counsel the client on the importance of close monitoring by the prescriber. Instruct the client to rotate and select injection sites and to report any signs of irritation at the injection sites or any symptoms of hyperglycemia or hypoglycemia.

■ **Evaluation.** The expected outcome of octreotide therapy as an antidiarrheal for gastrointestinal tumors or AIDS is that the client will experience fewer, firmer stools or a bowel elimination pattern that is normal for that client. If octreotide is administered for a pituitary tumor, there will be a reduction in the secretion of growth hormone as evidenced by suppressed tumor growth and a decrease in the client's symptoms of acromegaly.

POSTERIOR PITUITARY HORMONES

The posterior pituitary gland hormones are oxytocin and vasopressin (antidiuretic hormone [ADH]). Oxytocin is discussed in Chapter 53 with the drugs related to labor and delivery. Vasopressin is obtained from natural sources; lypressin and desmopressin are synthetic derivatives of vasopressin. Desmopressin has a longer duration of activity than the other agents.

✓ **vasopressin** [vay soe press′ in]) (Pitressin)
desmopressin [des moe press′ in] (DDAVP, Stimate)
lypressin [lye press′ in] (Diapid)

The ADH effect is the result of increasing water reabsorption in the collecting ducts of the nephron; this leads to a decreased urine volume with a higher osmolarity. At higher than physiologic dosages, vasopressin stimulates peristalsis through a direct effect on gastrointestinal motility; increases the secretion of corticotropin, growth hormone, and follicle-stimulating hormone; and may increase blood pressure secondary to a vasoconstrictive effect.

Vasopressin (Pitressin) is used to treat **diabetes insipidus,** a metabolic disorder characterized by extreme polyuria and polydipsia and caused by the deficient production or secretion of ADH centrally. It is not effective for polyuria induced by renal impairment, nephrogenic diabetes insipidus, psychogenic diabetes insipidus, or drug-induced (lithium or demeclocycline) diabetes insipidus.

The synthetic formulations (desmopressin [DDAVP] and lypressin [Diapid]) act as ADH with little vasopressor activity. Lypressin is used to treat clients with diabetes insipidus who are either nonresponsive to or cannot tolerate other interventions. This product prevents or controls the polydipsia, polyuria, and dehydration caused by insufficient ADH. Vasopressin, desmopressin, and lypressin are not effective for polyuria induced by renal impairment, nephrogenic diabetes insipidus, psychogenic diabetes insipidus, hypokalemia, hypercalcemia, or drug-induced diabetes insipidus (lithium).

Desmopressin intranasal is used for primary nocturnal enuresis and nocturnal polyuria in men (Cannon, Carter, McConnell, & Abrams, 1999). The oral, intranasal, and parenteral dosage forms are used to treat central diabetes insipidus, whereas only the parenteral dosage form of desmopressin is used for homeostasis in clients with hemophilia A and von Willebrand's disease.

Vasopressin administered intramuscularly or subcutaneously has a half-life of 10 to 20 minutes; the duration of effect is 2 to 8 hours. It is metabolized in the liver and kidneys and excreted by the kidneys.

Lypressin nasal spray has an immediate onset of antidiuretic activity, peaks in ½ to 1½ hours, and has a duration of action between 3 and 8 hours. Desmopressin nasal has a half-life of approximately 3.5 hours, and peak serum concentration is reached in 40 to 45 minutes; oral and intranasal dosage forms reach a peak serum level in 1 to 1½ hours. The onset of antidiuretic effects with desmopressin tablets is within 1 hour, with the maximum effect reached between 4 and 7 hours.

Table 47-1 lists the side effects/adverse reactions for these agents. No significant drug interactions have been reported.

The adult dosage of aqueous vasopressin injection (Pitressin) is 5 to 10 units IM or SC two or three times daily when needed to treat central diabetes insipidus. In children the dosage for the treatment of central diabetes insipidus is 2.5 to 10 units three or four times daily.

The adult dosage for lypressin nasal spray is 1 or 2 sprays to one or both nostrils when urinary frequency increases or when a significant thirst sensation occurs. The usual pediatric and adult dosage is 1 or 2 sprays in each nostril four times daily.

For primary nocturnal enuresis, the dosage of desmopressin intranasal for adults and children 6 years and older is 10 μg at bedtime, adjusted as necessary. The adult intranasal dosage for central diabetes insipidus is 0.1 to 0.4 mg daily as a single dose or in divided doses. The parenteral dosage is 0.5 to 1 mL SC or IV daily in 2 divided doses. The oral adult dosage starts with 0.05 mg twice daily and is adjusted according to response.

■ Nursing Management

Antidiuretic Hormone Therapy

■ **Assessment.** Use vasopressin with caution in clients with inadequate coronary circulation (the drug may precipitate anginal pain and myocardial infarction) and in clients with hypertension (the drug may increase blood pressure). Use with caution in older adults because of the risk of water intoxication and hyponatremia. Its use should be avoided if at all possible in clients who have chronic nephritis with nitrogen retention. Obtain a baseline ECG and fluid and electrolyte status determinations.

TABLE 47-1 Posterior Pituitary Hormones: Side Effects/Adverse Reactions

Drug	Side Effects*	Adverse Reactions†
desmopressin (DDAVP, Stimate)	Less frequent: headache, nausea, mild stomach cramps, vulval pain Injection: local redness, burning or swelling, facial flush, slight increase or decrease in blood pressure	Rare: severe allergic reaction, including anaphylaxis with parenteral administration
lypressin (Diapid)	Less frequent: abdominal distress, headache, heartburn, eye pain, nasal irritation or itching, runny nose, increase in bowel movements	Rare: continuous coughing, chest pain, shortness of breath, difficulty breathing
vasopressin (Pitressin)	Less frequent: abdominal distress, gas, sweating, nausea, vomiting, tremors, increased pressure for bowel evacuation, headache	Rare: chest pain due to angina or myocardial infarction; allergic reaction; increased or continuing headaches, confusion, coma, convulsions, weight gain, drowsiness, urinary difficulties (usually the result of water retention or intoxication)

*Inform the prescriber if side effects continue, increase, or disturb the client.
†If adverse reactions occur, contact the prescriber, because medical intervention may be necessary.

Lypressin and desmopressin have fewer pressor effects than vasopressin; therefore cardiovascular precautions are not as great for these two drugs. However, clients with allergic rhinitis, nasal congestion, or upper respiratory infection may experience less efficacy because of a decrease in absorption with the nasal form of these drugs.

▪ **Nursing Diagnosis.** The client receiving antidiuretic agents has the potential for the following nursing diagnoses: excess fluid volume related to water intoxication (confusion, drowsiness, increasing headache, weight gain, seizures); impaired tissue integrity at the injection site (pain); ineffective airway clearance with nasal dosage forms (runny or stuffy nose); impaired comfort (abdominal cramping, belching, nausea); diarrhea; and the potential complications of altered cardiac output related to increased fluid volume and the vasopressor effect of the drug; angina; and myocardial infarction (chest pain, shortness of breath).

▪ **Implementation**

▪ ***Monitoring.*** Obtain fluid and electrolyte determinations periodically during therapy. To evaluate the effectiveness of the drug, monitor the specific gravity of the client's urine, as well as the intake and output and daily weights. Monitor blood pressure because of the possible occurrence of hypertension or, in the case of nonresponse to the drug, hypotension. Factor VIII coagulant concentrations and other bleeding factors should be monitored if desmopressin is used for clients with hemophilia A or von Willebrand's disease.

Be alert for early signs of water toxicity—such as confusion, headache, drowsiness, and weight gain—which progress to seizures. Withdraw the drug and restrict fluid intake until the specific gravity of urine is at least 1.015 and polyuria occurs. Notify the prescriber immediately.

▪ ***Intervention.*** Vasopressin may be administered intramuscularly, subcutaneously, intravenously, or intraarterially. To allow for a precise intravenous or intraarterial flow rate, administer the vasopressin aqueous injection by an infusion pump. Avoid extravasation, because tissue necrosis and gangrene may result.

Lypressin is administered intranasally; it is not to be inhaled. If lypressin is not effective with 3 sprays, it is recommended to increase the frequency of administration rather than the number of sprays per dose.

Desmopressin is administered in a parenteral form for IV or SC use, as an intranasal dose to be administered as a spray, or through a flexible catheter known as a rhinyle.

▪ ***Education.*** Alert the client to the importance of taking the medication as prescribed and to maintain supervision by the prescriber. Instruct the client to hold the medication and report symptoms of water intoxication (e.g., weight gain, headache, confusion, and drowsiness). Fluid intake may need to be adjusted to decrease the risk for water intoxication, particularly in children and older adults.

With lypressin, the client may administer 1 to 2 sprays whenever the frequency of urination increases. An additional dose may be taken at bedtime if the daily dose does not control nocturia.

The dosage of desmopressin is adjusted to the diurnal pattern of response, with morning and evening doses adjusted separately. The initial goal is to control nocturia.

▪ **Evaluation.** The expected outcome for antidiuretic agents administered for diabetes insipidus is that the client will experience a decreased urinary output, and the client's urinalysis will indicate an increased osmolality and specific gravity. If desmopressin is administered for bleeding disorders, homeostasis will be maintained.

SUMMARY

Drugs affecting the pituitary gland are generally used as replacement therapy for hormone deficiency, as drug therapy for a specific disorder, or as diagnostic aids to diagnose hypofunctional or hyperfunctional hormone states. Somatrem is therapeutically equivalent to somatropin (the human growth hormone from the anterior pituitary); it is used for the treatment of growth failure in children caused by a deficiency of that hormone. Octreotide is used as a growth hormone–inhibiting agent.

The two posterior pituitary hormones are oxytocin and vasopressin. Oxytocin is discussed in Chapter 53. Vasopressin and the other antidiuretic agents (lypressin and desmopressin) are used for the treatment of diabetes insipidus, which results from a deficiency of ADH. The pituitary gland serves a major role in the regulation of the endocrine system.

Critical Thinking Questions

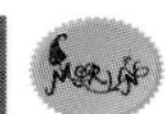

1. Timmy Johnson is receiving somatrem to enhance his growth process. In the last 6 months he has grown 3 cm; would you consider the drug to be effective? A current x-ray examination indicates epiphyseal closure. How does this impact his therapy?
2. Your client, Polly Jones, has been receiving vasopressin for her diabetes insipidus. Now she is disoriented, irritable, and short of breath. Her vital signs are stable on assessment: blood pressure, 124/70 mm Hg; pulse, 82 beats/min; respirations, 24 breaths/min; and temperature, 96.8° F (36° C). Her laboratory results are as follows:

Client	Normal Values
sodium, 116 mEq/L	135-145 mEq/L
chloride, 86 mEq/L	100-108 mEq/L
potassium, 3.6 mEq/L	3.5-5.0 mEq/L
blood urea nitrogen, 10 mg/dL	8-20 mg/dL
serum creatinine, 1 mg/dL	0.5-1.1 mg/dL for women
serum osmolality, 243 mOsm/kg H_2O	275-295 mOsm/kg H_2O
urine osmolality 1.541 mOsm/kg H_2O	300-1000 mOsm/kg H_2O
urine sodium, 320 mEq/24 hr	130-280 mEq/24 hr
urine specific gravity, 1.04	1.025-1.032

What is happening to Ms. Jones? How should the nurse intervene?

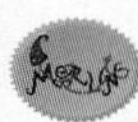

Collaborative Learning Activities

For Collaborative Learning Activities, go to mosby.com/MERLIN/McKenry/.

CASE STUDY

For a Case Study that will help ensure mastery of this chapter content, go to mosby.com/MERLIN/McKenry/.

BIBLIOGRAPHY

Ascoli, M. & Segaloff, D.L. (1996). Adenohypophyseal hormones and their hypothalamic releasing factors. In J.G. Hardman & L.E. Limbird (Eds.), *Goodman & Gilman's The pharmacological basis of therapeutics* (9th ed.). New York: McGraw-Hill.

American Hospital Formulary Service. (1999). *AHFS drug information '99*. Bethesda, MD: American Society of Hospital Pharmacists.

Anderson, K.N., Anderson, L.E., & Glanze, W.D. (Eds.). (1998). *Mosby's medical, nursing, & allied health dictionary* (5th ed.). St. Louis: Mosby.

Batcheller, J. (1992). Disorders of antidiuretic hormone secretion. *AACN Clinical Issues: Advanced Practice in Acute and Critical Care, 3*(2), 370.

Cannon, A., Carter, P.G., McConnell, A.A., & Abrams, P. (1999). Desmopressin in the treatment of nocturnal polyuria in the male. *British Journal of Urology, 84*(1), 20-24.

Drug Facts and Comparisons. (2000). St. Louis: Facts and Comparisons.

Haupt, H.A. (1993). Anabolic steroids and growth hormone. *American Journal of Sports Medicine, 21*(3), 468.

Jaffe, C.A. & Barkan, A.L. (1994). Acromegaly: recognition and treatment. *Drugs, 47*(3), 425-445.

United States Pharmacopeia Dispensing Information (USP DI): Drug information for the health care professional (19th ed.). (1999). Rockville, MD: United States Pharmacopeial Convention.

48 Drugs Affecting the Parathyroid and Thyroid Glands

Chapter Focus

Disorders of the parathyroid and thyroid have far-reaching effects because as part of the endocrine system they influence growth and development, metabolic rate, energy level, and reproductive systems. The nurse needs to be knowledgeable about the various drugs that affect the parathyroid and thyroid system in order to provide direct care to clients, as well as client education for the safe and accurate self-management of the therapeutic regimen.

Learning Objectives

1. Describe the clinical complications associated with hypothyroidism, hyperthyroidism, hypoparathyroidism, and hyperparathyroidism.
2. Describe the dose and action of calcium and vitamin D products in the treatment of hypoparathyroidism.
3. Implement the nursing management for clients receiving agents for the prophylaxis or treatment of osteoporosis.
4. Describe the primary therapy for and the agents available to treat hypothyroidism.
5. Describe the actions of iodine (iodide ion), radioactive iodine, and thioamide drugs in treating hyperthyroidism.
6. Implement the nursing management for clients receiving drugs affecting the parathyroid or thyroid gland.

Key Terms

iodine, p. 844
myxedema, p. 840
primary hyperparathyroidism, p. 837

Key Drugs [✓]

propylthiouracil, p. 847
thyroid, p. 840

This chapter will review the wide variety of medications available to treat the various conditions of the parathyroid and thyroid glands.

DRUGS AFFECTING THE PARATHYROID

In idiopathic hypoparathyroidism, serum calcium levels are decreased and serum phosphate levels are increased. Vitamin D levels are usually low. The administration of vitamin D and calcium supplements usually restore levels of calcium and phosphorus to normal (Table 48-1). Calcitriol (Rocaltrol) is an active metabolite form of vitamin D that is also used to elevate serum calcium levels. Table 48-2 lists the drugs used to treat hypocalcemia.

Primary hyperparathyroidism is a hyperactivity of the parathyroid glands. With this condition, the excessive secretion of parathyroid hormone results in increased resorption of calcium from the skeletal system and increased absorption of calcium by the kidneys and gastrointestinal system. The urine phosphate is high (the serum level is low to normal), which can lead to renal stones, bone pain with skeletal lesions, and possibly pathologic fractures. Because adenomas or tumors may cause this syndrome, surgery is usually the primary treatment. In clients with mild hypercalcemia or mild hyperparathyroidism, a thorough examination by a physician determines whether or not surgery is indicated. High serum levels of calcium may require immediate treatment. Table 48-3 describes typical recommendations for the treatment of hypercalcemia.

Calcitonin and Related Synthetic Drugs

Calcitonin and other synthetic drugs are used to treat hypercalcemia, osteoporosis, and Paget's disease. Two calcitonin products are available, salmon calcitonin (Calcimar) and human calcitonin (Cibacalcin); both products produce the same effect, but salmon calcitonin has a slightly longer half-life (70 to 90 minutes vs. 60 minutes). Calcitonin is indicated for the treatment of hypercalcemia (parenteral), Paget's disease (parenteral), postmenopausal osteoporosis, and osteoporosis in older men (nasal and parenteral) (*Drug Facts and Comparisons*, 2000).

The side effects/adverse reactions of calcitonin as a nasal spray (Miacalcin) include rhinitis, nasal irritation and redness, muscle and back pain, epistaxis, and headache. The parenteral dosage form of the drug may cause flushing or a tingling sensation of the face, ears, hands, and feet; gastric distress, anorexia, nausea, and vomiting; and pain or swelling at the injection site.

The usual adult dosage of salmon calcitonin for Paget's disease is 100 IU (IM or SC) daily, decreasing to 50 IU daily, every other day, and then three times weekly. For postmenopausal osteoporosis, the parenteral dosage is 100 IU (IM or SC) daily; the nasal dosage is 200 IU intranasally daily, alternating nostrils each day. To reduce the nausea or flushing side effects, bedtime administration is suggested, or a reduction in dosage may be required.

■ Nursing Management

Calcitonin Therapy

■ **Assessment.** Skin testing is recommended before initiating therapy to determine the client's sensitivity to calcitonin or foreign proteins. Serum calcium and serum alkaline phosphatase concentrations are usually determined. Urinary hydroxyproline (24-hour) levels may be determined but, as with all 24-hour urine samples, levels may be difficult to obtain with accuracy. A baseline assessment of the client's diet (sources of calcium and vitamin D) and underlying condition should be noted, such as bone pain, previous fractures, and bone loss.

TABLE 48-1 Calcium Supplements

The activity of calcium depends on calcium ion (elemental) content. The following calcium salts are listed by milligrams per gram, milliequivalents per gram, and the percentage of calcium in the preparations.

Preparation	Calcium (mg/g)	Calcium (mEq/g)	Percentage of Calcium	Calcium/Salt in Tablet (mg)	Number of Tablets Needed to Provide 1000 mg of Calcium
calcium carbonate	400	20.0	40	250/625	4
				500/1250	2
calcium chloride	272	13.6	27.2		
calcium citrate	211	10.5	21.1	200/950	5
calcium gluceptate	82	4.1	8.2		
calcium gluconate	90	4.5	9	45/500	22
calcium lactate	130	6.5	13	42/325	24
calcium phosphate				115/500	9
dibasic	230	11.5	23		
tribasic	400	20	38		

From Salerno, E. (1999). *Pharmacology for health professionals*. St. Louis: Mosby.

■ **Nursing Diagnosis.** The client receiving calcitonin is at risk for the following nursing diagnosis/collaborative problem: impaired comfort (anorexia; abdominal cramping; flushing or redness of the face, ears, hands, or feet; redness or swelling at the injection site; increased urinary frequency) and the potential complication of hypersensitivity.

TABLE 48-2 Drugs Used in the Treatment of Hypocalcemia

Drug	Usual Adult Dosage
calcium gluconate	IV: 970 mg given slowly at rate not exceeding 5 mL (47.5 mg) per minute
Vitamin D Analogues	
calcifediol (Calderol)	Oral: 50 μg daily per week; adjust dosage monthly if necessary
calcitriol (Rocaltrol)	Oral: 0.25 μg daily, increased every 2 to 4 weeks if necessary IV: 0.5 μg three times weekly, increased every 2 to 4 weeks if necessary
dihydrotachysterol (Hytakerol)	Oral: 0.125 to 2 mg daily
ergocalciferol (Calciferol)	Oral: individualized dosing; prophylaxis dosage is 5 to 10 μg daily

■ **Implementation**

■ ***Monitoring.*** Serum calcium, serum alkaline phosphatase, and urinary hydroxyproline (24-hour) concentrations are monitored periodically. The client should be monitored for the nursing diagnosis and potential complication mentioned previously, as well as for an improvement in baseline indicators. Monitor the client's diet for calcium and vitamin D intake.

■ ***Intervention.*** Administration at bedtime helps to reduce the nausea and facial flushing sometimes experienced with this drug. If using the nasal spray form of calcitonin, assemble the pump according to the manufacturer's instructions.

■ ***Education.*** Instruct the client how to manage, assemble, prime, use, and store the pump. Have the client blow his or her nose before administering the nasal spray; and instruct the client not to inhale while spraying. Advise the client on dietary sources of calcium and vitamin D.

■ **Evaluation.** The expected outcome of calcitonin therapy is that client will demonstrate increased bone mass, fewer fractures, and decreased bone pain. The client will also maintain a dietary intake adequate in calcium and vitamin D.

Bisphosphonates

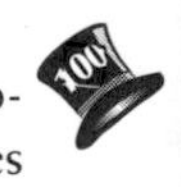

Alendronate (Fosamax ◆), etidronate (Didronel), pamidronate (Aredia), and tiludronate (Skelid) are bisphosphonates that are incorporated into bone to inhibit the normal and abnormal resorption of bone, primarily by decreasing the activity of osteoclasts. Etidronate also reduces bone forma-

TABLE 48-3 Hypercalcemia: Treatment Recommendations

Drug	Treatment
Increase Calcium Excretion	
saline hydration	Infuse normal saline (100 to 200 mL/hr) to increase calcium excretion. Monitor fluid intake, output, and electrolytes. Watch closely for evidence of fluid overload.
furosemide (Lasix)	Often used with the administration of normal saline as above. Usual dosage is 20 to 40 mg IV 2 to 4 times daily.
Inhibit Bone Resorption	
calcitonin-salmon (Calcimar)	IM or SC: 4 to 8 IU/kg q6-12h. Tolerance can develop in 24-72 hours; therefore corticosteroids may be prescribed concurrently.
etidronate (Didronel)	IV infusion: 7.5 mg/kg in 250 mL normal saline, administered over 2 hours daily until the calcium level is normal for 3 consecutive days. The dose may be repeated after a drug-free period of 1 week.
pamidronate (Aredia)	IV infusion: 60-90 mg in a liter of normal saline infused over 24 hours. The advantage of this product is that it is effective in a single dose.
plicamycin (Mithramycin)	More toxic than other agents. Reserve for individuals who do not respond to other therapies. Usual dosage is 25 μg/kg in 500 mL dextrose in water administered IV over 4-60 hours.

Information from Tang, I. & Lau, A.H. (1995). Fluid and electrolyte disorders. In L.Y. Young & M.A. Koda-Kimble (Eds.), *Applied therapeutics: The clinical use of drugs* (6th ed.). Vancouver, WA: Applied Therapeutics; and Shultz, N.J., & Slaker, R.A. (1999). Electrolyte homeostasis. In J. DiPiro, R.L. Talbert, G.C. Yee, G.R. Matzke, B.G. Wells, & L.M. Posey (Eds.), *Pharmacotherapy* (4th ed.). Stamford, CT: Appleton & Lange.

tion, but alendronate and pamidronate inhibit bone resorption without inhibiting bone formation.

Multiple mechanisms may be involved. Their action is postulated to result from binding to hydroxyapatite in bone, decreasing the dissolution of mineral bone content, or their effect on bone resorbing cells. For example, the incorporation of alendronate into bone decreases bone resorption by suppressing the number and action of osteoclasts. Tiludronate is the newest biphosphonate released that has an action similar to alendronate. It also decreases abnormal bone growth in Paget's disease because, unlike etidronate, it does not interfere with bone mineralization.

Alendronate is indicated for treating postmenopausal osteoporosis and Paget's disease and for reducing the risk of bone fractures; etidronate and pamidronate are indicated for the treatment of Paget's disease and the hypercalcemia associated with cancer. Etidronate is used for heterotopic ossification, whereas pamidronate is also used as a treatment adjunct for osteolytic metastases (bone metastases). Tiludronate is indicated for the treatment of Paget's disease. The bisphosphonates are also prescribed for osteoporosis in older men (Siddiqui, Shetty, & Duthie, 1999).

The side effects/adverse reactions of alendronate include gas production, acid regurgitation, esophageal ulcer, gastritis, dysphagia, muscle pain, headaches, constipation, or diarrhea. Bone pain (and perhaps bone fractures, osteomalacia), nausea, diarrhea, metallic taste and, rarely, hypersensitivity occur with etidronate. The side effects/adverse reactions of pamidronate include fever, nausea, vomiting, anorexia, leukopenia, hypocalcemia (more common with doses of 90 mg), and muscle stiffness. Tiludronate may cause an upper respiratory or flu-like syndrome (e.g., fever, nasal congestion, sore throat), back or body pain, abdominal distress, nausea, headache, diarrhea, arthralgia, conjunctivitis, pharyngitis, rash, nausea, vomiting, cataract, glaucoma, and chest pain.

The usual adult dosage of alendronate for Paget's disease is 40 mg PO daily before breakfast for 6 months. For etidronate, it is 5 mg/kg PO daily (2 hours before or after food) for 6 months or 7.5 mg/kg by IV infusion daily for 3 consecutive days. The adult dosage of pamidronate is 30 mg/day on 3 consecutive days by IV infusion, up to 30 mg weekly for 6 weeks (90 to 180 mg total dose per treatment) at a rate of 15 mg/hr. Refer to a current reference for other dosages, and see Table 48-3 for the treatment of hypercalcemia. For Paget's disease, the adult dosage of tiludronate is 400 mg PO at least 2 hours before or after food, beverages, or other medications.

■ Nursing Management

Bisphosphonate Therapy

■ **Assessment.** Etidronate and pamidronate therapy is contraindicated in clients with renal insufficiency when serum creatinine is >5 mg/dL; tiludronate is contraindicated when the creatinine clearance is <30 mL/min; and alendronate is contraindicated when the creatinine clearance is <35 mL/min. Caution is considered for any client with some degree of renal impairment. Clients with preexisting hypocalcemia or vitamin D deficiency should have these conditions corrected before beginning bisphosphonate therapy, because this therapy may worsen these conditions. The use of alendronate and tiludronate is contraindicated in clients with gastrointestinal diseases such as esophagitis, esophageal ulcers, or gastric ulcers. Sensitivity to any of the bisphosphonates should be determined. In clients with Paget's disease and bone fractures, etidronate therapy may be delayed until callus formation and calcification occur. Overhydration with the parenteral forms of etidronate and pamidronate is of concern for clients with cardiac failure. With etidronate, there is an increased risk of diarrhea in clients with enterocolitis.

Review the client's current drug regimen for potential drug interactions, such as would occur with calcium, iron, or other mineral supplements and antacids; these substances decrease the absorption of the bisphosphonates. Avoid the concurrent use of salicylates and alendronate or tiludronate because of the increased risk of upper GI irritation. Bisphosphonates and estrogen may be prescribed concurrently for significantly increased bone mass in postmenopausal osteoporosis (Lindsay et al., 1999).

A baseline assessment of the client with osteoporosis should include serum calcium levels and bone studies to determine bone mass. A history of fractures, particularly vertebral fractures, should be documented. Clients with Paget's disease require documentation of their symptoms (bone pain, headache, skull size) and serum alkaline phosphatase before beginning therapy. Assess for pain, weakness, and loss of function.

■ **Nursing Diagnosis.** Clients receiving bisphosphonate therapy may experience the following nursing diagnoses/collaborative problems: risk for injury related to the preexisting condition and the ineffectiveness of therapy; impaired comfort (headache, abdominal discomfort, bloating, nausea, heartburn, musculoskeletal pain, metallic taste, pain and swelling at injection site); diarrhea or constipation; impaired skin integrity (rash, erythema); and the potential complications of allergic reaction, hypercalcemia (nausea, vomiting, anorexia, weakness, constipation, thirst, cardiac dysrhythmias), hypocalcemia (paresthesia, muscle twitching, colic, cardiac dysrhythmias), and gastritis or esophageal ulceration. With tiludronate, the potential complications of cataracts and glaucoma may occur.

■ **Implementation**

■ ***Monitoring.*** Bone scans for bone density and serum calcium determinations should be performed periodically for clients being treated for osteoporosis. Clients with Paget's disease require periodic alkaline phosphatase determinations.

■ ***Intervention.*** Administer alendronate first thing in the morning with 8 ounces of water 30 minutes before meals or other medications. Have the client sit upright for 30 minutes after ingesting the drug to minimize esophageal irritation. The other oral bisphosphates are administered on an empty stomach at least 2 hours before or after food, milk or milk products, antacids, or other medications high in iron or other mineral supplements.

■ ***Education.*** Instruct the client to take the drug as previously discussed. Beverages other than water will decrease

TABLE 48-4 Thyroid Preparations: Equivalent and Usual Adult Dosages*

Drug	Equivalent Dose	Usual Adult Dosage
levothyroxine (Synthroid ◆, Levothroid ◆, Levoxyl ◆)	100 μg (0.1 mg)	Oral: 12.5-50 μg daily (dosage range for older adults or clients with cardiovascular disease is 12.5 to 25 μg daily); adjust dosage every 2 to 3 weeks as necessary. Injection: 50-100 μg IM or IV daily. The dosage is 200-500 μg IV initially for myxedema, stupor, or coma, even in older adults. If improvement is not noted by the second day, an additional 100-200 μg (0.1-0.3 mg) may be given. Switch to the oral dosage form as soon as possible.
liothyronine (Cytomel)	25 μg (0.025 mg)	Oral: 25-50 μg daily, adjusting the dosage every 1-2 weeks as needed. For myxedema and simple, nontoxic goiter, the dosage is 2.5-5 μg daily (increasing by 5- to 10-μg increments every 7 to 14 days) as necessary. The maintenance dosage for myxedema is 25-50 μg/day; for simple goiter it is 50-100 μg/day.
liotrix (Thyrolar)	50 to 60 μg of levothyroxine and 12.5 to 15 μg of liothyronine	Oral: For myxedema, 50-60 μg of levothyroxine and 12.5-15 μg of liothyronine daily; increase monthly if necessary. The dosage for older adults is 25%-50% of the usual adult dosage, adjusted as necessary at 6- to 8-week intervals.
thyroid	60 mg	Oral: 60-120 mg daily. For myxedema or hypothyroidism with cardiovascular disease, the initial dosage is 15 mg daily, increased as necessary every 2 weeks. Older adults: 7.5-15 mg daily, doubled every 6 to 8 weeks if necessary.

*Pregnancy safety for all thyroid products has been established as FDA category A.

absorption of the drug. Encourage the client to engage in supportive lifestyle changes, such as smoking cessation, reduction of alcohol intake, and participation in regular exercise with weight-bearing on the long bones (e.g., walking). Instruct the client in dietary sources of calcium and vitamin D. Consult with the prescriber about calcium and vitamin D supplementation.

▪ **Evaluation.** The expected outcome of biphosphonate therapy is that the client will experience a decrease in the progression of osteoporosis or Paget's disease and a reduction of the risk for vertebral and nonvertebral fractures (Hochberg et al., 1999; Meunier et al., 1999). Serum calcium and serum alkaline phosphatase determinations will be within the normal limits for age.

DRUGS AFFECTING THE THYROID

Thyroid Preparations

Individuals with hypothyroidism require thyroid replacement therapy. Natural or desiccated thyroid was used for replacement therapy for many years, but the synthetic thyroid preparations available today are more standardized and stable and therefore are usually prescribed. Thyroid USP is derived mainly from hog thyroid glands, but cattle and sheep thyroid glands have also been used.

The thyroid produces two iodine-containing active hormones, thyroxine (T_4) and triiodothyronine (T_3), which are essential for human growth and development and the maintenance of metabolic homeostasis. These hormones have been synthesized and are available as liothyronine (for T_3), levothyroxine (for T_4), and liotrix (both T_3 and T_4). (See Chapter 46 for further information on the functioning of the thyroid gland.) Table 48-4 summarizes the equivalent and usual adult dosages of the thyroid products.

The goal of treatment of clients with hypothyroidism or **myxedema** (adult hypothyroidism) is to eliminate their symptoms and restore them to a normal emotional and physical state. Table 48-5 lists the clinical features of hyperthyroidism vs. hypothyroidism. The clinical response is more important than the blood hormone level; nevertheless, laboratory assessments of T_3, T_4, serum cholesterol, and thyroid-stimulating hormone (TSH) are used as criteria for adequacy of therapy.

The hypothalamic-anterior pituitary and thyroid body feedback mechanism regulate thyroid hormone concentration (Box 48-1). Thyroid supplements are indicated for the

TABLE 48-5 Hyperthyroidism vs. Hypothyroidism: Clinical Features

	Hyperthyroidism	Hypothyroidism
Eyes	Prominent	Edematous eyelids, ptosis
Hair	Thin, fine texture	Dry, brittle, thin
Temperature	Intolerance to heat	Intolerance to cold
Weight	Appetite increases, weight loss	Appetite decreases, weight gain
Emotional state	Increased nervousness, irritability, insomnia	Lethargy, depression, increase in sleep needs
Gastrointestinal system	Diarrhea	Constipation
Neuromuscular system	Fast deep-tendon reflexes	Slow or delayed deep-tendon reflexes
Extremities	Hot, moist skin	Cold, dry skin

BOX 48-1

Thyroid Feedback Mechanism

Physiology of Influences on the Thyroid

When serum levels of T_3 and T_4 are increased, the release of thyrotropin-releasing hormone (TRH) from the hypothalamus and TSH from the anterior pituitary gland is reduced, thus inhibiting their effects on the thyroid gland.

When serum levels of T_3 and T_4 are decreased, TRH release triggers the release of TSH from the pituitary. TSH affects the thyroid by increasing the size and number of its follicular cells in the thyroid. The cells are then able to absorb more iodide and increase thyroglobulin breakdown, which releases T_3 and T_4 hormones from the thyroid gland into the bloodstream. This process increases the blood levels of the thyroid hormones.

treatment of hypothyroidism, the treatment and prevention of goiter, the treatment and prevention of thyroid carcinoma, and thyroid function diagnostic tests. Thyroid and levothyroxine are incompletely absorbed from the gastrointestinal tract (50% to 75%), whereas liothyronine is nearly completely absorbed (95%). Thyroid preparations are highly protein bound, with a peak effect in 3 to 4 weeks and a duration of action of 1 to 3 weeks for thyroid, thyroglobulin, and levothyroxine after withdrawing chronic therapy. Liothyronine peaks in 2 to 3 days and has a duration of action of up to 3 days after withdrawal. These agents are metabolized the same as endogenous thyroid hormone—some in peripheral tissues, smaller amounts in the liver—and are then excreted in bile.

The side effects of thyroid hormone therapy are dose related and may occur more rapidly with liothyronine than with the other products, mainly because it has a faster onset of action. The general signs of an underdose or hypothyroidism are dysmenorrhea, ataxia, coldness, dry skin, constipation, lethargy, headaches, drowsiness, tiredness, weight gain, and muscle aching. Hair loss may occur in children during the early period of treatment, but normal hair growth resumes with chronic therapy.

A rare adverse reaction is an allergic skin rash. An overdose of thyroid products results in hyperthyroidism—alterations in appetite and menstrual periods, elevated temperature, diarrhea, hand tremors, increased irritability, leg cramps, increased nervousness, tachycardia, irregular heart rate, increased sensitivity to heat, chest pain, respiratory difficulties, increased sweating, vomiting, weight loss, and insomnia.

■ Nursing Management

Thyroid Preparation Therapy

■ **Assessment.** Use thyroid preparations with care in older adults, because they are more sensitive to the effects of thyroid hormones. A 25% reduction in the dosage of the thyroid hormone replacement may be required for clients over 60 years of age (see the Special Considerations for Older Adults box on p. 842). The use of thyroid hormonal therapy is carefully considered if the client has preexisting adrenocortical or pituitary insufficiency (thyroid hormonal replacement increases the physiologic need for adrenocortical hormone), cardiovascular disease (too-rapid thyroid hormonal replacement increases metabolic demand), a history of hyperthyroidism, or thyrotoxicosis. An increased sensitivity may exist in cases of chronic hypothyroidism or myxedema. Pregnancy in women with previously diagnosed hypothyroidism may require an increased dosage of replacement therapy (Brent, 1999).

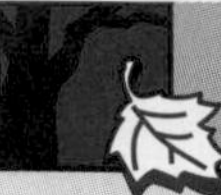

Special Considerations for Older Adults
Thyroid Hormones

Because older adults are usually more sensitive to thyroid hormones and experience more adverse reactions to them than other age-groups, it is recommended that the dosages of thyroid replacements be individualized. In some clients, the dosage should be 25% lower than the usual adult dosage.

Hypothyroidism, the second most common endocrine disease in older adults, is often misdiagnosed. Only one third of older adults exhibit the typical signs and symptoms of cold intolerance and weight gain. Most often the symptoms are nonspecific and include failure to thrive, stumbling and falling episodes, and incontinence; if neurologic involvement has occurred, the client may also be misdiagnosed with dementia, depression, or a psychotic episode (*United States Pharmacopeia Dispensing Information,* 1999).

Laboratory tests for serum T_4 and TSH are used to confirm hypothyroidism.

Levothyroxine (Synthroid, others) is usually the drug of choice for thyroid replacement.

Review the client's current medication regimen for the risk of significant drug interactions, such as those that may occur when thyroid preparations are given concurrently with the following drugs:

Drug	Possible Effect and Management
anticoagulants, oral (coumarins or indanediones)	May alter the therapeutic effects of the oral anticoagulant. An increase in thyroid hormone may require a decrease in the oral dosage of anticoagulant. Monitor coagulation time closely using the prothrombin time (PT) or International Normalization Ratio test.
cholestyramine (Questran) or colestipol (Colestid)	May bind thyroid hormones, delaying or decreasing their absorption from the gastrointestinal tract. A 4- to 5-hour interval is recommended between the administration of these drugs.
sympathomimetics	The effects of one or both medications may be increased. May result in an increased risk of coronary insufficiency if the client has coronary artery disease; if a thyroid preparation is given with tricyclic antidepressants, an increase in cardiac dysrhythmias may result from an increased receptor sensitivity to catecholamines. Monitor closely, because dosage adjustments may be necessary.

■ **Nursing Diagnosis.** The client receiving thyroid hormones is at risk for the following complications related to an underdose (hypothyroidism) or overdose (hyperthyroidism). Selected nursing diagnoses/collaborative problems associated with hypothyroidism are excess fluid volume, edema related to retention of fluids secondary to slowed metabolism; activity intolerance related to weakness and fatigue secondary to a decreased metabolic rate; imbalanced nutrition: more than body requirements related to decreased need; constipation related to decreased peristalsis; risk for ineffective breathing pattern, hypoventilation related to decreased respiratory drive; and the potential complication of myxedema coma. Selected nursing diagnoses/collaborative problems related to hyperthyroidism are imbalanced nutrition: less than body requirements related to hypermetabolism; disturbed sleep pattern; anxiety related to sympathetic nervous system stimulation; and the potential complication of thyrotoxic crisis. There is the potential complication of allergic reaction. (See the Nursing Care Plan on p. 843.)

■ Implementation

■ ***Monitoring.*** Assess the client for a decrease in the symptoms of hypothyroidism; the client should show weight loss, loss of constipation, and an increased activity level, appetite, sense of well-being, and pulse rate. Laboratory reports should indicate normal levels of T_3, T_4, and TSH.

Monitor thyroid function studies before and throughout therapy. Such studies may include free T_4 index determinations, TSH determinations, T_3 or T_4 resin uptake determinations, and total serum T_3 and T_4 determinations by radioimmunoassay. Assess children periodically for growth, bone age, and psychomotor development. Monitor apical pulse and blood pressure before and periodically during therapy.

Clients are at risk for altered cardiac output related to the thyroid's cardiovascular effects. If the resting pulse is over 100 beats/min, hold the dose and notify the prescriber. For clients with preexisting cardiovascular disease, observe closely for cardiac ischemia (chest pain) and tachydysrhythmias.

■ ***Intervention.*** Because clients with hypothyroidism respond rapidly to replacement doses, the client is started on the lowest possible dosage, with increases titrated over several weeks in accordance with the client's clinical response and laboratory data until the optimal clinical response is obtained. Once the maintenance dosage has been established, it is administered daily, preferably before breakfast. However, in neonates with congenital hypothyroidism, the full dosage of hormone replacement therapy should be started as soon as possible after birth. Replacement therapy started after 3 months of life may reverse many of the physical symptoms of hypothyroidism but not all of the mental effects.

Levothyroxine is preferred for thyroid replacement therapy. It is recommended that levothyroxine be taken on an empty stomach. In its parenteral form, levothyroxine sodium is reconstituted with sodium chloride injection (without preservative) to a solution of 100 μg (0.1 mg)/mL. It should be reconstituted immediately before use.

■ ***Education.*** Lifelong therapy is a possibility with thyroid hormonal replacement. Counsel the client accordingly. This means regular consultations with the prescriber to monitor the effectiveness of the therapy as well as compliance with the prescribed regimen. To simulate the natural process of the body, the client should take the medication at

Nursing Care Plan
Selected Nursing Diagnoses Related to Thyroid Therapy

Nursing Diagnosis	Outcome Criteria	Nursing Interventions
Deficient knowledge related to thyroid dysfunction	Client will: Express an understanding of normal thyroid function and the effects of altered thyroid function	Assess the client's level of understanding. Determine the educational needs of the client and family. Instruct the client in the function of the thyroid gland and thyroid hormones. Instruct the client in specific effects related to the client's alteration in thyroid function. Provide an opportunity for the client to ask questions and verbalize concerns.
Deficient knowledge related to drug regimen (thyroid drug)	Client will: Relate the purpose of drug therapy and identify side effects/adverse reactions of the medication	Teach the client the following: The purpose and action of the drug Proper administration The need for continued therapy throughout lifetime, even after a euthyroid state is obtained The signs and symptoms of hypothyroidism and hyperthyroidism Side effects/adverse reactions Provide the client with a list of drugs or conditions that interact with or alter the drug requirements. Explain the benefit of wearing or carrying a medical identification tag, bracelet, or card.
Disturbed body image related to thyroid dysfunction	Client and family will: Express concerns regarding body image changes State the basis for body changes related to thyroid function, and identify the benefit of drug therapy	Assess the client and family for perceptions and concerns related to body image. Encourage open communication and talking about perceived body image. Encourage adequate rest periods. Adjust calorie intake and diet to changing client needs. Encourage a high-bulk diet, fluids, and exercise to prevent or limit constipation. Encourage good grooming and attractive dress to promote self-confidence and a positive self-image.
Imbalanced nutrition related to altered metabolic needs	Client will: Maintain a stable body weight Show evidence of maintaining a well-balanced diet	Assess normal dietary patterns. Instruct the client to monitor his or her weight weekly. Instruct the client to adjust diet to match caloric needs. Assist the client in planning meals and dietary modifications.
Risk for impaired skin integrity related to altered thyroid function	Client will: Maintain intact skin Demonstrate proper skin care	Administer thyroid drugs as prescribed. Assess the skin for dryness, itching, or altered integrity. Monitor the client for the development of skin disruption. Keep the skin clean and well lubricated. Apply moisturizer as needed. Use skin massage and position changes. Instruct the client in proper skin care.

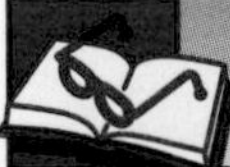

Case Study *The Client Receiving Thyroid Replacement Therapy*

Helen Hanson, a 47-year-old teacher, has been admitted to the hospital for a thyroidectomy. She noticed a lump in her neck 1 year ago. When she finally sought treatment, she was given a trial of sodium levothyroxine (Synthroid), 0.1 mg for 2 weeks, then 0.2 mg for 5 weeks. This treatment did not result in any decrease in the size of the nodule. Helen, a thin, active woman, did not note any changes in her weight, skin, or eyes. The only "hyperthyroid" symptoms noted were a heightened sense of "nervousness" and a fine tremor of her hands.

Helen and her health care provider decided on the surgical procedure because of the lack of definitive success with medical treatment and the need to identify the nature of the nodule. Before the surgery, the provider tried a short course of propylthiouracil, an antithyroid medication.

1. Why would the provider initially prescribe a thyroid replacement for Helen if her thyroid is already enlarged?
2. What are some key points that Helen needs to know about taking propylthiouracil?
3. What are the normal effects of propylthiouracil, and what side effects should Helen look for?
4. Helen will receive thyroid replacement therapy after surgery. What will be important to teach her about lifelong replacement therapy?

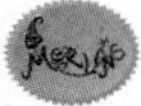

For answer guidelines, go to mosby.com/MERLIN/McKenry/.

the same time every day. Morning administration will help to prevent insomnia. (See the Case Study box above.)

Inform the client that a missed dose is to be taken as soon as possible. Caution the client not to take the missed dose if it is close to the next dose, because this will have the effect of doubling doses. Contact the prescriber if two or more consecutive doses are missed.

Tell the client to alert other health care providers about the thyroid hormonal replacement, particularly if any type of surgery is required (including dental surgery). A medical identification should be worn. Advise the client to consult with the prescriber before taking other medications concurrently with thyroid replacement.

Advise the client to inform the prescriber if the pulse rate increases or if palpitations or chest pain occur. Irritability, nervousness, heat intolerance, and excessive sweating may indicate the need for a dosage reduction; insomnia is usually the earliest sign. If such symptoms occur, drug withdrawal may be indicated for a few days before resuming it at a lower dosage.

Alert the parents of a child that a partial but temporary hair loss sometimes occurs during the first few months of therapy with children; the hair will usually return, even if hormonal replacement is continued.

Advise the client not to change brands of thyroid replacement therapy, because different brands of the same drug are not bioequivalent.

▪ **Evaluation.** The expected outcome of thyroid hormone replacement therapy is that the client is able to be independent in activities of daily living without becoming overtired. The client maintains a euthyroid state as evidenced by thyroid function studies within the normal limits.

Antithyroid Agents

An antithyroid drug is a chemical agent that lowers the basal metabolic rate by interfering with the formation, release, or action of thyroid hormones. Agents that interfere with the synthesis of the thyroid hormones are known as goitrogens. A variety of compounds are included in this category of antithyroid drugs; iodine (iodide ion), radioactive iodine, and thioamide derivatives are discussed in the following sections.

Iodine, Iodides

Iodine, an essential micronutrient, is the oldest of the antithyroid drugs. Almost 80% of the iodine in the body is found in the thyroid gland. Although a small amount of iodine is necessary for normal thyroid function and for the synthesis of thyroid hormones, the response of the client with thyrotoxicosis to iodine administration is inhibition of thyroid hormone synthesis and thyroid release from the hyperfunctioning thyroid gland.

Thyroid-Iodide Pump

Iodide from dietary sources is rapidly absorbed into the bloodstream. Approximately one third of it is removed from the blood by the iodide pump in the thyroid. The initial iodide removed from the blood is usually sodium or potassium iodide. The enzyme peroxidase converts the iodides to iodine; iodine is then used to form monoiodotyrosine (MIT) and diiodotyrosine (DIT), which are the components of T_3 and T_4. The synthesized hormones (T_3, T_4) are stored within thyroglobulin until they are released into the circulation.

These activities involve a complex negative feedback mechanism between the thyroid gland and the hypothalamus-pituitary gland. Low levels of circulating thyroid hormone increase the release of TSH from the pituitary and appear to influence the secretion of thyrotropin-releasing factor (TRF) from the hypothalamus. Increased levels of TSH increase iodide trapping by the gland, which results in an increase in synthesis and circulating thyroid hormones. As thyroid hormone levels increase, the hypothalamic and pituitary centers stop the release of TRF and TSH. This process is repeated if thyroid hormone levels decrease again in response to the declining levels of circulating thyroid hormones (see Box 48-1).

The inhibition of thyroid hormone release for several weeks leads to an increase in TSH secretion that can overcome this blockade. Thus large dosages of iodides are generally used for 7 to 14 days before thyroid surgery in order to decrease the size and vascularity of the thyroid, resulting in diminished blood loss and a less complicated surgical procedure.

Radioactive iodine (RAI) is preferred for clients with diffuse toxic goiter (Graves' disease) or toxic nodular goiter who are poor surgical risks (e.g., debilitated clients, clients with advanced cardiac disease, and older adults). It is the treatment of choice for clients with multinodular toxic goiter (Nygaard, Hegedus, Ulriksen, Nielsen, & Hansen, 1999). It is also used for clients who have not responded adequately to drug therapy or who have had recurrent hyperthyroidism after surgery. In addition to the risk involved with surgery and postsurgical complications, the primary disadvantage of surgery or RAI therapy is the induction of hypothyroidism (LeMoli, Wesche, Tiel-Van Buul, Wieringa, 1999).

Iodine Products

strong iodine solution (Lugol's solution)
potassium iodide (Thyro-Block)

Iodine is indicated to protect the thyroid gland from radiation before and after the administration of radioactive isotopes of iodine or in radiation emergencies; it may also be used with an antithyroid drug in clients with hyperthyroidism in preparation for thyroidectomy. Therapeutic effects may be noted within 24 hours, with the maximum effects achieved within 10 to 14 days of continuous therapy.

The side effects/adverse reactions of iodine therapy include diarrhea, nausea, vomiting, stomach pain, rash, and swelling of the salivary gland. With prolonged usage there may be severe headaches, sore gums or teeth, increased salivation, a burning sensation in the mouth or throat, or a metallic taste in the mouth.

Strong iodine solution is a combination of 5% iodine and 10% potassium iodide. The iodine is converted to iodide in the gastrointestinal tract before systemic absorption. The adult oral dosage is 2 to 6 drops three times daily.

Potassium iodide liquid or tablets are also commonly known as KI or SSKI. The adult oral dosage is 100 to 150 mg 24 hours before radiation, then daily for 3 to 10 days afterward. Children 1 year of age and older are given 130 mg PO daily for 10 days after exposure to radioactive iodine.

Although potassium iodide is unclassified regarding pregnancy safety, it does cross the placenta and may produce abnormal thyroid function in infants.

■ Nursing Management

Iodine Product Therapy

■ **Assessment.** Iodine products are contraindicated in clients who are sensitive to them. The initial assessment should determine if the client is allergic to seafood, because this may indicate a cross-sensitivity to iodine. Skin testing is recommended before administering parenteral doses. The earliest symptoms of hypersensitivity are irritation and swelling of the eyelids.

Be aware that iodine products are contraindicated in hyperkalemia because it might be exacerbated; checking serum potassium levels is advisable before administering iodine products. Pulmonary edema, acute bronchitis, and pulmonary tuberculosis are also contraindications to the use of iodines, because these drugs cause irritation and increase secretions. Ensure that the client has adequate renal function for potassium excretion. Iodine therapy during pregnancy can cause abnormal thyroid function or goiter in the newborn.

Review the client's medication regimen for the risk of significant drug interactions, such as those that may occur when iodine products are given concurrently with the following drugs:

Drug	Possible Effect and Management
antithyroid drugs	May increase the hypothyroid and goitrogenic effects of the drugs. Monitor closely for decreased metabolic activity.
diuretics, potassium-conserving type	If these diuretics are used concurrently with potassium iodide, increased levels of potassium may result in hyperkalemia, cardiac dysrhythmias, or cardiac arrest. Monitor serum potassium levels closely.
lithium	The hypothyroid and goitrogenic effects of both drugs may be potentiated. Obtain and monitor baseline thyroid status periodically to plan appropriate interventions.

Serum potassium concentrations and thyroid function studies should be ascertained as part of a baseline assessment.

■ **Nursing Diagnosis.** The client receiving iodine product therapy is at risk for the following nursing diagnoses/collaborative problems: diarrhea; impaired comfort (nausea and stomach cramps); and the potential complications of allergic reactions (angioedema, arthralgia, eosinophilia, urticaria), hyperkalemia (confusion, dysrhythmias, tingling or weakness of the hands and feet, tiredness, and weakness), and iodism (burning of the mouth and throat, gastric upset, increased salivation, metallic taste, headache, rhinitis).

■ **Implementation**

■ ***Monitoring.*** In addition to monitoring periodic serum potassium and thyroid function studies, assess the client's vital signs for a return to normal and the client's comfort status related to the gastrointestinal and dermatologic effects of iodine.

■ ***Intervention.*** To improve taste, dilute Lugol's solution and saturated solutions of sodium or potassium in 240 mL of fruit juice, carbonated beverage, broth, or other substance. Because the medication evaporates rapidly, do not leave it open to air for long periods before administration. Do not use if the solution has turned brownish yellow. If crystals form in the solution, warm the closed container and shake it gently until dissolved. Administer iodine products through a straw to prevent tooth discoloration. Administer after meals to minimize gastric irritation.

▪ ***Education.*** Instruct the client to discontinue use and notify the prescriber if any of the following occur: fever, skin rash, metallic/brassy taste, swelling of the neck and throat, burning soreness of the gums and teeth, head cold symptoms, or severe gastrointestinal distress. These symptoms are characteristic of iodism (chronic iodide poisoning). Stress the need for maintaining regular visits to the prescriber to monitor progress.

Advise the client to consult with the prescriber regarding the use of iodized salt and seafood in the diet. Iodine-rich foods such as soybeans, cabbage, kale, and other green leafy vegetables may need to be restricted.

Caution the client to maintain the prescribed dosage. Missing doses may precipitate a thyroid storm. Instruct the client to consult with the prescriber before taking over-the-counter (OTC) cold remedies—some contain iodides.

▪ **Evaluation.** The expected outcome of iodine product therapy is that the client will experience a decrease in the symptoms of hyperthyroidism. In clients receiving the drug as part of a preoperative course of therapy, there should be a decrease in the size and vascularity of the thyroid.

sodium iodide (^{131}I, Iodotope)

Sodium iodide, a radioactive isotope of iodine, accumulates in the thyroid tissue and selectively damages or destroys it. It is indicated for the treatment of hyperthyroidism and thyroid carcinoma.

Administered orally, this drug has an onset of effect within 2 to 4 weeks and a peak therapeutic effect between 2 and 4 months. It is mainly excreted by the kidneys. Up to 20% of the dose may appear in breast milk within 24 hours. Sodium iodide has a radionuclide half-life of approximately 8 days; the principal types of radiation are beta and gamma rays.

The side effects/adverse reactions of sodium iodide therapy may include a sore throat, a temporary loss of taste, nausea, vomiting, and painful and swollen salivary glands. Signs of hypothyroidism may follow treatment.

Although no significant drug interactions are noted with this product, many drugs are capable of interfering with test results. Refer to a current reference for possible drug interferences and current dosage recommendations. Pregnancy safety is classified as category X by the Food and Drug Administration (FDA).

▪ Nursing Management

Sodium Iodide ^{131}I Therapy

▪ **Assessment.** Thyroid function studies should be performed before and after therapy. Do not give radioactive iodine to pregnant women or nursing mothers. In women with childbearing potential, therapy begins the first few days after the onset of menses.

▪ **Nursing Diagnosis.** Most clients experience deficient knowledge and anxiety related to the administration of radioactive materials. The client may also experience temporary impaired comfort following a course of ^{131}I therapy as evidenced by a loss of taste, nausea and vomiting, and tenderness of the salivary glands. In addition, there is the potential complication of hypothyroidism with therapeutic dosages, the incidence of which should be 100% if the regimen has been successful. Potential complications may include leukopenia as evidenced by fever, chills, and sore throat, and thrombocytopenia with symptoms of unusual bleeding or bruising.

▪ **Implementation**

▪ ***Monitoring.*** After therapy, assess thyroid function with serum thyroxine examinations.

▪ ***Intervention.*** The client should take nothing by mouth after midnight before a morning dose, because food slows the absorption of the drug. Increase the fluid intake of the client to 2500 mL daily to enhance excretion of the isotope.

If the dose is administered for hyperthyroidism, institute full radiation precautions for 24 hours. If the dose is for thyroid cancer, isolate the client for 3 days. Check the institution's protocol for radiation precautions. Pregnant women (personnel or visitors) should not have contact with the client. Use disposable utensils with the client. Consult with nuclear medicine personnel about limitations for individual staff contact with the client. To avoid exposure to the radioactive products of the iodine, wear rubber gloves when giving ^{131}I to clients and when disposing of their excreta. Limit the exposure of individuals by limiting the time of contact with and increasing the distance from the source of radiation.

▪ ***Education.*** To prevent radiation contamination of others and the environment, instruct the client in the appropriate methods for disposing of urine and feces (e.g., double-flushing the toilet, washing hands after using the toilet) until radiation precautions are no longer needed. If the client is discharged but radiation precautions are still necessary, ensure that personnel from the nuclear medicine department provide the client with specific instructions for visitor contact and the disposal of utensils and excreta.

If the client received a dose of ^{131}I for the treatment of hyperthyroidism or thyroid carcinoma, 48- to 72-hour precautions may include the following: avoiding close contact with others, especially children; not kissing anyone or sharing other persons' eating or drinking utensils; not engaging in sexual activities; sleeping alone; washing the sink and tub after use; and using separate clothes, towels, and linens and washing them separately.

▪ **Evaluation.** The expected outcome of sodium iodide ^{131}I therapy is that the client will experience a euthyroid state as evidenced by thyroid function study values that are within the normal range.

Thioamide Derivatives

methimazole [meth im′ a zole] (Tapazole)
propylthiouracil [proe pill thye oh yoor′ a sill] (Propyl-Thyracil)

Thioamide derivatives, or antithyroid agents, inhibit thyroid hormone synthesis by inhibiting the incorporation of iodide into tyrosine and inhibiting the coupling of iodotyrosines. They do not affect exogenous thyroid hormones. Propylthiouracil (not methimazole) also inhibits the conversion of thyroxine (T_4) to triiodothyronine (T_3), which may make it more effective for the treatment of thyroid crisis or thyroid storm. These drugs are indicated for the treatment of hyperthyroidism, before surgery or radiotherapy, or as adjunct therapy for the treatment of thyrotoxicosis or thyroid storm (propylthiouracil is preferred for the latter indication).

The half-life of methimazole is 5 to 6 hours; the half-life of propylthiouracil is 1 to 2 hours. The peak effect is 7 weeks with methimazole and 17 weeks with propylthiouracil. Both substances are metabolized in the liver and excreted by the kidneys.

The side effects/adverse reactions of the thioamide derivatives include a loss of taste, nausea, vomiting, dizziness, skin rash, fever, and other signs of infection secondary to leukopenia or agranulocytosis.

The adult dosage of methimazole is 15 to 60 mg PO daily for hyperthyroidism; the maintenance dosage is 5 to 30 mg PO daily in 1 or 2 divided doses. To treat thyrotoxic crisis, the dosage is 15 to 20 mg PO every 4 hours for 24 hours as an adjunct to other therapies. The pediatric dosage for hyperthyroidism is 0.4 mg/kg PO daily; the maintenance dosage is 0.2 mg/kg PO daily.

The adult dosage of propylthiouracil is 300 to 900 mg PO daily in divided doses. Children between 6 and 10 years of age receive 50 to 150 mg PO daily, whereas children over 10 years of age receive 50 to 300 mg PO daily. For neonatal thyrotoxicosis, the dosage is 10 mg/kg PO daily in divided doses.

Both drugs cross the placenta and can cause fetal hypothyroidism and goiter; pregnancy safety has been established as FDA category D.

■ Nursing Management

Thioamide Derivative Therapy

■ **Assessment.** The client's health status should be reviewed to ascertain that he or she does not have a condition for which the administration of these drugs would entail a greater risk (e.g., infection, bone marrow depression, or hepatic function impairment). Determine if the client has a history of allergic reaction to these preparations. Monitor thyroid function studies before and periodically during therapy, and monitor leukocyte counts. Propylthiouracil is the drug of choice for pregnant women who require antithyroid therapy.

Review the client's drug regimen for the risk of significant drug interactions, such as those that may occur when methimazole or propylthiouracil is given concurrently with the following drugs:

Drug	Possible Effect and Management
amiodarone, iodinated glycerol, iodine, or potassium iodide	Amiodarone contains 37% iodine by weight. Increased or excess amounts of amiodarone, iodide, or iodine may result in a decreased response to the antithyroid drugs. However, iodine deficiency may result in an increased response to the antithyroid medications. Monitor closely.
anticoagulants (coumarins or indanediones)	As thyroid status approaches normal, the response to anticoagulants may decrease; if thioamide produces a drug-induced hypoprothrombinemia, the anticoagulant response may increase. Monitor closely, because dosages of anticoagulants are adjusted according to prothrombin time results.
digitalis glycosides	Serum levels of digoxin and digitoxin may increase as thyroid status approaches normal. Monitor closely, because dosage adjustments may be necessary.
sodium iodide ^{131}I	The thyroid uptake of ^{131}I may be decreased by the antithyroid agents. Monitor closely.

■ **Nursing Diagnosis.** The client receiving thioamide derivative therapy is at risk for the following nursing diagnoses/collaborative problems: impaired comfort (nausea, loss of taste, itching, stomach cramping, dizziness); ineffective protection related to the bone marrow depressant effects of the drug (delayed healing, gingival bleeding, leukopenia); and the potential complications of arthralgias, systemic lupus erythematous–like syndrome, and peripheral neuropathy, as well as hyperthyroidism as a result of ineffectiveness of the therapeutic regimen or hypothyroidism due to overdose.

■ **Implementation**

■ ***Monitoring.*** Observe the complete blood count periodically during therapy to detect blood dyscrasias such as agranulocytosis, leukopenia, or thrombocytopenia. Propylthiouracil may reduce thrombin and result in bleeding; monitor prothrombin time during therapy.

The client should be assessed for effectiveness of the therapeutic regimen. Signs of thyrotoxicosis (e.g., fever, tachycardia, irritability, weakness, diarrhea, and vomiting) indicate inadequate therapy. Signs of hypothyroidism (e.g., intolerance to cold, constipation, lethargy, weight gain) indicate overdose. TSH and T_4 assays are important in monitoring the client's status.

■ ***Intervention.*** Administer thioamide derivatives with meals to minimize gastric irritation. Use the smallest effective dose for pregnant clients. Propylthiouracil crosses the placental barrier; therefore large doses can cause goiter in the newborn or hypothyroidism in the fetus.

Because therapy to obtain a prolonged remission may last from 6 months to several years, client adherence may become an issue. For the greatest effectiveness, the doses should be divided into evenly spaced intervals throughout the day. To improve compliance and decrease the incidence of side effects, a once- or twice-daily dosage schedule may be used; however, this schedule is less effective. Antithyroid medications need to be taken at the same time every day in relation to meals, because food may alter the response to the drug by affecting its absorption.

Because of the risk of thyroid storm, the client should consult with the prescriber if his or her health status changes from infection, injury, or other illness, or if surgery, dental surgery, or emergency treatment is required.

■ ***Education.*** Instruct clients to report a sore throat, head cold, skin eruptions, or malaise immediately to their prescriber, because these symptoms signal the onset of agranulocytosis. This condition may occur too quickly to be determined by periodic blood testing. Instruct the client to consult with the prescriber about the restriction of iodized salt and seafood. Caution against taking OTC medications, because many contain iodine preparations. Alert breastfeeding mothers to take these drugs with caution and ensure thyroid function monitoring for their infants, because these drugs are excreted in the milk.

■ **Evaluation.** The expected outcome of thioamide derivative therapy is that the client will experience a euthyroid state with thyroid function study values that are within the normal range.

SUMMARY

As with other endocrine glands, parathyroid and thyroid functioning may increase or decrease, resulting in pathologic conditions for the client. With hypoparathyroidism, the administration of vitamin D and calcium supplements will usually restore the calcium and phosphorus levels to normal. Surgery is usually the primary treatment for hyperparathyroidism.

With hypothyroidism, the clinical goal is to eliminate the client's symptoms by thyroid replacement therapy, for which a number of preparations are available. Hyperthyroidism is managed by large doses of iodides, which inhibit the release of thyroid hormones and decrease the size of the thyroid; thioamide derivatives, which inhibit the synthesis of thyroid hormone; radioactive iodine; or surgery.

During all the therapies associated with hormonal replacement or inhibition, the client requires support and explanation to understand the many body and mood changes that may occur with these therapies. Because the clinical manifestations of the therapies are as important as laboratory studies in determining the efficacy of treatment, ongoing skilled assessment of the client's health status is essential.

Critical Thinking Questions

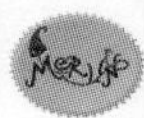

1. Grace Smith examines the label on the OTC calcium supplement she takes each day. It indicates that two tablets taken daily provide 3000 mg of calcium carbonate. How much elemental calcium is Grace taking?
2. Why is clinical response more important than blood hormone level in thyroid preparation therapy? What signs and symptoms should the nurse be monitoring to determine the effectiveness of the therapy?

Collaborative Learning Activities

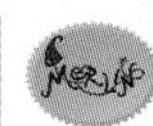

For Collaborative Learning Activities, go to mosby.com/MERLIN/McKenry/.

CASE STUDY

For a Case Study that will help ensure mastery of this chapter content, go to mosby.com/MERLIN/McKenry/.

BIBLIOGRAPHY

American Hospital Formulary Service. (1999). *AHFS drug information '99*. Bethesda, MD: American Society of Hospital Pharmacists.

Anderson, K.N., Anderson, L.E., & Glanze, W.D. (Eds.). (1998). *Mosby's medical, nursing, & allied health dictionary* (5th ed.). St. Louis: Mosby.

Angelucci, P.A. (1995). Caring for patients with hypothyroidism. *Nursing, 25*(5), 60-61.

Brent, G.A. (1999). Maternal hypothyroidism: Recognition and management. *Thyroid, 9*(7), 661-665.

Drug Facts and Comparisons. (2000). St. Louis: Facts and Comparisons.

Hochberg, M.C. Ross, P.D., Black, D., Cummings, S.R., Genant, H.K., Nevitt, M.C., Barrett-Connor, E., Musliner, T., Thompson, D. (1999). Larger increases in bone mineral density during alendronate therapy are associated with a lower risk of new vertebral fractures in women with postmenopausal osteoporosis. Fracture Intervention Trial Research Group. *Arthritis & Rheumatology, 42*(6), 1246-1254.

Katzung, B.G. (1998). *Basic and clinical pharmacology* (7th ed.). Stamford, CT: Appleton & Lange.

Kim, T.S. (1994). Primary hyperparathyroidism. *Orthopaedic Nursing, 13*(3), 17-28.

Kovacs, C.S., MacDonald, S.M., Chik, C.L., & Bruera, E. (1995). Hypercalcemia of malignancy in the palliative care patient: A treatment strategy. *Journal of Pain and Symptom Management, 10*(3), 224-232.

LeMoli, R., Wesche, M.F., Tiel-Van Buul, M.M., & Wieringa, W.M. (1999). Determinants of long-term outcome of radioiodine therapy of sporadic nontoxic goiter. *Clinical Endocrinology, 50*(6), 783-789.

Lindsay, R., Cosman, F., Lobo, R.A., Walsh, B.W., Harris, S.T., Reagan, J.E., Liss, C.L., Melton, M.E., Byrnes, C.A. (1999). Addition of alendronate to ongoing hormone replacement therapy in the treatment of osteoporosis: A randomized, controlled clinical trial. *Journal of Clinical Endocrinology & Metabolism, 84*(9), 3076-3081.

McCance, K.L. & Huether, S.E. (1998). *Pathophysiology: The biological basis for disease in adults and children* (3rd ed.). St. Louis: Mosby.

Melmon, K.L., Morrelli, H.F., Hoffman, B.B., & Nierenberg, D.W. (1992). *Melmon & Morrelli's clinical pharmacology: Basic principles in therapeutics* (3rd ed.). New York: McGraw-Hill.

Meunier, P.J., Delmas, P.D., Eastell, R., McClung, M.R., Papapoulos, S., Rizzoli, R., Seeman, E., Wasnich, R.D. (1999). Diagnosis and management of osteoporosis in postmenopausal women: Clinical guidelines. International Committee for Osteoporosis Clinical Guidelines. *Clinical Therapeutics, 21*(6), 1025-1044.

Nygaard, B., Hegedus, L., Ulriksen, P., Nielsen, K.G., & Hansen, J.M. (1999). Radioiodine therapy for multinodular toxic goiter. *Archives of Internal Medicine, 159*(12), 1364-1368.

Siddiqui, N.A., Shetty, K.R., & Duthie, E.H., Jr. (1999). Osteoporosis in older men: Discovering when and how to treat it. *Geriatrics, 54*(9), 20-22, 27-28, 30.

Tang, I. & Lau, A.H. (1995). Fluid and electrolyte disorders. In L.Y. Young & M.A. Koda-Kimble (Eds.), *Applied therapeutics: The clinical use of drugs* (6th ed.). Vancouver, WA: Applied Therapeutics.

Toft, A.D. (1994). Thyroxine therapy. *New England Journal of Medicine, 331*(3), 174-180.

United States Pharmacopeia Dispensing Information (USP DI): Drug information for the health care professional (19th ed.). (1999). Rockville, MD: United States Pharmacopeial Convention.

Watts, N.B. (1999). Postmenopausal osteoporosis. *Obstetrics & Gynecology Survey, 54*(8), 532-538.

49 Drugs Affecting the Adrenal Cortex

Chapter Focus

A number of pathologic conditions associated with hyposecretion or hypersecretion of the adrenal cortex are pharmacologically managed. The glucocorticoids are widely used in pharmacologic doses for their antiinflammatory and immunomodulating effects. However, clients receiving systemic corticosteroid preparations for nonendocrine disorders are at risk for adverse reactions. Nurses need to be skillful at assessing not only the steroid-responsive disorder but also the client's individual responses to corticosteroid therapy.

Learning Objectives

1. Compare and contrast glucocorticoids and mineralocorticoids.
2. Describe the major pharmacologic effects of the corticosteroids.
3. Discuss five significant drug interactions of the glucocorticoids.
4. Describe the advantages for an alternate-day dosing schedule.
5. Discuss a recommended method for corticosteroid drug withdrawal.
6. Name four major adverse reactions associated with the use of adrenocorticoids.
7. Implement the nursing management of drug therapy for the care of clients receiving agents affecting the adrenal cortex.

Key Terms

circadian rhythm, p. 852
corticosteroids, p. 851
glucocorticoid, p. 851
mineralocorticoids, p. 851, 857
septic shock, p. 851
ultradian rhythms, p. 852

Key Drugs [✔]

cortisone, p. 851
fludrocortisone, p. 858

The adrenal cortex secretes two classes of steroids: the corticosteroids (glucocorticoids and mineralocorticoids) and the androgens; androgens will be discussed in Chapter 54. In humans, hydrocortisone or cortisol is the primary (prototype) glucocorticoid, and aldosterone is the main mineralocorticoid.

The term **corticosteroids** refers to the adrenocortical hormones and the higher potency, synthetic formulations. The term **glucocorticoid** refers to the action of these drugs on glucose. **Mineralocorticoids** regulate mineral salts or electrolytes in the body. A physiologic effect is produced with low dosages of corticosteroids; larger dosages are necessary to produce a pharmacologic effect, such as for the treatment of asthma and inflammatory diseases. The pharmacologic actions are discussed in the following sections.

Corticosteroids, such as cortisol, have a profound effect on carbohydrate metabolism. Aldosterone, a mineralocorticoid, primarily affects mineral (or electrolyte) and water metabolism.

Cholesterol, which is used for the biosynthesis of corticosteroids, is synthesized and stored in the adrenal cortex. The synthesis of corticosteroids depends on pituitary adrenocorticotropic hormone (ACTH), which is governed by the corticotropin-releasing hormone (CRH) from the hypothalamus. Evidence suggests that increased levels of corticosteroids can inhibit the adrenal glucocorticoid system by inhibiting the release of CRH from the hypothalamus and by inhibiting the release of ACTH from the pituitary.

This chapter will review the pharmacology of the glucocorticoids (and the associated body rhythms), mineralocorticoids, and the antiadrenal agents.

BOX 49-1

Septic Shock

Septic shock usually results from a gram-negative bacteremia that leads to circulatory insufficiency. The inadequate tissue perfusion generally results in hypotension, oliguria, tachycardia, elevated temperature, and tachypnea.

Mechanism

Septic shock may be caused by bacterial substances that interact with body cell membranes and systems, especially coagulation and the complement system, which results in injury to cells and alterations in blood flow in the body.

Treatment

Treatment may consist of volume replacement, antibiotics, surgery (if the client has an abscessed or necrotic bowel or organs/tissues), vasoconstricting agents (dopamine, norepinephrine, or levarterenol), diuretics, and glucocorticoids (steroids). The use of steroids is somewhat controversial, but several published studies have reported a benefit with their use if used early in the treatment of shock.

Steroid Beneficial Effects

The beneficial effects of steroids include protecting cellular membranes from injury, decreasing platelet aggregation, reducing the extracellular release of leukocyte enzymes, and preventing the formation of vasoactive substances in the body.

GLUCOCORTICOIDS

Cortisone and prednisone are inactive substances until they are metabolized in the body to hydrocortisone and prednisolone, respectively.

Glucocorticoids are used in replacement therapy for adrenocortical insufficiency. They are also used to treat severe allergic reactions, anaphylactic reactions not responsive to other therapies, collagen disorders such as systemic lupus erythematosus, dermatologic conditions, hematologic disorders, neoplastic disease (adjunct treatment), ophthalmic disorders, respiratory disorders, rheumatic disorders, and shock and other conditions (Box 49-1).

Glucocorticoids have the following pharmacologic actions:

- *Antiinflammatory action.* Glucocorticoids, especially cortisol in larger than normal dosages, can stabilize lysosomal membranes and prevent the release of proteolytic enzymes during inflammation. They can also potentiate vasoconstrictor effects.
- *Maintenance of normal blood pressure.* Glucocorticoids potentiate the vasoconstrictor action of norepinephrine. When glucocorticoids are absent, the vasoconstricting action of the catecholamines is diminished, and blood pressure falls.
- *Carbohydrate and protein metabolism.* Glucocorticoids help to maintain the blood sugar level and the glycogen content of liver and muscle. They facilitate the breakdown of protein in muscle and extrahepatic tissues, which leads to increased plasma levels of amino acid. Glucocorticoids increase the trapping of amino acids by the liver and stimulate the deamination of amino acids. They also increase the activity of enzymes important to gluconeogenesis and inhibit glycolytic enzymes; this can produce hyperglycemia and glycosuria. They are diabetogenic (Hoogwerf & Danese, 1999); their effects can aggravate diabetes, bring on latent diabetes, and cause insulin resistance. The inhibition of protein synthesis can delay wound healing and cause muscle wasting and osteoporosis (Buckley, Marquez, Feezor, Ruffin, & Benson, 1999; Smith, Phillips, & Heller, 1999). These effects may inhibit growth in young persons (Van Bever, Desager, Lijssens, Weyler, & DuCaju, 1999).
- *Fat metabolism.* Glucocorticoids promote the mobilization of fatty acids from adipose tissue, increasing their concentration in the plasma and their use for energy. Despite this effect, clients taking glucocorticoids may

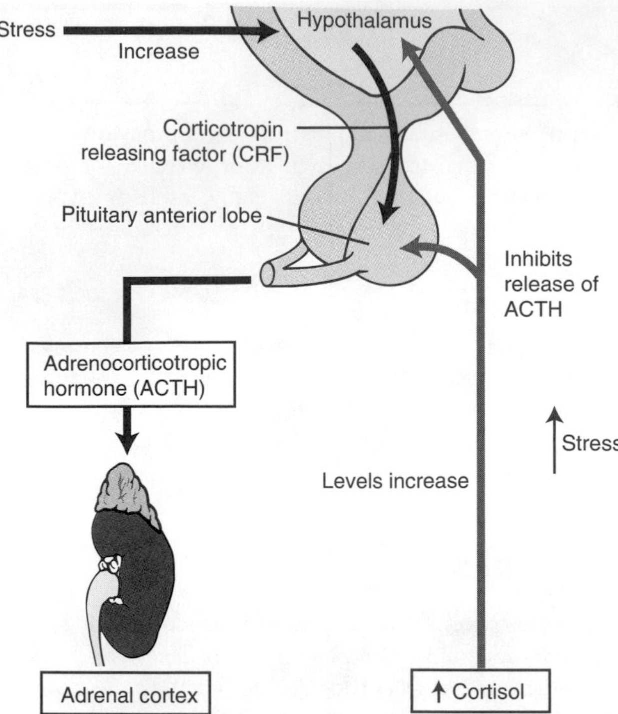

Figure 49-1 Glucocorticoid secretion.

accumulate fat stores (rounded face, buffalo hump). The effect of glucocorticoids on fat metabolism is complex and little known.

- *Thymolytic, lympholytic, and eosinopenic actions.* Glucocorticoids can cause atrophy of the thymus and decrease the number of lymphocytes, plasma cells, and eosinophils in the blood. By blocking the production and release of cytokines, corticosteroids interfere with the integrated role of T and B lymphocytes, macrophages, and monocytes in the immune response (Schimmer & Parker, 1996) and thus ultimately interfere with immune and allergic responses. This response, along with their antiinflammatory action, makes them useful immunosuppressants for delaying rejection in clients with organ or tissue transplants, as well as useful antiallergenics for the treatment of acute allergic reactions such as urticaria, bronchial asthma, and anaphylactic shock. However, steroids can also be a source of danger in infections by limiting useful protective inflammation (Kobashigawa, 1999). These hormones also inhibit the activity of the lymphatic system, causing lymphopenia and reducing the size of enlarged lymph nodes.
- *Stress effects.* During stressful situations (e.g., injury, major surgery), corticosteroids are suddenly released or are necessary to help maintain homeostasis (Figure 49-1). This sudden release is believed to be a protective mechanism. Hypotension and shock may occur without steroid administration. During stress, epinephrine and norepinephrine are released from the adrenal medulla, and these catecholamines have a synergistic action with the corticosteroids.
- *Central nervous system.* Corticosteroids affect mood and behavior and possibly cause neuronal or brain excitability. Some persons report euphoria, insomnia, anxiety, depression, or increased motor activity, or they may become psychotic.

Two rhythms appear to influence glucocorticoid function: circadian (daily) rhythm and ultradian rhythm. **Circadian rhythm** is a pattern based on a 24-hour cycle with the repetition of certain physiologic phenomena; it is controlled by the dark/light and sleep/wakefulness cycles. Sleeping in the dark at night normally increases plasma cortisol levels in the early morning hours. These levels reach a peak after awakening and then slowly fall to very low levels in the evening and during the early phase of sleep. The importance of this rhythm is emphasized by the finding that corticosteroid therapy is more potent when given at midnight than when given at noon.

Ultradian rhythms are periodic or intermittent functions with frequencies greater than once every 24 hours. In human beings, four to eight adrenal glucocorticoid bursts occur every 24 hours, which may follow bursts in the release of CRH and ACTH. These bursts are clustered close together and are very pronounced during the circadian rise in plasma glucocorticoid levels in the early morning hours. At other times these bursts are so widely spaced that adrenal secretion is zero. Consequently, the adrenal cortex secretes glucocorticoids only approximately 25% of the time in unstressed individuals.

The glucocorticoids are well absorbed orally. Parenterally (IM), the soluble esters (sodium phosphate, sodium succinate) are rapidly absorbed, whereas the poorly soluble agents (acetate, acetonide, diacetate, hexacetonide, tebutate) are slowly but completely absorbed. Topically, the soluble esters are less rapidly absorbed, whereas the poorly soluble agents are slowly but completely absorbed. Rectally, approximately 20% of the drug is absorbed normally; if the rectum is inflamed, absorption may increase up to 50%.

These agents are mainly metabolized in the liver and excreted by the kidneys. The fluorinated adrenocorticoids are more slowly metabolized than the other drugs. See Table 49-1 for the onset of action, peak effect, and duration of action for the glucocorticoids. See Table 49-2 for the relative potency of the major short-acting, intermediate-acting, and long-acting adrenocorticoids.

The side effects/adverse reactions of the glucocorticoids include euphoria, increased appetite, insomnia, restlessness, anxiety, gas, hyperpigmentation, hypotension, headache, hirsutism, lowered resistance to infections, visual disturbances (cataracts), increased urination or thirst, and decreased growth in children. Anorexia may occur with triamcinolone. Redness, swelling, rash, pain, tingling, or numbness may occur at the injection site. Chronic use may result in abdominal pain, acne, gastrointestinal bleeding,

TABLE 49-1 Adrenocorticoids/Corticotropin: Pharmacology

Drug	Onset of Action	Peak Effect	Duration of Action
betamethasone			
PO	—	1-2 hours	3.25 days
IM, IV	Rapid	—	—
betamethasone acetate/sodium phosphate (IM)	1-3 hours	—	7 days
corticotropin repository (IM)	—	—	12-24 hours
cortisone acetate			
PO	Rapid	2 hours	30-36 hours
IM	Slower	20-48 hours	—
dexamethasone			
PO	—	1-2 hours	66 hours
IM	—	8 hours	6 days
IV	Rapid	—	—
hydrocortisone			
PO	—	1 hour	30-36 hours
IM	—	4-8 hours	—
rectal enema (retention)	3-5 days	—	—
rectal foam	5-7 days	—	—
hydrocortisone cypionate			
PO	Slow	1-2 hours	—
IM	Rapid	1 hour	Varies
methylprednisolone			
PO	—	1-2 hours	30-36 hours
IM	6-48 hours	4-8 days	1-4 weeks
IA, IL, ST	Very slow	7 days	1-5 weeks
methylprednisolone sodium succinate (IV, IM)	Rapid	—	—
prednisolone (PO)	—	1-2 hours	30-36 hours
prednisolone acetate/sodium phosphate			
IM	—	—	Up to 4 weeks
IB, IS, IA, ST	—	—	3-28 days
prednisolone sodium phosphate (IV, IM)	Rapid	1 hour	—
prednisone (PO)	—	1-2 hours	30-36 hours
triamcinolone			
PO	—	1-2 hours	52 hours
IM	1-2 days	—	1-6 weeks

Information from *United States Pharmacopeia Dispensing Information (USP DI): Drug information for the health care professional* (19th ed.). (1999). Rockville, MD: United States Pharmacopeial Convention.
—, Not available; *PO*, orally; *IA*, intraarticularly; *IB*, intrabursal; *IL*, intralesional; *IM*, intramuscularly; *IS*, intrasynovial; *ST*, in soft tissue.

peptic ulcers, round face (Cushing's syndrome), hypertension, edema, weight gain, muscle cramps, weakness, irregular heart rate, nausea, vomiting, bone pain, increased bruising, and wounds that are difficult to heal.

The adult oral dosage of cortisone (Cortone) is 25 to 300 mg/day. The pediatric oral dosage for adrenocortical insufficiency is 0.7 mg/kg daily in divided doses. The adult oral dosage of betamethasone (Celestone) is 0.6 to 7.2 mg/day; the pediatric dosage for adrenocortical insufficiency is 18 μg/kg in 3 divided doses. The parenteral adult dosage for betamethasone is up to 9 mg/day (IM/IV/intraarticular/intralesional/soft tissue injections). The adult dosage of corticotropin (Acthar) as a diagnostic aid is 10 to 25 units in 500 mL D_5W.

When cortisone or hydrocortisone is used as replacement therapy, the drug should be scheduled according to the normal endogenous secretion of corticosteroid in the body; give ⅔ of the dose in the morning and ⅓ in the evening. Other corticosteroids have a longer duration of action, and therefore once-daily dosing is usually sufficient.

An alternate-day schedule may be used with chronic corticosteroid therapy to reduce the potential of suppressing the hypothalamic-pituitary-adrenal (HPA) axis and producing undesirable side effects. A short- or intermediate-acting cor-

TABLE 49-2 Major Adrenocorticoids: Relative Potency and Half-life

Adrenocorticoids	Equivalent Glucocorticoid Dose (mg)*	Relative Glucocorticoid Potency†	Relative Mineralocorticoid Potency‡	Half-life (hours)	
				Serum	Tissue
Short-Acting					
cortisone	25	0.8	2	0.5	8-12
hydrocortisone	20	1	2	1.5-2	8-12
Intermediate-Acting					
methylprednisolone	4	5	0§	>3.5	18-36
prednisolone	5	4	1	2.1-3.5	18-36
prednisone	5	4	1	3.4-3.8	18-36
triamcinolone	4	5	0§	2->5	18-36
Long-Acting					
betamethasone	0.6	20-30	0§	3-5	36-54
dexamethasone	0.5-0.75	20-30	0§	3-4.5	36-54

*Approximate dosages, applies to oral and IV only.
†Refers to antiinflammatory, immunosuppressant, and metabolic-type effects.
‡Potassium excretion, sodium and water retention.
§Some hypokalemia and/or sodium and water retention may occur, depending on the dose and individual response.

ticosteroid is used to stabilize the client's condition. The dosage on one day is tapered and the dosage on the alternate day is increased; this continues until the client is taking approximately two to three times the daily dose every other day (Small & Cooksey, 1995). A gradual dosage reduction is recommended when discontinuing these drugs. Table 49-3 provides additional information on corticosteroid drug dosing.

■ Nursing Management

Glucocorticoid Therapy

■ **Assessment.** Do not give glucocorticoids to clients with systemic fungal infections or tuberculosis, because these infections may be exacerbated. The prescriber should carefully consider the risk-benefit ratio before administering systemic corticosteroids to clients with acquired immunodeficiency syndrome (AIDS) or human immunodeficiency virus (HIV), or a predisposition to these conditions, because there is a risk for an uncontrollable infection. Clients with diabetes mellitus may experience an exacerbation of their condition. Symptoms of the progression or reactivation of active or latent esophagitis, gastritis, or peptic ulcer may be masked, and clients may bleed without warning. Clients for whom edema may be hazardous (e.g., those with cardiac disease, congestive heart failure, hypertension, or renal function impairment) should be monitored very carefully. Note that a myasthenic crisis may be induced if these drugs are administered to clients with myasthenia gravis. Clients with ocular herpes simplex are at risk for corneal perforation. The use of glucocorticoids in clients with existing or recent measles or chickenpox, including recent exposure, run the risk of contracting a generalized (potentially fatal) course of the disease.

Use glucocorticoids with caution in pregnant women, because adrenal insufficiency in both mother and child is possible at delivery. Fetal abnormalities can also occur. If the drug is administered maternally to help prevent neonatal respiratory distress syndrome, there is an increased risk of maternal infection (tuberculosis, herpes type II), uterine bleeding, placental insufficiency, and premature membrane rupture. Older adults are more likely to develop hypertension during glucocorticoid therapy, and postmenopausal women are more likely to develop osteoporosis.

If the corticosteroid is for an intraarticular injection, the joint should not be infected, bleeding, fractured, or have had recent surgery, because the condition will be aggravated and/or healing will be inhibited. Juxtaarticular nonarthritic osteoporosis may be worsened.

Rectal administration of the drug should be avoided in instances of bowel obstruction, recent gastrointestinal surgery, or infection, because healing will be delayed.

Because there is a risk for fluid volume excess related to sodium and fluid retention, obtain the client's baseline weight before initiating therapy. Obtain baseline data for hematologic values, serum electrolytes, and blood glucose. Check the stool for occult blood. If therapy is anticipated to last more than 6 weeks, the client should obtain a baseline ophthalmologic examination for the presence of cataracts, glaucoma, and ocular infections. These determinations should be monitored during therapy. Obtain a baseline assessment of the underlying condition for which the glucocorticoid is being prescribed.

Assess children for growth before and periodically during therapy, because there is a risk for altered growth and development with glucocorticoid therapy.

TABLE 49-3 Corticosteroid Preparations and Dosing*

Drug	Usual Dosage: Adult	Usual Dosage: Child
dexamethasone (Decadron and others)	PO: 0.5-9 mg daily	Adrenocortical insufficiency: 23.3 μg/kg daily in 3 divided doses
hydrocortisone (Cortef and others)	PO/IM: 15-20 mg, up to 240 mg daily	Oral: 0.56 mg/kg/day IM: 0.56-4 mg/kg/day
enema (Cortenema)	Rectal: 100 mg retention enema nightly for 3 weeks	Not established
methylprednisolone (Medrol)	PO: 4-48 mg daily	Adrenocortical insufficiency: 117 μg/kg daily in 3 divided doses
prednisolone (Delta-Cortef and others)	PO: 5-60 mg daily (maximum 250 mg/day)	Adrenocortical insufficiency: 140 μg/kg daily in 3 divided doses
prednisone (Deltasone and others)	PO: 5-60 mg daily	Dosage varies; refer to current drug references
triamcinolone (Aristocort, Kenacort)	PO: 4-48 mg daily	Adrenocortical insufficiency: 117 μg/kg daily

From Salerno, E. (1999). *Pharmacology for health professionals.* St. Louis: Mosby.
*Dexamethasone, methylprednisolone, prednisolone, and triamcinolone are also available in short-acting and long-acting preparations; refer to a current drug reference for dosing information.

Review the client's current medication regimen for significant drug interactions, such as those that may occur when corticosteroids are given concurrently with the following drugs:

Drug/Herb	Possible Effect and Management
Bold/color type indicates the most serious interactions.	
aminoglutethimide (Cytadren)	Suppresses adrenal function; therefore do not administer corticotropin concurrently. Glucocorticoid supplements are often prescribed when aminoglutethimide is given. Be aware that aminoglutethimide can increase the metabolism of dexamethasone and reduce its half-life significantly. Hydrocortisone is recommended, because its metabolism does not appear to be affected by aminoglutethimide.
amphotericin B parenteral (Fungizone)	May result in severe hypokalemia. If given concurrently, monitor serum potassium levels closely. May also decrease the adrenal gland response to corticotropin.
antacids	When given concurrently with prednisone or dexamethasone, a decrease in steroid absorption may result. Monitor closely, because steroid dosage adjustments may be necessary.
antidiabetic drugs (oral) or insulin	Glucocorticoids may elevate serum glucose levels (both during therapy and after, if the glucocorticoid is stopped); therefore a dosage adjustment of one or both drugs may be necessary.
digitalis glycosides	May result in an increased potential for toxicity (dysrhythmias) associated with hypokalemia.
diuretics	The sodium and fluid-retaining effects of the adrenocorticoids may reduce the effectiveness of the diuretic agents. Monitor closely for edema and fluid retention. Potassium-depleting diuretics given with adrenocorticoids may result in severe hypokalemia. Monitor potassium serum levels. The effects of potassium-sparing diuretics may be decreased. Monitor serum potassium levels and the client response closely.
hepatic enzyme-inducing agents	Barbiturates, carbamazepine, phenytoin, and others may decrease the adrenocorticoid effect because of increased metabolism. Dosage adjustments may be necessary. Monitor serum cortisol levels closely.
licorice, magnolia officinalis, Perilla frutescens, Saiboku-To, Scutellaria baicalensis, Zizyphus vulgaris	May enhance and prolong corticosteroid effects. Monitor.
mitotane (Lysodren)	Mitotane will decrease the response of the adrenal gland to corticotropin. Avoid concurrent use. Adrenocorticoids are usually necessary during mitotane administration because mitotane suppresses adrenocortical function. Higher than normal dosages of glucocorticoids are usually needed.
potassium supplements	The concurrent use of these drugs reduces the effect of the supplements and/or the corticosteroids on serum potassium levels. Monitor serum levels if given concurrently.

Drug/Herb	Possible Effect and Management
ritodrine (Yutopar)	When ritodrine is given to inhibit premature labor in the pregnant woman and the long-acting glucocorticoids are given to enhance fetal lung maturity, the result may be pulmonary edema in the mother. Monitor pregnant women closely for the first signs of pulmonary edema (shallow, rapid, difficult breathing; anxiety; restlessness; increased heart rate and blood pressure; enlarged peripheral and neck veins; edema of the extremities; lung rales; and diaphoresis); early detection and treatment are necessary to prevent a potentially serious adverse reaction or fatality.
sodium-containing foods or medications	Concurrent use may result in edema and hypertension. Monitor weight, intake and output, and blood pressure closely.
somatrem or somatropin	The growth response to somatrem or somatropin may be inhibited with concurrent chronic therapy with corticotropin or with daily doses of glucocorticoids above certain levels, such as daily doses of prednisone or prednisolone above 2.5 to 3.75 mg/m^2 of body surface. Refer to a current *USP DI* for the dosages of other glucocorticoids.
vaccines, live virus, and other immunizations	**In general, immunizations are not recommended for clients who are receiving pharmacologic or immunosuppressant doses of glucocorticosteroids. Because corticosteroids inhibit the antibody response, the immunization effect will be reduced or ineffective and the client may develop neurologic complications. Avoid concurrent use or a potentially serious drug interaction may occur. If live virus vaccines are given to individuals receiving immunosuppressant glucocorticoid therapy, the client may develop the viral disease or at least have a reduced response to the vaccine. Avoid concurrent use or a potentially serious drug interaction may occur. In addition, do not administer the oral polio vaccine to persons in close contact with someone who is receiving immunosuppressant glucocorticoid therapy.**

■ **Nursing Diagnosis.** Clients undergoing glucocorticoid therapy are at risk for the following nursing diagnoses/collaborative problems: disturbed sleep pattern due to drug-induced insomnia; disturbed body image related to physical changes with long-term therapy (moon face, central obesity, striae, acne, hirsutism); activity intolerance related to muscle wasting; sexual dysfunction related to physiologic limitations secondary to abnormal hormone levels; risk for infection related to immunosuppression; risk for trauma related to osteoporosis; disturbed thought processes related to the CNS effects (euphoria, psychotic behavior, restlessness); imbalanced nutrition: more than body requirements related to increased appetite; excess fluid volume related to sodium and water retention; and the potential complications of cataracts, mental depression, anaphylaxis, congestive heart failure and hypertension related to cardiovascular effects, peptic ulcer related to gastrointestinal effects, and hypokalemia, hyperglycemia, and hyperlipidemia related to metabolic effects.

■ Implementation

■ ***Monitoring.*** Weigh the client daily; report any sudden increases, which indicate fluid retention, to the prescriber. Monitor intake and output daily. Correlate these findings with physical findings of edema. Check the stool for occult blood. Assess for the following when long-term or excessive doses are given: CNS symptoms (anxiety, depression/stimulation), elevated blood pressure, hematologic values, serum electrolytes, and Cushing's syndrome. If therapy is more than 6 weeks, the client should obtain an ophthalmologic examination at periodic intervals.

Closely monitor the blood sugar of clients taking glucocorticoids, because these drugs can cause hyperglycemia. Clients with diabetes may need changes in diet or insulin dosage to maintain blood sugar control.

Remember that not only the total daily dose but also frequent individual doses during the day must be adjusted to meet the client's needs. Notify the prescriber of the client's varying responses to the drugs.

■ ***Intervention.*** Note that an alternate-day dosing regimen may be valuable when considering the long-term use of glucocorticoids in less severe disease processes, especially when an intermediate range–acting agent (methylprednisolone, prednisolone, prednisone) is used, because it diminishes suppression of the HPA axis. The alternate-day dose given every other morning before 9 AM is at least twice the daily dose equivalent. This therapy requires that a client's pituitary axis be responsive and stabilized initially on the alternate-day schedule.

Give glucocorticoids as a single daily dose in the morning (before 9 AM if possible) and with food or milk. Glucocorticoids suppress adrenal activity the least when it is at its peak, which is early morning.

Administer IM injections of suspensions deep in the gluteal muscle to avert local tissue atrophy at the injection sites. Note that injections into the deltoid muscle can cause atrophy.

Clients taking cortisone who require surgery should receive a preoperative dose of a rapid-acting corticosteroid. The drug is continued postoperatively in decreasing doses for several days. Clients with atrophy of the adrenal gland may be unable to cope with the stress of surgery if cortisone treatment is interrupted.

Be prepared to perform an HPA axis suppression test after high dosages or long-term therapy to determine the level of suppression. Withdrawal should be carried out slowly and under close supervision to avoid adrenal insufficiency. The usual rate of withdrawal of systemic corticosteroids is the steroid equivalent of 2.5 mg prednisone every 4 days when the client is under close and continuous medical supervision. When this is not possible, the withdrawal of systemic corticosteroids is slower, approximately 2.5 mg of prednisone (or an equivalent corticosteroid dose) every 10 days. If withdrawal symptoms such as weakness, lethargy, hypoglycemia, depression, anorexia, and nausea appear, the previous dose may be resumed for 7 days before continuing the decrease. If a medical-surgical emergency or stressful event occurs, the drug may be increased again to prevent the possibility of acute adrenal insufficiency.

Clients may require sodium restriction or potassium supplementation based on their serum electrolyte levels. An increased protein intake may also be necessary during long-term drug therapy because the drug promotes protein catabolism. Weight-bearing exercises (e.g., walking), and the administration of calcium and vitamin D may help to reduce the risk of drug-induced osteoporosis (Amin, LaValley, Simms, & Felson, 1999).

■ ***Education.*** Instruct the client not to overuse the injected joint after intraarticular injection. Weight-bearing joints should be rested 24 to 48 hours after injection.

With systemic administration, instruct clients to report any signs of infection, such as a sore throat, fever, and poor wound healing. Corticosteroids can mask infection and increase its spread. The client should avoid individuals with known contagious illnesses. Also advise clients to avoid any immunizations while taking glucocorticoids, because these agents impair the antibody response.

Instruct clients to report any visual disturbances. Long-term glucocorticoid therapy can cause cataracts, glaucoma, or optic nerve damage.

Because these drugs can cause gastric distress, instruct clients to report any persistent gastrointestinal symptoms. Instruct them to take the drug with meals or milk in the morning.

Warn the client and family that self-concept disturbances may occur as the result of changes in appearance (Box 49-2). Assist the client and family in dealing with the changes that occur, and reassure them that these changes will disappear when the drug is stopped.

Most clients receiving glucocorticoids should follow a high-potassium, low-sodium diet to counter the potassium-depleting and sodium-retaining effects of the drug. To minimize peptic ulceration, clients should limit their intake of alcohol, caffeine, aspirin, and other gastric irritants.

Inform female clients that they may experience menstrual irregularities while taking glucocorticoids. In addition, inform them that cortisone, dexamethasone, hydrocortisone, methylprednisolone, and prednisolone are unsafe to take during pregnancy because of their effects on the fetus. Have clients carry a card describing their medical condition and drug therapy. (See the Pregnancy Safety box above.)

Remember that any client who has received a significant amount of cortisone or related glucocorticoid is likely to experience some atrophy of the adrenal cortex. It is not known how much hormone produces atrophy and how long the atrophy persists, but acute adrenal insufficiency may result from too-rapid withdrawal of therapy. Instruct the client to report withdrawal symptoms, including weakness, lethargy, malaise, restlessness, hypoglycemia, psychologic despondency, anorexia, and nausea.

BOX 49-2

Body Image Alterations with Glucocorticoid Therapy

Alterations in body image may be a major concern in clients receiving glucocorticoid therapy. Among the body changes that may occur are the following:

- Abdominal distention
- Acneiform eruptions
- Fat deposits on the upper back ("buffalo hump")
- Fluid retention
- Hirsutism
- Hyperpigmentation
- Loss of muscle mass
- Systemic lupus erythematosus–like lesions
- Petechiae and ecchymosis
- Purpura
- Round face ("moon face")
- Striae
- Thin, fragile skin
- Thinning of extremities, thickening of torso
- Weight gain

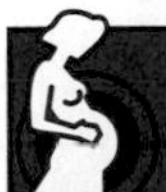

Pregnancy Safety
Drugs Affecting the Adrenal Cortex

Category	Drug
C	corticotropin, fludrocortisone
D	aminoglutethimide
Not established	other glucocorticoids

Because altered thought processes may occur, have the client report changes in mental status (euphoria, mood swings, depression) or insomnia to the prescriber. Caution the client to report any symptoms of abdominal pain, infection, bone pain, tiredness, bruising, or tarry stools.

■ **Evaluation.** The expected outcome of corticosteroid therapy is that the client will experience an improvement in the signs and symptoms of the underlying condition for which the glucocorticoid was administered without experiencing any adverse reactions to the drug.

MINERALOCORTICOIDS

Mineralocorticoids such as aldosterone are secreted by the adrenal cortex to increase the rate of sodium reabsorption by the kidneys, thereby increasing blood levels of sodium. This results in increased water reabsorption by the kidneys and increased blood volume. Mineralocorticoids also increase the excretion of potassium and hydrogen ions into the urine, thereby decreasing blood levels of potassium and hydrogen ions. In adrenal cortex insufficiency, it is necessary to replace a glucocorticoid and, in some individuals, a mineralocorticoid such as fludrocortisone.

fludrocortisone [floo droe kor′ ti sone] (Florinef)

Fludrocortisone has potent mineralocorticoid activity with some moderate glucocorticoid effects, but it is used primarily for its mineralocorticoid effects. It primarily acts on the renal distal tubule to reabsorb sodium and enhance the excretion of potassium and hydrogen, and it is indicated for the treatment of Addison's disease (chronic primary adrenocortical insufficiency) and congenital adrenogenital syndrome.

Fludrocortisone has good oral absorption, a half-life of approximately 3.5 hours in the plasma, and a biologic half-life of activity in the body of 18 to 36 hours. The duration of action is 24 to 48 hours. It is metabolized in the liver and kidneys and excreted by the kidneys.

The side effects/adverse reactions of fludrocortisone include severe or persistent headaches; hypertension; dizziness; edema of the lower extremities; joint pain; hypokalemia; increased weakness; tingling or numbness in legs that may progress to the arms, trunk, and face; congestive heart failure; and anaphylaxis. Such adverse reactions should be reported immediately to the prescriber.

The oral dosage for adults and adolescents is 0.1 mg daily. The usual dosage for children is 50 to 100 μg daily.

■ Nursing Management

Fludrocortisone Therapy

■ **Assessment.** Determine that the client does not have hypertension, congestive heart failure, cardiac disease, or renal function impairment (except for type IV renal tubular acidosis). Mineralocorticoid therapy is administered with caution in the presence of these conditions.

Because clients receiving mineralocorticoid therapy are at risk for fluid volume excess related to sodium and fluid retention, establish the client's baseline serum electrolytes, weight, and blood pressure.

Review the client's current medication regimen for the risk of significant drug interactions, such as those that may occur when fludrocortisone is given concurrently with the following drugs:

Drug	Possible Effect and Management
digitalis glycosides	Hypokalemic effect may potentiate the risk for cardiac dysrhythmias or digitalis toxicity. Monitor closely with electrocardiogram (ECG) and pulse readings.
diuretics, potassium-wasting hepatic enzyme inducers	The effectiveness of diuretics may be decreased with these medications. The concurrent use of potassium-depleting diuretics or hypokalemic-inducing medications may produce severe hypokalemia. Monitor serum potassium levels closely. The increased metabolism of mineralocorticoids may result in a decrease in the effectiveness of these drugs.
sodium in food or medications	In type IV renal tubular acidosis, the concurrent use of sodium with fludrocortisone may result in hypertension, hypernatremia, and edema. To avoid hypernatremia, monitor sodium intake closely and advise clients on the safe consumption of foods and medications. Instruct clients to read the labels on foods and medications.

■ **Nursing Diagnosis.** Clients receiving fludrocortisone are at risk for the following nursing diagnoses/collaborative problems: impaired comfort (headache); excess fluid volume (peripheral edema); and the potential complications of altered cardiac output related to congestive heart failure, anaphylaxis, and hypokalemic syndrome (weakness, anorexia, nausea, dysrhythmia, muscle cramps).

■ **Implementation**

■ ***Monitoring.*** Weigh the client daily, and report weight increases to the prescriber. Monitor intake and output. Periodically assess the client's blood pressure, and check for evidence of edema. If hypertension develops, adjust the salt intake and consult with the prescriber to modify the dosage of the steroid.

Periodic serum electrolyte determinations are recommended. Because there is a potential for hypokalemia, be aware that the excessive loss of potassium can cause dysrhythmias and sudden weakness, palpitations, paresthesia, or nausea.

■ ***Intervention.*** Provide the client with a diet that is low in sodium and high in potassium and protein.

■ ***Education.*** Advise the client to check serum electrolyte levels at periodic intervals, especially during prolonged therapy, and to implement dietary salt restrictions. The use of a potassium supplement may be necessary.

Instruct the client to weigh daily and to report a sudden weight gain to the prescriber. Consult with the prescriber for specific weight gain limitations for each client.

Advise the client to carry medical identification and to notify health care providers of the medication regimen.

■ **Evaluation.** The expected outcome of fludrocortisone therapy is that the client will not show any signs of fluid volume deficit, other signs and symptoms of mineralocorticoid insufficiency, or any adverse effects of fludrocortisone therapy.

ANTIADRENALS (ADRENAL STEROID INHIBITORS)

aminoglutethimide [a mee noe gloo teth′ i mide] (Cytadren)

Aminoglutethimide is an antiadrenal or adrenal steroid inhibitor that inhibits or suppresses adrenal cortex function. It inhibits the enzyme conversion of cholesterol or pregnenolone, thereby blocking the synthesis of adrenal steroids. It also may have other suppression effects in the synthesis and metabolism of the steroids. It also inhibits estrogen production from androgens by blocking an enzyme in the peripheral tissues and may also enhance the metabolism of estrone; thus it is investigationally used to treat breast cancer. It is indicated for the treatment of Cushing's syndrome associated with adrenal carcinoma, ectopic adrenocorticotropic hormone tumors, or adrenal gland hyperplasia.

Aminoglutethimide is absorbed orally and has a half-life of 13 hours, which is reduced to 7 hours after chronic therapy. The time to peak concentration is 1.5 hours, with adrenal function suppression occurring within 3 to 5 days of therapy. Aminoglutethimide is metabolized in the liver and excreted by the kidneys.

The side effects/adverse reactions of aminoglutethimide therapy include the CNS effects of ataxia, dizziness, sedation, loss of energy, uncontrolled eye movements, anorexia, nausea, vomiting, a measle-like rash on the face and/or the palms of the hands and, rarely, fever, chills, sore throat caused by leukopenia or agranulocytosis, jaundice of the eyes and skin, increased bleeding episodes, or unusual bruising (thrombocytopenia). The CNS effects are usually dose related and may decline in with 2 to 6 weeks of continuous therapy; however, the drug may need to be discontinued if these effects are severe.

The adult oral dosage of aminoglutethimide is 250 mg two or three times daily for approximately 14 days; the maintenance dosage is 250 mg every 6 hours four times daily. A pediatric dosage has not been established.

■ Nursing Management

Aminoglutethimide Therapy

■ **Assessment.** Because of the cortical hypofunction, use antiadrenals cautiously in clients undergoing stresses such as surgery, infection, trauma, and acute illness. Aminoglutethimide should not be administered to clients with chickenpox and herpes zoster or other infections (or who have had a recent exposure to these conditions), because the disease may become more generalized.

Do not give aminoglutethimide to pregnant women, because it causes increased fetal deaths and teratogenic effects. Older adults may be more sensitive to the CNS effects of the drug and become lethargic. Ensure that the client is not also taking dexamethasone. Aminoglutethimide increases the metabolism of dexamethasone, thus reducing its effectiveness. If a glucocorticoid is necessary for a client receiving aminoglutethimide, hydrocortisone is usually the drug of choice.

Obtain baseline lying and standing blood pressures, serum electrolyte levels, thyroid function studies, stool determinations for occult blood, and AST (SGOT) concentrations.

■ **Nursing Diagnosis.** The client receiving aminoglutethimide is at risk for the following nursing diagnoses/collaborative problems: risk for injury related to the CNS effects of hypotension, drowsiness, dizziness, and clumsiness; imbalanced nutrition related to gastrointestinal effects as evidenced by anorexia and nausea; disturbed body image related to masculinization and hirsutism in females; impaired comfort (measles-like rash, headache, and muscle pain); and the potential complications of allergic response, mental depression, hypothyroidism and goiter, thrombocytopenia, leukopenia, and agranulocytosis.

■ **Implementation**

■ ***Monitoring.*** Monitor thyroid function studies periodically during therapy. Because this drug can cause blood dyscrasias and liver and electrolyte abnormalities, routinely monitor serum electrolytes and hematologic and liver function studies. Monitor blood pressure, because hypotension (weakness, dizziness) is caused by aldosterone suppression. If aminoglutethimide is administered for adrenal disorders, plasma cortisol or 24-hour urinary 17-hydroxycorticosteroid concentrations should be monitored to determine if steroid supplementation is required. In prostatic carcinoma, serum acid phosphatase concentrations indicate the client's response to therapy; concentrations should decrease.

■ ***Intervention.*** Clients receiving aminoglutethimide should be under the care of an oncologist or endocrinologist. Consult with the prescriber about lowering the dosage if CNS side effects occur.

■ ***Education.*** Because the client may experience orthostatic hypotension, advise him or her to change position or to stand slowly to minimize this effect. Alert the client to avoid activities that require alertness until a response to the drug has been determined.

Instruct the client to carry a medical identification card and to alert other health care providers that the drug is being taken. The prescriber should be notified if injury, infection, or illness occurs, because a steroid supplement may be needed.

■ **Evaluation.** The expected outcome of aminoglutethimide therapy is that the client will experience an improvement in the signs and symptoms of Cushing's syndrome without any adverse reactions to the drug.

SUMMARY

Corticosteroids affect the adrenal cortex and are divided into two groups: glucocorticoids and mineralocorticoids. Glucocorticoids have many pharmacologic actions: antiinflammatory effects; maintenance of blood pressure; fat, carbohydrate, and protein metabolism; thymolytic, lympholytic, and eosinopenic actions; and stress effects. Mineralocorticoids act on the renal distal tubules to reabsorb sodium and enhance the excretion of potassium and hydrogen.

Because the actions of both of these groups affect all aspects of the body's physiology, it is particularly important to evaluate the client for the therapeutic effects and adverse reactions of their administration. Aminoglutethimide, an antiadrenal or adrenal steroid inhibitor, is used for the treatment of Cushing's syndrome and in some instances for the treatment of breast and prostate cancer; however, it is has not been approved by the Food and Drug Administration for oncology therapy.

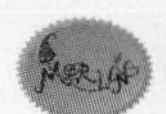

Critical Thinking Questions

1. A 28-year-old man is brought to the emergency department 2 hours after a motorcycle accident. He is conscious on admission, with stable vital signs and with minimal abrasions to the left side of his body. A neurologic examination reveals an absence of light touch and pinprick sensation in both lower extremities, lower-extremity paralysis, and no reflexes below the groin. High-dose IV methylprednisolone is initiated. Why is a corticosteroid indicated? What observations and interventions by the nurse will be necessary?
2. Bella (1992) reports that misunderstandings about steroid use, which have been generated by recent publicity about steroid abuse by athletes, have contributed to a widespread "steroid phobia." Why would that be so? How would you counter this impression in a newly diagnosed client with asthma who has been prescribed corticosteroid inhalers?

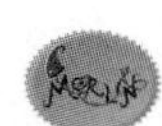

Collaborative Learning Activities

For Collaborative Learning Activities, go to mosby.com/MERLIN/McKenry/.

CASE STUDY

For a Case Study that will help ensure mastery of this chapter content, go to mosby.com/MERLIN/McKenry/.

BIBLIOGRAPHY

American Hospital Formulary Service. (1999). *AHFS drug information '99*. Bethesda, MD: American Society of Hospital Pharmacists.

Amin, S., LaValley, M.P., Simms, R.W., & Felson, D.T. (1999). The role of vitamin D in corticosteroid-induced osteoporosis: A meta-analytic approach. *Arthritis & Rheumatology, 42*(8), 1740-1751.

Anderson, K.N., Anderson, L.E., & Glanze, W.D. (Eds.) (1998). *Mosby's medical, nursing, & allied health dictionary* (5th ed.). St. Louis: Mosby.

Bella, L.A.D. (1992). Steroidphobia and the pulmonary patient. *American Journal of Nursing, 92*(2), 26.

Brus, R. (1999). Effects of high-dose inhaled corticosteroids on plasma cortisol concentrations in healthy adults. *Archives of Internal Medicine, 159*(16), 1903-1908.

Buckley, L.M., Marquez, M., Feezor, R., Ruffin, D.M., & Benson, L.L. (1999). Prevention of corticosteroid-induced osteoporosis: Results of a patient survey. *Arthritis & Rheumatology, 42*(8), 1736-1739.

Cron, R.Q., Sharma, S., & Sherry, D.D. (1999). Current treatment by United States and Canadian pediatric rheumatologists. *Journal of Rheumatology, 26*(9), 2036-2038.

Drug Facts and Comparisons. (2000). St. Louis: Facts and Comparisons.

Hoogwerf, B. & Danese, R.D. (1999). Drug selection and the management of corticosteroid-related diabetes mellitus. *Rheumatologic Disease Clinics of North America, 25*(3), 489-505.

Katzung, B.G. (1998). *Basic and clinical pharmacology* (7th ed.). Norwalk, CT: Appleton & Lange.

Kobashigawa, J.A. (1999). Postoperative management following heart transplantation. *Transplant Proceedings, 31*(5), 2038-2046.

Kuschner, W.G. (1999). Ten asthma pearls every primary care physician should know. *Postgraduate Medicine, 106*(3), 99-104.

Schimmer, B.P. & Parker, K.L. (1996). Adrenocorticotropic hormone: Adrenocortical steroids and their synthetic analogs; inhibitors of the synthesis and actions of adrenocortical hormones. In J.G. Hardman & L.E. Limbird (Eds.), *Goodman & Gilman's The pharmacological basis of therapeutics* (9th ed.). New York: McGraw-Hill.

Small, R.E. & Cooksey, L.J. (1995). Connective tissue disorders: The clinical use of corticosteroids. In L.Y. Young & M.A. Koda-Kimble (Eds.), *Applied therapeutics: The clinical use of drugs* (6th ed.). Vancouver, WA: Applied Therapeutics.

Smith, B.J., Phillips, P.J., & Heller, R.F. (1999). Asthma and chronic obstructive airway diseases are associated with osteoporosis and fractures: a literature review. *Respirology, 4*(2), 101-109.

Stein, R.B. & Hanauer, S.B. (1999). Medical therapy for inflammatory bowel disease. *Gastroenterology Clinics of North America, 28*(2), 297-321.

United States Pharmacopeia Dispensing Information (USP DI): Drug information for the health care professional (19th ed.). (1999). Rockville, MD: United States Pharmacopeial Convention.

Van Bever, H.P., Desager, K.N., Lijssens, N., Weyler, J.J., & Du-Caju, M.V. (1999). Does treatment of asthmatic children with inhaled corticosteroids affect their adult height? *Pediatric Pulmonology, 27*(6), 369-375.

Weltman, J.K. (1999). The use of inhaled corticosteroids in asthma. *Allergy & Asthma Proceedings, 20*(4), 255-260.

50 Drugs Affecting the Pancreas

Chapter Focus

Diabetes mellitus is the most important disease involving the pancreas. It affects approximately 5% of the U.S. population, half of whom are undiagnosed. The incidence is equal in males and females and increases with age. Clients with diabetes must manage their lives effectively to maintain a balance between lifestyle and treatment. To assist them in this process, nurses need to be knowledgeable about diabetes mellitus and the drugs affecting the disease process.

Learning Objectives

1. Describe type 1 (insulin-dependent) and type 2 (non–insulin-dependent) diabetes mellitus.
2. Compare and contrast the different insulin preparations.
3. Discuss oral hypoglycemic agents and the related nursing management of the client's therapeutic regimen.
4. List hyperglycemic agents and their mechanisms of action.
5. Implement the nursing management for clients receiving agents affecting the pancreas.

Key Terms

glucagon, p. 862
gluconeogenesis, p. 877
glycogenesis, p. 862
glycogenolysis, p. 862
insulin, p. 862
type 1 diabetes (insulin-dependent diabetes mellitus [IDDM]), p. 862
type 2 diabetes (non–insulin-dependent diabetes mellitus [NIDDM]), p. 862

Key Drugs [✓]

acarbose, p. 874
glucagon, p. 877
insulin, p. 863
tolbutamide, p. 872

Insulin and glucagon are the primary hormones released by the pancreas. When serum blood glucose declines, **glucagon,** which is synthesized in the alpha cells of the pancreatic islets, facilitates the catabolism of stored glycogen in the liver. The result is **glycogenolysis,** the conversion of glycogen to glucose; this leads to an increase in blood glucose (Figure 50-1). The release of glucagon stimulates the secretion of **insulin,** which then inhibits the release of glucagon. This feedback mechanism serves to keep glucose within a desired serum level. Alternately, the conversion of excess glucose to glycogen for storage in skeletal muscle and the liver (**glycogenesis**) occurs when blood glucose increases.

The most important endocrine disease involving the pancreas is diabetes mellitus, a disorder of carbohydrate metabolism that involves an insulin deficiency, insulin resistance, or both. All causes of diabetes lead to hyperglycemia (see Chapter 46).

DIABETES MELLITUS

Diabetes mellitus affects approximately 16 million Americans; nearly one half of this population has not been diagnosed (Beier, 1997). Uncontrolled diabetes is a devastating disease that is the leading cause of new cases of blindness, end-stage renal disease, and lower limb amputations. It is also the seventh leading cause of death in the United States (Baker, 1997). Diabetes mellitus affects males and females equally, and the incidence increases with age.

The two general classifications for diabetes mellitus are **type 1 (insulin-dependent diabetes mellitus [IDDM])** and **type 2 (non–insulin-dependent diabetes mellitus [NIDDM]).** Clients with type 1 diabetes have very little or usually no endogenous insulin capacity. This type of diabetes usually occurs before age 30 and was previously called juvenile-onset diabetes. Client with type 1 diabetes are prone to ketosis and require exogenous insulin therapy for survival.

Type 2 diabetes was previously known as maturity-onset diabetes because the age of onset is usually after 40 years of age. Approximately 90% of the diabetes cases are type 2 (Koda-Kimble & Carlisle, 1995). In general, clients with type 2 diabetes have some insulin function and thus are not fully dependent on insulin for survival. Weight reduction through dietary adjustments often helps to reduce hyperglycemia in clients with type 2 diabetes. The vast majority

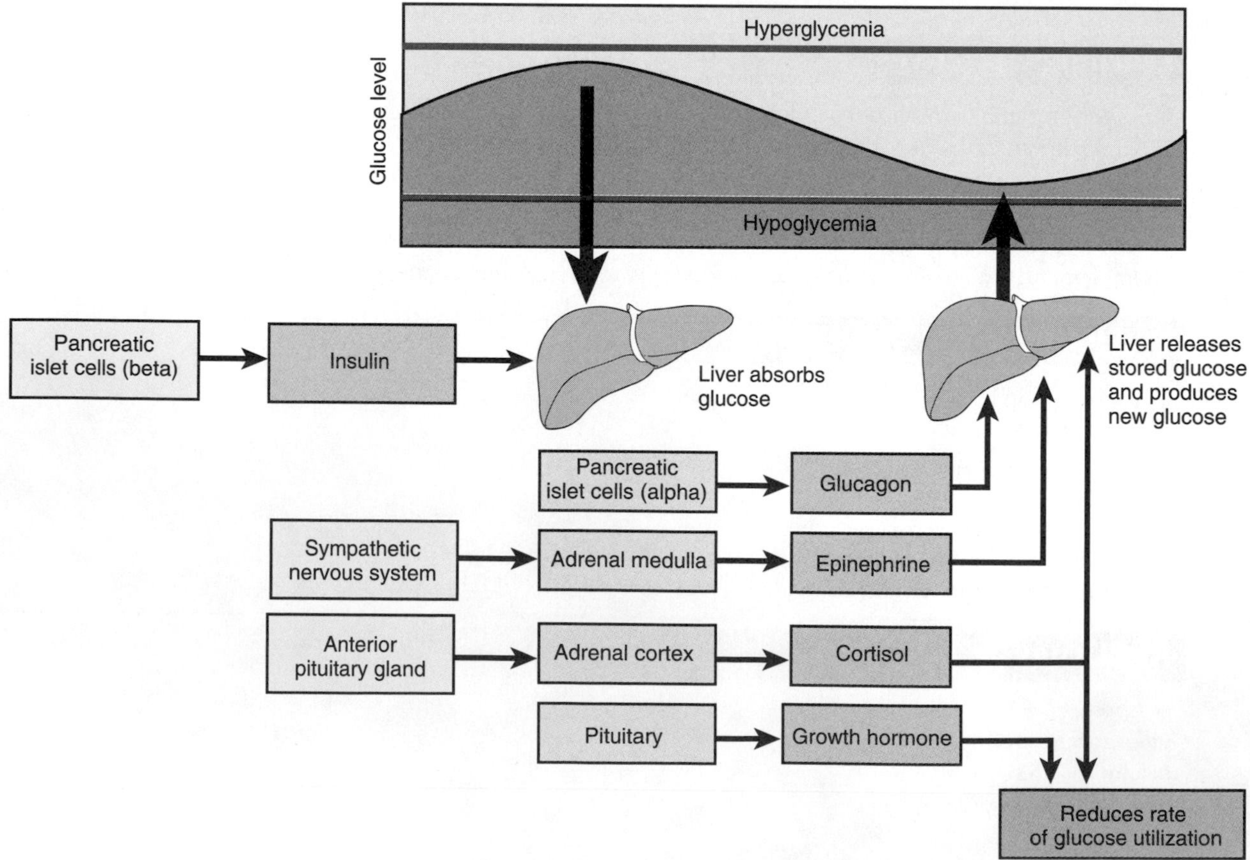

Figure 50-1 Insulin causes the liver to absorb excess blood glucose; when blood glucose levels are low, the alpha cells in the islets of Langerhans secrete glucagon, which stimulates liver glycogenolysis and gluconeogenesis. The sympathetic nervous system signals the adrenal medulla to secrete epinephrine, and the anterior pituitary gland stimulates the adrenal cortex to release cortisol. Both epinephrine and cortisol enhance gluconeogenesis; epinephrine also increases glycogenolysis, and cortisol slows down the rate of glucose utilization and also increases the plasma level of amino acids available for glucose production. The pituitary secretes growth hormone, which decreases the use of cellular glucose and promotes glycogenolysis.

of individuals with type 2 diabetes are obese, and ketosis is rare.

Although insulin resistance may occasionally occur with type 1 diabetes, it is believed to be more common in type 2 diabetes because of receptor and postreceptor defects. Table 50-1 compares the primary features of both types of diabetes. The treatment of diabetes mellitus usually includes diet, exercise and, if necessary, oral antidiabetic agent(s) or insulin to help control blood glucose levels.

INSULIN PREPARATIONS

Insulin is composed of two amino acid chains, A (acidic) and B (basic), which are joined together by disulfide linkages. It is synthesized in the beta cells of the pancreas, which are located in the islets of Langerhans; insulin is secreted by these cells when blood glucose levels are elevated.

Insulin preparations are derived from animals (extracted from beef or pork pancreas) or synthesized in the laboratory from either an alteration of pork insulin or a recombinant DNA technology that uses strains of *Escherichia coli* to form human insulin (a biosynthetic human insulin). Beef insulin differs from human insulin by three amino acids, whereas pork insulin differs from human insulin by only a single amino acid. Human (or recombinant) insulin is identical to the insulin produced by the pancreas.

Many individuals with diabetes do well with the beef-pork combination insulins if they have not developed insulin resistance, insulin allergies, or lipoatrophy (a breakdown of subcutaneous fat occurring after repeated injections) at the same insulin injection sites. There is a higher degree of immunogenicity reported with beef-pork insulin than with pork insulin (Koda-Kimble & Carlisle, 1995).

Pork insulin has been found to be useful for clients who have a short-term need for insulin or for clients with local or systemic allergies, insulin resistance, or lipoatrophy. Pure pork insulin is closer in composition to human insulin than is beef-pork combination insulin. Its use has resulted in a reduction of the insulin dosage (in insulin resistance) in many instances and in the improvement of local allergy (erythema, induration, and pruritus at injection site) in approximately 80% of clients with insulin allergies. However, its use is contraindicated for clients who are allergic to pork or who must avoid the use of pork for religious reasons.

Currently human insulin is substituted for the same reasons as pork insulin (especially in persons allergic to pork), because it is much less antigenic than the animal-based insulin. Subcutaneous human insulin may also be absorbed faster and has a shorter duration of action than the animal insulins. It is standard practice now to prescribe human insulin whenever possible. Clients who are switched from animal insulin to human insulin should be closely monitored initially, because a dosage adjustment may be necessary. As a result of the decreased allergenic effects, skin allergies, and resistance reported with human insulin, it is commonly prescribed for pregnant women and for clients who are newly diagnosed with diabetes (Davis & Granner, 1996).

A new, fast-acting insulin analogue, insulin lispro (Humalog), was approved for release in 1996. This insulin uses regular human insulin and reverses the sequence of two amino acids. The primary advantage of the new insulin is that it has a more rapid onset of action than regular insulin and therefore can be administered 15 minutes before a meal. Because it also has an earlier peak effect and a shorter duration of action, clients with type 1 diabetes mellitus usually require the concurrent use of a long-acting insulin product (Rodgers, 1996).

Insulin controls the storage and metabolism of carbohydrate, protein, and fat that binds to receptor sites on cellular plasma membranes, especially in the liver, muscle, and adipose tissues. Although the exact molecular mechanism of action for insulin is still being investigated, it is known that it influences cell membrane transport, cell growth, enzyme activation and inhibition, and the metabolism of protein and fats.

TABLE 50-1 Features of Type 1 and Type 2 Diabetes

	Type 1	Type 2
Synonym	Insulin-dependent diabetes mellitus (IDDM)	Non–insulin-dependent diabetes mellitus (NIDDM)
Age of onset	Usually <30 years	Usually >35 years
Onset of symptoms	Sudden (symptomatic)	Gradual (usually asymptomatic)
Body weight	Usually not obese	Obese (80%)
Family history	Usually negative	Often positive
Incidence	10%	90%
Insulin levels	Low, then absent	May be low, normal, or high (insulin resistance)
Insulin dependent	Yes	Usually not required
Insulin resistance	No	Yes
Receptors	Normal	Usually decreased or defective
Plasma insulin	Decreased	Normal or increased
Complications	Common	Common
Ketoacidosis	Prone to this condition	Usually resistant to this condition
Dietary modifications	Mandatory	Mandatory

Insulin is indicated for the treatment of type 1 diabetes mellitus and for the treatment of type 2 diabetes mellitus during emergencies or in specific situations, such as supplementation in the client with low physiologic endogenous insulin during high fevers, severe infection, ketoacidosis, severe burns, after major surgery and severe trauma, or during pregnancy.

The wide variety of available insulins (including combination mixtures) allow for sufficient blood glucose control to meet the need and lifestyle of a client with diabetes. Maintaining glucose levels as close as possible to normal will help to improve the client's quality of life and will also reduce the progression of complications associated with diabetes (Campbell, 1992).

Table 50-2 describes the pharmacokinetics of insulin.

There is no average dosage of insulin; each client's needs must be determined individually to attain euglycemia and avoid hypoglycemia and hyperglycemia. Box 50-1 lists the symptoms of hypoglycemia and hyperglycemia—the adverse effects of ineffective management of the therapeutic regimen.

Insulin dosages are expressed in units rather than in milliliters. Insulin injection is standardized so that each milliliter contains 100 USP units. Insulin is classified according to its duration of action (short- or rapid-acting, intermediate-acting, and long-acting) (Figure 50-2). In general, meals should occur at the same time that administered insulin reaches its peak effect. Insulin requirements can vary widely among clients, so dosages must be adjusted to individual need.

Clients with diabetes who become hyperglycemic, perhaps because of hospitalization or an infection, may need insulin coverage in addition to their regular insulin. The amount of insulin given will vary with the blood glucose values or, in some instances, with the glucose in the urine; this titration is known as the "sliding-scale" administration of insulin. Today urine testing is rarely used to monitor blood glucose. If at all possible, urine glucose tests should not be used to determine insulin dosages. Because there may be variations between urine glucose testing products, they should not be used interchangeably. Specific instructions for

BOX 50-1

Symptoms of Hypoglycemia and Hyperglycemia

Persons administering insulin should be aware of the symptoms of hypoglycemia and hyperglycemia and know what actions to take if they occur.

Hypoglycemia: Increased anxiety, blurred vision, chilly sensation, cold sweating, pallor, confusion, difficulty concentrating, drowsiness, headache, nausea, increased pulse rate, shakiness, increased weakness, increased appetite

Hyperglycemia: Drowsiness, red/dry skin, fruity breath odor, anorexia, abdominal pain, nausea, vomiting, dry mouth, increased urination, rapid/deep breathing, unusual thirst, rapid weight loss

TABLE 50-2 Insulin: Pharmacokinetics

Insulins*	Onset (hours)	Peak Effect (hours)	Duration of Action (hours)
Rapid Acting			
insulin injection (Regular Insulin, Humulin R)†	0.5-1	2-4	5-7
insulin aspart (NovoLog)	0.25	1-3	3-5
insulin lispro (Humalog)	0.25	1	4
Intermediate Acting			
isophane insulin suspension (NPH Insulin, Humulin N ◆)	3-4	6-12	18-28
insulin zinc suspension (Lente Insulin)	1-3	8-12	18-28
Long Acting			
extended insulin zinc suspension (Ultralente)	4-6	18-24	36
Combinations			
insulin glargine (Lantus)	1.1	5	24
isophane human insulin (50%) & human insulin (50%) (Humulin 50/50)	0.5	3	22-24
 isophane human insulin (70%) & human insulin (30%) (Humulin 70/30 ◆, Novolin 70/30)	0.5	4-8	24

*Semilente insulin is available in Canada but is no longer available in the United States. The onset of action of Semilente insulin is 1 to 3 hours, the peak effect is in 2 to 8 hours, and the duration of action is 12 to 16 hours.

†These insulins may be administered intravenously. Intravenously, the onset of action is within 1/6 to 1/2 hour, the peak effect is within 1/4 to 1/2 hour, and the duration of action is within 1/2 to 1 hour.

testing urine for glucose using a particular reagent is included with the testing kit.

The client's dietary intake, physical activity, ability to manage the therapeutic regimen, and glucose tolerance are taken into consideration when establishing insulin dosages. Insulin dosages should not be considered to be a fixed regimen; dosages may need to be adjusted as a result of physical growth (child growing into adulthood), illness, stress, the development of antiinsulin antibodies, concomitant administration of certain medications, or changes in exercise and diet. Specific instructions should be obtained regarding insulin administration for the preoperative client because of the alteration in the client's dietary patterns and metabolic requirements as the result of the surgical procedure. Treatment programs need to be reviewed and adjusted as necessary, with the prescriber, nurse, and client working closely to manage hypoglycemia and hyperglycemia and, if possible, avoid their complications. Research is supporting closer management for euglycemia (see the Nursing Research box below).

Insulin is given subcutaneously (or intravenously, regular insulin only). It cannot be given by mouth because digestive enzymes destroy it. Regular insulin is usually given approximately 15 to 30 minutes before meals.

Portable insulin pumps have improved the metabolic state of some clients with type 1 diabetes who do not have adequate diabetic control with intensive dietary restrictions and multiple daily insulin injections. The insulin pump is battery-operated and connected to a small computer that is programmed to release small amounts of in-

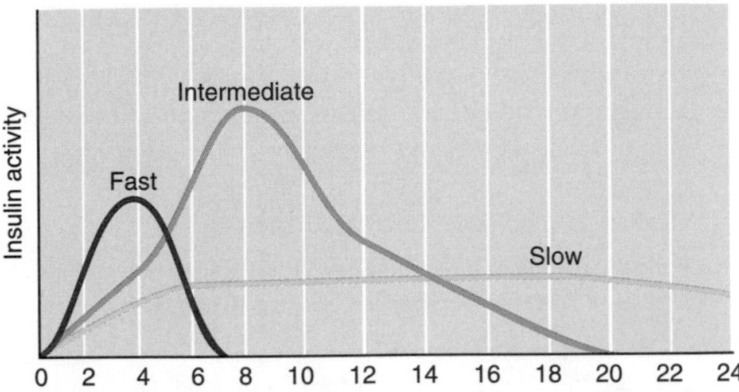

Figure 50-2 Insulin pharmacokinetics (see Table 50-1).

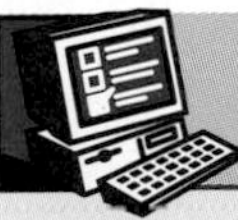

Nursing Research

The Effect of Long-Term Intensified Insulin Treatment on the Development of Microvascular Complications of Diabetes Mellitus

Citation: Reichard P., Nilsson B.Y., & Rosenquist U. (1993). The effect of long-term intensified insulin treatment on the development of microvascular complications of diabetes mellitus. *New England Journal of Medicine, 329,* 304.

Abstract: Microvascular complications develop in many clients with type 1 (insulin-dependent) diabetes mellitus, and the effect of intensified insulin treatment on these complications has not been established.

This study randomly assigned 102 individuals to intensified insulin treatment (48 participants) or standard insulin treatment (54 participants). All of these individuals had type 1 diabetes mellitus, nonproliferative retinopathy (a noninflammatory eye disorder resulting from changes in the retinal blood vessel), normal serum creatinine concentrations, and unsatisfactory blood glucose control. The participants were evaluated for microvascular complications after 18 months and at 3, 5, and 7.5 years.

The results of the study were as follows. The mean (± SD) glycosylated hemoglobin values were reduced from 9.5% (± 1.3%) to 7.1% (± 0.7%) in the group receiving intensified treatment and from 9.4% (± 1.4%) to 8.5% (± 0.7%) in the group receiving standard treatment (P = 0.001). Serious retinopathy requiring photocoagulation developed in 12 of the participants receiving intensified treatment (27% of those included in the analysis) and in 27 of those receiving standard treatment (52%) (P = 0.01). Visual acuity decreased in 6 participants receiving intensified treatment (14%) and in 18 receiving standard treatment (35%) (P = 0.02). Nephropathy (urinary albumin excretion >200 μg/min) developed in 1 participant receiving intensified treatment and in 9 participants receiving standard treatment (P = 0.01). No one in the intensified treatment group had neuropathy with subnormal glomerular filtration rates, but neuropathy did occur in 6 participants in the standard treatment group (P = 0.02). The conduction velocities of the ulnar, tibial, peroneal, and sural nerves decreased significantly more in the standard treatment group than in the intensified treatment group. The odds ratio for serious retinopathy was 0.4 (95% confidence interval, 0.2 to 1.0; P = 0.04) in the intensified treatment group as compared with the standard treatment group. The corresponding odds ratio for nephropathy was 0.1 (95% confidence interval, 0 to 0.8; P = 0.04).

The investigators concluded that long-term intensified insulin treatment, as compared with standard treatment, slows the development of microvascular complications in clients with type 1 diabetes.

Critical Thinking Questions

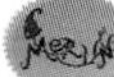

- How does this study support a "tight control" approach to the management of type 1 diabetes? What is its contribution to the importance of self-management of care by the client?
- All other things being equal, what was the difference in the treatment of the intensified vs. the standard treatment groups?
- What else may have been occurring during this study that might contribute to the findings?

sulin per hour. It does not analyze the blood glucose level, but it is programmed according to the client's daily insulin needs, diet, and physical exercise. The client can also push a button that releases a bolus dose to cover each meal consumed.

Although insulin pumps are effective and useful for clients who are properly trained, health care professionals need to be aware of several problems associated with them. Malfunction of the insulin infusion may occur because of battery failure, and defects in the tubing may cause leakage of insulin solution or blockage of the infusion tubing. Therefore it is vitally important to teach the client to change the infusion set and battery. Clients must be highly motivated and educated in the handling of insulin pumps. Clients should be capable of keeping records and following specific procedures and should be willing to perform blood tests daily or more often. These pumps are also very expensive. Therefore they are not recommended for every client with type 1 diabetes.

Needleless injectors, such as the Vitajet, Medi-Jector, and others are also available. These devices are expensive and appear to have limited usefulness in practice. Many devices are also available for the visually impaired client with diabetes. Information on injection aids for the blind may be obtained from state and national associations, such as the American Foundation for the Blind and the American Diabetes Association (ADA).

Insulin is the drug of choice to control diabetes during pregnancy. Insulin requirements may drop for 24 to 72 hours after delivery and slowly return to prepregnancy levels in approximately 6 weeks.

To maintain euglycemia, blood glucose levels are determined at frequent intervals by blood glucose monitoring. This process has been simplified by the availability of both visual test strips and strips used in blood glucose meters or instruments. Such devices allow clients to monitor their diabetes and make the necessary adjustments with medication, diet, and exercise as instructed by their physician or health care provider. The visual glucose testing strips are less expensive than the testing instruments, but the meter readings of the testing instruments are much more precise (assuming they are properly calibrated). Clients with visual problems or the need for a more accurate blood glucose reading benefit from using a blood glucose meter instrument.

Another evaluation test is involves determining the client's glycosylated hemoglobin (hemoglobin A_{1c}). The level of hemoglobin A_{1c} increases when individuals have prolonged hyperglycemic serum levels. Red blood cells have a life span of 4 months; therefore a measurement of hemoglobin A_{1c} will give the prescriber an evaluation of the client's long-term diabetic control. In other words, clients with diabetes may have undetected periods of hyperglycemia that alternate with a post-insulin time period of euglycemia or hypoglycemia. An elevated hemoglobin A_{1c} indicates inadequate diabetic control for the previous 3 to 5 weeks (Watson, 1995). For clients with diabetes, the usual target goal for hemoglobin A_{1c} is 7% or less.

BOX 50-2

Effects of Commonly Abused Drugs on Diabetes Management

Many drugs can increase or decrease blood glucose levels, but rarely are the commonly abused drugs reviewed in relation to diabetes. Because substance abuse by the client with diabetes can be very problematic, the most commonly abused drugs are reviewed here.

Alcohol

Alcohol promotes hypoglycemia and blocks the formation, storage, and release of glycogen. It may also interact with many other drugs, including oral hypoglycemic agents such as chlorpropamide. In alcoholics who have decreased their food intake, alcohol can cause a serious drop in blood glucose levels, which leads to a need for acute intervention.

CNS Stimulants

Amphetamines, sympathomimetics, anorexics, cocaine, psychedelic drugs, and others may result in hyperglycemia and an increase in the breakdown of liver glycogen. Large amounts of caffeine in products such as coffee, tea, and cola drinks can also increase blood glucose levels.

Marijuana

Marijuana may increase appetite and food consumption. Heavy use may produce a glucose intolerance, which leads to hyperglycemia.

Cigarettes

The nicotine in cigarettes is a potent vasoconstrictor. It can decrease the absorption of subcutaneous insulin or increase an individual's insulin requirements by 15% to 20%. Cigarette smoking can cause a drop of 1 to 2 degrees in skin temperature. It also is a risk factor for the development of diabetic nephropathy.

Abuse of CNS-Acting Drugs

CNS-acting drugs (e.g., stimulants, depressants, sedative-hypnotics, opiates, marijuana, alcohol) can impair judgment and alter perceptions (time, place) and thus interfere with the individual's control of the diabetic state.

Nursing Management

Insulin Therapy

▪ **Assessment.** A comprehensive nursing history is necessary in helping the client to manage the diabetic state. This assessment is as essential for clients newly diagnosed with diabetes as it is for clients who are seeking reassurance that they are managing their diabetes appropriately or for clients who have readjusted their insulin dosage because of stress, illness, change of lifestyle, or ineffective management of the

BOX 50-3

Sugar-Free Over-the-Counter Medications

Advise clients to always read bottle labels or check with their pharmacists before purchasing OTC medications. Manufacturers often change the sugar contents of OTC medications; therefore the best advice is to check the list of contents every time a medication is purchased. The following is a select listing of medications currently listed as sugar-free.

Antacids, Antiflatulents

Maalox Anti-Gas
Maalox Plus Extra Strength
Mylanta
Riopan
Titralac Extra Strength Antacid
Titralac Plus Tablets/Liquids

Antipyretics

Acetaminophen Solution
Bayer Aspirin
Motrin IB
Panadol Children's Liquid
Tempra 3 chewable tablets
Tylenol Children's Fruit Flavor

Cough-Cold Preparations

Benadryl Cold
Benylin Expectorant
Diabetic Tussin DM
Diabetic Tussin EX
Naldecon Senior DX and EX
Tussar-SF

Information from Covington, T.R. (Ed.). (1996). *Handbook of nonprescription drugs* (11th ed.). Washington, D.C.: American Pharmaceutical Association.

therapeutic regimen. A baseline assessment of the client's blood glucose level is obtained before beginning or adjusting insulin therapy.

Determine the client's ideal body weight, present weight, daily exercise, dietary management and preferences, and understanding of diabetes and its control. Also note any physical impairments (e.g., decreased manual dexterity and limitations of vision) that would impede the self-administration of insulin. Because the cost of insulin, injection equipment, and blood testing equipment can be considerable, assess the client's financial status and health insurance coverage, and locate alternative resources if necessary. Clients with certain religious affiliations (e.g., Jewish or Islamic clients) prefer not to use pork insulin because their dietary codes involve the avoidance of pork.

Many commonly abused substances can be very problematic for clients with diabetes (Box 50-2). Box 50-3 lists sugar-free over-the-counter (OTC) medications. Review the client's medication regimen for the risk of significant drug

BOX 50-4

Drugs Reported to Cause Hyperglycemia or Hypoglycemia

Hyperglycemia

baclofen
corticosteroids
diuretics
estrogens (oral contraceptives)
glucagon
NSAIDs
pentamidine
phenytoin
sympathomimetics
thyroid hormones

Hypoglycemia

ACE inhibitors
anabolic steroids
beta-adrenergic blocking agents
disopyramide
ethanol
lithium
monoamine oxidase inhibitors (MAO inhibitors)
NSAIDs
pentamidine (increases insulin release)
salicylates
sulfonamides

Information from *United States Pharmacopeia Dispensing Information (USP DI): Drug information for the health care professional* (19th ed.). (1999). Rockville, MD: United States Pharmacopeial Convention.

interactions, such as those that may occur when insulin is given concurrently with the following drugs and those listed in Box 50-4:

Drug	Possible Effect and Management
adrenocorticoids, glucocorticoids	Adrenocorticoids and glucocorticoids may increase blood glucose levels. A dosage adjustment of insulin may be necessary. Monitor closely.
alcohol	May increase the hypoglycemic effect of insulin. Monitor closely, because dosage adjustments may be necessary. If possible, avoid the concurrent use of alcohol.
beta-adrenergic blocking agents (including eye preparations)	These agents may mask symptoms of hypoglycemia, such as increased pulse rate and decreased blood pressure. They may also prolong hypoglycemia by blocking gluconeogenesis. Dosage adjustments of insulin may be necessary. Selective beta blockers in low dosages, such as metoprolol and atenolol, cause fewer problems than the other beta-adrenergic blocking agents. Propranolol may cause hyperglycemia or hypoglycemia when given concurrently with insulin. Periodic blood glucose tests are recommended to monitor the combined effects and allow for a dosage adjustment for insulin if necessary.

Drug	Possible Effect and Management
pentamidine (Pentam 300)	Pentamidine has a toxic effect on pancreatic beta cells, which results in a biphasic response to glucose concentrations. Initially there is insulin release with hypoglycemia, followed by hypoinsulinemia and hyperglycemia with continued use. The dosage of insulin should be reduced and then increased with continued use of pentamidine.

A baseline assessment includes skin (lesions and color), ophthalmologic testing, orientation, peripheral sensation, reflexes, blood pressure, pulse, respirations, lung sounds, urinalysis, and blood glucose levels.

▪ **Nursing Diagnosis.** See the Nursing Care Plan on p. 869 for nursing diagnoses that commonly apply to the client receiving insulin.

▪ **Implementation**

▪ ***Monitoring.*** Monitor the effectiveness of insulin therapy by obtaining blood glucose levels at frequent intervals—more often if the client is under stress, is pregnant, or has been recently diagnosed. Glucose-monitoring devices, such as Chemstrip and Dextrostix, allow for blood glucose monitoring at home and thus facilitate a tighter control of blood sugar levels.

Urine glucose testing is less commonly performed because it is an indirect measurement of the client's glycemic status secondary to individual differences in the renal threshold for glucose. The spillage of glucose into the urine usually occurs at blood levels of 160 to 180 mg/100 mL, but it may be higher in older adults or lower in children and pregnant women. Therefore it may not correlate well with serum glucose levels. The appropriate dosage of insulin for the client is indicated by the maintenance of normal fasting serum glucose levels within 70 to 105 mg/dL for adults under 60 years of age and 80 to 115 mg/dL for adults 60 years of age and over.

Hemoglobin A_{1c} determinations are performed to evaluate the adequacy of diabetic control more comprehensively and provide information not available in individual blood and urine glucose tests. Clients with diabetes may have undetected periods of hyperglycemia that alternate with post-insulin periods of euglycemia or hypoglycemia. High levels of hemoglobin A_{1c} indicate inadequate diabetic control for the previous 3 to 5 weeks (Watson, 1995).

Monitor the client for signs and symptoms of hyperglycemia and hypoglycemia. Observe injection sites for impaired tissue integrity, such as lipoatrophy or lipohypertrophy (a buildup of subcutaneous fat tissue).

Clients are evaluated periodically in the primary care setting for complications of diabetes mellitus related to the ineffectiveness of insulin therapy, including visual impairment (ophthalmic examination), nephropathy (complete urinalysis [including protein], blood urea nitrogen, serum creatinine), neuropathy (neurologic examination), increased atherosclerotic disease (serum cholesterol, high-density lipoprotein cholesterol, serum triglycerides, electrocardiogram, peripheral pulses, bruits), and foot and skin examinations for problem areas (American Diabetes Association, 1990).

▪ ***Intervention.*** Note that all insulin preparations are stable as long as the vials are protected from heat or cold; store them in a cool place, but do not freeze them. Regular (concentrated) Iletin II is available as U-500 for clients who have developed insulin resistance and require large dosages. Take care not to store U-500 insulin in the same area as other insulin preparations because of the possibility of a massive overdose if it is accidentally administered to a client.

Vials of insoluble preparations (all except regular insulin) should be rotated between the hands and inverted end-to-end several times before withdrawing a dose. The vial should not be shaken vigorously or the suspension will foam. Do not interchange human, beef-pork combination, or pork insulins, because species differences may require a dosage change. Do not use insulin that has become clumped or granular in appearance.

Use a properly calibrated syringe for insulin. For doses of less than 50 units of U-100, use a low-dose syringe (50 units of U-100/0.5 mL). The decreased diameter of the barrel of the syringe results in the calibrations being further apart, which enhances accuracy of the measurement. Avoid bubbles in the solution; the displacement of a few units of insulin, particularly with U-100 insulin, can alter the actual dose received by the client.

Administer insulin subcutaneously using a 25- or 26-gauge needle; the length of the needle is determined by the client's size. A ⅜- to ⅝-inch needle is usually used, with the injection administered at a 90-degree angle in a large fold of skin that has been gently pinched up. The injection may also be inserted at a 30- to 45-degree angle at the base of the fold of skin. Apply pressure after the injection; do not rub the site, because doing so alters the absorption rate. Rotate injection sites. Because of the differences in absorption from different anatomic sites, rotate injections with a pattern (e.g., morning injections rotated within the abdominal region, evening injections rotated in the thighs).

Understand that only the regular form of insulin may be injected by the IV route. Insulin adsorption onto plastic IV infusion administration sets removes up to 80% of an insulin dose; not less than 20% to 50% of a dose is most often removed by adsorption. Adsorption on the tubing surface occurs within 1 hour and requires individual client monitoring of insulin needs. Saturation of the adsorption sites on the tubing requires special care when changing the tubing, because exposure of the new tubing to insulin may result in decreased insulin dosing and the need for more frequent monitoring of client needs. Adsorption can be minimized by injecting directly into the vein, by using an intermittent infusion device, or by using a port close to the IV access site. Use an IV pump for accuracy when administering insulin as an infusion.

▪ ***Education.*** Instruct clients on the relationship of diabetes to the administration of insulin, blood glucose monitoring, and the necessity to maintain euglycemia. Teach clients about blood glucose monitoring so they can adjust insulin-dosages when their blood levels are above normal limits. To

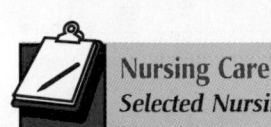

Nursing Care Plan

Selected Nursing Diagnoses for Clients Receiving Insulin

Nursing Diagnosis	Outcome Criteria	Nursing Interventions
Deficient knowledge related to newly diagnosed diabetes	Client and family will: Demonstrate an understanding of diabetes, its therapy and complications, and measures to minimize or prevent complications	Assess the understanding/learning ability of the client/family. Determine educational needs and desires. Provide information regarding the pathophysiology of diabetes and the function of insulin. Explain goals and methods of diet and drug therapy. Explain the function and purpose of tests. Answer questions and clarify misconceptions. Provide resources for further learning and support (American Diabetes Association [ADA], Juvenile Diabetes Foundation [JDF], and others).
Deficient knowledge related to newly prescribed diabetic medication (insulin)	Client and family will: Demonstrate correctly the appropriate storage, handling, and administration of insulin Be familiar with the signs and symptoms of insulin/hypoglycemic reaction and the appropriate response State the different insulin preparations and appropriate adjustment of drug therapy Be aware of possible side effects/adverse reactions of insulin	Teach the client and family: The function and importance of therapy and the name and dosage of insulin The technique of blood (or urine) glucose monitoring and adjusting insulin appropriately The proper technique of administration The need for lifelong dietary and drug management The differences between the three forms of insulin How to calculate dosages correctly The proper storage and handling of insulin The importance of rotating sites to minimize adverse local reactions The signs and symptoms of insulin/hypoglycemic reaction and appropriate management Help the client establish and maintain a monitoring record of blood (or urine) glucose and insulin administration. Advise the client to wear or carry a medical identification tag, bracelet, or card. Provide the client with a list of drugs and conditions that may alter insulin requirements.
Risk for injury related to hyperglycemia or hypoglycemia due to insulin administration	Client will: Achieve control of blood glucose and maintain desired nutritional intake Client and family will: Demonstrate knowledge of appropriate diabetic diet and modifications of dietary practices	Administer insulin as prescribed. Teach client and family: The correct method of blood (or urine) glucose monitoring The signs, symptoms, and treatment for hyperglycemia and hypoglycemia The importance of a balanced diabetic diet to control diabetes Provide dietary instruction and counseling regarding the appropriate diet; refer the client to a dietitian. Assist client and family in planning a sample diet.
Disturbed body image related to insulin dependence	Client and family will: Verbalize feelings and concerns Understand disease and measures of control Client will: Maintain, as much as possible, prediagnosis activities	Encourage the client and family to express feelings and concerns. Determine assets and strengths. With the client and family, determine strategies for managing areas of difficulty or concern. Provide resources for further learning and support (ADA, JDF, others). Be alert for signs of nonacceptance or difficulties such as denial or ineffective management of therapeutic regimen.
Powerlessness related to perceived lack of personal control	Client and family will: Identify those areas of diabetes that are possible to control, and participate in decision making related to diabetic management	Assess the client's and family's coping patterns and support mechanisms. Assess the client's and family's perceptions related to diagnosis. Allow and encourage the expression of concerns and fears. Encourage client and family participation in therapy planning and implementation.

help prevent soreness from daily finger sticks, instruct the client to use the left thumb on Monday, the left index finger on Tuesday, and so on through Friday. The right thumb can be used on Saturday and the right index finger on Sunday. The other three fingers can be used as alternates in case of an unsuccessful finger stick on another day. If finger sticks are performed twice daily, instruct the client to use the left thumb on Monday morning, the left index finger on Monday afternoon, the left middle finger on Tuesday morning, and so on. The client will use all of the fingers this way and by Saturday can start the sticks with the left thumb again (Vibulbhan, 1993).

Instruct the client in the administration of insulin, including the type of insulin, the proper storage of insulin, the disposal of syringes, and the rotation of injection sites.

Have the client agitate the vial (unless using regular insulin) and properly cleanse the top with 70% isopropyl alcohol. To draw insulin out of a vial, inject the vial with an amount of air equal to the insulin dose. This prevents a negative pressure from occurring in the vial, which would make the withdrawal of the insulin difficult. Teach the client to eliminate air bubbles from the syringe because they decrease the dose.

When mixing insulins, first inject air (equal to the dose to be withdrawn) into the vial of NPH insulin. Then inject air into the vial of the regular insulin. Keep the needle in the vial, and draw the regular insulin into the syringe first; this prevents contamination of the regular insulin vial with the other insulin admixture. Then return to the NPH vial and withdraw the dose of NPH insulin. The onset of action of regular insulin is delayed when mixed with other insulins. The interaction of regular and NPH insulin occurs within 15 minutes of mixing and remains at this stability for 30 days at room temperature and 90 days if refrigerated. The interaction of regular and Lente mixtures requires up to 24 hours before reaching a stable level of consistent response; if premixed in the same syringe, their activity is stable for 30 days at room temperature and 90 days under refrigeration. Clients stabilized on this premixed insulin will have a different response if they inject the insulin separately from each component (see the Community and Home Health Considerations box above). Different brands of syringes have sufficient differences in "dead space" (the unmeasured volume between the needle point and the bottom calibration) to cause improper dosages. Dosage errors are avoided by not changing the injection order of mixing insulins and by not changing the model of needles, brands of syringes, or sources of insulins.

Instruct the client in how to plan the rotation of injection sites and to observe for lipodystrophies, the occurrence of which may be minimized by rotation. Note that insulin is most rapidly absorbed from the abdomen, followed by the upper arm and then the thigh. Physical activity in the client accelerates absorption, especially in the injected limb; alert joggers and walkers.

Teach the client that alternating the insulin injection sites from the leg to the abdomen or arm has the effect of accelerating the absorption of insulin and diminishing the postprandial rise in plasma glucose. Varying injection sites within the same anatomic region rather than between different regions may diminish daily fluctuations or variations in insulin absorption and in metabolic control in clients who are insulin dependent. For example, if the abdomen is used for a morning injection, subsequent morning injections should also be given in the abdomen. Injections at another time of day should always be given in the same part of the body, for example, use thigh sites for before-dinner injections. Each injection should be administered an inch away from any previously used site, and a site should not be used more often than once a month (Box 50-5).

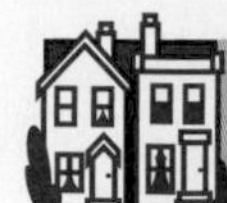

Community and Home Health Considerations

Prefilling of Insulin Syringes by Home Health Nurses

The timing of the chemical interaction following the combination of different types of insulins modifies the clinical effectiveness of the insulins by delaying the onset of action of regular insulin. Home health nurses who prefill insulin syringes with different insulins in the same syringe for future use by their clients should ensure that clients are not using insulin mixed the same day. The insulin should be administered so that there is a consistency of dosage in the insulin therapy. Administering a "fresh" syringe (one mixed within the previous 15 minutes) will produce the same reaction as administering the insulins separately, and this may significantly alter the client's blood glucose levels.

Be sure the client understands that frequent serum glucose monitoring is necessary to achieve insulin control. Stress compliance with the understanding that insulin helps to control hyperglycemia but is not a cure for diabetes.

Instruct clients about the signs and symptoms of hypoglycemia that can occur secondary to the dosage of insulin. A dosage adjustment downward may be necessary to prevent repeated episodes of hypoglycemia. A client with hypoglycemia should promptly ingest a carbohydrate with a high sugar content, and the prescriber should be notified. Orange juice, candy, a lump of sugar, or a complex carbohydrate such as milk or cheese and crackers can be given if the individual is conscious (Box 50-6). Early symptoms of hypoglycemia are fatigue, headache, drowsiness, lassitude, tremulousness, or nausea. Late symptoms are weakness, sweating, tremors, or nervousness. Observe the client at night for excessive restlessness and profuse sweating.

Teach clients to assess for signs of hyperglycemia: thirst, polyuria, flushed skin, fruity odor to the breath, and drowsiness that progresses to unconsciousness. Instruct the family to have regular insulin available for administration and to observe the client closely after insulin has been given.

Diabetic ketoacidosis is acidosis accompanied by an accumulation of ketones in the body, which results from faulty carbohydrate metabolism. It is evidenced by the symptoms of hyperglycemia (see Box 50-1) and, if left untreated, may

BOX 50-5

Intrasite Rotation of Insulin Injection Sites

A good approach to administering insulin is to instruct the client to mark the first injection site with a spot bandage and give future injections around the bandage. The client should imagine each circle as a clock, administering injections at the 12 o'clock, 3 o'clock, 6 o'clock, and 9 o'clock points before starting a new circle more than an inch away from the previous sites (see below).

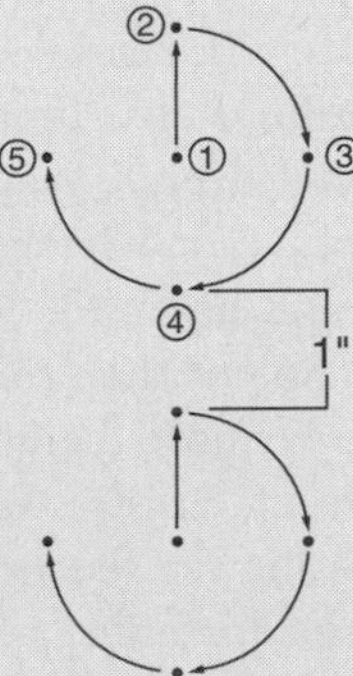

Following this plan, the client can administer five injections per circle. The spot bandage also works as a convenient memory jogger. After going through 2 or 3 showers, the bandage is usually ready to be removed and a new one applied; this occurs at the approximate time the circle is complete.

Figure modified from Drass, J. (1992). What you need to know about insulin injections. *Nursing*, 22(11), 40-43. Modified with permission from the December issue of *Nursing 92*, Springhouse.

BOX 50-6

Quick Fixes for Clients with Mild Hypoglycemia

Clients who have the potential to develop hypoglycemia should have ready access to a source of rapid-acting carbohydrate. The following substances contain 10 to 15 g of such a carbohydrate, which will stabilize a client who is having a mild hypoglycemic reaction—usually within 15 minutes. Some forms are easier to carry on a daily basis, such as the glucose tablets and cake frosting:

3 glucose tablets
4 ounces orange juice
6 ounces regular soda
6-8 ounces 2% fat or skim milk
6-8 Lifesavers
3 graham cracker squares
6 jelly beans
2 tablespoons of raisins
1 small (2-ounce) tube of cake frosting

From Macheca, M.J.K. (1993). Diabetic hypoglycemia: How to keep the threat at bay. *American Journal of Nursing*, 93(4), 26-30.

result in coma. Discuss the following with the client and family to prevent recurrences of ketoacidosis:

- Use a regimented pattern of diabetic control.
- Never omit antidiabetic drugs, particularly when a secondary illness is manifested.
- Consume clear liquids and eat smaller meals when illness occurs.
- When ill, test blood glucose levels at frequent intervals.
- Notify the prescriber of secondary illness, nausea and vomiting, fever, an inability to eat, or an inability to control blood glucose levels.

Inform the family and client that the following factors may lead to diabetic ketoacidosis: type 1 diabetes mellitus, omission of insulin, infections, cerebrovascular accidents (stroke), myocardial infarction, pregnancy, trauma, surgery, and stress (especially emotional).

Inform the client that diet therapy is an important part of glucose control. The dietitian and the meal preparer must be included in the total care of clients with diabetes. Before clients are discharged, they must be able to verbalize an understanding of their diet therapy and be willing to participate in meal planning.

Caution clients against the ingestion of alcohol, because hypoglycemia can result. If alcohol is consumed, the dosage of insulin may need to be reduced, because alcohol potentiates the hypoglycemic effect of insulin.

If the client is using urine testing to assess blood glucose, emphasize that it is important in determining the correct dosage of insulin. Whichever method of urine testing is used, the client should test the second voided specimen. Urine should be tested before each meal.

The client should carry medical identification at all times to identify himself or herself as diabetic and to describe the therapeutic regimen.

Refer to a general nursing text for other aspects of diabetes education not directly related to insulin therapy, such as skin care, foot care, stress reduction, and dietary regimen. (See also the Special Considerations for Children box on p. 872.)

■ **Evaluation.** The expected outcome of insulin therapy is that the client's blood glucose level will remain within normal limits and that the client will manage the therapeutic insulin regimen effectively (see the Case Study box on p. 872).

ORAL HYPOGLYCEMIC AGENTS

Clients with type 2 (non–insulin-dependent) diabetes mellitus are treated with the oral hypoglycemics, diet, exercise and, when necessary, insulin. Currently there are three classifications of oral agents: first- and second-generation sulfonylureas and a miscellaneous group that includes acarbose,

Special Considerations for Children
Diabetes

Children with type 1 diabetes produce little or no insulin; therefore they generally require a daily combination of regular insulin and NPH insulin.

Carefully planned and scheduled meals, exercise, and insulin dosages are necessary to control the child's blood glucose level.

Inform the child's teachers (including the gym teacher), teacher's aides, bus drivers, and anyone in regular contact with the child about diabetes and the signs, symptoms, and treatment of hypoglycemia. These people should also be aware that late or skipped meals or snacks or unplanned exercise can be potentially dangerous for the child.

Because many medications interact with insulin, check with the prescriber before administering any new prescription or nonprescription medications.

The child should carry or wear a MedicAlert identification tag at all times.

metformin (biguanide classification), repaglinide, and the glitazones.

Sulfonylureas

Although the sulfonylureas are sometimes called "oral insulins," this description is incorrect because chemically they are completely different from insulin. They also differ from insulin in their mode of action. See Table 50-3 for the pharmacokinetics and usual adult dosages of the sulfonylureas.

The first-generation sulfonylureas include acetohexamide (Dymelor), chlorpropamide (Diabinese), tolazamide (Tolinase), and ✔ tolbutamide (Orinase), which are considered to be equally effective but may differ in pharmacokinetics and some side effects/adverse reactions. The second-generation sulfonylureas include glimepiride (Amaryl), glipizide (Glucotrol), and glyburide (DiaBeta, Micronase), which are much more potent than the previous generation but have not proven to be more therapeutically or clinically effective (Koda-Kimble & Carlisle, 1995).

The advantages in using the second-generation sulfonylureas are that they have a long duration of action and fewer side effects/adverse reactions. Tolazamide, a first-generation

Case Study *The Client with Type 1 Diabetes Mellitus*

Edward Milton is 25 years old and has recently been diagnosed with type 1 diabetes mellitus. In addition to a 2300-calorie ADA diet, Mr. Milton was started on an insulin administration program that includes 5 U of regular insulin and 10 U of NPH insulin each morning, with 5 U of regular insulin and 5 U of NPH before the evening meal. He is also instructed in the procedure for self-monitoring blood glucose. Mr. Milton is advised to check his blood sugar in the morning before his insulin dose and in the late afternoon before dinner.

One month after beginning treatment, Mr. Milton comes to the emergency department at 6:00 PM with profuse sweating, tremors, headache, and an elevated blood pressure. His blood sugar by finger stick is 45 mg/dL. A serum blood sample confirmed the diagnosis of hypoglycemia. He is given an IV bolus of 50 mL of 50% dextrose. In interviewing Mr. Milton before releasing him from the emergency department, you discover that he had not eaten his usual meals that day because of a vague feeling of nausea, anorexia, and mild diarrhea. He also admits to not testing his blood sugar at home because he is too rushed in the morning. He often eats out in the evening with friends and is too embarrassed to test his blood sugar "in front of my friends." Mr. Milton says he does follow his diet and finds no problems in balancing his food intake.

1. What is significant about the time of day that Mr. Milton experienced his hypoglycemia?
2. Outline the instructions you will give Mr. Milton about managing his diabetes on days when he is sick.
3. Explain the importance of self-monitoring blood glucose for diabetes management.

After his first hypoglycemic episode, Mr. Milton began monitoring his blood glucose twice a day as instructed. One year later he reports that his sugars have been increasing in both the morning and the afternoon. He denies any change in food intake or activity and says he follows his diet faithfully. His insulin regimen is changed to add 5 U of regular insulin to the morning dose of NPH. He is also to take 10 U of NPH and 5 U of regular insulin before dinner in the evening. Although Mr. Milton agrees to the twice-daily insulin injections, he asks why he cannot take pills for diabetes the way his grandfather did for his diabetes.

4. How do you respond to Mr. Milton's questions about taking pills for his diabetes?
5. What does Mr. Milton need to learn about the differences between NPH and regular insulin?
6. List the steps you will teach Mr. Milton about preparing the two insulins for injection.

For answer guidelines, go to mosby.com/MERLIN/McKenry/.

TABLE 50-3 Hypoglycemic Agents: Pharmacokinetics and the Usual Adult Dosage

Generic (Brand Name)	Onset of Action (hours)	Peak Effect (hours)	Duration of Action (hours)	Usual Adult Dosage	Comments
Sulfonylureas					
First Generation					
acetohexamide (Dymelor, Dimelor ♣)	1	1.5-6*	8-24	250-1000 mg/day	Use with caution in older adults and in clients with renal insufficiency.
chlorpropamide (Diabinese)	1	2-4	24-72	250-500 mg/day	Longest acting hypoglycemic. More reported side effects than other agents.
tolazamide (Tolinase)	4-6	3-4	10-20	100-500 mg with breakfast	Active metabolites may be increased in renal impairment.
tolbutamide (Orinase, Mobenol ♣)	1	3-4	6-12	250-2000 mg daily in divided doses	Shortest acting agent. Rapidly metabolized to inactive metabolites.
Second Generation					
glimepiride (Amaryl ◆)	1	2-3	24	1-2 mg with breakfast	—
glipizide (Glucotrol)	1-1.5	1-3	12-24	5-40 mg before meals in divided doses	Administer 30 minutes before meals.
glipizide extended release (Glucotrol XL ◆)	—	6-12	24	5-20 mg with breakfast	—
glyburide nonmicronized (DiaBeta, Micronase)	2-4	4	24	1.25-20 mg with breakfast, divide dosages >10 mg	Use with caution in older adults with renal failure.
glyburide micronized (Glynase PresTab)	1	3	24	0.75-12 mg/day; doses >6 mg are divided and given with meals	Micronized formula has increased bioavailability; thus a lower dose is required.
Miscellaneous Hypoglycemics					
Alpha-Glucosidase Inhibitors					
acarbose	Not absorbed		—	50-100 mg with meals	Most effective if given with a high-fiber diet.
miglitol (Glyset)	N/A	2-3	N/A	25-100 mg 3 times daily	It reduces glycosylated hemoglobin in type 2 diabetes. Take with first bite of food.
Biguanides					
metformin (Glucophage ◆, Novo-Metformin ♣)	—	2-3	6-12	500 mg or 850 mg 2 or 3 times daily	Take with food to reduce nausea and vomiting.
Meglitinides					
nateglinide (Starlix)	—	1	1.5-3	120 mg 3 times daily before meals (1-30 minutes)	May be used alone or in combination with metformin.
repaglinide (Prandin)	—	1	N/A	0.5-2 mg before meals.	Take within 15 minutes of meals.
Thiazolidinediones (Glitazones)					
pioglitazone (Actos)	0.5	2	N/A	15-45 mg daily	Can be taken with/without meals.

Information from Davis, S.N. & Granner, D.K. (1996). Insulin, oral hypoglycemic agents, and the pharmacology of the endocrine pancreas. In J.G. Hardman & L.E. Limbird (Eds.), *Goodman & Gilman's The pharmacological basis of therapeutics* (9th ed.). New York: McGraw-Hill; *Drug Facts and Comparisons.* (2000). St. Louis: Facts and Comparisons; Koda-Kimble, M.A. & Carlisle, B.A. (1995). Diabetes mellitus. In L.Y. Young & M.A. Koda-Kimble (Eds.), *Applied therapeutics: The clinical use of drugs* (6th ed.). Vancouver, WA: Applied Therapeutics; *United States Pharmacopeia Dispensing Information (USP DI): Drug information for the health care professional* (19th ed.). (1999). Rockville, MD: United States Pharmacopeial Convention; and *Mosby's GenRx.* (1999). St. Louis: Mosby.
N/A, Not available.
*Includes the active metabolite hydroxyhexamide.

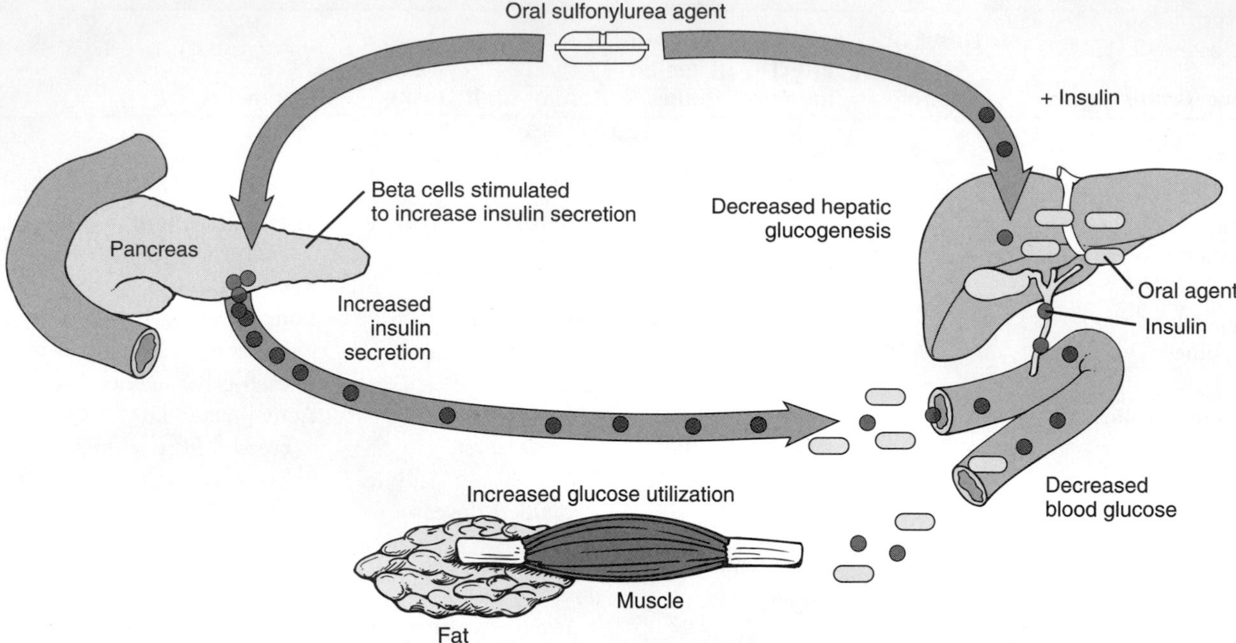

Figure 50-3 Mechanism of action of oral sulfonylurea agents. (From Beare, P.G. & Myers, J.L. [1994]. *Adult health nursing* [2nd ed.]. St. Louis: Mosby.)

sulfonylurea, also has similar advantages. However, Stahl and Berger (1999) reported a higher incidence of severe hypoglycemia leading to hospital admissions in older adults with type 2 diabetes mellitus treated with long-acting vs. short-acting sulfonylureas.

The sulfonylureas enhance the release of insulin from the beta cells in the pancreas, decrease liver glycogenolysis (the breakdown of glycogen stored in the liver to glucose) and gluconeogenesis (the formation of glycogen from fatty acids and proteins rather than from carbohydrates), and increase cellular sensitivity to insulin in body tissues. Therefore they reduce the concentration of blood glucose in people with a functioning pancreas (Figure 50-3). In addition, chlorpropamide has an antidiuretic effect; it increases the effect of low levels of antidiuretic hormone present in persons with central diabetes insipidus.

Oral hypoglycemic agents are indicated for the treatment of uncomplicated type 2 diabetes mellitus in those clients whose diabetes cannot be controlled by diet only.

The most common side effects of sulfonylurea therapy are diarrhea or constipation, dizziness, gas, anorexia, headache, nausea, vomiting, or abdominal distress; less common side effects are photosensitivity or rash. The prescriber should be notified of the following adverse reactions: respiratory difficulties (congestive heart failure), especially in persons with cardiac problems; sedation; muscle cramping; convulsions; edema of the face, hands, or ankles; comatose state, increased weakness (antidiuretic effect); pruritus, jaundice, light-colored stools, dark urine (impairment of liver function); or increased fatigue, sore throat, increased temperature, increased bleeding or bruising (blood dyscrasias).

Miscellaneous Hypoglycemics

The miscellaneous hypoglycemics include the alpha-glucosidase inhibitors (acarbose, miglitol), a biguanide (metformin), a meglitinide (repaglinide), and several thiazolidinediones or glitazones, such as rosiglitazone and pioglitazone.

Alpha-Glucosidase Inhibitors

acarbose [aye kar′ bohse] (Precose)
miglitol [mig le′ tol] (Glyset)

Acarbose and miglitol are oral alpha-glucosidase inhibitors that delay the digestion and absorption of carbohydrates in the small intestine, thereby causing a smaller rise in blood glucose levels after food is ingested. These agents are indicated as an adjunct to diet for the treatment of type 2 diabetes mellitus. These drugs do not increase insulin secretion or cause hypoglycemia, lactic acidosis, or weight gain. They may be given alone or in combination with a sulfonylurea to lower blood glucose.

The absorption of acarbose is minimal from the gastrointestinal tract. See Table 50-3 for the half-life, peak effect, and duration of action of this drug. Unabsorbed acarbose is primarily excreted in the feces.

The absorption of miglitol depends on the dose; for example, a 25-mg dose may be fully absorbed, but a 100-mg dose may be only 50% to 70% absorbed. Peak levels are reached in 2 to 3 hours. Miglitol is not metabolized; it is excreted unchanged by the kidneys.

The side effects/adverse reactions of the alpha-glucosidase inhibitors include, for miglitol, stomach pain, diarrhea, gas, and rash. Acarbose is poorly absorbed and therefore may cause the dose-related side effects of malabsorption, abdominal gas, stomach pain, bloating and, rarely, jaundice (Davis & Granner, 1996; *Drug Facts and Comparisons*, 2000).

See Table 50-3 for the dosage and administration of the alpha-glucosidase inhibitors.

Biguanides

metformin [met for′ min] (Glucophage, Novo-Metformin ♣)
glyburide/metformin [glye′ byoor ide met for′ min] (Glucovance)

Another non-sulfonylurea antihyperglycemic agent for the treatment of type 2 diabetes is metformin, which is chemically classified as a biguanide. The first drug released in this chemical category was phenformin, but it was withdrawn from the market because of its association with lactic acidosis. Metformin has been associated only rarely with this complication (Stang, Wysowski, & Butler-Jones, 1999).

Metformin decreases glucose absorption from the intestines and glucose production in the liver, and it also improves insulin sensitivity in the peripheral tissues. It does not affect the pancreatic beta cells; therefore it does not increase the release of insulin, nor does it cause hypoglycemia. It is an effective adjunct to other antidiabetic therapies (Aviles-Santa, Sinding, & Raskin, 1999).

See Table 50-3 for the pharmacokinetics and dosing of metformin and glyburide.

The most commonly reported side/adverse reactions of metformin include anorexia, abdominal gas or pain, headache, nausea, and vomiting.

Meglitinides

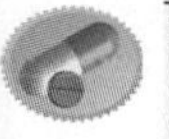

nateglinide [nat a gly′ nide] (Starlix)
repaglinide [rep a gly′ nide] (Prandin)

Nateglinide and repaglinide are nonsulfonylurea hypoglycemic agents that stimulate pancreatic beta cells to produce insulin. They also improve insulin secretion in response to increased glucose levels by regulating the ATP-sensitive K+ channels on pancreatic beta cells.

The drugs are shorter acting and are excreted faster than the oral sulfonylurea drugs; they produce a glucose control similar to therapy with glyburide.

Side effects/adverse reactions are similar to oral sulfonylureas with the exception of potential cardiovascular effects (e.g., hypertension, dysrhythmias) with repaglinide.

See Table 50-3 for pharmacokinetics and dosing of nateglinide and repaglinide.

Thiazolidinediones (Glitazones)

pioglitazone [pee oh glit′ a zone] (Actos)
rosiglitazone [roe zi glit′ a zone] (Avandia ◆)

Troglitazone was the first agent in a new classification of drugs that lowers insulin resistance in poorly controlled, type II diabetes mellitus. It was removed from the market because severe liver toxicity and fatalities were associated with its use. The other two drugs in this category, pioglitazone and rosiglitazone, appear to have the same benefits as troglitazone but produce less risk for severe liver toxicity (HHS News, 2000). Pioglitazone and rosiglitazone appear to resensitize the body to its own insulin; they decrease insulin resistance in the periphery and liver, which results in an increase in glucose processing in the body. Pioglitazone and rosiglitazone are potent agonists for peroxisome proliferator-activated receptors that are found in adipose tissue, skeletal muscle, and the liver. Activation of these receptors ultimately results in control of glucose production, transport and use in the body, and lipid metabolism.

This mechanism of action is totally different from all the other hypoglycemic agents. Be aware, however, that these agents are not indicated for clients with diabetes who cannot product insulin (type 1 diabetes).

Pioglitazone is rapidly absorbed orally in the fasting state. It reaches peak serum levels in 2 hours and is highly protein bound to serum albumin. It is metabolized in the liver, and the metabolites M-II and M-IV are active metabolites. Although a small amount of the drug is excreted by the kidneys unchanged, the primary source of excretion of the drug and metabolites is in bile and, ultimately, the feces. Rosiglitazone is well absorbed orally and reaches peak serum levels in approximately 1 hour. It has a half-life between 3 and 4 hours and is excreted primarily by the kidneys (*Mosby's GenRx*, 2000).

The side effects/adverse reactions of pioglitazone include edema, headache, myalgia, sinusitis, and upper respiratory infections. The side effects/adverse reactions of rosiglitazone include headache, edema, back pain, upper respiratory tract infection, and anemia (Allen, 1999). Blood testing for liver function should be performed before the start of therapy, every 2 months during the first year, and periodically thereafter (*Mosby's GenRx*, 2000).

The usual adult dosage of pioglitazone is 15 to 45 mg once daily. The usual adult monotherapy dosage for rosiglitazone is 4 mg daily or 2 mg twice daily. When rosiglitazone is combined with metformin, the initial dosage is 4 mg daily (or 2 mg twice daily), which may be increased if necessary after 3 months of therapy (Diabetes, 1999; *Mosby's GenRx*, 2000).

■ Nursing Management

Oral Hypoglycemic Agent Therapy

■ **Assessment.** The client's level of knowledge for health maintenance related to diabetes mellitus and the prescribed oral hypoglycemic agent should be assessed. Information is to be provided or reinforced related to compliance with the appropriate ADA diet for ideal weight attainment, weight monitoring, activity program, stress management, and adverse signs and symptoms to report to the health care provider.

Oral hypoglycemic agents are not administered to clients who require close control by titration of insulin, such as

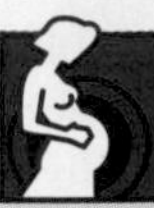

Pregnancy Safety
Drugs Affecting the Pancreas

Category	Drug
B	acarbose, glucagon, metformin
C	acetohexamide, chlorpropamide, diazoxide, glipizide, glyburide, nateglinide, pioglitazone, repaglinide, rosiglitazone, tolazamide, tolbutamide

those undergoing major surgery or those with diabetic coma, ketoacidosis, significant ketosis or acidosis, severe burns, infection, or trauma. The sulfonylureas are to be used with caution in debilitated or malnourished clients or in clients with adrenal or pituitary insufficiency, high fever, prolonged nausea and vomiting, or impairment of thyroid, renal, or hepatic function; these clients are predisposed to hypoglycemia. Because of the antidiuretic effects of chlorpropamide, consideration should be given to the use of oral hypoglycemic agents other than chlorpropamide in clients with cardiac impairment or fluid retention.

The client's sensitivity to sulfonylurea agents, sulfonamides, or thiazide-type diuretics needs to be determined because of their cross-sensitivity with the sulfonylureas. Determine the client's hypersensitivity to the oral hypoglycemic agent under consideration.

Because of its activity in the small bowel, acarbose should not be used in clients with intestinal disorders, such as inflammatory or ulcerative bowel disease or any condition of the bowel in which increased intestinal gas would be contraindicated. Acarbose may result in increased transaminase levels in clients with cirrhosis of the liver. Metformin should not be used in clients with any condition that may contribute to lactic acidosis, such as hepatic disease or decreased renal function. (See the Pregnancy Safety box above.)

Review the client's current medication regimen for the risk of significant drug interactions, such as those that may occur when the oral hypoglycemic agents are given with the following drugs (see Box 50-4):

Drug	Possible Effect and Management
Bold/color type indicates the most serious interactions.	
adsorbents, intestinal or digestive enzyme preparations	The use of acarbose with these agents will decrease the effectiveness of acarbose; avoid concurrent use.
alcohol	**May result in a disulfiram (Antabuse)-type reaction with the sulfonylureas, primarily chlorpropamide (Diabinese). The reaction may include stomach pain, nausea, vomiting, facial flushing, lowered blood glucose levels, and headaches. Avoid concurrent use or a potentially serious drug interaction may occur. This problem is reported less often with glipizide (Glucotrol) and glyburide (DiaBeta, Micronase).** In addition to the risk of hypoglycemia, the combination of alcohol and metformin may predispose the client to increased blood lactate levels.
anticoagulants, oral (coumarins or indanediones)	Initially, increased serum levels of sulfonylureas and anticoagulants may be seen, but a reduction in plasma levels and effectiveness of the anticoagulant is reported with chronic therapy. An increased serum level of the oral hypoglycemic agent may result in increased effects and toxicity because of a decrease in liver metabolism. Monitor closely, because one or both drugs may require a dosage adjustment.
beta-adrenergic blocking agents (including ophthalmics)	Increase the risk of hyperglycemia or hypoglycemia with the sulfonylureas or repaglinide. Refer to the drug interactions for insulin for further information.
chloramphenicol (Chloromycetin), guanethidine (Ismelin), insulin, monoamine oxidase (MAO) inhibitors, salicylates or sulfonamides	May result in an increase in the hypoglycemic effect of the sulfonylureas. Monitor closely, because dosage adjustments may be necessary.
cimetidine (Tagamet), and other drugs excreted by renal tubular transport, such as calcium channel blocking agents, digoxin (Lanoxin), morphine, ranitidine (Zantac)	These drugs have the potential to increase the serum levels of metformin. A dosage reduction of metformin may be necessary.
oral contraceptives, estrogen-containing	Concurrent use may induce drug metabolism, resulting in contraceptive failure. Alert the client to use barrier contraceptives.

A baseline assessment of the client is the same as for insulin administration.

▪ **Nursing Diagnosis.** Clients receiving sulfonylurea oral hypoglycemic agents may experience the following nursing diagnoses/collaborative problems: diarrhea or constipation; impaired comfort such as headache, heartburn, nausea, vomiting, abdominal discomfort, rash, and photosensitivity; and the potential complications of hypoglycemia, agranulocytosis, aplastic or hemolytic anemia, eosinophilia, thrombocytopenia, and hepatic function impairment. With chlorpropamide only, the client is at risk for excess fluid volume and altered cardiac output related to the antidiuretic effect of the drug as evidenced by weight gain, difficulty in breathing, oliguria, and edema of the face, hands, and feet. With acarbose, impaired comfort (abdominal pain, flatulence), diarrhea, and the potential complication of jaundice may occur. With metformin, impaired comfort (heartburn, flatulence, headache, metallic taste, anorexia) and the potential complications of anemia and lactic acidosis (diarrhea, shortness of breath, muscle pain, fatigue) may occur.

■ **Implementation**

■ ***Monitoring.*** Remember that the client with diabetes requires close supervision, especially when an oral hypoglycemic agent is tried for the first time. When converting from insulin to an oral hypoglycemic agent for the control of diabetic status, monitor the client's blood glucose levels at least three times daily before meals.

No transition period is usually required when changing from one sulfonylurea agent to metformin or another sulfonylurea agent (except with chlorpropamide). With chlorpropamide, caution should be exercised during the first 2 weeks because of its prolonged half-life of 25 to 60 hours. Older adults tend to be more sensitive to the effects of the sulfonylureas as oral hypoglycemic agents. Because hypoglycemia may be more difficult to recognize in these clients, they require lower dosages and closer monitoring.

Observe for hypoglycemia in the client who is taking sulfonylureas and has irregular meal patterns, exercises more than usual, or ingests significant amounts of alcohol; hypoglycemia is more likely in this client. A moderate lifestyle is essential to diabetes management. Periods of physiologic or psychologic stress may necessitate a temporary use of insulin.

Clients receiving acarbose should have their transaminase concentrations monitored at 3-month intervals during the first year of therapy and periodically after that time.

In addition to the other monitoring of a client with diabetes, the client taking metformin should also have renal function monitored. Metformin should be discontinued once or twice a year to see if it is contributing to the management of the client's diabetes.

See the section for client monitoring under Nursing Management: Insulin Therapy, p. 866.

■ ***Intervention.*** See Table 50-3 for recommended administration times. Acarbose is started at the lowest dosage and increased gradually to minimize the gastrointestinal effects of flatulence and diarrhea.

Metformin may be added to maximum-dose sulfonylurea therapy and vice versa, with the dosage of the new drug gradually titrated upward. If high-dose combination therapy is not effective in controlling the client's blood glucose in 3 months, oral hypoglycemic therapy should be discontinued and insulin started.

Repaglinide is to be taken 15 to 30 minutes before a meal.

■ ***Education.*** Recognize that the need for instruction that stresses dietary restriction is even greater for clients receiving oral hypoglycemic agents than for those taking insulin. Clients who are more than 20% over their ideal weight may not respond to oral hypoglycemic agents. The client should keep a weight record and weigh in once a week at the same time using the same scale. Remember that these clients should be taught how to test for blood glucose levels, proper skin care, and the signs and symptoms of hypoglycemia and hyperglycemia.

Caution clients about excessive alcohol intake (and medications containing alcohol) when sulfonylurea therapy is begun. Alcohol can increase the rate of metabolism of these drugs when there is long-term consumption of excessive quantities of these drugs. In addition, a disulfiram-like reaction may occur with the sulfonylureas.

Blood glucose testing should be performed at frequent intervals during the transition period when clients are switched from insulin to oral hypoglycemic agents. Teach clients to carry or have access to some form of glucose at all times.

Have the client administer the initial dosage of the sulfonylureas in the morning to decrease nocturnal hypoglycemia; they may be given with food to decrease any gastric upset. If the client is taking divided doses of the same sulfonylurea agent and omits a dose, advise that it be taken as soon as it is remembered; however, doses should not be taken together. Administering sulfonylureas before meals will maximize the release of postprandial insulin.

Acarbose is to be taken at the beginning of each meal. If the client completes the meal without taking the drug, skip that dose and take the next dose with the next meal. Metformin may be taken with food to minimize stomach upset.

Make the client aware that the administration of sulfonylurea agents has been associated with an increased incidence of death from cardiovascular disease compared with treatment with diet alone or diet plus insulin.

■ **Evaluation.** The expected outcome of oral hypoglycemic agent therapy is that the client's blood glucose level will remain within normal limits, and the client will manage the therapeutic oral hypoglycemic regimen effectively.

HYPERGLYCEMIC AGENTS

glucagon [gloo′ ka gon]

Glucagon (for injection) is a natural polypeptide hormone secreted by pancreatic alpha cells in response to hypoglycemia. It is released to maintain plasma levels of glucose by stimulating hepatic glycogenolysis and **gluconeogenesis** (the conversion of glycerol and amino acids to glucose) and by the inhibition of glycogen synthesis. The effect of glucagon is accelerated by stimulating the synthesis of cyclic adenosine monophosphate (cAMP). Hepatic and adipose tissue lipolysis is enhanced by activating adenyl cyclase, which produces free fatty acids and glycerol and stimulates ketogenesis and gluconeogenesis.

Glucagon is indicated for the treatment of severe hypoglycemia in clients with diabetes and as an adjunct for gastrointestinal radiography. It is useful in hypoglycemia only if liver glycogen is available; thus it is ineffective in chronic hypoglycemia, starvation, and adrenal insufficiency.

Glucagon is also used as an adjunct to barium in gastrointestinal radiography. It decreases peristalsis and produces relaxation of the esophagus, stomach, duodenum, small bowel, and colon (hypotonicity), thus improving outcome of the examination.

Parenterally administered (IM, IV, or SC), glucagon has a half-life of 10 minutes. The onset of action (hyperglycemic) depends on the route of administration: IV, 5 to 20 minutes; IM, 15 minutes; SC, 30 to 45 minutes. The duration of action is 1.5 hours. It is metabolized in the liver and excreted by the kidneys.

The side effects/adverse reactions of glucagon are not usually severe and may include nausea or vomiting and an allergic reaction. No significant drug interactions have been reported.

The adolescent and adult dosage of glucagon for hypoglycemia is 0.5 to 1 mg IM, IV, or SC, repeated in 20 minutes when necessary. The pediatric dosage is 0.025 mg/kg up to a maximum dose of 1 mg (IM, IV, or SC).

■ Nursing Management

Glucagon Therapy

■ **Assessment.** It is important to recognize the symptoms of hypoglycemia: anxiousness, irritability, altered mood, nervousness, weakness, shakiness, inability to concentrate, perspiration, cool/pale skin, hunger, nausea, headache, and unconsciousness. A rapid blood glucose level may be obtained to confirm the hypoglycemia.

If glucagon is being used for testing purposes, there is a risk for hyperglycemia in the client with diabetes mellitus. The risk-benefit ratio needs to be considered if the client has a history of insulinoma (a paradoxical decrease in blood glucose may occur) or pheochromocytoma (may cause hypertension as the result of the release of catecholamines).

■ **Nursing Diagnosis.** The client may develop impaired comfort (nausea and vomiting) as a result of the underlying hypoglycemia or glucagon overdose, and there is also the potential complication of allergic reaction or severe hypoglycemia due to ineffectiveness of the drug.

■ **Implementation**

■ ***Monitoring.*** Check the client's blood glucose level throughout the hypoglycemic episode, after administration, and for 3 to 4 hours after the client regains consciousness. Note the client's clinical response. Monitor the client's vital signs and level of consciousness.

■ ***Intervention.*** Glucagon is administered for hypoglycemia in the unconscious client as directed by the prescriber. After administering, turn the individual on one side to prevent choking and/or aspiration. Emergency medical assistance should be obtained as quickly as possible. Inform the prescriber of the client's status. If the client does not regain consciousness in 5 to 20 minutes, administer a second dose and transport the client to the hospital. IV glucose needs to be started if the individual does not respond to the second dose of glucagon. Glucagon and glucose may be given at the same time.

If the client does regain consciousness and can swallow, offer some oral form of sugar followed by a more complex carbohydrate, such as crackers and cheese or a glass of milk. This helps to prevent a recurrence of hypoglycemia before the next meal. Seek medical assistance if the client is experiencing nausea and vomiting that prevents food intake for more than an hour after the administration of glucagon.

Replace the client's supply of glucagon as soon as possible.

Medical follow-up is necessary for all clients who experience a hypoglycemic episode as a result of oral antidiabetic agents.

■ ***Education.*** Before the need arises to use glucagon, teach the family and the client how to mix the drug and how to inject it properly. A standard insulin syringe may be used for injection unless the dose is greater than the capacity of the syringe. The injection should be made at a 90-degree angle instead of the usual subcutaneous approach. Advise the client and family to keep supplies on hand and check the expiration dates frequently.

Instruct the client and family about the symptoms of hypoglycemia and the importance of ingesting some form of sugar when symptoms first occur, such as orange juice, honey, syrup, hard candy, sugar cubes, or milk.

■ **Evaluation.** The expected outcome of glucagon therapy is that the client's blood glucose level will be within normal limits. The client and family will state an understanding of the effective management of glucagon therapy and will successfully demonstrate administration techniques.

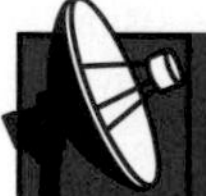

TechnologyLink

Drugs Affecting the Pancreas (Diabetes)

Video Resources

Nursing Management of Complications from Diabetes, ISBN 0-8151-6057-7 Mosby, Inc., 11830 Westline Industrial Drive, St. Louis, MO 63146; (800) 426-4545; www.mosby.com.

Web Resources

American Diabetes Association (www.diabetes.org/)
This site is dedicated to the prevention and cure of diabetes. It provides information for individuals with diabetes.

CDC's Diabetes and Public Health Resource (www.cdc.gov/diabetes/index.htm)
This site presents research findings, statistics, special projects, publications, and other information on diabetes.

Diabetes Exercise & Sports Association (www.diabetes-exercise.org/)
This site provides information on exercise and athletics for people with diabetes.

Diabetes Mall (www.diabetesnet.com/)
This site provides information on diabetes, including the latest technology, alternative approaches, and Internet resources.

For additional WebLinks, a free subscription to the "Mosby/Saunders ePharmacology Update" newsletter, and more, go to mosby.com/MERLIN/McKenry/.

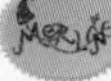

diazoxide [dye az ox′ ide] (Proglycem)

Oral diazoxide produces a prompt, dose-related increase in blood glucose levels by inhibiting the release of pancreatic insulin. It may also have an extrapancreatic effect. It is indicated for the treatment of hypoglycemia caused by hyperinsulinism, secondary to an inoperable islet cell adenoma or carcinoma, an extrapancreatic malignancy, or an islet cell hyperplasia. It is not indicated for treatment in functional hypoglycemia. It is also available in parenteral dosage form to treat hypertensive emergencies.

Under normal conditions, diazoxide is rapidly absorbed orally, has an onset of action within 1 hour, a duration of effect less than 8 hours, and a half-life between 20 and 36 hours. It is highly protein bound, metabolized in the liver, and excreted by the kidneys.

The side effects of diazoxide include taste alterations, constipation, anorexia, nausea, vomiting, and abdominal pain. With chronic use it may cause increased hair growth on the arms, legs, back, and forehead (hypertrichosis). The most commonly reported adverse reactions include a decrease in urine output that results in edema of the hands, feet, or lower extremities; weight gain; and possibly congestive heart failure in susceptible individuals. Hyperglycemia or ketoacidosis are typical symptoms of a diazoxide overdose.

The adult dosage of diazoxide is 1 mg/kg PO every 8 hours, with dosage adjustments as necessary. The maintenance dosage is 3 to 8 mg/kg PO daily, which is divided into 2 or 3 equal doses and administered every 8 or 12 hours. The maximum dosage is usually 15 mg/kg/day.

■ Nursing Management

Diazoxide Therapy

■ **Assessment.** Determine whether the client has a sensitivity to thiazide diuretics or other sulfonamide medication, because he or she may also be sensitive to diazoxide.

Carefully consider the use of diazoxide in clients with cardiovascular problems, such as acute aortic dissection, compensatory hypertension, coronary or cerebral insufficiency, or inadequate cardiac reserve, because there is a potential for fluid volume excess as a result of the drug's tendency to increase water and sodium retention.

Review the client's current medication regimen for the risk of significant drug interactions, such as those that may occur when diazoxide is given concurrently with the following drugs:

Drug	Possible Effect and Management
anticonvulsants, hydantoin (phenytoin)	May decrease or nullify the action of both drugs. Monitor the effects of both drugs, and adjust dosages accordingly.
medications that induce hypotension (alcohol, diuretics, calcium channel blocking agents, beta-adrenergic blocking drugs) and peripheral vasodilators	Concurrent use may cause an enhanced severe hypotensive effect. Monitor closely, because dosage adjustments may be necessary.

A baseline assessment of the client's urine and serum glucose and blood pressure should be obtained before initiating diazoxide therapy.

■ **Nursing Diagnosis.** Clients receiving diazoxide may experience the following nursing diagnoses/collaborative problems: excess fluid volume (rapid weight gain, swelling of the feet and ankles); impaired comfort (change in taste, nausea, vomiting, and abdominal pain); constipation; disturbed body image related to hypertrichosis; impaired physical mobility related to the drug's extrapyramidal effects as evidenced by stiffness of the limbs and trembling and shaking of the fingers and hands; and the potential complications of allergic reaction, angina pectoris, myocardial ischemia or infarction, thrombocytopenia, and transient cerebral ischemic attacks.

■ **Implementation**

■ ***Monitoring.*** Monitor blood glucose at least daily. Monitor the client's blood pressure, intake and output, and weight daily. Observe clients for swelling of the feet and lower legs, increased weight gain, and a decrease in urinary output as signs of excess fluid volume. Diuretics are sometimes given concurrently to avert these side effects. Observe for the signs and symptoms of hyperglycemia.

■ ***Intervention.*** Dosage forms vary in their ability to produce blood concentrations of diazoxide. The oral suspension dosage form produces higher concentrations than those of the capsule form. Caution needs to be taken when changing the client from one dosage form to the other.

After the IV administration of diazoxide, there is usually a transient hyperglycemia (24 to 48 hours), but this condition rarely progresses to ketoacidosis.

■ ***Education.*** Instruct clients about the importance of diet, blood glucose testing, regular visits to the prescriber, symptoms of hypoglycemia and hyperglycemia, and of not taking other medications unless discussed with the prescriber.

Advise the client to change positions from a lying to a sitting or standing position slowly to minimize lightheadedness and fainting.

■ **Evaluation.** The expected outcome of diazoxide therapy is that the client's blood glucose level will return to normal limits and that the client will not have fluid or sodium retention. The client and family will state an understanding of the effective management of diazoxide therapy. If the drug is not effective within 2 to 3 weeks in managing hypoglycemia, its use needs to be reevaluated.

glucose [gloo′ koes] (Glutose, Insta-Glucose)

Glucose is a monosaccharide that is absorbed from the intestine and then either used or stored by the body. It is indicated to treat or manage hypoglycemia. As a nutrient, glucose provides 4 cal/g.

The only side effects are some reports of nausea. No significant drug interactions have been reported.

In adults approximately 10 to 20 g PO are administered and repeated in 10 minutes if necessary.

Complementary and Alternative Therapies
Herbal Interactions with Hypoglycemics

Insulin, acetohexamide, chlorpropamide, glipizide, metformin, tolazamide, tolbutamide, and troglitazone may interact with the following to enhance hypoglycemic effects. Monitor closely:

bilberry
bitter melon
Coccinia indica
garlic
onion
Panax ginseng
Pterocarpus marsupium
saltbush
syzygium cucumi

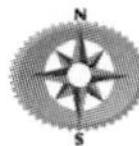
For a Concept Map on diabetes, go to mosby.com/MERLIN/McKenry/.

SUMMARY

The two primary hormones released by the pancreas are insulin and glucagon. When blood glucose falls, glucagon is released; this facilitates the catabolism of glycogen stored in the liver, which increases blood glucose. The release of glucagon stimulates the secretion of insulin, which inhibits the release of glucagon and maintains the homeostasis of carbohydrate metabolism.

Diabetes mellitus is a disorder of carbohydrate metabolism that is results from an insulin deficiency, a resistance, or both. Diabetes mellitus is classified as type 1 (insulin-dependent) diabetes mellitus (previously called juvenile-onset diabetes), and type 2 (non–insulin-dependent) diabetes mellitus (maturity-onset diabetes). Although type 2 may require insulin at some time, it is usually managed by dietary treatment, weight reduction, client education and, if necessary, oral hypoglycemic agents.

Insulin may be rapid-, intermediate-, or long-acting. Therapeutic dosages are not fixed but are set in response to blood glucose levels, considering the client's dietary intake and physical activity. Client education is essential so the client can participate in ascertaining the necessary insulin dosage through blood testing and can self-administer insulin safety and accurately. See the selected nursing diagnoses for clients receiving insulin on p. 869.

Oral hypoglycemic agents have a variety of mechanisms of action. They can encourage the release of insulin from the pancreas, decrease glycogenolysis and gluconeogenesis, increase the sensitivity of body tissues to insulin, and decrease the absorption of carbohydrates from the gastrointestinal tract, but all are used for type 2 diabetes mellitus.

Hyperglycemic agents are used in the treatment of hypoglycemia in which the client is unable to ingest sufficient amounts of glucose to meet body requirements.

Critical Thinking Questions

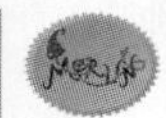

1. Sally Milton, age 59, was diagnosed with diabetes mellitus 6 years ago. In the past, her blood glucose control has been managed by weight loss and diet. She has just started treatment with glipizide (Glucotrol XL), 5 mg PO daily. She confides in you, "I'm pleased to be starting on the pills. I was tired of watching my diet." How should you respond?
2. Loretta Baxter, age 45, has recently been diagnosed with type 1 diabetes mellitus. She weighs 240 pounds when admitted to the hospital for additional testing. She is placed on a 1500-calorie ADA diet and prescribed 30 U of NPH insulin to be taken at 7 AM each morning. At 4 PM, she becomes diaphoretic, weak, and pale. What action should you take? What explanation will you provide Ms. Baxter about what has occurred?

Collaborative Learning Activities

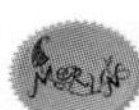

For Collaborative Learning Activities, go to mosby.com/MERLIN/McKenry/.

CASE STUDY

For a Case Study that will help ensure mastery of this chapter content, go to mosby.com/MERLIN/McKenry/.

BIBLIOGRAPHY

Allen, J. (1999). New drug: Pioglitazone (Actos). *Pharmacist's Letter/Prescriber's Letter.* Document #150802.

American Diabetes Association. (1990). *Physician's guide to non–insulin-dependent (type II) diabetes: Diagnosis and treatment.* Alexandria, VA: Author.

American Hospital Formulary Service (1999). *AHFS drug information '99.* Bethesda, MD: American Society of Hospital Pharmacists.

Anderson, K.N., Anderson, L.E., & Glanze, W.D. (Eds.). (1998). *Mosby's medical, nursing, & allied health dictionary* (5th ed.). St. Louis: Mosby.

Aviles-Santa, L., Sinding, J., & Raskin, P. (1999). Effects of metformin in patients with poorly controlled, insulin-treated type 2 diabetes mellitus: A randomized, double-blind, placebo-controlled trial. *Annals of Internal Medicine, 131*(3), 182-188.

Baker, D.E. (1997). Management of type 2 diabetes. *Clinical Pharmacy Newswatch, 4*(4), 1-6.

Beaulieu, J.A. (1989). Nursing diagnoses co-occurring in adults with insulin-dependent diabetes mellitus. *Classification of Nursing Diagnosis Proceedings Eighth Conference*. St. Louis: Mosby.

Beier, M.T.(1997) Incidence of NIDDM and impact of tight glucose control: Implication for long-term care. *The Consultant Pharmacist, 12*(suppl A), 3-6.

Betz, J.L. (1995). Pharmacy update: Fast-acting human insulin analogues: A promising innovation in diabetes care. *Diabetes Educator, 21*(3), 195, 197-198, 200.

Brown, J., Nichols, G.A., Glauber, H.S., & Bakst, A. (1999). Ten-year follow-up of antidiabetic drug use, nonadherence, and mortality in a defined population with type 2 diabetes mellitus. *Clinical Therapeutics, 21*(6), 1045-1057.

Campbell, R.K. (1992). The clinical use of insulin. *U.S. Pharmacist* (diabetes supplement), November.

Covington, T.R. (Ed.). (1996). *Handbook of nonprescription drugs* (11th ed.). Washington, D.C.: American Pharmaceutical Association.

Davis, S.N. & Granner, D.K. (1996). Insulin, oral hypoglycemic agents, and the pharmacology of the endocrine pancreas. In J.G. Hardman & L.E. Limbird (Eds.), *Goodman & Gilman's The pharmacological basis of therapeutics* (9th ed.). New York: McGraw-Hill.

DeFronzo, R.A. (1999). Pharmacologic therapy for type 2 diabetes mellitus. *Annals of Internal Medicine, 131*(4), 281-303.

Diabetes (1999). *Pharmacist's Letter, 15*(8), 43-44.

Drass, J. (1992). What you need to know about insulin injections. *Nursing, 22*(11), 40-43.

Drug Facts and Comparisons. (2000). St. Louis: Facts and Comparisons.

HHS News. (2000) Rezulin to be withdrawn from the market. Food and Drug Administration; www.fda.gov/bbs/topics/NEWS/NEW00721.html (4/23/00).

Katzung, B.G. (1998). *Basic and clinical pharmacology* (7th ed.). Norwalk, CT: Appleton & Lange.

Kitabchi, A.E. & Wall, B.M. (1999). Management of diabetic ketoacidosis. *American Family Physician, 60*(2), 455-464.

Koda-Kimble, M.A. & Carlisle, B.A. (1995). Diabetes mellitus. In L.Y. Young & M.A. Koda-Kimble (Eds.), *Applied therapeutics: The clinical use of drugs* (6th ed.). Vancouver, WA: Applied Therapeutics.

Kupecz, D. (1995). Metformin: An antihyperglycemic drug for non–insulin-dependent diabetes mellitus. *Nurse Practitioner, 20*(7), 70-72.

Macheca, M.J.K. (1993). Diabetic hypoglycemia: How to keep the threat at bay. *American Journal of Nursing, 93*(4), 26-30.

Mosby's GenRx (9th ed.). (1999). St. Louis: Mosby.

Reichard P., Nilsson B.Y., & Rosenquist U. (1993). The effect of long-term intensified insulin treatment on the development of microvascular complications of diabetes mellitus. *New England Journal of Medicine, 329*, 304.

Rodgers, K. (1996). New Ammon: Faster-acting insulin set to debut in August. *Drug Topics, 140*(13), 59.

Stahl, M. & Berger, W. (1999). Higher incidence of severe hypoglycemia leading to hospital admission in type 2 diabetic patients treated with long--acting versus short-acting sulfonylureas. *Diabetic Medicine, 16*(7), 586-590.

Stang, M., Wysowski, D.K., & Butler-Jones, D. (1999). Incidence of lactic acidosis in metformin users. *Diabetes Care, 22*(6), 925-927.

Turner, R.C., Cull, C.A., Frighi, V., & Holman, R.R. (1999). Glycemic control with diet, sulfonylurea, metformin, or insulin in patients with type 2 diabetes mellitus: Progressive requirement for multiple therapies (UKPDS 49). UK Prospective Diabetes Study (UKPDS) Group. *Journal of the American Medical Association, 281*(21), 2005-2012.

United States Pharmacopeia Dispensing Information (USP DI): Drug information for the health care professional (19th ed.). (1999). Rockville, MD: United States Pharmacopeial Convention.

Vaag, A. (1999). On the pathophysiology of late onset non–insulin-dependent diabetes mellitus: Current controversies and new insights. *Danish Medical Bulletin, 46*(3), 197-234.

Vibulbhan, S. (1993). Blood glucose sticks: A finger a day. *Nursing, 23*(5), 22.

Watson, J. (1995). *Nurse's manual of laboratory and diagnostic tests* (2nd ed.). Philadelphia: F.A. Davis.

Wilson, B.A. (1994). What nurses don't know about managing NIDDM. *MEDSURG Nursing 3*(2), 152-154.

51 Overview of the Female and Male Reproductive Systems

Chapter Focus

Because secrecy and cultural sensitivity often influence perceptions of reproductive disorders, caring for clients with dysfunctions of the reproductive system is particularly challenging for the nurse. The client may experience a disturbance of self-esteem, altered sexual patterns, and sexual dysfunction; this requires the nurse to apply his or her knowledge of reproductive anatomy and physiology and associated drugs for sensitive and appropriate teaching and counseling. This chapter reviews the anatomy and physiology of the female and male reproductive systems as background for the next four chapters, which discuss the drugs affecting the reproductive system.

Learning Objectives

1. Identify the anterior pituitary gland hormones that influence the female and male reproductive systems.
2. Describe hormonal influences on uterine function during the menstrual cycle.
3. Identify the primary male and female hormones.
4. Describe the effects of estrogen and progesterone during the proliferative stage.
5. Trace the transport of sperm in the male body from production to ejaculation.

Key Terms

androgen, p. 883
estrogen, p. 883
follicle-stimulating hormone (FSH), p. 883
luteinizing hormone (LH), p. 883
ovulation, p. 883
progestogen, p. 883
testosterone, p. 885

Reproduction is the sum of genetic and hormonal influences that originate from members of a species to perpetuate the species. In human beings, the reproductive process in both sexes is highly complex. It involves (1) follicle-stimulating hormone, which stimulates the growth and maturation of graafian follicles in the ovary and spermatogenesis in the testes; and (2) luteinizing hormone, which stimulates the secretion of sex hormones by the ovary and the testes and is involved in the maturation of the spermatozoa and ova. Both follicle-stimulating hormone and luteinizing hormone are secreted from the anterior pituitary gland. The hormones from the reproductive systems of the male (**androgens**) and the female (**estrogens** and **progestogens**) are also involved in the reproductive process.

ENDOCRINE GLANDS

The reproductive system of the human female consists of the ovaries, fallopian tubes, uterus, and vagina. The male reproductive system consists of the testes, seminal vesicles, prostate gland, bulbourethral glands, and penis. The reproductive organs of both the male and female are mainly under the control of the endocrine glands. The ovaries and testes, known as gonads, not only produce ova and sperm cells but also form endocrine secretions that initiate and maintain the secondary sexual characteristics of men and women. The structure and physiologic functions of the pituitary gland are reviewed in Chapter 47; the discussion of the pituitary gland in this chapter is limited to its effect on the female and male reproductive systems.

PITUITARY GONADOTROPIC HORMONES

The following gonadotropins or pituitary hormones are responsible for the development and maintenance of sexual gland functions:

1. **Follicle-stimulating hormone (FSH)** stimulates the development of the ovarian (graafian) follicles up to the point of ovulation in the female. In the male, FSH stimulates the development of the seminiferous tubules and promotes spermatogenesis.
2. **Luteinizing hormone (LH)**, or interstitial cell–stimulating hormone (ICSH), acts in the female to promote the growth of the interstitial cells in the follicle and the formation of the corpus luteum. In the male, LH stimulates the growth of interstitial cells in the testes and promotes the formation of the hormone androgen (testosterone).

In the female, FSH initiates the cycle of events in the ovary. Under the influence of both FSH and LH, the graafian follicle grows, matures, secretes estrogen, ovulates, and forms the corpus luteum. LH promotes the secretory activity of the corpus luteum and the formation of progesterone. In the absence of LH the corpus luteum undergoes regressive changes and fails to make progesterone.

FEMALE REPRODUCTIVE SYSTEM

The female reproductive system is illustrated in Figure 51-1. Figure 51-2 illustrates the effects of the pituitary hormones, ovarian hormones, and uterine functions during the menstrual cycle.

Day 1 of the menstrual cycle is the onset of menses, with day 5 usually signifying the end of menstruation. During this time, FSH stimulates follicular growth in the ovary and stimulates the ovary to produce estrogen, which is low at the beginning of the cycle. As estrogen levels increase, FSH levels decrease. The rising estrogen levels prepare the uterus for a fertilized ovum; this is known as the proliferative stage of the uterus and results in the following:

1. The growth of the glandular surface of the endometrium, or inner lining of the uterus
2. The production by the endocervical glands of a more plentiful and viscous mucus, which contains nutrients that can be used by the sperm

Increasing levels of estrogen also stimulate the pituitary gland to release LH. LH increases as FSH decreases. At this time (day 14), **ovulation** occurs when the mature follicle ruptures and releases its ovum. The ovum travels through the fallopian tube to the uterus.

Increasing levels of LH affect the ruptured follicle by changing the follicle capsule into the corpus luteum. Under the influence of LH, the corpus luteum releases estrogen and progesterone. In the second phase, or secretory phase, both uterine hormones increase the secretion of the endometrial glands. If the ovum is fertilized and reaches this area on approximately the eighteenth day of the cycle, it will be able to thrive on the nutrient secretions of the endometrium.

If fertilization does not occur, the pituitary responds to the increased levels of estrogen and progesterone by shutting off the release of FSH and LH. Without the central stimulation, the corpus luteum cannot produce estrogen or progesterone; the surface layer of the endometrium then sloughs off, resulting in menstruation. Figure 51-3 depicts the feedback mechanism of FSH and LH and their main effects on the ovaries.

Most women demonstrate month-to-month variations in their menstrual cycles; therefore ovulation is not always predictable. The previous description of the menstrual cycle is based on a 28-day cycle, but ovulation varies and occurs on different days in cycles of different lengths. Physiologically, this is the primary reason for the unreliability of the rhythm method of contraception, which depends on predicting the day of ovulation on the basis of previous menstrual cycles.

Female Sexual Response

For both males and females, psychologic stimulation and local sexual stimulation are necessary for a satisfactory sexual experience. Psychologic stimulation may be aided by an individual's erotic thoughts, but sexual desire is also affected by increasing levels of estrogen secretion, especially during the preovulatory period.

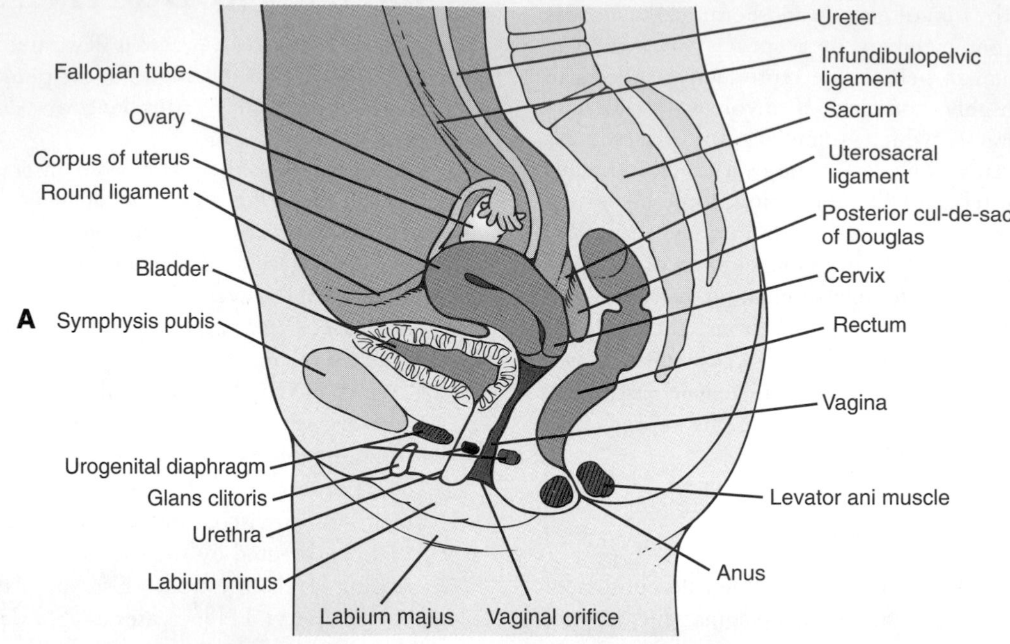

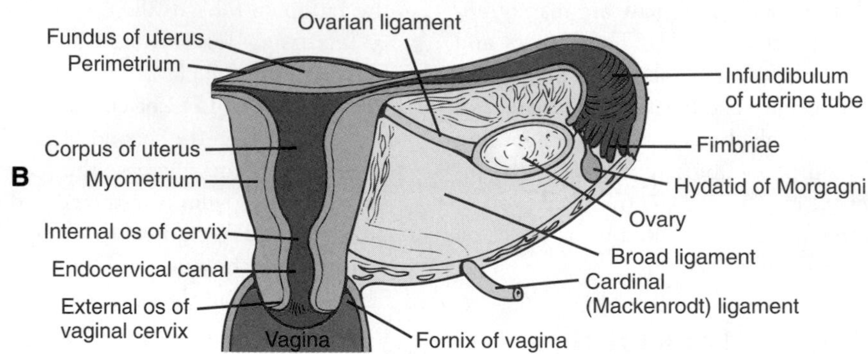

Figure 51-1 A, Female reproductive system. B, Cross section of the uterus, adnexa, and upper vagina. (B modified from Beare, P.G. & Myers, J.L. [1998]. *Adult health nursing* [3rd ed.]. St. Louis: Mosby.)

Local sexual stimulation causes similar responses in both sexes; massage, increasing stimulation, or irritation of the perineal region or sexual organs can result in an enhancement of sexual sensations. In the female, the clitoris is very sensitive, and its stimulation can initiate a sexual sensation. Erectile tissue is located in the introitus (vaginal opening) and clitoris. This tissue is under parasympathetic nerve control; in early stimulation, the parasympathetic nerves dilate the arteries in the erectile tissues. Blood collects in the erectile tissue so that the introitus tightens around the penis; this aids in male satisfaction of sexual stimulation, thus leading to ejaculation.

The parasympathetic nerves also signal the Bartholin's glands situated near the labia minora, which results in increased mucus secretion inside the introitus. This secretion, in addition to mucus from the vaginal epithelium, serves as a lubricant during sexual intercourse.

The female climax, or orgasm, is reached when the local sexual stimulation reaches the maximum sensation or intensity. It is considered similar to emission and ejaculation in the male and may also help to promote fertilization of the ovum. It has been theorized that orgasm produces a rhythm in the female tract from spinal cord reflexes; this rhythm increases both uterine and fallopian tube motility and may result in cervical canal dilation for up to 30 minutes. This allows for easy sperm transport in the female.

The intense sexual sensations that develop during orgasm also result in an increase in muscle tension throughout the body. After the sexual act, this tension subsides into relaxation or feelings of satisfaction, sometimes referred to as resolution.

MALE REPRODUCTIVE SYSTEM

The effects of FSH and LH in the male were described under Pituitary Gonadotropic Hormones. FSH from the anterior pituitary gland stimulates the seminiferous tubules to increase the production of spermatozoa, and LH stimu-

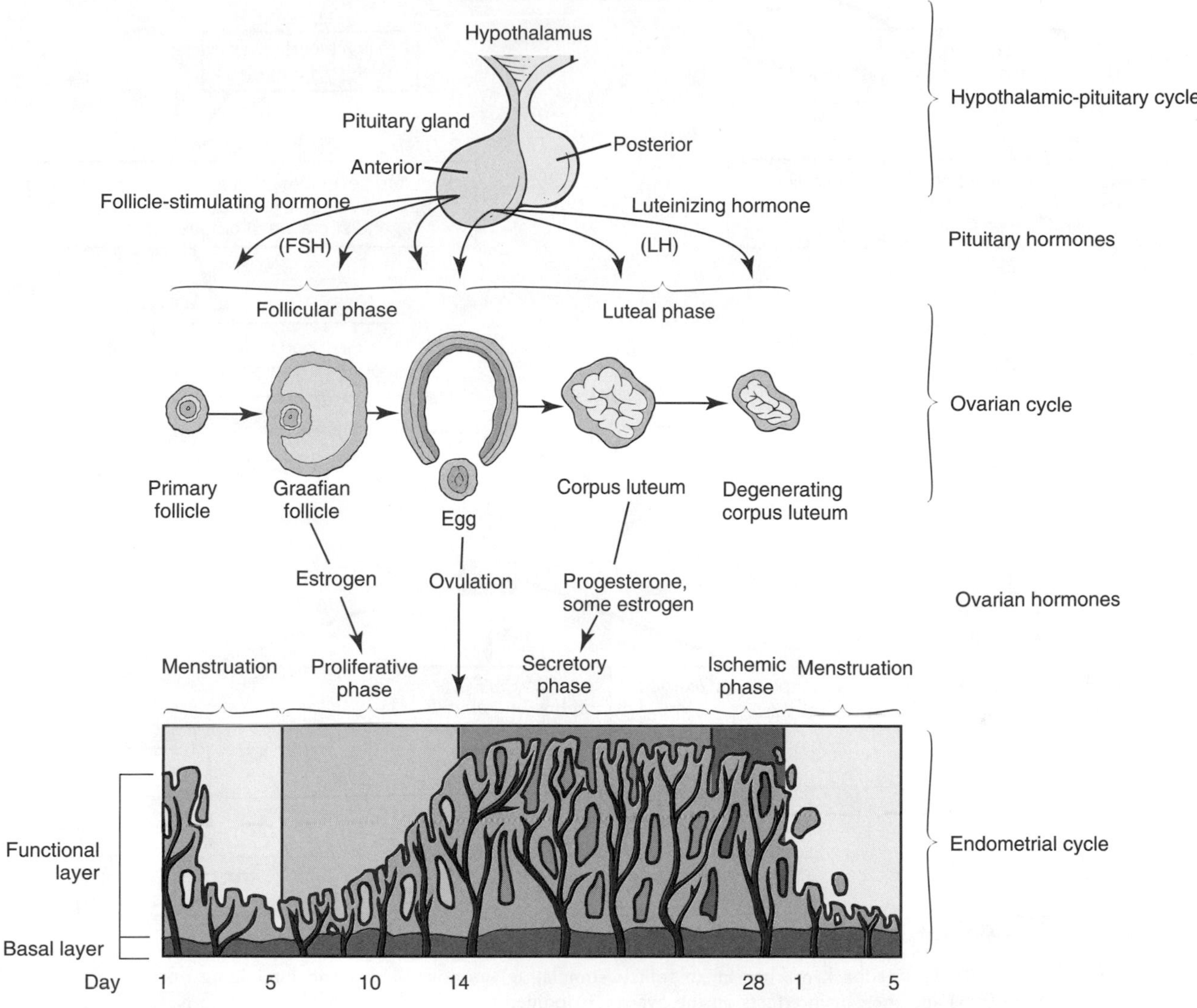

Figure 51-2 The menstrual cycle. (Modified from Lowdermilk, D.L., Perry, S.E., & Bobak, I.M. [1999]. *Maternity nursing* [5th ed.]. St. Louis: Mosby.)

lates the interstitial cells to increase the secretion of testosterone. A high level of testosterone inhibits the release of FSH and LH from the pituitary. Figure 51-4 illustrates the effects of LH on the secretion of testosterone.

Testosterone, an androgen, performs numerous functions in the male. It aids in developing and maintaining the male secondary sex characteristics and male accessory organs (e.g., prostate, seminal vesicles, and bulbourethral glands). Testosterone promotes adult male sexual behavior and regulates metabolism and protein anabolism, which results in the growth of bone and skeletal muscles. This hormone affects fluid and electrolyte metabolism by reabsorbing sodium and water and increasing the excretion of potassium. Testosterone also inhibits the secretion of FSH and LH from the anterior pituitary.

Transport of Sperm in the Male

Sperm is produced in the testes and matures by spending 1 to 3 weeks in the epididymis (ducts that lie around the top of the testes). The sperm, in seminal fluid, then travels through the epididymis to the vas deferens. The vas deferens, a duct extension of the epididymis, extends over the bladder surface (posteriorly) to the ampulla to form the ejaculatory duct. Depending on sexual activity, sperm can be stored in the vas deferens for more than 1 month without losing fertility. Thus a vasectomy, or a severing of the vas deferens, will produce sterility primarily by interrupting the journey of sperm to the ejaculatory duct and urethra. The male reproductive system is illustrated in Figure 51-5.

Male Sexual Response

Penile erection is a parasympathetic response that consists of dilation of the arteries and arterioles in the penis, which compresses the veins in this area. Because more blood is entering than leaving the penis, the penis becomes larger and erection occurs. Emission and ejaculation of the sperm and secretions (semen) is a reflex response. The stimulus that initiated the erection also helps to move the sperm and se-

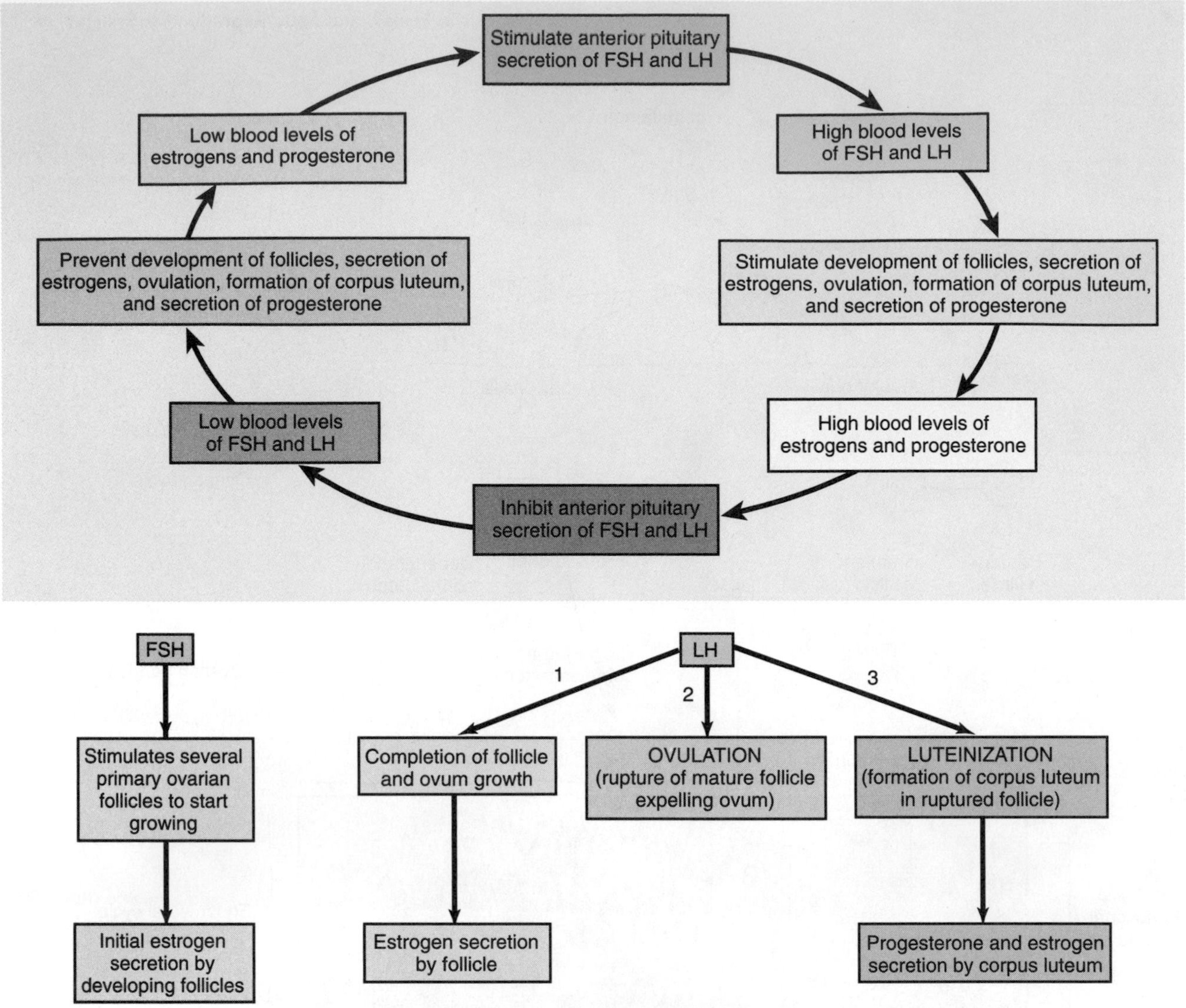

Stimulate anterior pituitary secretion of FSH and LH
High blood levels of FSH and LH
Stimulate development of follicles, secretion of estrogens, ovulation, formation of corpus luteum, and secretion of progesterone
High blood levels of estrogens and progesterone
Inhibit anterior pituitary secretion of FSH and LH
Low blood levels of FSH and LH
Prevent development of follicles, secretion of estrogens, ovulation, formation of corpus luteum, and secretion of progesterone
Low blood levels of estrogens and progesterone
FSH
Stimulates several primary ovarian follicles to start growing
Initial estrogen secretion by developing follicles
LH
1
2
3
Completion of follicle and ovum growth
Estrogen secretion by follicle
OVULATION (rupture of mature follicle expelling ovum)
LUTEINIZATION (formation of corpus luteum in ruptured follicle)
Progesterone and estrogen secretion by corpus luteum

Figure 51-3 Feedback mechanism of follicle-stimulating hormone (FSH) and luteinizing hormone (LH) and their main effects on the ovaries. (Modified from Thibodeau, G.A. & Patton, K.T. [1999]. *Anatomy and physiology* [4th ed.]. St. Louis: Mosby.)

Stimulates anterior pituitary secretion of LH
High blood concentration of LH
Stimulates interstitial cells of testes to secrete testosterone
High blood concentration of testosterone
Inhibits anterior pituitary secretion of LH
Low blood concentration of LH
Inhibits interstitial cell secretion of testosterone
Low blood concentration of testosterone

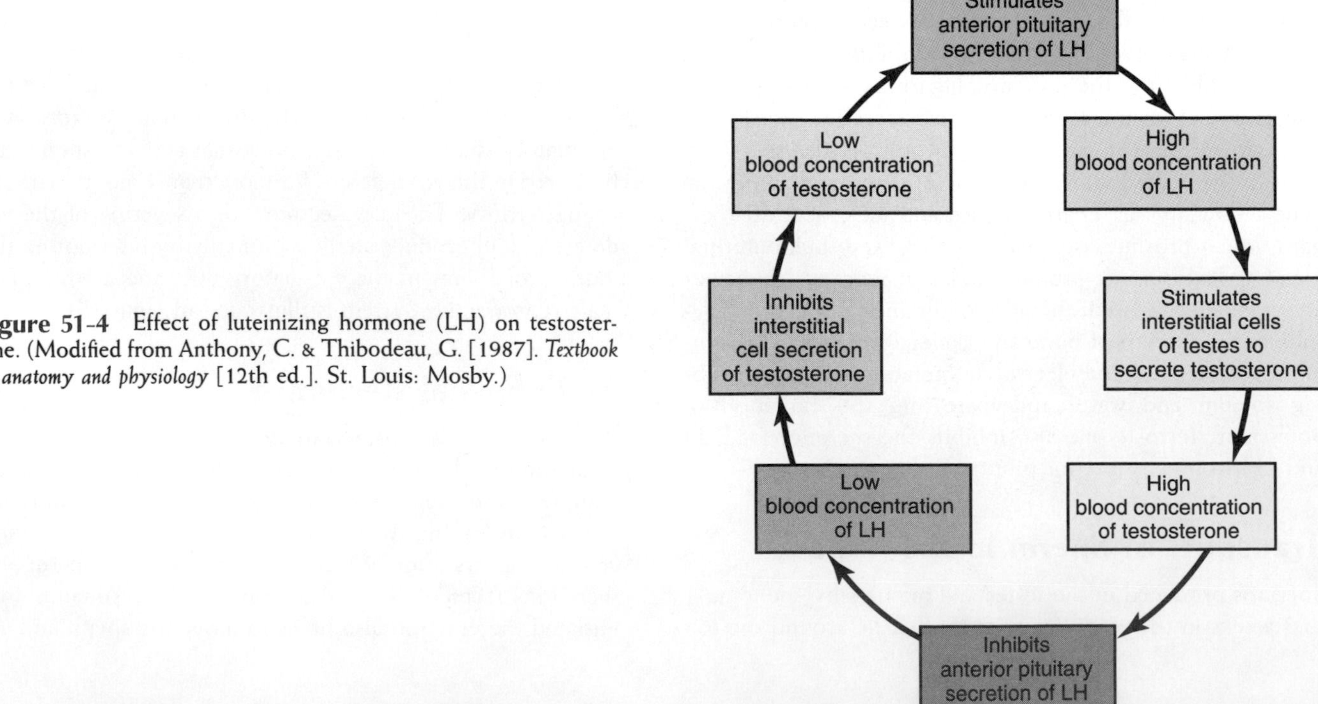

Figure 51-4 Effect of luteinizing hormone (LH) on testosterone. (Modified from Anthony, C. & Thibodeau, G. [1987]. *Textbook of anatomy and physiology* [12th ed.]. St. Louis: Mosby.)

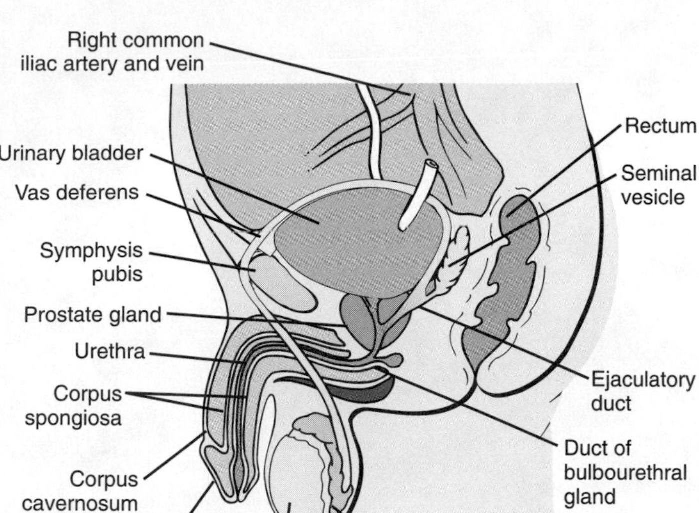

Figure 51-5 Male reproductive system. (Modified from Thibodeau, G.A. & Patton, K.T. [1999]. *Anatomy and physiology* [4th ed.]. St. Louis: Mosby.)

cretions from the genital ducts to the prostatic urethra. Orgasm, the climax of the sexual act, moves the semen through the ejaculatory ducts. Sperm can be transferred from the male to the female during coitus.

■ ■ ■

Gonadal function ceases later in life. Women undergo menopause (the cessation of menses), and men experience a decrease in the production of sex hormones (sometimes called the male climacteric).

SUMMARY

Disorders of the reproductive system of men and women result in acute and chronic physical and emotional stress. The nurse needs to have a sound knowledge of the anatomy and physiology of the reproductive system in order to assess clients for health adaptations and alterations and to assist them with complex health issues in this area.

Critical Thinking Questions

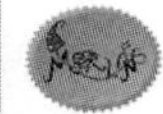

1. If you wanted to develop a birth control pill for men, how would you want that pill to influence the male hormonal system?
2. Because of the positive-feedback mechanism of hormonal influences in the menstrual cycle, what hormonal changes take place if fertilization does not occur?

Collaborative Learning Activities

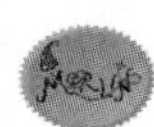

For Collaborative Learning Activities, go to mosby.com/MERLIN/McKenry/.

BIBLIOGRAPHY

Anderson, K.N., Anderson, L.E., & Glanze, W.D. (Eds.) (1998). *Mosby's medical, nursing, & allied health dictionary* (5th ed.). St. Louis: Mosby.

Gray, M. (1992). *Genitourinary disorders.* St. Louis: Mosby.

Guyton, A.C., & Hall, J.E. (2000). *Textbook of medical physiology* (10th ed.). Philadelphia: W.B. Saunders.

Thibodeau, G.A. & Patton, K.T. (1999). *Anatomy and physiology* (4th ed.). St. Louis: Mosby.

Van Wynsberghe, D., Noback, C.R., & Carola, R. (1995). *Human anatomy and physiology* (3rd ed.). New York: McGraw-Hill.

52 Drugs Affecting Women's Health and the Female Reproductive System

Chapter Focus

Drugs that affect the female reproductive system therapeutically are synthetic or natural analogues of homogenous hormones. They are administered to mimic the biologic effects of endogenous hormones, to supplement inadequate production (e.g., menopause), to correct hormonal balance (e.g., dysfunctional bleeding), to reverse an abnormal process (e.g., hirsutism), and for contraception. Whatever the indication, the nurse needs to be knowledgeable about these drugs to support the client's need for intervention and instruction.

Learning Objectives

1. List drugs affecting the female reproductive system.
2. Describe the source and action of chorionic gonadotropin.
3. Discuss the function of the primary female sex hormones.
4. Discuss the side effects/adverse reactions of estrogens and progestins.
5. Compare and contrast monophasic, biphasic, and triphasic oral contraceptives.
6. Implement the nursing management for the care of clients receiving drug therapy affecting the female reproductive system.

Key Terms

Key Drugs [✓]

Synthetic and natural substances that affect the female reproductive system include gonadotropin-releasing hormones, nonpituitary chorionic gonadotropin, menotropins, female sex hormones, oral contraceptives, ovulatory stimulants, and drugs used for infertility.

GONADOTROPIN-RELEASING HORMONE

Five preparations of gonadotropin-releasing hormone (GnRH) are available: leuprolide (Lupron) and goserelin (Zoladex), which are reviewed in Chapter 57; antineoplastic agents; and gonadorelin, nafarelin, and histrelin, which are discussed in this chapter. Ganirelix (Antagon), a GnRH antagonist, is also discussed in this section.

gonadorelin [goe nad oh rell′ in] (Factrel)

Gonadorelin is a synthetic GnRH used as an adjunct to other tests to diagnose hypogonadism in males and females. It is chemically identical to natural GnRH and stimulates the synthesis and release of luteinizing hormone (LH) and, to a lesser extent, follicle-stimulating hormone (FSH) from the anterior pituitary. When diagnosing hypogonadism, multiple dosing may be more valuable than a single-dose test in differentiating between hypothalamic function impairment and pituitary function impairment.

Intravenously, gonadorelin has an initial half-life of 2 to 10 minutes, followed by a terminal half-life of 10 to 40 minutes. It is metabolized rapidly in the body and excreted by the kidneys.

No significant drug interactions are reported with the use of gonadorelin. Adverse reactions include anaphylaxis, pain or inflammation at the injection site, and multiple pregnancies.

For adults and children 12 years of age and older, the dose for diagnosing hypogonadism is 100 μg SC or IV. In females, the drug should be administered in the early follicular phase of the menstrual cycle, preferably within the first week.

■ Nursing Management

Gonadorelin Therapy

■ **Assessment.** Before initiating gonadorelin testing, it should be determined that the client is in good general health and is not allergic to gonadorelin. The client should not have a preexisting GnRH adenoma or any other condition that might be worsened by reproductive hormones.

To determine a baseline serum concentration of LH, two samples of venous blood are drawn 15-20 minutes apart before administering gonadorelin, and the results are averaged. After administering the drug, multiple blood samples are drawn at regular intervals for diagnostic purposes (e.g., 15, 30, 45, 60, and 120 minutes). An ultrasound of the ovaries and a thorough health examination, including a gynecologic examination, are accomplished before drug administration.

■ **Nursing Diagnosis.** Once gonadorelin has been administered, the client should be assessed for the following nursing diagnoses/collaborative problems: impaired comfort (abdominal discomfort, transient flushing, headaches, lightheadedness, nausea); impaired skin integrity related to a generalized skin rash or itching and swelling at the injection site; and the potential complication of sensitization following multiple doses (anaphylaxis).

■ **Implementation**

■ ***Monitoring.*** When used to treat female infertility due to primary hypothalamic hypogonadism, pulsatile dosing may be used using a pump and a catheter, either IV or SC. The injection site should be monitored for symptoms of sepsis and hematoma, and the pump should be monitored for malfunction. The client should receive an ovarian ultrasound on the seventh and fourteenth day of treatment.

■ ***Intervention.*** Placing 8 mL of solution in the plastic reservoir of the pump will supply a pulsatile dose over 1 minute every 90 minutes for 7 consecutive days. Add the diluent supplied by the manufacturer immediately before use. Any unused reconstituted solution being used for diagnosis should be discarded after 24 hours.

■ ***Education.*** Explain the test procedure to the client. Alert the client to the symptoms of hypersensitivity reaction (e.g., hives, wheezing, and dyspnea), and indicate that these are to be reported immediately. For clients using the pumping device, provide an oral and written explanation on the proper use of the pump and proper care of the catheter site. Stress the need for regular visits to the prescriber for the necessary monitoring.

■ **Evaluation.** The expected outcome of gonadorelin therapy in postpubertal males and females and in premenopausal females is that the normal baseline serum LH concentration will be 5 to 25 mIU/mL depending on the laboratory. The test will determine the client's functional capacity and response to gonadotropic hormones without the client experiencing any untoward effects of the procedure. If used for infertility, the client will conceive.

GONADOTROPIN-RELEASING HORMONE AGONIST

nafarelin [naf′ a re lin] (Synarel)

Nafarelin is a potent agonist of GnRH that initially stimulates the release of LH and FSH but results in a decreased secretion of the gonadotropins with continued dosing. The continuous stimulation of the GnRH receptors results in desensitization and ultimately decreased production of LH and FSH. It is indicated for the treatment or management of endometriosis and central precocious puberty (CPP).

This product is administered nasally, with maximum serum levels reported in 10 to 40 minutes. It has a half-life of 3 hours and a maximum effect within 1 month.

There are no recorded significant drug interactions with the use of nafarelin. Side effects/adverse reactions include hot flashes, increased or decreased libido, vaginal dryness, headaches, insomnia, oily skin, acne, edema, hirsutism, hypersensitivity, and paresthesia.

The dosage for endometriosis is one nasal spray of 200 μg in one nostril in the morning and one spray in the other nostril at night. It is usually administered for a period of 6 months. For clients with CPP, the dosage is 2 sprays into each nostril two times daily; this dosage may be increased to a daily dose of 9 sprays (3 sprays into alternating nostrils three times daily) until puberty is desired.

■ Nursing Management

Nafarelin Therapy

■ **Assessment.** It should be determined before therapy that the client is not pregnant, breastfeeding, or experiencing any undiagnosed abnormal vaginal bleeding. Some bone density loss has been demonstrated with the use of this drug. Therefore caution should be used if more than one 6-month course is considered for women who are at high risk for osteoporosis (a strong family history of osteoporosis, chronic alcohol or tobacco use, or chronic use of drugs that can reduce bone mass [anticonvulsants or corticosteroids]). A baseline assessment of the client's endometriosis should be obtained before therapy.

CPP should be confirmed in children who develop secondary sex characteristics at an earlier stage than their cohorts and have significant advanced bone age. This diagnosis is confirmed by measuring serum sex steroids and basal levels of gonadotropins, testing the response to GnRH, assessing diagnostic imaging of the brain (including the pituitary and hypothalamus), and a pelvic ultrasound (in girls). Before initiating a course of therapy for clients with CPP, determine the parents' willingness to comply with dosing and the frequent monitoring by the prescriber, which is necessary for the first 6 to 8 weeks of therapy. Determine the client's sensitivity to nafarelin or any other gonadotropin-releasing agonists or hormones.

■ **Nursing Diagnosis.** The client with endometriosis should be assessed for the development of the following nursing diagnoses/collaborative problems related to adverse reactions to nafarelin: impaired comfort (hot flashes, headaches, eye pain, and galactorrhea); ineffective sexuality patterns related to a libido increase or decrease and vaginal dryness; disturbed sleep pattern (insomnia); fatigue; ineffective coping related to emotional lability or depression; disturbed body image related to acne, weight gain/weight loss, and hirsutism; and the potential complications of osteoporosis, arthralgia, ovarian enlargement or overstimulation, and breakthrough bleeding, menorrhagia, or amenorrhea.

The child being treated for CPP may experience several nursing diagnoses/collaborative problems. Girls may experience a situational low self-esteem related to changes in menstrual patterns, acne, hirsutism, or body odor; and ineffective coping related to emotional lability. Boys may experience a self-esteem disturbance related to the growth of pubic hair, body odor, acne, and dandruff.

All clients receiving nafarelin may experience impaired comfort (nasal irritation from the dosage form) and are at risk for the potential complication of allergic reaction.

■ **Implementation**

■ ***Monitoring.*** The client with endometriosis should be assessed at regular intervals for improvement of the condition. Pregnancy tests are required if therapy does not begin during menstruation or if the client has an irregular menses cycle. A bone density determination is recommended if a second course of therapy is considered.

For clients with CPP, bone linear growth and bone age velocity determinations, imaging studies of the left (or nondominant) hand and wrist, magnetic imaging of the brain, and pelvic sonography (for females) should be performed 3 to 6 after initiating therapy. Blood studies for various hormones are also performed.

Assess all clients receiving nafarelin for discomfort of the nasal passages, dryness, and irritation related to administration of the drug.

■ ***Intervention.*** Treatment is initiated between days 2 and 4 of the menstrual cycle for females. One spray of nafarelin is administered into one nostril in the morning and one spray into the other nostril in the evening.

Dietary calcium and calcium supplements have not been shown to help prevent bone calcium loss associated with the administration of GnRH.

■ ***Education.*** The client should be alerted that menstruation will cease with effective nafarelin therapy; the prescriber needs to be notified if regular menstruation continues. Although nafarelin will usually inhibit ovulation and menstruation, advise the client that it is not a reliable contraceptive and that a nonhormonal or barrier form of contraception should be used. The client should discontinue the drug and notify her prescriber immediately if she suspects she is pregnant.

The client with CPP and his or her parents need to be instructed to notify the prescriber if prepubertal symptoms are not suppressed within 6 to 8 weeks.

After administering the nasal dose, the client should tilt the head backwards for 30 seconds to allow the medication to reach the back of the nose. The client should try to avoid sneezing during or immediately after administration, because drug absorption may be decreased.

The prescriber may also recommend a nasal decongestant if the client develops rhinitis during therapy. The client should be instructed to use the decongestant at least 30 minutes after the nafarelin spray to minimize the possibility of decreasing drug absorption.

■ **Evaluation.** The expected outcome of nafarelin therapy is that the client with endometriosis will experience pain relief and a reduction in endometrial lesions. If administered for CPP, secondary sexual development of breasts in girls and genital enlargement in boys will diminish; in addition, linear bone growth will slow to 5 to 6 cm per year or less, thereby improving the possibility of attaining the predicted adult height.

histrelin [his' tre lin] (Supprelin)

Histrelin is a synthetic GnRH agonist that is more potent than the natural hormone. It controls the secretion of pituitary gonadotropin, which results in a decrease in sex steroid levels and a regression of secondary sexual characteristics in children with CPP. It is used only for clients with CPP—before age 8 in girls and age 9½ in boys. It decreases estradiol levels in females and inhibits testosterone in males. Decreases in LH, FSH, and sex steroid serum levels are noted within 3 months of therapy.

The side effects/adverse reactions of histrelin include vasodilation, vaginal dryness, breast edema and pain, gastric distress, headaches, fever, arthralgia, anxiety, and reactions at the site of injection. Transient vaginal bleeding usually occurs within the first 3 weeks of initial therapy.

The usual dosage for CPP is 10 μg/kg daily SC.

■ Nursing Management

Histrelin Therapy

■ **Assessment.** A thorough physical and endocrinologic evaluation should be performed before initiating histrelin therapy. This includes height and weight, a left (or nondominant) hand and wrist x-ray examination for bone age determination, and a determination of total sex steroid level (estradiol or testosterone) as a baseline for monitoring therapy. A GnRH stimulation test should be performed to establish that the client's pituitary response remains prepubertal. Assess whether the child and his or her parents will be able to maintain a daily regimen of injections.

■ **Nursing Diagnosis.** The child receiving histrelin therapy may experience the following nursing diagnoses/collaborative problems: impaired tissue integrity at the injection site (redness, swelling, itching [45%]); disturbed body image related to vaginal bleeding (usually only one episode after starting histrelin [22%]); impaired comfort (headache [22%], abdominal discomfort [3% to 10%], nausea, vomiting); diarrhea (3% to 10%); and the potential complications of hypersensitivity (2%), vasodilation (35%), and vaginal dryness (12%).

■ **Implementation**

■ ***Monitoring.*** The child is monitored after 3 months and every 6 to 12 months during therapy with height measurements, bone age determinations (yearly), and GnRH testing to ensure that the responsiveness of the pituitary remains prepubertal while undergoing therapy. Document evaluation of the secondary sex characteristics.

■ ***Intervention.*** Histrelin for injection contains no preservative; it is to be kept refrigerated. Inspect the vial for discoloration or particulate matter. Vials are used once, and any unused drug is discarded.

■ ***Education.*** Instruct the client and family in the proper administration of injections and the proper disposal of needles, syringes, and vials. The pubertal process may be reactivated if injections are not given daily. Stress the importance of administering the daily injection at the same time each day and in complying with daily administration. Instruct the client and family on the proper storage of the drug. The solution should come to room temperature before administration. Injection sites should be rotated between the upper arms, abdomen, and thighs.

Alert the client that she may experience a light menstrual flow during the first month of therapy because of the withdrawal of estrogen support from the endometrium. Advise the client that redness, swelling, and itching may occur at the injection site and to report it to the prescriber if the reactions become severe. Instruct the client to stop the drug and seek medical attention immediately if any signs of sensitivity occur.

■ **Evaluation.** The expected outcome of histrelin therapy for girls is that menses ceases, serum estradiol levels are decreased to prepubertal levels, linear growth velocities decrease, skeletal growth is slowed, and adult height predictions increase. In boys, growth is slowed, serum testosterone levels are decreased to prepubertal levels, and testicular volume is decreased.

ganirelix [gan i rel′ ix] (Antagon)

Ganirelix (Antagon) is a GnRH antagonist used to inhibit premature LH increase in women receiving controlled ovarian hyperstimulation. Adverse effects include abdominal pain, headache, vaginal bleeding, and nausea. It may cause fetal death and therefore should not be used during pregnancy. See package insert for additional information.

NONPITUITARY CHORIONIC GONADOTROPIN

Certain gonadotropic substances formed by the placenta during pregnancy are extracted from the urine of pregnant women. The action of human chorionic gonadotropin (HCG) is nearly equivalent to the that of LH in the pituitary, with little or no follicle-stimulating effects. Menotropins are discussed later in this chapter.

chorionic gonadotropin [goe nad′ oh troe pin] (APL, Pregnyl)

Chorionic gonadotropin is administered to make up for a deficiency in LH. Indications are as follows:

- Prepubertal cryptorchidism and hypogonadotropic hypogonadism. The stimulation of androgen production in the testes may enhance the descent of testes and increase the development of the secondary male sex characteristics.
- Treatment of male and female infertility. In females it is combined with other drugs, such as menotropins. Men may receive it alone or in combination.
- Stimulation of multiple oocytes in ovulatory women (used in conjunction with other procedures).

Administered intramuscularly, this drug has a half-life between 11 and 23 hours, and ovulation usually occurs within 32 to 36 hours of administration. It is excreted by the kidneys within 24 hours.

Chorionic gonadotropin has no significant drug interactions. The side effects/adverse reactions include headaches, anxiety, depression, breast enlargement, weakness, abdominal bloating/pain, increased incidence of multiple births, and possible arterial thromboembolism.

The adult dosage for male hypogonadotropic hypogonadism is 1000 to 4000 U IM two to three times weekly for several weeks or months (in some cases, indefinitely). For the induction of ovulation, 5000 to 10,000 U IM is administered after the last dose of menotropins or from 5 to 9 days after the last dose of clomiphene.

For children with prepubertal cryptorchidism, the dosage is 1000 to 5000 U IM two or three times weekly for a maximum of 10 doses; the therapy is discontinued when the desired response is achieved.

■ Nursing Management

Chorionic Gonadotropin Therapy

■ **Assessment.** It should be determined whether the client has a preexisting pituitary hypertrophy or tumor, because the medication will stimulate growth of the tumor. Chorionic gonadotropin should not be used for clients with precocious puberty, prostatic cancer, abnormal vaginal bleeding, fibroids, ovarian cysts, or active thrombophlebitis. In female clients an ultrasound examination is recommended before therapy to determine a baseline assessment of the ovaries. Baseline serum testosterone levels are determined for male clients.

Because of the potential for fluid volume excess due to fluid retention, this drug should be used with careful monitoring in clients with asthma, cardiac disease, epilepsy, migraine headaches, or renal dysfunction.

■ **Nursing Diagnosis.** The following nursing diagnoses may occur in clients receiving chorionic gonadotropin: impaired comfort (nausea, abdominal discomfort and distention, headache, or pain at the injection site); disturbed body image related to physical changes in the secondary sexual characteristics of young male clients, such as precocious puberty (rapid height increase, acne, growth of pubic hair, enlargement of penis or testes); excess fluid volume as evidenced by oliguria, rapid weight gain, shortness of breath, swelling of the feet and lower legs; and diarrhea. The potential complications of mental depression, ovarian cysts, or ovarian hyperstimulation syndrome (OHS) may also occur.

■ **Implementation**

■ ***Monitoring.*** The client's progress should be assessed periodically. Because the regimen is lengthy and time-consuming, the client should continue to be supported and encouraged to cooperate over the course of therapy.

Estradiol serum determinations should be performed to monitor the female client receiving chorionic gonadotropin for induction of ovulation. Hyperstimulation of the ovaries may be indicated by abdominal or pelvic pain and should be reported to the prescriber immediately. A pelvic examination and/or ultrasound examination may be performed to evaluate ovarian size and minimize the risk of OHS.

To monitor the male client receiving chorionic gonadotropin therapy for hypogonadism, inspect the genitalia for signs of puberty. Serum testosterone may be measured periodically to assess progress. If the drug is administered for male infertility, testosterone levels, sperm counts, and determinations of sperm mobility should also be performed.

■ ***Intervention.*** Reconstitute this drug with the diluent provided by the manufacturer.

■ ***Education.*** When used to treat infertility, provide support for the client and partner throughout their attempt to achieve fertility. Societal and familial pressures create stress for them both as a couple and individually. They should be advised that gonadotropin-induced ovulation is expensive and may result in multiple births. Because success is difficult to achieve, the couple should be counseled on alternatives such as adoption.

If the prescriber has requested a daily record of the woman's temperature, inform the client about the relationship of temperature to ovulation and its importance for the appropriate timing of intercourse to enhance the chance of pregnancy. Daily or every-other-day intercourse or insemination should be attempted beginning the day after chorionic gonadotropin is given until ovulation is thought to have occurred. Therapy should be reconsidered after three cycles of nonovulatory menses.

In treating prepubertal cryptorchidism, prepubertal males receiving chorionic gonadotropin should be prepared for an acceleration in sexual development and supported through self-image changes.

■ **Evaluation.** The expected outcomes of chorionic gonadotropin therapy for prepubertal cryptorchidism and hypogonadotropic hypogonadism is that the male experiences a descent of the testes into the scrotum and the normal development of secondary male sex characteristics. If administered for infertility, conception occurs.

MENOTROPINS

Menotropins is a human pituitary gonadotropin; it is a purified preparation of FSH and LH obtained from the urine of postmenopausal women. It is sometimes called human menopausal gonadotropins (HMG).

menotropins [men oh troe' pins] (Pergonal)

The mechanism of action of menotropins is equivalent to the effects produced by FSH and LH; menotropins stimulates the development of the ovarian follicle, causes ovulation, and may stimulate the development of the corpus luteum. It stimulates sperm production in males.

Menotropins is indicated for the treatment of the following conditions:

- It is administered in combination with chorionic gonadotropin for female infertility caused by ovulatory dysfunction. It is considered the treatment of choice for clients with hypothalamic hypogonadism or for those who did not respond to clomiphene.
- It is used in combination with chorionic gonadotropin for male infertility to stimulate spermatogenesis in primary or secondary hypogonadotropic hypogonadism (male infertility).
- It is used in combination with chorionic gonadotropin to stimulate multiple oocyte development in ovulatory clients who are using other technologies to conceive (e.g., gamete intrafallopian transfer or in vitro fertilization).

Menotropins are administered intramuscularly, and they are excreted by the kidneys.

There are no reported significant drug interactions. The side effects/adverse reactions of menotropins include gastric distress, severe pelvic pain, weight gain, edema, shortness of breath, decreased urine output, abdominal bloating or pain (usually in females), and breast enlargement and erythrocytosis in males.

The adult dosage of menotropins for the induction of ovulation is 1 ampule (75 units of FSH and LH activity) IM daily for one week or more; this is followed by 5000 to 10,000 U of chorionic gonadotropin 1 day after the last dose of menotropins. If necessary, the ampule dose may be increased every 4 to 5 days, up to a maximum of 6 ampules. For the treatment of male infertility, 1 ampule is administered intramuscularly three times weekly (in addition to chorionic gonadotropin twice weekly) for a minimum of 4 months after pretreatment with chorionic gonadotropin for 4 to 6 months.

The nursing management for menotropins is similar to that for chorionic gonadotropin, except that this preparation is reconstituted with 1 to 2 mL of sodium chloride injection USP.

FEMALE SEX HORMONES

In addition to providing ova, the ovaries manufacture and secrete female hormones that control secondary sex characteristics, the reproductive cycle, and the growth and development of the accessory reproductive organs in the female. Two main types of hormones are secreted by the ovary: (1) the follicular or estrogenic hormones **(estrogens)** produced by the cells of the developing graafian follicle, and (2) the luteal or progestational hormones **(progestogens)** derived from the corpus luteum that is formed in the ovary from the ruptured follicle. The periodic cycling of the female sex hormones depends on an interaction between FSH and LH and the ovarian hormones, estrogen and progesterone. This results in a menstrual cycle that normally continues throughout life until menopause (except during pregnancy). Estrogens are primarily secreted by the ovarian follicles, but some may also be secreted by the adrenals, corpus luteum, placenta, and testes.

Estrogens

Estrogens are available from natural sources (the urine of pregnant mares) in conjugated dosage forms and from synthetic formulations. Examples of natural steroidal estrogens include estradiol, estrone, and esterified estrogens; nonsteroidal estrogens include diethylstilbestrol (DES), dienestrol, and chlorotrianisene.

estrogen [ess' troe jen] (various manufacturers)

Estrogen increases the synthesis of DNA, RNA, and protein in estrogen-responsive tissues. Elevated estrogen serum levels inhibit the secretion of FSH and LH from the pituitary, which results in the inhibition of lactation and ovulation, as well as the development of a proliferative endometrium. Estrogen is indicated for the following conditions:

- Treatment of estrogen deficiency, atrophic vaginitis, female hypogonadism, insufficient primary ovarian function, abnormal uterine bleeding, severe vasomotor symptoms in menopause, and postmenopausal osteoporosis (McNagny, 1999)
- Treatment of selected metastatic breast carcinomas in postmenopausal women with tumor estrogen-negative receptors
- Treatment of selected male breast carcinomas and treatment of advanced prostatic carcinomas

The use of estrogen therapy in postmenopausal women has resulted in reports of a significant decrease in the risk of heart disease (Pharmacy Practice News, 1995), including a reduction in the death rate in women with coronary artery disease (Shoupe, 1999). Mosca et al. (1998) reported on an analysis of published studies in the United States indicating that the use of postmenopausal estrogen reduces the incidence of coronary heart disease by 35% to 50%. Several studies also indicated an increase in life expectancy secondary to postmenopausal estrogen use. Other studies reported a decrease in many diseases except breast cancer and venous thromboembolism (Mosca et al., 1998). Skin aging (Pierard-Franchimont et al., 1999) and lower urinary tract symptoms (Battaglia et al., 1999) have also responded positively to hormone replacement. Investigational studies are ongoing to help identify the unknown selection factors necessary to help determine who can take estrogen safely (Zeitoun & Carr, 1999). Until this is determined, prescribers weigh the risk-benefit ratio before prescribing estrogens during menopause. The nurse should be aware that the estrogen dose for postmenopausal hormone replacement is considerably less than the dose used in oral contraceptives (Williams & Stancel, 1996).

Estrogen is protein bound, metabolized in the liver, and excreted by the kidneys.

The side effects/adverse reactions of estrogen include stomach cramps or gas, anorexia, chloasma, headaches, nausea, vomiting, change in female libido, decrease in male sex drive, edema of the lower extremities, breast pain and enlargement, and changes in menstrual bleeding.

Precautions

1. The risk of endometrial cancer increases with prolonged use of estrogens in postmenopausal women. However, low-dose estrogen given cyclically or the use of a progestin (concurrently or sequentially) may reduce the risk of inducing endometrial cancer (Persson, Weiderpass, Bergkvist, Bergstrom, & Schairer, 1999; Weiderpass et al., 1999).
2. Estrogens, especially DES, should not be administered during pregnancy because there is an increased risk of congenital malformations (FDA category X). (See the Pregnancy Safety box on p. 897.)
3. Estrogens are excreted in breast milk and also inhibit lactation; therefore the administration of estrogens to nursing women is not recommended.

Dosage and Administration

1. The lowest effective dosage of estrogens should be administered for the shortest time period to reduce the possibility of serious adverse effects. When continuous therapy is required, the prescriber should reevaluate the client at least annually.
2. A cyclic dosing schedule of 3 weeks of estrogen administration and 1 week off or the addition of a progestin for the last 10 to 13 days of the cycle most closely approximates the natural hormonal cycle and prevents overstimulation of estrogen-sensitive tissues. This is not the schedule for clients who have had an oophorectomy or for clients who have cancer and are receiving hormonal therapy.
3. Estradiol and estrone are naturally occurring steroidal estrogens that are principal endogenous estrogens. Estradiol is available alone or synthetically as estradiol cypionate, estradiol valerate, ethinyl estradiol, and polyestradiol phosphate. The primary pharmacologic effects of all estrogens are similar.
4. Conjugated estrogens (Premarin ◆), a mixture of estrogenic substances (especially estrone and equilin), are available in oral, parenteral, and vaginal cream dosage forms. The dosage must be individualized according to diagnosis and therapeutic response (e.g., vasomotor symptoms associated with menopause). The usual oral adult dosage for esterified estrogens is 0.3 to 1.25 mg daily, either cyclically or continuously.  Some women may require higher dosages. Prempro ◆, a combination of conjugated estrogen and medroxyprogesterone, is indicated for the treatment of menopausal symptoms and vulval/vaginal atrophy.
5. DES is a synthetic nonsteroidal estrogen primarily used as an antineoplastic agent.
6. Transdermal estradiol (Estraderm) is as effective for women with estrogen deficiency as oral hormone replacement therapy (Mattsson et al., 1999). Applied topically to intact skin, the reservoir-type patch is available in 25 (Canada only), 50 (United States and Canada), and 100 μg (United States and Canada) and is replaced twice weekly. The matrix-type estradiol (Fem Patch, Climara) is available in 25, 50, or 100 μg for once-weekly dosing; the twice-weekly transdermal system (Vivelle, Alora) is available in 37.5, 50, 75, or 100 μg. The strengths listed are released daily from the transdermal patch. The patch should be replaced according to schedule. Usually no patch is worn on the fourth week, although continuous application may be appropriate for some clients.

■ Nursing Management

Estrogen Therapy

■ Assessment. Estrogen therapy is contraindicated if breast cancer is known or suspected, because there is the possible promotion of tumor growth. It is also contraindicated if the client has abnormal or undiagnosed vaginal bleeding; such bleeding may indicate endometrial hyperplasia or carcinoma, which would be promoted by estrogen use.

Estrogens are to be used with caution in clients who have hypercalcemia associated with metastatic breast disease, endometriosis, uterine fibroids, active thrombophlebitis, or a history of thrombophlebitis secondary to estrogen use; these conditions may be aggravated by estrogen use. In males for whom estrogens may be administered for the treatment of prostatic or breast cancer, there is an increased risk for myocardial infarction, pulmonary embolism, and thrombophlebitis; therefore care should be exercised in clients with a past or active history of these conditions.

Depending on the individual health status of the client, some of the following assessments are performed as a baseline before therapy: a physical examination that includes blood pressure, a serum lipid profile, and hepatic function determinations. In addition, a Papanicolaou (Pap) smear, breast examination, and mammogram are required for female clients; if appropriate, an endometrial biopsy is performed to rule out malignancy.

Review the client's current medication regimen for the risk of significant drug interactions, such as those that may occur when estrogens are given concurrently with the following drugs:

Drug	Possible Effect and Management
Bold/color type indicates the most serious interactions.	
bromocriptine (Parlodel)	Concurrent use may result in amenorrhea and may also interfere with the therapeutic effect of bromocriptine. Monitor closely, because a dosage adjustment may be required.
cyclosporine (Sandimmune)	Metabolism is inhibited, which may result in increased cyclosporine plasma levels and an increased risk of hepatotoxicity and nephrotoxicity. Use concurrently only with very close monitoring of cyclosporine serum levels and liver and kidney function.
hepatotoxic drugs, especially dantrolene	**Estrogens increase the risk of inducing hepatotoxicity, with women over 35 years of age at increased risk. Avoid concurrent use or a potentially serious drug interaction may occur.**
protease inhibitors, such as ritonavir (Norvir)	Decreases plasma levels of estrogens. Dosage adjustments may be necessary.
smoking tobacco	**Tobacco smoking increases the risk of serious cardiac adverse reactions, such as cerebrovascular accident (CVA), transient ischemic attacks (TIAs), thrombophlebitis, and pulmonary embolism. The risk is higher in women over 35 years of age who smoke. Avoid concurrent use or a potentially serious drug interaction may occur.**

■ Nursing Diagnosis. Clients receiving estrogen therapy may experience the following nursing diagnoses/collaborative problems: impaired comfort related to anorexia, nausea, vomiting, abdominal cramping, breast tenderness, headaches, or skin irritation (transdermal patches); impaired skin integrity related to the development of acne; disturbed sensory perception (vision) related to a steepening of the corneal curvature and contributing to an intolerance of contact lenses; excess fluid volume (peripheral edema, sudden weight gain); disturbed body image related to chloasma (brown, blotchy skin changes), gynecomastia (men), change in libido (women), or decreased libido (men); and the potential complications of hepatitis, hypercalcemia, chorea, irregular menses, breast tumors and, in men only, thrombophlebitis and thromboembolism.

■ **Implementation**

■ ***Monitoring.*** Blood pressure should be monitored periodically. Hepatic function studies should be performed every 6 to 12 months for clients with hepatic dysfunction. Males treated with estrogens should be checked regularly for the development of breast carcinomas. At least annually, females should undergo a physical examination that includes a Pap smear, mammogram, and serum lipid profile.

Bone age determinations are recommended every 6 months for children and adolescents.

■ ***Intervention.*** Estrogens are usually administered on a cycle of 3 weeks on and 1 week off, except in males, who take them continuously. Administer the IM forms slowly to minimize client discomfort. Large muscles, such as the gluteus maximus, should be used for injection to maximize absorption. For oil-based preparations, use at least a 21-gauge needle and a dry syringe.

Administer IV estrogens slowly; vaginal burning occurs if they are administered too rapidly.

Vaginal forms should be administered at bedtime to enhance absorption. Sanitary napkins or panty shields may be used to protect clothing from stains.

Clients who have been taking oral estrogens should wait a week after the last oral dose to start transdermal dosage forms.

■ ***Education.*** Assist the client in exploring concerns about the risks of taking estrogens. Provide the client with information regarding the occurrence of cardiovascular disease and cancer in relationship to age, smoking habits, and other health characteristics. Encourage the client to read the package insert carefully and then discuss any concerns. Advise the client to have regular physical examinations every 6 to 12 months during treatment, which for females should include a pelvic and breast examination, mammogram, and a Pap smear. Instructions should be provided for monthly self-examination of the breasts; any lumps found should be reported to the prescriber. The female client should be advised to stop the medication immediately and contact her prescriber if she suspects she is pregnant.

Caution the client that smoking increases the incidence of serious side effects, particularly in women over 35. Instruct the client to notify the health provider in the instance of severe headache, blurred or lost vision (which may signal possible stroke), or symptoms of chest pain, shortness of breath, or leg pain (which may indicate thromboembolism elsewhere in the body). The prescriber should also be informed of a severe abdominal pain or mass, jaundice, severe mental depression, or unusual bleeding.

Nausea often occurs at the beginning of therapy and usually ceases after 1 or 2 weeks. It is seldom severe and can be controlled by taking the medication with meals.

Advise the client to weigh one or two times weekly and to report a sharp increase in weight or other signs of fluid retention, such as swollen ankles, puffy eyelids, and "tight" rings. A low-sodium diet and diuretic may be prescribed to control these symptoms.

Encourage the client to maintain a program of good oral hygiene, including teeth cleaning by a professional and thorough brushing and plaque control by the client to minimize any gingival hyperplasia that may occur during estrogen therapy. Warn the client that exposure to the sun or tanning devices may result in a brown, blotchy discoloration of the skin. Bleeding after estrogen withdrawal is expected. Explain to postmenopausal women that such bleeding does not indicate that a state of fertility has returned.

Instruct clients with diabetes to report positive blood sugar tests so the dosage of their antidiabetic medications can be adjusted.

Forewarn male clients of estrogen-induced feminization and impotence, which will disappear when therapy terminates. Advise male clients of the increased risk of myocardial infarction, pulmonary embolism, and thrombophlebitis while undergoing estrogen therapy.

Instruct clients taking prescribed conjugated estrogens and esterified estrogens for osteoporosis prophylaxis to increase their intake of calcium and vitamin D and to engage in regular weight-bearing exercise such as walking (Watts, 1999).

When applying the transdermal form of the drug, the client should wash his or her hands before and after applying the patch. The system should be applied immediately after removing the pouch and its protective liner. It should be applied to the abdomen on clean, dry, intact skin without hair. The sites on the abdomen should be rotated to prevent application to any site more frequently than every 7 days. The patch should not be applied to the breasts or to the waistline, where clothing might cause the patch to become loose. The patch should be pressed into place for 10 seconds and then examined to ensure that all the edges are tight. The patch may be reapplied if it becomes loose, or a new one may be applied.

Clients using the estradiol vaginal insert should be instructed in the proper technique for insertion and removal.

■ **Evaluation.** The expected outcome of estrogen therapy is that the client will demonstrate an improvement in the underlying condition for which the drug was prescribed without experiencing any adverse reactions related to drug therapy.

Progesterone and Progestins

Progesterone produced by the ovaries is a naturally occurring progestin. The anterior pituitary LH stimulates the synthesis and secretion of progesterone from the corpus luteum, mainly during the latter half of the menstrual cycle. Progesterone may also be formed from steroid precursors available in the ovaries, testes, adrenal cortex, and placenta.

Progesterone and synthetic progestins have similar pharmacologic effects in the body. Progestins were developed because progesterone was not always therapeutically satisfactory. The following are advantages of progestins: (1) greater potency, which lowers the dosage necessary to produce an equivalent response to progesterone; (2) a longer duration of action; and (3) the availability of some products in an effective oral/sublingual dosage form.

progesterone [proe jess' ter one]
progestin [proe jess' tin] (various manufacturers)

Progesterone and progestins (hydroxyprogesterone, norethindrone, and others) produce biochemical changes in the endometrium to prepare for the implantation and nourishment of the embryo. They also perform the following functions: (1) supplement the action of estrogen in its effects on the uterus and mammary glands, (2) suppress ovulation during pregnancy, (3) cause relaxation of the uterine smooth muscles, (4) increase the synthesis of DNA and RNA, and (5) inhibit, in large doses, the secretion of LH from the anterior pituitary.

Progesterone/progestins are indicated for the treatment of female hormonal imbalance of amenorrhea, dysmenorrhea, endometriosis, and specific carcinomas. They are combined with estrogen to lower the risk of breast and endometrial cancer with hormone replacement therapy (Perrson et al., 1999). However, it is reported that the combination may diminish the cardiovascular benefits of estrogen hormone replacement therapy (Herrington, 1999). Progesterone/progestins are also used to diagnose endogenous estrogen deficiency and to prevent pregnancy (Box 52-1).

Progesterone/progestins are metabolized primarily in the liver and excreted by the kidneys.

Side effects/adverse reactions include weight gain, stomach pain/cramps, swelling of the face and lower extremities, headache, mood alterations, anxiety, increased weakness, amenorrhea, breakthrough bleeding, hyperglycemia, menorrhagia, galactorrhea, rash, acne, insomnia, and breast pain.

Dosage and Administration. Because the dosage and method of administration for progestins can vary according to indications and current standards of practice, the student is referred to a current package insert or *United States Pharmacopeia Dispensing Information (USP DI)* for the most recent recommendations. The following are examples of selected progestins and dosing regimens.

Hydroxyprogesterone [hye drox ee proe jess' ter one] (Hylutin and others). Indicated for amenorrhea, and dysfunctional bleeding of the uterus. The dosage is 375 mg IM as a single dose.

Megestrol [me jess' trole] (Megace). For breast cancer, the dosage is 40 mg PO four times daily or 160 mg as a single dose; to treat endometrial cancer, the dosage is 40 to 320 mg daily in divided doses. Allow 2 months of therapy with megestrol before evaluating its effectiveness.

Norethindrone [nor eth in' drone] (Micronor, Norlutate ✱). The dosage for contraception is 0.35 mg/day; for amenorrhea or dysfunctional uterine bleeding, the dosage is 2.5 to 10 mg PO from day 5 through day 25 of the menstrual cycle. For endometriosis, the dosage is 5 mg initially, which is increased by 2.5 mg daily at 2-week intervals until 15 mg/day is reached. This dosage is continued for 6 to 9 months.

Progesterone [proe jess' ter one] (Gesterol and others). When used to treat amenorrhea caused by female hormone imbalance, the dosage is 5 to 10 mg IM daily for 6 to 10 days. Bleeding will usually occur within 2 to 3 days after the last injection; normal menstrual cycles may then follow. Discontinue injections if menstrual bleeding occurs during the series of injections.

BOX 52-1

Abortion Drugs

Carboprost tromethamine (Hemabate) and dinoprostone or prostaglandin E_2 (Prepidil, Cervidil, Prostin E_2) are abortifacient prostaglandins used to induce abortion. Carboprost is used between 13 and 20 weeks of gestation, which is calculated from the first day of the last normal menstruation. It is an injectable for IM use only. The initial dose is 250 μg, followed by the same dose every 1.5 to 3.5 hours depending on the client's response.

Dinoprostone is used between 12 and 20 weeks of gestation, which again is calculated from the first day of the last normal menstruation. It is available as a 20-mg suppository (Prostin E_2), a gel (Prepidil), and a vaginal insert (Cervidil). These agents are inserted in the vagina following the specific instructions available in the package insert or *Drug Facts and Comparisons* (2000).

Abortifacient side effects/adverse reactions include leg cramps, fever, eye pain, rash, blurred vision, cardiac dysrhythmias, flushing nausea, vomiting, diarrhea and, possibly, uterine rupture.

■ Nursing Management

Progesterone/Progestin Therapy

■ **Assessment.** It should be determined that the client does not have preexisting cancer of the breast or reproductive tract, suspected pregnancy, incomplete abortion, abnormal and undiagnosed vaginal bleeding, a history of or active thrombophlebitis or thromboembolic disorder, hepatic dysfunction, or conditions for which progestins are contraindicated. Because of the tendency of progestins to cause fluid retention that might aggravate these conditions, these drugs should be used cautiously in clients with asthma, migraine headaches, epilepsy, cardiac insufficiency, or renal dysfunction. Hepatic disease may worsen, and/or the metabolism of

Pregnancy Safety
Drugs Affecting Women's Health/Female Reproductive System

Category	Drug
B	gonadorelin
C	chorionic gonadotropin, clomiphene
D	hydroxyprogesterone, progesterone
X	estrogens, ganirelix, histrelin, levonorgestrel, megestrol suspension, menotropins, nafarelin, norethindrone, norgestrel, oral contraceptives, urofollitropin

some progestins may be impaired. Clients with a history of ectopic pregnancy or diabetes should also be monitored carefully for any unusual symptoms. Because some progestins elevate levels of low-density lipoproteins (LDLs), hyperlipidemia may be aggravated. Mental depression may worsen. Determination of the client's sensitivity to progestins and to peanuts (for oral or parenteral progesterone) should be determined.

Congenital anomalies have been reported with the use of progestins during the first 4 months of pregnancy. They should not be used as diagnostic tests for pregnancy (see the Pregnancy Safety box above). Progestins are also excreted in breast milk and therefore are not recommended for use by nursing women.

When progestins are given concurrently with aminoglutethimide (Cytadren), the absorption of oral medroxyprogesterone may be decreased, and serum concentrations are significantly lowered. Hepatic enzyme-inducing drugs, such as carbamazepine (Tegretol), phenobarbital (Barbita), phenytoin (Dilantin), rifabutin (Mycobutin), or rifampin (Rifadin) may cause decreased serum concentrations of progestins; dosage adjustments may be necessary.

■ **Nursing Diagnosis.** Clients undergoing progesterone/progestin therapy are at risk for the following nursing diagnoses/collaborative problems: impaired comfort (headache, nausea, breast tenderness, hot flashes, or irritation at the injection site); excess fluid volume (peripheral edema, weight gain); disturbed sleep pattern (insomnia); fatigue; disturbed body image related to increased facial and body hair, loss of scalp hair, weight gain, or chloasma; impaired skin integrity (acne); disturbed sensory perception related to neuroocular lesions (double vision or loss of vision); and the potential complications of changed vaginal bleeding pattern, mental depression, hepatitis, ovarian enlargement or ovarian cyst formation and, in high-dose therapy for noncontraceptive uses, thrombophlebitis, retinal thrombosis, or thromboembolism.

■ **Implementation**

■ ***Monitoring.*** Undesirable effects are usually mild or absent during short-term use. However, the number and severity of adverse reactions increase as the duration of progestin therapy increases. An evaluation for these effects must continue as long as therapy continues. A physical examination at least every 6 to 12 months should include a breast and pelvic examination, Pap smear, and hepatic function studies.

■ ***Intervention.*** Give oil preparations by deep IM injection. A low-sodium diet and diuretic may be prescribed to control symptoms of fluid retention, such as swollen ankles and puffy eyelids.

■ ***Education.*** Regulations require that a package insert be given to every client who is dispensed a progestin unless the drug is being used as an antineoplastic adjunct. Encourage the client to read the package insert carefully and then discuss with the health care provider any concerns. Advise the client to have regular physical examinations as described previously.

Instruct the client to notify the prescriber in the instance of severe headache, blurred or lost vision (which may possibly signal stroke), and symptoms of chest pain, shortness of breath, or leg pain (which may indicate thromboembolism elsewhere in the body). The prescriber should also be informed of severe abdominal pain or mass, jaundice, severe mental depression, or unusual bleeding. Changes in vaginal bleeding may include irregular cycle time, spotting, breakthrough bleeding, or a complete lack of bleeding.

Instruction should be provided for monthly self-examination of the breasts; and any new lumps should be reported.

Because progestins may cause glucose intolerance, instruct users with diabetes to report positive glucose tests so that an adjustment in their insulin or oral hypoglycemic dosage may be prescribed.

If progestins are used for contraceptive purposes, instruct the client to take the drug at the same time of day, every day of the year. The tablets need to be kept in their original containers. It is best to keep an extra month's supply, replacing it with the new container of tablets purchased each month. This will always ensure a fresh supply.

The client should be advised to discontinue the medication immediately and notify the prescriber if she suspects she is pregnant. Pregnancy should be avoided during the first month of progestin administration and for at least 3 months after they are discontinued. Barrier contraceptives should be used during this time.

■ **Evaluation.** The expected outcome is that the client will demonstrate an improvement in the underlying condition for which the drug was prescribed without experiencing untoward effects. If the drug is taken for contraception, pregnancy will not occur.

ORAL CONTRACEPTIVES

The most effective form of birth control presently available is **oral contraception.** Millions of women have used oral contraceptives, and through experience an enormous amount of information about effectiveness, estrogen-progestin combination, and the relationship of risk factors to major side effects and mortality has been collected. The newer, low-dose oral contraceptives have (1) a lower risk for adverse cardiovascular effects; (2) an increased risk for a myocardial infarction, especially in smokers and women over 35 years of age; (c) a lower risk for stroke or thromboembolic disease than with the older oral contraceptives, although there is still a higher risk than with nonusers; (d) a decreased rate for ectopic pregnancies; (e) a decreased risk for ovarian cysts, epithelial ovarian cancer, and endometrial cancer; (f) an increased risk for cervical cancer, liver cancer, and possibly earlier onset of breast cancer after long-term use (Kenyon, 1995) (see the Nursing Research box on p. 899).

Performing a thorough history and physical examination, selecting an appropriate contraceptive method with the individual/couple, and instituting a client teaching and monitoring program are basic for the development of a good family planning program.

estrogens and progestins (oral contraceptives) (various manufacturers)

The combination oral contraceptives inhibit ovulation by increasing serum levels of estrogens and progestins that in turn inhibit the secretion of FSH and LH from the pituitary. In addition, changes in the endometrium impair ova implantation, and an increase in cervical mucus impedes the passage of sperm.

Estrogens and progestins are indicated for the prevention of pregnancy and for the treatment of hypermenorrhea. The oral contraceptives are protein bound, metabolized mainly in the liver, and excreted primarily by the kidneys.

Side Effects/Adverse Reactions. Hormone-related side effects are caused by an excess or a deficiency in estrogen or progestin or by an excess of androgen. Androgen effects are more common with norgestrel and levonorgestrel than with the other progestins. Reporting side effects to the prescriber is useful because it allows for the choice of a more appropriate oral contraceptive for the individual.

Excesses and deficiencies of estrogen and progestins produce a variety of symptoms. The side effects of an estrogen excess include nausea, dizziness, abdominal bloating, leg pain, chloasma, hypertension, cyclic weight gain, hypertension, breast tenderness, and an increase in breast size. A deficiency in estrogen may produce an increase in anxiety, hot flashes, midcycle spotting, a decrease in menstrual flow, and a possible decrease in libido. An excess in progestins may result in alopecia, oily skin (acne) and scalp, increased fatigue, increased appetite and weight gain that is noncyclic, decrease in length of menstrual flow, breast tenderness, and increased breast size. A progestin deficiency may manifest itself as dysmenorrhea, heavy menstrual flow, weight loss, and/or a delayed onset of menses. An excess of androgen may result in hirsutism, oily skin or skin rash, acne, pruritus, increased appetite and weight gain (noncyclic), and cholestatic jaundice.

Dosage and Administration

1. Although the use of exogenous estrogenic substances alone will inhibit ovulation, undesirable bleeding often occurs during the latter phase of the cycle. If estrogen levels are increased to prevent this, severe nausea and breast tenderness may occur. This is why estrogens are combined with progestins in oral contraceptives.
2. Progestins (steroidal compounds related to progesterone) were developed because naturally occurring progesterone is inactivated or extremely weak in its effect when taken orally and must be given by injection to be effective. The majority of the oral contraceptives contain a synthetic progestin—usually norethynodrel, norethindrone, or norgestrel.
3. Norethynodrel is a basic progestin, norethindrone is a more androgenic progestin, and norgestrel is a synthetic progestogen similar to norethindrone. Norethindrone is sometimes recommended for clients who are experiencing excess side effects from estrogen, such as greater weight gain and amenorrhea. Norethynodrel is good for clients with oily skin, acne, hirsutism, and breakthrough bleeding.
4. Levonorgestrel and ethinyl estradiol (Levlen, Levora 0.15/30, Nordette) or norgestrel and ethinyl estradiol (Lo/Ovral, Ovral) are used as systemic postcoital contraceptives. Four tablets (150 μg of levonorgestrel and 300 μg of ethinyl estradiol per tablet) are taken as soon as possible after unprotected coitus, preferably within 12 hours but no more than 72 hours later. Four more tablets are taken 12 hours after the first dose. With the norgestrel and ethinyl estradiol combination, two tablets (500 μg of norgestrel and 50 μg of ethinyl estradiol per tablet) or four tablets (300 μg norgestrel and 30 μg of ethinyl estradiol per tablet) are taken with the same timing as for postcoital contraception, but the second dose is the same as the first.
5. Several methods of oral contraception are available: combination estrogen and progestin, low-dose progestogens (minipill), and oral contraceptives with varying amounts of progestin (and sometimes estrogen) administered in 2 or 3 phases (biphasic or triphasic). The purpose of the phasic dosing was the belief that it might be less apt to interfere with women's normal metabolism. Clinically, however, this belief has not been substantiated. Table 52-1 lists the composition, doses, and brand names of the oral contraceptives used in these three methods.
6. Combination estrogen and progestin contraceptives are divided into three types:
   - **Monophasic** oral contraception is a fixed ratio of estrogen and progestin that is taken for 21 days of the normal menstrual cycle.
   - **Biphasic** oral contraception supplies two different amounts of progestin during the first and second phases of the menstrual cycle. Low levels of progestin are administered in the follicular phase (first 7 to 10 days) and are increased during the next 11 to 14 days of the luteal phase of the menstrual cycle. The 28-day biphasic cycle has placebo tablets of a third

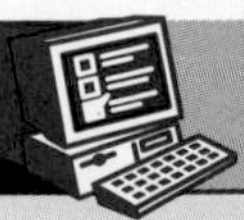

Nursing Research
The Controversy Surrounding Oral Contraceptive Use

Since its introduction the oral contraceptive pill has been a source of controversy, intense study, and media attention. It has probably been studied more extensively than any other medication. Despite this scrutiny, or perhaps because of it, "the pill" is widely misunderstood and feared. The risks of oral contraceptive use, including venous thromboembolism and myocardial infarction, have been known since the 1960s and are far less than those seen during pregnancy. In the widest clinical terms, most risks are not significant. For example, death from venous thromboembolism is less than 1% of total mortality in women between 15 and 44 years of age and is predominately associated with trauma, surgery, and major illness (Cohen & Edwards, 1999).

Over the years numerous studies have indicated that problems with the pill are dose related and that some underlying health problems can be potentiated with their use. However, the "great pill scare" of 1995 and 1996 seemed to indicate that second-generation OCPs were safer than the third-generation pills that had lower dosages (Jick, Jick, Gurewich, Myers, & Vasilakis, 1995; World Health Organization, 1995). The results of these studies were prematurely broadcast in the public media before being published in official journals for feedback from the scientific community. Bad news captures far more attention than good, and therefore these news stories added to the fear of many women regarding estrogen use and to their mistrust of information given by health care providers. Unanimity has not been reached by all epidemiologists; however, after reanalysis of the data and identification of bias and confounding factors, most agree there is equivalent safety of second- and third-generation OCPs. OCPs are very safe, especially in absolute terms, and women should use them consistently and not be afraid of using them if contraindications have been excluded (Cohen & Edwards, 1999).

Many clients believe that the use of estrogen increases the risk for cancer, particularly breast cancer. Henrich (1992) examined the postmenopausal estrogen/breast cancer controversy by reviewing 24 original articles and three meta-analyses, as well as five studies that minimized the influence of detection bias on risk estimates. Henrich found no compelling evidence that women who have ever used postmenopausal estrogens are at increased risk for breast cancer. Reports that women are at increased risk if they use estrogens over prolonged periods or have a surgical menopause, benign breast disease, or a family history of breast cancer are inconclusive and not consistent across studies.

The observation that estrogen effects predominate in lower-stage tumors and are associated with decreased mortality in current users only may reflect unique biologic characteristics of estrogen-associated tumors or be due to detection biases in studies that reported these effects. Detection bias relates to the issue that women diagnosed with breast cancer who had used estrogens were under closer medical surveillance and were more likely to have their disease detected at an earlier stage than women with breast cancer who had not used estrogens. Women who do not use estrogens are less likely than estrogen-treated women to be engaged in health promotion and disease prevention activities, such as breast cancer surveillance (Barrett-Connor, 1991). Henrich recognized that further research is required because the validity of the summary risk estimates are limited by the quality of the published data, some of which is based on the observation of antiquated medical knowledge and practice that involved unopposed, oral, conjugated estrogen use.

The pill offers protection against pelvic inflammatory disease, a major cause of infertility. Women who use the pill have a reduction in functional ovarian cysts, benign breast cysts, fibroadenomas of the breast, and iron-deficiency anemia. The incidence of ectopic pregnancy and rheumatoid arthritis is reduced (Dirubbo, 1992). Kritz-Silverstein & Barrett-Connor (1993) have examined the long-term consequences of prior contraceptive use for bone density in postmenopausal women. They found that women who had used oral contraceptives for 6 or more years had significantly higher bone density of the lumbar spine and femoral neck than women who had never used oral contraceptives; this higher bone density was not explained by age, body mass index, parity, cigarette smoking, years since menopause, or the use of estrogen and thiazide medications than women who had never used oral contraceptives. Higher lumbar spine bone mineral density related to OCP exposure continues to be demonstrated (Pasco et al., 2000).

Nurses play an important role in the prevention of unintended pregnancies and the use of hormonal replacement therapy by older women—therapies that might be influenced by misconceptions about estrogen use. Counseling and education are necessary to teach women of all ages about the effective management of estrogen therapy.

Critical Thinking Questions

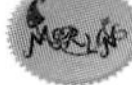

- How might you use this information about estrogen to assist your client in assessing the adverse risks associated with its use?
- If the use of oral contraceptives for 6 or more years reduces the risk of postmenopausal bone loss, what might be the impact on public health?

TABLE 52-1 Selected Oral Contraceptives

Brand Name	Estrogen Content (μg)	Progestin Content (mg)
Monophasic*		
Alesse-28 ◆	ethinyl estradiol 20	levonorgestrel 0.1
Necon 1/35 ◆	ethinyl estradiol 35	norethindrone 1
Ortho-Cyclen ◆	ethinyl estradiol 35	norgestimate 0.25
Lo-Ovral (21 & 28†)	ethinyl estradiol 30	norgestrel 0.3
Biphasic		
Ortho-Novum 10/11	Phase 1: ethinyl estradiol 35 (10 tablets)	norethindrone 0.5
	Phase 2: ethinyl estradiol 35	norethindrone 1
Triphasic		
Ortho-Novum 7/7/7 ◆	Phase 1: ethinyl estradiol 35	norethindrone 0.5
	Phase 2: ethinyl estradiol 35	norethindrone 0.75
	Phase 3: ethinyl estradiol 35	norethindrone 1
Triphasil ◆	Phase 1: ethinyl estradiol 30	levonorgestrel 0.05
	Phase 2: ethinyl estradiol 40	levonorgestrel 0.075
	Phase 3: ethinyl estradiol 30	levonorgestrel 0.125
Ortho Tri-Cyclen ◆	ethinyl estradiol 35	norgestimate 0.18-0.25

Information from *Drug Facts and Comparisons* (2000). St. Louis: Facts and Comparisons.
*Low-dose combination oral contraceptives.
†28s have 7 placebo tablets.

color to mark clearly the proper sequence and reduce any possibility of confusion.

- **Triphasic** oral contraception most closely simulates the normal estrogen and progesterone levels during the menstrual cycle. The dose of estrogen is kept at a low and constant level during the 21-day dosing period while the progestin is progressively increased (three times) to mimic the natural release of hormones in the female. Because the lowest possible doses of hormones are used in this type formulation, the incidence and severity of adverse reactions are considerably lower than with the monophasic or biphasic formulations.

7. Low-dose progestogens (mini-pill) oral contraceptives do not contain estrogen. They are generally prescribed for 28 days of the menstrual cycle and are usually less effective than the combination products. They also involve a higher incidence of spotting and breakthrough bleeding. One advantage is that they generally do not cause the more serious adverse reactions associated with estrogen therapy.
8. Long-acting progestin-only contraceptives include levonorgestrel implants (Norplant), intrauterine progesterone (Progestasert), and medroxyprogesterone injection (Depo-Provera). Side/adverse effects include vaginal bleeding, muscle pain, stomach distress, vaginitis, chloasma, breast discharge, and weight gain. Rarely reported is thrombus formation or thromboembolism.

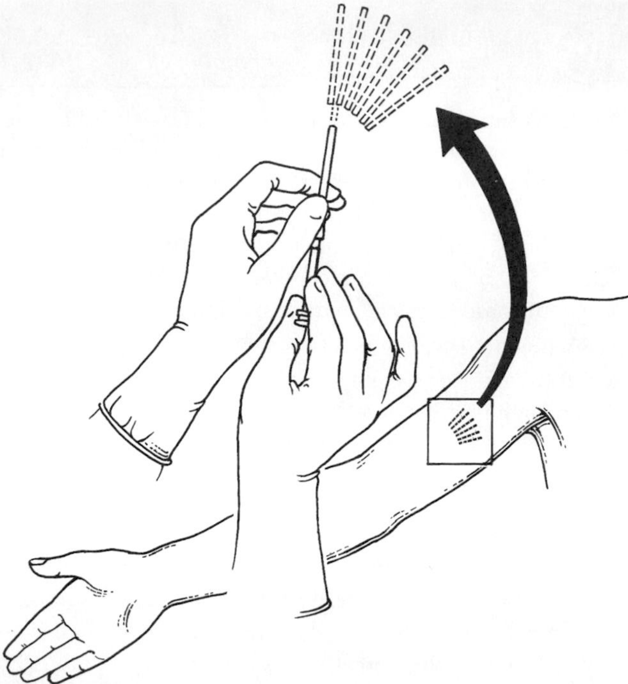

Figure 52-1 Norplant is another form of contraceptive therapy. Porous capsules containing progestin are placed just under the skin on the inside of the upper arm. (From Lowdermilk, D., Perry, S., Bobak, I. (2000). *Maternity & women's health care* (7th ed.). St. Louis: Mosby.)

The levonorgestrel system is a set of six silastic capsules; each capsule contains 36 mg of levonorgestrel and is implanted under the skin of the medial aspect of the upper arm (Figure 52-1). The progestin is released at a constant rate for approximately 5 years. It is then removed, and a new set is inserted if continuing contraceptive action is desired. Fertility returns after removal of the implants.

The intrauterine progesterone system is a unit that contains 38 mg of progesterone and is inserted in the uterine cavity. It is indicated for women in a stable, monogamous relationship who have had at least one child and do not have any history of pelvic inflammatory disease (PID). This system releases an average of 65 μg/day of progesterone for 1 year.

TABLE 52-2 Recommendations for the Selection of an Oral Contraceptive

Conditions	Contraceptive Management
Age	
Sexually active adolescents to women 35 years of age	Low estrogen (30-35 μg)/low progestin; discourage smoking
Women who are heavy smokers* and >35 years of age, or women who are nonsmokers and >40 years of age	Increased risk of serious cardiovascular side effects; use alternate methods of contraception
Concurrent Disease States	
Cancer (breast, uterus, cervix, liver)	Oral contraceptives contraindicated
Cerebrovascular disease, coronary artery disease, and thromboembolic disorders	
Liver impairment; smokers >35 years of age; history of cerebrovascular accident, uncontrolled hypertension, and migraine	Progestin only mini-pill
Management of Side Effects	
Acne, oily skin, hirsutism, sebaceous cysts, weight gain	Trial with oral contraceptives with a lower progestin dose
Breakthrough bleeding	Early to mid-cycle bleeding or bleeding that never completely stops after menses is usually due to an estrogen deficiency, whereas late breakthrough bleeding is due to a progestin deficiency; prescribers often continue with the same oral contraceptive for 3 to 4 months, because intermenstrual bleeding usually decreases with continued use; if bleeding continues, the dosage of estrogen and/or progestin may be adjusted to minimize the effects
Absence of withdrawal bleeding	First rule out pregnancy; if not pregnant, an oral contraceptive with a lower progestin dose may be prescribed; some prescribers use ethinyl estradiol 20 μg for 3 months in addition to the oral contraceptive (Ruggiero, 1995)

Information from *Drug Facts and Comparisons* (2000). St. Louis: Facts and Comparisons; Ruggiero, R. (1995). Contraception. In L.Y. Young, & M.A. Koda-Kimble (Eds.), *Applied therapeutics* (6th ed.). Vancouver, WA: Applied Therapeutics; and *United States Pharmacopeia Dispensing Information (USP DI): Drug information for the health care professional* (19th ed.). (1999). Rockville, MD: United States Pharmacopeial Convention.
*More than 15 cigarettes/day.

Medroxyprogesterone IM is administered to women every 3 months to inhibit gonadotropin secretion, thereby resulting in contraception.

Table 52-2 lists recommendations for the selection of an oral contraceptive.

Estrostep

Estrostep is a graduated estrophasic dosage form of an oral contraceptive. It contains norethindrone acetate and ethinyl estradiol and 20 μg of estrogen/1 mg progestin for the first 5 days, 30 μg/1 mg for days 6 through 12, and 35 μg/1 mg for days 13 through 21. A second formulation is a 28-day regimen that contains an additional 7 days of ferrous fumarate and is taken on days 22 through 28. The manufacturer reports that clinical studies found this product to be greater than 99% effective—more effective than other combination oral contraceptives (FDA News and Product Notes, 1997).

Nursing Management
Oral Contraceptive Therapy

■ **Assessment.** See the assessment for estrogens and progestins. Other drug interactions that need to be considered are corticosteroids (concurrent administration may decrease the clearance and increase the effects of corticosteroids and necessitate lower dosages) and theophylline (concurrent use increases serum concentrations of both drugs, but only the theophylline effect is clinically significant; lower dosages of theophylline may be required).

■ **Nursing Diagnosis.** In addition to the nursing diagnoses and collaborative problems previously cited in the material for estrogens and progestins, see the Nursing Care Plan on p. 902.

■ **Implementation**

■ ***Monitoring.*** Clients should be monitored for the development of side effects/adverse reactions. Among the more common reactions are fluid retention, breakthrough

Nursing Care Plan
Selected Nursing Diagnoses Related to Hormone Therapy and Oral Contraceptive Use

Nursing Diagnosis	Outcome Criteria	Nursing Interventions
Deficient knowledge related to female hormone therapy	Client will be able to verbalize action, use, dose, and side effects/adverse reactions of hormonal therapy. Client will demonstrate a reduction in symptoms without side effects/adverse reactions.	Instruct client to take the medication as prescribed. Advise the client using a vaginal cream form to administer at bedtime to increase absorption. Use a sanitary napkin, not tampons, to protect clothing. Advise the client that the medication may be taken with food to minimize or prevent nausea. Alert the client to stop taking her medication and consult with her prescriber if she suspects she is pregnant. Advise the client to report to the prescriber any symptoms of thromboembolism (sudden severe headache, sudden change in vision, sudden pain, weakness, or numbness), liver impairment (yellow eyes or skin, dark urine, pale stools), or mental depression. Alert the client that smoking cigarettes while taking this medication increases the risk of thromboembolism (deep vein thrombosis, pulmonary embolism, heart attack, stroke), particularly after age 35. Stress the importance of regular visits to the prescriber for follow-up care every 6-12 months.
Deficient knowledge related to the oral contraceptive regimen	Client will demonstrate compliance with the medication regimen (oral contraception) without experiencing side effects/adverse reactions.	Instruct the client to take the medication as prescribed. Advise the client to use an additional method of birth control during the first 3 weeks of the initial cycle. Encourage the client to take the medication at the same time each day, not more than 24 hours apart. Alert the client that although nausea may occur during the first few weeks of therapy, it is usually temporary and may be minimized by taking the dose with food. Advise the client to always keep a month's supply on hand. Replace the extra supply each month. Provide specific information regarding the appropriate action to be taken by the client when "missed" doses occur. Stress the importance of regular visits to the prescriber for follow-up care every 6-12 months. Advise the client to alert other health care providers that she is taking oral contraceptives, because they may cause serious symptoms and interact with other drugs to lessen the effectiveness of the contraceptive. Alert the client to stop taking her medication and consult with the prescriber if she suspects she is pregnant. Advise the client to report to the prescriber any symptoms of thromboembolism (sudden severe headache, sudden change in vision, sudden pain, weakness, or numbness), liver impairment (yellow eyes or skin, dark urine, pale stools), or mental depression. Alert the client that smoking cigarettes while taking this medication increases the risk of thromboembolism (deep vein thrombosis, pulmonary embolism, heart attack, stroke), particularly after age 35.

Case Study *The Client Taking Oral Contraceptives*

Linda Cosgrove is a 35-year-old woman who has been taking oral contraceptives for 5 years. She is currently using Ortho-Novum 7/7/7-28. On a recent routine physical examination the nurse notes that Linda's blood pressure has increased to 154/90 mm Hg from a previous range of 122/70 to 134/80 mm Hg. She has also experienced a recent 10-pound weight gain without a change in eating habits or activity.

1. Why might these symptoms be significant for this client?
2. What additional assessment data does the nurse need to gather from this client related to her drug therapy and her current status?
3. What elements of the physical examination are important for this client?
4. What information should the nurse provide this client regarding adverse reactions to oral contraceptives and her options for contraception?

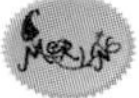

For answer guidelines, go to mosby.com/MERLIN/McKenry/.

bleeding, thromboembolic disorders, hypertension, and nausea. If significant adverse reactions occur, a different birth control pill formula or alternate birth control method should be used. For other monitoring considerations, see Nursing Management: Progesterone/Progestin Therapy, p. 896.

■ ***Education.*** Instruct the client to take the medications as prescribed. The tablets should be taken at the same time each day, preferably in association with another daily routine (e.g., brushing of teeth, cleansing of face in the morning or at night). Nighttime administration may be preferable to decrease nausea. Nausea occurs in some clients during the first cycle but tends to subside after the third or fourth month. It may be prevented or reduced by taking the medication with food.

Caution clients never to let their tablet supply run out and always to keep an extra month's supply on hand. The packages should be rotated by using the extra package after the pills currently being used and then replacing the extra supply each month on a regular basis.

Instruct the client to use the pills in the same sequence that they appear in the container.

Instruct clients who are beginning to use oral contraceptives to use a barrier method of birth control for the first cycle until the body adjusts to the medication. If the client misses a dose for 1 day of the 21-day schedule, she should take it as soon as she remembers. If she does not remember until the next day, tell her to take the missed tablet and the regularly scheduled one together. If she does not remember a dose for 2 days in a row, she should take 2 tablets a day for each of the next 2 days. In addition, she should use a second method of birth control for full protection. If she misses 3 or more doses in a row, she should stop taking the medicine and use another method of birth control until she menstruates or until it is determined she is not pregnant. She may restart the medication with the appropriate cycle.

If the client is using a 28-day schedule and misses any of the first 21 tablets, instruct her to follow the preceding instructions. If she misses any of the last 7 tablets, which are inactive, there is no hazard of pregnancy; however, the first tablet of the next month's series must be taken on the regularly scheduled day. Be sure to review the literature provided with the medication with the client to ensure understanding.

Assist the client in exploring her concerns about the risks of taking oral contraceptives. Provide her with information regarding the occurrence of cardiovascular disease and cancer in relationship to her age, smoking habits, and other health characteristics (Sherif, 1999). Encourage the client to read the package insert carefully and then to discuss with her health care provider any concerns she might have.

Advise the client to have physical examinations, which should include a pelvic and breast examination and a Pap smear, every 6 to 12 months during treatment.

Instruct the client to notify her prescriber immediately in the instance of severe headache, blurred or lost vision (which may signal possible stroke), and symptoms of chest pain, shortness of breath, or leg pain (which may indicate thromboembolism elsewhere in the body). The health care provider should also be informed of severe abdominal pain or mass, jaundice, severe mental depression, or unusual bleeding. Instructions should be provided for monthly self-examination of the breasts, and any lumps should be reported to the prescriber.

Medical intervention is necessary for various changes in menstrual bleeding pattern, increased and painful urination, jaundice, abdominal cramping, ocular changes (double vision, partial or complete loss of vision, bulging eyes), increased blood pressure, breast alterations (lumps, secretions), depression, or pain or numbness in the fingers or toes.

Compliance with therapy is especially important if oral contraceptives are to be effective. Periodically review with the client the appropriate use and importance of taking the drug daily. Ensure that the client knows the proper procedure to follow should one or more doses be missed.

■ **Evaluation.** The expected outcome of oral contraceptive therapy is that the client will not become pregnant and will not show evidence any untoward effects of the oral contraceptive. For further analysis of the client taking oral contraceptives, see the Case Study box above.

OVULATORY STIMULANTS AND DRUGS USED FOR INFERTILITY

Anovulation, the absence of ovulation, is physiologic in women who are pregnant, breastfeeding, or postmenopausal. It becomes a suspected pathologic condition in women with abnormal bleeding or infertility. The incidence of anovulation is unknown and cannot be ascertained, but diagnostic tests may determine its presence. Clomiphene and urofollitropin are ovulation stimulants used to treat infertility in the female.

clomiphene citrate [kloe′ mi feen] (Clomid, Serophene)

Clomiphene has antiestrogenic effects with some estrogen effects. Although its exact mechanism of action is unknown, it has been postulated that its competition with estrogen for receptor sites in the hypothalamus causes an increased secretion of FSH and LH. The result is ovarian stimulation, maturation of the ovarian follicle, and development of the corpus luteum.

Clomiphene is indicated to treat female infertility. It is well absorbed orally and recirculated in the enterohepatic system, which may account for its prolonged duration of action in the body. It has a plasma half-life of 5 to 7 days, with ovulation usually occurring between 4 to 10 days after the first day of treatment. It is metabolized in the liver and excreted in the feces and bile.

Clomiphene has no known significant drug interactions. Side effects/adverse reactions include hot flashes, abdominal pain or gas, visual disturbances, headache, nausea, vomiting, depression, anxiety, and weakness.

The adult dosage for female infertility is 50 mg PO daily for 5 days, starting on the fifth day of the menstrual period if bleeding occurs or at any time in women who have no recent uterine bleeding. This cycle is repeated until conception occurs, up to three or four cycles. If ovulation does not occur, the dosage is increased to 75 to 100 mg/day for 5 days, which may be repeated if necessary.

▪ Nursing Management

Clomiphene Therapy

▪ **Assessment.** It should be determined whether the client has preexisting conditions for which clomiphene would be contraindicated, such as abnormal and undiagnosed vaginal bleeding, endometriosis, fibroid tumors, mental depression, active hepatic dysfunction (or a history of it), or thrombophlebitis. If the client has ovarian cysts, clomiphene may cause them to enlarge. Clients with polycystic ovary syndrome may experience an exaggerated response to the drug. The presence of an ovarian cyst or ovarian enlargement not associated with polycystic ovarian disease is a contraindication for the use of this drug because of the risk of further enlargement.

▪ **Nursing Diagnosis.** Clients receiving clomiphene therapy are at risk for the following nursing diagnoses/collaborative problems: impaired comfort related to premenstrual syndrome (more than 5%), hot flashes (10%), headache, breast tenderness, nausea and vomiting; disturbed sleep pattern (insomnia); disturbed sensory perception (blurred vision, after-images, diplopia, floaters, phosphenes, scotoma, or photophobia); and the potential complications of development or enlargement of ovarian cysts, enlargement of uterine fibroids, mental depression, hepatotoxicity, or thromboembolism.

▪ **Implementation**

▪ ***Monitoring.*** A pelvic examination to assess ovarian size should be completed before each course of the drug. Immunologic assay for HCG is recommended for the detection of pregnancy if menses does not occur before the next course of clomiphene is to begin. Urinary LH surge testing may be used to predict ovulation. An ophthalmologic examination is recommended if treatment with clomiphene is continued for more than 1 year or if visual disturbances occur.

▪ ***Intervention.*** Women who have been hypoestrogenic for a long time may require pretreatment with estrogen therapy to ensure a better environment for ovum implantation. To increase the efficacy of clomiphene, a single injection of 5000 to 10,000 USP units of HCG may be given 5 to 9 days after the last dose of clomiphene to simulate the midcycle LH surge that results in ovulation. If three or four cycles of clomiphene therapy do not result in pregnancy, or if pregnancy does not occur after a treatment interval of 3 to 6 months with documented ovulation, review the course of therapy with the client and her partner to ensure understanding. If the regimen is being managed effectively by the client, the client's diagnosis should be reconsidered.

▪ ***Education.*** Coitus should occur at or around the time ovulation is anticipated, usually approximately 7 days (range 5 to 10 days) after the last dose of clomiphene to enhance fertilization.

If the medication is to start on day 5, count the first day of the menstrual period as day 1. Advise the client that taking the medication at the same time every day maintains drug levels and helps in remembering the daily dose. Advise the client to take a missed dose as soon as possible. If the dose is not remembered until it is time for the next dose, both should be taken together. If more than one dose is missed, the prescriber should be consulted.

Inform the client and her partner about the possibility of multiple births with this drug. Advise her that abdominal pain is an indication for immediate medical attention, because such pain may be symptomatic of the formation or enlargement of an ovarian cyst. Counsel the client to report visual disturbances to the prescriber at once. Alert her to be cautious with tasks that require alertness, because clomiphene may cause visual disturbances, vertigo, and lightheadedness.

▪ **Evaluation.** The expected outcome of clomiphene therapy is that the client will become pregnant without experiencing any adverse reactions to the drug.

urofollitropin [yoor oh foe′ li troe pin] (Metrodin)

Urofollitropin is used to treat female infertility. It is obtained from the urine of postmenopausal women and contains FSH. HCG (the action is very similar to LH) is administered after urofollitropin to simulate natural ovulation.

The most commonly reported side effects/adverse reactions of urofollitropin are ovarian cysts or ovarian enlargement, as well as pain and redness at the injection site. Other effects include severe stomach pain, bloating, decreased urination, severe nausea, vomiting or diarrhea, weight gain, swelling of the lower extremities, breathing difficulties, severe pelvic pain as a result of the syndrome of severe OHS, skin rash, elevated temperature, and chills.

The usual adult dosage is 75 units daily for a week or more, followed by 5000 to 10,000 units of HCG 1 day after the last dose of urofollitropin.

■ Nursing Management

Urofollitropin Therapy

■ **Assessment.** It should be ascertained that the client does not have a medical condition for which urofollitropin would be contraindicated, such as undiagnosed vaginal bleeding, ovarian cyst or enlargement not associated with polycystic ovary syndrome, or sensitivity to urofollitropin or other gonadotropins. No significant drug interactions have been reported with its use. A baseline ultrasound examination is recommended to determine the number and size of mature follicles.

■ **Nursing Diagnosis.** The woman receiving urofollitropin therapy is at risk for the following nursing diagnoses/collaborative problems: impaired comfort (breast tenderness, nausea, vomiting, chills, rash, mild diarrhea); imbalanced body temperature (fever); impaired tissue integrity (pain, swelling, and tenderness at the injection site); and the potential complications of ovarian enlargement or ovarian cysts (10% to 20%) and severe OHS.

■ **Implementation**

■ ***Monitoring.*** Serum estradiol concentrations are monitored to determine the best dosing levels and to decrease the risk of OHS. A periodic ultrasound examination to follow follicular development is recommended. Daily basal body temperatures may be taken to determine if ovulation has occurred.

■ ***Intervention.*** The dosage of urofollitropin varies considerably and is based on the client's clinical response.

■ ***Education.*** Intercourse or insemination should be performed daily beginning the day after the drug is administered until ovulation is thought to have occurred.

Instruct the client to take her basal body temperature daily and record it on a flow chart. This determines when ovulation occurs and assists in properly timing coitus to enhance fertilization. Easy-to-read oral thermometers are available that register 96° to 100° F; some prescribers prefer rectal temperatures for accuracy. The temperature is taken from day 1 of the menstrual period and every morning on awakening—before the client engages in any activity such as drinking coffee, brushing her teeth, smoking, or intercourse. Oral body temperature is low (approximately 97.5° F) and stable for 2 weeks after menstruation. There is a slight decrease at ovulation followed the next day by an increase (approximately 98.5° F), which continues if progesterone levels are normal. The temperature decreases again just before menstruation. If this decrease does not occur, the client may be pregnant.

■ **Evaluation.** The expected outcome of urofollitropin therapy is that the client will become pregnant without experiencing any ill effects of the drug.

SUMMARY

Drugs used for diagnostic purposes, to treat disorders, or to alter the normal functioning of the female reproductive system include many substances, such as GnRH, nonpituitary chorionic gonadotropin, menotropins, female sex hormones, oral contraceptives, ovulatory stimulants, and drugs used for infertility. GnRH, or gonadorelin, is used for the diagnosis of hypogonadism in both males and females and, investigationally, for the treatment of primary hypothalamic amenorrhea. Nafarelin, a GnRH agonist, is used in the management of endometriosis and CPP. A deficiency in LH is the indication for chorionic gonadotropin. Menotropins are used in the treatment of both male and female infertility.

Estrogens, progesterone, and progestins are the more commonly used drugs that affect the female reproductive system. Estrogen is used for hormonal replacement therapy, the treatment of breast and prostatic carcinomas, and the prevention of osteoporosis in postmenopausal women. Progesterone/progestins are indicated for hormonal replacement, the treatment of endometriosis and specific carcinomas, and the prevention of pregnancy.

Oral contraception with combinations of estrogen and progestin is the most effective form of birth control currently available. Because these drugs are primarily for self-administration, the emphasis for the nurse is on client education for safe and accurate administration and for early recognition of adverse reactions. Clomiphene and urofollitropin are indicated for the treatment of infertility.

Because all of these drugs affect sexual identity, the nurse must be sensitive to the client's needs as a sexual being and must be alert to cues that reflect problems such as a disturbance of self-concept.

Critical Thinking Questions

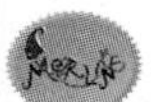

1. Lillian Taylor, a college freshman, was seen in the University Health Center in September by the nurse practitioner, who prescribed Ortho-Novum birth control pills for her. In February, Ms. Taylor calls the Center and states that she thinks she is pregnant even though she has consistently taken her birth control pills. What instructions should the nurse give her?
2. Mary Ann Gilbert, age 51, has been experiencing distressing menopausal symptoms for which her health care provider has prescribed estrogen replacement. As she is leaving the office, she seems concerned about filling her prescription because her neighbor has said that "those pills cause cancer." What action should the nurse take?

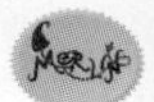

Collaborative Learning Activities

For Collaborative Learning Activities, go to mosby.com/MERLIN/McKenry/.

CASE STUDY

For a Case Study that will help ensure mastery of this chapter content, go to mosby.com/MERLIN/McKenry/.

BIBLIOGRAPHY

American Hospital Formulary Service. (1999). *AHFS drug information '99*. Bethesda, MD: American Society of Hospital Pharmacists.

Anderson, K.N., Anderson, L.E., & Glanze, W.D. (Eds.) (1998). *Mosby's medical, nursing, & allied health dictionary* (5th ed.). St. Louis: Mosby.

Barrett-Connor, E. (1991). Postmenopausal estrogen and prevention bias, *Annals of Internal Medicine 115*(6), 455-456.

Battaglia, C., Salvatori, M., Giulini, S., Primavera, M.R., Gallinelli, A., Volpe, A. (1999). Hormonal replacement therapy and urinary problems as evaluated by ultrasound and color Doppler. *Ultrasound Obstetrics & Gynecology, 13*(6), 420-424.

Brooks, T.L. & Shrier, L.A. (1999). An update on contraception for adolescents. *Adolescent Medicine, 10*(2), 211-219.

Cohen, C. & Edwards, R.G. (1999). Conclusions: The relative safety of modern oral contraceptives. *Human Reproduction Update, 5*(6), 756-771.

Dirubbo, N. (1992). Oral contraceptives still misunderstood. *Nurse Practitioner, 17*(8), 7.

Drug Facts and Comparisons. (2000). St. Louis: Facts and Comparisons.

FDA News and Product Notes. (1997). New formulations/combinations. *Formulary, 32*(1), 23.

Genazzani, A.R. & Gambacciani, M. (1999). Hormone replacement therapy: The perspectives for the 21st century. *Maturitas, 32*(1), 11-17.

Gold, M.A. (1999). Prescribing and managing oral contraceptives pills and emergency contraception for adolescents. *Pediatric Clinics of North America, 46*(4), 695-718.

Gordon, L. (1995). Cardiac benefits of ERT confirmed. *Medical Tribune for the Family Physician, 36*(1), 17.

Henrich, J.B. (1992). The postmenopausal estrogen/breast cancer controversy. *Journal of the American Medical Association, 268*(14), 1900-1902.

Herrington, D.M. (1999). The HERS trial results: Paradigms lost? Heart and Estrogen/Progestin Replacement Study. *Annals of Internal Medicine, 131*(6), 463-466.

Jick, H., Jick, S.S., Gurewich, V., Myers, M.W., & Vasilakis, C. (1995). Risk of idiopathic cardiovascular death and nonfatal venous thromboembolism in women using oral contraceptive with differing progestagen components. *Lancet, 346*(8990), 1589-1593.

Kenyon, J. (Ed.). (1995). Assessment of long-term risks and benefits of combined oral contraceptives. *Drugs & Therapeutic Perspectives, 6*(10), 9-11.

Kritz-Silverstein, D. & Barrett-Connor, E. (1993). Bone mineral density in postmenopausal women as determined by prior oral contraceptive use. *American Journal of Public Health, 83*(1), 100-102.

Mattsson, L.A., Bohnet, H.G., Gredmark, T., Torhorst, J., Hornig, F., & Huls, G. (1999). Continuous, combined hormone replacement: Randomized comparison of transdermal and oral preparations. *Obstetrics & Gynecology, 94*(1), 61-65.

McNagny, S.E. (1999). Prescribing hormone replacement therapy for menopausal symptoms. *Annals of Internal Medicine, 131*(8), 605-616.

Melmon, K.L., Morrelli, H.F., Hoffman, B.B., & Nierenberg, D.W. (Eds.). (1992). *Melmon and Morrelli's clinical pharmacology: Basic principles in therapeutics* (3rd ed.). New York: McGraw-Hill.

Moore, A.A. & Noonan, M.D. (1996). A nurse's guide to hormone replacement therapy. *Journal of Obstetrical, Gynecological & Neonatal Nursing, 25*(1), 24-31.

Mosca, L., Manson, J.E., Sutherland, S.E., Langer, A.D., Manolio, T., & Barrett-Connor, E. (1998). *Cardiovascular disease in women: A statement for healthcare professionals from the American Heart Association.* American Heart Association (www.americanheart.org/Scientific/statements/1997/109701.html [6/30/98]).

Pasco, J.A., Kotowicz, M.A., Henry, M.J., Panahi, S., Seeman, E., & Nicholson, G.C. (2000). Oral contraceptives and bone mineral density: A population-based study. *American Journal of Obstetrics & Gynecology, 182*(2), 265-269.

Persson, I., Weiderpass, E., Bergkvist, L., Bergstrom, R., & Schairer, C. (1999). Risks of breast and endometrial cancer after estrogen and estrogen-progestin replacement. *Cancer Causes & Control, 10*(4), 253-260.

Pharmacy Practice News. (1995). Hormone replacement scores in landmark trial. *Pharmacy Practice News, 22*(4), 43.

Pierard-Franchimont, C., Cornil, F., Dehavay, J., Deleixhe-Mauhin, F., Letot, B., & Pierard, G.E. (1999). Climacteric skin aging of the face: A prospective longitudinal comparative trial on the effect of oral hormone replacement therapy. *Maturitas, 32*(2), 87-93.

Qureshi, M. & Attaran, M. (1999). Review of newer contraceptive agents. *Cleveland Clinics Journal of Medicine, 66*(6), 358-366.

Recker, R.R., Davies, K.M., Dowd, R.M., & Heaney, R.P. (1999). The effect of low-dose continuous estrogen and progesterone therapy with calcium and vitamin D on bone in elderly women: A randomized, controlled study. *Annals of Internal Medicine, 130*(11), 897-904.

Ruggiero, R. (1995). Contraception. In L.Y. Young, & M.A. Koda-Kimble (Eds.), *Applied therapeutics* (6th ed.). Vancouver, WA: Applied Therapeutics.

Sherif, K. (1999). Benefits and risks of oral contraceptives. *American Journal of Obstetrics & Gynecology, 180*(6 pt 2), S343-S348.

Shoupe, D. (1999). Hormone replacement therapy: Reassessing the risks and benefits. *Hospital Practice, 34*(8), 97-103, 107-108, 113-114.

Sobel, N.R. (1994). Progestins in preventive hormone therapy, including pharmacology of the new progestins, desogestrel, norgestimate, and gestodene: Are there advantages? *Obstetrics & Gynecology Clinics of North America, 21*(2), 299-319.

United States Pharmacopeia Dispensing Information (USP DI): Drug information for the health care professional (19th ed.). (1999). Rockville, MD: United States Pharmacopeial Convention.

Watts, N.B. (1999). Postmenopausal osteoporosis. *Obstetric & Gynecology Survey, 54*(8), 532-538.

Wehrle, K.E. (1994). The Norplant system: Easy to insert, easy to remove. *Nurse Practitioner, 19*(4), 47-54.

Weiderpass, E., Adami, H.O., Baron, J.A., Magnusson, C., Bergstrom, R., Lindgren, A., Correia, N., Persson, I. (1999). Risk of endometrial cancer following estrogen replacement with and without progestin. *Journal of National Cancer Institute, 91*(13), 1131-1137.

Williams, C.L. & Stancel, G.M. (1996). Estrogens and progestins. In J.G. Hardman & L.E. Limbird (Eds.), *Goodman & Gilman's The pharmacological basis of therapeutics* (9th ed.). New York: McGraw-Hill.

World Health Organization. (1995). WHO Collaborative Study of Cardiovascular Disease and Steroid Hormone Contraception. Venous thromboembolic disease and combined oral contraceptives: Results of international multicentre case-control study. *Lancet, 347*(8990), 1575-1582.

Zeitoun, K. & Carr, B.R. (1999). Is there an increased risk of stroke associated with oral contraceptives? *Drug Safety, 20*(6), 467-473.

53 Drugs for Labor and Delivery

Chapter Focus

Labor and delivery are the culmination of the childbearing cycle and constitute an intense experience for all involved. To implement nursing care, the nurse must understand the essential processes of labor, maternal and fetal adaptations, and the effects of the drugs used for labor and delivery.

Learning Objectives

1. Describe the altered pharmacokinetic pattern of drugs during labor and delivery.
2. Discuss the pharmacologic action of oxytocics on the uterus.
3. Identify the three primary indications for the use of oxytocin.
4. Explain the two primary actions of ergonovine.
5. Discuss the mechanism of action and use of ritodrine.
6. Explain the action of lactation inhibitors.
7. Implement the nursing management for the drug therapy of a client experiencing labor and delivery.

Key Terms

Key Drugs [✔]

Because many drugs are available for use during labor and delivery, it is important to consider the benefit vs. the risk to the fetus. The pharmacokinetics of drugs may be altered during labor and delivery. For example, gastric emptying is delayed during labor, and vomiting may result; this alters drug absorption. Vomiting may also be exacerbated by the use of opioid analgesics. Because oral drug absorption is unpredictable at this time, parenteral routes should be used. Drug metabolism and excretion may be altered and prolonged during labor; and although clinical data are currently sparse, the potential for inducing adverse or undesirable effects is always a concern. If a drug such as an opioid analgesic or sedative may be potentially harmful to the fetus and if alternate methods are not available, then the smallest possible dose should be used.

Complications in pregnancy may also dictate the use of additional medications, such as those to treat diabetes, hypertension, preeclampsia, eclampsia, and systemic infections. These medications and their proper use are discussed in the appropriate pharmacologic sections of this text. For example, magnesium sulfate for toxemia of pregnancy is reviewed in Chapter 17. Discussion in this chapter is limited to the drugs used to induce labor (**oxytocics**), inhibit premature labor (**tocolytics**), and suppress lactation.

DRUGS THAT AFFECT THE UTERUS

The uterus is a highly muscular organ that exhibits a number of characteristic properties and activities. The smooth muscle fibers of the uterus extend longitudinally, circularly, and obliquely. The uterus has a rich blood supply; blood flow is diminished when the uterine muscle contracts. Profound changes occur in the uterus during pregnancy: it increases in weight from approximately 50 g to approximately 1000 g, its capacity increases tenfold in length, and new muscle fibers may be formed. These changes are accompanied by changes in the response to drugs.

Drugs that act on the uterus include oxytocics (which increase uterine contractility) and tocolytics (which decrease uterine contractility).

Oxytocics

Oxytocics are agents that stimulate contraction of the smooth muscle of the uterus, resulting in contractions and spontaneous labor. The most commonly used oxytocics are alkaloids of synthetic oxytocin and ergot, although many other drugs may have some effect on uterine contractility.

✔ **oxytocin** [ox i toe′ sin] (Pitocin, Syntocinon)

Oxytocin is one of two hormones secreted by the posterior pituitary, the other hormone being vasopressin, or antidiuretic hormone (ADH). Oxytocin means "rapid birth," a term derived from its ability to contract the pregnant uterus. It also facilitates milk ejection during lactation.

The nonpregnant uterus is relatively insensitive to oxytocin; uterine sensitivity to oxytocin gradually increases during pregnancy, with the uterus being most sensitive at term. The secretion of oxytocin may precede and possibly trigger delivery of the fetus. Large amounts of oxytocin have been detected in the blood during the expulsive phase of delivery. A positive feedback mechanism may be operating; more forceful contractions of uterine muscle and greater stretching of the cervix and vagina result in the release of more oxytocin. Oxytocin acts directly on the myometrium and has a stronger effect on the fundus than on the cervix. This activity is the rationale for its use for the induction of labor. Oxytocin has been associated with a significant shortening of labor without any demonstrable adverse fetal or neonatal effects or a significant difference in cesarean birth rates (Merrill & Zlatnik, 1999).

Oxytocin also transiently impedes uterine blood flow and stimulates the mammary gland to increase the excretion of milk from the breast; it does not increase the production of milk. This product is indicated for the control of postpartum and postabortion hemorrhage and for the stimulation of lactation.

This product is available parenterally and in a rapidly absorbed nasal dosage form (Syntocinon). Because the intranasal product may be erratic, it is primarily used before nursing or pumping of the breasts.

Oxytocin has a half-life of 1 to 6 minutes. The onset of action is as follows: nasal, within a couple of minutes; IM, within 3 to 5 minutes; IV, immediate, with uterine contractions increasing gradually over 15 to 60 minutes before stabilizing. The duration of action is as follows: nasal, 20 minutes; IM, 30 to 60 minutes; IV, within an hour after stopping the infusion. Oxytocin is metabolized and excreted by the kidneys.

The side effects/adverse reactions of parenteral oxytocin include nausea, vomiting, tachycardia, and an irregular heart rate. It may occasionally cause fetal bradycardia, dysrhythmias, neonatal jaundice, postpartum excessive bleeding and, rarely, hematoma in the pelvic area. Prolonged therapy may result in water intoxication and possible maternal death because of its slight antidiuretic effects.

The dosage to induce labor is 0.5 to 2 mU/min by IV infusion, increased every 15 to 60 minutes by 1 to 2 mU/min until a contraction pattern that simulates normal labor is established (up to a maximum of 20 mU/min).

For the control of postpartum uterine bleeding, the dosage is 10 units at a rate of 20 to 40 mU infused intravenously after birth of the infant. The dosage for the nasal solution is 1 spray in one or both nostrils 2 or 3 minutes before nursing or pumping the breasts.

▪ Nursing Management

Oxytocin Therapy

▪ **Assessment.** Before administering oxytocin, ascertain that the client in labor is not experiencing any contraindications to a vaginal delivery, such as cord presentation or prolapse, placenta previa or vasa previa, or fetal distress. Oxytocin is also contraindicated for clients with a history of

Pregnancy Safety
Drugs for Labor and Delivery

Category	Drug
B	ritodrine
X	oxytocin

Ergot products are contraindicated during pregnancy.

allergy to the drug and for clients with hypertonic uterine patterns. Prolonged use of oxytocin is not recommended for clients with uterine inertia; a course of oxytocin therapy is usually limited to 6 to 8 hours.

Oxytocin should be used cautiously if the client in labor exhibits grand multiparity (several prior births), overdistention of the uterus, or a past history of trauma or major surgery on the cervix or uterus (such clients are predisposed to uterine rupture); invasive cervical carcinoma (vaginal delivery is contraindicated); partial placenta previa; prematurity of the fetus; or an unfavorable fetal position. Caution is also recommended for women over 35 years of age or for those having an abortion using hypertonic saline because of the higher risk for water intoxication. When oxytocin is used as an adjunct to drugs that cause abortion (e.g., intraamniotic sodium chloride or urea or other oxytocics), it should not be administered until the oxytocic effect of the abortifacient has diminished to decrease the risk of uterine hyperactivity and cervical laceration. (See the Pregnancy Safety box above.)

Before administering the drug to induce labor, it should be determined that there is pelvic adequacy of the client in labor and that there is fetal maturity. Record baseline data, including blood pressure and other vital signs; the characteristics, frequency, and duration of the contractions; and fetal heart rate. If the nasal spray is indicated for pain related to postpartum breast engorgement, obtain a baseline assessment of the client's breastfeeding status before initiating therapy.

■ **Nursing Diagnosis.** Clients receiving oxytocin are at risk for the following nursing diagnoses/collaborative problems: excess fluid volume related to the antidiuretic effect of the drug (hypertension, water intoxication); impaired comfort with nasal use related to nasal irritation and tearing of the eyes; and the collaborative problems of anaphylaxis and other allergic reactions, cardiac dysrhythmias, hypotension, hypertension, or postpartum hemorrhage. The fetus may also be at risk because of the potential for injury related to fetal trauma (cardiac dysrhythmias, intracranial hemorrhage, asphyxia), fetal bradycardia, and neonatal jaundice.

■ **Implementation**

■ ***Monitoring.*** Check the client's blood pressure and pulse at least every 15 minutes, during the infusion; also assess the frequency, duration, and force of uterine contractions. Assess the myometrium for tonus during and between contractions, and report hypertonic uterine contractions or a period of uterine relaxation. Continuous fetal monitoring should be performed while the client is receiving oxytocin, and the infusion should be discontinued at any sign of uterine hyperactivity or fetal distress. The dosage is individualized for each client depending on maternal and fetal response.

Fluid intake and output determinations and the assessment of lung sounds are needed because oxytocin has a slight antidiuretic effect, which could result in severe water intoxication with prolonged IV infusion. Hypochloremia and hyponatremia may occur in the client because of water intoxication.

When the nasal spray is used for postpartum breast engorgement, monitor milk ejection and the client's comfort level.

■ ***Intervention.*** Parenteral administration should occur only in a hospital setting and under medical supervision. IV infusion is preferred for the induction or stimulation of labor because absorption from IM administration is difficult to regulate and could result in uterine hyperactivity and fetal distress. Accurate administration by infusion pump or microdrip regulator is mandatory, as is using a Y connection so the oxytocin solution may be discontinued while access to the vein is maintained. When preparing an oxytocin infusion, distribute the drug throughout the solution by gently rotating the bottle. Administer oxytocin for no longer than 6 to 8 hours in instances of uterine inertia. At the first sign of uterine hypertonicity or fetal distress, decrease the rate of oxytocin infusion, or discontinue it.

When oxytocin is administered by nasal spray, instruct the client to clear her nasal passages. Then, with the client's head in a vertical position and the bottle upright, spray the solution into the nostril. Use the spray before breastfeeding or pumping the breasts. Do not administer oxytocin by more than one route simultaneously.

■ ***Education.*** If oxytocin is being administered as a lactation stimulant, the client should be taught the proper technique for self-administration. She should also be aware of the possibility that oxytocin may not be effective.

■ **Evaluation.** When oxytocin is administered for postpartum breast engorgement, the expected outcome is that the client will experience pain relief and diminished swelling. When it is given to induce or stimulate labor, the client's labor will progress normally without indications of fluid volume excess, uterine hypertonicity, or fetal distress. When oxytocin is administered after expulsion of the placenta, postpartum bleeding will be reduced. For further analysis, see the Case Study box on p. 910.

ergonovine [er goe noe' veen] (Ergotrate)

Ergonovine increases the force and frequency of uterine contractions by direct stimulation of the smooth muscle of the uterine wall. It is indicated to prevent and treat postpartum hemorrhage.

Ergonovine is administered either orally or parenterally. The onset of action is as follows: orally, within 6 to 15 minutes; IM, within 2 to 3 minutes; and IV, within 1 minute. The duration of uterine contraction is as follows: orally and

Case Study *The Client in Labor*

Karen Evans has spent 12 hours in labor with her first pregnancy and has made little progress. She is becoming exhausted, and her uterine contractions have decreased in strength. Oxytocin is being considered as an alternative to improve the progress of her labor.

1. How might the oxytocin be administered?
2. What are the associated risks of the drug for both the mother and the fetus?
3. What physiologic signs and symptoms should be monitored in this client?
4. How should the nurse describe the drug therapy to this client?

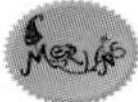

For answer guidelines, go to mosby.com/MERLIN/McKenry/.

IM, approximately 3 hours; and IV, approximately 45 minutes (rhythmic contractions can persist for up to 3 hours). This drug is metabolized in the liver and excreted by the kidneys.

Ergonovine has no significant drug interactions. The side effects/adverse reactions include nausea, vomiting, diarrhea, dizziness, tinnitus, increased sweating, confusion, hypertension, chest pain and, rarely, respiratory difficulties, pruritus, cold hands or feet, leg weakness, and pain in the arms, legs, or lower back.

The oral dosage for ergonovine maleate tablets is 0.2 to 0.4 mg two to four times daily (on a schedule of every 6 to 12 hours). The usual treatment course is 48 hours. Parenterally, 0.2 mg is administered intramuscularly or intravenously and repeated in 2 to 4 hours if necessary for up to five doses. The IV route is usually recommended only in emergencies or in cases of excessive uterine bleeding.

▪ Nursing Management

Ergonovine Therapy

▪ Assessment. If the client cannot tolerate other ergot derivatives, she may not tolerate ergonovine. Its use is contraindicated in clients with unstable angina or recent myocardial infarction, because ergonovine-induced vasospasm may precipitate another attack. Because ergonovine causes coronary vasospasm, it should be used cautiously in clients who have coronary artery disease, cardiovascular disease, mitral valve stenosis, or venoatrial shunts; ergonovine increases susceptibility to angina and myocardial infarction. Clients with occlusive peripheral vascular disease or Raynaud's phenomenon may experience an exacerbation of their ischemia. Ergonovine may also increase blood pressure; its use should be limited in clients with hypertension, preeclampsia, eclampsia, and a history of transient ischemic attacks and cerebrovascular accidents. As with most drugs, ergonovine is to be administered with care to clients with hepatic or renal function impairment. Clients who are septic may have an increased sensitivity to the drug.

The administration of ergonovine is contraindicated before delivery of the placenta, because it may result in entrapment of the placenta. It is not to be used for the induction of labor or in cases of threatened spontaneous abortion.

A baseline standard should be determined for the pulse, blood pressure, and uterine response. If indicated for the diagnosis of variant angina pectoris, a baseline blood pressure and electrocardiogram (ECG) should be obtained.

▪ Nursing Diagnosis. Clients receiving ergonovine are at risk for the following nursing diagnoses/collaborative problems: impaired comfort (severe uterine cramping, dizziness, sweating, nausea and vomiting); diarrhea; disturbed sensory perception (ringing in the ears); and the potential complications of severe hypertension, coronary vasospasm (chest pain), bradycardia, myocardial infarction, peripheral vasospasm, allergic reaction, and overdose (ergotism), with such symptoms as severe headache, diarrhea, nausea and vomiting, peripheral vasospasm, respiratory depression, and seizures.

▪ Implementation

▪ Monitoring. The client's blood pressure and pulse should be monitored, as well as fundal tone and placement; the character and amount of vaginal bleeding should also be assessed. If the client has chest pain, the physician or nurse-midwife should be notified immediately and an ECG obtained. ECG monitoring is essential if the drug is used for the diagnosis of variant angina pectoris.

If the client does not respond to the drug, tests to determine serum calcium levels should be performed. The correction of hypocalcemia with IV calcium salts will restore the oxytocic action of the drug.

The client should be observed for signs of ergotism, such as headache, nausea and vomiting, peripheral ischemia, and paresthesia.

▪ Intervention. When given intravenously, the drug should be administered slowly over a minimum of 1 minute.

▪ Education. Clients should be instructed to avoid smoking, because nicotine enhances the effects of ergonovine. The client should be alerted that discomfort may result from ergonovine-related uterine contractions and should be instructed about appropriate analgesics and nonpharmacologic methods to alleviate the discomfort.

▪ Evaluation. The expected outcome of ergonovine therapy is that the client will experience a reduction in or absence of uterine bleeding and will have stable vital signs.

methylergonovine [meth ill er goe noe' veen] (Methergine)

The mechanism of action is direct stimulation of the smooth muscle of the uterine wall, which results in hemostasis. Methylergonovine is indicated to prevent and treat postpartum hemorrhage. It may be administered orally or parenter-

BOX 53-1

Update: Terbutaline in Premature Labor

Terbutaline, a $beta_2$-adrenergic stimulant (betamimetic) is used investigationally for the inhibition of premature labor. Studies indicate that parenteral terbutaline is as effective as ritodrine, although the incidence of side effects/adverse reactions is significantly higher with terbutaline. The adverse effects of terbutaline may be dose related.

To prevent recurrent labor, oral terbutaline (30 mg/day) was more effective than oral ritodrine (120 mg/day) (Sagraves, Letassy, & Barton, 1995). Although terbutaline is being used for preterm labor inhibition, it is still not included as an indication for its use in U.S. drug labeling (*United States Pharmacopeia Dispensing Information,* 1999).

A meta-analysis of recent research (Sanchez-Ramos et al., 1999) does not support routine administration of maintenance tocolytic treatment after parenteral tocolytic therapy has halted acute preterm labor.

ally; the onset of a postpartum uterine contraction effect is as follows: orally, within 5 to 10 minutes; IM, 2 to 5 minutes; IV, immediately. The duration of action is approximately 3 hours for oral or IM dosage forms; the effect of the IV dosage form lasts approximately 45 minutes. This drug is metabolized in the liver and excreted by the kidneys.

Methylergonovine has no reported significant drug interactions; see the discussion of ergonovine for the side effects/adverse reactions of this drug.

The oral dosage of methylergonovine is 200 to 400 μg two to four times daily (spaced every 6 to 12 hours) until uterine bleeding and atony are under control. Oral dosing usually follows the administration of an initial parenteral dose.

Nursing management is the same as for ergonovine therapy.

Premature Labor Inhibitors

Preterm labor, or labor that occurs before the thirty-seventh week of pregnancy, is a major problem in obstetrics. It occurs in approximately 10% to 15% of all pregnancies. Premature birth increases the possibility of neonatal morbidity and mortality. Ritodrine is the prototype for premature labor inhibitors. Although terbutaline is being used to inhibit premature labor, its use is considered investigational (see Box 53-1).

ritodrine [ri' toe dreen] (Yutopar)

Ritodrine, a $beta_2$-adrenergic stimulant that relaxes uterine muscle by inhibiting uterine contractions, is indicated to prevent and treat uncomplicated premature labor in pregnancies of 20 or more weeks' gestation.

This drug is available orally and parenterally. With oral administration, the drug has an onset of action within ½ to 1 hour; the onset of action of the IV form is within 5 minutes. The time to peak serum concentration by both routes is within 1 hour. The half-life of the oral form is biphasic: 1.3 and 12 hours (in male testing); the IV half-life has three phases: 6 to 9 minutes, 1.7 to 2.6 hours, and 15 to 17 hours in nonpregnant females. This drug is metabolized in the liver and excreted by the kidneys.

The side effects/adverse reactions of IV ritodrine include increased maternal heart rate and increased systolic and decreased diastolic maternal blood pressure. The oral dosage forms may cause small increases in maternal heart rate but do not affect maternal blood pressure or fetal heart rate. Both dosage forms may cause trembling or tremors, anxiety, or restlessness. Nausea, vomiting, headaches, tachycardia, irregular heart rate and, rarely, chest pain and respiratory difficulties are reported with IV administration.

The IV dosage of ritodrine is 50 to 100 μg/min, which is increased in 50-μg increments every 10 minutes (as necessary) to an effective dosage. The maintenance dosage is 150 to 350 μg/min IV, which is continued for 12 to 24 hours after labor contractions have stopped. Oral ritodrine therapy is then instituted.

The initial oral dosage is 10 mg ½ hour before the ritodrine infusion is stopped, then 10 mg every 2 hours for 24 hours. The maintenance dosage is 10 to 20 mg PO every 4 to 6 hours until birth or as directed by the prescriber. The maximum recommended daily dose is 120 mg. Although the use of oral ritodrine for the treatment of preterm labor is approved in Canada, the USP Obstetrics and Gynecology Advisory Panel does not recommend its use because its efficacy has not been established. Bed rest at home and early admission are considered better alternatives than oral ritodrine. The results of a meta-analysis by Sanchez-Ramos, Kaunitz, Gaudier, & Delke (1999) do not support the use of maintenance tocolytic therapy after the successful treatment of preterm labor.

■ Nursing Management

Ritodrine Therapy

■ **Assessment.** The length of gestation should be determined, because ritodrine is not recommended for use before the twentieth week of pregnancy. Preterm labor should not have progressed more than 4 cm of cervical dilation or 80% effacement, or the drug may be ineffective. The use of ritodrine in clients with ruptured membranes may lead to intrauterine infection. The risk to the fetus must be considered because ritodrine crosses the placenta. Neonatal hypoglycemia, ketoacidosis, and tachycardia have been reported.

Ritodrine is contraindicated when the client has cardiovascular disorders or hyperthyroidism, because dysrhythmias or heart failure may occur. It is also contraindicated in clients with eclampsia, severe preeclampsia, or pulmonary hypertension. Immediate delivery is required for clients with intrauterine infection, nonreassuring fetal status, or intrauterine fetal death. Caution is indicated if the client has abruptio placentae, maternal hemorrhage, placenta previa, diabetes, or mild to moderate preeclampsia.

Review the client's current medication regimen for the risk of significant drug interactions, such as those that may occur when ritodrine is given concurrently with the following drugs:

Drug	Possible Effect and Management
Bold/color type indicates the most serious interactions.	
beta-adrenergic agonists	Concurrent use may cause an increased sympathomimetic response, such as hypertension or cardiac problems. Allow sufficient time after discontinuing one before beginning another.
beta-adrenergic blocking agents (labetalol nadolol, propranolol, and others)	Use is not recommended because the two drugs are antagonistic toward each other. Drugs with greater beta1 selectivity may be less antagonistic.
corticosteroids, long-acting (betamethasone, dexamethasone, paramethasone)	Concurrent drug use has resulted in pulmonary edema and death in pregnant women. Avoid concurrent use or a potentially serious drug interaction may occur. If concurrent drug administration is absolutely necessary, monitor closely and discontinue both drugs at the first sign of pulmonary edema.

A baseline assessment of the client's labor patterns should be obtained before initiating ritodrine therapy. A determination should be made of the client's beliefs, attitudes, and values regarding the possible premature birth in order to enhance the educational and emotional support provided by the nurse. See the Cultural Considerations box at right for a cultural perspective of premature birth.

■ **Nursing Diagnosis.** Clients receiving ritodrine are at risk for the following nursing diagnoses/collaborative problems: excess fluid volume (pulmonary edema [15% with IV use]); impaired comfort related to headache (10% to 15% with IV use), trembling (10% to 15%), or nausea and vomiting (10% to 15% with IV use, 5% to 8% with oral use); impaired skin integrity (rash [3% to 4% with oral use]); anxiety (5% to 8%); and the potential complications of altered cardiac output (tachycardia), which could result in angina (15% IV use); maternal hyperglycemia (80% to 100 % with IV use); decreased maternal diastolic blood pressure (80% to 100% with IV use); fetal and maternal cardiac dysrhythmias (80% to 100% with IV use); or hepatic function impairment.

■ **Implementation**

■ ***Monitoring.*** The client's blood pressure, heart rate, and uterine activity, as well as the fetal heart rate, should be monitored periodically. Increases in maternal heart rate and systolic blood pressure are common with IV ritodrine. Oral doses do not affect maternal blood pressure. If the maternal heart rate is greater than 120 beats/min or the fetal heart rate is greater than 170 or 180 beats/min, the IV rate may be slowed or the dosage decreased without reducing the effectiveness of ritodrine. It is recommended that ritodrine therapy be discontinued if labor persists after administration of the maximum dosage.

Blood glucose level, lung sounds, and fluid and electrolyte balance should be monitored in clients receiving prolonged IV therapy. Monitor fluids closely to prevent circulatory overload. Tachycardia and dyspnea may indicate impending pulmonary edema. Other side effects for which to observe are headache, nausea and vomiting, erythema, and trembling.

■ ***Intervention.*** When administering ritodrine intravenously, a controlled infusion device should be used to better enable dosage titration. Avoid the use of sodium chloride for infusion because of the risk of pulmonary edema. The client is placed on her left side to reduce blood pressure changes. IV administration is usually continued for 12 to 24 hours after contractions stop. If labor is irreversible, ritodrine is discontinued so that both the mother and the fetus can recover from hyperglycemia or other metabolic alteration before delivery.

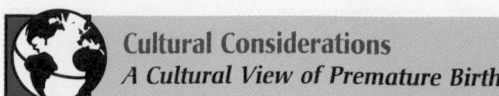

Cultural Considerations

A Cultural View of Premature Birth

In a recent article, Corrine, Bailey, Valentin, Morantus, and Shirley (1992) describe a situation involving Lily, a 30-year-old Haitian woman who has had a series of more than 11 miscarriages. A nurse visited her after her most recent miscarriage and found her very sad. Lily said, "I was almost seven months pregnant. I've never gotten that close before. I really thought I was going to have this baby." She continued, "You know, my husband's mother has hated me from day one. She promised that I would never have a child while she was alive. She sold my womb to the devil. But I kept praying to God that this condition would be reversed."

Many Haitian people are Roman Catholic but also practice voodoo, a religion of African origin in which the faithful congregate to worship the gods or spirits, known as loa. These spirits are believed to be angels who rebelled against God; they are thought to have great powers and provide favors related to protection, wealth, and health. Those who practice voodoo believe their sicknesses or problems are the result of an evil spirit. Western health services may be bypassed initially or are a second choice. The childbearing experience may be particularly culture bound.

Critical Thinking Question

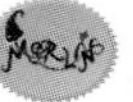

- How does a belief system such as Lily's influence the instruction the nurse provides related to ritodrine and the premature birth experience?

■ ***Education.*** The client should be cautioned to notify the prescriber if her water breaks or if her contractions begin again. If the client's contractions do not recur, she may gradually resume ambulation and other activities of daily living after 36 to 48 hours.

■ **Evaluation.** The expected outcome of ritodrine therapy is that the client will show evidence of the absence of premature labor.

DRUGS THAT INHIBIT LACTATION

Androgens have been used to treat postpartum breast engorgement (methyltestosterone, fluoxymesterone, and testosterone propionate) and to inhibit lactation (bromocriptine [Parlodel]). The use of estrogens for breast engorgement has declined over the years, mainly because the incidence of painful engorgement is considered low, and studies have indicated that analgesics or other supportive therapies are quite effective.

Bromocriptine directly inhibits the release of prolactin from the anterior pituitary gland, resulting in the suppression of lactation. For further information on bromocriptine, refer to the drug monograph for dopamine agonists in Chapter 23.

SUMMARY

Although many drugs are available for use during the process of labor and delivery, it is essential to consider the possible alteration of drug pharmacokinetics during labor and to weigh the risks and benefits to the fetus. The drugs discussed in this chapter focus on uterine contractility, which controls the labor process. Drugs that increase or decrease the contractility of the uterus also enhance or inhibit labor.

Oxytocics are drugs that increase uterine motility to induce labor, augment labor, control postpartum hemorrhage, and facilitate milk ejection during lactation. The most commonly used oxytocics are oxytocin, ergonovine, and methylergonovine. When oxytocics are used to induce or augment labor, the nurse should perform a baseline assessment of fetal heart tones, uterine status, and maternal vital signs. These indicators should be monitored every 15 to 30 minutes during the administration of these drugs.

Premature labor (labor that occurs before the thirty-seventh week of pregnancy) increases the possibility of neonatal morbidity and mortality. Ritodrine may be prescribed once a determination is made that it is in the best interest of the mother and the fetus to halt the labor process. Ritodrine, a $beta_2$-adrenergic stimulant that relaxes uterine muscle and inhibits uterine contractions, is used to prevent and treat premature labor in pregnancies of at least 20 weeks' gestation.

The role of the nurse in the administration of these drugs is to facilitate a healthy outcome for both the fetus and the mother.

Critical Thinking Questions

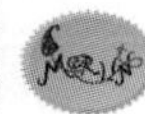

1. Shirley Demas is admitted to labor and delivery in possible preterm labor at 30 weeks' gestation. She is to be treated with ritodrine. What observations will be most relevant to determine the maternal side effects of this drug? Mrs. Demas' contractions do not abate, and betamethasone is ordered. The client asks you why she is receiving this drug. What is your response?
2. Lillian Chandler is admitted to the hospital for the birth of her first child. The nurse-midwife assesses that Mrs. Chandler is experiencing irregular contractions and decides to stimulate her labor by administering oxytocin. What assessments are required before such therapy can begin?

Collaborative Learning Activities

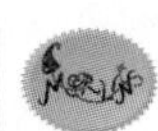

For Collaborative Learning Activities, go to mosby.com/MERLIN/McKenry/.

CASE STUDY

For a Case Study that will help ensure mastery of this chapter content, go to mosby.com/MERLIN/McKenry/.

BIBLIOGRAPHY

American Hospital Formulary Service. (1999). *AHFS drug information '99*. Bethesda, MD: American Society of Hospital Pharmacists.

Anderson, K.N., Anderson, L.E., & Glanze, W.D. (Eds.). (1998). *Mosby's medical, nursing, & allied health dictionary* (5th ed.). St. Louis: Mosby.

Bobak, I.M., Lowdermilk, D.L., & Jensen, M.D. (1995). *Maternity nursing* (4th ed.). St. Louis: Mosby.

Corrine, L., Bailey, V., Valentin, M., Morantus, E., & Shirley, L. (1992). The unheard voices of women: Spiritual interventions in maternal-child health. *Maternal Child Nursing, 17*(3), 141-145.

Cowam, M. (1993). Home care of the pregnant woman using terbutaline. *Maternal Child Nursing, 18*(2), 99-105.

Merrill, D.C. & Zlatnik, F.J. (1999). Randomized, double-masked comparison of oxytocin dosage in induction and augmentation of labor. *Obstetrics & Gynecology, 94*(3), 455-463.

Papke, K.R. (1993). Management of preterm labor and prevention of premature delivery. *Nursing Clinics of North America, 28*(2), 279-288.

Sagraves, R., Letassy, N.A., & Barton, T.L. (1995). Obstetrics. In L.Y. Young & M.A. Koda-Kimble (Eds.), *Applied therapeutics: The clinical use of drugs* (6th ed.). Vancouver, WA: Applied Therapeutics.

Sanchez-Ramos, L., Kaunitz, A.M., Gaudier, F.L., & Delke, I. (1999). Efficacy of maintenance therapy after acute tocolysis: A meta-analysis. *American Journal of Obstetrics & Gynecology, 181*(2), 484-490.

United States Pharmacopeia Dispensing Information (USP DI): Drug information for the health care professional (19th ed.). (1999). Rockville, MD: United States Pharmacopeial Convention.

54 Drugs Affecting the Male Reproductive System

Chapter Focus

Androgens are usually prescribed for androgen deficiency. When they are prescribed for other indications, their most common undesirable effect is virilism—the development of masculine characteristics. Body image disturbance may be of concern for clients who have an androgen deficiency or are receiving androgen therapy. The nurse must be prepared to encourage the client to express perceptions of self and provide reliable information about health concerns.

Learning Objectives

1. Compare the pharmacokinetics of three preparations of testosterone.
2. Discuss the approved indications for androgen (testosterone) therapy.
3. List the side effects/adverse reactions of androgen therapy.
4. Implement the nursing management for the care of clients undergoing androgen therapy.
5. Discuss the use of finasteride for benign prostatic hyperplasia.
6. Implement nursing management for the care of clients receiving finasteride therapy and other drugs affecting the male reproductive system.

Key Terms

androgens, p. 915
hypogonadism, p. 915
testosterone, p. 915

Key Drugs [✔]

testosterone, p. 915

Androgens, primarily testosterone, are male sex hormones necessary for the normal development and maintenance of male sex characteristics. Testosterone and its derivatives and synthetic agents are commonly used as replacement therapy for males who lack the hormone. In individuals with **hypogonadism** or eunuchoidism (a deficiency of male hormone), the androgens produce marked changes in the growth of the male sex organs, body contour, voice, and other secondary sex characteristics. Drugs that affect sexual behavior and impotence, such as sildenafil (Viagra), are reviewed in Chapter 55.

Hypertrophy of glandular and connective tissue in the portions of the prostate that surround the urethra, or benign prostatic hyperplasia (BPH), is considered a normal age-related change in men. Finasteride (Proscar) is a welcome addition to the treatment of BPH, which until recently had been almost exclusively surgical.

✔TESTOSTERONE

Testosterone, a naturally occurring androgenic hormone produced primarily by the testes, regulates male development. It is available in combination with esters to prolong its duration of action. For example, testosterone propionate is formulated in an oily solution that produces hormonal effects for 2 or 3 days. Testosterone cypionate and testosterone enanthate in oil are much longer acting and are usually administered once every 2 to 4 weeks. Testosterone pellets are available for subcutaneous implantation. This form also provides an extended duration of action; depending on the number of pellets used, replacement pellets may not be necessary for 2 to 6 months.

A transdermal testosterone system (Testoderm) was marketed in 1996. This system is applied to scrotal skin, where testosterone is highly absorbed at a rate at least five times greater than other skin sites. A second transdermal testosterone (Androderm) is also available and is applied to nonscrotal skin. This system requires the application of two patches nightly, every 24 hours. Either system requires an application at approximately 10 PM so that maximum serum concentrations are achieved in the morning; this simulates the normal circadian rhythm in healthy young males (*Drug Facts and Comparisons*, 2000).

Oral testosterone is absorbed but is highly metabolized by the liver before it reaches the systemic circulation. Administering methyltestosterone by the buccal route of administration increases its serum level and effectiveness. Fluoxymesterone is a synthetic androgen that is effective orally in tablet form.

Mechanism of Action. As a natural hormone in normal males, androgens are responsible for the stimulation of spermatogenesis, the development of secondary male sex characteristics and, at puberty, sexual maturity. Testosterone also stimulates the synthesis and activity of RNA, which results in increased production of protein. Androgens are also potent anabolic agents; they stimulate the formation and maintenance of muscular and skeletal protein. They bring about the retention of nitrogen (essential to the formation of protein in the body) and enhance the storage of inorganic phosphorus, sulfate, sodium, and potassium.

Athletes have used androgens to increase weight, musculature, and muscle strength. Weight gain may be caused by fluid retention, a side effect of androgen therapy. The potential risk of developing major serious adverse reactions from androgens far outweighs the advantages to be gained in athletic events. Many major sporting events disqualify athletes who have documented use of such products. Additional information on the abuse of androgens can be found in Chapter 9.

Indications. Testosterones are indicated for the following:

1. Treatment of androgen deficiency, such as testicular failure caused by cryptorchidism (failure of one or both testes to descend into the scrotum), orchitis (inflammation of the testes), orchidectomy (surgical removal of one or both testes), or pituitary-hypothalamic insufficiency
2. Treatment of delayed male puberty when not induced by a pathologic condition
3. Treatment of breast carcinoma; palliative or secondary treatment for inoperable metastatic breast cancer in postmenopausal women who have demonstrated a previous response to hormone therapy
4. Treatment of anemia; androgens stimulate erythropoiesis (production of erythrocytes) in certain types of anemia (primarily those that are refractory to other therapies), but this is not an approved indication for these products in the United States

Pharmacokinetics. The half-life of IM testosterone in plasma is 10 to 20 minutes; for oral fluoxymesterone, 9.2 hours; and for oral methyltestosterone, between 2.5 and 3.5 hours. The time to peak concentration for methyltestosterone, buccal tablet, is 1 hour; for the oral tablet, 2 hours. The duration of action depends on the dose and the ester formulation administered. The longest duration of action is for testosterone enanthate preparations, followed by cypionate and then propionate; the base form has the shortest duration of action. Testosterone is metabolized in the liver and excreted by the kidneys.

Side Effects/Adverse Reactions. The most common adverse reactions of testosterone in females are an increase in oily skin or acne, a deepening of the voice, increased hair growth or alopecia, an enlarged clitoris, and irregular menses. The deep voice or hoarseness may not reversed, even when the medication is stopped. The most common adverse reactions reported in males are urinary urgency, breast swelling or tenderness (gynecomastia), and frequent or continuous erections. Less common side effects of testosterone that occur in both sexes include abdominal pain, insomnia, diarrhea or constipation, dizziness, increased weakness, red skin or changes in skin color, redness at the site of injection, mouth soreness, frequent headaches, confusion, respiratory difficulties, depression, nausea, vomiting, pruritus, edema of the lower extremities, jaundice, an increase in bleeding episodes, and an unusual increase or decrease in libido.

Dosage and Administration

1. The choice of dosage and length of therapy depend on the diagnosis, the client's age and sex, and the intensity of the side effects/adverse reactions.
2. For delayed puberty and males with hypogonadism (a decrease in androgen secretion from the gonads), dosage regimens are started in the lower ranges and gradually increased according to the client's needs and response. With delayed puberty, androgens are discontinued for 1 to 3 months after 4 to 6 months of therapy, and x-ray examinations are evaluated to determine the drug's effect on bone growth. Males with hypogonadism will receive androgens throughout puberty, with dosage adjustments as required. Lower maintenance dosages are usually used after puberty.
3. Androgen antineoplastic therapy usually requires a 3-month period to evaluate effectiveness.
4. Temporary withdrawal of the drug is required if the male experiences priapism (persistent, abnormal penile erection). This is an indication of excessive dosing of the androgen.
5. Women with metastatic breast cancer should receive a shorter-acting androgen, especially during the initial therapies. It has been reported that androgens occasionally increase the progression of breast cancer.

Sterile Testosterone Suspension. The adult usual dosage is 25 to 50 mg IM two or three times weekly. Antineoplastic therapy for metastatic breast carcinoma in females is 50 to 100 mg three times weekly. The pediatric dosage for delayed puberty in males is 100 mg IM monthly for 4 to 6 months.

Testosterone Enanthate Injection. The usual adult dosage is 50 to 400 mg IM every 2 to 4 weeks. For antineoplastic therapy for inoperable breast cancer in females, the dosage is 200 to 400 mg every 2 to 4 weeks. The pediatric dosage for delayed puberty in males is 100 mg monthly for approximately 4 to 6 months.

Methyltestosterone Capsules (Metandren). The adult oral dosage for replacement therapy (hypogonadism, climacteric, or impotence) is 10 to 50 mg daily; for cryptorchidism, 10 mg PO three times daily; and for metastatic breast carcinoma in females, 50 mg one to four times daily. The pediatric dosage for delayed puberty in males is 5 to 25 mg/day for approximately 4 to 6 months.

Methyltestosterone Buccal Tablets (Metandren). The dosage is one half the capsule dosage previously noted.

Fluoxymesterone Tablets (Halotestin). The usual adult dosage is 5 mg one to four times daily. For metastatic breast carcinoma in females, the dosage is 20 to 50 mg daily for 2 to 6 months. The pediatric dosage for the treatment of delayed puberty in males is 2.5 to 10 mg daily for approximately 4 to 6 months.

■ Nursing Management

Testosterone Therapy

■ **Assessment.** Assess whether the male client has breast cancer or known or suspected prostatic cancer, because androgens will stimulate tumor growth and are thus contraindicated. These drugs should be used with caution in clients with cardiac impairment, severe cardiorenal disease, or nephrosis because they may cause fluid retention. Clients with prostatic hyperplasia may experience further enlargement. Impaired hepatic dysfunction may result in an increased half-life and so increase the incidence of gynecomastia. Because of the hypercholesterolemic effects of this drug, clients with a history of myocardial infarction or coronary artery disease may experience a worsening of their condition. Hypercalcemia secondary to metastatic breast cancer may be worsened.

Significant drug interactions have been reported with the concurrent administration of testosterone and oral anticoagulants (coumarin or indanedione) or other hepatotoxic medications. The anticoagulant effects are enhanced or increased, and the risk of inducing hepatotoxicity is increased.

A baseline assessment of children should include height, weight, and a description of their sexual development. For adults, a baseline description of the underlying condition for which the testosterone is being prescribed should be obtained.

■ **Nursing Diagnosis.** The client receiving androgen therapy is at risk for the following nursing diagnoses/collaborative problems: disturbed body image related to virilism in female clients and prepubertal males, gynecomastia and priapism in male clients, or increased or decreased libido in both sexes; excess fluid volume (rapid weight gain, edema of the feet and lower legs, shortness of breath); impaired comfort (headache, nausea, vomiting, and abdominal pain); disturbed sleep pattern (insomnia); impaired skin integrity (acne); impaired tissue integrity (pain, redness, and swelling at the injection site); and the potential complications of amenorrhea, oligomenorrhea, benign prostatic hyperplasia, hepatic impairment, hypercalcemia, erythrocytosis, and polycythemia.

■ **Implementation**

■ ***Monitoring.*** Monitor the client's serum calcium carefully. Promptly report indications of hypercalcemia: nausea and vomiting, lethargy, loss of muscle tone, polyuria, and increased urine and serum calcium levels. Hypercalcemia in clients with metastatic breast cancer usually indicates bone metastasis.

Serum cholesterol levels should be monitored to ascertain the client's risk of cardiovascular disease as the result of androgen administration. Hepatic function should also be monitored; hemoglobin and hematocrit should be evaluated for polycythemia. Bone age determinations should be performed every 6 months to assess the rate of bone maturation in children and adolescents. Tumor growth should be monitored by radiography. Older men should be observed for increasing difficulty or frequency of urination, which may indicate enlargement of the prostate secondary to the drug.

Total serum testosterone levels can help to determine appropriate dosages. When testing the testosterone levels of clients with transdermal systems, wait until the patch has been worn for 3 to 4 weeks. Draw the blood specimen 2 to 4 hours after patch application.

If androgens are administered for gender change androgen therapy, it is suggested that luteinizing hormone serum levels be determined every 6 months to monitor the success of therapy. ALTs should be monitored for adverse hepatic effects.

■ ***Intervention.*** Administer the oral preparations with food to minimize gastric distress. Administer IM testosterone deep within the gluteal muscle. Be aware that testosterone cypionate and testosterone enanthate are not interchangeable with testosterone propionate and suspension forms of the drug because of the difference in duration and action. With testosterone cypionate, the preparation may be warmed and shaken to dissolve the crystals. It may turn cloudy if a wet needle or syringe is used, but this does not affect its potency.

There is also a difference between the transdermal systems. The matrix type of patch is adhered to the scrotum and may be removed for swimming, bathing, or sexual activity. In contrast, the reservoir type of patch is placed on the abdomen, back, thighs, or upper arms and is not removed for those activities. Men over 65 years of age should not place patches on their backs, because doing so may cause a decrease in serum testosterone levels.

An implant form of testosterone can be inserted subcutaneously using local anesthesia. This implant is a crystallized form of testosterone that dissolves over 3 to 6 months.

The client should be encouraged to drink at least 3 to 4 L of fluids to ensure adequate urinary output to prevent urinary calculi. Active clients should be encouraged to perform weight-bearing exercise, such as walking daily. Clients confined to bed should perform range-of-motion exercises at least daily. This exercise inhibits the mobilization of calcium from bone.

Be sensitive to the emotional responses of clients taking androgens. Female clients may have changes in secondary sex characteristics, such as unnatural hair growth or heightened libido; these subside with cessation of the drug. Other changes that may occur, such as enlarged clitoris or hoarseness or deepening of the voice, may not be reversible. Adolescent male clients may need support to deal with deepening of the voice and rapid changes in height, size of sex organs, and hair growth patterns; these changes may occur more rapidly with testosterone than with normal growth and development. Frequent or continuing erection may be a concern.

■ ***Education.*** Work with the client and/or appropriate family member to develop a diet that is high in protein, calories, vitamins, and minerals and is individualized to the client's food preferences. Monitor the client with diabetes closely. Antidiabetic agents may require a dosage adjustment with concurrent administration of androgens. Instruct the client to weigh daily to monitor for fluid retention. Sodium restriction and/or diuretics may be required if edema occurs. Advise the client to maintain regular visits to the prescriber for monitoring progress.

Instruct the male client using the matrix type of transdermal patch to apply the patch to a clean, dry, and dry-shaved skin area of the scrotum. Caution the client not to use chemical depilatories. In addition, advise him that there is the potential to transfer testosterone to his female sexual partner, which might result in mild virilization. The reservoir-type patch site should be rotated between the abdomen, back, thighs, or upper arms and not applied to the scrotum, bony prominences, or any body area that would be subject to pressure when sitting or sleeping. If a patch from either system falls off and cannot be reapplied, do not use a new patch at that time, but return to the usual dosing schedule.

■ **Evaluation.** The expected outcome of testosterone therapy is that the client will show improvement of the underlying condition for which the drug has been prescribed.

BENIGN PROSTATIC HYPERPLASIA

Benign prostatic hyperplasia (BPH), the hypertrophy of the glandular and connective tissue in the portions of the prostate that surround the urethra, is considered a normal age-related change that begins in men around 40 years of age. By age 70, approximately 75% of males will develop BPH symptoms severe enough to require professional intervention (Thompson, 1995).

BPH obstructs the bladder neck and compresses the urethra, which results in urinary retention and increases the risk of bacteriuria. If left untreated, it may affect the ureters and kidneys and result in hydroureter, hydronephrosis, and renal impairment. Symptoms of BPH include hesitancy (difficulty starting the urinary stream), a decrease in the diameter and force of the stream, an inability to terminate urination abruptly that results in postvoid dribbling, and a sensation of incomplete bladder emptying that results in frequency and nocturia.

The pathophysiology of BPH may also include impaired detrusor contractility, sensory abnormalities of the bladder wall, and contractility of the smooth muscle of the prostatic urethra with functionally important alpha$_1$-adrenergic receptors; therefore pharmacologic treatment of BPH with nonselective adrenergic blockers has been tried. Prazosin (Minipress) has been used investigationally for this purpose, and terazosin (Hytrin) is approved for the treatment of BPH (*United States Pharmacopeia Dispensing Information*, 1999). (See Chapter 22 for a discussion of adrenergic blockers.) Finasteride, a 5-alpha reductase inhibitor, is also available for the treatment of BPH. (See the Complementary and Alternative Therapies box on p. 918.)

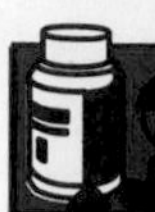

Complementary and Alternative Therapies
Saw Palmetto

Saw palmetto has been used traditionally to treat genitourinary problems such as chronic or subacute cystitis, decreased sperm production, and testicular atrophy. In recent years, saw palmetto has been investigated primarily for its therapeutic use in BPH. Increased DHT synthesis in the prostate and a shift in the androgen and estrogen ratio contributes to BPH. It is thought that the beneficial effects of saw palmetto—alleviating the symptoms of BPH—results from two actions: inhibition of the enzyme 5-alpha-reductase (inhibition prevents testosterone from converting to DHT) and the blocking of DHT binding at the androgen receptors. Use of the saw palmetto berry in clients with BPH has demonstrated improvements in urinary flow rates and ultrasound-determined residual urine volumes. Its use has also been demonstrated to decrease the frequency of nocturia.

Saw palmetto is considered safe when used in recommended dosages on a short-term basis. Side effects seem to be limited to headache and mild gastrointestinal upset. Because of its antiandrogenic and estrogenic properties, its use should be avoided in pregnancy and lactation and in clients taking oral contraceptives and hormone therapy. In client education, stress that urinary or prostate problems are not to be self-treated and that the diagnosis and management of therapy by a health care provider is essential.

The typical dosage of saw palmetto is 0.5 to 1 g of the dried berry or one cup of tea three times daily, which is prepared by simmering the dose of dried berry in 150 mL of boiling water for 5 to 10 minutes and then straining the solution before ingesting. Standardized extracts are available, which contain 80% to 95% fatty acids; the common dosage is 160 mg twice daily.

Information from Cirigliano, M.D. (1998). Ten most common herbs in clinical practice. In M.S. Micozzi (Ed.), *Current review of complementary medicine.* Philadelphia: Current Medicine; and Jellin, J.M., Batz, F., & Hitchens, K. (1999). *Pharmacist's letter/prescriber's letter natural medicines comprehensive database.* Stockton, CA: Therapeutic Research Faculty.

finasteride [fin ass' te ride] (Proscar)

Finasteride inhibits 5-alpha reductase, the enzyme that converts testosterone into the potent androgen 5-alpha dihydrotestosterone (DHT), a substance responsible for prostate gland growth. Finasteride decreases serum DHT by nearly 70%, which causes shrinkage of the enlarged prostate gland. It is the first of a new class of drugs approved by the Food and Drug Administration for the treatment of symptomatic BPH. Schafer et al. (1999) report that men treated with a daily dose of 5 mg of finasteride experienced a significant increase in urinary flow rate.

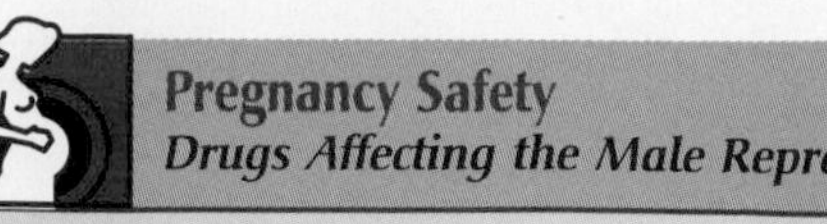

Pregnancy Safety
Drugs Affecting the Male Reproductive System

Category	Drug
C	terazosin
X	androgens, finasteride

Finasteride is 90% protein bound to plasma proteins, with maximum plasma concentrations reached 1 to 2 hours after oral administration. No dosage adjustments are required for older adults.

The side effects/adverse reactions of finasteride include decreased libido, impotency, and decreased amount of ejaculate. It is administered orally, 5 mg daily.

■ Nursing Management
Finasteride Therapy

■ **Assessment.** Finasteride is contraindicated in individuals with a hypersensitivity to any component of the drug. There is no indication for use in women and children. It should be used with caution in clients with liver function impairment. Determine whether the client has been evaluated for prostate cancer, because finasteride may interfere with the serum prostate-specific antigen (PSA) test, a test that may be used to screen for prostatic cancer. Drugs such as anticholinergics (or those with anticholinergic activity), adrenergic bronchodilators, and xanthine-derivative bronchodilators may precipitate or worsen urinary retention and so reduce the effectiveness of finasteride.

A baseline assessment of the client should include liver function studies, prostatic status, and an evaluation of the client's urinary elimination pattern.

■ **Nursing Diagnosis.** The client receiving finasteride is at risk for sexual dysfunction related to impotence and decreased libido; impaired comfort (headache, abdominal or back pain, dizziness, gynecomastia); diarrhea; and hypersensitivity reaction.

■ **Implementation**

■ ***Monitoring.*** Continue to monitor the client's urinary hesitancy, force of urinary stream, postvoid dribbling, nocturia, and frequency, urgency, and burning with urination. Periodic liver function studies should be accomplished. A periodic digital rectal examination will assist in detecting possible prostate cancer.

■ ***Intervention.*** Finasteride may be given with or without meals, because bioavailability is not affected by food. Women who are or may become pregnant should avoid handling the crushed tablets to avoid the possibility of transdermal absorption.

■ ***Education.*** Inform the client that 6 months of treatment may be necessary before the drug becomes effective in relieving symptoms. Alert the client that if his sexual partner is pregnant or to become pregnant, he should avoid exposing her to his semen because a small amount of the drug is present in semen (see the Pregnancy Safety box above).

Finasteride helps to control but does not cure BPH. Lifelong therapy may be necessary.

All clients with BPH should avoid drinking fluids, especially coffee and alcohol, in the evening to minimize nocturia. If the male client is using finasteride for male-pattern baldness, alert him that it will take at least 3 months to see an effect and that any improvement will only last as long as the medication is taken.

■ **Evaluation.** The expected outcome of finasteride therapy is that the client's prostate will decrease in size, and the client will not experience urinary hesitancy, urinary dribbling, nocturia, or frequency and urgency of urination. If finasteride is taken for male-pattern baldness, the client will experience hair growth.

SUMMARY

Androgens, the male sex hormones, are responsible for the normal development and maintenance of male sex characteristics. Testosterone is most commonly used for hormonal replacement therapy in males and is also indicated for the treatment of breast carcinoma and anemia. Clients receiving androgen therapy require additional support because of their risk for self-concept disturbance as a result of the drug's effects on secondary sex characteristics. Although testosterone may be essential for an improvement in health status, the development of virilism in female clients, gynecomastia and priapism in male clients, and a change in libido may be distressing for clients of both sexes.

Finasteride, a 5-alpha reductase inhibitor, is being used in the treatment of BPH and male-pattern baldness with positive results.

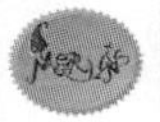

Critical Thinking Questions

1. Althea Johnson, who is 54 years old and 3 years postmenopause, has an estrogen-dependent tumor. The physician has prescribed testosterone for her condition. What do you need to teach Ms. Johnson about the effects of testosterone in women?
2. Ed Taylor, who is 56 years old and a widower of 2 years, has just been placed on finasteride. What assessments of his sexuality and sexual functioning pattern will be necessary?

Collaborative Learning Activities

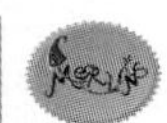

For Collaborative Learning Activities, go to mosby.com/MERLIN/McKenry/.

BIBLIOGRAPHY

American Hospital Formulary Service. (1999). *AHFS drug information '99*. Bethesda, MD: American Society of Hospital Pharmacists.

Anderson, K.N., Anderson, L.E., & Glanze, W.D. (Eds.) (1998). *Mosby's medical, nursing, & allied health dictionary* (5th ed.) St. Louis: Mosby.

Drug Facts and Comparisons. (2000). St. Louis: Facts and Comparisons.

Hardman, J.G. & Limbird, L.E. (Eds.). (1996). *Goodman and Gilman's The pharmacological basis of therapeutics* (9th ed.). New York: Macmillan.

Miller, C.A. (1993). New medication for the treatment of benign prostatic hyperplasia. *Geriatric Nursing, 14*(2), 111-112.

Monda, J.M. & Oesterling, J.E. (1994). Medical management of prostatic obstruction. *Journal of Urological Nursing, 13*(2), 717-738.

Schafer, W., Tammela, T.L., Barrett, D.M., Abrams, P., Hedlund, H., Rollema, H.J., Nordling, J., Andersen, J.T., Hald, T., Matos-Ferriera, A., Bruskewitz, R., Miller, P., Mustonen, S., Cannon, A., Malice, M.P., Jacobsen, C.A., Bach, M.A. (1999). Continued improvement in pressure-flow parameters in men receiving finasteride for 2 years: Finasteride Urodynamics Study Group. *Urology, 54*(2), 278-283.

Thompson, J.R. (1995). Geriatric urological disorders. In L.Y. Young & M.A. Koda-Kimble (Eds.), *Applied therapeutics: The clinical use of drugs*. Vancouver, WA: Applied Therapeutics.

United States Pharmacopeia Dispensing Information (USP DI): Drug information for the health care professional (19th ed.). (1999). Rockville, MD: United States Pharmacopeial Convention.

55 Drugs Affecting Sexual Behavior

Chapter Focus

Sexuality is an integral part of one's identity; it is a reflection of how one feels about oneself and how one interacts with others. Sexual function refers to the psychologic and physiologic ability to perform in a sexually satisfying manner, with or without a partner (Carpenito, 2000). Drugs can influence both sexuality and sexual function. The nurse should be able to discuss sexual health with the client and provide information about medications and their effects on sexual behavior.

Learning Objectives

1. Describe the effect of drugs on sexual behavior.
2. Identify the effect of commonly prescribed drugs, such as antihypertensives, antihistamines, antispasmodics, sedatives and tranquilizers, antidepressants, ethyl alcohol, barbiturates, steroid hormones, and methadone, on the libido.
3. Discuss drugs that may affect sexual behavior to enhance libido or sexual gratification.
4. Identify client cues about problems related to drug use and sexuality.
5. Provide appropriate client education about drugs that have the potential to cause sexual dysfunction.

Key Terms

impotence, p. 921
libido, p. 921
premenstrual syndrome (PMS), p. 923

Key Drugs [✔]

sildenafil, p. 925

Sexuality and sexual behavior have psychologic, social, and physiologic dimensions that reflect a complexity beyond drug-related effects. Contributing factors include self-esteem, general health, availability of a partner, appropriate environment, and perhaps age. Because drugs can affect sexual activities or sexual identity, nurses must be sensitive to their clients' needs as sexual beings and alert to cues that reflect problems. Clients may present these cues if given the chance, such as confusion or embarrassment about a lack of interest in sexual activities, about a lack of arousal despite desire, or about other phenomena they consider unusual. Nurses need to be aware of the potential sexual side effects of common drugs; with this knowledge, they can ask clients about sexual function as part of a routine drug history to determine issues that might influence the client's adherence to therapy (Kochar, Mazur, & Patel, 1999).

Certain drug therapies can produce one or more side effects/adverse reactions; among these are decreased levels of testosterone, which is normally present in both sexes and enhances **libido** or sexual drive; increased levels of estrogen; emotional depression that effectively limits interest or response to sexual stimuli; or autonomic nervous system blockade, which may interfere with tumescence, lubrication, erection, or ejaculation. The references at the end of this chapter and the information in Chapter 51 provide a better understanding of the structure and function of the reproductive systems.

Many physiologic functions significant to sexual pleasure are controlled by the psyche and the autonomic nervous system (see also Chapter 20). The autonomic nervous system comprises two parts—the sympathetic (adrenergic) and parasympathetic (cholinergic) systems—and its functional units are nerves, nerve plexuses, and ganglia. Although viewed as physiologic antagonists, the two systems often have synergistic effects on sexual functioning.

The male and female sexual organs are composed of homologous tissues; although the shapes of the organs differ, they correspond part for part in structure, position, and embryologic origin. The genital protuberance of the embryo appears identical in both sexes. The embryo is characteristically female initially and does not differentiate until fetal androgens begin to masculinize tissues (seventh to twelfth weeks of pregnancy). Thus it is not surprising that the mature analogous organs function similarly.

In the male, sympathetic (adrenergic) impulses produce ejaculation by causing contraction of the prostate and seminal vesicles along with effects on the bulbocavernous and ischiocavernous muscles. **Impotence,** or impotency, is the inability of the adult male to achieve or maintain a penile erection, along with decreased sexual function. Drugs that block adrenergic impulses may affect ejaculatory function through sympathetic blockade.

Parasympathetic (cholinergic) stimulation controls penile erection. This response results from congestion of the vascular sinuses in the penile corpora caused by parasympathetic nerve action in the venous channels. Drugs that interfere with parasympathetic nerve transmitters (cholinergic nerves) can cause defects in erection. Ganglionic blocking agents, which may block both sympathetic and parasympathetic nerve transmission, can cause complete impotence and impaired sexual functioning.

In the female, parasympathetic (cholinergic) impulses cause arterial dilation and venoconstriction, which produce clitoral erection and vasocongestion of the vulva, transudation (oozing of a fluid through pores) of lubricating secretions from the vaginal walls, and swelling of the introitus (vaginal opening). Continued stimulation of the clitoris and/or the Graefenberg spot, which is located on the anterior wall of the vagina, may then produce orgasm and, for some, a miniature facsimile of ejaculation from glands that surround the female urethra.

DRUGS THAT IMPAIR LIBIDO AND SEXUAL GRATIFICATION

Antihypertensives

Central-acting alpha$_2$ agonists such as methyldopa (Aldomet), clonidine (Catapres), guanabenz (Wytensin), and guanfacine (Tenex) have been associated with more frequent reports of impotence and sexual dysfunction. Difficulty in ejaculation has been reported with guanethidine (Ismelin), and reserpine (Serpasil) may induce impotence or a decreased interest in sex.

Anticholinergic drugs, especially those with ganglionic blocking activity, may also produce impotence and other untoward effects on sexual function. Guanethidine falls into this category. Other agents include mecamylamine (Inversine) and trimethaphan (Arfonad), which are used as antihypertensive agents. Because these drugs may block both sympathetic and parasympathetic innervation of the sex organs, both erectile capability and ejaculatory function may be affected during their use.

Diuretics

The thiazide diuretics may induce sexual dysfunction, and spironolactone (Aldactone) has been associated with a decrease in libido, impotence, and gynecomastia. Spironolactone is associated with considerably more reports of sexual dysfunction than the thiazides; this effect appears to be dose related.

Antihistamines

Antihistaminic drugs act as competitive inhibitors of histamine at physiologic receptor sites to prevent histaminic effects. Well-known examples of such drugs include diphenhydramine (Benadryl), promethazine (Phenergan), and chlorpheniramine (Chlor-Trimeton). These drugs are consumed by millions as antiemetics, as mild sedatives, and for the control of allergy symptoms. Most antihistamines display anticholinergic effects such as dry mouth, urinary retention, and constipation. Continuous use of these drugs may interfere with sexual activity. This effect is presumably mediated by the blockade of parasympathetic nerve impulses to the sex glands and organs.

Antianxiety and Psychotropic Drugs

A wide variety of central-acting agents affect sexual interest and capability both directly and indirectly (Gutierrez & Stimmel, 1999). The benzodiazepines, phenothiazines, and short-acting barbiturates are often associated with sexual dysfunction.

Phenothiazines such as chlorpromazine (Thorazine), prochlorperazine (Compazine), thioridazine (Mellaril), and mesoridazine (Serentil) are commonly prescribed agents that often induce a sedative effect that may partly account for the decreased sexual interest of persons undergoing phenothiazine therapy.

In addition to their central nervous system (CNS) effects, the peripheral effects of phenothiazines may contribute to the inhibition of sexual function. These drugs decrease skeletal muscle tone and block cholinergic synapses at both muscarinic and nicotinic receptors. Various adrenergic impulses may also be inhibited. Impotence, decreased libido, ejaculation disorders, and prolonged amenorrhea have been reported in individuals taking phenothiazines. Failure to ejaculate has been reported in men treated with thioridazine, but erection and orgasm do not appear to be affected. Thioridazine, which has a significantly greater peripheral alpha-adrenergic blocking effect than the other phenothiazines, results in a higher incidence of ejaculation failure. Ejaculation problems have also been reported with the use of chlorprothixene (Taractan) and mesoridazine (Serentil).

Benzodiazepine compounds are commonly prescribed antianxiety medications. Diazepam (Valium) is used for treating anxiety and alcoholism and as a skeletal muscle relaxant. The sedative and relaxing effects of this drug may account for the decreased interest in sexual activity. There have been several reports of anorgasmia in males and females, as well as ejaculation failure (Thompson, 1995). Alternatively, the judicious use of these tranquilizers has been considered to be of value in the treatment of sexual impotence and other problems involving sexual performance when excessive anxiety is a factor.

Several other types of drugs used in the treatment of psychologic problems depress sexual activity in human beings. Haloperidol (Haldol), an antipsychotic, can adversely affect libido in men. Failure to ejaculate without a concomitant alteration of erection or orgasm has been reported in individuals treated with phenoxybenzamine (Dibenzyline), an alpha-adrenergic blocking agent once used to supplement psychiatric therapy. This drug has been referred to as the male contraceptive. Interestingly enough, this product has been used successfully in males with problems of premature ejaculation (Ruggiero, 1995).

Antidepressants

Depression is often associated with diminished sexual interest, drive, and activity (see Chapter 19), and the drugs used to treat depression often compound the negative effects on sexual function. Although antidepressants generally elevate mood and thus increase sexuality, they can cause impotence and have an adverse effect on sexual behavior. The effect of tricyclic antidepressants on sexuality may be related to peripheral anticholinergic effects, such as those produced by some antihypertensives. Examples of these drugs include imipramine (Tofranil) and amitriptyline (Elavil). Although monoamine oxidase (MAO) inhibitors may be used as antihypertensives and antidepressants, the impotence that can result may be caused by their tendency to block peripheral ganglionic nerve transmission. The selective serotonin reuptake inhibitors are also known to decrease libido and sexual function (Landen, Eriksson, Agren, & Fahlen, 1999; Shen, Urosevich, & Clayton, 1999).

Ethyl Alcohol

As a drug of individual and unique notoriety, ethyl alcohol is considered for its effects on human sexual function and behavior. Revered for centuries as a sexual stimulant and a cure for all illnesses, alcohol is in fact a depressant and is recognized today to have far greater social than therapeutic value. Although a sedative, alcohol in moderate amounts may enhance sexual activity by relieving anxieties and loosening the inhibitions that often shroud sexual behavior.

Beyond a certain limit, however, neither desire nor potency overcome the depressed physical capability that occurs under its influence. Studies on the pharmacologic action of alcohol show that the CNS is more affected by alcohol than is any other system of the body. Electrophysiologic studies suggest that alcohol initially depresses the part of the brain responsible for integrating the various activities of the nervous system. The result is that various processes related to thought and motor activities become disrupted. The first mental processes affected are related to sobriety and self-restraint, which produces a less inhibited and less restrained approach to sexual behavior and other activities normally inhibited by previous training or experience. With continued alcohol consumption, the brain becomes narcotized, reflexes become slowed, blood vessels are dilated, and the capacity for sexual function is diminished. In addition, alcohol produces a severe diuretic effect, which may also interfere with sexual function.

Typically, the male alcoholic experiences delayed ejaculation during intoxication; impotence can occur after years of chronic alcoholism. Vascular changes, peripheral neuropathy, and lower testosterone levels because of liver damage are thought to cause the impotence. The problem is compounded by body image changes such as testicular atrophy and gynecomastia.

Barbiturates

Barbiturates, such as amobarbital (Amytal), pentobarbital (Nembutal), secobarbital (Seconal), and thiopental (Pentothal), are sedative-hypnotic drugs that have general depressant effects on all nervous tissues. As with alcohol, these drugs in their prescribed dosage produce relaxation, hypnosis, and sleep with depression of various body functions, including sexual performance and ability. Barbiturates can cause respiratory failure and death with prolonged use or overdose. Withdrawal after long-term, heavy consumption of barbiturates may result in convulsions. There is no rationale for their use in altering sexual behavior in human beings.

H_2 Receptor Antagonists

H_2 receptor antagonists such as cimetidine (Tagamet) and ranitidine (Zantac) have been reported to cause antiandrogenic effects (impotence, gynecomastia) when administered in high doses for a prolonged period.

Hormones and Derivatives

Sex hormones act on the CNS and other body organs to influence sexual and aggressive behavior, as well as mood and emotional outlook. Variations in female hormones may produce the anxiety, irritability, and depression associated with **premenstrual syndrome** (PMS), whereas male hormones are associated with aggression and increased sexual interest. Evidence indicates that sexual drive may be influenced by treatment with sex hormones.

The anabolic steroids are derived from or are related to the male sex hormone testosterone. They have been misused by athletes and other postpubertal persons to promote muscle growth and endurance. The effects of these drugs on strength and development are questionable when used by normally developed, well-nourished individuals. Considerable evidence indicates that these drugs cause (1) virilization, hirsutism, libido changes, and clitoral enlargement in females, and (2) testicular atrophy, impotence, chronic priapism, and oligospermia in males (see Chapter 9).

Additional Medications

A number of other medications have been reported to cause sexual dysfunction. Ketoconazole (Nizoral), an antifungal agent, may cause oligospermia and decreased libido in males (Cleary, Chapman, Clark, & Lucia, 1995). Propranolol (Inderal), a beta-blocking agent, has been associated with decreased libido and erectile dysfunction. Nifedipine (Adalat, Procardia), diltiazem (Cardizem), and verapamil (Calan, Isoptin) are calcium channel blocking agents that may cause erectile dysfunction. Opioids have also been associated with sexual dysfunction (Thompson, 1995).

DRUGS THAT ENHANCE LIBIDO AND SEXUAL GRATIFICATION

Substances to increase sexual potency or drive have been sought throughout history. Inscriptions in the ruins of ancient cultures have described the preparation of "erotic potions," and an endless number of "aphrodisiacs" have been described since then. In contemporary society many drugs and chemicals that modify mood and behavior are claimed to have aphrodisiac properties.

In reality, no known drugs specifically increase libido or sexual performance; chemicals taken for this purpose without medical advice (and especially in combination with other drugs) pose the danger of adverse reactions, drug interactions, or overdose. However, many pharmacologically active agents do temporarily modify both physiologic responsiveness and subjective perception to enhance the enjoyment, if not the fulfillment, of the sex act. Some of these agents are considered in this section.

cantharis [kan′ thar is]

Cantharis (cantharidin, Spanish fly), a legendary sexual stimulant, is a powerful irritant and potent systemic poison. This substance is a powder made from dried beetles (*Cantharis vesicatoria*) found in southern Europe, and it can produce severe illness characterized by vomiting, diarrhea, abdominal pain, and shock. When taken internally, it causes irritation and inflammation of the genitourinary tract and dilation of the blood vessels of the penis and clitoris, sometimes producing prolonged erections (priapism) or engorgement, usually without increased sexual desire. Deaths have been reported from the promiscuous use of cantharis as an aphrodisiac. It is currently recognized that cantharis is not an effective sexual stimulant.

yohimbine [yo him′ been]

Another natural substance with purported aphrodisiac properties is yohimbine, an alkaloid derived from the West African tree *Corynanthe yohimbe*. Yohimbine produces a competitive alpha-adrenergic block of limited duration and antidiuresis, probably from the release of antidiuretic hormone. Although yohimbine stimulates the lower spinal nerve centers controlling erection, there is no convincing evidence that it acts as a sexual stimulant. It currently has no therapeutic use.

opioids and psychoactive agents

The use of drugs such as morphine, heroin, cocaine, marijuana, lysergic acid diethylamide (LSD), and amphetamines as aphrodisiacs has become widespread in contemporary society. For some individuals, these agents can enhance the enjoyment of the sexual experience under certain circumstances. More commonly, however, sexual behavior decreases. Responsiveness varies because these agents have no particular properties that specifically increase sexual potency; instead they tend to affect the user according to expectations. Thus the user's state of mind and the amount consumed contribute considerably to the effect achieved. Like alcohol, these drugs act on the CNS to weaken inhibitions, which are often the cause of problems involving sexual behavior. If taken in excess or too often, these drugs have the opposite effect and inhibit sexual drive and function. Because of these variations, researchers are skeptical of their value.

Marijuana (cannabis), an extract of the *Cannabis sativa* plant, is considered by many to be a sexual stimulant. However, like alcohol, its effect results indirectly from relaxation and the release of inhibitions surrounding sexual activity. The active ingredient in marijuana is tetrahydrocannabinol (THC). The pharmacologic effects resulting from smoking marijuana depend on the expectations and personality of the user, the dose, and the prevailing circumstances. The usual effects of marijuana are time distortion and enhanced suggestibility, which produces the illusion that sexual climax is somewhat prolonged. The expectation that marijuana is an aphrodisiac may enhance enjoyment of the sex act. However, studies on the properties of marijuana for a specific effect on sexual behavior have revealed no such properties. On the contrary, there is evidence that marijuana smokers have a higher incidence of decreased libido and impaired potency than nonusers. In addition, chronic intensive use of marijuana depresses plasma testosterone levels in healthy males and produces gynecomastia in some users. Chromosomal breaks have also occurred.

LSD is another drug that, although considered an aphrodisiac by some, has potentially untoward effects on sexual function and behavior. As with marijuana, any alteration of sexual performance produced by LSD is principally subjective. This drug acts almost entirely on the CNS. Little response, if any, has been noted in other organ systems that can be attributed to the direct effect of LSD, and no biochemical or pharmacologic evidence supports the contention that LSD or similar drugs contain any sex-stimulating properties. In fact, the repeated use of LSD may produce serious psychologic problems, which overall could have an adverse affect on sexual interest or activity. Women who use LSD during pregnancy may have a higher rate of malformed babies or stillbirths than women who do not use LSD.

Amphetamines such as Dexedrine have also been used to stimulate sexual function. These drugs have a powerful central stimulant action in addition to peripheral alpha and beta sympathomimetic effects. Their main effects are wakefulness and alertness, mood elevation, increased motor and speech activity, and often elation and euphoria. Physical performance is usually improved, and fatigue can be prevented or reversed. The effects of amphetamines on sexual performance, however, are inconsistent.

Along with other psychoactive agents, amphetamines do little to promote the enjoyment of sexual activity and over time may produce adverse psychologic and physical effects that reduce sexual interest and capability.

DRUGS THAT STIMULATE SEXUAL BEHAVIOR

Various clinically used or experimental drugs enhance sexual interest or potency as a side effect in both humans and laboratory animals.

levodopa [lee voe doe′ pa] (L-dopa)

Levodopa (L-dopa) is a natural intermediate in the biosynthesis of catecholamines in the brain and peripheral adrenergic nerve terminals. In the biologic sequence of events it is converted to dopamine, which in turn serves as a substrate of the neurotransmitter norepinephrine. Levodopa is used successfully in the treatment of Parkinson's syndrome, a disease characterized by dopamine deficiency. When levodopa is administered to an individual with this syndrome, the symptoms of Parkinson's disease are ameliorated, presumably because the drug is converted to dopamine and thereby counteracts the deficiency.

Individuals treated with levodopa, especially older men, have been observed to experience a sexual rejuvenation. This effect has led to the belief that levodopa stimulates sexual powers. Consequently, studies with younger men complaining of decreased erectile ability have shown that levodopa increases libido and the incidence of penile erections. Overall, however, these effects are short-lived and do not reflect continued satisfactory sexual function and potency. Thus levodopa is not a true aphrodisiac. The increased sexual activity experienced by parkinsonian clients treated with levodopa may reflect improved well-being and partial recovery of normal sexual functions that were impaired by Parkinson's disease.

amyl nitrite [am′ il]

Amyl nitrite, a drug used in the past to treat angina pectoris, is alleged to enhance sexual activity in humans. As a vasodilator and smooth muscle stimulant, amyl nitrite has been reported to intensify the orgasmic experience for men if inhaled at the moment of orgasm. This effect is probably the result of relaxation of smooth muscles and consequent vasodilation of the genitourinary tract. No effects of amyl nitrite on libido have been reported, but a loss of erection or delayed ejaculation may result. Women generally experience negative effects on orgasm when taking this drug.

vitamin E

Much has been said about the positive effects of vitamin E (alpha tocopherol) on sexual performance and ability in human beings. Unfortunately, there is little scientific rationale to substantiate such claims. The primary reasons for attributing a positive role in sexual performance to vitamin E come from experiments on vitamin E deficiency in laboratory animals. In such experiments the principal manifestation of this deficiency is infertility, although the reasons for this condition differ in males and females. In female rats there is no loss in ability to produce apparently healthy ova, nor is there any defect in the placenta or uterus. However, fetal death occurs shortly after the first week of embryonic life, and fetuses are reabsorbed. This situation can be prevented if vitamin E is administered any time up to the fifth or sixth day of embryonic life. In the male rat the earliest observable effect of vitamin E deficiency is immobility of spermatozoa, with subsequent degeneration of the germinal epithelium. Secondary sex organs are not altered and sexual vigor is not diminished, but vigor may decrease if the deficiency continues.

Because of experimental results such as these, vitamin E has been conjectured to restore potency or to preserve fertility, sexual interest, and endurance in humans. No evidence supports these contentions, but because sexual performance is often influenced by mental attitude, a person who believes vitamin E may improve sexual prowess may actually find improvement. The only established therapeutic use for vitamin E is for the prevention or treatment of vitamin E deficiency, a condition that is rare in humans.

sildenafil [sil den′ afil] (Viagra ◆)

A new product sildenafil (Viagra) released in 1998 is the first oral medication approved by the Food and Drug Administration (FDA) to treat impotence. The mechanism of action is secondary to sexual stimulation, which increases the release of nitric oxide and increases the levels of cyclic guanosine monophosphate (cGMP), a smooth muscle relaxant. Sildenafil enhances the effects of nitric oxide by inhibiting phosphodiesterase 5, a substance found primarily in the penis that degrades cGMP. As a result, increased levels of cGMP in the corpus cavernosum enhance smooth muscle relaxation, the inflow of blood, and erection. Sildenafil has no effect in the absence of sexual stimulation (Viagra package information, 1998).

Since the release and public acceptance of sildenafil, postmarketing information indicates a number of reports of adverse reactions and approximately 16 reports of fatality associated with its use (Viagra Postmarketing Information, 1998). According to this report, the FDA still supports the safety of this drug, because concomitant medications and/or disease states may have been involved in the adverse outcomes. The manufacturer, Pfizer (1998), sent a letter to prescribers to warn them that "the only contraindication for taking Viagra is the concomitant administration of an organic nitrate." They also issued a list of organic nitrate products to remind the prescriber about products that should not be combined with sildenafil. This contraindication is based on the facts that the combination causes severe hypotension and possibly a decrease in coronary perfusion, which may result in myocardial ischemia and infarction.

Health care providers should be aware that a man without a history of angina who takes sildenafil for sexual impotence and develops his first angina attack should not receive any nitrate products in the emergency department. This includes nitroglycerin and nitroprusside.

The side effects/adverse reactions of sildenafil include headache, nausea, facial flushing, nasal congestion, gastric distress, back pain, flu syndrome, arthralgia, allergic reaction, and cardiovascular events (e.g., angina pectoris, tachycardia, hypotension). At higher doses, this drug may cause some visual changes, including a bluish tinge in the field of vision for some men. Although sildenafil has not been approved by the FDA for administration in women, it is categorized as pregnancy category B.

The usual adult dosage is 50 mg PO taken approximately 1 hour before sexual activity.

■ Nursing Management

Sildenafil Therapy

■ **Assessment.** Clients with cirrhosis or severe hepatic or renal function impairment should receive lower initial doses of sildenafil. Check the client's medication regimen for drugs that may cause serious drug interactions when administered concurrently, such as nitrates (for the reasons previously cited) and hepatic enzyme inhibitors for cytochrome P450, such as cimetidine (Tagamet), erythromycin (E-Mycin), itraconazole (Sporanox), ketoconazole (Nizoral), or mibefradil (Posicor). Both nitrates and hepatic enzyme inhibitors increase serum levels of sildenafil and necessitate lower doses of the drug. A thorough assessment of the client's cardiac status, including electrocardiogram (ECG), blood pressure, and cardiovascular risk factors and vision status is essential before the initiation of therapy. A baseline assessment of the client's underlying condition includes the frequency, firmness, and maintenance of erections; frequency of orgasm; frequency, satisfaction, and enjoyment of sexual activities; and satisfaction with the sexual relationship.

■ **Nursing Diagnosis.** The client taking sildenafil is at risk for the following nursing diagnoses/collaborative problems: sexual dysfunction related to ineffectiveness of drug; impaired comfort (heartburn, headache, flushing, nasal congestion); disturbed sensory perception (mild and transient blurred vision, sensitivity to light, color tinge to vision); diarrhea; risk for infection (urinary); risk for injury related to dizziness; and the potential complication of cardiac risk associated with sexual activity.

■ **Implementation**

■ ***Monitoring.*** Have the client maintain a diary related to the use of sildenafil and the client's sexual response to the drug, as well as any cardiovascular symptoms that may occur (transient chest pain, palpitations, throbbing headache). Monitor blood pressure and other cardiovascular risk factors on client visits.

■ ***Education.*** Advise the client that a delay in the response to the medication may occur when sildenafil is taken with a high-fat meal. Alert the client to seek emergency treatment for chest pain, severe palpitations, and a sudden, sharp headache and to report vision disturbances to the prescriber. The client should avoid activities that require alertness until the sensory-perceptual responses to the drug are known. Increasing fluid intake to 2000 mL daily may help prevent the adverse reaction of urinary tract infection.

▪ **Evaluation.** The expected outcome of sildenafil therapy is that the client will report satisfaction with the firmness and maintenance of erections, frequency of orgasm, and enjoyment of sexual activities without experiencing vision and adverse cardiac effects of the drug.

THE NURSE'S ROLE IN HUMAN SEXUALITY

An appreciation of the serious effects of sexual dysfunction on client's lives can produce a special sensitivity to their concerns. Clients often find it easier to confide in and discuss such important personal information with a nurse (male or female), than with anyone else.

Therefore high-quality professional nursing should be directed toward achieving the following goals:

- Gaining an understanding of and accepting feelings about one's own sexuality. It takes time and effort to be comfortable enough to be therapeutic with others who are having sexual problems.
- Being open to clients' discussions about sexual concerns.
- Allowing clients to hold any belief or sexual practice they choose that is not overtly harmful.
- Recognizing that it is probably impossible to be truly comfortable with all clients or all related topics. It may be necessary to refer some clients to more adequately prepared personnel. This might be a clinical nurse specialist or a social worker with expertise in dealing with sexual issues.
- Keeping current with the constantly changing data about drugs with the potential for causing sexual dysfunction. This becomes more complex with the discovery that certain combinations of drugs elicit unusual sexual responses. Drugs that are currently suspect include antihypertensives, antidepressants, antihistamines, sedatives and tranquilizers, ethyl alcohol, barbiturates, steroid hormones and derivatives, opioids and psychoactive drugs, and certain natural substances.
- Being able to identify and interpret client cues about problems dealing with sexuality, such as unexplained noncompliance with medication instructions, certain subjective data from the nursing history, avoidance of the topic, or other subtle cues.
- Discussing clients' medication with them (casual use of drugs and over-the-counter and prescribed drugs), including information about potential adverse reactions.
- Consulting with the prescriber when adverse reactions do appear and suggesting alternate forms or dosages of drug therapy, if feasible. Such changes may be the route to enhanced compliance.
- Listening with sensitivity to expressed feelings of frustration, anger, anxiety, or fear that may accompany body image changes or perceptions of aging and waning sexual ability and/or attractiveness; some of these feelings may result from the effects of prescribed drugs.

SUMMARY

Because drug therapy has many dimensions that affect sexuality and sexual behavior, nurses must be sensitive in their assessment of clients' needs as sexual beings and able to intervene to promote health in this area.

Critical Thinking Questions

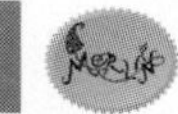

1. What are some appropriate assessment questions that will elicit client responses related to diminished libido secondary to a medication?
2. What would be your response if a nonnursing student at your school asked about the sexual effects of cannabis or alcohol?

Collaborative Learning Activities

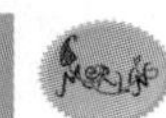

For Collaborative Learning Activities, go to mosby.com/MERLIN/McKenry/.

BIBLIOGRAPHY

Abramowicz, M. (Ed.). (1992). Drugs that cause sexual dysfunction: An update. *Medical Letter, 34*(876), 73.

Anderson, K.N., Anderson, L.E., & Glanze, W.D. (Eds.) (1998). *Mosby's medical, nursing, & allied health dictionary* (5th ed.). St. Louis: Mosby.

Carpenito, L.J. (2000). *Nursing diagnosis: Application to clinical practice* (8th ed.). Philadelphia: J.B. Lippincott.

Cleary, J.D., Chapman, S.W., Clark, A., & Lucia, H. (1995). Fungal infections. In L.Y. Young & M.A. Koda-Kimble (Eds.), *Applied therapeutics: The clinical use of drugs* (6th ed.). Vancouver, WA: Applied Therapeutics.

Gutierrez, M.A. & Stimmel, G.L. (1999). Management of and counseling for psychotropic drug-induced sexual dysfunction. *Pharmacotherapy, 19*(7), 823-831.

Kochar, M.S., Mazur, L.I., & Patel, A. (1999). What is causing your patient's sexual dysfunction? Uncovering a connection with hypertension and antihypertensive therapy. *Postgraduate Medicine, 106*(2), 149-152, 155-157.

Landen, M., Eriksson, E., Agren, H., & Fahlen, T. (1999). Effect of buspirone on sexual dysfunction in depressed patients treated with selective serotonin reuptake inhibitors. *Journal of Clinical Psychopharmacology, 19*(3), 268-271.

Nurnberg, H.G., Hensley, P.L., Lauriello, J., Parker, L.M., & Keith, S.J. (1999). Sildenafil for women patients with antidepressant-induced sexual dysfunction. *Psychiatric Services, 50*(8), 1076-1078.

Pfizer, Inc: U.S. Food and Drug Administration, retyped text of letter from Pfizer; www.fda.gov/medwatch/safety/1998/viagra.htm (7/4/98).

Ruggiero. R.J. (1995). Contraception. In L.Y. Young & M.A. Koda-Kimble, *Applied therapeutics: The clinical use of drugs* (6th ed.). Vancouver, WA: Applied Therapeutics.

Shen, W.W., Urosevich, Z., & Clayton, D.O. (1999). Sildenafil in the treatment of female sexual dysfunction induced by selective serotonin reuptake inhibitors. *Journal of Reproductive Medicine, 44*(6), 535-542.

Thompson, J.F. (1995). Geriatric urological disorders. In L.Y. Young & M.A. Koda-Kimble (Eds.), *Applied therapeutics: The clinical use of drugs* (6th ed.). Vancouver, WA: Applied Therapeutics.

Viagra Postmarketing Information: Sildenafil citrate (Viagra): Synopsis of fatal outcome reports submitted to the FDA regarding Viagra use; www.fda.gov/cder/news/viagrapostmarket.htm (7/4/98).

Viagra (sildenafil citrate), package information; www.viagra.com (7/4/98).

56 Principles of Antineoplastic Chemotherapy

Chapter Focus

Progress in antineoplastic chemotherapy has helped in providing palliation and a greater life expectancy for many persons with a diagnosis of cancer. Unfortunately, however, the cure for most cancers is unknown. Many of the commonly used antineoplastic agents also have undesirable side effects such as fatigue, nausea, vomiting, stomatitis, and bone marrow depression. Nurses not only administer antineoplastic agents as part of their role in many health care agencies but also are primarily responsible for providing care for clients receiving these agents, for promoting comfort, and for minimizing the risk for injury associated with these agents.

Learning Objectives

1. Identify four major developmental stages of normal and malignant cells.
2. List common antineoplastic drugs and their effects on the cell cycle.
3. Describe the major principles of chemotherapy.
4. Describe the common toxicities of antineoplastic chemotherapy.
5. Discuss age-related considerations for cancer in older adults and children.
6. Implement a plan of care using nursing management common to all antineoplastic drug therapy.

Key Terms

cancer, p. 929
combination chemotherapy, p. 931
dose-limiting effects, p. 931
Gompertzian growth, p. 930
metastasis, p. 930
micrometastases, p. 931

Cancer refers to a group of more than 300 diseases characterized by the uncontrolled growth and spread of abnormal cells. It has been estimated that approximately 40% to 45% of Americans will develop cancer during their lifetime (Finley, LaCivita, & Lindley, 1995). Many people fear cancer, and it is difficult to accept that a small lump or mole that has the potential for rapid growth may lead to serious illness or death. Therefore education and early treatment are imperative to win the battle against cancer, which is second only to cardiovascular disease as a cause of death.

Statistically, the chances of developing and dying from cancer are greater now than ever before. When a 20-year trend of cancer death rates from all sites was compared (from 1972 to 1974 and from 1992 to 1994), the death rate for males increased by 5%; for females, the rate increased by 7% (American Cancer Society, 1998). Although some decreases were noted for particular cancers (e.g., a 60% decrease in cancer death rate for Hodgkin's disease), the American Cancer Society (1998) reports that the death rate for lung cancer increased 147% in females and 49% in males. This explains the increase in the reported incidence of cancer deaths for particular cancers and for cancer overall as compared with past years.

This chapter discusses the principles of antineoplastic chemotherapy and the use of chemotherapeutic drugs in the treatment of cancer. To better understand the mechanisms and sites of action of the cancer chemotherapeutic agents, it is important to understand the kinetics of both normal cells and cancer cells.

CELL KINETICS

The reproductive cycles of normal and cancer cells are essentially the same (Figure 56-1). RNA and protein synthesis may occur during the presynthesis phase (G_1). The decision for cell replication or cell differentiation is also determined during this phase. The cell progresses to the synthesis phase (S), which is the replication phase; DNA doubles in preparation for cell division. DNA synthesis ceases during the postsynthesis or premitotic phase (G_2), but RNA and protein synthesis continues in order to prepare the cell for mitosis (M), or spindle formation. During the M phase, cells divide into two completely new cells. These two new cells may leave the cell cycle to do the following: (1) develop into differentiated cells that perform a specialized function (e.g., neuron, epithelium) and can no longer undergo cell division; or (2) become either temporarily or permanently nonproliferative (G_0 phase). Cells in the G_0 (or resting) phase may remain in this phase, reenter the cell cycle in time, or mature and die.

Anticancer agents have different sites of action on the dividing cell cycle. Agents that are most effective in one spe-

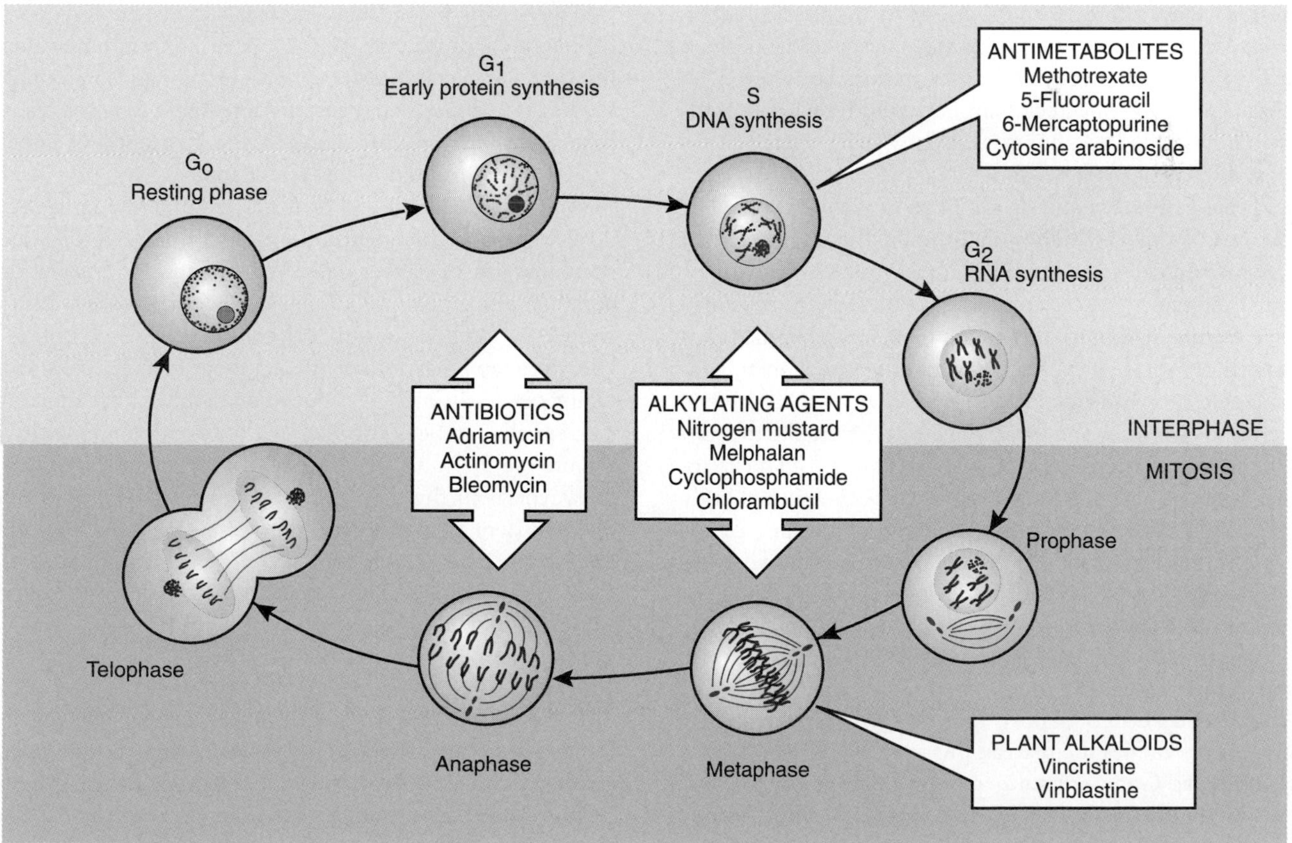

Figure 56-1 Phases of a cell cycle. Drugs are identified by where they exert their effect. (From Beare, P.G., & Myers, J.L. [1998]. *Adult health nursing* [3rd ed.]. St. Louis: Mosby.)

BOX 56-1

Cancer Cell Growth (Gompertzian)

	Number of Cells Present	
10^0	1	
10^1	10	
10^2	100	
10^3	1000	Subclinical disease (undetectable by physical examination)
10^4	10,000	
10^5	100,000	
10^6	1,000,000	
10^7	10,000,000	
10^8	100,000,000	
10^9	1,000,000,000	(1 g) Clinical symptoms appear
10^{10}	10,000,000,000	Regional spread
10^{11}	100,000,000,000	
10^{12}	1,000,000,000,000	Metastases (regional to advanced)
10^{13}	10,000,000,000,000	Possible lethal number of cancer cells

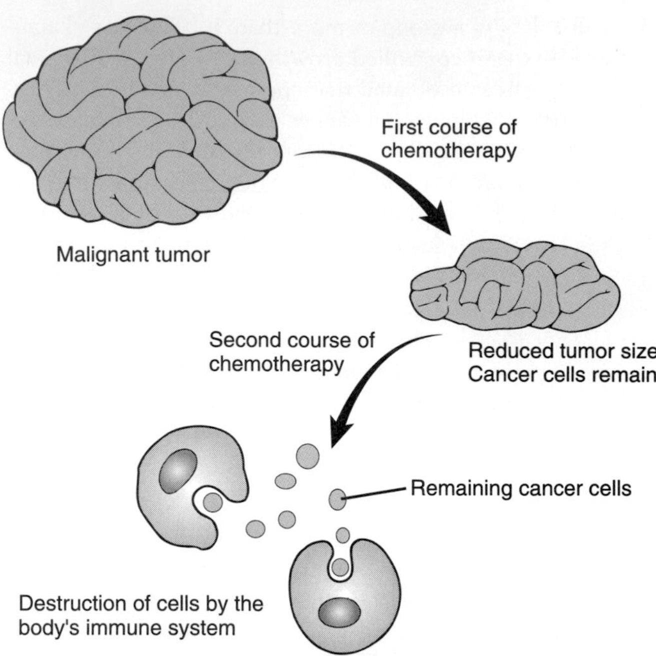

Figure 56-2 Cancer cell response to chemotherapy. (From Beare, P.G., & Myers, J.L. [1998]. Adult health nursing [3rd ed.]. St. Louis: Mosby.)

cific phase are referred to as cell cycle–specific agents. Antineoplastic agents that are active against both proliferating and resting cells are called cell cycle–nonspecific agents; alkylating agents are examples of this group (see Table 57-1). Antineoplastic classifications are an important consideration in selecting the appropriate drug(s) for the specific cancerous state. For example, methotrexate is more active in the S phase of the cell cycle and is therefore considered an S-phase cell cycle–specific agent; it would be much less effective in treating large tumor masses, which generally have slowly dividing cancer cells.

Normal cells grow and divide in an orderly fashion. The body process of cell adhesion inhibits the movement of newly formed cells, and the body's homeostatic mechanisms control the entire process of cell growth. Cancer cells may evolve from a hereditary or genetic predisposition plus contact with certain environmental conditions. In general, neoplastic cells lack the cellular differentiation of the tissues in which they originate and are unable to function like the normal cells around them. Cancer growth is enhanced by an increased rate of cell proliferation that lacks the normal body control system on cellular growth patterns. Because of the genetic differences, cancer cells lack the cell adhesive property of normal cells, which may lead to **metastasis,** or spreading of the cancer.

The growth of a cancer is usually rapid in the early stages. However, as the tumor enlarges, it nearly outgrows its blood and nutrient supply, and the growth rate pattern decreases or reaches the plateau phase for the tumor. This is referred to as **Gompertzian growth** kinetics (Box 56-1). A cell burden of 10^9 is usually the smallest tumor burden (quantitative size) that is physically detectable (palpated). At this point the client has approximately 1 billion cancer cells, which is equal to a tumor that is approximately the size of a small grape and weighs 1 g. This is the point at which clinical symptoms usually first appear.

The Papanicolaou (Pap) smear is a cytologic test capable of detecting carcinoma of the cervix and endometrium in the subclinical stages. The early detection and treatment of small cancer lesions that are not detectable by visual examination has dramatically reduced the mortality of cervical cancer in the United States and Canada.

Animal studies have shown that administering adequate doses of chemotherapeutic drugs to a host will kill a constant fraction of cancer cells. For example, a drug or drug combination capable of killing 99.9% of the cells would reduce a 10^{10} cell burden to 10^7 cancer cells. Each course of chemotherapy may reduce the number of cancer cells; eventually, cell levels may be reduced enough that the remaining cancer cells can be controlled by the client's immune system (Figure 56-2). This reduction may produce a remission. However, if further therapies are not instituted or the immune system is inadequate, the remaining cells may grow into another detectable tumor.

For a Concept Map on cancer, go to mosby.com/MERLIN/McKenry/. 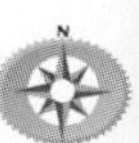

PRINCIPLES OF CHEMOTHERAPY

To obtain optimal therapeutic effects with an antineoplastic agent or with combination cancer chemotherapies, the following principles should be considered:

1. Cancer chemotherapy is most effective against small tumors because they usually have an efficient blood supply; an efficient blood supply increases drug deliv-

so that a higher cell-kill factor is possible.

ery to the cancer site. In addition, small tumors generally have a higher percentage of proliferating cells so that a higher cell-kill factor is possible.

2. The removal of large, localized tumors through surgery reduces the tumor cell burden and thus contributes to the success of the adjuvant chemotherapy. The major use of adjuvant chemotherapy is to help eradicate **micrometastases** (the migration of cancer cells via the bloodstream or lymphatic system to grow in organs, bone, or tissues—far from the primary site) after surgery or radiation.
3. In general, treatment with combination cancer chemotherapeutic agents produces a higher cancer cell–kill than treatment with a single drug agent.

COMBINATION CHEMOTHERAPY

In the late 1960s **combination chemotherapy** (the use of two or more anticancer drugs at the same time) was initiated for the treatment of acute lymphoblastic leukemia and Hodgkin's disease. When the complete response rates for single agents were compared with the response rates for combination drugs, the results were enlightening. The response rates for the "MOPP" treatment of advanced Hodgkin's disease is a classic illustration that is illustrated in the following list:

Drug	Complete Response Rates
M—mechlorethamine (Mustargen)	20%
O—vincristine (Oncovin)	<10%
P—procarbazine (Matulane)	<10%
P—prednisone	<5%
MOPP combination	80%

The following considerations are used to select the drugs for combination chemotherapy:

1. Each drug should be active against the specific cancer when used alone.
2. Each drug should have a different site of action and act at a different point of the cell cycle (specificity).
3. Each drug should have different organ toxicity or, if the toxic effect is similar, it should occur at different times for each drug.

When the preceding principles are applied to MOPP drug therapy, the concept of combination chemotherapy can be understood. First, the previous list illustrates the effectiveness of each single drug against Hodgkin's disease. Second, the sites of major activity are believed to be different for each antineoplastic agent used in MOPP therapy.

1. Mechlorethamine (Mustargen) is an alkylating agent that can interfere with the replication, transcription, and translation of DNA.
2. Vincristine (Oncovin) inhibits mitosis by interfering with the mitotic spindle.
3. Procarbazine (Matulane) is a weak monoamine oxidase (MAO) inhibitor, and its antineoplastic action is believed to occur during the S phase. It inhibits the synthesis of DNA, RNA, and protein.
4. Prednisone has lympholytic properties and may produce an antifibrotic effect that would be useful in treating cancer metastases surrounded by fibrous materials. It also improves appetite and general feelings of well-being.

The third principle, that of differing organ toxicities or toxicities that occur at different times, has also been substantiated for the MOPP combination. Many of these drugs have **dose-limiting effects**—drug responses that indicate that the maximum permissible dose has been reached and the drug should be decreased or discontinued. The dose-limiting toxicity of bone marrow suppression is a property of both mechlorethamine and procarbazine. However, the nadir (the lowest depression point for this effect) occurs approximately 10 days after the administration for mechlorethamine and 21 days after the administration of procarbazine. Thus additive myelosuppressive effects from this combination are essentially avoided. Vincristine does not have bone marrow suppression effects but does exhibit a dose-limiting neurotoxicity. Prednisone does not demonstrate bone marrow suppression or neurotoxicity.

Oncologists often use combination therapy for antineoplastic treatment. Table 56-1 lists other commonly prescribed combination chemotherapeutic regimens.

TABLE 56-1 Combination Chemotherapeutic Regimens

Cancer	Acronym	Drugs
Breast	CMF	cyclophosphamide methotrexate fluorouracil
	CFPT	cyclophosphamide fluorouracil prednisone tamoxifen
Colon	FLe	fluorouracil levamisole
	F-Cl	fluorouracil calcium leucovorin
Lung	CAV	cyclophosphamide doxorubicin (Adriamycin) vincristine
	COPE	cyclophosphamide vincristine (Oncovin) cisplatin (Platinol) etoposide

TOXIC EFFECTS OF CHEMOTHERAPY

Most of the currently available antineoplastic agents appear to act on similar metabolic pathways in both normal and malignant cells. A major limitation of cancer drugs is their lack of tumor specificity. Drug toxicities or side effects may be divided into (1) common side effects, (2) adverse reactions, and (3) specific dose-limiting drug effects.

The *most common side effects* of chemotherapeutic agents are alopecia (hair loss), nausea, vomiting, anorexia, diarrhea, and stomatitis (inflammation of the mouth). Cancer chemotherapy is most active or effective against dividing cells, but they are not capable of differentiating between cancer cells and normal dividing body cells. Therefore the most rapidly dividing cells in the body—which are in the bone marrow, hair follicles, and gastrointestinal tract—are generally those affected most by the anticancer drugs.

The *most common adverse reactions* that can lead to serious and even life-threatening infections are leukopenia, thrombocytopenia, and anemia. Bone marrow suppression is the major dose-limiting property most commonly encountered in cancer chemotherapy. Nursing assessment and monitoring are critical to improving client care and are reviewed in the nursing management section.

Specific *dose-limiting effects* are adverse reactions that should indicate to the prescriber that the maximum permissible dose has been delivered and that the drug needs to be discontinued. Fortunately, this occurs with only certain drugs. For example, drugs that can produce hepatotoxicity include methotrexate (Mexate, Folex), mercaptopurine (Purinethol), lomustine (CCNU, CeeNu), dacarbazine (DTIC-Dome), doxorubicin (Adriamycin), and carmustine (BCNU, BiCNU).

Cyclophosphamide (Cytoxan) is associated with hemorrhagic cystitis. (Because dehydration increases the risk factor, adequate fluid intake is important when this agent is administered.) Methotrexate is associated with tubular necrosis, which can be prevented by prehydrating with normal saline and alkalinizing the urine to increase elimination of the drug. Cisplatin (Platinol) is associated with tubular necrosis. Prehydration with 1 to 2 L of IV fluid and adequate fluids after drug administration help to reduce this adverse reaction. Nephrotoxicity, ototoxicity, and peripheral neuropathy have been reported with cisplatin.

Cardiac toxicity is reported with both doxorubicin (Adriamycin) and daunorubicin (Cerubidine). Cardiotoxicity increases in clients who receive more than 550 mg/m^2 of body surface (total accumulated dose given throughout therapy). Toxicity is also greater in older adults and in children under 2 years of age. Because this effect is cumulative if either drug is given, the amount of one drug already received by the client must be considered when planning therapy with the other drug.

Neurologic toxicity may range from tingling of the hands and feet and a loss of deep tendon reflexes to ataxia, footdrop, confusion, and personality changes. Drugs reported to produce neurologic effects include vincristine (Oncovin), vinblastine (Velban), and methotrexate (Folex).

AGE-RELATED CONSIDERATIONS IN CHEMOTHERAPY

Cancer in Older Adults

Cancer in older adults is a serious disease, and its incidence increases sharply with age. Approximately 50% of all cases of cancer in the United States occur in persons over 65 years of age (Patel & Koeller, 1993). When compared with younger cancer victims, older adults have more concurrent illnesses, which may decrease their ability to withstand the effects of cancer or the antineoplastic therapies. In addition, decreased pulmonary and renal function and decreased bone marrow cellularity may interfere with treatment. Other factors to consider when managing regimens for older adults are the possibility of reduced income and the loss of loved ones and family support.

Compromises in treatment are often made because of a client's advanced age; however, data suggest that a dosage reduction of chemotherapy based on age alone is not always appropriate. A treatment approach should be based on the individual cancer and the biologic and physiologic differences noted in the older adult. More clinical trials are needed to further examine the relationship between responsiveness to cancer chemotherapy and the person's age.

Cancer in Children

Although cancer in children is relatively uncommon, North American children (between the ages of 1 and 14 years) most commonly die of cancer. Acute leukemias are the most common cancers in children. Carcinomas, which are common in adults, are rare in children; sarcomas are much more common in children (Finley, Lindley, & Henry, 1995). Because tumors grow rapidly in children, childhood cancer is generally more responsive than adult cancer to chemotherapy. Children also tend to tolerate the acute side effects of chemotherapy better than adults. Fifty percent of children with cancer are long-term survivors or are actually cured. (See the Special Considerations for Children box on p. 933.)

■ Nursing Management

Antineoplastic Chemotherapy

The role of the nurse is to ensure safe and effective administration of antineoplastic agents. This responsibility becomes more complex as a greater proportion of these therapies is administered with shorter hospital admissions and within the client's home setting (Jacob, 1999). Because there is such a need to identify the knowledge and skills required of the nurse when administering and monitoring antineoplastic agents, nursing organizations such as the Oncology Nursing Society and the Intravenous Nurses Society have

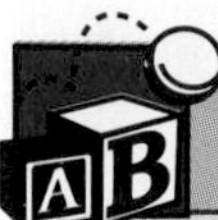

Special Considerations for Children
Antineoplastic Chemotherapy Agents

In 1997, cancer was the second leading cause of death among children ages 1 to 14 years of age (Greenlee, Murray, Bolden, & Wingo, 2000).

The leading cancers among children include leukemias (especially acute lymphocytic leukemia), Hodgkin's disease, neuroblastoma, non-Hodgkin's lymphoma, Wilms' tumor, central and sympathetic nervous system tumors, and soft tissue sarcomas (Greenlee et al., 2000).

Five-year cancer survival rates have improved tremendously. For example, from 1974 to 1976, the 5-year survival rate for acute lymphocytic leukemia, Hodgkin's disease, and Wilms' tumor was 53%, 78%, and 74%, respectively. From 1989 to 1995, the survival rates for the same cancers increased to 81%, 93%, and 93%, respectively (Greenlee et al., 2000).

Children have a greater risk of experiencing extrapyramidal symptoms than adults with the use of the antiemetics metoclopramide (Reglan), prochlorperazine (Compazine), and haloperidol (Haldol). Such agents should be avoided in this population. A combination of a selected serotonin receptor (5-HT_3) antagonist such as ondansetron (Zofran), granisetron (Kytril), or dolasetron (Anzemet) plus a corticosteroid is preferred (Holdsworth, 1998).

established recommendations and guidelines for practice (Box 56-2).

■ **Assessment.** Nursing care for clients receiving drug therapy with antineoplastic agents is complex and is inseparable from nursing care of the family. The client may be in any state of the disease process and may be facing impending death. In assessing the client and family, special considerations should be given to their coping abilities (Chrystal, 1997). The approach should be sensitive and appropriate to the individual needs of the client and family. The client's degree of acceptance of chemotherapy should be assessed, and the nurse may need to help the client deal with mixed emotions about the chemotherapy. The client's and family's knowledge of the chemotherapy and their expectations should also be assessed.

A baseline assessment includes a complete history and physical examination. Diagnostic procedures that are specific to the type of neoplasm and its location should be performed.

■ **Nursing Diagnosis.** See the Nursing Care Plan on p. 935 for selected nursing diagnoses related to the use of antineoplastic agents. Other nursing diagnoses related to chemotherapy might be imbalanced nutrition related to anorexia and gastrointestinal distress; impaired gas exchange related to anemia, cardiotoxicity, or pulmonary fibrosis; disturbed sensory perception (tactile, auditory) related to neurotoxicity; impaired skin integrity related to extravasation or drug-induced skin pathology; ineffective tissue perfusion (cardiopulmonary) related to drug-induced cardiotoxicity; and ineffective coping related to the stress of antineoplastic chemotherapy.

■ **Implementation**

■ ***Monitoring and Intervention.*** The nurse has many responsibilities in dealing with the inevitable side effects of antineoplastic drugs.

The potential for infection is increased because of bone marrow depression. Strict aseptic technique should be used during contact with the hospitalized client, who should also be protected from persons harboring harmful microorganisms. Monitor the client's temperature, and observe for signs of infection. Frequent blood counts are necessary, and the nurse is often responsible for ensuring that they are taken and that the results are monitored for early signs of bone marrow depression. A client with an absolute granulocyte count below 100 cells/mm^3 is at risk for infection. Clients with granulocytopenia should maintain scrupulous oral hygiene and receive topical antibiotics for abrasions and scratches. Encourage fluids and avoid indwelling catheters and other invasive procedures. Caution the client to avoid crowds and individuals with infectious diseases (e.g., colds, influenza, chickenpox, measles). No one in the client's household should be vaccinated with a live attenuated virus, such as polio. Clients should be instructed to report to the health care provider any signs of infection, such as elevated temperature, sore throat, cough, mouth ulcerations, or burning on urination.

Altered protection occurs for clients with thrombocytopenia when platelet levels fall below 50,000 cells/mm^3. Avoid taking rectal temperatures and administering suppositories to such clients. Protective care for these clients might include the administration of stool softeners and the use of soft-bristled toothbrushes and electric razors. Soft tissue injury should be avoided, and the use of padded side rails on beds should be considered. Oral preparations of analgesics and other medications should be used to avoid the tissue damage resulting from IM injections. Venipunctures should be performed carefully by experienced personnel using strict sterile technique. The client should be instructed to report signs that indicate decreased platelets, such as petechiae, easy bruising, hemorrhage, bleeding from the gums, epistaxis, and blood in the stool and urine.

The kidneys are at risk for injury because of the effectiveness of the antineoplastic agents. Purines are released through cell destruction and converted to uric acid. The possibility of renal failure may result from the precipitation of uric acid crystals in the kidneys. Monitor the client's intake and output, serum uric acid, blood urea nitrogen, serum creatinine, creatinine clearance, and serum electrolytes. Allopurinol may be prescribed to prevent the accumulation of uric acid in the kidneys. Fluid intake should be 3 L daily. Cold, clear liquids, such as tea, unsweetened apple juice or other juices, and soft drinks or carbonated beverages such as ginger ale may be well tolerated. Freezing a favorite beverage into ice cubes or popsicles is also recommended.

BOX 56-2

The Nurse's Role in the Administration of Antineoplastic Agents

The role of the nurse is dynamic, increasing in its competencies to meet the needs of increasing technology and the health care of society. Certainly this evolution of role is being demonstrated in the administration of antineoplastic agents and in the monitoring of clients receiving them. Because these types of changes in nursing responsibilities often come about by custom and practice rather than law, nurses must ensure that their health care agencies have policies and procedures in place to protect them and their clients. Nursing organizations often provide guidance for health care agencies by indicating their position in relation to the new responsibilities that nurses are to assume. The following Standard of Practice on the clinical management of oncology/antineoplastic therapy comes from the Intravenous Nurses Society and clearly states the requirement for safe and effective administration of these agents.

Standard

Administration of antineoplastic agents requires a physician's order. Knowledge and technical expertise of both administration and specific interventions is required to administer these agents.

Interpretation

The administration of antineoplastic agents should be established in organizational policy and procedure. Written consent by the patient or legally authorized representative should be obtained prior to the administration of these agents. This therapy requires patient education. The patient must be informed of all aspects of this therapy, including physical and psychologic effects, side effects, risks, and benefits. The administration of these agents requires knowledge and understanding of the cell cycle and malignant cell growth. Prior to administration, laboratory data should be reviewed and assessed for appropriateness of prescribed therapy. The nurse's responsibilities for administering these agents include knowledge of the disease process, drug classifications, pharmacologic indications, actions, side effects, adverse reactions, method of administration (i.e., intravenous push, continuous), rate of delivery, treatment goal (e.g., palliative or curative), and drug properties (e.g., vesicant, nonvesicant, and irritant).

The nurse must understand the vascular system. Preservation of venous access is crucial. To avoid serious complications of this therapy, technical expertise of cannula placement is mandatory. Selection of appropriate equipment will enhance therapy and help prevent potential complications. Cannula types should be selected based on the overall aspects of prescribed therapy and patient condition. Electronic infusion devices are a consideration in specific types of antineoplastic administration. When an electronic infusion device is indicated to administer a vesicant medication, a non-pressure device is the instrument of choice. A new access site is initiated immediately prior to any peripheral vesicant administration. Access device patency is verified prior to the administration of each antineoplastic agent. Knowledge of drug calculation as to dose and volume relative to age, height and weight, or body surface area is required.

Nurses must anticipate potential complications of administering this therapy and be skilled at performing immediate interventions. As with any intravenous drug administration, the possibility of extravasation should be anticipated, but not expected, and its occurrence requires immediate recognition with intervention and investigation. Decreasing extravasation and associated complications requires technical expertise in cannula placement and immediate recognition of drug extravasation.

Extravasation protocols for vesicants should be established in policy and procedure and administered when a vesicant infiltrates. Extravasation protocols should minimize further tissue damage, thus this protocol must be accomplished with technical expertise to obtain the desired outcome.

The discontinuation of antineoplastic agents is not considered life threatening. Therefore when an extravasation of a vesicant occurs, the extremity should not be used for subsequent cannula placement and alternative interventions should be explored such as termination of therapy, use of the other arm, or use of a central line.

Handling and mixing of these agents are not without risk. Nurses handling and mixing these agents should strictly adhere to protective protocols, such as mixing under vertical laminar flow hoods/biologic safety cabinets and wearing protective clothing. Pregnant women should not handle these agents, and consideration should be given to individuals of childbearing age. Organizational policy and procedure for the protection of personnel should be in keeping with the Occupational Safety and Health Adminstration's (OSHA's) guidelines. Disposal of these agents and associated equipment should be in keeping with the disposal guidelines for hazardous waste materials established by OSHA.

Critical Thinking Questions

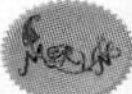

- How could a nursing standard statement such as this serve to protect the public? How would it serve to protect nurses?
- If you were the nurse manager on an oncology unit, how could you use this standard?

Standards reproduced by permission of the Intravenous Nurses Society. (1998). Intravenous nursing standards of practice. *Journal of Intravenous Nursing, 21*(1), supplement.

Nursing Care Plan
Selected Nursing Diagnoses Related to the Use of Antineoplastic Agents

Nursing Diagnosis	Outcome Criteria	Nursing Interventions
Impaired oral mucous membrane related to drug-induced stomatitis or poor oral hygiene	Client will: Demonstrate knowledge of oral hygiene Maintain adequate nutrition and hydration Maintain normal oral mucosa or have decreasing inflammation and/or ulceration	Instruct client to complete all dental work before beginning chemotherapy. Teach optimal oral hygiene to prevent stomatitis. Inspect the oral cavity with a tongue blade and light twice daily and before each administration of the antineoplastic drug. Implement appropriate mouth care if inflammation is present. Encourage soothing foods: bland foods, cool liquids, cool foods (popsicles). Instruct the client to avoid alcohol and tobacco, spicy or acidic foods, extremes in food temperature, and abrasive foods or those difficult to chew. Consult with the prescriber if oral pain relief solution is needed. Instruct the client to report any ulcers in or around the mouth.
Risk for infection related to bone marrow depression, leukopenia	Client will: Remain free of infection	Instruct the client in reading a thermometer. Teach the client to take temperature daily in the afternoon and report any elevation over 101° F. Teach the client to avoid being immunized with live virus vaccines and having contact with people with infections. Instruct the client to report any signs of infection, such as cough, sore throat, and burning on urination.
Risk for injury related to bone marrow depression, thrombocytopenia	Client will: Exhibit no signs of bleeding or excessive bruising	Avoid performing invasive procedures such as IM injections and rectal temperatures. Inspect IV sites, skin, and mucous membranes for signs of bleeding and bruising. Instruct the client to report easy bruising, bloody urine, and bleeding from the nose or gums. Test urine, emesis, and stool for occult blood. Instruct the client to exercise care in oral hygiene and in using safety razors and nail clippers. Teach the client to avoid constipation. Encourage the use of caution to prevent falls.
Risk for diarrhea or constipation	Client will: Maintain a normal bowel pattern Experience less constipation or diarrhea	Assess client's normal bowel pattern as a baseline. If the client is constipated, increase fluid intake and roughage in the diet. If the client has diarrhea, decrease roughage, increase fluids, and give small feedings. Consult with a prescriber if the stool softener, laxative, or antidiarrheal is needed. Assess the client for fluid and electrolyte status. Monitor bowel movements; record diarrhea as output. Clean and dry the perianal area after each bowel movement. Test stools for occult blood.
Disturbed body image related to alopecia	Client will: Demonstrate progress toward coping with disturbed body image	Allow the client to express apprehensions related to alopecia. Encourage the client to obtain cap or hairpiece before treatment begins. Reassure the client that hair growth should begin 8 weeks after therapy, but the new growth may be of a different color and texture.
Deficient fluid volume related to nausea and vomiting	Client will: Experience decreased incidence of nausea and vomiting	Administer antiemetic drugs 1-3 hours before administration of the antineoplastic drugs, or administer antineoplastic therapy before bedtime with an antiemetic and a sedative. Provide the client with frequent, small amounts of liquids of the client's preference (at least 3 L daily).

The client's body image may be disturbed as a result of alopecia. This side effect is extremely distressing to women, even when they have been prepared for it, have cosmetic aids available, and are aware that it is reversible. Clients, even those who experience only thinning of the hair, need to be assured that the hair will begin to grow back in approximately 6 to 8 weeks, although it may have a different texture or color. Treatment with hormones may necessitate support for the client in the event of effects such as masculinization in a female client or feminization in a male client. These clients need assistance in coping with body image problems.

Some clients lose their appetite or complain of a bitter or metallic taste in the mouth. Their desire for red meat or other protein foods may be reduced, because these foods are most commonly perceived as bitter tasting. Because protein is essential for good nutrition, alternative sources should be pursued. Cold cooked turkey, fish, eggs, and dairy products may be suitable substitutes. The biggest meal of the day should be planned for the time the client is usually hungriest, even if that time is early morning or midnight.

Nausea and vomiting that accompany the use of antineoplastic drugs can be relieved by (1) the administration of an antiemetic drug 1 to 3 hours before administration of the antineoplastic drugs, or (2) the administration of the antineoplastic drug at night with an antiemetic and a hypnotic, so that the client sleeps all night and experiences fewer side effects. Box 56-3 describes the emetic potential of chemotherapeutic agents. The antiemetic can be continued afterward as necessary. Speeding the passage of food through the stomach is sometimes the solution to the problem of nausea, vomiting, and feelings of fullness. Some quantities of carbohydrates eaten at frequent intervals help to achieve this effect. Weigh the client to monitor nutritional status.

Clients should not drink liquids at mealtime but instead should take them at frequent intervals throughout the day and up to 30 to 60 minutes before eating. Because hot foods have been reported to contribute to nausea, foods should be served at room temperature or cooler. Resting for 1 to 2 hours after eating is advised, because activity can slow the digestive process.

Stomatitis, oral ulcerations, xerostomia (dryness of the mouth), and other oral changes are common side effects of the potent antineoplastic agents and may interfere with the client's nutrition. Good oral hygiene is important to maintain a proper nutritional intake and decrease the possibility that oral infections will become systemic. The type of mouthwash solutions used depends on the status of the client's lesions. Small, frequent servings of cold or room-temperature, bland, nonirritating foods are best tolerated by the client. This type of diet also decreases the diarrhea that is a common side effect of cancer chemotherapy. Nystatin oral suspension or another antifungal agent may be prescribed to prevent infection with oral *Candida albicans*.

As a side effect of antineoplastic drugs, diarrhea results from the death of the rapidly dividing cells of the bowel mucosa. Assess the client's bowel status, hydration, and electrolyte levels, and record diarrhea as output. The intake of clear fluids should be encouraged between meals, although IV therapy may be needed to replace lost fluids if diarrhea is severe. Because of the client's frequent defecation, special attention should be given to skin care in the perianal area. Modification of the diet will prevent or decrease diarrhea. The client should be instructed to avoid foods that may cause gas and cramping, such as cabbage, beans, and highly spiced foods. Hot, spicy foods should be avoided because they increase peristalsis, which reduces nutrition absorption and may cause diarrhea. Reducing high-fiber foods in the diet (e.g., raw fruits and vegetables, bran, and whole grain cereals and bread) may help to control diarrhea. Foods that are high in potassium (to replace the potassium lost through diarrhea) and that usually do not worsen diarrhea include bananas, apricot or pear nectar, red meat, saltwater fish, boiled or mashed potatoes, and orange juice. Test stools for occult blood.

BOX 56-3

Selected Chemotherapeutic Agents: Emetic Potential

High Emetic Potential

cisplatin
dacarbazine (DTIC)
nitrogen mustard
streptozocin
actinomycin D
doxorubicin
daunorubicin
nitrosoureas (BCNU, CCNU)
procarbazine
cyclophosphamide (IV)
etoposide
mitomycin
methotrexate (high dose)

Low Emetic Potential

5-FU
vincristine
vinblastine
methotrexate
bleomycin
chlorambucil
melphalan
busulfan
cyclophosphamide (oral)
6-mercaptopurine

Information from Lane, M., Vogel, C.L., Ferguson, J., Krasnow, S., Saiers, J.L., Hamm, J., Salva, K., Wiernik, P.H., Holroyde, C.P., Hammill, S., et al. (1991). Dronabinol and prochlorperazine in combination for treatment of cancer chemotherapy–induced nausea and vomiting. *Journal of Pain and Symptom Management, 6*(6), 352-359.

Constipation may also be a problem with some clients. This may be an early symptom of central nervous system (CNS) toxicity or impaired intestinal motility from the drug therapy, or it may result from eating mostly soft and liquid foods. High-fiber foods and prune juice have a laxative effect; 1 or 2 tablespoons of bran may be added to cooked cereals, casseroles, and homemade baked goods. The client should be encouraged to drink plenty of fluids, preferably 8 to 10 glasses daily. Hot lemon water in the morning usually stimulates bowel activity. The prescriber may order a laxative or stool softener as needed. Avoid enemas, because they may injure the intestinal mucosa.

Pain commonly occurs in clients receiving antineoplastic drugs. The treatment of pain associated with cancer, especially chronic pain, requires a careful assessment of the client, consideration of appropriate nursing interventions, and skillful application of pharmacologic agents. Nonpharmacologic techniques for pain relief (e.g., relaxation therapy, guided imagery, aromatherapy, and diversional activities) may assist the client. Chronic pain may progress in a cycle to anxiety or depression, insomnia, fatigue, and increased pain. The factors that modify pain threshold are listed in Figure 14-1.

Nursing interventions may include physical activity to help prevent further deterioration resulting from inactivity. Deep breathing, turning the client, and skin care are some of the actions that reduce complications. In addition to physical and pharmacologic interventions, the client may need psychosocial, intellectual, and spiritual support. The holistic approach of carefully assessing the client's current needs and anticipating and planning for continued care is important in the care of many illnesses but is crucial for a client dying of a progressive illness. A variety of home-care programs are available. In addition, hospice programs have been developed throughout the United States and Canada to help provide the supportive and palliative services necessary for clients with life-threatening illness and their families. The American Cancer Society offers a variety of resources for the client with cancer and his or her family.

It must be remembered that anticancer drugs are potent drugs that are mutagenic and carcinogenic in animals and may be carcinogenic in humans. Nurses and pharmacists who prepare antineoplastic drugs should institute safety measures such as using proper technique; wearing gloves, mask, and protective clothing; and preparing the solutions in a vertical laminar flow, biologically safe hood whenever possible. All unused solutions, vials, needles, syringes, gloves, and materials used to clean up spills should be processed as hazardous materials; the waste should be properly incinerated. For further detail, check the policies related to hazardous waste for your health agency.

Although the development of cancer in professionals has not yet been directly related to the handling of materials, a relationship between fetal loss and occupational exposure to antineoplastic drugs in nurses has been reported. Governmental regulatory agencies have indicated that it is unacceptable to allow exposure to potential carcinogens to continue until cancer actually occurs. Regulatory agencies should not wait for epidemiologic evidence before taking action to limit exposure to chemicals considered to be carcinogenic.

■ ***Education.*** In addition to the client teaching discussed previously in relation to specific interventions, instruction about drug administration and drug effects may help to ease the client's anxiety. An assessment should reveal the expectations of the client and the family; they may need assistance in accepting a realistic view of the results of chemotherapy. Expectations of total cure may be unrealistic and should not be reinforced, whereas expectations of remission are often appropriate. One of the most important nursing interventions is providing emotional support to a client who is receiving physically and psychologically distressing therapy. The long periods of therapy, with frequent interruptions and sporadic progress, may compound the client's anxieties.

A client receiving cancer chemotherapy should be cautioned not to take any over-the-counter (OTC) medication before checking with the oncologist. Many OTC preparations contain aspirin, alcohol, or other substances that could interfere with the antineoplastic agents or increase the risk for toxicity. See the Nursing Care Plan on p. 935 for specific areas of client instruction related to selected nursing diagnoses.

Clients commonly return home after a few hours of receiving chemotherapy, or they receive chemotherapeutic agents at home administered by home health nurses. Home chemotherapy allows clients to be active participants in administering their own therapy, and it provides them the opportunity to regain the sense of control they may have believed they lost to their cancer (Cantania, 1999). In addition to learning the technical skills to maintain these therapies at home, the clients and their families need to practice the safe handling of cytotoxic drugs and body waste. The client and family need to know that these chemotherapeutic agents are eliminated from the body through vomitus, urine, and feces. Direct contact with these waste products can expose a person to the drug during the chemotherapy and for up to 48 hours after the drug has been discontinued. If precautions are not taken, the effects of these drugs may accumulate in the body of the caregiver who is routinely exposed over a period of time. For example, this may occur if the caregiver regularly changes and washes the bed linens of a client who is receiving these agents and is wetting the bed (Blecke, 1989). Soiled bedpans and containers contaminated with vomitus need to be handled with gloves, emptied directly into the toilet, and washed with detergent and water without splashing (with the rinse water discarded directly into the toilet); the toilet is then flushed three times. Hands are always washed after removing the gloves. Skin surfaces contaminated by body wastes or antineoplastic drugs should be washed with detergent and water for 5 minutes. If an eye is involved, it is washed with water for 10 to 15 minutes, and the oncologist is notified.

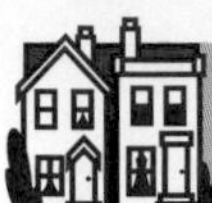

Community and Home Health Considerations
Home Spill Kit Procedure

A home spill kit that meets OSHA requirements usually contains 2 pairs of unpowdered surgical latex gloves, a disposable gown, chemical splash goggles, a respirator mask, 2 sheets (12 × 12) of disposable material, 2 spill control pillows, a small scoop and brush to collect glass fragments, a sharps container, 2 large chemotherapy waste disposal bags, and toxic waste labels. The following suggested procedure will need to be modified for spill kits containing other materials:

- Do not touch the spill with unprotected hands.
- Open the spill kit box and put on both pairs of gloves. If the bag or syringe with chemotherapy drugs has been broken or is leaking and you have a catheter or Port-A-Cath in place, first disconnect the catheter from the tubing and rinse and cap the catheter or Port-A-Cath according to normal procedure before cleaning the spill.
- Put on the gown (closes in back), splash goggles, and respirator.
- Use spill pillows to contain the spill; put them around the puddle to form a V.
- Use the absorbent sheets to blot up as much of the drug as possible.Put contaminated cleaning materials directly into the small plastic bag contained in the kit. Do not place them on unprotected surfaces.
- Use the scoop and brush to collect any broken glass, sweeping toward the V'ed spill pillows; dispose of the glass in the box of the kit (after emptying the box).
- While still wearing the protective gear, wash the area with detergent and warm water using paper towels, and put the paper towels in the small plastic bag with the other waste. Rinse the area with clean water, and dispose of the towels in the same plastic bag.
- Remove gloves, goggles, respirator, and gown and place them in the same plastic bag. Put all contaminated materials, including the spill kit box and the small plastic bag, into the second large plastic bag and label with the hazardous waste label in the kit.
- Wash your hands with soap and water.
- Call the home health nurse, clinic, or prescriber's office promptly to report the spill. Plans need to be made to have the waste material picked up or to have you bring it to the hospital for proper disposal.
- If upholstered or carpeted areas are contaminated, follow the above procedure—blot as much of the solution as possible with the absorbent sheets, wash the area with detergent, and follow with a clean water rinse. Do not use chemical spot removers or upholstery dry cleaners, because they may cause a chemical reaction with the drug.
- If the spill occurs on sheets or clothing, wash them in hot water separately from the other items. Wash clothing or bed linens contaminated with body wastes in the same manner.
- Clients on 24-hour infusions should use a plastic-backed mattress pad to protect the mattress from contamination.

Modified from Blecke, C. (1989). Home chemotherapy safety procedures. *Oncology Nursing Forum, 16*(7), 719-721, 201.

A spill of antineoplastic agents may occur in the home if IV fluid bags are defective or if IV lines leak or get disconnected accidentally. Although the client is usually provided a commercially available spill kit that fulfills the requirement of the Occupational Safety and Health Administration (OSHA), instruction on the spill kit procedure should be reinforced to prevent undue exposure of the client and caregivers (see the Community and Home Health Considerations box above).

■ **Evaluation.** Evaluation of drug effects is an integral nursing function in antineoplastic chemotherapy. Often no dosage schedule for antineoplastic agents is universally therapeutic, and the dosage is changed according to the client's response and the toxic effects of the drug. Thus it is essential that the nurse evaluate progress toward therapy goals and communicate both drug toxicity and client response. In evaluating toxic effects, the nurse should be vigilant for early signs, because the progression of toxic effects may have severe and irreversible consequences.

SUMMARY

Cancer is a major health issue today. Although many people fear cancer, more people are cured of cancer than ever before. Education for cancer prevention, early detection, and early treatment are essential to combating this disease. It is essential that nurses have knowledge of cell kinetics so they can understand the mechanisms and sites of action of the cancer chemotherapeutic agents and appropriately manage the nursing care of clients receiving such agents.

Critical Thinking Questions

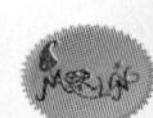

1. Mr. Matsui, a 56-year-old client with Hodgkin's disease, is questioning his MOPP therapy. He is concerned about the cost of his health care and wants to know why so many drugs are needed to treat him. What will be your response to Mr. Matsui?

2. Mrs. Hayes has been receiving a course of antineoplastic therapy. Her laboratory results show a platelet count of 46,000 cells/mm^3 and an absolute granulocyte count of 86 cells/mm^3. What assessments should be obtained? How should she be monitored on a daily basis? What safety precautions will you take with her care?

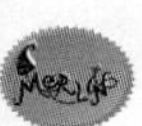

Collaborative Learning Activities

For Collaborative Learning Activities, go to mosby.com/MERLIN/McKenry/.

CASE STUDY

For a Case Study that will help ensure mastery of this chapter content, go to mosby.com/MERLIN/McKenry/.

BIBLIOGRAPHY

American Cancer Society. (1998). *Facts & figures: Cancer death rates, graphical data*, www.cancer.org/statistics/index.html (7/2/98).

Anderson, K.N., Anderson, L.E., & Glanze, W.D. (Eds.) (1998). *Mosby's medical, nursing, & allied health dictionary* (5th ed.). St. Louis: Mosby.

Belcher, A.E. (1992). *Cancer nursing*. St. Louis: Mosby.

Blecke, C. (1989). Home chemotherapy safety procedures. *Oncology Nursing Forum, 16*(7), 719-721, 201.

Carlson, P.A. (1995). Antineoplastic agents. *Critical Care Nursing Quarterly, 18*(4), 1-15.

Catania, P.N. (1999). When patients ask: Home chemotherapy: Basic concepts. *Home Care Provider, 4*(2), 60-61.

Chrystal, C. (1997). Administering continuous vesicant chemotherapy in the ambulatory setting. *Journal of Intravenous Nursing,* 20(2), 78-88.

Dodd, M.J., Thomas, M.L., Dibble, S.L. (1992). Self-care for patients experiencing cancer chemotherapy side effects: A concern for home care nurses. *Home Healthcare Nurse, 9*(6), 21-26.

Dose, A.M. (1995). The symptom experience of mucositis, stomatitis, and xerostomia. *Seminars in Oncology Nursing, 11*(4), 248-255.

Finley, R.S., LaCivita, C.L., & Lindley, C.M. (1995). Neoplastic disorders and their treatment: General principles. In L.Y. Young & M.A. Koda-Kimble (Eds.), *Applied therapeutics: The clinical use of drugs* (6th ed.). Vancouver, WA: Applied Therapeutics.

Finley, R.S., Lindley, C.L., & Henry, D.W. (1995). Solid tumors. In L.Y. Young & M.A. Koda-Kimble (Eds.), *Applied therapeutics: The clinical use of drugs* (6th ed.). Vancouver, WA: Applied Therapeutics.

Greenlee, R.T., Murray, T., Bolden, S., & Wingo, P.A. (2000). Cancer Statistics, 2000. *CA, A Cancer Journal for Clinicians, 50*(1), 7-33.

Hedges, C.B. (1994). Recognizing the patient at risk for opportunistic infections. *MEDSURG Nursing, 3*(6), 445-452.

Holdsworth, M.T. (1998). Selected issues in supportive care of pediatric cancer patients. *Highlights in Oncology Practice, 16*(3), 74-81.

Jacob, E. (1999). Making the transition from hospital to home: Caring for the newly diagnosed child with cancer. *Home Care Provider, 4*(2), 67-75.

McCance, K.L. & Huether, S.E. (1998). *Pathophysiology: The biological basis for disease in adults and children* (3rd ed.). St. Louis: Mosby.

Parker, G.G. (1992). Chemotherapy administration in the home. *Home Healthcare Nursing, 10*(1), 30.

Parker, S.L., Tong, T., Bolden, S., & Wingo, P.A. (1996). Cancer statistics: 1996. *Cancer Journal for Clinicians, 46*(1), 5-28.

Patel, N.H. & Koeller, J. (1993). Cancer chemotherapy in the elderly. *Highlights of Antineoplastic Drugs, 11*(4), 58-64.

Rhodes, V.A., Johnson, M.H., & McDaniel, R.W. (1995). Nausea, vomiting, and retching: The management of the symptom experience. *Seminar on Oncology Nursing, 11*(4), 256-265.

Rutherford, C. (1992). Position paper: Administration of antineoplastic agents. *Journal of Intravenous Nursing, 15*(1), 8-9.

Sansivero, G.E. & Murray, S.A. (1989). Patient education: Safe management of chemotherapy at home. *Oncology Nursing Forum, 16*(5), 711-713.

57 Antineoplastic Chemotherapy Agents

Chapter Focus

The efficacy of antineoplastic agents as both primary and adjunctive treatment for cancer has greatly increased the use of this therapy. The high level of toxicity associated with these agents requires that the nurse possess specialized knowledge and skills when administering them and monitoring the client who is receiving them.

Learning Objectives

1. Classify antineoplastic agents based on their major mechanism of action.
2. List the common side effects/adverse reactions of antineoplastic drugs.
3. Describe the use of "leucovorin rescue" with methotrexate treatments.
4. Discuss precautions in the preparation and administration of antineoplastic drugs.
5. Implement the nursing management for the care of clients receiving therapy with the various classifications of antineoplastic agents.

Key Terms

alkylating agents, p. 941
antibiotic antitumor agents, p. 941
antimetabolites, p. 941
immunomodulating agents, p. 961
leucovorin, p. 949
leucovorin rescue, p. 949
mitotic inhibitors, p. 941
nadir, p. 949

Key Drugs [✓]

cyclophosphamide, p. 952
doxorubicin, p. 956
methotrexate, p. 946
vincristine, p. 957

The antineoplastic agents do not directly kill tumor cells; they act by interfering with cell reproduction or replication at some point in the cell cycle. (See Chapter 56 for a discussion on cell cycle.) For cells to proliferate, DNA must be replicated once every cell cycle. DNA is the genetic substance in body cells that transfers information to produce RNA; RNA is needed to produce enzymes and synthesize protein (Figure 57-1). Enzymes determine the structure, biochemical activity, growth rate, and functions of the cell. These agents are divided into various classes based on their probable major mechanisms of action (Table 57-1).

OVERVIEW OF DRUG EFFECTS

The formation of the nucleic acids, DNA and ultimately RNA, requires pyrimidines and purines (nitrogen compounds) as the basic building block materials. **Antimetabolites** have a structure similar to a necessary building block for the formation of DNA. Antimetabolites are accepted by the cell as the necessary ingredient for cell growth but, because they are impostors, they interfere with the normal production of DNA.

Alkylating agents are drugs that substitute an alkyl chemical structure for a hydrogen atom in DNA. This results in a cross-linking of each strand of DNA, thus preventing cell division. Alkylator-like drugs are chemically different agents that are believed to have an action similar to the alkylating agents.

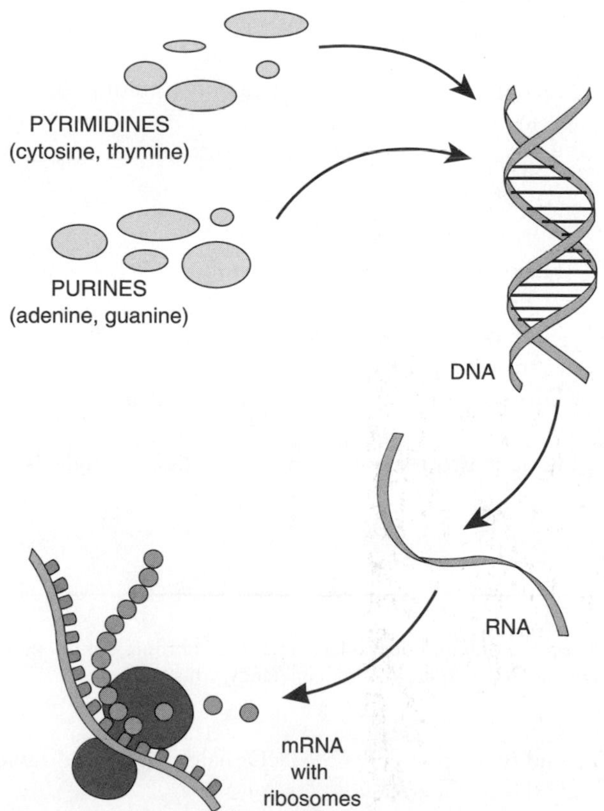

Figure 57-1 Protein synthesis.

Antibiotic antitumor agents interfere with DNA functioning by blocking the transcription of new DNA or RNA. They also delay or inhibit mitosis.

The **mitotic inhibitors,** vinblastine and vincristine, are plant alkaloids that block cell division in metaphase. Vinorelbine (Navelbine) is a semisynthetic vinca alkaloid that also has antitumor activity in metaphase. The mitotic inhibitors probably have other major sites of action, because these agents differ from each other pharmacologically and in therapeutic application. Vinblastine has been used in the treatment of various lymphomas and in carcinoma of the breast and testes, and vincristine is often used to treat acute leukemias and Hodgkin's disease. Vinorelbine is indicated for non–small-cell lung cancer.

Hormones, antihormones, corticosteroids, and various other agents are classified as miscellaneous in this chapter.

The health care professional should be aware that clinical trials are constantly being conducted to optimize drug combinations and treatment regimens for cancer. Current indications may not always be listed in the package insert of the drug or in the *Physician's Desk Reference,* but the *United States Pharmacopeia Dispensing Information (USP DI)* often lists unapproved indications (see Cancer Chemotherapy Research, p. 963).

ANTIMETABOLITE DRUGS

The antimetabolite classification contains capecitabine (Xeloda), fluorouracil (5-FU), floxuridine (FUDR), fludarabine (Fludara), methotrexate (Folex PFS), cytarabine (Cytosar-U), mercaptopurine (Purinethol), and thioguanine (TG). Two of the most common agents prescribed, fluorouracil and methotrexate, are reviewed in this section. The antidote leucovorin will also be discussed. The primary indications and major adverse effects of each drug are listed in Table 57-1. In this table the common side effects as noted in the previous chapter will be repeated only if the effect is considered to be a major problem.

fluorouracil [flure oh yoor′ a sill] (Adrucil, 5-FU)

Fluorouracil is a pyrimidine antagonist that interferes with the synthesis of DNA and RNA. It is a cell-cycle–specific agent that produces its effect in the S phase of cell division. It is indicated for palliative treatment of carcinomas of the colon, rectum, breast, stomach, and pancreas (Ghaneh, Kawesha, Howes, Jones, & Neoptolemos, 1999).

Fluorouracil is metabolized rapidly (within 1 hour) in the tissues to the active metabolite floxuridine. Final metabolic degradation occurs in the liver. This drug is distributed throughout the body and also crosses the blood-brain barrier. The half-life for the alpha phase is 10 to 20 minutes; the beta phase is prolonged up to 20 hours because of tissue storage of metabolites. Excretion is primarily respiratory as carbon dioxide (60% to 80%).

The side effects/adverse reactions of fluorouracil include diarrhea, esophagopharyngitis, leukopenia, thrombocytope-

TABLE 57-1 Antineoplastic Medications

Generic (Brand Name)	Indications	Major Toxicities
Alkylating Agents		
Nitrogen Mustards		
chlorambucil (Leukeran)	CLL, Hodgkin's & non-Hodgkin's lymphomas	Bone marrow suppression
cyclophosphamide* (Cytoxan)	See drug monograph in text	Bone marrow suppression, hemorrhagic cystitis
ifosfamide (IFEX)	Testicular tumors	Bone marrow suppression, nausea, vomiting, encephalopathy
mechlorethamine* (Mustargen)	See drug monograph in text	Bone marrow suppression, severe nausea, vomiting
melphalan (Alkeran)	Multiple myeloma, ovarian cancer	Bone marrow suppression, allergic reactions
uracil mustard (Uracil Mustard)	CLL, CML, non-Hodgkin's lymphomas, mycosis fungoides	Leukopenia, thrombocytopenia
Nitrosureas		
carmustine (BiCNU)	Primary brain tumors, multiple myeloma	Bone marrow suppression, lung fibrosis, nephrotoxicity
lomustine* (CeeNu)	See drug monograph in text	Bone marrow suppression, anorexia, nausea, vomiting
streptozocin (Zanosar)	Pancreatic cancer	Nephrotoxicity, nausea, vomiting
Other		
busulfan (Myleran)	CML	Bone marrow suppression, hyperpigmentation, gynecomastia
carboplatin (Paraplatin)	Ovarian carcinoma	Bone marrow suppression, nausea, vomiting, neurotoxicity, neuropathies, ototoxicity
cisplatin* (Platinol)	See drug monograph in text	Nephrotoxicity, severe nausea and vomiting, bone marrow suppression
thiotepa (Thioplex)	Breast, ovarian, and bladder cancers; lymphomas; malignant effusions	Bone marrow suppression
Antimetabolites		
capecitabine (Xeloda)	Breast cancer, metastatic	Hand and foot syndrome, lymphopenia, cardiotoxicity
cytarabine (Cytosar-U)	AML, ALL	Bone marrow suppression, anorexia, oral and gastrointestinal ulceration
fluorouracil* (Adrucil)	See drug monograph in text	Diarrhea, stomatitis, bone marrow suppression
floxuridine (FUDR)	Gastrointestinal adenocarcinoma with liver metastasis	Bone marrow suppression, stomatitis, anaphylaxis

*Drug monograph in text.
ALL, Acute lymphoblastic leukemia; *AML,* acute myelogenous leukemia; *ANLL,* acute nonlymphocytic leukemia; *CLL,* chronic lymphocytic leukemia; *CGL,* chronic granulocytic leukemia; *CML,* chronic myelocytic leukemia; *HIV,* human immunodeficiency virus.

nia, ulceration of the gastrointestinal tract (severe nausea and vomiting, black stools, abdominal cramps), dermatitis on the extremities (less often on the trunk), anorexia, weakness, loss of hair, and dry skin. A wide variety of doses and schedules of this agent is used, which often influences the extent and type of side effect (MacDonald, 1999). See Table 57-1 for the major toxicities.

The usual adult dosage is 7 to 12 mg/kg body weight IV daily for 4 days; if no toxicity occurs during the following 3 days, a dosage of 7 to 10 mg/kg body weight

TABLE 57-1 Antineoplastic Medications—cont'd

Generic (Brand Name)	Indications	Major Toxicities
Antimetabolites—cont'd		
fludarabine (Fludara)	CLL	Bone marrow suppression, fever, chills, nausea, vomiting, infection
mercaptopurine (Purinethol)	ALL, AML	Bone marrow suppression, anorexia, cholestasis
methotrexate* (Folex)	See drug monograph in text	Bone marrow suppression, diarrhea, stomatitis
thioguanine (6-Thioguanine)	ANLL	Bone marrow suppression
Antibiotics		
bleomycin (Blenoxane)	Squamous cell carcinoma, lymphomas, testicular cancer	Chills, fever, pneumonitis, mucositis, lung fibrosis, hyperpigmentation
dactinomycin (Cosmegen)	Wilms' tumor, Ewing's sarcoma, choriocarcinoma, rhabdomyosarcoma	Bone marrow suppression
daunorubicin liposomal (DaunoXome)	HIV-Kaposi's sarcoma	Bone marrow suppression, cardiomyopathy, severe mucositis
doxorubicin* (Adriamycin)	See drug monograph in text	Same as daunorubicin
idarubicin (Idamycin)	AML	Severe bone marrow suppression, infection, alopecia, nausea, vomiting, hemorrhage
mitomycin (Mutamycin)	Disseminated adenocarcinoma of pancreas or stomach	Bone marrow suppression
mitoxantrone (Novantrone)	ANLL	Cardiotoxicity, severe myelosuppression
pentostatin (Nipent)	Hairy cell leukemia	Bone marrow suppression, renal toxicity, rash
plicamycin (Mithracin)	Testicular tumors, hypercalcemia	Epistaxis, hemorrhage, nausea, bone marrow suppression, stomatitis, vomiting, diarrhea
valrubicin (Valstar)	Bladder cancer	Urinary tract infection, stomach pain, nausea, local adverse reactions (dysuria, bladder spasm and pain, hematuria, increased urination)
Mitotic Inhibitors		
etoposide (VePesid)	Refractory testicular tumors, small cell lung cancer	Bone marrow suppression, alopecia
teniposide (Vumon)	ALL	Bone marrow suppression, mucositis, alopecia
vinblastine* (Velban)	See drug monograph in text	Leukopenia, alopecia, muscle pain, hyperuricemia
vincristine* (Oncovin)	See drug monograph in text	Mild to severe paresthesias, jaw pain, ataxia, muscle wasting, constipation
vinorelbine (Navelbine)	Non–small-cell lung cancer	Bone marrow suppression, nausea, vomiting, asthenia

is administered every 3 to 4 days for a total course of 2 weeks. For alternate schedules, refer to a current package insert or drug reference. The maximum dosage for adults is 800 mg/day, or 400 mg/day for the high-risk client. Investigational protocols may use higher dosages than stated in the product's package insert (see Chapter 2 for legal implications).

Topical fluorouracil preparations (Efudex, Fluoroplex) are used for the treatment of skin cancer (basal cell carcinomas) and precancerous skin lesions.

■ Nursing Management

Fluorouracil Therapy

■ **Assessment.** Fluorouracil is contraindicated if the client presently has or recently has had chickenpox or herpes zoster, because there is a risk for the occurrence or exacerbation of these diseases. This contraindication also applies to clients who have had recent exposure to chickenpox or herpes zoster.

The use of fluorouracil is carefully considered when the client is pregnant or breastfeeding or has renal or hepatic function impairment, infection, bone marrow depression, or tumor cell infiltration of the bone marrow. A lower dosage is recommended if the client has had previous cytotoxic therapy with alkylating drugs or high-dose pelvic radiation. The client should not receive other bone marrow depressants concurrently unless they are part of an antineoplastic combination drug therapy regimen.

Review the client's medication regimen before initiating therapy. A significant drug interaction occurs if fluorouracil is administered with other bone marrow depressants; a dosage reduction of one or both drugs may be necessary. The administration of any live virus vaccine concurrently with fluorouracil should occur only with very close supervision of the oncologist. Fluorouracil will suppress the client's normal defense mechanisms and thus may increase the replication and adverse effects of the virus. It is usually recommended that live virus vaccines not be administered until months after chemotherapy has been discontinued.

Before beginning fluorouracil therapy, a baseline assessment of the client's overall health status, hematocrit or hemoglobin, total and differential white blood cell (WBC) count, platelet count, and renal and hepatic function studies should be obtained. The client's mouth is examined for ulceration with a tongue blade and flashlight before therapy is initiated and before each dose.

■ **Nursing Diagnosis.** Clients receiving fluorouracil are at risk for all of the nursing diagnoses discussed in Chapter 56. The following nursing diagnoses are more common: risk for infection related to the immunosuppression action of the drug (leukopenia); impaired oral mucous membrane (ulcerative stomatitis); impaired comfort related to anorexia, heartburn, nausea and vomiting, rash (dermatitis), or chest pain related to myocardial ischemia; diarrhea; ineffective protection related to an increased tendency for bleeding secondary to thrombocytopenia (unusual bleeding or bruising, petechiae, blood in urine or stool); or disturbed body image related to alopecia and palmar-plantar erythrodysesthesia syndrome or hand-foot syndrome (tingling, swelling, and reddening of the nail beds and the skin of the soles of the feet and the palms of the hands). The client is also at risk for the complication of gastrointestinal ulceration and complications related to the prolonged use of an arterial catheter to administer the drug, such as thrombosis, embolism, thrombophlebitis, abscesses, and bleeding, leakage, or infection at the catheter site.

■ Implementation

■ ***Monitoring.*** Monitor WBC and platelet counts, and watch the client for signs of bruising and bleeding, particularly gastrointestinal bleeding. Test stools for occult blood. In general, the lowest levels of WBC and platelet counts occur 9 to 14 days after the first day of fluorouracil therapy and recover by 30 days.

Monitor the client's temperature and observe for signs of infection, such as fever, chills, sore throat, low back pain, or painful urination.

Observe the client for skin rash and itching. Therapy should be discontinued but may be reinstated at a lower dosage when the side effects have subsided. Check also for oral candidiasis and herpes.

Gastrointestinal disturbances usually occur approximately the fourth day of therapy and subside 2 or 3 days after the medication is withdrawn. Weakness occurs immediately after the dose is administered and lasts for 12 to 36 hours or longer.

Watch for signs of toxicity and indications for discontinuing the drug, including intractable vomiting, diarrhea, severe stomatitis, a WBC count below 3500/mm^3, thrombocytopenia (below 10,000/mm^3), and gastrointestinal bleeding. The leukopenia and thrombocytopenia associated with the pharmacologic action of the drug are used as measures for the titration of each client's dosage.

■ ***Intervention.*** Dosages are determined by the client's weight. An estimated lean body mass is used with obese clients or in clients with edema or ascites. Administer antiemetics to reduce nausea and vomiting. If stomatitis occurs, use a topical oral anesthetic to reduce oral discomfort. Palmar-plantar erythrodysesthesia is usually treated with oral pyridoxine.

Fluorouracil may precipitate if exposed to low temperatures. Dissolve the crystals by warming them to 140° F (60° C), and allow them to cool before administering them. For administration by IV infusion, fluorouracil may be mixed with 5% dextrose injection or 0.9% sodium chloride injection. Vial entry is by a sterile dispensing device or transfer set; the use of a needle and syringe is contraindicated because of the risk of drug leakage.

Fluorouracil may be administered intraarterially by an infusion pump to ensure a consistent rate of infusion. The nurse should be knowledgeable about and skillful with the specific equipment being used. Special nursing management is required if the drug is administered intraperitoneally (Box 57-1).

Toxicity appears to be reduced by slow IV infusion (over 2 to 24 hours), but bolus injections (over 1 to 2 minutes) may be more effective. Because of the hazards in preparing the doses, consult the institution guidelines for the handling of antineoplastic agents (Box 57-2).

Take precautions against IV infiltration. Administration should be stopped immediately if extravasation occurs, with the remaining dose injected into another vein. Cold compresses may reduce local tissue damage.

Safety precautions should be taken if the platelet count is low. Precautions include avoiding invasive procedures or using extreme care in such procedures; regularly examining the skin, mucous membranes, and injection sites for bruising or bleeding; testing emesis, urine, and stool for signs of oc-

BOX 57-1

Nursing Management of Intraperitoneal Chemotherapy

During the last 20 years, intraperitoneal (IP) chemotherapy has developed as an accepted modality in the treatment of ovarian cancer. The possibility of its use for other cancers is also being explored, such as for gastric cancer (Yu et al., 1998) and colon cancer (Markman, 1999). Sound nursing management of clients receiving IP chemotherapy can minimize complications and thus improve quality of life.

The principles of IP chemotherapy are as follows: (1) tumor size should be small to ensure adequate drug penetration, (2) the drug needs to be mixed in large volumes of solution to allow maximum fluid distribution, and (3) the ratio of plasma drug clearance to peritoneal clearance should be high (i.e., it should clear the peritoneal cavity slowly to have as much tumor exposure as possible but then clear the systemic circulation as quickly as possible).

Ovarian cancer is most suited to IP chemotherapy because it metastasizes by IP seeding; the microscopic tumor breaks off and spreads to the serosal surfaces of the abdominal cavity. It is not until late in its course that it invades organs or spreads outside the peritoneal cavity.

Three drug delivery systems are being used. A temporary, single-use catheter can be placed percutaneously and then removed at the end of each infusion of chemotherapy. However, this can become technically difficult as the number of laparotomies increases, causing abdominal adhesions.

The Tenckhoff catheter is a silastic catheter with multiple holes at the distal end. It is placed through the anterior abdominal wall, tunneled subcutaneously, and enters the peritoneal cavity. It allows for rapid infusion rates and can be manipulated to dislodge fibrin deposits that may occur at the end of the catheter. Because it has an external component, it requires daily dressing changes and may decrease the client's acceptance of the catheter related to concept of altered body image.

The Port-A-Cath is totally implantable; a stainless steel port is attached to a silastic catheter tunneled the same way as the Tenckhoff catheter. Because the port lies subcutaneously, it needs to be accessed with a noncoring Huber needle each time the catheter is used. Although it has the advantage of lying completely under the skin, it has the disadvantages of decreased infusion rate because of the small lumen of the Huber needle and the requirement of surgical removal of the catheter and port.

Potential complications common to both catheters include decreased drainage owing to sheathlike fibrin deposits that develop around the end of the catheter (producing a one-way valve effect), catheter infections, and discomfort on infusion owing to distention of the abdomen and the stretching of adhesions formed from previous therapies.

Most health care facilities use a peritoneal dialysis set with a Y-tubing, with one end going to the client and the other two used for drug administration and drainage. Rapid infusion of the IP chemotherapy is important. Concurrent medications are given to protect specific organs or to prevent systemic toxicities similar to the administration of drugs concurrent with IV chemotherapy.

Nursing management of IP chemotherapy includes daily dressing of the Tenckhoff catheter site or accessing the Port-A-Cath, decreasing the discomfort involved with instillation of the drug, attempting to increase fluid return, and instructing the client related to the procedure and catheter used in the institution. Because peritoneal ports are usually placed over the lower edge of the rib cage, placing a pillow under the client on the same side as the port assists in access to the port. Because 2 L of fluid are needed to penetrate as much of the peritoneal cavity as possible, the client may experience abdominal pain, shortness of breath, anorexia, nausea, vomiting, diarrhea, constipation, esophageal reflux, and dysuria, which are treated symptomatically. Decreased return from both catheters occurs, and the nurse may be required to irrigate the catheter to dislodge fibrin deposits and turn the client to redistribute fluid. The nurse can educate the client and family to decrease their anxiety and to help them to understand potential problems and how to manage them when they do occur (Eriksson, 1998).

Information from Belcher, A.E. (1992). *Cancer nursing*. St. Louis: Mosby; and Hoff, S.T. (1991). Nursing perspectives on intraperitoneal chemotherapy. *Journal of Intravenous Nursing, 14*(5), 309-313.

cult bleeding; exercising care in the use of grooming implements, toothbrushes, toothpicks, razors, and nail clippers; preventing constipation; and preventing physical injury. Platelet transfusions may be required.

Protective isolation should be instituted if the WBC count falls below 3500/mm^3. Broad-spectrum antibiotics may be administered pending appropriate culture results.

For topical application, wear plastic gloves and wash hands immediately after handling the drug. Avoid occlusive dressings to minimize the reactions of normal skin around the affected area. Avoid contact with areas that are easily irritated, such as the eyes, nasolabial folds, and wrinkles. Alert the client that the treated area will become unsightly during therapy. After applying the drug, the skin becomes reddened, blisters, sloughs, and erodes before epithelialization occurs. Be aware that sun sensitivity may occur; the use of sun-blocking lotions may be advised.

■ ***Education.*** Clients should be instructed to avoid the intake of excessive amounts of alcohol and any aspirin because of the risk of gastrointestinal bleeding. The client should be

BOX 57-2

Precautions for Handling Antineoplastic Agents

All persons handling cytotoxic (hazardous) drugs, such as antineoplastic agents, should be properly trained in safety procedures and have access to policies and procedures that follow current standards of government and professional practice.

Drug Preparation and Administration

Wash hands thoroughly and wear a disposable gown, surgical latex gloves, and eye protection when preparing or administering cytotoxic drugs.

Whenever possible, it is highly recommended that injectable antineoplastic agents be prepared in the clean-air work station or biohazard cabinet.

Use drug preparation areas for that purpose only. Limit access to that area.

Remove only the required amount of the drug into the syringe. If more is withdrawn accidentally, inject the excess back into the vial and dispose of it properly.

Vent vials with a 20-gauge needle to avoid the creation of aerosol particles.

Nurses should not prepare or administer IV chemotherapy if they are pregnant because of suspected risk to the fetus.

Disposal of Antineoplastic Drugs and Equipment

All antineoplastic drugs and all vials, needles, syringes, tubing, and equipment used in their administration need to be discarded with caution. Special leakproof, puncture-proof, double-bagged containers should be used and labeled "Biohazard" for disposal by incineration.

Needles and syringes should not be broken and/or separated before disposal, because the medication may leak.

Spillage or Antineoplastic Drug Contact with Nurse or Client

Spillage

Wear two pairs of gloves when cleaning up an antineoplastic drug spill. Wash hands before and after.

Wear a mask and eye protection if the medication is powdered.

Place the spilled substance in a plastic bag. Wipe up the remainder with a damp cloth and place it in the plastic bag.

Seal the bag and place it inside of a second bag, and seal the second bag. Label it "Biohazard" and send it for disposal by incineration.

Drug Contact with the Nurse or Client

Thoroughly wash the affected area with soap and water. If clothing was contaminated, remove it immediately.

If eye contact was made, flush the eyes with copious amounts of water, holding the eyelids open during flushing.

Disposal of Client Excreta

Urine, vomitus, and other body fluids from clients receiving antineoplastic drugs should be handled with caution. Flush excreta down the toilet; wear gloves to avoid contact. Wash containers thoroughly.

cautioned against being immunized with live virus vaccines during fluorouracil therapy, because it may cause rather than prevent the disease. Persons in close contact with the client should not receive immunization with the oral poliovirus vaccine, because the live virus is excreted by the vaccine recipient and can be transmitted to the immunocompromised client. The client should avoid being exposed to infections. Inform the client that alopecia may occur but is reversible; hair regrowth may be different in texture or color. Instruct the client on the previously mentioned safety precautions. See the Community and Home Health Care Considerations box on p. 947 for a discussion about working with clients who are receiving antineoplastic agents at home.

■ **Evaluation.** The expected outcome of fluorouracil therapy is that the client will demonstrate signs of clinical improvement and decreased tumor mass without signs and symptoms of infection or bleeding. The client and family will demonstrate an understanding of fluorouracil therapy.

methotrexate [meth oh trex′ ate] (MTX, Folex PFS)

Methotrexate is an antimetabolite that is cell-cycle–specific for the S phase. To synthesize DNA, folic acid must be reduced to tetrahydrofolate by the enzyme dihydrofolate reductase. Methotrexate binds with dihydrofolate reductase, thereby inhibiting the synthesis of DNA and RNA. Because the growth of malignant cells is usually greater than the cell growth of normal tissues, cancer growth may be impaired by methotrexate.

Methotrexate is indicated for the treatment of the following conditions:

- Breast, head, neck, and lung cancers; trophoblastic tumors; renal, ovarian, bladder, and testicular carcinomas; acute lymphocytic leukemia and non-Hodgkin's lymphomas; and the prevention and treatment of meningeal leukemia
- Advanced cases of mycosis fungoides, osteosarcoma, and for the noncancerous, selected cases of severe pso-

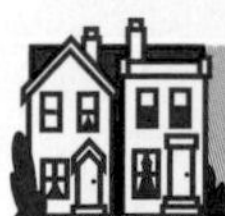

Community and Home Health Considerations
Home Administration of Antineoplastic Therapy

Home health care nurses are finding that the administration of antineoplastic chemotherapy has increased as oncologists have found it to be a cost-effective means of providing cancer care (Holdsworth, 1997). However, not all chemotherapeutic agents are appropriate for home administration. Some agents, such as L-asparaginase, have a high prophylactic potential; others (e.g., cisplatin) require rigorous hydration, which might not be feasible at home. Chemotherapeutic agents commonly administered at home include bleomycin, doxorubicin, etoposide, fluorouracil, methotrexate, plicamycin, and vincristine.

The nurse should be qualified to administer chemotherapy (see Chapter 56 for guidelines) and follow the specific policies established by the home health care agency. The client to receive home chemotherapy should also be carefully selected. Clients who are receiving an antineoplastic agent for the first time, are historically noncompliant, or have multiple, chronic, or unstable health problems are not good candidates for home chemotherapy. The client's support system and physical environment need to be adequate, with a qualified caregiver present should the client experience debilitating side effects and available plumbing and telephone services. All chemotherapeutic agents should be prepared by a pharmacist using established guidelines and packaged in a leakproof container for transport by the nurse. Supplies need to be available in the home to manage extravasation, anaphylaxis, or a chemical spill (see Chapter 56 for chemical spill instructions).

The nurse should review with the client and family the antineoplastic agent to be administered, the planned treatment schedule, the signs and symptoms to report, and how to care for the client should these signs and symptoms occur. Instruction should be provided about posttreatment care, such as hydration or medication administration. A 24-hour resource should be available in case the client requires assistance. All of this can be provided in written form to serve as a reference at home.

An environment conducive to safe administration, without distraction, should be established by the nurse. The client may be comfortably situated in bed or a reclining chair. If the client does not have an implanted venous access device, follow the instructions in Box 57-2. It is recommended that the nurse obtain written orders for the treatment of extravasation at the time the chemotherapy orders are received so that the antidote can be administered without delay.

Nurses should reduce their exposure to these agents as much as possible. Latex gloves are preferred to polyvinyl chloride gloves (if the nurse is not latex sensitive) because they are more resistant to needle punctures. Masks and gowns are not required for administration, but a plastic-backed barrier should cover the work surface. All used supplies should be bagged and labeled as toxic waste and returned to the agency or equipment supplier.

Documentation should be done in accordance with agency policy. It is particularly important that the site of the chemotherapy injection and its condition be recorded, because the effects of infiltration may not be evident until hours later. If extravasation occurs, record any actions taken to treat the infiltration and the client's response. Record any instructions provided to the client and family to care for the area. If possible, a photograph of the affected area should be obtained to document the degree of tissue damage and to provide a guideline for monitoring the site. Recording the client's and family's response to the therapies will assist in decision making regarding whether therapy should be continued in the home or moved to another setting.

Antineoplastic chemotherapy can be provided safely in the home through the preparation and knowledge of administration and symptom management for the benefit of clients and their families.

Information from Catania, P.N. (1999). When patients ask: Home chemotherapy: Basic concepts. *Home Care Provider, 4*(2), 60-61; Jaffee, M.S. & Skidmore-Roth, L. (1988). *Home health nursing care plans.* St. Louis: Mosby; and Parker, G.G. (1992). Chemotherapy administration in the home. *Home Healthcare Nursing, 10*(1), 30-36.

riasis and rheumatoid arthritis that are unresponsive to standard therapies

The side effects/adverse reactions of methotrexate include nausea, vomiting, anorexia, acne, boils, skin rash or itching, loss of hair, gastrointestinal ulcers and bleeding, leukopenia, infections, thrombocytopenia, stomatitis, pharyngitis and, with prolonged daily therapy, liver toxicity, pneumonitis, or pulmonary fibrosis. Renal failure, hyperuricemia, and cutaneous vasculitis may occur with high-dose therapy. See Table 57-1 for the indications and major toxicities of this drug.

Methotrexate is administered orally or parenterally (IM, IV, and intrathecal). The oral preparation reaches peak serum levels within 1 to 2 hours. Limited amounts of methotrexate can cross the blood-brain barrier, but significant quantities pass into the systemic circulation after intrathecal drug administration. It is metabolized intracellularly and in the liver, with the unchanged drug excreted by the kidneys.

The adult and pediatric dosage of methotrexate varies according to the indication and course of treatment. In general, the antineoplastic adult oral dosage is 15 to 30 mg daily for 5 days, repeated from three to five times with a 7- to 14-day interval between each course. The pediatric oral dosage is 20 to 40 mg/m^2 once weekly. For other indications and recommended parenteral dosages, refer to a current package insert or the *USP DI.*

▪ Nursing Management
Methotrexate Therapy

▪ **Assessment.** Methotrexate should not be administered if the client has immunodeficiency. Its use is not recommended when the client is pregnant or breastfeeding because of the risk to the fetus or infant. Methotrexate is to be used cautiously if the client has ascites, pleural effusion, or renal function impairment; there is an increased risk of drug toxicity because excretion is impaired and accumulation may occur. Caution is also used if there is bone marrow depression, infection, oral mucositis, peptic ulcer, or ulcerative colitis. With herpes zoster or an existing case of or recent exposure to chickenpox, there is the risk of generalized, more severe disease. The risk of hyperuricemia is increased if the client has a history of gout or urate renal stones. Caution should be used in clients with previous cytotoxic drug therapy or radiation therapy. Caution should be used with debilitated clients, very young children, or older adults.

Review the client's current medication regimen for the risk of significant drug interactions, such as those that may occur when methotrexate is given concurrently with the following drugs:

Drug	Possible Effect and Management
Bold/color type indicates the most serious interactions.	
acyclovir injection	**Neurologic complications may occur with the use of intrathecal methotrexate. Avoid concurrent use or a potentially serious drug interaction may occur.**
alcohol or hepatotoxic drugs	**Increases the risk of hepatotoxicity. Avoid concurrent use or a potentially serious drug interaction may occur.**
asparaginase	**Cell replication is inhibited by asparaginase, thus impairing the therapeutic effects of methotrexate. If asparaginase is administered 9 to 10 days before or within 24 hours after methotrexate, this effect is not reported. The major side effects of methotrexate—gastrointestinal and hematologic (blood component suppression)—may also be reduced with this drug administration schedule. Avoid concurrent use or a potentially serious drug interaction may occur.**
bone marrow depressants or radiation	Bone marrow depressant effects may be increased. A decrease in drug dosage is usually indicated.
nonsteroidal antiinflammatory drugs (NSAIDs)	**Concurrent administration may result in severe methotrexate toxicity. Avoid concurrent use or a potentially serious drug interaction may occur. Refer to the manufacturer's recommendations on individual NSAIDs to reduce this possibility.**
probenecid or salicylates	**May interfere with the excretion of methotrexate, which results in elevated serum levels. Salicylates may also displace methotrexate from its protein-binding sites, also resulting in increased, and possibly toxic, serum levels. Avoid concurrent use or a potentially serious drug interaction may occur. If necessary to use in combination, monitor serum methotrexate levels closely. The dosage of methotrexate should be decreased and the client closely monitored for signs of toxicity.**
vaccines, live oral	**May result in a decrease in antibody response along with an increase in side effects/adverse reactions. Avoid concurrent use or a potentially serious drug interaction may occur.**

Obtain a baseline assessment of the client's general health status, hematocrit or hemoglobin, platelet count, total and differential WBC count, blood urea nitrogen (BUN), serum creatinine concentration, serum uric acid levels, and hepatic function studies before initiating methotrexate therapy. If the client is to receive high-dose therapy with leucovorin rescue, a determination of urine pH is also included to ensure that its value remains above 7; this minimizes the risk of nephropathy and precipitation of the drug in the urine.

▪ **Nursing Diagnosis.** Clients receiving methotrexate are at risk for the following nursing diagnoses/collaborative problems: ineffective protection related to the thrombocytopenic effects of the drug (increased tendency to bleed); ineffective protection related to its immunosuppressive effects (leukopenia); impaired oral mucous membrane (ulcerative stomatitis); deficient fluid volume (anorexia, nausea or vomiting); disturbed body image related to alopecia; impaired comfort related to intrathecal administration (headache, back pain); disturbed sleep pattern (drowsiness); and the potential complications of dermatologic effects (cutaneous vasculitis or photosensitivity), gastrointestinal bleeding or ulceration, central nervous system (CNS) toxicity after intrathecal administration (confusion, convulsions), pneumonitis, nephrotoxicity, and hepatotoxicity.

▪ **Implementation**

▪ ***Monitoring.*** Serum methotrexate concentrations are usually monitored every 12 to 24 hours after methotrexate administration until concentrations are less than 5×10^{-8} Molar (M) to determine the leucovorin treatment needed to maintain rescue.

Because of the risk of injury related to nephrotoxicity, monitor BUN, serum creatinine, uric acid levels, and intake and output to ensure that the client is adequately hydrated; this will prevent hyperuricemia and uric acid nephropathy. Urine pH determinations are performed every 6 hours during leucovorin rescue until serum methotrexate concentrations are less than 5×10^{-8} M. Alkalinization of urine to pH greater than 7 is necessary to help prevent renal toxicity.

Monitor AST (SGOT), ALT (SGPT), lactate dehydrogenase (LDH), and serum bilirubin concentrations, and observe the client for signs of hepatotoxicity (yellowing of the eyes and skin, dark urine). Monitor complete blood count (CBC), and watch for signs of bruising and bleeding, particularly gastrointestinal bleeding. The **nadir** (lowest cell count) of the platelet count occurs after 7 to 10 days, with recovery approximately 7 days later. Antibiotics may be used for prophylaxis.

Because of the risk for infection related to immunosuppression, monitor the client's temperature and observe for signs of infection, fever, chills, or sore throat. The nadir of the WBC count also occurs after 7 to 10 days, with recovery approximately 7 days later.

The client's mouth should be examined for altered mucous membranes before the administration of each dose, because stomatitis is a sign of toxicity. Therapy should be discontinued but may be reinstated at a lower dosage when the side effects have subsided.

■ ***Intervention.*** Follow the policies and procedures of the health care agency for the administration of drugs that have a mutagenic, teratogenic, and carcinogenic risk.

Leucovorin calcium is administered 24 hours after methotrexate to block the systemic toxic effects of high-dose methotrexate (known as "**leucovorin rescue**"). High-dose methotrexate administration should not be initiated unless leucovorin is immediately available for administration.

For intrathecal use, reconstitute methotrexate with sterile, preservative-free sodium chloride for injection.

Safety precautions should be taken if the platelet count is low. Precautions include avoiding invasive procedures or using extreme care in such procedures; regularly examining the skin, mucous membranes, and injection sites for bruising or bleeding; testing emesis, urine, and stool for signs of occult bleeding; using care with grooming implements, toothbrushes, toothpicks, razors, and nail clippers; preventing constipation; and preventing physical injury.

The client should be maintained on an IV fluid intake of 3000 mL to ensure an increase in urinary output to prevent nephrotoxicity. If the serum uric acid level becomes elevated, allopurinol may be prescribed to reduce it, or sodium bicarbonate may be administered to alkalinize the urine.

Methotrexate should be withheld and the oncologist consulted if the WBC count falls below 1500/mm^3, if the neutrophil count is below 200/mm^3, the platelet count is below 75,000/mm^3, bilirubin is more than 1.2 mg/dL, ALT (SGPT) values are more than 450 units, the creatinine clearance increases by more than 50% from baseline, urine pH is below 7.0, or mouth ulcers or pleural effusion occur.

■ ***Education.*** Caution the client against being immunized with live virus vaccines during methotrexate therapy, because it may cause the disease rather than prevent it. Such immunizations are also contraindicated in family members and other persons in close contact with the client. The client should avoid being exposed to infections.

Instruct the client in the importance of continuing the medication despite gastric distress and of maintaining adequate fluid intake to prevent nephrotoxicity. Alcohol ingestion should be avoided, because it increases the hepatotoxicity associated with the drug. NSAIDs and salicylate products should be avoided because they increase drug toxicity. Instruct the client about the appropriate safety precautions discussed previously.

The client should be aware that skin sensitivity and photophobia may occur. Sun-blocking lotions and sunglasses may be advised. Inform the client that alopecia may occur but is reversible.

Instruct clients about the symptoms of toxicities to report to the prescriber.

■ **Evaluation.** The expected outcome of methotrexate therapy is that the client will demonstrate signs of clinical improvement without signs and symptoms of infection, bleeding, or drug toxicities. If administered as an antineoplastic, the client will experience a decrease in the malignant process, with a decrease in tumor size and metastases. In severe psoriasis, lesions will decrease in size and severity; for arthritis, the client will experience decreased joint swelling and increased mobility. The client and family will demonstrate an understanding of methotrexate therapy.

leucovorin [loo koe vor′ in] (folinic acid, Wellcovorin)

Leucovorin, or folinic acid, is a form of folic acid that does not require dihydrofolate reductase to produce folic acid. Therefore it is used to prevent or treat toxicity induced by folic acid antagonists. It is indicated for the following:

1. As an antidote (prophylaxis and treatment) for folic acid antagonists (e.g., methotrexate, pyrimethamine, and trimethoprim). *Leucovorin rescue* is a term used to describe high-dose methotrexate treatments that use leucovorin to reduce the time that sensitive (normal) cells are exposed to the toxic effects of methotrexate.
2. As a treatment for megaloblastic anemia caused by nutritional deficiencies, sprue, or pregnancy and whenever oral folic acid therapy is not appropriate.

Leucovorin is rapidly absorbed orally and converted by the intestinal mucous membrane and liver to 5-methyltetrahydrofolate, an active metabolite. The onset of action is as follows: oral, between 20 and 30 minutes; IM, 10 to 20 minutes; IV, less than 5 minutes. The duration of action by all routes is between 3 and 6 hours. It is primarily excreted by the kidneys.

The side effects/adverse reactions of leucovorin include allergic reactions (rash, hives, itching, wheezing) and convulsions. No significant drug interactions are reported with leucovorin.

As an antidote to the toxic effect of folic acid antagonists, the adult oral dosage is 10 mg/m^2 every 6 hours until blood levels of methotrexate fall to less than 5×10^{-8} M. For additional dosing recommendations, refer to a current drug reference or package insert.

■ **Nursing Management**

Leucovorin Therapy

All nursing management measures for methotrexate therapy should be observed. Leucovorin is administered after methotrexate rather than simultaneously with it. The first dose is usually administered within 24 to 42 hours of initiating high-dose methotrexate therapy. High-dose methotrexate therapy should not be initiated unless leucovorin is immediately available for administration, because rescue is critical. Leucovorin serves as an antidote that limits the time that normal cells are exposed.

ALKYLATING DRUGS

Alkylating drugs are often used as anticancer agents and are believed to be the first class of medications applied clinically in the modern era of antineoplastic drug therapy. Various groups of alkylating agents are available, including the nitrogen mustards and nitrosoureas. See Table 57-1 for the specific drugs, primary indications, and major toxicities of this classification.

This section reviews mechlorethamine (Mustargen) and cyclophosphamide (Cytoxan) from the nitrogen mustard category, lomustine (CeeNu) from the nitrosourea category, and cisplatin (Platinol), an alkylator-like drug.

mechlorethamine [me klor eth′ a meen] (Mustargen)

The cell-cycle–nonspecific agent mechlorethamine is an alkylating agent capable of cross-linking DNA and RNA and also inhibiting protein synthesis. It is indicated for the treatment of lung carcinoma, Hodgkin's and non-Hodgkin's lymphomas, chronic leukemia, malignant effusions, mycosis fungoides, and polycythemia vera. It may be administered intravenously or by intracavitary route (e.g., intrapleurally or intraperitoneally). A topical preparation is also available to treat cutaneous manifestations of mycosis fungoides.

The onset of action of mechlorethamine is nearly immediate (within seconds or minutes), and it is rapidly deactivated in body tissues.

The side effects/adverse reactions of mechlorethamine include nausea, vomiting, diarrhea, anorexia, a metallic taste in the mouth, neurotoxicity, weakness, alopecia, leukopenia, thrombocytopenia, precipitation of herpes zoster, ototoxicity, hyperuricemia, gonadal suppression, or missed menstrual periods. Peripheral neuropathy, allergic reaction, peptic ulcer, and liver toxicity are rarely reported. See Table 57-1 for the major indications and toxicities of this drug.

The usual adult total dosage is 0.4 mg/kg IV in single or divided doses. If clients have previously received drug chemotherapy or radiation, the dosage should not exceed 0.2 to 0.3 mg/kg body weight. For additional dosing recommendations, refer to a current drug reference or package insert.

■ **Nursing Management**

Mechlorethamine Therapy

■ **Assessment.** Carefully consider the use of mechlorethamine when the client is pregnant or breastfeeding or has bone marrow depression, infection, chickenpox, herpes zoster, tumor cell infiltration of the bone marrow, or a history of gout, urate renal stones, or previous cytotoxic drug therapy or radiation therapy.

Review the client's current medication regimen for the risk of significant drug interactions, such as those that may occur when mechlorethamine is given concurrently with the following drugs:

Drug	Possible Effect and Management
Bold/color type indicates the most serious interactions.	
bone marrow depressants or radiation	Increased bone marrow depression may occur. A decrease in drug dosage is usually indicated.
probenecid or sulfinpyrazone	Hyperuricemia and gout may occur. The prescriber may adjust the antigout medications or prescribe allopurinol. The latter is often preferred to prevent drug-induced hyperuricemia.
vaccines, live viral	Drug interactions are the same as for methotrexate.

A baseline assessment should be obtained for the client's general health status, hematocrit or hemoglobin, platelet count, total and differential WBC count, serum uric acid and creatinine levels, liver function studies, and sense of hearing by audiometric testing.

■ **Nursing Diagnosis.** Over the course of mechlorethamine therapy, the client should be assessed for the following nursing diagnoses/collaborative problems: disturbed sensory perception related to the ototoxic effects of the drug (hearing loss, tinnitus); ineffective protection related to thrombocytopenia (increased bleeding tendencies) and leukopenia (immunosuppression); impaired comfort (headache, rash, pain/redness at the injection site, metallic taste); deficient fluid volume related to anorexia, nausea, or vomiting; impaired oral mucous membrane (stomatitis); diarrhea; activity intolerance related to weakness; impaired tissue integrity related to extravasation of the drug (Box 57-3); disturbed sleep pattern (drowsiness); disturbed body image related to alopecia or menstrual irregularities; disturbed thought processes related to neurotoxicity (confusion); and the potential complications of peripheral neuropathy, allergic reaction, peptic ulcer, hepatotoxicity, ototoxicity, and uric acid nephropathy.

■ **Implementation**

■ ***Monitoring.*** During mechlorethamine therapy, continue to monitor laboratory studies as listed on the baseline assessment. Monitor serum uric acid levels as well as fluid intake and output. Adequate hydration will help to prevent renal complications, but alkalinization of the urine by the administration of sodium bicarbonate may be necessary if serum uric acid levels begin to increase.

Monitor the client's CBC, and monitor for the presence of fever, chills, and sore throat. Lymphocytopenia occurs within 24 hours of the first dose. Granulocytopenia occurs 6 to 8 days after the dose and lasts 10 days to 3 weeks. Monitor for signs of bleeding, such as hematuria, melena, epi-

BOX 57-3

Nursing Management of Extravasation of Vesicant/Irritant Agents

Try to prevent extravasation if at all possible. The best administration site is the forearm. Avoid sites in the hand, wrist, and other such areas; extravasation at these sites could permanently damage nerves, tendons, and muscles. Dilate veins by wrapping the extremity in warm towels or soaking it in warm water rather than using a tourniquet, particularly with older adults or frail clients; the pressure created by a tourniquet may cause the vein wall to rupture when the tourniquet is released. Avoid puncturing the same vein more than once; multiple venipunctures promote extravasation if the site used to administer the drug is distal to the previous site. If the venipuncture attempt is unsuccessful, select a different vein, preferably in the other arm. If the same vein must be used because no other vein is available, use an insertion site that is proximal to the previous one; this prevents extravasation from occurring at the so-called upstream venipuncture (Wood & Gullo, 1993).

If extravasation is suspected, stop administration of the chemotherapeutic agent immediately. Leave the IV in place and begin the extravasation procedure according to the protocol of the health care agency. Attempt to aspirate any residual vesicant agent and blood from the IV. Prepare and instill the antidote. Remove the needle. *If you are unable to aspirate any residual agent from the IV tubing, do not instill the antidote through the existing IV.* The amount of antidote used depends on the size of the extravasation and the amount of the drug thought to have been extravasated. Avoid applying direct pressure to the site; cover it lightly with a sterile occlusive dressing. Apply warm or cold compresses as discussed above. Take measurements of the affected area to use as a point of reference during the healing process. Elevate and rest the area. Notify the physician of the extravasation and the actions taken (Studva, 1993). The dose should be completed in another vein.

Information from *United States Pharmacopeia Dispensing Information (USP DI): Drug information for the health care professional* (19th ed.). (1999). Rockville, MD: United States Pharmacopeial Convention.

BOX 57-4

Double-Syringe Method of Drug Administration

Some antineoplastic agents have vesicant properties (causing blisters) and require careful handling. The following are common vesicant agents:

dactinomycin	mithramycin
carmustine (BiCNU)	mitomycin C
daunorubicin	vinblastine
doxorubicin	vincristine
mechlorethamine	

If these agents are administered by bolus dose, a double-syringe technique is used as follows:

1. Select the site for administration according to the following order of preference: forearm, dorsum of hand, wrist, or antecubital fossa.
2. Use a 20- or 21-gauge "butterfly" needle for drug administration. Use one syringe to administer 5 mL of normal saline solution; withdraw a small amount of blood into the tubing to test vein patency. If blood return is poor, select a site other than distal location.
3. Use another syringe to administer the vesicant agent for at least 3 minutes, drawing blood back into the tubing after every 2 to 3 mL of solution.
4. Flush with 3 to 5 mL of saline solution after administration.
5. If the client has pain at the site of injection or experience an unusual sensation during drug administration, extravasation may have occurred, in which case a new site for drug injection should be selected. The health care agency's procedure/protocol for extravasation should be followed.

staxis, hematemesis, and petechiae. Observe for extravasation during IV administration.

To detect the effects of ototoxicity as early as possible, periodic audiometric testing is required for clients who are receiving high doses of mechlorethamine.

■ ***Intervention.*** Do not use if the solution is discolored or if droplets of water appear in the vial before reconstitution. Reconstitute only with sterile water for injection or sodium chloride injection fluid. Reconstitute immediately before (or less than 15 minutes before) each dose. Discard any unused solution after neutralizing.

Avoid contact with the solution by wearing gloves while preparing and administering it. If contact with the skin, mucous membranes, or eye occurs, irrigate the affected area immediately with large amounts of water for 15 minutes; follow with an application of 2% thiosulfate solution. Neutralize all equipment used in the administration of the drug by soaking it for 45 minutes in a solution of equal parts of 5% sodium thiosulfate and 5% sodium bicarbonate. Box 57-4 explains the double-syringe method of administration.

When mechlorethamine is given by the intracavitary route, change the client's position (prone to supine to right side to left side to knee-chest) every 5 to 10 minutes for 1 hour to distribute the drug. Administer analgesics before the intracavitary administration of mechlorethamine to minimize the discomfort. Removing peritoneal fluid before intracavitary administration of mechlorethamine improves the contact of the medication with the cavity lining. Fluid is usually removed again from the cavity 24 to 36 hours after therapy (see Box 57-1).

Caution should be taken against IV infiltration. If extravasation occurs, promptly infiltrate the area with sterile isotonic sodium thiosulfate or 1% lidocaine, and apply ice compresses for 6 to 12 hours (see Box 57-3).

When applying mechlorethamine topically, follow the specific instructions for application for that client. Usually the client showers, rinses, and dries thoroughly before each treatment and does not shower until treatment the next day. Use plastic gloves to apply mechlorethamine, and avoid contact with the eyes, nose, and mouth. Treatment may be continued for months or even years.

Safety precautions should be taken regarding invasive procedures and the avoidance of infection as mentioned previously with the antimetabolite drugs. In particular, avoid invasive procedures such as IM injections when the platelet count is low. The nadir of thrombocytopenia usually occurs within 6 to 8 days, with recovery in 10 days to 3 weeks.

Nausea and vomiting occur in approximately 90% of clients, generally within 1 to 3 hours of the dose. Although vomiting usually lasts only 8 hours, nausea may persist for 24 hours. Symptoms may be decreased by the administration of antiemetics before mechlorethamine dosing. For the convenience of the client, mechlorethamine may be administered at night if sedatives are also required to control nausea and vomiting.

▪ ***Education.*** The client should be instructed not to be immunized with live virus vaccines during mechlorethamine therapy and to avoid contact with others receiving immunization during that time.

Female clients should be alerted that menstrual periods may become irregular. Alopecia may occur in clients, but they should be told that this effect is usually temporary.

The client should be instructed about the importance of adequate hydration in the prevention of complications. Allopurinol administration and/or alkalinization of the urine may also be prescribed to prevent uric acid nephropathy.

Clients receiving high doses of mechlorethamine should be instructed to report auditory disturbances to their prescriber and/or to receive audiometric testing at periodic intervals.

▪ **Evaluation.** The expected outcome of mechlorethamine therapy is that the client will demonstrate signs of clinical improvement, with the CBC within normal limits and no signs and symptoms of infection, bleeding, or drug toxicities. If administered as an antineoplastic, the client's tumor will diminish in size and the progression of metastases. The client and family will demonstrate an understanding of mechlorethamine therapy.

cyclophosphamide [sye kloe foss′ fa mide] (Cytoxan, Procytox ♣)

Cyclophosphamide is a cell-cycle–nonspecific agent that cross-links DNA and RNA strands and also inhibits protein synthesis. It is indicated for the following:

- Acute and chronic leukemias, carcinomas of the ovary and breast, neuroblastomas, retinoblastomas, Hodgkin's and non-Hodgkin's lymphomas, multiple myeloma, and mycosis fungoides
- As an immunosuppressant in corticosteroid-resistant nephrotic syndrome

Cyclophosphamide is well absorbed orally and has limited crossing of the blood-brain barrier. It undergoes hepatic metabolism to active and inactive metabolites, has a half-life between 3 and 12 hours, and is excreted primarily by the kidneys.

The side effects/adverse reactions of cyclophosphamide include nausea, vomiting, anorexia, darkening of the skin and nails, diarrhea, abdominal pain, flushing of the face, headache, increased sweating, swollen lips, rash, alopecia, gonadal suppression, missed menstrual periods, leukopenia, anemia, and thrombocytopenia. With high-dose therapies or long-term treatment, there may be cardiotoxicity, hemorrhagic cystitis, hyperuricemia, nephrotoxicity, pneumonitis or interstitial pulmonary fibrosis, and a condition that resembles the syndrome of inappropriate antidiuretic hormone (SIADH), with symptoms of confusion, agitation, increased weakness, and dizziness. See Table 57-1 for the primary indications and toxicities of cyclophosphamide.

The usual adult antineoplastic dosage is 1 to 5 mg/kg PO daily; the parenteral dosage is 40 to 50 mg/kg IV in divided doses over 2 to 5 days. The oral dosage for children is 2 to 8 mg/kg in divided doses for 6 or more days. The parenteral dosage for children is 2 to 8 mg/kg IV in divided doses for 6 or more days.

▪ Nursing Management

Cyclophosphamide Therapy

▪ **Assessment.** Carefully consider the use of cyclophosphamide when the client is pregnant (see the Pregnancy Safety box p. 953) or breastfeeding or has renal or hepatic function impairment, infection, bone marrow depression, tumor cell infiltration of the bone marrow, or previous cytotoxic drug or radiation therapy. It is not to be used if the client has herpes zoster or currently has, has recently had, or has been exposed to chickenpox because of the risk of exacerbation or increased severity of the disease.

Review the client's current medication regimen for the risk of significant drug interactions, such as those that may

occur when cyclophosphamide is given concurrently with the following drugs:

Drug	Possible Effect and Management
Bold/color type indicates the most serious interactions.	
bone marrow depressants or radiation	Increased bone marrow depression may occur. A decrease in drug dosage is usually indicated.
cocaine	**Inhibition of cholinesterase activity by cyclophosphamide reduces cocaine metabolism and excretion and may lead to cocaine toxicity. Avoid concurrent use or a potentially serious drug interaction may occur.**
cytarabine (Cytosar-U)	**Concurrent use in preparation for bone marrow transplant may result in increased cardiomyopathy with subsequent death. Avoid concurrent use or a potentially serious drug interaction may occur.**
immunosuppressant agents including azathioprine (Imuran), chlorambucil (Leukeran), corticosteroids, cyclosporine (Sandimmune), mercaptopurine (Purinethol), and muromonab-CD3 (Orthoclone OKT3)	**Increased risk of infections and further development of neoplasms. Avoid concurrent use or a potentially serious drug interaction may occur.**
probenecid (Benemid) or sulfinpyrazone (Anturane)	Hyperuricemia and gout may occur. The prescriber may adjust the antigout medications. Allopurinol is not indicated because it may increase the bone marrow toxicity of cyclophosphamide. If drugs are given concurrently, monitor closely for toxicity.
vaccines, live viral	**Drug interactions are the same as for methotrexate.**

A baseline assessment of the client's general health status, hematocrit or hemoglobin, platelet count, total and differential WBC count, serum uric acid and creatinine levels, BUN, and liver function studies should be obtained.

■ **Nursing Diagnosis.** Assess the client receiving cyclophosphamide therapy for the following nursing diagnoses: ineffective protection related to leukopenia and an increased tendency for bleeding related to thrombocytopenia; impaired tissue integrity related to extravasation; disturbed body image related to gonadal suppression, darkening of the skin and nails, or alopecia; activity intolerance related to anemia; impaired comfort (headache, rash); deficient fluid volume related to anorexia, nausea, and vomiting; diarrhea; impaired oral mucous membrane related to stomatitis; and the potential complications of allergic reaction, altered cardiac output (cardiotoxicity), hepatitis, SIADH-like syndrome (dizziness, confusion, edema, decreased urinary output), hemorrhagic cystitis, nephropathy (a result of hyperuricemia from rapid cell breakdown), pneumonitis, and interstitial pulmonary fibrosis.

Pregnancy Safety
Antineoplastic Chemotherapy Agents

Category	Drug
B	amifostine, mesna, trastuzumab
C	aldesleukin, anastrozole, asparaginase, dacarbazine, dactinomycin, dexrazoxane, interferon alfa-2a, interferon alfa-2b, levamisole, pegaspargase, rituximab, streptozocin, testolactone, valrubicin
D	altretamine, busulfan, capecitabine, carboplatin, carmustine, chlorambucil, cladribine, cyclophosphamide, cytarabine, daunorubicin, docetaxel, doxorubicin, etoposide, exemestane, fludarabine, fluorouracil, flutamide, goserelin, idarubicin, ifosfamide, lomustine, mechlorethamine, mercaptopurine, methotrexate, mitoxantrone, paclitaxel, pentostatin, pipobroman, procarbazine, tamoxifen, teniposide, thioguanine, toremifene, tretinoin, vinblastine, vincristine, vinorelbine
X	bexarotene, leuprolide, plicamycin, raloxifene

■ **Implementation**

■ ***Monitoring.*** Monitor BUN, serum uric acid and creatinine determinations, and perform a urinalysis for microscopic hematuria. A decrease in creatinine clearance and an increase in the other test values may indicate nephrotoxicity. Observe the client for symptoms of SIADH-like syndrome: reduced urinary output, weight gain over several days, and edema of the feet and lower legs, flank pain, pruritus, urine odor on the breath, anorexia, nausea, and vomiting.

Monitor for myelosuppression as evidenced by anemia and leukopenia. Monitor hematocrit, platelet count, and total and differential WBC count. Lowest levels of leukopenia generally occur 7 to 12 days after the first dose. The WBC count recovers 17 to 21 days after the last dose. Observe the client for fever of unknown origin, chills, sore throat, unusual bleeding, or bruising.

Monitor vital signs. Observe for cardiotoxicity, such as myopericarditis, as evidenced by tachycardia, fever and chills, and shortness of breath. Pneumonitis or other respiratory complications may result in a cough and shortness of breath.

■ ***Intervention.*** Reconstituted solutions may be stored for 24 hours at room temperature or 6 days if refrigerated. Antiemetics may be administered concurrently to reduce nausea and vomiting. Unless contraindicated, maintain the client's fluid intake at 3000 mL daily before treatment and for 72 hours following treatment to ensure frequent voiding, including at least once during the night; this minimizes the risk of hemorrhagic cystitis and promotes the excretion of uric acid. Adequate hydration minimizes uric acid nephropathy. Alkalinization of urine or allopurinol administration may also be used to prevent uric acid nephropathy.

The administration of cyclophosphamide is best accomplished early in the day so that most of the drug's metabolites have been excreted before bedtime; this prevents continued contact of the metabolites with the bladder mucosa. The drug should be discontinued at the first sign of hemorrhagic cystitis; symptomatic treatment may be instituted through routes such as blood replacement, cryosurgery, or formaldehyde bladder instillation.

▪ ***Education.*** Alopecia may occur but is reversible; the new hair may be different in color and texture. As with the antineoplastic agents previously discussed, instruct the client not to be immunized with live virus vaccines during the course of therapy. Advise the client of the safety precautions mentioned with previous antineoplastic agents.

Advise the client that nausea and vomiting often occur with cyclophosphamide therapy, but stress that the medication needs to be taken despite these symptoms.

▪ **Evaluation.** The expected outcome of cyclophosphamide therapy is that client will demonstrate signs of clinical improvement, including a decrease in tumor size and metastases and a normal CBC, without signs and symptoms of infection, bleeding, or drug toxicities. The client and family will demonstrate an understanding of cyclophosphamide therapy.

NITROSUREAS

Nitrosureas are highly lipophilic, alkylating agents that easily cross the blood-brain barrier. In general, these agents are very useful for the treatment of primary brain tumors. See Table 57-1 for other nitrosureas, their major indications, and their toxicities.

lomustine [loe mus′ teen] (CeeNu)

Lomustine is used to treat primary brain tumors and Hodgkin's lymphomas. It is well absorbed orally, has a half-life of approximately 90 minutes (the half-life of active metabolites is 16 to 48 hours), and is metabolized in the liver and excreted primarily by the kidneys.

The side effects/adverse reactions of lomustine include anorexia, nausea, vomiting, bone marrow depression (leukopenia, thrombocytopenia, anemia), neurotoxicity, nephrotoxicity and, rarely, hepatotoxicity, pulmonary infiltrates, and/or fibrosis. Drug toxicity is cumulative; thus drug dosage is adjusted regularly on the basis of the nadir blood count from the previous dose administered. Because of the seriousness of this effect, blood counts are closely monitored. Current reference sources should be reviewed when monitoring a client receiving these agents.

▪ Nursing Management
Nitrosurea Therapy

The nursing management of nitrosurea therapy is the same as that for the other antineoplastic agents. The nursing diagnosis/collaborative problems specific to this drug are ineffective protection related to immunosuppression (leukopenia) and bleeding tendencies (thrombocytopenia); activity intolerance related to anemia; impaired nutrition: less than body requirements related to anorexia, nausea, or vomiting; diarrhea; impaired skin integrity (skin rash, itching); disturbed body image related to alopecia; and the potential complications of neurotoxicity, renal toxicity, hepatotoxicity, or pulmonary fibrosis.

ALKYLATOR-LIKE DRUGS

cisplatin [sis′ pla tin] (Platinol)

Although the exact mechanism of action of cisplatin is unknown, it is believed to be a cell-cycle–nonspecific agent with an action similar to the alkylating agents. It cross-links DNA, thus interfering with its function. It is indicated for the treatment of bladder, ovarian, and testicular carcinomas.

The IV form of cisplatin does not significantly cross the blood-brain barrier; its half-life is biphasic. It is metabolized to inactive metabolites that are renally excreted after 5 days, although platinum has been detected in body tissues for 4 months or longer. See Table 57-1 for the major antineoplastic toxicities of cisplatin.

The side effects/adverse reactions of cisplatin include severe nausea and vomiting, anorexia, bone marrow suppression, nephrotoxicity, ototoxicity, neurotoxicity (peripheral neuropathies), anaphylaxis, and extravasation (pain or redness at the injection site, which can result in tissue cellulitis, fibrosis and necrosis). Rare adverse reactions include optic neuritis, blurred vision, and SIADH secretion. See Table 57-1 for primary indications and toxicities.

The adult dosage varies according to the site of cancerous growth; for example, the dosage for advanced bladder cancer is 50 to 70 mg/m^2 IV every 3 to 4 weeks. Recommended dosages vary according to the cancer, the protocol, and whether the therapy is initial or maintenance. Refer to a current drug reference for information.

▪ Nursing Management
Cisplatin Therapy

▪ **Assessment.** The use of cisplatin is not recommended when the client is pregnant or breastfeeding and should be carefully considered if the client has renal function impairment, infection, hearing impairment, bone marrow depression, or a history of gout, urate renal stones, or previous cytotoxic drug or radiation therapy. As with other antineoplastic agents, observe precautions for chickenpox, herpes zoster, and live viruses.

Review the client's current medication regimen for the risk of significant drug interactions, such as those that may occur when cisplatin is given concurrently with the following drugs:

Drug	Possible Effect and Management
Bold/color type indicates the most serious interactions.	
bone marrow depressants or radiation	Increased bone marrow depression may occur. A decrease in drug dosage is usually indicated.
nephrotoxic or ototoxic drugs	Concurrent or sequential administration is not recommended. The risk for nephrotoxicity and ototoxicity is increased, especially in clients with renal impairment. Avoid concurrent use or a potentially serious drug interaction may occur.
probenecid (Benemid) or sulfinpyrazone (Anturane)	Hyperuricemia and gout may occur. The prescriber may adjust the antigout medications or prescribe allopurinol. The latter is often preferred to prevent drug-induced hyperuricemia.
vaccines, live viral	Drug interactions are the same as for methotrexate.

A baseline assessment of the client's underlying condition, including hematocrit or hemoglobin, platelet count, total and differential WBC count, serum uric acid and creatinine levels, creatinine clearance, BUN, electrolytes, audiometric testing, and neurologic status should be obtained.

■ **Nursing Diagnosis.** Clients receiving cisplatin therapy are at risk for the following nursing diagnoses: activity intolerance related to anemia secondary to myelosuppression; ineffective protection related to leukopenia and thrombocytopenia; disturbed sensory perception related to ototoxicity (hearing loss, tinnitus, loss of balance) or to visual disturbances due to optic neuritis or papilledema; impaired oral mucous membrane (stomatitis); impaired comfort related to extravasation (pain/redness at injection site); deficient fluid volume related to anorexia, nausea, or vomiting; and the potential complications of anaphylactic reaction, SIADH secretion, nephrotoxicity/uric acid nephropathy, ototoxicity, optic neuritis, papilledema, and neurotoxicity (loss of reflexes, numbness of fingers and toes, ataxia, seizures).

■ **Implementation**

■ ***Monitoring.*** Evaluate for nephrotoxicity, hyperuricemia, and uric acid nephropathy. Nephrotoxicity is cumulative, and the effects may be irreversible with repeated or high dosages. Symptoms are reduced urinary output, weight gain over several days, edema of the feet and lower legs, flank pain, pruritus, urine odor on the breath, anorexia, nausea, and vomiting. Monitor BUN, creatinine clearance, and serum uric acid levels. A decrease in creatinine clearance and an increase in the other test values may indicate nephrotoxicity. General guidelines indicate that the drug is withheld until the creatinine clearance is greater than 90 mL/min, serum creatinine is less than 1.3 mg/100 mL, or BUN is under 20 mg/100 mL.

Test hearing status before the initial dose and each subsequent dose. Ringing in the ears and difficulty in hearing high frequencies may indicate ototoxicity. Hearing loss is cumulative and may be unilateral.

Monitor for myelosuppression as evidenced by anemia, leukopenia, and thrombocytopenia. Hematocrit, platelet count, and total and differential WBC count should also be monitored. The lowest WBC and platelet counts generally occur 18 to 23 days after a dose and recover within 39 days. Do not administer subsequent doses of cisplatin until platelet levels are over 100,000 cells/mm^3 and the WBC count is over 4000 cells/mm^3. The client should be observed for fever of unknown origin, chills, sore throat, unusual bleeding, or bruising.

Discontinue the administration of cisplatin at the first indication of peripheral neuropathy, because it may be irreversible. Symptoms to watch for are a loss of taste and numbness or tingling in the fingers, toes, or face. Perform regular neurologic examinations.

■ ***Intervention.*** Follow the health agency's policy for the handling of hazardous materials. Have available drugs and equipment available for the treatment of a possible anaphylactic reaction.

If the client is receiving a daily dose over a course of 1 to 5 days, the client may be hydrated with 1 to 2 L of IV infusion fluid 8 to 12 hours before the dose. The cisplatin infusion should be administered over 6 to 8 hours. Cisplatin may also be administered continuously over 24 hours to 5 days to reduce nausea and vomiting. Adequate IV hydration of 3000 mL daily should be maintained to reduce nephrotoxicity. Urinary output should be closely monitored. Alkalinization of urine and the administration of allopurinol may also be used to prevent uric acid nephropathy.

The total dose for a single course of cisplatin (whether given as a single daily infusion or as a continuous infusion over several days, to be repeated every 3 to 4 weeks) should not exceed 120 mg/m^2.

Reduce nausea and vomiting by administering a parenteral antiemetic ½ hour before administering cisplatin. Metoclopramide (Reglan) is usually indicated for cisplatin-induced emesis. Nausea and vomiting usually begin 1 to 4 hours after a dose. Antiemetic therapy is continued on a schedule as long as necessary. Cisplatin may be discontinued if nausea and vomiting are severe. As with the nursing management of the antineoplastic agents discussed in Chapter 56, observe safety precautions regarding invasive procedures.

Do not use aluminum needles or other equipment containing aluminum. Cisplatin is incompatible with aluminum; the interaction causes a black precipitate and a loss of potency.

■ ***Education.*** Instruct the client to record intake and output and to report any edema or decrease in urinary output. The client should report any numbness or tingling of the fingers or toes, any ringing in the ears, or hearing loss.

As with the other antineoplastic agents previously discussed, caution the client against being immunized with live virus vaccines, and alert the client to signs and symptoms to report to the prescriber. Instruct the client about safety measures to be taken while thrombocytopenia exists.

▪ **Evaluation.** The expected outcome is that the client will demonstrate signs of clinical improvement, with a decrease in tumor size and metastases and no signs and symptoms of infection, bleeding, tinnitus, or hearing loss. Renal function will be adequate. The client and family will demonstrate an understanding of cisplatin therapy.

ANTIBIOTIC ANTITUMOR DRUGS

The antitumor antibiotics are cytotoxic agents that directly bind DNA, thus inhibiting the synthesis of DNA and RNA. The early agents in this class cause the clinically limiting adverse effect of irreversible cardiomyopathy. Newer agents that lack this cardiac toxicity are being sought. See Table 57-1 for drugs in this classification, their primary indications, and their toxicities.

doxorubicin [dox oh roo′ bi sin] (Adriamycin)

Doxorubicin is an antineoplastic cell-cycle–specific agent for the S phase of cell division. It is indicated for the treatment of acute leukemia, Wilms' tumor, soft tissue and bone sarcomas, Hodgkin's disease, lymphomas, and breast and various other carcinomas.

Doxorubicin does not cross the blood-brain barrier and is highly tissue bound. It is metabolized in the liver to produce adriamycinol, an active metabolite. The half-life of doxorubicin is biphasic: 0.6 hours and 16.7 hours. The active metabolite has a half-life of 3.3 hours and 31.7 hours. It is metabolized in the liver and excreted primarily in the bile.

The side effects/adverse reactions of doxorubicin include severe nausea and vomiting; darkening of the soles, palms, or nails (especially in children and blacks); alopecia; diarrhea; red urine; leukopenia; thrombocytopenia; stomatitis; esophagitis; cardiotoxicity (usually congestive heart failure); extravasation leading to cellulitis or tissue necrosis; hyperuricemia; nephropathy; and dark or red skin. Be aware that liposomal doxorubicin is not interchangeable with doxorubicin (see Cancer Chemotherapy Research, p. 963).

The usual adult dosage is 60 to 75 mg/m^2 IV, repeated every 3 weeks. The pediatric dosage is 30 mg/m^2 daily on 3 consecutive days every month.

▪ Nursing Management

Doxorubicin Therapy

▪ **Assessment.** The use of doxorubicin is not recommended when the client is pregnant or breastfeeding. Its use is carefully considered if the client has bone marrow depression, tumor cell infiltration of the bone marrow, hepatic function impairment, or a history of gout, urate kidney stones, or cytotoxic drug or radiation therapy. The cardiotoxic effects of the drug may occur at lower levels if the client has heart disease or is over 70 years of age. Caution should be used with older adults because of their decreased bone marrow reserves. As with other antineoplastic agents, observe cautions for chickenpox and herpes zoster.

Significant drug interactions are reported with other bone marrow depressant drugs, irradiation, probenecid (Benemid), sulfinpyrazone (Anturane), and with live virus vaccines (see Mechlorethamine, p. 950, for comments regarding drug interactions). The use of doxorubicin in clients who have received daunorubicin (Cerubidine) increases the risk of inducing cardiotoxicity.

Before doxorubicin therapy, the client should have a baseline assessment that includes echocardiography, ECG, radionuclide angiography determination of ejection fraction, hematocrit or hemoglobin, platelet count, total and differential WBC count, serum uric acid levels, and liver function studies. The client's mouth should be examined for ulcerations.

▪ **Nursing Diagnosis.** Assess the client receiving doxorubicin for the possibility of the following nursing diagnoses/collaborative problems: impaired oral mucous membrane (stomatitis); ineffective protection related to immunosuppression (leukopenia) and an increased tendency to bleed due to thrombocytopenia; impaired tissue integrity related to extravasation or cellulitis at the injection site; diarrhea; deficient fluid volume related to anorexia, nausea, and vomiting; disturbed body image related to alopecia or darkening of nail beds or the skin of the soles of the feet or palms of the hands; and the potential complications of cardiotoxicity (pedal edema, dysrhythmias, shortness of breath), uric acid nephropathy, and allergic response.

▪ **Implementation**

▪ ***Monitoring.*** Monitor serum uric acid levels and intake and output to ensure that the client is adequately hydrated to prevent hyperuricemia. Allopurinol administration and urine alkalinization may be used to decrease serum uric acid levels.

Monitor hemoglobin, hematocrit, and platelets, and watch the client for signs of bruising and bleeding, particularly gastrointestinal bleeding. Monitor the client's temperature, and observe for signs of infection, fever, chills, or sore throat. Monitor the total and differential WBC count. The lowest WBC count usually occurs 10 to 14 days after dosage and recovers within 21 days.

Monitor echocardiography, ECG, and radionuclide angiography reports for evidence of cardiopathy; observe for swelling of the feet and lower legs and shortness of breath. Cardiotoxicity usually occurs within 1 to 6 months after initiating therapy and is more common in older adults over 70 years of age and in children under 2 years of age. The risk of cardiotoxicity is also dose related and is estimated to be 1% to 2% at a total cumulative dose of 300 mg/m^2 of body surface area, 3% to 5% at 400 mg/m^2, 5% to 8% at 450 mg/m^2, and 6% to 20% at 500 mg/m^2. Cardiotoxicity may develop suddenly and may be irreversible; it is critical that it be detected early, when it usually responds to therapy.

Examine the mouth for ulcerations before the administration of each dose, because stomatitis is a sign of toxicity. Stomatitis usually occurs 5 to 10 days after administration and may be severe enough to place the client at risk for infection.

▪ ***Intervention.*** Doxorubicin is usually administered slowly, over not less than 3 to 5 minutes, into the tubing of a freely running IV solution of 5% dextrose injection or 0.9% sodium chloride injection. Avoid venous sites over joints and sites in extremities with compromised venous and lymphatic circulation.

Avoid contact with the solution by wearing gloves during preparation and administration. If contact with the skin or mucous membranes occurs, wash thoroughly with soap and water. Refer to the guidelines of the institution for the safe handling of antineoplastic agents.

Take precautions against IV extravasation. If extravasation occurs, the IV line should be moved to another site for completion of the dose. Ice packs should be applied, and the extremity should be elevated to minimize injury. Surgical excision of the area may be required if inflammation is extensive. Do not administer doxorubicin intramuscularly or subcutaneously, because it will cause tissue necrosis.

As with the nursing management of other antineoplastic agents discussed in Chapter 56, observe safety precautions for invasive procedures.

■ ***Education.*** The client's urine may become reddish for 1 or 2 days after the administration of doxorubicin, but it generally clears in 48 hours. Teach that a discoloration of the skin and nails may occur, especially in children and blacks.

As with previously discussed antineoplastic agents, discuss with the client the importance of adequate hydration, the possibility of reversible alopecia, and the contraindication of being immunized with live virus vaccines during therapy. Instruct the client to report signs and symptoms of infection (fever, sore throat), bleeding, and congestive heart failure (pedal edema, shortness of breath).

■ **Evaluation.** The expected outcome of doxorubicin therapy is that the client will demonstrate signs of clinical improvement, with decreased tumor size and metastases and no bleeding, infection, local tissue damage at the infusion site, or signs and symptoms of cardiotoxicity. The client and family will demonstrate an understanding of doxorubicin therapy.

For information on epirubicin [ep i roo′ bi sin] (Ellence), a new drug in this classification, see Appendix E. 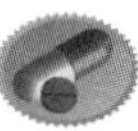

MITOTIC INHIBITORS

The primary mitotic inhibitors, vinblastine and vincristine (vinca alkaloids derived from a periwinkle plant), are cell-cycle–specific agents that inhibit mitosis during the M phase. Vinorelbine is a semisynthetic vinca alkaloid. These agents are similar chemically but have different therapeutic indications and different side effects/adverse reactions. See Table 57-1 for primary indications and toxicities.

vinblastine [vin blas′ teen] (Velban)
vincristine [vin kris′ teen] (Oncovin)

Vinblastine is used to treat breast and testicular carcinoma, Hodgkin's and non-Hodgkin's lymphomas, Kaposi's sarcoma, and mycosis fungoides. Vincristine is used to treat acute lymphoblastic leukemia, Hodgkin's and non-Hodgkin's lymphomas, rhabdomyosarcoma, neuroblastoma, Wilms' tumor, and various other carcinomas.

Vinblastine and vincristine are administered intravenously and do not cross the blood-brain barrier. They are highly tissue bound and have a triphasic half-life of 3.7 minutes, 1.6 hours, and 25 hours for vinblastine and of 0.07 hour, 2.27 hours, and 85 hours for vincristine. Both drugs are metabolized in the liver and excreted primarily in bile. (See the Case Study box below.)

The side effects/adverse reactions of the mitotic inhibitors include neurotoxicity (the major dose-limiting side effect for vincristine) and bone marrow suppression (the major undesirable effect for vinblastine). Muscle pain, nausea, vomiting, alopecia, extravasation at the injection site, cellulitis, hyperuricemia, stomatitis, rectal bleeding and hemorrhagic colitis have also been reported with vinblastine. Vincristine may also induce anorexia, nausea and vomiting,

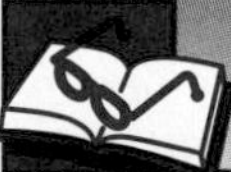

Case Study *The Client with Hodgkin's Disease*

Matthew Bennett is a 32-year-old, married salesperson who has been referred to an oncology clinic after a diagnosis of stage III-A Hodgkin's disease was confirmed by his primary physician. Mr. Bennett first went to his physician after finding a lump in his right axilla that persisted for several months. The oncologist has recommended a program of chemotherapy that includes the following drugs:

mechlorethamine (Mustargen)
vincristine (Oncovin)
prednisone (Deltasone)
procarbazine (Matulane)

1. How is each drug classified as a chemotherapeutic agent, and what is its effect on the cell cycle?
2. Why is prednisone used as part of the chemotherapy regimen?
3. What measures should the nurse implement before administering mechlorethamine to reduce nausea and vomiting?
4. What should the nurse do if the IV infusion infiltrates during the administration of mechlorethamine or vincristine?
5. During the course of therapy with vincristine, Mr. Bennett complains of numbness and tingling in his hands and feet. What is the significance of these symptoms?
6. What precautions should the nurse take when handling the equipment used for drug administration and body fluids?

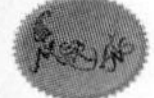

For answer guidelines, to to mosby.com/MERLIN/McKenry/.

rash, autonomic toxicity (abdominal cramping; constipation; bed-wetting; increased, decreased or painful urination; orthostatic hypotension; lack of sweating), hyperuricemia, a progressive neurotoxicity (blurred or double vision, difficulty in walking, drooping eyelids, headache, jaw pain, numbness and pain in the fingers and toes, weakness), and SIADH secretion.

The adult antineoplastic dosage for vinblastine is 0.1 mg/kg IV weekly, with dosages adjusted according to tumor size response and WBC count. The adult dosage of vincristine is 0.01 to 0.03 mg/kg as a single dose weekly. For various dosage schedules, refer to a current package insert or drug reference.

▪ Nursing Management

Vinblastine/Vincristine Therapy

▪ Assessment. Vinblastine and vincristine are not recommended when the client is pregnant or breastfeeding. The use of these drugs should be carefully considered if the client has hepatic function impairment, infection, bone marrow depression, tumor cell infiltration of the bone marrow, or a history of gout, urate kidney stones, or cytotoxic drug or radiation therapy. As with other antineoplastic agents, observe for contraindications for chickenpox and herpes zoster. The use of vincristine in clients with neuromuscular disease should be carefully considered.

Review the client's current medication regimen for drug interactions. Both drugs may have significant drug interactions with probenecid (Benemid), bone marrow depressants, sulfinpyrazone (Anturane), and live virus vaccines. See Mechlorethamine, p. 950, for a description of the interactions. In addition, significant drug interactions may occur when vincristine is given concurrently with the following antineoplastic drugs:

Drug	Possible Effect and Management
Bold/color type indicates the most serious interactions.	
asparaginase (Elspar)	**An increase in neurotoxicity may result when given concurrently with vincristine. To reduce the possibility of this interaction, asparaginase should be given only after vincristine is administered, not concurrently or before it.**
doxorubicin (Adriamycin)	**An increase in bone marrow depressant effects may occur if administered with vincristine and prednisone. Avoid concurrent use or a potentially serious drug interaction may occur.**

The client's baseline assessment should include the status of the underlying condition, bowel and bladder function, muscle tone and reflexes, serum uric acid concentrations, hematocrit, hemoglobin, platelet count, total and differential WBC count, and liver function studies.

▪ Nursing Diagnosis. Vinblastine or vincristine therapy places the client at risk for the following nursing diagnoses/collaborative problems: deficient fluid volume related to anorexia, nausea, and vomiting; impaired tissue integrity related to extravasation or cellulitis at the infusion site; impaired oral mucous membranes (stomatitis); ineffective protection related to leukopenia and thrombocytopenia; diarrhea or constipation; disturbed body image related to alopecia; and the potential complications of hyperuremia or uric acid nephropathy (joint pain, lower back pain) and neurotoxicity (numbness in fingers and toes, blurred vision). With vincristine, impaired urinary elimination related to autonomic toxicity is also a possibility and is evidenced by bed-wetting, increased or decreased urination, and painful or difficult urination; impaired comfort (headache, rash, bloating) is also possible. In addition, vinblastine has the potential complication of gastrointestinal bleeding.

▪ Implementation

▪ *Monitoring.* Monitor the client's CBC and observe for fever, chills, sore throat, bleeding, and bruising to assess the risk for infection or physical injury. With vinblastine, the lowest level of leukocytes occurs 5 to 10 days after the last day of administration, and recovery occurs within another 7 to 14 days. With vincristine, leukopenia is usually greatest within 4 days.

Monitor serum uric acid levels and the client's intake and output to ensure adequate hydration for the prevention of uric acid nephropathy and to detect early signs of urine retention.

Monitor the client's neuromuscular status. Watch for ataxia, numbness, tingling, or pain in the fingers or toes, headache, double vision, depression of deep tendon reflexes, and other early signs of neurotoxicity. Monitor the client's bowel status for early signs of autonomic toxicity, such as constipation.

Monitor the client's nutritional status, weight, and hydration if nausea and vomiting are adverse reactions.

Observe the injection/infusion site for extravasation and cellulitis.

▪ *Intervention.* Reconstitute vinblastine with sterile 0.9% sodium chloride injection. Only reconstituted vinblastine solution with preservatives can be refrigerated; the limit for such storage is 28 days.

Take precautions against IV infiltration. If extravasation occurs, stop the bolus injection immediately and administer the remaining dose into another vein. To alleviate discomfort and inflammation with vincristine extravasation, inject hyaluronidase locally and apply moderate heat or cold compresses according to protocol.

Administer vincristine and vinblastine by IV push, or inject into the tubing of a running IV infusion for 1 minute. Administer only intravenously; IM or SC administration will cause tissue necrosis, and intrathecal administration will cause death.

Intake should be 3000 mL daily. Urine may be alkalinized to promote the excretion of urinary uric acid if serum uric acid levels increase. The use of a laxative or stool softener will help to prevent upper colon impaction. Antiemetics are administered as needed.

As with the nursing management for the other antineoplastic agents discussed in Chapter 56, observe safety precautions for invasive procedures and the avoidance of infections.

■ ***Education.*** Stress the importance of adequate hydration, the possibility of alopecia, and the contraindication of being immunized with live virus vaccines during therapy (see Chapter 56).

■ **Evaluation.** The expected outcome of mitotic inhibitor therapy is that the client will demonstrate signs of clinical improvement with decreased tumor size and metastases, normal CBC, and no local tissue damage at the IV site, neuropathy, or nephropathy. The client and family will demonstrate an understanding of vinblastine/vincristine therapy.

MISCELLANEOUS ANTINEOPLASTIC AGENTS

Miscellaneous agents are those that cannot be classified by their mechanism of action into any of the previous groups. In this section, hormones, cytoprotective combinations, immunomodulator agents, and other agents are discussed.

Hormones

Hormonal agents are used in the treatment of neoplasms that are sensitive to hormonal growth controls in the body. The exact mechanism of action against neoplasms is unknown, but apparently they interfere with growth-stimulating receptors on target tissues. Such agents are more selective and less toxic than other antineoplastics and include corticosteroids, androgens and antiandrogens, estrogens and antiestrogens, progestins, and gonadotropin-releasing hormone.

Because corticosteroids slow lymphocytic proliferations, their greatest value lies in the treatment of lymphocytic leukemias and lymphomas. They are also used in conjunction with radiation therapy to decrease the occurrence of radiation edema in critical areas such as the superior mediastinum, brain, and spinal cord.

Prednisone and dexamethasone are corticosteroids that are often prescribed for clients with cancer. Prednisone has a demonstrated lympholytic and antiinflammatory effect that is useful in the treatment of leukemias, lymphomas, and breast carcinomas. Steroids, especially dexamethasone, are useful in reducing cerebral edema induced by the increasing growth of a brain tumor or from radiation therapy. Individual drugs belonging to this category are discussed in Chapter 49.

Androgens such as testosterone and fluoxymesterone (Halotestin) are used to treat advanced breast carcinoma if surgery, radiation, and other therapies are inappropriate or ineffective.

Antiandrogens

Bicalutamide [bik ah loot′ ah mide] (Casodex) competitively inhibits androgens from binding to receptors in target tissues. It is indicated in combination with a luteinizing hormone–releasing hormone for the treatment of advanced prostate cancer. Clinical trials indicate that it is comparable to flutamide combination in survival time *(Drug Facts and Comparisons,* 2000).

Flutamide [floo′ ta myde] (Eulexin), an oral antiandrogen product, inhibits the uptake and/or the binding of androgens at the target site. The result is suppression of ovarian and testicular steroidogenesis, which induces a medical castration. It is used in combination with leuprolide (Lupron), a luteinizing hormone–releasing hormone agonist, to treat metastatic prostate carcinomas. This combination has been reported to prolong survival by at least 25% as compared with leuprolide therapy alone. Side effects/adverse reactions include diarrhea, impotency, and hepatotoxicity.

Nilutamide [nye loot′ a mide] (Nilandron) is an antiandrogen used in conjunction with surgery or chemical castration for the treatment of metastatic prostate cancer. It blocks testosterone effects at the androgen receptor in vitro, and it interacts with the androgen receptor in vivo to prevent normal androgen responses. For maximum effect it must be started on the same day as surgical castration *(Drug Facts and Comparisons,* 2000).

Goserelin [goe′ se rel in] (Zoladex), a palliative agent used in the treatment of advanced prostate carcinoma, is also a luteinizing hormone–releasing hormone. It is a potent inhibitor of pituitary gonadotropins; the serum levels of testosterone usually drop to the range seen in surgically castrated men within 2 to 4 weeks of initiating drug therapy. A 3.6-mg dose is implanted subcutaneously in the upper abdominal wall every 28 days. Adverse reactions of goserelin are related to lowered testosterone levels and may include hot flashes, sexual dysfunction, and decreased erections.

For information on triptorelin [trip toe rel′ in] (Trelstar), a new drug in this classification, see Appendix E.

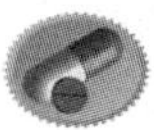

Estrogens

Estrogens may be used to treat androgen-sensitive prostatic carcinomas in men or advanced breast carcinoma in postmenopausal women. Estrogens such as diethylstilbestrol (DES, Stilphostrol), polyestradiol (Estradurin), ethinyl estradiol (Estinyl), and estramustine (Emcyt) are used to treat advanced prostatic carcinoma. The latter drug is a combination of estradiol and nitrogen mustard that provides both a weak hormone effect and an alkylating action. In this combination, estrogen helps to carry the drug into estrogen receptor cells, thus enhancing the nitrogen mustard cytotoxic effects in these cells.

The main precaution in monitoring estramustine is an increased risk of inducing thrombosis, especially in clients with a history of thrombophlebitis or thromboembolic disease. Avoid immunizations unless specifically ordered by the prescriber. The client and others in the household should avoid immunization with oral poliovirus vaccine.

Estramustine is taken orally with water (14 mg/kg/day in divided doses), preferably an hour before meals. Avoid concurrent consumption of milk, dairy products, or any calcium-containing products.

Antiestrogens

Tamoxifen [ta mox′ i fen] (Nolvadex, Nolvadex-D 🍁) an antiestrogen preparation, has replaced both androgens and estrogens as the initial approach in breast cancer therapy (Chabner, Allegra, Curt, & Calabresi, 1996). It has also been approved to prevent breast cancer in women who are at high risk. *High risk* is defined by the Gail Model Risk Assessment Tool* (*Drug Facts and Comparisons*, 2000). Tamoxifen is believed to bind to estrogen receptors in breast cancer cells and act as a competitive inhibitor of estrogen. It is effective for tumors that contain high concentrations of estrogen receptors. It is also an estrogen agonist in the liver, which has desirable effects on serum lipids in postmenopausal women; it also helps to preserve bone mineral density, which may decrease the risk for osteoporosis in these women (Robinson, Kimmick, & Muss, 1996). The side effects/adverse reactions of tamoxifen include hot flashes and weight gain in women; impotence in men, and nausea, vomiting, and headache in both men and women. Other rare adverse reactions include an increased risk for endometrial carcinoma, thromboembolism, and ocular toxicity (Robinson et al., 1996).

Raloxifene [ral ox′ ih feen] (Evista ◆) is currently used to prevent postmenopausal osteoporosis but is also being studied for the treatment of breast cancer. An initial study indicates it may have decreased the number of new breast cancer incidents by 50%, but further studies are necessary to validate these results and to compare raloxifene to tamoxifen (Tarlach, 1998).

Toremifene [tor em′ ih feen] (Fareston) is an antiestrogen product released in 1998 for the treatment of metastatic breast cancer in postmenopausal women. Toremifene is similar to tamoxifen chemically and has a similar pharmacologic effect. The major difference between the products is that the chronic use of large doses of tamoxifen is hepatotoxic in rats, whereas toremifene does not produce this effect. Both products have a hypocholesterolemic effect after chronic administration. The effect of toremifene on bone mineral density, thromboembolic events, and the risk for endometrial cancer is unknown because of the lack of long-term clinical studies (Buzdar & Hortobagyi, 1998). Toremifene is used to treat estrogen-receptor (ER) positive or ER unknown-type tumors.

Anastrozole [an a′ stroh zole] (Arimidex), letrozole [le′ troe zole] (Femara), and testolactone [tes tah lack′ tone] (Teslac) inhibit steroid aromatase, thereby reducing estrone synthesis in the adrenals, the major source of estrogen in postmenopausal women. These drugs are indicated as palliative therapy for advanced breast cancer in postmenopausal women. Testolactone is also used in premenopausal women with disseminated breast cancers that have a terminated ovarian function.

Exemestane [ex eh mes′ tane] (Aromasin) is an irreversible aromatase inactivator; that is, it reduces estrogen supplies to the cancer cells. It is indicated for advanced breast cancer in postmenopausal women who are responding to tamoxifen. The usual dosage is 25 mg daily PO after a meal.

*The Gail Model Risk Assessment Tool is available to health care professionals by calling (800) 456-3669, ext. 3838.

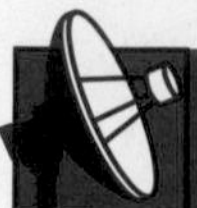

TechnologyLink
Antineoplastic Chemotherapy Agents

Video Resources

Mosby's Medical-Surgical Nursing Videotape Series
Mosby, Inc., 11830 Westline Industrial Drive, St. Louis, MO 63146; (800) 426-4545; www.mosby.com.
Nursing Management of Breast Cancer, ISBN 0-8151-6056-9
Nursing Management of Colon Cancer, ISBN 0-8151-6059-3

Web Resources

American Cancer Society (www.cancer.org/)
This site is a source of current cancer news, as well as information on types of cancer, cancer prevention, treatment options, chemotherapy, radiation therapy, alternative approaches, and much more.

Cancer News on the Net (www.cancernews.com/)
This site provides the most current information on the prevention, diagnosis, and treatment of cancer.

Quackwatch (www.quackwatch.com/)
The Quackwatch website provides information on alternative cancer treatments and cancer prevention.

National Guideline Clearinghouse (www.guideline.gov/body_home_nf.asp?view=home)
The National Guideline Clearinghouse is a site for evidence-based clinical practice guidelines and information on disease states, treatments, and nursing interventions.

For additional WebLinks, a free subscription to the "Mosby/Saunders ePharmacology Update" newsletter, and more, go to mosby.com/MERLIN/McKenry/.

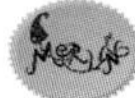

Progestins

Progestins such as medroxyprogesterone (Depo-Provera) and megestrol (Megace) are used to treat advanced endometrial cancer. It is primarily a palliative approach that seeks tumor regression and an increase in the client's survival time. Megestrol is also indicated for advanced carcinoma of the breast, and medroxyprogesterone is also used in clients with advanced renal carcinoma.

Cytoprotective Combinations

One antineoplastic drug combination is *ifosfamide* [eye foss′ fa mide] (IFEX) with *mesna* [mess′ na] (Mesnex). This product is used for the treatment of germ cell testicular tumors. Ifosfamide, an alkylating agent, has been studied since the early 1970s, but its adverse effect of hemorrhagic cystitis (urotoxicity) has limited its usefulness. Mesna has been found to be a specific antidote for this type of toxicity. Therefore using both drugs in combination allows for a more aggressive therapy while also reducing the potential of ifosfamide-induced hematuria and cystitis.

Amifostine [am i foss' teen] (Ethyol) is a cytoprotective agent administered before cisplatin to reduce the potential for renal toxicity. Dexrazoxane [dex ra zock' zain] (Zinecard) is a cardioprotective substance used with doxorubicin administration to reduce drug-induced cardiomyopathy. It is an intracellular chelating agent, but its mechanism of action is not clearly defined. There are some reports that the concurrent use of this product with the FAC (5-FU, doxorubicin [Adriamycin], and cyclophosphamide) regimen for breast cancer results in a lower response rate to therapy. For this reason, it is recommended that dexrazoxane be used only in clients who have received the cumulative 300 mg/m^2 dose of doxorubicin and are continuing to take this product (*Drug Facts and Comparisons*, 2000). The side effects/adverse reactions of dexrazoxane include the myelosuppression effects of alopecia, nausea, vomiting, tiredness, anorexia, stomatitis, fever, diarrhea, neurotoxicity, phlebitis, and dysphagia. Refer to a current package insert for more information.

Immunomodulator Agents: Interferons

Immunomodulating agents, agents that can either activate the body's immune defenses or modify a biologic response to an unwanted stimulus, such as an antitumor response, are used to assist the compromised immune system. See Chapter 64 for a further discussion of these agents and for nursing management.

Interferon alfa-2a, recombinant (Roferon-A), *interferon alfa-2b, recombinant* (Intron A), and *interferon alfa-n3* (Alferon N) are manufactured by the process of recombinant DNA technology. This process results in highly purified proteins that have an effect similar to natural interferon alfa subtypes.

Interferons are released in the body in response to viral infections or substances that induce their release. Interferons have several properties: antiviral (inhibit virus replication), antiproliferative (decrease cell proliferation), and immunomodulatory (enhance phagocyte activity and assist the cytotoxicity properties of lymphocytes for target cells). Their mechanism of action as antineoplastic agents is unknown but may be the result of one or more of the three properties identified. In some types of cancer, for example, interferon appears to have a dual effect of both cytotoxic and immune stimulation. Some clients demonstrate an increase in hematologic factors, granulocytes, platelets, and hemoglobin.

Interferon alfa-2a and alfa-2b are indicated for the treatment of hairy cell leukemia, genital warts, acquired immunodeficiency syndrome (AIDS)-related Kaposi's sarcoma, bladder cancer, and chronic active hepatitis. Toxicities reported include a flulike syndrome that includes fever, chills, muscle pain, loss of appetite, and lethargy. Myelosuppression, nausea, vomiting, neurotoxicity, and cardiotoxicity may occur at higher dosages.

Aldesleukin [al dess loo' kin] (Proleukin, interleukin-2) is another cytokine biologic product that stimulates immune function and is nearly identical in chemical structure and action to human interleukin-2. It is indicated for the treatment of renal cell carcinoma. This substance appears to stimulate T-cell proliferation and is a co-factor in developing cytotoxic T-lymphocyte activity against tumors. Its cytotoxic action may be caused by enhancing the growth of the body's natural killer cells and lymphokine-activated killer (LAK) cells. The side effects/adverse reactions of aldesleukin include edema, anemia, thrombocytopenia, and hypotension.

Granulocyte macrophage-colony stimulating factor (GM-CSF, sargramostim) and *granulocyte colony-stimulating factor* (G-CSF, filgrastim [Neupogen]) are immunomodulator agents with a variety of approved and investigational uses. GM-CSF is used to accelerate myeloid recovery in persons with acute lymphoblastic leukemia (ALL), Hodgkin's disease, and non-Hodgkin's lymphoma who are undergoing bone marrow transplantation. CBCs are performed to monitor the hematologic response to this drug. Investigationally this drug has been used to increase the WBC count in clients with AIDS who are receiving zidovudine (AZT) and to correct neutropenia in aplastic anemia. Closely monitor clients who are receiving lithium or corticosteroids concurrently, because the myeloproliferative action of this drug may be increased.

G-CSF (Neupogen) is used to decrease the potential for infection in clients receiving myelosuppressive agents that are associated with severe neutropenia and fever. Neutrophil counts are closely monitored; the drug should be discontinued when the absolute neutrophil count is 10,000/mm^3 or more after the nadir induced by the chemotherapy. The major side effects/adverse reactions of G-CSF include nausea, vomiting, alopecia, diarrhea, fevers, mucositis, anorexia, and fatigue. Bone pain is reported approximately 2 to 3 days before the increase in neutrophil count and is usually controlled with nonopioid-type analgesics. The usual starting dosage is 5 μg/kg/day by SC or IV injection.

Erythropoietin (epoetin alfa, recombinant [Epogen]) is used to treat the anemia associated with renal failure and AIDS. (See Chapter 36 for additional information on this drug.)

Rituximab [rit ux' ih mab] (Rituxan) is a genetically made monoclonal antibody that is directed against an antigen (CD20) located on the surface of both normal and malignant B lymphocytes. The CD20 antigen governs the early steps in cell-cycle initiation and differentiation and is found on more than 90% of B-cell non-Hodgkin's lymphomas. It is indicated for the treatment of clients who have relapsed or have a refractory low-grade or follicular, CD20-positive, B-cell, non-Hodgkin's lymphoma. Side effects/adverse reactions include fever, chills, weakness, headache, angioedema, hypotension, myalgia, nausea, vomiting, leukopenia, pruritus, and rash.

Other Agents

Altretamine [al tret' a meen] (Hexalen) is a cytotoxic agent for the palliative treatment of persistent or recurrent ovarian cancer. Its mechanism of action is unknown, but chemically it resembles the alkylating agents. Clinically, it is effective for ovarian tumors that are resistant to the previously marketed alkylating agents. The side effects/adverse reactions of altretamine include nausea and vomiting, neurotoxicity, myelosuppression, and CNS changes (ataxia, dizziness, mood alterations). The most significant drug interactions to avoid include cimetidine (increases the half-life of altretamine) and monoamine oxidase (MAO) inhibitors (severe hypotension).

Asparaginase [a spare' a gi nase] (Elspar, Kidrolase ♣) reduces asparagine to aspartic acid in the body. Asparagine is necessary for cell survival; because normal body cells are capable of synthesizing adequate supplies of asparaginase, they are not affected by an asparaginase deficiency. Certain cancer cells, however, depend on a circulating supply of asparaginase within the blood; when this supply is decreased, the cancer cells will die. Asparaginase is used to treat acute lymphocytic leukemia (ALL). The side effects/adverse reactions of asparaginase are hyperammonemia (headache, anorexia, nausea, vomiting, abdominal cramps), a decrease in the blood-clotting factors, allergic reactions, liver toxicity, pancreatitis, and anaphylaxis.

Cladribine [kla' dri been] (Leustatin) is used to treat hairy cell leukemia. Cladribine enters the cell and is phosphorylated to a deoxyadenosine concentration that accumulates in these cells, interfering with DNA repair and eventually causing cell death. The side effects/adverse reactions of cladribine include severe anemia, infection, skin rash, bleeding or bruising, anorexia, headache, nausea, vomiting, and fatigue.

Dacarbazine [da kar' ba zeen] (DTIC-Dome) is a cell-cycle–nonspecific agent that inhibits DNA and RNA synthesis and appears to be more active in the late G_2 phase of the cell cycle. It is indicated for the treatment of malignant melanoma and Hodgkin's disease. The side effects/adverse reactions of dacarbazine include flu-like syndrome, anorexia, nausea, vomiting, and diarrhea.

Denileukin diftitox [den ih loo' kin dif tee' tox] (Ontak) is a recombinant DNA-derived drug that is composed of diphtheria toxin fragments A & B amino acid sequences plus the sequence of interleukin-2. It is indicated for the treatment of persistent or recurrent cutaneous T-cell lymphoma.

Docetaxel [dok i tax' el] (Taxotere) is also a taxoid that is a semisynthetic product originating from the yew plant. It may produce its effect by binding and stabilizing microtubule bundles, thus inhibiting cell mitosis. It is indicated for the treatment of advanced breast cancer (Nabholtz et al., 1999; *Drug Facts and Comparisons,* 2000). The side effects/adverse reactions of docetaxel include bone marrow suppression, nausea, diarrhea, stomatitis, fever, skin reactions, and myalgia.

Gemcitabine [jem sit' ah been] (Gemzar) interferes with cell synthesis (S phase) and also blocks cell progression through the G_1/S part of the cycle. It is indicated for treatment of non–small-cell lung cancer and for adenocarcinoma of the pancreas in clients with nonresectable or metastatic pancreatic cancer who have been previously treated with 5-FU. The side effects/adverse reactions of gemcitabine include dyspnea, peripheral edema, flu-like syndrome, nausea, vomiting, diarrhea, rash, paresthesia, and stomatitis. Gemcitabine is administered intravenously; the adult dosage is 1000 mg/m^2 given over 30 minutes. Refer to the current literature for additional information (*Drug Facts and Comparisons,* 2000).

Hydroxyurea [hye drox' ee yoo ree ah] (Hydrea) inhibits DNA synthesis without affecting the synthesis of RNA or protein. It is indicated for the treatment of head, neck, and ovarian carcinoma; chronic myelocytic leukemia; and malignant melanoma. The side effects/adverse reactions of hydroxyurea include bone marrow suppression, diarrhea, anorexia, nausea, vomiting, and drowsiness.

Irinotecan [i rin' oe tee kan] (Camptosar) is the first of a new class of oncolytic agents indicated for the treatment of metastatic colorectal cancer or rectal cancer that has occurred or progressed after 5-FU chemotherapy. This product is a type 1 topoisomerase inhibitor that binds to the type 1 topoisomerase DNA complex, resulting in double-stranded DNA breaks that cause tumor cell death. Irinotecan may cause severe diarrhea, which requires immediate treatment with loperamide (Imodium). Severe myelosuppression, nausea, and vomiting may also occur (*Camptosar,* 1996).

Levamisole [lee vam' i sol] (Ergamisol), a biologic response modifier (immunostimulant), is used in combination with fluorouracil (5-FU) to treat colorectal carcinoma (Dukes stage C adenocarcinoma). This combination has resulted in an increased survival time (decreased mortality) and a decreased risk of cancer recurrence. Significant side effects/adverse reactions of levamisole include bone marrow suppression, nausea, diarrhea, metallic taste, arthralgia, and flu-like syndrome.

Mitotane [mye' toe tane] (Lysodren) is an adrenal gland suppressing agent indicated for the treatment of inoperable carcinoma of the adrenal cortex. Administered orally, it is distributed throughout the body but is mainly stored in fat. The onset of effect is reported within 48 to 72 hours of starting therapy; the tumor response is usually within 6 weeks. Significant side effects/adverse reactions of mitotane include adrenal gland insufficiency: dark skin, diarrhea, anorexia, depression, nausea, vomiting, weakness, drowsiness, and light-headedness.

Paclitaxel [pa kli tax' el] (Taxol) is a natural substance extracted from the yew tree and marketed for the treatment of metastatic ovarian cancer that is refractory to other drug treatments. It is an antimicrotubule agent that stabilizes microtubule bundles, thereby interfering with the late G_2 mitotic cell cycle and resulting in the inhibition of cell replication. It is also used for the treatment of metastatic breast cancer; some studies indicate it should be used earlier (e.g., immediately after surgery), because it then produces better effects than chemotherapy alone (Tarlach, 1998). The side effects/adverse reactions of paclitaxel include severe allergic reactions (to prevent such reactions, pretreat with a steroid and an H_1 and H_2 antagonist), bone marrow suppression, peripheral neuropathy, muscle pain, alopecia, and gastric distress.

Pegaspargase [peg as' per gase] (Oncaspar) is a modification of the L-asparaginase enzyme. It is used in combination chemotherapies for acute lymphoblastic leukemia in persons unable to take L-asparaginase. The side effects/adverse reactions of pegaspargase include hypersensitivity reactions, hepatotoxicity, and coagulopathies.

Procarbazine [pro kar' ba zeen] (Matulane) is an alkylating agent and a weak MAO inhibitor that is cell-cycle specific for the S phase of cell division and is believed to inhibit DNA, RNA, and protein synthesis. It is commonly prescribed for the treatment of Hodgkin's disease. Side effects/adverse reactions include bone marrow suppression, pneumonitis, nausea, vomiting, weakness, drowsiness, myalgia, muscle twitching, insomnia, nightmares, and nervousness.

Topotecan [toe poe' ti kan] (Hycamtin), a topoisomerase inhibitor, is indicated for the treatment of relapsed or refractory metastatic carcinoma of the ovary after the failure of other therapies. Its action may be due to inhibiting topoisomerase activity in DNA during DNA synthesis. This product should be administered only to women with adequate bone marrow reserves (i.e., neutrophils of at least 1500 cells/mm^3 and platelet counts of 100,000/mm^3 or greater). The side effects/adverse reactions of topotecan include neutropenia (a dose-limiting toxicity), leukopenia, thrombocytopenia, anemia, headache, diarrhea, stomach pain, nausea, vomiting, alopecia, tiredness, dyspnea, and neuromuscular pain. The usual dosage is 1.5 mg/m^2 by IV infusion over 30 minutes daily for 5 days. Refer to a current package insert for more information.

Trastuzumab [tra stoo' zoo mab] (Herceptin) is a monoclonal antibody that binds HER2, a growth factor identified in approximately 25% to 30% of women with breast cancer. The HER2 growth factor receptor was identified in certain types of breast cancer and may also be present in other cancers. The use of trastuzumab combined with chemotherapy for the treatment of breast cancer has resulted in an increase in clinical response rate and survival. The side effects/adverse reactions of trastuzumab include chills, fever (usually with the first infusion dose), diarrhea, leukopenia, and infections. One adverse reaction is an increased risk of cardiac dysfunction (congestive heart failure, tachycardia) in approximately 25% of women receiving the combination of trastuzumab and an anthracycline (e.g., doxorubicin [Adriamycin]) and in approximately 7% of women receiving only trastuzumab. Monitor closely for signs and symptoms of cardiovascular dysfunction (Food and Drug Administration Advisory Committee, 1999).

Tretinoin [tret' i noyn] (Vesanoid) is a retinoid that appears to enhance the maturation of primitive promyelocytes from the leukemic clone; this is followed by reseeding the bone marrow and blood with normal blood cells. It is used to treat acute promyelocytic leukemia. Side effects/adverse reactions include headaches, fever, increased weakness, malaise, shivering, infections, hemorrhage, and peripheral edema.

Bexarotene [bex aye' ro teen] (Targretin) is a retinoid indicated for advanced stage, cutaneous T-cell lymphoma. It may cause birth defects, and therefore contraception before, during, and for a month after its use is necessary. Avoid concurrent use of vitamin A.

For information on several new antineoplastic agents, including alemtuzumab [al em tuz' i mab] (Campath), arsenic trioxide (Trisenox), gemtuzumab ozogamicin [gem too' zoo mab] (Mylotarg), imatinib [i mat' i nib] (Gleevec), porfimer [pour' fih mur] (Photofrin), and temozolomide [tem oh zole' oh mide] (Temodar), see Appendix E.

CANCER CHEMOTHERAPY RESEARCH

Cancer chemotherapy research is a priority area of study in the United States and Canada. Many new drugs are being studied with the hope of improving the treatment and survival of clients with cancer and AIDS-induced cancer (see Chapter 64 for a review of AIDS). The reader is encouraged to monitor professional literature for information on the release of new drugs for the treatment of cancer and for other

BOX 57-5

Investigational Drug Classifications

Investigational drugs are agents that have not been released for marketing by the Food and Drug Administration (FDA). Although the responsibility for regulating drugs rests with the FDA, the National Cancer Institute (NCI) is the largest developer of antineoplastic agents in the United States. The NCI has established stringent regulations to monitor the receipt, use, and disposal of investigational drugs. It also requires that investigators report adverse reactions on an established time schedule. For example, anaphylactic reactions to an investigational drug must be reported by phoning a specific branch office (available on a 24-hour basis). This call must be followed up with a written report within 10 working days.

Investigational drugs are divided into three groups:

	Drug Group	Purpose
Phase I	A	To determine the maximum tolerated dosage To detect toxicities associated with various dosage schedules To determine pharmacokinetics and optimum dosing schedules
Phase II	B	To identify antineoplastic activity in specific cancers affecting humans To determine the client's response to various drug dosages and schedules
Phase III	C	The new agent is now compared with previously marketed drugs to ascertain effectiveness, and its effect on quality of life, mortality, and morbidity

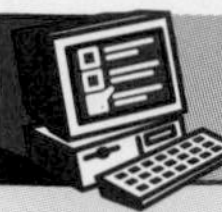

Nursing Research
Chemotherapy, Nausea, and Vomiting

Citation: Pickett, M. (1991). Determinants of anticipatory nausea and anticipatory vomiting in adults receiving cancer chemotherapy. *Cancer Nursing, 14*(6), 334-342.

Abstract: The chemotherapeutic treatment of cancer has become increasingly more successful in providing greater life expectancy and controlling the spread of disease. However, some persons receiving chemotherapy may choose to discontinue treatment based on their inability to tolerate the undesirable side effects, of which nausea and vomiting are among the most common and distressing. Pickett (1991) examined the relationship of anticipatory nausea and/or anticipatory vomiting (AN/AV) in adults receiving an initial course of cancer chemotherapy in an outpatient setting with the following set of variables: symptom distress, mood disturbance, stage of disease, sensitivity to conditioning cues, emetic potential of antineoplastic drugs, age, psychosocial stress, and ability to cope.

The setting for the study was seven outpatient chemotherapy clinics in the areas of the Northeast, Mid-Atlantic, and Southwest. Measures of selected variables were obtained with valid and reliable tools before the administration of chemotherapy on Day 1 of the first, fourth, and fifth consecutive treatment cycles. Episodes of AN/AV were assessed before the administration of chemotherapy. There was a significant difference between subjects who subsequently developed AN/AV and those who did not. Those who developed AN/AV were receiving a drug regimen higher in emetogenic potential, were younger, and were in an earlier stage of the disease than subjects who did not develop AN/AV.

This study suggests that it is possible to discriminate between those who will subsequently develop AN/AV and those who will not on the basis of data gathered before the administration of any chemotherapy. Multivariate analysis revealed a high degree of correlation between AN/AV and the following linear composite of variables: emetogenic potential of drug, symptom distress, psychosocial stress, ability to cope, and mood disturbance. This set of predictor variables correctly classified 100% of subjects who subsequently developed AN/AV.

Behavioral intervention strategies for anticipatory symptoms have achieved varying levels of success after the symptoms have become apparent. The findings of this study suggest that it might be possible to identify clients at high risk for anticipatory symptoms before they receive any chemotherapy.

Critical Thinking Questions

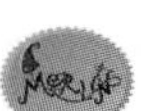

- What are the implications of these findings for nursing practice?

related research. Box 57-5 lists the classifications for investigational drugs.

Another promising area of study is the use of liposomes as a delivery system to hold lipid-soluble drugs. Drugs encapsulated in a liposome capsule can be distributed differently in the body than are free drugs. Liposomes accumulate at the sites of inflammation and infection, as well as in some solid tumors. Thus they are under study for the treatment of systemic fungal infections (amphotericin B) and for the treatment of specific cancers. Doxorubicin (Adriamycin), cisplatin (Platinol), and methotrexate (Folex) are just several of the antineoplastic agents currently undergoing clinical testing. Doxorubicin in liposome administration has been reported to deliver the drug more directly to the site of action, resulting in fewer cardiac effects and other side effects/adverse reactions. Cisplatin in liposomes has been reported to cause much less kidney damage than cisplatin alone. If studies of liposome drug therapy continue to report a decrease in side effects/adverse reactions as well as effective therapeutic outcomes, liposomes will have the potential of opening an exciting new avenue of drug delivery in the next few years. See the Nursing Research box above for other research in this area that influences nursing practice.

SUMMARY

The antineoplastic agents act by interfering with cell reproduction or replication at some point in the cell cycle. They are classified into various groups based on their probable mechanisms of action: antimetabolites, alkylating agents, mitotic inhibitors, antibiotic antitumor agents, hormones, cytoprotective and immunomodulator agents, and miscellaneous agents. Because the drugs are nonselective and affect all cells in the body as they replicate, there is always some degree of injury to normal cells. Cells with a high rate of growth (e.g., bone marrow, gastrointestinal epithelium, and hair follicles) are particularly susceptible. Bone marrow depression with the resultant anemia, leukocytopenia, and thrombocytopenia is unavoidable, and therefore laboratory values for blood counts are used to titrate the individual client's dosage and to determine when the client is most susceptible to infection and hemorrhage.

Much of the nursing management of antineoplastic therapy is to prevent injury and infection; promote comfort; provide care for the gastrointestinal effects of stomatitis, nausea, and vomiting and changes in bowel elimination; and assess for the development of nephrotoxicity, neurotoxicity, cardiotoxicity, pulmonary toxicity, and dermatologic effects. Although short-term toxicity and side effects occur, the potential for cure or a reduction of symptoms is a benefit that most often outweighs the risk and discomfort of the administration.

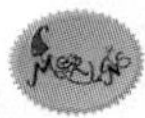

Critical Thinking Questions

1. Mr. Alan Hale, age 48, suddenly develops a high fever and petechiae on his chest and arms. After bone marrow aspiration, he is diagnosed with acute lymphocytic leukemia. The oncologist puts Mr. Hale on a regimen that contains vincristine (Oncovin). For what nursing diagnoses is Mr. Hale at risk? What laboratory values should the nurse be monitoring? If Mr. Hale develops a tingling in his fingers and toes, what might be occurring?
2. Mrs. Hextall is returning home after a series of antineoplastic chemotherapies. In discussing her home arrangements for care, she indicates that there should be no problem. Her daughter has moved back in with her, along with her 3-month-old granddaughter, and will care for her. Given Mrs. Hextall's altered protection status, what concerns might the nurse have about this arrangement?
3. Given that the antineoplastic agents have a number of potential complications, how would the nurse monitor the client receiving a relevant antineoplastic agent for cardiotoxicity? For neurotoxicity? For nephrotoxicity?

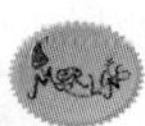

Collaborative Learning Activities

For Collaborative Learning Activities, go to mosby.com/MERLIN/McKenry/.

CASE STUDY

For a Case Study that will help ensure mastery of this chapter content, go to mosby.com/MERLIN/McKenry/.

BIBLIOGRAPHY

American Hospital Formulary Service. (1999). *AHFS drug information '99*. Bethesda, MD: American Society of Hospital Pharmacists.

Anderson, K.N., Anderson, L.E., & W.D. Glanze. (Eds.) (1998). *Mosby's medical, nursing, & allied health dictionary* (5th ed.). St. Louis: Mosby.

Belcher, A.E. (1992). *Cancer nursing*. St. Louis: Mosby.

Burris, H.A., III (1999). Single-agent docetaxel (Taxotere) in randomized phase III trials. *Seminars in Oncology, 26*(3 suppl 9), 1-6.

Buzdar, A.U., & Hortobagyi, G.N. (1998). Tamoxifen and toremifene in breast cancer: Comparison of safety and efficacy. *Journal of Clinical Oncology, 16*(1), 348-353.

Camptosar. (1996). Package insert. Pharmacia & Upjohn, #816 907 000.

Catania, P.N. (1999). When patients ask: Home chemotherapy: Basic concepts. *Home Care Provider, 4*(2), 60-61.

Chabner, B.A., Allegra, C.J., Curt, G.A., & Calabresi, P. (1996). Antineoplastic agents. In J.G. Hardman & L.E. Limbird (Eds.), *Goodman & Gilman's The pharmacological basis of therapeutics* (9th ed.). New York: McGraw-Hill.

Drug Facts and Comparisons. (2000). St. Louis: Facts and Comparisons.

Eriksson, J.H. (1998). Intraperitoneal chemotherapy. *Journal of Gynecologic Oncology Nursing, 8*(2), 22.

Food and Drug Administration Advisory Committee. (1999). *FDA Advisory Committee recommends Herceptin for metastatic breast cancer*; www.pslgroup.com/dg/ad566.htm (3/17/99).

Ghaneh, P., Kawesha, A., Howes, N., Jones, L., & Neoptolemos, J.P. (1999). Adjuvant therapy for pancreatic cancer. *World Journal of Surgery, 23*(9), 937-945.

Holdsworth, M.T., Raisch, D.W., Chevez, C.M., Duncan, M.H., Parasuraman, T.V., & Cox, F.M. (1997). Economic impact with home delivery of chemotherapy to pediatric oncology patients. *Annals of Pharmacotherapy, 31*(2), 140-148.

Jaffee, M.S. & Skidmore-Roth, L. (1988). *Home health nursing care plans*. St. Louis: Mosby.

MacDonald, J.S. (1999). Toxicity of 5-fluorouracil. *Oncology, 13*(7), 33-34.

Markman, M. (1999). Intraperitoneal chemotherapy in the management of colon cancer. *Seminars in Oncology, 26*(5), 536-539.

Marty, M., Espie, M., Cottu, P.H., Cuvier, C., & Lerebours, F. (1999). Optimizing chemotherapy for patients with advanced breast cancer. *Oncology, 57* (suppl 1), 21-26.

Nabholtz, J.M., Smylie, M., Mackey, J., Au, H.J., Tonkin, K., Au, R., Morrish, D., Salter, E. (1999). Docetaxel and anthracycline polychemotherapy in the treatment of breast cancer. *Seminars in Oncology, 26*(3 suppl 8), 47-52.

Parker, G.G. (1992). Chemotherapy administration in the home. *Home Healthcare Nursing, 10*(1), 30-36.

Pickett, M. (1991). Determinants of anticipatory nausea and anticipatory vomiting in adults receiving cancer chemotherapy. *Cancer Nursing, 14*(6), 334-342.

Robinson, E., Kimmick, G.G., & Muss, H.B. (1996). Tamoxifen in postmenopausal women: A safety perspective. *Drugs Aging, 8*(5), 329-337; www.medscape.com/server-java/MedPage?med95-97+593452+(tamoxifen+drug+review)(4/18/98).

Studva, K.V. (1993). Programmed instruction: Cancer chemotherapy. *Cancer Nursing, 16*(2), 145-159.

Tarlach, G.M. (1998). New advances hold promise in battle against cancer. *Hospital Pharmacist Report, 12*(6), 17, 20.

United States Pharmacopeia Dispensing Information (USP DI): Drug information for the health care professional (19th ed.). (1999). Rockville, MD: United States Pharmacopeial Convention.

Wood, L.S. & Gullo. (1993). IV vesicants: How to avoid extravasation. *American Journal of Nursing, 93*(4), 42-46.

Yu, W., Whang, I., Suh, I., Averbach, A., Chang, D., & and Sugarbaker, P.H. (1998). Prospective randomized trial of early postoperative intraperitoneal chemotherapy as an adjuvant to resectable gastric cancer. *Annals of Surgery, 228*(3), 347-354.

58 Overview of Infections, Inflammation, and Fever

Chapter Focus

Fever, inflammation, and infection have been a concern to those caring for the ill and injured since ancient times. The majority of clients have experienced these symptoms, not only as a direct result of their injuries or illnesses, but also as the indirect consequence of multiple invasive devices, surgical procedures, and immunosuppression. With these clients, nurses have the responsibility of assessment, palliation of symptoms, and the evaluation of therapies.

Learning Objectives

1. Describe the mediators of the inflammatory system.
2. Identify different types of fever.
3. Explain the body's set point temperature mechanism.
4. Describe the goal and mechanisms of action of antimicrobial therapy.
5. Identify the general adverse reactions to antimicrobial drugs.
6. Discuss general guidelines for the optimal use of antimicrobial agents.
7. Implement the nursing management for a client receiving antimicrobial therapy.

Key Terms

INFECTIONS

Infectious diseases comprise a wide spectrum of illnesses caused by pathogenic microorganisms. Some common pathogens and their most likely sites of infection in the body are listed in Table 58-1. These pathogens cause pneumonia, urinary tract infections, upper respiratory tract infections, gastroenteritis, venereal disease, vaginitis, tuberculosis, and candidiasis.

Infection is the invasion and multiplication of pathogenic microorganisms in body tissues; these microorganisms cause disease by local cellular injury, secretion of a toxin, or an antigen-antibody reaction in the host. An infection can be classified primarily as either local or systemic. A localized infection may involve the skin or internal organs and may progress to a systemic infection. A systemic infection involves the entire body rather than a localized area of the body. Several terms describe the degree of local or systemic infection.

Colonization is the localized presence of microorganisms in body tissues or organs, which can be pathogenic or part of the normal flora. Colonization alone is not necessarily an infection but rather signifies the potential for infection depending on the multiplication of the microorganisms or an alteration in the defense mechanisms of the host. When flora at their normal colonization site are altered (e.g., by the administration of an antibiotic that affects pathogens and some but not all normal microorganisms), unaffected-microorganisms within that environment may grow uninhibited and cause a secondary infection.

Inflammation is a protective mechanism of body tissues in response to invasion or toxins produced by colonizing microorganisms. This reaction consists of cytologic and his-

TABLE 58-1 Common Pathogens and Most Likely Sites of Infection

Organism	Infection Site
Gram-positive Cocci	
Staphylococcus aureus Non-penicillinase producing Penicillinase producing	Burns, skin, decubital and surgical wounds, paranasal and middle ear (chronic sinusitis and otitis), lungs, lung abscess, pleura, endocardium, bone (osteomyelitis), and joints
Staphylococcus epidermidis Non-penicillinase producing Penicillinase producing Methicillin resistant	
Streptococcus pneumoniae	Paranasal and middle ear, lungs, pleura
Streptococcus pyogenes (group A β-hemolytic)	Burns, skin infections, decubitus and surgical wounds, paranasal and middle ear, throat, bone (osteomyelitis), and joints
Streptococcus, viridans group	Endocardium
Gram-positive Bacilli	
Clostridium tetani (anaerobe)	Puncture wounds, lacerations, and crush injuries; toxins affecting nervous system
Corynebacterium diphtheriae	Throat, upper part of respiratory tract
Gram-negative Cocci	
Neisseria gonorrhoeae	Urethra, prostate, epididymis and testes, joints
Neisseria meningitidis	Meninges
Enteric Gram-negative Bacilli	
As a group (*Bacteroides, Enterobacter, Escherichia coli, Klebsiella pneumoniae, Proteus mirabilis,* other *Proteus, Salmonella, Serratia, Shigella*)	Peritoneum, biliary tract, kidney and bladder, prostate, decubital and surgical wounds, bone
Bacteroides	Brain abscess, lung abscess, throat, peritoneum
Enterobacter	Peritoneum, biliary tract, kidney and bladder, endocardium
Escherichia coli	Peritoneum, biliary tract, kidney and bladder
Klebsiella pneumoniae	Lungs, lung abscess
Other Gram-negative Bacilli	
Haemophilus influenzae	Meninges, paranasal and middle ear, lungs, pleura
Pseudomonas aeruginosa	Burns, paranasal and middle ear (chronic otitis media), decubital and surgical wounds, lungs, joints

Continued

TABLE 58-1 Common Pathogens and Most Likely Sites of Infection—cont'd

Organism	Infection Site
Acid-fast Bacilli	
Mycobacterium avium *Mycobacterium tuberculosis*	Lungs, pleura, peritoneum, meninges, kidney and bladder, testes, bone, joints
Mycoplasmas	
Mycoplasma pneumoniae	Lungs
Spirochetes	
Treponema pallidum (syphilis)	Any tissue or vascular organ of the body
Fungi	
Aspergillus	Paranasal and middle ear, lungs
Candida species *Cryptococcus*	Skin infections, throat, lungs, endocardium, kidney and bladder, vagina
Viruses	
Human immunodeficiency virus (HIV)	T cells and macrophages (see Chapter 64)
Herpes virus or varicella-zoster virus	Skin infections (herpes simplex or zoster)
Enterovirus, mumps virus, and others	Meninges, epididymis, and testes
Respiratory viruses (including Epstein-Barr virus)	Throat, lungs
Anaerobes	
Gram-positive *Clostridium difficile* *Clostridium perfringens* *Peptococcus* species *Peptostreptococcus* species Gram-negative *Bacteroides fragilis* *Fusobacterium* species	Deep wounds, gut

tologic tissue responses for the localization of phagocytic activity and the destruction or removal of injurious material, leading to repair and healing.

Bacteremia is the presence of viable bacteria in the circulatory system. **Septicemia** refers to a systemic infection caused by the multiplication of microorganisms in the circulation. Although bacteremia may lead to septicemia in the immunocompromised host, it is usually a short-lived, self-limited process (depending on the pathogen). In an immunocompromised host, bacteremia may rapidly produce an overwhelming systemic disease. **Sepsis** is a syndrome in which multiple organ systems are involved as a result of the circulation of microorganisms or their toxins in the blood.

In immunocompetent hosts, antibiotic therapy is rarely required to treat the colonization of nonpathogenic organisms or transient bacteremias without tissue invasion; however, prophylactic antibiotic therapy may be required in immunocompromised hosts. In most cases of localized inflammation (e.g., wound infections, pneumonia, or urinary tract infections), antimicrobials reduce the number of viable pathogens. This permits the immune system to eliminate the microorganisms. Antimicrobials are also an essential part of the treatment of septicemia and sepsis.

Microorganisms are divided into several groups: bacteria, mycoplasmas, spirochetes, fungi, and viruses. Bacteria are classified according to their shape (e.g., bacilli, spirilla, and cocci) and their capacity to be stained. The specific identification of bacteria requires a Gram stain and culture with chemical testing. A Gram stain is a sequential procedure that involves crystal violet and iodine solutions followed by alcohol. It allows the rapid identification of organisms into groups, such as gram-positive or gram-negative rods or cocci. Culture procedures require 24 to 48 hours for completion to identify specific organisms.

Often the initial or empiric antibiotic selection is based on the prescriber's clinical impression plus the Gram stain procedure; the antibiotic may be changed once culture and sensitivity results are available.

INFLAMMATION

Inflammation is the reaction of body tissues to injury, such as physical trauma, foreign bodies, chemical substances, surgery, radiation, and electricity. The affected area undergoes a series of changes as the body processes attempt to wall off, heal, and/or replace the injured tissue. For example, after an injury the body releases chemical substances into the tissue to form a wall called a chemotactic gradient. Fluids and cells begin to move toward this area.

Blood vessels dilate within 30 minutes of the insult, which provides for an increase in blood flow and the exudation of fluid from blood vessels into the injured tissues. The exudate includes protein-rich fluids that are high in fibrinogen and attract other substances to the area, such as complement, antibodies, and leukocytes. The collection of fluids in this area results in edema or swelling. In general, this occurs within 4 hours of the injury.

Neutrophils, monocytes (macrophages), and lymphocytes (which arrive later) are the granulocytes that affect the injured area. During the cellular phase, granulocytes migrate to the area from the dilated blood vessels at the site. They migrate toward the chemotactic site and accumulate in the area of injury. If the injury is a foreign substance or bacteria, they will engulf and destroy the foreign material (phagocytosis). The phagocytosis process tends to localize or wall off the foreign material to prevent its spread through the tissues. Large numbers of phagocytes lead to the accumulation of pus and the eventual destruction and removal of the foreign material.

Some pathogens are resistant to destruction and are only walled off; an example is the tuberculosis bacillus, which can live for many years within the confined cells in the body. Other pathogens may transform from a local infection into a systemic infection and require antimicrobial or antibiotic treatment.

Mediators of the Inflammatory System. The complement system is composed of complement components (18 distinct proteins and their cleavage products) that are present in the blood in the form of inactive proteins called zymogens. Complement is essential in reacting to an acute inflammatory reaction caused by bacteria, certain viruses, and immune complex diseases. Complement enhances chemotaxis, increases blood vessel permeability, and eventually causes cell lysis.

Histamine, prostaglandins, arachidonic acid, and leukotrienes are other mediators capable of producing local reactions, smooth muscle contraction, increased chemotaxis, blood vessel vasodilation, and other inflammatory effects. When the foreign agent is destroyed, the resulting debris are removed by the macrophages and neutrophils, and the inflammatory reaction is resolved.

FEVER

The hypothalamus sets the point at which body temperature is maintained, but body temperature regulation depends on a balance between heat production and heat loss. Fever may be the result of an infection or an inflammatory process. It may be caused by the release of endogenous pyrogens from the macrophages. These pyrogens, or fever-producing substances, interfere with the temperature-regulating centers located in the hypothalamus, which raises the thermostat set point. The body may respond to the pyrogens by increasing the formation of cytokines; this increases the synthesis of prostaglandin (PGE_2), which then increases the hypothalamic set point (Insel, 1996). The body reacts by conserving heat through vasoconstriction, piloerection (goose flesh), and shivering—all of which increase the body temperature.

Normal body temperature is 98.6° F (37° C); the normal range is 97° F to approximately 99° F when measured orally; it is 1° F higher when measured rectally. Hyperthermia occurs when the temperature of the body rises above normal. Convulsions may result when it reaches 106° F. If the body's thermoregulatory mechanisms have trouble returning the body temperature to a normal setting, body metabolism may increase so rapidly that the body cannot regulate its own heat production. At 108° F, tissue damage occurs and cells begin to die; this results in irreversible brain damage.

Several types of fever are known. For example, a constant fever that rises or falls only a few degrees above or below a specified point is seen with typhoid fever. An intermittent fever may return to normal once or several times in 24 hours. This type of fever is associated with pyogenic infections, abscesses, lymphomas, tuberculosis, and drug reactions. A remittent fever fluctuates but does not usually return to normal; this occurs in many viral and bacterial infections. A relapsing fever consists of afebrile episodes of one or more days between fevers, such as in malaria and Hodgkin's disease.

Fever of unknown origin (FUO) is described as a temperature greater than 103° F that is recorded daily for more than 2 weeks in a client with an uncertain diagnosis after a week's evaluation in a hospital setting. Most clients with FUO are later found to have an infection, neoplasm, or connective tissue disease.

Body temperature is regulated by feedback mechanisms of the nervous system through a temperature-regulating center in the hypothalamus. When the hypothalamus is no longer in contact with the pyrogens, it resets the temperature to the normal set point. Prostaglandins of the E series produced in response to endogenous pyrogens act on the anterior hypothalamus to increase the set point, resulting in fever. Drugs that inhibit the synthesis of E prostaglandins have antipyretic activity (e.g., acetaminophen, salicylates). Salicylates reduce raised body temperatures by causing the hypothalamic center to reestablish a normal set point. Heat production will not be inhibited, but heat loss will be increased by an increase in cutaneous blood flow and sweating caused by the lowered thermostat (Figure 58-1). Antibiotics indirectly reduce temperature by destroying the bacteria that are causing the fever.

ANTIMICROBIAL THERAPY

The treatment of an infectious disease depends on the microorganism; different groups of antimicrobial agents are

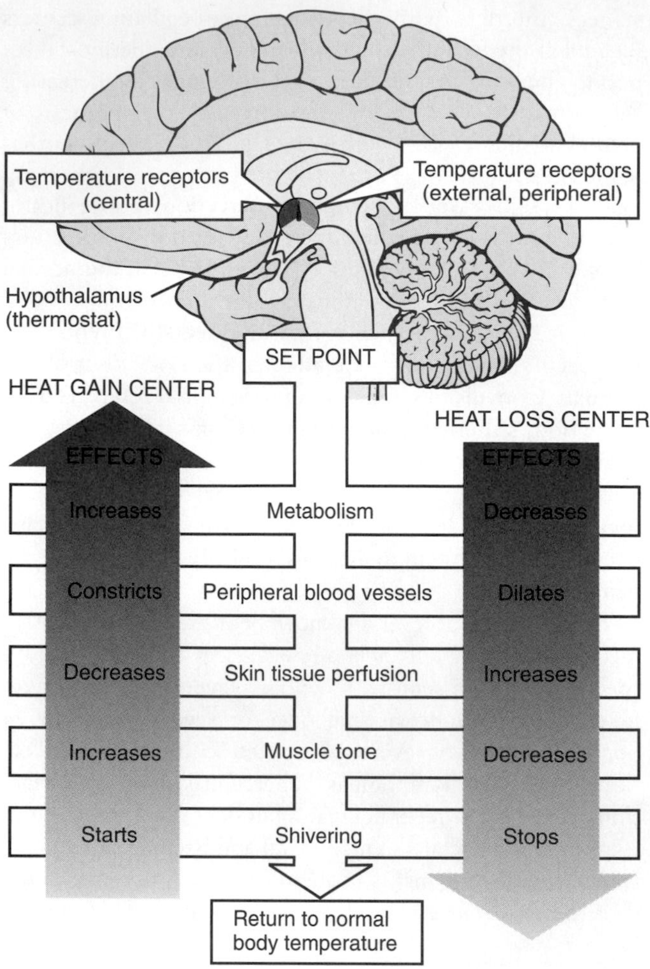

Figure 58-1 Set-point temperature mechanism.

used to treat different groups of microorganisms. Table 58-2 lists some antimicrobial agents used in the treatment of infectious diseases. Antimicrobial drugs can help cure or control most infections caused by microorganisms, but they alone do not necessarily produce the cure. They are adjuncts to methods such as surgical incision and drainage or wound debridement for the removal of nonviable, infected tissue.

The first major antimicrobial agents were the sulfonamides, and the second group of antimicrobials were true antibiotics such as penicillin. Antibiotics are natural substances derived from certain organisms (e.g., bacteria, fungus) that are used against infections caused by other organisms. As a result of research, there are now many synthetic and semisynthetic antibiotics. Other antimicrobial agents include the urinary tract antiseptics and the antimycobacterial, antifungal, and antiviral agents.

Mechanism of Action. The goal of antimicrobial therapy is to destroy or suppress the growth of infecting microorganisms so that normal host defense and other supporting mechanisms can control the infection, resulting in its cure. To exert their effects, antimicrobial agents must first gain access to target sites. Usually this can be accomplished by absorption and distribution of the drug into and by way of the circulatory system. More specific antibiotics or antimicrobial agents are capable of penetrating to the site and having an affinity for the bacterial target proteins. Local application to the infected area is sometimes necessary, such as with infections of the skin and eyes. Once the drug has reached its site of action, it can have bactericidal or bacteriostatic effects, depending on its mechanisms of action.

Bacteriostatic agents inhibit bacterial growth, which allows the host's defense mechanisms additional time to remove the invading microorganisms. In contrast, **bactericidal agents** cause bacterial cell death and lysis. Antimicrobial agents may be divided into bacteriostatic (e.g., sulfonamides) and bactericidal (e.g., penicillins) categories. However, such categorization is not always valid or reliable, because the same antimicrobial agent may have either effect depending on the dose administered and the concentration achieved at its site of action. For example, tetracycline is generally bacteriostatic but may be bactericidal in high concentrations. Chloramphenicol, which is often listed as a bacteriostatic drug, has bactericidal effects against *Streptococcus pneumoniae* and *Haemophilus influenzae* in the cerebrospinal fluid.

Antimicrobial agents may exert their bacteriostatic or bactericidal effects in one of four major ways:

1. Inhibit bacteria cell wall synthesis. Unlike host cells, bacteria are not isotonic with body fluids; therefore their contents are under high osmotic pressure and their viability depends on the integrity of the cell walls. Any compound that inhibits any step in the synthesis of this cell wall weakens it and causes the cell to lyse. Antimicrobial agents having this mechanism of action are bactericidal.
2. Disrupt or alter membrane permeability, resulting in the leakage of essential bacterial metabolic substrates. Agents causing these effects can be either bacteriostatic or bactericidal.
3. Inhibit protein synthesis. Antimicrobial agents may induce the formation of defective protein molecules; such agents are bactericidal in their action. Antimicrobial agents that inhibit specific steps in protein synthesis are bacteriostatic.
4. Inhibit the synthesis of essential metabolites. Antimicrobial agents that work in this manner structurally resemble physiologic compounds and act as competitive inhibitors in a metabolic pathway. In general, they are bacteriostatic agents (Box 58-1).

Side Effects/Adverse Reactions. Although the development of antimicrobial agents represents one of the most important advances in drug therapy, these drugs can have adverse and toxic effects. The list of side effects and toxic effects of each specific drug group is long and varied. Table 58-3 identifies some of the major allergic and toxic effects of a few antimicrobial agents. All antimicrobial agents are capable of producing two general types of adverse reactions of which the nurse must be aware: (1) allergic or hypersensitivity reactions, or (2) superinfection.

TABLE 58-2 Antimicrobial Agents Used to Treat Various Groups of Microorganisms

Organism	Antimicrobial Agent
Gram-positive Cocci	
Staphylococcus aureus	penicillin G or V, first-generation cephalosporins, vancomycin first-generation cephalosporins, cloxacillin, dicloxacillin, methicillin, vancomycin ± gentamicin ± rifampin
Non-penicillinase producing	
Penicillinase producing	
Methicillin resistant	
Streptococcus pneumoniae	penicillin G or V
Streptococcus pyogenes (Group A)	penicillin G or V
Streptococcus (Group B)	penicillin G, ampicillin
Streptococcus viridans	penicillin G ± gentamicin
Gram-positive Bacilli	
Bacillus anthracis	pencillin G, erythromycin
Corynebacterium diphtheriae	erythromycin
Corynebacterium, JK strain	vancomycin, erythromycin
Listeria monocytogenes	amikacin, gentamicin
Gram-negative Cocci	
Neisseria gonorrhoeae	ceftriaxone, cefixime
Neisseria meningitidis	penicillin G, cefotaxime
Gram-negative Enteric Bacilli	
Escherichia coli	cefotaxime, ceftizoxime
Klebsiella pneumoniae	same as *E. coli*
Proteus mirabilis	ampicillin, cephalosporin
Salmonella species	ceftriaxone, fluoroquinolone
Other Bacilli	
Pseudomonas aeruginosa	fluoroquinolone, carbenicillin
Anaerobes	
Gram-positive	
Clostridium difficile	metronidazole
Clostridium perfringens	penicillin G, metronidazole
Clostridium tetani	penicillin G, tetracycline
Gram-negative	
Bacteroides (gastrointestinal strains)	metronidazole, clindamycin
Mycoplasmas	
Mycoplasma pneumoniae	erythromycin, tetracycline, clarithromycin
Spirochetes	
Treponema pallidum (syphilis)	penicillin G
Fungi	
Aspergillus, Candida species	amphotericin B, fluconazole, itraconazole
Viruses	
Herpes simplex	vidarabine, acyclovir

Allergic or Hypersensitivity Reactions. Allergic or hypersensitivity reactions may occur with all available antimicrobial agents. Hypersensitivity is a state of altered reactivity in which the body reacts with an exaggerated immune response. Such responses include rash, fever, urticaria with pruritus, chills, a generalized erythema, anaphylaxis, and the Stevens-Johnson syndrome. Stevens-Johnson syndrome is a form of toxic epidermal necrolysis in which the epidermis separates from the dermis, leaving the client with a skin loss similar to a second-degree burn.

A minor rash may be easily tolerated, but a generalized rash or erythema accompanied by chills and fever needs

BOX 58-1

Antimicrobials: Classification by Mechanism of Action

Inhibit Cell Wall Synthesis

penicillins
cephalosporins
vancomycin
bacitracin
cycloserine

Alter Membrane Permeability

amphotericin B
nystatin
polymyxin
colistin

Inhibit Protein Synthesis

Impede Replication of Genetic Information

nalidixic acid
griseofulvin
novobiocin
rifampin
pyrimethamine

Impair Translation of Genetic Information

chloramphenicol
tetracycline
erythromycin
fluroquinolones
aminoglycosides
lincomycins

Antimetabolites

sulfonamides
paraaminosalicylic acid (PAS)
isoniazid (INH)
ethambutol

TABLE 58-3 Antimicrobial Drugs: Selected Allergic and Toxic Effects

Effect	Drug
Anaphylaxis	penicillin
Hematologic effects	chloramphenicol (low incidence but high mortality) sulfonamides (low incidence)
Nephrotoxicity	polymyxins aminoglycosides sulfonamides (low incidence with newer drugs)
Potential for neuromuscular blockade	polymyxins aminoglycosides
Injury to eighth cranial nerve	aminoglycosides
Photosensitivity	selected fluoroquinolones

medical intervention. For example, an allergic response to a rapid infusion of vancomycin can result in a generalized red skin reaction, fever, and chills; antihistamines need to be given to mitigate this reaction. Some rashes fade with continued treatment, as with some individuals receiving ampicillin; however, other symptoms may become more severe, which requires that the medication be discontinued. Respiratory distress (wheezing) or anaphylaxis is a medical emergency that requires immediate attention to prevent a fatal outcome.

Sensitization can occur through indirect exposure to a drug, such as drinking milk from cows treated with antibiotics or eating poultry or beef from livestock treated with antimicrobials. Previous topical application of antimicrobials may also cause sensitization.

The treatment of allergic reactions includes the use of antihistamines and epinephrine, which block or counteract the effects of the vasoactive mediators of allergy, and the use of corticosteroids, which may reduce tissue injury and edema in the inflammatory response. The use of steroids is controversial in the face of systemic infection because of their prolonged inhibition of normal host defense responses.

Superinfection. **Superinfection** is an infection that occurs during the course of antimicrobial therapy delivered for either therapeutic or prophylactic reasons. Most antibiotics reduce or eradicate the normal microbial flora of the body, which is then replaced by resistant exogenous or endogenous bacteria. If the number of these replacement organisms is large and the host conditions are favorable, clinical superinfection can occur.

Approximately 2% of persons treated with antibiotics get superinfections. The risk is greater when large doses of antibiotics are used, when more than one antibiotic is administered concurrently, and when broad-spectrum drugs are used. Superinfections are more commonly associated with certain antimicrobials than with others. For example, *Pseudomonas* organisms often colonize in and infect clients who are taking cephalosporins. In a similar manner, clients taking tetracyclines may become infected with *Candida albicans.*

In general, superinfections are caused by microorganisms that are resistant to the drug the client is receiving. In the past, penicillinase-producing staphylococci were the most common cause of superinfection. *Staphylococcus aureus* and *Staphylococcus epidermidis* superinfections, especially with methicillin-resistant strains, are again on the rise. Gram-negative enteric bacilli and fungi are the most common offenders. The proper management of superinfections includes the following: (1) discontinue the drug being given or replace it with another drug to which the organism is sensitive, (2) culture the suspected infected area, and (3) possibly, administer an antimicrobial agent effective against the new offending organism.

General Guidelines for Use. Several important principles guide the judicious and optimal use of the antimicrobial agents. Adverse reactions and therapeutic failures are often related to a lack of adherence to the following principles of antimicrobial therapy.

Identification of the Infecting Organism. Because most antimicrobial agents have a specific effect on a limited range of microorganisms, the prescriber must formulate a specific diagnosis about the potential pathogens or organisms most likely causing the infectious process. The drug most likely to be specifically effective against the suspected microorganism can then be selected.

This objective is most reliably accomplished by obtaining specimens from the infected area if possible (e.g., urine, sputum, wound drainage) or by obtaining venous blood specimens and sending them to the laboratory for culture and identification of the causative organism. The recovery of a specific microorganism from appropriate specimens is a significant factor in the determination of antimicrobial therapy. When a significant microorganism has been isolated, laboratory tests for antimicrobial susceptibility to various antimicrobial agents are performed.

It is desirable to receive culture and sensitivity reports before initiating antimicrobial therapy. In some situations, however, it is not practical to wait for these laboratory results. Antimicrobial therapy must be initiated without delay in acute, life-threatening situations such as peritonitis, septicemia, or pneumonia. In such situations the choice of antimicrobial agent for initial use must be based on tentative identification of the pathogen and a Gram stain. It is known, for example, that microorganisms commonly isolated in acute adult infections of the lung include pneumococci, *Haemophilus* strain streptococci, and staphylococci. Antimicrobial agents specifically toxic to those organisms may be administered temporarily. The drugs can be changed, if necessary, when laboratory reports are received.

When even tentative identification is difficult, broad-spectrum antibiotics (which are effective against a wide range of microorganisms) can be prescribed, or several antimicrobial agents may be prescribed for simultaneous administration.

Some infections are treated most effectively with the use of only one antibiotic. Combined antimicrobial drug therapy may be indicated for other situations. Indications for the simultaneous use of two or more antimicrobial agents include (1) the treatment of mixed infections, in which each drug may act on a separate portion of a complex microbial flora; (2) the need to delay the rapid emergence of bacteria that are resistant to one drug; and (3) the need to reduce the incidence or intensity of adverse reactions by decreasing the dosage of a potentially toxic drug. Indiscriminate use of combined antimicrobial drug therapy should be avoided because of expense, toxicity, and a higher incidence of superinfections and resistance.

Sensitivity and Resistance of Microorganisms. A discrepancy often exists between in vitro testing and the activity of the drug within the body. The activity of a drug in the body depends on a number of variables, such as affinity for antibiotic active sites and penetration into the bacteria, pH, temperature, and the ability of a drug to reach the site of an infection. For example, with meningitis it would be inappropriate to use a drug that does not cross the blood-brain barrier, even though the organism tested may be sensitive to the drug.

Resistance refers to the ability of a particular microorganism to resist the effects of a specific antibiotic. Resistance occurs in one of three ways:

1. The antibiotic is unable to reach the potential target site of its action. Some organisms, such as *Pseudomonas,* form a protective membrane (a glycocalyx or slime) that prevents the antibiotic from reaching the cell wall.
2. The microorganism may produce an enzyme that acts to reduce or eliminate the toxic effect of the antibiotic on the cell wall. Examples of these enzymes are the beta lactamases that cleave the beta-lactam ring on penicillins and cephalosporins, forming inactive compounds; acylases that acetylate chloramphenicol to yield inactive derivatives; and enzymes that inactivate aminoglycosides by phosphorylation, adenylation, and acetylation.
3. The microorganism may also be altered in the individual through several biochemical changes. The changes occur in such a way that the target site for the antibiotic no longer accommodates the drug. In this case a specific organism is said to have "become resistant" to a previously susceptible antibiotic. As a rule, microorganisms that are resistant to a certain drug will tend to be resistant to other chemically related antimicrobial agents; this phenomenon is known as *cross-resistance.* For example, bacteria that are unresponsive to tetracycline will also be resistant to oxytetracycline and chlortetracycline. Of major concern is the rapid, worldwide increase in multiple drug–resistant organisms in response to current antibiotic therapies (Ball, 1999).

Role of Host Defense Mechanisms. No antimicrobial agent will cure an infectious process if the host's defense mechanisms are inadequate. Such drugs act only on the causative organisms of infectious disease and have no effect on the defense mechanisms of the body, which need to be assessed and supported. Many infections do not require drug therapy and are adequately combated by individual defense mechanisms, including antibody production, phagocytosis, interferon production, fibrosis, or gastrointestinal rejection (vomiting, diarrhea). However, the host's defense mechanisms may be diminished, such as with diabetes mellitus, neoplastic disease, and immunologic suppression. A client who is very ill may require supportive care to ensure adequate oxygenation, fluid and electrolyte balance, and optimal nutrition so that antimicrobial therapy can be effective. Surgical intervention is also necessary in some situations. In general, in the presence of a substantial amount of pus, necrotic tissue, or foreign bodies, the most effective treatment is a combination of an antimicrobial agent and an appropriate surgical procedure.

The status of the host's defense mechanisms also influences the choice of therapy, route of administration, and dosage. For example, if an infection is fulminating, parenteral (preferably IV) administration of a bactericidal drug will be selected rather than the oral administration of a bacteriostatic drug. To achieve maximum blood concentrations rapidly, large "loading" doses of antimicrobial agents are often administered at the beginning of treatment for severe infections.

Factors influencing drug dosage are also related to the status of a client's renal function. Because many antimicrobial agents are metabolized and/or excreted by the kidneys, a major management problem exists in regard to individuals with compromised renal function. Drug dosages are then generally reduced in parallel with the client's creatinine clearance levels. Hemodialysis may further alter the therapeutic regimen. In some disease states (such as burns) the dosage of the antibiotic may need to be increased to achieve therapeutic levels.

In short, the administration of an antimicrobial agent specifically toxic to the isolated microorganism is not the only important measure in antimicrobial therapy. An additional and very important determinant of the effectiveness of an antimicrobial agent is the functional state of the host's defense mechanisms.

Dosage and Duration of Therapy. Administering antimicrobial drugs for therapeutic purposes in adequate dosages and for long enough periods of time is an important principle of infectious disease therapy. Fortunately, serum levels of some of the more potent antibiotics (e.g., aminoglycosides) can be monitored to prevent or minimize the risk of toxicity. The nurse should assess for alterations in renal and hepatic functions, because both can affect drug dosage, the dosing interval, and/or drug toxicity.

Failures in antimicrobial therapy are often the result of drug dosages that are too small or are given for too short of a time. In general, antimicrobial therapy should not be discontinued until the client has been afebrile and clinically well for 48 to 72 hours. Follow-up cultures should be obtained to assess the effectiveness of therapy.

Inadequate drug therapy may lead to remissions and exacerbations of the infectious process and may contribute to the development of resistance. When antibiotics are used prophylactically, they are usually given for short periods of time to enhance the host's defense mechanisms. With perioperative antibiotics, for example, a loading dose is given immediately before surgery and continued for 48 hours after surgery.

Antimicrobial agents in current use are discussed as chemically related groups of drugs. The nurse should be familiar with the general characteristics of each drug group or category and with one or two prototype drugs in each group. Because the dosage for any given antibiotic varies with the type of infection, the site of infection, and the age of the client, only general dosages or dosage ranges are given in this text. It is recommended that the reader consult the manufacturer's package insert or a formulary for specific dosages.

■ Nursing Management

Antimicrobial Therapy

Antimicrobial agents destroy or inhibit the growth of microorganisms. Some of these agents are derived from living organisms, whereas others are synthetic and semisynthetic chemical compounds. The goal of antimicrobial therapy for infectious diseases is to destroy or suppress the growth of infecting microorganisms so that normal host defense mechanisms can gain control and eliminate the infecting organisms. Among the microorganisms that can be controlled by these drugs today are most bacteria, many fungi, and a few viruses. It is necessary that the nurse have knowledge of host defenses and antimicrobial drugs for the safe and effective management of clients who are taking antimicrobials.

The primary defense mechanisms against infection are intact skin and mucous membranes, the chemical composition and pH of specific body secretions, phagocytic cells, mechanical movements of certain cells or tissues (e.g., cilia action, coughing, peristalsis), and the inflammatory process. Many factors can impair host defenses and thereby increase the risk for the development of infection by virulent organisms.

Any disruption in the integrity of skin or mucous membranes becomes a portal of entry for disease-producing organisms. Relatively minor breaks in the skin or mucosa can lead to fatal infections in very ill, hospitalized clients or in those who are immunocompromised (e.g., individuals who have acquired immunodeficiency syndrome [AIDS] or are receiving immunosuppressive therapies). Vigorous teeth cleaning, tube insertions, and injections should be avoided, if possible. Environmental hazards such as furniture obstructions, wet flooring, or the presence of irritating agents should be corrected so that injury is prevented. An impairment of blood supply to body tissues will also reduce host defenses by reducing the overall resistance of the tissues to injury and by preventing the migration of inflammatory cells to the area of injury. Other factors that impair the body's defenses against infection include neutropenia, anemia, protein malnutrition, and autoimmune and antiinflammatory agents such as antineoplastic agents and corticosteroids. Persons with chronic preexisting cardiopulmonary, renal, or metabolic disease and those at the extremes of age are susceptible to the development of infection because of altered organ function. Poor personal hygiene and the suppression of normal bacterial flora by antibiotics create conditions in which normal defenses are overwhelmed; this results in pathogen overgrowth (superinfection).

To exert their effects, antimicrobial agents must first gain access to target sites, usually by absorption of the drug into and distribution through the circulatory system. The drug then has bacteriostatic or bactericidal effects, depending on the mechanisms of action. Bacteriostatic agents such as sulfonamides inhibit bacterial growth, which allows the host's defense mechanisms additional time to remove the invading microorganisms. Bactericidal agents, such as the penicillins, cause bacterial cell death and lysis and superimpose this effect on the effects of host defenses. Antimicrobial agents may exert their bacteriostatic or bactericidal effects by inhibiting cell wall synthesis in bacteria, disrupting or altering membrane permeability, inhibiting protein synthesis, or synthesizing essential metabolites.

Hundreds of antimicrobial agents are marketed currently, and it is impossible for the nurse to have infinite knowledge about each drug. However, in spite of the numerous and varied drugs available, there are still only a few drug categories to remember. Knowledge of the general characteristics of each drug category and of the general principles of antimicrobial drug therapy should enable the nurse to function effectively.

In addition to the antibiotics, which include penicillins, cephalosporins, macrolides, lincomycins, vancomycin, aminoglycosides, tetracyclines, chloramphenicol, fluoroquinolones, and polymyxins, major groups of antiinfective drugs include sulfonamides, urinary tract antiseptics, and antimycobacterial, antifungal, and antiviral agents. See Table 58-3 for a brief summary of the major allergic and toxic effects of certain antimicrobial agents.

Nursing interventions in antimicrobial drug therapy generally relate to (1) assessing the client, (2) assisting in the identification of the infecting organism, (3) administering the drug, (4) monitoring the client's response to the drug, (5) educating the client, (6) providing comfort, and (7) preventing and treating adverse reactions, including pharmacologic and chemical drug interactions.

■ **Assessment.** In the initial assessment of the client, document the client's temperature, pulse, respiratory status, and blood pressure to detect fever and systemic responses to fever. Diaphoresis and flushing may also occur. Make note of the client's general behavior; a slumped posture, slow and unsteady posture, and careless grooming may indicate fatigue and malaise. Listen to the client's nonspecific symptoms, such as "aching all over," loss of appetite, headache, generalized discomfort, and "not feeling one's self" or "up-to-snuff." Ask the client about specific indicators, such as night sweats, pain, dyspnea, or arthralgia. Inspect the client's skin for heat, erythema, lesions, moistness, and swelling. Inspect and palpate the lymph nodes in the area of a suspected localized infection. Examine all the lymph nodes for a generalized infection. In addition, perform a history and physical examination, including a review of all systems (Grimes, 1991).

Cultures are obtained if an area of suspected infection is found. Obtaining cultures to determine the source and type of infection is often the nurse's responsibility. In the event that orders for an antimicrobial agent are given before an infective source is determined, obtain cultures before administering the first dose of the drug ordered.

Specimens obtained for culture should be taken directly to the laboratory and not allowed to stand. Delay may cause the death of fastidious organisms and allow contaminating organisms to overgrow the pathogen. Subsequent culture specimens obtained while the client is receiving antimicrobials should be sent to the laboratory with information regarding the drug(s) being administered. The appropriate selection of laboratory tests for the identification of offending organisms often depends on this knowledge.

The assessment of a client's previous reactions to drugs and to antimicrobial agents in particular is especially important in avoiding allergic reactions to drugs. Careful questioning of the individual regarding drugs previously taken and the client's exact clinical responses to them is an important part of the client's history. Some clients equate common side effects such as nausea and diarrhea with a drug allergy. Although these drug responses are important, their appearance may not be as sufficient a reason to withhold a specific antibiotic as would a true allergy. Once drug allergies are known, warnings should be prominently displayed on the client's record or hospital chart. The following actions are additional precautions: (1) ask the client if he or she has drug allergies before administering any medications; (2) tell the client what drug he or she is receiving; (3) observe the client for at least half an hour after drug administration (penicillin in particular), especially if the drug is administered parenterally and the client has never taken the drug previously; and (4) know what drugs are used for the treatment of allergic responses and where they are kept.

Because the administration of more than one drug to a client is the rule rather than the exception in current hospital practice, the possibility of drug interactions must be taken into account and the client's current medication regimen reviewed for significant interactions; this is necessary if antimicrobial therapy is to be optimally effective. Be alert to drugs that interact biologically with antimicrobial agents, as well as chemical incompatibilities between antimicrobial drugs and other agents when they are mixed for IV administration. The hospital formulary on each unit provides accurate and current information about these interactions.

In addition to the careful history of allergies and other adverse reactions to drugs and the review of the current medication regimen for potential significant drug interactions, the pre-therapy assessment should include the baseline signs and symptoms of the client's infection, as well as the white blood cell (WBC) count, serum electrolytes, and relevant culture and sensitivity.

■ **Nursing Diagnosis.** Clients receiving antimicrobial therapy are at risk for the following nursing diagnoses/collaborative problems: risk for infection and hyperthermia related to the ineffectiveness of antimicrobial therapy and/or the development of superinfection with another organism; risk for deficient fluid volume related to antimicrobial-induced adverse gastrointestinal reactions or anorexia, nausea, and vomiting related to gastric irritation by the drug; and the potential complications of allergic reaction, sepsis, ototoxicity, blood dyscrasias, and nephrotoxicity caused by specific antimicrobial agents.

■ **Implementation**

■ ***Monitoring.*** Assess for the effectiveness of drug therapy by monitoring the signs and symptoms of the client's infection, including WBC count and cultures. In most instances, the client's condition should improve within 48 hours after administration of the drug. Be alert for early signs of allergic or other adverse responses to therapy, as well as signs of superinfection, such as diarrhea and white patches in the oral cavity and vaginal area (see the following discussion of the management of adverse responses). Serum antibiotic concentrations can be monitored throughout therapy to assess for therapeutic and toxic levels of individual antimicrobials.

In addition to monitoring the therapeutic effects of antimicrobials, monitor the client for the development of common side effects of individual drugs. Fluid and electrolyte imbalances can occur during the course of administering many antibiotics, either from the drug itself, the mode of administration, or side effects such as diarrhea. For example, extracellular volume excess may result from administering multiple IV drugs, each of which is diluted in 100 mL of saline. Edema, pulmonary congestion with subsequent shortness of breath, and an increase in body weight indicate the presence of an extracellular volume excess.

Hypokalemia resulting from severe diarrhea or the IV administration of an antibiotic containing large quantities of sodium produces no obvious clinical signs or symptoms until the potassium deficit is significant. At this point, widespread muscular weakness and cardiac conduction abnormalities appear. In the client whose cardiac function is being monitored, the appearance of U waves may be an earlier indication of low serum potassium (McCance & Huether, 1998). Laboratory demonstration of hypokalemia is often the only way to detect this disorder.

Hypernatremia, another commonly seen disorder in clients receiving antimicrobial therapy, is also associated with few early clinical signs or symptoms, with the exception of a high serum sodium value, which is common because many antimicrobials have a sodium base. In general, it may be necessary to obtain periodic serum electrolyte studies in clients who must take prolonged courses of IV antimicrobials that can cause fluid and electrolyte imbalances.

■ ***Intervention.*** Because the constant and consistent administration of an antimicrobial drug at prescribed dosage intervals is necessary for maintaining therapeutic blood levels, administer such a drug according to the prescribed times as accurately as possible. This may mean awakening sleeping clients and ensuring that tests or therapies do not interrupt this schedule.

When antimicrobial agents are administered intravenously, observe the following additional precautions: (1) dilute the drugs in neutral solutions (pH 7.0 to 7.2) of isotonic sodium chloride (0.9%) or 5% dextrose in water, (2) administer the drugs without the admixture of any other drug to avoid chemical or physical incompatibilities, (3) administer the drugs by intermittent IV infusions to avoid inactivation (e.g., by temperature) and prolonged vein irritation from high drug concentration, (4) change the infusion site every 48 hours to reduce the risk of chemical phlebitis, and (5) inject IM antimicrobials deeply into large muscle masses (e.g., gluteal muscles), and rotate injection sites to prevent tissue irritation.

The establishment of automatic stop and renewal orders in many hospitals is another precaution against adverse reactions and for ensuring that the effectiveness of a particular drug is evaluated. Such orders restrict the administration of a prescribed antimicrobial agent to a definite time period (e.g., 7 days); its continued use past that time requires a new prescription.

■ ***Education.*** Clients should be taught principles of antimicrobial therapy clearly enough to understand that these drugs should never be taken without medical supervision and should be taken in strict accordance with their prescriptions. This is especially important because many individuals receiving antimicrobial drugs are not hospitalized and are responsible for self-medication. For example, clients should be taught the following:

- Not to stop taking these drugs as soon as symptoms abate, because an ineffective course of antimicrobial therapy will allow the opportunity for microbes to mutate and develop resistance to the drug.
- Not to share these drugs with family and friends, because they may have allergies and the drug may not be appropriate for their illness.
- Not to take "leftover" antimicrobial drugs for new illnesses, even if the symptoms appear similar. Many infections may have the same symptoms but are caused by different organisms or by organisms that have developed a resistance to the drug. In addition, some drugs become toxic as they degenerate past their expiration date.

Clients who are allergic to an antimicrobial agent should be taught how to protect themselves from future treatment with the drug in question, such as by using MedicAlert wallet cards or tags.

Special administration considerations, expected effects, side effects, and adverse reactions of individual antimicrobials could be appropriately described on "drug sheets" for clients to refer to at home while taking antimicrobial therapy. A telephone number to call when questions arise can also be written on the drug sheets to convey the message that it is expected and desirable for clients to discuss their medication concerns with health care workers.

Antimicrobials occasionally interfere with the results of home laboratory testing kits, and therefore clients must be cautioned. For example, the cephalosporins may produce a false-positive reading when individuals with diabetes use commercial chemical testing strips to monitor their urine glucose.

■ **Evaluation.** The expected outcome of antimicrobial therapy is a decrease in the severity or a disappearance of the clinical and laboratory manifestations of infection. Redness, heat, edema, and pain should decrease with local infections. In the case of a systemic infection, temperature, heart rate, respiratory rate, and WBC count should return to normal, and appetite and a sense of well-being should improve. Purulent drainage, if present, should decrease in amount and change to a more normal appearance and consistency. In clients who are seriously ill, an improvement in organ function should accompany other signs of infection resolution.

■ **Prevention and Management of Adverse Responses**

■ ***Anaphylaxis.*** The most serious allergic reaction to antimicrobials is anaphylaxis. This reaction can occur anywhere from a few seconds to 30 minutes after an antibiotic injection. The syndrome associated with this reaction usually begins with diffuse flushing, itching, and a feeling of warmth. Hives may appear on the client's face, neck, and chest. Generalized body edema develops as the syndrome progresses. Massive facial edema signals the possibility of upper airway edema, with impending obstruction and respiratory difficulty from pulmonary involvement. These problems are manifested as a choking sensation, stridor, chest tightness and pain, wheezing, shortness of breath, and restlessness.

The initial step in the emergent management of anaphylaxis is to stop the antibiotic immediately if it is still being infused. If the individual is not in a medical facility, immediate transport to one should be arranged, preferably by a vehicle staffed with paramedics, who can establish an artificial airway if client's airway becomes totally obstructed.

The reversal of anaphylaxis is accomplished by drug therapy. The antihistamine diphenhydramine (Benadryl) is administered parenterally or orally. Epinephrine 1 : 1000 can be injected subcutaneously and will reverse the vascular effects of anaphylaxis. Aminophylline or theophylline is administered if bronchospasm persists. If the individual is in anaphylactic shock, the concomitant administration of vasopressors and IV fluids may be necessary for the short-term management of hypotension. Corticosteroids (methylprednisolone) may be administered for the prevention of protracted symptoms in severe reactions.

■ ***Superinfection.*** The emergence of superinfection may be suspected in the presence of diarrhea or recurrent fever in clients who are taking antimicrobial drugs. Stomatitis is indicated by the presence of a sore mouth or white patches on the oral mucosa. Monilial vaginitis may produce a vaginal discharge or perineal rash. Increasing redness, heat, edema, pain, and possibly drainage may herald localized superinfections. *Clostridium difficile* as a nosocomial infection may manifest as a pseudomembranous colitis. Children, older adults, and others whose normal host defense mechanisms may be weakened should be especially observed for signs of superinfection. In the course of prolonged antimicrobial drug therapy, periodic cultures of the upper respiratory tract and of the feces may be indicated to determine changes in bacterial flora that may be subsequently responsible for secondary infection. Be careful not to introduce new microorganisms and should emphasize asepsis in those who are in contact with clients receiving antimicrobial therapy.

SUMMARY

Infectious disease has been a major health concern for humans even before recorded history. It comprises a variety of illnesses caused by pathogenic microorganisms, bacteria, fungi, and viruses. Inflammation is a reaction of the body tissues, not only to infection but also to physical, chemical, and thermal injuries. Fever is a sign of inflammation. All reactions present challenges for nursing care and antimicrobial therapy.

Depending on the concentration at the site of action, antimicrobial agents may be bacteriostatic (inhibiting bacterial growth), bactericidal (causing bacterial cell death and lysis), or both. These agents are effective by inhibiting synthesis of the bacterial cell wall, altering membrane permeability, inhibiting protein synthesis, or inhibiting the synthesis of essential metabolites. Antimicrobials are generally well tolerated by humans. However, with all antimicrobials there is the possibility of an allergic or hypersensitive response or a superinfection (an infection that occurs during the course of antimicrobial therapy because of a reduction in the normal microbial flora of the body).

The following are guidelines for the use of antimicrobials: identification of the infecting organism, which allows for the selection of the most effective antimicrobial for the specific infecting organism; determination of the ability of a specific antimicrobial to limit the growth of or kill microorganisms in vitro; supportive therapy for the host's defense mechanisms; and administration of the agent in an adequate dosage and for long enough periods to be effective. Nursing management of antimicrobial therapy includes the assessment of the client's ability to deal with the stressor of infection, the administration of antimicrobial drugs safely and accurately, the education of the client to do the same with regard to self-administration of the drug, the prevention and management of adverse responses, and the evaluation of the client's response to the drug and progress toward the goal of resolution of the infection.

Critical Thinking Questions

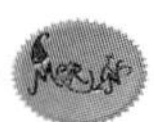

1. Susan Brooks is a 71-year-old resident of Laurelmont Nursing Home. She is fond of starting her day with an early morning cup of coffee. One morning she choked while trying to drink her coffee but seemed to recover fully. Some days later, however, you notice that Ms. Brooks has become more restless and agitated than usual and cannot sleep. She has no cough or sputum production, but her temperature is over 102° F. A chest x-ray examination shows right lower lobe infiltrate, a common finding in aspiration pneumonia. What nursing actions should occur before initiating antimicrobial therapy? After 3 days of antibiotic therapy, Ms. Brooks develops diarrhea. What do you suspect has occurred? How will you validate your suspicions? How will this change your plan of care for Ms. Brooks? What would be appropriate outcome criteria for her plan of care?
2. Nick Nicholson, a 78-year-old man with Alzheimer's disease, is also a resident of Laurelmont. He has fre-

quent urinary incontinence and wears an external catheter at night. One evening Mr. Nicholson vomits but otherwise does not seem unwell. The next day he has a fever of 101° F. He has no cough or sputum production, and his chest x-ray is negative. However, a urine culture shows greater than 100,000 colonies of *Escherichia coli* per millimeter, which indicates a urinary tract infection. What aspects of Ms. Brooks and Mr. Nicholson's plans of care will be the same, and how will they differ? How will you evaluate the effectiveness of your plan of care for Mr. Nicholson?

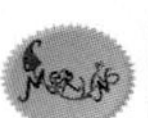

Collaborative Learning Activities

For Collaborative Learning Activities, go to mosby.com/MERLIN/McKenry/.

BIBLIOGRAPHY

Abramowicz, M. (Ed.) (1994). The choice of antibacterial drugs. *Medical Letter, 36*(925), 53-60.

Anderson, K.N., Anderson, L.E., & Glanze, W.D. (Eds.) (1998). *Mosby's medical, nursing, & allied health dictionary* (5th ed.). St. Louis: Mosby.

Balk, R.A. & Parrillo, J.E. (1992). Prognostic factors in sepsis: The cold facts. *Critical Care Medicine, 20*(10), 1373-1374.

Ball, P. (1999). Therapy for pneumococcal infection at the millennium: Doubts and certainties. *American Journal of Medicine, 107*(1A), 77S-85S.

Bergogone-Berezin, E. (1999). Current guidelines for the treatment and prevention of nosocomial infections. *Drugs, 58*(1), 51-67.

Bone, R.C. (1993). The search for a magic bullet to fight sepsis. *Journal of the American Medical Association, 269*(17), 2266.

Bruce, J.L. & Grove, S.K. (1992). Fever: Pathology and treatment. *Critical Care Nursing, 12* (1), 40-49.

Fraser, D. (1993). Patient assessment: Infection in the elderly. *Journal of Gerontological Nursing, 19*(7), 5-11.

Grimes, D. (1991). *Infectious diseases.* St. Louis: Mosby.

Insel, P.A. (1996). Analgesic-antipyretic and antiinflammatory agents and drugs employed in the treatment of gout. In J.G. Hardman & L.E. Limbird (Eds.), *Goodman & Gilman's The pharmacological basis of therapeutics* (9th ed.). New York: McGraw-Hill.

Lewis, S.L., Collier, I.C., Heitkemper, M.M., Dirksen, S.R. (2000) *Medical-surgical nursing: Assessment and management of clinical problems.* St. Louis: Mosby.

McCance, K.L. & Huether, S.E. (1998). *Pathophysiology: The biologic basis for disease in adults and children* (3rd ed.). St. Louis: Mosby.

Smeltzer, S.C. & Bare, B.G. (2000). *Brunner and Suddarth's textbook of medical-surgical nursing* (9th ed.). Philadelphia: J.B. Lippincott.

59 Antibiotics

Chapter Focus

Infectious disease has always held a special threat for humans. There have been eras in which uncontrolled plague and pestilence have shaped the course of humankind. It was not until Edward Jenner made his first public inoculation with the smallpox vaccine in 1796 that humans began to have some control over their experience with communicable diseases. The concept of asepsis was gradually accepted over the nineteenth century to help prevent the spread of infection. However, not until the advent of the sulfonamides, penicillin, and other antibiotics was there an effective treatment for those with infectious diseases. Today, with the occurrence of drug-resistant strains of microorganisms and the opportunistic bacterial infections that accompany the human immunodeficiency virus (HIV), the importance of disease prevention and the antibiotic agents cannot be overlooked.

Learning Objectives

1. Discuss the nursing management of antibiotic therapy.
2. Differentiate between peak, trough, and mean serum levels.
3. List four major classifications of antibiotics.
4. Differentiate between different antibiotics within the same general classification.
5. Compare the role of antibiotics, sulfonamides, urinary antiseptics, and urinary tract analgesics in the treatment of urinary tract infections.
6. Implement the nursing management for the care of clients receiving antibiotic therapy.

Key Terms

antibiotic, p. 980
cephalosporin, p. 988
fluoroquinolones, p. 1000
macrolide antibiotics, p. 991
penicillins, p. 982
superinfection, p. 980
tetracyclines, p. 997

Key Drugs [✔]

cefazolin, p. 988
ciprofloxacin, p. 1000
erythromycin, p. 991
gentamicin, p. 995
penicillin G, p. 982
trimethoprim-sulfamethoxazole, p. 1006
vancomycin, p. 994

Antibiotics are chemical substances produced from various microorganisms (bacteria, fungus) that kill or suppress the growth of other microorganisms. This term is also used for synthetic antimicrobial agents, such as sulfonamides and quinolones. Although hundreds of available antibiotics vary in antibacterial spectrum, mechanism of action, potency, toxicity, and pharmacokinetic properties, this chapter is divided into penicillins and related antibiotics, cephalosporins, macrolides, lincosamides, aminoglycosides, tetracyclines, quinolones, miscellaneous antimicrobials, and urinary tract antimicrobials. It is essential that the nurse understand the general principles of antibiotic therapy as discussed in Chapter 58. In addition, before administering an antibiotic, the nurse must be familiar with the specific drug and its actions and effects for the individual client.

■ Nursing Management

Antibiotic Therapy

■ **Assessment.** The nursing assessment is particularly important when an infection is suspected. Detailed information regarding the client's general health should be obtained, as well as the symptoms indicating an infection, such as elevated temperature, chills, sweats, redness, pain or swelling in a previously unaffected area, fatigue, anorexia, weight loss, cough, a change in the character or amount of sputum, increased white blood cell (WBC) count, and the amount and quality of pus or drainage.

Whenever possible, the infecting organism should be identified before drug therapy begins. The collection of specimens (blood, urine, sputum, wound drainage and discharge) and cultures should be completed before initiating antibiotic therapy. Specimens should be carefully obtained following agency guidelines to ensure test accuracy and to protect personnel from exposure to infectious organisms. Prompt treatment is imperative in serious infections; in such cases antimicrobial drugs should not be withheld pending laboratory study and culture results.

Antibiotics, particularly penicillins, have been associated with serious hypersensitivity and allergic reactions. A complete drug history of the client and family helps to identify possible hypersensitivity or cross-sensitivity to the drugs. Cross-sensitivity often exists between drugs of the same class (e.g., penicillins). Clients who are intolerant of one antibiotic may be intolerant of similar antibiotics. Information regarding possible contraindications, cautions, potential drug interactions, and drug-taking patterns is also obtained.

■ **Nursing Diagnosis.** Many antibiotics are administered prophylactically; in such cases, the nursing diagnosis of risk for infection would pertain. Once the client has an infection, risk for infection transmission is appropriate along with other nursing diagnoses specific to the client. See Chapter 58 and the Nursing Care Plan on p. 981 for other selected nursing diagnoses.

■ **Implementation**

■ ***Monitoring.*** When an antibiotic is administered for prophylaxis, the client should be monitored for signs indicating the absence or development of infection. When a specific infection is treated, a therapeutic response will be indicated by a decrease in the specific signs of infection identified in the baseline assessment (fever, malaise, elevated WBC count, redness, inflammation, drainage, pain, positive cultures). Evaluation of the therapeutic response is important, because antibiotic therapy may be ineffective for several reasons, including incorrect route of administration, inadequate drainage of abscesses, poor antibiotic penetration of infected tissues, subtherapeutic serum levels, or bacterial resistance to the antibiotic.

Reducing or eliminating normal flora by antibiotic therapy provides an environment conducive to the growth of undesirable bacteria, fungi, or yeasts in a condition known as **superinfection.** Examples commonly seen include diarrhea from altered intestinal flora or vaginal yeast infections resulting from a reduction in normal vaginal flora, which suppress yeast growth.

Adverse reactions vary widely and depend on the drug, dose, route of administration, and client-related factors. Refer to the nursing management sections of specific antibiotics for the side effects/adverse reactions and the nursing evaluation related to those drugs.

Allergic reactions are always possible following the first or successive doses. In general, it is important to monitor for allergic reactions such as anaphylaxis, skin rashes, urticaria, and bronchospasm. Administration should stop immediately at the first sign of an allergic reaction, and the prescriber should be notified (see Chapter 58 for more information).

■ ***Intervention.*** Dosages and routes of administration are highly individualized and are based on the organism or infection being treated and on a variety of individual client factors such as age, weight, general health, and preexisting diseases or organ or system dysfunction. Antibiotics are available in various dosage forms for topical, oral, or parenteral use. Dosage adjustments between different forms or routes of administration are necessary because of differences in absorption, distribution, metabolism, or excretion. For example, to achieve the same serum levels, an oral dose of penicillin G needs to be five times the amount of the parenteral dose.

Special attention must be given to the interactions of oral antibiotics with food or other drugs. Some antibiotics should not be administered with food. For example, tetracycline forms a nonabsorbable complex with dairy products. Other antibiotics are administered with food to minimize gastric irritation.

The times of antibiotic administration should be spaced as evenly as possible over a 24-hour period to ensure stable and consistent serum levels. Antibiotics that are to be given four times daily (qid) should be administered every 6 hours; antibiotics administered three times daily (tid) are given every 8 hours. It is important to administer antibiotics at the scheduled time to maintain a consistent blood level. Allowable variation differs with specific drugs and institutional policy. As a general rule, antibiotics should be administered within 15 minutes of the scheduled time.

Nursing Care Plan
Selected Nursing Diagnoses Related to Antibiotic Therapy

Nursing Diagnosis	Outcome Criteria	Nursing Interventions
Deficient knowledge related to antimicrobial drug therapy	Client will: Express an understanding of the purpose, function, and side effects/adverse reactions of drug therapy Demonstrate an understanding of proper handling and administration	Assess the client's level of knowledge and understanding. Determine the education needs of the client. Provide information related to the following: The specific problem being treated with the antimicrobial agent The purpose and function of drug therapy The side effects/adverse reactions of the drug The methods of reducing side effects Answer questions and clarify misconceptions. If drug the is to be self-administered, instruct the client in the following: The proper route and method of administration Proper storage and handling The importance of taking all of the prescribed drug Alert the client to possible drug interactions. Instruct the client not to take additional medications without first checking with the prescriber.
Imbalanced nutrition related to the gastrointestinal effects of antimicrobial drugs	Client will maintain desired nutritional status	Assess the client's normal dietary patterns and intake. Assess the normal pattern of bowel function. Emphasize the importance of adequate nutrition. Instruct the client to report any gastrointestinal changes (nausea, vomiting, cramping, gas, diarrhea, constipation). Administer the drug in relation to meals and food to minimize side effects (with meals, before or after, depending on the specific drug) yet maintain effectiveness of therapy. Encourage the intake of active culture yogurt or buttermilk to maintain or restore intestinal flora. Report adverse reactions to the prescriber.

The serum levels of many antibiotics are monitored to determine if the concentration is at the correct (therapeutic) level, a high (toxic) level, or a low (subtherapeutic) level. The timing of serum determinations is also important. To determine the lowest serum level, or trough concentration, the blood is drawn immediately before administering a dose. Mean serum levels are determined at some point between doses, and the highest serum level, or peak level, is determined shortly after dose administration. The desired serum concentration may vary with different drugs and the infecting organism. The exact timing of peak, mean, or trough serum concentrations is determined by each particular drug and route of administration.

■ ***Education.*** Clients should be fully informed about the nature of their condition and the treatment plan. They should understand the medication regimen, including the name of the medication (generic and trade names) and its general action, purpose, proper handling, dosage, and correct administration. Provide the client with a list of adverse reactions, drug-drug interactions, and food-drug interactions; advise the client of the proper response to take if these interactions occur.

Clients should be instructed to take the medication exactly as prescribed, at evenly spaced intervals, and for the full length of time prescribed or until all the drug is gone. Even if the client feels well, the infection may return if the full course of therapy is not completed. Any leftover medication should be appropriately discarded.

Rash, itching, hives, fever, chills, joint pain or swelling, difficulty breathing, or wheezing are signs of an adverse reaction. The drug should be stopped and the prescriber contacted immediately.

■ **Evaluation.** If the antibiotic therapy is administered prophylactically, the expected outcome is that the client will remain free of infectious processes and will demonstrate appropriate practices to prevent infection. If administered therapeutically, the client will maintain or achieve an infection-free state as evidenced by negative cultures, a body temperature within normal limits, a WBC count within the normal limits for age, and the resolution of any other infection-related symptoms that the client might be experiencing. The client will also manage the therapeutic regimen effectively and demonstrate practices to prevent the spread of infection.

PENICILLINS AND RELATED ANTIBIOTICS

Penicillins are antibiotics derived from a number of strains of common molds often seen on bread or fruit (Figure 59-1). Introduced into clinical practice in the 1940s, penicillin and related antibiotics constitute a large group of antimicrobial agents that remain the most effective and least toxic of all available antimicrobial drugs.

The cell walls of bacteria are permeable and rigid to protect cellular cytoplasm. Penicillins weaken the cell wall by inhibiting the transpeptidase enzymes responsible for cross-linking the cell wall strands, which results in cell lysis and death. Penicillins are therefore bactericidal because they inhibit the synthesis of the bacterial cell wall.

Penicillin is not useful in the presence of bacterial enzymes that are capable of destroying penicillins, such as penicillinase strains of the beta-lactamase enzymes. There are now four different classifications of antibiotics that contain the beta-lactam ring: penicillins, cephalosporins, monobactams, and carbapenems. Alteration of the beta-lactam rings (depending on the antibiotic and specific bacteria) has resulted in the formulation of drugs that are more active against gram-negative cell wall organisms and are less susceptible to beta-lactamases that inactivate the antibiotic. The beta-lactam–altered penicillins aztreonam and imipenem are stable in the presence of beta-lactamases, whereas ampicillin and/or amoxicillin must be combined with beta-lactamase inhibitors such as clavulanate, sulbactam, or tazobactam to improve their effectiveness.

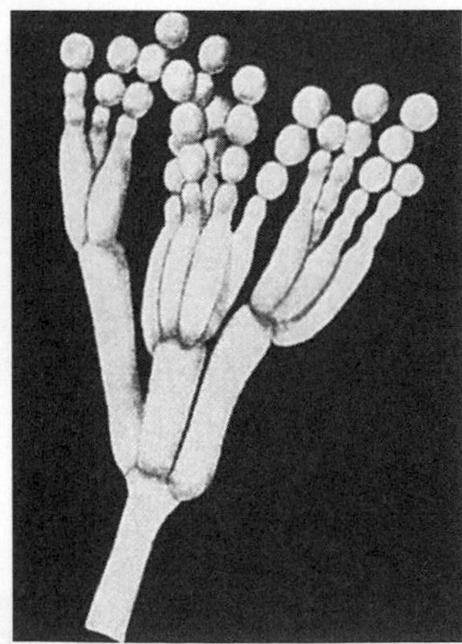

Figure 59-1 Typical penicillus of *Penicillus notatum*, Flemming's strain. (From Raper, K.B. & Alexander, D.F. [1945]. *J Elisha Mitchell Sc Soc*, 61, 74.)

Most penicillins are much more active against gram-positive than gram-negative bacteria. However, ticarcillin, carbenicillin, aztreonam, imipenem, and the combination of penicillins with beta-lactamase inhibitors are more effective against gram-negative bacteria (*Escherichia coli, Klebsiella pneumoniae,* and others). Prophylactically, penicillin is indicated for the prevention of diphtheria, bacterial endocarditis, and rheumatic fever. Penicillins are divided into the following categories:

1. *Natural penicillins.* This category includes penicillin G and penicillin V.

   Penicillin G and penicillin V are comparable therapeutically, but oral penicillin V is more stable in stomach acid and therefore reaches higher serum levels than oral penicillin G.

   Penicillin G is available in oral, IM, and IV dosage forms in various salt formulations: sodium penicillin G, potassium penicillin G, procaine penicillin G, benzathine penicillin G, and a parenteral combination of the latter two formulations. The active substance in all formulations is penicillin G.
2. *Penicillinase-resistant penicillins.* This category includes cloxacillin, dicloxacillin, methicillin, nafcillin, and oxacillin. A chemical alteration of the penicillin structure results in penicillins resistant to beta-lactamase inactivation; these penicillins are used to treat penicillinase-producing staphylococci. These antibiotics are not effective against methicillin-resistant bacteria.
3. *Aminopenicillins or broader-spectrum penicillins.* This category includes amoxicillin, amoxicillin and potassium clavulanate, ampicillin, ampicillin and sulbactam, and bacampicillin. Although these antibiotics have the spectrum of activity of penicillin in addition to efficacy against selected gram-negative bacteria, the single agents are usually not very effective against *Staphylococcus aureus* (beta-lactamase–producing) bacteria. The penicillin is protected from inactivation by beta-lactamase enzymes when combined with beta-lactamase inhibitors such as potassium clavulanate and sulbactam.
4. *Extended-spectrum penicillins.* This category includes carbenicillin, mezlocillin, piperacillin, piperacillin and tazobactam, ticarcillin, and ticarcillin and clavulanate potassium. These antibiotics have a broader spectrum of antimicrobial activity that includes *Pseudomonas aeruginosa, Enterobacter, Proteus,* and others. In this category, only the combination antibiotics are effective against *Staphylococcus aureus* (beta-lactamase–producing) bacteria.

The nurse should be aware that reducing or eliminating normal bacteria flora with antibiotic therapy may provide an environment that is conducive to the growth of undesirable microorganisms such as bacteria or fungus. This condition is known as superinfection and may present as diarrhea from an altered gastrointestinal flora or as a vaginal *Candida* fungal infection.

Table 59-1 summarizes pharmacokinetics and thc usual adult dosages of the penicillins.

The side effects/adverse reactions of penicillins include diarrhea, nausea, vomiting, headache, sore mouth or tongue, and oral and vaginal candidiasis. Less commonly reported are allergic reactions, anaphylaxis, serum sickness–type reaction (rash, joint pain, fever), hives, and pruritus.

■ Nursing Management

Penicillin Therapy

In addition to the following discussion, see Nursing Management: Antibiotic Therapy, p. 980, which also applies to the client receiving penicillin therapy.

■ **Assessment.** Ascertain the client's history of sensitivity to penicillins. Because allergic reactions are a significant problem in the use of penicillins, meticulous assessment of the client's previous drug experiences, with special attention given to the development of prior drug related rashes, is necessary. For infants less than 3 months of age, a history of penicillin allergy in the mother should be sought. If at all possible, no penicillin preparation of any type should be prescribed for or administered to an individual with a history of allergic reaction to the drug. Because of possible cross-sensitization, it is also wise to avoid the use of cephalosporins in clients with severe or immediate allergic reactions to penicillins. (See the Special Considerations for Children box on p. 986 regarding how to assess the appropriate antibiotic therapy in children.)

The client's health status should be assessed for conditions in which the administration of penicillin might be contraindicated or need cautious use. Clients with a history of bleeding disorders require monitoring for bleeding tendencies with the administration of carbenicillin, piperacillin, and ticarcillin because they may cause platelet dysfunction. Clients with a history of gastrointestinal disease, particularly ulcerative colitis and regional enteritis, are more at risk for pseudomembranous colitis as an adverse reaction. The sodium content of high doses of parenteral carbenicillin and ticarcillin should be considered with clients who may have sodium restrictions, such as those with congestive heart failure and hypertension. Skin rash may occur in 43% to 100% of clients who have infectious mononucleosis and are receiving ampicillin, bacampicillin, and pivampicillin. Clients with cystic fibrosis who are administered piperacillin are at greater risk for fever and skin rash. Clients with renal function impairment may require lower dosages. See the Pregnancy Safety box on p. 986 for the Food and Drug Administration (FDA) pregnancy categories for the penicillins.

Review the client's medications for the risk of significant drug interactions, such as those that may occur when penicillins are given with the following drugs:

Drug	Possible Effect and Management
Bold/color type indicates the most serious interactions.	
aminoglycosides	Mixing in vitro has resulted in significant inactivation of both drugs. Administer at separate sites at least 1 hour apart.
angiotensin-converting enzyme (ACE) inhibitors, potassium-sparing diuretics, potassium-containing drugs, or potassium supplements	If given concurrently with parenteral penicillin G potassium, serum potassium levels may increase, causing hyperkalemia. Monitor closely; dosage adjustments may be necessary.
anticoagulants, oral coumarin or indanedione, heparin or thrombolytic agent	**There is an increased risk of bleeding when given with high doses of parenteral carbenicillin, piperacillin, or ticarcillin, because these drugs inhibit platelet aggregation. Monitor closely for signs of bleeding. Concurrent use of these penicillins with thrombolytic agents also increases the risk for severe bleeding. Avoid concurrent use or a potentially serious drug interaction may occur.**
cholestyramine (Questran) or colestipol (Colestid)	May decrease the absorption of oral penicillin G if given concurrently. Advise clients to take the antibiotic first and other medications 3 hours later.
estrogen-containing contraceptives	When used concurrently with ampicillin, amoxicillin, or penicillin V, the effectiveness of the oral contraceptives may be decreased because of an increase in estrogen metabolism or a reduction in the enterohepatic circulation of estrogens. Advise clients to use an alternate method of contraception while taking these antibiotics.
methotrexate (Folex)	Concurrent use with penicillins decreases methotrexate clearance and may result in methotrexate toxicity. Monitor closely. Leucovorin rescue doses may need to be increased and given for a longer period of time.
nonsteroidal antiinflammatory drugs (NSAIDs), platelet aggregation inhibitors (e.g., salicylates, dextran, dipyridamole [Persantine], valproic acid [Depakote], and sulfinpyrazone [Anturane])	**An increased risk for bleeding or hemorrhage exists with high doses of carbenicillin, piperacillin, or ticarcillin (parenteral dosage forms). These drugs inhibit platelet function, and large doses of salicylates may induce hypoprothrombinemia and also gastrointestinal ulcers (from NSAIDs, salicylates, or sulfinpyrazone), all of which add to the potential risk of hemorrhage. Avoid concurrent use or a potentially serious drug interaction may occur.**

Continued

TABLE 59-1 Penicillins: Pharmacokinetics and Usual Adult Dosing

Classification	Pharmacokinetics			
Drug(s)	**Oral Absorption (%)**	**Peak Serum (hours)***	**Renal Excretion (%)†**	**Usual Adult Dosage**
Natural Penicillins				
penicillin G				
oral	15-30	1-2	20	200,000-500,000 U q4-6h
IV	—	—	60-90	1-5 mU q4-6h
IM	—	B: 24	60-90	1.2-2.4 mU single dose
		P: 4	60-90	600,000 U to 1.2 mU daily
penicillin V (Veetids ◆)				
oral	60-73	0.5-1	20-40	125-500 mg q6-8h
Penicillinase-Resistant Penicillins				
cloxacillin (Tegopen)				
oral	50	1-2	30-60	250-500 mg q6h
IV 🍁	—	E of I	30-60	250-500 mg q6h
dicloxacillin (Dynapen)				
oral	37-50	0.5-1	50-70	125-250 mg q6h
methicillin (Staphcillin)				
IM	—	0.5-1	60-80	1 g q4-6h
IV	—	E of I	60-80	1 g q6h
nafcillin (Unipen)				
oral	Erratic	1-2	10-30	250 mg to 1 g q4-6h
IM	—	0.5-1	10-30	500 mg q4-6h
IV	—	E of I	10-30	0.5-1.5 g q4h
oxacillin (Prostaphlin)				
oral	30-35	0.5-1	55-60	0.5-1 g q4-6h
IM	—	0.5-1	55-60	250 mg to 1 g q4-6h
IV	—	E of I	55-60	250 mg to 1 g q4-6h
Aminopenicillins (Broader-Spectrum)				
amoxicillin (Amoxil ◆)				
oral	75-90	1-2	60-75	250-500 mg q8h
amoxicillin + clavulanate (Augmentin ◆, Clavulin 🍁)				
oral	90	1-2	50-78	500 mg q8h

Information from *United States Pharmacopeial Dispensing Information (USP DI): Drug information for the health care professional* (19th ed.). (1999). Rockville, MD: United States Pharmacopeial Convention.
B, Benzathine dosage form; *P*, procaine dosage form; *mU*, million units; *E of I*, end of infusion.
*Time to peak serum level (hours).
†Renal excretion of active drug (percent excreted unchanged).
‡As ampicillin.

Drug	Possible Effect and Management
probenecid (Benemid)	Decreases renal tubular secretion of penicillins, resulting in elevated serum levels and an increase in half-life. It may also increase toxicity. Several combinations of penicillin and probenecid are marketed to take advantage of this effect.

A baseline assessment as described in Chapter 58 is necessary for clients who will be receiving penicillin therapy.

■ **Nursing Diagnosis.** Clients receiving penicillin therapy are at risk for the following nursing diagnoses/collaborative problems: ineffective protection related to a reduction in normal flora (superinfection) as evidenced by a darkened tongue (fungal superinfection) and white oral plaques and creamy vaginal discharge (*Candida* superinfec-

TABLE 59-1 Penicillins: Pharmacokinetics and Usual Adult Dosing—cont'd

Classification	Pharmacokinetics			
Drug(s)	Oral Absorption (%)	Peak Serum (hours)*	Renal Excretion (%)†	Usual Adult Dosage
Aminopenicillins (Broader-Spectrum)—cont'd				
ampicillin (Polycillin)				
oral	35-50	1-1.5	75-90	250-500 mg q6h
IM	—	1	75-90	250-500 mg q6h
IV	—	E of I	75-90	250-500 mg q6h
ampicillin + sulbactam (Unasyn)				
IM	—	—	75-85	1.5-3 g q6h
IV	—	E of I	—	1.5-3 g q6h
bacampicillin (Spectrobid)				
oral	35-50‡	0.5-1‡	70-75‡	400-800 mg q12h
Extended-Spectrum Penicillins				
carbenicillin (Geocillin)				
oral	30	0.5-1	36	0.5-1 g q6h
IM	—	0.5-1	—	50-83.3 mg/kg q4h
IV	—	E of I	75-95	50-83.3 mg/kg q4h
mezlocillin (Mezlin)				
IM	—	0.5-1	55-60	33.3-58.3 mg/kg q4h
IV	—	E of I	55-60	33.3-58.3 mg/kg q4h
piperacillin (Pipracil)				
IM	—	0.5	60-80	3-4 g q4-6h
IV	—	E of I	60-80	3-4 g q4-6h
piperacillin + tazobactam (Zosyn, Tazocin 🍁)				
IV	—	E of I	68	3.375-4.5 g q6-8h
ticarcillin (Ticar)				
IM	—	0.5-1	60-80	1 g q6h
IV	—	E of I	60-80	1-4 g q6h
ticarcillin + clavulanate (Timentin)				
IV	—	E of I	60-70	33.3-50 mg q4h

tion); diarrhea (watery and severe) related to the development of antibiotic-associated pseudomembranous colitis; deficient fluid volume related to nausea, vomiting, and/or diarrhea; impaired skin integrity (exfoliative dermatitis, urticaria [Figure 59-2], rash); and the potential complications of allergic response, interstitial nephritis, hepatotoxicity, leukopenia or neutropenia, thrombocytopenia, mental disturbances, seizures, or a cross-sensitivity to cephalosporins, cephamycins, griseofulvin, or penicillamine.

■ Implementation

■ ***Monitoring.*** Drug interactions with penicillins can increase or decrease the effectiveness of the penicillins and should be monitored. Gentamicin acts synergistically with penicillins against enterococci and *S. aureus* when used with nafcillin or methicillin. Acidifying agents such as ammonium chloride, ascorbic acid, methenamine, methionine, and citrus juice destroy oral penicillins, making them less effective. Tetracyclines slow bacterial multiplication and

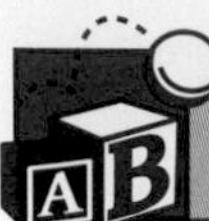

Special Considerations for Children
Antibiotic Therapy

To assess the appropriateness of antibiotic therapy in children, the following criteria are generally accepted:

1. In choosing empiric therapy, the selected antimicrobial should have documentation of both adequate penetration at the site and proven effectiveness against the common organisms usually isolated from that specific site.
2. Multiple drug therapy may be indicated if a broad range of possible microorganisms is suspected or if multiple organisms have been isolated from an infection site. However, the minimum number of drugs necessary to treat the infection should be used whenever possible.
3. If no contraindication is present, the drug of first choice should be selected. The drug dosage regimen should be within the accepted range of current usage for the individual client, taking into account the child's body surface area (height, weight), organ function, and concurrent disease processes.
4. Unless the benefit far outweighs the risk, no antibiotic should be used in clients who have prior documentation of an allergic or adverse reaction to the specific medication.
5. Children receiving potent and potentially dangerous drugs (e.g., gentamicin, amikacin, tobramycin, or vancomycin) for more than 2 days should have steady-state drug serum concentrations drawn at the appropriate times for evaluation.
6. Whenever possible, cultures should be drawn before the initiation of antibiotic therapy. The usual sites cultured include sputum, urine, blood, wound, or nonhealing topical sites.
7. Antibiotic therapy should be continued until the infection is no longer present. However, time periods should not exceed the usual treatment time established for the suspected infection. Prophylactic antibiotic therapy given after uncomplicated surgery is usually discontinued within 48 hours with few exceptions, such as cardiac surgery.

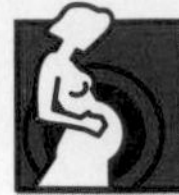

Pregnancy Safety
Antibiotics

Category	Drug
B	azithromycin, aztreonam, cephalosporins, metronidazole, nitrofurantoin, penicillins, phenazopyridine
C	cinoxacin, clarithromycin, dirithromycin, fluoroquinolones, gentamicin, imipenem/cilastatin, linezolid, methenamine, sulfonamides, vancomycin
D	amikacin, kanamycin, netilmicin, streptomycin, tetracyclines, tobramycin
Unclassified	chloramphenicol (not recommended at term or during labor), clindamycin, lincomycin, nalidixic acid (not recommended in pregnancy), spectinomycin, troleandomycin

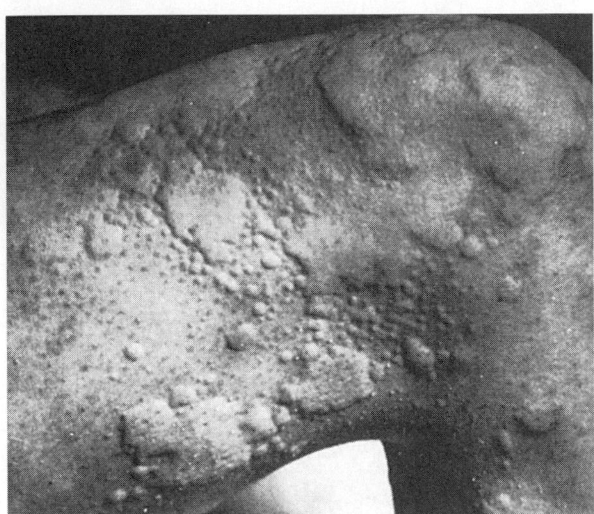

Figure 59-2 Urticaria such as that seen in individuals who are sensitive to penicillin.

thereby inhibit the penicillins that act against rapidly multiplying bacteria. Erythromycin inhibits the bactericidal activity of penicillins against most organisms.

Because of the possibility of bacterial and fungal superinfection, older adults and debilitated clients should be observed carefully for unusual weight loss (pseudomembranous colitis), abdominal cramps and diarrhea, a darkened or discolored tongue, and sore mouth. See Box 59-1 for a discussion of antibiotic-associated pseudomembranous colitis (AAPMC).

Serum electrolytes should be monitored for hyperkalemia and/or hypernatremia when the client is receiving carbenicillin (parenteral), mezlocillin, penicillin G (parenteral), piperacillin, and ticarcillin. Renal function studies may be required during prolonged therapy with methicillin, which causes interstitial nephritis in up to 33% of clients who are treated more than 10 days.

The client's vital signs, total and differential WBC count and culture results, and stool cytotoxin assays (if *Clostridium difficile* colitis occurs), should be monitored. Bleeding times (partial thromboplastin time [PTT] and prothrombin time [PT]) should be monitored with the administration of carbenicillin (parenteral), piperacillin, and ticarcillin.

■ ***Intervention.*** In addition to performing nursing measures common to all types of antibiotic drug therapy (as discussed previously in this chapter and Chapter 58), be especially cognizant of the following factors when penicillins are prescribed.

BOX 59-1

Antibiotic-Associated Pseudomembranous Colitis

Some clients may develop antibiotic-associated pseudomembranous colitis (AAPMC), which is caused by the *C. difficile* toxin, during or after treatment with penicillins, cephalosporins, lincomycins, and imipenem-cilastatin. This condition is characterized by inflammation and necrosis of the mucosal and submucosal layers of the bowel wall as evidenced by 2 to 5 semisolid or liquid stools per day in mild cases and 30 or more watery stools a day in severe disease. Fluid and electrolyte loss, abdominal tenderness, cramping, and fever also occur. AAPMC is fatal in 10% to 20% of cases in debilitated clients and older adults. It is called pseudomembranous because the inflammation causes the formation of exudative plaques, or "pseudomembranes," on the mucosal wall.

Two types of clients develop AAPMC: those who are carriers of *C. difficile* and are given antibiotics, and noncarriers who are given antibiotics and then exposed to the organism through environmental conditions. Spores of the organism have been known to exist for months after an infected client has been discharged (Doughty & Jackson, 1993).

Discontinuation of the causative drug is sufficient therapy for mild cases, but moderate to severe cases may require the replacement of fluid, electrolytes, and proteins. In clients nonresponsive to discontinuing the caustic antibiotic and in more severe cases, oral doses of metronidazole, bacitracin, vancomycin, or cholestyramine may be used. The antimicrobials are effective against the organism, and cholestyramine has been shown to bind the *C. difficile* toxin in vitro. If the cholestyramine is prescribed concurrently with vancomycin, the drugs should be administered several hours apart, because cholestyramine will also bind with oral vancomycin.

Recurrences are not uncommon and are treated with a second round of drugs. Watery diarrhea in AAPMC may occur during therapy and persist for several weeks after therapy. Antidiarrheals are not recommended because they retain the toxin within the bowel, thus prolonging and/or worsening the damage to the colon (*USP DI*, 1999).

When administering penicillins, remember that most oral penicillins are bound to food and are poorly absorbed in acid media. Therefore their administration should not be preceded or followed by food for at least 1 hour to minimize binding. Penicillin G should not be taken with acidic fruit juices, because this may facilitate decomposition of the penicillin. Table 59-2 lists the effect of food on oral penicillin absorption.

TABLE 59-2 Effect of Food on Oral Penicillin Absorption*

Drug	Food Effect
amoxicillin	None
amoxicillin and clavulanate	None
ampicillin	Decreased
bacampicillin tablet	None
carbenicillin indanyl sodium	Increased
cloxacillin	Decreased
dicloxacillin	Decreased
flucloxacillin	Decreased
nafcillin	Decreased
oxacillin	Decreased
penicillin G	Decreased
penicillin V potassium	Decreased slightly
pivampicillin	None
pivmecillinam	None

*Penicillins whose absorption decreases after food intake are generally acid labile; therefore they are administered with a full glass of water on an empty stomach 1 hour before or 2 hours after meals.

When administering penicillins intravenously, note that most penicillins in clinical use are sodium or potassium salts. Significant amounts of cations can be administered when these drugs are given intravenously in a massive dose. For example, 20 million units of potassium penicillin G contain 34 mEq of potassium ion. Fatalities have occurred because of the toxic effect of potassium on the heart following the administration of such large doses in the presence of renal insufficiency. Carbenicillin contains 4.7 to 6.5 mEq of sodium per gram and may be administered in doses of 30 to 40 g daily. Signs and symptoms of hyperkalemia and hypernatremia should be duly noted and reported.

When administering penicillins intravenously, do so intermittently to prevent blood vessel irritation and phlebitis. The IV site should be changed at least every 48 hours.

■ ***Education.*** Instruct the client to take the full course of medication, even if he or she is feeling better and is symptom free. Emphasize the importance of taking evenly spaced doses to maintain therapeutic blood levels. Prescriptions for antibiotics should never be shared with others or saved and taken for a different episode of illness.

Ampicillin, bacampicillin oral suspension, carbenicillin, cloxacillin, dicloxacillin, flucloxacillin, nafcillin, oxacillin, and penicillin G should be taken when the stomach is empty. Amoxicillin, bacampicillin tablets, penicillin V, pivampicillin, and pivmecillinam may be taken either on an empty stomach or with food to decrease gastrointestinal distress.

Women taking penicillins, especially ampicillin, amoxicillin, and penicillin V, should be cautioned to use an alternate form of contraception if they are using estrogen-containing contraceptives.

Clients with diabetes mellitus who use copper sulfate urine glucose tests (Clinitest) may have false-positive results while taking amoxicillin, ampicillin, bacampicillin, and penicillin G. Have the client use glucose-enzymatic tests, such as Clinistix or Keto-diastix.

Instruct clients to report to their prescriber if their condition fails to improve in a few days or if they develop severe diarrhea, rash, fever, or chills, which may indicate a delayed sensitivity reaction.

▪ **Evaluation.** The expected outcome of penicillin therapy is that the client will maintain or achieve an infection-free state as evidenced by negative cultures. If administered therapeutically, the client will have a body temperature within normal limits and a WBC count within the normal limits for age. The client will also experience the resolution of any other infection-related symptoms without adverse reactions to the drug. (See the Case Study box below.)

CEPHALOSPORINS AND RELATED PRODUCTS

Cephalosporins and related products are chemical modifications of the penicillin structure. These modifications create compounds with different microbiologic and pharmacologic activities. To classify the differences in antimicrobial activity, cephalosporins are divided into four generations. Loracarbef (Lorabid) is a beta-lactam antibiotic (carbacephem); it is chemically similar to second-generation cephalosporin and is included in this section.

Cephalosporins inhibit cell wall synthesis in a manner similar to penicillin; they are also bactericidal. They are effective in numerous situations, but until the third-generation cephalosporins were marketed the majority were not considered to be drugs of choice for any serious infection. First-generation cephalosporins are primarily active against gram-positive bacteria. The initial prototype drug for this category was cephalothin (Keflin), but it was taken off the market in 1998. Cefazolin (Ancef) is now referred to as the key or prototype drug. The second-generation cephalosporins (cefamandole and others) have increased activity against gram-negative microorganisms. The third generation is more active against gram-negative bacteria; ceftazidime and cefoperazone are also effective against *Pseudomonas aeruginosa*) and beta-lactamase–producing microbial strains. However, the third generation is less effective against gram-positive cocci. Cefepime (Maxipime) is a fourth-generation cephalosporin that has antimicrobial effects comparable to the third generation and is also more resistant to some beta-lactamases (Mandell & Petri, Jr, 1996).

The initial advantage of cephalosporins over penicillins was their resistance to enzymatic degradation by penicillinase (beta-lactamase). However, resistance has now been reported with drugs from the first three generations, possibly through four mechanisms: (1) the microorganisms lack an outer cell membrane permeability, which causes poor drug penetration in the bacteria; (2) the bacteria lack a receptor for the specific drug; (3) the bacteria produce a beta-lactamase enzyme that can split the beta-lactam ring in the cephalosporin (many such enzymes have been isolated); or (4) the bacteria develop a type of tolerance in which bacterial strains are inhibited but not killed by the cephalosporins. The reason for this effect is the lack of, or deficiency in, autolytic enzymes in the bacterial cell wall (Katzung, 1992). This class of drugs has been overused; as a result, reports of bacterial resistance have increased.

Cephalosporin antibiotics are often prescribed for clients who are allergic to penicillins. They should be used with caution, because the possibility of a cross reaction is 5% to 15%. The cephalosporins should not be used if the client reports a serious reaction or anaphylaxis to penicillin (Beringer & Middleton, 1995).

Because cephalosporins inhibit cell wall synthesis, cell division, and growth, rapidly dividing bacteria are most affected by them. These agents are indicated for the treatment of a variety of infections and as prophylactic agents before surgery. Combinations of third-generation cephalosporins and aminoglycosides are used synergistically to treat *P. aeruginosa, Serratia marcescens,* and other susceptible organisms.

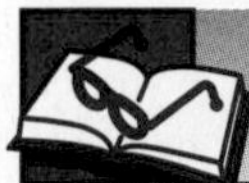

Case Study *The Client with a Bacterial Infection*

Gloria Lawton, a 42-year-old secretary, has come to the clinic complaining of a fever, sore throat, and cough for the past 24 hours. Her posterior pharynx is reddened, and there are patches of purulent exudate. She complains of pain with swallowing. Her cervical lymph nodes are enlarged and tender to touch. Based on the client's symptom history and physical examination, the nurse practitioner suspects a streptococcal infection. After a throat culture is obtained, Ms. Lawson is started on amoxicillin, 500 mg PO every 8 hours for 10 days.

1. Explain the rationale for obtaining a throat culture before administering the first dose of amoxicillin.
2. What additional assessment data does the nurse need to collect from the client before administering the first dose of amoxicillin?
3. What should Ms. Lawton be taught about taking the amoxicillin?
4. Ms. Lawton's upper respiratory symptoms resolve after completing the 10 days of drug therapy. However, she is now complaining of intense perineal itching and a vaginal discharge. How should the nurse respond to Ms. Lawton's questions about these symptoms?

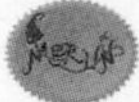

For answer guidelines, go to mosby.com/MERLIN/McKenry/.

The side effects/adverse reactions of cephalosporins include diarrhea, abdominal cramps or distress, oral and/or vaginal candidiasis, rash, pruritus, redness, or edema. An increase in bleeding episodes and bruising due to hypoprothrombinemia is reported with cefamandole, cefmetazole, cefoperazone, and cefotetan.

Table 59-3 summarizes the pharmacokinetics and usual adult dosages for the cephalosporins.

Nursing Management

Cephalosporin Therapy

In addition to the following discussion, see Nursing Management: Antibiotic Therapy, p. 980.

■ **Assessment.** The use of cephalosporins is contraindicated in clients with a history of sensitivity to cephalosporins, penicillin, penicillin derivatives, or penicillamine. Cephalosporins should be used with caution in clients who have a history of bleeding disorders, because all may cause hypoprothrombinemia and, potentially, bleeding. As with penicillins, clients with a history of gastrointestinal disease, particularly ulcerative colitis and regional enteritis, are at higher risk for pseudomembranous colitis. It is recommended that clients with renal and hepatic function impairment receive lower dosages. See the Pregnancy Safety box on p. 986 for FDA pregnancy safety categories for the cephalosporins.

Review the client's current medication regimen for the risk of significant drug interactions, such as those that may occur when cephalosporins are given concurrently with the following drugs:

Drug	Possible Effect and Management
Bold/color type indicates the most serious interactions.	
alcohol	**Not recommended with cefamandole, cefoperazone, or cefotetan. An increase in acetaldehyde in the blood may result, producing a disulfiram [Antabuse]–type reaction (e.g., stomach pain, nausea, vomiting, headaches, low blood pressure, tachycardia, respiratory difficulties, increased sweating, or flushing of the face). Clients should avoid the use of alcoholic beverages, medications containing alcohol, or IV alcohol solutions during the administration of these drugs and for 3 days afterward.**
anticoagulants, coumarin or indanedione, heparin, or thrombolytic agents	**There is an increased risk of bleeding and hemorrhage when given concurrently with cefamandole, cefoperazone, or cefotetan. These cephalosporins interfere with vitamin K metabolism in the liver, resulting in hypoprothrombinemia. Dosage adjustments of the anticoagulants may be necessary during and after the administration of these drugs. Avoid concurrent use of these drugs with thrombolytic agents because of the increased risk of serious bleeding and hemorrhage. An increased anticoagulant effect has been reported with the concurrent use of cefaclor and oral anticoagulants.**
NSAIDs, especially aspirin, inhibitors, and sulfinpyrazone (Anturane)	**When given with cefamandole, cefoperazone, or cefotetan, an increased risk of hemorrhage exists because of the additive effect on platelet inhibition. High doses of salicylates and/or the specified antibiotics may also induce hypoprothrombinemia, and the gastrointestinal potential for ulcers or hemorrhage with NSAIDs, salicylates, or sulfinpyrazone may increase when used with the previously mentioned cephalosporins. Avoid concurrent use or a potentially serious drug interaction may occur.**
probenecid (Benemid)	Probenecid decreases renal tubular secretion of the cephalosporins that are excreted by this mechanism, which can result in increased serum levels, an extended half-life, and an increased potential for toxicity. Probenecid does not affect the secretion of cefoperazone, ceftazidime, or ceftriaxone. Cephalosporins and probenecid are also used concurrently to treat specific infections in which a high serum level and prolonged effect are desirable, such as sexually transmitted diseases.

A baseline assessment as described in Chapter 58 should be obtained before initiating cephalosporin therapy.

■ **Nursing Diagnosis.** Clients receiving cephalosporins may experience any of the following nursing diagnoses/collaborative problems: impaired comfort (headache, abdominal cramping, mild diarrhea); diarrhea related to antibiotic-associated pseudomembranous colitis; risk for infection (oral or vaginal candidiasis); ineffective protection related to hypoprothrombinemia and superinfection; impaired tissue integrity (thrombophlebitis); deficient fluid volume related to nausea and vomiting; activity intolerance related to drug-induced immune hemolytic anemia; and the potential complications of hypersensitivity (fever, rash), allergic reactions (anaphylaxis, Stevens-Johnson syndrome, renal dysfunction, serum sickness–like reaction), and seizures (with high doses or renal impairment).

■ **Implementation**

■ ***Monitoring.*** Because of the possibility of superinfection, observe clients, particularly older adults and debilitated clients, for symptoms of bacterial and fungal overgrowth. Bleeding time and PT should be monitored, because hypoprothrombinemia may occur with cephalosporins, especially cefamandole, cefoperazone, or cefotetan. Many cephalosporins are excreted renally, and therefore most should be monitored by serum drug levels in clients with renal impairment. WBC counts and culture results should be monitored. Cytotoxin assays of stool samples to document the presence of *C. difficile* are needed if the client develops diarrhea.

■ ***Intervention.*** In addition to performing nursing measures common to all types of antimicrobial drug therapy (as discussed in Chapter 58), be aware of the following factors when cephalosporins are prescribed.

Most cephalosporins may be taken on a full or empty stomach. Taking them with food may help to prevent any gastrointestinal irritation. However, cefaclor extended-

TABLE 59-3 Cephalosporins: Pharmacokinetics and Usual Adult Dosage

Drug	Pharmacokinetics: Oral Absorption (%)	Pharmacokinetics: Peak Serum (hours)*	Pharmacokinetics: Renal Excretion (%/hours)†	Usual Adult Dosage
First Generation				
cefadroxil (Duricef)	95	PO: 1.5-2	93/24	500 mg q12h
cefazolin (Ancef)	—	IM: 1-2 IV: E of I	56-89/6 80-100/24	IM: 1 g presurgery IV infusion: 0.25-1.5 g q6-8h
cefmetazole (Zefazone)	—	IV: E of I	71/24	IV: 2 g q6-12h
cephalexin (Keflex)	95	PO: 1	80/6; 90/8	250-500 mg q6h
cephapirin (Cefadyl)	—	IM: 0.5-1 IV: E of I	70/6	IM/IV: 0.5-1 g q4-6h
cephradine (Velosef, Anspor)	95	PO: 1 IM: 0.8-2 IV: E of I	60-80/6	PO: 250-500 mg q6h IM/IV: 0.5-1 g q6h
Second Generation				
cefaclor (Ceclor)	95	PO: 0.5-1	60-85/8	250-500 mg q8h
cefamandole (Mandol)	—	IM: 0.5-2 IV: E of I	65-85/8	IM/IV: 500 mg q6h
cefonicid (Monocid)	—	IM: 1 IV: E of I	99/24	IM/IV: 0.5-1 g q24h
cefotetan (Cefotan)	—	IM: 1-3 IV: E of I	50-80/24	IM/IV: 1-2 g q12h
cefoxitin (Mefoxin)	—	IM: 0.3-0.5 IV: E of I	85/6	IV: 1-2 g q6-8h
cefprozil (Cefzil ◆)	95	PO: 1.5	60/8	500 mg q12h
cefuroxime (Zinacef, Ceftin ◆)	pc: 52 fasting: 37	PO: 2-3.6 IM: 0.75 IV: E of I	32-48/12	PO: 250-500 mg q12h IM/IV: 0.75-1.5 g q8h
loracarbef (Lorabid)	90	PO: 0.5-1.2	87-97	200-400 mg q12h
Third Generation				
cefdinir (Omnicef)	—	—	12-18/12	300 mg q 12h
cefixime (Suprax)	40-50	PO: 2-6	50/24	200 mg q12h
cefoperazone (Cefobid)	—	IM: 1-2 IV: E of I	20-30/12‡	IM/IV: 1-2 g q12h
cefotaxime (Claforan)	—	IM: 0.5 IV: E of I	60/6	IV infusion: 1-2 g q4-12h IM: 500 mg to 1g single dose for gonorrhea
cefpodoxime (Vantin)	50	PO: 2-3	29-33/12	200 mg q12h
ceftazidime (Fortaz)	—	IM: 1 IV: E of I	80-90/24	IM/IV: 0.5-2 g q8-12h
ceftibuten (Cedax)	—	PO: N/A	56%	400 mg daily
ceftizoxime (Cefizox)	—	IM: 1 IV: E of I	85-95/24	IV: 1-2 g q8-12h IM: 500 mg to 1 g q8-12h
ceftriaxone (Rocephin)	—	IM: 2-3 IV: E of I	33-67/24	IV: 1-2 g q24h IM: 1-2 g q24h
Fourth Generation				
cefepime (Maxipime)	—	IM: N/A IV: E of I	N/A	IM/IV: 0.5-1 g q12h

Information from *Drug Facts and Comparisons* (2000). St. Louis: Facts and Comparisons; and *United States Pharmacopeial Dispensing Information (USP DI): Drug information for the health care professional* (19th ed.). (1999). Rockville, MD: United States Pharmacopeial Convention.
E of I, End of infusion; *pc*, after meals, *N/A*, not available.
*Time to peak serum level (hours).
†Renal excretion, percent excreted unchanged/hr.
‡Majority excreted unchanged in bile.

release tablets, cefpodoxime proxetil, and cefuroxime axetil oral suspension should be taken with food. Ceftibuten oral suspension is the only cephalosporin that needs to be taken on an empty stomach, either 1 hour before or 2 hours after taking food.

IM cephalosporins should be given deeply into a large muscle mass, because they are irritating to tissues and can cause pain, induration, and sterile abscesses following injection.

The perioperative parenteral administration of cephalosporins for prophylaxis is usually discontinued 24 hours after surgery.

■ ***Education.*** Instruct the client to take the full course of medication, even though he or she may feel better and be symptom free. Stress the importance of taking evenly spaced doses to maintain therapeutic blood levels.

Clients with diabetes mellitus who are using copper sulfate urine glucose tests (Clinitest) may receive false-positive results while taking cephalosporins. Have the client use glucose-enzymatic tests such as Clinistix or Keto-diastix. The client should be cautioned not to drink alcoholic beverages or take alcohol-containing medications, because abdominal cramps, nausea, vomiting, hypotension, tachycardia, shortness of breath, sweating, and facial flushing may occur. Instruct clients to read the labels, because many cough and cold remedies contain alcohol.

■ **Evaluation.** The expected outcome of cephalosporin therapy is that the client will maintain or achieve an infection-free state as evidenced by negative cultures. If a cephalosporin is being administered therapeutically, the client will also have a body temperature within normal limits and a WBC count within the normal limits for age. The client with also experience a resolution of any other infection-related symptoms without adverse reactions to the drug.

MACROLIDE ANTIBIOTICS

The **macrolide antibiotics** are bacteriostatic because they inhibit RNA-dependent protein synthesis; they may be bactericidal in high concentrations with selected organisms. The macrolide antibiotics include azithromycin (Zithromax ◆, Zithromax Z-Pak ◆), clarithromycin (Biaxin ◆), erythromycin, dirithromycin (Dynabac), and troleandomycin (Tao). Dirithromycin is a pro-drug that is activated during intestinal absorption to erythromycylamine, an active metabolite. Erythromycin is the first macrolide and key drug for this classification.

With the exception of troleandomycin, these agents have similar antimicrobial action (against gram-positive and selected gram-negative microorganisms) and are used for respiratory, gastrointestinal tract, skin, and soft tissue infections when beta-lactam antibiotics are contraindicated (*Drug Facts and Comparisons*, 2000). Troleandomycin is the only macrolide drug indicated for the treatment of *Streptococcus pneumoniae* and *Streptococcus pyogenes*.

Significant side effects/adverse reactions include the following:

- azithromycin: stomach pain, nausea, vomiting and diarrhea; allergic reactions and acute interstitial nephritis are rare adverse reactions
- clarithromycin: anorexia, headache, nausea, vomiting, lethargy, severe anemia, fever, infection, rash, abnormal taste sensations and, rarely, *C. difficile* colitis, hepatotoxicity, hypersensitivity, and thrombocytopenia
- dirithromycin: stomach pain, headache, nausea, diarrhea, and *C. difficile* colitis
- erythromycin: abdominal cramps, diarrhea, nausea, vomiting, oral and/or vaginal candidiasis and, less commonly, hypersensitivity and hepatotoxicity
- troleandomycin: stomach cramps and discomfort, nausea, vomiting, diarrhea, skin rash, jaundice and, rarely, allergy or anaphylaxis

See Table 59-4 for the pharmacokinetics and usual adult dosages of the macrolides.

■ Nursing Management
Macrolide Antibiotic Therapy

In addition to the following discussion, see Nursing Management: Antibiotic Therapy, p. 980.

■ **Assessment.** Determine if the client has hepatic impairment, in which case erythromycin, particularly erythromycin estolate, is used with caution. Clients with a history of cardiac dysrhythmias may be at risk for a recurrence with high doses of erythromycin. Determine if the client has a sensitivity to any of the macrolides. The elimination of clarithromycin is reduced in clients with severe renal impairment.

Review the client's current medication regimen for the risk of significant drug interactions, such as those that may occur when macrolides are given concurrently with the following drugs:

Drug	Possible Effect and Management
Bold/color type indicates the most serious interactions.	
alfentanil (Alfenta)	Erythromycin may increase plasma levels and the action of alfentanil. Monitor closely if given in combination.
antacids, aluminum- and magnesium-containing antacids	The concurrent use of antacids with azithromycin decreases the peak antibiotic serum concentration. Administer azithromycin at least 1 hour before or 2 hours after antacids.
carbamazepine (Tegretol)	Carbamazepine metabolism may be inhibited by erythromycin and clarithromycin, leading to elevated serum levels and, possibly, toxicity. Monitor closely.
chloramphenicol (Chloromycetin) or lincosamides	Erythromycin may antagonize the therapeutic effects of chloramphenicol and lincomycin. Avoid concurrent administration.

Continued

TABLE 59-4 Macrolides: Pharmacokinetics and Usual Adult Dosage

	Pharmacokinetics			
Drug	**Oral Absorption (%)**	**Peak Serum (hours)***	**Renal Excretion (%/hours)†**	**Usual Adult Dosage**
azithromycin (Zithromax)	Good	2-4	4.5/72‡	500 mg first day, then 250 mg daily thereafter
clarithromycin (Biaxin)	Good	2-3	20-30/2	250-500 mg q12h
dirithromycin (Dynabac)	10	N/A	2/36‡	500 mg daily
erythromycin	30-65	2-4	2-5/—‡	PO: 250 mg q6h IV infusion: 250-500 mg q6h
troleandomycin (Tao)	N/A	2	20/2	250-500 mg 4 times daily

Information from *Drug Facts and Comparisons* (2000). St. Louis: Facts and Comparisons; and *United States Pharmacopeial Dispensing Information (USP DI): Drug information for the health care professional* (19th ed.). (1999). Rockville, MD: United States Pharmacopeial Convention.
N/A, Not available; —, unknown.
*Time to peak serum level (hours).
†Renal excretion, percent excreted unchanged/hr; balance excreted in feces/bile.
‡Primarily excreted unchanged in bile.

Drug	Possible Effect and Management
cyclosporine (Sandimmune)	Concurrent administration with erythromycin may increase cyclosporine serum levels and increase the risk for nephrotoxicity. Monitor closely if given concurrently.
digoxin (Lanoxin)	Concurrent use with clarithromycin increases the serum concentrations of digoxin. Monitor digoxin serum levels carefully.
hepatotoxic medications	There is an increased possibility for liver toxicity with erythromycin administration; monitor liver function studies closely if given concurrently.
rifabutin (Mycobutin), rifampin (Rifadin)	Concurrent use of clarithromycin with these drugs decreases the antibiotic serum level by more than 50%. Dosage adjustments may be necessary.
terfenadine* (Seldane), astemizole (Hismanal)	**Concurrent drug administrations with either erythromycin or clarithromycin may increase the risk of cardiotoxicity. Avoid concurrent use or a potentially serious drug interaction may occur.**
warfarin (Coumadin)	Concurrent use of erythromycin or clarithromycin may result in decreased warfarin metabolism and excretion, leading to an increased risk of bleeding or hemorrhage. Dosage adjustments of coumarin may be necessary during and after treatment with erythromycin. Monitor PT closely.
xanthines, such as aminophylline, caffeine, oxtriphylline, and theophylline (exception, dyphylline)	An increase in theophylline levels and/or toxicity is reported with this combination of drugs. This effect is usually seen at approximately the sixth day of erythromycin therapy, because it appears to be related to the peak serum levels of erythromycin. Monitor the serum levels of xanthines closely, because dosage adjustments of xanthines may be necessary during and after erythromycin therapy.
zidovudine (AZT)	Concurrent administration with clarithromycin may result in delayed time to peak zidovudine concentrations. Administer the doses of these two drugs at least 4 hours apart.

*No longer available in the United States but may be available in other countries.

A baseline assessment as described in Chapter 58 should be obtained before initiating macrolide antibiotic therapy.

■ **Nursing Diagnosis.** The client receiving erythromycin, azithromycin, or clarithromycin may experience the following nursing diagnoses/collaborative problems: diarrhea; impaired tissue integrity related to inflammation or phlebitis at the injection site; deficient fluid volume related to nausea and vomiting; impaired comfort (abdominal cramping); disturbed sensory perception related to hearing loss (erythromycin only); ineffective protection related to the loss of normal flora and the development of *Candida albicans* (sore mouth or tongue, vaginal itching and discharge); and the potential complications of hypersensitivity, hepatotoxicity (dark urine, pale stools, tiredness, and yellowing of the sclera and skin), acute interstitial nephritis (azithromycin only), thrombocytopenia (clarithromycin only), pancreatitis (erythromycin only), and cardiotoxicity (dysrhythmia, bradycardia, fainting, sudden death). With dirithromycin, impaired comfort (abdominal discomfort, nausea, vomiting, mild diarrhea) or the potential complication of *C. difficile* may be a problem.

■ **Implementation**

■ ***Monitoring.*** Periodic hepatic function studies and an electrocardiogram (ECG) may be required for clients who are receiving high-dose or prolonged erythromycin therapy. Temperature, WBC counts, cultures, and a focal examination of the infection should be performed.

■ ***Intervention.*** Macrolide antibiotics should be administered with a full glass of water on an empty stomach (1 hour before or 2 hours after meals) to obtain the maximum effect. Erythromycin enteric-coated tablets, delayed-release capsules, and estolate and ethylsuccinate preparations may be taken with meals and may be used with clients who have a gastrointestinal intolerance to other forms of oral erythromycin. Azithromycin (for adults) and clarithromycin may be taken with or without food. When administering oral suspensions, ensure that they have been refrigerated and shaken well and that the calibrated liquid-measuring device is used for accurate dosing.

Continuous infusion is preferable to intermittent infusion for the macrolide antibiotics. If intermittent infusion is considered, azithromycin should be administered over 1 to 3 hours and erythromycin over 20 to 60 minutes depending on the strength.

■ ***Education.*** The importance of complying with a full course of therapy, even though the client feels better or is symptom free, should be stressed. This course of therapy should continue at least 10 days in group A beta-hemolytic streptococcal infections to prevent the occurrence of acute rheumatic fever.

With most medications, a missed dose is omitted if it is almost time for the next dose. With erythromycin, however, the missed dose is to be taken as soon as possible. If it is almost time for the next dose of erythromycin and the dosing schedule is 2 doses daily, space the missed dose and the next dose 5 to 6 hours apart. If the dosing schedule is 3 doses daily, space the missed dose 2 to 4 hours apart or double the next dose.

The decreased frequency of dosing and fewer adverse gastrointestinal effects experience with the newer, longer-acting macrolide antibiotics (e.g., azithromycin, clarithromycin, and dirithromycin) may offset their higher prices and increase client adherence.

■ **Evaluation.** The expected outcome of macrolide antibiotic therapy is that the client will maintain or achieve an infection-free state as demonstrated by negative cultures. If administered therapeutically, the client will also demonstrate a body temperature within normal limits, a WBC count within the normal limits for age, and the resolution of any other infection-related symptoms without experiencing adverse reactions to the drug.

LINCOSAMIDES

clindamycin [klin da mye′ sin] (Cleocin, Dalacin C ✤)
lincomycin [lin koe mye′ sin] (Lincocin)

Lincomycin inhibits protein synthesis by binding to bacterial ribosomes and preventing peptide bond formation. It is primarily bacteriostatic but may be bactericidal in high doses with selected organisms. At one time it was used to treat serious streptococci, pneumococci, and staphylococci infections but has since been replaced by safer and more effective antibiotics.

Clindamycin, a semisynthetic derivative of lincomycin, has a mechanism of action similar to lincomycin but is more effective. It is indicated for the treatment of bone and joint infections, pelvic (female) and intraabdominal infections, bacterial septicemia, pneumonia, and skin and soft tissue infections caused by susceptible bacteria.

Oral clindamycin is well absorbed and should be administered with food or with a full glass (8 ounces) of water. It is rapidly distributed to most body fluids and tissues, with the exception of cerebrospinal fluid; the highest concentrations are noted in bone, bile, and urine. The half-life of clindamycin in adults is 2 to 3 hours. It reaches peak blood levels within 45 minutes to 1 hour after oral administration, 1 hour in children (IM), 3 hours in adults by IM injection, and by the end of the infusion with IV injection. It is metabolized in the liver and excreted primarily by the kidneys.

The most significant adverse and limiting effect for both clindamycin and lincomycin is AAPMC (see Box 59-1).

The usual adult dosage of clindamycin is 150 to 300 mg PO, IM, or IV every 6 hours. For infants 1 month of age and older, the oral dosage is 2 to 5 mg/kg body weight every 6 hours.

■ Nursing Management

Lincomycin and Clindamycin Therapy

In addition to the following discussion, see Nursing Management: Antibiotic Therapy, p. 980.

■ **Assessment.** Determine if the client has a history of gastrointestinal disease, particularly ulcerative colitis or regional enteritis, because pseudomembranous colitis may occur with therapy. Severe hepatic or renal function impairment will require a dosage reduction. Ascertain the client's sensitivity to lincomycins or doxorubicin.

Review the client's current medication regimen for the risk significant drug interactions, such as those that may occur when lincosamides are administered with the following drugs:

Drug	Possible Effect and Management
Bold/color type indicates the most serious interactions.	
anesthetics, such as chloroform cyclopropane, enflurane (Ethrane), halothane (Fluothane), isoflurane (Forane), methoxyflurane (Penthrane), trichloroethylene, or the neuromuscular blocking agents	**May result in enhanced neuromuscular blockade, skeletal muscle weakness, respiratory depression, or paralysis if this combination is used during or immediately after surgery. Avoid concurrent use or a potentially serious drug interaction may occur.**
antidiarrheals, adsorbent type (kaolins, attapulgite)	Decreases the absorption of oral lincomycins. Avoid concurrent use, or advise the client to take the antidiarrheal 2 hours before or 3 to 4 hours after the oral lincomycins.

Continued

Drug	Possible Effect and Management
antidiarrheals, antiperistaltic	May prolong pseudomembranous colitis by delaying toxin elimination.
chloramphenicol (Chloromycetin) or erythromycins	May antagonize the therapeutic effect of lincomycins. Avoid concurrent administration.

A baseline assessment as described in Chapter 58 should be performed before initiating lincomycin therapy. A cytotoxin assay of stool may be performed for the presence of *C. difficile*.

■ **Nursing Diagnosis.** The client receiving therapy with lincomycins should be assessed for the following nursing diagnoses/collaborative problems: diarrhea related to the development of AAPMC; deficient fluid volume related to nausea and vomiting; ineffective protection related to neutropenia (infection), thrombocytopenia (bleeding), and loss of normal flora (superinfection); and the potential complication of hypersensitivity.

■ **Implementation**

■ ***Monitoring.*** During therapy, observe the client for abdominal cramps, diarrhea, weight loss, or weakness, which might be indications of pseudomembranous colitis. In addition, monitor the client's temperature, WBC counts, cultures, and cytotoxin assays of stool samples. Perform a focal assessment related to the underlying infection.

■ ***Intervention.*** Administer clindamycin capsules with a full glass of water or with meals to prevent esophageal ulceration. To obtain optimum serum levels, lincomycin is taken on an empty stomach with a full glass of water (240 mL).

■ ***Education.*** Stress the importance of complying with a full course of the medication, even though the client feels well and is symptom free. Ten days is considered a minimal course of therapy for streptococcal infections. Instruct the client to take the medication at evenly spaced times to ensure that serum levels are maintained. Alert the client to adverse drug reactions and to report them to the prescriber.

■ **Evaluation.** The expected outcome of lincosamide therapy is that the client will maintain or achieve an infection-free state as evidenced by negative cultures. If administered therapeutically, the client will also demonstrate a body temperature within normal limits, a WBC count within the normal limits for age, and the resolution of any other infection-related symptoms without experiencing adverse reactions to the drug.

vancomycin [van koe mye' sin] (Vancocin)

Vancomycin inhibits bacterial cell walls by binding to a cell wall precursor, a mechanism that differs from penicillin or cephalosporins. This action leads to cell lysis, so it is bactericidal for many organisms. Vancomycin may also inhibit RNA synthesis. Oral vancomycin is indicated for the treatment of AAMPC (*C. difficile*) and the treatment of staphylococcal enterocolitis. Parenteral vancomycin is not recommended for use in AAPMC but is indicated for bone and joint infections, bacterial septicemia caused by *Staphylococcus* species, and for the prevention and treatment of bacterial endocarditis caused by staphylococcus, including methicillin-resistant strains.

The absorption of vancomycin from the intestinal tract is poor. It is excreted mainly in the feces. Parenteral vancomycin has a half-life of 6 hours in adults and approximately 2 to 3 hours in children. It is primarily excreted by the kidneys.

The significant side effects for oral doses include nausea, vomiting, and taste alterations. Less often or rarely, parenteral adverse reactions include ototoxicity and nephrotoxicity. The "red-neck syndrome" is reported after bolus or too-rapid drug injection, which results in histamine release and chills, fever, tachycardia, pruritus, rash, or a red face, neck, upper body, back, and arms (*United States Pharmacopeia Dispensing Information,* 1999).

The oral adult dosage of vancomycin for the treatment of *C. difficile* colitis or diarrhea is 125 to 500 mg every 6 hours for 7 to 10 days, repeated if necessary. In children, the dosage is 10 mg/kg (up to 125 mg) every 6 hours for 7 to 10 days, repeated if necessary. With IV infusion the adult dosage is 7.5 mg/kg every 6 hours. For IV dosing in children, refer to the package insert or a current reference.

■ Nursing Management

Vancomycin Therapy

In addition to the following discussion, see Nursing Management: Antibiotic Therapy, p. 980.

■ **Assessment.** Assess the client for hearing loss, because vancomycin has ototoxic properties. Clients with impaired renal function require reduced dosages. Ascertain if the client has a sensitivity to vancomycin.

Review the client's current medication regimen for the risk of significant interactions, such as those that may occur when vancomycin is given concurrently with the following drugs:

Drug	Possible Effect and Management
Bold/color type indicates the most serious interactions.	
aminoglycosides, amphotericin B parenteral (Fungizone), aspirin, bacitracin, parenteral bumetanide (Bumex), capreomycin (Capastat), cisplatin (Platinol), cyclosporine (Sandimmune), ethacrynate sodium parenteral (Edecrin), furosemide parenteral (Lasix), paromomycin (Humatin), polymyxins, or streptozocin (Zanosar)	**Increases the potential for ototoxicity and/or nephrotoxicity. In clients with pseudomembranous colitis or severe kidney impairment, the serum levels of vancomycin may be increased, thus leading to an increased potential for toxicity. Monitor serum levels closely. Avoid concurrent use or a potentially serious drug interaction may occur.**
cholestyramine (Questran) or Colestipol (Colestid)	**When given concurrently with the oral dosage form, a reduction in vancomycin antibacterial activity is reported. Avoid this combination if possible. If not, give oral vancomycin several hours apart from other medications.**

Drug	Possible Effect and Management
dexamethasone	May impair the penetration of vancomycin into the cerebrospinal fluid. If used as an adjunctive medication in bacterial meningitis, administer before the first dose of vancomycin.

In addition to the baseline assessment described in Chapter 58, a stool cytotoxin assay for the presence of *C. difficile* may be required before initiating vancomycin therapy.

■ **Nursing Diagnosis.** Clients receiving vancomycin therapy should be assessed for the following nursing diagnoses/collaborative problems: risk for injury related to histamine release common with bolus or rapid injection (chills, fever, tachycardia, flushing of the face and/or upper body, syncope, tingling, unpleasant taste); deficient fluid volume related to nausea and vomiting; ineffective protection related to neutropenia or thrombocytopenia; impaired tissue integrity related to extravasation; disturbed sensory perception related to ototoxicity (loss of hearing and tinnitus); and the potential complications of pseudomembranous colitis and nephrotoxicity (blood in urine, greatly increased or decreased frequency of urination and amount of urine).

■ **Implementation**

■ ***Monitoring.*** Because oral vancomycin is so poorly absorbed and used only for the treatment of *C. difficile*, the following discussion refers to the IV form of the drug. Renal function studies may be needed before and periodically during high-dose or prolonged therapy. Urinalyses should be monitored for the presence of albumin, casts, and cells in the urine, and for decreased specific gravity. Serum concentrations of vancomycin may need to be determined in clients with renal impairment or in clients over 60 years of age; peak concentrations should not exceed 40 μg/mL (trough, 10 μg/mL). Older adults excrete vancomycin more slowly and therefore should be assessed for hearing loss over the course of therapy. The IV site should be monitored for extravasation.

■ ***Intervention.*** Administer the oral liquid using the calibrated liquid-measuring device provided by the manufacturer. If the IV form is used for oral administration, each vial should be dissolved in 30 mL of water or juice. It may be administered straight or through a nasogastric tube to minimize the unpleasant taste.

Parenteral vancomycin is to be administered only intravenously because it is so irritating to the tissues. Care must be taken to avoid extravasation. To avoid side effects such as hypotension, thrombophlebitis, and "red-neck syndrome," do not administer this drug as a bolus injection. Vancomycin may be administered intermittently in at least 100 mL of 0.9% sodium chloride injection or 5% dextrose injection over 60 minutes. If intermittent IV administration is not feasible, vancomycin may be given by continuous IV infusion, 1 to 2 g in sufficient 5% dextrose injection or 0.9% sodium chloride to run over 24 hours. Rotation of the venous sites will help to prevent local irritation. Vancomycin is also incompatible with alkaline solutions, heavy metals, and a wide variety of substances. Consult the package insert before combining with other drugs, or administer it alone.

■ ***Education.*** Alert the client to possible side effects or adverse reactions, and instruct him or her to consult with the prescriber should they occur. Instruct the client to take the medication as prescribed and for the full course.

■ **Evaluation.** The expected outcome of vancomycin therapy is that the client will maintain or achieve an infection-free state as evidenced by negative culture results. If administered therapeutically, the client will also demonstrate a body temperature within normal limits, a WBC count within the normal limits, and the resolution of other infection-related symptoms without adverse reactions.

linezolid [lin i zole' id] (Zyvox)

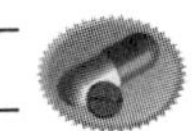

Linezolid (Zyvox) is an antibiotic indicated for vancomycin-resistant *Enterococcus* infections, nosocomial pneumonia, community-acquired pneumonia, and complicated and uncomplicated skin infections. It may cause pseudomembranous colitis and thrombocytopenia.

AMINOGLYCOSIDES

Aminoglycosides are potent bactericidal antibiotics that are usually reserved for serious or life-threatening infections. They are very effective against many bacteria (gram-positive and gram-negative) but are generally reserved for gram-negative infections. Safer and less toxic agents are available to treat the majority of gram-positive infections. Currently available aminoglycosides include the following:

amikacin [am ih kay' sin] (Amikin)
✔ **gentamicin** [jen ta mye' sin] (Garamycin)
kanamycin [kan ah mye' sin] (Kantrex)
netilmicin [ne til mye' sin] (Netromycin)
streptomycin [strep toe mye' sin]
tobramycin [toe bra mye' sin] (Nebcin)

The mechanism of action for aminoglycosides is to irreversibly bind ribosomes of the susceptible bacteria, thus inhibiting protein synthesis (interferes with the complex between messenger RNA and the bacteria ribosomes) and leading to eventual cell death (bactericidal). The aminoglycosides are indicated for the treatment of serious or life-threatening infections when other agents are ineffective or contraindicated. They are used with penicillins, cephalosporins, or vancomycin for their synergistic effects and are especially useful for the treatment of gram-negative infections such as those caused by *Pseudomonas* species, *E. coli*, *Proteus* species, *Klebsiella* species, *Serratia* species, and others.

Aminoglycosides are poorly absorbed from an intact intestinal tract but are rapidly absorbed intramuscularly. Local topical application or irrigation may lead to absorption from most areas of the body, with the exception of the bladder.

Therapeutic aminoglycoside serum levels (μg/mL) are as follows:

- amikacin: 15-25
- gentamicin: 4-10

- kanamycin: 15-30
- tobramycin: 4-10

Significant side effects/adverse reactions of the aminoglycosides include nephrotoxicity, neurotoxicity, ototoxicity (auditory and vestibular), and hypersensitivity.

The usual adult dosage of amikacin is 5 mg/kg IM, IV every 8 hours; for gentamicin, 1 to 1.7 mg/kg IM or by IV infusion every 8 hours; for kanamycin, 3.75 mg/kg IM every 6 hours; for netilmicin, 1.3 to 2.2 mg/kg IM, IV every 8 hours; for streptomycin (tuberculosis adult dosage), 1 g IM daily given in combination with other antimycobacterials; and for tobramycin, 0.75 mg to 1.25 mg/kg IM or IV infusion every 6 hours. For additional dosing recommendations, refer to a current package insert or reference.

■ Nursing Management

Aminoglycoside Therapy

In addition to the following discussion, see Nursing Management: Antibiotic Therapy, p. 980.

■ **Assessment.** Infants with botulism and clients with myasthenia gravis and parkinsonism may experience greater muscle weakness because of neuromuscular blockade with the aminoglycosides. Auditory and vestibular toxicity might occur in clients with impairment of the eighth cranial nerve. Renal function impairment increases the risk of toxicity. A previous history of an allergic response to one aminoglycoside would contraindicate the use of another because of cross-sensitivity.

Review the client's current medication regimen for the risk of significant drug interactions, such as those that may occur when aminoglycosides are given concurrently with the following drugs:

Drug	Possible Effect and Management
Bold/color type indicates the most serious interactions.	
other aminoglycosides (two or more concurrently) or capreomycin (Capastat)	Potential for ototoxicity, nephrotoxicity, and neuromuscular blockade is enhanced. Hearing loss may progress to deafness even after the drug is stopped. In some cases, hearing loss may be reversed. Avoid concurrent use or a potentially serious drug interaction may occur.
anesthetics (halogenated hydrocarbon) or citrate-anticoagulated blood by massive transfusions or neuromuscular blocking agents	May increase neuromuscular blockade. Avoid concurrent use or a potentially serious drug interaction may occur.
methoxyflurane (Penthrane) or polymyxins, parenteral	Increased possibility for nephrotoxicity and/or neuromuscular blockade. Avoid concurrent use or a potentially serious drug interaction may occur.
nephrotoxic drugs, other ototoxic drugs such as amphotericin B parenteral (Fungizone), aspirin, bacitracin parenteral, bumetanide parenteral (Bumex), cisplatin (Platinol), cyclosporine (Sandimmune), ethacrynate sodium parenteral (Edecrin), furosemide parenteral (Lasix), paromomycin (Humatin), streptozocin (Zanosar), or vancomycin (Vancocin)	Increased potential for ototoxicity and/or nephrotoxicity. Hearing loss may be permanent. If drugs are given concurrently, serial audiometric hearing determinations are suggested. Vancomycin and aminoglycosides may be ordered to prevent bacterial endocarditis or to treat specific infections (e.g., carditis caused by organisms such as streptococci and corynebacteria). Frequent determinations of drug serum levels and renal function are recommended in such instances, because dosage adjustments or other interventions may be necessary.

A baseline assessment as described in Chapter 58 should be performed before initiating aminoglycoside therapy. In addition, a urinalysis, audiogram, and renal and vestibular function determination should occur before the start of therapy. Before prolonged therapy with streptomycin, caloric stimulation tests are used to detect a baseline by which to measure the occurrence of vestibular toxicity.

■ **Nursing Diagnosis.** Clients receiving aminoglycoside therapy should be assessed for the following nursing diagnoses/collaborative problems: disturbed sensory perception related to auditory ototoxicity (loss of hearing and tinnitus), vestibular ototoxicity (dizziness and loss of balance) and, for streptomycin only, peripheral neuritis (tingling of the fingers and toes, facial burning); and the potential complications of hypersensitivity, nephrotoxicity (blood in urine, greatly increased or decreased frequency of urination and amount of urine), neurotoxicity (muscle twitching, numbness, or seizures), or neuromuscular blockade (weakness, difficulty breathing).

■ **Implementation**

■ ***Monitoring.*** Older adults are at greater risk of nephrotoxicity and ototoxicity because of reduced renal function, and they generally require smaller daily doses. However, a loss of hearing may occur in clients with normal renal function. Audiograms, renal function studies, and vestibular function studies should be performed periodically during high-dose therapy or therapy that lasts more than 10 days. Urinalyses should be monitored for the presence of albumin, casts, and cells, as well as for decreased specific gravity.

Monitor peak and trough drug levels routinely, because evidence suggests that the incidence of ototoxicity and nephrotoxicity with aminoglycosides correlates with slight elevations of either drug level but particularly with trough levels. The trough concentration is believed to be a more sensitive indicator of renal function than serum creatinine levels. Peak levels are drawn 30 minutes after a 30-minute infusion, and trough levels are drawn immediately before the next dose.

With streptomycin only, caloric stimulation tests may be required during and after prolonged therapy to detect vestibular toxicity.

■ ***Intervention.*** For IV administration, dilute appropriately and administer slowly over a 30- to 60-minute period to prevent neuromuscular blockade as the result of toxic serum levels. Clients should be well hydrated while taking these medications to minimize chemical irritation of the urinary tubules. Intake and output should be monitored. A

TABLE 59-5 Tetracycline: Half-life and Usual Adult Dosage

Drug	Half-life* Normal	Half-life* Anuric	Usual Adult Dosage
demeclocycline (Declomycin)	10-17	40-60	150 mg q6h
doxycycline (Vibramycin)	12-22	12-22	100 mg 2 times daily on first day, then 100 to 200 mg daily (PO or IV infusion)
minocycline (Minocin)	11-23	11-23	200 mg initially, then 100 mg q12h (PO or IV infusion)
oxytetracycline (Terramycin)	6-10	47-66	250-500 mg PO q6h, or 250-500 mg q12h by IV infusion
tetracycline	6-11	57-108	250-500 mg PO q6h, or 150 mg IM q12h

Information from *United States Pharmacopeial Dispensing Information (USP DI): Drug information for the health care professional* (19th ed.). (1999). Rockville, MD: United States Pharmacopeial Convention.
*Half-life in hours.

daily urinalysis may be required during therapy for signs of renal irritation.

Inject the IM dosage forms of these drugs deeply into the upper outer quadrant of the gluteal muscle.

■ ***Education.*** Instruct the client to report any loss of hearing or any ringing or buzzing in the ears, which indicates ototoxicity; any change in urinary pattern or blood in the urine, which indicates nephrotoxicity; dizziness, which indicates vestibular toxicity; or numbness, tingling, or twitching, which indicates neurotoxicity. Stress the importance of taking the full course of medication as prescribed.

■ **Evaluation.** The expected outcome of aminoglycoside therapy is that the client will maintain or achieve an infection-free state as evidenced by negative cultures. If administered therapeutically, the client will also demonstrate a body temperature within normal limits, a WBC count within the normal limits for age, and the resolution of any other infection-related symptoms without experiencing adverse reactions to the drug.

TETRACYCLINES

Tetracyclines were the first broad-spectrum antibiotics released in the United States. They include a large group of drugs that have a common basic structure and similar chemical activity.

demeclocycline [de me kloe sye′ kleen] (Declomycin)
doxycycline [dox i sye′ kleen] (Doxychel, Vibramycin)
minocycline [mi noe sye′ kleen] (Minocin)
oxytetracycline [ox i tet ra sye′ kleen] (Terramycin)
tetracycline [tet ra sye′ kleen] (Achromycin V, Novotetra ♣)

Tetracyclines are bacteriostatic for many gram-negative and gram-positive organisms; they exhibit cross-sensitivity and cross-resistance. Tetracyclines inhibit protein synthesis by blocking the binding of transfer RNA to the messenger RNA ribosome. Demeclocycline is also used to treat the syndrome of inappropriate diuretic hormone; it inhibits antidiuretic hormone (ADH)–induced water reabsorption in the kidneys, resulting in diuresis.

The tetracyclines are commonly used to treat many infections such as acne vulgaris, actinomycosis, anthrax, bacterial urinary tract infections, bronchitis, rickettsial infection (Rocky Mountain spotted fever, typhus, Q fever), Lyme disease, and numerous systemic bacterial infections sensitive to the tetracyclines (Smilack, 1999).

Oral tetracyclines are fairly well absorbed and distributed to most body fluids. Cerebrospinal fluid levels vary and can range from 10% to 25% of the plasma drug concentration following parenteral administration. Tetracyclines localize in the teeth, liver, spleen, tumors, and bone. Doxycycline can reach clinical concentrations in the eye and prostate, and minocycline results in high levels in saliva, sputum, and tears. Doxycycline and minocycline are inactivated in the liver, but most tetracyclines are excreted by the kidneys. Table 59-5 lists the half-life and usual adult dosages for the tetracyclines.

■ Nursing Management

Tetracycline Therapy

In addition the information provided in Nursing Management: Antibiotic Therapy, p. 980, observe the following measures with clients who are receiving drugs of the tetracycline family.

■ **Assessment.** Tetracyclines are contraindicated in pregnant women, breastfeeding women, and children under 8 years of age because they cause permanent mottling and discoloration of the teeth and decrease the linear skeletal growth rate in fetuses or children.

Clients who are hypersensitive to one tetracycline may also be hypersensitive to the others. In addition, clients with hypersensitivities to "caine-type" drugs, such as lidocaine or procaine, may be intolerant of the lidocaine in an oxytetracycline injection or to the procaine in a tetracycline IM injection.

With the exception of doxycycline and minocycline, the use of tetracyclines in clients with renal impairment is not recommended. Nephrogenic diabetes insipidus may worsen with the administration of demeclocycline.

Review the client's current medication regimen for the risk of significant drug interactions, such as those that may occur when tetracyclines are given concurrently with the following drugs:

Drug	Possible Effect and Management
antacids, calcium supplements, choline and magnesium salicylates, iron supplements, magnesium salicylate or magnesium laxatives, foods containing milk and milk products	May result in a nonabsorbable complex, thus reducing the absorption and serum levels of the antibiotic. Antacids may also increase gastric pH, which decreases the absorption of tetracyclines. If given concurrently, advise clients to separate medications by 1 to 3 hours from the oral tetracyclines.
colestipol (Colestid), cholestyramine (Questran)	May bind oral tetracyclines, thus decreasing their absorption. Separate drugs by at least 2 hours.
estrogen-containing oral contraceptives	Concurrent long-term therapy may reduce the effectiveness of contraceptives and may also result in breakthrough bleeding.

A baseline assessment as described in Chapter 58 should be performed before initiating tetracycline therapy.

■ **Nursing Diagnosis.** Clients receiving tetracycline therapy should be assessed for the following nursing diagnoses/collaborative problems: impaired comfort (heartburn and abdominal cramping); deficient fluid volume related to anorexia, nausea, and vomiting; diarrhea; ineffective protection related to the loss of normal flora (fungal overgrowth); and the potential complications of hypersensitivity, increased sensitivity of the skin to sunlight, central nervous system (CNS) toxicity (dizziness, syncope), nephrogenic diabetes insipidus, hepatotoxicity, and pancreatitis.

■ **Implementation**

■ ***Monitoring.*** Monitor the client's temperature, WBC count, cultures, and symptoms of the infection. Because the risk for superinfection is greater with tetracycline therapy than with other antimicrobial agents, observe clients carefully for signs and symptoms of secondary infections, especially *Candida* infections. Meticulous oral and perineal hygiene is helpful in preventing a *Candida* superinfection.

■ ***Intervention.*** Tetracyclines should be taken with a full glass of water to prevent esophageal erosion and gastrointestinal irritation. With the exception of doxycycline and minocycline, the tetracyclines should be taken on an empty stomach (1 hour before or 2 hours after meals) for maximum effectiveness. Administer the oral suspension using the calibrated liquid-measuring device provided by the manufacturer.

Doxycycline may be administered intravenously (not intramuscularly or subcutaneously) in concentrations not less than 100 μg/mL or greater than 1 mg/mL over a period of 1 to 4 hours. With IV oxytetracycline, dilute in at least 100 mL of the appropriate IV solution and avoid rapid administration; do not give the IV preparation intramuscularly or subcutaneously. Avoid the rapid administration of IV minocycline. Tetracycline may be administered intramuscularly but not intravenously or subcutaneously; the amount should not exceed 2 mL in each site. With IM preparations of oxytetracycline and tetracycline, serum levels are lower than with oral administration; the client should be switched to oral forms of the drugs as soon as possible.

■ ***Education.*** Stress the importance of taking the full course of the medication in evenly spaced doses to maintain serum levels. Photosensitivity may occur and persist for some time after discontinuing the drug. Instruct the client to avoid direct sunlight and ultraviolet light. If exposure is unavoidable, a sunscreen may help to prevent a reaction. Alert the client to the appropriate dosing schedule in relation to food and to drug-drug and drug-food interactions. Instruct the client to discard outdated tetracyclines (show the client where the expiration date is found), because they become toxic as they decompose.

■ **Evaluation.** The expected outcome of tetracycline therapy is that the client will maintain or achieve an infection-free state as evidenced by negative culture results. If administered therapeutically, the client will also demonstrate a body temperature within normal limits, a WBC count within the normal limits for age, and the resolution of any other infection-related symptoms without experiencing adverse reactions to the drug.

CHLORAMPHENICOL (CHLOROMYCETIN)

Chloramphenicol, a broad-spectrum antibiotic, is a potent inhibitor of protein synthesis. It is a bacteriostatic agent for a wide variety of gram-negative and gram-positive organisms. However, its approved indications are limited because it is potentially seriously toxic to bone marrow (aplasia leading to aplastic anemia and possibly death).

Although chloramphenicol is usually bacteriostatic, it may be bactericidal in high doses with highly susceptible organisms. It penetrates bacteria cell membranes and reversibly prevents peptide bond formation, thus inhibiting protein synthesis.

Chloramphenicol is indicated for the treatment of meningitis (*Haemophilus influenzae*, *S. pneumoniae*, and *Neisseria meningitidis*), paratyphoid fever, Q fever, Rocky Mountain spotted fever, typhoid fever (*Salmonella typhi*), typhus infections, brain abscesses, and bacterial septicemia.

Chloramphenicol has good oral and parenteral bioavailability, with highest concentrations reported in the liver and kidneys. Concentrations of up to 50% of serum levels have been noted in cerebrospinal fluid. Chloramphenicol is metabolized in the liver to glucuronide (an inactive metabolite). The immature liver of fetuses and neonates cannot conjugate chloramphenicol, which may result in toxic levels or an accumulation of the active drug ("gray syndrome"—blue-gray skin, hypothermia, irregular breathing, coma, cardiovascular collapse).

The half-life of chloramphenicol in an adult is 1.5 to 3.5 hours. In infants 1 to 2 days old, the half-life is 1 to 2 days or more; in infants 10 to 16 days old, the half-life is 10 hours. Peak serum levels are reached in 1 to 1.5 hours via the IV route or in 1 to 3 hours after an oral dose. Chloramphenicol is excreted mainly by the kidneys.

The uncommon side effects of chloramphenicol include diarrhea, nausea, or vomiting. Serious adverse reactions include blood dyscrasias, optic neuritis and, possibly, irreversible bone marrow depression that may result in aplastic anemia.

The oral dosage forms of chloramphenicol were withdrawn from the U.S. market in 1998. The IV adult dosage is 12.5 mg/kg every 6 hours. The pediatric IV dosage for premature and full-term infants up to 2 weeks old is 6.25 mg/kg every 6 hours. The dosage for infants 2 weeks old and older is 12.5 mg/kg every 6 hours. Chloramphenicol is not recommended for use during pregnancy or breastfeeding.

■ Nursing Management

Chloramphenicol Therapy

In addition to the following discussion, see Nursing Management: Antibiotic Therapy, p. 980.

■ **Assessment.** Consider carefully before using chloramphenicol in clients with bone marrow depression or in clients who have had previous cytotoxic drug or radiation therapy, because this drug may cause a dose-related bone marrow depression, aplastic anemia, and other blood dyscrasias. Complete blood counts (CBCs) are necessary for a baseline assessment before therapy. Clients with hepatic and renal function impairment require a dosage reduction. Chloramphenicol is a contraindication if the client has had a previous allergic or toxic response to the drug.

Review the client's current medication regimen for the risk of significant drug interactions, such as those that may occur when chloramphenicol is given concurrently with the following drugs:

Drug	Possible Effect and Management
alfentanil (Alfenta)	May result in increased alfentanil blood levels, prolonging its effect. Monitor closely.
anticonvulsants (hydantoins), blood dyscrasia–causing drugs, bone marrow depressants, radiation therapy	May result in enhanced bone marrow depressant effects. A dosage reduction may be necessary. Monitor CBCs closely for leukopenia.
clindamycin, erythromycin, or lincomycin	The therapeutic action of chloramphenicol and these drugs may be antagonized. Avoid this drug combination.
hypoglycemic oral agents	May inhibit the metabolism of antidiabetic drugs, resulting in increased serum levels and hypoglycemic effects of tolbutamide and chlorpropamide. Monitor blood glucose levels closely, because a dosage adjustment may be necessary.
phenobarbital (Luminal), phenytoin (Dilantin), or warfarin (Coumadin)	Concurrent drug administration may result in elevated drug serum levels and toxicity of these agents. Monitor all drugs metabolized by the liver enzyme system (chloramphenicol inhibits the cytochrome P-450 system), because toxicity may result.

A baseline assessment as described in Chapter 58 should be performed before initiating chloramphenicol therapy.

■ **Nursing Diagnosis.** Clients receiving chloramphenicol therapy should be assessed for the following nursing diagnoses: deficient fluid volume related to anorexia, nausea, and vomiting; ineffective protection related to dose-related bone marrow depression (leukopenia, thrombocytopenia, anemia); diarrhea; disturbed thought processes (confusion, delirium) related to neurotoxic reactions; disturbed sensory perception related to optic neuritis (blurred vision, loss of vision, eye pain) and peripheral neuritis (tingling, numbness, and burning pain of the hands and feet); and the potential complications of hypersensitivity (rash, fever, dyspnea) and "gray syndrome" in neonates only.

■ **Implementation**

■ ***Monitoring.*** Monitor periodic CBCs for dose-related, reversible bone marrow depression, reticulocytopenia, leukopenia, thrombocytopenia, and decreased red blood cells. Observe the client for pale skin, sore throat and fever, unusual bruising or bleeding, or unusual fatigue. CBCs are not helpful in predicting drug-related aplastic anemia, which usually occurs after the completion of treatment.

Monitor serum chloramphenicol levels, which should be in the range of 10 to 25 μg/mL (the most effective concentration). Concentrations higher than 30 μg/mL increase the risk for bone marrow depression and gray syndrome.

■ ***Intervention.*** Chloramphenicol that is administered intravenously should be infused over at least a 1-minute period. Check the IV site daily for local irritation. If chloramphenicol is administered intramuscularly, inject it deeply.

■ ***Education.*** Because the bone marrow depressant effects of chloramphenicol may increase gingival bleeding and delay healing, instruct the client to delay dental work until blood counts return to normal. Instruct all clients in proper oral hygiene and the cautious use of toothbrushes, dental floss, and toothpicks.

Advise the client to report to the prescriber immediately any symptoms of blood dyscrasia, such as sore throat, fever, extreme fatigue, or unusual bleeding or bruising. Alert clients to report activity intolerance and other signs of anemia that may occur weeks or months after therapy, because they are indicative of drug-related aplastic anemia.

Caution clients who test their urine with copper sulfate glucose tests (Clinitest tablets) that they may get false-positive results. Recommend the use of Clinistix or Keto-diastix during the course of antibiotic therapy.

■ **Evaluation.** The expected outcome of chloramphenicol therapy is that the client will maintain or achieve an infection free-state as evidenced by negative cultures. If administered therapeutically, the client will also demonstrate a body temperature within normal limits, a WBC count within the normal limits for age, and the resolution of any other infection-related symptoms without experiencing adverse reactions to the drug.

FLUOROQUINOLONES

Fluoroquinolones are synthetic, broad-spectrum agents with bactericidal activity. They alter DNA by interfering with the DNA gyrase, an enzyme necessary for duplication, transcription and repair of bacterial DNA. Examples of quinolones include the following:

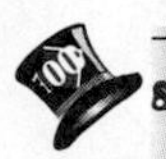

ciprofloxacin [sip ro flocks′ a sin] (Cipro ◆)
enoxacin [a nocks′ a sin] (Penetrex)
gatifloxacin [gat ih flocks′ a sin] (Tequin)
levofloxacin [lev o flocks′ a sin] (Levaquin ◆)
lomefloxacin [lome flocks′ a sin] (Maxaquin)
moxifloxacin [mox ih flocks′ a sin] (Avelox)
norfloxacin [nor flocks′ a sin] (Noroxin)
ofloxacin [o flocks′ a sin] (Floxin)
sparfloxacin [spar flocks′ a sin] (Zagam)
trovafloxacin/alatrofloxacin—pro-drug [tro va flocks′ a sin/a la troe flocks′ a sin] (Trovan)

Fluoroquinolones are indicated for the treatment of bone and joint infections, bronchitis, gastroenteritis, gonorrhea, pneumonia, urinary tract infections, and many other infections caused by susceptible microorganisms. Individual fluoroquinolones may vary in their spectrum of activity. For example, most of the drugs are indicated for the treatment of urinary tract infections, but only ciprofloxacin is approved to treat bone and joint infections. Therefore the nurse is referred to current references for approved individual drug indications.

The oral bioavailability of fluoroquinolones is good. They are widely distributed in the body and have the following half-lives: ciprofloxacin, 4 hours; enoxacin, 3 to 6 hours; levofloxacin, 6 to 8 hours; lomefloxacin, 7 to 8 hours; norfloxacin, 3 to 4 hours; ofloxacin, 4 to 7 hours, and sparfloxacin, 20 hours. Alatrofloxacin injection, which is measured as trovafloxacin, is administered intravenously; its half-life is 1 hour after the completion of infusion. Oral trovafloxacin has a half-life of 9 to 12 hours. These agents are metabolized in the liver (minimally for ofloxacin and lomefloxacin) and excreted primarily by the kidneys.

The significant side effects of fluoroquinolones include dizziness, drowsiness, restlessness, stomach distress, diarrhea, vaginitis (trovafloxacin), nausea, and vomiting. Rare adverse reactions include psychosis, confusion, hallucinations, tremors, hypersensitivity, and interstitial nephritis.

The usual adult dosage of ciprofloxacin is 500 to 750 mg PO, every 12 hours for 1 to 2 weeks; the IV dosage is 400 mg every 12 hours. For enoxacin, the dosage is 200 to 400 mg PO every 12 hours for 1 to 2 weeks; for gatifloxacin, 200 to 400 mg PO or by IV infusion daily for 7 to 10 days; for levofloxacin, 500 mg PO/IV daily; for lomefloxacin, 400 mg PO daily for 10 to 14 days; for moxifloxacin, 400 mg PO daily; for norfloxacin, 400 mg PO every 12 hours for 72 hours; for ofloxacin, 300 to 400 mg PO/IV every 12 hours for 10 days; for sparfloxacin, 400 mg PO the first day, then 200 mg daily every 24 hours for a total of 10 days; and for trovafloxacin, 100 to 200 mg PO daily. Fluoroquinolones are not recommended for use in infants and children.

■ Nursing Management

Fluoroquinolone Therapy

In addition to the following discussion, see Nursing Management: Antibiotic Therapy, p. 980.

■ **Assessment.** If a client has had an allergic reaction to any of the fluoroquinolones, all of them are contraindicated because of cross-sensitivity. Clients with hepatic or renal impairment may require reduced dosages. With CNS disorders such as cerebral arteriosclerosis or epilepsy, use the fluoroquinolones with caution because of the risk of CNS toxicity.

Review the client's current medication regimen for the risk of significant drug interactions, such as those that may occur when fluoroquinolones are given concurrently with the following drugs:

Drug	Possible Effect and Management
antacids, ferrous sulfate or sucralfate	May decrease the absorption of ciprofloxacin, enoxacin, levofloxacin, lomefloxacin, norfloxacin, and trovafloxacin/alatrofloxacin, which reduces drug effectiveness. Administer fluoroquinolones at least 2 hours before these medications.
caffeine	Ciprofloxacin, enoxacin, and norfloxacin significantly decrease the hepatic metabolism of caffeine, which increases its half-life and the risk for caffeine-related CNS stimulation. Avoid sources of caffeine while taking these drugs.
didanosine	Concurrent use decreases the absorption of ciprofloxacin. Do not use concurrently with any fluoroquinolone.
phenytoin	Concurrent administration of ciprofloxacin reduces phenytoin serum levels by 34% to 80%. Administering quinolones to clients who are stabilized on phenytoin may lower serum levels and result in seizures. Also monitor phenytoin levels when discontinuing these drugs.
theophylline and other xanthines	Fluoroquinolones (with the possible exception of lomefloxacin and ofloxacin) may result in increased theophylline plasma levels and toxicity. Monitor theophylline plasma levels closely, because dosage adjustments may be necessary.

Drug	Possible Effect and Management
warfarin (Coumadin)	May result in an increase in anticoagulant effect and the potential for bleeding. Although not currently reported with all quinolones, it is recommended that PT be monitored closely whenever these drugs are administered concurrently.

A baseline assessment as described in Chapter 58 should be performed before initiating fluoroquinolone therapy.

■ **Nursing Diagnosis.** Clients receiving fluoroquinolone therapy should be assessed for the following nursing diagnoses/collaborative problems: deficient fluid volume related to anorexia, nausea, and vomiting; impaired tissue integrity related to phlebitis (IV ciprofloxacin and ofloxacin only); diarrhea; disturbed thought processes related to CNS stimulation (confusion, acute psychosis, hallucinations); and the potential complications of hypersensitivity (rash, itching, swelling of face), interstitial nephritis (blood in the urine, lower back pain, rash, edema), photosensitivity (increased sensitivity of skin to sunlight), hepatotoxicity (dark urine, pale stools, anorexia, weakness), pseudomembranous colitis (severe watery stools, fever, abdominal pain), tendonitis or tendon rupture (pain and swelling in calves), and CNS toxicity (dizziness, headache, insomnia).

■ **Implementation**

■ ***Monitoring.*** Monitor the client for signs and symptoms of adverse reactions. Monitor urinary pH because ciprofloxacin becomes more insoluble in an alkaline medium (greater than 7.0), resulting in crystalluria. Monitor the client's temperature, WBC counts, cultures, and the symptoms of infection.

■ ***Intervention.*** Administer fluoroquinolones with a full glass of water. Ensure that the client maintains a urinary output of at least 1200 to 1500 mL daily (for adults) to minimize the occurrence of crystalluria. Enoxacin or norfloxacin are to be taken on an empty stomach; ciprofloxacin, lomefloxacin, ofloxacin, and sparfloxacin may be taken either with or without food.

IV ciprofloxacin and ofloxacin should be infused slowly into a large vein over 60 minutes to minimize discomfort and venous irritation.

■ ***Education.*** Stress the importance of taking a full course of therapy, taking all doses at evenly spaced intervals as prescribed to maintain therapeutic serum levels.

Advise the client to report dizziness, light-headedness, or depression; these signs indicate CNS toxicity. Visual disturbances such as blurred or double vision and increased light sensitivity should be reported for the same reason.

Take fluoroquinolones 2 hours before antacids. With ciprofloxacin and lomefloxacin, advise the client that photosensitivity is a possible effect of these drugs; avoid exposure to sun and sunlamps. Photophobia is a concern with norfloxacin; advise the client to wear sunglasses and avoid exposure to bright light.

Because visual disturbances, dizziness, light-headedness, or drowsiness may occur, advise the client to limit activities that require alertness and dexterity until his or her response to the drug has been determined.

■ **Evaluation.** The expected outcome of fluoroquinolone therapy is that the client will maintain or achieve an infection-free state as evidenced by negative cultures. If administered therapeutically, the client will also demonstrate a body temperature within normal limits, a WBC count within the normal limits for age, and the resolution of any other infection-related symptoms without experiencing adverse reactions to the drug.

MISCELLANEOUS ANTIBIOTICS

This section includes a monobactam (aztreonam), a carbapenem (imipenem-cilastatin), metronidazole, and spectinomycin. Other antibiotics in current use are primarily topical agents, which are discussed in Chapter 66.

aztreonam [az tree′ oh nam] (Azactam)

Aztreonam, the first drug in a monobactam class of antibiotics, is a synthetic bactericidal antibiotic with an activity similar to penicillin. It binds to the penicillin-binding protein, resulting in inhibition of bacterial cell wall synthesis, cell lysis, and death. It is active against many gram-negative microorganisms and is used in the treatment of urinary tract, bronchitis, and intraabdominal, gynecologic, and skin infections (Hellinger & Brewer, 1999).

The side effects/adverse reactions of aztreonam include gastric distress, diarrhea, nausea, vomiting, hypersensitivity, and thrombophlebitis at the site of injection.

Administered intravenously, the adult dosage is 0.5 to 2 g IV or IM every 8 to 12 hours.

The nursing management of aztreonam is the same as for the penicillins, except that there are no cautions for significant drug interactions.

imipenem-cilastatin [i mi pen′ em sye la stat′ in] (Primaxin IM; Primaxin IV)

Imipenem-cilastatin, a member of a new class of carbapenem antibiotics related to the beta-lactam antibiotics, has a wide spectrum of activity against gram-positive and gram-negative aerobic and anaerobic organisms. Imipenem binds to penicillin-binding proteins, thus inhibiting bacterial cell wall synthesis. It is very resistant to degradation by beta-lactamases. Cilastatin inhibits renal dehydropeptidase and blocks the tubular secretion of imipenem, thus preventing renal metabolism of this drug. Therefore cilastatin is combined with imipenem to prevent its inactivation by renal dehydropeptidase.

This antibiotic is indicated for the treatment of bone, joint, skin, and soft tissue infections, bacterial endocarditis, intraabdominal bacteria infections, pneumonia, urinary tract and pelvic infections, and bacterial septicemia when caused by susceptible bacterial organisms (Brismar & Nord, 1999).

When imipenem-cilastatin is administered intramuscularly, the time to peak serum level is within 2 hours, with a half-life of 2 to 3 hours. When administered intravenously, the half-life is approximately 60 minutes. Excretion is primarily by the kidneys. No significant drug interactions have been reported to date with this product.

The side effects/adverse reactions of imipenem-cilastatin include gastric distress, diarrhea, nausea, vomiting, allergic-type reactions, confusion, light-headedness, convulsions, and tremors. Pseudomembranous colitis has also been reported with this product.

The usual adult dosage for IV infusion is 250 to 500 mg every 6 hours for mild infections and 500 mg every 6 to 8 hours for moderate to severe infections. The maximum dosage is 50 mg/kg daily. The IM adult dosage is 500 to 750 mg every 12 hours, up to a maximum of 1500 mg/day. The dosage for children up to age 12 has not been determined; older children may receive the adult dosage.

■ Nursing Management

Imipenem-Cilastatin Therapy

In addition to the following discussion, see Nursing Management: Antibiotic Therapy, p. 980.

■ **Assessment.** Use imipenem-cilastatin with caution in clients who are allergic to imipenem, cilastatin, or other beta-lactams (e.g., penicillin and cephalosporins). Clients with CNS disorders, such as a history of seizures, are more likely to experience CNS side effects. Clients with renal function impairment require reduced dosages. No significant drug interactions have been reported.

■ **Nursing Diagnosis.** Clients receiving imipenem-cilastatin should be assessed for the following nursing diagnoses/collaborative problems: risk for injury related to a reaction to an infusion rate that is too rapid (dizziness, diaphoresis, fatigue, nausea and vomiting); impaired oral mucous membrane (glossitis); deficient fluid volume related to nausea, vomiting, and diarrhea; diarrhea; impaired tissue integrity related to thrombophlebitis at the infusion site; and the potential complications of allergic reactions (rash, hives, fever, dyspnea), CNS toxicity (confusion, dizziness, tremors, seizures), and pseudomembranous colitis (severe abdominal cramps and diarrhea, fever).

■ **Implementation**

■ ***Monitoring.*** Monitor for adverse reactions. Monitor clients receiving more than 2 g daily, because they are at higher risk for seizures. Observe the client's temperature, WBC counts, cultures, and symptoms related to the client's infection.

■ ***Intervention.*** To minimize the occurrence of an imipenem-cilastatin combination infusion rate reaction, doses of 250 to 500 mg of imipenem should be administered over 20 to 30 minutes, or 1 g over 40 to 60 minutes. In children, doses should be administered over a 20- to 30-minute period. Administer the IM preparation by deep injection into a large muscle mass, such as the ventrogluteal or vastus lateralis muscles.

■ ***Education.*** Alert the client to report early symptoms of adverse reactions.

■ **Evaluation.** The expected outcome of imipenem-cilastatin therapy is that the client will maintain or achieve an infection-free state as evidenced by negative cultures. If administered therapeutically, the client will also demonstrate a body temperature within normal limits, a WBC count within the normal limits for age, and the resolution of any other infection-related symptoms without experiencing adverse reactions to the drug.

meropenem [mer oh pen′ em] (Merrem IV)

Meropenem is a bactericidal, broad-spectrum carbapenem antibiotic. It inhibits cell wall synthesis and is indicated for the treatment of susceptible intraabdominal infections (complicated appendicitis and peritonitis) and bacterial meningitis.

Pseudomembranous colitis, hypersensitivity, and the side effects/adverse reactions of diarrhea, nausea, vomiting, headache, and rash have been reported.

The adult dosage is 1 g IV every 8 hours (*Drug Facts and Comparisons*, 2000).

The nursing management for imipenem-cilastatin is the same as for the penicillins, except there are no cautions for significant drug interactions.

metronidazole [me troe ni′ da zole] (Flagyl, Flagyl IV)

Metronidazole is reduced intracellularly to a short-acting, cytotoxic agent that interacts with DNA, thus inhibiting bacteria synthesis and resulting in cell death (microbicidal). It is active against many anaerobic bacteria and protozoa.

Metronidazole is indicated for the treatment of amebiasis (intestinal and extraintestinal), AAPMC, bone infections, brain abscesses, CNS infections, bacterial endocarditis, genitourinary tract infections, septicemia, trichomoniasis, and other infections caused by organisms susceptible to the action of metronidazole (Kasten, 1999).

Oral metronidazole is well absorbed and distributed throughout the body. It reaches peak serum levels within 1 to 2 hours and has a half-life of 8 hours. It is metabolized in the liver and primarily excreted in the kidneys.

The side effects/adverse reactions of metronidazole include dizziness, headache, gastric distress, diarrhea, anorexia, nausea, vomiting, peripheral neuropathy, CNS toxicity, leukopenia, thrombophlebitis, and vaginal candidiasis.

The usual oral adult dosage is 7.5 mg/kg, up to maximum of 1 g, every 6 hours for a week or longer. The adult dosage for IV infusion is 15 mg/kg initially, then 7.5 mg/kg up to a maximum of 1 g every 6 hours for a week or longer. The maximum daily dose is 4 g.

■ Nursing Management

Metronidazole Therapy

In addition to the following discussion, see Nursing Management: Antibiotic Therapy, p. 980.

■ **Assessment.** Because metronidazole may cause CNS toxicity, any individual with active organic CNS disease, such as epilepsy, should be carefully evaluated before treatment. The sodium content of the parenteral dosage forms should be considered if clients have a restricted sodium intake. Clients with a history of blood dyscrasias should be monitored carefully, because metronidazole may cause leukopenia. Reduced dosages may be required for clients with hepatic dysfunction. To use metronidazole for giardiasis, the *Giardia* organism should be identified. Metronidazole is contraindicated for clients who are hypersensitive to it.

Review the client's current medication regimen for the risk of significant drug interactions, such as those that may occur when metronidazole is given concurrently with the following drugs:

Drug	Possible Effect and Management
Bold/color type indicates the most serious interactions.	
alcohol	**Metronidazole interferes with the metabolism of alcohol, leading to an accumulation of acetaldehyde. This may result in disulfiram (Antabuse)-type effects: flushing, headaches, nausea, vomiting, and abdominal distress. Avoid concurrent use or a potentially serious drug interaction may occur.**
anticoagulants (coumarin or indanedione)	May enhance anticoagulant effects by inhibiting their metabolism. Monitor closely with prothrombin tests if given concurrently. Dosage adjustments may be necessary.
disulfiram (Antabuse)	**Avoid concurrent use, or use within 14 days of disulfiram administration in alcoholic clients. Adverse reactions such as confusion and psychosis have been reported.**

A baseline assessment as described in Chapter 58 should be performed before initiating metronidazole therapy.

■ **Nursing Diagnosis.** The client receiving metronidazole should be assessed for the following nursing diagnoses/collaborative problems: impaired comfort (headache and unpleasant metallic taste); deficient fluid volume related to anorexia, nausea, vomiting, and diarrhea; impaired tissue integrity related to the development of thrombophlebitis (IV administration only); ineffective protection related to leukopenia and the loss of normal flora (fungal overgrowth); disturbed sensory perception related to peripheral neuropathy (numbness, tingling, and pain in the hands and feet); disturbed thought processes related to CNS toxicity (confusion, mood changes); and the potential complications of hypersensitivity (rash, itching), seizures related to high doses, and pancreatitis (severe abdominal pain, nausea, and vomiting).

■ **Implementation**

■ ***Monitoring.*** Assess clients periodically for symptoms of peripheral neuropathy such as numbness and tingling of the hands or feet. Mood changes and irritability also indicate CNS toxicity.

Monitor CBCs at frequent intervals for blood dyscrasia, and instruct the client to report immediately to the prescriber any symptoms of sore throat, unusual tiredness or weakness, or unusual bleeding or bruising.

If metronidazole is administered for giardiasis, three stool examinations (taken several days apart) should be performed to determine the success of therapy; these should begin 3 to 4 weeks after treatment. Additional specimens may be required if symptoms persist.

■ ***Intervention.*** Administer the oral form of metronidazole with meals to minimize gastrointestinal irritation. Parenteral metronidazole is to be administered by slow IV infusion. It may be administered continuously or intermittently over a 1-hour period. If administered concurrently with a primary IV, the primary IV should be discontinued while the metronidazole is infused. The sodium content of the parenteral forms of the drug should be considered as part of sodium intake in clients for whom sodium intake is restricted.

■ ***Education.*** Advise the client that this drug may cause an unpleasant taste in the mouth, diminished taste sensation, and a dry mouth. The use of sugar-free candies, ice cubes, and frequent mouth rinses may bring some relief to the client. If therapy is long-term, dry mouth may contribute to dental caries and gum disease, and the client should receive regular dental checkups.

Stress the importance of completing a full course of therapy, even though the client may be feeling well and be symptom free. The doses should be evenly spaced to ensure that therapeutic serum levels are maintained.

Advise the client not to ingest alcoholic beverages while taking metronidazole, because a disulfiram-like effect may result (flushing, nausea and vomiting, and abdominal cramping).

If metronidazole is being prescribed for trichomoniasis, the client will need to prevent reinfection from her male partner. The partner will need to undergo concurrent drug therapy and use a condom until the infection is resolved in both partners.

Advise the client that the urine may turn a darker color but that this change is not medically significant.

■ **Evaluation.** The expected outcome of metronidazole therapy is that the client will maintain or achieve an infection-free state as evidenced by negative culture results. If administered therapeutically, the client will also demonstrate a body temperature within normal limits, a WBC count within the normal limits for age, and the resolution of any other infection-related symptoms without experiencing adverse reactions to the drug.

spectinomycin [spek ti noe mye' sin] (Trobicin)

The therapeutic indication for spectinomycin is the treatment of infections caused by *Neisseria gonorrhoeae.* It is bacteriostatic because it inhibits protein synthesis in the bacteria cell. It is for IM use only and generally is recommended as an alternate regimen for clients with gonorrhea who have antibiotic resistance or cannot take ceftriaxone.

Spectinomycin is not effective for treating syphilis and should not be used for mixed infections (gonorrhea and syphilis), because it can mask the symptoms of syphilis.

The side effects/adverse reactions of spectinomycin include chills, fever, nausea, dizziness, and urticaria.

The usual adult dosage is 2 g IM as a single dose.

▪ Nursing Management
Spectinomycin Therapy

In addition to the following discussion, see Nursing Management: Antibiotic Therapy, p. 980.

▪ **Assessment.** Spectinomycin is contraindicated for clients who are hypersensitive to this drug. This drug was formerly used for the treatment of gonococcal infections in children; however, the diluent to reconstitute spectinomycin contains 0.945% benzyl alcohol, which has been associated with fatal gasping syndrome in infants.

▪ **Nursing Diagnosis.** The client receiving spectinomycin therapy may experience the following nursing diagnoses/collaborative problems: risk for injury related to dizziness; impaired comfort (pain at the site of injection, abdominal cramping); deficient fluid volume related to nausea and vomiting; and the potential complication of allergic reaction (chills, fever, itching or redness of the skin).

▪ **Implementation**

▪ ***Monitoring.*** Observe the client for 45 to 60 minutes after injection, because anaphylaxis has been reported. At the beginning of therapy and after 3 months, perform a serologic examination to monitor the client with a gonococcal infection for concurrent syphilis. Obtain cultures of gonococcal infection sites to monitor for effectiveness of therapy.

▪ ***Intervention.*** Spectinomycin is for IM use only. Agitate the vial thoroughly to ensure even suspension of the drug. Administer the IM injection deep into the ventrogluteal site or vastus lateralis site. Inject the suspension using a 20-gauge needle, and inject only 5 mL in each site.

▪ ***Education.*** Caution the client that dizziness may occur and to avoid operating hazardous equipment until the vertigo effects of the drug are known. The client should be instructed to use a condom to prevent infection, and it may be necessary to treat the partner concurrently to prevent reinfection.

▪ **Evaluation.** The expected outcome of spectinomycin therapy is that the client's gonococcal infection sites will show negative culture results after 3 to 7 days.

URINARY TRACT ANTIMICROBIALS

Urinary tract infections (UTIs) are the most common bacterial infections reported in the United States. Between 10% and 20% of women experience at least one urinary tract infection in their lifetime. The incidence of UTIs increases in institutional settings—up to as much as 35% to 40% of the population in extended-stay hospitals (Sahai, 1995). Table 59-6 lists the predisposing risk factors for UTIs.

Differentiating between an upper UTI (pyelonephritis) and lower UTI (cystitis) is usually based on the presenting signs and symptoms. An upper UTI usually causes pain in the lower back, flank, or stomach, as well as fever, sweating, nausea, vomiting, weakness, and headache. A lower UTI leads to frequent but small amounts on urination, urgency, dysuria and, perhaps, incontinence. However, the infection may be present both in the upper and lower urinary tract in approximately one third of UTIs.

TABLE 59-6 Predisposing Risk Factors for Urinary Tract Infections

Risk Factors	Frequency Reported
Urinary tract instrumentation (urethral and ureteral catheterization)*	Up to 67%
Pregnant women	4%-10%
Nonpregnant women	2%-5%

Information from Ahronheim, J.C. (1992). *Handbook of prescribing medications for geriatric patients.* Boston: Little, Brown.
*After a week of indwelling catheterization, up to 100% colonization and bacteriuria.

UTIs are primarily caused by bacteria. In community-acquired infections, most UTIs are caused by gram-negative aerobic bacilli from the intestinal tract, such as *E. coli* (Rosenberg, 1999). It has been reported that *E. coli* may cause up to 90% of all community-acquired, uncomplicated UTIs (Sahai, 1995). Hospital-acquired infections are often complicated and difficult to treat. Organisms involved include *P. aeruginosa, Serratia, Enterobacter,* and other gram-negative microorganisms.

Drug therapies for lower UTIs are often started before culture and sensitivity reports are known. The most probable infecting organism and the antibiotic sensitivity can be predicted from the information discussed in the previous paragraph.

With today's increasing development of antibiotic resistance, the medications that are most effective for UTIs are the sulfonamides (e.g., trimethoprim-sulfamethoxazole [TMP-SMX]) and cephalosporins. Alternate medications include the urinary tract antiseptics, aztreonam, and fluoroquinolones; phenazopyridine (Pyridium) is used primarily as a urinary tract analgesic.

For a Concept Map on lower urinary tract infection, go to mosby.com/MERLIN/McKenry/.

▪ Nursing Management
Urinary Antimicrobial Therapy

▪ **Assessment.** The initial assessment of the client provides baseline information and includes the client's history of UTIs and the signs and symptoms of the current UTI. Drug allergies, concurrent drug therapy, or the altered function of any body system may affect the drug therapy.

Obtaining urine specimens to determine the causative organism for a UTI is often the nurse's responsibility. Through client education, most clients can obtain a clean-catch urine sample of the appropriate quantity and quality for laboratory testing. The health care provider will specify whether a midstream clean-catch or catheterized specimen is required. Specimens for culture should be taken directly to the

Nursing Care Plan
Selected Nursing Diagnoses Related to the Administration of Urinary Tract Antimicrobials

Nursing Diagnosis	Outcome Criteria	Nursing Interventions
Risk for infection	Infection is prevented or symptoms of infection are resolved: Temperature remains within the normal range. WBC count remains within the normal range. Urine cultures demonstrate no pathogens. Urine is clear and odorless. Fluid intake is 3000 mL/24 hr.	Monitor and record temperature at least every 4 hours. Report elevations. Monitor WBC count. Report significant changes. Culture urine as ordered, and monitor results. Use strict aseptic technique when inserting urinary catheters. Encourage a fluid intake of at least 3000 mL daily.
Deficient knowledge related to medication regimen	Client will describe underlying conditions and how the drug relates to the condition, how and when to take the medication, common drug interactions, safety precautions, common side effects/adverse reactions, and which of these warrant reporting. Client will self-administer medication safely and accurately.	Assess learning needs and learning readiness. Plan with the client for the achievement of realistic goals. Provide information to meet outcome criteria. Administer medication with food or milk to decrease gastrointestinal distress. Alert the client that medication may cause a discoloration of the urine. Instruct the client to take the medication as ordered and to consult with the prescriber if no improvement is seen within a few days.

laboratory to prevent the death of the suspect organisms and to prevent the growth of contaminating ones. However, there is economic value in empiric treatment without urine cultures in young women with dysuria and frequency (Andriole, 1999).

■ **Nursing Diagnosis.** The client receiving urinary antimicrobial therapy is at risk for the following nursing diagnoses: risk for injury related to a preexisting health condition, drug interaction, or side effect/adverse reaction of the drug; deficient knowledge related to the antimicrobial therapy; and ineffective therapeutic regimen management. (See the Nursing Care Plan above for other selected nursing diagnoses.)

■ **Implementation**

■ ***Monitoring.*** Periodic assessment should include the client's health status regarding fever, chills, flank pain, nausea and vomiting, frequency and urgency of urination, dysuria, costovertebral tenderness, gross hematuria and pyuria, and general well-being. Urinalyses should be monitored for WBCs, red blood cells, casts, protein, crystals, and bacteria. Urine culture and sensitivity examinations should indicate the efficacy of the drug. CBCs should also be monitored. Serum antibiotic concentrations can be monitored during the course of therapy to assess for therapeutic and toxic levels of specific antimicrobials. In addition to monitoring the therapeutic effects of these antimicrobials, assess the client for the development of common side effects/adverse reactions of individual drugs (see the discussions of specific drugs for these effects).

■ ***Intervention.*** Nursing interventions relative to antimicrobial drug therapy were discussed in greater detail in Chapter 58. In general, these interventions relate to (1) assistance in the identification of the infecting organism, (2) actual administration of the drug, (3) assessment of the client's response to the drug, (4) client education, and (5) prevention and treatment of adverse responses, including pharmacologic and chemical drug-drug interactions. If an antimicrobial agent is ordered before the infecting organism has been identified, it is important that the urine sample for initial culture be obtained before the first dose of the drug is administered. With subsequent specimens for culture, it is important to describe the client's antimicrobial regimen for the laboratory, because the selection and interpretation of laboratory tests often depend on this information.

Around-the-clock administration of antimicrobial drugs at prescribed intervals is required for maintaining therapeutic blood levels of these drugs, and it is the nurse's responsibility to see that this occurs. This is accomplished by providing the necessary client education, which may entail waking sleeping clients and ensuring that tests or therapies do not interrupt the dosing schedule.

■ ***Education.*** Clients should be taught the principles of antimicrobial therapy so that these drugs can be self-administered safely. The necessity of adhering to an incon-

BOX 59-2

Client Education to Reduce Occurrence of Urinary Tract Infections

UTIs often occur as a result of contamination of the lower urinary tract with perineal bacteria. Preventive measures attempt to (1) reduce perineal bacteria, and (2) prevent bacteria from entering the lower urinary tract. Client education should focus on these two measures and include the following instructions:

1. Good perineal hygiene helps to reduce bacterial growth.
2. Female clients should always wipe from the front to the back to prevent contamination of the urinary tract with fecal bacteria.
3. Emptying the bladder soon after intercourse helps to wash out bacteria that may have entered the urethra.
4. Cotton undergarments (or synthetics with a cotton crotch) that "breathe" are preferred to synthetics that foster bacterial growth.
5. Drinking six to eight glasses of fluids per day and urinating often helps to cleanse the urinary tract of bacteria.

venient around-the-clock schedule may require special reinforcement. Compliance for the full course of therapy is essential to prevent the possible development of resistant strains of microorganisms. "Leftover" antimicrobial medications should not be used for new bouts of UTI but disposed of properly. The prescriber should be consulted for any new bouts of infection. Refer to the text for specific instructions for each drug.

Instruct the client to avoid coffee, tea, juices with a high citric acid content, cola, alcohol, chocolate, and spices, which often irritate a sensitive bladder. The daily fluid intake for a client with a UTI should be at least 3000 mL (unless contraindicated) to help flush organisms from the urinary tract. The client should be taught health practices that may reduce the chance of developing another UTI (Box 59-2).

▪ **Evaluation.** Evaluation of the client for therapeutic responses to antimicrobial agents is a primary nursing responsibility. An expected outcome of urinary tract antimicrobial therapy is that the client will experience a decreased severity or a disappearance of the clinical and laboratory manifestations of the UTI (e.g., absence of pathogen on cultures, normothermia, WBC count within the normal range, and an absence of urgency, frequency, and burning of urination).

Sulfonamides

Sulfonamides are among the most widely used antibacterial agents in the world, particularly for UTIs; ✔ TMP-SMX is the most common sulfonamide. Rather than being bactericidal, these agents are primarily bacteriostatic in concentrations that are normally useful in controlling infections. All of the sulfonamides used therapeutically are synthetically produced.

Because the sulfonamides are structurally similar to paraaminobenzoic acid (PABA), they inhibit a bacterial enzyme (dihydropteroate synthetase) necessary to incorporate PABA into dihydrofolic acid. Blocking dihydrofolic acid synthesis results in a decrease in tetrahydrofolic acid, which interferes with the synthesis of purines, thymidine, and DNA in the microorganism. Therefore the bacteria most sensitive to sulfonamides are those that synthesize their own folic acid. The presence of pus, necrotic tissue, and serum interferes with the activities of the sulfonamides because PABA is present in such materials. Among the microorganisms highly susceptible to the sulfonamides are group A beta-hemolytic streptococci, pneumococci, *N. meningitides*, *N. gonorrhoeae*, *E. coli*, *Pasteurella pestis*, *Bacillus anthracis*, *Shigella* species, *H. influenzae*, and *Pneumocystis carinii*.

The absorption of sulfonamides is good. For most sulfonamides, peak serum levels are reached between 2 and 6 hours; for sulfamethoxazole, the intermediate acting sulfonamide, peak levels are reached in 6 to 12 hours. These agents are acetylated in the liver and excreted primarily by the kidneys.

Although the newer sulfonamides, such as sulfisoxazole and sulfacetamide, are quite soluble (even in acid urine), it is recommended that clients increase their fluid intake to maintain a urine output of at least 1200 mL/day (*USP DI*, 1999).

Table 59-7 describes the side effects/adverse reactions and usual adult dosage ranges for urinary tract agents.

▪ Nursing Management

Sulfonamide Therapy

In addition to the following discussion, see Nursing Management: Urinary Antimicrobial Therapy, p. 1004.

▪ **Assessment.** Although cross-sensitization with sulfonamides is not as severe as with penicillins, it is safer to avoid all sulfonamides in clients who develop a hypersensitivity to any one agent. Cross-sensitivity also exists with some diuretics (e.g., furosemide, acetazolamide, and the thiazides) and with sulfonylurea antidiabetic agents; therefore, as always, obtain an accurate history of the client's sensitivities. Avoid the use of sulfonamides in clients with hepatic and renal dysfunction, blood dyscrasias, glucose-6-phosphate dehydrogenase (G6PD) deficiency, and porphyria. The risk-benefit ratio should be considered for clients with blood dyscrasias and anemia due to folate deficiency, because these drugs may cause blood dyscrasias. The administration of sulfonamides is contraindicated in neonates. (See the Pregnancy Safety box on p. 986 for FDA categories of antimicrobials used for UTIs.)

Review the client's current medication regimen for the risk of significant drug interactions, such as those that may

TABLE 59-7 Urinary Tract Agents: Side Effects/Adverse Reactions and Usual Adult Dosage

Drug	Usual Adult Dosage	Side Effects/Adverse Reactions
Sulfonamides		Common: anorexia, diarrhea, nausea, vomiting, dizziness, headaches, pruritus, rash
sulfadiazine (generic)	2-4 g PO initially, then 1 g q4-6h	
sulfamethizole (Thiosulfil Forte)	0.5-1 g PO q6-8h	Less common: muscle and joint pain, fever, sore throat, Stevens-Johnson syndrome, pain on urination, increased bleeding tendencies
sulfamethoxazole (Gantanol)	2 g PO initially, then 1 g q8-12h	
sulfisoxazole (Gantrisin)	2-4 g PO initially, then 0.75-1.5 g q4h	
Antiseptics		
cinoxacin (Cinobac)	250 mg PO q hs	Less common: nausea, rash, pruritus, diarrhea, anorexia, vomiting, photosensitivity, tinnitus, insomnia
methenamine mandelate (Mandelamine)	1 g PO 4 times daily	Less common: nausea, rash, stomach distress, painful urination, low back pain
methenamine hippurate (Hiprex)	1 g PO 2 times daily	
nalidixic acid (NegGram)	1 g PO q6h	Common: diarrhea, nausea, vomiting, rash, pruritus, headache, drowsiness Less common: visual disturbances such as double or blurred vision, halos, or very bright appearance around lights
nitrofurantoin (Furadantin)	50-100 mg PO q6h	Common: stomach distress, diarrhea, anorexia, nausea, vomiting, and pneumonitis
Analgesic		
phenazopyridine (Pyridium, Phenazo ♣)	200 mg PO 3 times daily	Less common: stomach cramps or distress, headache Rare: hemolytic anemia, renal failure, hepatotoxicity, aseptic meningitis

occur when sulfonamides are given concurrently with the following drugs:

Drug	Possible Effect and Management
anticoagulants, such as coumarin or indanedione derivatives; anticonvulsants (hydantoin); oral antidiabetic agents; methotrexate	These agents are highly protein bound; concurrent drug administration may displace them from their protein-binding sites, resulting in increased serum levels and possible toxicity. The metabolism of these agents may also be inhibited by sulfonamides. Monitor closely for signs of toxicity, which indicate a need for dosage adjustments.
hemolytics, other hepatotoxic medications	Increased potential for toxicity. There is an increased risk of inducing liver toxicity. Monitor closely for symptoms such as yellow eyes or skin.
methenamine (Mandelamine)	Methenamine requires an acidic urine to be active and effective. It may precipitate if given with a sulfonamide and result in crystalluria. Do not administer concurrently.

A baseline assessment of the client's symptoms related to the UTI, as well as a CBC and urinalysis, should be obtained before initiating sulfonamide therapy.

■ **Nursing Diagnosis.** Clients receiving sulfonamide therapy should be assessed for the development of the following nursing diagnoses/collaborative problems: impaired comfort related to CNS effects (dizziness, headache); deficient fluid volume related to anorexia, nausea, vomiting, and diarrhea; diarrhea; and the potential complications of hypersensitivity (rash, fever), photosensitivity (increased sensitivity of skin to sunlight), blood dyscrasias (unusual bruising or bleeding, sore throat, fever, unusual fatigue), hepatitis (yellow eyes or skin), Lyell's syndrome (difficulty in swallowing, blistering of skin), Stevens-Johnson syndrome (aching joints and muscles, weakness, skin changes), goiter, interstitial nephritis, hematuria, or crystalluria.

■ **Implementation**

■ ***Monitoring.*** Because renal toxicity is a potentially serious problem, monitor the hospitalized client's urinary output and ensure that it totals at least 1200 mL in 24 hours. The maintenance of urinary output at this level decreases the tendency for crystals to form. The urine should be examined visually for the presence of crystals; periodic urinalyses should be performed with long-term sulfonamide therapy to determine if crystals are present. Monitor the urinalysis to determine the status of the UTI and for early detection of crystalluria. Carefully observe the client for toxic effects, such as a rash, sore throat, or purpura.

With prolonged sulfonamide therapy, the client requires periodic blood counts to assess for the occurrence of hematologic side effects (anemia, granulocytopenia, and thrombocytopenia).

■ ***Intervention.*** Administer sulfonamides on an empty stomach with a full glass of water to enhance absorption. If the common side effect of nausea and vomiting occurs, administer the drug with food to decrease gastrointestinal distress. Do not administer sulfonamides with antacids, because the latter inhibit their action by decreasing absorption.

■ ***Education.*** Clients should be instructed to drink at least 3 quarts of fluids per day unless contraindicated for renal or cardiac conditions. Liquids and vitamins that produce acid urine (e.g., ascorbic acid) should be avoided. Inform the client of the importance of completing a full course of drug therapy, even though he or she may feel better after several days of therapy. Instruct the client to observe for and report any dermatologic reactions after initiating the sulfonamide. Fever may occur after 7 to 10 days of therapy, indicating a serum sickness–like reaction. Fever may be accompanied by joint pain, urticaria, and leukopenia. All of these responses are indications for discontinuation of the drug and a follow-up referral to the prescriber. Advise the client to avoid direct skin exposure to the sun and sunlamps, because skin photosensitivity may be present. Alert clients with diabetes that sulfonamides may cause false-positive results of urine sugar and urine ketone tests.

■ **Evaluation.** The expected outcome of sulfonamide therapy is that the client will experience a decrease in the severity or a disappearance of the clinical and laboratory manifestations of the UTI (e.g., absence of pathogen on cultures, normothermia, WBC count within the normal range, and an absence of urgency, frequency, and burning of urination).

Urinary Tract Antiseptics

Cinoxacin, methenamine mandelate, nalidixic acid, and nitrofurantoin are the primary urinary tract antiseptics. Urinary tract antiseptics are drugs that exert antibacterial activity in the urine but have little or no systemic antibacterial effects. Their usefulness is limited to the treatment of UTIs.

cinoxacin [sin ox′ a sin] (Cinobac)

Cinoxacin inhibits the replication of bacterial DNA, thus producing bactericidal urinary effects. It is absorbed well orally. Its serum levels are usually low, and its urinary levels are high. This product does cross the placenta. The time for peak serum levels is between 2 and 3 hours. Cinoxacin is metabolized in the liver and excreted by the kidneys. See Table 59-5 for the side effects/adverse reactions and usual adult dosage ranges of the urinary tract agents.

methenamine mandelate [meth en′ a meen] (Mandelamine) **methenamine hippurate** (Hiprex, Urex, Hip-Rex ♣)

Methenamine, which is used to treat UTIs, combines the action of methenamine and mandelic acid or hippurate acid salts. Its effectiveness depends on the release of formaldehyde, which requires an acid medium. The acids released from the mandelate or hippurate salts contribute to this acidity. Formaldehyde may be bactericidal or bacteriostatic, and its effects are believed to be the result of denaturation of bacteria protein. It is ineffective in alkaline urine. Because of its fairly wide bacterial spectrum, low toxicity, and low incidence of resistance, methenamine is often the drug of choice for long-term suppression of infections.

Methenamine is absorbed orally and takes ½ to 2 hours to reach peak urinary formaldehyde levels at a urinary pH of 5.6; the enteric-coated methenamine mandelate reaches its urinary peak in 3 to 8 hours. Excretion is via the kidneys. See Table 59-5 for the side effects/adverse reactions and usual adult dosage ranges of the urinary tract agents.

The client's current medication regimen should be reviewed for significant drug interactions, such as those that may occur when methenamine is given concurrently with the following drugs:

Drug	Possible Effect and Management
Bold/color type indicates the most serious interactions.	
urinary alkalizers, such as antacids (calcium and/or magnesium), carbonic anhydrase inhibitors, citrates, sodium bicarbonate, or thiazide diuretics	May result in an alkaline urine, thus inhibiting the conversion of methenamine to formaldehyde and rendering it ineffective. Avoid concurrent drug administration.
sulfamethizole (Thiosulfil Forte)	In acid urine, the formaldehyde produced may precipitate with certain sulfonamides, which increases the potential for crystalluria. Avoid concurrent use or a potentially serious drug interaction may occur.

nalidixic acid [nal i dix′ ik] (NegGram)

Nalidixic acid appears to inhibit the synthesis of bacterial DNA by interfering with the polymerization of DNA. Resistance usually develops rapidly during treatment with this drug. This drug is indicated for the treatment of UTIs caused by *E. coli* and the *Proteus, Klebsiella,* and *Enterobacter* species.

Nalidixic acid is well absorbed orally and reaches peak serum levels in 1 to 2 hours and peak urine levels in 3 to 4 hours. This drug is metabolized in the liver, with approximately 30% converted to the active metabolite, hydroxynalidixic acid. It is excreted by the kidneys. See Table 59-5 for the side effects/adverse reactions and usual adult dosage ranges of the urinary tract agents.

When given with oral anticoagulants (e.g., coumarin), nalidixic acid may displace the anticoagulants from their protein binding sites, resulting in enhanced anticoagulant action. Dosage adjustments may be necessary if concurrent therapy is necessary, and the nurse should monitor the client's risk for injury related to an increase in bleeding tendency.

nitrofurantoin [nye troe fyoor′ an toyn] (Furadantin, Macrodantin, Macrobid ◆)

Nitrofurantoin is a broad-spectrum bactericidal agent at therapeutic serum levels. It is reduced by bacteria to reactive substances that inactivate or alter bacterial ribosomal proteins. It is indicated for the treatment of urinary tract infections caused by organisms such as *E. coli* and *S. aureus* or the *Klebsiella, Enterobacter,* and *Proteus* species.

After oral administration, nitrofurantoin is absorbed and has a half-life of 20 to 60 minutes. Approximately 65% of the drug is rapidly metabolized and inactivated in the liver and body tissues and excreted by the kidneys. See Table 59-5 for the side effects/adverse reactions and usual adult dosages of the urinary tract agents.

The client's current medication regimen should be reviewed for the risk of significant drug interactions, such as those that may occur when nitrofurantoin is given concurrently with the following drugs:

Drug	Possible Effect and Management
hemolytic agents	Increased possibility of toxic side effects. Monitor blood counts for anemia closely if concurrent therapy is necessary.
neurotoxic medications	Increased risk of inducing neurotoxicity. Monitor closely for dizziness, drowsiness, or headache if concurrent therapy is necessary.
probenecid (Benemid) or sulfinpyrazone (Anturane)	Tubular secretion of nitrofurantoin will be inhibited, leading to increased serum levels and possible toxicity. A decrease in urinary concentrations and effectiveness may also result. Dosage adjustments of probenecid may be required.

■ Nursing Management

Urinary Antiseptic Therapy

The following nursing measures include general ones for all urinary antiseptics and specific ones for particular antiseptics. For the general nursing care of these clients, see Nursing Management: Urinary Antimicrobial Therapy, p. 1004.

■ **Assessment.** Ascertain whether the client has preexisting hepatic or renal function impairment; urinary antiseptics are used cautiously in such instances. Use nitrofurantoin cautiously in clients with peripheral neuropathy (because it may be worsened) and also in clients with pulmonary disease (because the drug may cause a pulmonary reaction, including pneumonitis). CNS damage or a history of seizures is an indication to use caution with the administration of nalidixic acid. (See individual drug discussions of the urinary antiseptics for specific drug interactions to be assessed before initiating a specific medication regimen.)

■ **Nursing Diagnosis.** The client receiving urinary tract antiseptic therapy may experience the following nursing diagnoses: risk for injury related to a preexisting health condition, drug interaction, or side effect/adverse reaction of the drug; deficient knowledge, and ineffective therapeutic regimen management.

■ **Implementation**

■ ***Monitoring.*** The client's progress should be monitored periodically through client reports of decreased UTI symptoms, urinalysis, CBCs, and hepatic and renal function studies. With nitrofurantoin, pulmonary studies may be indicated.

■ ***Intervention.*** Acidification of the urine inhibits the growth of many urinary tract microorganisms and thereby enhances the effects of several urinary antiseptics. Thus when clients with UTIs are encouraged to consume large volumes of fluids, they should select fluids that increase urine acidity, such as cranberry juice or prune juice (Williams, 1995). Vitamin C will also acidify the urine and can enhance antiinfective therapy.

Methenamine is most effective when the urine pH is 5.5 or less. Urine pH is easily monitored at the bedside and at home with commercially available test strips.

Urinary antiseptics may be given with food or just after meals to prevent gastrointestinal distress. If oral solutions are used, ensure that they are shaken well and administered with the calibrated device provided by the manufacturer.

■ ***Education.*** The client should be instructed to complete a full course of therapy, even if marked improvement occurs within a few days. The prescriber should be notified if the client's symptoms do not significantly improve in the first 3 days of therapy. Cranberry juice contains a compound that prevents bacteria from anchoring themselves in the bladder. Suggesting cranberry sauce if the client considers cranberry juice unpalatable can increase compliance. Eating more protein, plums, or prunes will also help to make the urine more acidic (*USP DI,* 1999). Most fruits, particularly citrus fruits and juices, milk and other dairy products, and other alkalinizing foods should be avoided. Alka-Seltzer and sodium bicarbonate, which alkalinize the urine, should be avoided.

The client should be advised that dizziness and drowsiness may occur with these drugs and that these symptoms should be reported to the prescriber. Driving and other activities requiring alertness should be avoided until symptoms have resolved. With nalidixic acid, caution the client to report any visual disturbances to the prescriber.

Photophobia may occur during the use of cinoxacin. The client should be advised to avoid bright sunlight and to wear sunglasses. There is a possibility of photosensitivity during nalidixic acid therapy and for up to 3 months after it is discontinued. The client should be cautioned to avoid direct skin exposure to sunlight and sunlamps.

Clients with diabetes should use Clinistix, Diastix, or Tes-tape to test for glucosuria, because nitrofurantoin and nalidixic acid may produce a false-positive result with Clinitest. The client taking nitrofurantoin should be advised that urine may be brown in color. Nitrofurantoin is discolored by alkalis and strong light. The client should not use metal pillboxes unless they are stainless steel or aluminum, because this drug decomposes on contact with other metals.

▪ **Evaluation.** The expected outcome of urinary antiseptic therapy is that the client will experience an absence of urgency, frequency, and burning on urination, and the urine culture will show an absence of pathogen growth.

Aztreonam and the Fluoroquinolones

Aztreonam and fluoroquinolones (ciprofloxacin, norfloxacin, ofloxacin) are potent drugs used in the treatment of UTIs. Aztreonam is effective against many gram-negative bacteria and appears to be safer than aminoglycoside therapy in the seriously ill person. In general, the fluoroquinolones are preferred agents when antibiotic-resistant bacteria are suspected. Refer to the previous sections for information on these medications.

URINARY TRACT ANALGESIC

phenazopyridine [fen az oh peer′ i deen] (Pyridium)

The exact mechanism of action for phenazopyridine is unknown, but it appears to have a topical analgesic or local anesthetic effect on the mucosa of the urinary tract. Phenazopyridine is used for urinary tract irritation, such as urinary frequency and pain and burning on urination. It is indicated only for short-term use; the underlying reason for the irritation should be determined and treated appropriately.

Phenazopyridine is metabolized by the liver and other body tissues and is excreted by the kidneys. See Table 59-5 for the side effects/adverse reactions and the usual adult dosages of the urinary tract agents.

▪ Nursing Management

Phenazopyridine Therapy

▪ **Assessment.** Phenazopyridine is contraindicated in clients with G6PD deficiency, impaired renal or hepatic function, or a history of sensitivity to the drug.

▪ **Nursing Diagnosis.** The client receiving phenazopyridine therapy is at risk for the nursing diagnosis of impaired comfort (headache, heartburn, abdominal cramps) and the potential complications of hemolytic anemia (fatigue), renal function impairment, methemoglobinemia, allergic dermatitis, and hepatotoxicity (yellow eyes or skin).

▪ **Implementation**

▪ ***Monitoring.*** The client's progress should be monitored periodically through reports of decreased symptoms of urgency and burning on urination.

▪ ***Intervention.*** Phenazopyridine is usually prescribed in conjunction with an antimicrobial or urinary antiseptic. Administer with food to decrease gastrointestinal distress. Phenazopyridine may be discontinued after 2 days if the client's discomfort has resolved.

▪ ***Education.*** The client should be told that the urine will become reddish orange and may stain clothing. The client should be instructed to observe for yellowness of the skin and sclera, which may indicate an accumulation of the drug as a result of renal impairment. If this occurs, the drug is discontinued and the prescriber is notified. Clients with diabetes should use Clinistix, Diastix, or Tes-tape to test for glucosuria, because Clinitest may give a false-positive result during phenazopyridine therapy. Alert the client not to wear soft contact lenses during therapy or they may be permanently stained.

▪ **Evaluation.** The expected outcome of phenazopyridine therapy is that the client will experience an absence of urgency, frequency, and burning on urination.

SUMMARY

Antibiotics are chemical substances that kill or suppress the growth of microorganisms. Once the nurse has acquired an understanding of the principles of antibiotic therapy, the particular drugs may be classified by groups, actions, and effects for familiarization. Penicillins are derived from molds and inhibit the synthesis of bacterial cell walls; they are bactericidal for a wide range of gram-positive and some gram-negative organisms. Cephalosporins, now in their fourth generation, are chemical modifications of the penicillin structure and are bactericidal by inhibiting cell wall synthesis. Macrolide antibiotics, the most important of which is erythromycin, are bacteriostatic by inhibiting protein synthesis; they are bactericidal in higher concentrations with selected organisms. Lincosamides, which inhibit protein synthesis in bacteria by binding the ribosomes of susceptible organisms, are primarily bacteriostatic (except in higher concentrations with selected organisms, in which case they are bactericidal). Vancomycin is bactericidal for many organisms and bacteriostatic for enterococci by inhibiting RNA synthesis and bacterial cell wall synthesis, causing lysis. Aminoglycosides are potent bactericidal antibiotics that are usually held in reserve for serious or life-threatening infections. Tetracyclines block the binding of transfer RNA complex to the ribosome and are therefore bacteriostatic for a wide range of gram-positive and gram-negative organisms. Chloramphenicol inhibits protein synthesis and is bacteriostatic for a wide range of organisms; however, its use is limited because of its toxicity to bone marrow. Fluoroquinolones inhibit bacterial RNA synthesis and are bactericidal. Metronidazole, a short-acting cytotoxic agent that interacts with DNA, is effective against anaerobic bacteria and protozoa.

UTIs are a common reason for seeking medical care in the community as well as a major result of nosocomial infections in institutions; their incidence increases with age. Antimicrobial therapy for UTIs includes antibiotics (sulfonamides), urinary tract antiseptics, monobactams and fluoroquinolones, and urinary tract analgesics.

Although a repertoire of antibiotics can be used in the treatment of infections, health care professionals cannot become complacent in their use. The risk of infection in certain populations has increased with the emergence of newly recognized pathogens and drug resistance in known strains of organisms, the use of immunosuppressive agents, and the increase in invasive procedures for diagnosis and treatment.

Critical Thinking Questions

1. Why is the assessment stage so important in the nursing process for antibiotic therapy?
2. Kevin Reardon, age 27, has been prescribed oral ampicillin for otitis media. On the third day of ampicillin therapy, Mr. Reardon telephones the clinic to indicate he has developed diarrhea. What might be occurring with Mr. Reardon's therapy? What action should the nurse take?
3. In many countries where prescription regulations are not as restrictive as in the United States and Canada, many antibiotics are OTC drugs, including chloramphenicol. What might be the consequences of this lack of regulation?
4. Why is it important to monitor urinary output with the administration of the various antimicrobials?
5. Molly Ellis, age 22, has an acute lower urinary tract infection. Her health care provider prescribes the sulfonamide sulfisoxazole for 10 days. What instruction may be required to enable Ms. Ellis to manage her drug therapy effectively? What instruction should be reviewed with the client to assist her in preventing recurrences of the UTI?

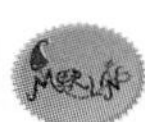

Collaborative Learning Activities

For Collaborative Learning Activities, go to mosby.com/MERLIN/McKenry/.

CASE STUDY

For a Case Study that will help ensure mastery of this chapter content, go to mosby.com/MERLIN/McKenry/.

BIBLIOGRAPHY

Ahronheim, J.C. (1992). *Handbook of prescribing medications for geriatric patients*. Boston: Little, Brown.

American Hospital Formulary Service. (1999). *AHFS drug information '99*. Bethesda, MD: American Society of Hospital Pharmacists.

Anderson, K.N., Anderson, L.E., & Glanze, W.D. (Eds.) (1998). *Mosby's medical, nursing, & allied health dictionary* (5th ed.). St. Louis: Mosby.

Andes, D.R. & Craig, W.A. Pharmacokinetics and pharmacodynamics of antibiotics in meningitis. *Infectious Disease Clinics of North America, 13*(3), 595-618.

Andriole, V.T. (1999). When to do culture in urinary tract infections. *International Journal of Antimicrobial Agents, 11*(3-4), 253-255.

Beringer, P.M. & Middleton, R.K. (1995). Anaphylaxis and drug allergies. In L.Y. Young & M.A. Koda-Kimble (Eds.), *Applied therapeutics: The clinical use of drugs* (6th ed.). Vancouver, WA: Applied Therapeutics.

Brismar, B. & Nord, C.E. (1999). Monobactams and carbapenems for treatment of intraabdominal infections. *Infection, 27*(2), 136-147.

Brumfitt, W. & Hamilton-Miller, J.M. (1999). Cefaclor into the millennium. *Journal of Chemotherapy, 11*(3), 163-178.

Carrie, A.G. & Zhanel, G.G. (1999). Antibacterial use in community practice: Assessing quantity, indications and appropriateness, and relationship to the development of antibacterial resistance. *Drugs, 57*(6), 871-881.

Cieslak, P.R., Strausbaugh, L.J., Fleming, D.W., & Ling, J.M. (1999). Vancomycin in Oregon: Who's using it and why. *Infection Control & Hospital Epidemiology, 20*(8), 557-560.

Cristino, J.M. (1999). Correlation between consumption of antimicrobials in humans and development of resistance in bacteria. *International Journal of Antimicrobial Agents, 12*(3), 199-202.

Danziger, L.H. & Itokazu, G.S. (1995). Gastrointestinal infections. In L.Y. Young & M.A. Koda-Kimble (Eds.). *Applied therapeutics: The clinical use of drugs* (6th ed.). Vancouver, WA: Applied Therapeutics.

Doughty, D.B. & Jackson, D.B. (1993). *Gastrointestinal disorders*. St. Louis: Mosby.

Drug Facts and Comparisons. (2000). St. Louis: Facts and Comparisons.

Fridkin, S.K., Edwards, J.R., Pichette, S.C., Pryor, E.R., McGowan, J.E. Jr., Tenover, F.C., Culver, D.H., Gaynes, R.P. (1999). Determinants of vancomycin use in adult intensive care units in 41 United States hospitals. *Clinical Infectious Diseases, 28*(5), 1119-1125.

Hellinger, W.C. & Brewer, N.S. (1999). Carbapenems and monobactams; imipenem, meropenem, and aztreonam. *Mayo Clinic Proceedings, 74*(4), 420-434.

Just, P.M. (1994). Overview of the fluoroquinolone antibiotics. *Pharmacotherapeutics, 13*(2 pt 2), 4S.

Kasten, M.J. (1999). Clindamycin, metronidazole, and chloramphenicol. *Mayo Clinic Proceedings, 74*(8), 825-833.

Katzung, B.G. (1992). *Basic and clinical pharmacology* (5th ed.). Norwalk, CT: Appleton & Lange.

Mandell, G.L. & Petri, Jr. W.A. (1996). Antimicrobial agents. In J.G. Hardman & L.E. Limbird (Eds.), *Goodman & Gilman's The pharmacological basis of therapeutics* (9th ed.). New York: McGraw-Hill.

Moore, P.A. (1999). Dental therapeutic indications for the newer long-acting macrolide antibiotics. *Journal of the American Dental Association, 130*(9), 1341-1343.

Mullenix, T., & Prince, R.A. (1997). Urinary tract infections and prostatitis. In J.T. DiPiro, R.L. Talbert, G.C. Yee, G.R. Matzke, B.G. Wells, & L.M. Posey (Eds.), *Pharmacotherapy: A pathophysiological approach* (3rd ed.). Norwalk, CT: Appleton & Lange.

Nelson, R.R. (1999). Intrinsically vancomycin-resistant gram-positive organisms: Clinical relevance and implications for infection control. *Journal of Hospital Infection, 42*(4), 275-282.

Rice, L.B. (1999). Successful interventions for gram-negative resistance to extended-spectrum beta-lactam antibiotics. *Pharmacotherapy, 19*(8 pt 2), 120S-128S.

Rosenberg, M. (1999). Pharmacoeconomics of treating uncomplicated urinary tract infections. *International Journal of Antimicrobial Agents, 11*(3-4), 247-251.

Sahai, J.V. (1995). Urinary tract infections. In L.Y. Young & M.A. Koda-Kimble (Eds.), *Applied therapeutics: The clinical use of drugs* (6th ed.). Vancouver, WA: Applied Therapeutics.

Semla, T.P., Beizer, J.L., & Higbee, M.D. (1993). *Geriatric dosage handbook.* Cleveland: American Pharmaceutical Association & Lexi-Comp.

Smilack, J.D. (1999) The tetracyclines. *Mayo Clinic Proceedings,* 74(7), 727-729.

United States Pharmacopeia Dispensing Information (USP DI): Advice for the patient: Drug information in lay language (19th ed.). (1999). Rockville, MD: United States Pharmacopeial Convention.

United States Pharmacopeia Dispensing Information (USP DI): Drug information for the health care professional (19th ed.). (1999). Rockville, MD: United States Pharmacopeial Convention.

Williams, S.R. (1995). *Basic nutrition and diet therapy* (10th ed.). St. Louis: Mosby.

60 Antifungal and Antiviral Drugs

Chapter Focus

Clients receiving broad-spectrum antibiotics for an infection, clients who are immunosuppressed as the result of a transplant or antineoplastic therapy, and clients with acquired immunodeficiency syndrome (AIDS) are all at risk for the development of superinfection with fungal or viral organisms. The growth of the AIDS epidemic has certainly fostered pharmaceutical research for agents to combat the diseases caused by these organisms. The last few years have seen the Food and Drug Administration approving these drugs in record time compared to past reviews. The nurse needs to remain current in the knowledge of old standards and newly approved antifungal and antiviral drugs.

Learning Objectives

1. List four commonly used antifungal agents.
2. Describe five side effects/adverse reactions of antifungal agents.
3. Implement the nursing management for the care of clients receiving antifungal agents.
4. State two reasons why effective antiviral drug therapy is more limited than antibacterial and antifungal therapy.
5. List four commonly used systemic antiviral agents.
6. Implement the nursing management for the care of clients receiving antiviral therapy.

Key Terms

candidiasis, p. 1014
chemoprophylactic, p. 1021
fungi, p. 1014
mycoses, p. 1014

Key Drugs [✔]

acyclovir, p. 1024
amphotericin B, p. 1014
indinavir, p. 1034
ketoconazole, p. 1016
zidovudine, p. 1033

ANTIFUNGAL DRUGS

Human infections with **fungi** can be caused by any of approximately 50 species of plantlike, parasitic microorganisms. These simple, parasitic plants lack chlorophyll; as a result, they are unable to make their own food and are dependent on other life forms. Infections with fungi, or **mycoses,** can range from mild and superficial to severe and life threatening. Infecting organisms can be ingested orally, implanted under the skin after injury, or inhaled if the fungal spores are airborne. One species of fungi, *Candida albicans,* is usually part of the normal flora of the skin, mouth, intestines, and vagina; overgrowth and systemic infection may result from antibiotic, antineoplastic, and corticosteroid drug therapy. This is referred to as an opportunistic infection. Oral **candidiasis** (thrush) is common in newborn infants and immunocompromised clients, whereas vaginal candidiasis is common in women who are pregnant, have diabetes mellitus, or take oral contraceptives. With the increase in the incidence of acquired immunodeficiency syndrome (AIDS), the prevalence of mycoses has increased as an opportunistic infection in clients with AIDS. Nonopportunistic fungal infections such as blastomycosis, histoplasmosis, and others are usually rare.

The lag in the development of antifungal chemotherapy is related to the high chemical antifungal concentrations that are necessary, which cannot be tolerated by the human host. Therefore only a few antifungal compounds are available for systemic use. The following discussions include only systemic agents. Topical antifungal preparations are discussed in Chapter 66.

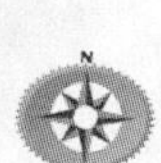

For a Concept Map on HIV, go to mosby.com/MERLIN/McKenry/.

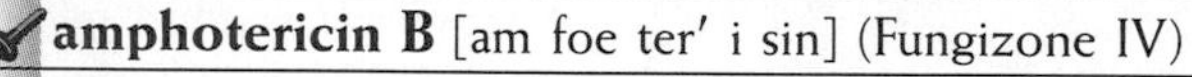

amphotericin B [am foe ter' i sin] (Fungizone IV)

Amphotericin B can be fungistatic or fungicidal depending on the concentrations achieved clinically. This drug does not have a therapeutic effect on bacteria or viruses. Amphotericin B binds to sterols in the fungus cell membrane, which increases cell permeability and results in a loss of potassium and other elements from the cell.

Amphotericin B is effective for treating aspergillosis, blastomycosis, candidiasis (moniliasis), coccidioidomycosis, cryptococcosis, fungal endocarditis, histoplasmosis, cryptococcal meningitis, fungal septicemia, and many other systemic fungal infections.

Administered parenterally, amphotericin B is widely distributed in the body. The initial half-life in adults is 24 hours, and the elimination half-life is approximately 15 days. The site of metabolism is unknown, but it is excreted by the kidneys. Approximately 40% of the drug is excreted over 7 days, but it can be detected in the urine for at least 7 weeks after it is discontinued.

The common side effects/adverse reactions with the IV infusion of amphotericin B include headache, gastrointestinal distress, anemia, hypokalemia, fever, chills, nausea, vomiting, and renal impairment.

The adult dosage for a systemic fungus infection is usually a 1-mg test dose in 5% dextrose solution administered over 10 to 30 minutes. This is followed by 5- to 10-mg increments of amphotericin B infusion (up to 50 mg/day), which are administered over 2 to 6 hours depending on the infection and the client's tolerance of the medication. The initial pediatric dosage is 0.25 mg/kg daily in 5% dextrose administered over 6 hours. The dosage may be increased gradually (up to 1 mg/kg/day), depending on the infection and the child's tolerance of the medication.

Amphotericin B lipid complex injection (Abelcet) is a liposomal encapsulation of amphotericin used to treat aspergillosis in clients who are refractory to or unable to tolerate standard amphotericin B therapy. The liposome formulation provides a therapeutic effect with significantly less nephrotoxicity than amphotericin B. The most common side effects/adverse reactions include fever, chills, nausea, hypotension, vomiting, dyspnea, and respiratory failure. The usual daily dose of Abelcet for adults and children is 5 mg/kg by a single infusion at a rate of 2.5 mg/kg/hr. See current drug references for additional information on this product (Abelcet, 1996).

■ Nursing Management

Amphotericin B Therapy

■ **Assessment.** Amphotericin B is used with caution if renal function is impaired. Although it is not renally excreted, amphotericin B is nephrotoxic and can worsen any preexisting renal pathologic condition. It is also administered with caution if there is intolerance to the drug or if the client is receiving other nephrotoxic agents. Leukocyte transfusions should not be administered concurrently with amphotericin B lipid complex (Abelcet); acute pulmonary toxicity has been reported.

Review the client's current medication regimen for the risk of significant drug interactions, such as those that may occur when amphotericin B is given concurrently with the following drugs:

Drug	Possible Effect and Management
adrenocorticoids, glucocorticoids, mineralocorticoids (ACTH)	May result in severe hypokalemia; if given concurrently, serum potassium determinations should be performed at frequent intervals. May decrease the adrenal cortex response to corticotropin (ACTH).
bone marrow depressants, radiation therapy	May produce increased bone marrow depressant effects; monitor blood cell counts closely because dosage adjustments may be necessary if anemia, leukopenia, or thrombocytopenia become extreme.
digitalis glycosides	Amphotericin B–induced hypokalemia may increase the potential for digitalis toxicity. Monitor closely for dysrhythmias, anorexia, nausea, vomiting, or other indications of possible toxicity.
nephrotoxic medications, potassium-depleting diuretics	Increased risk of nephrotoxicity; monitor closely for edema and oliguria, because dosage adjustments may be necessary.

A baseline assessment of the client's general health status should be obtained and include the underlying condition, weight, blood urea nitrogen (BUN), serum creatinine concentrations, electrolyte levels (particularly potassium), and complete blood and platelet counts. Appropriate specimens should be obtained before initiating therapy to identify the causative fungi.

■ **Nursing Diagnosis.** Clients receiving amphotericin B are at risk for the following nursing diagnoses/collaborative problems: deficient fluid volume related to anorexia, nausea, and vomiting; activity intolerance related to anemia or hypokalemia; hyperthermia; ineffective protection related to leukopenia and thrombocytopenia; impaired tissue integrity related to extravasation or thrombophlebitis at the infusion site; disturbed sensory perception related to polyneuropathy (numbness, tingling, or burning in the hands and feet), hearing loss, or a change in vision; and the potential complications of infusion-related reaction (fever, chills, nausea, vomiting, headache, hypotension), seizures, electrolyte imbalances (hypokalemia, hypomagnesemia), hypersensitivity, cardiac dysrhythmias, and nephrotoxicity (increased or decreased urinary output).

■ **Implementation**

■ ***Monitoring.*** Monitor vital signs and observe for adverse reactions (shortness of breath, fever, chills, nausea, and vomiting) during the test dose, which is usually administered when starting all new courses of therapy. A febrile response usually lasts for less than 4 hours after the infusion.

BUN and serum creatinine values should be determined every other day as the dosage is increased to its optimal level and then weekly once the maintenance dosage is achieved and until the drug is discontinued. If BUN levels exceed 40 mg/dL or serum creatinine increases to 3 mg/dL, the dosage should be decreased or discontinued until renal function improves. Serum potassium and magnesium levels should be monitored twice a week. Blood counts should be monitored weekly in anticipation of bone marrow suppression.

Pain at the site of infusion may indicate extravasation. Be cautious, because the drug causes local tissue irritation and thrombophlebitis.

Clients receiving amphotericin B intravenously should be assessed for gastrointestinal disturbances such as anorexia, indigestion, nausea and vomiting, and diarrhea. Daily weight monitoring will determine if these symptoms are associated with weight loss. Monitor fluid intake and output to determine fluid loss and renal status. Observe for signs of hypokalemia, such as muscle cramps, irregular pulse, and weakness or lethargy. Monitor for symptoms of bone marrow suppression (fever, sore throat, and unusual bleeding or bruising), and report them to the prescriber.

■ ***Intervention.*** Amphotericin B should not be used if there is any evidence of precipitate or foreign matter in the vial. Before administering, package inserts should be read for the major points of safe delivery. Because amphotericin B is incompatible with a wide range of drugs, confirm its compatibility with other drugs before preparing the infusion.

Reconstitute amphotericin B only with the diluents recommended; sodium chloride or bacteriostatic agents such as benzyl alcohol will cause the drug to precipitate. The pH of the dextrose injection should be above 4.2 before adding the drug. The manufacturer's package insert provides the aseptic procedure for testing and adjusting the pH if necessary. If in-line IV filters are used, they should have at least a 1-μm mean pore diameter, otherwise they may filter out clinically significant amounts of the drug. Gloves should be worn while preparing the drug. Because the reconstituted preparation is a colloidal suspension, the in-line membrane filter on the infusion should be no less than one micron mean pore diameter. Infuse slowly over 2 to 6 hours to minimize adverse cardiovascular reactions. In-line filters should not be used with the amphotericin B lipid complex (Abelcet) form of the drug. Shake the hanging solution every half hour during administration to keep it in suspension.

Administering amphotericin B on alternate days and over a 6-hour period may reduce the incidence of side effects. If therapy is interrupted for more than 7 days, the dosage should be restarted at the lowest level and increased to the appropriate therapeutic level. The duration of the course of amphotericin B should be sufficient to prevent a relapse.

Febrile reactions during administration may be minimized by administering a small dose of IV adrenocorticoid just before the infusion of amphotericin B. Antipyretics and antihistamines are also used. Nephrotoxicity may be minimized by sodium bicarbonate diuresis or salt loading just before the administration of amphotericin B. Heparin may be added to the IV infusion of amphotericin B to help prevent thrombophlebitis at the IV site. The infusion site should be changed with each dose to minimize the development of thrombophlebitis.

If the client has gastrointestinal symptoms during the administration of amphotericin B, a pleasant and relaxed atmosphere for mealtimes should be provided; small, frequent feedings of high-protein, high-calorie foods of the client's choice should be encouraged; and good oral hygiene should be maintained. Palliative medication may be necessary if the client is experiencing indigestion, vomiting, or diarrhea.

■ ***Education.*** The client should be advised to complete essential dental work before starting therapy with amphotericin B or to delay it until therapy is completed. The bone marrow suppressant effects of this drug may cause gingival bleeding and delay healing.

Appropriate oral hygiene should be taught, including the gentle use of soft toothbrushes and dental floss and the avoidance of toothpicks. Advise the client to alert the nursing staff at the first indication of pain at the IV site.

Alert the client to the side effects and adverse reactions of the drug and the need to report these promptly.

■ **Evaluation.** The expected outcome of amphotericin B therapy is that the client will experience symptomatic improvement, with clinical and laboratory evidence of decreased fungal infection, and will experience no adverse reactions to amphotericin B.

Azole Antifungals

fluconazole [floo koe' na zole] (Diflucan ◆)
itraconazole [eye trah koe' na zole] (Sporanox)
ketoconazole [kee toe koe' na zole] (Nizoral)
miconazole [my kon' a zole] injection (Monistat IV)

The azole antifungals may be fungistatic or fungicidal agents depending on the dosage and systemic levels achieved. Ergosterol is the primary sterol in fungus cell membranes. Azole antifungals affect the biosynthesis of the fungal sterols by interfering with the cytochrome P-450 enzyme system. The result is impaired or depleted ergosterol biosynthesis, which inhibits fungus growth.

Fluconazole and itraconazole have a greater affinity for fungal cytochrome P-450 activity than for the human liver cytochrome P-450 system. Fluconazole has good penetration in cerebrospinal fluid (CSF) and therefore is used for the treatment of cryptococcal meningitis; itraconazole has poor CSF penetration but is widely distributed in the body and is indicated for the treatment of aspergillosis, blastomycosis, and histoplasmosis (DeRosso & Gupta, 1999).

Ketoconazole is well distributed in body fluids (saliva, bile, urine, breast milk, and inflamed joint fluid), tendons, and other body tissues. It is indicated for the treatment of disseminated and mucocutaneous candidiasis, paracoccidioidomycosis, and recalcitrant tinea infections. Miconazole is also widely distributed in body tissues, but neither ketoconazole nor miconazole adequately crosses the blood-brain barrier. Miconazole is primarily indicated for the treatment of disseminated and chronic mucocutaneous candidiasis.

Pharmacokinetically, fluconazole, itraconazole, and ketoconazole are administered orally; fluconazole and miconazole may be administered intravenously. Oral administration rates are good if fluconazole is administered in the fasting state; itraconazole and ketoconazole should be administered with food. Ketoconazole requires an acid medium for dissolution and absorption; therefore achlorhydria, hypochlorhydria, or an increase in stomach pH caused by medications will impair the absorption of ketoconazole. Table 60-1 provides a summary of the pharmacokinetics and usual adult dosages of the azole antifungals.

The side effects/adverse reactions of the azole antifungals include nausea, vomiting, stomach distress, and diarrhea. Rash is more commonly reported with itraconazole. Ketoconazole can cause gynecomastia and impotency due to the inhibition of adrenal steroid and testosterone synthesis, but these reactions are rare. Menstrual irregularities have also been reported. Miconazole may cause phlebitis at the injection site; nausea, vomiting, and cardiorespiratory arrest have been reported with an injection that is too rapid.

■ Nursing Management

Azole Antifungal Therapy

■ **Assessment.** The risk of administering fluconazole should be considered for clients with impaired renal function; with these clients, the doses may need to be decreased or the dosage interval increased. There is no renal limitation for itraconazole. However, hypersensitivity to either drug or other azole antifungal agents may be a contraindication for use of the drug. Clients with achlorhydria or hypochlorhydria, which is common with AIDS, may experience a reduced absorption of these drugs. Use antifungals (especially ketoconazole) cautiously in clients with alcoholism or hepatic function impairment, because these clients are at risk for drug-induced hepatotoxicity. Ketoconazole has been known to cause a disulfiram-like reaction (flushing, rash, peripheral edema, headache, nausea, and vomiting) as a response to alcohol ingestion.

Review client's current medication regimen for the risk of significant drug interactions, such as those that may occur

TABLE 60-1 Azole Antifungals: Pharmacokinetics and Usual Adult Dosage

	Pharmacokinetics		
Drug	**Peak Serum (hours)***	**Half-life (hours)†**	**Usual Adult Dosage**
fluconazole (Diflucan)	1-2	Adults: 30 Children: 14-20	100-200 mg PO/IV daily
itraconazole (Sporanox)	3-4	Single dose: 21 Steady state: 64	200 mg PO once or twice daily
ketoconazole (Nizoral)	1-4	8	200 to 400 mg PO daily
miconazole (Monistat IV)	E of I	20-25	0.2 to 1.2 g IV infusion

Information from *Drug Facts and Comparisons* (2000). St. Louis: Facts and Comparisons; and *United States Pharmacopeia Dispensing Information (USP DI): Drug information for the health care professional* (19th ed.). (1999). Rockville, MD: United States Pharmacopeial Convention.
E of I, End of infusion.
*Time to peak serum concentration.
†Half-life for normal renal function.

when azole antifungals are given concurrently with the following drugs:

Drug	Possible Effect and Management
Bold/color type indicates the most serious interactions.	
alcohol or hepatotoxic drugs	Concurrent use increases the risk for hepatotoxicity. The use of alcohol and ketoconazole is reported to cause a disulfiram-like reaction.
antacids, anticholinergics, histamine H_2-receptor antagonists, omeprazole (Prilosec), sucralfate (Carafate), didanosine (Videx, ddI)	These drugs increase gastrointestinal pH, thereby reducing the absorption of itraconazole and ketoconazole. Administer the drugs at least 2 hours apart.
astemizole (Hismanal) or terfenadine* (Seldane)	**Concurrent use results in elevated plasma levels of astemizole or terfenadine by inhibiting their metabolic pathway, which may result in cardiac dysrhythmias and death. Avoid concurrent use or a potentially serious drug interaction may occur.**
carbamazepine (Tegretol)	Concurrent use decreases itraconazole levels and may lead to treatment failures.
cyclosporine (Sandimmune)	Monitor plasma cyclosporine levels closely, because they have been reported to increase in some clients receiving both cyclosporine and systemic azole antifungals.
didanosine (ddI, Videx)	Contains a buffer to increase gastrointestinal pH. Decreases the absorption of oral itraconazole and ketoconazole. Antifungals should be administered 2 hours before or after this drug.
digoxin (Lanoxin)	Itraconazole and ketoconazole increase serum digoxin levels, leading to digoxin toxicity. Monitor digoxin levels carefully.
hypoglycemic agents (oral chlorpropamide [Diabinese], glyburide [DiaBeta], glipizide [Glucotrol], tolbutamide [Orinase])	May result in increased serum concentrations of these antidiabetic agents, leading to hypoglycemia. Closely monitor blood glucose levels if drugs are given concurrently, because a dosage adjustment of the antidiabetic agents may be necessary.
indinavir (Crixivan)	Concurrent use with ketoconazole increases serum levels of this drug. A dosage reduction is recommended.
lovastatin (Mevacor) or simvastatin (Zocor)	Itraconazole inhibits the metabolism of these drugs, and the combination has been associated with rhabdomyolysis. Discontinue these drugs temporarily when administering itraconazole.
midazolam (Versed) or triazolam (Halcion)	Concurrent use with itraconazole or ketoconazole increases the sedative effects of these drugs. The oral forms of midazolam and triazolam should not be used concurrently with the antifungals.
phenytoin (Dilantin)	Concurrent use increases serum concentrations of phenytoin and decreases serum levels of the azole antifungals. The response to both medications should be monitored carefully.
rifampin (Rifadin) or isoniazid (INH, Laniazid)	Concurrent drug administration may result in increased fluconazole metabolism. Monitor closely; the dosage of fluconazole may need to be increased.
warfarin (Coumadin)	May result in a decrease in warfarin metabolism, resulting in an increase in prothrombin time (PT). Closely monitor PTs in clients who are receiving both drugs concurrently.

*No longer available in the United States but may be available in other countries.

A baseline assessment of the client's general health status is necessary and should include the underlying infection, weight, BUN and serum creatinine values, and liver function tests. Appropriate specimens should be taken to identify the causative fungi before initiating therapy.

■ **Nursing Diagnosis.** The client receiving azole antifungal agents is at risk for the following nursing diagnoses/collaborative problems: impaired tissue integrity due to IV administration (phlebitis); impaired comfort related to the central nervous system (CNS) effects of the drug (headache, dizziness, photophobia); sexual dysfunction (impotence); disturbed body image in male clients related to gynecomastia or impotence; deficient fluid volume related to anorexia, nausea, or vomiting; and the potential complications of anemia, agranulocytosis, thrombocytopenia, hypersensitivity (fever, chills, skin rash, and itching), Stevens-Johnson syndrome (blistering or peeling of skin), and hepatotoxicity.

■ **Implementation**

■ ***Monitoring.*** Monitor the site of the infection for improvement, because the dosage and length of treatment are determined by this and by the client's general response to therapy. Clients infected with human immunodeficiency virus (HIV) have a greater incidence of side effects with fluconazole (21%) than those who are HIV negative (13%); therefore they require closer management. BUN and serum creatinine values should be determined at routine intervals until the drug is discontinued.

Clients receiving azole antifungals should be assessed for gastrointestinal disturbances such as anorexia, indigestion, nausea and vomiting, and diarrhea. Daily weights will determine if these symptoms are associated with weight loss. Monitor fluid intake and output to determine fluid loss and renal status. Clients receiving itraconazole require periodic serum potassium determinations because hypokalemia can occur, leading to ventricular fibrillation.

The IV site for miconazole should be monitored periodically for pain and inflammation, which indicates phlebitis. Monitor complete blood counts (CBCs) for anemia and thrombocytopenia. Monitor serum electrolytes for hyponatremia and blood lipids for increases at periodic intervals.

Liver function studies need to be monitored; although a mild, transient increase in transaminases may occur with therapy, it may, on rare occasion, progress to hepatotoxicity.

Observe the client for dark urine, jaundice, and right upper quadrant abdominal pain.

▪ ***Intervention.*** Maintenance therapy with antifungals may be required with HIV-infected clients to prevent a relapse of their infection. Consult with the prescriber for an antiemetic prescription to manage nausea or vomiting or for an analgesic to treat a drug-induced headache.

The dosage for oral fluconazole is almost the same as the daily IV dosage because it is almost completely bioavailable. Itraconazole capsules and ketoconazole are administered with food to increase absorption; itraconazole solution is to be taken on an empty stomach for the same reason. If the client is receiving hemodialysis, fluconazole should be administered after dialysis so that plasma concentrations of the drug are not reduced. No change of therapy is required for clients who are undergoing continuous ambulatory peritoneal dialysis (CAPD).

Absorption may be decreased in clients who have achlorhydria and are taking ketoconazole tablets. To minimize this effect, the prescriber may prescribe that each tablet be dissolved in 4 mL of 0.2 N hydrochloric acid. The solution may be further diluted with a small amount of water and administered through a plastic or glass straw to prevent contact with the teeth. Have the client rinse his or her mouth with water and swallow the solution.

Administer IV fluconazole by continuous infusion; use an infusion pump and do not exceed 200 mg/hr. Do not mix other drugs with fluconazole.

The first dose of miconazole should be a test dose of 200 mg administered by IV infusion to determine whether the client is hypersensitive to the drug. Dilute each dose of miconazole in at least 200 mL of 0.9% sodium chloride solution or 5% dextrose injection for IV infusion. This solution will be stable at room temperature for 24 hours. The solution should be discarded if it darkens, because it has deteriorated. Do not mix with other medications. Administer IV infusions of miconazole over 30 to 60 minutes to prevent the dysrhythmias or increases in heart rate that can result from rapid administration. The nausea and vomiting secondary to the administration of miconazole may be minimized by reducing the dosage, slowing the infusion rate, or administering an antiemetic before beginning the infusion. To help prevent gastrointestinal effects, infusions should not be administered at mealtimes. Pruritus may be controlled by diphenhydramine. With mycoses of the bladder, IV administration of miconazole must be supplemented by bladder irrigation with miconazole solution; with fungal meningitis, IV administration must be supplemented by intrathecal administration, alternating the injections between cervical, lumbar, and cisternal punctures every 3 to 7 days.

▪ ***Education.*** Recommend that the client take ketoconazole with meals or food to minimize nausea and enhance absorption. Therapy is usually long term—in some cases months or years. Advise the client to complete the full course of medication even if he or she is feeling better, to maintain regular visits with the prescriber for monitoring, and to be alert for significant side effects/adverse reactions to report to the provider. Taking the drug at the same time every day increases compliance. Infected areas should be reevaluated periodically.

Caution the client to avoid alcoholic beverages while undergoing ketoconazole therapy. Advise the client to avoid exposure to bright light and to wear sunglasses because of the photophobic effects of the drug. Because ketoconazole causes drowsiness, caution the client to avoid activities that require mental alertness until his or her response has been determined.

With IV miconazole, instruct the client to alert the nurse if he or she has trouble breathing, a skin rash, or fever and chills; these are signs of hypersensitivity. Advise the client that it may take weeks or months for a therapeutic response to occur.

▪ **Evaluation.** The expected outcome of azole antifungal therapy is that the client will experience symptomatic improvement, with clinical and laboratory evidence of decreased fungal infection and without experiencing any adverse reactions to the specific agent.

flucytosine capsules [floo sye′ toe seen] (Ancobon, Ancotil 🍁)

Flucytosine enters fungus cells, where it is converted to fluorouracil, an antimetabolite. It interferes with the metabolism of pyrimidine, thus preventing the synthesis of nucleic acids and protein. It has selective toxicity against susceptible strains of fungi because the body cells do not convert significant quantities of this drug into fluorouracil.

Flucytosine is indicated for the treatment of fungal endocarditis caused by *Candida* species, fungal meningitis caused by *Cryptococcus* species, and fungal pneumonia, septicemia, or urinary infections caused by *Candida* or *Cryptococcus* species. It is well absorbed orally and widely distributed in the body, including the CSF; the CSF is approximately 60% to 90% of serum concentrations. Flucytosine, with a half-life of 2.5 to 6 hours, is not significantly metabolized but is excreted by the kidneys, mostly as unchanged drug.

The common side effects/adverse reactions of flucytosine include gastric distress, anemia, hepatitis, hypersensitivity, and bone marrow suppression. The adult and pediatric oral dosage is 12.5 to 37.5 mg/kg every 6 hours.

▪ Nursing Management

Flucytosine Therapy

▪ **Assessment.** Use flucytosine with caution if a client has preexisting bone marrow suppression, has had or is currently using a cytotoxic drug or radiation therapy, or has hepatic or renal function impairment. Renal impairment necessitates a dosage adjustment. This therapy is contraindicated if the client is allergic to flucytosine.

Administration of flucytosine concurrently with bone marrow depressants or radiation therapy may enhance the bone marrow suppressant effects; monitor CBCs closely, because dosage adjustments may be necessary.

A baseline assessment of the client's general health status, including the underlying infection, weight, CBC and platelet counts, BUN and serum creatinine values, and liver function values is necessary. Appropriate specimens should be taken to identify the causative fungi before initiating therapy.

■ **Nursing Diagnosis.** Clients receiving flucytosine should be assessed for the possibility of the following nursing diagnoses/collaborative problems: impaired comfort (headache, abdominal cramping); deficient fluid volume related to anorexia, nausea, or vomiting; activity intolerance related to anemia; ineffective protection related to leukopenia or thrombocytopenia; disturbed thought processes (confusion, hallucinations) related to CNS effects; and the potential complications of hypersensitivity and the development of hepatitis.

■ **Implementation**

■ ***Monitoring.*** Assess the client's fungal infection for improvement. Monitor intake and output to ensure adequate hydration and to minimize adverse renal reactions. Weigh the client daily to monitor nutritional status if the client has gastrointestinal side effects. Monitor the client for signs of bone marrow depression such as a sore throat and fever and signs of unusual bleeding, bruising, weakness, or tiredness.

Monitor blood counts and renal function studies during the course of therapy, as well as hepatic function studies (AST [SGOT]), (ALT [SGPT]), serum alkaline phosphatase, and serum bilirubin concentrations.

The serum level of flucytosine may be measured to ascertain whether it is being maintained in the therapeutic range (20 to 25 μg/mL). Serum concentrations are also used to assess renal excretion and prevent drug accumulation in clients with renal function impairment (creatinine clearance <40 mL/min).

■ ***Intervention.*** If multiple-dose units are prescribed as a single dose, administer them over 15 minutes to help prevent nausea and vomiting. Treat the client palliatively with antiemetics if these symptoms occur. Flucytosine is usually administered concurrently with parenteral amphotericin B to prevent the fungal resistance that may develop rapidly if it is used alone.

■ ***Education.*** Encourage the client to comply with the full course of therapy, even if he or she is feeling better. Progress should be monitored by regular visits to the health care provider. Advise the client to report any syncope, dizziness, or drowsiness to the health care provider.

As with amphotericin B, advise the client to complete dental work before or delay it until after a course of flucytosine. Recommend the gentle use of soft toothbrushes and dental floss and the avoidance of toothpicks because of the risk of gingival bleeding.

■ **Evaluation.** The expected outcome of flucytosine therapy is that the client will experience symptomatic relief and that therapeutic drug levels (20 to 25 μg/mL) are maintained without evidence of any adverse reactions to the drug.

griseofulvin microsize [gri see oh ful′ vin] (Grisactin, Grifulvin V, Fulvicin-U/F, Grisovin-FP ♣)
griseofulvin tablets, ultramicrosize (Fulvicin P/G)

Griseofulvin is a fungistatic agent; it inhibits fungus cell mitosis during metaphase. It is also deposited in the keratin precursor cells in the skin, hair, and nails, thus inhibiting fungal invasion of the keratin. When infested keratin is shed, healthy keratin replaces it. Griseofulvin is indicated for the treatment of susceptible organisms for onychomycosis, tinea barbae, tinea capitis, tinea corporis, tinea cruris, and tinea pedis.

The oral absorption of microsize griseofulvin varies from 25% to 70% of the oral dose, whereas the ultramicrosize form is nearly completely absorbed. Absorption is significantly enhanced if griseofulvin is administered with or after a fatty meal. Griseofulvin is distributed in keratin layers in the skin, hair, and nails; very little is distributed in body tissues and fluids. It has a half-life of 24 hours and reaches peak serum levels in approximately 4 hours. This drug is metabolized in the liver and excreted primarily unchanged in the feces.

The most commonly reported side effect of griseofulvin is headache; less commonly noted is hypersensitivity, confusion, gastric distress, oral thrush, weakness, and photosensitivity.

The oral adult dosage of microsize griseofulvin is 500 mg daily; the dose may be divided in 2 doses. To treat tinea pedis or onychomycosis, the dosage is 500 mg twice daily. The pediatric dosage is 5 mg/kg every 12 hours (*United States Pharmacopeia Dispensing Information*, 1999). The adult dosage for ultramicrosize is 250 to 375 mg daily.

■ **Nursing Management**

Griseofulvin Therapy

■ **Assessment.** Administer griseofulvin with caution if a client has preexisting porphyria, lupus erythematosus, hepatic function impairment, or sensitivity to griseofulvin.

Review the client's current medication regimen for the risk of significant drug interactions, such as those that may occur when griseofulvin is given concurrently with the following drugs:

Drug	Possible Effect and Management
anticoagulants, oral (coumarin or indanedione)	A decreased anticoagulant effect may be noted; monitor PT closely until a stable serum level is achieved. Dosage adjustments may be required during and after griseofulvin administration.
contraceptives, estrogen containing, oral	Chronic, long-term use of griseofulvin may decrease the effectiveness of oral contraceptives. Intercycle menstrual bleeding, amenorrhea, or pregnancy may occur. Advise the client to use an alternate method of contraception when taking griseofulvin.

The client's baseline assessment should include the underlying condition for which the griseofulvin is prescribed, a mental status examination, a CBC, serum creatinine concentration, urinalysis, and hepatic function studies. As with other antiinfectives, obtain specimens for culture before starting griseofulvin therapy.

■ **Nursing Diagnosis.** The client receiving griseofulvin should be assessed for the following nursing diagnoses/collaborative problems: impaired comfort (headache, abdominal cramping); fatigue; deficient fluid volume related to anorexia, nausea, or vomiting; risk for injury related to dizziness; ineffective protection related to leukopenia and agranulocytopenia; impaired oral mucous membrane related to oral thrush; disturbed sleep pattern (insomnia) related to CNS effects; disturbed sensory perception related to peripheral neuritis (numbness and tingling of the hands and feet); disturbed thought processes (confusion) related to CNS effects; and the potential complications of hypersensitivity, photosensitivity, or the development of hepatitis (jaundiced skin and sclera).

■ **Implementation**

■ ***Monitoring.*** Monitor blood counts and hepatic and renal function studies periodically during therapy. Therapy is continued until clinical signs or laboratory confirmation indicates that the causative organism has been eradicated.

■ ***Intervention.*** Administer griseofulvin with meals to help prevent gastrointestinal distress and to enhance absorption. Therapy is even more effective if the meal is fatty. Consult the prescriber if the client is on a low-fat diet. The concurrent use of an appropriate topical agent maximizes the therapeutic effect of griseofulvin and reduces the possibility of relapse. Administer the oral suspension using the calibrated measuring device provided by the manufacturer.

■ ***Education.*** Encourage the client to comply with the full course of therapy, even if he or she is feeling better. Regular visits to the prescriber are necessary to check progress. Advise the client that the treatment period is lengthy: 8 to 10 weeks for tinea capitis, 2 to 4 weeks for tinea corporis, and 4 to 8 weeks for tinea pedis. For onychomycosis, the treatment is at least 4 months for fingernails and at least 6 months for toenails. Even with treatment, the recurrence rate is very high for onychomycosis of the toenails. Concurrent use of a topical agent reduces the likelihood of relapse in tinea pedis.

Frequent shampoos and clipping of the hair and nails, as well as keeping affected skin areas clean and dry, will support the therapeutic effect of griseofulvin. Advise the client that skin may be more sensitive to sunlight; recommend that the client use sunscreen and avoid direct sunlight.

Advise the client to report any symptoms of fever and sore throat to the prescriber; such symptoms may indicate blood dyscrasias. Because the drug may cause dizziness, the client should avoid tasks that require mental alertness until the response to the drug can be ascertained. Instruct the client about good oral hygiene and to report any soreness or irritation of the mouth, which might indicate a fungal overgrowth (oral thrush). Advise the client not to ingest alcoholic beverages while taking griseofulvin, because it may potentiate the effects of alcohol, causing tachycardia and flushing.

■ **Evaluation.** The expected outcome of griseofulvin therapy is that the client will experience symptomatic improvement without evidence of any adverse reactions to the drug.

nystatin lozenges [nye stat′ in] (Mycostatin)
nystatin (Mycostatin, Nilstat, Nadostine ♣)

Nystatin is an antibiotic primarily used to treat cutaneous or mucocutaneous infections caused by the monilial organism *C. albicans.* Nystatin adheres to sterols in the fungal cell membrane, altering cell membrane permeability and resulting in the loss of essential intercellular contents.

Nystatin is not absorbed from the gastrointestinal tract, and therefore its antifungal effect is local. It is excreted in the feces.

In general, the side effects/adverse reactions of nystatin are rare; abdominal distress is reported but is uncommon.

The usual oral adult dosage for candidiasis is a lozenge of 200,000 to 400,000 U dissolved slowly in the mouth 4 or 5 times daily. The oral suspension dosage is a lozenge of 400,000 to 600,000 U four times daily; the tablet dosage is 500,000 to 1,000,000 U three times daily.

■ Nursing Management

Nystatin Therapy

■ **Assessment.** It should be determined if the client has an intolerance to nystatin. A baseline assessment of the client's candidiasis condition should be obtained and documented. There are no significant drug interactions.

■ **Nursing Diagnosis.** The client receiving nystatin should be assessed for the possibility of the following nursing diagnoses: deficient fluid volume related to anorexia, nausea, and vomiting; impaired comfort (abdominal cramping); and diarrhea.

■ **Implementation**

■ ***Monitoring.*** Nystatin is virtually nontoxic and is well tolerated by all age-groups. Monitor the client's infection throughout the course of therapy. Examine the client's mouth with a tongue blade and flashlight.

■ ***Intervention.*** Shake oral suspensions thoroughly before measuring dosages. With the prepared oral suspension, use the calibrated dosage-measuring device provided by the manufacturer. When mixing dry powdered nystatin, add the dose to 120 to 240 mL of water; administer it immediately because it contains no preservatives. Lozenges or pastilles are used to treat oral candidiasis because they are slow to dissolve and are in contact longer with the buccal mucosa. With infants, swab nystatin on the oral mucosa.

■ ***Education.*** Instruct the client to perform oral hygiene before taking each dose of nystatin. Half the dosage is placed in each side of the mouth. The medication is swished and held in the mouth for as long as possible. Lozenges are to be dissolved slowly in the mouth.

Caution the client to complete the full course of therapy even if he or she is feeling better. Therapy should be continued for at least 48 hours after normal culture results are obtained and symptoms have disappeared.

Alert the client to report to the prescriber symptoms of nausea, vomiting, diarrhea, or increased irritation at the site of infection.

■ **Evaluation.** The expected outcome of nystatin therapy is that the client's symptoms of infection will be alleviated without the client developing any adverse gastrointestinal effects from the drug therapy.

terbinafine [ter bin′ a feen] (Lamisil)

Terbinafine is an antifungal agent indicated for the treatment of onychomycosis (nail fungal infection), tinea capitis (ringworm of the scalp), tinea corporis (body ringworm), tinea cruris (groin ringworm or jock itch), and tinea pedis (ringworm of the feet, athlete's foot). This agent interferes with the biosynthesis of fungal ergosterol, which interferes with cell wall synthesis and results the death of fungal cells.

Terbinafine is well absorbed in the gastrointestinal tract and has an elimination half-life (plasma) of 11 to 17 hours. In sebum and stratum corneum, the elimination half-life is 3 to 5 days. It reaches a peak serum level in 2 hours and a steady state in 10 days to 2 weeks. It is metabolized in the liver and excreted primarily by the kidneys.

The side effects/adverse reactions of terbinafine include anorexia, skin rash, gastric distress (nausea, vomiting, pain, diarrhea) and, perhaps, taste alterations.

The usual dosage for adolescents and adults is 125 mg PO twice daily (or 250 mg daily). The course of therapy is 6 weeks to 3 months for onychomycosis, 4 to 6 weeks for tinea capitis, 2 to 4 weeks for tinea corporis and tinea cruris, and 2 to 6 weeks for tinea pedis.

■ Nursing Management

Terbinafine Therapy

■ **Assessment.** The risk of administering terbinafine should be considered for clients with impaired renal or hepatic function; dosages may need to be adjusted downward. Clients who have active alcoholism or liver function impairment or are in remission are at greater risk for hepatotoxicity. Terbinafine is contraindicated in clients who are sensitive to it. Assess the client's concurrent drug regimen for drug interactions. For example, alcohol and other hepatotoxic drugs increase the risk of hepatotoxicity; cytochrome P-450 enzyme inducers increase the clearance of terbinafine, and P-450 inhibitors decrease the clearance of terbinafine. A baseline assessment of the client's infection should be documented and include size, character, and location. Liver function tests are recommended before therapy.

■ **Nursing Diagnosis.** The client receiving terbinafine therapy should be assessed for the following nursing diagnoses/collaborative problems: impaired comfort (change or loss of taste, anorexia, mild stomach cramps, nausea, vomiting); diarrhea; ineffective protection (neutropenia); or the potential complications of hypersensitivity, Stevens-Johnson syndrome, or toxic epidermal necrolysis.

■ **Implementation**

■ ***Monitoring.*** Monitor the infection site for improvement. Hepatic function studies are recommended periodically throughout therapy.

■ ***Intervention.*** Terbinafine may be taken without regard to food.

■ ***Education.*** To prevent a relapse of the infection, it is important that the client adhere to the lengthy regimen. Doses are given once or twice daily at evenly-spaced intervals. A missed dose is taken as soon as it is remembered, but not if it is almost time for the next dose; doses are not to be doubled up. The client should maintain regular appointments with the prescriber to check progress.

■ **Evaluation.** The expected outcome of terbinafine therapy is that the client will have an absence of symptoms. For tinea corporis, tinea cruris, and tinea pedis, this assessment needs to occur 6 to 8 weeks after the cessation of therapy; for onychomycosis of the fingernails, 4 to 6 months after therapy; and for toenails, 6 to 9 months after therapy.

ANTIVIRAL DRUGS

Chemotherapy for viral diseases is more limited than chemotherapy for bacterial diseases because it is difficult to develop and clinically apply antiviral drugs. In many viral infections, virus replication in the body reaches its peak before any clinical symptoms appear. The multiplication of the virus is ending by the time signs and symptoms of illness appear, and the subsequent course of the illness has been determined. Thus, to be clinically effective in many viral conditions, antiviral drugs must be administered in a **chemoprophylactic** manner as preventive agents before disease appears.

A second factor limiting the development of antiviral drugs is that viruses are true parasites; they replicate within the mammalian cell and use the enzyme systems of the host cells. Drugs that would inhibit virus replication would also disturb the host cells and may therefore be toxic.

The protease inhibitors are currently the most potent antiviral agents available. These agents have suppressed viral replication for up to 1 year in clinical trials, and administering them in combination therapies has decreased viral loads and increased CD4 counts (MacDonald & Kazanjian, 1996). Palella (1999) has reported that the sickest ambulatory persons with an HIV infection (CD4 count of less than 100 cells/μL) demonstrated a reduced mortality and morbidity when given combination antiretroviral therapy that included a protease inhibitor. The conclusion of this study is that highly aggressive combination therapy with a protease inhibitor should be the standard of care for all clients with HIV infection. Figure 60-1 demonstrates the inhibition sites for drug therapy in HIV.

The antivirals reviewed here include acyclovir (Zovirax), amantadine (Symmetrel), famciclovir (Famvir), foscarnet (Foscavir), ganciclovir (Cytovene), ribavirin (Virazole), rimantadine (Flumadine), and valacyclovir (Valtrex). Antivirals in current use (alone or in combination) for the treat-

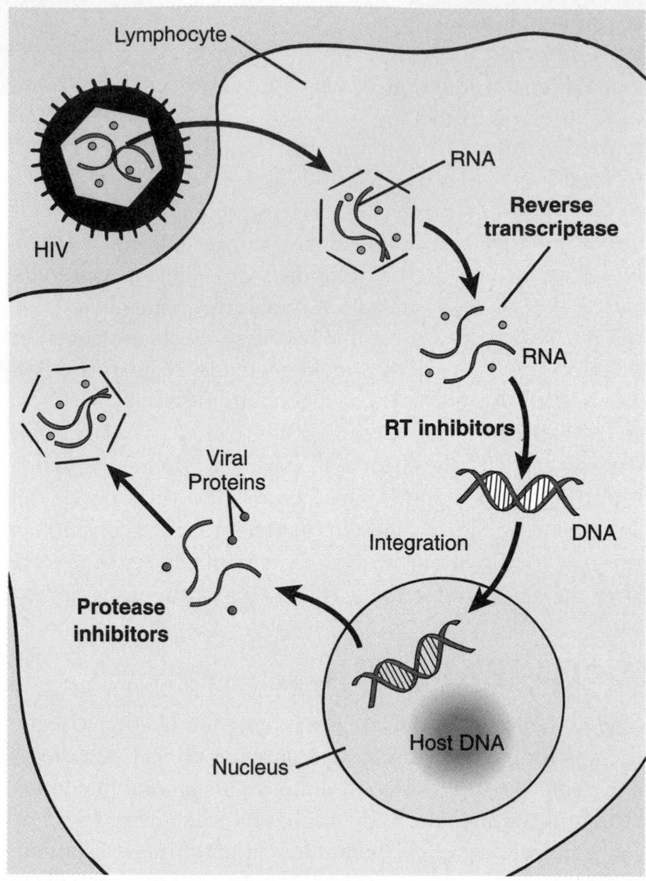

Figure 60-1 Inhibition sites for human immunodeficiency virus (HIV). The HIV genes are composed of RNA, which is translated to DNA by reverse transcriptase (RT) enzyme in order to reproduce. RT inhibitors interfere with virus production at this site. When integrated DNA becomes part of the cell, the cell produces viral proteins that require protease enzyme for the production of new HIV. The protease inhibitors block this enzyme to prevent the release of new viruses into the bloodstream. As a result, combination therapies can reduce the load of new HIV produced in the body.

ment of HIV infection are divided into three groups: (1) reverse transcriptase inhibitors (nucleoside analogues), (2) protease inhibitors, and (3) nonnucleoside reverse transcriptase inhibitors. The reverse transcriptase inhibitors include abacavir (Ziagen), didanosine (ddI, Videx), lamivudine (3TC, Epivir), stavudine (D4T, Zerit), zalcitabine (ddC, HIVID), and zidovudine (AZT, Retrovir). Protease inhibitors include indinavir (Crixivan), nelfinavir (Viracept), ritonavir (Norvir), and saquinavir (Invirase, Fortovase). The nonnucleoside reverse transcriptase inhibitors include delavirdine (Rescriptor), efavirenz (Sustiva), and nevirapine (Viramune). A combination reverse transcriptase inhibitor product available in the United States includes zidovudine and lamivudine (Combivir). Box 60-1 provides information on amprenavir, a new antiviral agent; Box 60-2 provides information on antiviral drugs for influenza.

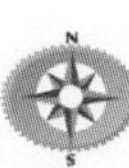
For a Concept Map on HIV, go to mosby.com/MERLIN/McKenry/.

BOX 60-1

Amprenavir (Agenerase)

Amprenavir (Agenerase) is used in combination with other antiretroviral agents in the treatment of HIV infection. It is not to be used concurrently with astemizole (Hismanal), bepridil (Vascor), dihydroergotamine (DHE 45), ergotamine, midazolam (Versed), or triazolam (Halcion); the inhibition of metabolism produced by these combinations may result in serious or life-threatening reactions. This agent may cause severe skin reactions, including Stevens-Johnson syndrome.

Numerous drug interactions have been reported with amprenavir; if this product is prescribed, review the client's entire medication regimen against the current literature or *USP DI.*

Amprenavir capsules and oral solution are not equivalent on a milligram-to-milligram basis. Follow the labeled directions carefully.

Information from *Drug Facts and Comparisons.* (2000). St. Louis: Facts and Comparisons.

■ Nursing Management

Antiviral Therapy

■ **Assessment.** An assessment would include the documentation of the client's physical and psychologic status. For some viral illnesses, such as herpes zoster or viral pneumonia, the disease episode is acute and self-limiting. Many emotional and social issues complicate a diagnosis of HIV. The baseline assessment includes nutritional, respiratory, neurologic, and fluid and electrolyte status; a description of the skin and mucous membranes; and the client's level of knowledge and emotional response to the diagnosis (Box 60-3). Potential risk factors need to be identified (e.g., sexual practices and IV drug use). A physiologic baseline includes a CBC with WBC differential and platelets, CD4 counts, measures of viral load, and renal and hepatic function studies. As with any medication, impaired renal and hepatic function places the client at higher risk for drug toxicities; this is especially true with the antivirals. The client's hypersensitivity to the drug should be determined and documented.

■ **Nursing Diagnosis.** Although many nursing diagnoses/collaborative problems are related to the viral diseases themselves, some are directly related to the antiviral medications: activity intolerance related to weakness and fatigue; ineffective protection related to blood dyscrasias (anemia, leukopenia, thrombocytopenia); and the potential complication of CNS toxicity (confusion, dizziness).

■ **Implementation**

■ ***Monitoring.*** See the unique monitoring for each of the antiviral agents.

BOX 60-2

Antiviral Drugs for Influenza

Zanamivir for inhalation (Relenza) and oseltamivir (Tamiflu) are members of a new drug classification—the neuraminidase inhibitors. These agents block the enzyme neuraminidase, which is located on the surface of the virus, thereby breaking the bond that typically holds new virus particles (A and B strains) in their cells of origin. This action prevents the release of the virion (virus) from infected cells, thus stopping its spread to other cells in the respiratory tract. Neuraminidase is necessary for the replication of the virus.

Zanamivir is a powder that is administered by oral inhalation, preferably within 2 days of the onset of symptoms of influenza (uncomplicated acute illness). Two separate 5-mg inhalations are given every 12 hours for 5 days. Oseltamivir is available as a 75-mg capsule; this agent must be started within 48 hours of the onset of influenza symptoms and is administered twice daily for 5 days.

The use of these agents does not eliminate the need for an influenza vaccine. Although these agents may help to reduce influenza symptoms, their impact on hospitalizations or economic savings has not been studied (Armstrong & Abarca, 2000).

■ ***Intervention.*** Timeliness is important in the administration of antiviral medications. Not only is it important to initiate the medications as soon as possible, but it is also necessary that they be administered on time and around-the-clock to maintain therapeutic serum levels.

■ ***Education.*** The client needs to be instructed to self-manage a complex medication regimen. A written drug regimen for the 24 hours and the use of an alarm clock assist in maintaining compliance. Stress the importance of not taking more medication than is prescribed. Many clients may increase their dosage with the erroneous belief that doing so will provide a "cure"; instead they experience greater drug toxicities. It is also important that the client not discontinue the antiviral medication without consulting with the prescriber. Many of the drugs have discomforting side effects but may be managed with changes of dosages, schedules, antiemetics, or other palliative measures. Stress to the client the importance of complying with the medication regimen, taking the drugs at evenly spaced times and not missing doses. Because many of the antivirals have serious drug interactions with a number of drugs, instruct the client not to take other medications, even over-the-counter medications, without checking with the prescriber.

Stress the importance of regular visits to the prescriber for blood tests to monitor the progress of therapy and to detect any adverse responses to drug therapy as early as possible. Encourage the client to report any adverse reactions to the prescriber as soon as possible.

Caution the client with HIV that antiviral therapy does not cure the disease or prevent its spread to others. Instruct in the avoidance of sexual contact, the possible use of con-

BOX 60-3

Assessment of the Client with AIDS

Nutritional Status

Height and Weight
Oral intake
Factors that could interfere with oral intake (anorexia, nausea, vomiting, mouth ulcers, difficulty swallowing)
Serum protein, BUN, albumin, transferrin levels

Respiratory Status

Presence and quality of breath sounds
Cough, sputum production, shortness of breath, tachypnea, chest pain
Chest x-ray examination findings, arterial blood gases, pulmonary function test results

Neurologic Status

Level of consciousness, orientation, memory lapses, mental status
Sensory deficits (visual disturbances, numbness and tingling in the extremities)
Motor involvement (weakness, altered gait, paralysis)
Seizure activity

Skin and Mucous Membranes

Evidence of breakdown, ulceration, infection
Mouth ulcerations, stomatitis, thrush
Perianal excoriation, infection
Wound cultures

Fluid and Electrolyte Status

Turgor and dryness of skin and mucous membranes
Thirst; urinary output; hypotension; irregular, weak, and rapid pulse
Nausea, vomiting, diarrhea
Decreased mental status, muscle twitching or cramps
Serum electrolytes: sodium, potassium, calcium, magnesium, chloride

Response to Diagnosis

Level of knowledge: disease and methods of transmission
Reaction to illness: denial, anger, fear, shame, depression
Identifiable sources of social support

Information from Smeltzer, S.C. & Bare, B.G. (2000). *Brunner and Suddarth's textbook of medical-surgical nursing* (9th ed.). Philadelphia: J.B. Lippincott.

doms, and the avoidance of sharing needles or giving blood to prevent the spread of the infection to others.

Advise clients, if appropriate, to delay dental work until therapy is complete, because bone marrow depressant effects may result in gingival bleeding and delayed healing. Teach appropriate oral hygiene, including the gentle use of toothbrushes and floss and the avoidance of toothpicks.

■ **Evaluation.** The expected outcome of antiviral therapy is that the client will experience a decrease in symptoms related to the underlying viral infection. Clients who are infected with HIV should experience a slowed progression of the HIV infection, increased CD4 counts, decreased viral loads, and an absence of opportunistic infections.

acyclovir [ay sye' kloe veer] (Zovirax)

Acyclovir is selectively taken up by herpes simplex virus (HSV)-infected cells and is eventually converted via a number of cellular enzymes to an active triphosphate form that is incorporated into growing DNA chains produced by the virus; this results in the inhibition of viral DNA replication.

Oral acyclovir is used in the prophylaxis and treatment of genital herpes infections in both immunocompromised and immunocompetent clients. It is also used to treat varicella (chickenpox) infections in immunocompetent children if used within 24 hours of the appearance of the rash. Injectable acyclovir is used to treat initial severe herpes genitalis in immunocompromised and immunocompetent clients who are unable to take or absorb the oral dosage form. The parenteral dosage form is also used to treat herpes simplex encephalitis and herpes zoster infections, the latter being caused by the varicella-zoster virus (VZV).

The oral dosage form of acyclovir is poorly absorbed (20%), but therapeutic serum levels are achieved. It is widely disseminated to various body fluids and tissues, including CSF and herpetic vesicular fluid. CSF levels are approximately 50% of the serum drug concentration. The half-life is approximately 2.5 hours; the drug is metabolized in the liver and excreted primarily in the urine.

The side effects/adverse reactions of the oral dosage form of acyclovir include nausea, headache, diarrhea, vomiting, and dizziness. When administered parenterally, phlebitis at the injection site or acute renal failure with rapid injection may occur.

The usual initial oral adult dosage for a herpes genital infection is 200 mg every 4 hours during the waking hours (five times daily) for 10 days. For a chronic suppressant, recurrent infection, the dosage is 400 mg twice daily. For children 2 to 12 years of age who weigh up to 40 kg, the varicella dosage is 20 mg/kg (up to 800 mg/dose) four times daily for 5 days.

The parenteral adult dosage for severe genital herpes is 5 mg/kg IV every 8 hours for 5 days. Refer to the current package insert for other dosage recommendations. A topical acyclovir is also available to treat herpes simplex infections, but the systemic dosage form is much more effective in immunocompromised persons.

■ Nursing Management

Acyclovir Therapy

■ **Assessment.** Use acyclovir with caution in clients with preexisting dehydration or renal function impairment; they are at greater risk for nephrotoxicity. A history of neurologic abnormalities or a previous neurologic reaction to cytotoxic agents may indicate a tendency for such responses to acyclovir. A hypersensitivity to acyclovir or ganciclovir requires special caution. With obese clients, the dosage is calculated on ideal body weight rather than actual weight.

Review the client's current medication regimen. The potential for nephrotoxicity is increased when acyclovir is given concurrently with other nephrotoxic drugs. Monitor renal function closely.

Assess lesions before administering the drug and daily throughout therapy. A baseline BUN and serum creatinine concentration should be determined, because the precipitation of acyclovir crystals in the renal tubules may result in renal tubular damage that progresses to acute renal failure.

■ **Nursing Diagnosis.** The client receiving acyclovir therapy should be assessed for the following nursing diagnoses/collaborative problems: impaired tissue integrity related to inflammation or phlebitis at the injection site; impaired comfort (headache); deficient fluid volume related to anorexia, nausea, and vomiting; risk for injury related to light-headedness; diarrhea; and the potential complications of acute renal failure (oliguria, thirst, anorexia, nausea, vomiting, fatigue) and encephalopathic effects (coma, confusion, seizures, tremors).

■ **Implementation**

■ ***Monitoring.*** Renal function studies, BUN levels, and serum creatinine concentrations should be obtained during therapy to monitor for the nephrotoxic effects of the drug. Fluid intake and output should be monitored, particularly if the client is receiving bolus injections of acyclovir; rapid bolus administration has been linked to precipitation of the drug in the renal tubules, resulting in acute renal insufficiency. Monitor the client's lesions for resolution.

■ ***Intervention.*** Acyclovir capsules may be administered with meals to minimize gastrointestinal distress. When dispensing the oral suspension, shake it well and use the calibrated measuring device supplied by the manufacturer.

IV acyclovir should be administered via an infusion pump at a constant rate for at least 1 hour; this prevents the precipitation of drug crystals in the renal tubules. The client should also receive hydration during the infusion and for 2 hours afterward to prevent this effect. Avoid rapid or bolus injection of the drug. Rotate infusion sites to prevent phlebitis. The IV solution is not to be used topically or orally or administered intramuscularly or subcutaneously.

■ ***Education.*** The client needs accurate information about herpes, its symptoms and transmission, and the course of the illness and treatment. Because herpes genitalis is sexually transmitted, misinformation about it is prevalent. The client should avoid sexual activity if either participant has symptoms of herpes. Condom use may help to prevent the spread of the infection, but spermicidal jellies or diaphragms probably will not. Acyclovir will neither prevent the transmission of the disease nor cure it.

The full course of therapy should be taken; however, caution the client not to take the drug longer than prescribed. Six months is generally the limit of long-term therapy. Instruct the client to report to the prescriber if symptoms do not subside.

The medication should be initiated as soon as possible after symptoms appear. To minimize the episode of herpes, the client should be instructed to begin taking the medication as soon as itching, tingling, or pain develops at the site.

Instruct the client regarding comfort measures, such as wearing loose-fitting clothing to minimize irritation of the lesions. The infected areas should be kept clean and dry.

Caution female clients to obtain a Papanicolaou (Pap) smear at least annually, because women with genital herpes are at higher risk for cervical cancer than women without genital herpes.

Because dizziness is an adverse effect of acyclovir, the client should be cautioned against performing tasks that require mental alertness (e.g., driving) until the response to the drug has been ascertained.

The client should be encouraged to maintain good dental hygiene, visit the dentist regularly for teeth cleaning, and monitor for the development of gingival hyperplasia.

■ **Evaluation.** The expected outcome of acyclovir therapy is that the client's infection will go into remission with a decrease in time to full crusting and a decrease in vesicles, ulcers, and crusts, and the client will not experience any adverse reactions to the drug.

amantadine [a man' ta deen] (Symmetrel, Symadine)

Amantadine appears to block the uncoating of the influenza A virus and the release of viral nucleic acid into the respiratory epithelial cells of the host. It also increases the release of dopamine and inhibits the reuptake of dopamine and norepinephrine centrally. Amantadine is therefore indicated for the prevention and treatment of influenza A and for treatment of Parkinson's disease and drug-induced, extrapyramidal reactions.

Amantadine is rapidly absorbed orally, distributed to saliva and nasal secretions, and crosses the blood-brain barrier. It has a half-life of 11 to 15 hours and reaches a peak serum level within 2 to 4 hours. Its onset of action as an antidyskinetic is usually within 2 days. It is excreted mostly unchanged by the kidneys.

The side effects/adverse reactions of amantadine include CNS toxicity, gastric distress and, with chronic therapy, livedo reticularis (a vasospastic disorder worsened by exposure to cold and evidenced by a reddish blue mottling of the legs and, sometimes, the arms). It also may cause anticholinergic side effects and orthostatic hypotension.

The adult dosage of the oral antiviral is 200 mg daily or 100 mg every 12 hours. The usual antidyskinetic dosage is 100 mg PO once or twice daily (up to 400 mg/day).

■ Nursing Management

Amantadine Therapy

■ **Assessment.** The following health problems necessitate the cautious use of amantadine: congestive heart failure and/or peripheral edema (because the drug may worsen the condition), epilepsy (because the drug may increase seizure activity), and renal impairment (because accumulation of the drug increases the risk of adverse CNS effects).

Older adults are more prone to confusion and difficulty in urination as common effects of amantadine because of its antimuscarinic activity.

Review the client's current drug regimen for the risk of significant drug interactions, such as those that may occur when amantadine is given concurrently with the following drugs:

Drug	Possible Effect and Management
Bold/color type indicates the most serious interactions.	
alcohol	**Increased risk for CNS side effects such as dizziness, fainting episodes, confusion, or circulatory problems. Avoid concurrent use or a potentially serious drug interaction may occur.**
anticholinergics	May result in an increase in anticholinergic side effects, such as hallucinations, dry mouth, blurred vision, confusion, and nightmares. Monitor closely, because a dosage adjustment of amantadine may be required.
CNS-stimulating agents	**May cause increased CNS stimulation, resulting in insomnia, increased irritability, and nervousness. Cardiac dysrhythmias and convulsions may also occur. Avoid concurrent use or a potentially serious drug interaction may occur. If given concurrently, be sure to monitor the client's pulse rate and neurologic status closely.**

A baseline assessment of the client's infection and neurologic status should be obtained before initiating amantadine therapy.

■ **Nursing Diagnosis.** The client receiving amantadine should be assessed for the possibility of the following nursing diagnoses/collaborative problems: impaired comfort (rash, headache, dry mouth, anorexia, and nausea); disturbed sleep pattern (insomnia); risk for injury related to the development of orthostatic hypotension; disturbed thought processes (confusion, hallucinations, severe mental or mood changes) related to the anticholinergic effects; impaired verbal communication related to the CNS effects; impaired urinary elimination (retention); constipation; and the potential complications of CNS toxicity (seizures), corneal deposits, congestive heart failure, and livedo reticularis (purplish spots on the skin; occurs with chronic therapy only).

■ **Implementation**

■ ***Monitoring.*** Closely monitor clients for side effects/adverse reactions if they are receiving dosages of more than 200 mg/day. Monitoring of blood pressure, temperature, pulse, and respirations is indicated, particularly for the first few days after a dosage increase.

The client should be monitored throughout the course of therapy if he or she is taking amantadine for parkinsonism or for dyskinetic symptoms such as tremors, rigidity, and gait disturbances.

Plasma concentrations need to be monitored in clients who are in end stage renal disease (ESRD); in such clients, a single dose may provide therapeutic levels for 7 to 10 days.

■ ***Intervention.*** If amantadine is administered as a chemoprophylactic agent, it should be started in anticipation of contact with, or as soon after exposure to, individuals with influenza A infections and continued for at least 10 days after exposure. Continue therapy for 2 to 3 weeks if given concurrently with the influenza vaccine.

Changing from a once-daily dosage to a twice-daily schedule may minimize syncope, insomnia, and nausea. Administering the last daily dose several hours before bedtime helps to minimize insomnia.

When administering the syrup form of the drug, use the calibrated measuring device provided by the manufacturer.

■ ***Education.*** Caution the client to avoid alcoholic beverages while taking amantadine, because alcohol increases the risk of CNS effects such as dizziness, syncope, and confusion.

The client should complete the full course of therapy and should notify the prescriber if viral infection symptoms do not decrease within a few days.

Clients taking amantadine as an antidyskinetic medication should complete the course of therapy as prescribed and not take more than the prescribed dosage. The client should be advised that it may require 2 or more weeks to obtain the full benefit of the drug. Counsel the client to resume physical activities gradually. The drug should be discontinued gradually.

Mental confusion, hallucinations, and difficulty sleeping are indications of CNS toxicity and should be reported to the prescriber promptly. Because amantadine may cause drowsiness or dizziness, caution the client to avoid tasks such as driving until his or her response to the drug has been determined. Because of the orthostatic effects of amantadine, advise clients to use caution when changing positions from lying to sitting or standing and from sitting to standing.

To decrease the discomfort of mouth dryness, clients may use ice, sugarless gum, or candy. Encourage oral hygiene to prevent caries and oral candidiasis.

Alert the client to the possible occurrence of a purplish red rash, which disappears 2 to 12 weeks after the medication is discontinued.

■ **Evaluation.** If amantadine therapy is administered for extrapyramidal symptoms, the expected outcome is that the client will experience improved motor control with decreased tremor. If administered for its antiviral effects, the expected outcome of amantadine therapy is influenza A prophylaxis and a decreased risk for infection of the susceptible client without adverse reactions to the drug.

famciclovir [fam sye' kloe veer] (Famvir)

Famciclovir, a pro-drug of penciclovir, the active antiviral substance, has inhibitory action against herpes simplex viruses (types 1 and 2) and varicella zoster virus. It is indicated for the treatment of genital herpes and acute herpes zoster.

Administered orally, famciclovir is well absorbed and converted in the intestinal wall to the active penciclovir. It reaches peak serum levels in approximately 1 hour and has a half-life of 2 to 3 hours. It is excreted primarily unchanged in the urine and feces.

The side effects/adverse reactions of famciclovir include headaches, weakness, gastric distress, and fatigue. The usual adult dosage for herpes zoster is 500 mg PO every 8 hours for 1 week.

■ Nursing Management

Famciclovir Therapy

■ **Assessment.** Famciclovir therapy is contraindicated for clients who are sensitive to the drug. Older adults and those with renal impairment may require a dosage reduction and careful monitoring. The concurrent administration of probenecid (Benemid) increases serum levels of penciclovir; dosage adjustments may be necessary.

A baseline assessment of the client's lesions should be documented.

■ **Nursing Diagnosis.** The client receiving famciclovir therapy may experience the following nursing diagnoses: fatigue, diarrhea, and impaired comfort (headache, nausea, vomiting).

■ **Implementation**

■ ***Monitoring.*** Assess the client's lesions during therapy. In addition, monitor for the presence of postherpetic neuralgia pain during and after therapy.

■ ***Intervention.*** Famciclovir therapy should be started as soon as herpes is diagnosed, preferably within 48 hours of its onset. It may be administered without regard to food.

■ ***Education.*** Review the client education for acyclovir.

■ **Evaluation.** The expected outcome of famciclovir therapy is that the client's lesions will be minimal, with decreased time to crusting; decreased vesicles, ulcers, and crusting; and decreased duration of neuralgia without any adverse reactions to the drug.

foscarnet [fos kar' net] (Foscavir)

Foscarnet is a virustatic agent; it inhibits viral replication of all known herpes viruses in vitro, including cytomegalovirus (CMV), herpes simplex virus types 1 and 2, Epstein-Barr virus, and varicella-zoster virus (Walmsley & Tseng, 1999). It acts by selective inhibition at the pyrophosphate-binding site of viral DNA polymerase. If the drug is discontinued, viral replication will resume. It is currently used to treat CMV retinitis in clients with AIDS.

This drug is administered by IV infusion, has an elimination half-life of 3.3 to 6.8 hours, reaches peak serum levels at the end of the infusion, is not metabolized, and is excreted primarily unchanged in the urine.

Common side effects/adverse reactions of foscarnet include nephrotoxicity, gastric distress, and neurotoxicity. It may also cause anemia and leukopenia.

For induction, the usual adult dosage by IV infusion is 60 mg/kg every 8 hours for 2 to 3 weeks. The maintenance dosage is 90 to 120 mg/kg daily.

■ Nursing Management

Foscarnet Therapy

■ **Assessment.** If the client has renal impairment, the dosage must be modified on the basis of the client's creatinine clearance. Dehydration will promote renal toxicity. A baseline assessment of the client's underlying infection and renal function should be ascertained. A baseline ophthalmologic examination is needed if the client is being treated for CMV retinitis.

Review the client's current medication regimen for the risk of significant drug interactions, such as those that may occur when foscarnet is given concurrently with the following drugs:

Drug	Possible Effect and Management
Bold/color type indicates the most serious interactions.	
acyclovir (Zovirax), aminoglycosides, amphotericin B (Fungizone), and other nephrotoxic medications	May result in an increased risk of renal toxicity. Monitor renal status closely if drugs are administered concurrently.
pentamidine (Pentam 300)	Concurrent administration of IV pentamidine with foscarnet may result in severe hypocalcemia, hypomagnesemia, and nephrotoxicity. Avoid concurrent use or a potentially serious drug interaction may occur.

■ **Nursing Diagnosis.** The client receiving foscarnet therapy should be assessed for the following nursing diagnoses/collaborative problems: impaired comfort related to phlebitis (pain at the site of infusion); ineffective protection related to anemia or leukopenia; deficient fluid volume related to anorexia, nausea, or vomiting; disturbed sensory perception related to CMV retinitis secondary to the ineffectiveness of the drug; and the potential complications of neurotoxicity (anxiety, confusion, dizziness, headache, tremor, seizures, pain or numbness in the hands and feet) and nephrotoxicity.

■ **Implementation**

■ ***Monitoring.*** Monitor the client's vision status, intake and output, serum electrolytes (calcium, magnesium, phosphate, potassium), BUN, serum creatinine concentration, and signs and symptoms of infection.

■ ***Intervention.*** The client must be adequately hydrated to prevent renal toxicity. Foscarnet is administered by slow IV infusion using a controlled infusion device over 1 hour for low doses and 2 hours for high doses. Rapid or direct IV injection may cause potentially toxic serum concentrations. It may be administered via a central or peripheral vein, but the solution for peripheral infusion must be diluted to 12 mg/mL to minimize local irritation.

An intravitreal injection may be used for the treatment of CMV retinitis in clients with an intolerance to acyclovir and advanced renal function impairment.

■ ***Education.*** Alert the client to report any change in urinary elimination pattern or a worsening vision pain in the involved eye(s).

■ **Evaluation.** The expected outcome of foscarnet therapy is that the client's CMV retinitis or other viral infection will be alleviated without the client experiencing any untoward effects of the drug.

ganciclovir [gan sye′ kloe vir] (Cytovene, Cytovene-IV)

Ganciclovir is a pro-drug; it is converted intracellularly to the active, antiviral triphosphate form. In the presence of the CMV, ganciclovir is rapidly phosphorylated to ganciclovir-triphosphate, which then inhibits viral DNA polymerase and suppresses viral DNA synthesis. If ganciclovir is discontinued, viral replication will resume.

Ganciclovir is administered by IV infusion or intravitreal injection. The serum half-life is 2.5 to 3.6 hours; the half-life in vitreous fluid is approximately 13 hours. This drug is primarily excreted unchanged by the kidneys.

Oral ganciclovir is indicated only for the maintenance of CMV retinitis in clients who have experienced a resolution of active retinitis after induction therapy with parenteral ganciclovir. The oral dosage form has a half-life of 3 to 5.5 hours and reaches peak serum concentrations in 3 hours if administered with food. An intravitreal ganciclovir implant (Vitrasert Implant) has been found to be more effective in delaying the progression of retinitis than IV ganciclovir (Hitchens, 1996). The implant releases ganciclovir for a period of 5 to 8 months.

The common side effects/adverse reactions of ganciclovir include granulocytopenia, thrombocytopenia and, possibly, gastric distress.

The usual adult dosage of ganciclovir by IV infusion for induction is 5 mg/kg every 12 hours for 2 to 3 weeks. The maintenance dosage is 5 mg/kg daily. With oral ganciclovir, the maintenance dosage is 1000 mg three times daily with food.

Box 60-4 provides information on cidofovir, another agent for the treatment of CMV retinitis.

■ Nursing Management

Ganciclovir Therapy

■ **Assessment.** The client should be assessed for any preexisting renal or hepatic function impairments that require dosage modification. A baseline assessment should also include the client's underlying condition, neurologic status, and CBC. The risk-benefit ratio must be determined for clients with an absolute neutrophil count <500 cells/mm^3 or a

BOX 60-4

Cidofovir (Vistide)

Cidofovir (Vistide) suppresses the replication of cytomegalovirus (CMV) by selectively inhibiting the synthesis of viral DNA. There are several advantages of cidofovir over other CMV drug therapies. For example, it is administered intravenously only once every 2 weeks; therefore the client does not need a surgically implanted catheter—often a major source of infections. Cidofovir has also been reported to be active against CMV that is resistant to either ganciclovir or foscarnet, although it may not be effective against CMV that is resistant to both drugs (Cidofovir approved, 1996). This product must be given with probenecid (Benemid) to reduce the clearance of cidofovir to approximately that of creatinine clearance.

The major dose-limiting adverse effect of cidofovir is severe nephrotoxicity; therefore clients should be closely monitored for renal function impairment changes, proteinuria, and changes in serum creatinine levels (≥0.4 mg per dL). Prehydration with normal saline and probenecid is required to help reduce this risk. The prescriber should follow carefully the recommended schedule for probenecid and hydration as noted in the package insert.

There are also special considerations for the preparation (class II laminar flow hood) and handling of this medication. The person preparing this product should wear surgical gloves and a closed-front, surgical-type gown with knit cuffs; in other words, do not expose skin to this product. If cidofovir comes in contact with the skin, wash it off thoroughly with soap and water. Any excess drug product should be placed in a leakproof, puncture-proof container and incinerated (*USP DI*, 1999).

platelet count <25,000/mm^3. The client's hypersensitivity to acyclovir or ganciclovir should be determined.

Review the client's current medication regimen for the risk of significant drug interactions, such as those that may occur when ganciclovir is given concurrently with the following drugs:

Drug	Possible Effect and Management
Bold/color type indicates the most serious interactions.	
bone marrow depressant drugs	Concurrent use may result in increased bone marrow depressant effects. Monitor CBC closely for neutropenia and thrombocytopenia.
nephrotoxic medications	**Concurrent use may increase the risk of renal function impairment. Avoid concurrent use.**
zidovudine (AZT)	**May result in severe hematologic toxicity. Avoid concurrent use or a potentially serious drug interaction may occur. Use extreme caution if used concurrently.**

▪ **Nursing Diagnosis.** The client receiving ganciclovir therapy should be assessed for the following nursing diagnoses/collaborative problems with IV administration: ineffective protection related to anemia, granulocytopenia, and thrombocytopenia; disturbed thought processes related to CNS toxicity (mood changes, nervousness); deficient fluid volume related to anorexia, nausea, or vomiting; impaired tissue integrity related to inflammation and phlebitis at the infusion site; and the potential complications of hypersensitivity, seizures, and coma. The client receiving intravitreal administration should also be assessed for the nursing diagnosis of disturbed sensory perception (visual) related to bacterial endophthalmitis, retinal detachment, scleral induration, or subconjunctival hemorrhage.

▪ **Implementation**

▪ ***Monitoring.*** The client's infection, CBC and platelet counts, BUN, and serum creatinine determinations should be monitored. If the client is receiving the drug for CMV retinitis, an ophthalmic examination should also be performed.

▪ ***Intervention.*** Ganciclovir is administered by slow IV infusion using a controlled infusion device. It may be administered via a central or peripheral vein. Rapid or direct IV injection may cause potentially toxic serum concentrations. Sterile water for injection, not bacteriostatic water, should be used to reconstitute the drug. Use the same precautions as when handling cytotoxic solutions; consult the procedure manual of the institution. All safety precautions should be taken with the client during periods of low blood counts.

Intravitreal injection is used for clients who are unresponsive to IV therapy or have severe myelosuppression due to ganciclovir therapy.

▪ ***Education.*** Alert the client to reportable drug-induced signs and symptoms, as well as signs of infection (fever or chills).

Instruct females of reproductive age who are taking ganciclovir to use effective contraception, because this drug has mutagenic and teratogenic potential (see the Pregnancy Safety box on p. 1029). Male clients should use barrier contraception during treatment and for at least 90 days after therapy.

▪ **Evaluation.** The expected outcome of ganciclovir therapy is the prevention of CMV retinitis in at-risk clients and a decrease in the progression of the disease in those clients already infected. The client will not experience any untoward effects.

ribavirin for inhalation [rye ba vye' rin] (Virazole)

Ribavirin is virustatic and has a mechanism of action that is diverse and not completely understood. It rapidly penetrates viral infected cells and is believed to reduce the storage of intracellular guanosine triphosphate (GTP). It inhibits viral RNA and protein synthesis, thus inhibiting viral duplication, viral spread to other cells, or both. It is indicated for serious viral pneumonia caused by respiratory syncytial virus (RSV).

Pregnancy Safety
Antifungal and Antiviral Drugs

Category	Drug
B	amphotericin B, didanosine, famciclovir, nelfinavir, ritonavir, saquinavir, valacyclovir
C	abacavir, acyclovir, amantadine, cidofovir, delavirdine, efavirenz, fluconazole, flucytosine, foscarnet, ganciclovir, indinavir, itraconazole, ketoconazole, lamivudine, miconazole, nevirapine, rimantadine, stavudine, zalcitabine, zidovudine
X	ribavirin

Pregnancy safety for griseofulvin has not been established, although it is recommended not to take this drug during pregnancy because of the reported teratogenic effects.

Following oral inhalation, ribavirin is well absorbed and rapidly distributed to plasma, respiratory tract secretions, and erythrocytes. The half-life is 9.5 hours after oral inhalation and approximately 40 days in erythrocytes. Ribavirin is metabolized in the liver and excreted primarily by the kidneys.

The side effects/adverse reactions of ribavirin are rare but may include skin rash or irritation with chronic administration.

The adult dosage of ribavirin for inhalation aerosol has not been established. For RSV infection in children, this drug is administered by oral inhalation via a Viratek small-particle aerosol generator, with a ribavirin concentration of 20 mg/mL in the reservoir. Administer over 12 to 18 hours per day for 3 to 7 days.

■ Nursing Management

Ribavirin Therapy

■ **Assessment.** Although not indicated for use in adults, health care workers and visitors who spend time at the bedside may become environmentally exposed. There is a risk of teratogenic and/or embryocidal effects in women who are pregnant. No significant drug interactions have been reported.

A baseline assessment of the client's infection and respiratory status should be obtained before initiating therapy.

■ **Nursing Diagnosis.** The child receiving ribavirin is at risk for impaired comfort related to direct contact chemical irritation as evidenced by conjunctivitis and/or rash. Health care workers in the client's environment may experience the same effects and headache.

■ **Implementation**

■ ***Monitoring.*** Monitor the child's respiratory status before and after the administration of ribavirin. If administered to clients receiving ventilation assistance, observe for increased positive-end expiratory pressure and increased positive inspiratory pressure, which occur if ribavirin precipitates within the ventilator apparatus. The equipment should be checked at least every half hour to prevent fluid accumulation in the tubing. Therapy is generally effective if begun within the first 3 days of RSV infection.

■ ***Intervention.*** Therapy with ribavirin may begin before the diagnosis is confirmed by diagnostic tests; however, treatment should not continue if the presence of RSV is not confirmed.

Ribavirin aerosol is to be administered only with the Viratek SPAG Model (SPAG-2); refer to the SPAG-2 manual for exceptions.

To prepare the solution for inhalation, add a measured quantity of sterile water for injection or inhalation to each 6-g vial, which is adequate to dissolve the drug. Do not use bacteriostatic water. Transfer the solution to a clean, sterilized SPAG-2 reservoir. Dilute the solution with sterile water to a total volume of 300 mL, with a final concentration of 20 mg/mL. Ensure that the final solution is free of particulate matter. Always discard the remaining solution when its level gets low and add freshly reconstituted solution to the reservoir. The solution retains its potency at room temperature for 24 hours. Do not administer ribavirin concurrently with any other medication by aerosolization.

■ ***Education.*** Instruct the parents about ribavirin therapy and its action, route of administration, equipment involved, frequency of treatments, and adverse effects.

■ **Evaluation.** The expected outcome of ribavirin therapy is that the client will experience improved airway clearance and that the RSV pneumonia will be resolved without producing adverse drug effects.

rimantadine [ri man′ ti deen] (Flumadine)

Rimantadine, an analogue of amantadine, inhibits viral replication by blocking or reducing the uncoating of viral RNA in host cells. It is indicated for the treatment and prevention of influenza type A respiratory tract infections.

This product is well absorbed orally and reaches a peak concentration in 1 to 4 hours. The half-life is 13 to 38 hours in children (4 to 8 years of age), 25 to 30 hours in younger adults (22 to 44 years of age), and 32 hours in older adults (71 to 79 years of age). It is metabolized in the liver and primarily excreted by the kidneys.

The side effects of rimantadine are uncommon, with older adults having a higher incidence of side effects than younger adults. The side effects/adverse reactions include CNS effects and gastric distress.

For adults and children over 10 years of age, the dosage of rimantadine for prophylaxis and treatment is 100 mg PO twice daily. The recommended dosage is 100 mg PO daily for older adults in nursing homes or in persons with severe liver or renal impairment.

▪ Nursing Management
Rimantadine Therapy

▪ **Assessment.** It should be determined if the client has a history of epilepsy or other seizure disorder, because rimantadine increases the risk of seizures. Clients with hepatic or renal function impairment have a reduced clearance of rimantadine. Hypersensitivity to amantadine or rimantadine precludes the use of this drug.

▪ **Nursing Diagnosis.** The client receiving rimantadine therapy is at risk for the following nursing diagnoses: deficient fluid volume related to anorexia, nausea, or vomiting; disturbed sleep pattern (insomnia); impaired comfort (headache); and risk for injury (dizziness).

▪ **Implementation**

▪ ***Monitoring.*** Monitor for the side effects of the drug and for the beginning symptoms of influenza A.

▪ ***Intervention.*** Administration should be continued for 10 days following exposure. It may be administered daily for 6 to 8 days during an influenza epidemic. Rimantadine that is administered concurrently with influenza A viral vaccine should be given for 2 to 3 weeks until protective antibodies have developed. Because it is only 70% to 80% effective in this instance, older adults and high-risk individuals may continue therapy longer.

▪ ***Education.*** Stress the importance of taking the drug every day and around-the-clock to maintain steady serum levels.

▪ **Evaluation.** The expected outcome of rimantadine therapy is that the client will not contract influenza A (or will have only mild symptoms) without experiencing any adverse effects of the rimantadine.

valacyclovir [va la sye′ kloe veer] (Valtrex)

Valacyclovir is a pro-drug that is converted to acyclovir by first-pass intestinal and liver metabolism. It is indicated for the treatment of herpes zoster (shingles) caused by VZV and herpes genitalis in immunocompetent persons. When compared to acyclovir, valacyclovir is reported to be more significant in reducing the pain and postherpetic neuralgia associated with herpes zoster in persons over 50 years of age. Valacyclovir has not been studied in children, immunocompromised individuals, or persons with disseminated zoster (*USP DI,* 2000).

Administered orally, valacyclovir is well absorbed and is converted to acyclovir, the active substance. It reaches peak serum levels in 1.6 to 2 hours and has a half-life of 2.5 to 3.3 hours. Valacyclovir is converted to inactive metabolites by alcohol and aldehyde dehydrogenase and is excreted primarily in the urine.

No serious adverse reactions of valacyclovir have been reported to date. Side effects include nausea, headache, weakness, gastric distress, and dizziness. The usual adult dosage for herpes zoster is 1 g three times daily for 1 week.

The nursing management for valacyclovir is the same as for acyclovir.

Reverse Transcriptase Inhibitors

abacavir [ah ba′ ka veer] (Ziagen)

Abacavir is a synthetic nucleoside with inhibitory effects against HIV. It is a pro-drug that is converted in the cell to carbovir triphosphate, an active metabolite. It inhibits reverse transcriptase by two mechanisms: (1) competing with the natural substrate dGTP, and (2) being incorporated into the viral DNA. The result is the termination of viral DNA growth.

Administered orally, abacavir is rapidly absorbed and is distributed in the blood and erythrocytes. It has an elimination half-life of 1 to 2 hours. It is metabolized by alcohol dehydrogenase and excreted primarily in urine.

The side effects/adverse reactions of abacavir in adults include nausea, vomiting, diarrhea, anorexia, insomnia, and hypersensitivity. Children have the same effects plus fever, headache, and rash.

The usual adult dosage is 300 mg PO twice daily in combination with other antiretroviral agents. Children 3 months to 16 years of age receive 8 mg/kg PO twice daily (up to a maximum of 300 mg twice daily) in combination with other antiretroviral agents.

▪ Nursing Management
Abacavir Therapy

In addition to the following discussion, see Nursing Management: Antiviral Therapy, p. 1022.

▪ **Assessment.** Hypersensitivity is a contraindication for the administration of abacavir; fatal reactions have occurred. Administer abacavir with caution to clients with hepatic function impairment. The concurrent use of ethanol increases the half-life of abacavir. A baseline assessment of the client's clinical status, including the signs and symptoms of HIV infection, CD4 count, viral load, and the presence of opportunistic infection, should be documented.

▪ **Nursing Diagnosis.** The client receiving abacavir is at risk for the following nursing diagnoses: impaired comfort (anorexia, nausea, vomiting); diarrhea; disturbed sleep pattern (insomnia); and for children, impaired comfort (rash, headache) and pyrexia. The potential complication of hepatotoxicity exists.

▪ **Implementation**

▪ ***Monitoring.*** Indicators included in the baseline assessment should be monitored to determine the therapeutic response to the abacavir.

▪ ***Intervention.*** Abacavir may be taken with or without food.

▪ ***Education.*** Alert the client to report to the prescriber immediately any symptoms of hypersensitivity, such as fever, rash, fatigue, and gastrointestinal symptoms (nausea, vomiting, abdominal pain); a hypersensitivity response to abacavir may result in death. Provide the client with the client medication guide that comes with each prescription and refill. Ensure that the client understands the information in the guide and carries a warning card that summarizes the symptoms of hypersensitivity. Advise the client that the long-term effects of abacavir are not yet known. Abacavir is not a cure for HIV, and the client may continue to experience illnesses associated with HIV (e.g., opportunistic infections). Stress the importance of taking the drug as prescribed.

■ **Evaluation.** The expected outcome of abacavir therapy is that the client will experience a decrease in symptoms related to HIV. The client will experience a slowing of the progression of the HIV infection, increased CD4 counts, decreased viral loads, and an absence of opportunistic infections.

didanosine [dye dah' noe seen] (ddI, Videx)

Didanosine is converted intracellularly to its active form, ddA-TP; this in turn inhibits HIV DNA reverse transcriptase and results in the suppression of HIV replication. Didanosine is indicated for the treatment of AIDS and advanced HIV in clients who are unable to take zidovudine or who exhibit a decreased response to it.

This product, which is available in oral dosage forms, is considered to be acid labile. Therefore oral formulations are buffered to increase gastric pH and thus protect this drug from gastric acid destruction. Didanosine crosses the blood-brain barrier, has a half-life of 1.5 hours in adults, and reaches peak serum concentrations in 30 to 60 minutes. It is excreted primarily by the kidneys.

The common side effects/adverse reactions of didanosine include peripheral neuropathy, CNS toxicity, gastric distress, and dry mouth.

The usual adult dosage for clients weighing less than 60 kg is 167 mg PO every 12 hours; for clients weighing more than 60 kg, the dosage is 250 mg PO every 12 hours. For the pediatric dosing schedule, check the current package insert or drug reference for didanosine (buffered oral suspension).

■ Nursing Management

Didanosine Therapy

In addition to the following discussion, see Nursing Management: Antiviral Therapy, p. 1022.

■ **Assessment.** It should be determined that the client does not currently have or have a history of pancreatitis, active alcoholism, or hypertriglyceridemia. Didanosine has caused pancreatitis, which on rare occasion has been fatal. These conditions place the client at higher risk for pancreatitis. The client with peripheral neuropathy may experience a worsening of the condition. Cautious use is required for clients on sodium restrictions, because each dose of 2 chewable/dispersible tablets contains 529 mg of sodium; each single-dose packet for powder for oral solution contains 1380 mg of sodium. A baseline assessment of the client's infection and serum amylase, lipase, and triglycerides should be obtained.

Review the client's current medication regimen for the risk of significant drug interactions, such as those that may occur when didanosine is given concurrently with the following drugs:

Drug	Possible Effect and Management
Bold/color type indicates the most serious interactions.	
alcohol, asparaginase (Elspar), azathioprine (Imuran), estrogens, furosemide (Lasix), methyldopa (Aldomet), nitrofurantoin (Furadantin), pentamidine IV (Pentam 300), sulfonamides, sulindac (Clinoril), tetracyclines, thiazide diuretics, valproic acid (Depakene), or other drugs associated with pancreatitis	**Concurrent drug use may result in pancreatitis. Avoid such use or a potentially serious drug interaction may occur. If combination therapy is necessary, use extreme caution.**
chloramphenicol, (Chloromycetin), cisplatin (Platinol), dapsone (Avlosulfon ♣), ethambutol (Myambutol), ethionamide (Trecator-SC), hydralazine (Apresoline), isoniazid (INH), lithium, metronidazole (Flagyl), nitrofurantoin (Furadantin), nitrous oxide, phenytoin (Dilantin), stavudine (Zerit), vincristine (Oncovin), zalcitabine (HIVID), or other drugs associated with peripheral neuropathy	**May increase the potential for peripheral neuropathy. Avoid concurrent use or a potentially serious drug interaction may occur. If it must be used, monitor closely for numbness and tingling in the fingers and toes.**
dapsone (Avlosulfon ♣), itraconazole (Sporanox), or ketoconazole (Nizoral)	May result in decreased absorption of dapsone or ketoconazole because they require an acidic media for absorption. Administer these drugs at least 2 hours before didanosine.
fluoroquinolone antibiotics (e.g., ciprofloxacin [Cipro], norfloxacin [Noroxin], and ofloxacin [Floxin]), tetracyclines	Concurrent drug administration may reduce the absorption of these antibiotics; didanosine chewable tablets and pediatric powder contain magnesium and aluminum antacids that may chelate the antibiotics, thus reducing absorption. If both drugs are prescribed, give antibiotics at least 2 hours before or 2 hours after these didanosine products. The buffered didanosine powder for oral solution has a citrate buffer that does not interfere with the antibiotics, thus its use reduces the potential for this interaction (*USP DI*, 1999).

■ **Nursing Diagnosis.** The client should be assessed for the possibility of the following nursing diagnoses/collaborative problems: disturbed sleep pattern (insomnia); impaired comfort (headache, restlessness, dry mouth); diarrhea; ineffective protection related to leukopenia, anemia, or granulocytopenia; risk for injury related to dizziness; and the potential complications of seizures, cardiomyopathy, hepatitis, retinal depigmentation, acute pancreatitis, and peripheral neuropathy.

■ **Implementation**

■ ***Monitoring.*** Observe the client for abdominal pain and numbness of the fingers and toes. Monitor serum amylase, lipase, and triglycerides over the course of the therapy. Ophthalmic examinations should be performed in children every 3 to 6 months to detect corneal pigmentation.

■ ***Intervention.*** Didanosine should be administered on an empty stomach at least 1 hour before or 2 hours after a meal. The tablets should not be swallowed whole but thoroughly chewed, crushed, or dissolved in water before administration. The tablets are hard and may need to be crushed by hand. Dissolve the tablets in at least 30 mL of water, stir, and have the client swallow the solution immediately. To produce adequate buffering and prevent gastric acid degradation, clients older than 1 year of age must take two tablets at each dose. Pediatric dosages are calculated according to body surface area, and adult dosages are calculated based on weight.

■ ***Education.*** Alert the client to report to the prescriber any abdominal discomfort, nausea and vomiting, or change of sensation in the fingers or toes. Caution clients with sodium restriction about the high sodium content of the drug.

■ **Evaluation.** The expected outcome of didanosine therapy is that the client will experience a decrease in symptoms related to HIV. The client will experience a slowing of the progression of the HIV infection, increased CD4 counts, decreased viral loads, and an absence of opportunistic infections.

lamivudine [la mi′ vue deen] (3TC, Epivir)

Lamivudine is used in combination with zidovudine for the treatment of HIV infection based on evidence of disease progression (it is currently available in combination dosage form as Combivir). Lamivudine is converted in the body to an active metabolite (L-TP) which then inhibits HIV reverse transcription by terminating the viral DNA chain. It also inhibits RNA and DNA-dependent DNA polymerase functions of reverse transcriptase.

This product is rapidly absorbed after oral administration. L-TP has an intracellular half-life of 10 to 15 hours and is excreted primarily unchanged by the kidneys.

The side effects/adverse reactions of lamivudine include headaches, fatigue, fever, nausea, vomiting, diarrhea, gastric pain or distress, anorexia, neuropathy, insomnia, depression, cough, and skeletal muscle pain.

The usual dosage of lamivudine for adolescents (12 to 16 years of age) and adults is 150 mg PO twice daily or, in combination form, 150 mg of lamivudine and 300 mg of zidovudine twice daily.

■ Nursing Management

Lamivudine Therapy

In addition to the following discussion, see Nursing Management: Antiviral Therapy, p. 1022.

■ **Assessment.** Lamivudine therapy is contraindicated for clients who are sensitive to the drug. Older adults and those with renal impairment may require a dosage reduction and careful monitoring. If children have a history of pancreatitis, use lamivudine only if there is no alternative and only with extreme caution.

Review the client's current drug regimen for potential drug interactions, such as with trimethoprim/sulfamethoxazole (Bactrim, TMP/SMX), which increases the blood levels of lamivudine; and zidovudine (AZT), which has its blood levels increased by lamivudine.

Obtain a baseline assessment of the client's HIV infection. CD4 levels, a CBC, serum lipase, serum amylase, BUN, serum creatinine, and liver function determinations should be obtained before initiating lamivudine therapy.

■ **Nursing Diagnosis.** The client receiving lamivudine therapy has the potential for the following nursing diagnoses/collaborative problems: fatigue; impaired comfort (headache, skin rash, nausea, vomiting); ineffective protection related to neutropenia and anemia; disturbed sleep pattern (insomnia); diarrhea; ineffective airway clearance (cough); and the potential complications of peripheral neuropathy and pancreatitis (children only).

■ **Implementation**

■ ***Monitoring.*** Monitor the client's CD4 levels, CBC with differential, serum amylase, serum lipase, serum creatinine, BUN, and liver function studies at periodic intervals throughout therapy. Assess the client for changes in symptoms of HIV infection, opportunistic infections, and peripheral neuropathy (tingling, burning, and weakness of the hands and feet). Monitor clients, particularly children, for symptoms of pancreatitis (e.g., nausea, vomiting, and abdominal pain); discontinue the drug and contact the prescriber immediately.

■ ***Intervention.*** Administer lamivudine without regard to food.

■ ***Education.*** Advise the client to take lamivudine as ordered (see the general discussion under Nursing Management: Antiviral Therapy, p. 1022). Encourage the client to report to the prescriber immediately any symptoms of neuropathy or pancreatitis.

■ **Evaluation.** The expected outcome of lamivudine therapy is that the client will experience a decrease in symptoms related to HIV. The client will experience a slowing of the progression of the HIV infection, increased CD4 counts, decreased viral loads, and an absence of opportunistic infections.

stavudine [stav′ yoo deen] (d4T, Zerit)

Stavudine is an antiviral agent indicated for the treatment of advanced HIV infection or AIDS in clients who have not responded to or are unable to take zidovudine and proven therapeutic agents. Stavudine is converted to stavudine triphosphate, which then competes with deoxythymidine triphosphate and results in the inhibition of HIV replication and DNA synthesis.

Oral stavudine is rapidly absorbed and reaches peak serum levels in 0.5 to 1.5 hours. It has a half-life of 1 to 1.6 hours and is excreted primarily unchanged by the kidneys.

The side effects/adverse reactions of stavudine include dose-related peripheral neuropathy and anemia.

The usual adult oral dosage of stavudine is 30 mg every 12 hours for persons weighing less than 60 kg; for persons weighing more than 60 kg, the dosage is 40 mg every 12 hours.

■ Nursing Management

Stavudine Therapy

In addition to the following discussion, see Nursing Management: Antiviral Therapy, p. 1022.

■ **Assessment.** Stavudine is contraindicated for clients who are hypersensitive to this drug or to didanosine, zalcitabine, or zidovudine. It is also contraindicated for clients with severe peripheral neuropathy. This drug is used with caution in clients with advanced HIV infections, bone marrow suppression, renal and hepatitis disease, or folic acid or B_{12} deficiency, or in women who are pregnant or lactating.

A review of the client's concurrent medication regimen is required. If the client is taking a drug that may cause peripheral neuropathy, such as chloramphenicol (Chloromycetin), cisplatin (Platinol), dapsone (Avlosulfon ♣), ethambutol (Myambutol), ethionamide (Trecator-SC), hydralazine (Apresoline), isoniazid (INH), lithium, metronidazole (Flagyl), nitrofurantoin (Furadantin), nitrous oxide, phenytoin (Dilantin), vincristine (Oncovin), or zalcitabine (HIVID), there is a greater risk of peripheral neuropathy occurring with the use of stavudine.

A baseline assessment of the client should include documentation of the client's symptoms, a neurologic examination, a CBC, and renal and liver function studies.

■ **Nursing Diagnosis.** The client receiving stavudine is at risk for the following nursing diagnoses/collaborative problems: ineffective protection related to bone marrow suppression (anemia); disturbed sensory perception (tactile) related to peripheral neuropathy; impaired comfort (headache, arthralgia, myalgia, anorexia, nausea, vomiting); disturbed sleep pattern (insomnia); and the potential complication of pancreatitis.

■ **Implementation**

■ ***Monitoring.*** Monitor the client's CBC, serum amylase, serum lipase, and renal and hepatic studies. Monitor the client's neurologic status, intake and output, and bowel pattern.

■ ***Intervention.*** This drug may be taken with or without food.

■ ***Education.*** Instruct the client to report symptoms of peripheral neuropathy (tingling, burning, or numbness of the extremities) or pancreatitis (severe and sharp abdominal pain). Advise the client to report to the prescriber other signs of infections, such as sore throat, cough, urinary burning, swollen lymph nodes, fever, and malaise.

■ **Evaluation.** The expected outcome of stavudine therapy is that the client will experience a decrease in symptoms related to HIV, such as diarrhea, fatigue, night sweats, and weight loss. The client will experience a slowing of the progression of the HIV infection, increased CD4 counts, decreased viral loads, and an absence of opportunistic infections.

zalcitabine [zal sit' ta been] (ddC, HIVID)

Zalcitabine, an antiviral agent, is converted by cellular enzymes to its active form (ddC-TP), which inhibits viral reverse transcriptase, thereby inhibiting viral replication. In vitro studies have shown zalcitabine to be approximately 10 times more potent than zidovudine against HIV (*USP DI*, 1999). Zalcitabine is indicated for the treatment of advanced HIV infection and AIDS in clients who either cannot take zidovudine or who experience a disease progression while taking zidovudine.

Administered orally, zalcitabine is metabolized intracellularly to ddC-TP; it reaches peak serum levels in 1 to 2 hours and has a half-life of 1 to 3 hours. It is excreted primarily by the kidneys.

The side effects/adverse reactions of zalcitabine include peripheral neuropathy, gastric distress, and headache.

The usual adult oral dosage of zalcitabine is 0.75 mg, alone or in combination with 200 mg of zidovudine every 8 hours.

■ Nursing Management

Zalcitabine Therapy

The nursing management of the client receiving zalcitabine is the same as didanosine except that zalcitabine should be administered 1 hour before or 2 hours after meals to enhance absorption. Zalcitabine is often administered in conjunction with zidovudine.

zidovudine [zye doe' vue deen] (AZT, Retrovir)

Zidovudine is an antiviral agent (virustatic) that intracellularly is converted to monophosphate, diphosphate, and then zidovudine triphosphate by cellular enzymes. The triphosphate form competes with natural thymidine triphosphate for incorporation into growing chains of viral RNA-dependent DNA polymerase (reverse transcriptase), thus inhibiting viral DNA replication. It has a greater affinity for retroviral reverse transcriptase than for the human alpha-DNA polymerase; thus it selectively inhibits viral replication.

Zidovudine is indicated for the treatment of HIV infection and AIDS in adults who have a CD4 lymphocyte count of $500/mm^3$ or less. Zidovudine may be used in combination with zalcitabine, especially when the CD4 count is $300/mm^3$ or less.

Administered orally, zidovudine is rapidly absorbed and distributed in the plasma and CSF. It reaches a peak serum level in 0.5 to 1.5 hours and has a half-life of approximately 1 hour (in serum, 3.3 hours intracellularly). It is metabolized in the liver and excreted by the kidneys.

The side effects/adverse reactions of zidovudine include nausea, myalgia, insomnia, severe headaches, and bone marrow depression.

The adult oral dosage for the treatment of symptomatic HIV infection is 100 mg every 4 hours around-the-clock (600 mg daily). For asymptomatic HIV infection, the adult dosage is 100 mg every 4 hours while awake (500 mg daily). For children 3 months to 12 years of age, the oral dosage 90 to 180 mg/m^2 every 6 hours.

The parenteral adult dosage for symptomatic HIV infection is 1 mg/kg by IV infusion, which is administered over 60 minutes every 4 hours around-the-clock until oral therapy can be used. The pediatric dosage is 120 mg/m^2 every 6 hours.

■ Nursing Management

Zidovudine Therapy

In addition to the following discussion, see Nursing Management: Antiviral Therapy, p. 1022.

■ **Assessment.** Assess the client's general health before initiating zidovudine therapy. The following health problems indicate that the drug is to be used with caution: bone marrow depression, which may result in blood dyscrasias; hepatic function impairment, which may affect metabolism of the drug, lead to drug accumulation, and cause toxicity; and folic acid or vitamin B_{12} deficiency, which may result in an increased risk of anemia and hypersensitivity to zidovudine.

Review the client's current medication regimen for the risk of significant drug interactions, such as those that may occur when zidovudine is given concurrently with the following drugs:

Drug	Possible Effect and Management
Bold/color type indicates the most serious interactions.	
bone marrow depressants, radiation therapy	May exacerbate bone marrow depression and toxicity. Dosage reductions may be necessary. Monitor CBCs closely for leukopenia and anemia.
clarithromycin (Biaxin)	Concurrent drug administration has been reported to result in a lower peak plasma level of zidovudine. Monitor serum concentrations of the drug closely.
ganciclovir (Cytovene)	**Concurrent use has been reported to result in synergistic myelosuppressive toxicity. Because this is a serious hematologic toxicity, avoid concurrent use or a potentially serious drug interaction may occur.**
probenecid (Benemid)	May result in decreased liver metabolism of zidovudine, resulting in increased serum levels and an increased risk of toxicity. There is also a high incidence of rash (*USP DI*, 1999). Monitor serum drug concentrations closely if drugs are administered concurrently.

A baseline assessment of the client should include the underlying condition, a CBC to detect anemia or granulocytopenia, and liver function tests.

■ **Nursing Diagnosis.** The client receiving zidovudine is at risk for the following nursing diagnoses/collaborative problems: impaired comfort (headache, myalgia); deficient fluid volume related to anorexia, nausea, or vomiting; disturbed sleep pattern (insomnia); ineffective protection related to leukopenia or anemia; anxiety; and the potential complications of hepatotoxicity (malaise, anorexia, nausea, abdominal discomfort), myopathy (muscle atrophy, weakness, and discomfort), and neurotoxicity (confusion, seizures).

■ **Implementation**

■ ***Monitoring.*** Monitor the client's underlying condition. Monitor the client's CBC at least every 2 weeks during therapy. Anemia usually occurs after 4 to 6 weeks of therapy and may be severe enough to reduce the dosage of zidovudine or require the administration of blood or epoetin. Observe the client for fever, sore throat, unusual bleeding or bruising, or unusual tiredness, all of which are symptoms of bone marrow depression. These symptoms may occur even after the medication is discontinued and should be reported to the health care provider. Liver function tests should also be monitored.

■ ***Intervention.*** Zidovudine should be diluted before administration to no greater than 4 mg/mL in 5% dextrose injection and given intravenously at a constant rate over 1 hour. It should not be administered intramuscularly, by IV bolus, or by rapid infusion.

The client may experience changes in taste, swelling of the lips and tongue, and mouth ulcers. These symptoms may affect the client's desire or ability to eat. The client must receive good oral hygiene to prevent infection and promote comfort. Food and fluid intake should be monitored to ensure adequate nutrition. Encourage the client to take small but frequent high-protein meals. Serve meals attractively, and offer foods that the client prefers. Bland and smooth-textured foods may be better tolerated.

■ ***Education.*** Advise the client to take the medication exactly as prescribed (see the general discussion under Nursing Management: Antiviral Therapy, p. 1022).

■ **Evaluation.** The expected outcome of zidovudine therapy is that the client will experience a decrease in symptoms related to HIV, such as diarrhea, fatigue, night sweats, and weight loss. The client will experience a slowing of the progression of the HIV infection, increased CD4 counts, decreased viral loads, and an absence of opportunistic infections.

Protease Inhibitors

Box 60-5 provides update information on the epidemic of AIDS.

indinavir [in din' a veer] (Crixivan)

Indinavir was released under the accelerated review of the Food and Drug Administration for the treatment of HIV infection in adults. Although its complete mechanism of action is unknown, indinavir appears to inhibit the replication

BOX 60-5

AIDS Update

AIDS Deaths Decline

The number of deaths of people with AIDS has decreased significantly since 1996. The Centers for Disease Control and Prevention (CDC) report a drop in AIDS-related infections, diseases, and deaths due to the new drug combinations, especially those that include a protease inhibitor (Reuters New Media, 1998).

Protease Inhibitor–Induced Lipodystrophy

Lipodystrophy related to the use of protease inhibitors was reported at the XIIth International Conference on AIDS (Geneva, Switzerland [June 28 to July 3, 1998]). Symptoms of lipodystrophy include the following (Norton, 1999):

- Swollen stomach
- Loss of fat in the face (with protruding cheekbones), arms, and legs
- Development of an upper dorsal fat pad (a "buffalo hump" at the back of the neck)
- Elevation of triglycerides and serum cholesterol
- Insulin resistance, high blood sugar, and diabetes

Some clients reported that switching to a different protease inhibitor improved or eliminated the symptoms of lipodystrophy (Side Effects of Anti-HIV Drugs, 1999).

Highly Active Antiretroviral Therapy (HAART)

Although the very effective combination therapies for the treatment of HIV are commonly referred to as HAART (Gilden, 1999), the potential side effects of the protease inhibitors have led to an interest in studying a protease-sparing HAART combination first, with the protease inhibitor saved for second-line therapy after the first drug combination becomes ineffective. Several studies presented at the Geneva conference reported good results with the protease-sparing HAART combination (Less pills, less doses, 1999).

of retroviruses (HIV types 1 and 2) by interfering with HIV protease. Indinavir affects the replication cycle of HIV and is active in both acute and chronically infected cells, which in general are not affected by dideoxynucleoside reverse transcriptase inhibitors (e.g., didanosine, lamivudine, stavudine, zalcitabine, and zidovudine). This inhibition results in the formation of immature, noninfectious viral particles.

Administered orally, indinavir reaches a peak serum level in approximately 1 hour; it is metabolized in the liver and excreted primarily by the kidneys.

The side effects/adverse reactions of indinavir include gastric distress, nausea, vomiting, diarrhea, headache, dizziness, fatigue, fever, flu-like syndrome, and chest pain.

The usual adult dosage of indinavir is 800 mg PO every 8 hours.

■ Nursing Management

Indinavir Therapy

In addition to the following discussion, see Nursing Management: Antiviral Therapy, p. 1022.

■ **Assessment.** Indinavir therapy is contraindicated for clients who are sensitive to this drug. Safety and efficacy have not been demonstrated for the use of this drug in children.

Review the client's current medication regimen for the risk of significant drug interactions, such as those that may occur when indinavir is given concurrently with the following drugs:

Drug	Possible Effect and Management
Bold/color type indicates the most serious interactions.	
didanosine (ddI, Videx)	The drugs have different requirements for gastric pH for absorption. Didanosine is buffered to increase gastric pH. Administer at least 1 hour apart on an empty stomach with a full glass of water.
ketoconazole (Nizoral)	This drug increases blood levels of indinavir. Monitor the client closely for adverse reactions to indinavir.
rifabutin (Mycobutin)	Concurrent use results in increased serum levels for both drugs. Decrease the dosage of rifabutin if administered with indinavir.
rifampin (Rifadin)	Decreases the serum levels of indinavir. Avoid concurrent use.
terfenadine* (Seldane), astemizole (Hismanal), cisapride* (Propulsid), midazolam (Versed), triazolam (Halcion)	**Indinavir may increase the blood levels of these drugs and increase the risk for cardiovascular toxicities. Avoid concurrent use or a potentially serious drug interaction may occur.**

Obtain a baseline assessment of the client's AIDS symptoms and opportunistic infections. A baseline assessment should include CBC, CD4 counts, viral load, and renal and hepatic function studies.

■ **Nursing Diagnosis.** The client receiving indinavir therapy has the potential for the following nursing diagnoses/collaborative problems: fatigue; impaired comfort (headache, nausea, vomiting, abdominal discomfort); diarrhea; activity intolerance related to weakness; disturbed sleep pattern (insomnia, sleepiness); disturbed sensory perception (taste perversion); and the potential complications of kidney stones and diabetes.

■ **Implementation**

■ ***Monitoring.*** The client's blood glucose, CBC, CD4 counts, viral load, and liver function studies should be monitored periodically throughout therapy. Assess the client for changes in symptoms of AIDS and opportunistic infections.

---

*No longer available in the United States but may be available in other countries.

■ ***Intervention.*** Administer indinavir 1 hour before or 2 hours after eating with a full glass of water (240 mL).

■ ***Education.*** Advise the client to take indinavir as ordered (see the general discussion under Nursing Management: Antiviral Therapy, p. 1022). Stress the importance of drinking 1.5 L of liquids over each 24-hour period to help prevent kidney stones. Encourage the client to report symptoms of diabetes (increased hunger, increased thirst, fatigue, unexplained weight loss, increased urination) and kidney stones (sharp back pain just below the ribs, blood in the urine).

■ **Evaluation.** The expected outcome of indinavir therapy is that the client will experience the slowing of the progression of the HIV infection and its sequelae, increased CD4 counts, decreased viral loads, and an absence of opportunistic infections.

nelfinavir [nel fin′ ah veer] (Viracept)

Nelfinavir is a protease inhibitor that inhibits HIV-1 protease, which results in the production of immature, noninfectious virus particles.

Nelfinavir is available as an oral powder and tablet. It has a half-life in plasma of 3.5 to 5 hours and reaches peak plasma levels in 2 to 4 hours. Nelfinavir is metabolized to active and inactive metabolites in the liver (cytochrome P-450) and is excreted primarily in the feces.

The side effects/adverse reactions of nelfinavir include diarrhea, gas, nausea, skin rash, hyperglycemia and, possibly, ketoacidosis.

The oral powder is for use in children only; children 2 to 13 years of age receive 20 to 30 mg/kg PO three times daily with food. The tablet dosage form is used for adolescents and adults; the dosage is usually 750 mg three times daily with food and in combination with other nucleoside agents.

■ Nursing Management

Nelfinavir Therapy

■ **Assessment.** Nelfinavir therapy is contraindicated for clients who are sensitive to it. The safety and efficacy has not been determined for use with children under 2 years of age.

Review the client's current medication regimen for the risk of significant drug interactions, such as those that may occur when nelfinavir is given concurrently with the following drugs:

Drug	Possible Effect and Management
Bold/color type indicates the most serious interactions.	
anticonvulsants	Avoid concurrent use, because it may result in decreased serum levels of nelfinavir.
contraceptives, estrogen-based, oral	Nelfinavir decreases the effects of oral contraceptives. Use alternative methods of contraception while taking nelfinavir.
rifabutin (Mycobutin)	Concurrent use results in an increased serum level of rifabutin. Decrease the dosage of rifabutin if administered with nelfinavir.
rifampin (Rifadin)	Decreases the serum levels of nelfinavir. Avoid concurrent use.
terfenadine* (Seldane), astemizole (Hismanal), cisapride* (Propulsid), midazolam (Versed), triazolam (Halcion)	**Indinavir may increase blood levels of these drugs and increase the risk of cardiovascular toxicities. Avoid concurrent use or a potentially serious drug interaction may occur.**

Obtain a baseline assessment of the client's AIDS symptoms and opportunistic infections. A baseline assessment should include CBCs, CD4 counts, viral load, and renal and hepatic function studies.

■ **Nursing Diagnosis.** The client receiving nelfinavir therapy has the potential for the following nursing diagnoses/collaborative problems: fatigue; impaired comfort (headache, nausea, vomiting, abdominal discomfort); diarrhea; activity intolerance related to weakness; ineffective protection (anemia, leukopenia, thrombocytopenia); disturbed sleep pattern (insomnia, sleepiness); disturbed sensory perception (taste perversion); and the potential complications of seizures and kidney stones.

■ **Implementation**

■ ***Monitoring.*** The client's CBC, CD4 counts, viral load and liver function studies should be monitored at periodic intervals throughout therapy. Assess the client for changes in symptoms of AIDS and opportunistic infections.

■ ***Intervention.*** Administer nelfinavir with food to enhance absorption. Mix the powder for reconstitution with a small amount of water, milk, formula or other non-acidic liquid. Mixing with acidic foods or juices (e.g., orange or apple juice) makes the preparation bitter.

■ ***Education.*** Advise the client to take nelfinavir as ordered (see the general discussion under Nursing Management: Antiviral Therapy, p. 1022). Stress the importance of drinking 1.5 L of liquids over each 24-hour period to help prevent kidney stones.

■ **Evaluation.** The expected outcome of nelfinavir therapy is that the client will experience the slowing of the progression of the HIV infection and its sequelae, increased CD4 counts, decreased viral loads, and an absence of opportunistic infections.

ritonavir [ri toe′ na veer] (Norvir)

Ritonavir is an inhibitor of HIV-1 and HIV-2 protease that interferes with the production of the HIV virus. The use of this product results in the production of noninfectious, immature HIV substances.

Administered orally, ritonavir reaches peak serum levels within 2 to 4 hours (fasting or nonfasting); five metabolites have been identified with ritonavir, but only the M-2 metabolite has antiviral activity. Most of this drug is excreted in the feces.

The side effects/adverse reactions of ritonavir include weakness, nausea, vomiting, diarrhea, stomach distress, taste alterations, peripheral paresthesias, allergic reactions, back

*No longer available in the United States but may be available in other countries.

or chest pain, chills, facial edema, flu-like symptoms, and many other potential adverse reactions. Refer to current references for a complete list of side effects/adverse reactions.

The usual dosage is 600 mg twice daily with meals.

The nursing management of the care of the client receiving ritonavir is the same as for indinavir, with a few exceptions. For example, ritonavir has significant drug interactions. It may produce large increases in the serum concentrations of the following drugs: amiodarone (Cordarone), astemizole (Hismanal), bepridil (Vascor), bupropion (Wellbutrin), clozapine (Clozaril), dihydroergotamine (DHE 45), flecainide (Tambocor), meperidine (Demerol), pimozide (Orap), piroxicam (Feldene), propafenone (Rhythmol), propoxyphene (Darvon), and rifabutin (Mycobutin). These drugs have known risks of cardiac dysrhythmias, hematologic abnormalities, CNS toxicity (seizures), and other serious adverse effects; do not administer them concurrently with ritonavir. In addition, concurrent administration with highly metabolized sedatives and hypnotics such as clorazepate (Tranxene), diazepam (Valium), estazolam (ProSom), flurazepam (Dalmane), midazolam (Versed), triazolam (Halcion), and zolpidem (Ambien) may result in extreme sedation and respiratory depression; do not coadminister. The concurrent use of oral ritonavir and estrogen-containing contraceptives may result in contraceptive failure; use alternative methods of contraception. Ritonavir is also taken with food to enhance its absorption.

saquinavir [sa kwin' a veer] (Invirase)

Saquinavir inhibits HIV protease and prevents the cleavage of viral polyproteins. It is used in combination with the nucleoside analogues to treat advanced HIV infection in selected individuals. For example, it may be prescribed concurrently with zidovudine (AZT) in untreated persons or with ddC in clients previously treated with extended AZT therapy. Clinical studies based on disease progression and survival are underway to determine the clinical benefits of combination therapy.

Administered orally, saquinavir has extensive first-pass metabolism, is highly protein bound, is metabolized in the liver, and is excreted primarily in the feces.

The side effects of saquinavir are usually mild and include diarrhea, abdominal distress, headache, and weakness. Serious adverse reactions are rare and may include confusion, Stevens-Johnson syndrome, seizures, thrombocytopenia, ataxia, anemias, and hepatotoxicity.

The usual dosage in combination with a nucleoside analogue is 200 mg 3 times daily, administered within 2 hours after a full meal.

■ Nursing Management

Saquinavir Therapy

In addition to the following discussion, see Nursing Management: Antiviral Therapy, p. 1022.

■ **Assessment.** Saquinavir therapy is contraindicated for clients with a sensitivity to this drug. Older adults and those with hepatic impairment may require a dosage reduction and careful monitoring. Safe use with children under 16 years of age has not been established.

Review the client's current medication regimen for the risk of significant drug interactions, such as those that may occur when saquinavir is given concurrently with the following drugs:

Drug	Possible Effect and Management
Bold/color type indicates the most serious interactions.	
rifampin (Rifadin), rifabutin (Mycobutin), carbamazepine (Tegretol), dexamethasone, phenobarbital, phenytoin (Dilantin)	**These drugs decrease saquinavir blood levels; concurrent use should be avoided.**
terfenadine* (Seldane), astemizole (Hismanal), ergot derivatives, midazolam (Versed), triazolam (Halcion)	**Saquinavir may increase blood levels of these drugs and increases the risk of cardiovascular toxicities. Avoid concurrent use or a potentially serious drug interaction may occur.**
calcium channel blockers, quinidine	Saquinavir may increase blood levels of these drugs. Monitor closely for drug toxicities.
delavirdine (Rescriptor)	Concurrent use elevates hepatic enzymes; monitor hepatic function at periodic intervals.

Obtain a baseline assessment of the client's AIDS symptoms and opportunistic infections. CBCs, CD4 counts, and liver function determinations should be obtained before initiating saquinavir therapy.

■ **Nursing Diagnosis.** The client receiving saquinavir therapy has the potential for the following nursing diagnoses/collaborative problems: fatigue; impaired comfort (headache, nausea, abdominal discomfort, rash); diarrhea; impaired oral mucous membrane (mouth ulcers); and the potential complications of diabetes and paresthesia (tingling or prickling sensations).

■ **Implementation**

■ ***Monitoring.*** The client's CBC, CD4 counts, viral load, and liver function studies should be monitored at periodic intervals throughout therapy. Assess the client for changes in symptoms of AIDS and opportunistic infections.

■ ***Intervention.*** Administer saquinavir with a full meal (or within 2 hours) for increased absorption.

■ ***Education.*** Advise the client to take saquinavir as ordered (see the general discussion under Nursing Management: Antiviral Therapy, p. 1022). Encourage the client to report symptoms of diabetes (fatigue, increased hunger, increased thirst, increased urination, unexplained weight loss).

■ **Evaluation.** The expected outcome of saquinavir therapy is that the client will experience a slowed progression of the HIV infection and its sequelae, increased CD4 counts, decreased viral loads, and an absence of opportunistic infections.

*No longer available in the United States but may be available in other countries.

Nonnucleoside, Reverse Transcriptase Inhibitors

delavirdine [deh lah vir' deen] (Rescriptor)

Delavirdine binds to HIV-1 reverse transcriptase to block RNA-dependent and DNA-dependent polymerase activities. It does not affect human DNA polymerase activities.

Administered orally, delavirdine is rapidly absorbed and is highly protein bound (98%). It reaches peak serum levels in 1 hour and has a half-life of approximately 6 hours (range 2 to 11 hours). It is metabolized in the liver by the cytochrome P-450 3A (CYP3A) system and can also reduce the action of CYP3A, which may be reversed in 7 days after discontinuing delavirdine therapy. It is excreted both in the feces (44%) and by the kidneys (51%).

The side effects/adverse reactions of delavirdine include nausea, vomiting, diarrhea, fatigue, skin rash, pruritus and, uncommonly or rarely, conjunctivitis, blisters, fever, joint and muscle pain, oral lesions, and dyspnea.

The usual adult dosage is 400 mg PO three times daily.

efavirenz [eh fah' vye renz] (Sustiva)

The mechanism of action of efavirenz is similar to delavirdine—non-competitive inhibition of HIV-1 reverse transcriptase.

Administered orally, efavirenz reaches peak plasma levels in 3 to 5 hours and steady-state plasma levels in 6 to 10 days. It is highly protein bound (99.5%) and is metabolized by the cytochrome P-450 system to inactive metabolites. Efavirenz can also increase P-450 enzyme activity, which results in an increase in its own metabolism (autoinduction). It has a half-life of 52 to 76 hours and is excreted in the urine and feces.

The side effects/adverse reactions of efavirenz include skin rashes (usually within the first 2 weeks of therapy), diarrhea, fatigue, headache, nausea, vomiting, insomnia, and diarrhea.

The usual adult dosage is 600 mg daily (at bedtime) in combination with other antiviral agents.

nevirapine [neh vye' rah peen] (Viramune)

Nevirapine is a nonnucleoside antiviral agent that binds directly to reverse transcriptase to block RNA-dependent and DNA-dependent DNA polymerase activity. This drug can cause resistant HIV if given alone; therefore it should be administered in combination with at least one other antiretroviral agent.

Administered orally, nevirapine is well absorbed, reaches peak serum levels in 4 hours, and is distributed in CSF (45% or serum concentration). Nevirapine is metabolized in the liver and is also an inducer of hepatic cytochrome P-450 metabolic enzymes; therefore autoinduction or an increased clearance and a decreased half-life occurs within 2 to 4 weeks of therapy.

The side effects/adverse reactions of nevirapine include nausea, headache, diarrhea, fever, and life-threatening skin reactions such as Stevens-Johnson syndrome. Discontinue this drug in clients who develop a severe rash or a rash accompanied by other symptoms such as fever, myalgia, fatigue, oral lesions, and conjunctivitis.

The initial therapy is 200 mg PO daily for 2 weeks; the maintenance dosage is 200 mg twice daily in combination with another antiretroviral agent.

▪ Nursing Management

Nonnucleoside, Reverse Transcriptase Inhibitor Therapy

In addition to the following discussion, see Nursing Management: Antiviral Therapy, p. 1022.

▪ **Assessment.** In addition to an assessment of the client's underlying condition, hepatic function studies should be completed as a baseline before initiating therapy, because hepatitis may occur as an adverse reaction to these drugs.

Review the client's current medication regimen for the risk of significant drug interactions, such as those that may occur when nonnucleoside, reverse transcriptase inhibitors are given concurrently with the following drugs:

Drug	Possible Effect and Management
Bold/color type indicates the most serious interactions.	
amphetamines, astemizole (Hismanal), benzodiazepines, calcium channel blocking drugs, cisapride* (Propulsid), ergot derivatives, terfenadine* (Seldane)	**Concurrent use with delavirdine may result in serious or life-threatening adverse reactions. Avoid the concurrent use of these medications.**
carbamazepine (Tegretol), phenobarbital, phenytoin (Dilantin)	Decreases the trough levels of delavirdine. Concurrent use is not recommended.
H_2 histamine blockers, such as cimetidine (Tagamet) and others	Increase gastric pH and reduce the absorption of delavirdine. Long-term concurrent use of these medications is not recommended.
clarithromycin (Biaxin)	Concurrent use of delavirdine increases serum levels for both drugs. Dosage adjustments may be necessary.
contraceptives, estrogen-containing, oral	Nevirapine reduces serum levels of oral contraceptives. Contraceptive failure may result. Alternative methods of contraception are recommended.
indinavir (Crixivan)	Delavirdine inhibits the metabolism of indinavir. Dosage adjustments may be necessary.
ketoconazole (Nizoral)	Concurrent use with nevirapine reduces serum levels of ketoconazole. Concurrent use is not recommended.
rifampin (Rifadin), rifabutin (Mycobutin)	**These drugs decrease blood levels of delavirdine and nevirapine; concurrent use should be avoided.**

*No longer available in the United States but may be available in other countries.

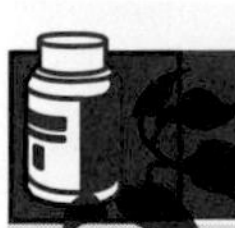

Complementary and Alternative Therapies
Cranberry Juice

Cranberry juice is widely used as a beverage and as a flavoring for sauces and jelly. For years it has been thought that cranberry juice reduces bacterial infections of the bladder. Recent studies now support that cranberry juice inhibits the adherence of *Escherichia coli* cells to cells of the urinary tract wall. Avorn, Monane, and Gurwitz (1994) studied 153 older women who drank 300 ml daily of cranberry juice or a placebo juice matched for taste, appearance, and vitamin C content. White blood cells and bacteria (signs of infection) appeared in the urine of those receiving the placebo twice as often as in the urine of those who drank the cranberry juice. However, there is no good evidence to suggest that cranberry juice is effective for the *treatment* of urinary infections (Jepson, Mihaljevic, & Craig, 2000). A number of juices have been tested to see how well they inhibit the adhesive ability of *E. coli*, the most common causative agent of urinary tract infections (Ofek, 1991). Only cranberry juice and blueberry juice were found to be beneficial. Because both berries belong to the genus *Vaccinium*, it makes sense that they would have a similar effect.

The usual dose has not been determined, but 30 to 300 ml daily as a juice has been used. Ensure that it is a juice and not a cranberry-flavored beverage. The latter beverages tend to have a minimal amount of the real juice as an ingredient. Clients with diabetes should be cautioned to avoid cranberry juice cocktail products sweetened with sugar and to use those sweetened with artificial sweeteners instead. Given the variation between juice products, cranberry capsules, 300 to 400 mg twice daily, may be more acceptable than cranberry juice, although the capsule-to-juice equivalency has also not been verified.

Information from Avorn, J., Monane, M., & Gurwitz, J.H. (1994). Reduction of bacteriuria and pyuria after ingestion of cranberry juice. *Journal of the American Medical Association*, 271(10):751-754; Jepson, R.G., Mihaljevic, L., Craig, J. (2000). Cranberries for treating urinary tract infections. *Cochrane Database of Systemic Reviews (computer file)*, 2:CD001322; and Ofek, I., Goldbar, J., Zafiri, D., et al. (1991). Anti-*Escherichia coli* adhesion activity of cranberry and blueberry juices. *New England Journal of Medicine*, 324(22):1599.

■ **Nursing Diagnosis.** The client undergoing nonnucleoside, reverse transcriptase inhibitor therapy has the potential for the following nursing diagnoses/collaborative problems: activity intolerance related to fatigue; diarrhea; impaired comfort (headache, muscle ache, nausea, vomiting); risk for imbalanced body temperature (fever); impaired skin integrity (skin rash, itching); impaired oral mucous membrane (mouth ulcers, conjunctivitis); and the potential complication of hepatitis.

■ **Implementation**

■ ***Monitoring.*** Hepatic function studies are continued throughout therapy for early detection of hepatitis.

■ ***Intervention.*** Administer without regard to meals; these drugs may be taken with or without food.

■ ***Education.*** Stress adherence to the medication regimen (see the general discussion under Nursing Management: Antiviral Therapy, p. 1022).

■ **Evaluation.** The expected outcome of nonnucleoside, reverse transcriptase inhibitor therapy is that the client will experience the slowing of the progression of the HIV infection and its sequelae, as well as increased CD4 counts, decreased viral loads, and an absence of opportunistic infections.

SUMMARY

Mycoses, infections of humans by fungi, range from very mild to life-threatening conditions. Some occur as the result of overgrowth during antibiotic, antineoplastic, or corticosteroid therapy.

Unfortunately, antifungal therapy is not as developed as antibacterial chemotherapy. Most agents are quite toxic to humans in concentrations that would be effective against most fungi; therefore most preparations are topical. Amphotericin B, fluconazole, flucytosine, griseofulvin, itraconazole, ketoconazole, miconazole, nystatin, and terbinafine are effective systemic fungistatic and fungicidal agents used for the treatment of a wide variety of mycotic infections.

Antiviral chemotherapy is even more difficult because, by the time symptoms of the illness appear, the course of the illness is set. Antiviral agents are best administered prophylactically to be most effective. Viruses are true parasites and use the enzyme systems of the host cells; for this reason, any effective therapy would also injure the host and thereby be too toxic for use. The general antiviral agents in use are acyclovir, amantadine, didanosine, famciclovir, foscarnet, ganciclovir, ribavirin, rimantadine, and valacyclovir. In addition, antivirals (alone or in combination) for the treatment of HIV infection are grouped in three categories: reverse transcriptase inhibitors, protease inhibitors, and nonnucleoside reverse transcriptase inhibitors; numerous agents are available in each of these categories. The prevention and management of adverse reactions are a major nursing responsibility for both antiviral and antifungal agents.

Critical Thinking Questions

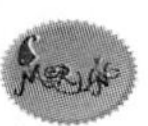

1. Why is antiviral therapy more limited than antibacterial or antifungal therapy?
2. Alice Mild, a 20-year-old college student, has been admitted to the hospital with histoplasmosis. The physician has prescribed amphotericin B to be administered 0.25 mg/kg IV. If Alice weighs 154 pounds, how many milligrams will her dose be? What precautions will the prescriber take before beginning the infusion

to minimize the adverse effects of the drug? How will the nurse monitor Alice's health status during the infusion?

Collaborative Learning Activities

For Collaborative Learning Activities, go to mosby.com/MERLIN/McKenry/.

CASE STUDY

For a Case Study that will help ensure mastery of this chapter content, go to mosby.com/MERLIN/McKenry/.

BIBLIOGRAPHY

Abelcet. (1996). *Abelcet package insert.* The Liposome Co. #1-1001-41-US-D.

American Hospital Formulary Service. (1999). *AHFS drug information: Current developments, Supplement A.* Washington, D.C.: American Society of Hospital Pharmacists.

Anderson. K.N., Anderson, L.E., & Glanze, W.D. (Eds.) (1998). *Mosby's medical, nursing, & allied health dictionary* (5th ed.). St. Louis: Mosby.

Armstrong, E.P., Abarca, J. (2000). Pharmacoeconomic model to evaluate new influenza treatments. *Formulary, 35*(2), 169-181.

Avorn, J., Monane, M., Gurwitz, J.H. (1994). Reduction of bateriuria and pyuria after ingestion of cranberry juice. *Journal of the American Medical Association, 271*(10):751-754.

Cidofovir Approved. (1996). *PI Perspective: Project Inform.* San Francisco: San Francisco Project Inform.

Cohen, B.A. & Brady, M. (1992). Practices surrounding ribavirin administration. *Pediatric Nursing, 18*(3), 253-257.

DeRosso, J.Q. & Gupta, A.K. (1999). Oral itraconazole therapy for superficial, subcutaneous, and systemic infections. *Postgraduate Medicine, 46*(6), 46-52.

Drug Facts and Comparisons. (2000). St. Louis: Facts and Comparisons.

Gilden, D. (1999). Absence makes the HAART grow fonder. *GMHC Treatment Issues, 13*(2), 1-12.

Hayden, F.G. (1996). Antimicrobial agents: Antiviral agents. In J.G. Hardman & L.E. Limbird (Eds.). *Goodman & Gilman's The pharmacological basis of therapeutics* (9th ed.). New York: McGraw-Hill.

Hitchens, K. (1996). New eye implant for treating cytomegalovirus. *Hospital Pharmacy Report, 10*(4), 20.

Jepson, R.G., Milhaljevic, L., Craig, J. (2000). Cranberries for treating urinary tract infections. *Cochrane Database of Systemic Reviews (computer file),* 2:CD001322.

Jury, D.L. (1993). More on RSV and ribavirin. *Pediatric Nursing, 19*(1), 89-91.

Less pills, less doses. (1999). *Simpler drug combinations for HIV: Internet updates from the AIDS Treatment Data Network;* 204.179.124.69/network/trs/aids98/rpt2.html (4/5/99).

MacDonald, L. & Kazanjian, P. (1996). Antiretroviral therapy in HIV infection: An update. *Hospital Formulary, 31*(9), 780-804.

Norton, M. (1999). Choosing the right initial antiretroviral regimens. *GMHC Treatment Issues, 13*(2), 7-10.

Ofek, I., Goldbar, J., Zafiri, D., et al. (1991). Anti-*Escherichia coli* adhesion activity of cranberry and blueberry juices. *New England Journal of Medicine, 324*(22):1599.

Pallela, F. (1999). Mortality and morbidity in HIV: Differences among therapeutic modalities. *Managed Care Interface Supplement,* pp. 10-14.

Podrasky, D.L. (1989). Amphotericin B: The nurse's role in controlling adverse reactions. *Focus Critical Care, 16*(3), 194.

Reuters New Media. (1998). *AIDS deaths drop for first time;* www.aegis.com/aegis/news/re/re1997/re970292.html (7/21/98).

Side effects of Anti-HIV drugs. (1999). *Internet update from the AIDS Treatment Data Network;* 204.179.124.69/network/trs/aids98/rpt3.html (4/5/99).

United States Pharmacopeia Dispensing Information (USP DI): Drug information for the health care professional (19th ed.). (1999). Rockville, MD: United States Pharmacopeial Convention.

United States Pharmacopeia Dispensing Information (USP DI): Drug information for the health care professional (20th ed.). (2000). Rockville, MD: United States Pharmacopeial Convention.

Walmsley, S. & Tseng, A. (1999). Comparative tolerability of therapies for cytomegalovirus retinitis. *Drug Safety, 21*(3), 203-224.

61 Other Antimicrobial Drugs and Antiparasitic Drugs

Chapter Focus

Many of the diseases discussed in this chapter were thought to be eradicable within this century. The teaching of good health practices and the use of effective drugs and insecticides held promise to end these diseases (e.g., malaria and tuberculosis), which are endemic in many parts of the world. The World Health Organization believed that malaria might be eradicated by 1964 with the combined use of DDT and antimalarial drugs; however, DDT was found to be harmful, and the *Anopheles* mosquito that carries the organism became resistant to the insecticide. In addition, the ability of pathogens to become drug-resistant to both tuberculosis and malaria has made health officials less optimistic. Tuberculosis has returned, with the resurgence of the disease peaking in 1992. Although rates remain high in the United States, there has been a decrease in the number of reported cases of tuberculosis (down 31% from 1992) (Centers for Disease Control and Prevention, 1999a). There has been a growth of ideal environments for the resurgence of tuberculosis—the homeless, the drug addicted, the impoverished, the immunosuppressed, and recent immigrants from countries where the disease is still endemic. These diseases will continue to challenge health care providers for some time.

Learning Objectives

1. Discuss the life cycle of the malarial parasite in the human body.
2. Implement the nursing management for the care of clients receiving antimalarial drug therapy.
3. Implement the nursing management for the care of clients receiving antituberculous drug therapy.
4. Describe the life cycle of the ameba, as well as intestinal and extraintestinal amebiasis in humans.
5. Discuss antiamebiasis agents and their nursing management.
6. Discuss other protozoan diseases and the drugs used in their treatment.

Key Terms

amebiasis, p. 1060
Hansen's disease, p. 1069
helminths, p. 1063
malaria, p. 1042
toxoplasmosis, p. 1062
trichomoniasis, p. 1063
tuberculosis, p. 1048

Key Drugs [✓]

chloroquine, p. 1044
isoniazid, p. 1056
rifampin, p. 1059
pyrazinamide, p. 1057

Antimicrobial and antiparasitic agents include antimalarial, antituberculous, amebicidal, anthelmintic, and leprostatic medications. Sulfonamides are reviewed in Chapter 59.

DRUGS USED IN THE TREATMENT OF MALARIA

Malaria is the most important of the parasitic diseases in humans; it affects 103 endemic countries with a population of more than 2.5 billion, and it causes 1 million to 3 million deaths each year (White and Breman, 1994). Although it is primarily endemic to the tropics, in 1995 the Centers for Disease Control and Prevention (CDC) received 1167 reports of malaria in the United States or its territories. This is an increase of 15% from the approximately 1000 cases reported in the United States in 1994; the cases in South America increased by 100% (Williams et al., 1999). Most U.S. cases involved persons who acquired this infection abroad because they either were not taking antimalarial chemoprophylaxis or were taking an inappropriate drug regimen. Four species of the genus *Plasmodium* are responsible for human malaria: *P. vivax*, *P. malariae*, *P. ovale*, and *P. falciparum* were identified in the U.S. cases, with *P. vivax* the most commonly reported. *P. falciparum* malaria is the most lethal form of malaria and is usually resistant to chloroquine.

Malaria may be transmitted to humans by the bite of an infected female *Anopheles* mosquito, by blood transfusion (usually *P. malariae*), congenitally, or by contaminated needles commonly used by substance abusers.

Life Cycle of the Malarial Parasite

To understand the chemotherapy of malaria, it is essential to review the life cycle of the malarial parasite, the plasmodium. Figure 61-1 presents the cycle in seven basic steps.

Plasmodia have two interdependent life cycles: (1) the sexual cycle, which takes place in the mosquito, and (2) the asexual cycle, which occurs in the human body.

Sexual Cycle. The sexual cycle is noted in step 7 of Figure 61-1. The female *Anopheles* mosquito becomes the carrier of the parasite by drawing blood that contains male and female forms from an infected person. These sexual forms of the parasite are known as gametocytes. The female gametocytes are fertilized by the male gametocytes in the stomach of the mosquito; zygotes form, which results in numerous cell divisions that develop into sporozoites. The formation of sporozoites in the mosquito completes the sexual cycle.

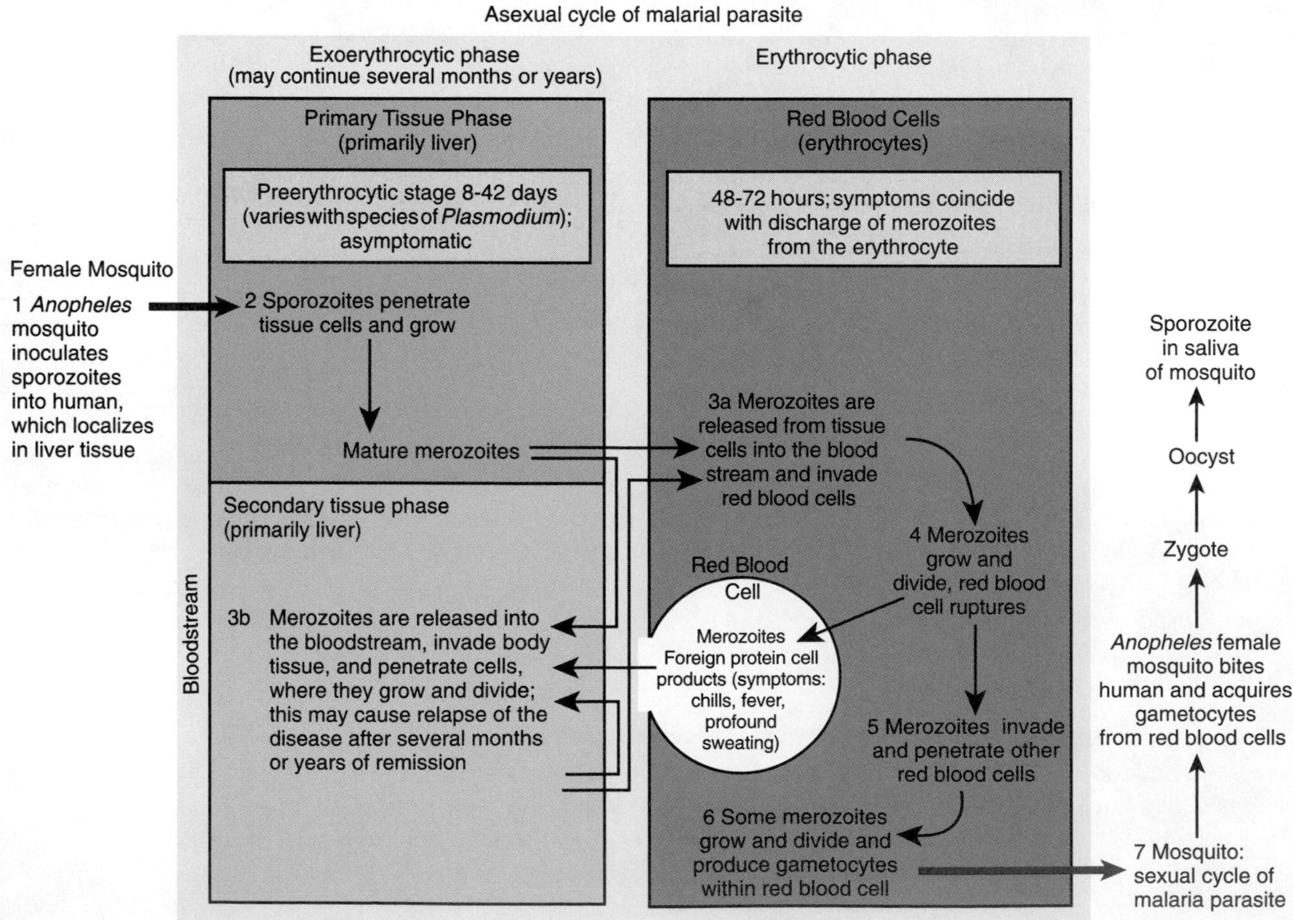

Figure 61-1 Life cycle of the malarial parasite.

Sporozoites then migrate to the salivary glands of the infected mosquito and are injected into the human bloodstream by the bite of the female insect (Figure 61-1, step 1).

Asexual Cycle. In the human, the asexual cycle of the plasmodium consists of the exoerythrocytic phase and the erythrocytic phase.

Exoerythrocytic Phase. Shortly after sporozoites are introduced into the circulation of the human, they leave the blood and enter the fixed tissue cells (reticuloendothelial cells) of the liver, where multiplication and maturation occur (step 2). For a period of time that varies with different plasmodia (8 to 42 days), the individual exhibits no symptoms, no parasites are found in the erythrocytes, and the blood is noninfective. This phase is known as the preerythrocytic stage. The parasites are called primary tissue schizonts, or preerythrocytic forms. After this stage, the young parasites burst from the liver cells as merozoites.

Erythrocytic Phase. When merozoites enter the bloodstream, they penetrate the erythrocytes and begin the erythrocytic phase of their existence (step 3a). In the case of *P. vivax* (but not *P. falciparum*), some of the merozoites invade other tissue cells to form secondary exoerythrocytic forms (step 3b). Relapses of *P. vivax* and other forms of malaria are believed to be caused by the successive formations of merozoites produced by various secondary exoerythrocytic forms of the parasite. Drugs affecting malarial parasites in the bloodstream do not always destroy those in the exoerythrocytic, or tissue, stage.

After the merozoites bore into red blood cells, they multiply again (this time asexually), and erythrocytic schizonts are formed. The erythrocytic phase is complete when the parasitized red blood cells rupture, setting free many more merozoites formed from the schizonts. Pyrogenic substances are also liberated, causing a rapid rise in body temperature (step 4). Some of the merozoites may be destroyed in the plasma of the blood by leukocytes and other agents, but some enter other erythrocytes to repeat the cycle (step 5). The recurring chills, fever, and prostration that are prominent clinical symptoms of malaria occur when the red blood cells rupture and release the young parasites with foreign protein and cell products. Depending on the plasmodium involved, the erythrocytic phase lasts from 48 to 72 hours. After a few cycles, some of the asexual forms of the malarial parasites develop into sexual forms called gametocytes (step 6). The cycle begins again when the mosquito bites a person infected with malarial parasites and ingests the sexual forms.

P. vivax is the most common form of malaria; this infestation is usually mild. Drug resistance is uncommon, and this form is suppressed easily with antimalarial medications. The *P. falciparum* strain of malaria is less common but is much more severe than *P. vivax*. Drug-resistant strains of *P. falciparum* are reported; symptoms of this infestation occur at irregular intervals and can cause very serious complications. If left untreated or if treatment is delayed, the disease may progress to irreversible cardiovascular shock and death. Relapses are reported with *P. vivax*, but no dormant forms remain in the liver once *P. falciparum* is eliminated; therefore no relapses are reported with *P. falciparum*.

Persons who harbor the sexual forms of plasmodia are called carriers; it is from carriers that mosquitoes receive the parasite forms that perpetuate the disease. The asexual forms cause the clinical symptoms of malaria. Carriers should avoid giving blood, because it is possible that the recipient of this blood will contract malaria or become a carrier. An increasing number of malaria cases (some fatal) have occurred from transfusions of infected blood. Some infected individuals who donated blood may have once lived in an area with malaria. Therefore any person who has had malaria or has been exposed to the disease by visiting a region where it is prevalent must be disqualified as a blood donor.

Antimalarial Medications

The choice of drug for treating malaria is based on the particular malarial strain involved and the stage of the *Plasmodium* life cycle. The drugs (schizonticides) are classified according to the type of therapy they provide, which is as follows:

1. Travelers to endemic areas should receive malaria chemoprophylaxis. They should call the CDC Division of Parasitic Diseases ([770] 488-7788) or the CDC Malaria Hotline ([888] 232-3228), which can verify if malaria prophylaxis and, also, if chloroquine (Aralen)-resistant *P. falciparum* has been reported in a specific country (Williams et al., 1999). Chloroquine, which suppresses the asexual erythrocytic forms, is effective against all species of malaria except the drug-resistant *P. falciparum*.
2. In areas containing chloroquine-resistant *P. falciparum*, mefloquine (Lariam) is used for prophylaxis; doxycycline is recommended if the client cannot take mefloquine.
3. Clinical cure of an acute malaria attack occurs when the multiplication of parasites within the erythrocyte is interrupted, thereby terminating the malarial symptoms of the attack. Fansidar (pyrimethamine-sulfadoxine) is recommended when a traveler develops a flu syndrome or fever and cannot reach medical care within 24 hours. Professional medical services should be obtained as soon as possible after treatment (CDC, 1999c).
4. Primaquine therapy may be recommended for the eradication of latent forms of *P. vivax* that persist and may cause an infection relapse. This drug is usually started after an acute attack or during the last few weeks of chloroquine prophylaxis. Inducing a radical cure requires medications that destroy both the exoerythrocytic and erythrocytic parasites to prevent relapsing malaria; therefore primaquine is given with chloroquine, which suppresses the erythrocytic cycle.

The emergence of drug-resistant strains of malaria, particularly that caused by *P. falciparum*, poses a major public health problem throughout the world (Bloland & Ettling,

1999). Despite the combined efforts of many countries to eradicate malaria, it remains the most devastating infectious disease in the world because of the many lives lost and the economic burdens it imposes. Fortunately, endemic malaria has been completely eradicated in the United States and Canada.

Malaria exists in Africa, Central and South America, the Middle East, Haiti, Mexico, and many other countries. It is essential that travelers contemplating a trip to malarious areas of the world be aware of the need to obtain information from their health care provider about measures for reducing exposure to the disease.

chloroquine [klor′ oh kwin] (Aralen)
hydroxychloroquine [hye drox ee klor′ oh kwin] (Plaquenil)

The mechanisms of action of chloroquine and hydroxychloroquine as antiprotozoals to treat malaria are unknown but may be a result of their ability to bind or alter DNA properties. They increase the pH of acid vesicles, thereby interfering with the functions of DNA. During suppressive therapy they inhibit the erythrocytic stage of development of plasmodia; during acute malarial attacks they interfere with the erythrocytic schizogony of parasites. As the drugs selectively accumulate in parasitized erythrocytes, they have a selective toxicity in the erythrocytic stages of plasmodial infestation.

These agents are indicated for the prevention and treatment of malaria for the four strains of plasmodium. Curing *P. vivax* and *P. ovale* malaria also requires the administration of primaquine. Hydroxychloroquine is also approved for the treatment of rheumatoid arthritis and for discoid and systemic lupus erythematosus.

Chloroquine and hydroxychloroquine are fairly well absorbed orally, are widely distributed in body tissues, and reach peak serum levels in approximately 3 to 3.5 hours. The terminal half-life of chloroquine is 1 to 2 months; the terminal half-life for hydroxychloroquine in blood is approximately 50 days (32 days in plasma). Both drugs are partially metabolized in the liver and excreted by the kidneys.

The side effects/adverse reactions of chloroquines are usually dose related and reversible. Gastric distress; headaches; pruritus; blurred vision; difficulty reading; headache and itching (reported mostly in black clients); hair loss or hair bleaching; blue-black discoloration of the skin, nails, or inside mouth; corneal opacities; and retinopathy have been reported. Blood disorders, cardiac dysrhythmia, mood alterations, ototoxicity, muscle weakness, and convulsions are rare.

The usual oral adult dosage of chloroquine to suppress malaria is 500 mg once every 7 days. The pediatric dosage is 8.3 mg/kg PO daily (not to exceed the adult dosage) every 7 days. The parenteral adult dosage is 200 to 250 mg IM repeated in 6 hours if needed. Do not exceed 1000 mg in the first day.

The adult oral dosage of hydroxychloroquine is 400 mg once every 7 days. The pediatric dosage is 6.4 mg/kg/day PO repeated weekly.

▪ Nursing Management

Chloroquine and Hydroxychloroquine Therapy

▪ **Assessment.** Chloroquine and hydroxychloroquine are used with caution in the presence of hypersensitivity to these substances, retinal or visual field changes, and pregnancy (to prevent retinal damage in the fetus). Long-term therapy in children is also contraindicated. These drugs are used with caution in clients with liver disease (who may require reduced dosages) and in clients with glucose-6-phosphate dehydrogenase (G6PD) deficiency and hematologic disorders (they may cause blood dyscrasias). Avoid the use of these drugs in clients with psoriasis or porphyria, because these conditions may become exacerbated. Polyneuritis, ototoxicity, seizures, or neuromyopathy from the administration of either of these two drugs may further compromise clients with severe neurologic disorders.

There are no drug interactions of clinical significance.

A baseline assessment of the client should include a history of foreign travel and exposure, the cyclic symptoms of fever and chills and other symptoms, and the findings of a complete blood count (CBC), ophthalmologic examination, and neuromuscular examination, including deep tendon reflexes of the knee and ankle reflexes.

▪ **Nursing Diagnosis.** The client receiving chloroquine and hydroxychloroquine therapy should be assessed for the following nursing diagnoses/collaborative problems: impaired comfort (headache and itching, particularly in black clients); deficient fluid volume related to anorexia, nausea, vomiting, and diarrhea; diarrhea; ineffective protection related to blood dyscrasias (agranulocytosis, aplastic anemia, neutropenia, thrombocytopenia); disturbed body image related to blue-black discoloration of the skin and fingernails or alopecia; disturbed sensory perception related to ototoxicity (tinnitus and hearing loss) or ocular toxicity (retinopathy, keratopathy, or cataracts evidenced by blurred vision); disturbed thought processes related to the development of psychosis (mood and mental changes); and the potential complications of cardiovascular toxicity (hypotension, QRS prolongation), neuromyopathy, or seizures.

▪ **Implementation**

▪ ***Monitoring.*** Obtain a baseline and periodic CBC, and test for G6PD deficiency to prevent the occurrence of hemolytic anemia (see the Cultural Considerations box on p. 1045). Signs of blood dyscrasia are fever, sore throat, fatigue, and easy bruising. Perform periodic tests of muscle strength and reflexes, particularly in clients who are undergoing long-term therapy. Consult with the prescriber to discontinue therapy if positive signs occur. Discontinue drugs at the first sign of retinal changes and/or visual disturbances, and continue to observe the client for possible progression even after therapy has been discontinued (Easterbrook, 1999).

Cultural Considerations

Glucose-6-Phosphate Dehydrogenase (G6PD) Deficiency and Antimalarial Agents

Approximately 10% of African Americans and 5% to 10% of Sephardic Jews, Greeks, Iranians, Chinese, Filipinos, and Indonesians have G6PD deficiency. This condition is transmitted as an X-linked trait. There is evidence that the enzyme G6PD in the red blood cells is essential for metabolism in the plasmodia; therefore persons with a genetic deficiency of G6PD in their red blood cells are believed to have some natural immunity to malaria.

Without G6PD, chloroquine and other antimalarial drugs impair the metabolism of red blood cells; therefore acute intravascular hemolysis may occur if these drugs are given. Treatment is by transfusion. Some blood banks test for G6PD deficiency in areas where malarial treatment is common.

Modified from Kuzma, E.C. (1992). Drug response: All bodies are not created equal. *American Journal of Nursing, 92*(12), 48.

Observe the client for drug resistance. Failure to prevent or cure clinical malaria may require treatment with other drugs if the person is infected with a resistant strain of the parasite.

■ ***Intervention.*** Administer oral drugs with milk or meals to minimize gastric irritation. If the client is undergoing parenteral therapy, substitute oral administration as soon as possible. For pediatric IV use, the drug should be diluted and administered very slowly, over at least 4 hours.

Hydroxychloroquine tablets may be crushed and placed in gelatin capsules or mixed with jam or gelatin to make them easier to swallow.

■ ***Education.*** Oral preparations are taken once a week. Suppressive therapy is initiated 2 weeks before exposure, and the medication is continued while the client is staying in the malarious area. Starting the drug in advance of travel also allows the client to determine his or her tolerance to the medication. Drug substitutions can be made before exposure if the client is intolerant. The client maintains the drug regimen for 4 weeks after leaving the region.

The client is to notify a health care provider if fever develops while traveling or within 2 months after leaving the endemic area. In addition to taking this medication to avoid contracting malaria, the client should also be instructed to stay indoors in well-screened areas after sundown, sleep under mosquito netting at night, wear trousers and long-sleeved shirts, and use mosquito repellent on exposed skin surfaces (Juckett, 1999).

Instruct the client to take the drug for the full course of treatment, even if he or she is feeling better. This will ensure that the infection is completely eradicated and that symptoms will not return. To obtain the full effect of the drug, inform the client to follow a regular schedule by taking it the same day each week. Keep this drug out of reach of children. Fatalities in children have occurred after the ingestion of one 300-mg tablet.

Instruct the client to keep regularly scheduled visits for ophthalmoscopic and audiometric examinations and to report to the prescriber any signs of visual and auditory disturbances. This is to prevent irreversible retinopathy, which may occur even after therapy is discontinued.

Explain to the client that the drug may cause a red or brown discoloration of the urine but that this is not medically significant.

When chloroquine and hydroxychloroquine are administered for rheumatoid arthritis, inform the client that therapeutic benefits usually do not occur until 6 to 12 months after initiating therapy.

Caution the client to avoid alcoholic beverages while taking this drug. Because the medication may cause dizziness, advise the client to avoid tasks that require mental alertness until his or her response to the medication has been determined.

■ **Evaluation.** The expected outcome of chloroquine and hydroxychloroquine therapy is that the client will be free of malarial infection (negative blood smears) without experiencing adverse reactions to the drug.

mefloquine [me′ floe kwin] (Lariam)

Mefloquine is a blood schizonticide; it prevents the replication of asexual erythrocytic parasites but has no effect on the gametocytes of *P. falciparum*. Its exact mechanism of action is unknown, but it is believed to inhibit protein synthesis (bind DNA), increase the intravascular pH of acid vesicles in the parasite, and have a variety of other actions. It is not effective in eliminating the exoerythrocytic or intrahepatic stages of *P. vivax* or *P. ovale* infections.

This drug is indicated for the prevention and treatment of chloroquine-resistant malaria and multiple drug-resistant strains of *P. falciparum*. It is also used to prevent malaria caused by *P. vivax*, *P. ovale*, and *P. malariae*.

Mefloquine is well absorbed orally. It is widely distributed in the body and reaches peak serum levels in 7 to 24 hours. It has an elimination half-life of 13 to 33 days, is partially metabolized in the liver, and is excreted primarily in the bile and feces.

The side effects/adverse reactions of mefloquine are uncommon and dose related. They occur more commonly in therapeutic than in prophylaxis drug regimens and include vomiting, headache, dizziness, insomnia, gastric distress, and visual disturbances.

The usual adult dosage for prophylaxis is 250 mg PO once weekly, beginning 1 week before travel, then weekly during traveling, and for 1 month after leaving the endemic areas. The therapeutic dosage for chloroquine-resistant *P. falciparum* malaria is 1250 mg PO as a single dose.

▪ Nursing Management

Mefloquine Therapy

Except for the following drug interactions, the nursing management of mefloquine therapy is essentially the same as that discussed for Nursing Management: Chloroquine and Hydroxychloroquine Therapy, p. 1044. This drug also has a neuropsychiatric toxicity that appears as anxiety, confusion, depression, hallucinations, psychoses, or seizures. It should be used carefully in clients who have a history of psychiatric disorders or in those whose occupation requires fine coordination and spatial discrimination, such as airline pilots or neurosurgeons.

Review the client's medication regimen for the risk of significant drug interactions, such as those that may occur when mefloquine is given with the following drugs:

Drug	Possible Effect and Management
Bold/color type indicates the most serious interactions	
beta blockers, calcium channel blocking agents, quinidine, or quinine	Concurrent use may result in an increased risk of dysrhythmias, cardiac arrest, and seizures (the latter especially with quinine). Avoid concurrent use or a potentially serious drug interaction may occur. If concurrent use cannot be avoided, monitor closely and also advise clients to take mefloquine at least 12 hours after a dose of quinidine or quinine.
chloroquine (Aralen)	May increase seizure activity. Monitor closely.
divalproex (Depakote) or valproic acid (Depakene)	Decreased serum levels of valproic acid are reported with a loss of seizure control. Monitor serum levels if concurrent drug therapy is necessary.

primaquine [prim′ a kween]

The mechanism of action of primaquine is unknown, but it can bind and alter DNA. It is very effective in the exoerythrocytic stages of *P. vivax* and *P. ovale* malaria and against the primary phase (exoerythrocytic stage) of *P. falciparum* malaria. It is also effective against the sexual forms (gametocytes) of plasmodia (especially *P. falciparum*). It is indicated to prevent malaria relapses (radical cure) caused by *P. vivax* and *P. ovale* and is also effective against gametocytes of *P. falciparum*.

Primaquine is absorbed orally and reaches a peak level within 2 to 3 hours. It has a half-life of approximately 6 hours and is rapidly metabolized in an unspecified site. A small amount is excreted by the kidneys.

The side effects/adverse reactions of primaquine include gastric distress, hemolytic anemia and, rarely, leukopenia.

The adult oral dosage of primaquine is 26.3 mg daily for 2 weeks. The pediatric dosage is 680 μg/kg daily for 2 weeks. Primaquine is not recommended for use during pregnancy.

▪ Nursing Management

Primaquine Therapy

▪ **Assessment.** The more serious adverse reactions to primaquine involve clients with a genetically determined G6PD deficiency, which can cause a lethal hemolysis of red blood cells.

Review the client's current medication regimen for the risk of significant drug interactions, such as those that may occur when primaquine is given concurrently with the following drugs:

Drug	Possible Effect and Management
Bold/color type indicates the most serious interactions.	
other hemolytic agents	May increase the risk for myelotoxic effects; monitor closely for muscle weakness and diminished deep tendon reflexes. Avoid concurrent use or a potentially serious drug interaction may occur.

A baseline assessment should include the client's history of exposure, underlying condition, CBC, hemoglobin, and G6PD determinations.

▪ **Nursing Diagnosis.** The client receiving primaquine should be assessed for the following nursing diagnoses/collaborative problems: deficient fluid volume related to anorexia, nausea, and vomiting; ineffective protection related to leukopenia; and the potential complications of hemolytic anemia and methemoglobinemia.

▪ **Implementation**

▪ ***Monitoring.*** Monitor CBCs and hemoglobin determinations weekly for a sudden decrease in hemoglobin concentration, erythrocyte count, or leukocyte count; discontinue medication if this occurs. Monitor for the signs of hemolytic anemia—fatigue, fever, pallor, anorexia, darkened urine, and back, leg, or abdominal pain. In addition, monitor for the less commonly occurring methemoglobinemia, with cyanosis, dizziness, dyspnea, and fatigue.

▪ ***Intervention.*** Gastric irritation can be minimized by administering primaquine with meals or antacids.

▪ ***Education.*** Encourage the client to comply with the full course of medication and to report promptly any symptoms of adverse reactions.

▪ **Evaluation.** The expected outcome of primaquine therapy is that client will be free of malaria infection (negative blood smears) without any experiencing adverse reactions to the drug.

quinine [kwye′ nine]

Quinine was the first drug used to treat malaria. As a schizonticidal agent it concentrates in parasitized erythrocytes, which may be why it has selective toxicity during the erythrocytic stages of plasmodial infections. It can also bind to DNA, thus inhibiting RNA synthesis and DNA replication.

Quinine sulfate was indicated for use in combination with other drugs for the treatment of chloroquine-resistant malaria caused by chloroquine-resistant *P. falciparum*, but today it is rarely used for malaria because more effective and less toxic drugs are available. Quinine has been reported to cause congenital malformations and stillbirths and therefore should not be taken by pregnant women (see the Pregnancy Safety box below).

■ Nursing Management

Quinine Sulfate Therapy

■ **Assessment.** Quinine is to be administered with caution to clients with G6PD deficiency because it may cause hemolytic anemia (see the Cultural Considerations box on p. 1045). Clients with hypoglycemia may experience a worsening of their condition, because quinine stimulates the release of insulin from the pancreas. Quinine may exacerbate muscle weakness in clients with myasthenia gravis and may cause thrombocytopenic purpura. Clients with a history of blackwater fever may be predisposed to the complications of this condition, including anemia and hemolysis with renal failure, when quinine is administered. Use quinine with caution in clients with cardiac dysrhythmias, because QT prolongation may occur. Note that quinine has quinidine-like activity. Hypersensitivity to quinine or quinidine would negate the use of this drug.

Review the client's medications for significant drug interactions. An increased incidence of convulsions and electrocardiogram (ECG) abnormalities have been reported when quinine is given with mefloquine. Administer mefloquine at least 12 hours after the last dose of quinine. If both drugs must be given concurrently, the client should be hospitalized and monitored closely for cardiac dysrhythmias and seizure activity.

Pregnancy Safety
Other Antimicrobial Drugs and Antiparasitic Drugs

Category	Drug
B	niclosamide, praziquantel, rifabutin
C	capreomycin, clofazimine, cycloserine, dapsone, isoniazid, mebendazole, mefloquine, oxamniquine, pyrazinamide, pyrimethamine, rifampin, thiabendazole
D	streptomycin
X	primaquine, quinine, thalidomide
Unclassified*	aminosalicylates, chloroquine, diethylcarbamazine, ethambutol, ethionamide, hydroxychloroquine, iodoquinol, paromomycin, piperazine, pyrantel

*The risk-benefit ratio should be carefully evaluated before use.

A baseline assessment should include a description of the client's disease symptoms, G6PD status, CBC and, if the client has an existing cardiovascular problem, an ECG.

■ **Nursing Diagnosis.** The client receiving quinine should be assessed for the following nursing diagnoses/collaborative problems: deficient fluid volume related to anorexia, nausea, vomiting, and diarrhea; ineffective protection related to agranulocytosis, hemolytic anemia, hypoprothrombinemia, and thrombocytopenia; disturbed sensory perception related to ocular toxicity (visual defects, blindness); and the potential complications of hypoglycemia, cardiovascular toxicity (hypotension, dysrhythmias, cardiac arrest), hypersensitivity (rash, fever, dyspnea), cinchonism (blurred vision, headache, ringing in ears), and hepatotoxicity.

■ **Implementation**

■ ***Monitoring.*** Observe for symptoms of cinchonism (tinnitus, dizziness, altered auditory acuity, visual disturbances, headache, gastrointestinal distress, nausea, and diarrhea). These symptoms disappear when the drug is discontinued. Monitor serum concentration levels; levels above 10 mg/100 mL may cause symptoms of cinchonism. Monitor CBC and liver function studies.

■ ***Intervention.*** Because quinine irritates the gastrointestinal mucosa, the capsule should be administered intact with food. Quinine has been replaced by more effective and less toxic drugs, except for its use in chloroquine-resistant falciparum malaria, for which it has been the traditional antimalarial remedy.

■ ***Education.*** Instruct the client to remain compliant with the antimalarial medication regimen for the full course of therapy. Instruct the client to report to the prescriber any side effects/adverse reactions, particularly any vision changes.

■ **Evaluation.** The expected outcome of quinine therapy is that the client is free of the malarial infection, with a negative blood smear and no adverse reactions to the drug.

pyrimethamine tablets [peer i meth′ a meen] (Daraprim)
pyrimethamine with sulfadoxine (Fansidar)

Pyrimethamine is an antiprotozoal agent used to treat malaria and toxoplasmosis. It binds to and inhibits the protozoal enzyme dihydrofolate reductase, thus inhibiting the conversion of dihydrofolic acid to tetrahydrofolic acid. This results in a depletion of folate, which is essential for nucleic acid synthesis and protein production. Pyrimethamine in combination with mefloquine and sulfadoxine is indicated for the treatment of chloroquine-resistant *P. falciparum* malaria. This drug is also combined with a sulfonamide to treat toxoplasmosis caused by *Toxoplasma gondii*.

Pyrimethamine is absorbed orally and is widely distributed in the body; it concentrates mainly in the blood cells, kidneys, liver, and spleen. It reaches peak plasma levels in 3 hours and has a half-life of 80 to 123 hours. It is metabolized in the liver and excreted by the kidneys.

The side effects/adverse reactions of pyrimethamine are usually rare, but gastric distress, atrophic glossitis, and blood dyscrasias are reported with high dosages.

The adult oral dosage in specific world areas (e.g., Southeast Asia, East Africa, or the Amazon) is 75 mg of pyrimethamine in combination with 750 mg mefloquine and 1.5 g of sulfadoxine as a single dose. For additional dosing recommendations, refer to a current package insert or the *United States Pharmacopeia Dispensing Information*.

▪ Nursing Management

Pyrimethamine Therapy

▪ **Assessment.** The risk-benefit ratio must be considered in nursing mothers, because pyrimethamine may disrupt the metabolism of folic acid in a nursing infant.

Use pyrimethamine with caution in clients with anemia or bone marrow depression, because it may cause folic acid deficiency and result in megaloblastic anemia and blood dyscrasias. Do not use this drug for the treatment of resistant forms of the parasite.

An increase in leukopenia and/or thrombocytopenia may occur when pyrimethamine is administered concurrently with other bone marrow depressants. A baseline assessment should include a CBC and platelet count, as well as a history of exposure and a description of the client's disease symptoms.

▪ **Nursing Diagnosis.** The client receiving pyrimethamine should be assessed for the following nursing diagnoses/collaborative problems: deficient fluid volume related to anorexia, nausea, vomiting, and diarrhea; ineffective protection related to blood dyscrasias (agranulocytosis, megaloblastic anemia, thrombocytopenia); impaired oral mucous membrane related to folic acid deficiency (pain and inflammation of the tongue [atrophic glossitis]); and the potential complications of hypersensitivity (rash) and neurotoxicity (excitability, seizures).

▪ **Implementation**

▪ ***Monitoring.*** The high dosage required for treating toxoplasmosis could approach the toxic level. Monitor CBCs and platelet counts. The dosage may be reduced if folic acid deficiency develops. The clinical symptoms of folic acid deficiency are soreness, redness, or burning of the tongue; pharyngitis; mouth ulcers; or diarrhea. Therapy should be discontinued if these symptoms occur; folic acid deficiency may be prevented by the administration of leucovorin. The administration of folinic acid (leucovorin) restores the depressed platelet or white blood counts to normal levels.

▪ ***Intervention.*** Administer pyrimethamine with milk or food to minimize gastric irritation. For children, tablets may be crushed to prepare 1% solution in normal saline; use within 24 hours at room temperature. If mixed with cherry syrup National Formulary (NF), use immediately after preparation. To prevent possible central nervous system (CNS) toxicity in clients with convulsive disorders, use a small initial dose for the treatment of toxoplasmosis.

If used to prevent malaria, pyrimethamine should be taken 2 weeks before entering a malarious area and continued for 6 weeks after leaving it. Besides building tissue stores of the drug, early administration allows assessment of the client's tolerance of the drug.

▪ ***Education.*** Advise the client to have weekly blood counts and platelet counts if undergoing high-dose therapy. If taken as a malaria suppressant, instruct the client to follow the dosage schedule as prescribed by taking the drug on the same day each week.

Advise the client to sleep under mosquito netting to avoid being bitten by malaria-carrying mosquitoes while in endemic areas. Advise the client to wear proper clothing so that arms and legs are covered, especially at dawn and during the evening hours, when mosquitoes are out. The use of mosquito repellent on uncovered areas of the skin may help to protect the client from the bites of infected mosquitoes.

Instruct the client to report to the prescriber any signs of possible blood dyscrasia (fever, sore throat, unusual bleeding or bruising, extreme weakness, and fatigue). Alert the client to use caution when performing dental hygiene, such as using soft toothbrushes, no dental floss, and no toothpicks. Dental work is postponed until blood counts are within normal limits.

Because of the risk of severe skin reactions, Fansidar (pyrimethamine with sulfadoxine) should be used only when the client is planning to stay longer than 3 weeks in an area where chloroquine-resistant malaria is prevalent. The drug should be discontinued and a health care provider notified at the first sign of a rash.

▪ **Evaluation.** The expected outcome of pyrimethamine therapy is that the client is free of infection, with negative blood smears and no adverse reactions to the drug.

DRUGS USED IN THE TREATMENT OF TUBERCULOSIS

Tuberculosis (TB) is a chronic granulomatous infection caused by the acid-fast bacillus *Mycobacterium tuberculosis*. It declined in incidence in the United States until 1985, when an increased incidence was noted in native-born Americans. Approximately 8 million new cases of TB are diagnosed worldwide, with 2.9 million dying annually from this disease (Cali, 1995). In 1998, 18,361 cases of TB were reported in the United States; this represents a decrease of 7.5% and 31% when compared to 1997 and 1992 reports, respectively. Approximately 24% of the cases involved individuals 65 years of age and older (Surveillance Report, 1999). The decrease in TB has occurred primarily in persons born in the United States, whereas an increase has been reported in foreign-born individuals. TB is largely attributed to high-risk individuals, such as those with acquired immunodeficiency syndrome (AIDS), those living on the street, homeless persons, substance abusers, undernourished or malnourished persons, or those taking immunosuppressant drugs or suffering from cancer.

M. tuberculosis, the bacteria that causes TB, most commonly affects the lungs, but other body areas can also be infected, such as the bones, joints, skin, meninges, or genitourinary tract. This bacterium is an aerobic bacillus that needs a highly oxygenated organ site for growth; thus the lungs, the growing ends of the bones, and the cerebral cortex are ideal sites. Tubercle bacilli may be transmitted by airborne droplets but cannot be transmitted on objects such as dishes, clothing, or sheets and bedding (Figure 61-2). Sharing an enclosed environment with an infected person is associated with a high risk of developing this infection, especially in facilities that provide less than optimum health care (Posey, 1996).

The development of drug-resistant TB is a major concern today. It is estimated that there is approximately a 9% incidence of drug-resistant organisms in the United States (Ward, 1995). Resistance to two or more drugs (multidrug-resistant TB [MDR TB]) has resulted in outbreaks in institutional facilities. Fortunately, a decrease in the development of MDR TB was reported in 1997; however, a stable resistance level is still present with isoniazid (Surveillance Report, 1999). This may indicate progress in early detection and the use of appropriate therapies as factors that contributed to this decline.

Pathogenesis

Tubercle bacilli droplets are transmitted when an infected person coughs or sneezes. In general, persons who produce sputum have many bacilli and are more infectious than infected persons who do not cough. The three primary types of tubercle bacilli that are pathogenic to humans are human to human, bovine to human, and avian to human. Avian TB is rare in the United States and Canada; bovine TB is much less prevalent with the pasteurization of milk and testing of cows. Thus the primary source of transmission is human to human.

When tubercle bacilli enter the lungs, infection can spread to other body organs through the blood and lymph system. Usually, however, the infection becomes dormant and is walled off by calcified and fibrous tissues. The bacilli become inactive, perhaps for the lifetime of the host. How-

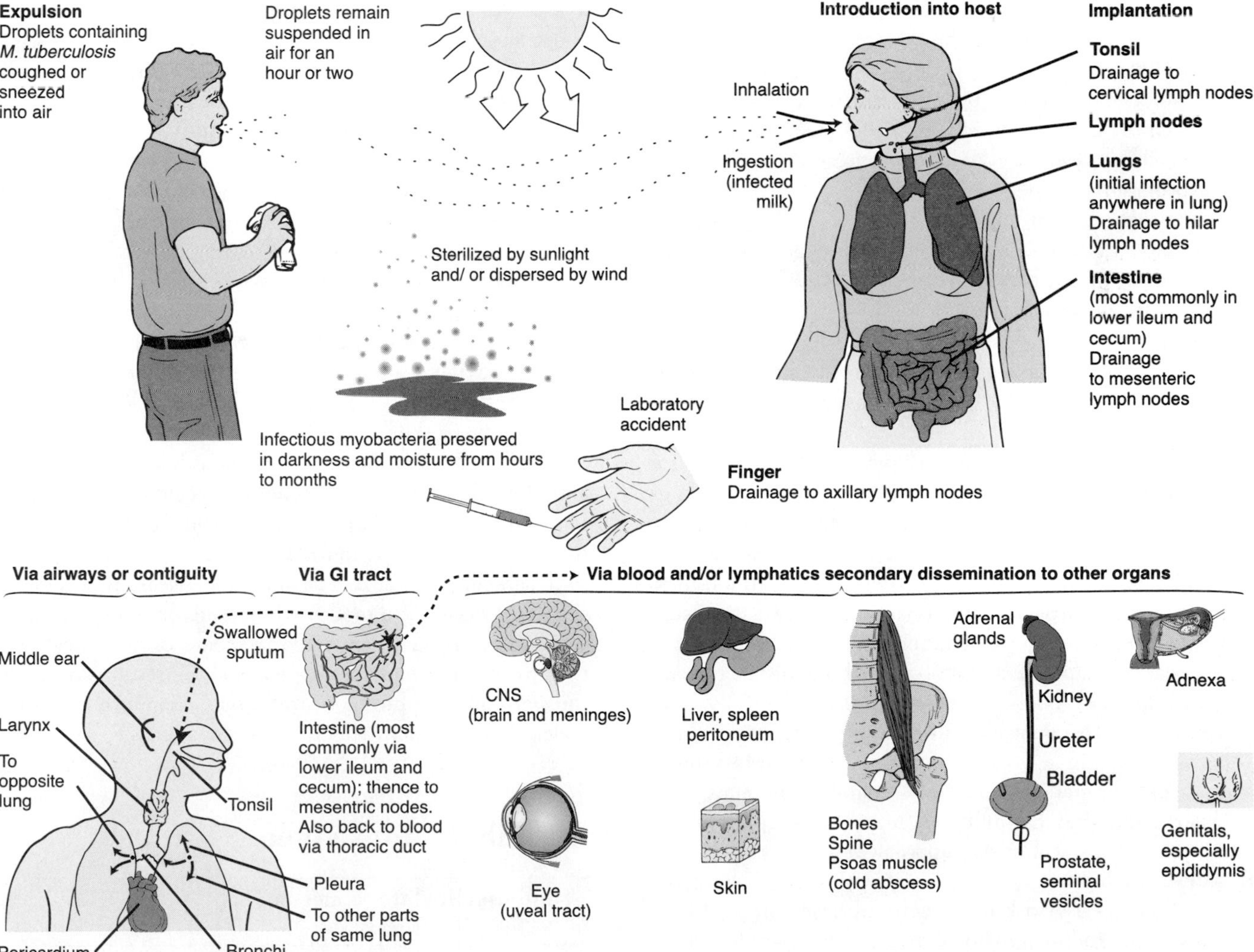

Figure 61-2 Dissemination of tuberculosis.

ever, the bacilli may be reactivated if host defenses break down or if the host receives an immunosuppressive drug.

Drug Treatment Regimens

Effective drug regimens are available to prevent and treat TB. Drug selection is based on the development of drug-resistant organisms and drug toxicity. General guidelines include the following:

1. To avoid the development of drug-resistant organisms, all individuals diagnosed with TB (isolated *M. tuberculosis*) should undergo drug susceptibility tests on their first isolation.
2. In most instances drug therapy is started before the results of the in vitro susceptibility test are known. It is recommended that a four-drug regimen be instituted (especially in areas where primary isoniazid resistance occurs), because this regimen provides adequate therapy that will be at least 95% effective, even in the presence of drug-resistant organisms (Table 61-1). The recommended drugs are INH, rifampin, pyrazinamide (PZA), and ethambutol or streptomycin (Table 61-2) (CDC, 1999b; Mandell & Petri, 1996).
3. The drug regimen can be adjusted when drug susceptibility results are available.
4. Monitor the prescribed therapy regimen closely to support client compliance, detect side effects or adverse reactions, and register progress of the treatment program.

The usual regimen for the prevention of TB is isoniazid given daily for 6 months; HIV-infected clients receive 12 months of isoniazid preventive therapy (CDC, 1999b).

▪ Nursing Management

Antituberculous Therapy

This general nursing management for antituberculous agents will be supplemented by specific considerations for each agent.

▪ **Assessment.** Cultures for *Mycobacterium* and tests for the organism's susceptibility to the antituberculous drugs should be obtained before and periodically during the course of drug therapy. Sputum specimens can help confirm active TB and help to estimate the degree of infectiousness. If the client has suspected pulmonary TB, at least three sputum specimens should be examined by smear and culture. The smear test can detect mycobacterial organisms, but culture testing takes much longer—from 2 to 12 weeks (Boutotte, 1993). The client may also exhibit nonspecific symptoms, such as fatigue, weakness, anorexia, weight loss, night sweats, or low-grade fever. X-ray examinations may show nodular lesions, patchy infiltrates (many in the upper lobes), cavity formation, scar tissue, and calcium deposits.

▪ **Nursing Diagnosis.** The client with TB will have the nursing diagnosis of risk for infection transmission (at least initially). The following should also be considered: ineffective airway clearance related to copious tracheobronchial secretions; risk of infection related to the ineffectiveness of the antituberculous drug; risk for infection transmission; deficient knowledge related to unfamiliarity with the disease process and treatment methods; ineffective therapeutic regimen management; and any collaborative problems that might relate to complications of the disease.

▪ **Implementation**

▪ ***Monitoring.*** Sputum cultures and x-ray examinations are used to monitor the client's status and the general health status of the client. Monitor the client for symptoms that indicate resolution of the infection: diminished cough and sputum production, decreased fever and night sweats, reduction of cavitation on x-ray examination, reduction of anorexia with concomitant weight gain, and decreased acid-fast bacteria (AFB) in sputum specimens. (See the Community and Home Health Considerations box on p. 1052 for information regarding medication monitoring in the community.)

▪ ***Intervention.*** Attempt to administer these drugs with consideration for the client's comfort. For example, gastrointestinal disturbances following administration can be reduced by the concurrent administration of food or antacids.

Some settings have instituted directly observed therapy (DOT) to prevent multidrug-resistant therapy (CDC, 1999b; Iseman, 1999; Yew 1999).

▪ ***Education.*** For maximum therapeutic effectiveness, the client must take prescribed medications regularly and without interruption. A client who is responsible for self-medication should be instructed about the necessity of taking these drugs (two or more concurrently) according to the prescribed regimen and not discontinuing them when feeling better. Alert the client to the adverse effects of the specific drugs and the need to report these effects immediately. Instruct clients who are self-medicating about the necessity for periodic medical evaluations to evaluate the effectiveness of therapy.

Remind the client to get sufficient rest. Stress the importance of having a well-balanced diet. The client should eat small, frequent meals if he or she is anorexic. Record the client's weight weekly.

When peripheral neuritis appears as a side effect of the antituberculous drugs, teach clients precautionary strategies to avoid injury from burning agents and sharp objects until the alteration in sensation is remedied.

Teach clients measures to minimize disease transmission, such as covering the mouth when coughing and sneezing.

▪ **Evaluation.** The expected outcome of antituberculous therapy is that the client's sputum culture result is negative, the signs and symptoms of the disease diminish or do not appear, and the client effectively self-manages the therapeutic regimen.

Antituberculous Agents

aminosalicylate [a mee noe sal i′ si late] (PAS, Tubasal, Nemasol 🍁)

Aminosalicylate is a bacteriostatic agent closely related to paraaminobenzoic acid (PABA); thus it competitively inhibits folic acid formation and results in the suppression of the

TABLE 61-1 Treatment Regimens and Dosages for Tuberculosis: Six-Month Regimen Options[a] for Pulmonary and Extrapulmonary Tuberculosis in Adults and Children

	Initial Phase		Continuation Phase		
	Drugs	**Interval and Duration**	**Drugs**	**Interval and Duration**	**Comments**
1	INH, RIF, PZA[f], EMB[b], or SM[f]	Daily for 8 weeks	INH, RIF	Daily or 2 or 3 times weekly[c] for 16 weeks[d]	EMB or SM[f] should be continued until susceptibility to INH and RIF is shown. In areas where fewer than 4% of cases are resistant to INH (first drug susceptibility test only), EMB or SM[f] may not be necessary for clients with no individual risk factors for drug resistance.
2	INH, RIF, PZA, EMB[b], or SM[f]	Daily for 2 weeks, then 2 times weekly[c] for 6 weeks	INH, RIF	2 times weekly[c] for 16 weeks[d]	Clients prescribed this regimen should be given directly observed therapy. After the initial phase, EMB or SM[f] should be continued until susceptibility to INH and RIF is shown, unless drug resistance is unlikely.
3	INH, RIF, PZA[f], EMB[b], or SM[f]	3 times weekly[c] for 6 months[d]			Clients prescribed this regimen should be given directly observed therapy. Continue all four drugs for 6 months.[e] This regimen has been shown to be effective for INH-resistant TB.

INH, Isoniazid; *RIF,* rifampin; *PZA,* pyrazinamide; *SM,* streptomycin; *EMB,* ethambutol.

NOTE: Consult a TB medical expert if a client's drug susceptibility results show resistance to INH, RIF, PZA[f], EMB, or SM[f], or if the client has symptoms, positive smears, or positive cultures after 3 months.

[a]Different regimen options are necessary for adults who have smear- and culture-negative pulmonary TB and for adults and children for whom PZA[f] is contraindicated. Consult a medical expert for further information.

[b]Ethambutol is not recommended for children who are too young to be monitored for vision changes. However, ethambutol should be considered for all children who have TB that is resistant to other drugs but susceptible to ethambutol.

[c]All clients who are prescribed an intermittent regimen should be given directly observed therapy.

[d]Treatment should last at least 12 months for infants and children with miliary TB, bone and joint TB, or TB meningitis. Responses to therapy should be monitored closely in adults with these forms of extrapulmonary TB. If the response is slow or inadequate, treatment may be prolonged on a case-by-case basis.

[e]There is some evidence that SM[f] may be discontinued after 4 months if the isolate is susceptible to all drugs.

[f]PZA and SM should *not* be used by pregnant women. There is not enough information about how PZA affects the fetus, and SM has been shown to have harmful effects on the fetus.

TABLE 61-2 Dosage Recommendations for the Treatment of Tuberculosis in Children* and Adults

	Dosage in mg/kg (maximum dose)					
	Daily		2 times/week†		3 times/week†	
Drug	**Children**	**Adults**	**Children**	**Adults**	**Children**	**Adults**
isoniazid (INH)	10-20 (300 mg)	5 (300 mg)	20-40 (900 mg)	15 (900 mg)	20-40 (900 mg)	15 (900 mg)
rifampin (RIF)	10-20 (600 mg)	10 (600 mg)	10-20 (600 mg)	10 (600 mg)	10-20 (600 mg)	10 (600 mg)
pyrazinamide (PZA)‡	15-30 (2 g)	15-30 (2 g)	50-70 (4 g)	50-70 (4 g)	50-70 (3 g)	50-70 (3 g)
ethambutol (EMB)§	15-25	15-25	50	50	25-30	25-30
streptomycin (SM)‡	20-40 (1 g)	15 (1 g)	25-30 (1.5 g)	25-30 (1.5 g)	25-30 (1.5 g)	25-30 (1.5 g)

From Centers for Disease Control and Prevention. *Treatment of tuberculosis infection and disease;* www.cdc.gov/phtn/tbmodules/modules1-5/m4/4-m-04c.htm (2/15/00).

NOTE: Dosages are based on weight must be adjusted as the client's weight changes.

*Children younger than 12 years of age.

†All clients who are prescribed an intermittent regimen should be given directly observed therapy.

‡Pyrazinamide and streptomycin should not be used to treat pregnant women.

§Ethambutol is not recommended for children who are too young to be monitored for vision changes. However, ethambutol should be considered for all children who have TB that is resistant to other drugs but susceptible to ethambutol.

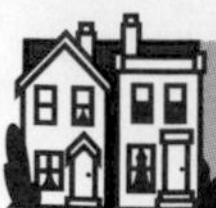

Community and Home Health Considerations
Antituberculous Medication Management in the Community

Nursing management of an antituberculous therapeutic regimen has the following expected outcomes: completion of an effective course of therapy that consists of at least two drugs to which the organism is susceptible; keeping the course of therapy as short as possible to promote client adherence; and preventing the transmission of outbreaks (Boutotte, 1993):

1. Monitor the client's response to therapy. A client with pulmonary TB should have his or her sputum tested at least monthly until the culture results are negative. Follow-up sputum testing is necessary to determine the client's response to therapy and how long therapy should last. Once effective antituberculous therapy begins, the number of organisms in the smear tests will decrease, and the client's symptoms will improve. If specimens remain positive after 3 months of therapy, the disease may be the result of a drug-resistant organism, or the client is not taking his or her medications as prescribed.
2. Ensure client adherence. Instruct the client in the importance of taking the medication for the duration of therapy, even if he or she is feeling better. Assess for adherence at every follow-up visit. Pill counts are helpful. Urine tests are available as a dipstick test that can detect INH in the urine 24 to 48 hours after the drugs are taken. Rifampin also turns the urine orange-colored for several hours after a dose.

   The most effective way to ensure client compliance is "directly observed therapy." DOT requires that someone actually observe the client take every dose of medication for the entire therapeutic regimen. DOT programs increase adherence in both rural and urban settings. One hospital in New York City reported that only 11% of clients under care for TB reported to an outpatient clinic for further treatment when discharged from the hospital. In contrast, a program in which DOT is routinely used for all clients had a completion rate of 98%. Although an expanded use of DOT may require additional resources, intermittent and directly observed regimens are cost-effective (CDC, 1999b). DOT can be conducted with regimens given once daily, 2 times weekly, or 3 times weekly.
3. Monitor for adverse drug reactions. Because of the long-term nature of drug therapy for TB, clients may need support in maintaining the therapeutic regimen and in managing the side effects of the TB drugs.

growth and reproduction of *M. tuberculosis*. It is indicated for the treatment of pulmonary and extrapulmonary *M. tuberculosis* in combination with other antituberculous drugs.

Aminosalicylate is well absorbed orally and distributed to various body fluids, with high levels accumulating in the pleural fluids, kidney, lungs, and liver tissues. The half-life is between 45 and 60 minutes, although it may extend up to 23 hours in clients with impaired renal function. Peak serum levels are reached within 1 to 2 hours. This drug is metabolized in the liver and excreted by the kidneys.

The side effects/adverse reactions of aminosalicylate therapy include a hypersensitivity reaction and gastric distress.

The adult oral dosage given in combination with other antimycobacterials is 3.3 to 4 g every 8 hours. The maximum daily dose is 20 g. The pediatric dosage in combination with other antimycobacterials is 50 to 75 mg/kg PO every 6 hours.

■ Nursing Management
Aminosalicylate Therapy

In addition to the following discussion, see Nursing Management: Antituberculous Therapy, p. 1050.

■ **Assessment.** A history of allergic reaction to other salicylates and sulfonamides may indicate a cross-intolerance for aminosalicylate, in which case the drug is contraindicated. Aminosalicylates should be used with caution if the client has any of the following preexisting conditions: anemia (this drug competes successfully with vitamin B_{12} and worsens anemias) or severe renal or hepatic function impairment (reduced dosages are required). Aminosalicylate in the Paser granule form has no significant drug interactions.

A baseline assessment is to be performed as described in the previous section on antituberculous drug therapy.

■ **Nursing Diagnosis.** The client receiving aminosalicylates should be assessed for the following nursing diagnoses/collaborative problems: deficient fluid volume related to anorexia, nausea, vomiting, and diarrhea; ineffective protection related to leukopenia or thrombocytopenia; activity intolerance related to hemolytic anemia or an infectious mononucleosis-like syndrome (fever, headache, rash, sore throat, fatigue); and the potential complications of hepatitis (yellow sclera and skin) and crystalluria.

■ **Implementation**

■ ***Monitoring.*** Monitor the client for adverse reactions to the drug therapy as noted in the Nursing Diagnosis section. Urinalyses should be performed at periodic intervals during drug therapy to monitor for crystals, casts, cells, and decreased specific gravity.

■ ***Intervention.*** The Paser extended-release granules may be administered by sprinkling them on applesauce or yogurt or by mixing them in a glass to suspend them in an acidic drink such as orange, grapefruit, grape, cranberry, apple or tomato juice, or fruit punch. The client should have a fluid intake of 3000 mL daily, and the urine should be maintained at a neutral or alkaline pH to minimize crystalluria.

■ ***Education.*** Therapy may need to continue for 1 to 2 years or longer; and therefore the client's ability to manage the therapeutic regimen effectively is extremely important. Alert the client to discontinue the drug and contact the prescriber at the first sign of hypersensitivity, such as rash, fever, and gastrointestinal symptoms. Advise the client that the skeleton of the granules may be seen in the stool but that this is not significant.

Aminosalicylate should not be used if the packets are swollen or if the granules have changed from tan to dark brown or purple.

■ **Evaluation.** The expected outcome of aminosalicylate therapy is that the client will eventually be free of infection (negative sputum or other culture for AFB) without experiencing any adverse reactions to the drug.

capreomycin [kap ree oh mye′ sin] (Capastat)

Capreomycin is an antimycobacterial agent with an unknown mechanism of action. It is indicated in combination therapy for the treatment of pulmonary TB caused by *M. tuberculosis* after primary medications (streptomycin, isoniazid, rifampin, pyrazinamide, and ethambutol) fail or when these medications cannot be used because of resistant bacilli or drug toxicity.

Administered intramuscularly, capreomycin has a half-life between 3 and 6 hours and reaches peak serum levels in 1 to 2 hours. It is excreted primarily unchanged by the kidneys.

The side effects/adverse reactions of capreomycin include nephrotoxicity, hypokalemia, neuromuscular blockade, ototoxicity, and hypersensitivity.

The adult dosage in combination with other antituberculous agents is 1 g IM daily for 2 to 4 months, followed by 1 g two or three times weekly.

■ Nursing Management

Capreomycin Therapy

In addition to the following discussion, see Nursing Management: Antituberculous Therapy, p. 1050.

■ **Assessment.** The health assessment should determine if the client has the following preexisting conditions: dehydration (increases the risk of toxicity due to increased serum levels of the drug), myasthenia gravis and parkinsonism (neuromuscular deficits may increase), impairment of the eighth cranial nerve (may cause increased auditory and vestibular toxicity), and renal impairment (may increase because of the nephrotoxic effects of this drug). Because of these effects, fluid balance, audiograms, and vestibular and renal function determinations should be assessed before therapy. Hypersensitivity to the drug should be determined.

Review the client's medication regimen for the risk of potentially life-threatening drug interactions. When capreomycin is administered with any of the following drugs, very serious reactions may result. Avoid the following combinations if possible:

Drug	Possible Effect and Management
Bold/color type indicates the most serious interactions.	
aminoglycosides, parenteral	**Increased risk for developing ototoxicity, nephrotoxicity, and neuromuscular blockade. Hearing loss may progress to deafness, even after the drug is stopped. This can be a very dangerous combination. Avoid concurrent drug administration.**
methoxyflurane (Penthrane) or polymyxins, parenteral	**The potential for nephrotoxicity and/or neuromuscular blockade is increased, which may lead to respiratory depression or paralysis. Avoid concurrent or sequential drug administration.**
nephrotoxic or ototoxic medications, such as amphotericin B parenteral, bacitracin parenteral, bumetanide parenteral (Bumex), cisplatin (Platinol), cyclosporine (Sandimmune), ethacrynic acid (Edecrin), furosemide parenteral (Lasix), paromomycin (Humatin), or vancomycin (Vancocin)	**Concurrent or even sequential use of capreomycin with any of these drugs can increase the risk of ototoxicity and/or nephrotoxicity. Hearing loss may occur and progress to deafness, even if the drugs are stopped. Avoid concurrent or sequential use if at all possible.**
neuromuscular blocking agents	**May result in increased neuromuscular blocking effects, resulting in respiratory depression or paralysis. Monitor closely, especially during surgery or in the postoperative period. Avoid this combination if possible. If not, closely monitor and keep anticholinesterase agents or calcium salts on hand to reverse the blockade.**

■ **Nursing Diagnosis.** The client receiving capreomycin should be assessed for the following nursing diagnoses/collaborative problems: impaired tissue integrity related to the injection of capreomycin (pain, bleeding, or induration at the injection site); disturbed sensory preception related to auditory ototoxicity (tinnitus or hearing loss) or vestibular ototoxicity (dizziness or unsteadiness); and the potential complications of hypersensitivity (rash, swelling, fever), hypokalemia (dysrhythmia, anorexia, nausea and vomiting, muscle cramps, fatigue), nephrotoxicity (increased or decreased frequency of urination or amount of urine), and neuromuscular blockade (fatigue, weakness, drowsiness, dyspnea).

■ **Implementation**

■ ***Monitoring.*** Weekly renal function studies should be performed; the medication should be stopped if the blood urea nitrogen (BUN) is above 30 mg/dL. Fluid intake and output should be monitored throughout therapy. In addition, liver function studies and serum potassium levels should be performed at periodic intervals. Weekly or twice-weekly audiograms and periodic vestibular function determinations should be monitored.

■ ***Intervention.*** To prepare for IM administration, add 2 mL of 0.9% sodium chloride injection or sterile water for injection to the vial. Allow 2 to 3 minutes for dissolution to occur. Reconstituted solutions may darken, but this does not affect their potency. These solutions are stable for 48 hours at room temperature or for 14 days if refrigerated.

Administer capreomycin intramuscularly deep into a large muscle mass to increase absorption and minimize pain and the risk of sterile abscesses.

■ ***Education.*** The client should maintain regular contact with the health care provider to monitor his or her condition. Symptoms of tinnitus, hearing deficits, and/or vertigo should be reported to the prescriber.

■ **Evaluation.** The expected outcome of capreomycin is that the client will be free of infection (negative sputum culture for AFB) without experiencing any adverse reactions to the drug. The client will manage the therapeutic regimen effectively.

cycloserine [sye kloe ser′ een] (Seromycin)

Cycloserine is a broad-spectrum antibiotic that can be bacteriostatic or bactericidal depending on drug concentration at the infection site and the susceptibility of the organism. It is an antimycobacterial agent that interferes with synthesis of the bacterial cell wall. In combination with other drugs, it is indicated for the treatment of active pulmonary and extrapulmonary TB after failure of the primary antituberculous medications.

Cycloserine is well absorbed orally and is widely distributed in body tissues and fluids. It reaches peak serum levels between 3 and 4 hours and has a half-life of 10 hours. Approximately 35% of cycloserine is metabolized, with excretion primarily via the kidneys.

The side effects/adverse reactions of cycloserine include headache and dose-related CNS toxicity.

The adult oral dosage used in combination with other drugs is 250 mg every 12 hours for 2 weeks; the dosage is then increased as necessary up to 250 mg every 6 to 8 hours. The maximum daily dose is 1 g. The pediatric dosage is 10 to 20 mg/kg daily in divided doses.

■ Nursing Management

Cycloserine Therapy

In addition to the following discussion, see Nursing Management: Antituberculous Therapy, p. 1050.

■ **Assessment.** Cycloserine should be used with caution if the client has the following preexisting conditions: severe renal impairment, alcoholism, or seizure disorders (the risk for seizures is greater); or severe anxiety, depression, or psychosis (these conditions may be worsened). Hypersensitivity to cycloserine should be determined.

BUN and serum creatinine concentrations should be determined before administering cycloserine. The CBC will serve as a baseline, because this drug has been associated with deficiencies of vitamin B_{12} and/or folic acid, resulting in anemia.

Review the client's current medication regimen for the risk of significant drug interactions, such as those that may occur when cycloserine is given concurrently with the following drugs:

Drug	Possible Effect and Management
Bold/color type indicates the most serious interactions.	
alcohol	**In chronic alcohol abusers, cycloserine may increase the risk of seizures. Avoid concurrent use or a potentially serious drug interaction may occur.**
ethionamide (Trecator-SC)	May increase CNS side effects such as seizures. Monitor closely, because dosage adjustments may be necessary.

■ **Nursing Diagnosis.** The client receiving cycloserine should be assessed for the following nursing diagnoses/collaborative problems: impaired comfort (headache); disturbed sensory perception related to peripheral neuritis (numbness, tingling in the fingers and toes); and the potential complications of hypersensitivity (rash) and CNS toxicity (anxiety, confusion, dizziness, drowsiness, irritability, depression, nightmares, mood swings, suicidal ideation, seizures).

■ **Implementation**

■ ***Monitoring.*** Renal function studies and CBCs may be required periodically. Serum cycloserine levels may also be required; levels should be 25 to 30 μg/mL, and levels above 30 μg/mL are to be avoided.

■ ***Intervention.*** Administer cycloserine after meals if the client experiences gastrointestinal irritation. Therapy may be continued for 1 to 2 years or longer. The daily administration of pyridoxine will help to prevent drug-related neurotoxicities.

■ ***Education.*** Caution the client to avoid alcohol while taking this medication, because it increases the risks of CNS toxicity such as dizziness, mental disturbances, and seizures. Advise the client to report immediately to the prescriber any signs of dizziness, drowsiness, numbness or tingling of the fingers and toes, or thoughts of suicide.

■ **Evaluation.** The expected outcome of cycloserine therapy is that the client will manage the therapeutic regimen effectively and eventually be free of infection (negative sputum or other culture for AFB) without experiencing any adverse reactions to the drug.

ethambutol [e tham′ byoo tole] (Myambutol, Etibi 🍁)

Ethambutol is a bacteriostatic antituberculous agent; it is believed to diffuse into the mycobacteria bacilli and suppress RNA synthesis. It is effective only against actively dividing mycobacteria. It is indicated in combination with other drugs for the treatment of TB.

Ethambutol is absorbed orally and distributed to most body tissues and fluids (with the exception of cerebrospinal fluid). High concentrations are found in the kidneys, lungs, saliva, urine, and erythrocytes. The time to peak serum levels is 2 to 4 hours, and the half-life is between 3 and 4 hours. Ethambutol is metabolized in the liver and excreted by the kidneys.

The side effects/adverse reactions of ethambutol include gastric distress, confusion, disorientation, headache, and optic neuritis.

The adult oral dosage in combination with other agents is 15 to 25 mg/kg daily.

■ Nursing Management

Ethambutol Therapy

In addition to the following discussion, see Nursing Management: Antituberculous Therapy, p. 1050.

■ **Assessment.** Use ethambutol with caution in clients with preexisting optic neuritis and/or renal impairment. Ethambutol may also increase uric acid concentrations, and therefore care must be taken in clients with gout. Weigh clients carefully, because the dosage is based on weight. The client's hypersensitivity to the drug should be determined.

The risk for neurotoxicity (e.g., optic and peripheral neuritis) is increased if ethambutol is administered concurrently with other neurotoxic agents. A baseline ophthalmic examination should be performed before initiating ethambutol therapy.

■ **Nursing Diagnosis.** The client receiving ethambutol should be assessed for the following nursing diagnoses/collaborative problems: impaired comfort (headache); disturbed thought processes (confusion); deficient fluid volume related to anorexia, nausea, and vomiting; disturbed sensory perception related to retrobulbar optic neuritis (red-green color blindness, blurred vision, or vision loss); and the potential complications of hypersensitivity (rash, fever, arthralgia), hyperuricemia and gout (pain and swelling of joints, particularly the big toe, ankle, and knee), and peripheral neuritis (numbness, tingling of the fingers and toes).

■ **Implementation**

■ ***Monitoring.*** Ethambutol is known to decrease visual acuity and the ability to see red and green. This presents a safety hazard, especially in driving motor vehicles, and clients should be tested for these visual disturbances at frequent intervals during drug therapy. Discontinuation of the drug is usually indicated when visual acuity is disturbed.

Uric acid determinations are required periodically during the course of therapy, because elevated levels may result in gout.

■ ***Intervention.*** Administer ethambutol with food to minimize gastrointestinal distress. Administer it in a single daily dose; divided doses may not result in therapeutic serum levels. Ethambutol is administered concurrently with other antituberculous agents because of the tendency for bacterial resistance to occur when it is used alone.

■ ***Education.*** Encourage the client to visit the health care provider regularly to monitor progress. Therapy may need to continue for 1 to 2 years or longer. The prescriber should be notified if no improvement occurs in 2 to 3 weeks. Report promptly signs of optic neuritis (blurred vision, any loss of vision or red-green perception, or eye pain) or peripheral neuritis (numbness, tingling, or weakness in the hands and feet).

■ **Evaluation.** The expected outcome of ethambutol therapy is that the client will effectively manage the therapeutic regimen and eventually be free of infection (negative sputum or other cultures for AFB) without experiencing any adverse reactions to the drug.

ethionamide [e thye on am′ ide] (Trecator-SC)

Ethionamide is an antimycobacterial agent indicated for the treatment of TB after failure of the primary antituberculous agents (streptomycin, isoniazid, rifampin, and ethambutol). Its mechanism of action is unknown, but it is believed to inhibit peptide synthesis.

Ethionamide is well absorbed orally and is distributed to most body tissues and fluids, including cerebrospinal fluid. It has a half-life of 2 to 3 hours and may be metabolized in the liver and excreted primarily by the kidneys.

The side effects/adverse reactions of ethionamide include gastric distress, orthostatic hypotension, and peripheral neuritis.

The adult oral dosage in combination with other agents is 250 mg every 8 to 12 hours. The pediatric dosage is 4 to 5 mg/kg PO every 8 hours.

■ Nursing Management

Ethionamide Therapy

In addition to the following discussion, see Nursing Management: Antituberculous Therapy, p. 1050.

■ **Assessment.** Ethionamide is administered cautiously to clients with diabetes mellitus because hypoglycemia related to its administration makes the management of diabetes more difficult. Clients with severe hepatic dysfunction have a higher risk of adverse hepatic reactions. Determine the client's tolerance for ethionamide.

The concurrent use of cycloserine will increase the risk for CNS toxicity, especially seizures. Dosage adjustments may be necessary, and the client should be monitored closely for CNS toxicity.

A baseline assessment should include cultures, an ophthalmologic examination, a neurologic examination, and hepatic function determinations.

■ **Nursing Diagnosis.** The client receiving ethionamide should be assessed for the following nursing diagnoses/collaborative problems: impaired comfort (rash and metallic taste); deficient fluid volume related to anorexia, nausea, and vomiting; risk for injury related to orthostatic hypotension (dizziness upon standing); disturbed thought processes related to CNS toxicity (psychiatric disturbances, mood and mental changes, confusion); disturbed body image related to gynecomastia (in males); disturbed sensory perception related to optic neuritis (blurred vision or loss of vision) or peripheral neuritis (numbness or tingling of the fingers and toes); and the potential complications of hepatitis (yellow sclera and skin), hypoglycemia (tachycardia, shakiness, confusion), mental depression, and goiter/

hypothyroidism (weight gain, dry, puffy skin, lethargy, coldness).

■ **Implementation**

■ ***Monitoring.*** Although its incidence is rare, optic neuritis (blurred vision, vision loss, and/or eye pain) does occur. The client should have a thorough ophthalmologic examination at periodic intervals and at the first indication of symptoms related to vision changes. To monitor for hepatotoxic effects, AST (SGOT) and ALT (SGPT) should be performed at least monthly during the course of therapy. Observe the client for jaundice. Cultures should be performed periodically throughout therapy to monitor progress.

■ ***Intervention.*** Administer ethionamide with meals to minimize gastrointestinal distress. Gastrointestinal upset may be minimized by a divided dosage schedule, but serum concentrations may not be adequate. Pyridoxine may be prescribed concurrently to prevent peripheral neuritis.

Bacterial resistance develops rapidly if this drug is administered alone; therefore it is administered in combination with other antimycobacterial drugs.

■ ***Education.*** Advise the client about the importance of complying with the medication regimen, particularly when such a course may be continued for 1 to 2 years or more. Regular visits to the health care provider are necessary to monitor progress and to receive periodic eye examinations. Any symptoms related to changes in vision should be reported to the prescriber promptly.

Advise the client that ethionamide may cause dizziness, drowsiness, or weakness; hazardous activities requiring mental alertness (e.g., driving) should be avoided until the response to the medication has been ascertained. Alert the client to other potential side effects, such as mental depression or mood changes.

■ **Evaluation.** The expected outcome of ethionamide therapy is that the client will manage the therapeutic regimen effectively and will eventually be free of infection (negative sputum or other culture for AFB) without experiencing any adverse reactions to the drug.

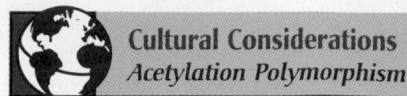

Cultural Considerations
Acetylation Polymorphism

Acetylation polymorphism, a well-known example of a genetic defect in drug metabolism, was first studied when isoniazid therapy was introduced for the treatment of TB. Individuals were classified as fast or slow eliminators of isoniazid on the basis of a metabolic defect in their ability to metabolize the drug. This polymorphism is especially important in the study of ethnic and racial drug responses, because the proportions of rapid acetylators (RAs) and slow acetylators (SAs) vary dramatically in different ethnic and/or geographic populations (Meyer, 1992). For example, both Caucasian and black populations have approximately equal numbers of SAs and RAs, whereas in Eskimo or Japanese populations the percentage of SAs is particularly low (7% to 22%) and that of RAs is high (Levy, 1993).

Critical Thinking Question

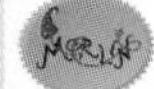

- How would knowing whether your client was an RA or an SA affect your clinical management of his or her isoniazid therapy?

isoniazid [eye soe nye' a zid] (Nydrazid, INH)

Isoniazid is an antimycobacterial (bactericidal) agent that affects mycobacteria in the division phase. The exact mechanism of action is unknown, but it is believed to inhibit mycolic acid synthesis and cause cell wall disruption in susceptible organisms. Isoniazid is indicated for the treatment and prevention of TB.

Isoniazid is well absorbed orally and is widely distributed throughout the body. The time to peak serum levels is 1 to 2 hours for fast drug acetylators (metabolism) or 4 to 6 hours for slow drug acetylators. The half-life in fast acetylators is 0.5 to 1.6 hours; the half-life in slow acetylators is 2 to 5 hours. Isoniazid is metabolized in the liver, primarily by acetylation to inactive metabolites, some of which may be hepatotoxic. The rate of acetylation by the liver is genetically determined; slow acetylators have a decrease in hepatic *N*-acetyltransferase (see the Cultural Considerations box above). Excretion is primarily by the kidneys.

The side effects/adverse reactions of isoniazid include gastric distress, anorexia, nausea, vomiting, weakness, hepatitis, and peripheral neuritis.

The adult oral and parenteral (IM) prophylactic dosage of isoniazid is 300 mg daily. When administered in combination with other agents, the parenteral (IM) treatment dosage is 5 mg/kg, up to 300 mg once daily. When given in combination with other agents to treat TB, the oral dosage is 300 mg daily. The pediatric dosage for prophylaxis orally and parenterally (IM) is 10 mg/kg, up to 300 mg daily.

isoniazid combinations

For ease of drug administration, isoniazid has been combined with rifampin (Rifamate) and is available in dual packs (Rimactane/INH). A three-drug combination is available that contains rifampin, isoniazid, and pyrazinamide (Rifater). The marketing of combination antituberculous products may help to improve compliance with drug therapy. See the sections on isoniazid, pyrazinamide, and rifampin for additional information.

■ Nursing Management

Isoniazid Therapy

In addition to the following discussion, see Nursing Management: Antituberculous Therapy, p. 1050.

■ **Assessment.** Isoniazid should be administered cautiously to clients who have a history of alcoholism and/or hepatic function impairment, because there is increased risk of hepatitis. Clients who are hypersensitive to niacin, ethionamide, and pyrazinamide may also be intolerant of isoniazid.

Review the client's current medication regimen for the risk of significant drug interactions, such as those that may occur when isoniazid is given concurrently with the following drugs:

Drug	Possible Effect and Management
Bold/color type indicates the most serious interactions.	
alcohol	Daily use of alcohol may result in increased isoniazid metabolism and an increased risk of hepatotoxicity. Monitor clients, because a dosage adjustment may be necessary.
alfentanil (Alfenta)	Isoniazid inhibits liver metabolism, which may decrease alfentanil metabolism and lead to increased serum levels of alfentanil and prolong its duration of action. Monitor serum levels closely.
carbamazepine (Tegretol)	May result in increased carbamazepine serum levels and toxicity. Monitor serum levels closely.
disulfiram (Antabuse)	May increase the incidence of CNS side effects, such as ataxia, irritability, dizziness, or insomnia. Monitor closely for these symptoms, because a dosage reduction or even the discontinuation of disulfiram may be required.
hepatotoxic drugs	May increase the potential for hepatotoxicity. Avoid concurrent use or a potentially serious drug interaction may occur.
ketoconazole (Nizoral)	Isoniazid with ketoconazole may decrease serum levels of ketoconazole. Combining isoniazid with ketoconazole is not recommended.
phenytoin (Dilantin)	May result in impaired phenytoin metabolism, leading to increased serum levels and toxicity. The dosage of phenytoin may need to be adjusted. Monitor serum phenytoin closely.
rifampin (Rifadin)	Rifampin with isoniazid may increase the potential for hepatotoxicity, especially in clients with liver impairment. Monitor closely for hepatotoxicity, especially during the first 90 days of therapy.

Mycobacterial cultures and sensitivities should be performed before therapy. Hepatic function determinations and the status of the underlying TB should also be documented in the baseline assessment.

■ **Nursing Diagnosis.** The client receiving isoniazid should be assessed for the following nursing diagnoses/collaborative problems: deficient fluid volume related to anorexia, nausea, vomiting, and diarrhea; disturbed sensory perception related to peripheral neuritis (numbness and tingling of the fingers and toes) and optic neuritis (blurred vision or loss of vision); ineffective protection related to leukopenia, thrombocytopenia, and anemia (fever, sore throat, fatigue, unusual bruising, or bleeding); impaired tissue integrity related to IM injection (local irritation); and the potential complications of hepatitis (yellow skin and sclera), neurotoxicity (depression, psychosis, seizures), and hypersensitivity (fever, rash, arthralgia).

■ **Implementation**

■ ***Monitoring.*** AST (SGOT) and ALT (SGPT) determinations should be performed at least monthly during the course of therapy to monitor for hepatotoxic effects. The client should be observed for symptoms of jaundice and hepatitis prodromal syndrome (anorexia, nausea, or fatigue). Clients over 50 years of age are more prone to the development of hepatitis. Isoniazid should be discontinued at the first signs of hepatotoxicity.

Although its incidence is rare, optic neuritis (blurred vision, vision loss, and/or eye pain) does occur. The client should undergo an ophthalmologic examination at the first indication of symptoms related to vision changes. AFB cultures are performed periodically throughout therapy to monitor the effectiveness of the drug.

■ ***Intervention.*** Administer oral preparations with meals or antacids to minimize gastrointestinal distress. If aluminum-containing antacids are required, administer them at least 1 hour after isoniazid. Oral absorption may be decreased if the drug is taken with food or antacids.

Pyridoxine may be prescribed concurrently to help prevent peripheral neuritis. This may not be required for children if their dietary intake of vitamins is adequate.

There are slow and fast acetylators of isoniazid. Slow acetylators may require lower dosages and are more apt to develop adverse reactions, particularly peripheral neuritis. The highest prevalence of slow acetylators is found in Egyptian, Israeli, Scandinavian, and other Caucasian and black populations; the lowest prevalence of slow acetylators is found in Eskimo, Oriental, and Native American populations. (See the Cultural Considerations box on p. 1056.)

■ ***Education.*** Encourage the client to comply with the full course of isoniazid therapy. Regular visits to the health care provider are necessary for monitoring progress and for periodic eye examinations. Any symptoms related to changes in vision should be promptly reported to the prescriber.

Because alcohol decreases the effects of isoniazid by increasing its metabolism, it should not be used in combination with isoniazid.

Clients with diabetes who test their urine with copper sulfate tests (Clinitest) may obtain false-positive test results. Other tests for urine glucose (Clinistix, Tes-tape) are unaffected.

■ **Evaluation.** The expected outcome of isoniazid therapy is that the client will be able to manage the therapeutic regimen effectively, with the client's sputum or other culture result negative. The client will not experience any adverse reactions to the drug.

pyrazinamide [peer a zin' a mide]
(pms-Pyrazinamide ♣, Tebrazid ♣)

Pyrazinamide is an antimycobacterial agent with an unknown mechanism of action. This drug can be bacteriostatic or bactericidal depending on its concentration at the site of action and the susceptibility of the mycobacteria. It is indicated in combination with other agents for the treatment of TB.

Pyrazinamide is well absorbed orally and is widely distributed in the body. The time to peak serum levels is 1 to 2 hours; the elimination half-life is 9 to 10 hours. Pyrazinamide is primarily metabolized in the liver and is excreted by the kidneys.

The side effects/adverse reactions of pyrazinamide include arthralgia related to hyperuricemia.

When given in combination with other agents, the adult oral dosage of pyrazinamide is 15 to 30 mg/kg daily, up to a maximum dosage of 2 g daily.

■ Nursing Management

Pyrazinamide Therapy

In addition to the following discussion, see Nursing Management: Antituberculous Therapy, p. 1050.

■ **Assessment.** Specimens for mycobacterial cultures and sensitivity testing should be acquired before initiating pyrazinamide therapy. This drug is hepatotoxic, and therefore clients with impaired hepatic function should not receive pyrazinamide unless it is absolutely essential. Hepatic function studies should be performed before initiating therapy.

Because pyrazinamide increases serum uric acid concentrations, use them with caution in clients who have a history of gout. It should be determined whether or not the client has a hypersensitivity for ethionamide, niacin, isoniazid, or other chemically related drugs, because there may be a cross-intolerance with pyrazinamide.

■ **Nursing Diagnosis.** The client receiving pyrazinamide should be assessed for the following nursing diagnoses/collaborative problem: impaired skin integrity (rash and itching); impaired comfort related to hyperuricemia (gouty arthritis [pain and swelling of joints, especially the big toe, ankle, and knee]); and the potential complication of hepatotoxicity (anorexia, fatigue, yellow skin, and sclera).

■ **Implementation**

■ ***Monitoring.*** Cultures should be performed periodically throughout therapy to monitor progress, and serum uric acid levels should be monitored to help prevent an acute episode of gout. AST (SGOT) and ALT (SGPT) determinations should be performed every 2 to 4 weeks to monitor for hepatotoxicity. Observe clients for jaundice and symptoms of acute gouty arthralgia (pain and swelling of joints such as the big toe, knee, and ankle).

■ ***Intervention.*** Pyrazinamide should be administered concurrently with other antituberculous drugs to minimize bacterial resistance. Isoniazid, rifampin, pyrazinamide, and streptomycin or ethambutol are usually given together daily or 2 or 3 times a week for 2 months, followed by isoniazid and rifampin for 4 months. The regimen is altered as appropriate when the results of susceptibility for these medications are available. All of these dosages are taken under the direct observation of a health care provider to ensure compliance.

■ ***Education.*** Encourage the client to remain compliant with the full course of therapy, which is long term. Regular visits to the health care provider are essential for monitoring progress. Alert clients with diabetes who test their urine for ketones that the test results may be unreliable.

Teach clients measures to prevent gout, such as maintaining a fluid intake of 2500 mL daily, adjusting to an optimum weight, and limiting the intake of alcohol and foods high in purines, such as organ meats (liver, kidneys, hearts, sweetbreads), shellfish, and sardines.

■ **Evaluation.** The expected outcome of pyrazinamide therapy is that the client will manage the therapeutic regimen effectively and have negative sputum or other cultures without experiencing any adverse reactions to the drug.

rifabutin [riff′ a byoo tin] (Mycobutin)

Rifabutin is an antimycobacterial indicated for the prophylaxis for disseminated *Mycobacterium avium* complex (MAC) in persons with advanced human immunodeficiency virus (HIV) infection. It inhibits DNA-dependent RNA polymerase in susceptible *Escherichia coli* and *Bacillus subtilis* microorganisms.

This drug is absorbed from the gastrointestinal tract, reaches peak serum levels in 2 to 4 hours, and has a terminal half-life of 45 hours. It is metabolized in the liver and primarily excreted by the kidneys.

The side effects/adverse reactions of rifabutin include nausea, vomiting, and skin rash. The usual adult dosage is 300 mg daily.

■ Nursing Management

Rifabutin Therapy

■ **Assessment.** It should be determined that the client does not have a hypersensitivity to rifabutin or rifampin. Rifabutin is not administered to clients with active TB; they are better treated with the therapies previously described. If rifabutin is administered to active TB as a prophylaxis of MAC, there is the risk of the TB becoming resistant to both rifabutin and rifampin.

A CBC with a white blood cell differential and platelets are required as a part of the baseline assessment, because this drug may cause blood dyscrasias. The concurrent administration of zidovudine and rifabutin does increase the clearance of zidovudine, but in vitro studies have indicated that rifabutin does not affect the inhibition of HIV by zidovudine.

■ **Nursing Diagnosis.** The client undergoing rifabutin therapy has a potential for developing the following nursing diagnoses/collaborative problem: deficient fluid volume related to a change in taste, nausea, or vomiting; impaired comfort related to arthralgia (joint pain), myalgia (muscle pain), and eye pain (uveitis); impaired skin integrity (rash); ineffective protection related to neutropenia; and the potential complication of pseudojaundice.

■ **Implementation**

■ ***Monitoring.*** Platelet counts and white blood cell counts should be performed at periodic intervals to monitor for neutropenia and, rarely, thrombocytopenia. Monitor the client for the development of MAC.

■ ***Intervention.*** Rifabutin is absorbed more quickly if administered on an empty stomach; administer the drug with food if gastrointestinal distress occurs. The contents of the capsules may be mixed with applesauce or pudding for clients who have difficulty swallowing.

■ ***Education.*** Alert the client that body secretions and excretions (urine, feces, saliva, perspiration, and tears) will turn a reddish orange to reddish brown. Discolored tears may also stain soft contact lenses.

Stress the need for regular visits to the prescriber to monitor progress.

■ **Evaluation.** The expected outcome of rifabutin therapy is that the client will manage the therapeutic regimen effectively and will not contract MAC.

rifampin [rif′ am pin] (Rifadin, Rofact ♣)

Rifampin is a broad-spectrum bactericidal antibiotic (antimycobacterial) that blocks RNA transcription. It is indicated for the treatment of TB and for asymptomatic meningococcal carriers of *Neisseria meningitidis*.

This drug is well absorbed orally and is widely distributed in the body. It is lipid soluble and therefore may reach and kill intracellular and extracellular susceptible bacteria. The time to peak serum levels is 1.5 to 4 hours, and the elimination half-life is up to 5 hours. It is metabolized in the liver and excreted primarily in the feces.

The side effects/adverse reactions of rifampin include gastric distress, hypersensitivity, and a flu-like syndrome.

The adult oral dosage of rifampin in combination with other agents (for TB) is 600 mg daily. To treat asymptomatic meningococcal carriers, the dosage is 600 mg PO twice daily for 2 days. For children 1 month and older, the dosage to treat TB (with other antituberculous drugs) is 10 to 20 mg/kg PO daily. For asymptomatic meningococcal carriers, the dosage is 5 mg/kg PO every 12 hours for 2 days.

■ Nursing Management

Rifampin Therapy

In addition to the following discussion, see Nursing Management: Antituberculous Therapy, p. 1050.

■ **Assessment.** Because of the high risk for hepatotoxicity, clients with impaired hepatic function and/or active alcoholism (or a history of it) should not receive rifampin unless absolutely essential. The client's hypersensitivity to rifampin should be determined. Specimens for mycobacterial cultures and sensitivity testing and hepatic function studies (ALT [SGPT], AST [SGOT], serum alkaline phosphatase, serum bilirubin levels) should be obtained before initiating rifampin therapy.

Review the client's current medication regimen for the risk of significant drug interactions, such as those that may occur when rifampin is given concurrently with the following drugs:

Bold/color type indicates the most serious interactions.

Drug	Possible Effect and Management
alcohol	Daily use of alcohol may increase the risk of rifampin-induced hepatotoxicity and increase the rate of rifampin metabolism. Monitor hepatic function studies closely, because dosage adjustments may be necessary.
corticosteroids, glucocorticoids, mineralocorticoids, anticoagulants, oral warfarin (Coumadin) or indanedione, digitalis glycosides, disopyramide (Norpace), mexiletine (Mexitil), tocainide (Tonocard), quinidine, azole antifungals, phenytoin (Dilantin), chloramphenicol (Chloromycetin)	Rifampin increases levels of hepatic enzymes and therefore may decrease the effectiveness of these medications, which are metabolized by the liver. Monitor the serum levels of these drugs closely to ensure therapeutic levels, because dosage adjustments may be necessary.
estrogen-containing oral contraceptives, estramustine, or estrogens	Decreases effectiveness due to increased liver metabolism of estrogen. May result in menstrual irregularities, spotting, and unplanned pregnancies. Advise clients of the possible effects when these drugs are combined, and advise alternative contraception.
hepatotoxic drugs, other	**Increases the risk of hepatotoxicity. Avoid concurrent use or a potentially serious drug interaction may occur.**
HIV protease inhibitors	**Rifampin increases the metabolism of HIV protease inhibitors, resulting in subtherapeutic levels of the drug. In addition, these drugs increase serum levels of rifampin and increase the risk of toxicity. Concurrent use is not recommended.**
hypoglycemic agents (oral)	Concurrent use enhances the metabolism of the antidiabetic drugs; dosage adjustments may be indicated.
isoniazid (INH)	**Increased risk for hepatotoxicity (see Isoniazid, p. 1056). Avoid concurrent drug administration if possible.**
methadone	May decrease the effectiveness of methadone and may induce methadone withdrawal in dependent clients. Monitor closely; dosage adjustments may be necessary during and after rifampin therapy.
verapamil, oral	Accelerates the metabolism of oral verapamil, decreasing blood levels and decreasing its cardiovascular effects.
xanthines, aminophylline, oxtriphylline, theophylline	Increases the metabolism of these drugs, which increases drug clearance. Monitor with serum levels of the client's xanthine drug.

■ **Nursing Diagnosis.** The client receiving rifampin should be assessed for the following nursing diagnoses/collaborative problems: impaired comfort related to rash (hypersensitivity) and flu-like syndrome (chills, fever, headache, generalized discomfort); diarrhea; ineffective protection related to fungal overgrowth (sore mouth and tongue) and blood dyscrasias; deficient fluid volume related to nausea and vomiting; impaired urinary elimination related to interstitial nephritis as evidenced by greatly decreased frequency of urination and amount of urine; and the potential complications of hepatitis and Redman syndrome (red-orange discoloration of the skin, mucous membranes, and sclera).

■ **Implementation**

■ ***Monitoring.*** As with other antituberculous drugs, cultures should be performed periodically throughout rifampin therapy to monitor progress. In addition, hepatic function studies are required intermittently during therapy. The client should be monitored for anorexia, nausea, fatigue, jaundice, yellow sclera, and dark urine, which may indicate hepatotoxicity.

■ ***Intervention.*** Clients with hepatic impairment may require as much as a 50% reduction in dosage.

For optimal absorption, administer rifampin with a full glass of water on an empty stomach; rifampin may be given with food if the client experiences dyspepsia. The contents of the capsule may be mixed with applesauce or jam for clients who have difficulty swallowing.

Rifampin is administered concurrently with other antituberculous drugs to minimize bacterial resistance. The treatment period may be 6 months to 2 years.

■ ***Education.*** Encourage the client to complete the full course of therapy, which may take years. Regular visits to the health care provider are essential for monitoring progress.

Alert the client that there may be a reddish brown discoloration of urine, feces, saliva, sputum, sweat, and tears but that this effect is not hazardous. However, clients who wear soft contact lenses should be cautioned that this same effect may permanently discolor the lens.

Women taking oral contraceptives who are also receiving rifampin should be cautioned to use an alternate form of contraception.

Clients should be advised to avoid alcoholic beverages while taking rifampin because it increases the risk of hepatotoxicity.

■ **Evaluation.** The expected outcome of rifampin therapy is that the client will effectively manage the therapeutic regimen and eventually be free of infection (negative sputum or other cultures) without experiencing any adverse reactions to the drug.

streptomycin injection [strep toe mye′ sin]

Streptomycin is an aminoglycoside antibiotic that is poorly absorbed from the gastrointestinal tract; therefore it is given intramuscularly. It was one of the first effective agents used in the late 1940s to treat TB, and it remains an important agent in managing severe TB.

As with other aminoglycosides, the major toxicities of streptomycin include ototoxicity and nephrotoxicity, especially when given to clients with impaired renal function or with other medications with the same toxicities. See Chapter 59 for detailed information on the aminoglycosides and their nursing management.

The adult dosage for streptomycin is 1 g IM daily. As soon as possible, reduce the dosage to 1 g two or three times weekly. The dosage for older adults is 500 to 750 mg daily in combination with other antituberculous agents. The dosage for children is 20 mg/kg daily in combination with other antituberculous agents. The maximum daily dose is 1 g.

DRUGS USED IN THE TREATMENT OF AMEBIASIS

Amebiasis is an infection of the large intestine produced by a protozoan parasite, *Entamoeba histolytica*. This infestation is found worldwide but is prevalent and severe in tropical areas. It has been detected in poorly sanitized areas, including some rural communities, Native American reservations, and migrant labor farm camps; it is also common in homosexual males (Anandan, 1995). Transmission is usually through the ingestion of cysts (fecal to oral route) from contaminated food or water or from person-to-person contact. Poor personal hygiene can increase the spread of this parasite.

Life Cycle of the Ameba

The protozoan has two stages in its life cycle: (1) the trophozoite (vegetative ameba), which is the active, motile form; and (2) the cyst, or inactive, drug-resistant form that appears in intestinal excretion. The *trophozoite stage* is capable of ameboid motion and sexual activity. Because of its susceptibility to injury, it generally succumbs to an unfavorable environment. The trophozoite protects itself under certain circumstances by entering the *cystic stage*. During this phase the protozoan becomes inactive by surrounding itself with a resistant cell wall within which it can survive for a long time, even in an unsuitable environment.

The complete life cycle of the ameba occurs in humans, the main host. It begins when the human ingests cysts that are present on hands, in food, or in water contaminated by feces. The hydrochloric acid of the stomach does not destroy the swallowed cysts; they pass unharmed into the small intestine. The digestive juices penetrate the cystic walls, and the trophozoites are released. The motile amoebae later pass into the colon, where they live and multiply for a time, feeding on the bacterial flora of the gut. The presence of bacteria is essential for the survival of amoebae.

Before excretion, the trophozoites move toward the terminal end of the bowel and again become encysted. The cysts remain viable and infective after being eliminated in the feces. The cycle may begin again when the cysts that appear in fecal excretion are ingested through the contamination of food or water.

The parasite causing amebiasis replicates in three major locations: (1) the lumen of the bowel, (2) the intestinal mucosa, and (3) extraintestinal sites. Amebiasis is classified according to its primary site of action: intestinal amebiasis, where amebic activity is restricted to the bowel lumen or intestinal mucosa; or extraintestinal amebiasis, where parasitic invasion occurs outside the intestine.

Intestinal Amebiasis. Intestinal amebiasis may be manifested as an asymptomatic intestinal infection or as a symptomatic intestinal infection that may be mild, moderate, or severe.

Asymptomatic Intestinal Amebiasis. In asymptomatic intestinal amebiasis the action of the parasite is restricted to the lumen of the bowel. The individual is asymptomatic but becomes a carrier of the disease by passing mature cysts of the parasite in formed stools. The cysts can live for several weeks outside the body and can survive dry, freezing, or high-temperature conditions. The infection is transmitted from person to person by flies or contaminated food or water. Ordinary concentrations of chlorine in water purification do not destroy the cysts. Serious gastrointestinal pathologic problems eventually develop if the carrier fails to follow any drug treatment. Mild symptoms occasionally exist and include vague abdominal pain, nausea, flatulence, fatigue, and nervousness.

Symptomatic Intestinal Amebiasis. Symptomatic amebiasis occurs when the trophozoites in the lumen of the bowel penetrate the mucosal lining of the colon. After they multiply and thrive on bacterial flora, a large infestation occurs and produces diarrhea and abdominal pain. The increased loss of fluid may cause prostration. Ulcerative colitis may also result. This state of the disease is called intestinal amebiasis and is usually diagnosed as mild, moderate, or severe according to the intensity of the symptoms and the extent of the disease.

Extraintestinal Amebiasis. The term *extraintestinal amebiasis* means the parasites have migrated to other parts of the body, such as the liver or occasionally the spleen, lungs, or brain. When the parasites are in the liver, necrotic foci develop because of the parasites' destructive effect on tissues. The terms *liver abscess* and *hepatic amebiasis* are usually used when there is liver involvement.

Antiamebiasis Agents

Drugs for the treatment of amebiasis are classified according to the site of the previously described amebic action. Luminal amebicides act primarily in the bowel lumen and in general are ineffective against parasites in the bowel wall or tissues. Tissue amebicides are drugs that act primarily in the bowel wall, liver, and other extraintestinal tissues. No single drug is effective for both types of amebiasis, and therefore a luminal and extraluminal (tissue) amebicide or combination therapy is often prescribed. The intestinal amebicides are considered to be iodoquinol, metronidazole, and paromomycin; the extraintestinal amebicides are chloroquine and metronidazole.

iodoquinol [eye oh do kwin' ole]
(diiodohydroxyquin, Yodoxin)

Iodoquinol is an antiprotozoal with an unknown mechanism of action. It is poorly absorbed from the intestinal tract; thus it produces its effect against the trophozoites of *E. histolytica* at the site of intestinal infestation. It is indicated for the treatment of intestinal amebiasis in asymptomatic carriers of *E. histolytica*.

Following administration and local effect, iodoquinol is excreted in the feces.

The side effects/adverse reactions of iodoquinol include gastric distress, hypersensitivity, fever, and chills.

The adult oral dosage is 650 mg three times daily after meals for 20 days. The pediatric dosage is 40 mg/kg PO in three divided doses after meals for 20 days.

■ Nursing Management

Iodoquinol Therapy

■ **Assessment.** Iodoquinol should be used with caution if the client has the following preexisting conditions: intolerance to iodoquinol, chloroxine, iodine, pentaquine, or primaquine; optic neuropathy; or thyroid, hepatic, or renal disease.

A baseline assessment as described in Chapter 58 should be performed. Stool specimens should be collected and taken directly to the laboratory for the detection of parasites. Clients should undergo an ophthalmologic examination before initiating iodoquinol therapy.

■ **Nursing Diagnosis.** The client receiving iodoquinol should be assessed for the following nursing diagnoses/collaborative problem: impaired comfort (rash, itching of rectal area, or headache); deficient fluid volume related to nausea, vomiting, and diarrhea; hyperthermia; diarrhea; disturbed sensory perception, such as visual disturbances related to optic atrophy, optic neuritis, or subacute myelooptic neuropathy, or sensory disturbances related to numbness and tingling of the fingers and toes from the development of peripheral neuropathy; and the potential complication of thyroid enlargement.

■ **Implementation**

■ ***Monitoring.*** Intake and output, as well as the frequency and character of stools, should be documented. Fresh, warm stools should be monitored for the presence of amoebae. Diarrhea may occur during the first few days of therapy with iodoquinol. Alert the prescriber if it continues for more than 3 days. Ophthalmologic examinations are required periodically during long-term therapy.

The development of neurologic disorders such as myelooptic neuropathy, optic atrophy, optic neuritis, and peripheral neuropathy has been implicated in treatment with prolonged high doses.

Iodoquinol may cause thyroid enlargement and interferes with certain thyroid function tests by increasing protein-bound serum iodine levels for as long as 6 months after discontinuing therapy. This drug contains approximately 64% iodine.

In children, the administration of iodoquinol for chronic diarrhea has been responsible for causing optic atrophy and permanent vision loss. Thus the administration of this drug is not advocated for the treatment or prophylaxis of "traveler's diarrhea" or for use in chronic nonspecific diarrhea.

■ ***Intervention.*** Administer iodoquinol after meals to minimize gastrointestinal irritation. This course of therapy may be repeated if necessary after a 2- to 3-week rest period.

Tablets may be crushed and mixed with applesauce, gelatin dessert, or ice cream for ease of administration to children and to clients who may have difficulty swallowing.

■ ***Education.*** Clients should be instructed in proper hygiene to prevent reinfection. Inform the client that any results of thyroid function studies completed within 6 months of discontinuing iodoquinol may be distorted.

■ **Evaluation.** The expected outcome of iodoquinol is that the client will be free of amoebae in stools at the end of the year following therapy.

paromomycin [par oh moe mye' sin] (Humatin)

Paromomycin is both an amebicidal and an antibacterial agent. The drug is an aminoglycoside antibiotic with antibacterial properties similar to that of neomycin. Paromomycin acts directly on intestinal amoebae and on bacteria such as *Salmonella* and *Shigella*. Because the drug is poorly absorbed from the gastrointestinal tract, it exerts no effect on systemic infections such as extraintestinal amebiasis. It is indicated for the treatment of acute and chronic intestinal amebiasis and for adjunct therapy in the management of hepatic coma.

Paromomycin is poorly absorbed from the intestinal tract; thus most of the drug is excreted in the feces.

The side effects/adverse reactions of paromomycin include nausea, diarrhea, and gastric distress. Paromomycin is an aminoglycoside, and the drug interactions possible with this family of medications may also occur with paromomycin. (See the discussion of aminoglycoside antibiotics in Chapter 59.)

The adult and pediatric dosages to treat intestinal amebiasis is 25 to 35 mg/kg daily, administered in 3 divided doses with meals for 5 to 10 days. To manage hepatic coma, the adult dosage is 4 g daily in divided doses at regular intervals for 5 or 6 days.

■ Nursing Management

Paromomycin Therapy

In addition to the following discussion, see Nursing Management: Aminoglycoside Therapy, Chapter 59.

■ **Assessment.** Paromomycin is contraindicated for use in intestinal obstruction and in ulcerative bowel lesions because of possible systemic absorption. It is to be used only for luminal amebiasis.

■ **Nursing Diagnosis.** The client receiving paromomycin should be assessed for the following nursing diagnoses: deficient fluid volume related to nausea, vomiting, and diarrhea; diarrhea; activity intolerance related to lightheadedness and dizziness; and disturbed sensory perception (auditory disturbances) related to tinnitus and hearing loss.

■ **Implementation**

■ ***Monitoring.*** After the end of therapy, examine fresh, warm stools for the presence of amoebae at weekly intervals for 6 weeks, then monthly for 2 years to indicate that the client is not harboring the parasite. Notify the prescriber of any ringing in the ears or dizziness, because this drug is ototoxic.

■ ***Intervention.*** Administer paromomycin after meals to minimize gastrointestinal distress.

■ ***Education.*** Teach the client proper personal hygiene to prevent reinfection.

■ **Evaluation.** The expected outcome of paromomycin therapy is that the client will manage the therapeutic regimen effectively and be free of amoebas in stools for 1 year.

OTHER DRUGS USED IN AMEBIASIS

Metronidazole (Flagyl) is an antibacterial, antiprotozoal, and anthelmintic agent. It is used for the treatment of extraintestinal and intestinal amebiasis. When used for the treatment of invasive amebiasis, it is recommended that it be administered with a luminal amebicide, such as iodoquinol or paromomycin.

The mechanism of action appears to result from an interaction between the intracellular reduced metronidazole (which is cytotoxic) and DNA, which results in the inhibition of nucleic acid synthesis and cell death. (See Chapter 59 for additional information.)

Chloroquine (Aralen) is used to treat amebic liver abscess, usually in combination with other drugs. See the discussion of chloroquine earlier in this chapter for further information.

Dehydroemetine (Mebadin) and diloxanide furoate (Furamide) are additional antiinfective agents used to treat amebiasis. However, these are available only from the CDC,* because they are considered investigational agents.

DRUGS USED IN THE TREATMENT OF OTHER PROTOZOAN DISEASES

Several other protozoan diseases are widespread throughout the world and may be encountered in clinical practice in the United States and Canada. This following sections describe these diseases and the primary antiprotozoan agent used in their treatment.

Toxoplasmosis

Toxoplasmosis is caused by an intracellular parasite, *T. gondii*, which is found worldwide and infests a variety of animals, including humans. It is often harbored in the host, and there is no evidence of the disease. Toxoplasmosis is contracted by ingesting the cysts found in inadequately cooked raw meat or by accidentally ingesting the cysts from cat feces.

The most common form of toxoplasmosis in the United States and Canada is usually subclinical. Symptomatically the individual may experience lymphadenopathy, fever, and

*Parasitic Disease Drug Service, Division of Host Factors, Center for Infectious Disease, Atlanta, GA, 30333.

occasionally a rash on the palms and soles. The most serious complication of toxoplasmosis is meningoencephalitis. Toxoplasmosis is treated with a combination of sulfadiazine and pyrimethamine, both of which alter the folic acid cycle of the *Toxoplasma* organism, resulting in its death. The oral dosage of pyrimethamine is 25 mg/day for 3 to 4 weeks; the dosage of sulfadiazine is 1 to 4 g/day for 1 to 3 weeks.

Trichomoniasis

Trichomoniasis is a vaginal disease caused by *Trichomonas vaginalis*. Its characteristic presentation consists of a wet, inflamed vagina, a "strawberry" cervix, and a thin, yellow, frothy malodorous discharge. Both sexual partners are usually infected by this organism, which can be identified microscopically in the semen, prostatic fluid, or exudate from the vagina. Infections often recur, which indicates that the protozoans persist in the extravaginal foci, male urethra, or periurethral glands and ducts of both sexes. Metronidazole (Flagyl) is the drug of choice, and treatment must be given simultaneously to both partners involved.

DRUGS USED IN THE TREATMENT OF HELMINTHIASIS

The disease-producing **helminths** are classified as metazoa, or multicellular animal parasites. Unlike the protozoa, they are large organisms that have a complex cellular structure and feed on host tissue. They may be present in the gastrointestinal tract, but several types also penetrate the tissues; some undergo developmental changes, during which they wander extensively in the host. Because most anthelminthics used today are highly effective against specific parasites, the organism must be accurately identified before treatment is started, usually by finding the parasite ova or larvae in the feces, urine, blood sputum, or tissues of the host.

Parasitic infestations do not necessarily cause clinical manifestations, but they may be injurious for a number of reasons:

1. Worms may cause mechanical injury to the tissues and organs. Roundworms in large numbers may cause obstruction in the intestine; filariae may block lymphatic channels and cause massive edema; and hookworms often cause extensive damage to the wall of the intestine and considerable loss of blood.
2. Toxic substances produced by the parasite may be absorbed by the host.
3. The tissues of the host may be traumatized by the presence of the parasite and made more susceptible to bacterial infections.
4. Heavy infestation with worms will rob the host of food. This is particularly significant in children.

Helminths that are parasitic to humans are classified as (1) *Platyhelminthes* (flatworms), which include two subclasses: cestodes (tapeworms) and trematodes (flukes); and (2) *Nematoda* (roundworms).

Platyhelminthes (Flatworms)

Cestodes

Cestodes are tapeworms, of which there are four varieties: (1) *Taenia saginata* (beef tapeworm), (2) *Taenia solium* (pork tapeworm), (3) *Diphyllobothrium latum* (fish tapeworm), and (4) *Hymenolepis nana* (dwarf tapeworm). As indicated by the name of the worm, the parasite enters the intestine by way of improperly cooked beef, pork, or fish or, in the case of the dwarf tapeworm, contaminated food.

Cestodes are segmented flatworms with a head or scolex (which has hooks or suckers used to attach to tissues) and a number of segments, or proglottids, which in some cases may extend for 20 to 30 feet in the bowel. Drugs affecting the scolex allow the organisms to be expulsed from the intestine. Each of the proglottids contains both male and female reproductive units. Fertilized eggs are expelled from the worm into the environment. Upon ingestion, the infected larvae develop into adults in the small intestine of the human. The larvae may travel to extraintestinal sites and enter other tissues such as the liver, muscle, and eye. With the exception of the dwarf tapeworm, tapeworms spend part of their life cycle in a host other than humans—pigs, fish, or cattle. Dwarf tapeworms do not require an intermediate host.

The tapeworm has no digestive tract; it depends on the nutrients intended for the host. The host suffers by eventually developing a nutritional deficiency.

Trematodes

Trematodes, or flukes, are flat, nonsegmented parasites with suckers that attach to and feed on host tissue. The life cycle begins with the egg, which is passed into fresh water following fecal excretion from the body of the human host. The egg containing the embryo forms into a ciliated organism (the *miracidium*). In the presence of water the miracidium escapes from the egg and enters the intermediate host—the freshwater snail, which exists extensively in rice paddies and irrigation ditches. After entry, the fluke forms a cyst in the lungs of the snail, and many organisms develop in this cyst. The organisms can penetrate other parts of the snail and grow into worms called *cercariae*. Eventually the cercariae are released from the snail into the water, where they attach themselves to blades of grass to encyst. A human, the final host, then becomes infected by the parasite.

When humans swallow encysted organisms in snails (or even in fish and crabs), they develop into adult flukes in different structures of the body. The flukes are classified according to the type of tissues they invade. Following ingestion, the eggs of *Schistosoma haematobium* appear in the urinary bladder and cause inflammation of the urogenital system. This can result in chronic cystitis and hematuria. Infestations with *Schistosoma japonicum* and *Schistosoma mansoni* produce intestinal disturbances with resultant ulceration and necrosis of the rectum. *S. japonicum* is more concentrated in the veins of the small intestine. If the liver and spleen become infected, the disease is usually fatal. *S. mansoni* prefers the portal veins that drain the large intestine, particularly the sigmoid colon and rectum. Unlike the other parasites, the cercariae of *S. mansoni* are not ingested but burrow through the skin, especially between the toes of a human host who is standing in contaminated water. They then make their way to the portal system, where they mature into adult flukes.

Schistosomiasis (bilharziasis) is endemic to Africa, Asia, South America, and the Caribbean islands. The disease can be controlled largely by eliminating the intermediate host, the snail. Travelers to these areas must avoid contact with contaminated water for drinking, bathing, or swimming. Unfortunately, immigrants or individuals who have traveled to the endemic areas have introduced the disease in the United States and Canada.

Nematoda (Roundworms)

Nematoda are nonsegmented, cylindrical worms that consist of a mouth and complete digestive tract. The adults reside in the human intestinal tract; there is no intermediate host. Two types of nematode infection exist in the human: the egg form and the larval form.

Egg Infective Form. *Ascaris lumbricoides* is a large nematode (approximately 30 cm in length) that is known as the "roundworm of humans."

The adult *Ascaris* usually resides in the upper end of the small intestine of the human, where it feeds on semidigested foods. When excreted with feces, the fertilized egg can survive in the soil for a long time. When inadvertently ingested by another host, the embryos escape from the eggs and mature into adults in the new host. To prevent the disease, proper sanitary conditions and meticulous personal habits must be observed.

Infection with *Enterobius vermicularis*, or pinworm, is highly prevalent among children and adults in the United States. Adult pinworms reside in the large intestine. The female migrates to the anus and deposits her eggs around the skin of the anal region. This causes intense itching and can be noted especially in children.

Diagnosis is made by finding the eggs deposited in the perianal region; these eggs are detected by applying clear cellulose acetate tape to the perianal region in the morning. The ingestion of excreted eggs can infect an individual. In addition, eggs that contaminate clothing, bedding, furniture, and other items may be responsible for reinfecting an individual and initiating the infection of others.

Larval Infective Form. *Necator americanus* (New World) or *Ancylostoma duodenale* (Old World) hookworms are somewhat similar in action. They reside in the small intestine of humans. When the eggs are excreted in the feces, the larvae hatch in the soil. The larvae can penetrate the skin of humans, particularly through the soles of the feet, and produce dermatitis (ground itch). On entry into the small intestine, they develop into adult worms. During this process they extravasate blood from the intestinal vessels and cause a profound anemia in the victim. The presence of eggs in the feces indicates a positive test for hookworm disease. This type of infection can be avoided by wearing shoes.

Trichinella spiralis is a small pork roundworm that causes trichinosis. In humans the disease begins by ingesting insufficiently cooked pork or bear meat. After the entry of encysted meat into the small intestine, the larvae are released from the cysts.

Following maturation, the females develop eggs that later form into larvae. The larvae migrate through the bloodstream and lymphatic system to the skeletal muscles, where they encyst. Encapsulation and eventually calcification of the cysts occur. Diagnosis of trichinosis is made by muscle biopsy, in which microscopic examination reveals the presence of larvae. This disease is prevented by cooking pork and bear meat thoroughly before eating.

Anthelmintic Agents

Anthelmintic drugs are used to rid the body of worms (helminths). Anthelmintics are among the most primitive types of chemotherapy. It has been estimated that one third of the world's population is infested with these parasites.

diethylcarbamazine [dye eth il kar′ ba ma zeen] (Hetrazan)

Diethylcarbamazine has microfilaricidal and macrofilaricidal effects. The microfilaricidal action increases the loss of microfilariae and inhibits the rate of embryogenesis from nematodes. It has no sterilizing effect on adult worms. It is indicated for the treatment of Bancroft's filariasis, loiasis, onchocerciasis, and tropical eosinophilia.

This drug is absorbed after oral administration and is distributed to nonfatty tissues. Peak serum levels are reached in 1 to 2 hours, and the half-life is 8 hours. Excretion is via the kidneys.

The side effects/adverse reactions of diethylcarbamazine include joint pains, fever, increased weakness, headache, dizziness, nausea and vomiting, facial swelling (especially around the eyes), and pruritus. Less often reported are a rash and painful, tender glands (especially in the neck, armpits, or groin area).

The adult dosage of diethylcarbamazine is 2 to 3 mg/kg PO three times daily. For tropical eosinophilia the dosage is 6 mg/kg PO daily for 4 to 7 days.

■ Nursing Management

Diethylcarbamazine Therapy

■ **Assessment.** The treatment of pregnant clients should be deferred until after delivery. Treatment is also contraindicated with ocular onchocerciasis, because long-term therapy may cause inflammation and then degenerative changes in the optic disc and retina. Ophthalmologic examinations should be part of the baseline assessment. In addition, microfilarial blood concentrations and skin biopsy for intradermal microfilariae should be obtained before therapy if diethylcarbamazine is administered for Bancroft's filariasis and loiasis.

■ **Nursing Diagnosis.** The client receiving diethylcarbamazine should be assessed for the following nursing diagnoses: impaired comfort (headache, itching, swelling of the face, rash, lymphadenopathy, and arthralgia); fatigue; hyperthermia; deficient fluid volume related to nausea and vomiting; risk for injury related to light-headedness and dizziness; and disturbed sensory perception related to night blindness, tunnel vision, and vision loss.

■ **Implementation**

■ ***Monitoring.*** Contact the prescriber if allergic reactions (swelling and itching of the skin, fine papular rash, tenderness of lymph nodes, headache, fever, tachycardia, conjunctivitis, uveitis) occur as the result of the substances released when the microfilariae are destroyed. Microfilarial blood concentrations are used to monitor this effect, and antihistamine therapy or corticosteroids are usually prescribed to relieve these symptoms. Ophthalmoscopic examinations are performed on clients treated for onchocerciasis. Report immediately any signs of itching or swelling of eyes. Corticosteroid eye drops may be administered for the treatment of this condition. Blood and skin samples are obtained periodically to monitor the client's progress.

■ ***Intervention.*** For ease of administration, the tablet may be chewed, swallowed whole, or crushed and mixed with food. Dietary restrictions, laxatives, or posttreatment purging are not required. A second course of therapy is required if the client is not cured in 3 weeks.

If a severe reaction occurs after a single dose, discontinue use. For intense infestations, one dose may be given on the first day, two doses the second day, and three doses daily thereafter for 30 days.

■ ***Education.*** Emphasize the importance of following meticulous hygiene, such as washing hands before eating and after going to the toilet and keeping hands or objects out of the mouth.

Stress the importance of remaining under the prescriber's care during the treatment of filariasis. Failure to follow the drug regimen can eventually obstruct lymph flow, thereby producing hydrocele, elephantiasis of the limbs, an enlarged scrotum or breasts, and chyluria (milk-like urine).

■ **Evaluation.** The expected outcome of diethylcarbamazine therapy is that the client will have three negative stool samples after the completion of therapy. For pinworms, the client will have negative perianal swabs for 7 days. The client/caregiver will be able to manage the therapeutic regimen effectively.

mebendazole [me ben′ da zole] (Vermox)

Mebendazole is vermicidal and may also be ovicidal for most helminths. It causes degeneration of a parasite's cytoplasmic microtubules, which results in blocking glucose uptake in the helminth and leads to the death of the parasite. It is indicated for the treatment of single or mixed infestations of *Trichuris* (whipworm), *Enterobius* (pinworm), *Ascaris* (roundworm), *Ancylostoma* (common hookworm), and *Necator* (American hookworm).

The oral absorption of mebendazole is increased if given with fatty foods. It is distributed to the serum, cyst fluid, liver, hepatic cysts, and muscle tissues, and it has a half-life of 2.5 to 5.5 hours. It is metabolized in the liver and excreted primarily in the feces.

The side effects of mebendazole are uncommon and include gastric distress, diarrhea, nausea, and vomiting.

The adult and pediatric dosage (children 2 years of age and over) is 100 mg PO twice daily for 3 days. This dosage may be repeated in 2 to 3 weeks if necessary.

■ Nursing Management
Mebendazole Therapy

■ **Assessment.** Clients with Crohn's ileitis and ulcerative colitis may have increased absorption with mebendazole and therefore be at greater risk for toxicity. Those with hepatic function impairment may require lower dosages.

A CBC is required as a baseline before therapy, because mebendazole may cause leukopenia.

Collect pinworm specimens for a baseline assessment. To do so, wrap a transparent strip of cellophane tape (sticky side out) around a tongue blade and press it against the perianal area. Place the sticky side of the tape on a glass slide and send it to the laboratory. The female worm emerges from the rectum during the night to lay eggs in the perianal area. This causes the client to become restless during sleep. The emerging worms can be seen at night with a flashlight.

For roundworm and whipworm specimens, send a baseline, warm stool sample to the laboratory.

■ **Nursing Diagnosis.** The client receiving mebendazole should be assessed for the following nursing diagnoses/collaborative problem: impaired comfort (headache) deficient fluid volume related to nausea, vomiting, and diarrhea; diarrhea; ineffective protection related to neutropenia (sore throat, fever, and fatigue); disturbed body image related to alopecia; and the potential complication of hypersensitivity.

■ **Implementation**

■ ***Monitoring.*** Continue to monitor the client's progress with perianal or stool examinations. Collect the stool specimen in a clean, dry, and properly labeled container, and send it to the laboratory. Do not contaminate the specimen with water, urine, or chemicals, because the parasite may be destroyed. Review the CBC for neutropenia.

■ ***Intervention.*** For ease of administration, tablets may be crushed and mixed with applesauce or other food. No dietary restrictions, laxatives, or posttreatment enemas are necessary.

Treat all family members for pinworm infestation, because it is readily transmitted from person to person. Clients with heavy infestation may require more prolonged therapy.

■ ***Education.*** Stress the importance of handwashing and sanitary disposal of the feces. Avoid walking barefoot to prevent hookworm infestation; the larvae hatch in the soil and penetrate through the skin. Instruct the client to take frequent showers rather than baths; to change underclothes, nightclothes, bedclothes, and towels daily; and to disinfect toilet facilities daily. Instruct the client to wash the perianal area daily to prevent reinfestation.

For pinworm infestation, instruct the client to wash (not shake) all the bedclothing and nightclothes after treatment.

For hookworm or whipworm infestation, instruct the client to take iron supplements during treatment and for up to 6 months afterward if he or she is anemic.

■ **Evaluation.** The expected outcome of mebendazole therapy is that the client will have three negative stool samples after completion of the therapy. For pinworms, the client will have negative perianal swabs for 7 days. The client will be able to manage the therapeutic regimen effectively.

niclosamide [ni kloe′ sa mide] (Niclocide)

Niclosamide is an anthelmintic that affects the mitochondria of the cestode, inhibiting aerobic metabolism and possibly anaerobic metabolism, on which many cestodes depend for survival. Contact with the drug results in destruction of the scolex and proximal segments of the organism, the proglottids. When loosened from the intestinal wall, the scolex is usually digested in the intestine. Consequently, the worm cannot be identified in the feces.

Niclosamide is indicated for the treatment of *T. saginata* (beef tapeworm), *D. latum* (fish tapeworm), *H. nana* (dwarf tapeworm), *Dipylidium caninum* (dog and cat tapeworm), and *T. solium* (pork tapeworm) infestations.

Because niclosamide is poorly absorbed from the intestinal tract, it can exert its effect on intestinal helminths, the site of its action. Excretion is in the feces.

The side effects/adverse reactions of niclosamide include stomach pain or distress, anorexia, nausea, vomiting and, uncommonly or rarely, gastric distress, dizziness, sedation, pruritus of the rectum, rash, and a bad taste in the mouth.

Niclosamide tablets should be thoroughly chewed and taken with water. The adult dosage for fish and beef tapeworms is four tablets (2 g) as single dose; for dwarf tapeworm the dose is four tablets (2 g) daily for 1 week. Refer to a current package insert or drug reference for additional dosing recommendations.

■ Nursing Management

Niclosamide Therapy

■ **Assessment.** Niclosamide should not be administered to clients who are hypersensitive to this drug.

■ **Nursing Diagnosis.** The client receiving niclosamide should be assessed for the following nursing diagnoses: impaired comfort (headache, unpleasant taste, rash, and itching of the perianal area); deficient fluid volume related to nausea, vomiting, and diarrhea; diarrhea; and risk for injury related to drowsiness, light-headedness, and dizziness.

■ **Implementation**

■ ***Monitoring.*** Stress the importance of follow-up studies; the client is considered cured only if stool examination results are negative for a minimum of 3 months. A stool examination is required 1 month and 3 months following drug therapy.

■ ***Intervention.*** Administer niclosamide after a light meal such as breakfast. No dietary restrictions are required before or after treatment. Instruct the client to chew the tablet thoroughly and swallow it with a small amount of water. For children, crush the tablet to a fine powder and mix it with a small amount of water to form a paste. If the client is constipated, a mild laxative should be prescribed to ensure a normal bowel movement. Treatment may be administered on an outpatient basis.

■ ***Education.*** Advise the client to take the drug for the full course of therapy to prevent the infection from returning. Stress the importance of reporting progress to the prescriber. A second course of therapy may be required if there is no improvement. Niclosamide destroys the tapeworm on contact while in the intestine. The killed worms (including the scolex) are passed in the stool and may not be seen.

In the treatment of *T. solium* (pork tapeworm), a saline purge such as magnesium sulfate should be given 1 or 2 hours after the administration of niclosamide to prevent the development of cysticercosis in the intestinal tract. Moreover, the procedure provides a good possibility of expulsion of an intact scolex. Note that niclosamide has no effect on cysticercosis.

Because the drug may cause dizziness, warn the client about driving a motor vehicle or operating dangerous machinery.

Instruct the client to observe strict hygiene (both personal and environmental) to prevent reinfection. This observance applies particularly to *H. nana* (dwarf tapeworm).

■ **Evaluation.** The expected outcome of niclosamide therapy is that the client will have three negative stool samples over a period of 3 months after completion of the therapy.

oxamniquine [ox am′ ni kwin] (Vansil)

Oxamniquine is schistosomicidal against both immature and mature worms, and it produces its effect by causing worms to shift from the mesenteric veins to the liver, where they are destroyed. Although male schistosomes appear to be more susceptible to this drug than female schistosomes, female schistosomes do stop laying eggs after successful treatment with this agent. Oxamniquine is indicated for the treatment of schistosomiasis.

Oxamniquine is well absorbed orally, with a time to peak serum levels of 1 to 1.5 hours. It is metabolized in the liver and excreted by the kidneys.

Oxamniquine is usually well tolerated; side effects are uncommon and include gastric distress, dizziness, sedation, and headaches.

The adult oral dosage is 12 to 15 mg/kg as a single dose for *S. mansoni*. The pediatric dosage is 20 mg/kg administered in 2 divided doses approximately 2 to 8 hours apart (*Drug Facts and Comparisons*, 2000).

■ Nursing Management

Oxamniquine Therapy

■ **Assessment.** Use oxamniquine with caution in individuals who have a history of convulsive disorders, because seizures are more apt to occur.

■ **Nursing Diagnosis.** The client receiving oxamniquine should be assessed for the following nursing diagnoses/collaborative problem: impaired comfort (headache, rash); deficient fluid volume related to anorexia, nausea, vomiting, and diarrhea; diarrhea; hyperthermia (particularly in Egyptian clients); risk for injury related to drowsiness, dizziness, and seizures; disturbed thought processes related to auditory and visual hallucinations; and the potential complication of hypersensitivity.

■ **Implementation**

■ ***Monitoring.*** Monitor the client's temperature, and observe for signs and symptoms of side effects/adverse reactions.

■ ***Intervention.*** Administer oxamniquine after meals to minimize side effects such as dizziness, drowsiness, and gastrointestinal distress. Oxamniquine therapy does not require special preparation such as fasting, dietary restrictions, or enemas.

■ ***Education.*** Caution the client to avoid hazardous tasks that require mental alertness (e.g., driving) until the response to the drug has been ascertained.

Advise the client that oxamniquine causes a harmless reddish orange discoloration of the urine.

Encourage the client to complete the full course of therapy and to check with the prescriber if there is no improvement after completing a full course of therapy.

■ **Evaluation.** The expected outcome of oxamniquine therapy is that the client will effectively manage the therapeutic regimen and be free of infection without experiencing any adverse reactions to the oxamniquine.

piperazine [pi′ per a zeen]

Piperazine is an anthelmintic that affects the worm muscle (paralysis), possibly by blocking the stimulating effects of acetylcholine at the myoneural junction. The muscle paralysis of roundworms makes them unable to maintain their position in the host; they are dislodged and expelled as a result of normal peristalsis.

Piperazine is indicated for the treatment of enterobiasis (pinworms) and ascariasis (roundworm). It is absorbed orally and reaches peak serum levels in 2 to 4 hours. It is partially metabolized in the liver and primarily excreted by the kidneys.

The side effects/adverse reactions of piperazine include gastric distress and CNS effects (headaches, dizziness, ataxia, trembling).

The adult dosage for ascariasis is 3.5 g PO daily for 2 days. For children the dosage is 75 mg/kg (up to 3.5 g) daily for 2 days. For enterobiasis, the dosage for adults and children is a single daily dose of 65 mg/kg for 7 consecutive days; the maximum daily dose is 2.5 g.

■ Nursing Management

Piperazine Therapy

■ **Assessment.** Observe clients with renal insufficiency for signs of neurologic symptoms. This drug is contraindicated for use in renal or hepatic impairment and in convulsive disorders.

■ **Nursing Diagnosis.** The client receiving piperazine should be assessed for the following nursing diagnoses/collaborative problems: impaired comfort (headache); deficient fluid volume related to nausea, vomiting, and diarrhea; diarrhea; hyperthermia (hypersensitivity); risk for injury related to drowsiness or dizziness; disturbed thought processes (memory defect); and the collaborative problems of hypersensitivity and seizures.

■ **Implementation**

■ ***Monitoring.*** Continue to monitor progress with perianal or stool examinations.

■ ***Intervention.*** Piperazine may be taken with food. Some prescribers prefer single-dose therapy with mebendazole or pyrantel pamoate. Dietary restrictions, laxatives, or enemas are not required with piperazine.

■ ***Education.*** Stress the importance of handwashing and of sanitary disposal of feces. Instruct the client to wash the perianal area daily to prevent reinfection. Underwear and bed linens should be changed daily to prevent reinfection. Wash (not shake) all bedding and nightclothes after treatment to prevent reinfection. All family members should be treated at the same time.

■ **Evaluation.** The expected outcome of piperazine therapy is that the client will have three negative stool samples after completing therapy. For pinworms, the client will have negative perianal swabs for 7 days.

praziquantel [pray zi kwon′ tel] (Biltricide)

Praziquantel is an anthelmintic that penetrates cell membranes and increases cell permeability in susceptible worms. This results in an increased loss of intracellular calcium, contractions, and muscle paralysis of the worm. The drug also disintegrates the schistosome tegument (covering). Subsequently, phagocytes are attracted to the worm and ultimately kill it.

Praziquantel is indicated for the treatment of schistosomiasis, opisthorchiasis (liver flukes), and clonorchiasis (Chinese or Oriental liver fluke) infestations. Praziquantel is absorbed orally and reaches peak serum levels in 1 to 3 hours. The half-life is 0.8 to 1.5 hours for praziquantel and 4 to 6 hours for its metabolites. It is excreted by the kidneys and is generally well tolerated.

The side effects/adverse reactions of praziquantel include headache, light-headedness, gastric distress, sweating, and fever.

For clonorchiasis, the dosage for adults or children 4 years of age and older is 25 mg/kg three times daily for 1 day.

■ Nursing Management

Praziquantel Therapy

■ **Assessment.** Praziquantel is contraindicated in clients with ocular cysticercosis because the destruction of the parasites in the eye by the medication may cause severe ocular damage. Use with caution in clients with liver disease. Document the client's hypersensitivity to the drug.

▪ **Nursing Diagnosis.** The client receiving praziquantel should be assessed for the following nursing diagnoses/collaborative problem: impaired comfort (headache); deficient fluid volume related to nausea, vomiting, and diarrhea; diarrhea; hyperthermia; risk for injury related to lightheadedness, weakness, and dizziness; and the potential complication of hypersensitivity (rash).

▪ **Implementation**

▪ ***Monitoring.*** Urine examinations for the eggs of *S. haematobium* are necessary at 1, 3, and 12 months after therapy to provide proof of a cure. Examinations of stool specimens for tapeworms, flukes, and other *Schistosoma* are required at 1, 3, and 12 months after treatment to determine the efficacy of the drug.

▪ ***Intervention.*** No special preparations such as fasting, dietary restrictions, or laxatives are necessary for the administration of praziquantel. However, the tablets should be taken with meals and swallowed whole with a small amount of fluid to avoid the extremely bitter taste. Chewing the tablets may cause gagging and vomiting.

▪ ***Education.*** The client should be encouraged to comply with the medication regimen and to visit the prescriber regularly to monitor progress. Because of the side effects of dizziness and drowsiness, caution the client to avoid hazardous activities such as driving until the response to the medication has been ascertained.

▪ **Evaluation.** To monitor the expected outcomes of praziquantel therapy, stool examinations are completed at specific intervals depending on the parasite. These examinations should be negative for eggs or worm segments:

- Intestinal, liver, and blood flukes: 1 week and 1, 6, and 12 months after treatment
- Lung flukes: 1 month after treatment
- Tapeworms: 1 and 3 months after treatment

For *Schistosoma haematobium* and *Schistosoma mekongi*, urine examinations are required at 1, 3, and 6 months to determine proof of a cure. A client is not considered cured unless examination results have been negative for several months.

pyrantel [pi ran' tel] (Antiminth, Combantrin ♣)

Pyrantel is an anthelmintic that is a depolarizing neuromuscular blocking agent; it causes contraction and then paralysis of the helminth muscles. The helminths are dislodged and expelled from the body by peristalsis. Pyrantel is indicated for the treatment of ascariasis, enterobiasis, and helminth infestations.

This product is poorly absorbed from the gastrointestinal tract. Pyrantel reaches peak serum levels in 1 to 3 hours and is primarily excreted in the feces.

Side effects/adverse reactions include gastric distress and CNS side effects.

For ascariasis and enterobiasis, the dosage for adults and children 2 years of age and over is 11 mg/kg PO as a single dose. This may be repeated in 2 to 3 weeks if necessary.

▪ Nursing Management

Pyrantel Therapy

▪ **Assessment.** Use pyrantel with caution in clients who are hypersensitive to it. Perianal swabs and stool examinations confirm the presence of the helminth. Concurrent use of piperazine is not recommended because it antagonizes the anthelmintic effects of pyrantel.

▪ **Nursing Diagnosis.** The client receiving pyrantel should be assessed for the following nursing diagnoses/collaborative problem: impaired comfort (headache); deficient fluid volume related to anorexia, nausea, vomiting, and diarrhea; diarrhea; risk for injury related to CNS effects (drowsiness, light-headedness, and dizziness); and the potential complication of hypersensitivity.

▪ **Implementation**

▪ ***Monitoring.*** For pinworms, monitor the perianal area with cellophane tape swabs starting 1 week after treatment; this should be performed every morning before bathing or defecation. For roundworms, stool examinations are checked 2 weeks after therapy.

▪ ***Intervention.*** The administration of pyrantel does not require any special preparation such as fasting, dietary restrictions, laxatives, or enemas. It may be taken with or without food or at any time of day. Shake well and use the calibrated measuring device provided to measure the dosage accurately.

▪ ***Education.*** Encourage the client to take the full course of therapy and to visit the prescriber on a regular basis to monitor progress. Alert the client to avoid hazardous tasks that require mental alertness (e.g., driving) until the response has been determined.

For pinworm infestation, it is important to wash (without shaking) all of the bed linens and nightclothes to prevent reinfestation. All household members should be treated simultaneously. Stress proper hygiene, both personal and environmental, with the client.

▪ **Evaluation.** The expected outcome of pyrantel therapy for pinworms is that the client's perianal examinations using cellophane tape swabs will demonstrate negative results for 7 consecutive days. For roundworms, stool examination results should be negative for ova, larvae, or worms 2 to 3 weeks after the completion of therapy.

thiabendazole [thye a ben' da zole] (Mintezol)

The mechanism of action of thiabendazole is unknown but has been reported to inhibit specific enzymes (fumarate reductase) in the helminth. It is vermicidal. Thiabendazole is indicated for the treatment of cutaneous and visceral larva migrans (creeping eruption), strongyloidiasis, and trichinosis.

Thiabendazole is rapidly absorbed orally and reaches peak serum levels in 1 to 2 hours. The half-life ranges from 0.9 to 2 hours, with metabolism in the liver and excretion by the kidneys.

The side effects/adverse reactions of thiabendazole include a dry mouth and eyes, gastric distress, and neuropsychiatric and CNS adverse effects.

For cutaneous larva migrans, the dosage of thiabendazole for adults and children weighing 13.6 kg and over is 25 mg/kg PO twice daily for 2 days. If lesions are still present, the dosage may be repeated 2 days after completion of the initial treatment. For other dosing recommendations, see a current package insert or the *United States Pharmacopeia Dispensing Information*.

■ Nursing Management

Thiabendazole Therapy

■ **Assessment.** Thiabendazole should be used with caution in clients with hepatic or renal dysfunction or a hypersensitivity to thiabendazole. Concurrent administration with theophylline decreases theophylline clearance, which may result in elevated serum levels and toxicity. Monitor theophylline levels.

■ **Nursing Diagnosis.** The client receiving thiabendazole should be assessed for the following nursing diagnoses/collaborative problems: deficient fluid volume related to anorexia, nausea, vomiting, and diarrhea; diarrhea; disturbed sensory perception—visual (blurred vision), and tactile (numbness or tingling in the hands and feet); disturbed thought processes related to neuropsychiatric toxicity (irritability, disorientation, hallucinations); and the potential complications of hypersensitivity, Stevens-Johnson syndrome, crystalluria, and CNS toxicity (seizures).

■ **Implementation**

■ ***Monitoring.*** Sputum examinations will monitor the progress of treatment of strongyloidiasis; for all other organisms, monitor stool examinations approximately 2 to 3 weeks after therapy. Observe the client for hypersensitivity reactions to detect severe erythema multiforme (Stevens-Johnson syndrome).

■ ***Intervention.*** Thiabendazole should be administered after meals to minimize anorexia, nausea, and vomiting; no dietary restrictions, laxatives, or enemas are required with this drug. For the oral suspension form, shake well and use the calibrated measuring device provided to ensure accurate dosage. Chew or crush the tablet form before swallowing.

■ ***Education.*** Encourage the client to comply with the full course of treatment and to visit the prescriber to monitor progress. Because of the side effects of dizziness and drowsiness, caution the client to avoid hazardous activities that require alertness, such as driving. Teach proper hygiene, both personal and environmental.

■ **Evaluation.** The expected outcome of thiabendazole therapy is that the client will manage the therapeutic regimen effectively and have a negative sputum examination for strongyloidiasis or a negative stool examination for eggs, larvae, or worms.

DRUGS USED IN THE TREATMENT OF LEPROSY

Leprosy, or **Hansen's disease**, is a chronic infectious disease that is caused by *Mycobacterium leprae* in humans. In 1985 the World Health Organization estimated 10 to 12 million leprosy cases worldwide; this figure has declined to under 1 million registered cases in 1998 as a result of effective, multidrug therapy. Each year approximately 500,000 new cases are identified, primarily from countries that have a public health problem (Spiegel & Perkins, 1999).

Although the precise mode of transmission is unknown, the incubation period for leprosy is a few months to decades. Large numbers of leprosy bacilli are generally shed from skin ulcers, nasal secretions, the gastrointestinal tract and, perhaps, biting insects.

M. leprae is a bacillus that in humans first presents as a skin lesion—a large plaque or macule that is erythematous or hypopigmented in the center. More numerous lesions, peripheral nerve trunk involvement, and the common complications of plantar ulceration of the feet, footdrop, loss of hand function, and corneal abrasions may follow.

Most cases can be arrested, if not cured, by appropriate therapy and management. The drugs of choice are dapsone and clofazimine. Thalidomide (Thalomid) was approved in 1998 for the treatment and prevention of cutaneous manifestations of erythema nodosum leprosum (ENL).

dapsone [dap′ sone] (DDS, Avlosulfon ♣)

Dapsone is an antibacterial (antileprosy) agent that is bacteriostatic and has an action similar to that of the sulfonamides. It may also be a dihydrofolate reductase inhibitor. Dapsone is effective against *M. leprae* (the cause of leprosy) and therefore is indicated for the treatment of all types of leprosy and for dermatitis herpetiformis.

Dapsone is absorbed orally, distributed throughout the body, and found in fluids and in all body tissues. The time to peak serum levels is 2 to 6 hours; the half-life is approximately 30 hours. It is acetylated by *N*-acetyltransferase in the liver; thus slow acetylators are more apt to develop higher serum levels and adverse reactions than fast acetylators. Excretion is via the kidneys.

The side effects/adverse reactions of dapsone include hypersensitivity, hemolytic anemia, and methemoglobinemia.

The adult dosage for leprosy (given in combination with other antileprosy drugs) is 50 to 100 mg PO daily. As a suppressant for dermatitis herpetiformis, the adult dosage is 50 mg PO daily initially, which is increased as necessary until symptoms are controlled. As an antileprosy agent, the dosage for children is 1.4 mg/kg PO daily.

■ Nursing Management

Dapsone Therapy

■ **Assessment.** Administer dapsone cautiously in clients with severe anemia, G6PD deficiencies, and methemoglobin reductase, because hemolytic anemia may occur. Use caution in clients with hepatic or renal function impairment. This drug is also contraindicated with clients who are hypersensitive to dapsone and sulfonamides. A CBC and platelet count, as well as ALT (SGPT) and AST (SGOT) levels, should be completed before dapsone therapy for a baseline assessment.

Review the client's current medication regimen for the risk of significant drug interactions, such as those that may occur when dapsone is given with the following drugs:

Drug	Possible Effect and Management
Bold/color type indicates the most serious interactions.	
didanosine (ddI)	Concurrent drug administration may reduce the absorption of dapsone. Dapsone requires an acid media for absorption, whereas didanosine is given with a buffer to neutralize stomach acid to increase absorption. Administer dapsone at least 2 hours before ddI.
hemolytic agents	Increases the potential for serious adverse reactions. Avoid concurrent use or a potentially serious drug interaction may occur.

▪ **Nursing Diagnosis.** The client receiving dapsone therapy should be assessed for the following nursing diagnoses/collaborative problems: impaired comfort (headache); deficient fluid volume related to anorexia, nausea, and vomiting; disturbed thought processes (mood and mental changes); ineffective protection related to leukopenia, thrombocytopenia, and anemia; and the collaborative problems of methemoglobinemia (bluish discoloration of the skin and lips), exfoliative dermatitis, peripheral neuritis (numbness and tingling of the hands and feet), hypersensitivity (rash), hepatic damage, and a "sulfone syndrome"—a hypersensitivity reaction that occurs after 6 to 8 weeks of therapy with fever, malaise, lymphadenopathy, exfoliative dermatitis, and anemia.

▪ **Implementation**

▪ ***Monitoring.*** Once therapy has started, a CBC should be determined monthly for 1 to 3 months and then semiannually for the remainder of dapsone therapy. The dosage may be reduced or suspended if CBC values are diminished: RBCs, below 2.5 million/mm^3; hemoglobin, below 9 g/dL; WBCs, below 5000/mm^3. In addition, the client should be observed for the development of hemolytic anemia; symptoms are pale skin, fever, and unusual tiredness and weakness.

Hepatic function studies should be performed if the client develops anorexia, nausea, vomiting, or jaundice. Peripheral neuritis (numbness and tingling of the hands and feet) and exfoliative dermatitis (itching and scaling of the skin and loss of hair) are also indications for dosage interruption.

▪ ***Intervention.*** Because of bacterial resistance, dapsone is usually given with other antimycobacterial agents. Therapy is continued for 6 months to 3 years or more for indeterminate and tuberculoid leprosy, 2 to 10 years for borderline (dimorphous) leprosy, and 2 years to life for lepromatous leprosy.

▪ ***Education.*** Encourage the client to comply with the dapsone regimen, and stress that the use of the drug is long-term or indefinite. Taking the medication at the same time each day will assist in compliance. Stress the importance of regular visits to the prescriber to monitor progress.

▪ **Evaluation.** The expected outcome of dapsone therapy is that the client will effectively manage the therapeutic regimen and that the infection will be arrested without experiencing any adverse reactions to the drug.

clofazimine [kloe fa' zi meen] (Lamprene)

The antileprosy mechanism of action for clofazimine is unknown; it has a slow bactericidal effect on *M. leprae*, inhibits mycobacterial growth, and tends to bind preferentially to mycobacterial DNA. It is indicated as a secondary drug for the treatment of leprosy, especially for the dapsone-resistant type of leprosy.

Clofazimine has a variable oral absorption and is distributed primarily in fatty tissues and cells. Macrophages take up this drug and further distribute it throughout the body. The half-life is approximately 2 to 3 months with chronic therapy, with time to peak serum levels between 1 and 6 hours. It is excreted primarily in the feces.

The side effects/adverse reactions of clofazimine include gastric distress, ichthyosis, and discoloration of the skin, feces, sweat, tears, and urine.

The adult dosage in dapsone-resistant leprosy, in combination with one or more other agents, is 50 to 100 mg PO daily.

▪ Nursing Management

Clofazimine Therapy

In addition to the following discussion, see Nursing Management: Dapsone Therapy, p. 1069.

Clients with gastrointestinal problems are at risk for gastrointestinal bleeding, bowel obstruction, splenic infarction, and enteritis. There are no significant drug interactions with this drug.

The client receiving clofazimine should be assessed for the following nursing diagnoses/collaborative problems: impaired comfort (photosensitivity, rash and itching, and change in taste); deficient fluid volume related to anorexia, nausea, and vomiting; disturbed thought processes (mood and mental changes, especially depression and suicidal thoughts related to skin discoloration); disturbed body image related to pink, red, or brownish-black discoloration of the skin and lips; and the potential complications of gastrointestinal bleeding, clofazimine toxicity, and hepatitis.

thalidomide [tha lid' oh myde] (Thalomid)

Despite its history of causing thousands of deformed infants (birth defects) in the 1960s and being withdrawn from the market in Germany, Great Britain, Japan, Canada, and many other countries, thalidomide has been studied as an investigational drug for the past 30 years. As a result, thalidomide has exhibited some promising new uses for clinical practice. It is now approved in the United States for the treatment and prevention of a painful skin problem caused by leprosy (erythema nodosum leprosum).

Thalidomide reaches peak serum levels in approximately 3 to 5.7 hours. It has a half-life of 5 to 7 hours and is excreted primarily in urine.

The side effects/adverse reactions of thalidomide include sedation, peripheral neuropathy, hypotension, hypersensitivity, rash, and bradycardia (*Drug Facts and Comparisons*, 2000). The most serious toxicity is its human teratogenic effects (the Food and Drug Administration pregnancy safety category is X). It is recommended that women who take this medication during their childbearing years use two reliable methods of birth control for 1 month before taking thalidomide, during therapy, and for 1 month after the last dose. Men should use a latex condom even if they have had a vasectomy, and they should continue using condoms for at least 30 days after taking their last dose of thalidomide. Advise clients that they cannot donate blood while taking this drug (New Drug Checklist, 1998).

The usual dosage of thalidomide is 100 to 300 mg/day initially and is adjusted or tapered by 50 mg every 2 to 4 weeks when the symptoms subside. It is recommended the dose be taken with water at bedtime (Davis & Waters, 1999).

■ Nursing Management

Thalidomide Therapy

Thalidomide is contraindicated for clients with peripheral neuropathy because that condition is a serious adverse reaction of the drug. For this same reason, concurrent administration of other medications associated with peripheral neuropathy is contraindicated. Thalidomide has CNS depressant effects; therefore use caution whenever other CNS depressants are prescribed. Other nursing management is similar to that for dapsone therapy.

SUMMARY

Malaria is still prevalent despite the World Health Organization's attempts to eradicate it by controlling the insect vector and the causative parasite. Although it is essentially considered a tropical disease, nurses in the United States and Canada may come into contact with imported cases; both countries have populations that travel extensively, and both countries provide havens for refugees and immigrants from areas in which the disease is endemic. Chloroquine, hydroxychloroquine, mefloquine, primaquine, quinine, and other drugs are commonly used for the prevention and treatment of malaria.

The incidence of TB is increasing because of the increasing numbers of persons with AIDS, persons who are living in the street or are homeless, substance abusers, malnourished individuals, and those taking immunosuppressant drugs. In general, three or more antituberculous agents are administered concurrently for their additive effect and to minimize the risk of the organism becoming drug resistant. Aminosalicylates, capreomycin, cycloserine, ethambutol, ethionamide, isoniazid, pyrazinamide, rifampin, and streptomycin are commonly used antituberculous agents.

Amebiasis, an infection of the large intestine by *E. histolytica*, is prevalent in tropical areas and is again imported by travel; it is also found in poorly sanitized areas of Canada and the United States. Transmission is fecal to oral and occurs through the ingestion of cysts from contaminated food and water. Antiamebiasis agents in current use are iodoquinol and paromomycin. Other protozoan diseases of concern are toxoplasmosis and trichomoniasis.

Helminths (worms parasitic to man) may be flatworms (platyhelminthes) or roundworms (nematodes). There are two types of flatworms: tapeworms (cestodes) and flukes (trematodes). They cause injury to the host in a variety of ways: by causing damage to and loss of blood from the intestinal wall, by producing toxic substances absorbed by the host, by traumatizing the host's tissues and making the host more susceptible to infection, and by competing with the host for sustenance within the bowel. The anthelmintic agents most commonly used are diethylcarbamazine, mebendazole, niclosamide, oxamniquine, piperazine, praziquantel, pyrantel, and thiabendazole.

Leprosy, or Hansen's disease, is caused by *M. leprae* and is treated with dapsone, clofazimine, and thalidomide.

Although these diseases and the therapeutic agents used in their prevention and treatment are not commonly dealt with by most U.S. and Canadian nurses, familiarity with them is necessary to manage them appropriately when they do occur.

Critical Thinking Questions

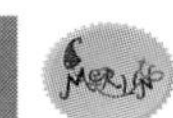

1. Why is it necessary to determine whether an antimalarial is being used prophylactically, for the suppression of symptoms, or for the acute phase of malaria?
2. Why are three or more antituberculous drugs administered concurrently?
3. What advice would you provide for someone who was traveling to a place where malaria is endemic? Amebiasis? Leprosy?

Collaborative Learning Activities

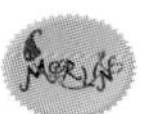

For Collaborative Learning Activities, go to mosby.com/MERLIN/McKenry/.

CASE STUDY

For a Case Study that will help ensure mastery of this chapter content, go to mosby.com/MERLIN/McKenry/.

BIBLIOGRAPHY

American Hospital Formulary Service. (1999). *AHFS: drug information '99*. Bethesda, MD: American Society of Hospital Pharmacists.

Anandan, J.V. (1995). Parasitic infections. In L.Y. Young & M.A. Koda-Kimble (Eds.), *Applied therapeutics: The clinical use of drugs* (6th ed.). Vancouver, WA: Applied Therapeutics.

Anderson, K.N., Anderson, L.E., & Glanze, W.D. (Eds.) (1998). *Mosby's medical, nursing, & allied health dictionary* (5th ed.). St. Louis: Mosby.

Bloland, P.B., & Ettling, M. (1999). Making malaria-treatment policy in face of drug resistance. *Annals of Tropical Medicine & Parasitology, 93*(1), 5-23.

Boutotte, J. (1993). T.B. the second time around...and how you can help to control it. *Nursing, 23*(5), 42-50.

Cali, T.J. (1995). Tuberculosis: Implications for the 1990s and beyond. *Clinical Consultant, 14*(12), 1-12.

Centers for Disease Control and Prevention. (1999a). *Executive Commentary of 1998 Tuberculosis Surveillance Report.* Atlanta: Centers for Disease Control and Prevention, Division of Tuberculosis Elimination; www.cdc.gov/nchstp/tb/surv/surv98/surv98pdf/exesum98.pdf (12/7/99).

Centers for Disease Control and Prevention. (1999b). *TB facts for health care workers: Treatment of tuberculosis.* Atlanta: Centers for Disease Control and Prevention, Division of Tuberculosis Elimination; www.cdc.gov/nchstp/tb/faqs/tbfacts/treatment.htm (12/6/99).

Centers for Disease Control and Prevention. (1999c). *CDC travel information for health care providers;* www.cdc.gov/travel/malariadrugs2.htm (5/21/99).

Centers for Disease Control and Prevention. (1996). *Prescription drugs for malaria.* CDC Doc. No. 221010, pp. 1-3; Atlanta: Author.

Davis, W.M. & Waters, I.W. (1999). New drug approvals of 1998, Part 2. *Drug Topics, 143*(5), 68-71.

Drug Facts and Comparisons. (2000). St. Louis: Facts and Comparisons.

Easterbrook, M. (1999). Detection and prevention of maculopathy associated with antimalarial agents. *International Ophthalmology Clinics, 39*(2), 49-57.

Elpern, E.H. & Girzadas, A.M. (1993). Tuberculosis update: New challenges of an old disease. *MEDSURG Nursing, 2*(3), 176-183.

Iseman, M.D. (1999). Management of multidrug resistant tuberculosis. *Chemotherapy, 45*(suppl 2), 3-11.

Juckett, G. (1999). Malaria prevention in travelers. *American Family Physician, 59*(9), 2523-2530, 2535-2536.

Kuzma, E.C. (1992). Drug response: All bodies are not created equal. *American Journal of Nursing, 92*(12), 48.

Levy, R.A. (1993). *Ethnic and racial differences in response to medicines: Preserving individualized therapy in managed pharmaceutical programs.* Reston, VA: National Pharmaceutical Council.

Lordi, G.M. & Reichman, L.B. (1993). Drug-resistant tuberculosis: The new face of an old enemy. *Drug Therapy,* (March):17-28.

Mandell, G.L. & Petri, Jr., A.W. (1996). Drugs used in the chemotherapy of tuberculosis, *Mycobacterium avium* complex disease, and leprosy. In J.G. Hardman & L.E. Limbird (Eds.), *Goodman & Gilman's The pharmacological basis of therapeutics* (9th ed.). New York: McGraw-Hill.

Meyer, U.A. (1992). Drugs in special patient groups: Clinical importance of genetics in drug effects. In Melmon, K.L., Morrelli, H.F., Hoffman, B.B., & Nierenberg, D.W. (Eds.), *Melmon and Morrelli's clinical pharmacology: Basic principles in therapeutics* (3rd ed.). New York: McGraw-Hill.

New Drug Checklist. (1998). Thalidomide, UltiMedex Integration Services division of Micromedex, Inc. *Drug Topics, 142*(21), 30.

Posey, L.M. (1996). Tuberculosis: New problems from an old disease. *The Consultant Pharmacist, 11*(1), 27-28, 31.

Spiegel, R.A. & Perkins, B.A. (1999). Leprosy in Annex A: Fact sheets for candidate diseases for elimination or eradication. *MMWR Supplement, 48*(SUO1), 154-203; www.cdc.gov/epo/mmwr/preview/mmwrhtml/su48a26.htm (5/28/00).

Surveillance Report. (1999). Reported tuberculosis in the United States, 1997. Atlanta: Centers for Disease Control and Prevention, Division of Tuberculosis Elimination; www.cdc.gov/nchstp/tb/surv/surv97/surv97.htm (5/26/99).

United States Pharmacopeia Dispensing Information (USP DI): Drug information for the health care professional (19th ed.). (1999). Rockville, MD: United States Pharmacopeial Convention.

Ward, Jr., E.S. (1995). Tuberculosis. In L.Y. Young & M.A. Koda-Kimble (Eds.), *Applied therapeutics: The clinical use of drugs* (6th ed.). Vancouver, WA: Applied Therapeutics.

White, N.J. & Breman, J.G. (1994). Malaria and babesiosis. In K.J. Isselbacher, E. Braunwald, J.D. Wilson, J.B. Martin, A.S. Fauci, & D.L. Kasper (Eds.), *Harrison's principles of internal medicine* (13th ed.). New York: McGraw-Hill.

Williams, H.A., Roberts, J., Kachur, S.P., Barber, A.M., Barat, L.M., Bloland, P.B., Ruebush II, T.K., & Wolfe, E.B. (1999). *Malaria Surveillance: United States, 1995.* Epidemic Intelligence Service, CDC Division of Parasitic Diseases; www.cdc.gov/epo/mmwr/preview/mmwrhtml/00056518.htm (5/13/1999).

Yew, W.W. (1999). Directly observed therapy, short course: The best way to prevent multidrug-resistant tuberculosis. *Chemotherapy, 45*(suppl 2), 26-33.

Yoshikawa, T.T. (1995). Tuberculosis in the nursing home. *Nursing Home Medicine, 3*(9), 207-213.

mosby.com/MERLIN/McKenry/

62 Overview of the Immunologic System

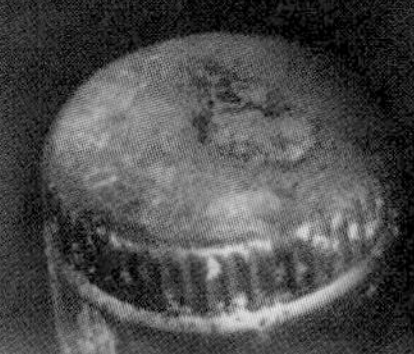

Chapter Focus

The immunologic system is composed of cells and organs that defend the body against invasion by foreign biologic and/or chemical substances. The immunocompetent cells in the body have an inherent ability to distinguish foreign protein substances from the body's own cells. This chapter reviews the organs and tissues of the immune system, the immunocompetent cells, and the types of immunity.

Learning Objectives

1. Identify the lymphoid organs of the immune system.
2. Describe the role of each of the lymphoid organs in defending the body against foreign biologic and/or chemical substances.
3. Identify the immunocompetent cells involved in the immune response.
4. Compare and contrast the functions of the three major groups of T cells.
5. Describe the action of B cells in responding to foreign antigens.
6. Identify the five classes of antibodies and their functions.
7. Compare and contrast humoral immunity and cell-mediated immunity.
8. Describe the two types of active immunity and two types of passive immunity.

Key Terms

antibodies, p. 1076
B lymphocytes (B cells), p. 1075
complement system, p. 1076
immunity, p. 1076
immunocompetent cells, p. 1075
polymorphonuclear leukocytes (PMLs), p. 1075
T lymphocytes (T cells), p. 1074

THE IMMUNE SYSTEM

The lymphoid organs consist of the spleen, tonsils, lymph nodes, and thymus. The lymphoid tissues are mainly lymphocytes and plasma cells that travel freely throughout the human system. The two major classes of lymphocytes are T cell and B cell lymphocytes, which are discussed under Immunocompetent Cells. Figure 62-1 identifies the organs and tissues of the immune system.

Spleen

The spleen, the largest lymphatic organ in the body, is located on the left side of the body in the extreme superior, posterior corner of the abdominal cavity. It has two main functions: (1) a storage site or reservoir for blood, and (2) a processing station for red blood cells (i.e., red blood cells break down in the spleen near the end of their life cycle). The spleen intercepts foreign matter or antigens that have reached the bloodstream. Macrophages lining the pulp and sinuses of the spleen remove cellular debris and process hemoglobin in the red pulp area of the spleen. The white pulp area of the spleen contains lymphocytes and plasma cells that are involved in the immune process.

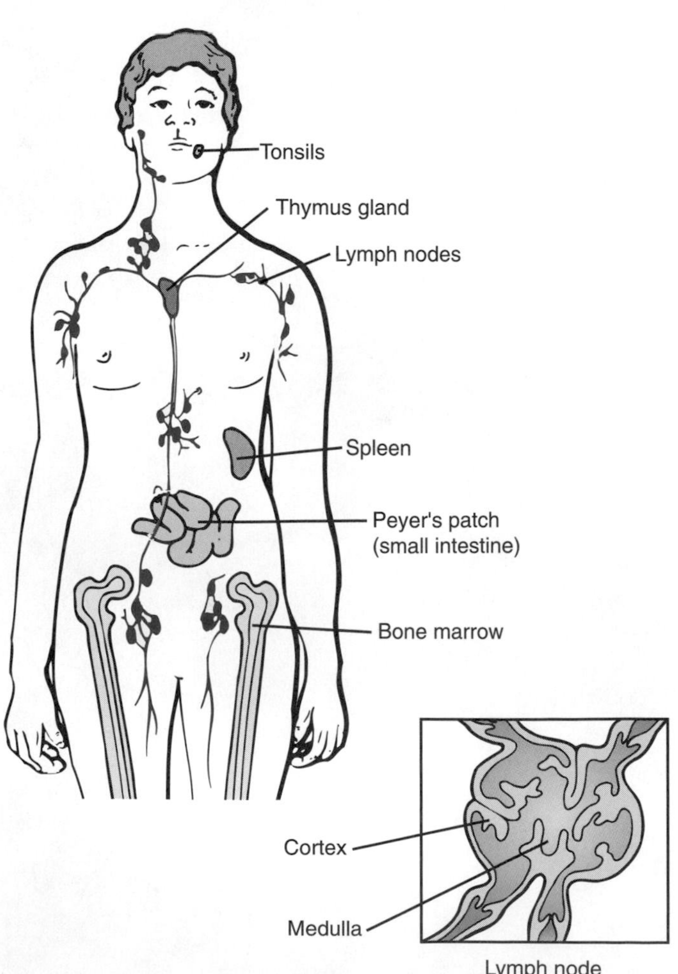

Figure 62-1 Location of organs and tissues of the immune system; insert shows cross-section of lymph node.

Tonsils

The tonsils are an accumulation of lymphoid tissue and are named according to their location: lingual, palatine, and pharyngeal tonsils. They intercept foreign bodies or antigens that enter the body by way of the respiratory tract. Similar lymphoid tissue is located in the submucosal areas of the gastrointestinal tract (Peyer's patches) to intercept antigens (bacteria and viruses) entering from the gut. Other lymphoid tissues are located in the bone marrow and help to intercept antigens in the blood and in the lymph nodes.

Lymph Nodes

The lymph nodes are capsulated organs that are located throughout the body and are involved with lymph circulation. The outer portion of the lymph node is the cortex, and the inner portion is the medulla. The thymus-dependent zone exists in the deep area or middle cortex. This area contains mainly **T lymphocytes (T cells)**; T cells are lymphocytes formed or seeded from the thymus gland that when exposed to an antigen divide rapidly and produce large numbers of new T cells sensitized to that antigen.

Lymph nodes are essentially a row of in-line filters that screen the lymph flowing through it. Many lymphocytes and macrophages are located throughout the lymph nodes, especially in the cortical, paracortical, and medullary areas. T lymphocytes are located mainly in the paracortical region, whereas plasma cells are found in the medullary sinuses.

Thymus Gland

The thymus gland is located in the mediastinal area. It processes lymphocytes and, in the early years up to puberty, it rapidly produces lymphocytes. The immune system is developed when immature lymphocytes from the bone marrow are processed in the thymus gland and then sent to the spleen, lymphatic system, and other tissues and organs in the body to mature. The lymphocytes are active against some bacteria and viruses, allergens, fungus infections, and foreign tissue.

At birth, the thymus gland is larger than it is in an adult. By the time a person reaches puberty, the thymus has grown to nearly six times its original size. After puberty, this gland undergoes involution; in older adults, it is usually a small mass of reticular fibers with some lymphocytes and connective tissue. Although its importance was largely discounted over the years, today it is one of the most important areas for medical research. Scientists are searching for answers to the many questions about the thymus gland and its relationship to the other tissues and organs in the immune system.

IMMUNOCOMPETENT CELLS

Mononuclear T cells and B cells and the **polymorphonuclear leukocytes (PMLs)** are involved in the immune response. However, only mononuclear T cells and B cells are **immunocompetent cells**—cells with the ability to mobilize and deploy antibodies and other responses to stimulation by an antibody. The PMLs are nonspecific cells that interact with lymphocytes to produce an inflammatory response, whereas T cells and B cells are capable of recognizing specific antigens and initiating the immune response.

In humans, stem cells from the bone marrow are transformed to T cells (T lymphocytes) in the thymus gland and B cells (B lymphocytes) elsewhere in the body. As stated in the previous section, the T lymphocytes then migrate to lymphoid tissue and organs. When in contact with an antigen, T lymphocytes form specialized cells to provide cellular immunity. **B lymphocytes (B cells)** are small, agranulocytic leukocytes that form antibodies to search out, identify, and bind with specific antigens to provide humoral immunity.

T Lymphocytes (T Cells)

T cells are generally long-lived. When they are not in their special areas, they circulate continuously through the body by way of the bloodstream and lymphatic system. They are involved with the B lymphocytes (B cells) in that they can cooperate with them (helper T cells) or inhibit them (suppressor T cells). The B cells do not interact with the thymus. Clones are groups of lymphocytes capable of forming one specific antibody (B cell or T cell) to respond to a specific type of antigen; only the specific antigen can activate the specialized clones.

When the T cells first contact an antigen, the lymphocytes that recognize the foreign substance proliferate, which gives rise to larger numbers of cells that have the capacity to recognize and respond to this antigen. Some of the cells produce antibodies or cell-mediated immune-type responses, whereas others increase the population of antigen-sensitive memory cells. This is called acquired immunity, an immunity that is not innate but is obtained during life. A second exposure to this antigen will provoke a more powerful response by the specific T cells.

Three major groups of T cells identified in the past few years include (1) cytotoxic T cells, (2) helper T cells, and (3) suppressor T cells.

Cytotoxic T Cells. Cytotoxic T cells can bind tightly to organisms or cells that contain their binding-specific antigen, and they release cytotoxic (probably lysosomal) enzymes directly into the cell. Cytotoxic T cells are capable of killing microorganisms, cancer cells, viruses, heart transplant cells, and other cells that are foreign to the body. Body tissue that contains viruses or foreign cells may also be attacked by the killer cells.

Helper T Cells. Helper T cells account for the majority of T cells and help the immune system in many ways. They increase the activation of B cells, cytotoxic T cells, and suppressor T cells by antigens. Helper T cell clones are activated by very small amounts of antigens, quantities that may not activate B cells, cytotoxic T cells, or suppressor T cells. Once helper T cells are activated, they secrete lymphokines; these chemical factors attract macrophages to the site of infection or inflammation and increase the response of the B cells, cytotoxic T cells, and suppressor T cells to the antigen.

Helper T cells may also secrete interleukin-2, a lymphokine that is capable of stimulating the action of other T cells, such as cytotoxic T cells and some suppressor T cells. Helper T cells also secrete macrophage migration inhibition factor, another lymphokine. This substance slows or stops the migration of macrophages into the affected area and also activates the macrophages that are present to be more effective phagocytotic agents. The activated macrophages can attack and destroy a vastly increased number of invading organisms.

Acquired immunodeficiency syndrome (AIDS) is the final outcome of an infection with the human immunodeficiency virus (HIV). This virus binds to protein on the cell membranes of the helper T lymphocytes (T4 cells), monocytes, macrophages, and colorectal cells. The helper T cells are destroyed by the virus, which leads to the immunodeficiency syndrome known as AIDS. (See Chapter 64 for additional information on this disease and its treatment.)

Suppressor T Cells. Less is known about suppressor T cells, but it is known that they can suppress the function of both cytotoxic and helper T cells. This suppression may be useful in preventing excessive immune reactions that can cause severe body damage. These cells are often called regulatory T cells.

B Lymphocytes (B Cells)

B lymphocyte clones lie dormant in lymphoid tissue until a foreign antigen appears. The macrophages in the lymphoid tissue phagocytize the foreign substance, and the adjacent B lymphocytes and perhaps the T cells are activated. B cells specific for the antigen enlarge, and some differentiate to form plasmablasts (a plasma cell precursor) and memory cells. The plasmablasts proliferate and divide, and in 4 days approximately 500 plasma cells are present for each original plasmablast. The plasma cells rapidly produce gamma globulin antibodies that are secreted into the lymph and transported by the blood.

Cells similar to those in the original clone are called memory cells. The first response to an antigen may be slow, weak, and of short duration. The second response is much more rapid and far more potent and prolonged, and antibodies are formed for months rather than only for a few weeks. This is why vaccinations that use several doses given weeks or months apart are so effective (Figure 62-2).

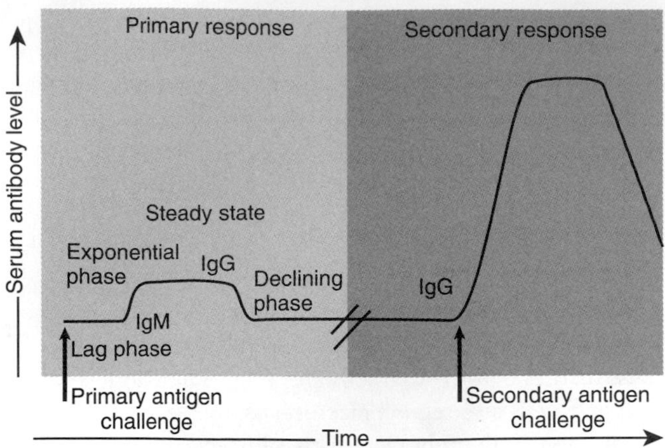

Figure 62-2 Primary and secondary immune responses. (From Mudge-Grout, C.L. [1993]. *Immunologic disorders*. St. Louis: Mosby.)

ANTIBODIES

Antibodies are gamma globulins (a type of protein) called immunoglobulins. They are specific for particular antigens and are produced by lymphoid tissue in response to antigens. At the present time, five classes of antibodies have been identified: IgG, IgM, IgA, IgD, and IgE. (The "Ig" stands for immunoglobulin, and the other letters designate the classes.)

IgG is the major immunoglobulin in the blood (approximately 75% to 80% of the total antibodies in the normal person) and is capable of entering tissue spaces, coating microorganisms, and activating the complement system, thus accelerating phagocytosis. It is the only immunoglobulin capable of crossing the placenta to provide the fetus with passive immunity until the infant can produce his or her own immune defense system.

IgM is the first immunoglobulin produced during an immune response. It is located primarily in the bloodstream and develops in response to an invasion of bacteria or viruses. IgM activates complement and can destroy foreign invaders during the initial antigen exposure. Its level decreases in approximately 1 week, whereas IgG levels progressively increase.

IgA is located primarily in external body secretions—saliva, sweat, tears, mucus, bile, and colostrum—and it is found in respiratory tract mucosa and in plasma. It helps to provide a defense against antigens on exposed surfaces and antigens that enter the respiratory and gastrointestinal tracts. The plasma cells in the intestinal area secrete IgA and secretory components to defend the body against bacteria and viruses.

The function of IgD is unknown. It is found in the plasma and has been located on lymphocyte surfaces together with IgM; therefore it may be associated with binding antigens to the cell surface. Although levels of IgD are increased in chronic infections, IgD does not appear to have a particular affinity for specialized antigens.

IgE binds to histamine-containing mast cells and basophils. It can mediate the release of histamine in the immune response to parasites (helminths) and in some allergic conditions. It is often called the *reaginic antibody* because of its involvement in immediate hypersensitivity reactions. Serum concentrations are low because the antibody is firmly fixed on tissue surfaces. Once activated by an antigen, IgE triggers the release of the mast cell granules, resulting in the signs and symptoms of allergy and anaphylaxis.

IMMUNITY

Links in the chain of infectious disease may be broken at many points. One link can be broken by attacking the pathogen (human disease–causing organism) with antimicrobial or antiinfective therapy. Another can be broken by augmenting human resistance with biologic agents such as vaccines and serums, which artificially supply antibodies or catalyze the ability of the immune system to produce its own. An immunologic reaction that destroys or resists foreign cells or their products (antigens) is termed **immunity.** The most successful antigens, or immunogens, are protein or polysaccharide macromolecules that are usually bacterial, viral, fungal, or rickettsial in origin.

The primary types of immunity are humoral immunity and cell-mediated immunity.

Humoral Immunity

Antigens may be recognized by T-helper cells that activate specific B cells, by a strong B-cell response to the invasion of certain antigens (e.g., large polymers, *Escherichia coli,* dextrans), or by a macrophage intermediary. Macrophage interactions often enhance the antigen recognition by both T cells and B cells in the body. Humoral response is described as a primary or secondary immune response.

Primary Response. A foreign antigen in the body will bind to specific B cells to produce specialized antibody-producing plasma cells. Antibodies specific to the antigen can be found in the blood, usually within 6 days. The initial immunoglobulin is IgM, which increases in quantity for up to 2 weeks; production then declines so that very little IgM is present in a few weeks. After the initial IgM elevation, IgG antibodies start to appear at approximately day 10; these levels peak in several weeks and maintain high levels for a much longer time period (see Figure 62-2).

Secondary Response. The secondary response is often called the *memory response* because the immune system responds so much faster to a second exposure to the same antigen. Both T and B memory cells are involved in beginning the immediate production of antibodies in large amounts.

The second part of humoral immunity is activation of the **complement system,** a series of approximately 20 proteins that circulate in the blood in an inactive form. When an antigen-antibody complex triggers complement, each component in the cascade is activated in precise order. This reaction causes the mast cells to release substances that produce redness, increased heat, and the edema of inflammation. It may also cause bacterial cell death and damage to normal tissue that surrounds the affected area.

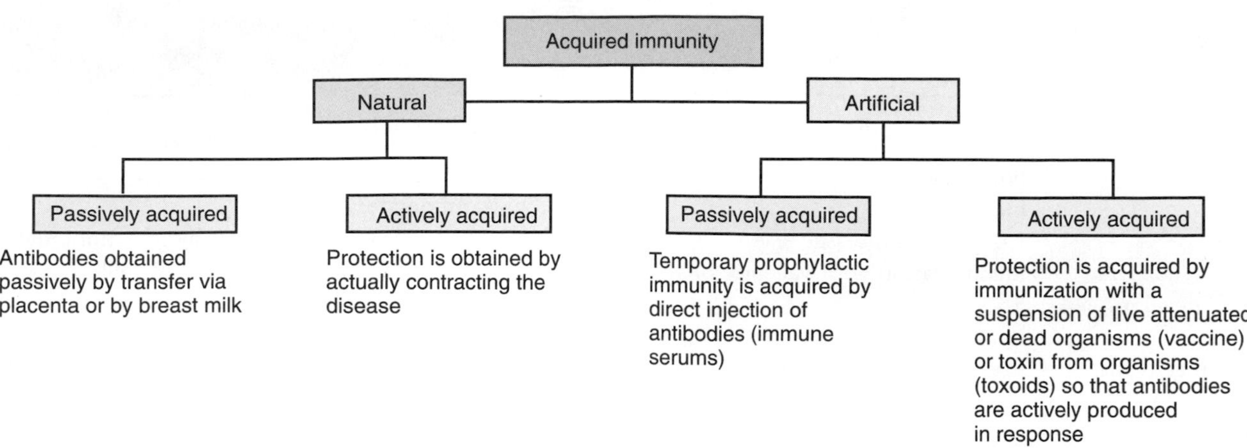

Figure 62-3 The process of acquired immunity.

Cell-Mediated Immunity

Cell-mediated immunity is the result of contact between T cells and antigens. Receptors on the T-cell surface are capable of recognizing foreign antigens, and antigen destruction may occur through one of two processes: (1) directly, by injecting chemical compounds into the target cell membrane (killer activity by cytotoxic T cells); or (2) by secreting lymphokines. The lymphokines can enhance or suppress the action of other lymphocytes, or they can create a chemotactic gradient in the area that will attract macrophages (and eosinophils, basophils, and neutrophils) to the site. Cell-mediated immunity (delayed hypersensitivity) involves only the direct action of T cells without humoral assistance.

Natural and Acquired Immunity

The body has certain inherited and innate abilities to resist encounters with antigens. This ability is known as *natural resistance* or *natural immunity,* which is not to be confused with naturally acquired immunity. Some general defenses inherent to natural resistance come from factors familiar to the focus of nursing, such as adequate rest, nutrition, exercise, and freedom from undue stress. Others are physiologic factors that discourage the proliferation of microbes, including the acidity of gastric secretions, respiratory tract cilia, and bactericidal lysozymes in tears. During his or her lifetime, an individual may also acquire further immune capabilities through both natural and artificial means. This type of acquired immunity is conferred by either active or passive action (Figure 62-3).

Unbroken skin is extremely effective in barring entry to microorganisms. If invasion does succeed, a barrage of defenses is mounted by the inflammatory response. The immune system identifies the threatening antigens or allergens and creates specific gamma globulins destructive to the particular species of antigen. These gamma globulins, or antibodies or immunoglobulins, are proteins that are chemically complementary and specifically configured to lock into the foreign antigen and inactivate it.

Antibodies also activate cellular defenses to phagocytize invading microorganisms. Custom-made gamma globulins, or antibodies, provide acquired immunity to the specific antigen for varying lengths of time. Those antibodies will gradually disappear from the serum, but the potential for their rapid replication in response to a repeat challenge by that specific antigen continues to exist after the initial exposure. Consequently, the result is known as *naturally acquired immunity,* which is a process of *naturally acquired active immunity* because of the body's active involvement in creating the antibodies. Naturally acquired immunity can also result from a process of passive immunity when antibodies made by the mother's body are passively transferred through the placenta or breast milk (especially colostrum, the breast milk produced shortly after delivery) to the fetus or infant.

Artificial induction of the immune state, *artificially acquired immunity,* is initiated purposefully to protect the susceptible individual. It may also be induced either actively or passively. Artificially acquired *active* immunity is evoked by the deliberate administration of antigens, either live partially modified organisms, killed organisms, or their toxins. The parenteral route is the predominant mode of administration. Periodic reactivation of actively acquired artificial immunity against certain organisms by booster doses (e.g., tetanus) is sometimes necessary. Artificially acquired *passive* immunity is conferred by the parenteral administration of antibody-containing immune serum from immune humans or animals (see Figure 62-3).

In general, artificially acquired active immunity secures protection for a longer duration than any type of passive immunity and is usually the prophylactic treatment of choice for populations at risk. Side effects may include local pain at the injection site and headache with mild to moderate fever. Because of the agents used, *active* immunity results in fewer adverse reactions than passive immunity. Artificially acquired *passive* immunity is often chosen for susceptible individuals following a known exposure. A combination of active and passive approaches is also occasionally used. A number of products used in artificial passive immunization cause adverse reactions because of individual hypersensitivi-

TABLE 62-1 Comparison of Active and Passive Immunity

	Active Immunity	Passive Immunity
Source	Individual	Other human or animal
Efficacy	High	Low to moderate
Method	Contracting disease Immunization with vaccines or toxoids	Administer preformed antibody by injection, maternal transplacental transfer, or in breast milk
Time to develop	5-21 days	Immediate effect
Duration	Long, up to years	Usually shorter in time
Ease of reactivation	Easy with booster dose	Can be dangerous; anaphylaxis may occur, especially if animal sources are used
Purpose	Prophylaxis	Prophylaxis and therapy

ties to animal products (especially horse serum or eggs), to the preservative used in a medication, or to an antibiotic. The products of bacterial metabolism are the agents responsible for other adverse reactions.

The presence of mild to moderate upper respiratory tract infection or pregnancy does not always prohibit immunization. However, an immunosuppressed state (as a result of cancer chemotherapy or disease) may prohibit immunization. Current manufacturers' instructions should always be consulted. Table 62-1 compares the capabilities and effects of active and passive immunity.

SUMMARY

The immunologic system consists of lymphoid organs (the spleen, tonsils, lymph nodes, and thymus) and immunocompetent cells known as T lymphocytes (T cells) and B lymphocytes (B cells). All of these components defend the body against the invasion of foreign biologic and chemical substances. Antibodies are immunoglobulins that are specific for particular antigens. Immunity is the immunologic reaction that destroys or resists foreign cells or their products. It may be natural or artificial and actively or passively acquired. Pharmacologic therapy is usually aimed at strengthening the body's immunologic status for the prevention of disease.

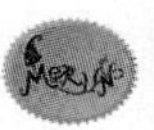

Critical Thinking Questions

1. As a bacterium entering a human body, what do you anticipate will be your experience when encountering T cells? You have invited a friend, a virus, to meet you by entering via the respiratory system. What will be her experience with the various antibodies?
2. What type of immunity do the following have:
   a. A child recovering from the measles?
   b. A 6-week-old nursing infant?
   c. A first-grader with a DPT (diphtheria, polio, tetanus) and polio vaccine booster?
   d. A nurse who receives hepatitis B immune globulin after exposure to hepatitis B?
3. Suppose you had an additive that could be used with injectable solutions to delay but not stop the release of the drug from an injection site into the blood. If you injected an antigen into one injection site and injected into another site an antigen mixed with the additive to cause delay of absorption for 2 to 3 weeks, which injection would result in the greater response of antibody production? Why?*

Collaborative Learning Activities

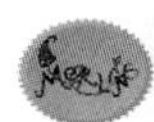

For Collaborative Learning Activities, go to mosby.com/MERLIN/McKenry/.

BIBLIOGRAPHY

Anderson, K.N., Anderson, L.E., & Glanze, W.D. (Eds.) (1998). *Mosby's medical, nursing, & allied health dictionary* (5th ed.). St. Louis: Mosby.

Klein, D.M. & Witek-Janusek, L. (1992). Advances in immunotherapy of sepsis. *Dimensions of Critical Care Nursing, 11*(2), 75.

McCance, K.L. & Huether, S.E. (1998). *Pathophysiology: The biological basis for disease in adults and children* (3rd ed.). St. Louis: Mosby.

McIntyre, W.J. & Tami, J.A. (1993). Immunology for the consultant pharmacist. *Consultant Pharmacist, 8*(4), 376.

Mudge-Grout, C.L. (1992). *Immunologic disorders.* St. Louis: Mosby.

Thibodeau, G.A. & Patton, K.T. (1999). *Anatomy and physiology* (4th ed.). St. Louis: Mosby.

Van Wynsberghe, D., Noback, C.R., & Carola, R. (1995). *Human anatomy and physiology* (3rd ed.). New York: McGraw-Hill.

*Question from Seeley, R.S. & Tate, P. (1995). Anatomy and physiology (3rd ed.). St. Louis: Mosby.

63 Serums, Vaccines, and Other Immunizing Agents

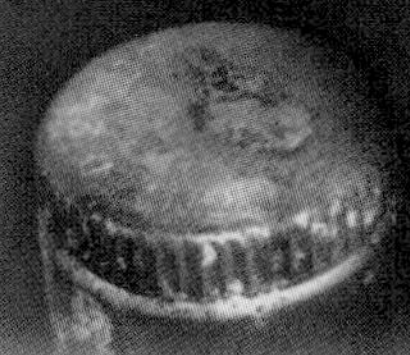

Chapter Focus

More than 200 years ago, Edward Jenner observed that milkmaids who developed cowpox were rarely victims of smallpox; this prompted him to develop the first vaccine. A modern version of this vaccine led to the eradication of smallpox in 1980—a health success for the world. The development of vaccines against more than 20 infectious diseases has revolutionized the approach to public health. Nine new or improved vaccines have become available in the last two decades alone. Today advances in molecular biology are enabling scientists to develop new vaccines against diseases that continue to plague the world.

Learning Objectives

1. Discuss the present status of immunization and anticipated future developments.
2. State the appropriate immunization schedule for children 2 years of age and under.
3. Identify immunizations recommended for adults.
4. Describe the recommended use of tetanus toxoid and tetanus immune globulin in wound management.
5. Discuss the nursing management of immunotherapy.
6. List the side effects/adverse reactions of immunizations, and correlate them with client education.
7. Compare the advantages and disadvantages of live attenuated and inactivated biologic products.

Key Terms

active immunity, p. 1080
antibody titer, p. 1081

The body's first defense against invasion by potentially lethal microorganisms is intact skin and mucous membranes. The antiinflammatory process and/or a competent immune system are the body's defense against microbes that break this barrier.

Active immunity exists when the body is capable of producing specific antibodies to combat infections caused by specific antigens or microbes. This immunity may be referred to as *naturally acquired immunity,* because a person who recovers from an infectious disease produces antibodies and memory cells against that specific antigen. The next time the body is in contact with the same antigen, the immune system will be primed to destroy the antigen.

Passively acquired immunity occurs when antibodies are transferred from a human or animal to a susceptible person. Newborn infants usually have passively acquired immunization that is naturally acquired from their mothers. However, this type of immunity protects for only short periods of time (weeks to several months).

Vaccines and toxoids are available to provide artificially acquired active immunity; vaccines contain whole microbes (dead or attenuated) that are not pathogenic but can induce the formation of antibodies. Toxoids contain detoxified microbe by-products, which are antigenic and also induce antibody production. Sera and antitoxins contain exogenous antibodies and are used to provide artificially acquired passive immunity (Box 63-1).

OVERVIEW

The critical age period for immunization is from birth through grade school entry and during the school years (many states now require maintenance of immunizations as a criterion for retention in the school system). Certain groups are found to be at high risk: adolescents, new parents (if they are unimmunized or have waning immunity, because they are exposed to childhood illness or vaccines), debilitated persons, and health care providers. Other groups such as migrant workers and recent immigrants to the United States and Canada are predictably at high risk for infectious diseases. (See the Cultural Considerations box below for a discussion of risk factors for *Haemophilus influenzae* type b [Hib] meningitis.)

International political and economic upheavals and the refugee influx to the United States and Canada have illustrated the major problems encountered in other countries: diphtheria, measles, hepatitis B, tuberculosis, and malaria carrier status. Immunization programs that are taken for granted in the United States, Canada, and other countries are not as well funded in developing countries.

As a group, adolescents also seem to be at high risk for preventable infections. Of these, certain subgroups may be

BOX 63-1

Live vs. Inactivated Products

The advantages of a live attenuated-type immunization are the long-lasting immunity and the similarity of the resistance that occurs to that which is produced by the natural disease. The disadvantages of a live immunization are an increased risk of inducing disease plus the fact that a mild disease state is usually needed in order to induce immunity. There also is a higher risk of the vaccine being contaminated; finally, the product is more labile and requires special storage.

The inactivated (killed) biologic product is easier to ship and store. It is usually highly purified, and there is little risk of inducing a disease from infection. The disadvantage is that it provides a short-acting immunity, and therefore the client often needs reimmunization. It may or may not simulate protective-type factors, and it may not prevent a reinfection without the actual disease having been present.

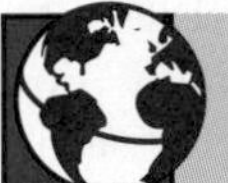

Cultural Considerations

Ethnicity as a Risk Factor: Implications for Immunization

In planning for immunization programs, populations are examined for their risk of having the disease. These groups are then targeted for intensive immunization efforts. In the case of *Haemophilus influenzae* type b, inoculation with the Hib vaccine has been demonstrated to provide high immunogenicity in all age-groups. But what groups should be targeted for immunization?

Reece (1991) reports that, in addition to age (i.e., younger than 18 months), day-care placement is an important risk factor. Infants less than 1 year of age who are placed in day-care facilities have an attack rate 10 times that of infants who do not attend day-care programs.

In general, ethnicity is not considered a risk factor in and of itself. However, Reece reports that Native Americans and Eskimos from Alaska are at greater risk for contracting invasive Hib infections. Navajo Indians have an annual Hib-meningitis infection rate of 173 per 100,000 in children less than 5 years of age, and Alaskan Eskimos have a rate of 409 per 100,000. Black and Hispanic children may also be at increased risk. Children who have a household contact with an index case of invasive disease are also at a substantial risk for infection—585 times the rate of same-age individuals within the general population.

Critical Thinking Questions

- What other factors besides ethnicity have contributed to the infection rates of the groups mentioned above?
- Given the information above, how would you develop an immunization program if all of these groups were found within your community?

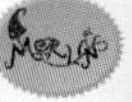

particularly in need of immunization, such as athletes, heavy substance users, runaways, foreign travelers, and those isolated from or rejecting allopathic health care. Several million children are not immunized against measles, polio, rubella (German measles), mumps, diphtheria, pertussis (whooping cough), and tetanus.

Newspapers and television news programs have reported the adverse reactions associated with the pertussis vaccine and other vaccines; such reports have served to bias some individuals against vaccination. (See the Nursing Research box at right about the perceptions of vaccine efficacy among inner-city parents.) It is important to stress that, although vaccines are not without some risks, the risks associated with not being vaccinated and actually contracting the disease are even more serious. Table 63-1 illustrates the impact of diseases before immunizations. Diphtheria, tetanus, polio, and other diseases can cause crippling and death, and most of these diseases are very contagious.

Other perceived barriers to immunization are living in medically underserved areas, not having health insurance, having problems accessing immunization clinics (Gore et al., 1999), and having insufficient information about the value of immunizations (Freeman & Freed, 1999). The incidence rates of traditional vaccine-preventable diseases are at an all-time low, and corresponding vaccination coverage rates are at an all-time high; however, a system to ensure the timely vaccination of newborn infants that also incorporates newly recommended vaccines is incomplete (National Vaccine Advisory Committee, 1999). Schedules for immunizations for these diseases have been developed as guidelines for the practitioner and for parents to ensure adequate protection for their children (Figure 63-1).

With some of these diseases, obtaining a valid history of clinical disease or an **antibody titer** (the concentration of antibodies in the serum) is useful in determining disease exposure and immunity. Proven exposure to the disease does not always guarantee immunity. Therefore timely immunizations are even more important if the potential for developing the disease is imminent or increased, such as with persons traveling to foreign countries where some diseases are endemic or indigenous to a geographic area or population. Required and recommended immunizations for foreign travel are constantly changing and are best obtained before travel from the local public health department.

The client's tetanus immunization status must be assessed any time a traumatic wound (especially a puncture wound) is encountered. A booster dose of tetanus toxoid may be in order if the client has not been fully immunized within the past 10 years or if the wound is contaminated and an immunization is more than 5 years old. Tetanus and diphtheria toxoid is recommended for adults, because diphtheria protection is enhanced by this combination (McCormack & Brown, 1996).

Most new parents today are too young to remember the fear engendered by the very mention of childhood illnesses a few decades ago. For example, measles, the most common childhood disease, can cause pneumonia, encephalopathy, deafness, blindness, and seizures in 1 out of every 1000 children (McCormack & Brown, 1996). If parents are not convinced, outbreaks of communicable diseases (e.g., poliomyelitis) may make the argument for us. Complacency about childhood illnesses and their current and potential threats

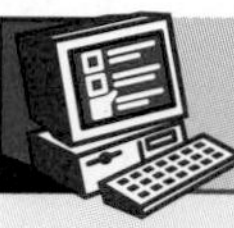

Nursing Research

Misperceptions of Parents Concerning Vaccination

Citation: Keane, V., Stanton, B., Horton, L., Aronson, R., Galbraith, J., Hughart, N. (1993). Perceptions of vaccine efficacy, illness, and health among inner-city parents. Clinical Pediatrics, 32(1), 2–7.

Abstract: A resurgence of measles in the past decade has focused attention on the limitations of current immunization programs, particularly for inner-city, low-income populations. As part of a larger study of immunization rates, Keane et al. (1993) discussed perceptions of disease severity and vaccine efficacy, as well as the prioritization of the tasks of parenthood, with 40 parents of infants living in inner-city Baltimore to discover their beliefs about immunization.

The focus group approach was used. A focus group usually consists of 4 to 12 people and is a group interview technique that relies on the interaction between group members rather than between an interviewer and a respondent. All parents/guardians of infants 18 to 24 months of age who attended the Pediatric Ambulatory Center (the community-based health center of the Department of Pediatrics, University of Maryland School of Medicine) were invited by letter to participate in a 2-hour discussion of why parents do or do not use health care services, including immunizations. Forty parents participated in the focus group discussions.

Vaccines were considered only partly successful; susceptibility to chickenpox after vaccination was repeatedly cited as evidence of vaccine failure. Fever was seen as a primary indicator of illness; thus vaccines were believed to cause, rather than prevent, illness. Immunization was not considered a high-priority parental responsibility. These findings suggest that future interventions should be aimed at changing parental perceptions of vaccines as ineffective and of fever after immunization as an indicator of illness. Educational strategies building on local perceptions may be more effective than external perceptions. Finally, immunizations should be made easily available, even during clinic visits for a child's illness.

Critical Thinking Questions

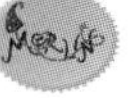

- What misconceptions did the parents in this study have?
- If you were working at the Pediatric Ambulatory Center, how would you conduct an educational program to provide information to parents?

TABLE 63-1 Impact of Selected Diseases Before Immunizations

Disease	Comments
Measles	Before vaccinations, nearly everyone in the United States contracted measles (an estimated 3 to 4 million cases annually). The average annual number of measles-related deaths was 450 (1953 to 1963). A low rate of vaccination in preschool children in 1995 resulted in >55,000 cases, 11,000 hospitalizations, and 120 deaths. The risk for measles in African-American and Hispanic children was 8 to 10 times greater than in white children, because vaccination rates in African-American and Hispanic children were lower.
H. influenzae type b (Hib) meningitis	Before the release of this vaccine in December 1987, Hib was the most common cause of meningitis in infants and children in the United States. Approximately 8000 new cases were seen annually (with 600 deaths), and many survivors were left with deafness, convulsions, or mental retardation. Since the release of the vaccine, the incidence of Hib meningitis has decreased 97% to 99% from previous reports.
Pertussis (whooping cough)	Before this vaccine, 150,000 to 260,000 children had pertussis annually, and there were approximately 9000 deaths. Pertussis is a serious illness; it can cause weeks of prolonged coughing and vomiting. Infants may contract pneumonia. Pertussis may also cause convulsions, brain damage, and mental retardation. The new acellular pertussis (DTaP) vaccine is safer than the older, whole-cell DTP vaccine; it has been available in the United States since 1991. Countries have reported epidemics of pertussis that correspond to decreased immunization levels; for example, Japan's immunization dropped from 80% to 20% from 1974 to 1979, and in 1979 a pertussis epidemic resulted in 13,000 new cases and 41 deaths.
Rubella	This is usually a mild disease in children and adults but is a serious problem in pregnant women during the first trimester. Adverse reactions may occur in up to 90% of the exposed infants; that is, they may contract congenital rubella syndrome (CRS), which causes heart defects, cataracts, deafness, and mental retardation. A rubella epidemic occurred during 1964 and 1965 (before rubella vaccinations were used regularly in the United States). Nearly 20,000 infants were born with CRS, 2100 died, and 11,250 miscarriages were reported. Of the 20,000 infants with CRS, 11,600 were born deaf, 3580 were blind, and 1800 were mentally retarded.

Information from Centers for Disease Control and Prevention. (2000). What would happen if we stopped vaccinations; www.cdc.gov/nip/publications/fs/gen/whatifstop.htm (7/15/00).

must be shaken. The initial effects of childhood illnesses can be very serious, and more potential future hazards are currently being discovered (e.g., the possible association of mumps with eventual diabetes and of chickenpox with shingles).

A request for exemption from the immunizations required for school entry on medical grounds can be obtained from the child's physician. A model form for exemption on religious grounds can be obtained from the Christian Science Committee on Publications. However, it is *theoretically* possible that the right to exempt certain children could interfere with "herd immunity" by sustaining a continued pool of susceptibles, thereby maintaining a hazard that would be unacceptable to other parents, who might apply legal and other pressures.

Community health nurses, school nurses, teachers, local public health departments, the Department of Health and Human Services, and the World Health Organization need to work together to share expertise in educating the public, in case finding and reporting, in screening, and in mass immunization programs.

CURRENT ISSUES

Refinements and developments in the field of clinical immunology are advancing, with the Centers for Disease Control and Prevention (CDC) (1994) issuing the general recommendations discussed in the following sections.

Spacing of Immunizations

When multiple doses of a particular immunization are recommended to achieve an adequate antibody response, the recommended time interval between doses should be followed. Although an interval that is longer than recommended is acceptable and does not require starting over,

Recommended Childhood Immunization Schedule United States, 2002

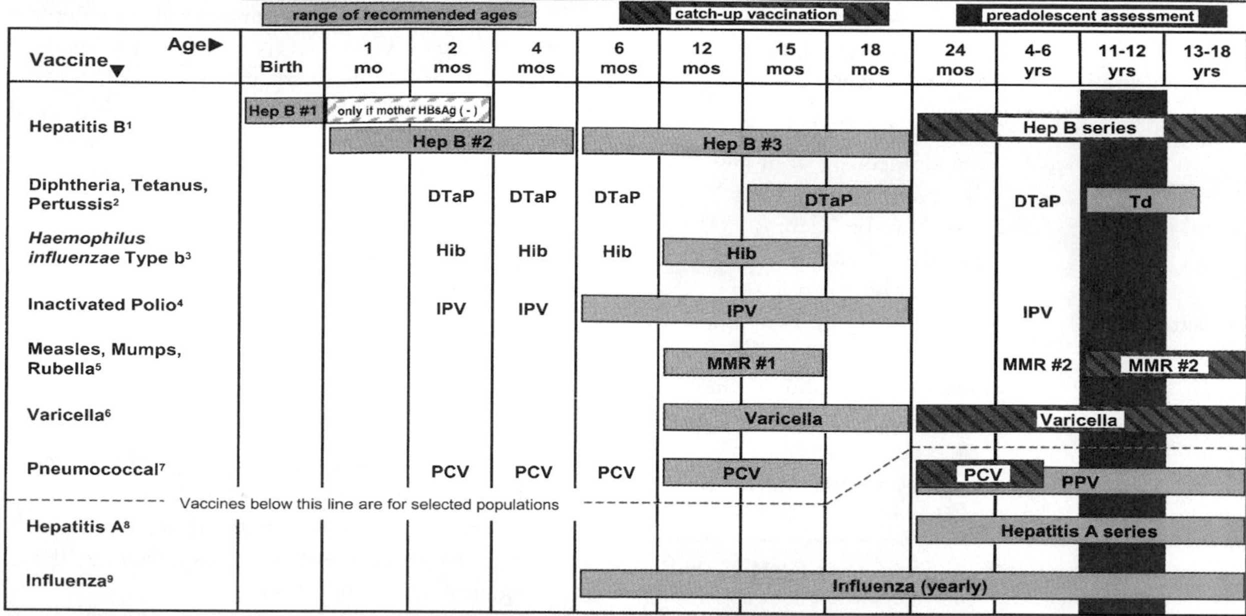

range of recommended ages | catch-up vaccination | preadolescent assessment

Vaccine ▼ / Age ▶	Birth	1 mo	2 mos	4 mos	6 mos	12 mos	15 mos	18 mos	24 mos	4-6 yrs	11-12 yrs	13-18 yrs
Hepatitis B[1]	Hep B #1	only if mother HBsAg (-)										
		Hep B #2			Hep B #3						Hep B series	
Diphtheria, Tetanus, Pertussis[2]			DTaP	DTaP	DTaP		DTaP			DTaP	Td	
Haemophilus influenzae Type b[3]			Hib	Hib	Hib	Hib						
Inactivated Polio[4]			IPV	IPV	IPV					IPV		
Measles, Mumps, Rubella[5]						MMR #1				MMR #2	MMR #2	
Varicella[6]							Varicella				Varicella	
Pneumococcal[7]			PCV	PCV	PCV	PCV			PCV	PPV		
Vaccines below this line are for selected populations												
Hepatitis A[8]											Hepatitis A series	
Influenza[9]									Influenza (yearly)			

This schedule indicates the recommended ages for routine administration of currently licensed childhood vaccines, as of December 1, 2001, for children through age 18 years. Any dose not given at the recommended age should be given at any subsequent visit when indicated and feasible. ▨ Indicates age groups that warrant special effort to administer those vaccines not previously given. Additional vaccines may be licensed and recommended during the year. Licensed combination vaccines may be used whenever any components of the combination are indicated and the vaccine's other components are not contraindicated. Providers should consult the manufacturers' package inserts for detailed recommendations.

1. Hepatitis B vaccine (Hep B). All infants should receive the first dose of hepatitis B vaccine soon after birth and before hospital discharge; the first dose may also be given by age 2 months if the infant's mother is HBsAg-negative. Only monovalent hepatitis B vaccine can be used for the birth dose. Monovalent or combination vaccine containing Hep B may be used to complete the series; four doses of vaccine may be administered if combination vaccine is used. The second dose should be given at least 4 weeks after the first dose, except for Hib-containing vaccine which cannot be administered before age 6 weeks. The third dose should be given at least 16 weeks after the first dose and at least 8 weeks after the second dose. The last dose in the vaccination series (third or fourth dose) should not be administered before age 6 months.

Infants born to HBsAg-positive mothers should receive hepatitis B vaccine and 0.5 mL hepatitis B immune globulin (HBIG) within 12 hours of birth at separate sites. The second dose is recommended at age 1-2 months and the vaccination series should be completed (third or fourth dose) at age 6 months.

Infants born to mothers whose HBsAg status is unknown should receive the first dose of the hepatitis B vaccine series within 12 hours of birth. Maternal blood should be drawn at the time of delivery to determine the mother's HBsAg status; if the HBsAg test is positive, the infant should receive HBIG as soon as possible (no later than age 1 week).

2. Diphtheria and tetanus toxoids and acellular pertussis vaccine (DTaP). The fourth dose of DTaP may be administered as early as age 12 months, provided 6 months have elapsed since the third dose and the child is unlikely to return at age 15-18 months. **Tetanus and diphtheria toxoids (Td)** is recommended at age 11-12 years if at least 5 years have elapsed since the last dose of tetanus and diphtheria toxoid-containing vaccine. Subsequent routine Td boosters are recommended every 10 years.

3. *Haemophilus influenzae* type b (Hib) conjugate vaccine. Three Hib conjugate vaccines are licensed for infant use. If PRP-OMP (PedvaxHIB® or ComVax® [Merck]) is administered at ages 2 and 4 months, a dose at age 6 months is not required. DTaP/Hib combination products should not be used for primary immunization in infants at ages 2, 4 or 6 months, but can be used as boosters following any Hib vaccine.

4. Inactivated polio vaccine (IPV). An all-IPV schedule is recommended for routine childhood polio vaccination in the United States. All children should receive four doses of IPV at ages 2 months, 4 months, 6-18 months, and 4-6 years.

5. Measles, mumps, and rubella vaccine (MMR). The second dose of MMR is recommended routinely at age 4-6 years but may be administered during any visit, provided at least 4 weeks have elapsed since the first dose and that both doses are administered beginning at or after age 12 months. Those who have not previously received the second dose should complete the schedule by the 11-12 year old visit.

6. Varicella vaccine. Varicella vaccine is recommended at any visit at or after age 12 months for susceptible children, i.e. those who lack a reliable history of chickenpox. Susceptible persons aged ≥ 13 years should receive two doses, given at least 4 weeks apart.

7. Pneumococcal vaccine. The heptavalent **pneumococcal conjugate vaccine (PCV)** is recommended for all children age 2-23 months. It is also recommended for certain children age 24-59 months. **Pneumococcal polysaccharide vaccine (PPV)** is recommended in addition to PCV for certain high-risk groups. See *MMWR* 2000;49(RR-9);1-35.

8. Hepatitis A vaccine. Hepatitis A vaccine is recommended for use in selected states and regions, and for certain high-risk groups; consult your local public health authority. See *MMWR* 1999;48(RR-12);1-37.

9. Influenza vaccine. Influenza vaccine is recommended annually for children age ≥ 6 months with certain risk factors (including but not limited to asthma, cardiac disease, sickle cell disease, HIV, diabetes; see *MMWR* 2001;50(RR-4);1-44), and can be administered to all others wishing to obtain immunity. Children aged ≤12 years should receive vaccine in a dosage appropriate for their age (0.25 mL if age 6-35 months or 0.5 mL if aged ≥ 3 years). Children aged ≤ 8 years who are receiving influenza vaccine for the first time should receive two doses separated by at least 4 weeks.

For additional information about vaccines, vaccine supply, and contraindications for immunization, please visit the National Immunization Program Website at www.cdc.gov/nip or call the National Immunization Hotline at 800-232-2522 (English) or 800-232-0233 (Spanish).

Approved by the Advisory Committee on Immunization Practices (www.cdc.gov/nip/acip), the American Academy of Pediatrics (www.aap.org), and the American Academy of Family Physicians (www.aafp.org).

OSP 02 64574

Figure 63-1 Recommended childhood immunization schedule, United States. (From Centers for Disease Control and Prevention, National Immunization Program. Available at www.cdc.gov/nip/recs/child-schedule.pdf.

TABLE 63-2 Guidelines for Spacing the Administration of Live and Killed Antigens

Antigen Combination	Recommended Minimum Interval Between Doses
≥2 killed antigens	None. May be administered simultaneously or at any interval between doses.*
Killed and live antigens	None. May be administered simultaneously or at any interval between doses.†
≥2 live antigens	4-week minimum interval if not administered simultaneously.‡ However, oral polio vaccine can be administered at any time before, with, or after measles-mumps-rubella, if indicated.

From Centers for Disease Control and Prevention (1994). General recommendations on immunization: Recommendations of the Advisory Committee on Immunization Practices (ACIP). *MMWR: Morbidity & Mortality Weekly Report, 43*(RR-1), 1-38.

*If possible, vaccines associated with local or systemic side effects (e.g., cholera, parenteral typhoid, and plague vaccines) should be administered on separate occasions to avoid accentuated reactions.

†A cholera vaccine with yellow fever vaccine is the exception. If time permits, these antigens should not be administered simultaneously, and at least 3 weeks should elapse between the administration of the yellow fever vaccine and the cholera vaccine. If the vaccines must be administered simultaneously or within 3 weeks of each other, the antibody response may not be optimal.

‡If an oral live typhoid vaccine is indicated (e.g., for international travel taken on short notice), it can be administered before, simultaneously with, or after the oral polio vaccine (OPV).

shorter intervals are not acceptable because the overall antibody response will be decreased, and some persons will experience an increased frequency in local or systemic adverse reactions (Centers for Disease Control and Prevention, 1994). Although live vaccines such as the oral polio and yellow fever vaccines can be given at any time with an immune globulin, there is some evidence that high doses of immune globulin can inhibit the immune response to a measles vaccine for more than 3 months. There are instances in which an inactivated vaccine interferes with other killed or live antigens. Tables 63-2 and 63-3 list the recommended guidelines for spacing the administration of live and killed antigens and immune globulin.

Vaccination in Special Situations

- Premature infants should be vaccinated on the same chronologic age schedule as full-term infants and with the same recommended vaccine dose.
- There is no contraindication to breastfeeding and vaccinations.
- Vaccinations during pregnancy depend on weighing the potential risk of the vaccine against the result of disease exposure. For example, tetanus and diphtheria toxoids are routinely used for susceptible pregnant women; hepatitis B vaccine, influenza, and pneumococcal vaccines are also recommended for pregnant women at risk for the infection or complications of the disease.
- Contraindications to all vaccines include a history of anaphylaxis to the individual vaccine or a component of it, or the presence of moderate to severe illness with or without a fever. In general, immunocompromised individuals should not receive any live vaccines. Special exceptions for immunocompromised clients and specific recommendations for their household contacts are available (CDC, 1994).

AIDS Vaccine

Acquired immunodeficiency syndrome (AIDS) often results in fatal and unusual malignancies and opportunistic infections. It is recognized as an immunodeficiency state that results from an infection with a human retrovirus, the human immunodeficiency virus (HIV).

Various kits have been investigated by the Food and Drug Administration (FDA) to detect HIV. For example, the Home Access HIV Test provides a kit to test blood for HIV. This is considered a reliable test and is currently the only home HIV test approved by the FDA (Home Health Testing, 2000). Vaccines for AIDS are also in various stages of development (investigational studies). The HIV immune globulin (HIVIG) is in phase III testing as an immunomodulator to prevent maternal-to-fetal transfer of HIV. HIV immunotherapeutic vaccine is in phase II/III as an antiviral to treat asymptomatic HIV. There are also a number of other vaccines under study, but the majority of them are in phase I/II studies (*Drug Facts and Comparisons*, 2000).

Many viral vaccines work by preventing the acute illness from developing—not by preventing the infection itself. This method may be risky with HIV, but investigators are currently looking into this possibility by testing in primates (Santiago, 1996). (See Chapter 64 for more information.)

SIDE EFFECTS/ADVERSE REACTIONS

Although being protected from debilitating infectious disease is important, immunization is not without some risk. Side effects (e.g., slight fever, sore injection site, or minor rash) are usually mild and transient; more serious effects (i.e., encephalitis and convulsions) are occasionally reported.

Although serious, the incidence of these effects usually tips the balance in favor of immunization when weighed against the effects of diseases preventable through immunization, particularly for individuals at high risk.

Joint pains and malaise may also be seen, especially with certain live and inactivated vaccines. Although rare, an allergy to the egg protein providing the culture medium for the organism involved, to antiserums or antitoxins, to the

TABLE 63-3 Guidelines for Spacing the Administration of Immune Globulin Preparations* and Vaccines

Simultaneous Administration		Nonsimultaneous Administration		
		Immunobiologic Administered		
Immunobiologic Combination	Recommended Minimum Interval Between Doses	First	Second	Recommended Minimum Interval Between Doses
Immune globulin and killed antigen	None. May be given simultaneously at different sites or at any time between doses.	Immune globulin Killed antigen	Killed antigen Immune globulin	None None
Immune globulin and live antigen	In general, should not be administered simultaneously.† If simultaneous administration of measles-mumps-rubella (MMR), measles-rubella, and monovalent measles vaccine is unavoidable, administer at different sites and revaccinate or test for seroconversion after the recommended interval.	Immune globulin Live antigen	Live antigen Immune globulin	Dose related†,‡ 2 weeks

From Centers for Disease Control and Prevention (1994). General Recommendations on Immunization: Recommendations of the Advisory Committee on Immunization Practices (ACIP). *MMWR: Morbidity & Mortality Weekly Report, 43*(RR-1), 1-38.
*Blood products containing large amounts of immune globulin, such as serum immune globulin, specific immune globulins (e.g., tetanus immune globulin [TIG] and hepatitis B immune globulin [HBIG]), IV immune globulin (IVIG), whole blood, packed red cells, plasma, and platelet products.
†Oral poliovirus, yellow fever, and oral typhoid (Ty21a) vaccines are exceptions to these recommendations. These vaccines may be administered at any time before, after, or simultaneously with an immune globulin–containing product without substantially decreasing the antibody response.
‡The duration of interference of immune globulin preparations with the immune response to the measles component of the MMR, measles-rubella, and monovalent measles vaccine is dose related (Table 8 of original document).

mercury preservative, or to contained antibiotics causes a reaction that is usually controllable by antihistamines. When any unusual or severe reaction occurs, the nurse should contact the prescriber, and an informational form should be sent to the CDC. Vaccinees should be given a contact's name in case they become sick, and they should visit a health care provider, hospital, or clinic within 4 weeks of immunization.

Monitoring for adverse reactions is part of a surveillance system to detect uncommon, severe, previously unrecognized, and rare reactions to vaccination. Past examples are the Guillain-Barré syndrome (which accompanies a small percentage of influenza vaccinations), encephalitis following a measles vaccine, and peripheral neuropathy after rubella vaccinations. All of these occurrences are very rare.

Although uncommon, a large number of benign, expected reactions could indicate a "hot" lot of vaccine. Data are collected by the CDC for comparison with national data and are published in the *Quarterly Adverse Reaction Report*.

Minor expected reactions can be treated with acetaminophen (with prescriber approval) and rest. Severe fevers (temperatures more than 103° F) can be treated with acetaminophen and sponge baths to reduce body temperature; occasionally a convulsion may accompany a high temperature, and parents need to be advised. Serum sickness sometimes occurs after repeated serum injections and consists of a rash, urticaria, arthritis, adenopathy, and fever that starts hours or even days after the injection. Treatment consists of analgesics, antihistamines, or corticosteroids.

Rare but serious anaphylactic reactions can cause urticaria, dyspnea, cyanosis, shock, or unconsciousness that occurs within minutes of injection. This is not normal; it is an emergency situation. Therefore a nurse or someone responsible should observe any recipient of immunotherapy for up to half an hour after therapy. Treatment for anaphylaxis may require the administration of epinephrine. Vasopressors and intermittent positive-pressure breathing (IPPB) oxygen, antihistamines, and corticosteroids may help. Immunization therapy may be resumed with caution after all signs of anaphylaxis are gone.

Nurses often find themselves in charge of vaccination programs and clinics. Because nurses are often the first to be consulted by clients, keeping current on the changes in immunizations is important. A description of biologic agents (active and passive) used for immunization and their secondary effects may be found in Table 63-4. Box 63-2 on p. 1092 provides information on RespiGam.

Text continued on p. 1090

TABLE 63-4 Biologic Agents for Active Immunization

Active immunization uses either inactivated (killed [K]) material or live (L) attenuated agents.
Advantages: Higher levels of antibody are usually induced, and frequent immunizations are not necessary.
Disadvantages: Adverse reactions (e.g., allergic reactions) may occur; these are not usually seen with passive immunization.
See Box 63-1 for the advantages and disadvantages of live attenuated and inactivated biologic products.

Product	Route of Administration	Primary Immunization Schedule	Comments	Nursing Assessment for Contraindications and Side Effects/Implementation
Cholera vaccine	K bacteria: SC, IM	Two doses 1-4 weeks apart (adult dosage)	Provides 50% protection for approximately 6 months.	*Assessment.* Contraindications: acute illness; severe reaction or allergic response to previous dose; pregnancy evaluated individually. Precautions: review of hypersensitivity history. Side effects: redness, induration, pain at site; occasionally malaise, headache, mild to moderate temperature elevations. *Implementation.* Administer SC or IM (in the deltoid muscle) to adults and children over 3 years of age. Have epinephrine 1:1000 on hand.
Hemophilus influenzae	IM	See Figure 63-1	Efficacy improved if given to children under 2 years of age.	*Assessment.* Contraindicated in immunosuppression, acute illnesses, and febrile states. *Implementation.* Shake vial well and store in medical refrigerator. May be given at the same time as the diphtheria, tetanus, pertussis vaccine (DTP) but at different sites. Reconstitute with diluent provided. Record date on vial. Refrigerate; stable 30 days. Have epinephrine 1:1000 available.
Hepatitis B	K: IM	See Figure 63-1	Provides >90% protection.	*Assessment.* Contraindications/precautions: hypersensitivity. Safety and efficacy not yet established for children under 3 months of age or for pregnant or breastfeeding women. Clinical judgment would probably weigh the risk of the disease higher than the potential risks caused by the secondary effects of the vaccine. Delay giving this vaccine in the presence of serious active infection or severely compromised cardiopulmonary status. Frequent handwashing, gloving (especially if there are any breaks in the skin), and isolation modalities are essential for nurses in particular. Side effects: 50% report various degrees of temporary injection site soreness; temperatures of 101° F are occasionally reported; malaise, headache, nausea, myalgias, and arthralgias are uncommon.

TABLE 63-4 Biologic Agents for Active Immunization—cont'd

Product	Route of Administration	Primary Immunization Schedule	Comments	Nursing Assessment for Contraindications and Side Effects/Implementation
				Implementation. Shake before drawing up the suspension; inspect for particles; do not dilute. Store opened and unopened vials in the refrigerator. Have epinephrine 1:1000 available.
Influenza	K: IM	One dose; split doses used in persons under 13 years of age (lower incidence of side effects)	Give annually by November.	*Assessment.* Contraindications: hypersensitivity to egg products; clients who are immunosuppressed; acute febrile illness; do not inject intravenously. Precautions: pregnancy; not effective against all possible strains of influenza virus; complete immunizations by November. Toxic drug reactions may occur (especially with phenytoin, warfarin, or theophylline) following viral infection or vaccination. Side effects: local tenderness, redness, induration, fever, malaise, myalgia; allergic skin, respiratory reactions, and Guillain-Barré syndrome are rare; encephalopathy is very rare. *Implementation.* Inject IM into deltoid or lateral mid-thigh or gluteus. Refrigerate. Have epinephrine 1:1000 available.
Measles virus vaccine	L: SC	One dose at 12 to 15 months of age; earlier if epidemic occurs See Figure 63-1	May need to reimmunize if given before 15 months of age. May also prevent disease if given within 72 hours of exposure to measles.	*Assessment.* Contraindications: neomycin or chicken product hypersensitivity; active febrile infection; active, untreated tuberculosis (TB); immunosuppression or immunodeficiency; bone marrow or lymphatic deficiencies; pregnancy (pregnancy should also be avoided for 3 months after vaccination). Precautions: give no sooner than 3 months after transfusion of blood/plasma/human ISG of more than 0.02 mL/lb body weight. Give with or after a TB skin test. Do not give the vaccine within 1 month of immunization by other live virus vaccines, except one of the MMR types or combinations. Side effects: moderate fever to 102° F, rash (in 5-12 days); a temperature more than 103° F with convulsions is rare; encephalitis or subacute sclerosing panencephalitis occurs in 1 out of 1 million clients. Previous recipients of killed virus vaccine may experience local swelling, redness, and vesiculation.

Continued

TABLE 63-4 Biologic Agents for Active Immunization—cont'd

Product	Route of Administration	Primary Immunization Schedule	Comments	Nursing Assessment for Contraindications and Side Effects/Implementation
				Implementation. A 25-gauge ⅝-inch needle is recommended. Refrigerate before reconstitution and afterward. Use within 8 hours, and avoid light at all times. Inject 0.5 mL reconstituted vaccine subcutaneously. The solution may be pink or yellow but must be clear; discard cloudy solutions. Have epinephrine 1:1000 available.
Meningococcal meningitis vaccine	SC	One dose; if a household disease, antibiotic prophylaxis (rifampin) should be given for several days, because the antibody response requires at least 5 days	Used in epidemics.	*Assessment.* Obtain immunization and allergy history. Contraindications: immunosuppression; acute illness. Precautions: pregnancy. Side effects: mild, local erythema. *Implementation.* Administer in a single parenteral dose. Do not give IV. Have epinephrine 1:1000 available.
Mumps vaccine	L: SC	One dose	Reimmunization may be necessary if administered before 1 year of age.	*Assessment.* Contraindications and precautions: same as for measles vaccine, with the following exceptions in side effects. Side effects: mild fever (a temperature more than 103° F is uncommon); low incidence of parotitis, orchitis, purpura, allergic reactions (urticaria); encephalitis and other nervous system reactions are very rare. *Implementation.* Same as measles vaccine.
Pertussis (in DTP or DTP-HbOC)	K: IM	As per DTP	Use only whole cell DTP for the first 3 doses. See Figure 63-1.	*Assessment.* Contraindications: acute infection; previous reactions to an initial dose (all 3 antigens or only pertussis may then be omitted), such as temperature greater than 103° F (39° C), convulsions, altered consciousness, focal neurologic signs, "screaming fits," shock/collapse, purpura; preexisting neurologic disorder; immunosuppression; older than 6 years of age (give Td instead). Precautions: reactions to DTP or DTP-HbOC call for reevaluation and possible administration of Td only.

TABLE 63-4 Biologic Agents for Active Immunization—cont'd

Product	Route of Administration	Primary Immunization Schedule	Comments	Nursing Assessment for Contraindications and Side Effects/Implementation
				Side effects: usually include local redness, induration, and possible tenderness; possible abscess; mild to moderate fever. *Implementation.* Administer IM into deltoid or thigh, varying site each time. Shake before using. Refrigerate. Have epinephrine 1:1000 available.
Pneumococci vaccine	SC, IM	See current literature	Not used in children under 2 years of age.	*Assessment.* Contraindications: hypersensitivity, revaccination, pregnancy, intradermal administration, and IV administration. Will not protect against specific antigens not included. Vaccine is contraindicated within 10 days of initiating chemotherapy for Hodgkin's disease. Precautions: active infection; under 2 years of age; immunosuppression; severely compromised cardiac or pulmonary function; history of pneumococcal infection. Side effect: local redness and soreness, induration, temperature above 100.9° F; anaphylactoid reactions are rare. *Implementation.* Keep refrigerated. Inject into deltoid or midlateral thigh. Have epinephrine 1:1000 available.
Poliomyelitis vaccine	L: Oral	See Figure 63-1		*Assessment.* Contraindications: never administered parenterally or in the presence of acute illness, advanced/debilitated condition, persistent vomiting or diarrhea, or immunodeficient or immunosuppressed states. Precautions: will not modify/prevent existing or incubating disease. Side effect: paralytic disease is rare after vaccination or after contact with vaccinee (advise unimmunized close contacts of vaccinee to seek immunization as needed). *Implementation.* Store frozen, thaw before use, and administer (using disposable pipette) directly into the mouth of the vaccinee. See package insert for specific storage advice. Change of color from pink to yellow is not remarkable.

Continued

TABLE 63-4 Biologic Agents for Active Immunization—cont'd

Product	Route of Administration	Primary Immunization Schedule	Comments	Nursing Assessment for Contraindications and Side Effects/Implementation
Rabies vaccine	K: IM	Preexposure: 2 doses 1 week apart followed by a third dose between 21 and 28 days. Postexposure: see current literature for guidelines		*Assessment.* History of hypersensitivity dictates cautious use of rabies vaccine. *Implementation.* Flush and cleanse wound; possible initial prophylaxis with tetanus and antibiotic therapy. Have epinephrine 1:1000 available. Discontinue corticosteroids during immunization.
Rubella vaccine	L: SC	One dose See Figure 63-1	Give between 12 and 15 months of age. Do not give during pregnancy. Woman must not become pregnant for 3 months after injection. Contraceptive counseling may be needed.	*Assessment.* Contraindications and precautions are the same as for Attenuvax, with the following exceptions. Contraindications: postpubertal females with rubella titers of more than 1:8; pregnancy (pregnancy also to be avoided for 3 months after the vaccine). Precautions: theoretical possibility of live virus transmission from nose/throat of vaccinees. Side effects: mild symptoms of naturally acquired rubella occasionally occur (lymphadenopathy, urticaria, rash, malaise, sore throat, fever, headache, polyneuritis, arthralgias, local pain, swelling, redness); a temperature higher than 103° F is rare; encephalitis is very rare. *Implementation.* Same as for measles vaccine.

■ Nursing Management

Immunotherapy

▪ **Assessment.** The client and family should be interviewed before an immunization is given. The individual's age, current physical condition and general resistance to disease, history of exposure to infectious diseases (both past and potential), and previous immunizations should be assessed. Providers are required to provide detailed information on the risks and benefits of immunization. Before immunization, a signed consent form or a note indicating that the individual has read and understood the information regarding the specific immunization may be obtained. Printed information can be shared at this time to ensure that the parent/client is aware of the side effects/adverse reactions and how to manage them (Merenstein, Kaplan, & Rosenberg, 1994). The following is a list of general contraindications to immunization:

- Current acute or febrile illness
- Immunosuppressive therapy in progress or an immunodeficient state
- Recent immune serum globulin (ISG), plasma, or blood transfusions
- Certain malignancies that leave the client susceptible to infection (e.g., leukemias, lymphomas)
- Simultaneous administration of another single live virus, unless proved safe
- Prior unusual or allergic reaction to the same vaccine or a similar vaccine

TABLE 63-4 Biologic Agents for Active Immunization—cont'd

Product	Route of Administration	Primary Immunization Schedule	Comments	Nursing Assessment for Contraindications and Side Effects/Implementation
Tetanus toxoid	IM	Included in DTP See Figure 63-1	DTP is preferred for children; tetanus and diphtheria (Td) is preferred for adults. Tetanus toxoid is usually used to test cell-mediated immunity.	*Assessment.* Contraindication: not for treatment of an actual tetanus infection; any acute infection; immunosuppression. Precautions: hypersensitivity; history of cerebral damage, neurologic disorders, or febrile convulsions. Keep epinephrine on hand. Side effects: occasional Arthus-type reaction to high levels of tetanus antibody (antitoxin) in those receiving regular or frequent tetanus toxoid boosters (thus the recommended 10-year interval between Td boosters). Response may include significant local symptoms of redness, edema resembling a giant "hive," axillary lymphadenopathy; systemic symptoms can include low fever, malaise, aches and pains, general urticaria, tachycardia, and hypotension. Prolonged intervals between primary immunizing doses has no effect on eventual immunity status. *Implementation.* Shake well and administer a deep IM injection, avoiding blood vessels. Refrigerate, but do not freeze. Have epinephrine 1:1000 available.

- Allergy to antibiotics in the vaccine, thimerosal as a preservative, or other constituents

Minor afebrile infections such as the common cold are not usually contraindications to immunization.

Assess clients (especially children) for immune status at routine intervals. High-risk groups include adolescents, new parents, individuals not vaccinated with the live measles vaccine, migrant workers, and recent immigrants. Older adults (especially those in nursing homes) and anyone with chronic health problems are at particular risk for respiratory infections and should be encouraged to obtain an annual influenza virus vaccination.

Individuals are also candidates for immunization if they have been exposed to or are at risk of exposure to one of the childhood diseases or serious communicable diseases or if they have incurred a traumatic wound.

Be aware that a history of hypersensitivity reactions to the biologic agent or to any contained antibiotics or preservatives is a contraindication to immunotherapy.

Always assess the client's allergy history carefully and test for hypersensitivity before administering animal sera. Keep epinephrine on hand to counter any potentially dangerous event (e.g., anaphylaxis).

■ **Nursing Diagnosis.** The client receiving immunotherapy has the potential for the following selected nursing diagnoses/collaborative problems: impaired comfort (malaise, headache, rash, lymphadenopathy, and pain and tenderness at the injection site); imbalanced body temperature

BOX 63-2

RespiGam

Respiratory syncytial virus IV immune globulin (RespiGam) protects against the serious lower respiratory tract infection caused by respiratory syncytial virus (RSV) in children under 2 years of age who were either born prematurely or have bronchopulmonary dysplasia. RSV is potentially life threatening for more than 90,000 infants.

RespiGam reduces the incidence and duration of RSV hospitalizations as well as the severity of the disease in high-risk infants. RespiGam is infused at a dosage of 750 mg/kg once a month during the RSV period from November through April (Pharmacy News, 1996; Significant Protection, 1999).

Be aware that infants with pulmonary disease may experience fluid overload with the administration of RespiGam. A loop diuretic such as furosemide or bumetanide may be necessary before, during, and after infusion. Serious allergic reactions such as anaphylaxis or angioneurotic edema are rare but may occur during drug infusion. If hypotension or a severe reaction occurs, stop the infusion and administer epinephrine as necessary (RespiGam, 1999).

(fever); and the potential complications of allergic reaction and encephalopathy.

▪ **Implementation**

▪ ***Monitoring.*** Because of the risk of anaphylaxis after any immunization, ask clients to remain in the immediate area for up to half an hour for observation of any developing adverse reactions. Be alert for the early symptoms of such a reaction—hives, shock-like appearance, confusion, and hypotension.

▪ ***Intervention.*** Immune antisera and globulin are administered intramuscularly unless otherwise noted. Passive immunization or immunoprophylaxis should always be administered as soon as possible after exposure to the agent.

Almost all immunotherapy is parenteral and must be given by the specified route and with the specified diluent to avoid local reactions (especially when the intracutaneous route is used) or possible anaphylaxis (especially when the IV route is used). All needles should be changed after the vaccine is withdrawn from the vial, if possible. Aspiration after insertion is, of course, also necessary to prevent the danger of depositing the dose into the bloodstream.

Be aware that a crying, wriggling baby or child presents a challenging moving target for injection, and therefore they must be restrained temporarily. This can often be accomplished just as effectively in the warmth and security of another's arms (the parent's, if feasible) rather than on a hard table surface. Taking out the needle and syringe and explaining that "this may hurt for only a minute" *just before* the actual injection will lessen the fear of pain.

Record immunization dates at the time of administration, and give a copy to the recipient or parents for permanent safekeeping. Explain that this record may be invaluable later, when these dates may be required on applications to school, summer camp, college, or visas for travel to other countries.

Be aware that most products lose their potency at temperatures higher than 35.6° to 46.4° F (2° to 8° C); trivalent oral polio vaccine (TOPV) must be kept frozen. Therefore most immunization agents should be stored in a medical refrigerator and replaced immediately after use. They should not be stored near a heat source, on a windowsill, or on a refrigerator door shelf because of unpredictable temperatures.

▪ ***Education.*** Perceptions and misconceptions concerning immunization must be clarified. The relative safety and merits of immunization vs. the risks of the disease process itself (both short-range and long-range) should be discussed, and statistics should be used where appropriate. The client and/or family should be told that a repeat immunization is usually not contraindicated if records are unclear; the risk with the repeat immunization is usually minimal, and in this way future protection is ensured. Unimmunized parents should be identified and probably immunized before their children, especially when an oral polio vaccine is administered.

Noncompletion of an immunization series may occasionally be prevented if vaccinees or their parents know that a prolonged period between phases of immunization makes no difference to eventual antibody levels as long as they have the entire series. Giving a copy of the immunization schedule to the client or family also enhances compliance with the immunization series.

Complete, written, and accurate documentation of immunizations with dates is rare even in office records. Nonetheless, having access to these data is important. Therefore it is crucial to teach parents or vaccinees to keep careful written records for each vaccination, especially in view of the high mobility of today's population. Simple blank forms are available for this purpose and should be given to parents or the vaccinee with an explanation and advice to keep them updated and in a safe place (e.g., with health record files at home or in the family Bible) and to bring them to each child's appointment.

Teach clients or their parents how to recognize and differentiate between anticipated side effects and serious adverse reactions. Acetaminophen may be taken for the not uncommon aches, local pain and swelling, or mild temperature elevations, which may occur within 24 hours. Recipients of immunotherapy should understand who they are to contact if complications later occur.

▪ **Evaluation.** The expected outcome of immunotherapy is that the client will receive immunity without experiencing adverse reactions to the drug.

▪ ▪ ▪

Primary sources of information on immunization include the Public Health Service Advisory Committee on Immunization Practices (ACIP), which advises public health agencies; and the Committee on Control of Infectious Diseases (the Red Book Committee), which is drawn from the members of the American Academy of Pediatrics and advises the private health sector. The ACIP can be contacted through the CDC. Because the two groups maintain a slightly different perspective, minor inconsequential variations in recommendations may occasionally be noted. Other sources include local public health departments and printed package inserts included with the vaccine or serum. Biologic preparations and the accompanying inserts are regulated by the Bureau of Biologics of the FDA.

The state of the art of immunotherapy is in rapid flux. The only constant in immunization practice is change itself. To read, attend seminars, and consult with experts is to keep pace.

SUMMARY

Immunization is available for a number of diseases whose prevalence has abruptly declined because of the availability of vaccines and sera; such diseases include measles, polio, rubella, mumps, diphtheria, and tetanus. Vaccines are also available for yellow fever, hepatitis B, influenza, rabies, cholera, typhoid, plague, and other diseases. Smallpox has been eradicated because of a World Health Organization campaign of near-universal vaccination. Although such preparations are available, nurses must still educate the public to minimize complacency regarding the diseases for which they provide protection and to promote immunization.

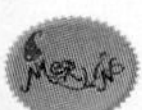

Critical Thinking Questions

1. An adolescent mother brings her infant to the clinic for its first well-baby checkup at 6 weeks. What would you include when teaching her about her infant's immunizations?
2. As an adult and as a nursing student, what immunizations should you have and why?

Collaborative Learning Activities

For Collaborative Learning Activities, go to mosby.com/MERLIN/McKenry/.

CASE STUDY

For a Case Study that will help ensure mastery of this chapter content, go to mosby.com/MERLIN/McKenry/.

BIBLIOGRAPHY

Anderson, K.N., Anderson, L.E., & Glanze, W.D. (Eds.) (1998). *Mosby's medical, nursing, & allied health dictionary* (5th ed.). St. Louis: Mosby.

Centers for Disease Control and Prevention (1994).General Recommendations on Immunization: Recommendations of the Advisory Committee on Immunization Practices (ACIP). *MMWR: Morbidity & Mortality Weekly Report, 43*(RR-1), 1-38.

DiPiro, J.T., Talbert, R.L., Yee, G.C., Matzke. G.R., Wells, B.G., & Posey, L.M. (Eds.). (1997). *Pharmacotherapeutics: A pathophysiological approach* (3rd ed.). Norwalk, CT: Appleton & Lange.

Drug Facts and Comparisons. (2000). St. Louis: Facts and Comparisons.

Freeman, V.A., & Freed, G.L. (1999). Parental knowledge, attitudes, and demand regarding a vaccine to prevent varicella. *American Journal of Preventive Medicine, 17*(2), 153-155.

Gore, P., Madhavan, S., Curry, D., McClung, G., Castiglia, M., Rosenbluth, S.A., Smego, R.A. (1999). Predictors of childhood immunization completion in a rural population. *Social Science & Medicine, 48*(8), 1011-1027.

Home Health Testing (2000). Home HIV test, Home Access HIV Test Kit; www.homedrug-test.com/hdt04.htm (5/28/00).

Keane, V., Stanton, B., Horton, L., Aronson R., Galbraith, J., & Hughart, N. (1993). Perceptions of vaccine efficacy, illness, and health among inner-city parents. *Clinical Pediatrics, 32*(1), 2-7.

McCann, J. (1994). Researchers tout triple therapy for HIV/AIDS. *Hospital Pharmacy Reports, 8*(9), 18.

McCormack, J.P. & Brown, G. (1996). Traumatic skin and soft tissue infections. In L.Y. Young & M.A. Koda-Kimble (Eds.), *Applied therapeutics* (6th ed.). Vancouver, WA: Applied Therapeutics.

Merenstein, G.B., Kaplan, D.W., & Rosenberg, A.A. (1994). *Handbook of pediatrics* (17th ed.) Norwalk, CT: Appleton & Lange.

National Institutes of Allergy and Infectious Diseases (NIAID). (1992). Evolution of vaccine development. *Neonatal Network, 11*(4), 43-44.

National vaccination coverage levels among children aged 19-35 months: United States, 1998. (1999). *MMWR: Morbidity & Mortality Weekly Report, 48*(37), 829-830.

National Vaccine Advisory Committee. (1999). Strategies to sustain success in childhood immunizations. *Journal of the American Medical Association,* 282(4), 363-370.

Pharmacy News. (1996). Drug updates. *Journal of American Pharmacy, NS36*(4), 225.

Reece, S.M. (1991). New protection against *Haemophilus influenzae* type b infections in infants and young children. *Nurse Practitioner, 16*(11), 27, 31-36.

RespiGam. (1999). Respiratory Syncytial Virus Immune Globulin Intravenous (Human) [TRS-IGIV], RespiGam package insert; www.medimmune.com/medimmune/products/respi.htm (7/16/00).

Santiago, L. (1996). Slow progress on HIV vaccines. *GMHC Treatment Issues, 10*(4), 1-4.

Significant Protection. (1999). *Significant protection for infants at risk;* www.medimmune.com/medimmune/respigam/index.htm (7/16/00).

Task Force on Community Preventive Services. (1999). Vaccine-preventable diseases: Improving vaccination coverage in children, adolescents, and adults. *MMWR: Morbidity & Mortality Weekly Report, 48*(RR-8), 1-15.

64 Immunosuppressants and Immunomodulators

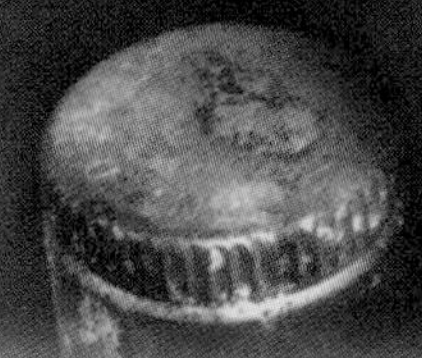

Chapter Focus

As client acuity levels increase and treatments become more complex, nurses are increasingly aware of the impact of the immune system on the treatment regimens of clients. Because nurses administer treatments that decrease immunity (immunosuppressants) or enhance immune function (immunoglobulin), they need to maintain a working understanding of the immune system, how it relates to the clinical picture of clients, and the agents that affect it.

Learning Objectives

1. Identify the four factors relating to the immune system that can lead to an immunocompromised state.
2. Discuss the general nursing management of the immunosuppressed client.
3. Compare and contrast the nursing management of clients receiving azathioprine, basiliximab, cyclosporine, daclizumab, muromonab-CD3, mycophenolate mofetil, and tacrolimus therapy.
4. Implement the nursing management for the care of clients receiving immunosuppressant and immunomodulator agents.

Key Terms

acquired immunodeficiency syndrome (AIDS), p. 1104
human immunodeficiency virus (HIV) , p. 1104
immunocompromised state, p. 1095
immunomodulating agents, p. 1104
immunosuppressant agents, p. 1095

Key Drugs [✐]

azathioprine, p. 1097

The rejection of kidney, liver, and heart allogenic transplants has led to the development of **immunosuppressant agents**—agents that decrease or prevent an immune response. A foreign substance or organ transplant in the body activates an immune response by releasing macrophages to phagocytize and process the foreign substance. In addition, interleukin-1 (IL-1) production increases, which activates helper T cells containing a surface receptor or CD3. The activated T cell stimulates the production of killer or cytotoxic T lymphocytes and B lymphocytes, in part by producing interleukin-2 (IL-2). T cells are necessary for cellular immunity (attack the foreign substance directly and with released toxic substances), and the B lymphocytes are responsible for humoral immunity or the production of antibodies. The primary sites of action of the immunosuppressant agents are noted in Figure 64-1.

Immunodeficiency or immunosuppression may also occur from a genetic or an acquired disorder of the immune system. Although genetic disorders such as agammaglobulinemia or severe combined immune deficiency syndrome (SCIDS) are usually diagnosed shortly after birth, acquired disorders may occur at any time throughout life. Acquired immunodeficiency may be induced by a variety of drugs, such as chemotherapeutic and immunosuppressant agents or radiation therapy, or through viral infections such as acquired immunodeficiency syndrome (AIDS). Because AIDS often has devastating complications and a fatal outcome, much research interest has been directed toward the development of immunomodulating or immunostimulating medications.

An **immunocompromised state** may result from one or more of the following: (1) inhibition of granulocyte formation leading to severe neutropenia; (2) impairment of synthesis and antibody production; (3) loss of mucocutaneous barriers that permit bacteria or microorganisms access to internal organs, which may occur in a variety of therapeutic situations, such as after the use of medical devices (central venous catheters, Foley catheters, endotracheal tubes) or after chemotherapy; and (4) impairment of cellular immunity such as macrophages and T-cell lymphocytes (usually seen in clients who receive immunosuppressive agents such as corticosteroids or cyclosporine, clients with certain types of cancer [Hodgkin's lymphoma], or organ transplant recipients).

In the majority of clients, combinations of these defects are common because several immune functions may be affected at the same time. For example, chronic therapy with antineoplastic medications will affect granulocytes and cellular immunity. Chemotherapy may result in the loss of mucocutaneous barriers or the development of mucositis and ulcers in the mouth and gastrointestinal tract. These individuals are at greater risk for the development of bacterial, fungal, or viral infections. This chapter reviews some of the primary agents that suppress, modify, or stimulate the human immune system.

■ Nursing Management

The Immunosuppressed Client

The care of the client with a secondary immunodeficiency, which is immunosuppression caused by the therapeutic regi-

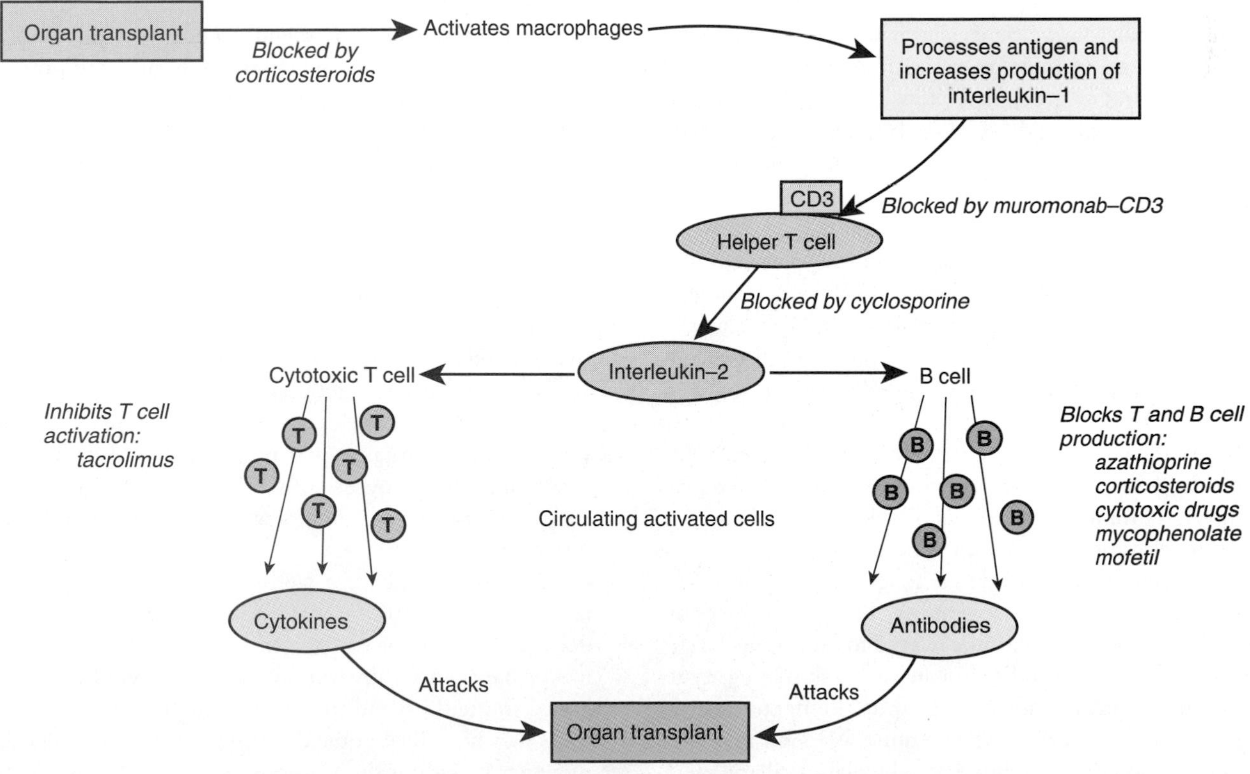

Figure 64-1 Sites of action for immunosuppressive agents.

men, focuses on immunotherapy and on treatment of the underlying condition.

■ **Assessment.** The client should be assessed for his or her understanding of the condition and his or her feelings about the illness. The availability of a support system should be considered.

It should be determined that the client does not have or has not recently had or been exposed to either chickenpox or herpes zoster, because there is the risk for the occurrence of severe generalized disease when an immunosuppressing drug is administered. Determine if the client has a history of malignancy, because there is an increased incidence of certain malignancies with immunosuppression.

Nutritional status and the client's likes and dislikes should be assessed so that nutritional counseling will be effective; these clients usually have had some weight loss or require a modified diet. Level of comfort should be determined with regard to activity tolerance and participation in therapies.

Assess the client for opportunistic infections. The head, eyes, ears, neck, and throat should be examined for white patches on the tongue and oral mucosa (thrush), pulling at the ears, tympanic membrane inflammation, impaired hearing, purulent nasal drainage, and tender sinuses. The need for nutritional, renal, and gastrointestinal assessment is indicated by decreased weight and height in children, chronic diarrhea, and/or malabsorption. An examination of the mucous membranes of the mouth, vagina, and perianal areas might indicate the presence of ulcers, thrush, and/or herpetic lesions. The client's skin and nails may have recurrent infections. The cardiovascular system is usually within normal limits, except for tachycardia with severe infections. The respiratory tract may be unremarkable, but if pneumonia is present there may be dyspnea, tachypnea, nasal flaring, use of accessory muscles, retractions, decreased breath sounds, rales, and/or green or yellow sputum. Neuromuscular development may be delayed in children. Psychosocially, the client may be irritable, and children may demonstrate failure to thrive. Perform an initial age-appropriate developmental screening.

■ **Nursing Diagnosis.** The administration of immunosuppressive agents increases the client's risk for the following nursing diagnoses/collaborative problems: anxiety related to actual or perceived threat to biologic integrity, self-concept, or unfamiliar people or surroundings; diarrhea; activity intolerance related to weakness and fatigue; impaired comfort (headache, muscle aches); ineffective protection related to immunodeficiency; risk for infection related to inadequate immunity; risk for injury related to bleeding/hemorrhage secondary to thrombocytopenia; imbalanced nutrition (less than body requirements) related to decreased intake secondary to anorexia, nausea, vomiting, or chronic infection; impaired oral mucous membrane related to drug-induced stomatitis or mycotic superinfection; impaired skin integrity related to cutaneous reactions to the drug; ineffective airway clearance related to excessive sputum caused by infection; impaired gas exchange related to alveolar-capillary membrane changes secondary to inflammation; imbalanced body temperature (fever) related to infection; risk for delayed growth and development related to prolonged illness and hospitalization; social isolation related to altered health status and prolonged hospitalization; and the potential complications of neurologic sequelae and fluid and electrolyte imbalances.

■ **Implementation**

■ ***Monitoring.*** Assess for symptoms of opportunistic infections, such as night sweats, fever, fatigue, involuntary weight loss, persistent diarrhea, headache, persistent cough, and the presence of green or yellow sputum. Monitor the client's temperature and the results of any cultures at frequent intervals. Auscultate the lungs for rales, consolidation, and pleural friction rub. Monitor arterial blood gases (ABGs) and the complete blood count (CBC). White blood cell counts indicate the effectiveness of the drug; drug dosage is usually titrated on the leukocyte and platelet counts.

Assess nutritional status daily; note weight, fluid intake and output, caloric intake, hematocrit, hemoglobin, and serum protein and albumin values. Monitor the client for dehydration (decreased urine output, increased specific gravity, poor skin turgor, confusion). Assess stool, urine, emesis, and secretions for the presence of occult blood. Assess and document skin for redness and purulent drainage, and mucous membrane integrity for redness, creamy white patches, and a black furry tongue. Monitor skin color and capillary refill. Assess the client's tolerance to activity by assessing blood pressure, respiratory rate, and pulse rate before and immediately after activity. Monitor the client for verbal or nonverbal indications of anxiety and social isolation.

■ ***Intervention.*** Careful medical asepsis is a priority with the immunosuppressed client. Thorough handwashing, avoiding other persons with infection, and promoting the client's own resources to prevent infection are essential nursing interventions. Provide meticulous mouth, skin, and perianal care. Proper mouth care with a topical antifungal agent will help to prevent oral candidiasis.

Injections should be avoided when possible; if necessary, the skin should be cleansed with povidone-iodine and allowed to dry for 30 seconds. Clean all cuts and scrapes immediately with antiseptic soap. Avoid unnecessary and invasive procedures (e.g., biopsy, barium enemas); when they are necessary, prophylactic antibiotic coverage is required. Irrigating solutions, vases, and other standing collections of water in which organisms may breed should be avoided.

Administer antipyretics as ordered and monitor the client's response. In children, acetaminophen should be used instead of aspirin.

■ ***Education.*** Advise a well-balanced diet and a fluid intake of at least 1500 mL daily to minimize the risk of tissue dehydration and of urinary tract infection associated with low urinary output. Instruct the client to avoid trauma (e.g., breaks in the skin) and to seek medical treatment for wounds that do not heal quickly. Encourage meticulous oral hygiene, including the cautious use of toothbrushes, dental floss, and toothpicks, as well as regular dental care to minimize gingival inflammation and for early detection of altered oral mucous membranes. Promote pulmonary toilet by encouraging the client to perform frequent breathing or incentive spirometry exercises. Encourage ambulation; if the client is unable to ambulate, reposition him or her at frequent intervals. The ingestion of alcohol and aspirin should be avoided to minimize the risk of gastrointestinal bleeding.

Instruct the client to report any signs and symptoms of infection (sore throat, malaise, headache, fever, dysuria, urinary frequency), bleeding gums, bruising, or signs and symptoms of hepatic dysfunction (abdominal pain, jaundice, pruritus, clay-colored stools). Advise the client to consult with the prescriber before taking any over-the-counter (OTC) medications (including aspirin) or receiving any vaccinations while taking immunosuppressant medications. Live viral vaccines should not be given to the client, and no one in the household should receive an oral polio vaccine. Reinforce the importance of keeping appointments with the health care provider for follow-up care and laboratory examinations.

The client and family should be taught to monitor the client's blood pressure at home. Instruct the client to report any significant changes in blood pressure, hematuria, cloudy urine, decreased urinary output, sudden weight gain, edema of the face or ankles, headache, or unusual fatigue.

Caution the client that raw oysters or other shellfish may contain microbes that can cause serious illness. Even though such seafood comes from a good restaurant or "clean" water, there is the possibility that it may be contaminated. Although eating this seafood is not risky for most healthy individuals, clients with immunosuppression are at risk for serious disease.

If the client is taking the immunosuppressant to prevent transplant rejection, emphasize the importance of lifelong therapy.

■ **Evaluation.** The expected outcome is that immunosuppression of the client will occur without rejection of the transplanted tissue, the presence of infection, or impaired skin integrity. The client/caregiver should also be able to describe methods of preventing infection, the need to maintain optimal nutrition, and other issues for effective management of the therapeutic regimen.

IMMUNOSUPPRESSANTS

The primary immunosuppressant drugs are azathioprine (Imuran), basiliximab (Simulect), cyclosporine (Neoral, Sandimmune), daclizumab (Zenapax), muromonab-CD3 (Orthoclone OKT3), mycophenolate mofetil (CellCept), and tacrolimus (FK 506, Prograf).

✓ azathioprine [ay za thye' oh preen] (Imuran)

Azathioprine is indicated as an adjunct medication to prevent rejection in renal organ transplants and for severe, active rheumatoid arthritis in clients who have not responded to other therapies. The mechanism of action for azathioprine is unknown, but it appears primarily to suppress T cell and B cell production; that is, it suppresses cell-mediated hypersensitivity and antibody production. In combination with steroids, this drug appears to have a steroid-conserving effect; a lower dosage of steroid may be used to treat chronic inflammatory processes when given with azathioprine.

Azathioprine is available in oral and parenteral dosage forms. The oral dosage form is well absorbed from the intestinal tract and has a half-life of 5 hours and an onset of action of 6 to 8 weeks for rheumatoid arthritis and perhaps 4 to 8 weeks for other inflammatory disease states. It is metabolized in the liver to active metabolites (6-mercaptopurine and 6-thioinosinic acid), with further metabolism by xanthine oxidase. It is primarily excreted via the biliary system.

The side effects/adverse reactions of azathioprine include anorexia, nausea, vomiting, leukopenia or infection, megaloblastic anemia (usually asymptomatic, but the client may also have fever, chills, cough, low back or side pain, pain on urination, or increased weakness), hepatitis, hypersensitivity, pneumonitis, sores in the mouth and on the lips, and skin rash. The risk of hepatotoxicity is greater when the dosage of azathioprine exceeds 2.5 mg/kg/day.

The immunosuppressant dosage for adults and children is 3 to 5 mg/kg PO 1 to 3 days before or at the time of surgery; if administered intravenously, this dose is given before, during, or immediately after surgery. The maintenance dosage is 1 to 3 mg/kg/day. For rheumatoid arthritis, the adult oral dosage is 1 mg/kg daily and is adjusted every 1 to 2 months as necessary.

■ Nursing Management

Azathioprine Therapy

In addition to the following discussion, see Nursing Management: The Immunosuppressed Client, p. 1095.

■ **Assessment.** It is essential to assess exposure to or the presence of infection, especially chickenpox or herpes zoster. Any infection that the client might have may become life threatening with the administration of azathioprine. Caution should also be used with clients who have undergone previous cytotoxic drug and radiation therapy. Clients with renal or hepatic function impairment or severe xanthine oxidase deficiency will experience reduced metabolism/excretion of the drug with an increased risk for azathioprine toxicity; dosages may need to be reduced.

If azathioprine is administered for rheumatoid arthritis, assess the client's range of motion, status of affected joints (swelling, pain, and strength), and ability to accomplish activities of daily living before and at periodic intervals during therapy. Hematologic function should be monitored via complete cell counts before initiating therapy.

Review the client's current medication regimen for the risk of significant drug interactions, such as those that may occur when azathioprine is given with the following drugs:

Drug	Possible Effect and Management
Bold/color type indicates the most serious interactions.	
allopurinol	Allopurinol inhibits xanthine oxidase, which may result in increased azathioprine activity and toxicity. Avoid concurrent use or a potentially serious drug interaction may occur. If it is absolutely necessary to give both drugs concurrently, reduce the dosage of azathioprine to one fourth or one third of the usually prescribed dosage; monitor closely and adjust the dosage as needed.
immunosuppressant agents, other (glucocorticoids, cyclophosphamide, cyclosporine)	May increase the risk for developing infections and/or neoplasms. Avoid concurrent use or a potentially serious drug interaction may occur.
vaccines, live virus	Immunization with live vaccines should be postponed in clients receiving this drug and in close family members. The use of a live virus vaccine in immunosuppressed clients may result in increased replication of the vaccine virus, may increase side effects/adverse reactions to the vaccine virus, and possibly cause a decrease in the client's antibody response to the vaccine. Avoid concurrent use or a potentially serious drug interaction may occur.

▪ **Nursing Diagnosis.** In addition to the earlier discussion, the client receiving azathioprine may experience the following nursing diagnoses/collaborative problems: impaired mucous membranes (mouth ulcers); and the potential complications of hepatitis, pancreatitis, and skin rash.

▪ **Implementation**

▪ ***Monitoring.*** CBCs should be performed weekly during the first month, twice a month for the next 2 to 3 months, and monthly thereafter. Notify the prescriber if the leukocyte count is less than 3000/mm^3 or if platelets are less than 100,000/mm^3; therapy will be reinstituted at reduced dosages when these counts reach an acceptable level, usually after 7 to 10 days. A decrease in hemoglobin may indicate bone marrow suppression. Renal and hepatic function studies should be monitored with the same frequency. Increased alkaline phosphatase, bilirubin, SGOT (AST), SGPT (ALT), and amylase concentrations may indicate hepatotoxicity. Because of the delayed action of azathioprine, the dosage will be reduced at the first indication of serious bone marrow depression (leukocyte count $<$3000/mm^3 or platelet count $<$100,000/mm^3).

▪ ***Intervention.*** Azathioprine is usually started 1 to 5 days before transplantation and restarted within 24 hours after transplantation. Administer oral doses of azathioprine with or after meals to minimize gastrointestinal distress. Reconstitute each 100 mg for IV use by adding 10 mL of sterile water for injection to the vial and swirling to dissolve. It may be administered by IV push or further diluted with 0.9% sodium chloride injection or 5% dextrose and 0.9% sodium chloride injection for IV infusion. It may be administered over a time period of 5 minutes to 8 hours. Once reconstituted, azathioprine is stable at room temperature for 24 hours.

Handle this drug with caution because of its potential mutagenicity, teratogenicity, and carcinogenicity. Consult the policies and procedures of the health care agency.

▪ ***Education.*** If azathioprine is being administered for rheumatoid arthritis, the client should be advised to continue physical therapy and other concurrent therapy (salicylates, nonsteroidal antiinflammatory drugs, glucocorticoids) as prescribed. Because azathioprine has teratogenic effects, advise female clients who are of childbearing age to practice contraception during the course of therapy and for at least 4 months after its completion (see the Pregnancy Safety box below).

Alert the client to report to the prescriber unusual bleeding or bruising; blood in the urine or stools; black, tarry stools; or pinpoint red spots on the skin.

▪ **Evaluation.** The expected outcome of azathioprine therapy prescribed for rheumatoid arthritis is that the client will experience decreased pain, stiffness, and swelling of the affected joints in 6 to 8 weeks. If administered to prevent transplant rejection, the client will not experience rejection of the transplanted organ and will manage the therapeutic regimen effectively.

basiliximab [bas i licks' i mab] (Simulect)

Basiliximab is an immunosuppressant used in combination with cyclosporine and corticosteroids to prevent kidney transplant rejection. This product is an IL-2 receptor antagonist; it binds to the alpha subunit on the IL-2 receptor to inhibit IL-2 binding. This binding prevents IL-2–mediated lymphocyte activation, thus impairing the response of the immune system to antigens.

Basiliximab is administered by IV infusion; it has a half-life of 7.2 ± 3.2 days in adults and 11.5 ± 6.3 days in children. The duration of action is 36 ± 14 days.

The side effects/adverse reactions of basiliximab include weakness, stomach and/or back pain, candidiasis, cough,

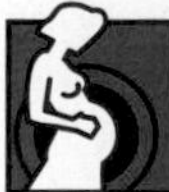

Pregnancy Safety
Immunosuppressants and Immunomodulators

Category	Drug
B	basiliximab
C	cyclosporine, daclizumab, muromonab-CD3, mycophenolate mofetil, tacrolimus
D	azathioprine

shortness of breath, dysuria, edema, fever, hypertension, infection, pharyngitis, nausea, vomiting, tremors, acne, headache, insomnia, and weight gain.

The usual adult dosage is 20 mg administered by IV infusion 2 hours before the transplantation surgery and repeated 4 days later. The pediatric dosage is 12 mg/m^2 of body surface area by IV infusion administered 2 hours before the transplantation surgery. This dose is repeated 4 days later.

■ Nursing Management

Basiliximab Therapy

In addition to the following discussion, see Nursing Management: The Immunosuppressed Client, p. 1095.

■ **Assessment.** In clinical trials, basiliximab was used concurrently with clients receiving other immunosuppressants. No drug interactions have been reported with its use.

■ **Nursing Diagnosis.** The client receiving basiliximab may experience the following nursing diagnoses/collaborative problems: impaired skin integrity (acne, rash); diarrhea; constipation; impaired comfort (headache, heartburn, arthralgia, myalgia); disturbed sleep pattern (insomnia); disturbed body image (hypertrichosis, weight gain); fatigue; risk for injury due to orthostatic hypotension (dizziness); and the potential complications of candidiasis, neuropathy, pulmonary edema (shortness of breath), and urinary retention.

■ **Implementation**

■ ***Monitoring.*** Observe closely and measure vital signs at frequent intervals to detect an anaphylactoid reaction during IV infusion. Clients undergoing long-term therapy should be monitored for infection and malignancy.

■ ***Intervention.*** Vials of basiliximab should be used within 4 hours of preparation, because basiliximab does not contain preservatives. Avoid shaking the vial of basiliximab because doing so may cause foaming. Medications and equipment for the emergency management of acute hypersensitivity reactions should be in the immediate area.

■ ***Education.*** Advise women of childbearing age to use effective contraception before, during, and for 2 months after receiving basiliximab.

■ **Evaluation.** The expected outcome of basiliximab therapy is that the client will not experience transplanted organ rejection and will manage the drug regimen effectively.

cyclosporine [sye' klow spor een] (Neoral, Sandimmune)

Cyclosporine is a potent immunosuppressant used for the prevention of organ transplant rejection (renal, hepatic, or cardiac allografts). It is usually administered in combination with corticosteroids. Its mechanism of action is unknown, but studies indicate it inhibits the formation and release of IL-2, the substance necessary to induce the response of cytotoxic T lymphocytes to an antigenic challenge. It does not cause significant myelosuppression or bone marrow depression.

Cyclosporine is available in oral and parenteral dosage forms. Orally, its bioavailability is variable (approximately 30%) and may improve with increasing dosages and chronic administration. Absorption may decrease after a liver transplant or in clients with liver impairment or gastrointestinal dysfunction (e.g., diarrhea or vomiting). It has a half-life of approximately 7 hours in children and 19 hours in adults; orally it reaches peak serum levels in 3.5 hours. It is metabolized extensively in the liver and excreted primary in the bile and feces.

The side effects of cyclosporine are dose related and include hirsutism, leg cramps, nausea, vomiting, acne or oily skin, and tremors. Adverse reactions include nephrotoxicity, gingival hyperplasia (bleeding, swollen gums), and severe hypertension; the latter is usually associated with 25 to 50 mg/kg doses of cyclosporine. Lymphomas and other lymphoproliferative-type disorders have been reported; some regress when the drug is stopped (*United States Pharmacopeia Dispensing Information*, 1999). Gingival hyperplasia, a common problem with the use of this drug, is generally reversible approximately 6 months after discontinuing cyclosporine.

The oral dosage for adults and children is 12 to 15 mg/kg daily, starting 4 to 12 hours before surgery and continuing for 7 to 14 days afterward. The dosage is then decreased weekly until a maintenance dosage of 5 to 10 mg/kg daily is reached. Children may need higher or more frequent dosing because they seem to metabolize this drug rapidly. The IV adult dosage is 2 to 6 mg/kg daily until the client can take the oral medication.

■ Nursing Management

Cyclosporine Therapy

In addition to the following discussion, see Nursing Management: The Immunosuppressed Client, p. 1095.

■ **Assessment.** As with azathioprine therapy, determine that the client does not have and has neither recently had nor been exposed to chickenpox or herpes zoster because of the risk for severe generalized disease. Any infection that the client might have may become life threatening with the administration of cyclosporine. Determine the client's history of malignancy, because the use of cyclosporine is associated with an increased risk or worsening of malignancies. Clients with an impairment of renal and hepatic function may require a reduced dosage.

Review the client's current medication regimen for the risk of significant drug interactions, such as those that may occur if cyclosporine is given concurrently with the following drugs:

Drug	Possible Effect and Management
androgens, allopurinol (Zyloprim), bromocriptine (Parlodel), cimetidine (Tagamet), clarithromycin (Biaxin), danazol (Danocrine), diltiazem (Cardizem), erythromycin, estrogens, itraconazole (Sporanox), ketoconazole (Nizoral), nefazodone (Serzone), nicardipine (Cardene), or verapamil (Calan)	May result in increased serum levels of cyclosporine, increasing the potential risk for hepatotoxicity and nephrotoxicity. If drugs must be administered concurrently, use extreme caution and monitor closely.

Drug	Possible Effect and Management
coal tar, methoxsalen (Oxsoralen), radiation therapy, or trioxsalen (Trisoralen)	Clients with psoriasis previously treated with cyclosporine or any of these therapies are at increased risk of skin malignancy.
diuretics, potassium-sparing (amiloride, spironolactone, or triamterene) or potassium supplements or salt substitutes	May increase the risk of hyperkalemia. Monitor serum levels and signs and symptoms of hyperkalemia (confusion; irregular heart rate; paresthesias of hands, feet, or lips; respiratory difficulties; increased weakness; feeling of weak or heavy legs).
immunosuppressants, other	Increases the risk of developing infection or lymphoproliferative-type disorders (e.g., lymphomas). Use extreme caution if given concurrently.
lovastatin (Mevacor), simvastatin (Zocor)	When used in heart transplant clients, lovastatin or simvastatin may increase the risk of developing rhabdomyolysis and acute renal failure. Monitor closely if concurrent therapy is necessary.
vaccines, live virus	See azathioprine.

For the treatment of psoriasis and rheumatoid arthritis, two baseline serum creatinine determinations should be performed before initiating therapy. Blood pressure, blood urea nitrogen (BUN), cholesterol, CBC, serum magnesium, serum potassium, and uric acid should also be documented. Hepatic function studies are performed before initiating therapy. The results of a dental examination should be documented for baseline data.

▪ **Nursing Diagnosis.** In addition to the nursing diagnoses cited earlier in the chapter, the client taking cyclosporine has the potential for disturbed body image related to acne, gingival hyperplasia, and hirsutism, as well as the potential complications of hypertension, post-transplant lymphoproliferative disorder (PTLD), nephrotoxicity, hepatotoxicity, and pancreatitis.

▪ **Implementation**

▪ ***Monitoring.*** Baseline assessments, except for hepatic studies and dental examinations, should be performed every 2 weeks during the first 3 months of therapy; after this time they should be performed monthly with clients who have stabilized. Serum cyclosporine levels are evaluated periodically during a course of therapy, and dosages are adjusted accordingly. Significant changes in renal and hepatic function may necessitate a reduction in dosage or a discontinuation of cyclosporine. Dental examinations should be performed at 3-month intervals for the early detection and treatment of gingival hyperplasia.

Monitor the client for signs and symptoms of hypersensitivity (dyspnea, wheezing, hypotension), and have resuscitation equipment near when the drug is administered intravenously.

▪ ***Intervention.*** When administering the oral solution, use the calibrated measuring device supplied by the manufacturer. Because cyclosporine is a mixture of alcohol and vegetable oil and has an unpleasant taste, mix it thoroughly with milk, chocolate milk, or orange juice at room temperature, and drink it at once. Use a glass container to prevent adherence, and rinse with additional juice or milk to ensure that the entire dose is taken. Wipe the measuring device dry; do not wash it after use.

The IV infusion is begun 4 to 12 hours before surgery and continued postoperatively until the client can tolerate an oral dosage form. The drug is prepared for IV infusion by diluting each 1 mL in 20 to 100 mL of 0.9% sodium chloride injection or 5% dextrose injection. Glass containers are preferred to prevent the leaching of diethylhexylphthalate (DEHP) from the polyvinyl chloride (PVC) infusion bags into the cyclosporine solution. However, some agencies will use PVC containers and prepare the drug just before it is administered. Significant amounts of the drug are lost when administered through PVC tubing. The solution is stable for 24 hours in 5% dextrose injection. In 0.9% sodium chloride injection at room temperature, cyclosporine is stable for 6 hours in a PVC container and for 12 hours in a glass container. Infuse over 2 to 6 hours using an infusion pump, or continuously over 24 hours.

▪ ***Education.*** Advise the transplant client about the need to adhere to the drug regimen to prevent rejection. Advise all clients about the need for close monitoring by the prescriber. Warn the client to avoid immunizations unless approved by the prescriber and to avoid others who have been immunized with oral poliovirus vaccine. Alert the client to report any signs of infection as soon as noted. Instruct the client of the need to maintain good dental hygiene and to visit a dentist frequently for teeth cleaning to help prevent gingival hyperplasia.

Alert the client not to drink grapefruit juice or eat grapefruit; it inhibits the metabolism of cyclosporine, resulting in toxic blood levels of the drug.

Clients receiving cyclosporine therapy for rheumatoid arthritis may continue to take corticosteroids, nonsteroidal antiinflammatory drugs (NSAIDs), and salicylates. For clients with psoriasis, any skin lesion that is not typical of that condition should be biopsied for malignancy.

▪ **Evaluation.** The expected outcome of cyclosporine therapy for clients being treated for psoriasis is that they will experience some improvement within 2 weeks; satisfactory control of symptoms may take 12 to 16 weeks. The client taking cyclosporine as part of the therapeutic regimen for transplantation will not demonstrate signs of organ rejection and will remain free of hepatotoxicity and nephrotoxicity. The client will also manage the therapeutic regimen effectively.

daclizumab [dak′ lih zoo mab] (Zenapax)

Daclizumab is an immunosuppressant agent combined with cyclosporine and corticosteroids to prevent kidney transplant rejection. Its mechanism of action is the same as basiliximab.

This drug is administered by IV infusion and has a half-life of 11 to 38 days. The therapeutic serum level is between 5 and 10 μg/mL.

Side effects/adverse reactions of daclizumab include headache, muscle and/or joint pain, dizziness, weakness, insomnia, nausea, vomiting, gas, constipation, diarrhea, shortness of breath, hypertension or hypotension, peripheral edema, tachycardia, tremor, and wound infection.

The adult dosage is 1 mg/kg body weight administered over 15 minutes every 2 weeks for 5 doses. The first dose should be administered no earlier than 24 hours before the transplantation.

The nursing management of the client receiving daclizumab therapy is the same as for basiliximab.

muromonab-CD3 [myoo roe moe' nab-CD3] (Orthoclone OKT3)

Muromonab-CD3 is a monoclonal antibody that reacts with CD3 receptors on the surface of T lymphocytes. It blocks the activation and functions of the T cells in response to an antigenic challenge. Thus it functions as an immunosuppressant and does not cause myelosuppression.

Muromonab-CD3 is indicated for the treatment of acute renal organ transplant rejection and is usually given in combination with azathioprine, cyclosporine, and/or corticosteroids. It is also administered to treat steroid-resistant acute rejection in cardiac and hepatic transplants. Available parenterally, it acts to reduce activated T cells within minutes of administration. It reaches steady-state plasma levels in approximately 3 days and has a duration of action of approximately 7 days. In other words, the number of circulating CD3-positive T cells will return to baseline levels within a week of discontinuing muromonab-CD3.

The most common adverse reactions of muromonab-CD3 occur with the first course. The first-dose effect consists of light-headedness, elevated temperature, chills, nausea, vomiting, diarrhea, headache, dyspnea, chest pain, and tremors and trembling. These effects may be repeated to a lesser degree after the second dose but are rarely encountered with later doses. Fever and chills that occur later may be caused by infection. Anaphylaxis, hypersensitivity, encephalopathy, convulsions, cerebral edema, and aseptic meningitis syndrome are reported less frequently.

The adult IV dosage is 5 mg daily for 10 to 14 days. Children under 12 years of age receive 0.1 mg/kg/day for 10 to 14 days.

■ Nursing Management

Muromonab-CD3 Therapy

In addition to the following discussion, see Nursing Management: The Immunosuppressed Client, p. 1095.

■ **Assessment.** The client's temperature should be taken before drug administration. A temperature above 100° F (37.8° C) should be lowered with antipyretics, and infection should be ruled out before muromonab-CD3 is administered. Uncompensated heart failure or fluid volume excess is a contraindication for this drug because of the risk of life-threatening pulmonary edema if administered. There is an increased risk of hypersensitivity to muromonab-CD3 if the anti-mouse titer is 1:1000 or more.

The most significant drug interactions for which the client's current drug regimen should be reviewed occur with other immunosuppressant agents and live virus vaccines. (See the drug interactions listed for azathioprine for a description of these interactions.)

■ **Nursing Diagnosis.** In addition to the nursing diagnoses/collaborative problems cited in the general nursing management for immunosuppressed clients, the client receiving muromonab-CD3 has the potential for the following: hyperthermia; risk for injury related to cytokine release syndrome (chest pain, dizziness, fever and chills, tachycardia, dyspnea, tremors); impaired comfort (headache); risk for infection (fever, chills); and the potential complication of anaphylaxis, aseptic meningitis syndrome, cerebral edema, pulmonary edema, and encephalopathy (confusion, hallucinations, coma, seizures).

■ **Implementation**

■ ***Monitoring.*** Monitor the client's temperature at frequent intervals for several hours after administration, especially with the first two doses. A cytokine release syndrome may occur as evidenced by the symptoms listed in the previous section. These symptoms occur in most clients 30 minutes to 48 hours after the first dose and may last several hours; they may occur to a lesser extent with each subsequent dose. Fever and chills occurring later in therapy may be caused by infection. The client should also be assessed for headache, stiff neck, and photosensitivity, because aseptic meningitis syndrome may occur in the first 3 days of therapy. CBCs should be monitored periodically throughout the course of treatment.

Observe the client for fluid volume excess: auscultate the lungs, check for peripheral edema, monitor daily weights, and monitor fluid intake and output. Monitor vital signs and observe for signs of infection.

Muromonab-CD3 serum concentrations may be monitored to ensure that they are at least 800 ng/mL.

■ ***Intervention.*** Cardiopulmonary resuscitation equipment and medications should be immediately available during the administration of the first dose. Muromonab-CD3 should be administered by IV push over a period of less than 1 minute by a health care provider who is experienced in immunosuppressive therapy.

Methylprednisolone may be administered intravenously before the first dose to minimize cytokine release syndrome. IV hydrocortisone sodium succinate may be given 30 minutes after the first dose (and possibly the second dose) for the same reason. Antihistamines may also be used to minimize this reaction. The client's temperature should be maintained below 100° F (37.8° C) with acetaminophen.

Muromonab-CD3 is prepared for IV administration by drawing the solution through a low protein-binding 0.2- or 0.22-μm filter, then discarding the filter and attaching the appropriate needle for administration. The drug is not administered by IV infusion or with other drug solutions. Do not shake.

■ ***Education.*** The client should be prepared for the possibility of the cytokine release syndrome and asked to report any of the adverse signs and symptoms of that reaction or of aseptic meningitis syndrome.

■ **Evaluation.** The expected outcome of muromonab-CD3 therapy is that the client will not experience transplanted organ rejection and will be able to manage the therapeutic regimen.

mycophenolate mofetil [mye koe fee′ noe late moe′ fe tyl] (CellCept)

Mycophenolate is used in conjunction with cyclosporine and corticosteroids and is indicated for the prophylaxis of renal transplant and allogeneic cardiac rejection. Mycophenolate is metabolized to MPA, an active metabolite that inhibits the response of T and B lymphocytes to mitogenic and allospecific stimulation. Therefore this drug has a cytostatic effect on lymphocytes. It also suppresses antibody formation by B lymphocytes and may inhibit the influx of leukocytes into inflammatory and graft rejection sites.

Available orally, mycophenolate is rapidly metabolized to the active metabolite MPA and other inactive metabolites. The half-life of MPA is 18 hours, with excretion primarily in the kidneys.

The major side effects/adverse reactions of mycophenolate include diarrhea, vomiting, and respiratory infections (leukopenia, sepsis). Peripheral edema, urinary tract infections, anemia, hypertension, and abdominal pain are also reported.

For renal transplant prophylaxis, an oral dosage of 1 g twice daily is administered as soon as possible after surgery in combination with cyclosporine and corticosteroids (European Mycophenolate Mofetil Cooperative Study Group, 1999). For cardiac transplant rejection prophylaxis, the dosage is 1.5 g twice daily in combination with cyclosporine and corticosteroids.

■ Nursing Management

Mycophenolate Therapy

In addition to the following discussion, see Nursing Management: The Immunosuppressed Client, p. 1095.

■ **Assessment.** It is essential to assess exposure to or the presence of infection. Although mycophenolate mofetil has enhanced immunosuppression for both acute and chronic rejection, the client is at higher risk for infection than with other similar agents (Kim, Moon, Kim, & Park, 1999; Rothwell, Gloor, Morgenstern, & Milliner, 1999). Any infection that the client might have may become life threatening with the administration of mycophenolate. This drug is contraindicated for clients who are hypersensitive to the drug. Caution should also be used for clients with serious disease of the gastrointestinal tract or a history of ulcer disease or gastrointestinal bleeding. Clients with renal function impairment will experience a reduced excretion of the drug with an increased risk of mycophenolate toxicity; dosages may need to be reduced.

CBCs and electrolytes should be determined before initiating therapy. Baseline renal and hepatic function studies should be obtained.

Review the client's current medication regimen for the risk of significant drug interactions, such as those that may occur when mycophenolate is given concurrently with the following drugs:

Drug	Possible Effect and Management
other immunosuppressant agents, such as anti-thymocyte globulin, azathioprine (Imuran), chlorambucil (Leukeran), glucocorticoids, cyclophosphamide (Cytoxan), cyclosporine (Sandimmune), mercaptopurine (Purinethol), muromonab-CD3 (Orthoclone OKT3), tacrolimus (Prograf)	May increase the risk for developing infections and/or neoplasms.

■ **Nursing Diagnosis.** Clients receiving mycophenolate may experience the following nursing diagnoses/collaborative problems: impaired comfort (headache, heartburn, nausea, vomiting); disturbed sleep pattern (insomnia); impaired skin integrity (acne, rash); diarrhea; constipation; ineffective protection related to leukopenia or thrombocytopenia; activity intolerance related to anemia; ineffective airway clearance (cough); excess fluid volume (dyspnea, peripheral edema); risk for infection; and the potential complications of gastrointestinal bleeding, congestive heart failure, and increased risk of malignancy.

■ **Implementation**

■ ***Monitoring.*** CBCs should be performed weekly during the first month, twice a month for the next 2 to 3 months, and monthly thereafter. Notify the prescriber if the absolute neutrophil count is less than 100,000/mm^3. Renal and hepatic function studies and electrolytes should be monitored periodically during therapy. Increased alkaline phosphatase, bilirubin, AST, ALT, and amylase concentrations may indicate hepatotoxicity. Increased serum creatinine, hypercalcemia, hypocalcemia, hyponatremia, hyperglycemia, hypoglycemia, and hyperlipidemia may occur.

■ ***Intervention.*** Mycophenolate is given within 72 hours of transplantation. Administer oral doses on an empty stomach, 1 hour before or 2 hours after meals. Capsules should be swallowed whole, not opened, crushed, or chewed.

■ ***Education.*** Female clients who are of childbearing age need to practice two reliable forms of contraception or abstinence both during the course of therapy and for 6 weeks following the end of therapy.

Instruct the client to take mycophenolate as directed. Stress the need for lifelong therapy to prevent transplant rejection. Emphasize the need to seek medical attention if symptoms of organ rejection occur. Advise avoiding others with infectious diseases. Encourage the client not to take other medications without consulting with the prescriber and to maintain follow-up appointments for laboratory work and clinical monitoring.

■ **Evaluation.** The expected outcome of mycophenolate mofetil therapy is that the client will not experience transplanted organ rejection and will be able to manage the therapeutic regimen effectively.

tacrolimus [tak roe lye' mus] (FK 506, Prograf)

Tacrolimus in conjunction with corticosteroids is indicated for the prophylaxis of organ rejection (kidney, liver and, investigationally, other organs). It inhibits the activation of T lymphocytes. Although its exact mechanism of action is unknown, it is believed to bind to FKBP-12 protein and form complexes that prevent the activation of T lymphocytes.

This drug is available orally and parenterally. Oral absorption is variable, with peak blood levels reached in 1.5 to 3.5 hours. It is metabolized in the liver (primarily by the cytochrome P-450 system) to a number of metabolites, including several active ones; less than 1% is excreted in the urine.

The side effects/adverse reactions of tacrolimus include headaches, nausea, diarrhea, hypertension, tremors, and renal dysfunction. Hyperkalemia, hypomagnesemia, hyperuricemia, and hyperglycemia that require insulin therapy have also been reported (*Drug Facts and Comparisons*, 2000).

The initial adult dosage by IV infusion is 0.03 to 0.05 mg/kg/day; the client is converted to the oral dosage form as soon as possible, usually in 2 to 3 days of therapy. The initial oral adult dosage is 0.1 to 0.2 mg/kg/day (American Hospital Formulary Service, 1999).

■ Nursing Management

Tacrolimus Therapy

In addition to the following discussion, see Nursing Management: The Immunosuppressed Client, p. 1095.

■ **Assessment.** The use of tacrolimus is contraindicated for clients with hypersensitivity to the drug or to HCO-60 polyoxyl hydrogenated castor oil (which is contained in the injection solution). Use the drug cautiously in clients with renal and hepatic impairment. This drug has been associated with increased susceptibility to malignancy.

Review the client's current drug regimen for the risk of significant drug interactions, such as those that may occur when tacrolimus is given concurrently with the following drugs:

Bold/color type indicates the most serious interactions.

Drug	Possible Effect and Management
bromocriptine (Parlodel), cimetidine (Tagamet), clarithromycin (Biaxin), danazol (Danocrine), erythromycin, itraconazole (Sporanox), ketoconazole (Nizoral), nifedipine (Procardia)	Concurrent use increases tacrolimus blood levels. Monitor tacrolimus blood levels at frequent intervals. Dosage adjustments may be necessary.
rifampin (Rifadin)	Concurrent use decreases blood levels of tacrolimus.
cyclosporine (Sandimmune)	Concurrent use increases the risk of nephrotoxicity. Allow 24 hours to pass after discontinuing cyclosporine before starting tacrolimus. Monitor renal function studies carefully.
potassium-sparing diuretics	Concurrent use increases the risk of hyperkalemia. Monitor serum potassium levels.
vaccines, live	**Avoid concurrent use. Vaccines other than live ones may be less effective if given concurrently.**

A baseline assessment should include serum creatinine, serum electrolytes, CBC and platelet counts, and blood glucose. The client's clinical status should be documented.

■ **Nursing Diagnosis.** The client receiving tacrolimus may experience the following nursing diagnoses/collaborative problems: impaired comfort (headache, abdominal pain, generalized aches); impaired skin integrity (rash, pruritus); disturbed sleep pattern (insomnia); deficient fluid volume related to anorexia, nausea, and vomiting; diarrhea; ineffective protection related to anemia, leukopenia, and thrombocytopenia; and the potential problems of nephrotoxicity (hypertension, peripheral edema, ascites), neurotoxicity (paresthesia, tremor, neuropathy, seizures), gastrointestinal bleeding, hepatotoxicity, pleural effusion, hypertension, PTLD (fever, fatigue, weight loss), and electrolyte imbalances (hyperglycemia, hyperkalemia, hypomagnesemia).

■ **Implementation**

■ ***Monitoring.*** Observe the client for a hypersensitivity response for at least 30 minutes after IV tacrolimus and frequently thereafter. Monitor blood pressure closely during therapy. Monitor CBCs and platelet counts, blood glucose, serum electrolytes, serum creatinine levels, and tacrolimus blood levels. Assess the client for symptoms of the nursing diagnoses mentioned previously. Monitor children closely, because higher dosages are necessary to maintain adequate blood levels.

■ ***Intervention.*** Tacrolimus therapy should be initiated no sooner than 6 hours after transplantation. Concurrent glucocorticoid therapy may occur. IV administration is by continuous infusion over 24 hours. The client should be changed to oral administration of tacrolimus as soon as possible to reduce the risk of adverse reactions to IV tacrolimus—usually 8 to 12 hours after the last IV dosing.

■ ***Education.*** Instruct the client to take tacrolimus at the same time each day and as directed, emphasizing the need for lifelong therapy to prevent rejection. Inform the client of symptoms of organ rejection and the need to seek medical attention at once if they occur. Reinforce the importance of keeping appointments for laboratory work and follow-up care. Advise clients of childbearing age of the risks of taking tacrolimus while pregnant, and instruct them about contraception as needed.

Alert the client to avoid grapefruit and grapefruit juice; both increase the serum levels of tacrolimus and may result in drug toxicity.

▪ **Evaluation.** The expected outcome of tacrolimus therapy is that the client will not experience transplanted organ rejection and will manage the therapeutic regimen effectively.

IMMUNOMODULATORS

Biotechnology refers to the development of new agents that can either activate the body's immune defenses or modify a biologic response to an unwanted stimulus, such as an antitumor response. These agents are called **immunomodulating agents.** With the advent of recombinant DNA technology in the early 1980s, new agents were made available in larger quantities for clinical trials and investigations. Although still in its infancy, this area of study has the potential for solving some of the mysteries about disease that have eluded researchers for centuries and may also provide pharmaceuticals that control the devastation, pain, and suffering induced by many viral diseases, AIDS, and cancer. (See the Complementary and Alternative Therapies box at right.)

Acquired Immunodeficiency Syndrome

A pathogenic retrovirus known as **human immunodeficiency virus (HIV)** is the etiologic agent in **acquired immunodeficiency syndrome (AIDS)** (Box 64-1). AIDS is one of the leading causes of death in Americans between 25 and 44 years of age. From 1987 to 1994, deaths associated with the AIDS virus increased an average of 16% per year; in 1995 and 1996, AIDS-related deaths dropped by 26% (Atlanta, 1997). This change in AIDS-related deaths is largely a result of new drugs (especially the protease inhibitors) and, perhaps, more effective prevention programs.

According to the Reuters Health Information Systems (1998), the Centers for Disease Control and Prevention (CDC) reported a decline of 15% in deaths in males but an increased death rate in females (3%). In addition, AIDS deaths have decreased by 18% in homosexual males, but an increase has been reported in persons infected through heterosexual contacts.

The early spread of HIV disease was primarily among homosexual men, IV substance abusers, and persons receiving contaminated blood products. However, in the last few years the progression of disease in these populations has declined, and an increased incidence has been reported in heterosexuals, especially females and infants. Most AIDS cases in children are a result of perinatal transmission. Although AIDS can affect all racial groups, current statistics indicate that the incidence of cases in children is much more common in black and Hispanic children than in Caucasian children (Morse, Shelton, & O'Donnell, 1996).

HIV is transmitted sexually via blood and blood products or from a mother with AIDS to her child during birth. Transmission through commercial blood transfusion is considered rare today, but transmission via IV substance abusers is still very common. Current evidence indicates that shaking hands, hugging, socially kissing, coughing, sneezing, or sharing meals will not transmit HIV. It is also not contracted from swimming pools, toilet seats, hot tubs, dishes, or via food prepared by persons infected with HIV. HIV is transmitted by intimate contact with the body fluids of an infected person, which can occur through sex, sharing of con-

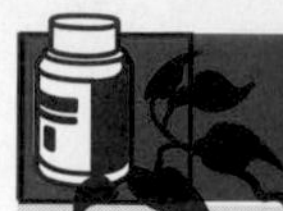

Complementary and Alternative Therapies
Echinacea

Echinacea is the most popular herb in the United States and Canada. It is commonly used orally for its immunostimulant activity in the treatment of colds and other upper respiratory diseases. Echinacea extracts demonstrate antiviral activity and increase phagocytosis—effects that tend to increase the body's resistance to microbial activity. Although much of the clinical trial work with this drug is inconclusive or inadequate because of variations in the species, plant part, or dosage form, a few studies appear to demonstrate that it reduces the severity and duration of cold symptoms and is considered to be possibly effective for this use. Its use should not be encouraged to prevent colds but rather to treat them once they begin.

Echinacea is considered safe when used appropriately. The German Commission E, a major authoritative reference on herbal remedies, advises limiting the use of echinacea to 8 continuous weeks of use. There is concern that long-term daily use may actually depress immunity. Side effects appear to be rare, but short-term fever, nausea and vomiting, and allergic reactions are possible. Avoid use in pregnancy and lactation. The use of echinacea is contraindicated in clients with immune disorders (e.g., AIDS and HIV infection) and tuberculosis, multiple sclerosis, and other progressive systemic diseases because of its potential for stimulating the autoimmune process. There is cross-allergenicity with echinacea in clients sensitive to ragweed, marigolds, chrysanthemums, and other flowers and herbs. Although there are no known drug interactions with echinacea, theoretically it might interfere with immunosuppressant therapy.

The typical oral dosage of echinacea is 1 g of dried root three times daily, or one cup of tea made by steeping 1 g of root in 5 ounces of boiling water for 5 to 10 minutes, three times daily. Echinacea liquid extract and tinctures are also used for oral dosing. The usual dosage of liquid extract is 0.25 to 1 mL of a 1 : 1 preparation in 45% alcohol three times daily; for the tincture, 1 to 2 mL (1 : 5 in 45% alcohol) is usually given three times daily. (See Chapter 12 for more information.)

Information from Cirigliano, M.D. (1998). Ten most common herbs in clinical practice. In M.S. Micozzi (Ed.), *Current review of complementary medicine.* Philadelphia: Current Medicine; and Jellin, J.M., Batz, F., & Hitchens, K. (1999). *Pharmacist's letter/prescriber's letter natural medicines comprehensive database.* Stockton, CA: Therapeutic Research Faculty.

BOX 64-1

AIDS Overview

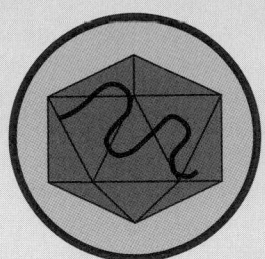

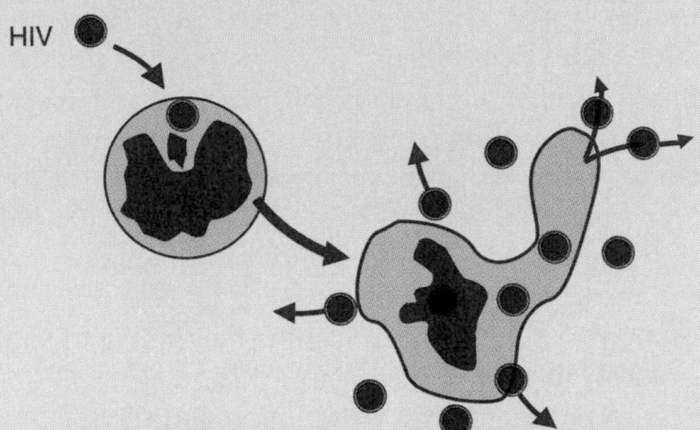

The HIV virus enters T cells and macrophages which, ironically, are the cells the body sent to destroy the virus. By reproduction the virus eventually kills them.

AIDS has no cure. Note the following:

- HIV reproduces faster than any other virus.
- It is present in the bloodstream in very small amounts and therefore is currently hard to target with medications.

AIDS has been diagnosed in the following:

- All races
- Men, women, and children
- Homosexuals and heterosexuals

AIDS in Older Adults

10% of cases are persons over 50 years of age; 10,000 were over 60 years of age in 1992.

The majority of clients between ages 50 and 59 are homosexual/bisexual; older persons were infected by blood transfusions.

Older adults diagnosed with AIDS have much shorter life spans after diagnosis than younger persons.

Nearly 50% of all older adults with AIDS develop symptoms of dementia (e.g., personality changes, impaired concentration, apathy) (Cowan, 1993).

AIDS Infection

AIDS may be acquired in the following ways:

- IV drug use with an infected or contaminated needle.
- Sexual contact with an infected person. The virus is transmitted in blood products, semen, breast milk, and vaginal secretions. A small tear in the rectum lining or in the vagina can provide an entrance for the virus.
- AIDS can be transmitted during birth or during breastfeeding.
- HIV-infected persons are not always sick, but they can still transmit the AIDS virus.

Client Counseling

The following precautions should be followed to reduce the possibility of infection:

- Allow no exchange of body fluids.
- Do not share needles.
- Recommend the use of latex condoms or nonoxynol-9 cream with a condom.

Symptoms of HIV Infection

Fever
Chills
Skin rash
Sore or aching muscles
Enlarged glands
Headache
Weight loss
Women: chronic vaginal infections; may not present with fever, chills, or weight loss

taminated needles and syringes (drug addicts), blood or blood product transfusions, and from mother to child, before, during, or shortly after birth.

Health care workers with documented invasive exposure to the HIV virus may test positive for the HIV antibody. The CDC has issued guidelines for health care workers to follow to minimize the possibility of virus exposure and transfer (Gilden, 1996; Reuters Health Information Systems, 1998). The following is a summary of these recommendations:

1. Chemoprophylaxis is recommended when health care personnel are exposed to HIV in the workplace and it is a high-risk exposure (punctured skin). Zidovudine should be included in any antiretroviral regimen, with treatment starting promptly, preferably within an hour or two of exposure.

2. A three-drug combination—zidovudine, lamivudine, and indinavir—is recommended after exposure to HIV-contaminated blood. Two drugs (zidovudine and lamivudine) may be used if the exposure presents a lower degree of risk, such as contact with the mucous membranes or skin or exposure to contaminated body fluids other than blood.
3. Information is limited on effectiveness and toxicity with the use of drugs in postexposure prophylaxis. A consultation with a health care professional who is knowledgeable about these drugs and HIV transmission is suggested to ascertain the risk-benefit ratio.

The virus that caused the global AIDS-epidemic is HIV-1, group M. Of special concern is the finding of a rare AIDS strain (HIV-1, group O) in an African woman in California (Cooper, 1996). This is the first time this strain was discovered in the United States; fewer than 100 cases known worldwide have this strain or have been infected with this strain. This strain has mostly been identified in infected people from western or central Africa. When compared to the group M population, the group O strain does not appear to be different in mode of transmission, disease progression, or the types of opportunistic infections reported. However, additional information about this strain is limited.

AIDS is a deadly disease and there is no known cure for it at this time; therefore client teaching should focus on disease prevention.

HIV Life Cycle

Although the pathogenesis of AIDS is not fully understood, HIV is an intracellular infection that primarily infests CD4 T lymphocytes. The virus is a retrovirus that has RNA in its core; after it binds to CD4 T lymphocyte receptor cells in the body, it releases its RNA into the cytoplasm. It also has the potential of infecting monocytes and macrophages. Reverse transcriptase, an enzyme carried by HIV, assists in transcribing the HIV RNA into viral DNA strands in the host body. Thereafter, activation of this DNA will result in the production of viral substances that infect other CD4 T lymphocyte cells; this leads to the eventual loss of functioning CD4 lymphocytes.

The CD4 helper cells are destroyed by the virus, which eventually leads to the immunodeficiency disease known as AIDS. The CD4 cells are needed directly and indirectly for proper functioning of the human immune system. Both the humoral immune response, which involves antibodies produced by B lymphocytes, and the cellular immune response involving stimulation of the cytotoxic T cells (or T8 cells) are mediated by the helper-inducer T cells (Wong, 1993). Therefore a severe decline or destruction of CD4 cells by HIV is responsible for the multiple symptoms of AIDS—severe suppression of the immune system leading to opportunistic infections and cancers. See Box 64-2 for functions of a T4 helper cell and Figure 64-2 for T4 cell effects in the body.

BOX 64-2

Functions of a T4 Helper Cell

T4 cells are responsible for a variety of immune functions, some of which include the following:

1. Release of colony-stimulating factors and lymphokines to stimulate the production of leukocytes, such as macrophages and eosinophils
2. Activation of the natural killer cells (cytotoxic NK cells), which are large lymphocytes in the blood that have non–antigen-specific antitumor and antibacterial properties
3. Activation of T8 suppressor cells by T4 helper-inducer cells can, which will stop antibody production, or activation of T8 cytotoxic T cells and stimulation of B cells by T4 suppressor-inducers to increase the production of antibodies.

The revised CDC classification for HIV infection emphasizes the importance of the CD4 T lymphocyte count. This system includes all symptomatic and asymptomatic persons with a CD4 count <200 CD4 T lymphocytes/μL or a CD4 T lymphocyte percentage of total lymphocytes of <14. This expanded definition has been estimated to result in an increased number of AIDS cases reported initially, thus allowing for better surveillance and earlier interventions for this devastating disease state.

As CD4 T lymphocytes decline, the risk and severity of opportunistic infections increases; therefore the use of this system helps to identify persons in need of close medical attention. Instituting antiviral therapy and antimicrobial prophylaxis in correlation with HIV immunosuppression levels as measured by CD4 T lymphocytes has slowed the rate of progression from HIV status to AIDS-defined clinical conditions (Centers for Disease Control and Prevention, 1992). Zidovudine (AZT) was the first antiretroviral agent for the treatment of AIDS, but mutations of HIV have developed and are resistant to this drug. The second class of antiretrovirals, the protease inhibitors, includes ritonavir (Norvir), indinavir (Crixivan), and saquinavir (Invirase). (See Chapter 60 for the pharmacologic review of antiviral agents.)

Ongoing trials with drug combinations (e.g., AZT and saquinavir or AZT/ddC and a protease inhibitor) appear to be more effective than individual drugs alone and may help to delay resistance to the individual agents. Unusual symptoms have been reported since protease inhibitors were added to the HIV drug regimen. These symptoms include hyperglycemia or exacerbated cases of diabetes, elevated levels of triglycerides and cholesterol (in some cases, excessive elevations), and changes in body composition, such as lipodystrophy or abnormal fat accumulations in the back (buffalo hump), breast, and stomach. Affected individuals typically appear to have muscle wasting in the arms, chest, and legs, along with fatty growths such as lipomas of the

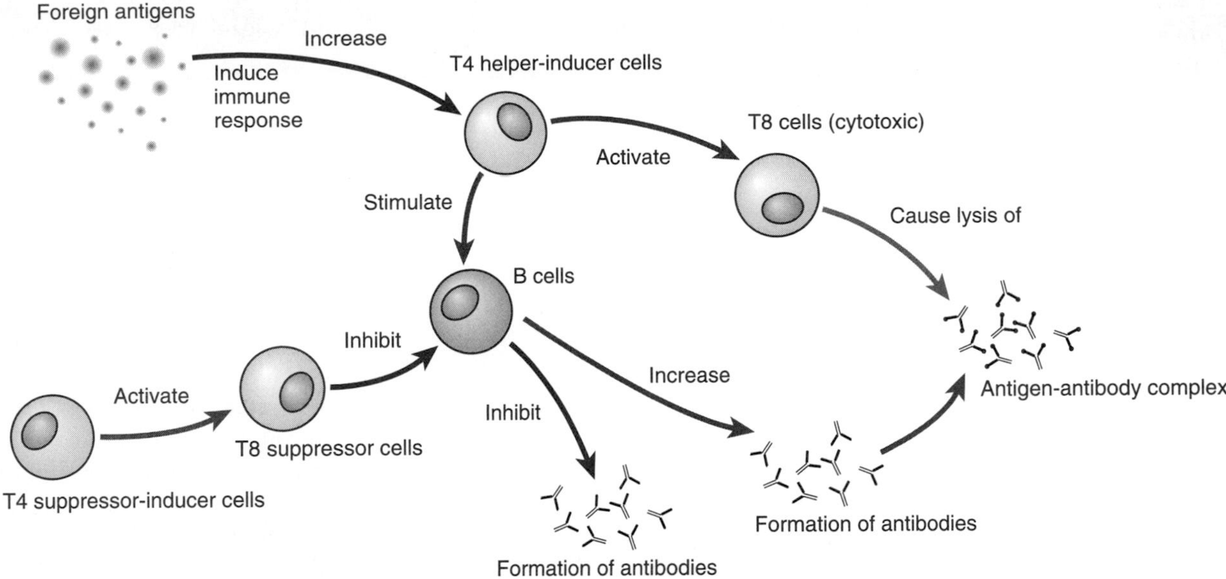

Figure 64-2 T4 cell effects in the body. T4 cells are mainly the helper-inducer type of cells and increase when antigens are present. T4 suppressor-inducer cells do not respond to antigens. They act indirectly to suppress antibody formation.

upper back and neck. Most clients start to develop this condition soon after starting the triple combination drug regimen with protease inhibitors, especially indinavir. Approximately 20 cases of hemolytic anemia have also been reported with indinavir (Huff, 1997/1998). Additional studies are necessary to determine the short-term and long-term effects of these agents.

The prognosis of HIV disease is variable, with some clients remaining in a fairly stable state for many years. In the later stages the breakdown in cellular immunity results in the development of opportunistic infections in the body. See Box 64-3 for the recommended antiretroviral drugs to treat HIV infection. Guidelines have been propagated for prophylaxis to prevent the first episode of opportunistic disease in adults and adolescents (Table 64-1) and for prophylaxis to prevent the recurrence of opportunistic disease after chemotherapy for acute disease in adults and adolescents infected with HIV (Table 64-2). The rating system shown in Appendix H is used to evaluate the HIV treatment recommendations in Tables 64-1 and 64-2.

Most clients in the advanced stages of AIDS have a very low helper T cell count, with the majority usually dying within a few years. Box 64-4 discusses the most common opportunistic infection, *Pneumocystis carinii* pneumonia (PCP). For further analysis, see the Case Study box on p. 1113.

Immunotherapy

Lymphokines (IL-1 and IL-2), interferons (primarily alpha) and granulocyte or granulocyte-macrophage colony-stimulating factors (G-CSF or filgrastim [Neupogen] and sargramostim [GM-CSF; Leukine]) are being used to help

Text continued on p. 1113

BOX 64-3

Recommended Antiretroviral Drugs to Treat HIV Infection

Drug regimens include one drug from Column A and one combination from Column B.

Preferred Recommendations

Column A	Column B
efavirenz	stavudine + didanosine
indinavir	stavudine + lamivudine
nelfinavir	zidovudine + zalcitabine
ritonavir	zidovudine + lamivudine
ritonavir + saquinavir	didanosine + lamivudine

Alternative Regimens

abacavir + didanosine + lamivudine
delavirdine or nevirapine + selection from Column B

Not Recommended

All drug monotherapies

Column A	Column B
saquinavir	stavudine + zidovudine
	zalcitabine + lamivudine
	zalcitabine + didanosine
	zalcitabine + stavudine

Information from Guidelines for the Use of Antiretroviral Agents in HIV-Infected Adults and Adolescents, Department of Health & Human Services & Henry J. Kaiser Family Foundation; www.hivatis.org/guidelines/adult/pdf/A&ajani.pdf (5/5/99).

TABLE 64-1 Prophylaxis to Prevent First Episode of Opportunistic Disease in Adults and Adolescents Infected with Human Immunodeficiency Virus

Pathogen	Indication	Preventive Regimens: First Choice	Preventive Regimens: Alternatives
I. Strongly Recommended as Standard of Care			
Pneumocystis carinii[a]	CD4+ count <200/μL or oropharyngeal candidiasis	trimethoprim-sulfamethoxazole (TMP-SMZ), 1 DS PO q.d. (AI) TMP-SMZ, 1 SS PO q.d. (AI)	dapsone, 50 mg PO b.i.d. *or* 100 mg PO q.d. (BI); dapsone, 50 mg PO q.d. *plus* pyrimethamine, 50 mg PO q.w. *plus* leucovorin, 25 mg PO q.w. (BI); dapsone, 200 mg PO *plus* pyrimethamine, 75 mg PO *plus* leucovorin, 25 mg PO q.w. (BI); aerosolized pentamidine, 300 mg q.m. via Respirgard II nebulizer (BI); atovaquone, 1500 mg PO q.d. (BI); TMP-SMZ, 1 DS PO t.i.w. (BI)
Mycobacterium tuberculosis Isoniazid-sensitive[b]	TST reaction ≥5 mm or prior positive TST result without treatment *or* contact with case of active tuberculosis	isoniazid, 300 mg PO *plus* pyridoxine, 50 mg PO q.d. × 9 months (AII) or isoniazid, 900 mg PO *plus* pyridoxine, 100 mg PO b.i.w. × 9 months (BI); rifampin, 600 mg *plus* pyrazinamide, 20 mg/kg PO q.d. × 2 months (AI)	rifabutin 300 mg PO q.d. *plus* pyrazinamide, 20 mg/kg PO q.d. × 2 months (BIII); rifampin 600 mg PO q.d. × 4 months (BIII)
Isoniazid-resistant	Same; high probability of exposure to isoniazid-resistant tuberculosis	rifampin 600 mg *plus* pyrazinamide, 20 mg/kg PO q.d. × 2 months (AI)	rifabutin, 300 mg *plus* pyrazinamide 20 mg/kg PO q.d. × 2 months (BIII); rifampin, 600 mg PO q.d. × 4 months (BIII); rifabutin, 300 mg PO q.d. × 4 months (CIII)
Multidrug-(isoniazid and rifampin) resistant	Same; high probability of exposure to multidrug-resistant tuberculosis	Choice of drugs requires consultation with public health authorities	None
Toxoplasma gondii[c]	IgG antibody to *Toxoplasma* and CD4+ count <100/μL	TMP-SMZ, 1 DS PO q.d. (AII)	TMP-SMZ, 1 SS PO q.d. (BIII); dapsone, 50 mg PO q.d. *plus* pyrimethamine, 50 mg PO q.w. *plus* leukovorin, 25 mg PO q.w. (BI); atovaquone, 1500 mg PO q.d. with or without pyrimethamine, 25 mg PO q.d. *plus* leukovorin, 10 mg PO q.d. (CIII)
Mycobacterium avium complex[d]	CD4+ count <50/μL	azithromycin, 1200 mg PO q.w. (AI) or clarithromycin, 500 mg PO b.i.d. (AI)	rifabutin, 300 mg PO q.d. (BI); azithromycin, 1200 mg PO q.w. *plus* rifabutin, 300 mg PO q.d. (CI)

From 1999 USPHS/IDSA Prevention of Opportunistic Infections Working Group, U.S. Public Health Service and Infectious Diseases Society of America. (1999). *USPHS/IDSA guidelines for the prevention of opportunistic infections in persons infected with human immunodeficiency virus.* 48(RR10), 1-59; www.cdc.gov/epo/mmwr/preview/mmwrhtml/rr4810al.htm (2/17/00).

TABLE 64-1 Prophylaxis to Prevent First Episode of Opportunistic Disease in Adults and Adolescents Infected with Human Immunodeficiency Virus—cont'd

Pathogen	Preventive Regimens: Indication	Preventive Regimens: First Choice	Preventive Regimens: Alternatives
I. Strongly Recommended as Standard of Care—cont'd			
Varicella zoster virus (VZV)	Significant exposure to chickenpox or shingles for patients who have no history of either condition or, if available, negative antibody to VZV	Varicella zoster immune globulin (VZIG), 5 vials (1.25 mL each) IM, administered ≤96 hours after exposure, ideally within 48 hours (AIII)	
II. Generally Recommended			
Streptococcus pneumoniae[e]	All patients	Pneumococcal vaccine, 0.5 mL IM (CD4+ ≥ 200/µL [BII]; CD4+ <200/µL [CIII]—might reimmunize if initial immunization was given when CD4+ <200/µL and if CD4+ increases to >200/µL on HAART (CIII)	None
Hepatitis B virus[f]	All susceptible (anti-HBc-negative) patients	Hepatitis B vaccine: 3 doses (BII)	None
Influenza virus[f]	All patients (annually, before influenza season)	Whole or split virus, 0.5 mL IM/year (BIII)	rimantadine, 100 mg PO b.i.d. (CIII), or amantadine, 100 mg PO b.i.d. (CIII)
Hepatitis A virus[f]	All susceptible (anti-HAV-negative) patients with chronic hepatitis C	Hepatitis A vaccine: two doses (BIII)	None
III. Not Routinely Indicated			
Bacteria	Neutropenia	Granulocyte colony-stimulating factor (G-CSF), 5-10 µg/kg SC q.d. × 2-4 weeks or granulocyte-macrophage colony-stimulating factor (GM-CSF), 250 µg/m² IV over 2 hours q.d. × 2-4 weeks (CII)	None
Cryptococcus neoformans[g]	CD4+ count <50/µL	fluconazole, 100-200 mg PO q.d. (CI)	itraconazole, 200 mg PO q.d. (CIII)
Histoplasma capsulatum[g]	CD4+ count <100/µL, endemic geographic area	itraconazole capsule, 200 mg PO q.d. (CI)	None

Continued

TABLE 64-1 Prophylaxis to Prevent First Episode of Opportunistic Disease in Adults and Adolescents Infected with Human Immunodeficiency Virus—cont'd

	Preventive Regimens		
Pathogen	**Indication**	**First Choice**	**Alternatives**
III. Not Routinely Indicated—cont'd			
Cytomegalovirus (CMV)[h]	CD4+ count <50/μL and CMV antibody positivity	Oral ganciclovir, 1 g PO t.i.d. (CI)	None

From 1999 USPHS/IDSA Prevention of Opportunistic Infections Working Group, U.S. Public Health Service and Infectious Diseases Society of America. (1999). *USPHS/IDSA guidelines for the prevention of opportunistic infections in persons infected with human immunodeficiency virus.* 48(RR10), 1-59; www.cdc.gov/epo/mmwr/preview/mmwrhtml/rr4810al.htm (2/17/00).

NOTES: Information included in these guidelines might not represent Food and Drug Administration (FDA) approval or approved labeling for the particular products or indications in question. Specifically, the terms "safe" and "effective" might not be synonymous with the FDA-defined legal standards for product approval.

The Respirgard II nebulizer is manufactured by Marquest, Englewood, Colorado. Letters and Roman numerals in parentheses after regimens indicate the strength of the recommendation and the quality of evidence supporting it.

Anti-HBc, Antibody to hepatitis B core antigen; *b.i.w.*, twice a week; *DS*, double-strength tablet; *HAART*, highly active antiretroviral therapy; *HAV*, hepatitis A virus; *HIV*, human immunodeficiency virus; *IM*, intramuscular; *IV*, intravenous; *PO*, by mouth; *q.d.*, daily; *q.m.*, monthly; *q.w.*, weekly; *SS*, single-strength tablet; *t.i.w.* three times a week; *TMP-SMZ*, trimethoprim-sulfamethoxazole; *sc*, subcutaneous; and *TST*, tuberculin skin test.

[a] Prophylaxis should also be considered for persons with a CD4+ percentage of <14%, for persons with a history of an AIDS-defining illness, and possibly for those with CD4+ counts 200 but <250 cells/μL. TMP-SMZ also reduces the frequency of toxoplasmosis and some bacterial infections. Patients receiving dapsone should be tested for glucose-6 phosphate dehydrogenase deficiency. A dosage of 50 mg q.d. is probably less effective than that of 100 mg q.d. The efficacy of parenteral pentamidine (e.g., 4 mg/kg/month) is uncertain. Fansidar (sulfadoxine-pyrimethamine) is rarely used because of severe hypersensitivity reactions. Patients who are being administered therapy for toxoplasmosis with sulfadiazine-pyrimethamine are protected against *Pneumocystis carinii* pneumonia and do not need additional prophylaxis against PCP.

[b] Directly observed therapy is recommended for isoniazid, 900 mg b.i.w.; isoniazid regimens should include pyridoxine to prevent peripheral neuropathy. Rifampin should not be administered concurrently with protease inhibitors or nonnucleoside reverse transcriptase inhibitors. Rifabutin should not be given with hard-gel saquinavir or delavirdine; caution is also advised when the drug is coadministered with soft-gel saquinavir. Rifabutin may be administered at a reduced dose (150 mg q.d.) with indinavir, nelfinavir, or amprenavir; at a reduced dose of 150 mg q.o.d. (or 150 mg three times weekly) with ritonavir; or at an increased dose (450 mg q.d.) with efavirenz; information is lacking regarding coadministration of rifabutin with nevirapine. Exposure to multidrug-resistant tuberculosis might require prophylaxis with two drugs; consult public health authorities. Possible regimens include pyrazinamide plus either ethambutol or a fluoroquinolone.

[c] Protection against toxoplasmosis is provided by TMP-SMZ, dapsone plus pyrimethamine, and possibly by atovaquone. Atovaquone may be used with or without pyrimethamine. Pyrimethamine alone probably provides little, if any, protection.

[d] See footnote b regarding the use of rifabutin with protease inhibitors or nonnucleoside reverse transcriptase inhibitors.

[e] Vaccination should be offered to persons who have a CD4+ T-lymphocyte count <200 cells/μL, although the efficacy might be diminished. Revaccination 5 years after the first dose or sooner if the initial immunization was given when the CD4+ count was <200 cells/μL and the CD4+ count has increased to >200 cells/μL on HAART is considered optional. Some authorities are concerned that immunizations might stimulate the replication of HIV. However, one study showed no adverse effect of pneumococcal vaccination on patient survival (McNaghten AD, Hanson DL, Jones JL, Dworkin MS, Ward JW, and the Adult/Adolescent Spectrum of Disease Group. Effects of antiretroviral therapy and opportunistic illness primary chemoprophylaxis on survival after AIDS diagnosis. AIDS 1999 [in press]).

[f] These immunizations or chemoprophylactic regimens do not target pathogens traditionally classified as opportunistic but should be considered for use in HIV-infected patients as indicated. Data are inadequate concerning clinical benefit of these vaccines in this population, although it is logical to assume that those patients who develop antibody responses will derive some protection. Some authorities are concerned that immunizations might stimulate HIV replication, although for influenza vaccination, a large observational study of HIV-infected persons in clinical care showed no adverse effect of this vaccine, including multiple doses, on patient survival (J. Ward, CDC, personal communication). Hepatitis B vaccine has been recommended for all children and adolescents and for all adults with risk factors for hepatitis B virus (HBV). Rimantadine and amantadine are appropriate during outbreaks of influenza A. Because of the theoretical concern that increases in HIV plasma RNA following vaccination during pregnancy might increase the risk of perinatal transmission of HIV, providers may wish to defer vaccination until after antiretroviral therapy is initiated. For additional information regarding vaccination against hepatitis A and B and vaccination and antiviral therapy against influenza, see CDC. Prevention of hepatitis A through active or passive immunization: recommendations of the Advisory Committee on Immunization Practices (ACIP). MMWR 1996;45(No. RR-15); CDC. Hepatitis B virus: a comprehensive strategy for eliminating transmission in the United States through universal childhood vaccination: recommendations of the Advisory Committee on Immunization Practices (ACIP). MMWR 1991;40(No. RR-13); and CDC Prevention and control of influenza: recommendations of the Advisory Committee on Immunization Practices (ACIP). MMWR 1999;48(No. RR-4).

[g] In a few unusual occupational or other circumstances, prophylaxis should be considered; consult a specialist.

[h] Acyclovir is not protective against CMV. Valacyclovir is not recommended because of an unexplained trend toward increased mortality observed in persons with AIDS who were being administered this drug for prevention of CMV disease.

TABLE 64-2 Prophylaxis to Prevent Recurrence of Opportunistic Disease (After Chemotherapy for Acute Disease) in Adults and Adolescents Infected with Human Immunodeficiency Virus

		Preventive Regimens	
Pathogen	**Indication**	**First Choice**	**Alternatives**
I. Recommended for Life as Standard of Care			
Pneumocystis carinii	Prior *P. carinii* pneumonia	trimethoprim-sulfamethoxazole (TMP-SMZ), 1 DS PO q.d. (AI); TMP-SMZ 1 SS PO q.d. (AI)	dapsone, 50 mg PO b.i.d. *or* 100 mg PO q.d. (BI); dapsone, 50 mg PO q.d. *plus* pyrimethamine, 50 mg PO q.w. *plus* leucovorin, 25 mg PO q.w. (BI); dapsone, 200 mg PO *plus* pyrimethamine, 75 mg PO *plus* leucovorin, 25 mg PO q.w. (BI); aerosolized pentamidine, 300 mg q.m. via Respirgard II nebulizer (BI); atovaquone, 1500 mg PO q.d. (BI); TMP-SMZ, 1 DS PO t.i.w. (CI)
Toxoplasma gondii[a]	Prior toxoplasmic encephalitis	sulfadiazine, 500-1000 mg PO q.i.d. *plus* pyrimethamine, 25-75 mg PO q.d. *plus* leucovorin, 10-25 mg PO q.d. (AI)	clindamycin, 300-450 mg PO q6-8h *plus* pyrimethamine, 25-75 mg PO q.d. *plus* leucovorin, 10-25 mg PO q.d. (BI); atovaquone, 750 mg PO q6-12h with or without pyrimethamine, 25 mg PO q.d. *plus* leucovorin, 10 mg PO q.d. (CIII)
Mycobacterium avium complex[b]	Documented disseminated disease	clarithromycin, 500 mg PO b.i.d. (AI) *plus* ethambutol, 15 mg/kg PO q.d. (AII); with or without rifabutin, 300 mg PO q.d. (CI)	azithromycin, 500 mg PO q.d. (AII) *plus* ethambutol, 15 mg/kg PO q.d. (AII); with or without rifabutin, 300 mg PO q.d. (CI)
Cytomegalovirus	Prior end-organ disease	ganciclovir, 5-6 mg/kg IV 5-7 days/wk or 1000 mg PO t.i.d. (AI); or foscarnet, 90-120 mg/kg IV q.d. (AI); or (for retinitis) ganciclovir sustained-release implant q 6-9 months *plus* ganciclovir, 1.0-1.5 g PO t.i.d. (AI)	cidofovir, 5 mg/kg IV q.o.w. with probenecid 2 g PO 3 hours before the dose followed by 1 g PO given 2 hours after the dose, and 1 g PO 8 hours after the dose (total of 4 g) (AI). Fomivirsen 1 vial (330 μg) injected into the vitreous, then repeated every 2-4 weeks (AI)
Cryptococcus neoformans	Documented disease	fluconazole, 200 mg PO q.d. (AI)	amphotericin B, 0.6-1.0 mg/kg IV q.w.-t.i.w. (AI); itraconazole, 200 mg PO q.d. (BI)
Histoplasma capsulatum	Documented disease	itraconazole capsule, 200 mg PO b.i.d. (AI)	amphotericin B, 1.0 mg/kg IV q.w. (AI)
Coccidioides immitis	Documented disease	fluconazole, 400 mg PO q.d. (AII)	amphotericin B, 1.0 mg/kg IV q.w. (AI); itraconazole, 200 mg PO b.i.d. (AII)
Salmonella species, (non-typhi)[c]	Bacteremia	ciprofloxacin, 500 mg PO b.i.d. for several months (BII)	antibiotic chemoprophylaxis with another active agent (CIII)

From 1999 USPHS/IDSA Prevention of Opportunistic Infections Working Group, U.S. Public Health Service and Infectious Diseases Society of America. (1999). *USPHS/IDSA guidelines for the prevention of opportunistic infections in persons infected with human immunodeficiency virus.* 48(RR10), 1-59; www.cdc.gov/nchstp/tb/pubs/mmwr/rr4810.pdf

Continued

TABLE 64-2 Prophylaxis to Prevent Recurrence of Opportunistic Disease (After Chemotherapy for Acute Disease) in Adults and Adolescents Infected with Human Immunodeficiency Virus—cont'd

		Preventive Regimens	
Pathogen	**Indication**	**First Choice**	**Alternatives**
II. Recommended Only if Subsequent Episodes Are Frequent or Severe			
Herpes simplex virus	Frequent/severe recurrences	acyclovir, 200 mg PO t.i.d. or 400 mg PO b.i.d. (AI) famciclovir 500 mg PO b.i.d. (AI)	valacyclovir, 500 mg PO b.i.d. (CIII)
Candida (oropharyngeal or vaginal)	Frequent/severe recurrences	fluconazole 100-200 mg PO q.d. (CI)	itraconazole solution, 200 mg PO q.d. (CI); ketoconazole, 200 mg PO q.d. (CIII)
Candida (esophageal)	Frequent/severe recurrences	fluconazole 100-200 mg PO q.d. (BI)	itraconazole solution, 200 mg PO q.d. (BI); ketoconazole, 200 mg PO q.d. (CIII)

From 1999 USPHS/IDSA Prevention of Opportunistic Infections Working Group, U.S. Public Health Service and Infectious Diseases Society of America. (1999). *USPHS/IDSA guidelines for the prevention of opportunistic infections in persons infected with human immunodeficiency virus.* 48(RR10), 1-59; www.cdc.gov/epo/mmwr/preview/mmwrhtml/rr4810al.htm (2/17/00).

NOTES: Information included in these guidelines might not represent Food and Drug Administration (FDA) approval or approved labeling for the particular products or indications in question. Specifically, the terms "safe" and "effective" might not be synonymous with the FDA-defined legal standards for product approval.

The Respirgard II nebulizer is manufactured by Marquest, Englewood, Colorado. Letters and Roman numerals in parentheses after regimens indicate the strength of the recommendation and the quality of evidence supporting it.

ABBREVIATIONS: *b.i.d.*, twice a day; *DS*, double-strength tablet; *PO*, by mouth; *q.d.*, daily; *q.m.*, monthly; *q.w.*, weekly; *q.o.w.*, every other week; *SS*, single-strength tablet; *t.i.d.*, three times a day; *t.i.w.*, three times a week; and TMP-SMZ, trimethoprim-sulfamethoxazole.

[a] Pyrimethamine-sulfadiazine confers protection against PCP as well as toxoplasmosis; clindamycin-pyrimethamine does not.

[b] Many multiple-drug regimens are poorly tolerated. Drug interactions (e.g., those seen with clarithromycin and rifabutin) can be problematic; rifabutin has been associated with uveitis, especially when administered at daily doses of >300 mg or concurrently with fluconazole or clarithromycin. Rifabutin should not be administered concurrently with hard-gel saquinavir or delavirdine; caution is also advised when the drug is coadministered with soft-gel saquinavir. Rifabutin may be administered at reduced dose (150 mg q.d. with indinavir, nelfinavir, or amprenavir; or 150 mg q.o.d. with ritonavir) or at increased dose (450 mg q.d. with efavirenz); (CDC. Prevention and treatment of tuberculosis among patients infected with human immunodeficiency virus: principles of therapy and revised recommendations. MMWR 1998;47[RR-20]). Information is lacking regarding coadministration of rifabutin with nevirapine.

[c] Efficacy of eradication of *Salmonella* has been demonstrated only for ciprofloxacin.

BOX 64-4

Pneumocystis carinii Pneumonia

Pneumocystis carinii pneumonia (PCP) is a common infection in persons with bone marrow transplants and AIDS. Untreated PCP has a high mortality rate.

Symptoms

Fever
Dry, persistent, nonproductive cough
Shallow breathing
Progressive shortness of breath
Weight loss
Night sweats

Treatment

Active Infection

TMP-SMX, IV or PO, 15 to 20 mg/kg/day TMX and 75 to 100 mg/kg/day SMX in 4 divided doses for 2 to 3 weeks

Pentamidine IV (Pentam 300): 4 mg/kg/day administered over 60 to 90 minutes for 2 to 3 weeks

Atovaquone (Mepron): 750 mg every 8 hours for 3 weeks

Trimetrexate (Neutrexin), a dihydrofolate reductase inhibitor: 45 mg/m^2 every 6 hours for 3 weeks; may be given with sulfadiazine, 1 g every 6 hours for 3 weeks

Prophylaxis

TMP-SMX, PO: 160 mg TMP with 800 mg SMX daily or three times a week

Pentamidine inhalation (NebuPent): 300 mg once a month

Information from *Drug Facts and Comparisons.* (2000). St. Louis: Facts and Comparisons.
TMP-SMX, Trimethoprim-sulfamethoxazole (Cotrimoxazole).

Case Study *Home Treatment of the Client with AIDS*

Robbie Parks is a 21-year-old construction worker and has a history of heroin abuse. He has been experiencing fever, weight loss, and diarrhea and has been diagnosed as having AIDS. At this time he has a low-grade fever, severe diarrhea, and a productive cough. He is admitted to the hospital with *P. carinii* pneumonia. While hospitalized, he develops systemic candidiasis and is treated symptomatically. The symptoms resolve somewhat, and he is discharged. He is sent home on fluconazole (Diflucan), 400 mg IV daily the first day and then 200 mg IV daily for the following 4 weeks.

1. Describe the postulated mechanism of action for fluconazole.
2. What medication side effects should this client be taught to look for?
3. What substance has the potential for interacting with the drug?
4. Robbie's symptoms have completely resolved, and he wonders how much longer he must receive the drug. What should you tell him?

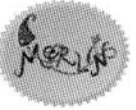

For answer guidelines, go to mosby.com/MERLIN/McKenry/.

the compromised immune system. Lymphokines are protein substances released by sensitized lymphocytes when in contact with specific antigens to activate macrophages to stimulate humoral and cellular immunity for the host. Interleukins have been called the chemical messengers of immune cell communication. IL-2 is believed to be a T cell growth factor that promotes the long-term survival and growth of the T lymphocytes, which is necessary for the continuation of the immune response and is also involved in the rejection of transplanted organs. Although some persons have been helped with these therapies, to date the data on therapy effectiveness is conflicting; adjuvant therapies were required in at least some instances (Morse et al., 1996).

■ Nursing Management

Colony Stimulating Factor Therapy

In addition to the following discussion about clients receiving filgrastim or sargramostim (as examples of CSF therapy), see Nursing Management: The Immunosuppressed Client, p. 1095.

■ Assessment. CSF therapy is used in clients with serious underlying disease. A causal relationship between the drug and the adverse effects is not clear, because many adverse reactions have been reported in both clients receiving this drug and in clients not receiving the drug. A complete baseline assessment should be performed with the client to facilitate the monitoring of any change in signs and symptoms that may occur.

If the client has excessive leukemic myeloid blasts in the bone marrow or peripheral blood (10% or more), more growth may be stimulated by CSF agents. For filgrastim, sensitivity to *Escherichia coli*–derived proteins must be determined; with sargramostim, a sensitivity to yeast-derived proteins needs to be determined.

■ Nursing Diagnosis. The client receiving CSF agents is at risk for the following nursing diagnoses: impaired comfort (pain at injection site, headache, arthralgias, myalgias, first-dose reaction for sargramostim [hypotension, flushing, syncope]); impaired tissue integrity (thrombophlebitis at the infusion site); and the potential complications of allergic reaction, dysrhythmias, and pericarditis.

■ Implementation

■ *Monitoring.* CBCs and platelet counts should be performed twice weekly. CSF therapy is usually discontinued if the absolute neutrophil count (ANC) exceeds 10,000/mm^3. Be alert to the development of adult respiratory syndrome. Check the client's blood pressure, because a transient hypotension may occur. Monitor the client's general health status to provide for supportive care.

■ *Intervention.* If administered to a client receiving chemotherapy, immunomodulator therapy is usually begun at least 24 hours after the last dose of chemotherapy and is discontinued at least 24 hours before the next dose of chemotherapy. With radiotherapy, the timing is 12 hours before and after therapy.

Examine the vial to ensure that the solution is clear and does not contain particulate matter. Do not shake the vial. Keep the medication refrigerated, although it is stable for 24 hours at room temperature.

■ *Education.* If it is determined that the client or caregiver can administer the drug in the home safely and effectively, they should be given the client information supplied by the manufacturer. They should also receive instructions on the proper dosage and administration of the drug, including aseptic technique. Instruction should be provided on the proper safe disposal of needles, syringes, and any unused drug.

■ Evaluation. The expected outcome of CSF therapy is that the client's ANC will exceed 10,000/ mm^3. The client or caregiver will manage the therapeutic regimen effectively.

SUMMARY

Immunosuppressants and immunomodulators are relatively new products used to lessen or modify an immune system response. Research is extensive, and many new pharmacologic products are likely to be developed in the next few years. Nursing management centers on careful medical asepsis, proper diet and oral hygiene, and prevention of infection. As new drugs continue to be introduced, the nurse's role in this important new therapy is likely to continue to expand.

Critical Thinking Questions

1. Susan Goode, age 35, has just received a kidney transplant. Her physician has prescribed cyclosporine, 15 mg/kg PO daily. What is the mechanism of action by which cyclosporine prevents transplant rejection? What nursing care is required to support Susan's cyclosporine regimen?
2. Herman Myers, age 45, is receiving cyclic antineoplastic chemotherapy. He has been prescribed filgrastim to combat his chemotherapy-induced neutropenia. What is special about the timing of the administration of the two medications? Why is that timing important?

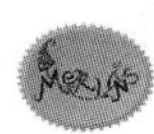

Collaborative Learning Activities

For Collaborative Learning Activities, go to mosby.com/MERLIN/McKenry/.

CASE STUDY

For a Case Study that will help ensure mastery of this chapter content, go to mosby.com/MERLIN/McKenry/.

BIBLIOGRAPHY

American Hospital Formulary Service. (1999). *AHFS drug information '99*. Bethesda, MD: American Society of Hospital Pharmacists.

Anderson, K.N., Anderson, L.E., & Glanze, W.D. (Eds.) (1998). *Mosby's medical, nursing, & allied health dictionary* (5th ed.). St. Louis: Mosby.

Atlanta. (1997). AIDS Study Shows Drop of 26% in Mortality Rate. Wall Street Journal, September 23, 1997; www.aegis.com/aegis/news/wsj/wj970902.html (7/21/98).

Centers for Disease Control and Prevention. (1992). 1993 revised classification for HIV infection and expanded surveillance case definition for AIDS among adolescents and adults. *MMWR: Morbidity & Mortality Weekly Report, 41*(RR-17), 1.

Cooper, M. (1996). Rare AIDS strain found for first time in U.S., AEGIS (AIDS Education Global Information System); www.aegis.com/aegis/news/re/re1996/re960729.html (7/21/98).

Cowan, K. (1993). AIDS in the elderly. *Geriatric Medicine Currents, 14*(1), 4.

Drug Facts and Comparisons. (2000). St. Louis: Facts and Comparisons.

European Mycophenolate Mofetil Cooperative Study Group. (1999). Mycophenolate mofetil in renal transplantation: 3-year results from the placebo-controlled trial. *Transplantation, 68*(3), 3916.

Fletcher, C.V. & Collier, A.C. (1996). Principles and management of the acquired immunodeficiency syndrome. In J.T. DiPiro, R.L. Talbert, G.C. Yee, G.R. Matzke, B.G. Wells, & L.M. Posey (Eds.), *Pharmacotherapy: A pathophysiologic approach* (2nd ed.). Norwalk, CT: Appleton & Lange.

Gilden, D. (1996). Protease inhibitor new math. *GMHC Treatment Issues: Newsletter of Experiments in AIDS Therapy, 10*(5), 3-6.

Hengster, P., Pescovitz, M.D., Hyatt, D., & Margreiter, R. (1999). Cytomegalovirus infections after treatment with daclizumab, an anti IL-2 receptor antibody, for prevention of renal allograft rejection. Roche Study Group. *Transplantation, 68*(2), 310-313.

Huff, A. (1997/1998). Protease inhibitor side effects take people by surprise. *GMHC Treatment Issues, 12*(1), 25-27.

Jain, A. Reyes, J., Kashyap, R., Rohal, S., Abu-Elmagd, K., Starzl, T., Fung, J. (1999). What have we learned about primary liver transplantation under tacrolimus immunosuppression? Long-term follow-up of the first 1000 patients. *Annals of Surgery, 230*(3),441-448.

Kim, Y.S., Moon, J.I., Kim, S.I., & Park, K. (1999). Clear benefit of mycophenolate mofetil-based triple therapy in reducing the incidence of acute rejection after living donor renal transplantations. *Transplantation, 68*(4), 578-581.

Morse, G.D., Shelton, M.J., & O'Donnell, A.M. (1996). Human immunodeficiency virus (HIV) infection. In L.Y. Young, & M.A. Koda-Kimble, (Eds.), *Applied therapeutics* (6th ed.). Vancouver, WA: Applied Therapeutics.

Project Inform. (1996). The new era in AIDS treatment. *PI Perspective, 18*, 1-8.

Reichenspurner, H., Kur, F., Treede, H., Meiser, B.M., Deutsch, O., Welz, A., Vogelmeier, C., Schwaiblmair, M., Muller ,C., Furst, H., Briegel, J., Reichart, B. (1999). Optimization of the immunosuppressive protocol after lung transplantation. *Transplantation, 68*(1), 67-71.

Reuters Health Information Systems. (1998). New CDC Guidelines for Occupational HIV Exposure, AEGIS (AIDS Education Global Information System (from *MMWR* 1996; 45:468-472); www.aegis.com/aegis/news/re/re1997/re970294.html and www.aegis.com/aegis/news/re/re1997/re970292.html (7/21/98).

Roberti, I. & Reisman, L. (1999). A comparative analysis of the use of mycophenolate mofetil in pediatric vs. adult renal allograft recipients. *Pediatric Transplant, 3*(3), 231-235.

Rothwell, W.S., Gloor, J.M., Morgenstern, B.Z., & Milliner, D.S. (1999). Disseminated varicella infection in pediatric renal transplant recipients treated with mycophenolate mofetil. *Transplantation, 68*(1):158-161.

United States Pharmacopeia Dispensing Information (USP DI): Drug information for the health care professional (19th ed.). (1999). Rockville, MD: United States Pharmacopeial Convention.

USPHS/IDSA Guidelines Virus (1999). Guidelines for the prevention of opportunistic infections in persons infected with human immunodeficiency. *MMWR, 48*(RR-10):1-59.

U.S. Renal Transplant Mycophenolate Mofetil Study Group. (1999). Mycophenolate mofetil in cadaveric renal transplantation. *American Journal of Kidney Disease, 34*(2), 296-303.

Wiesner, R.H., Batts, K.P., & Krom, R.A. (1999). Evolving concepts in the diagnosis, pathogenesis, and treatment of chronic hepatitis allograft rejection. *Liver Transplant Surgery, 5*(5), 399-400.

Wong, R.J. (1993). Treating HIV infection: What pharmacists need to know. *American Pharmacist, NS33*(5), 57.

65 Overview of the Integumentary System

Chapter Focus

The skin is the body's largest organ and forms a protective boundary between the internal environment and external world. Drugs are applied to the skin in the case of impaired skin integrity, and the skin is also being increasingly used for the administration of drugs for systemic purposes. The nurse must know the structure and function of the skin in order to administer drugs for both purposes.

Learning Objectives

1. Describe the two layers of the skin.
2. Differentiate between the three types of exocrine glands.
3. Explain five major functions of the skin.
4. Name three appendages of the skin.

Key Terms

apocrine glands, p. 1116
dermis, p. 1116
eccrine glands, p. 1116
epidermis, p. 1116
exocrine glands, p. 1116
melanin, p. 1116
sebaceous glands, p. 1116

The skin (or integument) has been described as the largest organ in the body. In most disease states, medications are administered at a site that is distant from the target organ. In dermatology, medications can be applied directly to the target site; some skin conditions, however, may require systemic medications. Because skin functions are vital to survival and are also quite diverse, this chapter reviews the structure of the skin, functions of the skin, and skin appendages (Figure 65-1).

STRUCTURE OF THE SKIN

The skin is made up of two layers: the epidermis and the dermis. The **epidermis,** or outer skin layer, consists of four strata or layers:

1. *Stratum corneum (horny layer).* This layer contains dead outer cells that have been converted to keratin, a water-repellent protein. This layer forms a protective cover for the body; it will desquamate or shed and be replaced by new cells from the bottom layers.
2. *Stratum lucidum or clear layer.* This area contains translucent flat cells; keratin is formed here.
3. *Stratum granulosum or granular layer.* Granules are located in the cytoplasm of these cells. Cells die in this layer of skin.
4. *Stratum germinativum.* This layer has been divided into two layers in some references; the top layer is the stratum spinosum, and the innermost layer is the stratum basale. The latter two names were devised to describe the cellular structure of the two layers; the stratum spinosum contains spinelike cells, whereas the stratum basale has column-shaped cells. The cells in the latter area germinate; they undergo cellular mitosis to generate new cells for the skin.

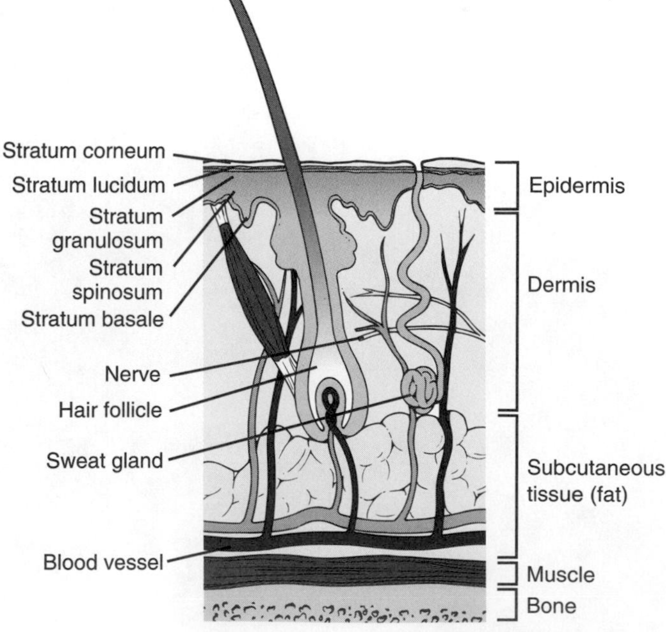

Figure 65-1 Structures of the skin.

Melanocytes, which are responsible for synthesizing **melanin,** a skin color pigment that occurs naturally in the hair and skin, are also located deep in the stratum germinativum. The more melanin that is present, the deeper the brown skin color. Melanin also is a protective agent; it blocks ultraviolet rays, thus preventing injury to the underlying dermis and tissues.

The epidermis has no direct blood supply of its own; it is nourished only by diffusion. The **dermis** lies between the epidermis and subcutaneous fat. It is approximately 40 times thicker than the epidermis, and it contains and provides skin support from its blood vessels, nerves, lymphatic tissue, and elastic and connective tissues. The two main divisions of the dermis are the papillary dermis and the reticular dermis. Sweat glands, sebaceous glands, and hair follicles originate in the reticular dermis, and their structures branch out in the papillary dermis.

Below the dermis layer is the hypodermis or subcutaneous layer, which contributes flexibility to the skin. Subcutaneous fat tissue is an area for thermal insulation, nutrition, and cushioning or padding.

The skin contains three types of **exocrine glands**: sebaceous, eccrine, and apocrine. These exocrine glands are multicellular glands that open on the surface of the skin through ducts in the epithelium.

Sebaceous glands are large, lipid-containing cells that produce sebum, the oil or film layer that covers the epidermis; these glands are especially abundant in the scalp, face, anus, and external ear. Sebum protects and lubricates the skin; it is not only water repellent but also has some antiseptic effects. The sebaceous fluid travels by way of a short duct (sebaceous duct) to the hair follicles in the upper dermis. Therefore hair, which is located everywhere on the skin except the palms of the hands, soles of the feet, and mucous membrane tissues, is lubricated.

The **eccrine glands,** or sweat glands, are also widely distributed on the skin surface, including the soles and palms. These glands help to regulate body temperature by promoting cooling through evaporation of their secretion; they also help to prevent excessive skin dryness.

The **apocrine glands** are located mainly in the axillae, genital organs, and breast areas. They are odoriferous and are believed to represent scent or sex glands.

Normal skin is weakly acidic, with a pH of 4.5 to 5.5. This acid mantle is a protective mechanism, because microorganisms grow best at a pH 6.0 to 7.5. Infected areas of the skin usually have a higher pH.

FUNCTIONS OF THE SKIN

The skin serves many functions in the body. The following are some of the major functions:

- **Protector.** The skin forms a protective covering for the entire body. It protects the internal organs and their environment from external forces. Thus it is a barrier against invasion by microorganisms and chemicals.

- **Organ of sensation.** Nerve endings permit the transfer of stimuli sensations, such as heat, cold, pressure, and pain.
- **Body temperature regulator.** The skin maintains body temperature homeostasis by regulating heat loss or heat conservation. Blood vessels in the dermis area can dilate, and perspiration increases when body temperature is elevated. If the body temperature is below normal, the skin blood vessels constrict, and perspiration is decreased to conserve body heat.

Skin excretes fluid and electrolytes (sweat glands), stores fat, synthesizes vitamin D (when skin is exposed to sunlight or ultraviolet rays, 7-dehydrocholesterol—a steroid normally present in the skin—is converted to vitamin D_3), and provides a site for drug absorption. Fat-soluble vitamins (A, D, E, and K), estrogens, corticoid hormones, and some chemicals can be absorbed through the skin.

Skin contributes to the concept of body image and a feeling of well-being. A disfiguring skin condition can lead to emotional problems, and a chronic skin condition may also lead to depression.

APPENDAGES OF THE SKIN

The appendages of the skin are the hair, nails, and skin glands. These areas are discussed with the drug therapy specific for these sites.

SUMMARY

The skin, the largest organ of the body, consists of two layers: the epidermis and the dermis. The pharmacologic activity of dermatologic agents occurs at the target site. Skin injuries, lesions, and disorders result in a variety of dermatologic problems for the client, as well as various nursing care issues for the health care provider. Major skin problems are discussed in the next chapter.

Critical Thinking Questions

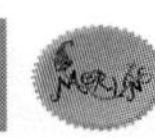

1. Johnny, age 10, is outside playing ball on a hot summer day. How does his skin serve to regulate his body temperature?
2. In what other ways does the skin function to protect the body?

Collaborative Learning Activities

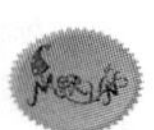

For Collaborative Learning Activities, go to mosby.com/MERLIN/McKenry/.

BIBLIOGRAPHY

Anderson, K.N., Anderson, L.E., & Glanze, W.D. (Eds.) (1998). *Mosby's medical, nursing, & allied health dictionary* (5th ed.). St. Louis: Mosby.

McCance, K.L., & Huether, S.E. (1998). *Pathophysiology: The biologic basis for disease in adults and children* (3rd ed.). St. Louis: Mosby.

Seeley, R.R., Stephens, T.D., & Tate, P. (1995). *Anatomy and physiology* (3rd ed.). St. Louis: Mosby.

Thibodeau, G.A. & Patton, K.T. (1999). *Anatomy and physiology* (4th ed.). St. Louis: Mosby.

66 Dermatologic Drugs

Chapter Focus

The integumentary system is the largest organ system in the body. The skin performs a number of vital functions, such as protecting internal structures from mechanical and chemical damage, preventing the entry of infectious agents, providing protection against ultraviolet radiation from the sun, preventing dehydration, regulating temperature, producing vitamin D, and detecting stimuli. In addition, the skin often contributes to our definition of who we are through color, aging processes, scarring, and other conditions. Clients with skin disorders may experience body image disturbance along with their physical conditions. The nurse needs to be not only skilled at various procedures related to treatment of skin disorders but also sensitive to the client as a whole.

Learning Objectives

1. State the principles of skin absorption.
2. Describe different types of lesions and some of the conditions associated with them.
3. Identify common drug-induced dermatologic conditions.
4. Identify life-threatening, drug-induced skin eruptions.
5. Describe the general goals of dermatologic therapy.
6. Describe the general dermatologic preparations and their indications: baths, soaps, solutions, lotions, and cleansers.
7. Implement the nursing management for the care of clients receiving therapy with topical antiinfectives, antiinflammatory corticosteroids, topical anesthetics, and acne and burn products.
8. Discuss ectoparasitic diseases and the use of topical ectoparasiticidal drugs in their treatment.

Key Terms

ectoparasite, p. 1136
keratolytic, p. 1130
sun protection factor (SPF), p. 1126

Many dermatologic preparations are available to treat the numerous and common skin disorders. Certain ointments, creams, powders, or specific vehicles often provide a desired effect without the addition of an active ingredient. For example, an ointment with an occlusive emollient effect (e.g., lanolin or a synthetic base) is desired for clients with the dry, scaly skin found in psoriasis or dry eczema. Clients with a moist or dry skin condition may receive a cooling emollient preparation that is also moisturizing, such as a cream formulation.

Clients with an acute inflammation that is weeping or oozing often need a drying and soothing lotion, such as a saline solution, aluminum acetate solution, or calamine lotion. A lichenified, oozing skin problem (eczema) may need a protective and drying agent, such as coal tar paste, Lassar's paste, or zinc compound paste. If the skin problem is sore, wet, and located on an elbow or knee, a dusting powder such as talcum or starch may be appropriate to reduce friction and help to dry the area.

SKIN DISORDERS

Reactions or disorders of the skin are manifested by symptoms such as itching, pain, or tingling, and by signs such as swelling, redness, papules, pustules, blisters, and hives. Common dermatologic disorders in the United States and Canada include acne vulgaris (cystic acne and acne scars), atopic dermatitis, eczema, folliculitis, fungus infections, herpes simplex, lichen simplex chronicus, psoriasis, seborrheic dermatitis, verruca (warts), and vitiligo.

A skin reaction that makes the client uncomfortable or unsightly may be due to a drug sensitivity, allergy, infection, emotional conflict, genetic disease (e.g., atopic eczema, psoriasis), hormonal imbalance, or degenerative disease. Sometimes the cause of the skin disorder is unknown; in such cases treatment may be empiric in the hope that the right remedy is found.

Dermatologic diagnosis includes physical assessment, personal and family medical history, drug history (including over-the-counter [OTC] medications), and laboratory tests, biopsy, and cytodiagnosis.

When the nature of the lesion has been established, its characteristics should be defined according to size, shape, surface, and color (Box 66-1).

The next step is to discover the distribution of the condition; sometimes the diagnosis can be made from the distribution alone. However, a disease should not be ruled out as a possible diagnosis just because it is not found in its usual pattern of distribution. For example, psoriasis is commonly found on the extensors, but occasionally it is seen as a solitary lesion in the external ear. A basal cell carcinoma is most common on the face, but occasionally it occurs on the trunk. On the other hand, rosacea attacks only those areas of the face that flush.

Box 66-2 is a summary of common drug-induced dermatologic conditions. Some may even be life-threatening. See Table 66-1 for the drugs most commonly involved in life-threatening, drug-induced skin eruptions.

The nurse always needs to be cognizant of a client's drug history and current therapy in order to relate such lesions and sequelae to the appropriate cause; simply discontinuing a particular drug can often resolve a complicated dermatologic problem or sequelae of unknown origin.

The following are some dermatologic conditions for which drugs may be indicated:

1. Eczema and dermatitis are noninfectious inflammatory dermatoses. Contact dermatitis has clinical features that include a skin rash with eczema (red, thick, crusty, fissured, suppurating area) in various stages. The causes may be from contact with a primary irritant (acids, oils, soaps) in the environment, home, or work place or from a delayed allergic reaction (as seen with poison ivy contact).
2. Atopic dermatitis appears as general eczema dermatitis, usually on the flexor body surfaces; it has genetic associations with hay fever or asthma.
3. Seborrheic dermatitis often appears on the scalp, eyebrows, ears, or sternum as a brown to red scaly rash.
4. Stasis dermatitis often preceding a venous stasis ulcer is found on the lower legs secondary to venous stasis and poor vascularity; it is brown and eczematous in appearance.
5. Papulosquamous eruptions are noninfectious inflammatory dermatoses that include urticaria (hives), psoriasis, pityriasis rosea, lichen planus, and exfoliative dermatitis. The nurse will see acute urticaria as an insidious, itchy erythematous wheal resulting from an allergen. Chronic urticaria appears as a large hive without the sensation of itch or pruritus, and it is often accompanied by angioneurotic edema.
6. Psoriasis often appears as erythematous plaques and orange-red-brown lesions covered with silvery scales. Psoriasis is often found on the scalp and extensor surfaces of the limbs and neck. The nails often become thick and irregular.
7. Pityriasis rosea is a self-limited, oval salmon-colored patch that follows the axis of the skin cleavage lines. The major patches appear on the trunk, and smaller scales appear on the peripheral areas.
8. Infectious inflammatory dermatoses include viral diseases (verruca [wart], herpes simplex, varicella zoster/chickenpox), bacterial diseases (impetigo, folliculitis, furuncle [boil]), and fungal diseases. Herpes simplex and infectious inflammatory dermatoses appear as vesicles with an inflamed base and have an incubation period of up to 2 weeks in the primary infection. Late antibody development occurs. The herpes virus type 1 affects the skin and the oral cavity, whereas herpes virus type 2 affects the skin of neonates and genital mucosa. A recurrent infection is a reactivation of the older infection or new infection; antibodies appear early.
9. Fungal diseases, which include tinea or dermatophytosis, appear in the following various clinical clas-

BOX 66-1

Different Types of Lesions and Some Conditions Associated with Them

Macule—flat; nonpalpable; circumscribed; less than 1 cm in diameter; brown, red, purple, white, or tan in color
Examples: Freckles; flat moles; rubella; rubeola; drug eruptions

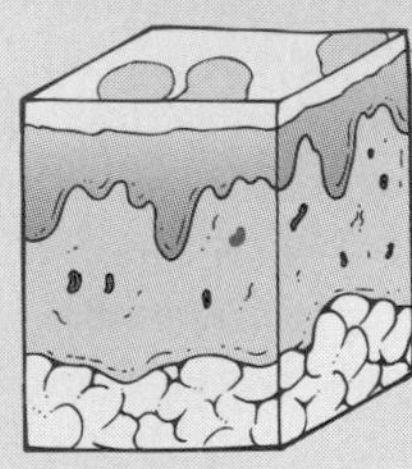

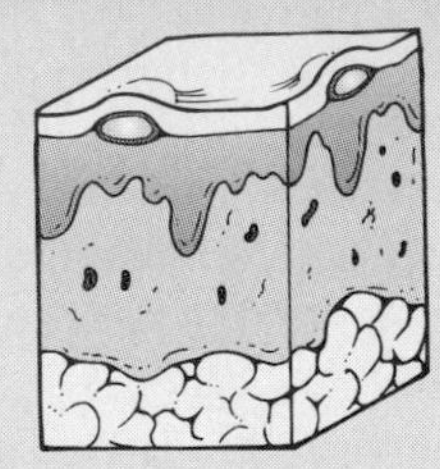

Vesicle—elevated; circumscribed; superficial; filled with serous fluid; less than 1 cm in diameter
Examples: Blister varicella

Papule—elevated; palpable; firm; circumscribed; less than 1 cm in diameter; brown, red, pink, tan, or bluish red in color
Examples: Warts; drug-related eruptions; pigmented nevi; eczema

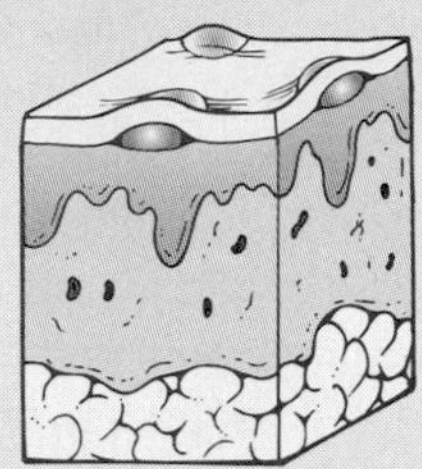

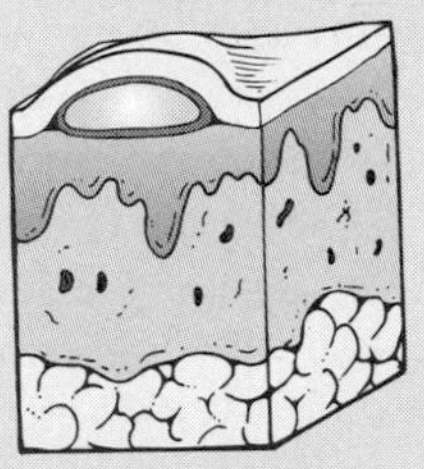

Bulla—vesicle greater than 1 cm in diameter
Examples: Blister; pemphigus vulgaris

Plaque—elevated; flat topped; firm; rough; superficial papule greater than 1 cm in diameter, may be coalesced papules
Example: Psoriasis; seborrheic and actinic keratoses; eczema

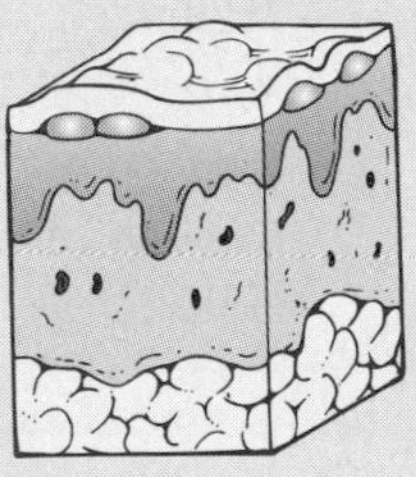

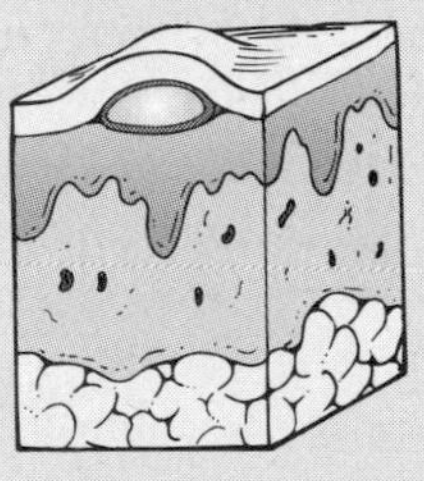

Pustule—elevated; superficial; similar to vesicle but filled with purulent fluid
Examples: Impetigo; acne; variola; herpes zoster

Wheal—elevated, irregular-shaped area of cutaneous edema; solid, transient, changing variable diameter; pale pink in color
Examples: Urticaria; insect bites

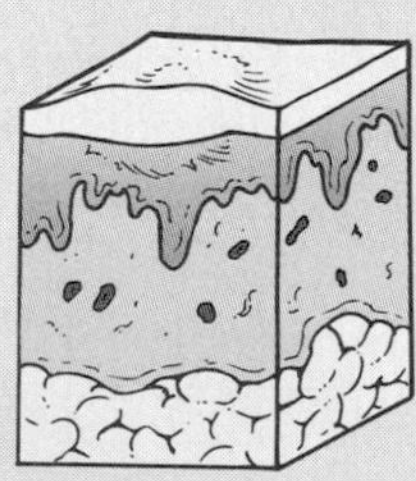

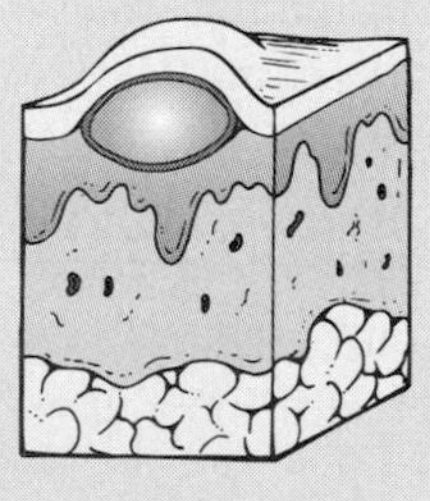

Cyst—elevated; circumscribed; palpable; encapsulated; filled with liquid or semi-solid material
Example: Sebaceous cyst

Nodule—elevated; firm; circumscribed; palpable; deeper in dermis than papule; 1 to 2 cm in diameter
Examples: Erythema nodosum; lipomas

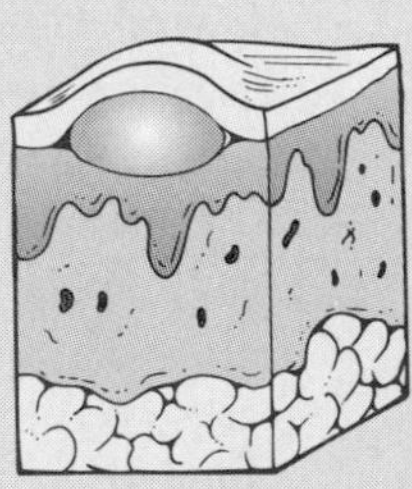

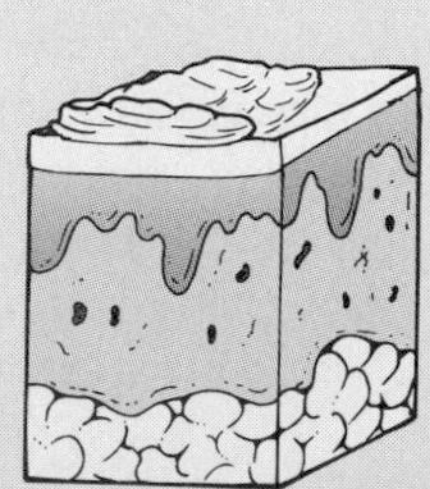

Scale—heaped-up keratinized cells; flaky exfoliation; irregular; thick or thin; dry or oily; varied size; silver, white, or tan in color
Examples: Psoriasis; exfoliative dermatitis

Tumor—elevated; solid; may or may not be clearly demarcated; greater than 2 cm in diameter; may or may not vary from skin color
Example: Neoplasms

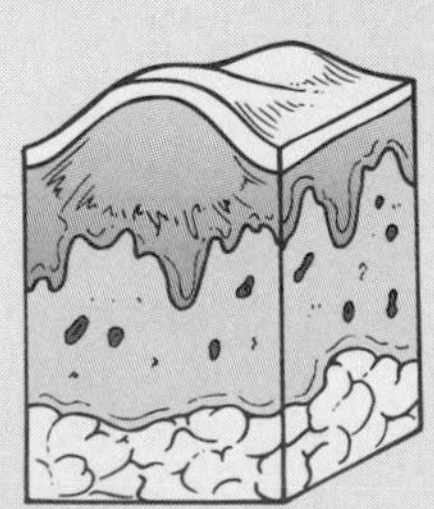

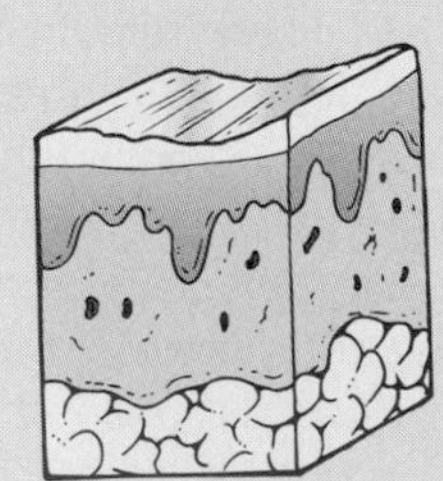

Lichenification—rough, thickened epidermis; accentuated skin markings due to rubbing or irritation; often involves flexor aspect of extremity
Example: Chronic dermatitis

From Beare, P.G. & Myers, J.L. (1998). *Adult health nursing* (3rd ed.) St. Louis: Mosby.

BOX 66-2

Common Drug-Induced Dermatologic Conditions

Drugs Causing an Acneform Reaction

ACTH
androgenic hormones
corticosteroids
cyanocobalamin
hydantoins
iodides
methyltestosterone
oral contraceptives

Drugs Causing Purpura

ACTH
allopurinol
amitriptyline
anticoagulants
barbiturates
carbamides
chloral hydrate
chlorothiazide
chlorpromazine
chlorpropamide
corticosteroids
digitalis
fluoxymesterone
gold salts
griseofulvin
iodides
meprobamate
penicillin
quinidine
rifampin
sulfonamides
thiazides
trifluoperazine

Drugs Causing Urticaria

ACTH
amitriptyline
barbiturates
chloramphenicol
dextran
enzymes
erythromycin
griseofulvin
hydantoins
insulin
iodides
meperidine
meprobamate
mercurials
nitrofurantoin
opioids
penicillin
penicillinase
pentazocine
phenolphthalein
phenothiazines
propoxyphene
rifampin
salicylates
serums
streptomycin
sulfonamides
tetracyclines
thiouracil

Drugs Causing Alopecia

alkylating agents
anticoagulants
antimetabolites
bleomycin
mephenytoin
methimazole
methotrexate
norethindrone acetate
quinacrine
oral contraceptives
warfarin
trimethadione

Drugs Causing Morbilliform Reactions

anticonvulsants
anticholinergics
antihistamines
barbiturates
chloral hydrate
chlordiazepoxide
chlorothiazide
gold salts
griseofulvin
hydantoins
insulin
meprobamate
mercurials
para-aminosalicylic acid
penicillin
phenothiazines
quinacrine
salicylates
serums
streptomycin
sulfonamides
sulfones
tetracyclines
thiouracil

Drugs Causing Lichenoid Reactions

chloroquine
gold salts compounds
para-aminosalicylic acid
quinacrine
quinidine
thiazides

Drugs Causing Fixed Eruptions

acetylsalicylic acid
amphetamine sulfate
anthralin
antipyrine
barbiturates
belladonna
bismuth salts
chloral hydrate
chloroquine
chlorothiazide and sun
chlorpromazine
chlortetracycline
dextroamphetamine
diethylstilbestrol
digitalis
dimenhydrinate
diphenhydramine
disulfiram and alcohol
ephedrine
epinephrine
ergot alkaloids
erythromycin
eucalyptus oil
gold compounds
griseofulvin
iodine
ipecac
karaya gum
magnesium hydroxide
meprobamate
mercury salts
methenamine
opioids
oxytetracycline
para-aminosalicylic acid
penicillin
phenobarbital
phenytoin
potassium chlorate
quinidine
quinine
reserpine
salicylates
saccharin
scopolamine
sodium salicylate
streptomycin
sulfadiazine
sulfapyridine
sulfathiazole
sulfisoxazole
sulfonamides
tetracyclines
tripelennamine
vaccines and immunizing agents

Drugs Causing Contact Dermatitis

antihistamine
bacitracin
balsam of Peru
benzocaine
bleomycin
chloramphenicol
chlorhexidine
chlorphenesin
chlorpromazine
diphenhydramine
ephedrine
formaldehyde
iodine
isoniazid
lanolin
meprobamate
mercurials
neomycin
nitrofurazone
novobiocin
para-aminosalicylic acid
penicillin
phenindamine
phenol
procaine and other anesthetics
promethazine
quinacrine
quinine

Continued

BOX 66-2

Common Drug-Induced Dermatologic Conditions—cont'd

Drugs Causing Contact Dermatitis—cont'd

resorcin
streptomycin
sulfonamides
tetracyclines
thiamine
thimerosal

Photosensitizers

acetohexamide
aminobenzoic acid
anesthetics (procaine group)
antimalarials
barbiturates
benzene
bergamot (perfume)
carbamazepine
carbinoxamine d-form
carrots, wild
cedar oil
celery
chlorophyll
citrus fruits
clover
coal tar
corticosteroids, topical
cyproheptadine
desipramine
diethylstilbestrol
digalloyl trioleate (sunscreen)
dill
diphenhydramine
disopyramide
dyes (methylene blue, toluidine blue)
estrone
fennel
fluorescein dyes
5-fluorouracil
gold salts
grass (meadow)
griseofulvin
haloperidol
lavender oil
lime oil
6-mercaptopurine
methotrimeprazine
methoxsalen
8-methoxypsoralen
mustards
nalidixic acid
naphthalene
oral contraceptives
parsley
parsnips
phenolic compounds
phenothiazines
phenytoin
porphyrins
promethazine
pyrazinamide
quinethazone
quinidine
quinine
salicylanilides
salicylates
sandalwood oil (perfume)
silver salts
sulfonamides
sulfonylureas (antidiabetics)
tetracyclines
thiazide diuretics
tolbutamide
toluene
tricyclic antidepressants
trimethadione
vanillin oils
xylene

TABLE 66-1 Life-Threatening, Drug-Induced Skin Eruptions

Skin Eruption	Description	Drugs Involved
Exfoliative dermatitis	Entire surface of skin is red and scaly and eventually sloughs off. Hair and nails may also be affected. Eruption may take weeks or months to resolve after causative agent is stopped. If not resolved, it may be fatal.	barbiturates, carbamazepine, demeclocycline, furosemide, gold, griseofulvin, penicillin, phenothiazines, phenytoin, sulfonamides, tetracyclines
Stevens-Johnson syndrome (erythema multiforme)	Severe form that involves widespread eruptions or lesions, usually on the face, neck, arms, legs, hands, and feet. May also involve mucosa, and may produce fever and malaise. Syndrome may last for months and is life threatening.	May result from the use of many drugs, especially carbamazepine, penicillin, phenytoin, sulfonamides, tetracyclines
Lupus erythematosus	Erythematous rash that may be flat or elevated (butterfly) on cheek (malar), and across nose. Joint swelling and pain, rash, oral ulcers, serositis, renal, hematologic, pulmonary, and other systems may be affected. Condition is reversible when drug is stopped.	hydantoins, hydralazine, isoniazid, procainamide, quinidine, trimethadione

sifications: tinea capitis (caused by either a *Trichophyton* or *Microsporum* fungal infection in children or adults); tinea corporis (or *Microsporum* in children; *Trichophyton* in adults); tinea cruris (*Epidermophyton* or *Trichophyton*); and tinea pedis; onychomycosis (*Trichophyton*); and tinea versicolor (*Malassezia furfur*). Tinea or dermatophytosis often appears as a scaly, erythematous circular lesion. Tinea versicolor appears as a brown discoloration. Hair breakage is seen in tinea capitis or tinea barbae. The client with onychomycosis has thick, discolored nails.

▪ Nursing Management

Dermatologic Agent Therapy

▪ **Assessment.** Both a thorough history and an objective examination of the dermatologic condition are essential for the initial assessment and ongoing evaluation of nursing

BOX 66-3

Principles of Skin Absorption

Keratin in the outer skin layer provides a waterproof barrier. To enhance drug absorption, the epidermis (keratin skin layer) needs to be hydrated. Therefore some medications are placed under an occlusive dressing (e.g., plastic wrap) or administered in an occlusive type of ointment (petroleum jelly), because both trap and prevent the loss of water (sweat) from the skin, thus increasing epidermis hydration.

Fat- or lipid-soluble drugs are better absorbed through the skin than water-soluble drugs.

In specific body areas, the skin is very thin (eyelids, scrotum area, or the skin of a child) or very thick. The palms of the hands and soles of the feet are nearly impenetrable by topical agents.

Products with alcohol content may be administered for drying effects.

Steroid products thin the skin, and many are contraindicated for the face, groin, and axillae. Fluorinated steroids should not be used for these areas. Hydrocortisone is generally recommended if a steroid is necessary.

care. Elicit information regarding the onset of the problem, changes in the condition since onset, specific cause if known (or if not, recent exposures to new or different activities that might provide a clue about cause), client-determined or prescriber-prescribed factors that may have alleviated the condition, and the client's psychologic response to the problem. Direct inspection and observation should be accomplished with a good light source. Palpation may be necessary, particularly when assessing dark skin, where erythema may not be noticeable but warmth and edema can be determined. Observations should be systematic and thorough, and the left side should be compared with the right. Descriptions need to be specific, using the metric system for measurement, and recorded. It may be helpful to take a Polaroid photo of the affected area as a baseline observation. Recorded changes determine the client's progress toward the desired outcome of resolution of the dermatologic problem.

■ **Nursing Diagnosis.** Clients receiving care with dermatologic agents are at risk for the following nursing diagnoses: impaired skin integrity; impaired comfort (pain, burning, or itching of the affected areas); risk for infection related to open skin areas; self-care deficits related to the location of the affected areas; deficient knowledge related to new or altered dermatologic therapy; and disturbed body image related to perceived and actual disfigurement of the affected areas.

■ **Implementation**

■ ***Monitoring.*** Observation and palpation are essential in evaluating the client's progress toward resolving the dermatologic condition. The description of the dermatologic condition, including its area, body part involvement, depth, surface appearance, color, drainage, sensation, and healing should be monitored and documented along with any systemic effects such as fever. The effectiveness of the prescribed therapy should also be documented.

BOX 66-4

General Goals of Dermatologic Drug Therapy

- Identify and remove the cause of the skin disorder, if possible.
- Institute measures to restore and maintain the structure and normal function of the skin.
- Relieve symptoms that are produced by the disorder, such as itching, dryness, pain, and infection.

■ ***Intervention.*** The manufacturer's instructions should be followed in detail for application of the various preparations used for dermatologic conditions. In addition, some conditions may be severe enough to require supportive therapy that is more systemic in nature. See also Boxes 66-3 and 66-4 regarding skin absorption principles and the general goals of dermatologic drug therapy.

■ ***Education.*** If the etiology of the condition is known, counsel the client on avoiding exposure to the causative agent to prevent future episodes (unless the condition is genetic). Advise the client to maintain good hygiene of the unaffected areas of the body and to cleanse the affected area only in the prescribed fashion. Instruct the client not to touch the affected areas and to dress to avoid or minimize contact with the involved area. Apply only prescribed preparations to the area and follow through with therapy, even when the improvement may not be immediate. Avoid exposing the involved areas to direct sunlight unless advised as part of therapy. The client should be instructed to report any side effects/adverse reactions to the prescriber.

■ **Evaluation.** The expected outcome for therapy with dermatologic agents is that the client's lesions will decrease in size and eventually disappear.

■ ■ ■

As previously stated, so many dermatologic products are available that it would be difficult to discuss all of them in this chapter. For the sake of simplicity, this chapter discusses three selected groups of dermatologic products: general products, prophylactic agents, and therapeutic agents.

General dermatologic products include those previously discussed plus solutions, baths, soaps, wet dressings, and soaks. Prophylactic agents include sunscreens, protectives, and antiseptics and disinfectants. Therapeutic agents include antiinfectives, antiinflammatory corticosteroids, keratolytic agents, acne products, stimulants and irritants, topical anesthetics, products for second- and third-degree burns, antiaging products, and ectoparasiticidal topical drugs.

GENERAL DERMATOLOGIC PREPARATIONS

This section refers to single and combination formulations used as bath preparations, cleansers, soaps, solutions and lotions, emollients, skin protectants, wet dressings and soaks, and rubs and liniments.

Baths

Baths may be used to cleanse the skin, medicate, or reduce temperature. The usual method of cleansing the skin is by the use of soap and water, but this may not be tolerated in skin diseases. In some cases even water is not tolerated; in such cases inert oils must be substituted. Persons with dry skin should bathe less frequently than those with oily skin. Frequent bathing tends to stimulate oil production, causing oily skin to remain oily. It is possible to keep the skin clean without a daily bath. Nurses are sometimes accused of overbathing hospitalized clients, causing their skin to become dry and itchy. For dry skin, an oily lotion is preferable to alcohol (isopropyl or ethyl).

To render baths soothing in irritative conditions, oatmeal, starch, or gelatin may be added—usually 1 to 2 ounces per gallon of water. Oils such as Alpha-Keri and oilated oatmeal (in a proportion of 1 ounce to a tub of water) decrease the drying effect of water and help to relieve the itching of sensitive, xerotic skin. A lubricating topical medication or bland emollient should be applied immediately after the bath while skin is still moist; this increases absorption and hydration.

Soaps

Ordinary soap, the sodium salt of palmitic, oleic, or stearic acids alone or in a mixture, is made by saponifying fats or oils with alkalies. The oil used for castile soap is supposed to be olive oil; some soaps are made with coconut oil. The consistency of the soap depends on the major acid and alkali used.

Although all soaps are relatively alkaline, an excess of free alkali or acid is a potential source of skin irritation. Medicated soaps contain antiseptics, but soaps per se are antiseptic only to the degree that they mechanically clean the skin. Many people believe that soap and water are bad for the complexion; this belief is erroneous, because clean skin helps to promote healthy skin. The soap used in maintaining clean skin should be mild and contain a minimum of irritating materials. Perfumed or medicated soaps may be harmful if the skin is extra sensitive to soap products or if the soap is not adequately rinsed off the skin, stimulates excess production of natural skin oils, or dries the skin excessively. Soaps are irritating to mucous membranes; they are used in enemas mainly because of this action.

Solutions and Lotions

Soothing preparations may be liquids that carry an insoluble powder or suspension, or they may be mild acid or alkaline solutions, such as boric acid solution, limewater, or aluminum acetate used as wet dressings and soaks. Bismuth salts and starch are also commonly used for their soothing effect.

Aluminum Acetate Solution (Burow's Solution, Modified Burow's Solution). This solution is a mild astringent that coagulates bacterial and serum protein. It is diluted with 10 to 40 parts of water before application.

Calamine Lotion. Calamine lotion contains calamine, zinc oxide, bentonite magma, and glycerin in a calcium hydroxide solution. It is a soothing lotion used for the dermatitis caused by conditions such as poison ivy, insect bites, and prickly heat.

Cleansers

Cleansers are usually free of soap or are modified soap products recommended for clients with sensitive, dry, or irritated skin or for clients who may have had a previous reaction to a soap product. These cleansers are less irritating, may contain an emollient substance, and may also have been adjusted to a slightly acidic or neutral pH. Included in this category are Aveeno Cleansing Bar, Lowila Cake, and others.

Emollients

Emollients are fatty or oily substances that may be used to soften or soothe irritated skin and mucous membranes. An emollient is often used as a vehicle for other medicinal substances. Examples of emollients include lanolin, petroleum jelly (Vaseline), vitamin A and D ointment, vitamin E, and cold cream. Examples of emollient products on the market include Panthoderm, vitamin E topical products, vitamin A and D topicals, Lubriderm, Dermassage, Nivea Skin, and many more.

Skin Protectants

Skin protectants are used to coat minor skin irritations or to protect the person's skin from chemical irritants. Some commercially available products include AeroZoin, Benzoin, and Benzoin Compound.

Wet Dressings and Soaks

Wet dressings and soaks include some of the preparations discussed under Solutions and Lotions. These liquids are either a wet or an astringent type of dressing used to treat inflammatory skin conditions such as insect bites and poison ivy. Aluminum acetate solution, Domeboro Powder, and others are available for this use.

Rubs and Liniments

Rubs and liniments are indicated for pain relief for intact skin. Pain caused by muscle aches, neuralgia, rheumatism, arthritis, and sprains are the types of pain that usually respond to these products. The ingredients in the preparations may include a counterirritant (e.g., camphor, oil of cloves, methyl salicylate), an antiseptic (chloroxylenol, eugenol, thymol), a local anesthetic (benzocaine), or analgesics (salicylate-containing substances). Examples from this category include Aspercreme, Ben-Gay, and Icy Hot. See Chapter 14 for information on capsaicin topical.

PROPHYLACTIC AGENTS

Protectives

Protectives are soothing, cooling preparations that form a film on the skin. To be useful, they must not macerate the skin, must prevent drying of the tissues, and must keep out light, air, and dust. Nonabsorbable powders are usually listed as protectives, but they are not particularly useful because they stick to wet surfaces and need to be scraped off, and they do not stick to dry surfaces at all. Nonabsorbable powders include zinc stearate, zinc oxide, certain bismuth preparations, talcum powder, and aluminum silicate.

Collodion is a 5% solution of pyroxylin in a mixture of ether and alcohol. When collodion is applied to the skin, the ether and alcohol evaporate, leaving a transparent film that adheres to the skin to protect it. Flexible collodion is a mixture of collodion with 2% camphor and 3% castor oil. The addition of the latter makes the resulting film elastic and more tenacious. Styptic collodion contains 20% tannic acid and therefore is both astringent and protective.

Although it is safe to say that no substances known at present can stimulate healing at a more rapid rate than is normal under optimal conditions, preparations that act as bland protectives may help by preventing crusting and trauma. In some instances they may reduce offensive odors.

Sunscreen Preparations

Extended exposure to the sun, whether from sunbathing or as a normal consequence of an outdoor occupation, may lead to sunburn and/or premature aging of the skin (photoaging). Certain chemicals (e.g., tetracyclines, sulfonamides, thiazides, phenothiazines), plants, cosmetics, and soaps may cause photosensitivity or phototoxicity when an ultraviolet wavelength substance (UVA-absorbing compound) is present on the skin in sufficient amounts and is also exposed to a particular sunlight wavelength. The substance absorbs the offending wavelength, and energy is transferred; as a result, it becomes destructive to surrounding tissues. The exposed skin rapidly becomes red, painful, prickling, or burning, with a peak skin reaction reached within 24 to 48 hours of exposure. This reaction does not involve the immune system.

A photoallergy reaction is different from a phototoxic reaction; it is less common and requires prior exposure to the photosensitizing agent. The immune system is involved; a delayed hypersensitivity reaction occurs when the photosensitizers react with UVA. The reaction occurs several days after exposure and presents as severe pruritus and a rash that can spread to skin areas that were not exposed to sunlight (Mailloux, 1995).

Excessive exposure to ultraviolet rays (UVRs) may result in skin damage that progresses from minor irritation to a precancerous skin condition and, perhaps, to skin cancer later in life. Cutaneous malignant melanoma has been associated with excessive sun exposure, especially during childhood, whereas large cumulative UVR doses over a lifetime appear to increase the incidence of nonmelanoma skin cancers (Box 66-5).

Sunscreen preparations are applied either to absorb or to reflect the sun's harmful rays. Absorbing agents are chemicals such as aminobenzoic acid (para-aminobenzoic acid [PABA]), benzophenones, cinnamates, and anthranilates; reflectors are physical agents such as titanium dioxide and zinc oxide. The latter agents are opaque (i.e., look like thick paste) and must be applied heavily; thus they are not cosmetically acceptable to most persons. The Food and Drug Administration (FDA) has approved 16 active ingredients in sunscreens (Sunscreen drug products, 1999).

The spectrum for ultraviolet radiation includes UVA, UVB, and UVC. UVA, or long-wave radiation, has a wavelength of 320 to 400 nm and is the closest to visible light. UVB has also been determined to be responsible for inducing skin cancer, although the carcinogenic properties of UVB appear to be augmented by UVA. Approximately 90%

BOX 66-5

Skin Cancer

Incidence

Nonmelanoma skin cancer is the most prevalent cancer in the United States. Skin cancers are composed essentially of nonmelanoma (basal and squamous cell carcinomas) and malignant melanoma. The American Cancer Society has predicted 1 million cases of skin cancer for 1998 (Hill, Ferrini, 1998; McDonald, 1998). Melanoma is the most common cause of death from skin cancer.

Preventive Measures

Sun protection is necessary because of the 10- to 20-year period between the ultraviolet (UV) light exposure (especially UVB) and the appearance of the skin cancer.

The primary source of protection is to avoid sunburns, especially in childhood and adolescence. If possible, avoid outdoor activities when the sun is strongest (10 or 11 AM to 3 PM), wear protective clothing (hat and long sleeves) and, if exposed to sun, use a sunscreen that blocks exposure to UV light (SPF 15 or 30). Reapply every 1 to 2 hours and after swimming.

UV radiation can also affect the eyes, increasing the risk for cataracts and other eye disorders, and it can also suppress the immune system. It is recommended that sunglasses that block 99% to 100% of UV radiation be worn (Strange, 1998).

From Salerno, E. (1999). *Pharmacology for health professionals.* St. Louis: Mosby.

of UVB radiation is blocked by the earth's ozone layer, with the balance absorbed by the epidermal skin layer. UVB has a wavelength between 290 and 320 nm, which causes erythema and is also associated with the synthesis of vitamin D_3. The UVC radiation from the sun does not appear to reach the earth's surface; therefore this type of radiation is usually emitted by artificial ultraviolet sources. UVC can cause some erythema but will not stimulate tanning.

The **sun protection factor (SPF)** is a ratio between the exposures to ultraviolet wavelengths required to cause erythema with and without a sunscreen. This is expressed as the minimal erythema dose (MED), which has been defined as "the quantity of erythema-effective energy (expressed in Joules per square meter) required to produce the first perceptible redness reaction with clearly defined borders." (Sunscreen drug products, 1999). Therefore if a person experiences 1 MED with 25 units of UV radiation (in an unprotected state) but requires 250 units of radiation to produce 1 MED after applying a sunscreen, then this sunscreen is given an SPF rating of 10. In general, the higher the SPF, the longer it takes to develop a tan. If a person normally burns within 30 minutes with 1 MED, then applying a sunscreen with an SPF of 6 allows that person to stay in the sun six times longer, or for nearly 3 hours, before reaching 1 MED. The following are current SPF values according to individual requirements (Sunscreen drug products, 1999):

Sun Protection Required	SPF Recommended
Minimal	2 to 11
Moderate	12 to 29
High	30 or above (30+)

The FDA has limited the highest SPF category to 30 plus (or 30+) for any SPF values above 30 (Sunscreen drug products for over-the-counter human use, 1999). The testing methods used for establishing the higher SPFs are in question. In the future, the consumer will no longer find sunscreen products with an SPF of 40, 50, 60 or more on sunscreen product labels; such products will need to be labeled 30+. Manufacturers have been given 24 months to comply with these requirements.

The best way to choose a sunscreen agent is according to skin type, the length of time spent in the sun, the usual intensity of the sun's rays in the particular geographic area, and the preferred type of preparation or formulation. For example, if an individual's skin turns red after being in the sun for 10 minutes, then an SPF of 15 may permit him or her to stay in the sun 15 × 10, or 150 minutes. A SPF of 30 is recommended for use in the tropics (Weil, 1999).

A sunscreen that contains ingredients that absorb at least 85% of the radiation in the UV range of 290 to 400 nm is known as a sunscreen with active ingredients. According to the FDA, the previous category of opaque sunblock is no longer an acceptable term for label use (Sunscreen drug products, 1999). The term *sunblock* implies an agent that blocks all sun rays (e.g., titanium dioxide), which the product does not do; therefore the term *sunblock* cannot appear on the label of a product.

A topical sunscreen can be either chemical (absorbs and blocks UV radiation) or physical (opaque; reflects and scatters UV radiation but does not absorb it). Most products are a combination of these categories. The primary difference between a preventive agent and a suntanning agent might be the concentration of the active ingredient.

The effectiveness of a sunscreening agent depends on its ability to remain effective during vigorous exercise, sweating, and swimming. Two categories with SPF values of 30 or above may also be labeled water-resistant and very water-resistant if they meet the following criteria:

- Water-resistant products maintain their SPF after 40 minutes in the water.
- Very water-resistant products maintain their SPF after 80 minutes of water activity or sweating.

The nurse should advise clients on the appropriate selection and use of a sunscreen. To achieve maximum effectiveness, sunscreens should be applied liberally to all exposed body areas (except eyelids) and reapplied as frequently as recommended.

The nurse should teach clients to do the following:

- Reapply the sunscreen every 2 to 3 hours.
- Refrain from being in the sun between 10 AM and 3 PM, when the sun's rays are most direct and damaging.
- Wear sunscreen and limit exposure on overcast or cloudy days. Very little UV radiation is blocked by cloud cover, although the infrared radiation that contributes to the sensation of heat is usually reduced. This heat reduction might give a false sense of security against sunburn.
- Be aware of reflective surfaces; the sun's rays can be reflected on skin from water, concrete, snow, and sand.
- When practical, wear a broad-brimmed hat, a long-sleeved shirt, and long pants.
- Keep infants out of the sun, and always use sunscreens on children over 6 months of age.

It has been projected that the use of an SPF 15 from 6 months of age through 18 years of age will result in a 78% reduction in the incidence of skin cancer over a person's lifetime (DeSimone, 1996). See Table 66-2 for examples of sunscreen preparations, including their SPFs.

TABLE 66-2 Selected Sunscreen Preparations

Name	Sun Protection Factor (SPF)
Hawaiian Tropic Baby Faces Sunblock	25
Coppertone Moisturizing Sunblock	30 or 45
PreSun Active	15 or 30
Blistex Ultra Protection	30
Coppertone Sport	4, 8, 15 or 30

From Salerno, E. (1999). *Pharmacology for health professionals.* St. Louis: Mosby.

THERAPEUTIC AGENTS

Topical Antiinfectives

Antiinfectives include topical antibiotics, antiviral agents, and antifungal agents.

Antibiotics

The most common causative organisms of skin infections (exodermas) are *Streptococcus pyogenes* and *Staphylococcus aureus*. Folliculitis, impetigo, furuncles, carbuncles, and cellulitis often result from these organisms. These common skin disorders are infections for which topical prophylaxis antibiotics may be applied. Some of these agents are discussed next; other topical antibiotics are discussed in sections on acne products, antifungals, and antivirals.

bacitracin [bass i tray′ sin]

Bacitracin is very useful in the local treatment of infectious lesions. The ointment form (Baciguent) is most commonly used, although it has also been used in solution to moisten wet dressings or as a dusting powder. It is odorless and nonstaining, and its use seldom results in sensitizing; however, allergic contact dermatitis has occurred.

neomycin [nee oh mye′ sin]

Neomycin has been used successfully in the treatment of infections of the skin and mucous membranes. Applied topically, it occasionally irritates the skin; allergic contact dermatitis has been reported, especially when neomycin is used on stasis ulcers. An ointment (Mycitracin), which combines *neomycin, bacitracin,* and *polymixin B,* may be more efficacious in mixed infections than when these agents are used singly.

In conditions where the absorption of neomycin may occur (including burns and trophic ulceration), there is the potential for nephrotoxicity, ototoxicity, and neomycin hypersensitivity reactions. This risk is seen more often in clients with compromised renal function, in clients with extensive burns, and in clients using other aminoglycoside antibiotics. Sensitization may occur to any of the antibiotic ingredients, and prolonged use may produce a superinfection as an overgrowth of nonsusceptible organisms such as fungi. Photosensitivity is reported with topical gentamicin.

TABLE 66-3 Antimicrobial Activity of Topical Antibiotics

	Spectrum of Activity		
Antibiotic	**Gram-positive**	**Gram-negative**	**Broad Spectrum**
bacitracin ointment		X	
chlortetracycline ointment			X
chloramphenicol cream			X
erythromycin liquid or ointment	X		
gentamicin cream and ointment			X
neomycin cream and ointment			X

■ ■ ■

The possibility of hypersensitivity occurs when chloramphenicol is used topically, as does the additional risk of bone marrow hypoplasia, blood dyscrasias, itching, burning, angioneurotic edema, urticaria, and vesicular and maculopapular dermatitis. Tetracyclines may stain clothing and cause local erythema, irritation, and swelling. See Table 66-3 for a list of topical antibiotics and their spectrum of activity. Although erythromycin generally has activity against gram-positive organisms, it is also approved for the treatment of acne vulgaris.

Mupirocin [myoo peer′ oh sin] (Bactroban ◆) is a topical antibacterial preparation indicated for the treatment of impetigo caused by *S. aureus* and other beta-hemolytic streptococci. It is usually applied to affected areas three times daily.

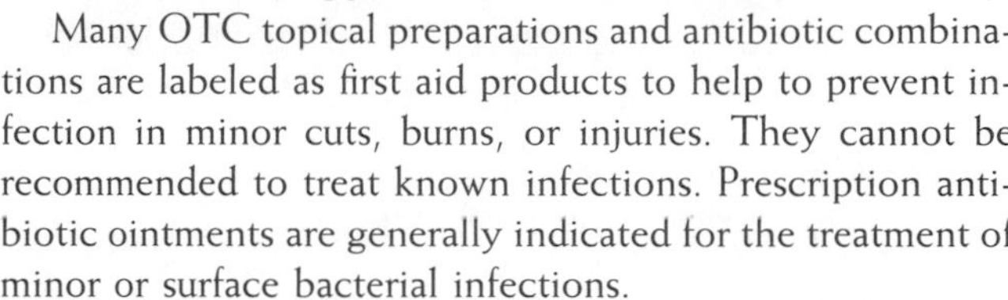

Many OTC topical preparations and antibiotic combinations are labeled as first aid products to help to prevent infection in minor cuts, burns, or injuries. They cannot be recommended to treat known infections. Prescription antibiotic ointments are generally indicated for the treatment of minor or surface bacterial infections.

Antivirals

acyclovir [ay sye′ kloe ver] (Zovirax Ointment 5%)

Acyclovir inhibits the viral enzymes necessary for DNA synthesis. Topical acyclovir is used for the treatment of initial episodes of herpes genitalis and for herpes simplex in immunocompromised clients. In many instances systemic acyclovir is much more effective and may be the preferred formulation.

The more common side effects/adverse reactions of acyclovir include local pain, pruritus, or stinging. The dosage is adequate covering of the lesions with ointment every 3 hours six times daily for 7 days.

■ Nursing Management

Acyclovir Therapy

In addition to the following discussion, see Nursing Management: Dermatologic Agent Therapy, p. 1122.

The dose per application will vary depending on the lesion area; a 1/2-inch ribbon of ointment covers approximately 4 inches of surface area. Store the ointment at 15° to 25° C (59° to 78° F).

Instruct the client to use a finger cot or rubber glove when applying the ointment to prevent autoinoculation to other sites. It is applied as soon as symptoms of herpes infection begin. Avoid contact with eyes. Advise an annual or more frequent Papanicolaou (Pap) smear, because women with herpes genitalis are more likely to develop cervical cancer. Recommend that the client wear loose clothing and keep the affected areas clean and dry to prevent further irritation. Advise the client to avoid sexual activity if either partner has active lesions. The disease can still be sexually transmitted even if the partner is asymptomatic; depending on the location of the lesion, the use of a condom may help to prevent the transmission of herpes.

Antifungals

A few fungi produce keratinolytic enzymes to provide for their existence on the skin. Three infectious fungi can cause local fungal infections without producing systemic effects: *Microsporum*, *Trichophyton*, and *Epidermophyton*. The possibility of a mixed infection with these fungi must never be overlooked.

Fungi exist in a moist, warm environment, preferably in dark areas such as skin areas covered by shoes and socks (tinea pedis or athlete's foot). Immunologic mechanisms may have an important role in fungal control. The triad of suspicion for fungal infections is an immunologic deficit, a specific fungal involvement, and the skin condition.

The stratum corneum is a layer of dead, desquamated cells that are shed normally or are dissolved in sebum. The fungi invade this layer and cause inflammation and induce sensitivity when they penetrate the epidermis and dermis. Because the stratum corneum is shed daily, the ability to spread or transmit the fungi is by contact.

The most commonly reported side effects/adverse reactions with the use of topical antifungals include local irritation, pruritus, a burning sensation, and scaling. Erythema, blistering, stinging, peeling, urticaria, pruritus, and general irritation may occur with products such as clotrimazole.

The primary topical antifungal agents include undecylenic acid products (Desenex and others), clioquinol (Vioform), miconazole (Micatin), econazole (Spectazole), ciclopirox (Loprox), clotrimazole (Lotrimin), oxiconazole (Oxistat), triacetin (Fungoid), haloprogin (Halotex), tolnaftate (Tinactin), nystatin, gentian violet, and a variety of antifungal combination ointments, powders, and liquids. See Table 66-4 for the generic name, trade name,

TABLE 66-4 Topical Antifungal Agents

Name	Prescription Drug	Over-the-Counter	Special Comments
amphotericin B (Fungizone)	X		Equivalent to nystatin against *Candida albicans* (Monilia) infections.
 betamethasone and clotrimazole (Lotrisone ◆)	X		Combination of corticosteroid and antifungal.
ciclopirox olamine (Loprox)	X		Broad-spectrum antifungal. Used for tinea pedis, tinea cruris, tinea corporis, candidiasis caused by *C. albicans*, and tinea versicolor caused by *M. furfur*.
clioquinol (Vioform)		X	Antibacterial and antifungal. May cause staining of clothes, skin, or hair.
clotrimazole (Lotrimin, Mycelex)	X	X	Broad-spectrum antifungal agent.
econazole nitrate (Spectazole)	X		Broad-spectrum antifungal agent.
haloprogin (Halotex)	X		Synthetic antifungal agent. Broad-spectrum antifungal agent.
ketoconazole (Nizoral)	X		Broad-spectrum synthetic antifungal agent.
miconazole (Micatin)		X	Used for tinea pedis (athlete's foot), tinea cruris, tinea corporis, and tinea versicolor. Lotion is preferred for intertriginous areas.
(Monistat-Derm)	X		
nystatin (Mycostatin, Nilstat)	X		Antifungal antibiotic with both fungicidal and fungistatic effects.
tolnaftate (Tinactin, Aftate)		X	Used for topical fungus skin infections.
triacetin (Fungoid)	X		Treats athlete's foot and other topical fungus infections.
undecylenic acid (Desenex)		X	Antifungal and antibacterial for athlete's foot and ringworm, with the exception of nails and hairy sites. Also used for diaper rash, prickly heat, minor skin irritations, jock itch, excessive perspiration, and skin irritation in the groin area.

status of (OTC or prescription), and comments on these products.

■ Nursing Management

Antifungal Agent Therapy

In addition to the following discussion, see Nursing Management: Dermatologic Agent Therapy, p. 1122.

Carefully note skin characteristics, symptoms, and predisposing factors such as trauma, suppressed immunity, general health, hygiene practices, or exposure to an infecting agent. Laboratory tests to be obtained (e.g., cultures of exudate or tissue) should be obtained before the topical agent is applied.

The use of these agents may lead to skin sensitization and result in symptoms of hypersensitization, increasing redness and swelling, weeping, and itching and burning not present at the beginning of therapy.

Topical substances for antifungal purposes should be applied liberally to a clean, dry, affected skin area. An occlusive dressing should not be applied unless directed by the prescriber. Avoid contact of these substances with the eyes. Store them below 30° C (85° F), but do not freeze them.

Encourage the client to comply with the full course of therapy. In general, fungal infections require prolonged therapy. Encourage the client with a superficial fungal infection to practice adequate hygiene to discourage growth. Principles of hygiene include the following: (1) keeping the affected areas dry and aerated, and avoiding clothing that is warm or that causes an occlusive environment of moisture; (2) keeping body areas dry with powders (with or without antifungal ingredients) to prevent maceration; (3) before applying the antifungal medication, washing the area with mild soap and water and then drying it; (4) avoiding friction or trauma of the area by not wearing tight-fitting clothing, which causes friction; clothing should be laundered daily. For infants with anogenital lesions, avoid tight diapers, disposable diapers, and plastic pants. Advise clients with foot infections to wear cotton socks and well-ventilated shoes or sandals.

The expected outcome of topical antifungal therapy is that the client will experience a resolution of the fungal infection. The client needs to be reevaluated if no improvement is seen within 4 weeks.

Corticosteroids

Topical corticosteroids are generally indicated for the relief of inflammatory and pruritic dermatoses (Correale, Walker, Murphy, Craig, 1999). They also offer the benefit of fewer systemic side effects, and they allow direct contact with the localized lesion.

The effectiveness of topical corticosteroids is a result of their antiinflammatory, antipruritic, and vasoconstrictor actions. Topical corticosteroids may also stabilize epidermal lysosomes in the skin, and fluorinated steroids are antiproliferative.

Fluorinated topical corticosteroids (fluocinonide, betamethasone, and others) are used for the treatment of dermatologic disorders such as psoriasis because of their antiinflammatory, antipruritic, and vasoconstrictive actions, as well as their ability to decrease cell proliferation. They are very potent agents and are less likely to cause sodium retention.

A correlation exists between the potency and the therapeutic efficacy of corticosteroids (Box 66-6). The vehicle in which the corticosteroid is placed (aerosol, cream, gel, lotion, ointment, solution, or tape) may alter the vasoconstrictor property and therapeutic efficacy. Corticosteroid skin penetration is enhanced by the following vehicles (in decreasing order of effectiveness): ointments, gels, creams, and lotions.

Ointment bases and propylene glycol both enhance the penetration of the corticosteroid and its vasoconstrictor effects. As a result of their occlusive nature, ointments hydrate the stratum corneum, permitting granular steroid penetration. Lotions are well suited for hairy areas or for lesions that are oozing and wet. Creams and ointments are well suited for dry, scaling, thickened, and pruritic areas. Sprays, lotions, and gels are suited for the scalp or for hairy areas. Sprays are aesthetically suitable for acute weeping lesions; they are cooling and have antipruritic effects. All of these vehicles influence absorption and have a therapeutic effect.

The rate of percutaneous penetration after application also influences therapeutic efficacy. The percutaneous penetration of a steroid increases with its vehicle base solubility. It is limited by three factors: rate of dissolution, rate of pas-

BOX 66-6

Potencies of Topical Steroid Products

The following list compares the relative potencies of topical corticosteroid products.

Most Potent

clobetasol (Temovate 0.05%)
halobetasol (Ultravate 0.05%)

High Potency

amcinocide (Cyclocort)
betamethasone dipropionate (Diprosone 0.05%)
desoximetasone (Topicort 0.25%)
fluocinolone (Lidex 0.05%)

Moderate Potency

betamethasone (Benisone 0.025%)
betamethasone valerate (Valisone 0.1%)
desoximetasone (Topicort 0.05%)
flurandrenolide (Cordran 0.025%)
triamcinolone (Aristocort)

Less Potent

desonide (Tridesilon)
fluocinolone acetonide (Synalar 0.01%)
hydrocortisone 0.25% to 2.5%

sive diffusion, and rate of drug penetration (the skin itself is a barrier, and the stratum corneum is a rate-limiting membrane). The skin is selectively permeable by regional variations in absorptive capacity. Because most topical corticosteroids are in suspension vehicles (ointments, creams, lotions), the addition of a solvent (propylene glycol) to the product can enhance drug dissolution, which may improve absorption. Sebum, enzymes, and perspiration partially convert topical suspensions to solutions; thus they need the inclusion of a solvent, surfactant, or emulsifier in the vehicle to increase the rate of dissolution and distribution. Inflamed skin absorbs topical steroids to a greater degree than thick or lichenified skin.

The side effects/adverse reactions of topical corticosteroids include acneiform eruptions, allergic contact dermatitis, burning sensations, dryness, itching, hypopigmentation, purpura, hirsutism (usually facial), folliculitis, a round and swollen face, alopecia (usually of the scalp), immunosuppression, and overgrowth of bacteria, fungi, and viruses.

The adult dosage is one or two applications daily as directed. The frequency of application depends on the site, response of the cutaneous eruption to medication, and application technique.

▪ Nursing Management

Topical Corticosteroid Therapy

In addition to the following discussion, see Nursing Management: Dermatologic Agent Therapy, p. 1122.

The age of the skin affects absorption of the potent fluorinated corticosteroids; the very young and the very old have skin that is more permeable.

To help prevent adverse reactions if prolonged treatment is required, treatment may be interrupted periodically, small amounts of the drug can be applied, or one area of the body can be treated at a time. Most side effects are temporary and are resolved when the topical steroid is discontinued.

Gradual withdrawal of therapy may be indicated after high-dose or prolonged therapy to help prevent a rebound flare-up of psoriasis.

Occlusive dressings may cause folliculitis from a bacterial or candidal infection, hyperthermia from heat retention, or systemic effects related to increased drug absorption. Do not use an occlusive dressing if the client has a fever. If the site becomes infected, discontinue the use of topical corticosteroids, and initiate the appropriate treatment.

To enhance client compliance, the reasons for the occlusive dressing procedure should be explained to the client. This technique intensifies percutaneous penetration of the topical steroid and concentrates the medication in the area where it is most needed. Check with the prescriber if no improvement is noticeable after 1 week.

The expected outcome of topical corticosteroid therapy is that the client will experience resolution of the skin lesions with diminished weeping, itching, redness, and size.

Keratolytics

Keratolytics (keratin dissolvers) are drugs that soften scales and loosen the outer horny layer of the skin. Salicylic acid and resorcinol are the drugs of choice. Their action makes the penetration of other medical substances possible by cleaning the involved lesions. Salicylic acid is particularly important for its keratolytic effect in the local treatment of scalp conditions, warts, corns, fungous infections, acne, and chronic types of dermatitis. It is used up to 20% in ointments, plasters, or collodion for this purpose. Examples of salicylic acid products include Panscol Ointment, Wart-Off and Dr. Scholl's Corn/Callus Remover.

Acne Products

Acne vulgaris is a skin disease that involves increased sebum production and abnormal keratinization and leads to the formation of a keratin plug at the base of the pilosebaceous follicle; it affects up to 90% of adolescents (Seaton, 1995). The reduction and removal of sebum and bacteria, specifically *Propionibacterium acnes,* is the goal of acne vulgaris therapy.

Treatment of acne therapy may include (1) removing keratin plugs, (2) decreasing the amount of *P. acnes*, (3) lowering the amounts of free fatty acid and formation, (4) decreasing sebum production, and (5) effectively improving the appearance of the client for psychosocial benefits.

Of the many treatment modalities in acne therapy, only the topical forms of benzoyl peroxide, tetracycline, erythromycin, clindamycin, tretinoin, and isotretinoin are discussed here.

benzoyl peroxide [ben' zoe ill per ox' eyde]

Benzoyl peroxide slowly and continuously liberates active oxygen to produce an antibacterial, keratolytic, and drying effect in the treatment of acne vulgaris. The release of oxygen into the pilosebaceous and comedone area creates unfavorable growth conditions for *P. acnes* and reduces the release of fatty acids from the sebum. In addition, the drying vehicle aids in shrinking the papules or pustules but does not have an effect on comedones or cysts.

Benzoyl peroxide is absorbed and metabolized in the skin to benzoic acid. Approximately 5% of the benzoic acid is absorbed and excreted by the kidneys. Acne improvement is usually noted after 4 to 6 weeks of therapy.

Side effects/adverse reactions are uncommon and include dry or peeling skin, red skin, a sensation of warmth of the skin, severe redness, pruritus, blisters, and burning or swelling of the skin caused by an allergic reaction. No significant drug interactions are reported.

In adults and children 12 years of age and older, benzoyl peroxide lotion (5% or 10%) is applied one to four times daily.

Topical Antibiotics

Topical and systemic antibiotics used in the treatment of acne have an unknown mechanism of action. Acne is not an infection nor is it contagious, but *P. acnes* appears to convert comedones to inflamed pustules or papules. Antibiotics may decrease the colonization of *P. acnes*, thus decreasing the formation of sebaceous fatty acid byproducts and preventing the formation of new acne lesions. The antibiotics used include clindamycin, erythromycin, and tetracycline. Topical erythromycin and clindamycin are most commonly prescribed for mild to moderate acne, whereas oral antibiotics (tetracyclines) are generally reserved for severe acne and for clients who are intolerant of or did not respond to topical agents. Treatment failures have been associated with antibiotic resistance (Seaton, 1995).

clindamycin [klin da mye' sin] (Cleocin T topical solution)

Topical clindamycin may be as effective as low-dose, oral tetracycline therapy for inflammatory acne. It is believed to lower the free fatty acid concentration on the skin and to suppress the growth of *P. acnes*. It has an antibacterial effect. By hydrolysis, skin phosphatases convert inactive clindamycin phosphate to active clindamycin base, which is excreted by the kidneys.

Clindamycin is one of the most widely used topical antibiotics indicated for the treatment of acne vulgaris.

Side effects/adverse reactions include dry, scaly and/or peeling skin, a stinging or burning sensation, and a hypersensitive skin reaction.

■ Nursing Management

Clindamycin Therapy

In addition to the following discussion, see Nursing Management: Dermatologic Agent Therapy, p. 1122.

Cross-resistance exists with lincomycin. Contraindications demonstrated by hypersensitivity to any form of clindamycin or lincomycin may apply to the topical preparation. During the client interviews, inquire about any previous sensitivity not only to clindamycin but also to other antibiotics or allergens, as well as a history of regional enteritis. Atopic clients should be questioned, because some absorption may occur through the skin.

Some clients develop antibiotic-associated pseudomembranous colitis caused by *Clostridium difficile* during or following topical clindamycin therapy. The client should report any diarrhea to the prescriber. Mild cases may resolve by discontinuing the clindamycin; more severe cases may require fluid and electrolyte replacement.

For adults and children, the dosage is an application of a thin film twice daily to the affected area. Shake the topical suspension well before applying.

erythromycin topical solution [er ith roe mye' sin] (A/T/S, EryDerm)

Erythromycin topical solution is also indicated for the treatment of acne vulgaris. Side effects/adverse reactions include skin reactions such as erythema, desquamation, tenderness, dryness, pruritus, burning, oiliness, and acne.

■ Nursing Management

Erythromycin Topical Solution Therapy

In addition to the following discussion, see Nursing Management: Dermatologic Agent Therapy, p. 1122.

Hypersensitivity to erythromycin or the other components of the solution (alcohol, propylene glycol, or acetone) is a contraindication to its use. A cumulative irritant effect may occur with the concomitant use of peeling, desquamating, or abrasive agents.

Noticeable improvement may be seen in 3 to 4 weeks, but the maximum effects may take 8 to 12 weeks.

Erythromycin topical solution is applied to the affected areas morning and evening. Wait at least 1 hour before applying any other topical preparation to the skin.

Caution the client that erythromycin solution should not be used near the eyes, nose, mouth, and other mucous membranes.

tetracycline topical solution [tet ra sye' kleen] (Topicycline)

Topical tetracycline, which is believed to suppress *P. acnes* growth, is applied directly to the pilosebaceous units (hair follicle and sebaceous gland), which are most numerous on the face, back, chest, and upper arms.

Side effects/adverse reactions of topical tetracycline include dry/scaly skin, stinging, pain, and redness or swelling at the site of application. Low-dose, oral tetracycline (usually 250 mg/day) is usually reserved for severe acne as reviewed previously. This dose may be increased for acute acne flare-ups but should be decreased to maintenance dosing within a month or so. Although low-dose therapy has been continued for years, it has been recommended that the antibiotic be discontinued periodically (Seaton, 1995). This may help reduce the potential for side effects/adverse reactions and possible drug resistance.

■ Nursing Management

Topical Tetracycline Therapy

In addition to the following discussion, see Nursing Management: Dermatologic Agent Therapy, p. 1122.

Tetracycline is generously applied twice daily (morning and evening) to affected areas until the skin is wet. Wait an hour before applying other agents. Because of the 40% ethanol and other components, the eyes, nose, mouth, and mucous membrane areas should be avoided. Because of the alcohol content, avoid open flames or smoking while applying the medication. The normal use of cosmetics is permitted, but avoid other agents that would dry the skin. A gauze dressing may be used with tetracycline ointment to avoid staining clothing. (See Chapter 59 for a more complete discussion of tetracycline.) Transient stinging or burning may often occur with application. The slight yellow superficial coloring of the skin of light-complected clients may be washed off. Treated areas will fluoresce under a source of ultraviolet light (sun, sunlamp).

tretinoin [tret' i noyn] (retinoic acid, vitamin A acid, Retin-A)

Tretinoin is an irritant that stimulates the turnover of epidermal cells, which causes skin peeling. The primary effect of tretinoin is to reduce the hyperkeratinization that results in

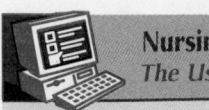

Nursing Research
The Use of Topical Tretinoin for Photoaging

Citation: Dickens C.H., Edwards, L., Ellis, C.N., & Shalita, A.R. (1992). Retinoids: What role in your practice? *Patient Care, 26*(10), 18–45.

Abstract: In practice, topical tretinoin is probably used more often to treat aging skin than to treat acne. Ortho has reformulated the agent as 0.05% tretinoin in an emollient cream base (Renova). Although tretinoin has been promoted in the lay media as a cure for wrinkles, the effects of therapy involve the whole range of photodamage. Tretinoin not only improves fine and coarse wrinkling cosmetically, but it also decreases skin laxity, roughness, sallowness, and hyperpigmentation. This agent reduces the number of precancerous skin lesions and stimulates new collagen and possibly the production of new elastin. It increases the thickness of epidermal and granular layers, decreases melanin content, and makes the stratum corneum more compact (Bhawan et al., 1991).

The use of topical tretinoin must be discussed with the client in the context of a complete program of photoprotection. Instruct the client to use sunscreens, to wear hats and protective clothing when in the sun, and to avoid sun exposure between 10 AM and 2 PM (standard time), when the greatest damage can occur. Ensure that the client understands that shade does not offer protection from ultraviolet radiation.

Despite the desirability of some of the positive skin changes, the use of tretinoin to treat photodamaged skin remains highly controversial. Many physicians see the benefits as cosmetic rather than medical. The FDA Advisory Committee shared some of this concern in recommending that the labeling for Renova indicate that tretinoin improves the appearance of the skin but does not actually repair sun-damaged skin. On the other hand, many dermatologists advocate a different perspective—that tretinoin is a medical treatment for a serious medical condition. The client has suffered environmental exposure to a harmful substance, which has caused damage and can benefit from therapy. Helping clients look better is as legitimate a goal as reducing cancer risk, and positive psychologic effects have been documented with such therapy (Gupta et al., 1991).

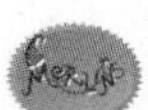

Critical Thinking Questions

- Do you believe that photoaging therapy, such as tretinoin therapy, is beneficial for clients?
- Is this therapy for cosmetic reasons justifiable in a health system with scarce resources?
- If the treatment of mildly to moderately photoaged skin with topical tretinoin has a favorable psychosocial effect on a client, wouldn't this enhance the client's health from a holistic perspective?

comedone formation, a lesion in acne. Tretinoin is used for the treatment of acne vulgaris in which comedones, pustules, and papules are predominant (see the Nursing Research box at left).

The side effects/adverse reactions of tretinoin include red and edematous blisters; crusted, stinging, or peeling skin; and temporary alterations in skin pigmentation. Concomitant topical use with drying or peeling agents such as benzoyl peroxide, resorcinol, salicylic acid, and sulfur may result in excessive keratolytic and peeling effects.

Tretinoin emollient cream (Renova) is used to treat facial wrinkles caused by aging or sun exposure. This product contains 0.05% tretinoin and is the first prescription drug with this indication (*Drug Facts and Comparisons,* 2000).

▪ Nursing Management
Tretinoin Therapy

In addition to the following discussion, see Nursing Management: Dermatologic Agent Therapy, p. 1122.

Irritation and desquamation are most likely during the first 1 to 3 weeks of treatment. For acne, therapeutic results can be seen after 2 to 3 weeks of therapy, with an optimal response after 3 months. If used for the effects of photoaging, the improvement continues for 2 months after therapy, with a partial and gradual regression.

Apply this drug each night by covering the area lightly at bedtime. Some clients require less frequent applications or the use of a lower-percentage strength, whereas others may respond to the higher percentage forms. Tretinoin should be applied after a thorough cleansing of area. Allow a minimum of 30 minutes for the skin to dry before applying tretrinoin, because an increased drying effect and redness may occur if it is applied to wet skin. After application, wait 1 hour before applying any other preparation to the same area.

Clients with sunburned skin, skin that is sensitive to ultraviolet light, or skin exposed to weather extremes must exercise caution and avoid tretinoin until the skin has recovered. The client must avoid medicated or abrasive cleansers, astringents, soaps, and cosmetics that have a drying effect and a high alcohol concentration. The client will be excessively sensitive to the sun and should wear a sunscreen of at least 15 SPF during therapy.

isotretinoin [eye soe tret′ i noyn] (Accutane)

Isotretinoin is an oral product indicated for the treatment of severe, recalcitrant, cystic acne. This product inhibits sebaceous gland activity, thereby decreasing the formation and secretion of sebum. It also has antikeratinizing and antiinflammatory effects. It is reserved to treat severe acne and has induced prolonged remissions in severe cystic acne.

Women who are pregnant or are planning to become pregnant should not use this drug. Many spontaneous abortions have been reported in pregnant women, as well as major abnormalities (hydrocephalus, microcephalus, external ear, and cardiovascular problems) in the fetus at birth.

Pregnancy Safety
Dermatologic Drugs

Category	Drug
B	topical clindamycin, erythromycin, meclocycline, and tetracycline; lindane, malathion topical, permethrin, silver sulfadiazine
C	benzoyl peroxide, corticosteroids (topical), crotamiton, mafenide, tretinoin
X	isotretinoin

■ Nursing Management

Isotretinoin Therapy

In addition to the following discussion, see Nursing Management: Dermatologic Agent Therapy, p. 1122.

■ **Assessment.** Because isotretinoin has been demonstrated to cause fetal abnormalities, a negative pregnancy test and an appropriate history and physical examination should be used to determine that the client is not pregnant. Clients of childbearing age should be assessed for a capability to comply with mandatory contraceptive measures; these should be accomplished for at least 1 month before therapy, during therapy, and for 1 month after the end of therapy (see the Pregnancy Safety box above).

Review the client's medication regimen. Isotretinoin is not recommended to be taken concurrently with acitretin, oral tretinoin, or vitamin A, because additive toxic effects may result. The use of tetracyclines with isotretinoin increases the risk for the development of pseudotumor cerebri—a condition characterized by increased intracranial pressure, headache, blurring of the optic disc margins, vomiting, and papilledema without neurologic findings (except palsy of the sixth cranial nerve).

The client should receive a baseline complete blood count (CBC), blood lipid levels, blood glucose levels, and hepatic function studies. These should also be monitored throughout therapy.

■ **Nursing Diagnosis.** The client receiving isotretinoin is at risk for the following nursing diagnoses/collaborative problems: impaired comfort (headache; heartburn; inflammation of the eye; pain, tenderness, and stiffness of the muscles, bones, or joints; dryness of the mouth, skin, and eyes; difficulty wearing contact lenses); fatigue; impaired skin integrity (scaling, redness, inflammation of the skin); and the potential complications of mental depression, nosebleeds, cataracts, optic neuritis, corneal opacities, pseudotumor cerebri, hepatitis, and inflammatory bowel disease.

■ **Implementation**

■ ***Monitoring.*** Monitor laboratory reports, nursing diagnoses, and potential complications as mentioned previously.

■ ***Education.*** The client is to receive both oral and written instructions regarding the hazards of pregnancy, and she should indicate her understanding and acceptance of the written warnings. The client receiving isotretinoin should be alerted not to donate blood during or for 30 days after therapy, because there is a risk to the fetus of a pregnant woman who may receive the blood. Because isotretinoin may increase concentrations of plasma triglycerides, clients at particular cardiovascular risk should be cautioned; this includes clients with a history of high alcohol intake or obesity or a history or family history of hypertriglyceridemia or diabetes mellitus.

To minimize additive toxic effects, alert the client to avoid the concurrent use of vitamin A unless prescribed by a physician. Avoid the ingestion of alcohol because of possible hypertriglyceridemia and consequent cardiovascular risks. Caution the client about a decrease in night vision; the client should alert the prescriber if this occurs. The client may also be intolerant of contact lenses because of dryness of the eyes. Contact lens use may need to be discontinued during therapy if an ocular lubricant is not successful in relieving dryness. Ice or sugar-free gum or candies may be recommended to relieve mouth dryness.

Advise the client to contact the prescriber if there is no improvement in 1 to 2 months; full improvement may take 5 to 6 months. Skin irritation may occur during the first several weeks of therapy. Stress the need for protection from exposure to wind and sun, with the use of protective clothing and a sunscreen of at least 15 SPF at all times.

Advise the client that dental problems may occur from mouth dryness; regular dental appointments are necessary to minimize dental complications.

■ **Evaluation.** The expected outcome of isotretinoin therapy is that cystic acne should improve after 1 to 2 months; 5 to 6 months of therapy may be required.

■ ■ ■

Several other acne products are available, including azelaic acid (Azelex Cream) and tazarotene (Tazorac). Azelaic acid has a low pH, and therefore skin irritation (burning, stinging, or pruritus) may occur if it is applied on broken skin. Tazarotene is a retinoid pro-drug that is converted to its active form (cognate carboxylic acid of tazarotene) after application to the skin. This product is used to treat mild to moderate facial acne vulgaris and psoriasis.

Burn Products

Burn injuries range from mild and superficial to very severe, with extensive skin loss associated with systemic and metabolic complications. Approximately 12,000 Americans die from thermal injury each year (Mailloux, 1995). The chief cause of death is shock; this fact is of considerable significance in any effective plan of treatment.

Burns cause skin lesions accompanied by pain. The burn may be caused by heat (thermal burn), chemical cauterizing agents (chemical burns), or electricity (electrical burns). Sources may be friction, lightning, or electromagnetic energy (ultraviolet light, x-rays, lasers, or atomic explosion). The types of burns that result from various sources are relatively specific and diagnostic.

A consideration of what takes place in the damaged tissues clarifies many points of treatment. Capillary permeability is initially altered in the local injured area; permeability is increased, which results in plasma loss and weeping of the surface tissues. If the burn is at all extensive, considerable amounts of plasma fluid may be lost in a relatively short time.

This plasma loss depletes blood volume and causes a decreased cardiac output and diminished blood flow. Unless the situation is brought under control quickly, irreparable damage may result from rapidly developing tissue anoxia. The lack of sufficient oxygen and accumulation of waste products from inadequate oxidation results in a loss of tone in the small blood vessels. Increased capillary permeability then extends to tissues remote from those suffering the initial injury. A generalized edema often develops; once established, the vicious cycle tends to be self-perpetuating. One of the aims of the treatment of burns is to stop the loss of plasma and to replenish that which is lost as quickly as possible.

Partial- or full-thickness burns must be thought of as open wounds with the accompanying danger of infection. The infection must be prevented or treated. The treatment, however, must not cause any further destruction of tissue or of the small islands of remaining epithelium from which growth and regeneration can take place.

Burns are classified by degree, which is determined by the depth of skin involved within a geographic designation. First-degree burns involve only the epidermis, causing erythema with characteristic dry, painful reddening and edema without blistering or vesiculation (e.g., overexposure to sun or a flash burn). Second-degree burns involve the epidermis and extend into the dermis; they may be superficial or involve a deep dermal necrosis. Epithelial regeneration may extend from deep skin appendages, such as hair follicles and sebaceous glands that penetrate the dermis. This burn is characterized by a moist, blistered, very painful surface (e.g., flash or scald burns from nonviscous liquids). Third-degree burns involve destruction of the entire dermis and epidermis and are characterized by white, lustrous, or opaque skin; dry, leathery skin; or coagulated, charred skin without sensation as a result of the destruction of nerve endings (e.g., flame burns or hot, viscous liquids). Fourth-degree burns extend into subcutaneous fat, muscle, or bone; they appear black and dry in appearance and cause scarring.

The severity of electrical burns depends on the amount of voltage received, the condition of the skin (e.g., cuts, abrasions, and moisture, which lower resistance), and the contraction of flexor muscles, which inhibits release from the power source. Electrical burns result in the necrosis of more tissue than thermal burns and are of three types:

Type I. The electrical current causes effects on blood vessels such as occlusion, thrombosis, or tissue destruction.

Type II. Electrical burns from high-tension currents (e.g., an electrical arc) produce a crater in the skin.

Type III. These burns are similar to flame burns because the arc flame ignites the victim's clothes.

Chemical burns occur after contact with an acid or alkali; the initial treatment is water irrigation of the affected area followed by neutralization. Chemical burns may occur in the mouth and appear as a white slough because of necrosis of the epithelium and underlying connective tissues.

Regardless of the cause (chemical, electric, thermal), an important first-aid treatment for minor and major burns is to cool the wound immediately to remove irritants, decrease inflammation, and constrict blood vessels; this reduces the permeability of the blood vessels and checks the formation of edema. Cold tap water can be used to flush the wound thoroughly and to cool hot clothing. The more quickly the wound is cooled, the less tissue damage there is likely to be, and the more rapid the recovery. Greasy ointments, lard, butter, or dressings should not be applied, because they inhibit the loss of heat from the burn and increase both discomfort and tissue damage. The burn may be left exposed to the air, or cold, wet compresses may be applied until the victim can be transported for medical attention.

Burn victims treated in an emergency department or burn unit are stabilized with IV fluids, given analgesics for pain, and sedated if necessary. These individuals are immunized with tetanus toxoid and/or tetanus immunoglobulin depending on their immunization status. Depending on their status, catheterization may be necessary to measure urinary output. Following stabilization, the burn wound is cleaned with a mild soap and water, and a sterile, nonadherent gauze dressing with hydrophilic petrolatum is applied. In some settings, synthetic dressings (Duoderm, Opsite) may be used. Topical antiinfective therapy may also be indicated. Silver sulfadiazine is usually preferred because of its broad-spectrum activity; this product is easy and painless to apply and remove from the burn. Povidone-iodine penetrates eschar and was commonly used in some centers. However, it also causes pain on application and hardens the eschar area when dry (Mailloux, 1995).

silver sulfadiazine [sul fa dye′ a zeen] (Silvadene)

Silver sulfadiazine is an antiinfective agent with broad antimicrobial activity against many gram-negative and gram-positive bacteria (similar to mafenide). It acts only on the cell membrane and cell wall to produce its bactericidal effect.

Silver sulfadiazine is used in second- and third-degree burns for the prevention and treatment of sepsis. It softens eschar, facilitating its removal and preparation of the wound for grafting.

Silver sulfadiazine is available as a 1% cream to be applied topically to cleansed, debrided burn wounds once or twice daily. It should be applied with a sterile gloved hand to a thickness of approximately 1.5 mm. Burn wounds should be continuously covered with the cream. Daily bathing and debriding are important, and a dressing may or may not be used.

Therapy is usually continued until satisfactory healing has occurred or until the wound is ready for grafting. Because silver sulfadiazine inhibits bacterial growth, delayed eschar separation may occur, which necessitates an escharotomy to prevent contractures. Pain, burning, and itching occur infrequently after application of the silver sulfadiazine cream.

Silver sulfadiazine may cause a hypersensitivity reaction, in which case the drug should be discontinued. Hemolysis may occur in persons with glucose-6-phosphate dehydrogenase (G6PD) deficiency. When silver sulfadiazine is applied to extensive areas of the body, significant amounts of the drug may be absorbed, reaching therapeutic serum levels and producing adverse reactions characteristic of the sulfonamides. Renal function in these clients should be monitored and the urine examined for sulfa crystals.

Consult Chapter 71 for the nursing management of the client undergoing silver sulfadiazine therapy.

mafenide [ma′ fe nide] (Sulfamylon)

Mafenide (sulfonamide), a broad-spectrum, antibacterial (bacteriostatic) topical agent, penetrates eschar even in the presence of pus and serum. It is a carbonic anhydrase inhibitor that can alter acid-base balance, resulting in metabolic acidosis. In contrast to silver sulfadiazine, it is usually painful on application.

On application, mafenide rapidly diffuses through partial (second-degree) and full-thickness (third-degree) burns and has proved to be an effective means for preventing and slowing bacterial invasion in burn wounds. It is relatively nontoxic, but burning or pain on application and allergic reactions have been reported. It is rapidly metabolized to a metabolite and eliminated by way of the kidneys.

■ Nursing Management

Mafenide Therapy

In addition to the following discussion, see Nursing Management: Dermatologic Agent Therapy, p. 1122.

Ascertain the client's sensitivity to sulfites before using this product. Because this drug and its metabolite are strong carbonic anhydrase inhibitors, acidosis (metabolic) may occur and is usually compensated by hyperventilation. The client should be observed carefully for any signs resulting in respiratory alkalosis. If rapid or labored respirations occur, the ointment should be washed off the wound.

Bathe the burned area daily; whirlpools and showers are helpful. Mafenide may cause some discomfort when first applied (in a 1/16-inch layer once or twice daily); a burning or pain sensation may occur that lasts from a few minutes to as long as an hour. Keep the affected areas covered with the cream at all times; reapply it to burned areas from which it has been removed by client activity. It is not necessary to discontinue mafenide therapy if infection occurs.

Therapy can be interrupted for 2 to 3 days without impairing bacterial control of the wound while continuing fluid therapy and acid-base restoration.

Mafenide is a highly stable drug. It remains active for several years and does not need to be refrigerated except in tropical countries.

The expected outcome of mafenide therapy is that the client's wound will show granulation and healing by primary intention or split-thickness skin grafting within an acceptable time frame.

nitrofurazone [nye troe fyoor′ an zohn] (Furacin)

Nitrofurazone is a broad antibacterial topical agent and is active against many bacteria that cause local infections, including *S. aureus, Streptococcus, Escherichia coli,* and others. It is indicated as adjunct therapy to clients with second- and third-degree burns when bacterial resistance to other agents is a problem; it is also used during skin grafting when bacterial contamination may result in graft rejection or a donor site infection.

Rash, itching, local edema (dermatitis), and allergic reactions have been reported. Hypersensitivity occurs early in the treatment of a few individuals. Bacterial and fungal superinfections may occur. Furacin is not absorbed significantly through mucosal or burned tissues, and systemic toxicity is rare. However, its polyethylene glycol base may be absorbed and may challenge the client with renal dysfunction.

The 0.2% cream, ointment, or solution may be applied directly on the area or to a gauze dressing for application. Efficacy is reduced in the presence of heavy microbial contamination, plasma, or blood. Resistance seldom develops.

■ Nursing Management

Nitrofurazone Therapy

■ **Assessment.** Determine that the client has not had a previous sensitivity reaction to the drug. Pregnant women should avoid using this product unless the potential benefits outweigh the possible risks to the fetus. Judgment should be used in treating a client with these preparations if he or she has a renal disorder; these preparations include polyethylene glycol and may produce adverse effects. Older adults are at a higher risk for allergic responses to nitrofurazone.

■ **Nursing Diagnosis.** The client is at risk for impaired skin integrity related to allergic contact dermatitis (erythema, pruritus, and burning), which occurs in approximately 1% of those treated.

■ **Implementation**

■ ***Monitoring.*** Evaluate the affected areas daily. If areas do not seem to be responding to treatment by nitrofurazone, consider the possibility of overgrowth by nonsusceptible organisms such as fungi and *Pseudomonas* or an allergic response. Watch for dermatitis or other manifestations of hypersensitivity to this product.

■ ***Intervention.*** Cleanse the affected area before each dressing change. Treatment by nitrofurazone may be suggested in instances of burn or wound infections that are resistant to other medications. As a solution, nitrofurazone may be sprayed directly on the wound. If the solution is cloudy, it may be warmed to restore clarity. To apply the ointment, use sterile gloves and cover the affected areas with a thin layer. Meticulous sterile technique is essential during dressing changes and when opening and withdrawing nitrofurazone-saturated dressings from their sterile packets. Nitrofurazone darkens on exposure to light, but such discoloration does not affect the potency of the drug.

Severe skin reactions to nitrofurazone may require topically applied steroids or the short-term administration of systemic corticosteroids.

■ ***Education.*** Clients should be instructed how to apply nitrofurazone correctly, and they should be alerted to its adverse reactions.

■ **Evaluation.** The expected outcome of nitrofurazone therapy is that the client's wound will evidence granulation and healing by primary intention or split-thickness skin grafting within an acceptable time frame.

Topical Antipruritics

Antipruritic agents are given to allay itching of the skin and mucous membranes. There is less of a need for these preparations, because the constitutional treatment of clients with skin disorders is better understood. Dilute solutions containing phenol have been widely used. Dressings wet with potassium permanganate 1 : 4000, aluminum subacetate 1 : 16, boric acid, or physiologic saline solution may cool and soothe and thus prevent itching. Lotions such as calamine or calamine with phenol (phenolated calamine), as well as cornstarch or oatmeal baths, may also be used to relieve itching.

Local anesthetics such as dibucaine and benzocaine may decrease pruritus, but their use is not recommended because of their high sensitizing and irritating effects. The application of hydrocortisone in a lotion or ointment in a strength of 0.5% to 1% has proved to be one of the best methods of relieving pruritus and decreasing inflammation. An additional advantage is its low sensitizing index.

Topical Ectoparasiticidal Drugs

Ectoparasites are insects that live on the outer surface of the body, and ectoparasiticides are drugs used against those animal parasites. For human use, these drugs are more commonly referred to as *pediculicides* and *scabicides (miticides)*; these names reflect the parasite treated with each group.

Pediculosis is a parasitic infestation of lice on the skin of a human. Lice are transmitted from one person to another by close contact with infested persons, clothing, combs, and towels. There are three different varieties of infestations: (1) pediculosis pubis, caused by *Phthirus pubis* (pubic or crab louse); (2) pediculosis corporis, caused by *Pediculus humanus corporis* (body louse), and (3) pediculosis capitis, caused by *Pediculus humanus capitis* (head louse) (Figure 66-1). Except in individuals with heavy infestation, a characteristic finding of pediculosis corporis is that the parasite is absent from the body but inhabits seams of clothing that come in contact with the axillae or that are in the beltline or collar.

Common findings in a person who is infested include pruritus, nits (eggs of louse) on hair shafts, lice on skin or clothes and, with pubic lice, occasional sky-blue macules on the inner thighs or lower abdomen. The drug of choice is the pediculicide lindane (gamma benzene hexachloride).

Scabies is a parasitic infestation caused by the itch mite *Sarcoptes scabiei*. It is transmitted from one person to another by close contact, such as sleeping next to an infested individual. It bores into the horny layers of the skin in cracks and folds, causing irritation and pruritus. Itching occurs almost exclusively at night. The adult infestation is usually generalized over the body, especially in the webbed spaces between the fingers, wrists, elbows, and buttocks. The drug of choice is permethrin cream because it is considered to be more effective than crotamiton and lindane (Anandan, 1995).

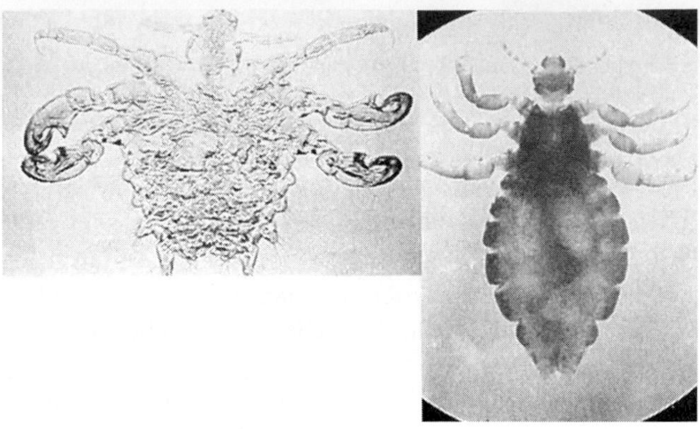

Figure 66-1 Pubic louse *(Phthirus pubis), left,* and body louse *(Pediculus humanus), right.* Notice that the first pair of legs on the pubic louse are thinner than the second and third pairs, and the abdomen is shorter. On the body louse, all legs are approximately the same length, and the abdomen is longer.

■ Nursing Management

Topical Ectoparasiticidal Therapy

The first approach to the treatment of both pediculosis and scabies is identification of the source of infestation. Decontamination of the clothing and personal articles used by the infested person is also necessary. This can be performed by washing clothing and bedding with hot, soapy water or by dry cleaning items that cannot be washed. Usually all persons involved (e.g., the entire family) are treated to prevent reinfestation.

lindane [lin' dane] (gamma benzene hexachloride [Kwell])

Lindane is both a scabicide and a pediculicide because it is effective in the treatment of both lice and mite infestations. It is available in a 1% cream, lotion, and shampoo. To treat pediculosis pubis and infestations of *P. humanus capitis,* the cream or lotion is applied in a sufficient quantity to cover the skin and hair of the infected and surrounding areas; it is left on for 12 hours and then washed out thoroughly. It seldom needs to be applied more than once. The shampoo is worked into the hair and left on for 4 minutes. The hair is then rinsed and dried, and the nits (eggs) are combed from the hair shafts. Retreatment is usually not necessary.

Lindane cream or lotion is used for the treatment of scabies. If crusted lesions are present, a warm bath preceding the application of lindane is recommended. Lindane is applied over the entire body from the neck down. It is left on for 8 hours and then washed off. One application is usually sufficient. It is common to have pruritus after application, but this does not indicate a need for reapplication unless live mites can be demonstrated.

Lindane occasionally will cause an eczematous skin rash. It penetrates human skin and has a potential for producing

TABLE 66-5 Miscellaneous Topical Agents

Generic (Trade Name)	Indication(s)	Comment(s)
becaplermin (Regranex)	diabetic neuropathic ulcers	Advise the client to wash his or her hands thoroughly before applying this drug. Avoid allowing the tip of the tube to come into contact with the ulcer or any other surface. Apply once daily as ordered by the prescriber.
imiquimod (Aldara)	external genital and vaginal warts	Concurrent use with a condom or diaphragm is not recommended. Avoid sexual contact when cream is on skin. Wash treatment area with a mild soap and water 6 to 10 hours after application. Local skin reaction may occur (e.g., redness, flaking, erosion, pruritus, and edema).
masoprocol (Actinex)	actinic keratoses	Do not apply near the eyes or the mucous membranes of the nose or mouth. Apply morning and evening for 28 days. Transient burning, flaking, pruritus, and dryness have been reported.
minoxidil (Rogaine)	androgenetic alopecia	Advise the client that hair growth usually takes up to 4 months to appear. If treatment is stopped, new growth will probably shed in a couple of months. Do not use on an irritated or sunburned scalp. Do not use with other topical medications on the scalp.
podofilox (Condylox)	external genital and perianal warts	Do not use to treat mucous membrane warts. Adverse reactions include burning, pain, inflammation, and pruritus.

Information from *Drug Facts and Comparisons* (2000). St. Louis: Facts and Comparisons.

central nervous system toxicity (e.g., seizures, increased irritability, dizziness), especially in children.

crotamiton [kroe tam′ i ton] (Eurax)

Crotamiton is indicated for the treatment of scabies; it is rubbed into the skin from the chin down, particularly in the folds and creases of the body and moist areas, such as the underarms and groin. It is reapplied in 24 hours and is washed from the body surface 48 hours after the second application. Two applications of crotamiton usually eradicate most infestations. In resistant cases it may be reapplied in 1 week.

Crotamiton is available as a 10% cream or lotion and may cause an occasional skin rash on application.

permethrin [per meth′ rin] (Nix)

Permethrin acts on the nerve cell membranes of lice, ticks, mites, and fleas. It disrupts sodium channel repolarization, thus paralyzing the parasites. Although it has a high cure rate after only a single application, head lice in children who reside where pediculicides are readily available are less susceptible to permethrin (Pollack et al., 1999).

The most common side effects/adverse reactions of permethrin include pruritus, mild burning on application, transient erythema, edema, and rash.

malathion [mal i thye′ on] (Ovide)

Malathion is an organophosphate cholinesterase inhibitor available for the treatment of head lice and ova. This product is usually effective in lice-infested individuals within 24 hours and is well tolerated. Malathion lotion is rubbed into the scalp and left to air dry. Because the drug is flammable, the client must be warned to avoid open flames and warned not to smoke or use a hairdryer. The hair is shampooed 8 to 12 hours after application, and the dead lice are combed out.

Miscellaneous Therapeutic Agents

Numerous other topical products are available alone or in combination. An example of an older product is coal tar or its derivatives, which are antipruritic and antieczematous and therefore are used to treat psoriasis and other skin conditions. Examples of products with coal tar as an ingredient include Medotar, Tegrin Lotion for Psoriasis and PolyTar. See Table 66-5 for other miscellaneous topical agents.

SUMMARY

Many dermatologic agents are available and are used to treat numerous skin disorders. Three major groups of preparations were discussed: general products, prophylactic agents, and therapeutic agents. General dermatologic preparations include bath substances, cleansers, soaps, solutions and emollients, skin protectants, wet dressings and soaks, and rubs and liniments. Many are soothing and are used to promote the comfort of clients who have a dermatologic condition. Prophylactic agents form a film on the skin to keep out sun, light, air, or dust. Therapeutic agents may be anti-infectives (antibiotics, antivirals, and antifungals), corticosteroids, keratolytics, acne products, burn products, antipruritics, and ectoparasiticidal drugs. The nurse must apply these preparations correctly and safely and instruct the client to do likewise if they are to be self-administered. Evaluating the effectiveness of dermatologic agents is based on improvement without adverse reactions.

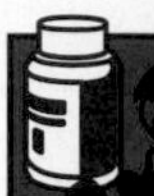

Complementary and Alternative Therapies
Aloe Vera Gel

Aloe vera gel is taken orally as a general tonic and for arthritis, gastroduodenal ulcers, diabetes, hyperlipidemia, and asthma. However, there is insufficient reliable information about its effectiveness for these uses, and it may be unsafe for these uses because its constituents act as a stimulant laxative. Topically, aloe gel is used for burns, wound healing, and inflammation. There is some evidence from randomized, double-blind trials to show that aloe vera is effective for psoriasis and genital herpes, although the results were based on few patients. There is no high-quality evidence of the effectiveness of aloe vera for wound healing or radiation-induced skin injury, although it is considered to be possibly effective when applied topically for reducing pain and inflammation and enhancing the healing of burns and other alterations of the skin. The usual topical dosage of aloe vera gel is liberal application to the affected area three to five times daily.

Information from Vogler B.K., Ernst, E. (1999). Aloe vera: A systematic review of its clinical effectiveness. *British Journal of General Practice 49*(447): 823-828.

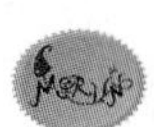

Critical Thinking Questions

1. Ronald Jones, age 48, comes to the clinic with a superficial skin infection as the result of an abrasion he received on the job as a construction worker. The health care provider orders the wound to be cleansed and dressed with bacitracin ointment (500 units/g, which the client is to continue three times daily) and also orders a culture and sensitivity tests. As the nurse, what action will you take and in what sequence?
2. What teaching would you provide to a mother who has discovered a pediculosis infestation in one of her children?

Collaborative Learning Activities

For Collaborative Learning Activities, go to mosby.com/MERLIN/McKenry/.

CASE STUDY

For a Case Study that will help ensure mastery of this chapter content, go to mosby.com/MERLIN/McKenry/.

BIBLIOGRAPHY

Anandan, J.V. (1995). Parasitic infections. In L.Y. Young & M.A. Koda-Kimble (Eds.), *Applied therapeutics: The clinical use of drugs* (6th ed.). Vancouver, WA: Applied Therapeutics.

Anderson, K.N., Anderson, L.E., & Glanze, W.D. (Eds.) (1998). *Mosby's medical, nursing, & allied health dictionary* (5th ed.). St. Louis: Mosby.

Bhawan, J., Gonzalez-Serva, A., Nehal, K., Labadie, R., Lufrano, L., Thorne, E.G., Gilchrest, B.A. (1991). Effects of tretinoin on photodamaged skin: A histologic study. *Archives of Dermatology, 127* (5), 666-672

Correale, C.E., Walker, C., Murphy, L., & Craig, T.J. (1999). Atopic dermatitis: A review of diagnosis and treatment. *American Family Physician, 60*(4), 1191-1198, 1209-1210.

DeSimone, II, E.M. (1996). Sunscreen and suntan products. In T.R. Covington (Ed.), *Handbook of nonprescription drugs* (11th ed.). Washington, D.C.: American Pharmaceutical Association.

Dickens C.H., Edwards, L., Ellis, C.N., & Shalita, A.R. (1992). Retinoids: What role in your practice? *Patient Care, 26*(10), 18-45.

Drug Facts and Comparisons. (2000). St. Louis: Facts and Comparisons.

Freedburg, I.M., Eisen, A.Z., & Wolff, K. (1998). *Fitzpatrick's dermatology in general medicine,* volumes I & II (5th ed.). New York: McGraw-Hill.

Gupta, M.A., Goldfarb, M.T., Schork, N.J., Weiss, J.S., Gupta, A.K., Ellis, C.N., Voorhees, J.J. (1991). Treatment of mildly to moderately photoaged skin with topical tretinoin has a favorable psychosocial effect: A prospective study. *Journal of the American Academy of Dermatology, 24*(5 pt 1), 780-781.

Hanifin, J.M. & Chan, S. (1999). Biochemical and immunologic mechanisms in atopic dermatitis: New targets for emerging therapies. *Journal of the American Academy of Dermatology, 41*(1), 72-77.

Hart, R., Bell-Syer, S.E., Crawford, F., Torgerson, D.J., Young, P., Russell, I. (1999). Systematic review of topical treatments for fungal infections of the skin and nails of the feet. *British Medical Journal, 319*(7207), 79-82.

Hill, L., Ferrini, R.L. (1998). Skin cancer prevention and screening: Summary of the American College of Preventive Medicine's Practice Policy Statements. *CA: A Cancer Journal for Clinicians, 48,* 232-235.

Mailloux, A.T. (1995). Photosensitivity and burns. In L.Y. Young & M.A. Koda-Kimble (Eds.), *Applied therapeutics: The clinical use of drugs* (6th ed.). Vancouver, WA: Applied Therapeutics.

McDonald, C.J. (1998). American Cancer Society perspective on the American College of Preventive Medicine's Policy Statements on Skin Cancer Prevention and Screening. *CA: A Cancer Journal for Clinicians, 48,* 229-231.

Pollack, R.J., Kiszewski, A., Armstrong, P., Hahn, C., Wolfe, N., Rahman, H.A., Laserson, K., Telford, S.R. 3rd, Spielman, A. (1999). Differential permethrin susceptibility of head lice sampled in the United States and Borneo. *Archives of Pediatric & Adolescent Medicine, 153*(9), 969-973.

Seaton, T.L. (1995). Acne. In L.Y. Young & M.A. Koda-Kimble (Eds.), *Applied therapeutics: The clinical use of drugs* (6th ed.). Vancouver, WA: Applied Therapeutics.

Strange, C.J. (1998). Thwarting skin cancer with sun sense. *FDA Consumer,* 29(6), July-Aug 1998; www.fda.gov/fdac/features/695_skincanc.html; 7/23/98.

Sunscreen drug products for over-the-counter human use. (1999). *Federal Register, 64*(98), Rules and Regulation (21 CFR Parts 310, 352, 700 and 740).

United States Pharmacopeia Dispensing Information (USP DI): Drug information for the health care professional (19th ed.). (1999). Rockville, MD: United States Pharmacopeial Convention.

Vogler, B.K., & Ernst, E. (1999). Aloe vera: A systematic review of its clinical effectiveness. *British Journal of General Practice 49*(447) 823-828.

Weil, A. (1999). Best method to block out sunburn; cgi.pathfinder.com/drweil/archiveqa/1,2283,1313,00.html (6/4/99).

Wright, J.B., Lam, K., Hansen, D., & Burrell, R.E. (1999). Efficacy of topical silver against fungal burn wound pathogens. *American Journal of Infection Control, 27*(4), 344-350.

67 Debriding Agents

Chapter Focus

Nurses have the major responsibility of assessing the client's risk for pressure sores and planning for the care needed to prevent them. Cleansing, debridement, and dressing of the wounds are necessary when pressure sores do occur. A knowledge of the various debriding agents will allow the nurse to apply the most appropriate agent for the client's pressure sores according to their location, size, presence of eschar, or state of granulation.

Learning Objectives

1. Use preventive and treatment measures to reduce the occurrence of decubitus ulcers.
2. Describe a classification system for grades of decubitus ulcers.
3. State the purpose of proteolytic enzyme preparations in the treatment of decubitus ulcers.
4. Implement the nursing management for the care of clients receiving topical enzymatic agents.
5. Describe the mechanism of action of nonenzymatic agent therapy for decubitus ulcers.
6. Implement the nursing management for the care of clients receiving nonenzymatic agent therapy for decubitus ulcers.

Key Terms

debridement, p. 1144
eschar, p. 1145
granulation tissue, p. 1145
pressure sore, p. 1140
proteolytic enzyme, p. 1144

This chapter covers debriding agents, which are agents used to remove dirt, foreign objects, damaged tissue, and cellular debris from a wound or burn to prevent infection and promote healing. When treating a wound, debridement is the first step in cleansing it; it also allows examination of the extent of the injury.

OVERVIEW OF PRESSURE SORES

The **pressure sore** (bed sore or decubitus ulcer) is a break in the skin and underlying subcutaneous and muscle tissue. It is caused by abnormal, sustained pressure or friction exerted over the bony prominences of the body by the object on which the body part rests. It results in vascular insufficiency and ischemic necrosis, and it most commonly affects debilitated, comatose, immobilized, or paralyzed clients.

According to the Agency for Health Care Policy and Research (AHCPR), the prevalence of pressure ulcers ranges from 9.2% in acute care facilities, to 33% in critical care clients, and up to 23% in skilled care facilities and nursing homes (Bergstrom et al., 1994). In addition to the human suffering of clients and their families, the total cost of treating such wounds was estimated to exceed $1.335 billion (Bergstrom et al., 1994).

Many causes contribute to this condition and must be treated. Among the local and systemic causes are the following: obesity or malnutrition; debilitation; a pressure and shearing force on the lower body if the head of the bed is raised more than 30 degrees; a loss of sensation of pressure or pain; muscle atrophy and motor paralysis; a reduction in the amount of adipose tissue between the skin and underlying bone; emaciation and dehydration; poor nutrition because of an inadequate intake of vitamins, minerals, and trace elements (such as copper and zinc); friction; local anatomic defects; trauma; incontinence; edema; infections; heat and moisture (maceration); hypertension; septicemia; and local circulatory interference.

The bacterial flora of pressure sores (present in stages II, III and IV) are both gram-negative and gram-positive organisms and include *Staphylococcus aureus, Streptococcus* groups A and D, *Escherichia coli, Clostridium tetani,* and *Bacteroides, Proteus, Pseudomonas, Klebsiella,* and *Citrobacter* organisms. Parenteral antibiotics (as adequate levels in granulating wounds are not reached) may be needed in infected pressure sores that are difficult to treat; these antibiotics are used as an adjunct to surgical management just before and at the time of surgery.

A client with a full-thickness loss of skin may be a candidate for surgical intervention either to cover the ulcer area or to stabilize the wound. Surgical decisions include the underlying disease, the ability of the client to withstand surgery, and the condition or prognosis of the pressure sore (especially those in which all soft tissue is destroyed and bone is exposed).

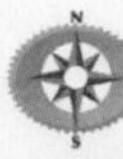

For a Concept Map on pressure sores, go to mosby.com/MERLIN/McKenry/.

■ Nursing Management

Pressure Sores

■ **Assessment.** To assess the client's risk for developing pressure sores, know their causes. Most health care agencies have assessment guides by which to assess the client's risk (Figure 67-1). These assessment guides address common risk factors such as mobility, activity, mental status, medications that affect blood circulation or cognition, incontinence, nutritional status, and other current illnesses. Clients are assessed and given a score; the higher the score, the higher the risk. These assessment guides are usually completed during admission of the client to the agency; continue to monitor the client for the risk of impaired skin integrity during his or her stay with the health care agency. If the client has an ulceration, accurate assessment determines the intervention. See the clinical guideline algorithm for the treatment of pressure ulcers developed by the Agency for Healthcare Research and Quality (formerly the Agency for Health Care Policy and Research) (Figure 67-2).

■ **Nursing Diagnosis.** The pertinent nursing diagnosis is either risk for impaired skin integrity (given the client's assessment score) or actual impairment of skin integrity if the client demonstrates skin changes such as erythema that does not resolve in 30 minutes, blisters, or tissue erosion. Risk for infection and impaired comfort (pain) may also occur.

■ **Implementation**

■ ***Monitoring.*** Monitor the bony prominences of the ankles, coccyx, elbows, heels, hips, knees, shoulders, and other areas having thin layers of subcutaneous tissue. Continue to assess the client for the presence or worsening of the risk factors previously discussed. If a pressure sore occurs, assess the wound on a daily basis for a gradual reduction in size; measure and record the size at its greatest length, width, and depth. Determine the stage of the wound and describe its appearance regarding necrotic debris, eschar, granulation tissue, drainage, color, and odor. Assess for pockets, tracts, and undermining. Observe the wound margins for induration or tenderness.

■ ***Intervention.*** The prevention and treatment of pressure sores are centered around treating the underlying causes, providing a well-balanced nutritional state, and minimizing or eliminating the pressure or friction that is causing the tissue damage. The following are some preventive and treatment measures that can be used to reduce the occurrence of impaired skin integrity:

1. Change the client's position frequently (every 1 to 2 hours day and night) for pressure relief.
2. Maintain a clean, dry, and wrinkle-free bed. Bedclothes should be smooth rather than coarse and should be changed frequently.
3. Provide active and passive exercise to increase muscle and skin tone and to improve vascularity, or use a whirlpool for hydrotherapy.
4. Position the client with pillows and pads; do not exceed a 30-degree elevation of the head.
5. Use hydrofloat devices, silica gel pads, polystyrene, and convoluted foam pads and heel protectors to re-

SKIN INTEGRITY HIGH RISK FORM

	PARAMETERS	0	1	2	3	4	5	SCORE
1.	General state of health	Good	Fair	Poor	Moribund			
2.	Predisposing diseases	Absent	Slight	Moderate	Severe			
3.	Mental status	Alert	Lethargic	Semicoma	Comatose			
4.	Nutrition	Good	Fair	Poor	None			
5.	Fluid intake	Good	Fair	Poor	None			
6.	Activity	Ambulates	Needs help			Chairfast	Bedfast	
7.	Mobility	Full	Limited			Very limited	Immobile	
8.	Incontinence	None	Occasional			Frequent	Total	
							TOTAL	

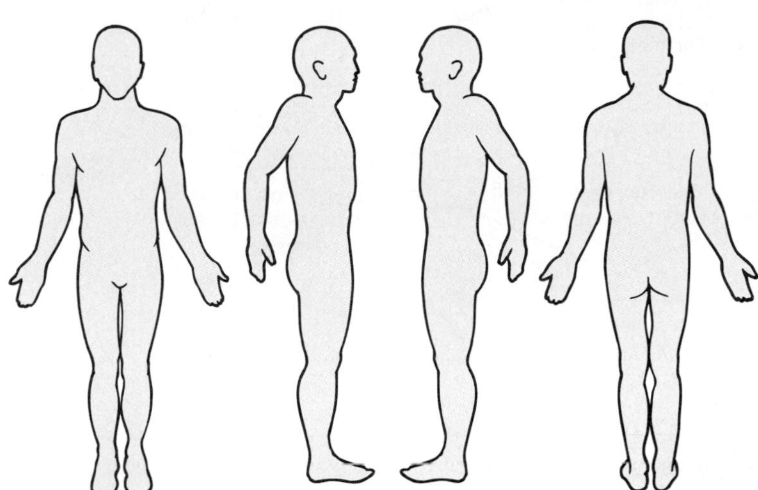

Draw and Number Impairments

	#1
Stage:	
Size:	
Shape:	
Drainage:	
	#2
Stage:	
Size:	
Shape:	
Drainage:	
	#3
Stage:	
Size:	
Shape:	
Drainage:	

Date/Signature:

PARAMETERS:

1. GENERAL STATE OF HEALTH:
   - 0–Good: injury limited to one area, no major health problems
   - 1–Fair: minor surgery or controlled health problems
   - 2–Poor: major surgery or serious health problems
   - 3–Moribund: prognosis fatal, death within 3 months
2. PREDISPOSING DISEASE:
   - 0–Absent: no vascular disease, anemia, diabetes, neuropathies
   - 1–Slight: controlled diabetes, anemia, mild vascular diseases, mild skin disorder
   - 2–Moderate: brittle diabetes, advanced vascular disease, unhealed ulcers, absent peripheral pulses
   - 3–Severe: uncontrolled diabetes/anemia, severe vascular disease manifested by decreased sensation, edema of ankles and feet, thin atrophic skin, brown pigmentation with stasis dermatitis
3. MENTAL STATUS:
   - 0–Alert: oriented, communicates appropriately
   - 1–Lethargic: listless, sluggish, slow to respond
   - 2–Semicoma or confused: responds to painful stimuli, unable to cooperate with pressure relief
   - 3–Comatose: no verbal response, no response to pain
4. NUTRITION:
   - 0–Good: weight within normal limits
   - 1–Fair: under or overweight, enternal or parenteral nutrition meeting RDA
   - 2–Poor: losing weight slowly or obese, seldom eats 1/2 served portion, enteral feeding tolerated poor, i.e., high gastric residual, diarrhea
   - 3–None: losing weight rapidly, emaciated, unable to eat, refuses to eat, no nutritional support
5. FLUID INTAKE:
   - 0–Good: 1500 mL, skin warm resilient, normal turgor
   - 1–Fair: 1000-1500 mL, dry skin and flaccid, concentrated urine output
   - 2–Poor: ↓1000 mL, skin dry, cracked and flaky, mouth dry, lips parched, decreased urine output in the absence of renal disease
   - 3–None: no fluid intake
6. ACTIVITY:
   - 0–Ambulates: walks without help
   - 1–Needs help: requires assistance, uses crutch, walker
   - 2–Chairfast: cannot ambulate, confined to chair
   - 3–Bedfast: remains in bed constantly
7. MOBILITY:
   - 0–Full: voluntarily changes position
   - 1–Limited: cannot voluntarily move all extremities, cast on arm or leg, pain with movement
   - 2–Very limited: move only with assistance, severe pain with movement, body cast, paraplegia, hemiparesis
   - 3–Immobile: never voluntarily changes position, contractures prevent movement, quadriplegia
8. INCONTINENCE:
   - 0–None: control of bowel and bladder
   - 1–Occasional: stress incontinence, occasional diarrhea with the continent patient
   - 2–Frequent: usually of urine and/or bowels
   - 3–Total: no control of bowel or bladder

Figure 67-1 Assessment guide. A score of 12 or greater is an indication that the client is at risk for impaired skin integrity. This nursing diagnosis should be included in the client's care plan.

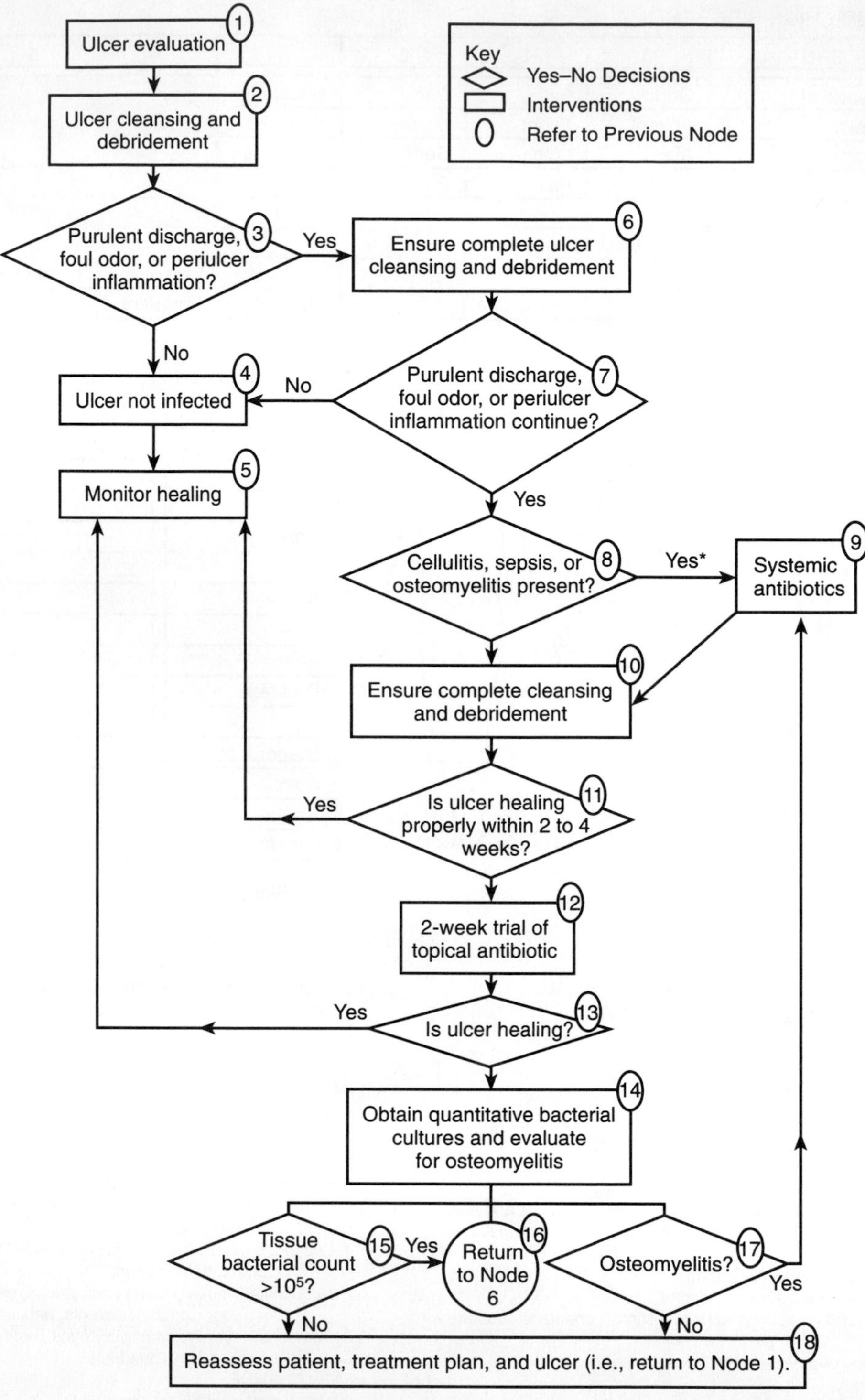

Figure 67-2 Clinical guideline algorithm for the treatment of pressure ulcers. *Suspicion of sepsis requires urgent medical evaluation and treatment. The treatment of sepsis is not discussed in this guideline. (From Agency for Health Care Policy and Research [1994]. *Pressure ulcer treatment: Quick reference guideline.* No. 15. AHCPR Pub. No. 95-0653. Rockville, MD: Agency for Health Care Policy and Research, Public Health Service, U.S. Department of Health and Human Services.)

duce pressure. Place them on a mattress in direct contact with the client's skin. The mattress should be free of surface bulges and indentations and should have a uniform, flat surface to prevent friction or wrinkles.

6. Use an alternating pressure mattress pad covered with one layer of sheet to promote circulation and to reduce the occurrence of tissue ischemia.
7. Provide meticulous skin hygiene, with frequent inspections for abnormal alterations. Wash the skin

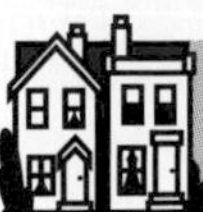

Community and Home Health Considerations
Wound Care at Home

Instruction should be provided for the caregiver if decubitus care is to be performed in the home. This should include all of the supportive care to the client, such as positioning, nutrition, and hydration discussed in the interventions. Pressure sore dressings should be changed as ordered by the prescriber or when soiled.

Dressing supplies, the debriding agent, gloves, and a bag for disposal of the soiled dressings should be gathered together before the dressing change is begun. The client should be positioned for comfort and for good access to the pressure sore. The pressure sore should be assessed each time the dressing is changed; the size and character of the wound is recorded to monitor progress. Any increase in drainage or foul smell should be reported to the nurse.

Expose the pressure sore, and drape the client for modesty as much as possible. Glove hands and remove the soiled dressing, pulling the adhesive tape in the direction of the pressure sore. Mineral oil may be used to loosen the adhesive tape. Discard the old dressings and gloves in the bag. Glove hands to clean the wound from the center out, using one stroke each time until crusting and old drainage are removed. Apply a pharmacologic agent as ordered using swabs, a tongue blade, or gloved fingers. Apply outer dressings. Remove gloves, and secure dressing with tape. Discard soiled gloves in the bag.

gently with warm water and, if needed, mild nondetergent soap; rinse the skin and blot it dry with a soft towel. An emollient lubricating lotion may be used after washing to keep the skin soft.

8. Keep the skin of incontinent clients dry and clear of urine and fecal contamination, because maceration from moisture promotes tissue breakdown and predisposes clients to infection. Perspiration in the continent client is also a cause of maceration. Trimmed nails prevent self-inflicted injury caused by scratching of the skin.
9. Maintain nutritional support for a positive nitrogen balance, tissue turgor, and adequate fluid intake with 3800 to 4600 cal/24 hours and a diet high in protein, vitamins, minerals, and trace elements. The client's hemoglobin level should be at least 12 g/100 mL, and serum protein levels should be above 6 g/100 mL.
10. Necrotic pressure sores often require meticulous wound care and debridement by surgical or drug methods.
11. Clients should be offered analgesics before pressure sore care depending on the extent of the wound and the client's preferences.
12. Treatment regimens are based on the extent of skin involvement.

■ ***Education.*** Preventive measures should be taught to clients, family members, or other caregivers of bedridden clients or other clients who are at risk for developing pressure sores. If a pressure sore is present, inform the client that the preparations used are to promote healing, and describe the procedure involved in cleansing and dressing the wound (see the Community and Home Health Considerations box at left).

■ **Evaluation.** The expected outcome of pressure sore care is that the client's skin will remain warm, without erythema, and intact. If a pressure sore exists, the wound will diminish in size and form a healthy, clean surface.

PHARMACOLOGIC MANAGEMENT OF PRESSURE SORES

A treatment plan for pressure sores should take into consideration four basic principles: (1) providing assessment and interventions to improve the client's general health, which may help to reduce factors contributing to the problem, such as incontinence, anemia, or edema; (2) reducing pressure sites through positioning or the use of padding, special beds, and other items, thus increasing blood flow to the site; (3) maintaining a clean wound site; and (4) using an appropriate agent for treatment or stimulation of granulation tissue.

The treatment of pressure sores depends on the stage of the ulcer and the condition of the wound bed. In many instances, cleansing and debridement prevents bacterial colonization from progressing to an infection. A 2-week trial with topical antibiotics should be considered if a clean ulcer has exudate or does not heal after 2 to 4 weeks of treatment. The topical agent should be effective against gram-positive, gram-negative, and anaerobic bacteria, such as triple antibiotic or silver sulfadiazine (Bergstrom et al., 1994).

If the ulcerated area does not respond, a tissue biopsy and bacterial culture are recommended in addition to an evaluation for osteomyelitis. Systemic antibiotics are necessary for sepsis, osteomyelitis, bacteremia, and advancing cellulitis (Bergstrom et al., 1994).

Saline solutions are considered safe and effective in cleaning most pressure sores. Avoid the use of povidone-iodine, iodophor, Dakin's solution, acetic acid, and hydrogen peroxide, because they are reported to be cytotoxic (i.e., toxic to fibroblasts) and interfere with the granulation process (Eastman, 1995).

Pressure sores are classified into four grades or stages (Figure 67-3):

Stage I: A red area that overlies a bony or tendinous (tendons) site that remains even when the pressure is relieved

Stage II: A partial-thickness skin loss that involves the epidermis and/or dermis

Stage III: A skin ulcer that extends into exposed subcutaneous tissue; it may include necrotic tissue, sinus tract formation, exudate, and/or infection

Stage IV: A deep skin ulcer that exposes muscle and bone; the body enzymes usually separate the eschar.

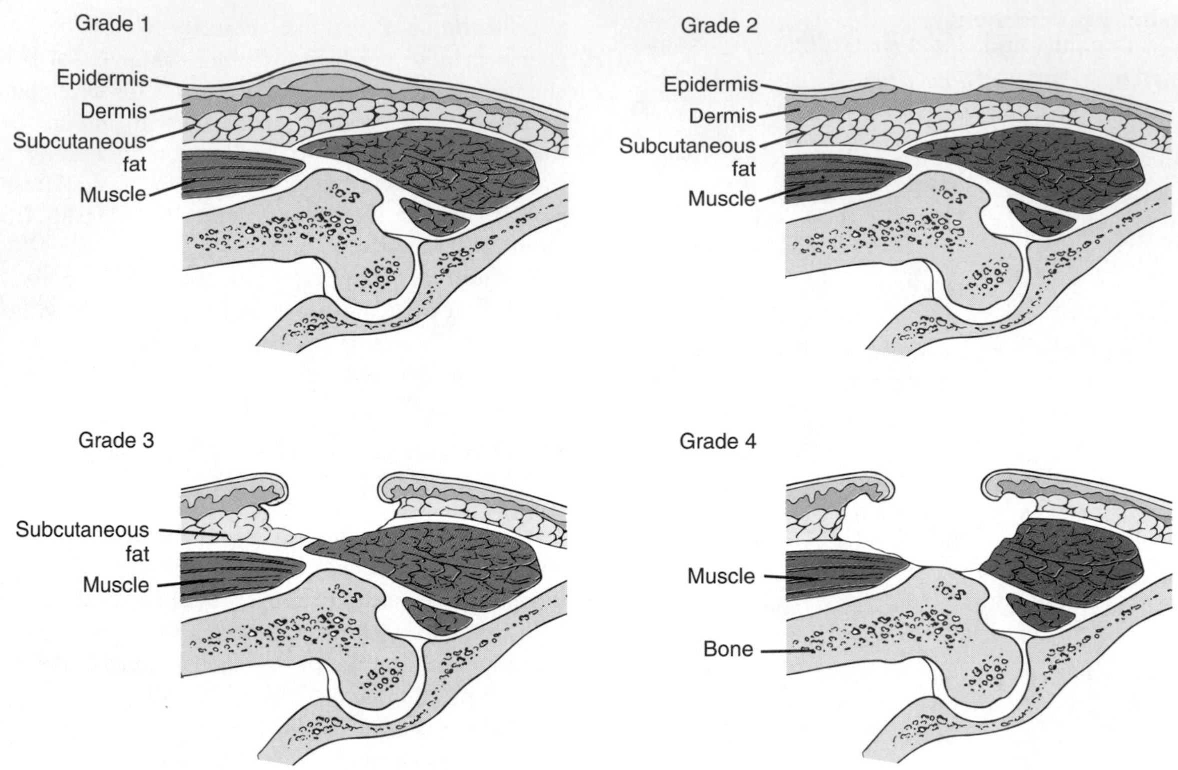

Figure 67-3 The four grades of pressure sores.

TABLE 67-1 Decubitus Ulcers: Recommended Treatment Protocol

Staging	Typical Treatment Modalities
Stage I or II	Silicone spray, transparent or hydrocolloidal dressing
Stage III	Wet-to-dry dressings, enzymatic debridement, hydrocolloidal dressing
Stage IV	Wet-to-dry dressings, enzymatic debridement, surgical debridement

The sloughing of tissue results in an ulcer and may include necrotic tissue, sinus tract formation, exudate, and/or infection

In addition to the nursing management previously reviewed, numerous treatment protocols have been applied. The treatment approach can vary considerably depending on the evaluation of the wound, the physician, the nurse, and local practice. Table 67-1 is a recommended treatment protocol based on the staging system previously noted.

Proteolytic (Debriding) Enzymes

Debridement is used to remove necrotic and sloughing tissue in a pressure ulcer. This tissue delays healing and provides a media for bacterial infestation. Although commonly used for debridement, wet-to-dry saline dressings can be irritating, painful, and disruptive to healthy tissue. **Proteolytic enzymes** are used for chemical debridement; they digest or liquefy necrotic tissue. The drawback with these preparations is that 2 or 3 days are usually needed to get rid of an eschar. However, their use is appropriate for noninfected necrotic sites and for clients unable to tolerate surgical intervention. If these preparations are used for infected necrosis tissue, a systemic antibiotic may also be necessary.

The enzyme preparation should be discontinued when granulation tissue is evident or if bleeding occurs during gentle cleansing (Chamberlain et al., 1992). Surgical debridement may be required for very serious ulcerations or if complications (e.g., osteomyelitis) are present.

Most enzymes contain the suffix "ase" in their name plus the name of the substrate on which they act. For example, collagenase acts on and degrades collagen, and hyaluronidase acts on hyaluronic acid (a ground substance of connective tissue). Enzymes are also grouped according to the reactions they catalyze. For example, proteolytic enzymes hasten the hydrolysis of proteins. Because enzymes are proteins, they may be antigenic and cause immunologic-type toxic reactions.

The enzymes discussed in this chapter are used topically for *medical* or *chemical debridement*—the removal, by enzymatic digestion, of necrotic and injured tissue, clotted blood, purulent exudates, or fibrinous accumulations in wounds. This action cleans the wounds and facilitates healing.

■ Nursing Management

Proteolytic Enzyme Therapy

The following are aspects of care for clients being treated with topically applied enzymatic drugs (not the nonenzymatic agents). These are in addition to the aspects of care previously discussed under Nursing Management: Pressure Sores, p. 1140. Before the topical aseptic application of enzymes, the wound should be thoroughly cleansed (flushing away necrotic debris and fibrinous exudates) with a solution that does not inactivate the enzyme (e.g., physiologic saline or sterile distilled water). Healing wounds should be cleansed gently; high-pressure irrigation or aggressive scrubbing with gauze pads should be avoided, because tissue will be traumatized and healing will be delayed. Solutions containing heavy metals, detergents, and antiseptics should be avoided to prevent inactivation of the enzymes. As much necrotic tissue as can be readily removed should be removed with forceps and scissors. All previously applied ointment should be removed before new ointment is applied to the substrate.

Dense, dry, and thick **eschar,** or crust, should be cross-hatched by the physician with a No. 10 or No. 11 blade for adequate contact of the enzyme with the substrate of necrotic debris. Ointment should be applied directly to the wound with a sterile tongue depressor or spatula and then covered with sterile petrolatum gauze or sterile gauze (or other nonadhering dressing); ointment can also be applied with a sterile gauze pad that is then placed over the wound. A bandage and/or tape should be used to hold the dressing in place.

Ointment or jelly preparations should be confined to the wound. The surrounding healthy tissue (or skin) should be protected from the enzyme (e.g., zinc oxide paste can be used). The treated lesion should be kept moist and protected from drying. The enzyme must be in direct contact with the wound for a sufficient length of time—usually about 4 days. To avoid delayed healing, the enzyme should be discontinued when the wound is cleaned and debrided and when **granulation tissue** (healthy pink, soft new tissue) is evident. Secondary skin closure or grafting may follow debridement.

Topical enzymes used for debriding may increase the risk of bacteremia in the debilitated client; this may necessitate monitoring these clients for systemic bacterial infections. Clients should be observed for allergic or sensitivity reactions (e.g., dermatitis and febrile reactions).

collagenase [kole′ a jen aze] (Santyl)

Collagenase is an enzymatic debriding agent capable of degrading both native and denatured collagen. Other proteolytic enzymes act only on denatured collagen. Thus it is claimed that collagenase produces more effective debridement by acting on collagen at the wound edges, where necrotic slough is anchored. This product is used to debride necrotic lesions and severe burns.

This ointment should be applied only within the area of the lesion; a transient erythema has been reported as a cutaneous reaction on the wound surface or the area adjacent to the lesion. Applying a protectant (e.g., zinc oxide paste) may prevent this reaction around the lesion.

■ Nursing Management

Collagenase Therapy

In addition to the following discussion, see Nursing Management: Pressure Sores, p. 1140 and Nursing Management: Proteolytic Enzyme Therapy, at left. Determine that the client is not sensitive to collagenase before initiating therapy.

Review the client's current medication regimen for the risk of significant drug interactions, such as those that may occur if collagenase is given concurrently with the following drugs:

Drug	Possible Effect and Management
Burow's solution and other acidic solutions	Collagenase can be inactivated by irrigating the lesion with acidic solutions such as Burow's solution (pH 3.6 to 4.4). The optimal pH range for collagenase is 6 to 8; an alteration outside this range decreases the activity of the enzyme.
detergents, soaps, cleansing agents, heavy metal ions (mercury, silver), antiseptics (e.g., iodine, hexachlorophene, benzalkonium chloride), nitrofurazone (Furacin)	The activity of collagenase is inhibited.

The wound area is cleansed of debris by gentle irrigation with sterile normal saline. The ulcer should be patted dry with a sterile gauze pad. If infection is present, a topical antibacterial agent (e.g., neomycin, bacitracin-polymyxin B solution or powder) is applied directly to the ulcer surface before the collagenase.

Collagenase should be applied once daily. If the wound is deep, collagenase should be applied directly with a wooden tongue depressor or spatula. The application should be repeated if the dressing area becomes soiled (e.g., because of incontinence).

The average time for complete debridement of dermal ulcers and decubiti with collagenase is approximately 11 days. This time permits debridement of necrotic tissue and the establishment of granulation tissue. Careful observation of the wound bed is indicated. The enzyme should be stopped when granulation tissue is evident. The ointment does not need to be refrigerated; it is stored at room temperature.

fibrinolysin and desoxyribonuclease [fye bri nol′ ih sin/des ock see rye bo nu′ klee aze] (Elase)

The proteolytic enzymes fibrinolysin and desoxyribonuclease have individual effects; fibrinolysin digests fibrin or blood clots, and desoxyribonuclease digests deoxyribonucleic acid (nucleic acids). Because purulent exudates are composed mainly of fibrin and nucleic acids, this product produces its effects on denatured proteins (devitalized tissue); the protein elements of living cells remain unaffected.

An ointment that contains the two enzymes in combination with chloramphenicol is also available. The added antibiotic bacteriostatic properties inhibit the synthesis of bacterial protein in infected lesions. Systemic antibiotics are also indicated when clinical infection has been verified by positive culture results.

This product is used to debride inflamed and/or infected lesions, including surgical wounds, ulcerative lesions, second- and third-degree burns, and wounds resulting from circumcision or episiotomy. The combination product with antibiotic is preferred for infected lesions. This product is also used for the treatment of vaginitis and cervicitis (intravaginal use) and for the irrigation of infected wounds and superficial hematomas not adjacent to or near fatty tissue.

▪ Nursing Management

Fibrinolysin and Desoxyribonuclease Therapy

In addition to the following discussion, see Nursing Management: Pressure Sores, p. 1140, as well as Nursing Management: Proteolytic Enzyme Therapy, p. 1145.

Obtain the client's sensitivity history, because allergic reactions have been observed in clients who are sensitive to bovine source materials or mercury compounds (thimerosal, a mercury derivative, is used as a preservative in the ointment base of Elase). When using the ointment formulation containing chloramphenicol, monitor the wound for superinfection.

This preparation is available as an ointment or as a dry powder in vials, in which case it will need to be reconstituted with 10 to 50 mL of 0.9% sodium chloride for injection. The solution may then be used as a spray or for a wet dressing. Saturate strips of fine-mesh gauze or unfolded sterile gauze pads in the solution; pack the ulcerated area with the gauze to ensure that it is in contact with the necrotic substrate. The dressing should be allowed to dry in contact with the tissue, which may take 6 to 8 hours. Remove the gauze three or four times daily. As the gauze dries, the necrotic tissues slough, become enmeshed in the gauze, and are removed from the wound. After 2 to 4 days the wound should become clean and begin to evidence granulation tissue. Mix the preparation on a daily basis because it becomes inactive after 24 hours, even if refrigerated.

sutilains [soo′ ti layns] (Travase)

Sutilains is a sterile preparation of proteolytic enzyme that digests necrotic soft tissues and purulent exudates. It aids in the selective removal of only nonviable protein in necrotic soft tissue and of purulent exudate from open wounds and ulcers resulting from second- and third-degree burns, decubiti, peripheral vascular disease, and wounds (incisions, trauma, pyogens).

The side effects are mild and include mild, transient pain (managed with a mild analgesic), local paresthesia, bleeding, and transient dermatitis.

▪ Nursing Management

Sutilains Therapy

In addition the following discussion, see Nursing Management: Proteolytic Enzyme Therapy, p. 1145 and Nursing Management: Collagenase Therapy, p. 1145.

Sutilains should not be applied to wounds that communicate with major body cavities, wounds with exposed major nerves or nerve tissue, neoplastic ulcers, or wounds in women of childbearing age. Because its use causes increased fluid and blood loss, it should be used with caution in clients with limited cardiac and pulmonary reserves.

Review the client's wound therapy for significant drug interactions, which may occur if sutilains is used concurrently with the drugs discussed for collagenase therapy.

Monitor the client as described under the general nursing management for pressure sores. Sutilains should be discontinued if bleeding or dermatitis occurs. Although systemic allergic reactions have not been reported, this drug is capable of causing an antibody response.

Sutilains is prepared as an ointment containing 82,000 casein units/g ointment base (15-g tubes). It must be refrigerated at a temperature between 2° and 10° C.

The wound should be cleansed thoroughly (including the removal of antiseptics) with water or isotonic sodium chloride solution and left moist or wet before a thin layer of sutilains ointment is applied in a thin layer (⅛ inch) up to ½-inch beyond the area needing debriding. When used for extensive burns, the ointment should be used only on 10% to 15% of the burned skin area at one time. The area should be covered with loose, wet dressings. This process should be repeated 3 to 4 times daily, although adequate responses have occurred with 1 to 2 changes daily. A moist environment is necessary for the enzymatic activity of this agent. Apply sutilains first when used concurrently with topical antibiotics.

Sutilains must be kept away from the eyes; if contact occurs, the eyes should be rinsed with copious amounts of sterile water.

This drug should be discontinued if dissolution does not occur in 24 to 48 hours.

Topical Enzyme Combination Products

Trypsin and papain (proteolytic enzymes), balsam of Peru (a mild antibacterial agent that aids in improving circulation in the wound area by stimulating the capillary bed), castor oil (provides protective covering and improves epithelialization), urea (emollient and keratolytic), and chlorophyll derivatives (aid in controlling wound odor and healing) have been formulated into various combinations and marketed. For example, Granulex contains trypsin, balsam of Peru, and castor oil, whereas Panafil contains papain, urea, and chlorophyll derivatives.

Such products may be ordered for administration once or twice daily. The wound area should be cleansed by flushing it with physiologic saline before each application. Be aware that hydrogen peroxide solution can inactivate papain.

Nonenzymatic Agents

dextranomer [dex tran' oh mer] (Debrisan)

Dextranomers are hydrophilic beads placed in the wound to absorb exudate, bacteria, and other matter. They are used for cleansing only a wet or secreting wound (not dry wounds); the action continues until all the beads are saturated. The assumption of a grayish-yellow color by the beads indicates that they are saturated and ready for removal.

■ Nursing Management

Dextranomer Therapy

In addition to the following discussion, see Nursing Management: Pressure Sores, p. 1140.

Dextranomer is available in 4-g packages; in 25-, 60-, and 120-g containers; and in paste form. The contents of each container should be used for only one client to limit cross-contamination.

Initially preparation of the wound involves irrigation with sterile water or saline; the area should be left moist. A whirlpool bath will assist in removing persistent patches of beads. To achieve the desired suction effect, the beads should cover the wound surface to a depth of 6 mm (¼ inch) (e.g., 4 g of beads covers a wound or ulcer 1½ × 1½ inches). A paste mixture is often used for areas that consist of irregular body surfaces or are difficult to reach. If the premade paste dosage form is not available (10-g foil packets), mix the beads with glycerin (only glycerin), and dress the wound in the usual manner. The beads or paste must be reapplied every 12 hours or more often while reducing the number of applications as the exudate diminishes. If the wound is a cratered pressure sore, allow for expansion of the beads by not packing the wound tightly. Dextranomer should be used only in body areas where complete removal is possible (not deep fistulas or sinus tracts). Be aware that the floor becomes slippery if the beads are spilled on the floor, thus creating a work hazard.

The wound should be lightly bandaged on all four sides to hold the beads in place and prevent maceration from occlusion. The degree of wound secretion determines the number of dressing changes (one or two daily profuse secretions may necessitate three or four dressing changes). Dressings are changed before encrustation or full saturation of the beads (grayish yellow color) to prevent drying and to facilitate bead removal by irrigation (e.g., sterile water, saline). These moisture-reactive dressings for pressure sores and leg ulcers may remain in place for 1 to 7 days; by interacting with the available skin moisture, a bond is created that keeps them in place. While in place over the wound, the moisture-reactive particles embedded in a polymer base interact with the wound fluid exudate, creating a soft moist gel over the wound; this eases removal of the dressing, with minimal damage to newly formed regenerating tissues.

As the edema reduces during the first few days, the wound itself may appear larger in size than it did before treatment. Therapy should be discontinued when healthy granulation is established. Treatment of an underlying pathologic condition (e.g., impaired venous or arterial flow or pressure) is concurrent. Clients with diabetes mellitus and immunosuppression may be susceptible to severe infections. A client may experience some occasional minor pain during dressing changes.

Consult with the prescriber if the condition worsens or persists beyond 14 to 21 days.

flexible hydroactive dressings and granules (DuoDerm)

Controlling the absorption of wound fluid exudate is a function of the rate at which the dressing interacts with the exudate. Flexible hydroactive dressings are indicated for necrotic wounds only after the thick eschar at the wound margin is removed. They provide local management of venous stasis ulcers, ulcers secondary to arterial insufficiency, diabetes mellitus, trauma, pressure sores, and superficial wounds. The granule form is for the local management of exudating dermal ulcers in association with the dressings.

■ Nursing Management

Flexible Hydroactive Dressings and Granules

In addition to the following discussion, see Nursing Management: Pressure Sores, p. 1140.

The use of flexible hydroactive dressings and granules should be avoided with the following dermal conditions: tissue of muscle, tendon, or bone; ulcers with infection (tuberculosis, syphilis, or deep fungal infections); and active vasculitis (periarteritis nodosa, systemic lupus erythematosus, and cryoglobulinemia).

During the initial phase of treatment, the wound increases in size and depth because of the cleaning away of necrotic debris.

The liquefied material left in the wound, which is seen when the dressing is removed, has the appearance of pus and should be washed away before proceeding with further wound evaluation.

Clean the wound site before applying this product, and follow the specific instructions outlined in the package labeling. Dressings are designed to remain in place from 1 to 7 days. The characteristic disagreeable dermal ulcer odor, which is apparent when the dressing is removed or when the wound leaks, may be diminished with the use of the granule dosage form during periods of excess exudation.

During periods of infection, the dressings or granules should be discontinued and antibiotic treatment started until the infection is completely treated.

The presence of excessive exudate may necessitate application of the granule dosage form into the wound to prevent leakage, to allow the dressing to remain in place longer, and to reduce dressing changes.

metronidazole [me troe ni' da zole] (Flagyl)

Metronidazole is an antiinfective systemic agent used investigationally to treat grades III and IV anaerobically infested, decubitus ulcers (*Drug Facts and Comparisons,* 2000). An approved topical metronidazole (MetroGel) is used to treat acne rosacea in adults (*United States Pharmacopeia Dispensing Information,* 1999).

SUMMARY

Pressure sores add greatly to the length and cost of a hospital stay. They are best prevented; when they do occur they are treated with proteolytic enzyme or nonenzymatic preparations depending on the cause and extent of the wound.

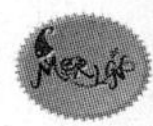

Critical Thinking Questions

1. How do the indications for the use of proteolytic enzyme preparations differ from the uses for flexible hydroactive dressings and granules?
2. How might a nurse determine that it is time to discontinue the use of proteolytic enzyme preparations?

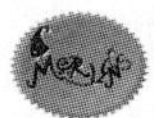

Collaborative Learning Activities

For Collaborative Learning Activities, go to mosby.com/MERLIN/McKenry/.

BIBLIOGRAPHY

Agency for Health Care Policy and Research. (1994). *Pressure ulcer treatment: Quick reference guideline, No. 15.* AHCPR Pub. No. 95-0653. Rockville, MD: Agency for Health Care Policy and Research, Public Health Service, U.S. Department of Health and Human Services.

Anderson, K.N., Anderson, L.E., & Glanze, W.D. (Eds.). (1998). *Mosby's medical, nursing, & allied health dictionary* (5th ed.). St. Louis: Mosby.

Bergstrom, N., Bennett, M.A., Carlson, C.E., et al. (1994). *Treatment of pressure ulcers: Clinical practice guidelines, No. 15.* AHCPR Pub. No. 95-0652. Rockville, MD: Agency for Health Care Policy and Research, Public Health Service, U.S. Department of Health and Human Services.

Chamberlain, T.M. et al. (1992). Assessment and management of pressure sores in long-term care facilities. *Consultant Pharmacist, 7*(112), 1328-1340.

Drug Facts and Comparisons. (2000). St. Louis: Facts and Comparisons.

Eastman, S.R. (1995). Prevention and treatment of pressure ulcers; Interpretation and practical application of AHCPR Guidelines, Part 1. *Clinical Consultant, 14*(10), 1-8.

Jaffee, M.S. & Skidmore-Roth, L. (1993). *Home health nursing care plans* (2nd ed.). St. Louis: Mosby.

United States Pharmacopeia Dispensing Information (USP DI): Drug information for the health care professional (19th ed.). (1999). Rockville, MD: United States Pharmacopeial Convention.

Zanowiak, P. (1992). Safe and effective management of pressure ulcers. *US Pharmacist,* Skin care supplement 6, 6.

68 Vitamins and Minerals

Chapter Focus

Over-the-counter vitamin and mineral preparations are very popular in the United States and Canada. However, these dietary supplements possess the capacity for producing toxic reactions if used inappropriately. Consumers often do not perceive vitamins and minerals as being drugs. It is imperative that nurses incorporate the assessment and instruction of vitamin therapy into their practice to be supportive of appropriate nutrient management for their clients.

Learning Objectives

1. Review the recommended daily allowances of vitamins and minerals.
2. Discuss factors that might contribute to the inadequate intake of vitamins and minerals.
3. Describe the difference between fat-soluble and water-soluble vitamins.
4. Cite the results of a deficiency or excess of each vitamin.
5. Implement the nursing management essential for the care of clients receiving vitamin therapy.
6. Compare the contents of over-the-counter vitamin and mineral preparations with recommended daily allowances.

Key Terms

avitaminosis, p. 1150
fat-soluble vitamins, p. 1151
hypervitaminosis, p. 1151
vitamins, p. 1150
water-soluble vitamins, p. 1151

The nutritional needs of the individual are best met by adequate oral ingestion of fluids and regular, balanced meals. There is a growing body of research that demonstrates that the prevalence of vitamin deficiency in usual Western diets is higher than generally believed. Subtle deficiencies in several vitamins (at levels below that which cause classic vitamin deficiency syndromes such as scurvy or pellagra) put the individual at risk for chronic degenerative diseases such as atherosclerosis, cancer, and osteoporosis.

Breast milk or formula meets the normal nutritional needs of the infant, and strained and chopped table foods are added to the diet as tolerated by the growing child. Throughout life, challenges to nutrition status can occur and necessitate the replacement or supplementation of nutrients, vitamins, minerals, electrolytes, and fluids. Debilitation from nutritional deprivation may impair wound healing; reduce collagen, hormone, and enzyme synthesis; and decrease essential protein production, reducing circulating albumin, fibrinogen, and hemoglobin. Malnutrition or mild-to-moderate starvation produces serious cellular biochemical changes, including diminished liver glycogen stores that start the first day of deprivation. Protein stores are more diminished via gluconeogenesis because amino acids are converted into glucose as an energy source. Tissue proteins are depleted and short-lived in the intestinal mucous membranes, liver, pancreas, and kidney tubular epithelia. Muscle proteins are converted to provide energy, and adipose tissues are metabolized to produce free fatty acids for energy substrates. The byproducts of fatty acid oxidation (ketones) are used as energy for the brain if starvation is prolonged.

Unusual or abnormal circumstances that necessitate the administration of various nutritional modalities (e.g., vitamin replacement and enteral or parenteral feedings) are discussed in the following sections.

VITAMINS

Vitamins are organic compounds that help to maintain normal metabolic functions, growth, and tissue repair. Mechanisms of action, specific indications for use, and pharmacokinetics are not well understood for all vitamins, nor have dosages been established for all vitamins. However, vitamin supplement therapy may be essential during periods of nutritional challenge, typically during rapid growth, pregnancy, lactation, or convalescence. Other challenges to nutrition occur with inadequate nutrient ingestion, malabsorption syndromes, and increased nutrient requirements caused by specific disease states, such as celiac sprue and ulcerative colitis. An increase in cellular proliferation in the latter conditions may result in the depletion of key nutrients, such as folic acid.

Insufficient dietary intake of vitamins and other essential nutrients may be occasionally traced to impoverished diets resulting from cultural, religious, or personal beliefs; fad diets; alcoholism; poverty; ignorance; or a lack of available food. Mild forms of **avitaminosis** (vitamin deficiency) are more common in the United States and Canada (often as a result of alcoholism) than are the pronounced deficiency states of beriberi, pellagra, rickets, or scurvy. The potential for iatrogenic starvation exists because of ignorance or oversight on the part of health care personnel who routinely fail to assess their clients' nutrition status or do not know how to correct it when necessary. Many medical procedures, such as nothing by mouth (NPO) orders to prepare the person for various gastrointestinal x-rays and procedures, may also potentiate client malnutrition.

A commonly prescribed IV solution of dextrose 5% in water delivers only 170 calories/L, and it is delivered purely in the form of a carbohydrate. Multiple cleansing enemas or prolonged gastrointestinal suction robs the body of essential electrolytes. Only a perfunctory medical assessment may be made of the effects of intraoperative blood losses or of wound drainage on nutrition needs, and surgery is always accompanied by increased nitrogen excretion. Common nursing problems that result when the client does not, cannot, or will not eat are often not given adequate medical attention to enable satisfactory nursing care.

Vitamin preparations and other more aggressive and supportive nutrition therapies are needed for the hospitalized client more often than is recognized, because only a few vitamins are synthesized in the body—bacteria in the gut form vitamin K, vitamin D is produced when skin is exposed to sunlight, and small and insufficient amounts of vitamin B are made in the gut. Most vitamins must either be ingested in food or taken as dietary supplements. There are two schools of thought concerning the consumption of vitamin supplements. In the past it was generally believed that the average American diet contains adequate vitamins and that additional supplements are unnecessary. Achievement of the recommended daily allowances (RDAs) was considered appropriate. However, the RDAs are established by the National Academy of Sciences and National Research Council as the amount necessary to prevent gross deficiency syndromes. It is now becoming apparent that some vitamins aid in preventing chronic disease. There is also concern regarding surveys that indicate specific segments of our society—older adults, smokers, nursing home residents, and teenagers—who reportedly do not consume the RDA levels of all vitamins and minerals. The most effective approach to correct such deficiencies is through diet, perhaps with the help of a dietitian.

A strong rationale for a daily multivitamin for all adults is developing. Homocystinemia, a major risk factor for cardiovascular disease, can be lowered by one RDA of folic acid daily (Robinson et al., 1998). Vitamin D deficiency is common in older adults; supplements of vitamin D with calcium have been shown to reduce fracture sites (Dawson-Hughes, Harris, Krall, & Dallal, 1997). Vitamin B_{12} deficiency in older adults may account for some cases of neurologic disease, such as dementia (Lindenbaum et al., 1988). Antioxidant supplements may reduce coronary events, improve immune function, and prevent dementia and macular degeneration (Box 68-1) (Fletcher, 1999). Multivitamins are inexpensive, convenient, and safe. Table 68-1 reviews vitamins and recommended their RDAs.

Hypervitaminosis is also of concern today, especially with the large consumption of vitamins in the United States. Hypervitaminosis is defined as an abnormal condition that results from the consumption of high or excessive amounts of one or more vitamins, usually over an extended period. The effects produced are discussed under the each vitamin monograph in the later sections.

Vitamins are important components of enzyme systems that catalyze the reactions for protein, fat, and carbohydrate metabolism. They are classified as being fat-soluble or water-soluble. The **fat-soluble vitamins** are A, D, E, and K. They are stored in the liver and fatty tissue in large amounts. A deficiency in these vitamins occurs only after a long deprivation from an adequate supply or as a result of disorders that prevent their absorption. **Water-soluble vitamins** include the B-complex group and vitamin C. These vitamins are not stored in the body in large amounts, and short periods of inadequate intake can lead to a deficiency.

BOX 68-1

Antioxidant Recommendations

The Institute of Medicine (2000) has issued recommendations on vitamin antioxidants that include higher RDAs for vitamin C and vitamin E from food sources, not supplements. The recommendation for vitamin C is 75 mg/day for females and 90 mg/day for males—up from the previously recommended 60 mg/day for adults. Smokers should take an additional 35 mg/day to compensate for vitamin C depletion as a result of smoking. The maximum intake recommended for vitamin C from food and supplements is 2000 mg/day for adults. Natural sources of vitamin C include citrus fruit, broccoli, strawberries, potatoes, and green leafy vegetables.

Vitamin E recommendations for adults are 15 mg/day of alpha-tocopherol, which is equivalent to 22 International Units (IU) of natural vitamin E or 33 IU of synthetic vitamin E (dl-alpha-tocopherol). The maximum adult dosage recommended is 1000 mg of alpha-tocopherol daily. Natural food sources of vitamin E include nuts, seeds, liver, vegetable oil, and green leafy vegetables.

This report also states that evidence regarding megadoses of antioxidants to prevent chronic disease has not been established. Instead this report warns that very large doses of vitamins may cause adverse side effects and health problems.

Information from Institute of Medicine (2000). Dietary intakes for vitamin C, vitamin E, selenium, and carotenoids. The National Academy Press. Washington, D.C. *Pharmacist's Letter, 16*(5), 26-27.

Many multivitamin capsules and tablets vary in their contents. "Optional vitamins" (E, B_6, folic acid, pantothenic acid, and B_{12}) may or may not be included as ingredients in over-the-counter (OTC) multivitamin preparations. The most popular OTC multivitamin preparations contain all of the vitamins needed by humans. Most OTC vitamin preparations are designed to meet the daily needs of the body completely without regard for the amounts of various vitamins contained in the daily diet.

■ Nursing Management

Vitamin and Mineral Therapy

Good nutrition is essential for good health. The nurse's participation in health promotion includes providing information regarding all aspects of nutrition. With the many misconceptions regarding vitamins and minerals and their function in health, as well as the prevention of illness prevalent today, the nurse has an important role in providing accurate dietary counseling with regard to vitamins and minerals.

■ **Assessment.** A dietary history for the client provides the nurse with insights into the client's eating patterns (e.g., in the last 24 hours). In addition, obtain information related to food source and preparation, living arrangements, financial status, coping patterns, knowledge of nutrition, and physiologic alterations that the client is experiencing as background for client teaching. This will also provide the client with more specifics regarding his or her dietary planning. Obtain the client's height and weight. Assess for signs of the specific vitamin or mineral deficiency throughout therapy. (Refer to the specific vitamin for relevant nursing management.) Consider that vitamin and mineral requirements may change with age and health status (e.g., in pregnancy). (See the Pregnancy Safety box below for the Food and Drug Administration's (FDA's) categories for vitamins). Baseline diagnostic studies can be obtained for the specific vitamin or mineral deficiency (e.g., serum folic acid and hemoglobin determinations).

■ **Nursing Diagnosis.** The general nursing diagnosis for clients with vitamin and mineral deficiencies is imbalanced nutrition: less than body requirements. Depending on the

Text continued on p. 1156

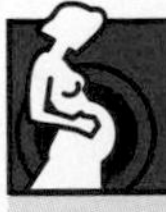

Pregnancy Safety
Vitamins

Category	Drug
A	folic acid, thiamine, pyridoxine
C	ascorbic acid (vitamin C), cyanocobalamin (vitamin B_{12}), vitamin D, iron
X	vitamin A
Unclassified	niacin, riboflavin, vitamin E, vitamin K

TABLE 68-1 Vitamin Review

Vitamin	Sources	Adverse Effects*
Fat-Soluble Vitamins		
A	Fish-liver oil, liver, butter, yellow fruit, green leafy vegetables, milk	*Acute:* confusion, irritation, diarrhea, dizziness, visual alterations, skin peeling, severe vomiting *Chronic:* Bone pain, dry/cracked skin or lips; fever, increased urination, anorexia, hair loss, seizures, vomiting
D	fish-liver oil, fortified milk, fish, exposure to sunlight	*Early with hypercalcemia:* constipation (mostly in children), diarrhea, headache, increased thirst and urination, metallic taste, nausea, vomiting
E	Nuts, green leafy vegetables, wheat and rice germ	*Acute:* Visual disturbances, headache, nausea, stomach pain, weakness, blurred vision *Chronic:* Increased bleeding tendencies in vitamin K–deficient clients, altered thyroid metabolism, impaired sexual function
K	Liver, green leafy vegetables	Hypersensitivity (flushing, dyspnea, chest pain), taste alterations
Water-Soluble Vitamins		
B_1 (thiamine)	Whole grain and enriched cereals, beef, pork, peas, beans, nuts	Low oral toxicity
B_2 (riboflavin)	Milk, cheese, eggs, green leafy vegetables, whole grain and enriched cereals and breads, organ meats	Low toxicity

Information from Allen, Jr., L.V. (1996). Nutritional products. In T.R. Covington (Ed.), *Handbook of nonprescription drugs* (11th ed.). Washington, D.C.: American Pharmaceutical Association; Marcus, R., & Coulston, A.M. (1996). Water-soluble vitamins; Fat-soluble vitamins. In J. G. Hardman, & L. E. Limbird, (Eds.), *Goodman & Gilman's The pharmacological basis of therapeutics* (9th ed.). New York: McGraw-Hill; and *United States Pharmacopeia Dispensing Information (USP DI): Drug information for the health care professional* (19th ed.). (1999). Rockville, MD: United States Pharmacopeial Convention.

**Adverse effects* include acute and chronic early and late overdose symptoms, when available.

†RDA is the daily allowance recommended from dietary sources.

‡RNIs by Health and Welfare Canada.

Deficiency Effects	Individuals	U.S. RDA†	Canadian RNI‡
Night blindness, xerophthalmia, keratomalacia, skin lesions	Infants and children		
	Birth to 3 years of age	375-400 μg	400 μg
	4 to 6 years of age	500 μg	500 μg
	7 to 10 years of age	700 μg	700-800 μg
	Adolescent and adult males	1000 μg	1000 μg
	Adolescent and adult females	800 μg	800 μg
	Pregnant females	800 μg	900 μg
	Breastfeeding females	1200-1300 μg	1200 μg
Bone-muscle pain, pain, weakness, and softening of the bones that may result in fractures	Infants and children		
	Birth to 3 years of age	7.5-10 μg	5-10 μg
	4 to 6 years of age	10 μg	5 μg
	7 to 10 years of age	10 μg	2.5-5 μg
	Adolescents and adults	5-10 μg	2.5-5 μg
	Pregnant and breastfeeding females	10 μg	5-7.5 μg
Hyporeflexia, ataxia, myopathy, anemia; may increase cancer risk	Infants and children	**mg of alpha-TE**	**mg of alpha-TE**
	Birth to 3 years of age	3-6 mg	3-4 mg
	4 to 6 years of age	7 mg	5 mg
	7 to 10 years of age	7 mg	6-8 mg
	Adolescent and adult males	10 mg	6-10 mg
	Adolescent and adult females	8 mg	5-7 mg
	Pregnant females	10 mg	8-9 mg
	Breastfeeding females	11-12 mg	9-10 mg
Increased bleeding (e.g., ecchymoses, hematuria, gastrointestinal bleeding)	Infants	5-10 μg	
	Children	15-30 μg	
	Males	45-80 μg	
	Females	45-65 μg	
	Pregnant females	65 μg	
Peripheral neuritis, loss of muscle strength, depression, memory loss, anorexia, poor memory, dyspnea	Infants and children		
	Birth to 3 years of age	0.3-0.7 mg	0.3-0.6 mg
	4 to 6 years of age	0.9 mg	0.7 mg
	7 to 10 years of age	1 mg	0.8-1 mg
	Adolescent and adult males	1.2-1.5 mg	0.8-1.3 mg
	Adolescent and adult females	1-1.1 mg	0.8-0.9 mg
	Pregnant females	1.5 mg	0.9-1 mg
	Breastfeeding females	1.6 mg	1-1.2 mg
Sore throat; stomatitis; red, painful, or swollen tongue; facial dermatitis; anemia	Infants and children		
	Birth to 3 years of age	0-4-0.8 mg	0.3-0.7 mg
	4 to 6 years of age	1.1 mg	0.9 mg
	7 to 10 years of age	1.2 mg	1-1.3 mg
	Adolescent and adult males	1.4-1.8 mg	1-1.6 mg
	Adolescent and adult females	1.2-1.3 mg	1-1.1 mg
	Pregnant females	1.6 mg	1.1-1.4 mg
	Breastfeeding females	1.7-1.8 mg	1.4-1.5 mg

Continued

TABLE 68-1 Vitamin Review—cont'd

Vitamin	Sources	Adverse Effects*
B_3 (niacin)	Meats, eggs, milk, dairy products	Flushing, pruritus, feelings of warmth *High doses:* Dizziness, dysrhythmias, dry skin, hyperglycemia, myalgia, nausea, vomiting, diarrhea
B_6 (pyridoxine)	Liver, meats, whole grain breads and cereals, soybeans, eggs, vegetables	*Acute:* Low toxicity *Chronic high doses:* neurotoxicity—ataxia, numb feet, clumsiness
B_9 (folic acid)	Liver, fresh green vegetables, yeast, some fruits	Allergic reaction, red skin, fever, skin rash, pruritus
B_{12} (cyanocobalamin)	Fish, egg yolk, milk, fermented cheeses	No toxicity
C (ascorbic acid)	Citrus fruits, tomatoes, potatoes, strawberries, cabbage	Kidney stones, dizziness *High doses:* diarrhea, red skin, headache, nausea, vomiting

Information from Allen, Jr., L.V. (1996). Nutritional products. In T.R. Covington (Ed.), *Handbook of nonprescription drugs* (11th ed.). Washington, D.C.: American Pharmaceutical Association; Marcus, R., & Coulston, A.M. (1996). Water-soluble vitamins; Fat-soluble vitamins. In J. G. Hardman, & L. E. Limbird, (Eds.), *Goodman & Gilman's The pharmacological basis of therapeutics* (9th ed.). New York: McGraw-Hill; and *United States Pharmacopeia Dispensing Information (USP DI): Drug information for the health care professional* (19th ed.). (1999). Rockville, MD: United States Pharmacopeial Convention.

**Adverse effects* include acute and chronic early and late overdose symptoms, when available.

†RDA is the daily allowance recommended from dietary sources.

‡RNIs (Recommended Nutrient Intake) by Health and Welfare Canada.

Deficiency Effects	Individuals	U.S. RDA†	Canadian RNI‡
Skin eruptions, stomatitis, diarrhea, enteritis, headache, dizziness, insomnia, memory impairment, dementia	Infants and children		
	Birth to 3 years of age	5-9 mg	4-9 mg
	4 to 6 years of age	12 mg	13 mg
	7 to 10 years of age	13 mg	14-18 mg
	Adolescent and adult males	15-20 mg	14-23 mg
	Adolescent and adult females	13-15 mg	14-16 mg
	Pregnant females	17 mg	14-16 mg
	Breastfeeding females	20 mg	14-16 mg
Seborrhea-like skin lesions, stomatitis, seizures, peripheral neuritis	Infants and children		
	Birth to 3 years of age	0.3-1 mg	0.3-1 mg
	4 to 6 years of age	1.1 mg	1.1 mg
	7 to 10 years of age	1.4 mg	1.4 mg
	Adolescent and adult males	1.7-2 mg	1.7-2 mg
	Adolescent and adult females	1.4-1.6 mg	1.4-1.6 mg
	Pregnant females	2.2 mg	2.2 mg
	Breastfeeding females	2.1 mg	2.1 mg
Megaloblastic anemia	Infants and children		
	Birth to 3 years of age	25-50 μg	50-80 μg
	4 to 6 years of age	75 μg	90 μg
	7 to 10 years of age	100 μg	125-180 μg
	Adolescent and adult males	150-200 μg	150-220 μg
	Adolescent and adult females	150-180 μg	145-190 μg
	Pregnant females	400 μg	445-475 μg
	Breastfeeding females	260-280 μg	245-275 μg
Irreversible nervous system damage (paresthesia, ataxia), memory loss, confusion, dementia, abnormal hematopoiesis	Infants and children		
	Birth to 3 years of age	0.3-0.7 μg	0.3-0.4 μg
	4 to 6 years of age	1 μg	0.5 μg
	7 to 10 years of age	1.4 μg	0.8-1 μg
	Adolescent and adult males	2 μg	1-2 μg
	Adolescent and adult females	2 μg	1-2 μg
	Pregnant females	2.2 μg	2-3 μg
	Breastfeeding females	2.6 μg	1.5-2.5 μg
Scurvy (loosening of teeth, gingivitis), anemia *Infants:* irritability, pain if touched	Infants and children		
	Birth to 3 years of age	30-40 mg	20 mg
	4 to 6 years of age	45 mg	25 mg
	7 to 10 years of age	45 mg	25 mg
	Adolescent and adult males	50-60 mg	24-40 mg
	Adolescent and adult females	50-60 mg	25-30 mg
	Pregnant females	70 mg	30-40 mg
	Breastfeeding females	90-95 mg	55 mg
	Smokers	100 mg	45-60 mg

type and severity of the deficiency and the nature of the client's signs and symptoms, other nursing diagnoses or collaborative problems are also relevant.

■ **Implementation**

■ ***Monitoring.*** A food diary will assist in monitoring the client's effective management of the therapeutic regimen. A regression of the client's symptoms should be noted. Weight should be recorded at every visit; height should also be recorded for children.

■ ***Intervention.*** Use the calibrated measuring device provided by the manufacturer for accurate dosing. Chewable tablets should be chewed or crushed thoroughly before swallowing. Use caution in administering fat-soluble vitamins to children, because they are more sensitive to high doses.

■ ***Education.*** Discussions with the client regarding vitamins should cover their function in the body, signs of vitamin deficiency, and unproven uses. Diet is the treatment of choice for vitamin deficiencies; vitamins are not a substitute for a balanced diet.

Instruct the client about the food pyramid with its six food groups and, in particular, about specific foods that supply the vitamin in which he or she is deficient. Encourage a diet with at least five fruits and vegetables a day; fruits and vegetables not only provide known vitamins, they also contain fiber and other poorly defined nutrients. They may also be filling and limit the individuals' intake of meat and animal fats. Advise that the client take a daily multivitamin that meets the RDA for all adults. Megadoses are not recommended, and there is the risk of toxicity with chronic overdoses; the RDA should not be exceeded. There is a great deal of ongoing research about the prophylactic role for vitamins.

■ **Evaluation.** The expected outcome of vitamin and mineral therapy is that the client will not demonstrate any signs or symptoms of vitamin or mineral deficiency or hypervitaminosis.

Fat-Soluble Vitamins

vitamin A [Aquasol A]

Vitamin A, the fat-soluble, growth-promoting vitamin, is essential for growth in the younger age groups, for normal function of the retina, and for health maintenance at all ages. Vitamin A (retinol) is derived from animals, whereas the provitamin A carotenoids are found in plants. Beta-carotene, the most active carotenoid from plants, is hydrolyzed in the body to form two molecules of vitamin A. Animal fats, such as those found in butter, milk, eggs, and fish liver, are sources of carotenoids that were originally derived from plants and stored in animal tissues.

Vitamin A is essential for promoting normal growth and the development of bones and teeth and for maintaining the health of epithelial tissues of the body. Its function in relation to normal vision and the prevention of night blindness has been studied carefully. Vitamin A actually is part of one of the major retinal pigments, rhodopsin, and thus is required for normal "rod vision" in the retina of human beings and many animals.

Vitamin A has the following indications:

1. It is used to treat or relieve symptoms associated with a deficiency of vitamin A, such as night blindness (nyctalopia), hyperkeratosis, delayed growth, xerophthalmia, keratomalacia, weakness, and increased susceptibility of the mucous membranes to infection.
2. Certain analogues (e.g., tretinoin) are used to treat acne (see Chapter 66).
3. Vitamin requirements increase during pregnancy and during breastfeeding; when possible, these needs are best met with food rather than with drugs. However, prescribers may recommend vitamin supplementation, especially for women who may not consume a proper diet or for those in a high-risk category, such as heavy cigarette smokers, alcohol or substance abusers, or women pregnant with more than one fetus. Consuming excessive amounts of vitamins, especially fat-soluble vitamins, may be dangerous to both the mother and the fetus. Large doses of vitamin A may cause neurologic and skin damage in adults, and excessive doses are known to produce highly toxic effects in rats and in young children. (See the Nursing Research box on p. 1157.)

Vitamin A and carotene are readily absorbed from the normal gastrointestinal tract. Efficient absorption depends on fat absorption and therefore on the presence of adequate bile salts in the intestine. Certain conditions, such as obstructive jaundice, some infectious diseases, and the presence of mineral oil in the intestine, may result in vitamin A deficiency even if a normal amount is ingested.

Vitamin A is stored to a greater extent in the liver than elsewhere. The liver also functions in changing carotene to vitamin A; this function is inhibited by liver diseases and diabetes. The amount of vitamin A stored depends on dietary intake. When intake is high or excessive, the stores formed in the liver may be sufficient enough to last several years. Vitamin A is metabolized by the liver and excreted by the feces and kidneys. Table 68-1 provides the RDA, adverse reactions, and deficiency effects for vitamin A.

The dosage for vitamin A depends on the age, sex, purpose (prophylaxis or treatment), and condition of the individual. Refer to a current reference for dosing information.

■ Nursing Management

Vitamin A Therapy

In addition to the following discussion, see Nursing Management: Vitamin and Mineral Therapy, p. 1151.

■ **Assessment.** Obtain a baseline of the client's vision, including night blindness, and the appearance of the eyes, skin, and mucous membranes. In addition to dry skin and corneal changes, infants may show failure to thrive and apathy. Serum vitamin A levels less than 20 μg/dL in adults and 10 μg/dL in children indicate a vitamin A deficiency.

Vitamin A is contraindicated for clients with hypervitaminosis A and is administered cautiously to clients with re-

Nursing Research
High-Dose Vitamin A in Children with Measles

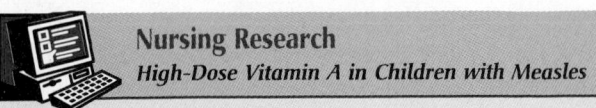

Citation: Fawzi, W.W., Chalmers, T.C., Herrera, M.G., Mosteller, F. (1993). Vitamin A supplementation and child mortality: A meta-analysis. *Journal of the American Medical Association, 269*(7), 898-903.

Abstract: According to a study conducted by Frederick Mosteller, Ph.D., and his colleagues from the Harvard School of Public Health, large doses of vitamin A are clearly lifesaving when given to children with measles. Measles is responsible for approximately 1.5 million deaths worldwide each year, and children in developing countries are particularly susceptible because of problems in obtaining and distributing the measles vaccine in these areas. Vitamin A supplements may also benefit children in developed countries. In another recent study, American children with measles had lower blood levels of vitamin A than children who did not have measles.

The Harvard study conducted a meta-analysis of findings from four hospital-based studies and eight community-based studies of children (mainly from developing countries) and found that large doses of vitamin A lowered the risk of death by 60% in hospitalized children and 90% in hospitalized infants—even in populations in which vitamin A deficiency was not a problem. Ordinarily, the risk of measles-related diarrhea was less severe in children who took vitamin A supplements, and there were 70% fewer deaths among children receiving supplements who developed measles-related pneumonia either before or during their hospital stay.

The investigators concluded that vitamin A supplements should be given to all clients with measles in developing countries, whether or not they have symptoms of vitamin A deficiency. They call for further research on the effects of vitamin A as a supplement to conventional therapy for other serious childhood diseases, such as diarrhea and lower respiratory infections.

Critical Thinking Questions

- Given that there is at present only one approved use for vitamin A—for vitamin A deficiency—how do you explain these findings?
- Which would be more cost-effective or have the better risk-benefit ratio, vitamin A therapy or immunization for measles? Under what circumstances?

nal function impairment, because serum vitamin A levels are increased.

An increase in toxic side effects may result when vitamin A is given concurrently with etretinate (Tegison) or isotretinoin (Accutane). Avoid concurrent administration if possible. If concurrent administration cannot be avoided, monitor closely for retinoid toxicity (headache, nausea, vomiting, elevated liver enzymes, hair loss, hepatomegaly, and dry, fissured skin).

■ **Nursing Diagnosis.** The client undergoing vitamin A deficiency therapy is at risk for the following nursing diagnoses: disturbed sensory perception (night blindness), fatigue, impaired skin integrity, and impaired oral mucous membrane. Nursing diagnoses associated with vitamin A toxicity are impaired comfort (headache, bone or joint pain, general feeling of discomfort, irritability); impaired oral mucous membrane (dry mouth, drying or cracking of lips); imbalanced body temperature (fever); deficient fluid volume (anorexia, nausea, vomiting); disturbed body image related to hair loss or yellow-orange patches on the palms of the hands, soles of the feet, or skin around the nose and mouth; hyperthermia; impaired urinary elimination (frequency); and fatigue. With infants there is the potential complication of bulging fontanel.

■ **Implementation**

■ ***Monitoring.*** Monitor the client's diet and serum levels of vitamin A. Monitor for signs and symptoms of vitamin A deficiency, hypercarotenemia (orange coloration of the skin and eyes), and hypervitaminosis A (see the Nursing Diagnosis section for this vitamin). Plasma levels of vitamin A may not be indicative of vitamin A status because of significant hepatic storage; however, a vitamin A deficiency does correlate with low serum levels.

■ ***Intervention.*** Administer oral vitamin A with or after meals.

■ ***Education.*** Provide the client with nutritional counseling. The best sources of dietary vitamin A are fish liver oil, liver, kidney, egg yolk, butter, milk, cream, cheese, and fortified margarine, as well as its precursor carotene, which is found in dark green leafy vegetables and yellow and orange fruits and vegetables. Water-miscible products are available for clients with fat malabsorption.

If administered intravenously, vitamin A is adsorbed by polyvinyl chloride (PVC) containers and tubing. Exposure to light causes vitamin A to degrade, and therefore total parenteral solutions containing vitamin A should be protected from the light.

■ **Evaluation.** The expected outcome of vitamin A therapy is that the client will achieve adequate serum concentrations of vitamin A, consume adequate dietary vitamin A, and maintain normal vision and intact skin.

vitamin D

The term *vitamin D* is applied to two substances that affect the proper use of calcium and phosphorus in the body. Both substances have the ability to prevent or cure rickets. The plant vitamin D is referred to as vitamin D_2, or ergocalciferol; the natural form of vitamin D is produced in the skin by ultraviolet irradiation of 7-dehydrocholesterol and is referred to as vitamin D_3, or cholecalciferol. Although ergocalciferol contains a chemical double bond and an extra methyl group, the difference between these two substances is not physiologically significant.

Both cholecalciferol and ergocalciferol are metabolized in the liver to calcifediol. Calcifediol is transported to the kidney and converted to calcitriol, which is believed to be the most active analogue (Marcus, 1996).

Calcitriol appears to bind to a receptor in the intestinal mucosa; it is incorporated into the cell nucleus, which results in the formation of a calcium-binding protein that increases calcium absorption from the intestine. Parathyroid hormone and calcitriol act to control the transfer of calcium ions from bones into the extracellular fluid; therefore they maintain calcium homeostasis in the extracellular fluid. Although an essential vitamin, vitamin D is found in only a few foods in the average diet of Americans and Canadians (see Table 68-1).

Other available vitamin D analogues include alfacalcidol (One-Alpha ♣), calcitriol (Rocaltrol), and dihydrotachysterol (Hytakerol). They are preferred in certain situations, such as renal failure, because they do not require conversion for their action. They also have shorter half-lives, which makes any toxic adverse reactions easier to manage. Calcifediol (Calderol) appears to have some vitamin D activity in addition to its conversion to the active metabolite calcitriol.

Vitamin D is necessary for the absorption and use of calcium and phosphorus in the body and for the normal calcification of bone. Rickets in children and osteomalacia in adults may result in the absence of vitamin D—even if the intake of calcium and phosphate is adequate. Vitamin D is used to treat and prevent nutritional rickets, osteomalacia, hypoparathyroidism, and osteoporosis (Marcus, 1996).

The incidence of rickets is low in the United States and Canada but can occur in young children who are restricted to vegetarian diets without milk supplementation or in infants who are breastfed by mothers who did not take prenatal vitamins or drink milk. Vitamin D deficiency results in an inadequate intake and perhaps an excessive loss of calcium from the body. The prevalence of vitamin D deficiency is high in older adults as a result of a combination of decreased dietary intake, diminished absorption, and limited exposure to sunlight.

Vitamin D is absorbed from the small intestine (ergocalciferol requires the presence of bile salts for absorption). It is protein bound and is stored mainly in fat and in the liver. The serum half-life for calcifediol is approximately 16 days; for calcitriol, from 3 to 6 hours; and for ergocalciferol, within 19 to 48 hours. Ergocalciferol can be stored in fat sites for longer periods. For calcitriol, the onset of hypercalcemic effects is within 3 to 6 hours; for dihydrotachysterol, within hours (although the maximum effect is seen in 7 to 14 days); for ergocalciferol, within 12 to 24 hours (although the therapeutic response may not be seen until 10 to 14 days later).

The duration of effect after oral administration is calcifediol, 15 to 20 days; calcitriol, 3 to 5 days; dihydrotachysterol, up to 9 weeks; and ergocalciferol, up to 6 months. Excretion is via the bile and kidneys.

See Table 68-1 for adverse reactions, deficiency effects, and the RDA of vitamin D.

The usual adolescent and adult dosage for alfacalcidol is 1 μg/day; for calcifediol, 50 to 100 μg/day; for calcitriol, 0.25 mg/day, and for dihydrotachysterol, 125 μg to 2 mg/day. Dosages are adjusted periodically as necessary. Pediatric dosages vary. Refer to a current reference for recommendations.

■ Nursing Management

Vitamin D Therapy

In addition to the following discussion, see Nursing Management: Vitamin and Mineral Therapy, p. 1151.

■ **Assessment.** The administration of vitamin D is contraindicated in clients with hypercalcemia, hypervitaminosis D, or renal osteodystrophy with hyperphosphatemia because of the risk for metabolic calcification. Hyperphosphatemia must be controlled before the start of vitamin D therapy. The nurse's assessment should rule out these conditions before initiating vitamin D therapy. Other conditions for which caution should be used in the administration of vitamin D are arteriosclerosis, hyperphosphatemia, hypersensitivity to vitamin D, and renal or cardiac impairment.

A baseline assessment of the client's skeletal status by x-ray examination and the appearance of bone malformations should be obtained. Serum calcium levels under 7.5 mg/dL, serum inorganic phosphorus levels under 3 mg/dL, serum citrate levels under 2.5 mg/dL, and elevated serum alkaline phosphatase levels indicate a vitamin D deficiency.

Review the client's current medication regimen for the risk of significant drug interactions, such as those that may occur when vitamin D products are given concurrently with the following drugs:

Drug	Possible Effect and Management
Bold/color type indicates the most serious interactions.	
antacids containing magnesium	May result in hypermagnesemia, especially in clients with chronic renal failure. Avoid concurrent administration if possible; if not, monitor closely for diminished reflexes, muscle weakness, drowsiness, confusion, lethargy, bradycardia, and hypotension.
calcium preparations in high doses or thiazide diuretics	Increases the risk for hypercalcemia. Monitor closely for drowsiness, lethargy, weakness, muscle flaccidity, hypertension, anorexia, nausea, constipation, polyuria, and flank pain.
vitamin D, other products	**Increased risk for toxicity. Avoid concurrent use or a potentially serious drug interaction may occur.**

■ **Nursing Diagnosis.** Clients receiving vitamin D therapy may experience the following nursing diagnoses because of their underlying vitamin D deficiency: impaired comfort related to ineffective drug therapy (pain in the legs and lower back); risk for injury related to motor deficits resulting from skeletal deformities and weakness; and impaired physical mobility related to poorly developed muscles. Nursing diagnoses related to the drug toxicity itself are constipation; diarrhea; fatigue; deficient fluid volume related to anorexia, nausea, or vomiting; and impaired comfort (headache, metallic taste).

■ **Implementation**

■ ***Monitoring.*** Because vitamin D has a narrow therapeutic range, serum calcium levels should be monitored weekly during early therapy along with periodic evaluations of renal function; this will help to establish the dosage. Serum calcium values should be in the 8 to 9 mg/dL range, and the product of calcium and phosphorus (Ca × P [mg/dL]) should not be greater than 60. Other examinations may be required according to the client's response to therapy.

Children should have their growth monitored during therapy, because growth may be inhibited by prolonged administration of vitamin D. X-ray studies are recommended every 3 to 6 months until the client is stable. In addition, assess for signs of toxicity as described in the Nursing Diagnosis section for this vitamin.

■ ***Education.*** Stress the importance of regular visits to the health care provider to monitor progress. Review with the client any instructions for a special diet or for a calcium supplement if prescribed. Foods high in vitamin D include fish and fish liver oils, egg yolks, and vitamin-D–fortified milk. Judicious exposure to sunlight is helpful. Vitamin D content is not altered with cooking.

The daily intake of vitamin D in older adults should be at least 800 IU, with at least 1.2 g of elemental calcium in the diet or as a supplement. If prescribed a supplement, the client should be cautioned not to use any OTC products that contain calcium, phosphorus, or vitamin D unless approved by the prescriber. Clients taking calcifediol or calcitriol should avoid the use of antacids containing magnesium.

■ **Evaluation.** The expected outcome of vitamin D therapy is that the client will consume adequate dietary vitamin D and remain pain free. The child or infant will maintain adequate growth.

vitamin E (α-tocopherol)
vitamin E capsules (Aquasol E)

Vitamin E is a fat-soluble vitamin that is present in margarine made from plant oils such as cottonseed oil; it is also present in green, leafy vegetables and whole grains. Although a number of compounds have been found to exhibit vitamin E activity, the most active of these is α-tocopherol; it is the substance used to calculate the food content of vitamin E.

Studies have reported a significant decrease in coronary artery disease in persons consuming large doses of vitamin E. The hypothesis is that the oxidation of lipoproteins reduces atherogenesis (Steinberg, 1993).

Rimm et al. (1993) studied 39,910 male health care professionals in the United States for 4 years and assessed their intake of various nutrients, including vitamin E. They found that males who consumed a high intake of vitamin E had a lower risk of developing coronary artery heart disease. Stampfer et al. (1993) followed 87,245 female nurses between the ages of 34 and 59 years for up to 8 years and reported similar findings; middle-aged women using vitamin E supplements for more than 2 years had a reduced risk for developing coronary heart disease. In both studies anyone with a history of cardiovascular disease was excluded. Further studies are necessary to evaluate the vitamin E dosages necessary to produce this effect and also to evaluate the potential risk of toxicity from the long-term consumption of large doses of vitamin E.

Vitamin E is an essential nutrient, but its exact function is unknown. It has been reported to have antioxidant properties when used in conjunction with dietary selenium, to prevent the effects of peroxidase on unsaturated bonds in the cell membranes, and to protect red blood cells (RBCs) from hemolysis. It is also known to be a cofactor for several enzyme systems in the body.

The absorption of vitamin E from the gastrointestinal tract requires the presence of bile salts, dietary fats, and normal pancreatic functioning. Vitamin E binds to beta lipoproteins in the blood and is stored in all body tissues, especially in fat deposits (which contain up to a 4-year requirement of this vitamin). It is metabolized in the liver and excreted in the bile and kidneys.

See Table 68-1 for adverse reactions and deficiency effects for vitamin E.

The oxidation of vitamin E increases when given concurrently with large doses of iron supplements; this increases the daily requirement for vitamin E. If given concurrently, monitor closely to determine an appropriate intervention.

The usual adult dosage for vitamin E deficiency is 100 to 400 units daily. Pediatric dosages vary. Refer to a current reference for recommendations.

■ **Nursing Management**

Vitamin E Therapy

In addition to the following discussion, see Nursing Management: Vitamin and Mineral Therapy, p. 1151.

■ **Assessment.** Before the initiation of vitamin E therapy, it should be ascertained whether the client has hypoprothrombinemia as a result of vitamin K deficiency; vitamin E in doses over 400 U will aggravate this condition. Clients who are taking anticoagulants should be advised against taking high doses of vitamin E.

A baseline assessment should include the presence or absence of edema, skin condition, and extent of muscle weakness. A serum α-tocopherol level below 0.5 mg/dL in adults and below 0.2 mg/dL in infants confirms a vitamin E deficiency.

■ **Nursing Diagnosis.** The client with a vitamin E deficiency may experience the following selected nursing diagnoses: excess fluid volume; impaired skin integrity; and impaired physical mobility. Nursing diagnoses associated with vitamin E toxicity are disturbed sensory perception (visual) related to blurred vision; diarrhea; fatigue; impaired comfort (headache, nausea or stomach cramps, dizziness); and risk for injury related to increased bleeding tendencies.

■ **Implementation**

■ ***Monitoring.*** Monitor the client's dietary intake, regression of symptoms, and serum α-tocopherol levels.

■ ***Intervention.*** Water-miscible forms are more readily absorbed from the gastrointestinal tract. The client taking large doses of vitamin E for prolonged periods should be assessed for signs of toxicity (see the Nursing Diagnosis section for this vitamin).

▪ ***Education.*** Although a vitamin E deficiency is uncommon, dietary instruction for clients may be necessary. Foods high in vitamin E are vegetable oils, wheat germ, whole-grain cereals, egg yolks, and liver.

▪ **Evaluation.** The expected outcome of therapy is that the client will maintain a diet adequate in vitamin E and will experience normal muscle strength, intact skin, and α-tocopherol levels within normal limits.

vitamin K

Vitamin K is a fat-soluble vitamin. Because of its importance in blood coagulation, it is covered in detail in Chapter 31 (see Table 68-1 for a review of this vitamin).

Water-Soluble Vitamins

The water-soluble vitamins are ascorbic acid (vitamin C) and B vitamins. The B vitamins are often found together in food and are referred to as vitamin B complex. However, they are chemically dissimilar and have different metabolic functions. This B grouping is largely based on their having been discovered in sequential order. A sensible and increasingly popular trend promotes discarding names such as vitamin B_1 and B_2 and referring to these vitamins as thiamine and riboflavin, respectively. The vitamin B complex includes thiamine, riboflavin, nicotinic acid, pyridoxine, folic acid, pantothenic acid, biotin, choline, inositol, and vitamin B_{12} (cyanocobalamin).

This discussion will be limited to the B vitamins that are associated with deficiency states and for which information on therapeutic application is available: thiamine (vitamin B_1), riboflavin (vitamin B_2), niacin (nicotinic acid), pyridoxine (vitamin B_6), vitamin B_{12} (cyanocobalamin), and folic acid.

thiamine [thye' a min] (vitamin B_1, Biamine, Bewon ✱)

Thiamine in combination with adenosine triphosphate (ATP) results in thiamine pyrophosphate coenzyme, a substance necessary for carbohydrate metabolism. Thiamine is used to prevent and treat thiamine deficiencies, which can result in beriberi or Wernicke's encephalopathy.

Thiamine is well absorbed from the gastrointestinal tract, except in malabsorption syndrome or in the presence of alcohol, which inhibits absorption. It is metabolized in the liver and excreted by the kidneys.

Side effects with thiamine use are usually rare. Skin rash, pruritus, or respiratory difficulties (wheezing) may occur after a large IV dose is administered (anaphylactic reaction) but are rare.

The usual adult dosage is determined by the age, sex, and degree of vitamin deficiency and ranges from 5 to 30 mg/day. Refer to a current reference for recommended pediatric dosages.

▪ Nursing Management

Thiamine Therapy

In addition to the following discussion, see Nursing Management: Vitamin and Mineral Therapy, p. 1151.

▪ **Assessment.** Thiamine rarely causes toxicity in clients who have normal renal function. Because a deficiency of a single B vitamin is uncommon, the client needs to be assessed for multiple deficiencies.

A baseline assessment of the client should include neurologic and mental status, pulse rate, blood pressure, and 24-hour urinary thiamine levels. Deficiency levels vary by age; less than 27 μg/dL indicates a deficiency in adults.

▪ **Nursing Diagnosis.** The client with a thiamine deficiency may exhibit the following nursing diagnoses: disturbed thought processes (confusion, psychosis); decreased cardiac output (tachycardia, palpitations); and disturbed sensory perception (neuropathy, ataxia, nystagmus). The only potential complication with the administration of thiamine is an anaphylactic reaction (rare), usually after a large IV dose.

▪ **Implementation**

▪ ***Monitoring.*** Continue to monitor the client with the indicators in the baseline assessment.

▪ ***Intervention.*** In most instances thiamine is administered as an oral preparation; if this is not acceptable or possible, parenteral forms are available.

▪ ***Education.*** Instruction for the client should include sources that are high in thiamine, such as whole grain or enriched cereals and meats, particularly pork, nuts, fish, organ/muscle meat, poultry, rice bran, legumes, and green vegetables. Nutritional loss during cooking is variable and may be as high as 50%.

▪ **Evaluation.** The expected outcome of thiamine therapy is that the client will maintain a diet adequate in thiamine, a normal neurologic and cardiovascular status, and normal levels of urinary thiamine.

riboflavin [rye' boo flay vin] (vitamin B_2)

Riboflavin is converted in the body into two coenzymes: flavin mononucleotide (FMN) and flavin adenine dinucleotide (FAD). Both of these substances are necessary for normal tissue respiration. Riboflavin is also necessary to activate pyridoxine and to convert tryptophan to niacin, and it may be associated with the maintenance of erythrocyte integrity.

Riboflavin is indicated for the prevention and treatment of riboflavin deficiency; usually this deficiency does not occur in healthy persons, but it may be detected as a result of malnutrition or intestinal malabsorption.

Riboflavin is well absorbed in the gastrointestinal tract and has a half-life of approximately 1 to 1.5 hours. It is metabolized in the liver and excreted by the kidneys.

Side effects are rare with riboflavin. No significant drug interactions have been reported.

The usual adult dosage to treat riboflavin deficiency ranges from 5 to 10 mg. Refer to a current reference for additional dosing information.

■ Nursing Management

Riboflavin Therapy

In addition to the following discussion, see Nursing Management: Vitamin and Mineral Therapy, p. 1151.

■ **Assessment.** A baseline assessment of the client with riboflavin deficiency should include examining the skin and mucous membranes, checking the appearance of the eyes and the client's vision status, and monitoring levels of RBCs, hemoglobin, and hematocrit. Riboflavin deficiency may be detected by measuring erythrocyte or urinary riboflavin concentrations.

■ **Nursing Diagnosis.** The client with a riboflavin deficiency and ineffective riboflavin therapy may experience the following nursing diagnoses: impaired oral mucous membrane (cracking of the lips and corners of the mouth, glossitis); impaired skin integrity (seborrheic dermatitis in nasolabial folds, scrotum, labia; generalized dermatitis); and disturbed sensory perception (light sensitivity, burning of the eyes).

■ **Implementation**

■ ***Monitoring.*** Water-soluble vitamins rarely cause toxicity in clients with normal kidney function. Monitor indicators within the baseline assessment.

■ ***Education.*** Alert the client that large doses of riboflavin may cause the urine to become yellow in color. The best food sources of riboflavin are milk and dairy products, meats, eggs, fish, poultry, enriched grains/cereals, and green, leafy vegetables (see Table 68-1). There is little loss of riboflavin with cooking.

■ **Evaluation.** The expected outcome of riboflavin therapy is that the client will maintain an adequate dietary intake of riboflavin and will have intact skin and mucous membranes, normal vision, and urinary riboflavin concentration values within the normal range.

niacin [nye' a sin] (nicotinic acid)
niacin extended-release (Nicobid, Slo-Niacin)
niacinamide tablets/injection

Niacin is converted to niacinamide in the body and is part of two coenzymes: nicotinamide adenine dinucleotide (NAD) and nicotinamide adenine dinucleotide phosphate (NADP), which are necessary for glycogenolysis, tissue respiration, and lipid, protein, and purine metabolism. As an antihyperlipidemic agent, niacin lowers serum cholesterol and triglyceride levels by reducing the synthesis of very-low-density lipoproteins (VLDLs). VLDL is the precursor to low-density lipoprotein, the main carrier of cholesterol in the blood.

Niacin and niacinamide are indicated for the prevention and treatment of vitamin B_3 deficiency conditions. A niacin deficiency may result in pellagra. Only niacin is indicated as a treatment adjunct for hyperlipidemia, but its usefulness may be limited by its side effects, especially its vasodilating effects. Niacinamide does not cause direct peripheral vasodilation.

With the exception of the malabsorption syndromes, both niacin and niacinamide are readily absorbed orally and have a half-life of 45 minutes. The onset of action to reduce triglyceride serum levels is several hours, whereas reducing cholesterol levels takes several days. Niacin is metabolized by the liver and excreted in the kidneys.

See Table 68-1 for the side effects/adverse reactions of niacin. No significant drug interactions are reported with their use.

For antihyperlipidemia, the usual adult dosage for niacin is 1 g PO daily, increased every 2 to 4 weeks as necessary. Refer to a current reference for additional information, because the dosages of niacin and niacinamide vary according to age and sex of the client.

■ Nursing Management

Niacin and Niacinamide Therapy

In addition to the following discussion, see Nursing Management: Vitamin and Mineral Therapy, p. 1151.

■ **Assessment.** Before large doses are administered, it should be determined if the client has arterial bleeding, diabetes mellitus (niacin only), peptic ulcer, or hepatic disease; all of these conditions will be aggravated by niacin and niacinamide.

A baseline assessment should include activity tolerance, skin status, bowel status, and neurologic and mental status.

■ **Nursing Diagnosis.** The client with a niacin deficiency and ineffective niacin therapy may experience the following nursing diagnoses: activity intolerance (fatigue, muscle weakness); impaired comfort (headache, indigestion); impaired skin integrity (dermatitis); impaired mucous membranes (red and sore mouth, tongue, and lips); diarrhea; and disturbed thought processes (confusion, disorientation, hallucinations). Clients undergoing niacin and niacinamide therapy may experience impaired comfort (flushing, headache [niacin only]); risk for injury (dizziness); impaired skin integrity (pruritus); and the potential complication of hepatitis (with the long-term use of extended-release niacin).

■ **Implementation**

■ ***Monitoring.*** Monitor the client's progress by indicators within the baseline assessment. Blood glucose and hepatic function should be monitored if clients are receiving large doses of niacin or niacinamide for prolonged periods.

■ ***Intervention.*** Administer with milk or food to help prevent gastrointestinal distress. Oral administration of niacin is preferred. Parenteral niacin is used only when the oral route is not acceptable or possible. If administered intravenously, do not exceed a rate of 2 mg/min.

■ ***Education.*** Alert the client to expect a feeling of warmth and a flushing of the skin of the face and neck shortly after taking the tablets for the first 2 weeks of therapy. This sensation may be reduced by starting with a low dosage and gradually increasing it to the therapeutic level. Niacinamide is preferred because it lacks this blushing effect.

Stress the importance of regular visits to the health care provider to monitor the effectiveness of the medication and the client's progress.

Because one of the adverse reactions is dizziness, caution the client to avoid hazardous tasks that require mental alertness until the response to the medication has been determined.

The best food sources of niacin are meats, eggs, whole grain and enriched cereal/bread/flour, milk, and other dairy products (see Table 68-1).

■ **Evaluation.** The expected outcome of niacin and niacinamide therapy is that the client will maintain an adequate dietary intake of niacin and will not show any signs of niacin deficiency.

pyridoxine [peer i dox′ een] (vitamin B_6)
pyridoxine extended-release (Rodex)

Pyridoxine is taken up by erythrocytes and converted into pyridoxal phosphate, a coenzyme necessary for many metabolic functions that affect proteins, carbohydrates, and lipid use in the body. Pyridoxine is also involved with converting tryptophan to niacin or serotonin.

Pyridoxine is indicated to treat or prevent pyridoxine deficiency. A deficiency state can lead to sideroblastic anemia, neurologic disturbances, seborrheic dermatitis, cheilosis, and xanthurenic aciduria. Vitamin B_6, folic acid, and vitamin B_{12} are required for the metabolism of homocysteine; an increased level of homocysteine is a major risk factor for vascular disease. Selhub, Jacques, Wilson, Rush, & Rosenberg (1993) evaluated a cohort of 1041 older adults and determined that two thirds of those with elevated levels of homocysteine had a subnormal plasma concentration of folate, vitamin B_{12}, or the coenzyme form of B_6 (pyridoxal-5-phosphate).

Oral pyridoxine is well absorbed from the jejunum and is converted in the erythrocytes to pyridoxal phosphate, which is totally protein bound in the plasma. It has a half-life of 15 to 20 days and is metabolized by the liver and excreted in the kidneys.

The side effects/adverse reactions of pyridoxine are very rare. Side effects are seen only when dosages of 200 mg/day are given for more than a month, leading to a dependency-type syndrome. Megadoses can cause problems (see Table 68-1).

The usual dosage of pyridoxine varies according to age, sex, and degree of vitamin deficiency. Refer to a current reference for dosing recommendations.

■ Nursing Management

Pyridoxine Therapy

In addition to the following discussion, see Nursing Management: Vitamin and Mineral Therapy, p. 1151.

■ **Assessment.** The initial assessment should determine whether the client has Parkinson's disease, which is treated with levodopa. A significant drug interaction occurs when pyridoxine is given with levodopa—the antiparkinsonian effects of levodopa may be reduced or reversed. This effect is not reported with the carbidopa-levodopa combination.

A baseline assessment of the client with a pyridoxine deficiency should include an inspection of the skin and mucous membranes and neurologic status. A pyridoxine deficiency is indicated by decreased serum transaminase and RBC levels and reduced urinary excretion of pyridoxic acid.

■ **Nursing Diagnosis.** The client with a pyridoxine deficiency and ineffective pyridoxine therapy may experience the following nursing diagnoses: impaired skin integrity (dermatitis); fatigue; activity intolerance related to anemia (weakness); risk for injury related to unsteady gait; and disturbed sleep pattern (drowsiness).

■ **Implementation**

■ ***Monitoring.*** Observe for improvement of deficiency symptoms. Evaluate the client for nutritional adequacy.

■ ***Intervention.*** IV pyridoxine may be administered undiluted at a rate of 50 mg/min and may be added to most IV solutions.

■ ***Education.*** Large doses of pyridoxine for a period of several months may result in sensory neuropathy, which affects gait and causes numbness of the hands and feet.

The best food sources of pyridoxine are meats, poultry, fish, eggs, bananas, potatoes, sweet potatoes, lima beans, and whole grain cereals.

■ **Evaluation.** The expected outcome of pyridoxine therapy is that the client will maintain an adequate dietary intake of pyridoxine, intact skin and mucous membranes, and a normal neurologic and mental status.

cyanocobalamin [sye an oh koe bal′ a min] (vitamin B_{12})
hydroxocobalamin [hye drox oh koe bal′ a min] (Alphamin)

Cyanocobalamin is a coenzyme for a variety of metabolic functions, including protein synthesis and fat and carbohydrate metabolism. It is also needed for growth, cell replication, hematopoiesis, and nucleoprotein and myelin synthesis. A deficiency of vitamin B_{12} (along with folic acid and pyridoxine [vitamin B_6] deficiencies) is a cause of abnormal homocysteine metabolism.

Cyanocobalamin is used to treat pernicious anemia (caused by a lack of intrinsic factor) and to prevent and treat vitamin B_{12} deficiency caused by malabsorption or strict vegetarianism. Vitamin B_{12} deficiency can lead to macrocytic megaloblastic anemia and irreversible neurologic damage.

Intrinsic factor must be present in the intestinal tract in order for vitamin B_{12} to be absorbed orally. It is highly protein bound, has a half-life of 6 days, and reaches peak serum levels in 8 to 12 hours. It is metabolized (and stored) by the liver and excreted in the bile and urine.

Anaphylactic reactions are possible but are rare after a parenteral injection (see Table 68-1). No significant drug interactions are reported.

The usual dosage of vitamin B_{12} varies according to age, sex, and degree of vitamin deficiency. See Box 68-2 for information on the nasal spray form of vitamin B_{12}. Refer to a current reference for dosing recommendations.

BOX 68-2

Vitamin B_{12} Nasal Spray

Nascobal, a vitamin B_{12} nasal spray, was approved as a maintenance drug for persons in remission after undergoing IM therapy for conditions such as pernicious anemia. The dose is usually 500 μg intranasally once weekly. A warning on the product states that the resumption of IM vitamin B_{12} is necessary if the client is not properly maintained on the nasal spray. Side effects/adverse reactions include infection, headache, glossitis, nausea, and rhinitis.

Information from FDA News and Product Notes. (1997). New formulations/combinations. *Formulary*, 32(1), 23-24.

■ Nursing Management

Cyanocobalamin/Hydroxocobalamin Therapy

In addition to the following discussion, see Nursing Management: Vitamin and Mineral Therapy, p. 1151.

■ **Assessment.** Cyanocobalamin is contraindicated for Leber's disease (a rare type of blindness resulting from an autosomal recessive trait); cyanocobalamin levels are already elevated in this condition, and optic nerve atrophy can occur rapidly after the administration of more cyanocobalamin. Ascertain the client's sensitivity to cyanocobalamin before initiating therapy.

Plasma levels of vitamin B_{12} should be determined before initiating therapy and on approximately the sixth day of therapy. A diagnosis of vitamin B_{12} deficiency should be confirmed by the laboratory (serum B_{12} levels under 150 pg/mL); otherwise the initiation of B_{12} therapy may mask pernicious anemia or a folic acid deficiency.

A baseline assessment should include activity tolerance, neurologic status, RBC count, hemoglobin, hematocrit, and serum cobalamin levels.

■ **Nursing Diagnosis.** The client with a cyanocobalamin deficiency and ineffective cyanocobalamin therapy may experience the following nursing diagnoses: activity intolerance related to anemia; and disturbed sensory perception (peripheral neuritis, hyperactive reflexes). Clients undergoing cyanocobalamin therapy may also experience diarrhea, impaired comfort (pruritus), and the potential complication of anaphylaxis.

■ **Implementation**

■ ***Monitoring.*** During the first 48 hours of therapy, serum potassium levels should be monitored closely for the possibility of severe hypokalemia. Hypersensitivity, which is rare, is demonstrated by a skin rash and, after parenteral administration, wheezing. Serum B_{12} levels should be obtained on the fifth and seventh days of therapy.

■ ***Intervention.*** Administer oral forms of cyanocobalamin with meals to enhance absorption. Parenteral cyanocobalamin is administered intramuscularly or subcutaneously, not intravenously. Small amounts are sometimes included in total parenteral nutrition (TPN).

■ ***Education.*** Stress compliance with the medication regimen if the client is undergoing life-long therapy following a gastrectomy or ileal resection or for pernicious anemia. For these conditions the drug is administered intramuscularly because of the absence of intrinsic factor.

The best food sources of vitamin B_{12} are meats, seafood, poultry, egg yolk, milk, and fermented cheeses. There is little loss of the vitamin with ordinary cooking, but severe heating may cause its destruction.

■ **Evaluation.** The expected outcome of cyanocobalamin therapy is that the client will maintain an adequate dietary intake of B_{12}, a normal neurologic status, serum B_{12} levels above 150 pg/mL, and RBC, hemoglobin, and hematocrit values that are within normal limits.

folic acid (vitamin B_9, Folvite, Apo-Folic ♣)

Folic acid is converted to tetrahydrofolic acid in the body, which is necessary for normal erythropoiesis, the metabolism of amino acids, and nucleoprotein synthesis.

Folic acid is used to treat and prevent folic acid deficiency. Folic acid should not be administered until pernicious anemia has been ruled out as a potential diagnosis. If administered to clients with undiagnosed pernicious anemia, folic acid will correct the hematologic changes and mask pernicious anemia while the underlying neurologic damage progresses.

Folic acid and vitamins B_6 and B_{12} supplements lower plasma homocysteine levels by 25% to 50% in clients with normal levels of homocysteine and in clients with hyperhomocystinemia (den Heijer et al., 1998; Woodside et al., 1998).

A folic acid deficiency may result in megaloblastic and macrocytic anemias and glossitis. A deficiency of maternal folic acid is associated with neural tube defects. The U.S. Preventive Services Task Force (1996) recommends a folic acid supplement of 400 μg daily for all women in the child-bearing years.

Folic acid is absorbed mostly from the upper duodenum; it is highly protein bound, metabolized (and stored) in the liver, and excreted by the kidneys. In the presence of vitamin C, folic acid (ascorbic acid) is converted in the liver and serum to its active form, tetrahydrofolic acid, by dihydrofolate reductase.

Side effects/adverse reactions are rare. An allergic reaction (elevated temperature and rash) or yellow discoloration of urine may occur.

The usual dosage of folic acid varies according to age, sex, and degree of vitamin deficiency. Refer to a current reference for dosing recommendations.

■ Nursing Management

Folic Acid Therapy

In addition to the following discussion, see Nursing Management: Vitamin and Mineral Therapy, p. 1151.

■ **Assessment.** It should be determined if the client has pernicious anemia, because folic acid will reverse hematologic abnormalities while the neurologic aspects of the disease continue to progress. No significant drug interactions are reported. Ascertain if the client has a sensitivity to the vitamin before initiating therapy.

A baseline assessment should include the client's activity tolerance, RBC count, hemoglobin, and hematocrit.

■ **Nursing Diagnosis.** Clients with folic acid deficiency will probably experience activity intolerance and ineffective protection secondary to anemia. Those receiving folic acid may experience the potential complication of anaphylaxis.

■ **Implementation**

■ ***Monitoring.*** Monitor the client's progress using the indicators in the baseline assessment.

■ ***Intervention.*** Folic acid is available as oral tablets or may be given undiluted intravenously over 1 minute. It may be added to most IV solutions. The injection preparation contains benzyl alcohol as a preservative and should not be administered to newborns and immature infants.

■ ***Education.*** Alert the client that large doses of folic acid may turn the urine yellow. The best food sources of folic acid are yeast, liver, whole grains, bran, fresh leafy vegetables, fruits, nuts, dried beans, and lentils.

■ **Evaluation.** The expected outcome of folic acid therapy is that the client will maintain an adequate dietary intake of folic acid, a tolerance for desired activities, and an RBC count, hemoglobin, and hematocrit within normal limits. If the client is pregnant, the infant will be born without a neural tube defect.

ascorbic acid (vitamin C)

Ascorbic acid is necessary for collagen formation in fibrous tissue (including bone) and in the development of teeth, blood vessels, and blood cells. It also plays a role in carbohydrate metabolism. It is believed to stimulate the fibroblasts of connective tissue and thus promote tissue repair and wound healing. It may also help to maintain the integrity of the intercellular substance in the walls of blood vessels; the capillary fragility associated with scurvy is explained on this basis. Ascorbic acid may be necessary for the metabolism of phenylalanine, tyrosine, folic acid, norepinephrine, histamine, and iron.

The effectiveness of ascorbic acid in preventing or relieving cold symptoms or in treating cancer, infertility, aging, or peptic ulcer is primarily unproven. Studies performed over the years have not substantiated these claims (*United States Pharmacopeia Dispensing Information*, 1999).

Ascorbic acid is well absorbed from the gastrointestinal tract and is stored in the plasma and cells, with the highest concentration found in glandular sites. It is metabolized in the liver and excreted by the kidneys (see Table 68-1).

High doses of ascorbic acid may cause diarrhea, cramps, headache, nausea, vomiting, and red skin.

The adult dosage as a nutritional supplement is 50 to 100 mg daily. The dosage to treat a vitamin C deficiency varies according to the age of the client and the severity of the vitamin deficiency.

■ Nursing Management

Ascorbic Acid Therapy

In addition to the following discussion, see Nursing Management: Vitamin and Mineral Therapy, p. 1151.

■ **Assessment.** It should be determined that the client does not have cystinuria, oxalosis, or a history of gout or urate renal stones, because there is a risk for the formation of urinary stones when large doses of vitamin C are given to clients with these conditions. Large doses may also precipitate a crisis in sickle cell anemia. Clients with diabetes mellitus may find that large doses of vitamin C interfere with glucose testing.

The concurrent use of ascorbic acid with deferoxamine (Desferal) may enhance tissue iron toxicity in tissues, especially in the heart, causing cardiac decompensation. The oral dose of ascorbic acid should be given 1 to 2 hours after the initiation of a deferoxamine infusion, when adequate levels of deferoxamine have been achieved.

If the purpose of administering vitamin C is to acidify the urine, urinary pH needs to be monitored to determine the effectiveness of the drug.

A baseline assessment of the client should include an inspection of the skin and mucous membranes, comfort levels, mental status, and serum levels of ascorbic acid. Check the bowel status and temperature in children. Serum ascorbic acid levels less than 0.2 mg/dL confirm a deficiency.

■ **Nursing Diagnosis.** The client with a vitamin C deficiency and ineffective ascorbic acid therapy may experience the following nursing diagnoses: impaired comfort (limb and joint pain); impaired oral mucous membrane (swollen or bleeding gums); ineffective protection related to capillary fragility (petechiae, ecchymoses); and disturbed thought processes (irritability, depression, hysteria). Clients receiving ascorbic acid therapy may experience diarrhea; impaired comfort (headache, flushing of the skin, stomach cramps); deficient fluid volume related to nausea and vomiting; and the potential complication of oxalate kidney stones.

■ **Implementation**

■ ***Monitoring.*** Monitor the client using the indicators in the baseline assessment.

■ ***Intervention.*** Ascorbic acid can be can be added to IV solutions and given as a continuous infusion. Bolus therapy that is administered too rapidly may cause dizziness and syncope. Ensure that the oral effervescent tablet form is dissolved in water just before administering.

■ ***Education.*** Clients taking more than 600 mg of ascorbic acid daily may experience a small increase in urination; with more than 1 g daily, diarrhea; and with more than 2 to 3 g daily of prolonged therapy, withdrawal scurvy.

The best food sources of vitamin C are citrus fruits, tomatoes, strawberries, cantaloupe, potatoes, and green vegetables (green peppers, broccoli, cabbage). Cooking destroys the vitamin C content of food by 30% to 50%, especially if copper pots are used. A gradual loss occurs in fresh foods in storage, but not with freezing unless over prolonged periods. Chopping fresh vegetables also causes some loss.

■ **Evaluation.** The expected outcome of ascorbic acid therapy is that the client will maintain an adequate intake of dietary vitamin C; healthy skin, mucous membranes, and mental state; and serum levels of ascorbic acid that are within the normal limits.

Multivitamin Preparations

Numerous multivitamin preparations are available in the United States and Canada. Supplemental preparations should provide 100% of the United States RDA to meet the needs of the vast majority of clients. Extra-potency or high-potency vitamins are rarely necessary for routine supplementation. In addition, the nurse should be aware that many preparations contain chemicals not yet known to be associated with any deficiency states.

MINERALS

Although many minerals are available, the discussion in this chapter is limited to iron—the most commonly prescribed mineral for iron-deficiency anemia. Other minerals are reviewed in other sections of this text.

iron supplements

Iron is an essential mineral for the proper functioning of many biologic systems in the body. It functions as an oxygen carrier in hemoglobin and myoglobin and is also involved in tissue respiration and in many enzyme reactions in the body. It is also stored in various body sites such as the liver, spleen, and bone marrow.

Iron deficiency is the most common nutritional deficiency in the United States and Canada that results in anemia. Young children and women, especially pregnant women, are most commonly affected.

Iron is supplied through diet (lean red meats) and iron supplements. Ingested iron is converted to the ferrous state by gastric juices; it is then more readily absorbed in the body. The absorption of iron is increased if it is taken with ascorbic acid (vitamin C), orange juice, veal, and other animal tissues. Coffee, tea, milk, eggs, whole grain breads and cereals decrease iron absorption.

Iron is indicated for the treatment of iron-deficiency anemia. In iron deficiency, between 10% to 30% of iron is absorbed; in normal individuals, approximately 5% to 15% is usually absorbed. Ferrous iron is absorbed better than the ferric dosage form. Iron binds to transferrin and is transported to bone marrow to aid in RBC production. Iron is not eliminated physiologically by the body. Excess iron intake can result in accumulation and iron toxicity. Small amounts are lost daily in the shedding of skin, nails, and hair; in breast milk; in urine; and in menstrual blood. The daily iron loss in healthy adults is approximately 1 mg/day for males and postmenopausal females and 1.5 to 2 mg/day in healthy premenopausal females.

The most common side effects of iron therapy include nausea, vomiting, constipation (diarrhea is less commonly reported), and abdominal cramps. For the treatment of iron toxicity, see the Management of Drug Overdose box below).

■ Nursing Management
Iron Therapy

In addition to the following discussion, see Nursing Management: Vitamin and Mineral Therapy, p. 1151.

■ **Assessment.** Complete a thorough dietary history, and assess the client's nutritional status to ascertain the possible causes of anemia and the need for client education. See Table 68-2 for the daily recommended requirements of elemental iron.

Iron should be administered for iron-deficiency anemias specifically rather than for all anemias in general. Some anemic conditions, such as thalassemia, may actually result in excess deposits of iron in the body.

It should be determined that the client does not have a disorder of iron metabolism such as hemochromatosis, which causes an excess deposition of iron in the tissues, skin pigmentation, cirrhosis of the liver, and decreased carbohydrate tolerance; or hemosiderosis, an increase in tissue iron stores without associated tissue damage. Porphyria cutanea tarda may be caused by an excess accumulation of iron in the liver. All of these conditions contraindicate the use of iron. Clients receiving repeated blood transfusions are also at risk for iron overload as a result of the addition of a high erythrocytic iron content.

Some older adults may need larger doses of iron than the usual daily adult dose for iron deficiency anemia, because

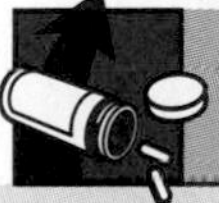

Management of Drug Overdose
Iron Supplements

- **Early signs of acute toxicity:** diarrhea that may contain blood, fever, severe abdominal cramps/pain, vomiting
- **Late signs:** pale, cold skin; convulsions; increased weakness; sedation; blue-tinted lips, fingernails, and palms of hands; irregular heart beat; hypotension, metabolic acidosis; cardiovascular collapse

Treatment

- Seek medical attention immediately.
- Induce emesis with ipecac syrup or a lavage containing sodium bicarbonate, depending on the client's condition.
- Maintain fluid and electrolyte balance.
- An antidote (deferoxamine) is used for severe iron toxicity. Avoid using the antidote if the client has renal failure.
- Monitor laboratory tests (e.g., serum iron, hemoglobin, hematocrit, electrolytes, blood gases, blood glucose, total iron-binding capacity, complete blood counts) closely.
- An exchange transfusion may be used if necessary.

TABLE 68-2 Daily Recommended Requirements for Elemental Iron

Individuals	United States (mg)	Canada (mg)
Infants and children		
Birth to 3 years of age	6-10	0.3-6
4 to 6 years of age	10	8
7 to 10 years of age	10	8-10
Adolescent and adult males	10	8-10
Adolescent and adult females	10-15	8-13
Pregnant females	30	17-22
Breastfeeding females	15	8-13

Information from *United States Pharmacopeia Dispensing Information (USP DI): Drug information for the health care professional* (19th ed.). (1999). Rockville, MD: United States Pharmacopeial Convention.

the reduction of gastric secretions and achlorhydria that accompanies aging also inhibits the ability to absorb iron.

A baseline assessment of the client should include activity tolerance; a hemoglobin, hematocrit, and reticulocyte count; and plasma iron and ferritin values.

Review the client's current medication regimen for the risk of significant drug interactions, such as those that may occur when iron salts are given concurrently with the following drugs:

Drug	Possible Effect and Management
Bold/color type indicates the most serious interactions.	
acetohydroxamic acid (Lithostat)	Iron may be chelated by acetohydroxamic acid, resulting in reduced absorption of both drugs. If iron therapy is necessary for a client receiving acetohydroxamic acid, it is suggested that iron be administered parenterally.
antacids, calcium supplements, milk or dairy products, coffee, fiber or selected food products (see previous discussion on p. 1165)	Decreased iron absorption may result. Schedule iron supplements at least 1 hour before and 2 hours after the administration of these substances.
dimercaprol (BAL in oil)	A toxic complex may result if iron and dimercaprol are given concurrently. Postpone the daily administration of iron for at least 24 hours after discontinuing dimercaprol. A blood transfusion may be indicated if a severe iron deficiency occurs while the client is receiving dimercaprol.
etidronate (Didronel)	May result in decreased absorption of oral etidronate. Teach clients to avoid the consumption of iron products within 2 hours of etidronate.
fluoroquinolones	Iron may reduce the absorption of these antibiotics; take fluoroquinolones at least 2 hours before or 2 hours after iron supplements.
tetracyclines, oral	Decreases the absorption of tetracycline, which may result in reduced antibiotic effectiveness. May impair hematologic effectiveness of the iron supplement. Administer iron supplements 2 hours after tetracyclines.
vitamin E	Concurrent administration with iron may reduce the client's hematologic response to iron therapy. If larger iron doses are administered, vitamin E requirements may also need to be increased. Close monitoring is suggested when concurrent therapy is administered.

▪ **Nursing Diagnosis.** The client receiving iron therapy is at risk for the following nursing diagnoses/collaborative problems: activity intolerance related to ineffectiveness of the therapy (anemia); constipation; diarrhea; impaired comfort (heartburn); impaired tissue integrity (pain, redness at the injection or infusion site); disturbed body image related to stained teeth from liquid forms of iron; deficient fluid volume related to nausea and vomiting; and the potential complications of allergic reaction (backache, chills, dizziness, fever, headache, nausea, tingling of the hands or feet) or toxicity (fever, nausea, stomach pain, vomiting, and diarrhea, sometimes with blood).

▪ **Implementation**

▪ ***Monitoring.*** The hemoglobin, hematocrit, reticulocyte count, and plasma iron values should be monitored every 3 weeks during the first 2 months of oral iron therapy or for a few days after the initiation of parenteral therapy. It usually takes 1 to 2 months of oral therapy for the hemoglobin concentration of a client with iron deficiency anemia to reach normal levels. The client's diagnosis should be reconsidered if a 1 g/100 mL increase in hemoglobin does not occur during the first 2 weeks of therapy.

▪ ***Intervention.*** The ferrous rather than ferric preparation of iron provides for the most efficient absorption of iron. Iron is best administered on an empty stomach. When taken with food, its absorption may be decreased by as much as one half to one third.

Administer liquid iron preparations with a full glass of water to prevent staining of the teeth. A drinking straw or a dropper may be used to place the dose far back on the tongue to prevent contact with the teeth. Oral preparations of iron should be discontinued before parenteral iron therapy begins.

Anaphylaxis has been known to occur up to 24 hours after parenteral administration. Epinephrine should be available during the injection of iron dextran, particularly in clients with asthma and known allergies. A test dose of 25 mg should be administered intramuscularly or intravenously to all clients at least 1 hour before their first therapeutic parenteral dose.

Do not mix the IV administration of iron dextran with other medications or add it to parenteral nutrition solutions. It should be administered undiluted and at a rate of no more than 1 mL/min. Flush the IV line with normal saline for injection. Maintain the client in a recumbent position for 30 minutes in case orthostatic hypotension should occur.

It is recommended that iron dextran be administered into the muscle mass of the upper outer quadrant of the buttock using the Z-track technique (see Chapter 5) and a 2- to 3-inch, 19- or 20-gauge needle. The preparation should never be injected into the upper arm or any other exposed area because of the possibility that it will stain the skin dark brown. To minimize staining of the flesh, use a separate needle to withdraw the drug from the vial.

■ ***Education.*** The client should be alerted that iron preparations cause black stools, which are medically insignificant. However, the prescriber should be notified if the client experiences other symptoms of internal blood loss, such as bloody streaks in the stool, abdominal tenderness, cramping, or pain. If the client experiences dental discoloration from iron therapy, recommend a baking soda toothpaste or one that contains 3% hydrogen peroxide.

Instruct the client to maintain a diet rich in sources of iron, such as liver, green leafy vegetables, potatoes, dried peas and beans, dried fruit, and enriched flour, breads, and cereals.

■ **Evaluation.** The expected outcome of iron therapy is that the client will maintain an adequate dietary intake of iron, tolerate activities as desired, and maintain hemoglobin, hematocrit, reticulocyte count, and plasma iron values within normal limits.

SUMMARY

Nutritional requirements are best met by the oral ingestion of adequate fluids and regular, balanced meals. When clients experience altered nutrition: less than body requirements, the nurse may participate in various nutritional modalities, such as vitamin replacement and enteral or parenteral feedings. Vitamins are essential to help maintain normal metabolic functions, growth, and tissue repair.

Most vitamin deficiencies are not singular but are multiple and result from impoverished diets due to alcoholism, poverty, fads, or ignorance. Replacement therapy is available for the water-soluble vitamins (vitamin C and the B-complex groups) and the fat-soluble ones (vitamins A, D, E, and K). Because water-soluble vitamins are not stored in the body, deficiencies can appear after short periods of inadequate intake. Fat-soluble vitamins, on the other hand, are stored in the liver and fatty tissue in large amounts; deficiencies occur only after a long period of deprivation. However, toxic levels are easier to reach with supplements of fat-soluble vitamins. Iron deficiency is the most common nutritional deficiency in the United States and Canada, especially in young children and women. Supplement therapy is practical but, as in all nutritional deficiencies, the best remedy is dietary intake.

Critical Thinking Questions

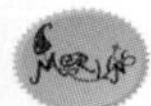

1. How would you plan to incorporate the U.S. RDA requirements for vitamins and minerals into a day's diet for a vegetarian? For a Puerto Rican client? For an edentulous client? For an older adult on a limited income with only biweekly access to transportation?
2. Take 10 minutes and write down your diet for the last 24 hours. Using your nutrition books, analyze the diet's vitamin and mineral content. Did you meet the U.S. RDA requirements for vitamins and minerals? How would you modify your diet to do so? What are the barriers to these modifications?

Collaborative Learning Activities

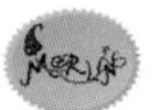

For Collaborative Learning Activities, go to mosby.com/MERLIN/McKenry/.

BIBLIOGRAPHY

Allen, Jr., L.V. (1996). Nutritional products. In T.R. Covington (Ed.), *Handbook of nonprescription drugs* (11th ed.). Washington, D.C.: American Pharmaceutical Association.

American Hospital Formulary Service. (1999). *AHFS: Drug information '99*. Bethesda, MD: American Society of Hospital Pharmacists.

Anderson, K.N., Anderson, L.E., & Glanze, W.D. (Eds.). (1998). *Mosby's medical, nursing, & allied health dictionary* (5th ed.). St. Louis: Mosby.

Covington, T.R. (Ed.) (1996). *Handbook of nonprescription drugs* (11th ed.). Washington, D.C.: American Pharmaceutical Association and The National Professional Society of Pharmacists.

Dawson-Hughes, B., Harris, S.S., Krall, E.A., & Dallal, G.E. (1997). Effect of calcium and vitamin D supplementation on bone density in men and women 65 years of age or older. *New England Journal of Medicine, 337*(10), 670-676.

Dawson-Hughes B., Harris S.S., Krall E.A., Dallal G.E., Falconer G., Green C.L. (1997). Rates of bone loss in postmenopausal women randomly assigned to one of two dosages of vitamin D. *American Journal of Clinical Nutrition, 61*(5), 1140-1145.

den Heijer, M., Brouwer, I.A., Bos, G.M., Blom, H.J., van der Put, N.M., Spaans, A.P., Rosendaal, F.R., Thomas, C.M., Haak, H.L., Wijermans, P.W., Gerrits, W.B. (1998). Vitamin supplementation reduces blood homocysteine levels: A controlled trial in patients with venous thrombosis and healthy volunteers. *Arteriosclerosis, Thrombosis, and Vascular Biology, 18*(3), 356-361.

Fawzi, W.W., Chalmers, T.C., Herrera, M.G., Mosteller, F. (1993). Vitamin A supplementation and child mortality: A meta-analysis. *Journal of the American Medical Association, 269*(7), 898-903.

FDA News and Product Notes. (1997). New formulations/combinations. *Formulary, 32*(1), 23-24.

Fletcher, R.H. (1999). Vitamin supplementation in disease prevention. In *UpToDate: Electronic Textbook of Medicine.*

Institute of Medicine (2000). Dietary intakes for vitamin C, vitamin e, selenium, and carotenoids. The National Academy Press. Washington, D.C. *Pharmacist's Letter, 16*(5), 26-27.

Katzung, B.G. (1998). *Basic and clinical pharmacology* (7th ed.). Norwalk, CT: Appleton & Lange.

Lindenbaum, J., Healton, E.B., Savage, D.G., Brust, J.C., Garrett, T.J., Podell, E.R., Marcell, P.D., Stabler, S.P., Allen, R.H. (1988). Neuropsychiatric disorders caused by cobalamin deficiency in the absence of anemia or macrocytosis. *New England Journal of Medicine, 318*(26), 1720-1728.

Linderborn, K.M. (1993). Independently living seniors and vitamin therapy: What nurses should know. *Journal of Gerontological Nursing, 19*(8), 10-20.

Marcus, R. (1996). Agents affecting calcification and bone turnover. In J.F. Hardman & L.E. Limbird (Eds.), *Goodman & Gilman's The pharmacological basis of therapeutics* (9th ed.). New York: McGraw-Hill.

Marcus, R. & Coulston, A.M. (1996). Water-soluble vitamins and fat-soluble vitamins. In J.G. Hardman & L.E. Limbird (Eds.), *Goodman & Gilman's The pharmacological basis of therapeutics* (9th ed.). New York: McGraw-Hill.

Rimm, E.B., Stampfer, M.J., Ascherio, A., Giovannucci, E., Colditz, G.A., Willett, W.C. (1993). Vitamin E consumption and the risk of coronary heart disease in men. *New England Journal of Medicine, 328*(20), 1450-1456.

Robinson, K., Arheart, K., Refsum, H., Brattstrom, L., Boers, G., Ueland, P., Rubba, P., Palma-Reis, R., Meleady, R., Daly, L., Witteman, J., Graham, I. (1998). Low circulating folate and vitamin B_6 concentrations: risk factors for stroke, peripheral vascular disease, and coronary artery disease. European COMAC Group. *Circulation, 97*(5), 437-443.

Selhub, J., Jacques, P.F., Wilson, P.W., Rush, D., Rosenberg, I.H. (1993). Vitamin status and intake as primary determinants of homocystinemia in an elderly population. *Journal of the American Medical Association, 270*(22), 2693-2698.

Sharts-Hopko, N.C. (1993). Folic acid in the prevention of neural tube defects. *Maternal Child Nursing, 18*(4), 232.

Stampfer, M.J., Hennekens, C.H., Manson, J.E., Colditz, G.A., Rosner, B., Willett, W.C. (1993). Vitamin E consumption and the risk of coronary disease in women. *New England Journal of Medicine* 328(20):1444-1449.

Steinberg, D. (1993). Antioxidant vitamins and coronary heart disease. *New England Journal of Medicine* 328(20):1487-1489.

United States Pharmacopeia Dispensing Information (USP DI): Drug information for the health care professional (19th ed.). (1999). Rockville, MD: United States Pharmacopeial Convention.

United States Preventive Services Task Force. (1996). *Guide to clinical preventive services* (2nd ed.). Baltimore: Williams & Wilkins.

Woodside, J.V., Yarnell, J.W., McMaster, D., Young, I.S., Harmon, D.L., McCrum, E.E., Patterson, C.C., Gey, K.F., Whitehead, A.S., Evans, A. (1998). Effect of B-group vitamins and antioxidant vitamins on hyperhomocystinemia: A double-blind, randomized, factorial-design, controlled trial. *American Journal of Clinical Nutrition, 67*(5), 858-866.

69 Fluids and Electrolytes

Chapter Focus

The concept of fluid and electrolyte balance cuts across the nursing care of all clients. It is essential that nurses have an understanding of the physiology involved. With this knowledge, nurses can accurately identify clients at risk for specific imbalances so that derangements can be detected early and corrective measures taken.

Learning Objectives

1. Identify the various therapeutic reasons for the infusion of IV solutions.
2. Describe the role of water in human physiology.
3. Explain water transport in the body.
4. Describe the four categories of parenteral solutions, and give examples of particular solutions in each category.
5. Identify abnormal states of fluid-electrolyte balance.
6. Describe the symptoms of hypertonic dehydration by clinical grading.
7. State the normal requirements, dietary sources, specific functions, and problems associated with an excess or deficiency of sodium, potassium, calcium, and magnesium.
8. Implement the nursing management for the care of clients receiving IV therapy.

Key Terms

dehydration, p. 1171
extracellular fluid, p. 1170
intracellular fluid, p. 1170
milliequivalent (mEq), p. 1179
osmosis, p. 1171
overhydration, p. 1171

The IV administration of parenteral fluids has become more prevalent during the past 50 years. The problems initially associated with the use of unsafe solutions were a result of pyrogens. Once this issue was resolved, advances in the technology of IV therapy resulted in products that have significantly improved client safety (Box 69-1).

There has also been a vast increase in outpatient and home administration of IV medications, hyperalimentation, and fluids. New and sophisticated delivery systems have been developed, and different methods of application are constantly being conceived. IV solutions are infused for various therapeutic reasons, including the following:

- Replacing fluids and electrolytes
- Correcting acid-base imbalance
- Administering medications
- Maintaining ready access to the venous system if any of the first three measures is anticipated
- Measuring changes in venous pressure
- Measuring the kidneys' excretory capabilities by diagnostic test
- Administering essential nutrients

Blood and its components are transfused intravenously to (1) replace blood volume or plasma fractions; (2) restore the blood's capabilities for carrying oxygen, clotting, or oncotic pressure; or (3) cleanse the plasma of harmful constituents by exchanges. IV hyperalimentation or parenteral nutrition solutions are infused to complement or supplement the dietary intake of clients in deprived nutrition states.

FLUIDS

Depending on the amount of adipose tissue present, water accounts for 45% to 75% of the total body weight in humans. Infants and young children have more water per unit of body weight than adults, and female adults have less water content than male adults. The greatest amount of body water (up to 45% of body weight) is to be found in the intracellular fluid; the remainder of body water is located in the extracellular fluid. **Intracellular fluid** is the fluid inside the cells, where the chemical reactions of all metabolism essential to life occur. **Extracellular fluid** is the fluid surrounding the cells—plasma, interstitial fluid, and lymph—as well as extracellular portions of dense connective tissue, cartilage, and bone. The volume of fluid in the two body fluid compartments varies with age and differs in the sexes. Metabolic exchanges between the cells and tissues and the external environment occur in this fluid.

The importance of body water is highlighted by two facts: (1) it is the medium in which all metabolic reactions occur, and (2) the precise regulation of volume and compo-

BOX 69-1

Intravenous Therapy: 1930s to Today

Early 1930s

IV injections are reserved only for seriously ill clients.
Only a physician can perform venipuncture.

1940s

Massachusetts General Hospital becomes one of the first hospitals to assign a nurse to IV therapy.
The job description includes administering IV solutions and blood transfusions, cleaning the infusion sets for reuse, and cleaning and sharpening needles for reuse.
The primary responsibility is of a technical nature: administering and maintaining the infusions and keeping the equipment clean and functional.

1950s

Improvements and innovations in equipment (e.g., pumps and monitors), needles (e.g., Intracaths), and tubing; the development of plastic and disposable equipment; and an increased variety of commercially prepared IV fluids increase the safety of IV therapy.

1960s

A variety of IV solutions are developed.
In addition to IV fluids, the IV route is used to administer many medications and hyperalimentation fluids.

1970s

The Centers for Disease Control (CDC) develop standards for infection control related to IV therapy.
Hickman-Broviac and Groshong tunneled catheters are developed for long-term access.
IV nurse specialists, IV departments or teams in the hospital, standards for client care, and professional organizations to promote IV therapy as a specialty area in nursing are developed.

1980s

The National Intravenous Therapy Association (NITA) publishes recommended practices for therapy.
Implantable ports are developed for long-term access.

1990s

The role of the nurse is to incorporate IV skills in all settings, including community.
The role for IV therapy is extended to LPNs/LVNs.

Information from Phillip, L.D. (1997). *Manual of IV therapeutics* (2nd ed.). Philadephia: F.A. Davis.

sition of body fluid is essential to health. In healthy individuals, body water remains remarkably constant and is maintained by a balance between intake and excretion—the water gained each day is equal to the water lost. If the water gained exceeds the water lost, fluid volume excess (**overhydration**) and edema occur. If the water lost exceeds the water gained, fluid volume deficit (**dehydration**) occur. If 20% to 25% of body water is lost, death usually occurs.

Water is an excellent solvent that permits many substances to be dispersed through it; it also has a high dielectric constant that permits the ionization of electrolytes. These electrolytes are important in maintaining physiologic processes and the volume and distribution of body fluid. These electrolytes include the cations sodium (Na^+) for extracellular fluid and potassium (K^+) and magnesium (Mg^{++}) for intracellular fluid; and the anions chloride (Cl^-) and bicarbonate (HCO_3^-) for extracellular fluid and phosphate (PO_4^{--}) and protein for intracellular fluid. Intracellular ions also occur in the extracellular fluid but in smaller amounts.

Water is also an excellent lubricant between membranes, and it functions well as a heat insulator and heat exchanger.

The daily intake of water in some form is essential to maintain water balance. Human beings can go several weeks without food but can survive only a few days without water. The average volume of water consumed daily is 120 to 150 mL/kg body weight in neonates and infants, 120 to 130 mL/kg in children, and 30 mL/kg in adults.

Thirst, the subjective desire to ingest water, helps to maintain water balance. Although thirst is complex and not well understood, it is induced by a decrease in saliva and dryness of the mouth and throat. The dehydration of thirst receptors may lead to their stimulation.

Water intake occurs primarily by (1) drinking fluids, (2) ingesting food containing moisture (most foods contain a high percentage of water), and (3) absorbing water formed by the oxidation of hydrogen in the food during metabolic processes. This third process produces approximately 0.5 L of water per day.

Water is lost from the body in five principal ways: (1) through the kidneys as urine, (2) through the skin as insensible perspiration and sweat, (3) through expired air as water vapor, (4) through feces, and (5) through the excretion of tears and saliva. Urine excretion accounts for 50% to 60% of the total daily water loss. Urine output, of course, varies with the amount of water ingested.

Water loss by the kidney varies with the solute (molecular ions or particles) load and the antidiuretic hormone (ADH or vasopressin) level. If an increase in solute load occurs, such as with diabetes mellitus or following the ingestion of excessive amounts of food (especially those that generate solutes, such as sodium from salty foods), the kidney excretes sufficient urine to transport the solutes into the bladder. The reabsorption of water in the distal convoluted tubules is controlled by vasopressin (ADH). An increase in ADH levels leads to an increase in water reabsorption, which produces more concentrated urine. ADH is secreted by the posterior pituitary gland; this secretion is regulated by osmoreceptors located in the supraoptic nucleus. ADH acts on specific vasopressin receptors on the medullary tubular cell to stimulate the production of cyclic adenosine monophosphate (cAMP). cAMP activates an enzyme that alters the structure of protein in the cell membrane to increase the permeability of the tubular cell to water. This increases water resorption and urine osmolality.

Water Transport in the Body

Water travels from less concentrated areas to areas with higher concentrations of solutes or dissolved substances by **osmosis.** The solutes may be electrolytes (e.g., potassium chloride or sodium chloride), which yield potassium cations and chloride anions when dissolved in water (a chemical balance is maintained); or nonelectrolytes such as dextrose, urea, or creatinine. Each fluid compartment in the body—intracellular and extracellular compartments—has its own electrolyte composition (Table 69-1). Disturbances in electrolyte composition can be reflected in clinical symptoms in the client.

Osmolality refers to the total solute concentration usually expressed per liter of serum. The number of solutes in solution decides the osmotic pressure. For example, if the extracellular fluid contains a large amount of dissolved particles and the intracellular fluid has a small amount of dissolved particles, then the osmotic pressure from the intracellular fluid forces water to pass from the less concentrated intracellular area to the more concentrated extracellular area. This process occurs until both concentrations are equal.

Deciding on the appropriate IV therapy for a client necessitates knowing the electrolyte values. Knowing the level of sodium, the principal electrolyte in the extracellular fluid, is essential; potassium levels, serum osmolality, current disease state or illness, specific laboratory values (if appropriate), and the initial signs and symptoms are also important.

TABLE 69-1 Normal Distribution of Electrolytes in the Body*

	Extracellular (mEq/L)		Intracellular
Electrolytes	**Plasma**	**Interstitial**	**(mEq/L)**
sodium (Na^+)	142	146	15
potassium (K^+)	5	5	150
calcium (Ca^{++})	5	3	2
magnesium (Mg^{++})	2	1	27
chloride (Cl^-)	103	114	1
bicarbonate (HCO_3^-)	27	30	10

*In addition, phosphates, sulfates, and other substances are located in the extracellular and intracellular fluids.

Parenteral Solutions

In general, parenteral solutions may be divided into four categories: (1) hydrating solutions, (2) isotonic solutions, (3) maintenance solutions, and (4) hypertonic solutions (Table 69-2).

Hydrating solutions include dextrose 2.5%, 5%, or higher in water, or 0.2% to 0.5% in normal saline. (Hypotonic saline—note that full strength normal saline is not included in this category.) Hydrating solutions are used to hydrate or to prevent dehydration. They are often used to assess kidney status before specific electrolytes are ordered as replacement and maintenance therapy and also to help increase diuresis in dehydrated clients.

Dextrose is a source of calories (1 L of 5% dextrose = approximately 170 calories) that is rapidly metabolized in the body. Dextrose solutions are considered isotonic or more than isotonic in the bottle. Dextrose is metabolized internally, which leaves water that decreases the osmotic pressure of the plasma, easily transfers to body cells, and provides water immediately to dehydrated tissues.

Isotonic solutions are usually prescribed to replace extracellular fluid losses that occur from blood loss, severe vomiting episodes, or any situation in which the chloride loss is equal to or greater than the sodium loss. Isotonic or normal saline is also used before and after a blood transfusion, because the hemolysis of red blood cells, which occurs with dextrose in water, is avoided by using this product.

Isotonic sodium chloride is also used to treat metabolic alkalosis, especially when it occurs in the presence of fluid loss. The increased administration of chloride ions helps to decrease the number of bicarbonate ions in the client. Other solutions that are considered isotonic include Ringer's injection and lactated Ringer's injection. A major difference between Ringer's injection and lactated Ringer's injection is the 28 mEq of lactate (a precursor of bicarbonate) in the lactated injection. Therefore lactated Ringer's is preferred for clients with metabolic acidosis perhaps caused by burns or infections. Ringer's injection has more chloride ions and is more useful in treating dehydration from reduced water intake, vomiting, or diarrhea or for clients with hypochloremia.

Maintenance solutions or multiple electrolyte solutions have been formulated to replace daily electrolyte and extracellular needs and water. Such solutions may also be indicated to replace electrolytes and water loss from severe vomiting or diarrhea. With these preparations, the extracellular replacement is usually achieved within 2 days (usually 1 to 3 L/day is administered); this should be closely monitored by laboratory tests. If maintenance solutions are continued after the client's deficits have been corrected, the excess sodium may lead to circulatory overload, pulmonary edema, and heart failure. Examples of maintenance solutions include Plasma-Lyte and Normosol.

Hypertonic solutions are used to treat hypotonic expansion (water intoxication) when increased body fluid volume is caused by water only. This can happen under several different circumstances: (1) hospitalized clients who receive large amounts of dextrose 5% in water or electrolyte-free solutions to replace fluid and electrolytes lost from vomiting, diarrhea, diuresis, or gastric suction, or (2) most likely in older adults during the postoperative period, when water is retained in response to stress (endocrine response to stress).

Overhydration or hypotonic expansion should be considered when behavioral changes such as lethargy, confusion

TABLE 69-2 Four Categories of Parenteral Solutions*

	Na^+	K^+	Mg^{++}	Ca^{++}	Cl^-	Osmolarity
Hydrating Solutions						
dextrose 2.5%, 5%, 10%						126, 252, 505
dextrose 2.5% in 0.45% NaCl injection†	56				56	280
dextrose 5% in 0.45% NaCl injection‡	7				77	405
Isotonic Solutions						
normal saline or sodium chloride injection (0.9% NaCl)	154				154	310
Ringer's injection	147	4		4	155	310
lactated Ringer's injection	130	4		3	109	275
Maintenance Solutions						
Plasmalyte 56	40	13	3		40	111
Plasmalyte 148 (or Normosol-R, Isolyte S)	140	5		3	98	295
Hypertonic Solutions						
sodium chloride, 3% injection	513				513	1025
sodium chloride, 5% injection	855				855	1710

*Normal plasma contains Na^+ (136-145 mEq/L), K^+ (3.5-5 mEq/L), Mg^{++} (1.5-2.5 mEq/L), Ca^{++} (4.3-5.3 mEq/L), Cl^- (100-106 mEq/L), HCO_3^- (27 mEq/L); normal osmolarity is 280-300 mOsm/L.

†Dextrose 2.5% = 25 g dextrose/L or 85 calories.

‡Dextrose 5% = 50 g dextrose/L or 170 calories.

and, perhaps, disorientation occur postoperatively in an older adult. Central nervous system signs and symptoms such as increased tiredness, muscle twitching, headaches, nausea, vomiting, and even seizures have been noted. Weight gain is always present, and the blood pressure may be normal or elevated.

In milder cases of overhydration, the treatment usually includes withholding all fluids until excess fluids are excreted. In severe cases of hyponatremia, small quantities of hypertonic sodium chloride are administered to (1) increase the osmotic pressure, (2) increase the water flow from body cells to the extracellular compartment, and (3) to enhance the excretion of fluids by the kidneys.

The typical hypertonic saline is a 3% or 5% solution that must be administered slowly with close supervision to prevent pulmonary edema. Close monitoring of laboratory tests for electrolytes is also required.

Fluid-Electrolyte Balance and Dehydration

A dynamic relationship exists in the body between water and sodium. Abnormal states of hydration can be classified as (1) dehydration (volume depletion), (2) overhydration (hypervolemia or volume excess), (3) loss of water in excess of sodium (hypernatremia), and (4) loss of sodium in excess of water (hyponatremia). Overhydration was reviewed in the preceding section under the description of hypertonic solutions. The other three abnormal states may be viewed as various types of dehydration.

Table 69-3 illustrates the differences between the three types of dehydration. Note that the causes of the three dehydration states are different, as are the effects on fluid compartments in the body and some of the initial signs and laboratory values, especially sodium concentration. This is very important information because it aids the provider not only in diagnosing the initial condition but also in choosing the appropriate IV therapy.

Hypertonic dehydration caused by heat exhaustion and resulting from water depletion can occur on land or sea. Many boaters lost at sea or refugees fleeing their countries for another country run out of water for days before being rescued or reaching land. Such persons require intensive care for their dehydration, and some may die from this deprivation (Table 69-4).

The nurse should be aware that older adults with decreased renal function are more vulnerable to dehydration and electrolyte imbalance. The additional physiologic changes experienced by older adults as a result of the aging process may also make them more susceptible to the adverse effects of fluid and electrolyte administration, such as overhydration or decreased renal excretion of exogenous potassium or magnesium, with resultant toxic accumulation in the body.

ELECTROLYTES

The major electrolytes in the body are sodium, potassium, calcium, and magnesium. This section reviews the normal requirements, sources, and specific functions of these elec-

TABLE 69-3 Differences Among the Three Types of Dehydration

	Hypotonic	Isotonic	Hypertonic
Cause	Loss of salt (NaCl)	Blood loss	Water loss or lack of sufficient fluid intake
Effect on ICF and ECF compartments	Volume ICF↑ Volume ECF↓	Decrease in ECF volume	Decrease in ICF and ECF volume
Significant signs:			
Rate of water elimination	Increased	Decreased	Decreased
Thirst			Early warning because of cell dehydration
Pulse rate	Increased, weak, thready	Regular	Regular in early stages
Behavioral signs	May see vomiting, abdominal cramps		Confusion, irritability, agitation
Late stages	Skin turgor Weak pulse, lethargy, confusion, death owing to circulatory failure	Shock, weak Weak, thready pulse	Skin turgor Dry, furrowed tongue; death
Clinical laboratory results			
Hematocrit	Increased	Increased	Increased
Hemoglobin	Increased	Increased	Increased
Sodium levels	Decreased		Increased

ECF, Extracellular fluid; *ICF*, intracellular fluid.

TABLE 69-4 Symptoms of Hypertonic Dehydration

Clinical Grading	Symptoms
Mild or early	Increased thirst. Usually a 2% loss in body weight.
Moderate to severe	Very dry mouth, difficulty swallowing, scant urine output (highly concentrated urine), increased pulse rate and body temperature, poor skin turgor, an approximate 6% body weight loss.
Extreme or very severe	All previous symptoms plus impaired mental and physical capabilities, very high rectal temperature, respiratory difficulties (hyperventilation that may lead to tetany), cyanosis, severe oliguria or anuria, circulatory failure, loss of more than 7% in body weight. Coma and death usually occur when approximately 15% of body weight is lost.

trolytes, as well as the problems associated with their excess or deficiency.

Sodium

Sodium is the major electrolyte in the extracellular fluid; the normal range is from 136 to 145 mEq/L of plasma. Sodium content in the body is regulated by sodium consumption (dietary) and sodium excretion by the kidneys. In the average person with normal renal function, sodium excretion closely matches sodium intake. This helps to keep sodium content in the body at a constant level, even if sodium intake is somewhat varied. Major dietary sources of sodium are table salt (sodium chloride), catsup, mustard, cured meats and fish, cheese, peanut butter, pickles, olives, potato chips, and popcorn. The typical American diet provides between 3 to 6 g of sodium per day (Johnson, Parker, & Geraci, 1999), even though the recommended dietary sodium allowance is much less. Sodium is necessary for the control of body water; for the electrophysiology of nerve, muscle, and gland cells; and for the regulation of pH and isotonicity.

Hyponatremia

Hyponatremia may be detected when serum levels fall below 135 mEq/L. This condition may be induced by excessive sweating when only the water is replaced, by the infusion of large quantities of nonelectrolyte parenteral fluids, by syndrome of inappropriate antidiuretic hormone (SIADH), and by adrenal insufficiency or gastrointestinal suctioning with replacement fluids limited to water by mouth.

Symptoms include lethargy, hypotension, stomach cramps, vomiting, diarrhea and, possibly, seizures. Deficiency states are usually treated with Ringer's solution or normal saline injection.

Hypernatremia

Hypernatremia is seen when serum sodium levels are higher than normal (usually >150 mEq/L). This excess may be induced by the excessive use of saline infusions, inadequate water consumption (as described previously), or excess fluid loss without a corresponding loss of sodium.

The signs and symptoms of hypernatremia include edema; hypertonicity; red, flushed skin; dry and sticky mucous membranes; increased thirst; elevated temperature; and a decrease in or absence of urination. Treatment includes reducing salt intake and using dextrose in water intravenously to promote diuresis and increase the excretion of both salt and water from the blood.

Potassium

Potassium is the major electrolyte in the intracellular fluids. The amount of potassium in the intracellular fluid is approximately 150 mEq/L, whereas the amount in the plasma is between 3.5 and 5 mEq/L. Even though this plasma amount appears to be low, it is of great importance—serum potassium must be maintained between 3.5 and 5 mEq/L for survival. The diet of most individuals contains from 35 to 100 mEq of potassium daily, with any excess potassium normally excreted by the kidney in the urine. Potassium plays an important part role in (1) muscle contraction, (2) conduction of nerve impulses, (3) enzyme action, and (4) cell membrane function.

Hypokalemia

Hypokalemia, or a potassium deficit, may be caused by the chronic administration of IV solutions containing little or no potassium; diuretic therapy with potassium-depleting medications; reduced dietary intake (e.g., in persons on "starvation diets"); poor absorption because of steatorrhea, regional enteritis, or short bowel syndrome; loss of gastrointestinal secretions (which are very rich in potassium) due to vomiting, diarrhea, gastrointestinal suction, or fistula drainage; extensive burn conditions; or the presence of excessive amounts of adrenocorticotropic hormone (ACTH).

Unlike sodium, which is reabsorbed when the serum sodium level is low, potassium ions continue to be excreted in the urine even when the serum potassium level is low. As potassium loss continues, the individual's condition deteriorates unless potassium intake is increased and normal levels are reestablished.

With hypokalemia, impaired skeletal muscle function may cause profound weakness or paralysis, including paralysis of the respiratory muscles. Impaired smooth muscle function may result in ileus. The cardiac effects of hypokalemia include an increased sensitivity to digitalis with potential toxicity and electrocardiogram (ECG) changes. Early potassium deficiency may be detected by the use of the ECG, because the T wave tends to flatten when serum potassium levels are below 3.5 mEq/L and tends to elongate vertically when the serum potassium level is 5.8 mEq/L or higher. Atrioventricular block and cardiac arrest may occur.

Hypokalemia also causes the movement of Na^+ and H^+ from the extracellular fluid and the excretion of H^+, which may elevate plasma pH and result in metabolic alkalosis. Other effects include increased risk of electrolyte abnormalities, elevated serum enzymes, and other systemic effects (Johnson et al., 1999).

Treat hypokalemia by replacing potassium orally or parenterally. Be aware, however, that one hazard of parenteral correction is potassium poisoning, or hyperkalemia.

Parenteral or IV Supplementation. The dosage of potassium supplements depends on the individual requirement and requires close supervision. *IV potassium must always be diluted* and administered slowly. In general, potassium is given only to clients with a documented adequate urine flow. In dehydrated clients, it is best to administer a potassium-free fluid first to hydrate the client and determine urinary output.

It is recommended that parenteral fluids not contain more than 40 mEq/L of potassium, and the rate of administration should not be more than 20 mEq/hour (American Hospital Formulary Service, 1999). Whenever possible, the oral preparations or the consumption of foods high in potassium should replace the IV potassium solutions (see Chapter 34).

Parenteral potassium salts are available as acetate, chloride, and phosphate salts. In general, potassium chloride is the preferred preparation, because the chloride helps to correct the hypochloremia often seen with hypokalemia. In general, the alkalinizing potassium salts (acetate, bicarbonate, citrate, or gluconate) may be necessary to treat the hypokalemia associated with metabolic acidosis (a rare situation).

Oral Supplementation. The potassium salts available for oral administration include acetate, bicarbonate, chloride, citrate, and gluconate, either alone or in combination. Liquid preparations are generally preferred for oral therapy, and most contain 10, 20, or 40 mEq of potassium/15 mL. These preparations must be diluted with fruit juice or water before ingestion and taken after meals with a full glass of water to minimize gastrointestinal irritation. For powder preparations, follow the manufacturer's instructions closely. Uncoated and enteric-coated (no longer available in the United States) dosage forms of potassium have caused intestinal and gastric ulcers with bleeding episodes (AHFS, 1999). Although still available, they are rarely used medically; liquids, effervescent forms, powders, and extended-release dosage forms (wax matrix, microencapsulated) are the currently preferred products. Ulceration has been reported with the extended-release products, although much less often than with the other products; therefore these preparations should be reserved for clients who cannot or will not take the liquid or effervescent potassium.

Extended-release potassium should be discontinued immediately and the prescriber contacted if the client complains of stomach pain, swelling, or severe vomiting, or if gastrointestinal bleeding is noted. Potassium supplements are contraindicated with severe renal impairment, untreated chronic adrenocortical insufficiency (Addison's disease), hyperkalemia, and severe burn conditions or acute dehydration. They should also be avoided or used with extreme caution in clients who are taking potassium-sparing diuretics or angiotensin-converting enzyme (ACE) inhibitors. Solid dosage forms of potassium should not be administered to clients with esophageal compression caused by an enlarged left atrium or other anatomic variation that results in increased compression in this area. In such cases, the ingestion of potassium-rich foods may also be helpful (see Table 34-2).

K-Dur20 ◆ (controlled release) and Klor-Con ◆ (potassium chloride powder) are commonly prescribed. The dosage of potassium supplements depends on individual requirements. The approximate daily allowance for adults is 40 to 50 mEq; for infants, approximately 1 to 3 mEq/kg body weight daily.

Hyperkalemia

Hyperkalemia, or potassium excess, can be caused by acute or chronic renal failure; the release of large amounts of intracellular potassium in burns, crush injuries, or severe infections; overtreatment with potassium salts; or metabolic acidosis, including diabetic ketoacidosis, which causes a shift of potassium from the cells into the extracellular fluids.

Hyperkalemia interferes with neuromuscular function and may result in abdominal distention, diarrhea, weakness, and paralysis. The cardiac effects caused by hyperkalemia result from impaired conduction. The ECG shows a widening and slurring of the QRS complexes, peaked T waves, depressed ST segments and, possibly, a disappearance of P waves. Ventricular fibrillation and cardiac arrest may occur.

The treatment of hyperkalemia depends on the serum level of potassium and on the ECG patterns. Mild hyperkalemia usually involves serum levels below 6.5 mEq/L, with ECG changes limited to peaking of the T waves. Moderate hyperkalemia involves potassium serum levels between 6.5 and 8 mEq/L, and severe hyperkalemia involves serum levels above 8 mEq/L with an ECG pattern of absent P waves, widened QRS complexes, or ventricular dysrhythmias. (See the Management of Drug Overdose Box on p. 1176 for the treatment of hyperkalemia.)

Calcium

Calcium (Ca^{++}) is essential for the growth and ossification of bones, neuromuscular transmission, cell membrane permeability, the maintenance of excitability in nerve fibers, hormone secretion and action, muscle contraction, maintenance of cardiac and vascular tone, many enzyme activities, and the normal coagulation of blood.

Almost all of the 1000 to 1200 g calcium in the normal adult is found in the skeletal tissue; only about 1% of the total body calcium is in solution in body fluids. Approximately

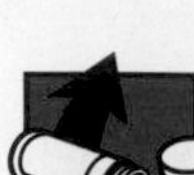

Management of Drug Overdose
Hyperkalemia

- For mild hyperkalemia, remove or treat the cause. For example, if the client is receiving potassium supplements or an ACE inhibitor, stop the medications. If metabolic acidosis is present, treat this condition.
- Moderate to severe hyperkalemia may require infusing hypertonic dextrose solutions with insulin to shift potassium into the cells. Parenteral sodium bicarbonate may be used to correct acidosis and also to help shift serum potassium into cells. Calcium gluconate is administered intravenously under constant ECG monitoring for severe cardiac toxicity. Calcium counteracts the adverse effects of potassium on the neuromuscular membranes, but this is only a temporary measure. Lowering potassium levels is critical to reversing this situation.
- The above methods do not remove potassium from the body. Sodium polystyrene sulfonate (Kayexalate), a cation exchange resin, can be given orally or rectally to remove potassium from the body.
- The oral adult dose of sodium polystyrene sulfonate is 15 g one to four times daily in water or, preferably, a 70% sorbitol solution to reduce the possibility of constipation. The rectal (retention enema) adult dosage is 25 to 100 g of resin suspended in 100 to 200 mL of sorbitol or 10% dextrose in water. This dose may be administered every 6 hours.
- Laxatives must be used when the drug is given orally. Because its action is considered slow, the previously discussed treatments are indicated if ECG changes indicate severe potassium intoxication. Administration should be discontinued when serum potassium levels fall to 4 or 5 mEq/L.
- The side effects of sodium polystyrene sulfonate treatment include anorexia, nausea, vomiting, constipation, hypokalemia, and hypocalcemia. Fecal impaction has also been reported; it can be prevented with the use of laxatives (*USP DI,* 1999).

half the calcium in plasma is bound to complex organic anions (e.g., bicarbonate and phosphate). Nearly all unbound serum calcium is ionized. The normal serum concentration of calcium is 4.5 to 5.5 mEq/L or 9 to 11 mg/100 mL.

The recommended dietary allowance of calcium for adults is 0.8 to 1.2 g daily. Pregnant or lactating women need 1.2 g; children 1 to 3 years of age, 0.4 to 0.8 g; and children 4 to 10 years of age, 0.8 g. Although many individuals have sufficient calcium from dietary sources, calcium supplementation to prevent bone loss seems reasonable for women. Early evidence that a high calcium intake reduces the risk for colon cancer has not been confirmed in subsequent studies. At most, calcium reduces the risk for colon cancer only slightly (Martinez et al., 1996).

The absorption of calcium depends on how well it is kept in solution in the digestive tract; an acid medium favors calcium solubility and absorption in the upper intestinal tract. Absorption is decreased by the presence of alkalis and large amounts of fatty acids. Adequate intake of vitamin D appears to promote calcium absorption. Calcium is excreted in the urine and feces and in perspiration. Estrogen deficiency promotes calcium loss.

The maintenance of normal concentrations of serum calcium depends on the interactions of three agents: parathyroid hormone, vitamin D, and calcitonin (Mundy & Guise, 1999). Parathyroid hormone and vitamin D mobilize the removal of calcium from bone—the principal source of calcium for extracellular fluids. Parathyroid hormone also promotes renal tubular reabsorption of calcium and a slight increase in intestinal absorption of calcium. Calcitonin synthesized in the thyroid gland moderates or decreases the rate of removal of calcium from the bone.

Hypocalcemia

Hypocalcemia, or a decrease in serum calcium, results from (1) hypoparathyroidism, (2) chronic renal insufficiency, (3) hypoalbuminemia, (4) malabsorption syndrome, and (5) a deficiency of vitamin D. Hypoparathyroidism may follow a thyroidectomy, because several parathyroid glands are often removed with this surgery. If the function of the remaining gland(s) is impaired, the result is depressed parathyroid activity.

Clients who are bedridden tend to develop a negative calcium balance—the ion is lost from the bones and excreted. This effect is likely to be serious when the client needs to be immobilized for long periods.

Hypocalcemia increases the excitability of the nerves and neuromuscular junction; this leads to muscle cramps, muscle twitching, and tetany. Numbness and tingling of the fingers, toes, and lips occurs. Hypertonicity of muscle may cause tonic contractions of the hands and feet (carpopedal spasm), whereas increased neural excitability may cause convulsions, abnormal behavior, and personality changes. Prolonged hypocalcemia in children has resulted in mental retardation. The ECG shows a prolonged QT interval and an inverted T wave. In prolonged hypocalcemia, defects can occur in the nails, skin, and teeth; cataracts may appear; and calcification of the basal ganglia may occur.

Regardless of the underlying cause, severe hypocalcemia is treated initially with the IV administration of rapidly available calcium ions. An oral calcium salt is administered for latent tetany, mild symptoms of hypocalcemia, and maintenance therapy. Vitamin D may also be prescribed. An overdose of calcium may cause hypercalcemia, which results in anorexia, nausea, vomiting, weakness, depression, polyuria, and polydipsia.

Calcium must be administered cautiously to clients undergoing digitalis therapy, because calcium potentiates the effect of digitalis and may precipitate dysrhythmias. ECG

TABLE 69-5 Calcium Content of Various Calcium Salts

	Percentage of Calcium	Amount of Calcium per Tablet	Tablets Needed for 1 g Calcium
calcium carbonate	40	260 mg/650 mg	4
calcium gluconate	9	45 mg/500 mg	22
calcium lactate	13	42 mg/325 mg	24
calcium phosphate tribasic	39	600 mg/1565 mg	1.66

monitoring of the client is recommended when parenteral calcium is administered.

Calcium salts are used as a nutritional supplement, particularly during pregnancy and lactation. They are specific in the treatment of hypocalcemic tetany. They have also been used for their antispasmodic effects in cases of abdominal pain, tenesmus, and colic resulting from disease of the gallbladder or painful contractions of the ureters. The basic salts of calcium are also used as antacids. Approximately 1 to 1.5 g calcium per day has been recommended to prevent postmenopausal bone loss or osteoporosis.

The most widely used calcium salt is calcium carbonate, which requires an acid medium to form soluble calcium salts because it is nearly insoluble in water. The absorption or dissolution of calcium phosphate and calcium sulfate is also pH dependent, whereas calcium lactate, calcium citrate, and calcium gluconate are considered pH independent. Impaired stomach acid production is common in older adults and postmenopausal women; the high stomach pH or achlorhydric state results in a decreased solubility of pH-dependent calcium salts.

Because the different calcium salts contain different amounts of calcium, many professionals choose the calcium salt with the highest percentage of calcium per gram; in this way, a smaller quantity of drug may be administered. For example, if the recommended daily dose of calcium is 1000 mg/day, it would be necessary to administer nearly 10 g of calcium gluconate to reach this amount, whereas only 2.5 g of calcium carbonate per day would be required. This would require the consumption of smaller quantities of tablets to obtain the same amount of calcium, assuming of course that the calcium is soluble under the conditions present in the client (Table 69-5).

To improve the solubility of calcium carbonate tablets, especially in achlorhydric conditions, it is recommended the tablets be taken with meals, when acid secretion is highest. Avoid taking the tablets on an empty stomach or at night, because acid secretions are minimal at these times. Calcium phosphates and tricalcium phosphate have little usefulness in possible achlorhydric states and, perhaps, even in individuals with normal production of stomach acid. Both products have a very poor dissolution rate or pattern, thus reducing the possibility of calcium absorption. Soluble calcium salts (lactate or citrate) might be the appropriate form to use in clients with known achlorhydric states, even though it is necessary to use more tablets to provide sufficient quantities of calcium. Selected food consumption is another source for calcium (Table 69-6).

TABLE 69-6 Foods with High Calcium Content

Food	Calcium Content
Yogurt, low fat (1 cup)	275-400 mg
Skim milk (1 cup)	300 mg
Cheese, Swiss (1 ounce)	272 mg
Cheese, cottage (1 cup)	215 mg
Cheese, cheddar (1 ounce)	200 mg
Broccoli, raw (1 cup)	100 mg
Ice cream (1/2 cup)	100 mg
Ice milk (3/4 cup)	132 mg

Hypercalcemia

Neoplasms with or without bone metastases may cause hypercalcemia, or elevated serum calcium levels (Barnett, 1999). Carcinoma of the ovary, kidney, or lung can synthesize and secrete a parathyroid-like hormone, causing hypercalcemia. Other common causes are hyperparathyroidism, thiazide diuretic therapy, multiple myeloma, sarcoidosis, and vitamin D intoxication.

The clinical manifestations of hypercalcemia are highly variable and involve many organ systems, because calcium may be deposited in various body tissues. Symptoms may include the following:

- Gastrointestinal: anorexia, nausea, vomiting, constipation, and abdominal pain.
- Neurologic: weakness, apathy, depression, amnesia, confusion, stupor, and coma may occur.
- Renal: polyuria and nephrocalcinosis may occur, seriously impairing renal function; this may lead to edema, uremia, and hypertension, which may be irreversible.
- Cardiovascular: increased cardiac contractility, ventricular extrasystoles, and heart block. ECG changes include a short QT segment and characteristic signs of heart block.

Treatment is variable and aimed at controlling the underlying disease. For dehydrated clients, restore extracellular fluid volume with normal saline infusions; this also increases calcium excretion. Furosemide may be prescribed to enhance diuresis, but thiazide diuretics should be avoided because they block or lower calcium excretion. Chelating (binding) agents, such as disodium edetate, have been used to treat acute hypercalcemia in selected individuals. It increases the renal excretion of calcium by forming soluble complexes with the calcium that is not reabsorbed by the renal tubules.

Bisphosphonates are analogues of pyrophosphate (normal component of bone); these drugs are incorporated into bone, where they inhibit bone resorption by decreasing the activity of osteoclasts, resulting in a decrease in serum calcium (Brown & Robbins, 1999). The currently available bisphosphonates include alendronate (Fosamax), etidronate (Didronel), pamidronate (Aredia), risedronate (Actonel), and tiludronate (Skelid).

These agents are used to treat Paget's disease and hypercalcemia of malignancy. For hypercalcemia of malignancy, pamidronate is more potent and is usually the preferred agent. Parenteral etidronate is also used as adjunct therapy to treat hypercalcemia associated with neoplasms; alendronate is also indicated for the prevention and treatment of osteoporosis in postmenopausal women. An antineoplastic drug, plicamycin (Mithracin) also reduces serum calcium levels (*Drug Facts and Comparisons*, 2000; Tang & Lau, 1995; *USP DI*, 1999).

Oral alendronate has a low bioavailability (0.7%), which can be negligible if given with meals or up to 2 hours after breakfast. Therefore it should be administered on an empty stomach with 8 ounces of water and at least 30 minutes before the consumption of any food, beverage, or other medication. Etidronate is available orally and parenterally; absorption of the oral dosage form is approximately 1% in doses of 5 mg/kg, and up to 2.5% to 6% in doses of 10 to 20 mg/kg taken on an empty stomach. Pamidronate is available parenterally, whereas risedronate and tiludronate are oral dosage forms that also require an empty stomach for absorption.

See Table 69-7 for the pharmacokinetics and dosing of the bisphosphonates.

The side effects/adverse reactions of the bisphosphonates include the following:

- The effects of alendronate include dysphagia, heartburn, headache, muscle pain and, the most serious effect, esophagitis (pain and ulceration).
- Etidronate may cause an altered taste sensation, anorexia, nausea, diarrhea, bone pain (especially in clients with Paget's disease), and osteomalacia (bone fractures, especially of the femur), which usually occurs if clients are taking doses higher than 20 mg/kg or if therapy is continued longer than 6 months.
- The effects of pamidronate include nausea, fever, pain, and edema at the injection site; muscle stiffness, hypocalcemia (stomach cramps, confusion, muscle spasms), and leukopenia (chills, fever, or sore throat).

TABLE 69-7 Bisphosphonates: Pharmacokinetics and Dosing

Name	Pharmacokinetics	Adult Dosage
alendronate (Fosamax)	D of A: 6 weeks after single dose of 5 mg for osteoporosis; 6 months in PD Excretion: primarily in urine	PO: PD, 40 mg daily in morning (empty stomach); PMO, 10 mg daily in morning (empty stomach)
etidronate (Didronel)	O of A: PD, 1 month; hypercalcemia, 24 hours. Peak effect: hypercalcemia, decrease in serum calcium peaks after third infusion. D of A: PD, up to 1 year after drug is stopped Hypercalcemia: about 11 days Excretion: primarily in urine	PO: PD, 5 mg/kg/day for 6 months; hypercalcemia, 20 mg/kg/day for 1-3 months IV infusion: hypercalcemia 7.5mg/day for 3 days
pamidronate (Aredia)	Half-life: 1.6 hours (alpha), 27.2 hours (beta) Excretion: primarily in urine	IV infusion: 60 mg given over 4-24 hours for hypercalcemia or 90-180 mg total dose for PD
risedronate (Actonel)	Absorption: rapid Half-life: initial 1.5 hours, terminal 220 hours Excretion: primarily in urine	PO: PD, 30 mg daily for 2 months, taken in morning (empty stomach); supplements or calcium and vitamin D necessary if dietary intake insufficient
tiludronate (Skelid)	Half-life: elimination 50 hours in healthy persons; 150 hours in PD clients Excretion: primarily in urine	PO: PD, 400 mg daily on empty stomach

Information from Salerno, E. (1999.). *Pharmacology for health professionals*. St. Louis: Mosby; *Drug Facts and Comparisons*. (2000). St. Louis: Facts and Comparisons; and *United States Pharmacopoeia Dispensing Information (USP DI): Drug information for the health care professional* (19th ed.). (1999). Rockville, MD: United States Pharmacopeial Convention.
D of A, duration of action; *O of A*, onset of action; *PD*, Paget's disease; *PMO*, postmenopausal osteoporosis.

- The effects of risedronate include dizziness, headache, chest or stomach pain, nausea, diarrhea, constipation, arthralgia, bone pain, leg cramps, weakness, peripheral edema, a flu-like syndrome, and rash.
- The effects of tiludronate include generalized body pain, back pain, gastric distress, vomiting, joint pain, conjunctivitis, cough, pharyngitis, rhinitis, upper respiratory tract infection, a flu-type syndrome, rash, dizziness, chest pain, glaucoma, and cataracts.

See Chapter 48 for the nursing management of bisphosphonate therapy.

Magnesium

Magnesium (Mg^{++}) is an important ion for the function of many enzyme systems.

Hypomagnesemia

Hypomagnesemia, a deficit of magnesium, may be encountered in chronic alcoholism, severe malabsorption, starvation, diarrhea, prolonged gastrointestinal suction, vigorous diuresis, acute pancreatitis, and primary aldosteronism (Agus, 1999). Magnesium, the second most abundant intracellular cation, plays an important role in regulating the function of the sodium-potassium adenosine triphosphatase (ATPase) pump, neuromuscular transmission, cardiovascular function, and mitochondrial and other cellular functions in the body.

A magnesium deficiency may result in additional electrolyte problems (hypokalemia, hypocalcemia), cardiac dysrhythmias, and neurotoxicity. It may also cause an increase in neuromuscular irritability and contractility, coarse tremors, muscle spasm, delirium, athetoid movements, nystagmus, and tetany. It also causes tachycardia, hypertension, and vasomotor changes and increases the risk of digitalis toxicity in clients who are taking cardiac glycosides.

Hypomagnesemia may be treated with IV fluids containing magnesium (10 to 40 mEq/day for a severe deficit) followed by 10 mEq/day for maintenance. The use of IV fluids containing from 3 to 5 mEq magnesium/L may avert a magnesium deficiency that arises from the prolonged administration of IV solutions that do not contain magnesium.

Hypermagnesemia

Hypermagnesemia occurs primarily in clients with chronic renal insufficiency. The adverse effects of hypermagnesemia include flushing, sweating, hypothermia, areflexia, paralysis, and the depression of cardiac, CNS, and respiratory functions. Decreased muscle cell excitability is caused by blockade of the myoneural junction (inhibition of acetylcholine release). Cardiac depression effects result in an increase in conduction time, with the ECG showing a lengthened PR segment and a prolonged QRS complex. If the Mg^{++} concentration continues to increase, third-degree atrioventricular block and cardiac arrest may occur.

An excess of Mg^{++} may require dialysis. Because calcium acts as an antagonist to Mg^{++}, calcium salts may be given parenterally. Normal serum concentration is 1.5 to 2.5 mEq/L, with one third bound to protein and two thirds free. A toxic blood level involves a magnesium level greater than 4 mEq/L. Magnesium has physiologic effects on the nervous system that are similar to those of calcium.

Monitoring Electrolytes

Laboratory tests are used to monitor the client's electrolyte levels and to help determine replacement therapies when necessary for electrolyte deficiency. The normal plasma values are listed in the notes of Table 69-2. Health care professionals should be aware of the difference between milligrams (mg), which reflects weight, and milliequivalents (mEq), which measures the number of chemically active ions in solution. A **milliequivalent (mEq)** is the number of grams of solute or electrolyte that is dissolved in one milliliter of a normal solution. It is a more precise measure of the relative potency of an electrolyte solution and is the method the prescriber uses to order electrolytes.

Additional Single-Salt Solutions

In addition to the previously discussed salt preparations, ammonium chloride injection and sodium lactate injection are also available for use.

Ammonium chloride injection is indicated to treat hypochloremia and metabolic alkalosis (not associated with severe liver disease) to prevent tetany or renal damage. Most cases respond to sodium chloride solution, but ammonium chloride is available for the rare, nonresponsive situation. Ammonium chloride has been used as a urinary acidifier to promote the excretion of alkaline substances.

This product is available in 20-mL vials (100 mEq). The dose selected depends on the client—usually 1 to 2 vials, which is added to normal saline and infused slowly.

Sodium lactate injection available as a ⅙ molar solution contains 167 mEq/L each of sodium and lactate ions. It is used to treat metabolic acidosis when no evidence of an elevated level of lactic acid exists. Sodium lactate is converted to sodium bicarbonate in the liver. Sodium bicarbonate is preferred for clients with lactic acidosis or impaired liver function.

■ Nursing Management

Intravenous Therapy

IV fluid and dextrose or electrolyte replacement by infusion continues to be the most common application of intravascular therapy. Although the dosage and choice of solution is tailored to the client's needs by the prescriber according to the disorder and body surface area, monitoring the therapy is the nurse's responsibility. With the increasing prevalence of clients receiving some type of intravascular therapy in hospitals, as well as in home settings, the role of the nurse in IV therapy has also grown and developed. See the Community and Home Health Considerations box on p. 1180 for additional information on IV therapy in the home.

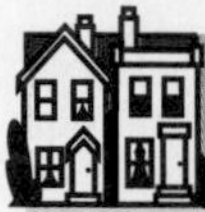

Community and Home Health Considerations
Clients Receiving Home IV Therapy

The provision of IV therapy to clients in their homes is growing in practice. It allows the client to remain in a home setting, to be more comfortable, and to perform many daily activities. There may also be cost benefits for clients and health care agencies.

Clients should be carefully selected to receive home IV therapy. Instruction should begin in the hospital and be completed before the client is discharged. If the nurse is to provide IV therapy on a home visit, all of the nursing processes applicable to institutional care are adapted for the home setting. If the IV therapy is to be self-administered or administered by a caregiver in the home, it should be determined that the client/caregiver is willing and capable of administering the therapy safely. This capability includes the economics and transportation to obtain supplies; fine movement coordination to manipulate the equipment; and an understanding of asepsis, the rationale for therapy, the interventions, the potential complications, and whom to contact in case of emergency.

Instruct the client in any activity limitations; how to check the venipuncture site for complications; and what to do if redness/swelling/pain occurs, if the dressing becomes soiled, if blood appears in the tubing, or if the alarm sounds on the electronic infusion device. If the client is using a heparin lock, teach the client how and when to flush it. Have the client document a daily check of the venipuncture site. Have the client/caregiver perform return demonstrations. Develop a number of "what if . . . " scenarios to test the client's understanding and decision-making skills before an urgent situation occurs. Encourage the client/caregiver to contact the health care provider for assistance if required.

Consider intravascular therapy as a closed-system, sterile procedure. It is invasive, and its effects are relatively irreversible; therefore take care to perform and maintain it precisely.

■ **Assessment.** Assessment begins with an understanding of the purpose of the particular client's IV therapy and the potential risks to the client. Clients who are debilitated, have a renal or cardiovascular problem, are prone to infection, or have very sclerotic veins are particularly at risk for complications related to IV therapy.

Factors to be considered for site selection include the following: suitable location, purpose of infusion, expected duration of therapy, condition of veins, restrictions imposed by the client's current health status and past health history, and the dominant extremity (Metheny, 1996). Unless contraindicated, it is most appropriate to use veins in the nondominant upper extremity. When more than one puncture is anticipated, it is better to make the first venipuncture distally and work proximally. Avoid venipuncture in the affected arm of clients who have undergone axillary dissection (as in radical mastectomy) or have impaired mobility of the upper extremity (as in unilateral paralysis secondary to a cerebrovascular accident). In both instances circulation may not be adequate and affects the flow of the infusion, causing increased edema.

■ **Nursing Diagnosis.** Every client with an IV infusion is at risk for the following nursing diagnoses: impaired tissue integrity related to infiltration, thrombosis, thrombophlebitis, and necrosis; pain at the administration site; and the potential complications of pulmonary edema, pyrogenic reaction, speed shock, and sepsis. Because of their smaller body size, infants and children are especially at risk for overhydration.

■ **Implementation**

■ ***Monitoring.*** Continued reassessments of laboratory data reports are essential for clients who are receiving electrolyte replacement therapy. Serum electrolytes should not exceed the following accepted ranges during IV therapy:

Sodium	135 to 145 mEq/L
Chlorides	95 to 108 mEq/L
Potassium	3.5 to 5 mEq/L
Calcium	4.5 to 5.8 mEq/L
Magnesium	1.5 to 2.5 mEq/L

Note that fluctuations in potassium, calcium, and magnesium must be watched carefully during IV electrolyte therapy, because even a small deviation in these electrolytes creates a much greater risk than in those electrolytes with a wider range of normal values. Understanding that milliequivalents (mEq) are not related to milligrams also is important; "mEq" does not reflect a measure of weight.

Milliequivalents measure the number of chemically active ions in solution, which is a more precise measure of the relative potency of an electrolyte solution than weight-by-volume measurements. (See Chapter 5 for the equipment and technical aspects of IV therapy.)

Remember that an ongoing assessment of client response is essential to preventing complications from IV therapy (Powers, 1999). The entire IV system should be monitored—from the fluid container to the client's infusion site. Such assessments should be made at frequent intervals. Flow rates may change 20% to 40% during an infusion; check the flow rate every hour if not using an infusion pump. The nurse may be responsible for calculating the need for hourly changes in IV flow rates based on individual fluid output. The nurse may titrate infusion fluid intake according to the amount of urine, gastric, or other outputs over specified periods.

Ongoing assessment of the client receiving IV therapy should include observations for the complications described in the following sections.

■ *Infiltration.* Infiltration occurs when the needle is dislodged from the vein; this permits the solution to enter the surrounding tissues and causes pain and edema. Check the infusion site at frequent intervals for signs of infiltration (painful, blanched, cool swelling at infusion site without blood return). There may also be a significant decrease in flow rate, or it may stop altogether if the infiltration is extensive.

To detect infiltration in a questionable IV site, locate the vein in which the parenteral solution is infusing. Place two fingers on the vein, approximately 3 to 4 inches above the injection, depending on the length of the needle or catheter that is in place. Observe the drip chamber while applying digital pressure. If the flow of solution in the drip chamber stops, the needle is in the vein. If there is no alteration of flow in the drip chamber, the needle is probably in the tissue, because flow continues into the tissues even if the vein is occluded (Metheny, 1996). If infiltration is confirmed, stop the infusion.

■ *Thrombosis.* An intravascular blood clot occurs when platelets agglutinate and fibrin strands and red and white blood cells adhere to the platelet mass. A thrombus may form any time a blood vessel is injured, including injury by venipuncture. A thrombus may form in or around the needle or catheter, plugging the lumen; if this occurs, the infusion stops.

■ *Thrombophlebitis.* Formation of a blood clot and inflammation of the vein may result from several factors: chemical as a result of the pH of the solution or the toxicity of the drug being administered; mechanical as a result of injury of the vein by movement of the cannula; and septic as a result of contamination. Thrombophlebitis is manifested by pain, heat, swelling, and redness along the course of the vein, as well as loss of motion of the affected part.

■ *Pain at Administration Site.* Pain occurs when (1) the needle touches the venous wall, (2) too much tension is put on the needle or tubing, and (3) irritating drugs are administered too rapidly.

■ *Necrosis.* Death and sloughing of tissue can occur when irritating drugs or solutions, such as epinephrine or norepinephrine, infiltrate into the tissues.

■ *Pulmonary Edema.* Pulmonary edema occurs when the circulatory system is overloaded with fluids. Careful monitoring of flow rate and urinary output is necessary. Central venous pressure monitoring, particularly in clients with cardiac disease, can help to prevent this hazardous complication. The client will exhibit dyspnea on exertion, orthopnea, and coughing. Tachycardia, tachypnea, dependent crackles, neck vein distention, and diastolic (S_3) gallop may be heard. Coughing produces frothy, bloody sputum. Dysrhythmias may occur. The client becomes cold, clammy, sweaty, and cyanotic; blood pressure falls, and the pulse becomes thready.

■ *Pyrogenic Reactions.* Pyrogenic reactions occur when pyrogens, or fever-producing substances, are introduced into the circulatory system. Bacterial pyrogens are filterable, thermostable products of bacterial origin and activity that may accumulate and tend to cause a severe rigor when injected into the body. Pyrogenic reactions are characterized by fever and chills, malaise, headache, backache, nausea, vomiting and, if severe, vascular collapse with hypotension.

■ *Air Emboli.* Although they rarely occur, air emboli have a 40% to 50% mortality rate (McConnell, 1986). Cannulation of the central veins is far more likely to be associated with air embolism than is cannulation of the peripheral veins (Thielen, 1990). The occurrence of the following symptoms in a client receiving an infusion may indicate the presence of an air embolism: dyspnea, cyanosis, hypotension, weak/rapid pulse, loud and continuous churning sound over the precordium (not always present), and loss of consciousness.

The assessment for some clients may include whether IV fluids should be used at all (Box 69-2).

■ ***Intervention.*** Maintain a steady, even flow at the rate ordered; do not speed up rates to make up for lost time (watch the literature, however, for a resolution of the question about slowed rates being more compatible with basal metabolic rates during the before-dawn hours). Use every aid to facilitate therapy, such as calculating drops to be infused per minute and then time-taping the container. The use of an electronic infusion device (EID) is the standard for practice in many institutions, with either a controller that regulates IV flow rates by gravity or a controller that uses positive pressure to maintain flow (Box 69-3). Avoid using restraints and checking blood pressures on the arm receiving the infusion; the cuff interferes with fluid flow, forces blood back into the needle, and may cause clot formation. See Chapter 5 for techniques associated with IV therapy.

Changes in solutions may require changes in equipment. Be aware of the options available in selecting a filter for the specific IV infusion. Several different IV filter products are designed for different filtration needs. Filters are available in a range of sizes and in add-on or in-line form:

- A 5-μm filter removes *particulate* material and is designed to filter gross particulate matter. The smallest particle visible to the unaided eye is approximately 30 μm in diameter.
- A 0.5-μm filter is considered a *bacteria-retention* filter, which is designed to prevent the passage of most particulate matter and certain fungi and bacteria. A yeast cell is approximately 3 μm in diameter.
- The 0.22-μm filter is called a *sterilizing* filter, because it is designed to prevent the passage of virtually all particulate matter and most bacteria for at least 24 hours. Bacteria range in size from 0.2 to 2 μm in diameter. Travenol Laboratories and other manufacturers provide these filters for use with the add-on or in-line systems. Select a 0.22-μm filter for parenteral nutrition solutions.

Tightly secure all connections in the administration setup to prevent air from being drawn in. Do not allow containers to empty completely, because air in the tubing could be driven into the vein when another full container is attached. Keep containers approximately 3 feet above the site during all client activities. If not using an infusion device, a higher position will cause the solution to infuse too rapidly; if too low, blood may find its way into the needle or tubing and clot there. Avoid using areas of flexion (e.g., the wrist or antecubital fossa); if such a site must be used, use an armboard.

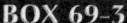

BOX 69-2

Should IV Fluids be Given to the Dying?

IV fluids are often provided to terminally ill clients in the belief that electrolyte imbalance and dehydration are painful, agonizing events. It is also feared that the lack of medical intervention may be interpreted as abandonment, provoking familial condemnation and raising the specter of malpractice (Rousseau, 1992).

From a legal standpoint, however, IV fluids may be withheld or withdrawn in the same manner as other medical treatments with the proviso that the client requests such limitations. A study by Andrews and Levine (1989) reports that dehydration is not painful and may even be beneficial to a dying client. Although the administration of IV fluids may produce a temporary sense of well-being, it often aggravates the client's symptoms. Hydration increases urinary output, often necessitating the insertion of an indwelling catheter and exposing the client to infection. Pulmonary and pharyngeal secretions increase and precipitate a cough, dyspnea, and pulmonary edema; pulmonary symptoms also increase. Increased gastrointestinal secretions exacerbate nausea and vomiting. IV fluids may also produce peripheral edema and increase the risk for skin breakdown. All of these symptoms increase the client's discomfort, and the IV fluids may prolong the dying process.

Fluid deprivation reduces these symptoms. The fluid and electrolyte imbalance produced by dehydration may be a natural anesthetic, thereby reducing the discomfort associated with the dying process (Rousseau, 1992).

Once a client decides to undergo terminal dehydration, the nurse's role is to provide scrupulous oral hygiene to reduce inflammation and minimize discomfort and to provide the client and family emotional support.

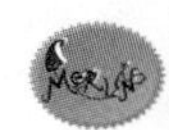

Critical Thinking Questions

- As a nurse, what feelings do you have about participating in the care of a dying client for whom IV rehydration is being withheld?
- How would you respond when asked about the rationale for this approach to the care of a dying client?

BOX 69-3

Recognizing a Hazard of Electronic Infusion Devices

Accidental, uncontrolled free flow of medication may occur when an IV administration set is removed from an electronic infusion device (EID). Although EIDs have been on the market for a number of years, only in the last few years have incidents of overdosing as the result of free flow begun to be reported anecdotally. This scarcity of information may be due to health care professionals blaming themselves rather than considering the overdoses to be the result of an EID design flaw. Many EID manufacturers are recognizing the problem and modifying their equipment to correct it.

Because the switch to safer equipment takes time, nurses need to be alert to ways to protect their clients from this hazard. Ensure that only health care providers who are fully prepared in EID technology be authorized to set up, adjust, or remove IV administration sets. Some instances of overdose have occurred when clients, nursing assistants, or x-ray technicians remove a pump to undress or ambulate. Check that the infusion is not running when the pump is removed, and be sure to check or recalculate the infusion rate.

Visible labels should be applied to EIDs that do not prevent free flow; this will alert staff to the possible occurrence of free flow with that equipment. Limit the use of one type of EID to each unit to increase staff familiarity with a particular EID. Use only protected EIDs in critical care units or with critical care drugs (Cohen & Davis, 1993).

Although the technology with which nurses practice is created to facilitate the provision of more effective nursing care, nurses need to remain vigilant as they apply it to clinical practice.

Take the necessary precautions to prevent thrombophlebitis by doing the following: using sterile aseptic technique with proper cleansing of skin before inserting the needle; checking solutions for precipitation, debris, sediment, or color changes before and during IV therapy; ascertaining that no IV bottle or tubing is left in place for more than 24 hours, because some organisms proliferate at room temperature in IV fluids; and changing and dating the IV setup and site dressings every 24 hours to reduce the possibility of sepsis. In addition, especially with the administration of irritating drugs, use veins with ample blood volume, use a cannula smaller than the vein to provide for greater hemodilution, administer irritating drugs slowly, rotate venipuncture sites every 48 to 72 hours, and avoid injecting IV infusions into leg veins or small veins.

The infusion should be discontinued and restarted at another site if infiltration, thrombus, thrombophlebitis, or necrosis occur. If the IV has infiltrated, elevate the arm and apply heat to promote absorption of the infiltrated solution. Infiltration is especially serious when infusions of vasopressors (e.g., norepinephrine, dopamine) or vesicants (e.g., many antineoplastic agents) are involved; this is usually known as extravasation. If extravasation occurs, the infusion should be stopped *immediately* and the known antidote injected immediately and subcutaneously in small amounts at many sites in the edematous area. Dress the wound, elevate the extremity, and apply heat or cold (depending on the infiltrated agent) for the client's comfort. See Chapter 57 for specific antineoplastic agents and their antidotes.

If a thrombus has occurred, the infusion should be restarted at a new site with a new needle or catheter. It is unwise and unsafe to attempt to unplug the needle by forcing a bolus of solution in a syringe through the needle into the vein. Theoretically, the thrombus may become an embolus and lodge in a vital organ, causing more serious complications (e.g., pulmonary embolus). Although most hospital policies discourage irrigating, this practice is widespread; no confirmed pulmonary embolism has been reported; this would seem to support the justification for irrigating (Wong, 1999). Elevate the affected extremity and apply heat to enhance resorption of the thrombus.

When thrombophlebitis occurs, the infusion should be stopped, the needle withdrawn, and the condition reported and recorded immediately. Treatment usually consists of applying moist heat to the affected area and resting the body part; anticoagulant therapy may also be ordered.

If pain occurs at the venipuncture site in the absence of other symptoms, adjust the needle and relieve the tension by readjusting the needle support or relaxing the pull on the tubing, and administer irritating drugs at a slow rate. These actions may alleviate the pain and discomfort.

Pulmonary edema is considered to be a medical emergency; the prescriber needs to be notified as soon as the client's fluid volume excess is noted. The IV infusion is slowed to a "keep open" (KVO, keep vein open) rate to provide access for emergency medications. Oxygen can be started to improve gas exchange. Vital signs are monitored every 15 to 30 minutes; arterial blood gases and intake and output are also monitored. The following may be ordered: bronchodilators to decrease bronchospasm; diuretics to mobilize extravascular fluid; digitalis or pressor agents to increase cardiac contractility; nitroprusside to decrease peripheral vascular resistance, preload, and afterload; and morphine to reduce anxiety and dyspnea. Provide support for the client, who will be fearful due to decreased respiratory capacity.

If a pyrogenic reaction is suspected, the infusion should be stopped *at once.* The solution should not be discarded but instead sent to the pharmacist. Pyrogenic reactions are treated symptomatically but must be reported and recorded. The stock number should be noted, because an entire batch of solutions may be contaminated.

When difficulties are encountered, consult agency infusion specialists, such as members of the IV therapy team, when available.

▪ ***Education.*** Clients or family members should be informed to notify the nurse if pain or swelling occurs at the infusion site or if any symptoms of the previously mentioned complications occur. Instruct the ambulatory client to ambulate with the involved arm held lightly at the waist and with the unaffected arm guiding the IV pole. Advise the client to avoid actions that elevate the arm with the venipuncture, such as using that arm to comb the hair or to shave.

▪ **Evaluation.** The expected outcome of IV therapy is that the client will receive fluid and electrolyte therapy as ordered, with serum electrolyte determinations returning to or remaining within the normal limits; the client will not experience any adverse reactions to IV therapy.

SUMMARY

The administration of IV fluids and electrolytes has become commonplace in the experience of hospitalized clients. IV fluids are administered for a variety of reasons: to replace fluids and electrolytes, to correct acid-base imbalance, to administer medications, to maintain access to the venous system, to measure changes in venous pressure, to measure renal function, and to administer essential nutrients. With the increased prevalence of intravascular therapy, the role of nursing management in IV therapy has also grown and developed.

Critical Thinking Questions

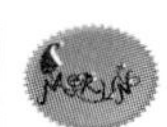

1. How do water, potassium, sodium, calcium, and magnesium contribute to survival?
2. How would you minimize the risk of the various complications of IV therapy?

Collaborative Learning Activities

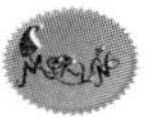

For Collaborative Learning Activities, go to mosby.com/MERLIN/McKenry/.

BIBLIOGRAPHY

Agus, Z.S. (1999). Hypomagnesemia. *Journal of the American Society of Nephrology, 10*(7), 1616-1622.

American Hospital Formulary Service. (1999). *AHFS drug information '99.* Bethesda, MD: American Society of Hospital Pharmacists.

Anderson, K.N., Anderson, L.E., & Glanze, W.D. (Eds.) (1998). *Mosby's medical, nursing, & allied health dictionary* (5th ed.). St. Louis: Mosby.

Andrews, M.R. & Levine, A.M. (1989). Dehydration in the terminal patient: Perception of hospice nurses. *American Journal of Hospice Care 6*(1), 31-34.

Barnett, M.L. (1999). Hypercalcemia. *Seminars in Oncology Nursing, 15*(3), 190-201.

Brown, D.L. & Robbins, R. (1999). Developments in the therapeutic applications of bisphosphonates. *Journal of Clinical Pharmacology, 39*(7), 651-660.

Brown, R.G. (1993). Disorders of water and sodium balance. *Postgraduate Medicine, 93*(4), 227-246.

Brown, R.O. (1993). Hypomagnesemia in critically ill patients: Issues in pharmacotherapy. *The American College of Chest Physicians Report, 13*(3), 6.

Cohen, M.R. & Davis, N.M. (1993). Recognizing the dangers of free flow from an EID. *Nursing, 23*(6), 56-59.

Drug Facts and Comparisons. (2000). St. Louis: Facts and Comparisons.

Johnson, J.A., Parker, R.B., & Geraci, S.A. (1999). Heart failure. In J.T. DiPiro, R.L. Talbert, G.C., Yee, G.R. Matzke, B.G. Wells, & L.M. Posey, (Eds.), *Pharmacotherapy: A pathophysiological approach* (4th ed.). Norwalk, CT: Appleton & Lange.

Keenan, A.M. (1999). Syndrome of inappropriate secretion of antidiuretic hormone in malignancy. *Seminars in Oncology Nursing, 15*(3), 160-167.

Latzka, W.A. & Montain, S.J. (1999). Water and electrolyte requirements for exercise. *Clinical Sports Medicine, 18*(3), 513-524.

Martinez, M.E., Giovannucci, E.L., Colditz, G.A., Stampfer, M.J., Hunter, D.J., Speizer, F.E., Wing, A., & Willett, W.C. (1996). Calcium, vitamin D, and the occurrence of colorectal cancer among women. *Journal of the National Cancer Institute, 88,* 1375-1382.

McConnell, E. (1986) Preventing air embolism in patients with central venous catheters. *Nursing Life 6*(2), 47-49.

Mendyka, B.E. (1992). Fluid and electrolyte disorders caused by diuretic therapy. *AACN Clinical Issues: Advanced Practice in Acute and Critical Care, 3*(3), 672-680.

Metheny, N.M. (1996). *Fluid and electrolyte balance: Nursing considerations.* (3rd ed.). Philadelphia: Williams & Wilkins.

Mundy, G.R. & Guise, T.A. (1999). Hormonal control of calcium homeostasis. *Clinical Chemistry, 45*(8 pt 2), 1347-1352.

Phillips, L.D. (1997) *Manual of IV therapeutics* (2nd ed.). Philadelphia: F.A. Davis.

Powers, F.A. (1999). Your elderly patient needs i.v. therapy . . . can you keep her safe? *Nursing, 29*(7), 54-55.

Rousseau, P.C. (1992). Why give IV fluids to the dying? *Patient Care, 26*(10):71-74.

Tang, I. & Lau, A.H. (1995) Fluid and electrolyte disorders. In L.Y. Young & M.A. Koda-Kimble (Eds.), *Applied therapeutics: The clinical use of drugs* (6th ed.). Vancouver, WA: Applied Therapeutics.

Thielen, J. (1990). Air emboli: A potentially lethal complication of central venous lines. *Focus on Critical Care, 17*(5), 374.

Understanding imbalances caused by GI fluid loss. *Nursing, 29*(8), 72.

United States Pharmacopeia Dispensing Information (USP DI): Drug information for the health care professional (19th ed.). (1999). Rockville, MD: United States Pharmacopeial Convention.

Wong, D.L., Hockenberry-Eaton, M., Wilson, D., Winkelstein, M.L., Ahmann, E., DiVito-Thomas, P.A. (1999). *Whaley & Wong's nursing care of infants and children* (6th ed.). St. Louis: Mosby.

Wood, L.S. & Gullo, S.M. (1993). IV vesicants: How to avoid extravasation. *American Journal of Nursing, 93*(4), 42-46.

70 Enteral and Parenteral Nutrition

Chapter Focus

Enteral and parenteral feedings are commonly used to provide nutritional support to clients who, for some reason, cannot consume adequate nutrients through the normal processes of ingestion. The nursing focus for the nursing diagnosis "impaired nutrition" is on assisting the client or family to improve nutritional intake; this diagnosis should not be used to describe clients who are prescribed nothing by mouth (NPO) or cannot ingest food (Carpenito, 1999). Because enteral and parenteral nutrition is used most commonly for clients who are NPO or cannot ingest food, this chapter considers the potential complications of electrolyte imbalances and negative nitrogen balance.

Learning Objectives

1. Describe the techniques commonly used to deliver enteral feedings.
2. Distinguish among elemental, polymeric, modular, and altered amino acid formulations for enteral feedings.
3. Identify major drug-food interactions to be aware of when administering enteral nutrient formulations.
4. Implement the nursing management for the care of clients receiving enteral formulations.
5. Discuss parenteral protein-sparing nutrition, peripheral-vein parenteral nutrition, and central hyperalimentation and the indications for their use.
6. Describe the components of total parenteral nutrition solutions and the function of each element in the attainment of body requirements.
7. Cite the possible complications of parenteral nutrition therapy.
8. Implement the nursing management for the care of clients receiving parenteral nutritional therapy.

Key Terms

amino acid, p. 1192
enteral nutrition, p. 1186
essential amino acids, p. 1192
hyperalimentation, p. 1191
negative nitrogen balance, p. 1189
nonessential amino acids, p. 1192
protein-sparing nutrition, p. 1193
semiessential amino acids, p. 1192
total parenteral nutrition (TPN), p. 1191

To achieve and maintain good health requires a regular intake of sufficient amounts of protein (amino acids), carbohydrates, fats, vitamins, and minerals. Under normal conditions adequate nutrition can be achieved by the ingestion of a balanced diet, but there are situations in which the nutritional needs of the body are not met. Such conditions include malnutrition, severe inflammatory bowel disease and other gastrointestinal diseases, coma, postsurgical complications, major burns, and others. Nutritional support is necessary for such persons.

Over the past 30 to 40 years many advances have been recorded in the fields of both enteral and parenteral nutrition. Clinical nutrition is now a recognized and active entity for improving health care in all settings, including the client's home, long-term care facilities, and hospitals. Today nutritional programs or specific products have been developed for clients with specific disease states or illnesses. In this chapter, enteral and parenteral nutrition are reviewed along with selected disease states and criteria for the use of specific nutritional products.

ENTERAL NUTRITION

Malnutrition among hospitalized persons and nursing home residents is associated with complications such as muscle atrophy, slow wound healing, impaired immunocompetence, infection, and death. Other complications include peripheral edema caused by reduced plasma proteins and its resultant decreased oncotic pressure, dry and flaky skin, and hair loss.

Malnutrition is also reflected in reduced total lymphocyte count, serum albumin, and transferrin levels (or iron-binding capacity). An increase in the concentration of 24-hour urine urea nitrogen reflects the protein catabolism that occurs with malnutrition.

Stress in relation to hospitalization may alter a client's usual eating habits. Unfamiliar foods and the general malaise resulting from illness also may cause clients to lose their appetites. An inadequate oral intake may result from oropharyngeal surgery, trauma, neoplasm, paralysis, or esophageal fistula. Fasting before surgery or for a diagnostic workup may also be nutritionally depleting. Energy needs may be doubled when sepsis, trauma, major surgery, inflammation, infection, or severe burns supervene. Enteral or tube feedings may effectively supply essential nutrition if the gastrointestinal tract is functional.

Enteral nutrition is the oral or tube feeding of a client, usually via a nasogastric, nasoduodenal, nasojejunal, gastrostomy, or jejunostomy tube (Figure 70-1). The cost per person for tube feedings is approximately equal to a regular hospital diet and provides more complete control and assessment of intake. Tube feedings may also be used to supplement inadequate oral intake and parenteral nutrition as it is being tapered.

Enteral feedings may be administered by bolus doses, typically 250 to 400 mL of formula every 4 to 6 hours; by intermittent feedings using a 20- to 30-minute drip; or by continuous gravity or enteral pumps. The continuous method over 16 to 24 hours has had more success because it helps to prevent complications such as dumping syndrome and avoids the need for frequent tube irrigations. Dumping syndrome is the result of a sudden influx of feeding and the creation of a high osmotic gradient within the small intestine; this causes a sudden shift of fluid from the vascular compartment to the intestinal lumen. Plasma volume decreases, causing vasomotor responses such as increased pulse rate, hypotension, weakness, pallor, sweating, and dizziness. Rapid distention of the intestine produces a feeling of fullness, cramping, nausea, vomiting, and diarrhea.

Enteral feedings can be administered by the following routes: nasogastric, nasoduodenal, esophagostomy, gastrostomy, and jejunostomy. The last three are more invasive and require surgically created stomas; therefore they are less preferred routes for short-term enteral feeding. Nasogastric, esophagostomy, and gastrostomy feedings allow for more natural digestion in the stomach. Aspiration is a risk with nasogastric tubes because incomplete closure of the esophageal sphincter may result in gastric reflux.

Administering feedings directly into the small intestine reduces the risk of aspiration, but gastrointestinal distress and diarrhea may develop because of the sudden influx. Skin excoriation and infection are potential risks with gastrostomies and jejunostomies, because the surgical opening penetrates the peritoneum. These complications are avoided in the cervical esophagostomy, which is a surgically created, skin-lined canal that is tunneled from the lower neck border and extends to below the cervical esophagus.

The selection of a tube feeding formula depends on the client's nutritional needs, concomitant disease states, lactose intolerance, and gastrointestinal competence, as well as on convenience, feasibility, and cost. Nutritional assessment may be based on anthropometric parameters, biochemical data, and physical findings, as well as on medical, diet, drug, and socioeconomic histories. Ideal body weight (IBW) can be obtained from tables or by estimation as shown below. IBW can be used instead of actual weight for determining nutritional requirements, because adipose tissue requires less energy for maintenance; if actual weight is used in the calculations, a client who is obese would receive excessive calories:

- *Men:* 106 pounds (48 kg) for the first 5 feet (150 cm) plus 6 pounds (2.7 kg) per inch (2.5 cm) over 5 feet (plus or minus 10%)
- *Women:* 100 pounds (45 kg) for the first 5 feet plus 5 pounds (2.2 kg) per inch over 5 feet (plus or minus 10%)

Enteral Formulations

Numerous different enteral formulations are available, and they can be broadly divided into oligomeric, polymeric, modular, and specialized formulations (Rollins, 1996).

1. *Oligomeric formulations* are chemically defined formulations that require minimum digestion and produce minimal residue in the colon. The two oligomeric sub-

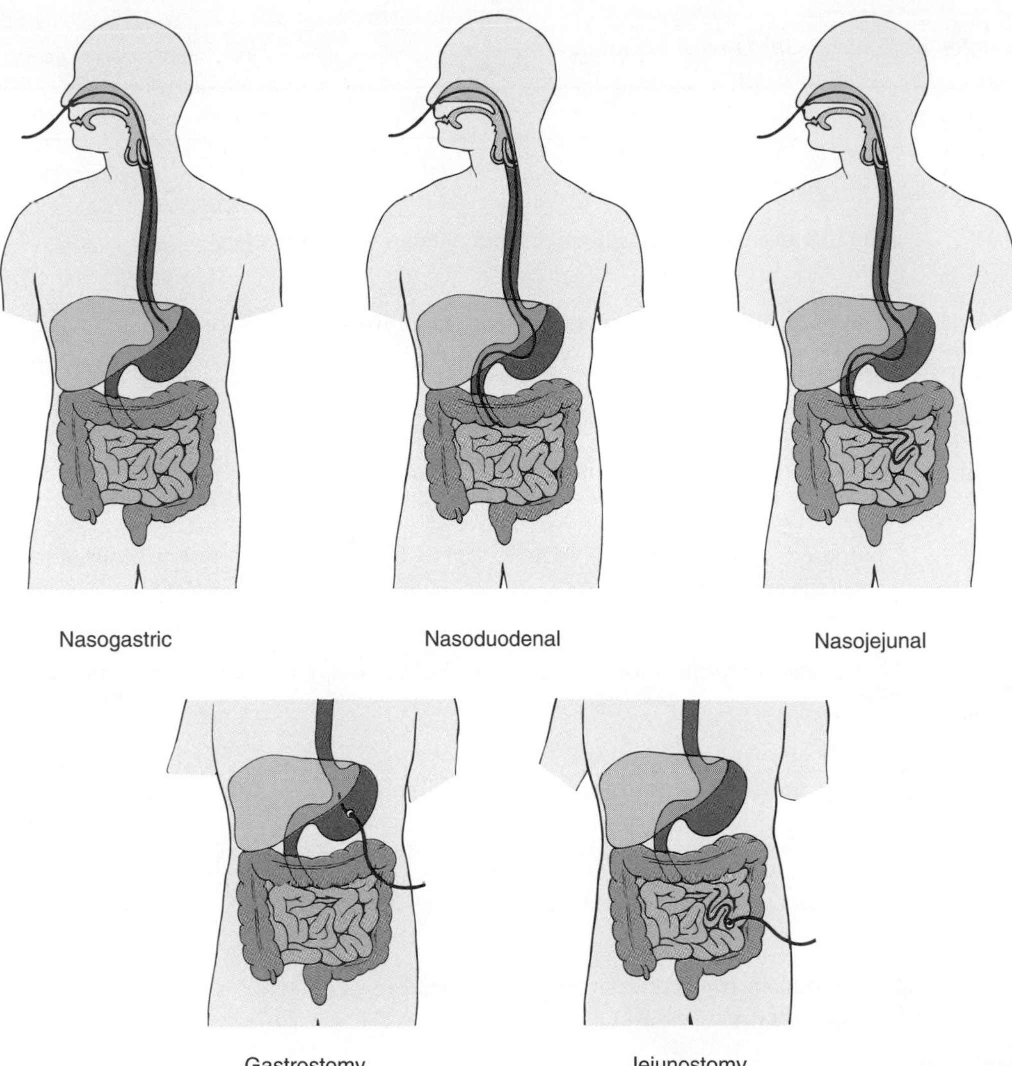

Figure 70-1 Tube feeding routes. (Modified from Beare, P.G. & Myers, J.L. [1998]. *Adult health nursing* [3rd ed.]. St. Louis: Mosby.)

groups include true elemental formulations that contain free amino acids and peptide-based formulations that contain dipeptides and tripeptides and/or crystalline amino acids. These formulations are indicated for clients with partial bowel obstruction, inflammatory bowel disease, radiation enteritis, bowel fistulas, and short bowel syndrome.

2. *Polymeric formulations* are the most commonly prescribed complete formula, enteral preparations. Such formulations contain complex nutrients: protein (e.g., casein and soy protein), carbohydrates (e.g., corn syrup solid, maltodextrins), and fat (vegetable oil or milk fat) and are preferred for clients who have a fully functional gastrointestinal tract and few or no specialized nutrient requirements. They should not be used in clients with a malabsorption problem. These formulations are preferred because the hyperosmolarity of the oligomeric preparations causes more gastrointestinal problems than the polymeric formulations.
3. *Modular formulations* are single-nutrient formulas (i.e., protein, carbohydrate, or fat). Such a formula can be added to a monomeric or polymeric formulation to provide a more individualized and specialized nutrient formulation.
4. *Specialized formulations* are indicated for clients with specific disease states such as genetic errors of metabolism (e.g., phenylketonuria, homocystinuria, maple syrup urine disease) or acquired disorders of nitrogen accumulation (e.g., cirrhosis or chronic renal failure), as well as for clients who are catabolic because of injuries or infection (Table 70-1).

Drug-Food Interactions

A number of drug–enteral nutrient interactions have been identified, and these interactions can be clinically significant. However, this possibility is often overlooked when enteral nutrient formulations are being administered. The ma-

TABLE 70-1 Examples of Commercial Enteral Formulations

Formulations	Comments
Oligomeric	
Elemental	
Vivonex T.E.N.	Contains free amino acids, linoleic acid, vitamins, and minerals
Peptide-Based	
Peptamen Liquid	Composed of hydrolyzed whey proteins, carbohydrates, fat, vitamins, and minerals
Polymeric	
Nutrient Source	
Blenderized Compleat Regular	Has beef, fruits, vegetables, nonfat milk, vitamins, and minerals; tube feeding preparation
Milk-Based	
Sustacal powder	Composed of nonfat and whole milk, sugars, butter, vitamins, and minerals; contains high protein content and lactose
Lactose-Free	
Ensure-Plus	Higher caloric formulation of protein, carbohydrates, fat, vitamins, and minerals; lactose-free
Modular Components	
Carbohydrates	
Polycose	Glucose polymers derived from cornstarch; high source of calories from carbohydrates
Proteins	
Amin-Aid	Contains essential amino acids, carbohydrates, and fat; has high caloric formula and is indicated for acute or chronic renal failure
Fats	
MCT Oil	Medium-chain triglycerides (MCTs) that need less bile acid for digestion; does not provide any essential fatty acids
Specialized Formulations	
Renal Failure	
Amin-Aid	See above
Hepatic Failure	
Hepatic-Aid II	Contains amino acids (approximately 50% protein as branched-chain amino acids [BCAAs]), carbohydrates, and fat; hepatic encephalopathy reportedly improved by increased serum levels of BCAAs (Rollins, 1996); used for chronic liver disease
Pulmonary Disease	
Pulmocare	Composed of calcium and sodium caseinate, amino acids, carbohydrates, fats, vitamins, minerals; has high caloric content; the fat in this preparation is primarily from canola oil and corn oil (60%) plus 40% from MCT; persons with respiratory disease that received high fat, low carbohydrate diets demonstrated improvement in respiratory monitoring parameters (Rollins, 1996)

jor drug interactions with enteral or tube feedings are listed in Table 70-2.

■ Nursing Management
Enteral Nutrition Therapy

■ **Assessment.** A baseline assessment of the client should include body weight, weight loss history, and any clinical manifestations of undernutrition. The nutritional history should include (along with the cause if possible) inadequate nutrient intake, excessive nutrient losses or a failure to absorb nutrients, increased metabolic requirements, or medications that might have a catabolic effect, such as corticosteroids or antineoplastic agents. Baseline laboratory determinations, such as serum albumin, serum electrolytes, serum transferrin, serum prealbumin, urine creatinine clearance, and total lymphocyte count are indicators of protein nourishment. Hemoglobin, hematocrit, mean corpuscular

TABLE 70-2 Drug Interactions with Enteral and Tube Feedings*

Drug	Comments
carbamazepine (Tegretol)	Bioavailability of carbamazepine suspension is affected if given through a polyvinyl nasogastric feeding tube. Serum levels also decreased when administered during enteral feedings. Recommended that suspension be diluted and given as described in phenytoin below.
phenytoin (Dilantin)	Lower serum phenytoin levels are reported. Recommended approach is to stop enteral feeding for 2 hours before and after phenytoin administration; flushing tubing with 2 ounces of water before giving phenytoin suspension is recommended.
warfarin (Coumadin)	Warfarin resistance is reported when drug is administered with an enteral preparation. Interaction may be due to vitamin K in the feeding or due to warfarin binding to protein ingredients in the formulation.

*Closely monitor clients receiving the above and any other drugs in combination with enteral formulations. Laboratory tests such as serum drug levels or prothrombin time, when appropriate, may be ordered (Estoup, 1994). (For additional information, see Miyagawa, 1993.)

volume (MCV), mean corpuscular hemoglobin (MCH), mean corpuscular hemoglobin concentration (MCHC), and the various blood levels of specific vitamins and minerals are indicators of vitamin and mineral nourishment.

In general, enteral feedings are contraindicated for clients who are capable of oral intake or who have adynamic ileus, intestinal obstruction, intractable vomiting, or esophageal fistulas.

▪ **Nursing Diagnosis.** See the Nursing Care Plan on p. 1190 for nursing diagnoses related to a client with enteral tube feedings. In addition, the potential complications of **negative nitrogen balance** (a condition in which more nitrogen is excreted than is taken in, indicating the wasting of tissue) and electrolyte imbalances exist.

▪ **Implementation**

▪ ***Monitoring.*** Monitor the client's nutritional status using the indicators mentioned in the baseline assessment. Assess the client for respiratory distress, frothy sputum, abnormal lung sounds, or new pulmonary infiltrates on x-ray examination. Tinting the formula with blue food coloring assists in the assessment for aspiration.

When tube feedings are prescribed, monitor the temperature, volume, and flow rate of the feeding.

Assess periodically for residual gastric volume and tube placement, particularly before each feeding or before administering a dose of a medication into the feeding tube. Monitor continuous feedings every 4 to 8 hours; simply stop the feeding and measure the residual by aspirating the stomach contents with a syringe. This aspirate is readministered to the client. It is not necessary to clamp off the tube and wait for an interval of time, because these feedings should move through the system continuously. If the residual is more than 10% to 20% above the volume of 1 hour of continuous feeding, delay the feeding and reassess in 1 hour. If this occurs twice, consult with the prescriber. For intermittent administration, measure the residual volume halfway between feedings. If the residual is greater than 50% of the previous feeding, return the aspirate, hold the feeding, and notify the physician. In both of these instances, a reduction in the volume of the feeding may be necessary.

Monitor bowel sounds to ensure that the client has good bowel function. Bowel elimination patterns and fluid intake and output should be carefully documented.

Many types of enteral formulas are lactose-free (nonmilk proteins are the base) for clients who lack sufficient lactase in intestinal microvilli for lactose absorption. Blacks, Asians, American Indians, and Jews are particularly prone to lactase deficiency. Lactose ingestion causes varying degrees of diarrhea, abdominal cramps, bloating, and flatulence. Isotonic formulas may be useful in preventing dumping syndrome. Commercially prepared enteral formulas have been developed and are designed for specific disease states (Varella & Young, 1999).

▪ ***Intervention.*** Although the gastrointestinal tract is the optimal route for nutrient administration, in many ill clients the normal ingestion of food is difficult, if not nearly impossible, to achieve. Enteral nutrient preparations were designed for such clients. These formulations may be administered by the nasoenteral route through thin, flexible tubing that is generally well tolerated by clients. These feeding tubes are now made from silicone or polyurethane compounds and have much smaller lumen sizes (5 to 10 French). These tubes are much preferred to the older, thicker rubber or polyvinyl chloride types (Salem pump, Levin tube) that stiffen in contact with digestive juices. However, aspirating for residual gastrointestinal contents and irrigating may be more difficult with these small-lumen tubes than with the older, larger tubes.

Small-diameter feeding tubes also get clogged more easily. To prevent the buildup of formula residue, flush the tubes every 4 hours (and each time feeding is interrupted) with 20 mL of cranberry juice followed by 10 mL of water. The acidity of the juice breaks up the formula residue, and the water prevents sugar from crystallizing.

Transnasal tube placement in the intestine requires the use of longer, mercury- or tungsten-weighted feeding tubes

Nursing Care Plan

Selected Potential Nursing Diagnoses for the Client with Enteral Tube Feedings

Nursing Diagnosis	Outcome Criteria	Interventions
Diarrhea	The client will have soft, formed stools fewer than 3 times daily.	Record the frequency and consistency of stools. If not contraindicated, decrease the hypertonicity of the feedings by diluting. Check the client's medication regimen for diarrhea-causing drugs. Assess the hygiene used in the administration of the feedings. Perform a digital examination to ensure that the client does not have a fecal impaction. Administer antidiarrheals as prescribed.
Risk for aspiration	The client will not experience aspiration.	Assess the client for respiratory distress, frothy sputum, abnormal lung sounds, and new infiltrates on x-ray examination. Tinting formula with blue food coloring assists assessment. Elevate the head of bed at least 30 degrees during and for 1 hour after feeding. Verify placement of the nasogastric or nasojejunal feeding tube with air auscultation. Aspirate for residual contents every 4 to 8 hours or before each residual feeding. Hold the feeding and notify the prescriber if residuals are greater than the amount of 2 hours of continuous feeding or 50% of the volume of the previous intermittent feeding.
Deficient fluid volume	Fluid balance will be maintained. Hematocrit, BUN, and urine specific gravity will be within normal limits.	Assess the client for poor skin turgor, dry mucous membranes, and thirst. Monitor fluid intake and output. Monitor laboratory values for increases in BUN, hematocrit, and urine specific gravity. Provide increased amounts of water through feeding tube.

that gradually advance by peristalsis. This process takes approximately 24 hours, and radiographic confirmation of tube placement must be made.

Surgical placement of a gastrostomy (G) tube or a jejunostomy (J) tube can be instituted if tube feedings must be administered for long periods of time. This helps to reduce the need for frequent flushing and replacement of the nasoenteral tube, and it is more comfortable for the client. A more common procedure in use today is the placement of a G tube percutaneously using endoscopic guidance; this is known as percutaneous endoscopic gastrostomy (PEG).

Initially, the infusion of enteral formulas is begun at half-strength concentrations at a rate of 50 mL/hr. The rate and strength of these infusions can be titrated according to the client's tolerance to the formulation. For example, the rate may be increased by 25 mL/hr and the concentration increased to three-quarters strength, which eventually is increased to the full-strength formulation. The desired calories and total volume ordered will then be administered, assuming the client can tolerate the full-strength preparation. To avoid inducing vomiting or diarrhea, increases in rate and fluid concentration should not be made simultaneously.

The more rapid the feeding, the more likely complications such as hyperglycemia or dumping syndrome may occur. However, nursing efforts should be maintained to encourage intake; milk-based formulas, for example, contain 1 kcal/mL, and the client must take 1000 to 2000 mL of formula to achieve their caloric needs and to obtain the Recommended Dietary Allowance (RDA) or Reference Nutrient Intake (RNI) for vitamins and minerals. Elevate the head of the bed at least 30 degrees during and for 1 hour after the feeding. Warm the feeding to room temperature before administering.

The enteral preparation may be given continuously or by cyclic administration. Cyclic feedings are similar to a person's normal feeding cycle and are the preferred method in some settings. Additional water may be added to the enteral formulations if the client cannot or does not drink additional water while receiving the formulations. In general, enteral formulations that have 1 kcal/mL usually contain approximately 80% water, whereas the formulations

TABLE 70-3 Most Common Secondary Effects of Tube Feedings

Condition	Cause	Preventive Action
Aspiration	Impaired gag reflex	Position head of bed at 30-60 degrees for feedings and for 1 hour after.
	Uncuffed tracheostomy tube	Stop; suction trachea; inflate cuff before feedings.
	Decreased gastric motility	Check for residual of feedings and tube placement.
	Misplaced tube	Check taping and placement of tube. Advance tube through pyloric sphincter. Add blue food coloring to tube feeding to monitor for aspiration.
Obstructed tube	Plugged tube end-ports	Flush tubing before and after feedings or instillation of medications. Shake or mix formula well.
Hyperglycemia, dumping syndrome: nausea, vomiting, diaphoresis, cramping	Osmotic intolerance to hyperosmolar load of feeding, rapid rate, or high concentration; ice-cold feeding	Change volume or rate of delivery, and dilute feeding temporarily. Allow feedings to warm slightly.

with more concentrated kcal/mL contain less than 70% water.

If the client still develops diarrhea after the nurse has slowed the rate of administration, lowered the concentration by diluting the formula, and had the solutions at room temperature, then the prescriber needs to be consulted regarding the osmolality of the formula. Antidiarrheal preparations may also be helpful in controlling diarrhea.

In the case of accidental aspiration after a tube feeding into the stomach, the tube may be advanced through the pyloric sphincter to prevent future regurgitation. However, the resultant hyperosmolality in the small intestine potentiates hyperglycemia or the dumping syndrome. Physiologic osmolality is approximately 280 mOsm/L, but some preparations are greater than 400 mOsm/L.

State-of-the-art enteral feedings are in rapid evolution. One source for current information is Ross Laboratories, Columbus, OH, 43215-1724.

■ ***Education.*** The self-administration of tube feedings is now possible with the advent of smaller tubes and infusion instrumentation that incorporates improved human engineering features. The necessary preparation of the client and another family member should begin as soon as possible after admission. Individualized instruction with return demonstrations of learning take approximately 3 to 6 hours, perhaps more if insertion and removal of the tube is learned. Coughing, choking, difficulty speaking, or cyanosis signifies incorrect tube placement. The concept of correct tube placement cannot be overemphasized. Written and verbal instructions related to possible secondary effects are also necessary (Table 70-3). Resuming daily activities at home is more inconvenient for the tube-fed ostomy client who must loosen clothing or undress for each feeding.

Clients receiving tube feedings are deprived of the usual personal and social gratifications of the eating act. They may feel "different" and alienated from others. To some, it may be symbolic of a rapidly deteriorating state of health and a last resort for survival. They especially need to understand the procedure, its rationale, and what to expect from it. Once given the opportunity to discuss its meaning, many can go on to participate actively in their own feedings and express greater satisfaction.

■ **Evaluation.** The expected outcome of enteral nutrition therapy is that the client will experience adequate nutrition as evidenced by blood urea nitrogen (BUN), serum protein, hemoglobin, and hematocrit levels that are within normal limits. The client will maintain or progress to a weight-for-height ratio normal for age and will not experience diarrhea, aspiration, or fluid volume deficit.

PARENTERAL NUTRITION

Parenteral nutrition is the treatment of choice for selected clients who are unable to tolerate and maintain adequate enteral intake. Often called **hyperalimentation** or **total parenteral nutrition** (TPN), it is the IV approach to complete nutrition. TPN is the administration of a nutritionally adequate hypertonic solution that consists of glucose, protein hydrolysates, minerals, and vitamins. Fat is also provided in a three-in-one solution or "piggy-backed." TPN can supply all of the calories, dextrose, amino acids, fats, trace elements, and other essential nutrients needed for growth, weight gain, wound healing, convalescence, immunocompetence, and other health-sustaining functions. It provides these components in the ratio of a regular diet, and it promotes anabolism by supplying all necessary nutrients in excess of those needed for energy expenditure. TPN may be infused through a central vein, a peripheral vein, or both simultaneously.

Although the related nomenclature has not yet been standardized, partial parenteral nutrition has come to denote parenteral nutrition therapy with IV solutions that are lacking some essential elements, notably fats. Although insulin and heparin (and several other medications) have been added to parenteral nutrition preparations for specific clients, the addition of medications to TPN solutions should generally be avoided because of the potential incompatibilities of the medication with the nutrients in the solution (Holcombe, 1996). The following are the major parenteral systems for nutritional support:

1. Peripheral vein total parenteral nutrition
2. Central-line venous hyperalimentation

Peripheral Vein Total Parenteral Nutrition

Peripheral vein total parenteral nutrition (PTPN) is prescribed for clients who need nutritional support and for whom insertion of a central venous line for total parenteral nutrition may not be possible or necessary. The client may be nutritionally healthy or have slight to moderate nutritional deficits without being in a hypermetabolic state. The client's current health status indicates that a nutritional deficit will probably occur if nutritional therapy is not instituted.

PTPN is considered a temporary measure to provide an appropriate nitrogen balance in clients who have mild deficits or are NPO with a slightly elevated metabolic rate. It may be prescribed to precede a procedure that imposes restrictions on oral feedings; for gastrointestinal illnesses that prevent oral food ingestion; for anorexia caused by radiation or chemotherapy in cancer treatment programs; or following surgery if the client's nutritional deficits are minimal but oral food consumption will not be instituted for 5 or more days. It is not indicated for nutritionally depleted clients in a hypermetabolic state. If used for such clients, it should be a temporary measure until central vein hyperalimentation can be initiated.

PTPN solution is composed of 3% to 5% isotonic amino acids mixed with a carbohydrate solution (usually dextrose 5% to 7%), vitamins, minerals, and electrolytes for administration through a peripheral vein. The solution will provide between 500 and 700 calories/day. The major advancement in this therapy is the use of a lipid as a nonprotein source of calories. When administered peripherally, dextrose must be limited to a 10% solution to avoid sclerosing of the veins. For the same reason, some institutions also limit the concentration of electrolytes to be infused.

Peripherally administered lipid preparations or IV fat emulsions (Liposyn, Intralipid, and others) are a source of additional calories for the client.

Central Hyperalimentation

In central hyperalimentation, a catheter is placed in a central vein, most commonly the subclavian vein, in order to administer solutions that contain hypertonic glucose and amino acids. Because of its blood flow, the central vein can accept the high-osmolar concentrated solutions. Central hyperalimentation or TPN is usually composed of the three major nutrients—dextrose, crystalline amino acids, and lipid emulsions—plus vitamins, minerals, trace elements, electrolytes, and water. The solutions may vary according to the client's requirements and, in general, according to the supplier of the basic amino acid solution. Special preparations of amino acids are also available for the client with a specific disease state.

Central hyperalimentation is used primarily for clients with nonfunctioning gastrointestinal tracts, those that should not use the oral route for more than 5 to 7 days, or for clients who either have a limited peripheral access or whose needs cannot be met by peripheral formulations (Holcombe, 1996). For example, clients with conditions of short bowel syndrome, acute pancreatitis, enteric or enterocutaneous fistulas, active inflammatory process, gastrointestinal tract obstruction, major trauma, or burns—with whom enteral feedings are not possible—may need central hyperalimentation for survival.

Solution Formulations

The basic total parenteral solution contains amino acids, carbohydrates (dextrose), lipids, and micronutrients (e.g., trace elements, vitamins).

See Box 70-1 for information on a potentially life-threatening drug interaction associated with TPN.

Amino Acids

Amino acids are necessary to promote the production of proteins (anabolism), to reduce protein breakdown (catabolism), and to help promote wound healing. Protein is composed of essential and nonessential amino acids. The body cannot synthesize **essential amino acids**, but **nonessential amino acids** can be synthesized from a nitrogen source (amino acids, ammonium salts, urea). A negative nitrogen balance is a situation in which more nitrogen is excreted than taken in, which leads to a wasting of body tissue.

All natural amino acids are needed for growth and development and must be present concurrently in the proper amounts for protein synthesis to occur. Adults can synthesize all but eight of these amino acids; these eight are considered essential in adults. To the extent that the oral intake of amino acids is limited, protein synthesis depends on an exogenous source. The **semiessential amino acids** (histidine, arginine) are not synthesized in adequate amounts during growth periods; thus 10 amino acids are considered essential in infants.

At a minimum, a healthy adult usually requires approximately 0.9 g protein/kg, whereas an infant or child needs

BOX 70-1

Potentially Life-Threatening Drug Interaction in Total Parenteral Nutrition

The amount of calcium and phosphorus (or phosphates) in a TPN admixture must be closely monitored, because life-threatening events and deaths have been reported from the precipitation of calcium phosphate. The Food and Drug Administration (FDA) issued warnings concerning this drug interaction, and they include the following:

- Use an in-line filter whenever infusing TPN solutions centrally or peripherally.
- Start TPN admixtures within 24 hours after mixing, or keep them at room temperature. If refrigerated, start within 24 hours of rewarming.
- *Stop the infusion immediately* if acute respiratory distress symptoms occur.

Special compounding instructions were issued to pharmacists regarding this safety alert.

Information from Mirtallo, J.M. (1994). The complexity of mixing calcium and phosphate. *American Journal of Hospital Pharmacy, 51*(6), 1535-1536; and Food and Drug Administration. (1994). Safety alert: Hazards of precipitation associated with parenteral nutrition. *American Journal of Hospital Pharmacy, 51*(6), 1427-1428.

between 1.4 and 2.2 g protein/kg. This requirement can increase substantially in undernourished or traumatized clients; for example, it can increase up to sixfold in a traumatized or seriously ill client, because his or her daily need is approximately 3 g/kg body weight. A nonprotein source of calories must be provided with the amino acids to offset their use as an energy source.

Amino acid solutions contain crystalline amino acid (Aminosyn and many others); solutions are also available with electrolytes. Amino acid crystalline solutions contain synthetic amino acids but not peptides. This is the preferred form of amino acid, because most clients are able to tolerate this formulation. Dextrose usually is administered with these solutions because of the protein-sparing action of carbohydrates. If the protein is administered without adequate calories in the form of carbohydrates, the protein will be used for the body's caloric needs rather than for the repair and regeneration of tissue.

Protein-sparing nutrition is usually reserved for clients who have minimal protein deficiencies and sufficient fat stores. A 3% to 5% isotonic amino acid is mixed with carbohydrate-free fluids, vitamins, minerals, and electrolytes that are administered by peripheral vein. The solution will provide approximately 400 to 600 calories/day. The client will meet many energy requirements by using the free fatty acids and ketones derived from their endogenous adipose tissue, thereby preserving their protein compartment in the body. This type is usually used for short-term periods for clients who are not nutritionally compromised and are not in a hypermetabolic state.

Carbohydrates

Carbohydrates and lipids are used as the primary source of calories for the client. One gram of D-glucose provides 3.4 calories, whereas fat supplies 9 cal/g and protein supplies 4 cal/g. Concentrations of dextrose solutions above 10% are hyperosmolar and are too irritating to be given continuously peripherally; thus they should be administered through central venous catheters. Centrally, the concentration of infused dextrose solutions is usually between 25% and 35%.

Hyperglycemia usually occurs when dextrose is administered without lipids as the primary source of calories. Because dextrose requires insulin for utilization, a combination of caloric sources, dextrose, and lipids will help to decrease the potential for hyperglycemia and the extra need for insulin in some clients. Dextrose alone also increases the rate of metabolism and production of carbon dioxide, which may increase the client's respiratory demands. Administering a combination caloric preparation of dextrose and lipids will reduce the increase in respiratory demands.

Although not as prevalent in usage, other sources of available calories include alcohol in dextrose solution and invert sugar and electrolytes solution (*Drug Facts and Comparisons*, 2000). The dextrose used in formulations is derived from corn sugar; invert sugar derived from cane or beet sugar is an alternative for the very small portion of the population who may be sensitive to corn derivatives. Alcohol is another substrate that provides 7 kcal/g, and it does not require insulin for peripheral utilization. However, providing enough calories would necessitate a quantity of alcohol that would produce a potential for intoxication and hepatotoxicity.

Because dextrose is inexpensive and readily available, it is almost always the preferred product for administration.

Fats

lipid emulsions (Intralipid; Liposyn)

Fat constitutes 40% to 50% of the total calories supplied in the average North American diet. The American Heart Association recommends the following: fat should constitute 30% or less of total calories in the diet; carbohydrates, 55% or more; and protein, approximately 15%. Fat emulsions are derived from either soybean or safflower oil, which provides a mixture of neutral triglycerides and unsaturated fatty acids. The two functions of IV fat emulsions in parenteral nutrition are to supply essential fatty acids and to be a source of energy or calories (9 cal/g).

Linoleic, linolenic, and arachidonic acids are essential in humans. Linoleic acid cannot be synthesized in the body, and it is the precursor to both linolenic and arachidonic acid. If linoleic acid is either unavailable or deficient, the enzyme system will act on oleic acid to synthesize eicosatrienoic acid, which is incapable of functioning like arachidonic

TABLE 70-4 Trace Elements

Elements	Dose*	Deficiency Symptoms
copper	0.5-1.5 mg	Decrease in red and white blood cells; hair and skeletal abnormalities; defective tissue growth
chromium	10-15 μg	Neuropathy, confusion, impaired glucose tolerance, ataxia
manganese	150-800 μg	Defective growth, nausea, vomiting, weight loss, skin rash, CNS alterations (ataxia, seizures)
selenium	40-80 μg	Muscle aches, pain or tenderness, cardiomyopathy, kwashiorkor
zinc	2.5-4 mg	Nausea, vomiting, diarrhea, weakness, anorexia, growth retardation, anemia, hypogeusia, rash, depression, eye lesions, defective wound healing, and hepatosplenomegaly

*Recommended daily adult dose.

acid. Essential fatty acid deficiency (EFAD) is noted with clinical signs of hair loss, scaly dermatitis, slowed growth, reduced wound healing, decreased platelets, and fatty liver. This necessitates the IV administration of a fat emulsion to correct the biochemical alteration.

The fat emulsions currently available are either safflower oil (Liposyn) or soybean oil (Intralipid) or a combination of both (Liposyn II). Fat emulsion particles are thought to be metabolized from the bloodstream in a manner similar to that of the chylomicrons, which appear in the blood postprandially. Fat emulsions may minimize hyperglycemia, hyperinsulinemia, and hyperosmolar syndrome, which often occurs in clients who are given dextrose as the only source of parenteral caloric nutrition. Fat emulsions pose some dangers for clients with severe liver disease, pulmonary disease, anemia, or blood coagulation disorders and for acutely ill clients with elevated serum concentrations of C-reactive protein. Fat emboli and the accumulation of intravascular fat may occur in the lungs of premature, preterm, or low-birth-weight infants (the infusion rate is not to exceed 1 g/kg in 4 hours).

Trace Elements and Electrolytes

Although some of the commercial parenteral nutrition solutions contain trace elements, or minerals, clients who are placed on long-term administration should be evaluated for deficiencies in trace elements. Trace element solutions are available individually (zinc, copper, manganese, chromium, and selenium) and in combination formulations (M.T.E. formulations and others). Several trace metal formulations are also available in combination with electrolytes [Tracelyte and others].

Examples of the signs and symptoms of trace element deficiency, normal serum levels, and primary excretion sites are noted in Table 70-4. It is also critical to monitor serum electrolyte levels, especially the cations of sodium, potassium, calcium, and magnesium and the anions of chloride, phosphate, bicarbonate, and acetate. In general, serum levels of trace elements are not routinely monitored.

If iron replacement is necessary, oral replacement is the preferred route of administration. If iron cannot be administered orally, it can be given by IM Z-track injection or by IV injection or infusion. Do not mix iron with other drugs or add it to parenteral nutrition solutions. For additional information on iron [Iron Dextran], refer to a current package insert or current drug reference book.

Vitamins

The client receiving parenteral feedings will also need additional vitamins. A combination of multivitamin infusion (MVI) and, perhaps, additional vitamins is usually given on alternate days to meet the client's needs for fat-soluble vitamins A and D and the water-soluble vitamins B and C. Such preparations, if prescribed, can be added to the parenteral nutrition solution. Vitamin K is usually administered weekly by IM or SC injection. The specific dosage and frequency for vitamin regimens depend primarily on the individual client's needs and on the usual protocols of the prescriber.

Special Formulations or Administration

Specially formulated amino acid preparations are available for clients with special disease conditions, such as renal failure, high metabolic stress, encephalopathy, and liver failure. For example, formulas such as HepatAmine are used for hepatic failure, and Nephramine and others are used for renal failure.

Parenteral nutrition is often administered in a home setting, usually in one single container per day. Whenever possible, all the necessary nutrients are combined and administered on a cycling basis, depending on the client. Cyclic therapy is the infusion of the feeding over less than 24 hours; this frees the client from constant therapy. Such preparations are often administered during the evening and night hours (Holcombe, 1996).

■ Nursing Management

Parenteral Nutrition Therapy

■ **Assessment.** A baseline assessment of the client should include body weight, weight loss history, and any clinical manifestations of undernutrition. The nutritional history should include, with cause if possible, inadequate nutrient intake, excessive nutrient losses or failure to absorb nutrients, increased metabolic requirements, or medications that might have a catabolic effect, such as corticosteroids or antineoplastic agents. Baseline laboratory determinations, such as serum albumin, serum electrolytes, serum transferrin, serum prealbumin, urine creatinine clearance, and the total lymphocyte count are indicators of protein nourishment. Hemoglobin, hematocrit, MCV, MCH, MCHC, and the various blood levels of specific vitamins and minerals are indicators of vitamin and mineral nourishment.

▪ **Nursing Diagnosis.** The client receiving parenteral nutrition therapy may experience the following nursing diagnoses/collaborative problems: risk for infection; deficient fluid volume; excess fluid volume; and the potential complications of negative nitrogen balance related to the underlying condition, hyperglycemia/hypoglycemia, depressed levels of the electrolytes potassium/phosphate/calcium/magnesium, trace element deficiencies, and essential fatty acid deficiency (EFAD) caused by prolonged fat-free hyperalimentation therapy (Box 70-2).

▪ **Implementation**

▪ ***Monitoring.*** Close, ongoing reassessment of clients' responses to this complex therapy is essential. In particular, the development of circulatory fluid overload or electrolyte imbalance should be monitored through assessments of vital signs, fluid intake and output, and electrolyte studies. A uniform infusion rate should be maintained at all times as prescribed by the prescriber. Infusion instrumentation does not eliminate the need for alert nursing care, because this equipment has the same potential for malfunction as all other equipment.

Some level of glucosuria may occur, particularly at the initiation of therapy, because insulin response is challenged by the glucose load. The urine may be tested at 6-hour intervals for glucose, acetone, and protein. The client should be weighed on a daily basis (preferably the first thing in the morning after voiding) and at the same time of day, wearing the same type of clothing, and on the same scale. BUN is tested daily for 3 to 5 days, then every other day as needed. A sequential multichannel autoanalyzer (SMA) 12/60 procedure should be performed weekly, as well as tests for protein, partial thromboplastin time (PTT), and complete blood count (CBC). Serum electrolytes should be monitored daily. Monitor serum triglycerides closely if lipid formulations are used. There is less aggressive monitoring of the long-term stable client receiving TPN.

Monitor clients with diabetes mellitus carefully; insulin may be required to control hyperglycemia. Clients with cardiac insufficiency need to be watched closely for fluid volume excess. Observe the infusion site regularly for inflammation and infection, and monitor the peripheral infusion lines for phlebitis.

It is critical to record daily the following data and to notify the prescriber of abnormal values: blood glucose in excess of 200 mg/100 mL; weight loss; change in pulse and blood pressure; sweating; elevated temperature; swelling and edema over the puncture site or on the head, neck, or face; abnormal serum electrolytes; distended veins in the neck, arms, and hands; convulsions; coma; or other radical changes in the client's condition.

▪ ***Intervention.*** Because these balanced nutritional solutions provide an excellent medium for the growth of microorganisms, strict asepsis must be used when preparing solutions (usually done by pharmacists, and ideally under a laminar flow hood) and when handling solutions or the insertion site.

BOX 70-2

Complications of Parenteral Nutrition

Complications Arising from Infection and Sepsis

Catheter seeding from bloodborne or distant infection
Contamination of catheter entrance site during insertion or long-term catheter placement
Solution contamination

Complications That Are Metabolic in Origin

Azotemia
Cholelithiasis
Dehydration from osmotic diuresis
Electrolyte imbalance
Hyperammonemia
Hyperosmolar, hyperglycemic, nonketotic coma (HHNC)
Hyperphosphatemia and hypophosphatemia
Hypocalcemia
Hypomagnesemia
Rebound hypoglycemia or sudden cessation of parenteral nutrition
Trace element deficiencies

Complications Arising from Subclavian Catheterization

Air embolism
Arteriovenous fistula
Brachial plexus injury
Cardiac perforation, tamponade
Catheter embolism
Catheter misplacement
Central vein thrombophlebitis
Endocarditis
Hemothorax
Hydromediastinum
Hydrothorax
Pneumothorax
Subclavian artery injury
Subclavian hematoma
Subcutaneous emphysema
Tension pneumothorax
Thoracic duct injury

Hickman or Broviac catheters are two central venous catheters that can be used for intermittent infusions of drugs, parenteral feedings, and other adjunctive therapies. These catheters are designed so that the ends may be capped between infusions. Heparinized saline is instilled at the completion of infusions, and the tube is recapped. Except during lipid infusions, in-line filters may be used to trap air and bacteria. Parenteral lines are reserved for hyperalimentation.

Fat emulsions may be administered either peripherally or centrally. If fat emulsions are co-infused from separate containers that flow into the same vein as the dextrose and amino acid solutions, a Y-connector is used and is positioned just in front of the infusion site. The lipid infusion line should be at least 6 inches higher than the dextrose–amino acid line, because the lipid emulsion has a lower specific gravity. If not administered in this order, the lipid emulsion may flow backward into the amino acid-dextrose line.

The intake of parenteral nutrition may begin at a rate less than 1 L/12 hr for the first 2 days. If tolerated, the rate may be increased gradually during the first 5 days to the final goal rate. Ideally, the rate of parenteral nutrition solutions should be regulated by an infusion pump to maintain a steady flow.

Peripheral infusions are limited to amino acids 2.5% and dextrose 10%.

Do not shake lipid emulsion infusions that have separated in solution to mix them; instead discard them according to agency policy. In addition, the fats in lipid emulsions have been found to leach out the plasticizer di(2-ethylhexyl) phthalate (DEHP) in polyvinyl chloride tubing. Because the toxic potential for DEHP is not known, it is wise to use the administration sets provided by the manufacturer for fat emulsions in parenteral nutrition therapy.

Dressings should be changed if they become wet or dislodged; they are designed to be air-occlusive. Specific protocols for dressing changes can be found in selected references. Report any elevation of the client's temperature to the physician. Cultures (fungal, bacterial) should be taken of the insertion site, tubing, parenteral solutions, and the client's blood. In general, peripheral vein sites are changed routinely every 10 to 12 hours.

Air embolism is a potential hazard with central venous lines because of the low pressure in the venous system. Tubing connections must be kept taped to prevent their separation. When necessary, tubing should be changed quickly while the client is in a supine position and is executing a Valsalva's maneuver (forced exhalation against a closed glottis). Central line insertions should be accomplished with the client in Trendelenburg's position.

▪ ***Education.*** Parenteral nutrition can now be continued at home for indefinite periods of time for those who need ongoing nutritional support and who meet the criteria. Education of the client and family is essential with regard to the purposes and techniques of the following: preventing infection, caring for the solution, regulating flow rate, recording daily weights, recording intake and output, monitoring urine for glycosuria, and keeping close contact with community health nurses and other personnel. The client and family/caregiver must understand infusion pump monitoring before assuming full responsibility for this technology. Every attempt should be made to resume the usual activities of daily living and to integrate this therapy into the client's lifestyle. See the Community and Home Health Considerations box above for the nursing care of a client who is receiving TPN in the home.

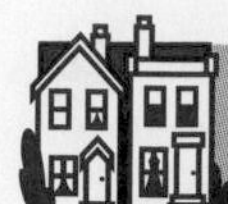

Community and Home Health Considerations

Total Parenteral Nutrition in the Home Setting

The client and family/caregiver should have the opportunity to practice the procedures in the hospital under nursing supervision. Review the procedures for storage of the solution, which should be picked up or delivered every day for the client. Instruct the client to keep the containers refrigerated but to allow them to come to room temperature before administering the solution. Advise the client to check the expiration date, the label of contents, and the appearance of the solution.

The dressing is to be changed at least every 2 days. Instruct the family/caregiver to use aseptic technique when changing the dressing. The site should be inspected for swelling, redness, or drainage; these should be reported to the health care provider if found. Demonstrate to the family how to irrigate the catheter. Instruct the client in how to set the pump to the appropriate settings, how the infusion pump works, how to care for the pump, and what to do if the alarm sounds. Also demonstrate how to change the solution bag, tubing, and filter.

Explain that the client should be weighed daily and the client's intake and output monitored. Ask the client and family to observe for edema, and show them how to check urine glucose levels. Review the potential complications of TPN, such as chills, fever, dyspnea, chest pain, and coughing as an adverse reaction to lipid infusion; dyspnea, chest pain, and coughing with air embolism; nervousness, faintness, and tachycardia with hypoglycemia; and nausea, vomiting, polyuria, polydipsia, and positive urine glucose or acetone with hyperglycemia. Instruct the client to discontinue the infusion and to contact the prescriber if any of these occur. Recommend that the client keep the telephone number of the prescriber, nursing service, and community emergency services within easy reach.

▪ **Evaluation.** The expected outcome of parenteral nutrition therapy is that the client's nutritional status will be improved. If therapy is successful, weight increases of 2 to 3 pounds a week can be expected until the client's weight is within the normal limits for height and age. The client should also demonstrate improved strength and activity tolerance and healthy gums and oral mucous membranes. Laboratory values should be within the normal limits for BUN and serum albumin, protein, hematocrit, hemoglobin, vitamin B_{12}, folic acid, cholesterol, lymphocytes, and transferrin.

SUMMARY

Nutrition in the form of enteral or parenteral solutions plays a vital role in the treatment of clients. Enteral nutrition bypasses the upper gastrointestinal tract and introduces liquid enteral formula or pureed foods directly into the stomach or small intestine by way of a feeding tube. Enteral feeding is indicated for clients who have a functional gastrointestinal tract but cannot take sufficient food by mouth. The complications of enteral nutrition may be mechanical or metabolic.

Parenteral nutrition refers to the IV administration of a solution containing dextrose, proteins, electrolytes, vitamins, and trace elements in amounts that exceed the client's energy needs. It is used for instances in which enteral feeding is contraindicated or ineffective. In both enteral and parenteral nutrition, the nurse has an important role to ensure that clients are nourished adequately and safely.

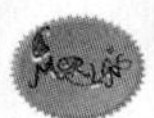

Critical Thinking Questions

1. Jean Sims, age 76, has been admitted to the hospital because of several chronic ailments, including asthma, emphysema, and esophageal motility problems. She has been losing weight rapidly because she is having trouble swallowing and is working so hard to breathe that she is not getting enough to eat. Rather than insert a nasogastric tube, the physician has inserted a gastrostomy tube percutaneously. What are the advantages for this client of the PEG compared to a nasogastric tube?
2. Would TPN have any advantages for Mrs. Sims? Why or why not?

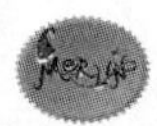

Collaborative Learning Activities

For Collaborative Learning Activities, go to mosby.com/MERLIN/McKenry/.

BIBLIOGRAPHY

American Hospital Formulary Service. (1999). *AHFS drug information '99*. Bethesda, MD: American Society of Hospital Pharmacists.

Anderson, K.N., Anderson, L.E., & Glanze, W.D. (Eds.). (1998). *Mosby's medical, nursing, & allied health dictionary* (5th ed.). St. Louis: Mosby.

Beare, P.G. & Myers, J.L. (1998). *Adult health nursing* (3rd ed.). St. Louis: Mosby.

Beizer, J. (1992). Enteral feeding in the LTC setting. *Long Term Care Forum, 2*(2), 8.

Carpenito, L.J. (1999). *Nursing diagnosis: Application to clinical practice* (8th ed.). Philadelphia: J.B. Lippincott.

Drug Facts and Comparisons. (2000). St. Louis: Facts and Comparisons.

Estoup, M. (1994). Approaches and limitations of medication delivery in patients with enteral feeding tubes. *Critical Care Nurse, 14*(2), 68-78.

Food and Drug Administration. (1994). Safety alert: Hazards of precipitation associated with parenteral nutrition. *American Journal of Hospital Pharmacy, 51*(6), 1427-1428.

Holcombe, B.J. (1996). Adult parenteral nutrition. In L.Y. Young & M.A. Koda-Kimble (Eds.), *Applied therapeutics: The clinical use of drugs* (6th ed.). Vancouver, WA: Applied Therapeutics.

Lipman, T.O. (1993). Total parenteral nutrition: Indications for hospitalized adults. *Drug Therapy,* 17(3):199-200.

Matlow, A.G., Kitai, I., Kirpalani, H., Chapman, N.H., Corey, M., Perlman, M., Pencharz, P., Jewell, S., Phillips-Gordon, C., Summerbell, R., Ford-Jones, E.L. (1999). A randomized trial of 72-versus 24-hour intravenous tubing set changes in newborns receiving lipid therapy. *Infection Control Hospital Epidemiology, 20*(7), 487-493.

McCloskey, J.C. & Bulechek, G.M. (Eds.). (1996). *Nursing interventions classification (NIC)* (2nd ed.). St. Louis: Mosby.

Meteney, N. (1993). Minimizing respiratory complications of nasoenteric tube feedings: State of the science. *Heart Lung, 22*(3), 213-222.

Metheny, N.M. (1996). *Fluid and electrolyte balance: Nursing considerations*. (3rd ed.). Philadelphia: Williams & Wilkins.

Mirtallo, J.M. (1994). The complexity of mixing calcium and phosphate. *American Journal of Hospital Pharmacy, 51*(6), 1535-1536.

Miyagawa, C.I. (1993). Drug-nutrient interactions in critically ill patients. *Critical Care Nurse, 13*(10), 69-90.

Phillips, L.D. (1997) *Manual of IV therapeutics* (2nd ed.). Philadelphia: F.A. Davis.

Rollins, C.J. (1996). Adult enteral nutrition. In L.Y. Young & M.A. Koda-Kimble (Eds.), *Applied therapeutics: The clinical use of drugs* (6th ed.). Vancouver, WA: Applied Therapeutics.

Tokars, J.I., Cookson, S.T., McArthur, M.A., Boyer, C.L., McGeer, A.J., & Jarvis, W.R. (1999). Prospective evaluation of risk factors for bloodstream infection in patients receiving home infusion therapy. *Annals of Internal Medicine, 131*(5), 340-347.

United States Pharmacopeia Dispensing Information (USP DI): Drug information for the health care professional (19th ed.). (1999). Rockville, MD: United States Pharmacopeial Convention.

Varella, L.D. & Young, R.J. (1999). New options for pumps and tubes: Progress in enteral feeding techniques and devices. *Current Opinion in Clinical Nutrition & Metabolic Care, 2*(4), 271-275.

71 Antiseptics, Disinfectants, and Sterilants

Chapter Focus

Most infectious diseases are transmitted in one of four ways: airborne transmission (inhalation of contaminated, evaporated droplets); vector-borne transmission of an organism by an intermediate carrier, such as a mosquito; contact transmission (direct or indirect contact with the source); and enteric transmission (oral-fecal transmission through direct or indirect contact with feces or objects heavily contaminated with feces). To inhibit the transmission of infection, nurses both practice and teach good aseptic and sterile technique. Nurses work to break the cycle of contact and enteric transmission by using antiseptics, disinfectants, and sterilant agents to decontaminate surfaces and equipment to prevent the spread of infection.

Learning Objectives

1. Compare nosocomial infections and community- or home-acquired infections.
2. Differentiate between medical asepsis and surgical asepsis.
3. Describe the characteristics of an ideal antiseptic/disinfectant.
4. Discuss the mechanisms of action of antiseptics and disinfectants.
5. List the indications for use of common antiseptics and disinfectants.
6. Discuss the uses and limitations of silver nitrate and silver sulfadiazine.
7. Describe the effectiveness of iodine compounds and iodophors.
8. Explain the mechanism of action of oxidizing agents.
9. Discuss the current uses of sterilants.
10. Implement nursing management for the safe and effective use of antiseptics, disinfectants, and sterilants.

Key Terms

Infections and infectious diseases, although differing in type and character, occur in people in all settings—hospitals, institutions, the community at large, and the home.

Community-acquired infections in usually healthy individuals are often benign and are relatively responsive to treatment. *S. pneumoniae* or *M. pneumoniae* infections are common in this population. **Nosocomial infections** are acquired in the hospital and most commonly result from gram-negative infections—*Pseudomonas, Proteus, Serratia, Providencia,* and others (Bailey & Powderly, 1992). Nosocomial infections have been called one of the most significant current ecologic problems in North America. They are occasionally caused by virulent microorganisms resistant to antibiotics.

Urinary tract infections and postoperative wound infections account for the majority (approximately 70% or more) of the nosocomial infections detected in a hospital setting. High-risk areas, such as critical care units, burn units, and dialysis units, usually have the highest incidence of infection outbreaks and antibiotic resistance. Nurses must be aware of this problem and of the methods used to reduce the incidence of nosocomial infections in their practice (Cheung, Ortiz, & DiMarino, 1999).

MEDICAL AND SURGICAL ASEPSIS

Medical asepsis (the absence of pathogenic organisms) and **surgical asepsis** (the absence of all microorganisms) are used in health care to reduce the number and spread of organisms. These approaches presume the presence of pathogens (organisms capable of inducing disease or infection in human beings) or potential pathogens in the immediate environment and seek to limit their transmission.

Methods in surgical asepsis destroy *all* microorganisms, including spores; in medical asepsis, only *pathogens* are destroyed or inhibited. The focus in surgical asepsis is to keep all organisms out of a designated area (e.g., fresh wound), whereas in medical asepsis the goal is to remove or destroy the pathogens in the area and to contain the remaining nonpathogens by conscious efforts. Surgical asepsis uses "sterile technique" (the use of sterile equipment or sterile fields), and medical asepsis uses "clean technique" (e.g., hygienic measures, cleaning agents, antiseptics, disinfectants, and barrier fields). The technique used in a given situation depends largely on the susceptibility of the host, the organism's virulence, and other factors in the infectious cycle.

An object is sterile if it is free of all forms and types of life. **Sterilization** is a process that destroys all forms of life on an instrument or utensil, in a liquid, or within a substance. Living tissue (of clients, nurses, or surgeons) cannot be sterilized by any known means without damaging that tissue; therefore sterilization is applied only to objects. It is also important to grasp the concept put forth by the Council on Pharmacy and Chemistry that the terms *sterile, sterilizer,* and *sterilization* can be used only in the absolute sense—there is no acceptable concept of relative sterility. However, just because a piece of equipment is labeled "sterilizer" does not mean that it is totally and permanently effective for sterilizing. Nor does the term *sterilized* testify to an object's current condition of purity.

Several acceptable and practicable sterilization methods now exist. Steam under pressure (autoclaving) is preferred as the most effective method. Ethylene oxide is a gas sterilant used for heat-labile materials, for sharp-edged instruments that could be dulled by steam, for electrical and anesthesia equipment, and for bedding. Hot air ovens are used to sterilize glassware. Chemical sterilants are also used when necessary.

ANTISEPTICS AND DISINFECTANTS

Antiseptics and **disinfectants** are chemical agents used to kill many pathogens within a given population of microorganisms. In general, their mechanisms of action are not very effective against spores of bacteria and fungi, many viruses, and some very resistant bacterial strains. As a group, the effects of disinfectants and antiseptics differ from sterilization largely in the type of organisms destroyed and the degree to which they are destroyed. Disinfectants and antiseptics kill only pathogens, but sterilizing kills all types of organisms.

Although some of the literature uses the terms *disinfectant* and *antiseptic* interchangeably, such use is erroneous and confusing. Disinfectants differ from antiseptics in the matter on which they are used and in their ability to destroy organisms. Disinfectants are used only on nonliving objects; they are toxic to living tissue. Antiseptics are typically applied only to living tissue; they must be less potent or made more dilute to prevent cell damage. Such lessening of potency, although crucial to viable tissue, decreases effectiveness accordingly. Some definitions of antiseptics emphasize their inhibiting rather than their destructive effects. The narrow range of tolerance by tissues to antiinfective topical preparations tends to limit the variety and number of acceptable antiseptic agents available. Antiseptics may differ markedly from disinfectants in chemical composition or may simply be a dilute version of a disinfectant for use on intact tissue. Thus some chemical substances may be used either as an antiseptic or as a disinfectant, depending on concentration.

Antiseptics and disinfectants are further categorized as bacteriostatic or bactericidal in character. Antiseptics are most often **bacteriostatic**; they slow the growth and replication of bacteria but do not kill off the entire bacteria population. Disinfectants are **bactericidal** (bactericides); they actually kill bacteria, but perhaps not all types (depending on the disinfectant, its specificity, and so on) and often not fungi, viruses, or spores. Other disinfectants—fungicides, virucides, and sporicides—act specifically on these organisms. *Germicides* is an all-encompassing term for agents that work against many types of "germs"—bacteria, fungi, viruses, and spores.

Organisms vary in their sensitivity to disinfectants and antiseptics (Box 71-1). However, factors such as the dormant and impervious spore forms of some bacteria; the waxy envelopes of the tubercle bacilli; and certain properties of

BOX 71-1

Sensitivity of Organisms to Disinfectants and Antiseptics*

Least resistant
- Bacteria
  - Gram-positive and gram-negative
  - Vegetative forms
- Fungi
- Viruses, lipophilic
  - Influenza
  - Herpes
  - Vaccinia
  - Rubella
  - Mumps
  - Varicella
- Tubercle bacilli
- Viruses, hydrophilic
  - Enteroviruses
  - Rhinoviruses
  - Hepatitis viruses A and B
- Bacterial and fungal spores

Most resistant

*May vary with concentration of compound and other factors.

some types of gram-positive bacteria (staphylococci and enterococci), some gram-negative bacteria (*Salmonella* and *Pseudomonas* species), and hepatitis viruses make them highly refractory to many forms of disinfectants or antiseptics.

The ideal all-around antiseptic/disinfectant does not yet exist. Such an ideal agent would need to do the following:

- Be destructive to all forms of microorganisms without being toxic to human cells
- Have a low incidence of hypersensitivity
- Be active in the presence of organic matter and soaps
- Be stable, noncorrosive, nonstaining, and inexpensive

The current criteria for an effective disinfectant includes the ability to destroy within 10 minutes all vegetative bacteria (not spores) and fungi, tubercle bacilli, animal parasites, and viruses (not hepatitis viruses). Many variables affect the relative efficiency of a product, including the ingredients' ability to dissolve, mix, and work in the presence of organic matter such as blood or other exudate and its ability to penetrate into recesses. Other properties include chemical composition, concentration, pH, ionization, surface tension, temperature, and length of time required for action. In actual clinical use, there may be extreme variability in the effectiveness of any given product; this variability depends on the specific application and situation. Although several standard tests for the efficacy of these products are available, the results are subject to the same variables and may also be difficult to administer.

Currently, there are few established guidelines for specific approved use of any particular disinfectant—a disinfectant is considered a disinfectant whether it is to be used on corridor floors or on surgical instruments. This method of classifying permits widespread practices such as the common use of iodophor solutions as disinfectants when they have earned approval by the Food and Drug Administration (FDA) as antiseptics. Antiseptics are not required to be as potent as disinfectants.

The relative usefulness of various antiseptics can be compared based on their therapeutic index. This index is the relationship between the specific antiseptic concentration proved to be effective against microorganisms without irritating tissues or interfering with healing. Other decisive factors are the potential for causing hypersensitivity reactions or systemic absorption. *Thorough handwashing still predominates as the most effective measure for controlling the spread of infection.*

To place the concepts of sterilization, disinfection, and antisepsis in perspective, it should be made clear that these processes differ in the degree to which they destroy organisms. Anything that is sterile can also be considered both disinfected and antiseptic. (The converse is, of course, not true.) All of these processes correctly begin with handwashing, even when gloves are to be worn. It has been repeatedly demonstrated that clean, washed hands are crucial deterrents to the growth, reproduction, and transmission of microorganisms in any environment.

Antiseptics and disinfectants may act in three ways:

1. They may bring about a change in the structure of the protein of the microbial cell (denaturation), which often proceeds to coagulation of protein with increased concentration of the chemical agent.
2. They may lower the surface tension of the aqueous medium of the parasitic cell, which increases the permeability of the plasma membrane. This results in the lysis or destruction of cellular constituents. (The surface-active agents are thought to act this way.)
3. They may alter a metabolic process in the microbial cells, which interferes with the cell's ability to survive and multiply.

Phenols

Phenol was used for more than 100 years as an antiseptic and disinfectant, but today it may be used in some facilities as a disinfectant. All phenols are deadly poisons if taken internally or applied topically to abraded skin. Phenol itself is no longer used because of its toxicity on absorption, its carcinogenic effect, and its corrosive effect on equipment. Its derivatives are used, and these compounds disrupt cell walls and membranes, precipitate proteins, and inactivate enzymes; this makes them bactericidal, fungicidal, and capable of inactivating lipophilic viruses.

▪ Nursing Management

Phenols

Phenol and phenolic compounds are intended for disinfectant use only. These disinfectants should not come in contact with the skin in concentrations stronger than 2%, and they should never come in contact with broken skin. If accidental skin contact is made or if a burning sensation is noted, the area should be washed with copious amounts of water. Phenolic disinfectants used to clean bassinets and mattresses in poorly ventilated nurseries have produced epidemics of neonatal hyperbilirubinemia, and fatalities have been documented in infants. Phenol in concentrations above 5% has been implicated in the promotion of tumor growth, and therefore studies are underway to determine the carcinogenic, mutagenic, and teratogenic safety of this agent.

hexachlorophene [heks' a klo roe feen] (pHisoHex, Septisol)

Hexachlorophene is a bacteriostatic agent that at one time was incorporated into detergent creams, soaps, lotions, shampoos, and other topical products to reduce the incidence of pathogenic bacteria on the skin. Because of its toxicity, especially in infants, it is currently available only by prescription for surgical scrub purposes and as a bacteriostatic skin cleanser against staphylococci and other gram-positive bacteria. It is used as a surgical scrub and bacteriostatic skin cleansing agent, although other antiseptics such as chlorhexidine are more effective and are safer to use.

A single skin washing with hexachlorophene is no more effective than soap in reducing the number of bacteria; however, this product has a cumulative antibacterial property and steadily decreases bacterial flora with repeated use. Cleansing with alcohol and repeated washing with soap removes its antibacterial residue.

Hexachlorophene is a toxic agent that can be absorbed through the skin, causing gastric symptoms and central nervous system (CNS) toxicity. Daily topical use on newborns or application several times daily to the skin or vagina in adults has resulted in confusion, diplopia, lethargy, convulsions, respiratory arrest, and death. Hexachlorophene is usually not used routinely or recommended for use in bathing infants. It also should not be used on mucous membranes or burned or denuded skin or for any prolonged skin contact without rinsing. Dermatitis and photosensitivity have also been reported.

■ Nursing Management

Hexachlorophene

Most authoritative sources recommend against the use of pHisoHex for use in bathing infants or for use by pregnant or hypersensitive persons.

There is a potential for poisoning; a resultant CNS toxicity may occur if there is accidental excessive exposure to or ingestion of these agents. Observe clients with prolonged exposure for signs of CNS toxicity: a change in sensorium, double vision, lethargy, and seizures.

These products are highly toxic if ingested and are easily absorbed (even through intact skin) if not thoroughly rinsed. Do not leave these substances in contact with the skin or mucous membranes, such as in occlusive dressings, wet packs, lotions, or vaginal packs. Avoid contact with the eyes. Use should be discontinued if gastric or CNS signs appear.

pHisoHex is most effective for handwashing when no other antiseptic or solvent follows the rinse, because its antibacterial effects are progressive and cumulative with repeated use. It is available by prescription for home preparations for surgeries. If used for a preoperative preparation, scrub the operative site and surrounding areas every day for 3 days for optimal effectiveness. pHisoHex may turn brown when exposed to light, but this does not affect its action. Dispensers should be cleaned every 1 to 2 weeks.

hexylresorcinol [hex ill re sore' sin ole]

Hexylresorcinol is a stainless and odorless antiseptic. Although quite irritating to body tissues, diluted solutions of hexylresorcinol are used to cleanse skin wounds and are also used in mouthwashes or pharyngeal antiseptic preparations. Occasionally a marked hypersensitivity reaction may occur.

■ Nursing Management

Hexylresorcinol

Watch for signs of inflammation or irritation. Advise that this product be discontinued if such signs are evident, because they may indicate hypersensitivity rather than simple dermal irritation.

Dyes

Rosaniline dyes are a group of basic dyes used only occasionally today as antibacterial and antifungal agents. Most of these dyes (gentian violet, methyl violet, and others) have been removed from the market or have been replaced by other topical products.

Mercury Compounds

The FDA has banned all first aid antiseptic mercury products, including thimerosal (Merthiolate) and merbromin (Mercurochrome), because they lack evidence of safety and effectiveness (Federal Register, 1998).

Silver Compounds

silver nitrate; silver protein, mild

Many inorganic silver compounds have antiseptic qualities when applied locally. Silver salts that are highly ionizable and soluble produce astringent or caustic actions. Free silver ions precipitate bacterial cellular proteins, which results in bactericidal effects. The effectiveness of these agents is directly proportional to their concentration and duration of contact time. An immediate bactericidal effect occurs when silver solutions are applied to tissue. The silver proteinate that is formed slowly liberates small amounts of ionic silver, which provides continued bacteriostatic action. An unexplained and strongly bactericidal quality resides in distilled water when it is in contact with metallic silver.

Silver nitrate reacts with soluble chloride, iodides, and bromides to form insoluble salts, which stops the action of silver nitrate. Therefore its action can be halted if necessary by irrigating the area with sodium chloride solutions. This chemical characteristic explains why solutions of silver salts penetrate tissues slowly; chlorides apparently precipitate the silver ions and inactivate them.

Silver protein, mild (Argyrol S.S. 10%) is used to treat local and mild inflammation in the eye, nose, and throat. *Silver sulfadiazine (Silvadene)* is bactericidal for many gram-positive and gram-negative organisms and yeast, and it also inhibits bacteria that are resistant to other agents (see Chapter 66). It is used to prevent and treat infections in second- and third-degree burns.

With silver nitrate 1% solution, eye redness or irritation is the primary adverse reaction; with other silver nitrate preparations, it is skin irritation. The long-term use of silver salts can permanently discolor the skin because of the deposit of reduced silver (argyria). Prolonged use of mild silver protein can result in permanent skin discoloration and conjunctival argyria.

With silver nitrate 1% solution, 2 drops are instilled and allowed to remain in the eyes for no more than 30 seconds. The American Academy of Pediatrics has endorsed a recommendation to eliminate eye irrigation after instillation of silver nitrate (*Drug Facts and Comparisons*, 2000). In many hospitals, topical erythromycin or tetracycline ophthalmic ointments have replaced silver nitrate because they are effective against chlamydia and gonococcus eye infections (DiPiro et al., 1993).

For infections, instill 1 to 3 drops of silver protein, mild (Argyrol S.S.) in the eye(s) every 3 to 4 hours for several days; for preoperative use, place 2 or 3 drops in the eye(s) and then rinse with a sterile irrigating solution.

▪ Nursing Management
Silver Compounds

See Chapter 66 for the nursing management of silver sulfadiazine.

▪ **Assessment.** Question the client about hypersensitivity to silver, blood dyscrasias, porphyria, or a glucose-6-phosphate dehydrogenase deficiency; these conditions may preclude treatment with silver compounds. The effects in children and in pregnant or breastfeeding women are not known.

▪ **Nursing Diagnosis.** The client receiving silver compound therapy may be at risk for impaired comfort (an itching or burning feeling on treated areas).

▪ **Implementation**

▪ ***Monitoring.*** Evaluate the affected mucous membranes daily, and note any changes. Perform an ongoing evaluation of clients treated with these compounds to limit the adverse reactions related to hypersensitivities.

▪ ***Intervention.*** Store silver nitrate solutions at temperatures between 15° and 30° C (59° and 86° F), and protect them from light. Use only the appropriate concentrations for antiseptic purposes to avoid irritation and burns to tissue. Sodium chloride can be used to flood the area should this occur accidentally.

Take care with silver solutions to keep spills and stains to a minimum. Gloves are advised when working with silver solutions. Most tissue stains gradually disappear. Stains may be removed from linens, clothing, and shoes by applying household chlorine bleach.

▪ ***Education.*** Alert the client that rarely the skin may stain a brownish black. Instruct in the proper application technique. Instruct the client to store silver nitrate solutions out of reach of children and never to take them internally.

▪ **Evaluation.** The expected outcome of silver compound therapy is that the client's mucous membrane will be moist, pink, and intact without drainage or other signs of inflammation or infection.

Halogens

Chlorine Compounds

Although chlorine can be bactericidal (it is ineffective against acid-fast bacteria), sporicidal, viricidal, and amebicidal, the elemental form of chlorine itself has limited usefulness as a disinfectant because the gas is difficult to handle. The antibacterial action of chlorine is said to be caused by the formation of hypochlorous acids, which results when chlorine reacts with water. Therefore chlorine-containing products that can release hypochlorous acid are in use today:

1. *Sodium hypochlorite solution, 1%* is used to sterilize equipment; the 0.5% solution is used as an antiseptic for wound irrigation. This solution is of limited usefulness for wound irrigations, except for debridement purposes, because they are irritating to the skin and delay the clotting process. Common household bleaches are usually 5% solutions of sodium hypochlorite. Therapeutic solutions are unstable and must be freshly prepared before use. See the Nursing Research box on p. 1203 for information on the use of hypochlorite solutions for preventing the spread of AIDS among IV drug users.
2. Oxychlorosene (Clorpactin WCS-90) is a combination product that contains hypochlorous acid, which when released is effective (bactericidal) against both gram-negative and gram-positive organisms, fungi, yeast, viruses, molds, and spores. It is indicated for the treatment of localized infections, especially if caused by resistant organisms, and for cleansing and irrigating necrotic debris, wounds, sinus tracts, and empyemas. Dilutions of this product are also used in urology and ophthalmology.

▪ Nursing Management
Chlorine Compounds

Dakin's solution, a diluted 0.5% sodium hypochlorite solution adjusted to a neutral pH with sodium bicarbonate, was once widely used to treat suppurating wounds, but its solvent action delays clotting.

Store chlorine products in marked containers and out of the reach of children. If a chlorine agent is swallowed, a poison control center should be contacted and emergency treatment sought. Store these products away from light and in airtight containers if possible. Avoid spills on skin or delicate tissues because it will cause irritation. Avoid spills on clothing or contact with hair because of its bleaching properties. Rinse thoroughly with clear water if a spill occurs.

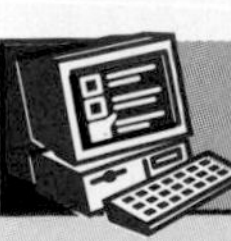

Nursing Research
Effectiveness of Bleach Distribution to Prevent HIV Transmission

Citation: Romanelli, F., Smith, K.M., & Pomeroy, C. (2000). Reducing the transmission of HIV-1: needle bleaching as a means of disinfection. *Journal of the American Pharmaceutical Association 40*(6):812-817; and Siegel, J.E., Weinstein, M.C., Fineberg, H.V. (1991). Bleach programs for preventing AIDS among IV users: Modeling the impact of HIV prevalence. *American Journal of Public Health, 81*(10), 1273-1279.

Abstract: IV drug users risk HIV infection from sexual contact and from sharing injection equipment—needles, syringes, or other items—with infected individuals. Although protective changes in behavior have been reported among homosexuals, most IV drug users continue to place themselves at risk. The growing importance of drug use as a mode of HIV transmission has led to increased attention to AIDS prevention among IV drug users.

Siegel and others (1991) examined the effectiveness of bleach distribution, which is a program to prevent HIV transmission via shared needles. Bleach programs employ outreach workers to distribute small bottles of bleach, which IV drug users use to disinfect their injection equipment. An important argument for the implementation of bleach programs has been that they are more politically feasible than needle exchange programs. They examined whether and to what extent the initial HIV prevalence among IV drug users influences program effectiveness. Because the difficulty of conducting longitudinal surveys of transient populations of IV drug users prevents studies of existing programs, they used a Markov model to provide a practical means for studying the conditions that determine the success of bleach programs.

This model incorporates survey data on risk behaviors and published information describing HIV incubation andmortality. It predicts life expectancy for cohorts of IV drug users with and without a bleach program to estimate program effectiveness.

They found that bleach programs can produce the greatest life-year savings in areas of low HIV prevalence. In the lowest-prevalence scenario (0.02 initial prevalence), initiation of the program resulted in a projected savings of 2.3 life years per HIV-negative drug user, compared with 1.7 and 1.3 years under medium- (0.25) and high- (0.60) prevalence scenarios, respectively. The investigators concluded that bleach programs are beneficial to all groups of IV drug users and that these results highlight the advantages of introducing bleach programs early—when prevalence is still comparatively low in a drug-user population.

In 2000, Romanelli and others reviewed controlled studies cited in MEDLINE between 1966 and 1999 to review the efficacy, safety, and proper methods for the use of bleach for needle disinfection. They concluded that, used properly, undiluted bleach still appears to be an effective disinfection solution for used needles and that proper needle disinfection with undiluted bleach reduces the risk of HIV transmission from needle sharing among IV drug users.

Critical Thinking Questions

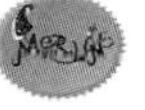

- Because HIV prevalence among drug users can increase rapidly, what do you think the opportunities are for early intervention with bleach programs?
- In your own community, what types of programs are available for IV drug users to prevent the spread of HIV? If a bleach program is not available, how would you go about instituting one?

Iodine and Iodophors

iodine tincture; povidone-iodine solution (Betadine)

Iodine is slightly soluble in water but is soluble in alcohol and in aqueous solutions of sodium and potassium iodide. Iodine is volatile, and solutions should not be exposed to air except during use. In its elemental or free form, iodine is very rapidly bactericidal, viricidal, fungicidal, and lethal to protozoa; it is less effective against spores. It is one of the most efficient chemical disinfectants and antiseptics currently in use.

Some iodine compounds are believed to be superior to other antiseptics, because all types of bacteria may be destroyed with a single concentration of iodine and because it is effective over a wide pH range. Organic matter interferes with the potency of iodine only when it is first applied; effectiveness later increases because of diffusion as the iodine complexes dissociate. This initial delayed effect in the presence of organic material may also be offset by the increased strengths of solution concentrations now on the market.

Iodine solution is used for the treatment of minor wounds, abrasions, and infected wounds; iodine tincture is preferred for intact skin procedures, such as skin preparation before invasive procedures, Hickman catheter and parenteral nutrition dressing changes, and IV needle insertions. Aqueous solutions are thought to be as effective as tincture of iodine for similar therapeutic purposes; because they are less irritating, they are used for abraded skin areas.

An aqueous solution of 5% iodine and 10% potassium iodide (Lugol's solution) can also be given orally for the treatment of goiter (see Chapter 48). The various iodine compounds marketed for antisepsis and disinfection include Iodine Topical and Iodine Tincture (the most commonly used iodine antiseptic). Although they both contain 2% iodine and 2.4% sodium iodide, the solution is in water, whereas the tincture has 47% alcohol.

iodophor: povidone-iodine (Betadine, Operand)

Iodophors have become widely used as *antiseptics*. This is the only purpose for which they have been approved by the FDA, although in practice they continue to be used to disinfect certain equipment. Iodophors are a group of iodine compounds combined with povidone (carrier), which increases the water solubility of iodine and provides a slow release of iodine. It has the same germicidal action of iodine without irritating the skin and mucous membranes. Povidone-iodines are available in many formulations, such as solution, 2% scrub, spray, foam, vaginal gel and suppositories, ointment, mouthwash, or perineal wash.

Iodine is toxic if taken internally. It is locally corrosive to gastrointestinal tissues but is inactivated by gastrointestinal contents. Iodine tincture may be transiently quite painful when applied to open skin areas, but the aqueous solution form stings only slightly. These agents may be absorbed through the skin and may affect thyroid function with chronic use. Neonates have developed hypothyroidism following the topical application of povidone-iodine. Marked hypersensitivity reactions occasionally occur, even with topical application; they are manifested by severe systemic reactions of fever and generalized skin eruptions.

■ Nursing Management
Iodine Compounds and Iodophors

■ **Assessment.** Before applying iodine compounds and iodophors, ask the client about any past allergic reactions to iodine, shellfish, or iodine-containing diagnostic agents. If there is any doubt, substitute another product. Do not use povidone-iodine as a vaginal douche during pregnancy.

■ **Nursing Diagnosis.** The client is at risk for impaired skin integrity related to hypersensitivity or local irritation, as well as impaired comfort with iodine tincture related to pain and stinging on application of the agent.

■ **Implementation**

■ ***Monitoring.*** Observe the area for irritation not present at the initiation of therapy. Monitor the lesions on a periodic basis for healing.

■ ***Intervention.*** Iodine compounds and iodophors are exceptionally valuable because of their efficiency, low toxicity, and low cost.

Do not bandage or tape areas treated with tincture of iodine. A cover dressing may be applied if necessary after treatment with povidone-iodine. Wash the skin if irritation develops.

Artificially elevated blood glucose determinations have been noted when povidone-iodine swabs are used for skin preparation. Soap and water cleansing of the fingertips before skin puncture for blood glucose monitoring by some reagent strips is recommended.

Iodophors will stain only starched linen or clothing. Tinctures and solutions of iodine may stain more freely.

■ ***Education.*** Advise the client to purchase iodine preparations in very small quantities and to discard them routinely after a short time, because evaporation of the solvent or vehicle will leave a concentrated iodine preparation that may burn tissues on application.

■ **Evaluation.** The expected outcome of using iodine compounds and iodophors is that the client will demonstrate signs of wound healing within an appropriate time frame. If the agent is used as an antiseptic to prepare for a procedure, there will be no evidence of sepsis following the procedure.

Oxidizing Agents

hydrogen peroxide

Hydrogen peroxide is a weak antiseptic; when in contact with a tissue enzyme (catalase), it is converted to effervescent oxygen to produce an antibacterial action and cleansing effect on the wound. The presence of blood and pus decreases the efficacy of hydrogen peroxide (American Hospital Formulary Service, 1999). The antiseptic action of hydrogen peroxide is fairly fast acting and short-lived; it acts as an antibacterial agent only as long as the bubbling action continues.

The oxygen that is released is particularly suited for destroying aerobic microorganisms in wounds, but as an antibacterial it is weak and slow. However, its effervescent action provides a mechanical effect to aid in removing foreign tissue debris. Several products containing hydrogen peroxide are marketed.

Hydrogen peroxide topical solution is available in a 3% solution in water and is used to irrigate suppurating wounds and some extensive traumatic wounds. It should be used in areas where the oxygen can escape and therefore should not be instilled into closed body spaces or abscesses (AHFS, 1999). It is not recommended for use in pressure ulcers, because it and many other antiseptic agents are considered to be cytotoxic to normal tissues (Clinical Practice Guide Panel, 1994).

The official hydrogen peroxide solution has been further diluted with water into a ½ or ¼ strength for most applications. The mouth rinse or mouthwash (Peroxyl) is a 1.5% solution.

Side effects/adverse reactions. If a small amount of diluted hydrogen peroxide solution is swallowed, it rapidly decomposes in the stomach into relatively harmless molecular oxygen and water. Repeated use as a mouthwash may cause hypertrophied papillae of the tongue ("hairy tongue"), a reversible condition. The concentrated solutions used for hair bleaching may cause skin irritation and contact dermatitis.

■ Nursing Management
Oxidizing Agents

To delay deterioration of the contents, solutions are stored in tightly capped, amber containers to protect them from light and air. Solutions in containers should be discarded frequently, and fresh solutions should be used. The rapidity and vigor with which bubbling occurs may be used as a general guide to the freshness of the solution. The bubbling action makes hydrogen peroxide useful for removing mucus secretions from equipment (i.e., inner cannulae of tracheostomy tubes).

Do not leave paper cups containing hydrogen peroxide where clients can reach them. Because the solution looks like water, clients have mistakenly drunk it despite the unusual taste. Although very small amounts are not harmful, large amounts in the stomach can be harmful because of the resultant effervescence in the stomach, a closed cavity. As with all medications, these compounds should be kept secured and out of children's reach.

Biguanides

chlorhexidine [klor hex′ i deen] (Hibiclens)

Chlorhexidine is a biguanide with antiseptic action against both gram-positive and gram-negative bacteria, such as *Pseudomonas aeruginosa.* Chlorhexidine acts by disrupting the plasma membrane of the bacterial cell (particularly gram-positive organisms).

A bactericidal skin cleansing solution containing chlorhexidine (Hibiclens) is useful as a surgical scrub, as a hand-washing agent for personnel, and as a skin wound cleanser. Chlorhexidine oral rinse (Peridex, PerioGard) is also used as an antibacterial dental product to treat gingivitis between dental visits.

Chlorhexidine is a relatively safe antiseptic. There have been reports of deafness occurring when these products came into contact with the middle ear through a perforated eardrum. Rare secondary effects include dermatitis, photosensitivity, and irritation of mucosal tissue. The physiochemical properties of these agents suggest that absorption through the skin is minimal.

As a handwash, Hibiclens is applied, water is added, and friction is applied for 15 seconds. Skin wounds should be washed gently with Hibiclens and rinsed. For surgical scrubs, a brush or sponge is used to scrub the hands and forearms with approximately 5 mL Hibiclens for 3 minutes without water. After the hands and forearms are rinsed, the washing is repeated for 3 more minutes.

■ Nursing Management

Chlorhexidine

Use judgment when diluting these agents, because their effectiveness may be greatly reduced in proportion to the dilution. Certain solutions less than 4% may actually support bacterial growth. Chlorhexidine-treated areas should not be wiped with alcohol; this will neutralize the intended residual action. Do not use chlorhexidine on delicate tissues such as eyes and mucous membranes; these areas should be rinsed promptly if contact occurs. Advise clients not to swallow chlorhexidine compounds (especially when used for mouth care).

Surface-Active Agents

benzalkonium chloride [benz al koe′ nee um] (Zephiran Chloride)

As wetting agents, emulsifiers, or detergents, surface-acting agents are considered superior to soap because they can be used in hard water, are stable in acid or alkaline solutions, decrease surface tension more effectively, and are less irritating to the skin.

Benzalkonium chloride is a cationic (has a positive electric charge on the active portion of the agent) quaternary ammonium compound used in solution as a topical antiseptic or as a disinfectant. In general, it is believed that benzalkonium chloride is not very reliable in either role. As an antiseptic it has a limited antibacterial spectrum, because it lacks fast action and has a potential for inducing toxicity. As a disinfectant, it must be changed regularly to maintain concentration and effectiveness. It is also inactivated by anionic substances such as soap and organic materials.

The mechanism of action is not known for certain, but it may be due to the inactivation of bacterial enzymes.

Chemical burns may occur if benzalkonium chloride is allowed to stay in contact with tissues, as in wet packs or occlusive dressings. Delicate tissues may be injured if specified dilution recommendations are not used. Ingestion only rarely causes toxicity. Hypersensitivity reactions can occur. The tincture and the spray formulations are flammable.

Benzalkonium chloride is slow acting in comparison to iodine. The therapeutic effects are thought to be in direct relation to the concentration of the solution used. Depending on the purpose and tissues or equipment to be treated, recommended dilutions range from 1 : 750 (tincture or aqueous solutions) on intact skin, minor wounds, and abrasions to 1 : 5000 or 1 : 10,000 (aqueous solution) for mucous membranes and broken or diseased skin. A variety of gram-positive and gram-negative organisms and many fungi and viruses (not hepatitis) are said to be susceptible to this agent. Tap water that contains metallic ions, organic matter, or resin-deionized water may reduce its effectiveness.

■ Nursing Management

Benzalkonium Chloride

If any of these compounds have been used, continue to monitor the area or utensil critically for contamination. In view of the highly questionable efficacy of surface-active agents, especially benzalkonium chloride, question an order or a suggestion to use them as antiseptics or disinfectants. Suggest the substitution of an iodophor, alcohol, or other compound. Use only the concentration recommended for each specified area. Do not use them with occlusive dressings.

Do not apply these compounds to areas previously treated with soaps or anionic agents. Do not apply them to delicate tissues. Flood the area with water if these agents are accidentally introduced. Do not reuse solutions after soaking cotton balls, dressings, or instruments.

Avoid using benzalkonium chloride to disinfect thermometers. If it must be used, use not less than the recommended 1:750 concentration. Do not use the tincture of spray formulation near an open flame.

Miscellaneous Agents

Alcohols

ethanol [eth′ a nole] (ethyl alcohol)
isopropanol [eye soe proe′ pa nole] (isopropyl alcohol)

A 70% alcohol solution is antiseptic. The 70% aqueous solution is more effective than absolute alcohol in reducing the surface tension of bacterial cells, which precipitates protoplasm at the periphery of the cell and thus tends to inhibit penetration of the agent. Alcohol also inhibits the growth of bacteria, and thus it is often used as a preservative of biologic specimens and in some prepackaged injectables and medications. Alcohols are potent viricidal agents and may precipitate cellular proteins.

Alcohol is used topically as a bactericidal agent; to prepare skin for minor invasive procedures (using commercially packaged skin wipes); and for disinfection of heat-labile instruments, polyethylene tubing, catheters, implants, prostheses, smooth/hard-surfaced objects, hinged instruments, and inhalation and anesthesia equipment. Because of their rapid evaporation rate, dilute solutions of alcohols are still used occasionally as sponge baths to reduce fever, although systemic absorption may be especially harmful to neonates and children. Alcohols are also used as preservatives in solutions, as diluents, to dissolve other drugs, and in combination with many other drugs for over-the-counter purchase (often without rationale). Ethyl alcohol is also ingested purposefully as an intoxicating beverage.

Depending on the dose, essentially all alcohols are poisonous drugs when taken internally. Isopropyl alcohol is inherently highly poisonous. Ethyl alcohol is pure alcohol made from vegetables, fruits, canes, and grains, and it is used in alcoholic beverages. The degree to which fractional distillation is carried out determines the resultant concentration.

Alcohols can cause intoxication when continuously inhaled or absorbed through the skin. Ethyl alcohol is irritating if left in contact with the skin for prolonged periods. If ethyl alcohol is applied to open skin, a film develops and can harbor microorganisms. Isopropyl alcohol causes subcutaneous vasodilation, which can cause needle sites and incisions to bleed somewhat more freely.

Ethyl alcohol is slightly less effective as an antiseptic than isopropyl alcohol. Its efficacy may depend on the concentration used and the amount of mechanical friction applied. The most effective solutions of ethyl alcohol are concentrations of 50% to 70%; stronger solutions are less effective. At concentrations of 70%, almost 90% of the bacteria on the skin are killed within 2 minutes if the wet surface is allowed to dry naturally. Inadequate disinfection may occasionally result, even if friction is conscientiously applied to surfaces.

Isopropyl alcohol is used in aqueous solutions of 70% concentration or undiluted as 99% concentration (isopropyl rubbing alcohol). It may be combined with other disinfectants such as iodine and formaldehyde to improve efficiency.

▪ Nursing Management

Ethanol and Isopropanol

▪ **Assessment.** Alcohols should not be used to disinfect wounds, because they cause tissue irritation with painful burning and stinging and because they precipitate protein in which bacteria may grow. Use alcohols as a rub with caution for children, because the inhalation of fumes may be intoxicating.

▪ **Nursing Diagnosis.** There is a risk for poisoning in children and debilitated clients, because they are at risk for accidental exposure to or ingestion of these agents.

▪ **Implementation**

▪ ***Monitoring.*** If alcohol is applied externally to reduce fever, the client's temperature should be monitored regularly.

▪ ***Intervention.*** The antiseptic action of alcohols can be enhanced by mechanically cleansing the skin with water and a detergent before applying them, by gently rubbing the skin with a sterile gauze during application, and by allowing the area to dry for 2 minutes without fanning. Be prepared to apply more pressure and possibly a small pressure dressing after giving an injection or discontinuing an IV infusion if alcohol has been applied to the site, because evaporation of the alcohol may cause localized surface vasodilation. If the client is also receiving anticoagulant therapy, the bleeding may be extensive.

If alcohol is used in a home setting to disinfect thermometers, cleanse them with detergent and tepid water before placing them to soak in an alcohol solution; any adherent organic matter will inhibit the action of the solution. Alcohol solutions themselves may harbor organisms and may rust instruments; therefore they are often not the best solution for disinfecting or for sterile storage of equipment.

Applying an emollient alleviates the dry feeling of the skin after an alcohol rub.

▪ ***Education.*** Alert personnel, clients, and parents that all alcohols are inherently or potentially poisonous and that intoxication or dangerous poisoning can occur as a result of their absorption, inhalation, or ingestion. Keep alcohols secured and out of the reach of children.

▪ **Evaluation.** If alcohol is used for fever reduction, the expected outcome is that the client's temperature will be within normal limits. If it is used as an antiseptic to prepare the skin for a procedure, there will be no evidence of sepsis following the procedure.

Acids

acetic acid (vinegar); benzoic acid; lactic acid; boric acid

Various acids have been used as antiseptics or as cauterizing agents; of these, vinegar is the most commonly used, especially in community health nursing, because of its practicality, availability, and low cost. Other acids used as antiseptics include benzoic acid (0.1%), which prevents bacterial and fungous growth; lactic acid, which is used primarily as a component of spermatocides in the United States; and boric acid, which is so mild that it is used in eye and ear preparations. Of these other acids, most have lost credibility as effective antiseptics; for example, boric acid has been implicated in cases of serious systemic intoxication by absorption.

Acetic acid provides an acid medium that inhibits the growth of organisms dependent on a neutral or alkaline medium. In a 5% concentration, acetic acid is germicidal to many organisms and is bacteriostatic at lower concentrations. A mild vinegar solution is often recommended as a vaginal douche for antisepsis in the prevention or suppression of vaginal infections. Acetic acid may also be used as a mild antiseptic-deodorant for many other applications, such as bladder irrigation (0.25% concentration) and diaper soaks.

■ Nursing Management

Acetic Acid

A mildly effective, soothing vaginal douche can be prepared by adding 1 to 2 tablespoons of white household vinegar (5%) to 1 quart of warm water. Stronger concentrations are no more effective and may irritate mucosal tissues. The residual pungent odor of acetic acid may be a deterrent to its use.

The use of aseptic technique is essential when irrigating solutions are used for urethral catheters. The solution should not be used unless it is clear and the container is undamaged and has an intact seal. To minimize bacterial growth, the solution is to be used promptly after opening the container. Unused portions of the solutions should be discarded. Antiseptics instilled in urinary collection bags should be of concentrations that are not injurious to bladder mucosa in case the bag is inadvertently raised so that contents reflux into the bladder.

STERILANTS

Aldehydes

formaldehyde solution

Formaldehyde solution is a 37% concentration of formalin (by weight). It is a clear, colorless disinfectant liquid that liberates a pungent, irritating gas on exposure to air. In a concentration of 1% to 10%, it kills microorganisms and spores within 1 to 6 hours. It is effective against bacteria, fungi, and viruses and acts by combining with them to precipitate protein. It has been widely used as a disinfectant for instruments.

glutaraldehyde [gloo tuh ral′ dah hyde] (Cidex)

Glutaraldehyde (Cidex), 2% alkaline solution, is a liquid disinfectant used as a germicidal agent to disinfect and sterilize some rigid optical instruments and prosthetic equipment. It kills some microorganisms in 10 minutes and kills spores in 10 hours. However, the solution is unstable, and contact with skin should be avoided.

SUMMARY

Medical asepsis and surgical asepsis are used in health care settings to reduce the number and spread of organisms. Although thorough handwashing is still the best method for accomplishing this reduction, antiseptics, disinfectants, and sterilants need to be used. Antiseptics are chemicals typically applied to living tissue to decrease the microbial population; disinfectants are used only on nonliving objects because they are caustic to living tissue. Antiseptics and disinfectants may be bacteriostatic, bactericidal, or both depending on the concentrations used. Sterilants free objects of all forms and types of life. Although these substances are used for therapeutic purposes, they still are caustic and therefore require careful handling to prevent irritation and injury.

Critical Thinking Questions

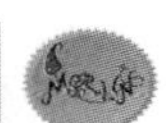

1. Given the criteria for the ideal antiseptic/disinfectant, which of the agents in this chapter would be closest to the ideal? Why?
2. Mrs. Taylor, age 24, was prescribed pHisoHex for her preoperative facial scrubs for the rhinoplasty she was having as a day-stay case. When she comes to the clinic for a postoperative follow-up visit, she asks about using the leftover pHisoHex for her baby's diaper rash. How do you respond?

Collaborative Learning Activities

For Collaborative Learning Activities, go to mosby.com/MERLIN/McKenry/.

BIBLIOGRAPHY

American Hospital Formulary Service. (1999). *AHFS drug information '99*. Bethesda, MD: American Society of Health-System Pharmacists.

Anderson, K.N., Anderson, L.E., & Glanze, W.D. (Eds.) (1998). *Mosby's medical, nursing, & allied health dictionary* (5th ed.). St. Louis: Mosby.

Bailey, T.C. & Powderly, W.G. (1992). Treatment of infectious disease. In M. Woodley & A. Whelan (Eds.), *The Washington manual: Manual of medical therapeutics* (27th ed.). Boston: Little, Brown.

Cheung, R.J., Ortiz, D., & DiMarino, A.J. Jr. (1999). GI endoscopic reprocessing practices in the United States. *Gastrointestinal Endoscopy, 50*(3), 362-368.

Clinical Practice Guide Panel. (1994). *Treatment of pressure sores: Clinical practice guideline,* No. 15. AHCPR Pub. No. 95-0652. Rockville, MD: U.S. Department of Health and Human Services. Public Health Service. Agency for Health Care Policy and Research.

DiPiro, J.T., Talbert, R.L., Yee, G.C., Matzke, G.R. Wells, B.G., & Posey, L.M. (Eds.). (1993). *Pharmacotherapy: A pathophysiologic approach* (2nd ed.). New York: Elsevier.

Drug Facts and Comparisons. (2000). St. Louis: Facts and Comparisons.

Federal Register. (1998). *Status of certain additional over-the-counter drug category II and III active ingredients. 63*(77), 19799-19802. Department of Health and Human Services, Food and Drug Administration.

Jones, R.D. (1999). Bacterial resistance and topical antimicrobial wash products. *American Journal of Infection Control, 27*(4), 351-363.

Katzung, B.G. (1998). *Basic and Clinical Pharmacology* (7th ed.). Norwalk, CT: Appleton & Lange.

Siegel, J.E., Weinstein, M.C., Fineberg, H.V. (1991). Bleach programs for preventing AIDS among IV users: Modeling the impact of HIV prevalence. *American Journal of Public Health, 81*(10), 1273-1279.

United States Pharmacopeia Dispensing Information (USP DI): Drug information for the health care professional (19th ed.). (1999). Rockville, MD: United States Pharmacopeial Convention.

72 Diagnostic Agents

Chapter Focus

Diagnostic and laboratory tests are one more source of information for the nurse in the assessment and ongoing monitoring of clients. The nurse is also responsible for preparing the client for diagnostic studies and for coordinating the completion of these tests. Many of these examinations require diagnostic agents with which the nurse needs to be knowledgeable in order to provide appropriate instruction and care for clients undergoing diagnostic testing.

Learning Objectives

1. Describe the mechanism of action of radiopaque contrast medium.
2. State the method of absorption, metabolism, and excretion of barium sulfate and iodinated contrast media.
3. Discuss the nursing assessments necessary to detect side effects/adverse reactions of iodinated contrast medium and the appropriate nursing interventions to manage the initial symptoms.
4. Explain the pharmacokinetics of diagnostic agents used as radioactive tracers and imaging agents.
5. State the indications, secondary effects, and nursing management of common nonradioactive agents used for evaluating organ function and challenging glandular response.
6. Discuss the common tests used to screen selected health conditions.

Key Terms

computed tomography (CT), p. 1214
diagnostic agents, p. 1210
nuclear magnetic resonance imaging (MRI), p. 1214
radionuclides, p. 1212
radiopharmaceutical agents, p. 1212
ultrasonography, p. 1214

Diagnostic agents are chemical substances used to diagnose or monitor a client's condition or disease. With diagnostic agents, certain secondary chemical characteristics are used to confirm a diagnosis or prognosis or to guide therapy. One type of diagnostic agent may interact with a bodily fluid specimen as a reagent to produce a color as an indicator, whereas another may induce an inflammatory response or enhance the functioning of a particular gland.

Other agents may act by contrasting and enhancing visibility on an x-ray film of the lumens or cavities of internal body structures. Some permit critical assessment of organ function because of a special affinity and uptake by certain organs. As with any drug, diagnostic agents may have side effects and adverse reactions. Thus it is necessary that the nurse know the agent used, its mechanism of action, and its indications for use. Secondary effects are equally important, because many agents have a somewhat narrow range of safety. In some instances, nurses are responsible for correctly collecting and testing specimens and interpreting the results. Specialized training and professional education are necessary to administer some types of agents; others are packaged in simple kit form for over-the-counter sale. Because the field of diagnostics and its products is burgeoning, manufacturers' instructions should always be consulted to ensure that the most current information is obtained.

RADIOPAQUE AGENTS FOR VISUALIZING ORGAN STRUCTURE

When injected or instilled, radiopaque agents make the body cavity or compartment more radiographically dense or opaque than neighboring anatomic structures. They are used when the structural integrity of a soft-tissue organ system is under study. Ordinary x-ray examinations are useful only for studies of dense materials such as bone. Radiopaque contrast media may also permit visualization of the functional dynamics of organs as part of associated diagnostic tests.

Many of these agents contain molecular iodine in the radiopaque contrast medium to provide the opacity necessary for outlining internal organ cavities, lumens, or ducts that would otherwise be invisible by x-ray study or fluoroscopy.

Barium contrast media consist of barium sulfate powder and a vehicle such as hydrosol gum, which are mixed with a prescribed volume of water to provide a suspension for oral or rectal administration. Iodinated radiopaque agents consist of substituted, triiodinated, benzoic acid derivatives or water-soluble, triiodinated, benzoic acid salts. Check the manufacturers' instructions for ingredients.

The prescriber should be consulted when a client reports a history of idiosyncratic response; a hypersensitivity to iodine, shellfish, or contrast media; or a history of multiple radiographic or radionuclide studies. The most common radiopaque contrast agents are barium sulfate suspensions and iodinated contrast materials. Table 72-1 lists the iodine content of and indications for selected medications.

Indications

1. Barium-containing preparations are typically used to opacify the gastrointestinal (GI) tract. In general, these preparations are used when ulcers, inflammatory bowel disease, or cancer is suspected. One of the most common uses of barium contrast media is in "double-contrast" studies for gastrointestinal tract evaluation. "Double contrast" is a method of making an x-ray image by using two contrast agents—usually a gaseous medium and a water-soluble radiopaque agent.
2. The most common clinical use of iodinated contrast media includes IV urography and angiography. Iodinated contrast media are often used during computed tomography (CT) of the head and body to visualize vascular structures and to detect tumors.

Pharmacokinetics. Radiopaque agents may be administered by the oral, vaginal, rectal, IV, or intraarterial routes, or they may be instilled into other body cavities. Orally administered iodinated agents for visualization of the gallbladder are absorbed across the GI mucosa and enter the systemic circulation through the portal venous system. Orally or rectally administered iodinated media for delineation of the GI tract are absorbed only minimally but are absorbed enough that the renal tract may also be visualized. Barium sulfate preparations are not absorbed. They are metabolized by the liver and gallbladder and excreted by the kidneys.

Side Effects/Adverse Reactions. Radiopaque agents are not without risk. The effects are diverse, mild to moderate in severity, and usually occur within 1 to 3 minutes. Delayed reactions may occur up to 1 hour after injection. Anaphylaxis and hypersensitivity reactions are also reported.

IV cholangiography has caused the highest number of reactions and has therefore been largely replaced by radionuclide diagnostics and retrograde duodenal examination. Excretory urography is commonly performed, and serious reactions are rare. Milder reactions result from the administration of oral cholecystographic agents. Certain agents are more likely to cause secondary effects than others; the manufacturers' information should be consulted.

A history of allergy puts the client at twice the risk of reaction to contrast media although, paradoxically, these are not true hypersensitivity reactions. Clients with a previous anaphylactoid reaction to contrast media may have an increased risk of tenfold or more (*Drug Facts and Comparisons*, 2000).

Because they are not absorbed internally, barium sulfate preparations are only potentially hazardous when administered to persons with bowel perforations or fistulas. Barium sulfate may cause constipation if allowed to remain in the colon. Hospitalization and close observation during the procedures are recommended for clients who have a high potential for reactions or complications.

The most commonly reported side effects are nausea or flushing, with feelings of warmth over the abdomen and chest. Severely dehydrated clients, older adults, infants, and the seriously ill tolerate these hemodynamic and hyperosmolar changes less well than others do.

TABLE 72-1 Medications, Iodine Content, and Indications

Medication	Indications	Iodine Content
Contrast Media		
diatrizoate sodium injection (Hypaque Sodium)	Cerebral angiography Aortography Cholangiography	150 mg/mL (25% solution) 300 mg/mL (50% solution)
iocetamic acid (Cholebrine)	Oral cholecystography	465 mg/750 mg tablet
iopanoic acid (Telepaque)	Oral cholecystography	333 mg/500 mg tablet
ipodate (Oragrafin)	Oral cholecystography	3 g contains 61.7% iodine
tyropanoate (Bilopaque)	Oral cholecystography	430 mg/750 mg capsule
Other Agents		
amiodarone (Cordarone)	Antidysrhythmic	74 mg/200 mg tablet
iodoquinol (Yodoxin)	Antiprotozoal	134-416 mg/tablet
echothiophate iodide ophthalmic (Phospholine Iodide)	Antiglaucoma Cyclostimulant Diagnostic aid	5-41 μg/drop
idoxuridine ophthalmic (Herplex, Stoxil)	Antiviral	18 μg/drop

Information from Farwell, A.P. & Braverman, L.E. (1996). Thyroid and antithyroid drugs. In J.G. Hardman & L.E. Limbird (Eds.), *Goodman & Gilman's The pharmacological basis of therapeutics* (9th ed.). New York: McGraw-Hill; and *United States Pharmacopeia Dispensing Information (USP DI): Drug information for the health care professional* (19th ed.). (1999). Rockville, MD: United States Pharmacopeial Convention.

Diazoate salts may inhibit blood coagulation, which can cause a severe thromboembolic event. Platelet aggregation is inhibited by several agents. Exacerbations of sickle cell disease may result from intravascular injections of contrast media.

Rare adverse reactions include cerebral hematomas, hemodynamic alterations, sinus bradycardia, transient ECG changes, ventricular fibrillation, and petechiae.

Renal system involvement may be manifested by nephrosis of the proximal tubular cells in excretory urography; this condition may proceed to renal failure. Altered respiratory status may include rhinitis, cough, dyspnea, bronchospasm, asthma, laryngeal or pulmonary edema, and subclinical pulmonary emboli.

The senses may be impaired (e.g., distorted taste sensations; irritated, itching, tearing eyes; conjunctivitis). Hypersensitivity reactions and anaphylaxis may occur. A history of allergy predisposes the client to reactions to contrast media.

■ Nursing Management

Radiopaque Agents

■ **Assessment.** Radiographic examinations are not without hazard to the client or to personnel. The risk-benefit ratios must be established on an individual basis. Reactions may arise from either the physical or the chemical properties of the compounds used. Almost any organ system may be affected (see Side Effects/Adverse Reactions). Conduct a careful history related to kidney, thyroid, or liver disease. Obtain an allergy history, and pay particular attention to the client's previous reactions to tartrazine, contrast media, or iodine-containing foods (e.g., shellfish or iodized table salt). For clients with a history of iodine hypersensitivity and those with a generally positive allergy history, pretreatment with prednisone, diphenhydramine (Benadryl), and ephedrine may minimize but not prevent hypersensitivity reactions. This pretreatment regimen reduced the incidence of adverse reactions in one study from 35% to 3%. Do not mix these pretreatment medications for concurrent administration with the contrast media; they are incompatible.

It is recommended that radiography, fluoroscopy, or CT not be performed on female clients if they are pregnant or if it has been 10 days since their last menstrual period.

Medications should be held during the preparation period for examinations using radiopaque agents. Consult with the prescriber for instructions for essential medications, such as antivirals or medications for epilepsy.

Perform a baseline assessment of the client's vital signs, mental status, and level of consciousness before testing.

■ **Nursing Diagnosis.** The client receiving radiopaque agents for diagnostic testing should be assessed for the following nursing diagnoses/collaborative problems: impaired comfort (flushing of the skin, nausea); impaired tissue integrity related to irritation or extravasation at the injection site; ineffective protection related to leukopenia, thrombocytopenia, and anemia; constipation; and the potential complications of hypersensitivity to the agent, nephrotoxicity, and adverse cardiovascular and CNS effects of the agent.

■ **Implementation**

■ ***Monitoring.*** Monitor levels of consciousness and vital signs during the procedure as feasible and after the procedure for at least 1 hour. Monitor for flushing of the skin, nausea, and other untoward effects of the agents.

■ ***Intervention.*** Prepare clients appropriately for their examinations using protocols from the radiology department. A repeat preparation and examination may be necessary if visualization was sufficiently impaired. Such impairment results if the bowels are inadequately prepared, if tablets are not taken as directed, or if foods and fluids other than water are not withheld. The manufacturers' instructions for dose preparation and administration should be followed. Iodinated radiopaque agents may be instilled or administered orally (tablets, paste, granules, or suspensions), rectally (enema), or parenterally. If tablet form of the agent is used, 4 to 6 tablets may need to be taken over a short interval the morning before the test, with the client ingesting nothing else but water after their administration.

Barium sulfate compounds are noniodinated, and most are prepared from powders for suspensions to be taken orally or instilled rectally. The volume of orally administered reconstituted agents is approximately 8 ounces; the enema volume may range from 500 to 1500 mL. IV injection volumes vary according to the agent—from 20 to 300 mL. Certain high concentrations of iothalamate solutions should never be directly injected into carotid or vertebral arteries. Older adults should be hydrated before barium tests to help prevent posttest constipation.

Nurses should ask for lead shielding devices and client-supporting devices before participating in radiographic examinations. Nurses who are often involved in such examinations should monitor their cumulative exposure by wearing a film badge that is checked monthly or quarterly. It is worn outside any shields, and reports are obtained. A bedpan, an emesis basin, tissues, and a warm blanket are transported with the patient to the client to the radiology department (the room temperature and the equipment in radiologic units are often noted to be cold).

Have drugs, equipment, and medical assistance readily available in case of an emergency such as cardiac arrest.

Obtain an order for a laxative to prevent constipation after a barium enema, or similarly instruct the client.

■ ***Education.*** Apprise clients and all those working in an environment of ionizing radiation that there may be current and long-term effects of radiation, which are cumulative. There is no established safe dosage, single or cumulative; therefore keep exposure to a minimum. The risks and benefits of each procedure should be weighed carefully by the clinician and the informed client.

Instruct the client, as appropriate, to prepare for the specific examination. This may require the client to take the agent with water the night before the procedure, to receive an enema, or not to ingest anything but water until the test is completed. Explain as appropriate that the procedure may include the administration of approximately 8 ounces of a fairly thick oral suspension or a retention enema and that position changes may be necessary during the procedure.

■ **Evaluation.** The expected outcome of the use of radiopaque agents is that client will complete the diagnostic procedure successfully without experiencing any adverse reactions to the agents.

AGENTS FOR EVALUATING ORGAN FUNCTION

Some diagnostic agents can be used to track and visualize the functional processes of organ systems. Inferences can be made about organ function by measuring the degree to which or the rate at which the agent is distributed, taken up, sequestered, secreted, or excreted from the target organ system or by measuring the volume or flow rates. Some diagnostic agents are **radionuclides** (a species of radioactive atom characterized by a higher atomic number than bodily tissues) whose gamma-ray emissions can be tracked or whose residues can be sampled. Other nonradioactive agents are dyes, polysaccharides, or other substances whose dissemination may be traced by color changes or chemical analysis.

Radioactive Agents

A radionuclide is an unstable form of a chemical element. **Radiopharmaceutical agents** are those in which one of the nonradioactive atoms has been replaced by a radioactive atom. They are either of natural origin or are produced by particle accelerators or generators. The process of neutron activation used in nuclear medicine to produce radionuclides describes the capture of a slow neutron into a stable nucleus with the subsequent emission of a gamma ray. Transmutation is a similar operation but uses a fast neutron. After the injection or ingestion of the resultant nuclide, its distribution can be followed by a gamma-ray detector combined with a rectilinear scanner, scintillation camera, or other radiation-display device. Substances such as glucose, ^{14}C, air, blood, lymph, spinal fluids, urine, or biopsy specimens may be collected and the residual radioactivity analyzed or counted as it is excreted. These data are used to make inferences about organ disorders and the body's ability to absorb, metabolize, or excrete substances.

Ionizing Radiation. Through the use of radiation, much can be learned that could not otherwise be discovered or diagnosed. As with any other diagnostic technique, a risk-benefit ratio must be determined. Ionizing radiation has the ability to knock electrons out of atoms to create electrically charged ions. This radiation may be defined as electromagnetic radiation (x-rays and gamma rays) or particulate radiation (electrons, occasionally beta particles, protons, neutrons, or atomic nuclei with kinetic energy).

Impact by emitted radiation energy may disrupt bonds between atoms in crucial biologic molecules such as DNA. Disruption can lead to cell death, mutations, or defective mitosis. Energy that is absorbed by tissues can lead to acute effects (as in radiotherapy or radiation accidents) or chronic effects (as from multiple low-radiation doses). Effects such as cataracts may appear only after long periods or in subsequent generations.

The amount of radiation absorbed by the tissues during radiologic tests is determined by the dose administered, the half-life of the radionuclide, the energy, the mode of decay, and the length of time the agent dwells in the body. There is no known safe dosage of ionizing radiation, despite limits set by the Nuclear Regulatory Commission and the National Council on Radiation, Protection and Measurements.

Estimations of the amount of radiation emitted, the effect, and the dose absorbed may be denoted by the following terms:

- *Roentgen:* the amount of gamma or x-ray radiation that creates 1 electrostatic unit of ions in 1 mL of air at 0° C
- *Rem:* the predicted effect on the human body of a 1-roentgen dose
- *Rad:* a unit of measurement of absorbed ionizing radiation energy; one rad = 100 ergs of radiation energy per gram of matter

Although arbitrary, the annual limits of radiation for the general population and for any single gestational period are set at 0.5 rem (for x-rays, 1 rem is equal to 1 rad) and for closely monitored occupational workers at approximately 3 rem/year. Most nurses, physicians, and other health care personnel are not routinely monitored for radiation exposure unless assigned to an area with a high potential for exposure. Their risk for cumulative exposure is nonetheless higher than that of the general population (see the Nursing Research box at right).

Very little is known about the full effects of radiation. Certain increased risks are associated: infertility, birth defects, potential for certain malignant neoplasms, and manifestations of aging. Exposure to low-level ionizing radiation (e.g., from radiographic examinations) and agents containing radionuclides add to the individual's total radiation history. The effects may be insidious, perhaps manifesting themselves in crucial enzyme defects many years after exposure. There is some evidence of the body's ability to repair chromosomal damage, but the scope of this ability is unknown.

The term *excessive radiation exposure* describes any unnecessary exposure above natural background levels. Although natural background radiation adds to the cumulative risk, medical and dental therapies account for the largest proportion of artificially generated exposure.

Indications. Most radionuclides in use today in radiology are for imaging organs, evaluating organ function, or detecting or treating cancer. The role of nuclear imaging is gradually diminishing because of increased reliance on CT, ultrasound, and magnetic resonance imaging.

Radionuclides are used as tracers to evaluate the physiologic and biochemical functioning of organ systems. With imaging methods, extremely sensitive radioactivity sensing devices make it possible to detect, count, visualize, and analyze minute amounts of radionuclides. Uniquely useful applications of nuclear imagery include the following:

1. Assessing thyroid enlargement or disease. Agents currently used include ^{131}I and ^{123}I. These iodine isotopes emit a type of radiation that can be mapped externally. A 24-hour uptake study is usually used to determine the extent and areas of thyroid activity. A scan is then performed to evaluate any thyroid mass or enlargement. "Cold" tumors have a 20% to 25% probability of representing a thyroid cancer. Tumors that localize the radionuclide well are usually benign.

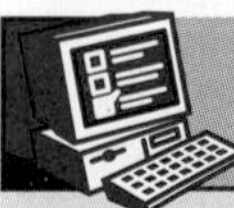

Nursing Research

Radiation Hazard in the Health Care Environment

Citation: Dewey, P., & Incoll, I. (1998). Evaluation of thyroid shields for reduction of radiation exposure to orthopedic surgeons, *ANZ Journal of Surgery 68*(9):635-636; Muller, L.P., Suffner, J., Wenda, K., Mohr, W., & Rommens, P.M. (1998). Radiation exposure to the hands and thyroid of the surgeon during intramedullary nailing, *Injury 29*(6):461-468; and Singer, C.M., Baraff, L.J., Benedict, S.H., Weiss, E.L., Singer, B.D. (1989). Exposure of emergency medicine personnel to ionizing radiation during cervical spine radiography. *Annals of Emergency Medicine, 18*(8), 822-825.

Abstract: There is a risk of ionizing radiation exposure to health care workers who routinely function in areas where x-ray studies are performed outside of radiology departments. To study the exposure of health workers who stabilized the necks of trauma clients during cervical spine radiography, Singer et al. (1989) used an artificial torso and placed a radiation monitor where a health worker's fingers, hands, arms, and thyroid gland would be while standard cervical spine radiographs were taken. If the simulated exposures were indicative of actual client situations, a health care worker who holds the head of a trauma client four times each week with unshielded hands would receive more than twice the maximum allowable annual occupational radiation exposure to the extremities as recommended by the National Council of Radiation Protection and Measurements. It was concluded that health workers who routinely stabilize the necks of trauma clients during cervical spine radiography may incur a radiation risk and that 0.5-mm lead-equivalent gloves provide an effective barrier to ionizing radiation (Singer et al., 1989). Muller and others (1998) looked at radiation exposure to the hands and thyroid area of orthopedic surgeons. They found the average registered ionizing dosage without a thyroid shield to be approximately 70 times higher than with thyroid lead protection. Although the risk of radiation exposure is known, Dewey and Incoll (1998) found the availability and usage of thyroid shields to be low.

The rules and regulations of federal agencies and state radiation protection programs provide the basis for hospital policy regarding radiation safety for nurses. Each agency with radiology services has a radiation safety officer to ensure that radiation exposures to health care personnel are as low as reasonably achievable and that special considerations are given to pregnant nurses (Jankowski, 1992).

Critical Thinking Questions

- Why is it particularly important that pregnant women be protected from radiation?
- Many nurses and other health care providers have a strong fear—almost a phobia—of radiation. Why might that be so? What could be done to minimize this fear?

For answer guidelines for these *new Critical Thinking Questions,* go to mosby.com/MERLIN/McKenry/. 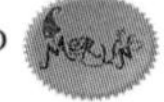

2. Screening clients with diagnosed malignancies for metastases. Many clients treated for breast cancer, colon cancer, malignant melanoma, lymphoma, prostate cancer, lung cancer, and other cancers are often successfully evaluated by periodic scintigrams of the liver, spleen, and skeletal system. A scintigraph is a photographic recording that shows the distribution and intensity of radioactivity in various tissues and organs following the administration of a radiopharmaceutical. The risk-benefit ratio is very high, and information about new or recurrent disease can help the oncologist and the client make crucial decisions about goals, management, prognosis, and so forth.
3. Evaluating heart disease. This is a primary application of nuclear imagery. Computers are used to analyze data from the images to detect the extent of myocardial damage and wall motion abnormalities and to estimate the ejection fraction of the ventricles. Underlying coronary artery disease can also be estimated with radionuclides before catheterization or other invasive procedures.
4. Tracking physiologic substances and assessing the status of an organ (e.g., renal function, biliary excretion). In addition to diagnostic uses, some radiopharmaceuticals may be administered therapeutically to deliver radiation to internal body tissues (e.g., ^{131}I for the destruction of thyroid tissue in hyperthyroidism). Radioactive tracer substances may also be incorporated into a nonradioactive drug to track the pharmacokinetics of the second drug for research purposes.

Computed tomography scans body parts in a series of contiguous slices with pencil-thin x-ray beams; after these beams pass through the body, they produce data from detectors positioned diametrically across from the beam source. Huge amounts of data are integrated and displayed by the computer as a video image. CT presents a series of two-dimensional images that represent a reconstructed "slice" in the axial plane. By viewing a series of these images, the anatomy can be perceived in a three-dimensional sense. CT therefore often conveys more information than other modalities about lesion density, location, and size.

CT has largely replaced older techniques such as pneumoencephalography and angiography in the diagnosis of intracranial disease, although angiography is still used for this application. CT may eliminate the need for other x-ray examinations, but it is not considered a first-line or screening technique. Radionuclide scans continue to be used for initial diagnostic screening and for specific tests where their results are more fruitful. Radiation exposure from CT varies depending on the equipment used and the frequency of testing, but it is said to be equal to or sometimes considerably higher than ordinary x-ray techniques or radionuclides. Although CT is considered to be a noninvasive procedure, IV contrast material is often injected to enhance structures for differential diagnosis. This is referred to as CT with infusion.

Ultrasonography is a nonradioactive diagnostic modality with cardiovascular, abdominal, obstetric, and other applications. It is used with anatomic and physiologic information obtained by other nuclear medicine techniques. Ultrasound examinations yield data about organ contours and tissue consistency or, in the case of Doppler scanning, blood flow patterns. Results can be distorted by the presence of bone or gases in the body. The secondary effects of high-frequency sound waves on cellular structures and functions are not fully known, but such tests are considered to be noninvasive and innocuous by many in the field.

Nuclear magnetic resonance imaging (MRI) is a diagnostic modality that uses radio waves and a magnet, not radiation, drugs, biopsy specimens, or body fluids. Like CT, MRI provides sectioned imagery but gives more than the gross anatomic information gained by CT scanning. MRI supplies extremely detailed images of internal heart and brain structures, and it is capable of imaging areas of the spine, abdomen, and extremities. It can differentiate between lesions and normal tissue. Persons ineligible for diagnosis with MRI include those with metal prostheses or pacemakers, because the strong magnetic field surrounding the client may move some metallic devices, or the metallic object may result in a distorted test image.

Pharmacokinetics. Each type of radionuclide emits alpha or beta particles or gamma rays or a combination of these. This spontaneous emission of charged particles is termed *radioactive decay* and eventually results in disintegration of the nucleus. The time it takes for the original radioactivity to decay to one half its original value is known as the physical or radioactive *half-life* of the particular radionuclide. As with drugs, the rate at which a tracer substance is excreted from the body also influences its effects, both valuable and undesirable.

Dosage and Administration. The manufacturers' current directions should be reviewed. Dosages are not detailed here because they vary with the needs of the client.

The major considerations in radionuclide dosing are the amount of radioactivity that is administered to produce effective readings and secondary radionuclide effects. Although the radioactive material is in the body, it irradiates even after the study has been completed; in contrast, x-rays irradiate from an external source and do so only while the body is exposed during the examination. The radionuclide dosage unit for imaging or nonimaging doses of radionuclide is a *microcurie* (one millionth of a curie). A *curie* is a specified measure of radioactivity associated with a specific amount of a radioactive substance (e.g., a radionuclide). Recommended dosages are spelled out in the manufacturers' literature. The client's absorbed dose of each radionuclide has been predicted for each procedure, with the following three factors being considered: (1) the biologic parameters that describe the uptake, distribution, retention, and release of the radiopharmaceutical in the body; (2) the energy released by the radionuclide and whether it is penetrating or nonpenetrating; and (3) the fraction of emitted energy that is absorbed by the target.

The ultimate radiation dose to both the target organ and the entire body is somewhat less in radionuclide nonimaging procedures than in imaging procedures. It is considerably more in radiation therapy, which is not discussed here.

Shielding is a practical method to prevent or reduce the excess radiation exposure of staff or clients during certain diagnostic examinations. Shielding reduces the intensity of radiation to acceptable limits in body areas not intended for exposure during the radiologic examination. Alpha and beta radiation require very little shielding. An alpha particle can be blocked by the thickness of a sheet of paper, and a beta particle can be blocked by an inch of wood; however, several feet of concrete or several inches of lead are necessary to stop gamma ray or x-ray radiation. *Half-value layer* is the term describing the thickness of any material required to reduce the intensity of an x-ray or gamma-ray beam to half its original value. Because of its characteristic density, lead is the material typically used for radiation shielding equipment and for coverings such as aprons and gloves.

■ Nursing Management

Radioactive Agents

In addition to the following discussion, see Nursing Management: Radiopaque Agents, p. 1211.

The basic principles of radiation exposure safety are relative to the source of radiation, the *time* spent in the radioactive field, the *distance* from the source, and *shielding*. The amount of radiation absorbed is directly proportional to the time spent in a radioactive field and inversely related to the distance from the source of radioactive emission. Thus quality nursing care requires careful planning so that limitations on time spent in the radioactive field do not reduce the quality of client care.

Wear rubber or plastic gloves when handling bedpans, urine specimens, or continuous drainage bags of clients within a day or two after nuclear medicine procedures. Wherever radionuclides are used, one person (designated the radiation safety officer) has the responsibility for safety in case of spills or accidents with radioactive materials. This officer should be consulted if there is a break in safety procedures or if, for example, linen has been contaminated by vomitus or excreta within 24 hours of administration of a radiopharmaceutical. Although it may be determined that unusual precautions are not needed, it is wise to seek consultation as needed.

Follow the instructions of the radiopharmaceutical manufacturers about radionuclide storage (some require refrigeration), dosage, and technique. Errors in technique must not be tolerated, especially with regard to handling radiopharmaceuticals, disposing of contaminated equipment, and properly shielding all who are present for radiologic and imaging procedures. Monitoring badges should be worn by those who regularly participate in these procedures. Protection should be ensured for those who are unfamiliar with these procedures. Women of childbearing age who had their last menstrual period more than 10 days ago or who are pregnant should not assist. (*Radiation therapy* requires other precautions.)

The client's anxiety may be heightened by the uncertainty of unknown diagnosis, a fear of radiation, and cold or unfamiliar surroundings. Clients may be introduced to the personnel, surroundings, and large equipment some time before the scheduled examination and given the opportunity for questions and explanations.

Clients should be taught that there may be some discomfort at the site of injection, taste alterations, or a feeling of warmth or discomfort in various parts of the body if the administered agent contains an iodine preparation. If a counter or rectilinear scanner is used, clients should be advised that it may typically emit irregular clicks as it collects data; it does not emit radiation. Clients may be required to maintain a single position on a hard surface for extended periods, or they may be restrained for a brief period; supply foam wedge supports and coverings as necessary. Explain that personnel may wear strange-looking gray or green apparel to shield them from excess radiation and that clients will also be protected according to established protocols.

Give clients written instructions, especially about the specific time they should return for the examination after the nuclide dose. Explain that the test must be performed at a very specific time after the medication is administered (at the point of a specific half-life).

Follow the policies of the health care agency regarding the length, frequency, and duration of exposure to clients in the posttest period. In addition, provide instructions for caring for the client at home.

Nonradioactive Agents

Nonradioactive Agents for Evaluating Organ Function via Volumes and Flows

These relatively biologically inert and nonradioactive substances are commonly used to measure flow rates, fluid volumes, diffusion, concentration ability, and organ function. These compounds are mostly dyes, polysaccharides, or other substances that can be assayed chemically or detected by characteristic colors after administration. Many of the dye tests determine the rate of plasma clearance of the dye by the organ under study. The ability to measure certain parameters against known normal values at defined points in the procedure makes these compounds useful as diagnostic aids. They are used variously to evaluate processes such as cardiac output, liver or kidney function, blood flow, circulation time, and intestinal absorption (Table 72-2).

These compounds are administered primarily by the IV or IM routes. They are rapidly absorbed by the organ system under examination and are usually excreted by that system. These drugs are relatively pharmacologically inert and are used to measure specific physiologic functions without themselves significantly altering those functions (Table 72-3).

Nonradioactive Agents for Challenging Glandular Response

Certain compounds are used diagnostically to challenge a particular system (often glandular) to produce measurable responses. Secretory responses indicate whether or not

TABLE 72-2 Multiple Urine Test Products*

Product & Distributor	Glucose	Protein	pH	Blood	Ketones	Bilirubin	Urobilinogen	Nitrite	Leukocytes
Chemstrip 2 GP (Boehringer Mannheim)	X	X							
Uristix (Bayer Corp)	X	X							
Combistix (Bayer Corp)	X	X	X						
Hema-Combistix (Bayer Corp)	X	X	X	X					
Uristix 4 (Bayer Corp)	X	X						X	X
Chemstrip 4 the OB (Boehringer Mannheim)	X	X		X					X
Chemstrip uGK (Boehringer Mannheim)	X				X				
Keto-Diastix (Bayer Corp)	X				X				
Chemstrip 6 (Boehringer Mannheim)	X	X	X	X	X				X
Labstix (Bayer Corp)	X	X	X	X	X				
Bili-Labstix (Bayer Corp)	X	X	X	X	X	X			
Chemstrip 7 (Boehringer Mannheim)	X	X	X	X	X	X			X
Multistix (Bayer Corp)	X	X	X	X	X	X	X		
Multistix SG† (Bayer Corp)	X	X	X	X	X	X	X		
Multistix 7 (Bayer Corp)	X	X	X	X	X			X	X
Multistix 8 SG† (Bayer Corp)	X	X	X	X	X			X	X
Chemstrip 8 (Boehringer Mannheim)	X	X	X	X	X	X	X		X
N-Multistix (Bayer Corp)	X	X	X	X	X	X	X	X	
N-Multistix SG† (Bayer Corp)	X	X	X	X	X	X	X	X	
Multistix 9 SG† (Bayer Corp)	X	X	X	X	X	X		X	X
Multistix 10 SG† (Bayer Corp)	X	X	X	X	X	X	X	X	X
Chemstrip 10 With SG† (Boehringer Mannheim)	X	X	X	X	X	X	X	X	X
Chemstrip 9 (Boehringer Mannheim)	X	X	X	X	X	X	X	X	X
Multistix 9 (Bayer Corp)	X	X	X	X	X	X	X	X	X
Chemstrip 2 LN (Boehringer Mannheim)								X	X
Multistix 2 (Bayer Corp)								X	X
Biotel Kidney (Biotel)		X		X					

*To make simultaneous determinations of two or more urine tests.

†Also tests specific gravity.

there is functional integrity within the secreting gland or system. Many of these testing agents are protein substances that mimic the action of naturally occurring bodily chemicals, such as secretagogues for exocrine gland response and stimulants for endocrine secretion. Because most of these agents are administered intramuscularly or intravenously, they move rapidly to the site of action. The degradation of these agents is equally rapid.

Nonradioactive agents are used to evaluate or enhance capabilities such as thyroid secretion, gallbladder contraction, insulin response, and gastric acid secretory function. These testing agents act on the targeted gland or site as releasing factors. Thus the secondary effects may be as widespread and disruptive to bodily chemical balance as a large dose of the secretion or hormone itself (Table 72-4).

Epinephrine, antihistamines, corticoids, and a tourniquet should be readily available for all tests in case of severe reactions. Analgesics, nasogastric suction equipment, vasodilators (for histamine agents), IV glucose solutions (for tolbutamide), and atropine (for edrophonium) should also be kept available. The manufacturers' instructions should be followed very closely, because nearly all of these compounds are administered parenterally and in very small doses.

AGENTS FOR SCREENING AND MONITORING IMMUNE DISORDERS AND IMMUNE STATUS

Screening and monitoring agents may be extracts of common allergens (ragweed, grasses, trees, molds, animal dander, and foods); purified derivatives or concentrates of microbial antigens, hormones, or animal cellular antigens; or

TABLE 72-3 Selected Nonradioactive Agents for Evaluation of Organ Function

Agent	Indication(s)	Secondary Effects	Nursing Management
aminohippurate sodium	Measures renal plasma flow and tubular secretory mechanism	Nausea, vomiting, cramping, flushing, and tingling	Give IV at a constant rate. Use caution with clients with low cardiac reserve; may precipitate congestive heart failure. Have atropine at hand to relieve severe anticholinergic reactions.
D-xylose (Xylo-Pfan)	Evaluates intestinal absorption	Infrequent: nausea, vomiting, cramps, and diarrhea	A number of medical conditions give false-positives with this test; check the literature.
indocyanine green (CardioGreen)	Measures cardiac output and hepatic function; used for ophthalmic angiography	Low incidence of side effects	Use caution with clients who have a history of iodide allergy. IV via cardiac catheter.
inulin	Diagnostic for renal function	Minimal side effects	IV injection.
mannitol (Osmitrol)	Diuretic, antiglaucoma, antihemolytic	Dry mouth, thirst, headache, acidosis, dehydration; contraindicated in anuria, intracranial bleeding, severe dehydration, and pulmonary edema	IV infusion. Monitor vital signs and urinary output closely.

Information from American Hospital Formulary Service. (1999). *AHFS drug information '99*. Bethesda, MD: American Society of Hospital Pharmacists; and *United States Pharmacopeia Dispensing Information (USP DI): Drug information for the health care professional* (19th ed.). (1999). Rockville, MD: United States Pharmacopeial Convention.

chemical reagents. Many chemical reagents for common diagnostic purposes are packaged in simple kit form for over-the-counter or prescribed purchase; they may also be used routinely in institutions and in primary health care settings.

Mechanism of Action and Pharmacokinetics. Antigens applied topically or intradermally cause antigen-antibody reactions, which may be manifested by a local inflammatory response at the test site. The test site is assessed after a prescribed time interval. A positive response is indicated by the presence of erythema and induration (a firm lump under the skin). In the case of microbial antigen challenge, this positive response may merely indicate a previous exposure to the microbe or its products; it does not necessarily indicate the presence of an active disease process. False negative results may also occur, and further investigation may be necessary. The size of the erythematous area or induration may be measured to estimate the degree of the client's sensitivity or immune response. These responses may be short lived or of lifelong duration. (See also Chapter 63.)

Clients who are immunosuppressed because of cancer chemotherapy or radiation treatments, malnutrition, debilitation, or congenital or acquired immunodeficiency syndrome (AIDS) may demonstrate no response (anergy) when tested with a prescribed battery of antigen challenges. These clients are extremely vulnerable to infection and may need metabolic support and precautions to avoid infection. Test results may not be reliable in those who have viral infections, are febrile or uremic, or have recently received live viral vaccinations.

Indications. Some diagnostic agents measure a client's physiologic response or hypersensitivity to the agent as a specific chemical challenge. These agents are typically used in simple baseline screening procedures as part of an initial diagnostic workup. Some are used in skin tests by patch, prick, scratch, or intradermal injection to assess hypersensitivity (allergy), anergy (congenital or acquired inability to develop a cell-mediated reaction), cellular immunity, or antibody response (Table 72-5). Others are used as reagents in specimens of blood, urine, and bodily discharges to detect the levels of certain components to facilitate diagnosis or to monitor known conditions (Table 72-6; see also Table 72-2).

Side Effects/Adverse Reactions. Local reactions to skin tests do not usually cause discomfort. Occasionally a highly positive reaction will result in vesiculation and necrosis of the overlying skin, and corticosteroids may be ordered. Transient tachycardia, malaise, or low-grade fever may occur separately from a local reaction. Occasionally a client may report systemic allergic reactions of urticaria, sneezing, or dyspnea. An overwhelming antigen-antibody response (anaphylactic response) is rare but can occur; such

TABLE 72-4 Common Nonradioactive Agents for Evaluation of Body Response

Agent	Indications/Secondary Effects	Nursing Management
edrophonium (Tensilon)	Indications: myasthenia gravis, cholinergic stimulant Secondary effects: severe cholinergic reaction, bradycardia or cardiac standstill, dysrhythmias	Have 1 mg IV atropine available to relieve the adverse muscarinic effects of edrophonium. Monitor vital signs carefully. Have facilities available for CPR, cardiac monitoring, and respiratory assistance. A placebo may be administered first as if it were the test dose to evaluate baseline muscular capabilities. A number of drugs may be withheld for at least 8 hours; check with the prescriber.
histamine	Indications: gastric function Secondary effects: flushing, dizziness, headache, dyspnea, asthma, urticaria, hypotension or hypertension, tachycardia, gastrointestinal distress, convulsions	Withhold food for 12 hours and fluids and smoking for 8 hours before the test. Withhold medications: antacids, anticholinergics, alcohol, histamine, histamine receptor antagonists, insulin, parasympathomimetics, adrenergic blockers, and corticosteroids. Keep epinephrine available for severe hypotension.
pentagastrin (Peptavlon)	Indications: gastric function in pernicious anemia, Zollinger-Ellison syndrome, and other gastrointestinal conditions Secondary effects: hypersensitivity, stimulation of pancreatic secretion, gastrointestinal distress or bleeding	This is the drug of choice for gastric secretion testing. Withhold food, liquids, and smoking after midnight before the test. Inform the client that a nasogastric tube will be passed. Withhold medications as above with histamine. Observe for gastrointestinal distress after the test. Resume usual diet and medications.
protirelin (Thypinone)	Indications: thyroid function Secondary effects: blood pressure alterations, breast enlargement, nausea, increased urination, dizziness, dry mouth, headache	Have client urinate and assume a supine position. Drug is administered as a bolus over 15-30 seconds. Measure blood pressure at frequent intervals for the first 15 minutes. Increases in blood pressure (less than 30 mm Hg) are more common than decreases. Use caution in clients for whom rapid changes in blood pressure would be dangerous.
sincalide (Kinevac)	Indications: gallbladder and pancreatic function Secondary effects: hypersensitivity, nausea, cramps, dizziness, flushing	Administered IV. Adverse effects usually occur immediately after the injection and last for a few minutes.
tolbutamide (Orinase Diagnostic)	Indications: pancreatic islet cell function Secondary effects: severe hypoglycemia	Instruct the client to adhere to a 150-300 g/day carbohydrate diet for 3 days before the test and to fast overnight. Avoid smoking during fasting and during the test. Tolbutamide is not administered to clients who have known sensitivities to the drug or other sulfonylurea drugs. For 3 days before the examination, withhold salicylates and other drugs known to potentiate the hypoglycemic action of tolbutamide (see Chapter 50). If severe hypoglycemia occurs during the test, administer 12.5-25 g of glucose in a 25%-50% IV.

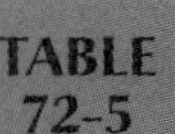

TABLE 72-5 Biologic Agents Used for Diagnostic Tests

Biologic Product*	Indication/Adult Dosage
Tuberculin (purified protein derivative, PPD, Mantoux test) (Aplitest, Tuberculin PPD Tine Test)	Indication: tuberculosis. Adult dosage: 5 U.S. units, intradermal; special instructions for application of the Tine Test should be followed.
Tuberculin (PPD) (Aplisol, Tubersol)	Indication: tuberculosis. Adult dosage: 5 U.S. units, intradermal following specific instructions as noted by manufacturer or *United States Pharmacopeia Dispensing Information.*
Allergenic extracts	Several hundred individual purified fluid allergens are available for diagnosis and hyposensitization of allergies: pollens, poison ivy, foods, dusts, yeast, and other allergens. Treatment: periodic SC injection of gradually increasing potent dilutions of a specific allergen.

*See the nursing management for each of these agents.

TABLE 72-6 Common Tests for Screening Selected Conditions

Identifies/Detects	Test(s)	Available Forms
Ketones in blood or urine	Acetone tests: Acetest, KetoStix	Tablets, strips
Protein in urine	Albumin tests: Albustix	Strips
Nitrates, uropathogens, bacteria	Microstix-3, Uricult	Culture paddles, strips
Bilirubin in urine	Ictotest	Tablets
Urea nitrogen in blood	Azostix	Strips
Candida albicans, vaginal	Isocult for Candida, CandidaSure	Culture paddles, reagent slides
Chlamydia trachomatis	Chlamydiazyme, Sure Cell Chlamydia	Kits
Cholesterol	Advanced Care Cholesterol Test—for home use	Kits
Cryptococcus neoformans in cerebrospinal fluids and serum	Crypto-LA	Slide tests
Gastrointestinal duodenal fluid stomach acid	Entero-Test Gastro-Test	String capsules String capsules
Glucose in blood	Chemstrip bG, Dextrostix, Diascan, Glucometer Encore, and others	Strips
Glucose in urine	Clinitest, Chemstrip bG, Clinistix, TesTape	Tablets, strips
Gonorrhea	Biocult-GC, Gonozyme Diagnostic, others	Kits
Human immunodeficiency virus (HIV) tests	HIV-1 LA Recombigen, HIV-1 Latex Agglutination test, HIVAB HIV-1 EIA, others	Kits
Meningitis	Bactigen N Meningitidis	Slide tests
Mononucleosis	Mono-Diff, Mono-Latex, others	Kits
Occult blood screening	ColoCARE, Colo-Screen, others	Kits
Ovulation tests	Answer Ovulation, ClearplanEasy, Ovu-Quick Self-Test, others	Kits
Human chorionic gonadotropin pregnancy tests	Advance, Answer Plus, Answer Quick & Simple, Fact Plus, others	Kits
Rheumatoid factor	Rheumatex, Rheumaton	Slide tests
Hemoglobin S sickle cell test	Sickledex	Kit
Staphylococcus aureus	Isocult for Staphylococcus	Culture paddles
Streptococci tests	Sure Cell Streptococci, Bactigen B Streptococcus-CS, others	Kits
Virus tests, miscellaneous	Human T-Lymphotropic Virus Type, Sure Cell Herpes, Rubazyme for Rubella, others	Kits

a reaction calls for emergency measures such as the administration of epinephrine and respiratory and circulatory support. These secondary effects are more likely to occur if hyposensitization therapy is begun, because this includes a well-controlled program of increasing dosages of the allergen in question.

Dosage and Administration. For certain standardized tests such as that for coccidioidomycosis, the dosage is fixed (0.1 mL of a 1 : 100 dilution). Dosages for allergy testing are also very small (0.02 to 0.05 mL) but may be individualized. The manufacturers' instructions for all these diagnostic agents should be followed carefully.

Nursing Management

Screening Agents

Administer screening agents with care because of their propensity to trigger allergic reactions. Question the client regarding any previous reactions to skin testing. If the client responds positively, dilute test doses of less than one tenth the usual concentration may be administered.

Be prepared for major allergic manifestations such as angioedema, urticaria, serum sickness, or anaphylactic shock, which can occur. Have the client wait for 30 minutes to observe for development of an allergic reaction.

Inspect the liquid extract of the antigen for clarity; do not use it if particles are seen. As appropriate, administer these diagnostic test agents using one of the methods described in the following paragraphs.

A sterile needle or other instrument may be used to prick or scratch the skin after a drop of the extract is placed on the skin. Depending on the approach used, the results may be read directly or after removing the testing patch.

Intradermal injections are commonly administered on the ventral surface of the forearm. Use a tuberculin syringe with a 25- to 27-gauge needle. Inject intradermally with the needle nearly parallel to the skin surface, making certain that the needle does not penetrate deeper into subcutaneous tissue. This intradermal insertion will increase the precision with which the results may be interpreted; it will also prevent febrile reactions to tuberculin tests.

Stop inserting the needle as soon as the tip of the needle, with its bevel up, has entered the skin but is still visible. Inject the antigen with steady pressure. A correctly administered intradermal injection will immediately raise a small, colorless bleb or lump.

Have medications available for emergency administration, such as antihistamines (e.g., diphenhydramine and epinephrine, 0.2 mL for subcutaneous use). Equipment for full circulatory and respiratory support should also be available.

After the injection there is a prescribed wait—often 20 minutes or several days (depending on the antigen)—before the local reaction is assessed for erythema and induration. A positive reaction to some antigens is determined by the presence of induration alone; erythema is not always a criterion. *Erythema* (redness) is categorized as follows:

Trace	Faint discoloration
+ (one plus)	Pink
++	Red
+++	Purplish red
++++	Vesiculation or necrosis

Measure the single largest induration (area of hardness) or the largest coalesced induration. Induration can be measured with precision by using the following technique:

1. Place your index, middle, and ring fingers together, and stroke the test site to determine the presence of induration.
2. To delimit the indurated area, use a ballpoint pen to draw a line toward the indurated area in four directions. The edges of the induration can easily be perceived as the ballpoint tip touches them; stop each marking when the edge is perceived.
3. Measure the diameter of the remaining unmarked indurated area in millimeters, or use the following criteria for indurations:

Trace	Barely palpable
+	Palpable, but not visible
++	Easily palpable and visible; indurated area buckles when squeezed gently
+++	Easily palpable and visible; does not buckle when squeezed gently
++++	Vesiculation or necrosis

Criteria used to categorize Mantoux tuberculin test results according to the induration diameter are as follows: less than 5 mm is a negative result; 5 to 9 mm is a questionable result (retesting by another method may be necessary), and more than 9 mm is a positive result.

Indurations resulting from multiple-puncture tuberculin testing devices are interpreted as positive if they have a diameter of more than 2 mm. Results from multiple-puncture tuberculin tests are considered less reliable than the results of Mantoux tests.

SUMMARY

Diagnostic agents are chemical substances used to diagnose or monitor a condition or disease. As with other drugs, they may also produce side effects/adverse reactions. Radiopaque agents are used for visualizing organ structure. Examinations used for evaluating organ function involve radioactive agents, computed tomography, ultrasonography, and nuclear magnetic resonance imaging. Nonradioactive agents may be used for evaluating organ function via volumes and flows and for challenging a glandular response. Other agents are available for screening and monitoring immune status and disorders. It is essential that the nurse know the agent used, its mechanism of action and indications, and how to prevent or minimize any adverse reactions.

Critical Thinking Questions

1. Bobby Brown, age 24, a newly hired teacher, is required by the school board to have a medical history and physical examination, including diagnostic skin testing with tuberculin (the PPD test), before his employment is finalized. Why would the PPD be included? What would constitute a positive response for a PPD? What would a positive response indicate? Suppose Mr. Brown tells the nurse who is about to administer his PPD that he has had a positive response to the test in the past. What action should the nurse take?
2. Sally Grey, age 54, has been advised by her health care provider to get a mammogram every year. She confesses to you that she is concerned about excessive radiation exposure. How will you respond?

Collaborative Learning Activities

For Collaborative Learning Activities, go to mosby.com/MERLIN/McKenry/.

BIBLIOGRAPHY

American Hospital Formulary Service. (1999). *AHFS drug information '99*. Bethesda, MD: American Society of Hospital Pharmacists.

Anderson, K.N., Anderson, L.E., & Glanze, W.D. (Eds.) (1998). *Mosby's medical, nursing, & allied health dictionary* (5th ed.). St. Louis: Mosby.

DiPiro, J.T., Talbert, R.L., Yee, G.C., Matzke, G.R., Wells, B.G., & Posey, L.M. (Eds.). (1997). *Pharmacotherapy: A pathophysiologic approach*. (3rd ed.). Norwalk, CT: Appleton & Lange.

Drug Facts and Comparisons. (2000). St. Louis: Facts and Comparisons.

Early, P.J. & Sodee, D.B. (1991). *Principles and practice of nuclear medicine* (2nd ed.). St. Louis: Mosby.

Farwell, A.P. & Braverman, L.E. (1996). Thyroid and antithyroid drugs. In J.G. Hardman & L.E. Limbird (Eds.), *Goodman & Gilman's The pharmacological basis of therapeutics* (9th ed.). New York: McGraw-Hill.

Haaga, J.R. & Alfidi, R.J. (1988). *Computed tomography of the whole body* (2nd ed.). St. Louis: Mosby.

Jankowski, C.B. (1992). Radiation protection for nurses: Regulations and guidelines. *Journal of Nursing Administration, 17*(2), 30-34.

Kee, J.L. (1999). *Laboratory and diagnostic tests with nursing implications*. Stamford, CT: Appleton & Lange.

Pagana, K.D. & Pagana, T.J. (1997). *Mosby's diagnostic and laboratory test reference* (3rd ed.). St. Louis: Mosby.

Singer, C.M., Baraff, L.J., Benedict, S.H., Weiss, E.L., Singer, B.D. (1989). Exposure of emergency medicine personnel to ionizing radiation during cervical spine radiography. *Annals of Emergency Medicine, 18*(8), 822-825.

United States Pharmacopeia Dispensing Information (USP DI): Drug information for the health care professional (19th ed.). (1999). Rockville, MD: United States Pharmacopeial Convention.

Watson, J. & Jaffee, M.S. (1995). *Nurse's manual of laboratory and diagnostic tests* (2nd ed.). Philadelphia: F.A. Davis.

73 Poisons and Antidotes

Chapter Focus

As with most critical illnesses, an assessment followed by the appropriate interventions will influence the ultimate outcome for the client with poisoning. The role of the nurse is important not only in the treatment of such clients but also in the teaching of safety promotion and accident prevention to keep poisonings from occurring.

Learning Objectives

1. Discuss the major causes of poisoning in children of various ages.
2. List at least five objective and/or subjective nursing assessments of a client presenting with a suspected poisoning.
3. Describe the four grades of drug overdose–induced coma.
4. Discuss the major drugs causing organ or tissue damage resulting from chemical poisoning.
5. Implement the nursing management for the care of a client with suspected poisoning.
6. Implement the nursing management for the pharmacologic treatment of acetaminophen, cyanide, iron, and insecticide overdose.

Key Terms

acute poisoning, p. 1223
chronic poisoning, p. 1223
gastric lavage, p. 1230
poison, p. 1223
toxicology, p. 1223
toxidromes, p. 1225

Regional poison control centers reported nearly 2.2 million calls concerning human drug or chemical exposures in the United States during 1996. Of this number, approximately 53% of the reports involved children younger than 6 years of age. There were also 726 deaths documented that included 4% of children under 6 years of age. Although the incidence of poisoning in children is high, the mortality rate in this population is usually low. The majority of ingestion cases in children are accidental, whereas most drug overdoses in adults are intentional and are the result of a suicide attempt or substance abuse. Drug overdoses resulting from substance abuse are reviewed in Chapter 9.

An unusual type of poisoning has resulted from the proliferation of battery-operated games, cameras, hearing aids, calculators, and watches. Each year an estimated 500 to 600 miniature button or disk batteries are swallowed by persons of all ages. Their major component is aqueous potassium hydroxide, which also is used to unclog pipes. Children can mistake small batteries for candy, and adults may mistake them for medication tablets. Batteries that lodge in the esophagus, cecum, or other areas of the gastrointestinal tract present two problems: (1) they are locally corrosive to mucosa, causing ulceration or perforation in 1 to 2 hours; and (2) they may cause mercury poisoning when certain battery contents leak. Endoscopic or surgical removal is necessary if the battery remains in the stomach for more than 24 hours, if gastric or peritoneal irritation develops, if radiologic evidence shows the battery lodging or leaking in the gastrointestinal tract, or if the particular type of battery is prone to leakage.

See the Cultural Considerations box on p. 1224 for a discussion of the poisoning associated with the use of traditional ethnic remedies.

DETECTION OF POISONS

Toxicology is the study of poisons and their action and effects, methods of detection, and diagnosis and treatment. A **poison** is defined as any substance that in relatively small amounts can cause death or serious bodily harm. All drugs are potential poisons when used improperly or in excess doses. Poisoning may be acute or chronic. In **acute poisoning** the effects are immediate, whereas in **chronic poisoning** the effects are insidious because of the cumulative effects of small amounts of poison absorbed over a prolonged period. Chronic poisoning causes chronic illness, which may or may not be reversible.

Nurses may be confronted with a suspected poisoning in many ways. A mother may call, upset that her small child has taken one of her contraceptive pills; a nursing home resident may accidentally drink the glass of peroxide mixture intended as a mouthwash; or an adolescent who cannot be aroused may be brought into the emergency department.

Cues that typically point to poisoning include sudden, violent symptoms of severe nausea, vomiting, diarrhea, collapse, or convulsions. If possible, it is important to find out what poison has been taken and how much. Additional information that might prove helpful to the health care provider in making a diagnosis includes answers to questions or reports of observed phenomena, with the nurse noting the following:

- Any reports of poison contact by the victim
- Poisoning in the "at-risk" age-group (1 to 5 years of age)
- Report of a history of previous poisonings or the ingestion of foreign substances
- Diverse symptoms or signs indicating multiple organ system involvement that defy diagnosis
- A history of suicidal intent or thought
- Symptoms that appear suddenly in an otherwise healthy individual or in a number of persons who become ill at approximately the same time, as might occur in food poisoning
- Anything unusual about the individual, his or her clothing, or the surroundings; evidence of burns around the lips and mouth; discolored gums; needle (hypodermic) pricks, pustules, or scars on the exposed and accessible surfaces of the body or dilated or constricted pupils, as may be seen in drug addicts; any skin rash or discoloration
- The odor of the breath, the rate of respiration, any difficulty in respiration, and cyanosis
- The quality and rate of the pulse
- The appearance and odor of vomitus, if any, as well as accompanying diarrhea or abdominal pain
- Any abnormalities of stool and urine; any change in color or the presence of blood
- For signs of involvement of the nervous system, the presence of excitement, muscular twitching, delirium, speech difficulty, stupor, coma, constriction or dilation of the pupils, and elevated or subnormal temperature

Coma caused by a drug overdose is characterized by the following categories:

Grade I. The individual is asleep but is easily aroused and reacts to painful stimuli. Deep tendon reflexes are present, pupils are normal and reactive, ocular movements are present, and vital signs are stable.

Grade II. Pain response is absent, deep tendon reflexes are depressed, pupils are slightly dilated but reactive, and vital signs are stable.

Grade III. Deep tendon and pupillary reflexes are absent, and vital signs are stable.

Grade IV. Respiration and circulation are depressed.

All specimens of vomitus, urine, or stool for examination and possible submission to the proper authority for analysis *should be refrigerated in a covered container.* This is of particular importance not only in making or confirming a diagnosis but also in the event that the case has medicolegal significance.

Any of the signs listed earlier should be noted carefully for reporting to the poison control center or physician in charge. However, a complete reliance on the signs and symptoms for a clear-cut diagnosis and poison identification is fraught with danger, because these incidents may occur concurrently with an episode of acute disease, especially in

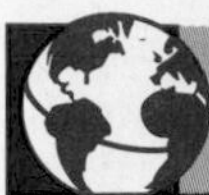

Cultural Considerations
Poisoning Associated with the Use of Traditional Ethnic Remedies

Traditional herbal products are widely available in the United States and Canada. The consumption of these traditional ethnic remedies can have adverse health effects. However, because they are not marketed as a drug, these products have not been subjected to standard tests for safety and effectiveness.

Kwan, Paiusco, and Kohl (1992) reported a case of digitalis toxicity in a 90-year-old Chinese man after he took a nonprescription Chinese medication, Yixin Wan; this product contains several ingredients, including toad venom, ginseng, pearl, and musk. According to the package, it has been shown to be helpful for clients with coronary artery disease and congestive heart failure. Cardiac glycosides are present in a large number of plant extracts and in the venom of toads, and the clinical toxicity of toad venom has been described.

As the result of publicly funded childhood blood lead screening tests in California, Flattery et al. reported 40 cases of elevated blood lead levels in children who had received traditional ethnic remedies. For 36 of the 40 cases, the traditional remedies reported were azarcon or greta—the Hispanic remedies used for digestive problems. Other remedies were paylooah (Southeast Asia) used for rash or fever, surma (India) used to improve eyesight, and an unnamed ayurvedic substance from Tibet used to improve slow development. In many cases, family members initially denied the use of these remedies, but they later reported their use with subsequent case follow-up efforts. The reluctance of family members to report the use of traditional ethnic remedies during initial interviews may reflect factors such as uncertainty about the legality of using such medicines, a belief in the effectiveness of these remedies, and concerns regarding responsibility for the child's illness. In addition, some persons may not consider these substances to be "remedies" or "medicines"; therefore health care providers should ask about the use of these substances by their common names (Public Health Service, U.S. Department of Health and Human Services, 1993).

Horowitz et al. report life-threatening bradycardia with rapid onset and CNS and respiratory depression that developed in three unrelated children in Colorado following the ingestion of Jin Bu Huan tablets, a Chinese herbal medicine used for relieving pain. On analysis the active ingredient was determined to be levo-tetrahydropalmatine (L-THP), a naloxone-resistant substance that results in sedation, analgesia, neuromuscular blockade, and dopamine receptor antagonism. The hazard of this particular substance was a combination of factors: the extreme potency of L-THP, the misidentification of the source plant, the false and potentially misleading medical claims, the availability of the product, and the lack of childproof packaging. (Public Health Service, U.S. Department of Health and Human Services, 1993).

To prevent cases of unintentional poisoning associated with herbal and other botanical products, such products should be sold in childproof packaging and kept in childproof containers, and parents should be informed about the potential toxicity of these products. In addition, accurate labeling of the active ingredient is critical to enable prompt and proper medical treatment for unintentional poisoning (Public Health Service, U.S. Department of Health and Human Services, 1993).

The use of traditional ethnic remedies in the United States and Canada is quite common. Older adults in ethnic populations and newly arrived immigrants have a strong cultural belief in traditional medicines and less confidence in "modern" medicine. These traditional remedies are easily obtained in ethnic stores and pharmacies. With a rapidly growing, culturally diverse population, health care providers must be alert for the potential toxicity of the nonstandard therapies that these individuals may be taking.

Critical Thinking Questions

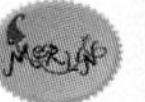

- In your own community, how could you increase your skill in taking drug histories to identify traditional ethnic remedies?
- How could you work within your community to help prevent the poisonings described above?

children (e.g., aspirin intoxication), and the symptoms may be similar or otherwise confusing. In addition, more than one substance may be responsible for the signs of poisoning observed.

Not all substances commonly and accidentally ingested are toxic if small amounts are taken only once. Poison control centers define a small amount as the quantity of a substance contained in "a taste," "one bite," or "a small piece," as opposed to "a mouthful." Although subjective, this is typical of the data received when taking a poisoning history. The following is a list of some commonly ingested products that are usually systematically nontoxic if taken in small amounts:

- Abrasives, bleaches (sodium hypochlorite, less than 5%)
- Chalk
- Cigarettes, cigarette ash, cigars
- Cosmetics, perfume, cologne, deodorants
- Crayons (if labeled C.P., A.P., or C.S., 2 130-46)
- Glues, rubber cement
- Hydrogen peroxide (medicinal, 3%)
- Indelible pen or magic markers

BOX 73-1

Toxidromes*

atropine, scopolamine, anticholinergics: dry skin, tachycardia, beet-red skin color, agitation, dilated pupils, delirium, hyperthermia, hallucinations, coma
barbiturates, sedative-hypnotics, tranquilizers: ataxia, drowsiness, slurred speech (without an alcohol breath odor), respiratory depression, hypotension
cholinergics (such as organophosphates), mushrooms (Amanita or Galerina): salivation, lacrimation, involuntary urination and defecation, miosis, pulmonary congestion, seizures
opioids: miosis, respiratory depression, hypotension, slow respiration, coma
salicylates: fever, vomiting, hyperglycemia, mixed respiratory alkalosis and metabolic acidosis, hyperpnea
tricyclic antidepressants: anticholinergic signs and symptoms, plus dysrhythmias (prolonged QRS duration on ECG report), convulsions, coma

*The drugs or drug types in bold are followed by clusters of signs of poisonings.

- Ink in full cartridge of a ballpoint pen
- Paint (latex)
- Pencil (graphite or coloring)
- Saccharin and cyclamates
- Safety matches
- Soaps, liquid shampoos, household detergents (except dishwasher detergents)
- Toothpaste (unless there is a heavy ingestion of fluorides)
- Vitamins (in amounts usually available for a single overdose, unless containing iron)

The ingestion of small amounts of these nonedible substances may produce mild gastric irritation but not systemic poisoning. However, contact with a poison control center or physician is important—and essential if symptoms exist—because no product or drug is entirely safe for ingestion, and hypersensitivity reactions can occur.

In assisting with the poisoning diagnosis and in the identification of a toxic substance, nurses (especially emergency department nurses and nurse practitioners) should familiarize themselves with certain clusters of signs associated with common drug poisonings or overdoses. These clusters are called **toxidromes** and are listed in Box 73-1. Other common single signs and their associated causative toxins are listed in Table 73-1.

POISON CONTROL CENTERS

There are approximately 600 poison control centers in the United States, with the majority located near hospitals or in the emergency departments of large community hospitals. Their telephone numbers are listed in the local telephone book or may be obtained from a pharmacist. The *United States Pharmacopeia Dispensing Information (USP DI)*, *Mosby's GenRx*, and the *Physician's Desk Reference (PDR)* include a list of certified poison control centers that are open 24 hours a day. These centers are staffed to answer specific questions from the public or other professionals about the identification of ingredients in trade-named products, estimate their toxicity, and suggest specific treatment for poisonings.

CLASSIFICATION OF THE ACTION OF POISONS

The classification of poisons is as broad as the classification of drugs, because any drug is a potential poison when used in excess. Poisons may be classified in various ways. They may be grouped according to chemical classifications as organic and inorganic poisons; as alkaloids, glycosides, and resins; or as acids, alkalis, heavy metals, oxidizing agents, halogenated hydrocarbons, and so on. Poisons may also be classified according to the organ or tissue of the body in which the most damaging effects are produced. Some poisons injure all cells they contact; these are sometimes called protoplasmic poisons or cytotoxins. Others have a greater effect on the kidney (nephrotoxins), the liver (hepatotoxins), or the blood-forming organs.

Poisons that mainly affect the nervous system are called neurotoxin poisons. They must be studied separately, because different symptoms characterize each one. Symptoms of toxicity are mentioned with each of these drugs in previous chapters. Although the symptoms of this group of poisons are specific to some extent, certain symptoms are encountered repeatedly and are associated with many poisons. Drowsiness, dizziness, headache, delirium, coma, and convulsive seizures always indicate central nervous system (CNS) involvement. On the other hand, dry mouth, dilated pupils, and difficulty swallowing are associated with an overdose of atropine or one of the atropine-like drugs. Ringing in the ears, excessive perspiration, and gastric upset may be associated with an overdose of salicylate.

Often the precise mechanism of action is not known; death may be caused by respiratory failure, but exactly what happens to cause depression of the respiratory center may not be known. The human body depends on a constant supply of oxygen if various physiologic functions are to proceed satisfactorily. Anything that interferes with the use of oxygen by the cells or with the transportation of oxygen will produce damaging effects faster in some cells than in others. Carbon monoxide from automobile engines and unvented gas heaters is one of the most widely distributed toxic agents. It poisons by producing hypoxia and finally asphyxia. Carbon monoxide has a great affinity for hemoglobin and forms carboxyhemoglobin; this interferes with the production of oxyhemoglobin and the free transport of oxygen, and oxygen deficiency soon develops in the cells.

TABLE 73-1 Single Signs That Suggest the Presence of Certain Toxins

Sign	Inference
Abdominal colic	Black widow spider bite
	Heavy metals
	Withdrawal from narcotic depressant
Ataxia	Alcohol
	Barbiturates
	Bromides
	Carbon monoxide
	Hallucinogens
	Heavy metals
	Organic solvents
	Phenytoin (Dilantin)
	Tranquilizers
Coma and drowsiness	Alcohol (ethyl)
	Antihistamines
	Barbiturates, other hypnotics
	Carbon monoxide
	Opiates
	Salicylates
	Tranquilizers
Convulsions or muscle twitching	Alcohol
	Amphetamines
	Antihistamines
	Boric acid
	Camphor
	Chlorinated hydrocarbon insecticides (DDT)
	Cyanide
	Lead
	Organophosphate insecticides
	Plants (azalea, iris, lily-of-the-valley, water hemlock)
	Salicylates
	Strychnine
	Withdrawal from drugs: barbiturates, benzodiazepines (Valium, Librium), meprobamate
Paralysis	Botulism
	Heavy metals
	Plants (e.g., poison hemlock)
	Triorthocresyl phosphate (plasticizer)
Oliguria/anuria	Carbon tetrachloride
	Ethylene glycol (antifreeze)
	Heavy metals
	Hemolysis caused by naphthalene, plants, and so on
	Methanol
	Mushrooms
	Oxylates
	Petroleum distillates
	Solvents
Oral signs	
Breath odors	
Acetone	Acetone
	Alcohol (methyl or isopropyl)
	Phenol
	Salicylates
Alcohol	Ethyl alcohol
Bitter almonds	Cyanide
Coal gas	Carbon monoxide
Garlic	Arsenic
	Dimethyl sulfoxide (DMSO)
	Phosphorus
	Organophosphate insecticides
	Thallium
Salivation	Arsenic
	Corrosive substances
	Mercury
	Mushrooms
	Organophosphate insecticides
	Thallium

Anoxia may produce serious brain damage unless exposure to the carbon monoxide is terminated before 40% of hemoglobin has been changed to carboxyhemoglobin. Death occurs when 60% of the hemoglobin has been changed to carboxyhemoglobin.

The cyanides act somewhat similarly in that they bring about cellular anoxia, but they do so differently. They inactivate certain tissue enzymes so that cells are unable to use oxygen. Death may occur very rapidly. Curare and the curariform drugs in toxic amounts bring about paralysis of the diaphragm, and again the victim dies from lack of oxygen.

Certain drugs have a direct effect on muscle tissue from the body, such as that of the myocardium or the smooth muscle of the blood vessels. Death results from the failure of circulation or cardiac arrest. The nitrites, potassium salts, and digitalis drugs may exert such toxic effects. Strong acids and alkalis denature and destroy cellular proteins. Examples of corrosive acids are hydrochloric, nitric, and sulfuric acids. Sodium, potassium, and ammonium hydroxides are examples of strong and caustic alkalis. Locally, these substances cause destruction of tissue, and death may result from hemorrhage, perforation, or shock. Corrosive poisons may also cause death by altering the pH of the blood or

TABLE 73-1 Single Signs That Suggest the Presence of Certain Toxins—cont'd

Sign	Inference
Pupillary changes	
Dilated	Amphetamines
	Antihistamines
	Atropine
	Barbiturates (when combined with coma)
	Cocaine
	Ephedrine
	LSD (occasionally)
	Methanol
	Withdrawal from narcotic depressants (occasionally)
Constricted, pinpoint pupils	Mushrooms (muscarinic)
	Opiates
	Organophosphate insecticides
Nystagmus on lateral gaze	Barbiturates
	Minor tranquilizers (meprobamate, benzodiazepines), phenytoin (Dilantin)
Respiratory alterations	
Increased	Amphetamines
	Barbiturates (early sign)
	Carbon monoxide
	Methanol
	Petroleum distillates
Paralysis	Botulism
	Salicylates
Slowed or depressed	Organophosphate insecticides
	Alcohol (late sign)
	Barbiturates (late sign)
	Opiates
	Tranquilizers
Wheezing/pulmonary edema	Mushrooms (muscarinic)
	Opiates
	Organophosphate insecticides
	Petroleum distillates
Skin color changes	
Jaundice	Aniline dyes/coal tar colors
	Arsenic
	Carbon tetrachloride
	Castor bean
	Fava bean
	Mushroom
	Naphthalene (moth repellent/insecticide)
Red flush	Yellow phosphorus
	Alcohol
	Antihistamines
	Atropine
	Boric acid
	Carbon monoxide
	Nitrites
	Tricyclic antidepressants
Cyanosis	Aniline dyes
	Carbon monoxide
	Cyanide
	Nitrites
	Strychnine
	Tricyclic antidepressants
Violent emesis (with or without hematemesis)	Aminophylline
	Bacterial food poisoning
	Boric acid
	Corrosives
	Fluoride
	Heavy metals
	Phenol
	Salicylates

other body fluids, or they may produce marked degenerative changes in vital organs such as the liver or kidney.

SPECIFIC POISONS, SYMPTOMS, AND SUGGESTED EMERGENCY TREATMENT

Because the emphasis is on *prompt* treatment, health care may be best served by the quick action of informed bystanders at the scene who administer first aid while help is sought from the poison control center and while transportation to a hospital or other health care setting is arranged. Box 73-2 provides first aid instructions for possible poisoning.

The caller to the poison control center should have the following information, if available:

1. Physical appearance of the substance
2. Odor, color, texture, and distinguishing characteristics of the substance
3. Trade name or chemical name, if known
4. Purpose of the substance or how the substance was meant to be used
5. Label statements relating to "poison" content or flammability

BOX 73-2

First Aid for Possible Poisoning

Remember: any nonfood substance may be poisonous.

1. Keep all potential poisons—household products and medicines—out of children's reach.
2. Use "safety caps" (child-resistant containers) to avoid accidents.
3. Have 1 ounce of ipecac syrup in your home and in your first aid kit for camping, travel, and so on.
4. Keep the phone number of your poison center and your physician handy.

If you think an accidental ingestion has occurred, do the following:

1. Keep calm. Do not wait for symptoms. Call for help promptly.
2. Find out if the substance is toxic; your poison control center or your physician can tell you if a risk exists and what you should do.
3. Have the product's container or label with you at the phone.
   a. If a poison is on the skin:
      Immediately remove affected clothing.
      Flood involved body parts with water, wash with soap or detergent, and rinse thoroughly.
   b. If a poison is in the eye:
      Immediately flush the eye with water for up to 20 minutes.
   c. If a poison is inhaled:
      Immediately get the victim to fresh air. Give mouth-to-mouth resuscitation if necessary.
   d. If vomiting has been recommended:
      Give the appropriate dose of ipecac syrup as instructed, followed by at least one glass (8 ounces) of clear liquid. If the client does not vomit within 15 to 20 minutes, give 1 more tablespoon of ipecac and more water. Do not use salt water.

Never induce vomiting in the following situations:

1. The victim is in a *coma* (unconscious).
2. The victim is *convulsing* (having a seizure).
3. The victim has swallowed a caustic or corrosive substance (e.g., lye).

For reemphasis:

1. Always call to be certain of possible toxicity before undertaking treatment.
2. Never induce vomiting until you are instructed to do so.
3. Do not rely on the label's antidote information, because it may be out of date. Call instead.
4. If you need to go to an emergency department, take the tablets, capsules, capsules, container, and/or label with you.
5. Do not hesitate to call your poison center or your physician a second time if the victim seems to be getting worse.

Information from Covington, T.R. (1996). *Handbook of nonprescription drugs* (11th ed.). Washington, D.C.: American Pharmaceutical Association and The National Professional Society of Pharmacists; and Vale, J.A., & Proudfoot, A. (1997). Drug overdosage and poisoning. In T.M. Speight & N.H.G. Holford (Eds.), *Avery's drug treatment* (4th ed.). Auckland, New Zealand: Adis International.

After the events of the suspected poisoning have been assessed, prompt medical interventions must be instituted. Nursing management is therefore guided by the four major goals:

1. Vital functions (respirations, circulation, and others) will be maintained, supported, or restored.
2. The toxic substance will be removed or eliminated from the system as soon as possible.
3. The action of certain specific poisons may be counteracted, reversed, or antagonized by specific antidotes.
4. Recurrences will be reduced or prevented.

Support of Vital Functions

Basic to the treatment of poisoning is intensive supportive therapy, good nursing care, and minimal dangerous invasive interventions. Nursing care of the poisoned client should focus on the restoration, support, and maintenance of vital functions such as ventilation, circulation, and acid-base and fluid-electrolyte balance. Emotional support for the client and others involved in this crisis is crucial.

A general assessment and history should be performed quickly and competently to determine the extent of any impairments of body systems or particular susceptibilities. Expert nursing care is essential for observing the following for information that indicates impending complications:

1. Level of consciousness.
2. Vital signs. Temperature may be elevated with certain CNS stimulants and salicylates and depressed with others. Transient cardiac dysrhythmias may occur; anticipate obtaining an electrocardiogram (ECG). Pulmonary congestion, airway obstruction, or apnea is common; aspiration of vomitus can occur.

Implemented plans may include the following:

1. Turning, deep breathing, coughing, and suctioning
2. Auscultation to demonstrate a need for chest x-ray examination, suctioning, tracheostomy, endotracheal in-

tubation, blood gas determinations, supplemental oxygen, and a respirator/ventilator

It is also essential that the victim be positioned to prevent aspiration of vomitus and that mouth care be provided promptly after emesis. Moderate amounts of plain water by mouth (if a gag or swallow reflex is present) may be all that is needed to dilute or effectively inactivate many ingested poisons. Close attention to developing problems and responsive interventions can often prevent the need for more aggressive medical therapies that tax the already tenuous condition of the poisoned individual.

Removal or Elimination of Poison

Careful evaluation of the client who has been affected by a toxic substance is essential to determine which of the foregoing steps take priority and by which route the poison should be removed or eliminated, if necessary. The route is largely determined by the manner of the poisoning. The removal of ingested substances can be attempted in several ways: (1) by directly removing it from the stomach, if the poisoning is discovered early; (2) by increasing the rate of transit of the poison through the colon, even though little or no absorption occurs there and thus may not be effective; or (3) by attempting to remove or filter it from the bloodstream if the substance has probably already been assimilated into the system or was injected. Contact poisons may be flushed from the skin, eyes, and other external areas with copious volumes of plain, flowing water from a pitcher or other container. Inhaled toxins are treated by placing the individual in fresh air and by administering artificial respiration or oxygen and other supportive measures as necessary.

Various methods exist for the removal or elimination of poisons from the gastrointestinal tract or systemic circulation: emesis, gastric lavage, cathartics, diuretics, dialysis or, occasionally, blood exchange transfusions or hemoperfusion through charcoal or exchange resins.

Emesis

The most effective method for removing ingested toxins is usually the most natural one—emesis, which is done as soon as possible. In general, emptying the stomach is ineffective if more than 4 hours have elapsed since the poison was ingested. Exceptions are poisonings by anticholinergic drugs, which slow gastric motility, and by salicylates, which promote pyloric spasm. Some drugs, such as ethanol, are absorbed too rapidly to be recovered after 1 hour. However, when situations have warranted emptying the stomach, whole tablets have occasionally been recovered even a day later. Because of such findings, some physicians recommend emptying the stomach even after a delay. In some instances, however, emesis is contraindicated (Box 73-3).

Ipecac syrup is usually administered if vomiting does not or cannot occur naturally. Apomorphine is no longer recommended for emesis because ipecac syrup is safer and is more convenient to use (*United States Pharmacopeia Dispensing Information*, 1999). However, neither emetic may be effective if the ingested substance is a sedative-hypnotic, a phenothiazine, or a tricyclic antidepressant; all of these substances have antiemetic properties.

BOX 73-3

Contraindications for Induced Emesis in Poisonings

Infants up to 1 year of age
Comatose or convulsing clients
Absent gag and cough reflexes
Ingestion of the following:
- Convulsion-inducing substances
- Sharp objects (e.g., glass, nails) along with the toxic substance
- CNS poisons (e.g., camphor, strychnine), which must be removed more quickly by lavage

Acids, alkalis, or petroleum distillates, such as kerosene, gasoline, or paint thinner
Presence of hematemesis

Information from Wuest, J.R. & Gossel, T.A. (1992). A primer for pharmacists on treatment of poisoning. *Florida Pharmacy Today, 56*(3), 22.

ipecac syrup [ip' e kak]

The most commonly used emetic is ipecac syrup, which acts both centrally and locally by stimulating the vomiting center and by irritating the gastric mucosa. The usual dosage for adults is 15 to 30 mL, which is followed immediately by 240 mL of water. Four to eight ounces of water is given with the following dosages: children 6 months to 1 year of age, 5 to 10 mL (under special circumstances only); and children 1 to 12 years of age, 15 mL. Vomiting usually occurs in 15 to 30 minutes. The dose may be repeated once after 20 minutes if the first dose is not effective.

Ipecac syrup is available without a prescription in 1-ounce (30-mL) bottles that bear the following instructions:

1. For emergency use to cause vomiting in poisoning. Before using, call the physician, poison control center, or hospital emergency department immediately for advice.
2. Warning—Keep out of reach of children. Do not use if strychnine, corrosives such as alkalis (lye) and strong acids, or petroleum distillates such as kerosene, gasoline, fuel oil, coal oil, paint thinner, or cleaning fluid have been ingested.

Gastric lavage should be performed if vomiting does not occur within 30 minutes. Ipecac syrup is cardiotoxic if absorbed and may cause conduction disturbances, atrial fibrillation, or myocarditis.

Gastric Lavage

If the individual is conscious, drug-induced vomiting is usually preferable to gastric lavage, particularly in children, because the aspiration of vomitus is less likely to occur. Nurses should use the necessary measures to reduce the likelihood of aspiration of vomitus (e.g., proper positioning of client). Stimulating the pharynx may occasionally facilitate the induction of vomiting, but time should not be wasted in repeated futile attempts.

Except under most of the same contraindicating conditions (e.g., untreated convulsions, absent reflexes, corrosives), gastric lavage should be begun if emesis cannot be induced. **Gastric lavage** involves washing out the stomach with sterile water or a saline solution. (Refer to a basic nursing text for the procedure.) Lavage may be the preferred treatment for pregnant women and for individuals who have ingested more than 2 mL/kg body weight of a petroleum distillate and who should have an endotracheal intubation to protect the airway. Lavage may be contraindicated in the presence of cardiac dysrhythmias.

An Ewald orogastric tube, No. 16 to 30 French, may be used for lavage in children; tube sizes for an adult lavage range from No. 34 to 42 French. The newer, clear-plastic Levacuator tube also may be used. A standard nasogastric tube is too narrow for the extraction of particulate matter such as intact tablets (Figure 73-1). Stomach contents should be aspirated first and saved for toxicologic analysis if necessary.

Several liters of half-strength saline solution may be used in increments of 50 to 100 mL for children and 150 to 200 mL for adults during repeated lavages until return flows are clear. (Remember that dead space in the tube itself accounts for 20 to 25 mL of the fluid instilled.) Neither emesis nor lavage is guaranteed to empty the stomach completely.

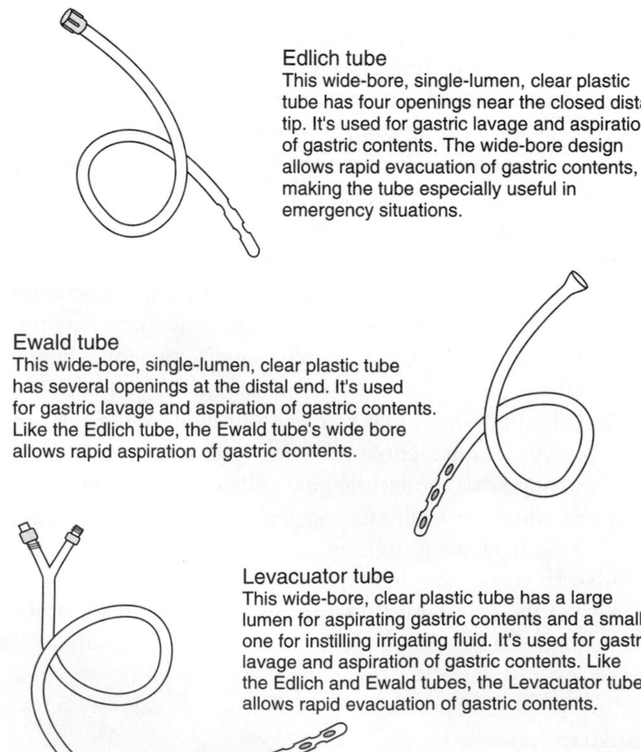

Edlich tube
This wide-bore, single-lumen, clear plastic tube has four openings near the closed distal tip. It's used for gastric lavage and aspiration of gastric contents. The wide-bore design allows rapid evacuation of gastric contents, making the tube especially useful in emergency situations.
Ewald tube
This wide-bore, single-lumen, clear plastic tube has several openings at the distal end. It's used for gastric lavage and aspiration of gastric contents. Like the Edlich tube, the Ewald tube's wide bore allows rapid aspiration of gastric contents.
Levacuator tube
This wide-bore, clear plastic tube has a large lumen for aspirating gastric contents and a small one for instilling irrigating fluid. It's used for gastric lavage and aspiration of gastric contents. Like the Edlich and Ewald tubes, the Levacuator tube allows rapid evacuation of gastric contents.

Figure 73-1 Various tubes used for lavage.

Activated Charcoal

Following emesis or gastric lavage, activated charcoal prepared as an aqueous slurry may be administered to act as an absorbent. Activated charcoal should be given as soon after poison ingestion as feasible, but not immediately after ipecac and emesis, because it will adsorb the ipecac. It is recommended 1 to 2 hours after ipecac-induced vomiting.

Activated charcoal adsorbs many substances and therefore is used as an adjunct in the treatment of oral poisonings with heavy metals, mercuric chloride, strychnine, phenol, atropine, phenolphthalein, oxalic acid, poisonous mushrooms, aspirin, and most drugs. It is not effective for poisoning with ethanol, methanol, caustic alkalis, ferrous sulfate, boric acid, gas, kerosene, lithium, and mineral acids. The charcoal mixture need not be removed from the stomach afterward because no known adverse effects exist. Activated charcoal can also serve as a stool marker to indicate when further gastrointestinal absorption of the ingested poison has ended. Tablets or capsules of charcoal should not be used to treat poisoning, because they are less effective than the powder.

Other Treatments

Other methods to block or eliminate toxins from the system include forced diuresis, cathartics and enemas, dialysis, hemoperfusion, and exchange transfusions. These methods should be reserved as treatment under certain conditions and for specific poisons because they are not universally effective and are much less commonly used than emesis or lavage.

Changing the pH of the urine by alkalinization (sodium bicarbonate) may enhance the excretion of certain drugs, such as salicylates and, possibly, tricyclic antidepressants. Forced acid diuresis is probably more potentially hazardous but is often recommended for poisoning with amphetamines and fenfluramine (Pondimin).

Poisons are occasionally cleared directly from the bloodstream by peritoneal dialysis or hemodialysis, hemoperfusion, or transfusion to augment the other measures previously discussed. Peritoneal dialysis is less effective than hemodialysis or hemoperfusion. The degree to which these methods may be useful depends in part on the properties of the substance (i.e., whether it freely circulates or whether it is bound to plasma proteins or to tissues). Various lists of substances amenable to dialysis exist; some substances for which hemodialysis has *not* proved useful are as follows: cefixime (Suprax), clindamycin (Cleocin), diazepam (Valium), cyclosporine, digoxin (Lanoxin), phenytoin (Dilantin), propranolol (Inderal), and zidovudine (Retrovir) (*USP DI*, 1999; Aweeka, 1996).

Antidotes

The number of antidotes for specific toxins is minimal; no widely accepted "universal antidote" exists. Nevertheless, some general statements can be made about antidotes. Antidotes are more effective after the stomach is empty. The correct dosage to reverse toxicity depends on the specific drug involved, its half-life, and the severity of toxicity shown.

Antidotes work by any of the following mechanisms: (1) antagonizing or stimulating receptor sites that have been rendered hyperfunctional or dysfunctional by the poison, (2) interfering with enzyme inhibition, (3) administering the product of metabolism that has been interfered with, (4) inhibiting the biotransformation of a substance to a poisonous metabolite, (5) giving an agent that inactivates the toxic product, (6) chelation (forming highly stable complexes, tying up the substance—usually a heavy metal such as iron), and (7) producing immunotherapy—the use of antidrug antibodies to bind and inactivate drugs (e.g., severe digoxin poisoning reversed with sheep digoxin-specific antibodies).

PREVENTION OF POISONING

The focus of nursing on primary care and its corollary, prevention, applies readily to poisonings. The nursing profession has always emphasized prevention, and now other disciplines are beginning to take part. Combined efforts with drug information centers and other health care professionals and creative approaches have already had an impact on the frequency of certain categories of drug poisoning, notably aspirin poisoning.

Various creative graphic symbols appear on the labels of poisonous substances to alert the adult and/or nonreading child to the potential hazard contained therein. "Mr. Yuk," an ugly, green-faced, scowling image, is one of these. Tricky-to-open caps appear to delay if not completely prevent children's indiscriminate use of medicines. Others who have no need for these caps can request medication in the familiar easy-to-open caps.

There is much to learn about both apparent and potential toxins in the environment, and there is much to do in the way of poison prevention. Concerted, thoughtful efforts have already had a positive effect on statistics.

■ Nursing Management

Care of the Client with Poisoning

■ **Assessment.** An assessment should be performed quickly to determine what substance is involved so that immediate action can be taken to prevent or minimize its effects. Depending on the causative agent, symptoms may include nausea and vomiting, abdominal cramping, convulsions, a change in the level of consciousness, and decreased rates of pulse and respiration. Assess cardiopulmonary and respiratory function. Poisoning should be suspected in any unconscious individual with no history of diabetes, seizure disorders, or trauma.

To assist in determining the agent, the lips and mouth are checked for excessive salivation, burns, or difficulty swallowing. The breath should be assessed for its odor. Some petroleum and cleaning products have distinct smells that can be identified.

The pupils should be checked for dilation or constriction, which may also help to indicate the substance.

If the individual is conscious, he or she should be questioned about what substance was taken and in what quantity. If the individual is unconscious, identification of the substance is facilitated by clues in the environment. Empty containers, open bottles or medication containers, or syringes should be gathered and taken to the hospital with the victim. Containers often list the ingredients of the substance to assist the health care provider in choosing the treatment or antidote.

Toxicologic studies, which include drug screens, can determine poison levels in the mouth, vomitus, urine, feces, or blood or on the individual's hands and clothing and confirm the diagnosis. For inhalation poisoning, chest x-ray studies might show pulmonary infiltrates or edema.

■ **Nursing Diagnosis.** The client receiving care for poisoning is at risk for the following nursing diagnoses/collaborative problems: disturbed thought processes (confusion); risk for aspiration; risk for self-harm (suicide attempt); and the potential complications of seizures, coma, and death.

■ **Implementation**

■ ***Monitoring.*** Carefully monitor the client's vital signs and level of consciousness. Observe the client for nausea, vomiting, diarrhea, and abdominal cramping. The client's vomitus, stool, and urine should be observed for abnormalities such as the presence of blood. These body substances need to be retained for analysis for both medical and legal reasons.

■ ***Intervention.*** With poisoning, immediate action is required to prevent the absorption of the substance. If the individual is unconscious, he or she should be transported as soon as possible to a hospital. If the individual is conscious, a physician and/or the poison control center should be contacted immediately. The telephone number of the nearest poison control center is usually listed in the front of the telephone directory with other emergency numbers for the community.

If the poison has been inhaled (e.g., a toxic gas or carbon monoxide), the individual should be removed from the source to the fresh air, and oxygen should be administered if available. Cardiopulmonary resuscitation should be started if indicated. Call 911; the victim will need to be transported to the hospital.

If the substance is a contact poison absorbed through the skin and mucous membranes, the individual should be rinsed off immediately with copious amounts of water. The clothing should then be removed, and the skin is rinsed again. A shower is the best method for removing the agent from the skin.

If the poison is ingested, the objective is to prevent absorption of the substance either by inducing vomiting or by lavage to remove the agent or by administering an agent to inactivate the poisonous substance. The most recommended method of inducing vomiting is to have the client take 15 mL ipecac syrup followed by a full glass of water. This procedure may be repeated in 20 minutes if necessary. Lavage that is attempted in an unconscious individual should be performed with a cuffed endotracheal tube in place to prevent aspiration. Vomiting or lavage should not be attempted for the ingestion of caustic substances or hydrocarbons (found in petroleum products). Care for the ingestion of these substances is to give nothing by mouth and to seek urgent medical assistance.

If the substance has a known antidote, the physician will administer it.

Other nursing interventions relate to the supportive care of the acutely ill client. Monitor vital signs and report any changes immediately. Administer oxygen and suction if respirations are depressed. Maintain IV fluids as ordered. Keep the client warm and turn him or her at frequent intervals to promote drainage from the respiratory tract.

If the poisoning was intentional, such as a suicide attempt, safety precautions should be instituted to protect the client from further self-destructive behavior. In addition, a psychiatric referral should be considered.

■ ***Education.*** To prevent accidental poisoning, families should be assisted to evaluate environmental hazards in the home. Toddlers are at the greatest risk. Cleaning agents, especially furniture polish and products containing caustic agents, should be stored in high cabinets with childproof locks. In homes where children live or visit, all medications should be stored in locked cabinets or boxes. Remind parents that pocketbooks containing medications should be kept out of the reach of youngsters. Substances such as insecticides or alcohol should be inaccessible to children. All medications should be clearly labeled with the type, dosage, and storage requirements. In addition, the client's ability to safely self-medicate should be assessed before there is an expectation for self-medication.

Clients should be cautioned not to store toxic substances in food containers or improperly labeled containers or in a place that is accessible to children. Medications should not be stored beyond the date of expiration. Poisonous plants should not be kept in households where there are small children.

Ipecac syrup, as well as the appropriate directions for its use, is a necessary ingredient in a household first aid container.

When interacting with clients, nurses should be alert to the presence of anger, depression, withdrawal, and faulty judgment, which may precede intentional or unintentional poisoning.

■ **Evaluation.** The expected outcome of antidote use in poisoning is that the client will experience a regression of symptoms, which indicates the successful elimination and inactivation of the poison.

COMMON POISONS

Alcohols (ethanol, isopropyl, and methyl) are reviewed in Chapter 9, and acetaminophen is covered in Chapters 11 and 14. Carbon monoxide, iron, and organophosphate insecticides are reviewed here.

Carbon Monoxide

Carbon monoxide (CO) is an odorless gas produced by the incomplete combustion of carbon or carbonaceous materials. Sources of this gas include improperly maintained heating systems, improperly ventilated charcoal cookers or fireplaces, and industrial furnaces, such as those in steel mills. Automobile exhaust contains 3% to 7% CO. CO causes more deaths in the United States and Canada than any other poison. The inhalation of automobile exhaust is a common method of suicide, and accidental home and industrial exposure to CO is much more common than generally appreciated.

Poisoning by CO results from pulmonary absorption of the gas, which readily combines with hemoglobin to form carboxyhemoglobin. The oxygen in hemoglobin is replaced, thus lowering the available oxygen carried by the blood to the body tissues. With the addition of each CO molecule the oxygen molecules remaining on the hemoglobin become so tightly bound that they are not readily released to the oxygen-starved tissues. CO is measured in the blood as the percent carboxyhemoglobin (%HbCO). In addition, CO gas that is dissolved in blood but not bound to hemoglobin diffuses into the body tissues and poisons the cytochrome enzymes necessary for the use of oxygen by cells.

In general, the symptoms of CO poisoning are related to %HbCO. Clinically, only mild (if any) symptoms occur at 10% HbCO; cigarette smokers may have a CO level of this percentage. The initial signs of poisoning usually occur at 10% to 30% HbCO and include a throbbing headache, nausea, vomiting, dizziness, weakness, and visual disturbances. These early symptoms of intoxication are nonspecific and may be attributed to a number of other causes unless a history of CO is available or laboratory tests demonstrate an elevated %HbCO. At 40% to 50% HbCO, syncope, tachycardia, tightness in the chest, and tachypnea occur. HbCO has a cherry pink color rather than the red color of oxyhemoglobin; therefore the client may have a cherry pink coloration to the skin. A level of HbCO in excess of 50% causes life-threatening convulsions, coma, dangerously compromised cardiopulmonary function, and possible death. Fatalities in victims of suicide or fire often have a %HbCO of 60% to 80%.

Treatment for CO poisoning is based on the client's symptoms and %HbCO. Hyperbaric oxygen is the antidote of choice, because oxygen under pressure is capable of replacing CO from hemoglobin and from the iron containing respiratory cytochrome enzymes in the tissues.

Ninety-five percent of absorbed CO is excreted by the lungs; once removed from the source of exposure, the half-life of CO in normal ambient air is 4 hours. If 100% oxygen is administered, the half-life ($t^{1/2}$) decreases to 40 minutes. Hyperbaric oxygen at 3 atmospheres of pressure decreases the $t^{1/2}$ of CO to only 23 minutes. In severe poisoning, cardiopulmonary support is maintained throughout therapy. Additional drug therapy to control dysrhythmias, cerebral edema, and convulsions may be indicated.

■ **Nursing Management**

Carbon Monoxide Poisoning

The nursing management for carbon monoxide poisoning is the same as for poisoning.

Iron

Iron supplements are a leading cause of pediatric poisoning deaths in the United States. Since 1986, more than 110,000 accidental ingestions of iron preparations have been reported, with 33 deaths (Food and Drug Administration, 1997). Iron overdoses have also been noted to result in profound mental retardation; therefore such products should be dispensed in child-resistant containers and stored in an area that is not readily accessible to small children.

Iron deficiency is a primary cause of anemia in both infants and adults. Thus iron is often added to infant formulas and foods and is available in more than 100 commercial products for adults, including multiple and prenatal vitamins. Available products use a number of forms of iron and various salts and chelates. The toxic effects of iron are caused by its elemental form; therefore the relative toxicity of iron salts is related to the percentage of elemental iron in the substance. For example, ferrous fumarate (33% iron) is more toxic on a weight basis than ferrous gluconate (12% iron).

On ingestion, large amounts of iron cause local corrosive actions on the gastric and duodenal mucosa and upper gastrointestinal tract. Initial symptoms of iron poisoning include nausea, vomiting, upper abdominal pain, and bloody diarrhea. The corrosive action destroys the normal mucosal barrier to iron absorption, allowing the rapid absorption of large amounts of iron into the general circulation. These overdose concentrations of iron exceed the binding capacity of transferrin, the iron-carrying protein of the blood. The excess free iron readily diffuses into various tissues and binds to the sulfhydryl (SH) radicals of numerous enzymes and structural proteins. This binding of iron to compounds necessary for normal cellular function poisons the tissue cells.

Symptoms of systemic intoxication—cyanosis, pulmonary edema, and possible cardiovascular collapse—start to occur within 6 to 24 hours after ingestion. Coagulation defects, hepatic necrosis, and renal failure may develop within a few days. As with adults, the initial symptoms of pediatric iron poisoning are characterized by repeated vomiting, abdominal pain, and diarrhea. A latent phase often occurs—the initial symptoms abate and the child appears well for a 6- to 12-hour period; this is followed by rapid illness and the development of shock. The determination of serum iron value will indicate the severity of the intoxication and prevent the possible dangerous misinterpretation of this latency period.

In addition, serum iron values indicate the necessity of initiating antidotal therapy. Serum iron concentrations of 350 μg/dL or less are rarely associated with clinical illness. Concentrations between 350 and 500 μg/dL call for observation of the client for the development of clinical signs of intoxication. Deferoxamine (an iron chelating agent) therapy is recommended for concentrations above 500 μg/dL. Deferoxamine is a specific chelator that binds free serum iron and the iron associated with hepatic and splenic stores. It does not bind with zinc, copper, or other trace metals. The deferoxamine-iron complex is nontoxic and is freely excreted by the kidneys.

The treatment for iron poisoning includes general supportive measures, as well as a specific antidote to bind the ingested iron. Emesis may be induced to expel unabsorbed iron tablets in the stomach; a sodium bicarbonate lavage is also indicated, because bicarbonate converts ferrous iron to ferrous carbonate, which is poorly absorbed. After lavage, 200 to 300 mL of the bicarbonate solution should be left in the stomach.

■ **Nursing Management**

Iron Poisoning

In addition to the following discussion, which is specific to iron poisoning, see Nursing Management: Care of the Client with Poisoning, p. 1231.

Obtain a careful history to elicit the possibility of pregnancy. Advise against the use of deferoxamine if the client is pregnant or may have a severe renal impairment.

Institute emesis or gastric lavage as soon as possible. Initiate supportive measures, including maintaining a clear airway and providing interventions related to the presence of shock and to acidosis. Administer deferoxamine using a long needle and the Z-track method; 0.2 to 0.3 mL of air may be added to the medication in the syringe to prevent pain and induration at the site of injections. Carefully controlled, slow IV infusion rates may be equally effective in preventing infusion pain.

Tell the client to expect a reddish brown coloration of urine and stools.

Organophosphate Insecticides

Organophosphate compounds are highly effective insecticides. Their chemical structure is unstable, which results in their disintegration into nontoxic radicals within days of their application. Therefore they do not persist or accumulate in the environment or animal tissues as do the chlorinated insecticides such as DDT. This accounts for their addition to numerous commercial products—from flea collars, bug bombs, and flypapers to most home and commercial insect sprays. Their popularity accounts for their high potential for accidental poisoning.

Organophosphate compounds are powerful inhibitors of the enzyme acetylcholinesterase (AChE), which breaks down the neurotransmitter acetylcholine (ACh) (see Chapter 21). In general, organophosphates are rapidly absorbed in the body by all routes. Individual organophosphates display a wide variation in their ability to penetrate the skin, in oral absorption, and thus in their toxicity. For example, malathion does not penetrate the skin well and its oral toxicity is low; this makes it a popular insecticide for use in home products.

The signs and symptoms of organophosphate insecticide poisoning are related to inhibition of AChE, which results in an accumulation of ACh in the parasympathetic nervous system. As a result, all organs affected by ACh are overstimulated. The expected results of organophosphate poisoning are as follows: bradycardia, hypotension, dyspnea, wheezing, miosis, blurred vision, convulsions, muscular fasciculations, and profuse sweating. A common mnemonic for symptoms of organophosphate intoxication is SLUDGE: salivation, lacrimation, urination, defecation, gastrointestinal distress, and emesis. The usual mode of death is respiratory arrest caused by bronchospasm, decreased pulmonary muscle strength, and finally depression of the CNS control of respiration. The sequence in which specific systems develop is related to the route of exposure. Respiratory tract effects appear first after inhalation, whereas gastrointestinal effects appear initially after ingestion. Skin absorption results in immediate profuse sweating and muscle weakness.

Therapy for organophosphate poisoning involves the support of cardiopulmonary function, the clearance of respiratory tract secretions to maintain a clear airway, and the use of appropriate antidotes, atropine and pralidoxime (2-PAM, Protopam). Atropine competitively antagonizes the action of ACh at muscarinic receptors on the organs innervated by postganglionic parasympathetic nerves and cholinergic sympathetic nerves (Chapter 21).

Although atropine is effective in blocking the muscarinic symptoms of bradycardia, bronchoconstriction, and excess secretions, muscular fasciculations are refractory to this antidote. These involuntary contractions and twitchings and respiratory paralysis are best treated with 2-PAM, a cholinesterase reactivator that removes organophosphates bound to AChE. This frees AChE to break down the accumulated ACh, thereby resuming normal activity at the neuromuscular junction. 2-PAM also directly detoxifies certain organophosphates. The side effects of 2-PAM include dizziness, nausea, headache, and tachycardia.

▪ Nursing Management

Organophosphate Poisoning

In addition to the following discussion, see Nursing Management: Care of the Client with Poisoning, p.1231.

If there is cyanosis, establish and maintain an airway first. Document the extent of SLUDGE symptoms.

Closely monitor both respiratory status and the production of secretions, because doses of atropine may be predicated on this information. Plan to monitor client's status closely for 72 hours.

Copious secretions may initially necessitate nearly continuous suctioning; anticipate supplemental oxygen therapy. Induce vomiting or perform a gastric lavage if the poison was ingested. Cleanse the skin if any insecticide contaminant is present. If signs of excessive atropinization appear, plan for treatment with physostigmine to antagonize atropine. Anticipate the need to administer pralidoxime (Protopam) if poisoning is severe.

SUMMARY

Poisoning, either accidental or intentional, is a commonplace reason for admission to a hospital emergency department. Children make up the majority of the accidental poisoning population, whereas intentional poisoning is more likely to be the result of a suicide attempt or an overdose of an abused substance. No matter how poisonings are classified, the care provided focuses on prompt treatment, identification of the substance (if possible), the support of vital functions, the removal or elimination of the poison, and the prevention of future occurrences.

Critical Thinking Questions

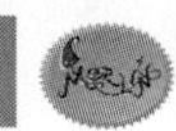

1. In what poisoning situations would the following be the most appropriate therapy: Emesis? Gastric lavage? Refraining from induced vomiting?
2. Two-year-old Samantha Rogers has been brought to the emergency department by her mother, who found Samantha in the bathroom with a container of toilet bowl cleaner (alkali base) in her hands. She is crying and her lips are swollen and excoriated. Mrs. Rogers believes that Samantha has ingested some of the liquid. What sequence of actions should the nurse take?

Collaborative Learning Activities

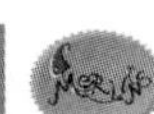

For Collaborative Learning Activities, go to mosby.com/MERLIN/McKenry/.

BIBLIOGRAPHY

Anderson, K.N., Anderson, L.E., & Glanze, W.D. (Eds.) (1998). *Mosby's medical, nursing, & allied health dictionary* (5th ed.). St. Louis: Mosby.

Aweeka, F.T. (1996). Dosing of drugs in renal failure. In L.Y. Young & M.A. Koda-Kimble (Eds.), *Applied therapeutics: The clinical use of drugs* (6th ed.). Vancouver, WA: Applied Therapeutics.

Chyka, P.A. (1999). Clinical toxicology. In J.T. DiPiro et al (Eds.), *Pharmacotherapy: A pathophysiologic approach* (4th ed.). Norwalk, CT: Appleton & Lange.

Covington, T.R. (1993). *Handbook of nonprescription drugs* (10th ed.). Washington, D.C.: American Pharmaceutical Association and The National Professional Society of Pharmacists.

Drug Facts and Comparisons. (2000). St. Louis: Facts and Comparisons.

Food and Drug Administration (FDA). (1997). *Protect children from iron poisoning*. Rockville, MD: Author; vm.cfsan.fda.gov/~dms/fdairon.html (6/6/99).

Kwan, T., Paiusco, A.D., Kohl, L. (1992). Digitalis toxicity caused by toad venom. *Chest, 102*(3), 949-950.

Lammon, C.A. & Adams, M.H. (1992). Organophosphate overdose: Nursing strategies. *DCCN, 11*(6):310-317.

Litovitz, T.L., Klein-Schwartz, W., Caravati, E.M., Youniss, J., Crouch, B., & Lee, S. (1999). 1998 annual report of the American Association of Poison Control Centers toxic exposure surveillance system. *American Journal of Emergency Medicine, 17*(5), 435-487.

Melmon, K.L., Morrelli, H.F., Hoffman, B.B., & Nierenberg, D.W. (Eds.). (1992). *Melmon and Morrelli's clinical pharmacology: Basic principles in therapeutics* (3rd ed.). New York: McGraw-Hill.

Oderda, G.A. & Jennings, J.C. (1996). Emetic and antiemetic products. In T.R. Covington (Ed.), *Handbook of nonprescription drugs* (11th ed.). Washington, D.C.: American Pharmaceutical Association.

Physicians' Desk Reference (53th ed.). (1999). Oradell, NJ: Medical Economics.

Public Health Service, U.S. Department of Health and Human Services. (1993). Jin bu huan toxicity in children—Colorado. *MMWR: Morbidity and Mortality Weekly Report, 42*(33), 633-636.

Public Health Service, U.S. Department of Health and Human Services. (1993). Lead poisoning associated with use of traditional ethnic remedies—California, 1991-1992. *MMWR: Morbidity and Mortality Weekly Report, 42*(27), 521-524.

United States Pharmacopeia Dispensing Information (USP DI): Drug information for the health care professional (19th ed.). (1999). Rockville, MD: United States Pharmacopeial Convention.

Vale, J.A. & Proudfoot, A. (1997). Drug overdosage and poisoning. In T.M. Speight & N.H.G. Holford (Eds.), *Avery's drug treatment* (4th ed.). Auckland, New Zealand: Adis International.

Watson, W.A. (1996). Clinical toxicology. In L.Y. Young & M.A. Koda-Kimble (Eds.), *Applied therapeutics: The clinical use of drugs* (6th ed.). Vancouver, WA: Applied Therapeutics.

Wong, D.L., Hockenberry-Eaton, M., Wilson, D., Winkelstein, M.L., Ahmann, E., DiVito-Thomas, P.A. (1999). *Whaley & Wong's nursing care of infants and children* (6th ed.). St. Louis: Mosby.

Wuest, J.R. & Gossel, T.A. (1992). A primer for pharmacists on treatment of poisoning. *Florida Pharmacy Today, 56*(3), 22.

Appendix

A Sugar-Free Products*

The following is a selection of sugar-free products by therapeutic categories. However, check the labels, because some of these medications may contain sorbitol, alcohol, or other sources of carbohydrate.

ANTACIDS

Alka-Seltzer Original
Alka-Seltzer, Lemon-Lime
Aluminum Hydroxide Gel
Gaviscon Liquid
Gelusil Liquid
Maalox
Maalox HRF
Riopan
Riopan Plus
Titralac
Titralac Plus

ANALGESICS

Acetaminophen Oral solution, USP, Cherry
Arthritis Pain Formula
Aspirin, Delayed-Release
Bayer Aspirin
Bufferin Arthritis Strength
Bufferin Extra Strength
Excedrin Aspirin Free
Feverall Sprinkle Caps
Motrin IB
Nuprin
Panadol
Tempra
Tylenol

*Check label ingredients because manufacturers may alter or reformulate their products.

COUGH, COLD, AND ANTIHISTAMINES

Benadryl Dye-Free
Benylin Adult Cough Formula
Benylin Expectorant Cough Formula
Cheracol Sore Throat
Diabetic Tussin Allergy Relief
Diabetic Tussin DM
Guaifenesin CF
Guaifenesin DM
Naldecon DX Adult Liquid
Naldecon DX Children's Syrup
Naldecon EX Children's Syrup
Naldecon EX Pediatric Drops
Naldecon Senior DX Liquid
Naldecon Senior EX Liquid
Robitussin Pediatric Cough
Tussar SF

FOOD SUPPLEMENTS

Criticare HN
Fibersource
Fibersource HN
Impact
Impact with Fiber
Isocal
MCT Oil
Vivonex T.E.N.

LAXATIVES

Doxidan
Dulcolax
Fiberall, Natural
Haley's M-O
Konsyl
Metamucil Sugar Free
Milk of Magnesia
Surfak

Appendix

B Alcohol-Free Products*

ANALGESICS

Acetaminophen
Liquiprin Drops
Mapap Infant Drops
Panadol, Children's
Panadol, Infants'
Silapap, Infants'
Tylenol, Children's Cherry Flavor
Tylenol, Children's Liquid
Tylenol, Infants'

ANTIASTHMATIC PRODUCTS

Aerolate Oral Solution
Alupent Syrup
Dilor G Liquid
Slo-Phyllin Syrup
Slo-Phyllin GG Syrup
Theolair Liquid

COUGH, COLD, AND ANTIHISTAMINES

Benadryl Allergy Decongestant Liquid
Benylin Adult Liquid
Benylin Pediatric Liquid
Benylin Expectorant
Diabetic Tussin DM
Diabetic Tussin EX
Dimetapp Elixir
Dimetapp DM Elixir
Drixoral Cough & Congestion Liquid Caps
Naldecon CX Adult Liquid
Naldecon DX Adult Liquid
Naldecon DX Children's Syrup
Naldecon DX Pediatric Drops
Naldecon EX Pediatric Drops
Naldecon Senior DX Liquid
NyQuil Children's Cold/Cough Liquid
PediaCare Cough-Cold Liquid
Robitussin Pediatric Cough & Cold Liquid
Robitussin Night Relief
Triaminic AM Cough & Decongestant Formula
Triaminic AM Decongestant Formula
Triaminic Expectorant Liquid
Tussar-DM Syrup
Tylenol Children's Cold Multi-Symptom
Vicks Pediatric Formula 44E
Vicks DayQuil Liquid

GARGLE/MOUTHWASHES

Chloraseptic Gly-Oxide Liquid
Orabase-O
Orabase Plain
Oral-B Anti-Cavity Rinse

PSYCHOTROPICS

Haldol Concentrate
Stelazine Concentrate
Thorazine Syrup

*Check label ingredients because manufacturers may alter or reformulate their products.

Appendix

C Drugs That Change Urine or Stool Color

Medications That May Alter Urine Color

Drug	Possible Color Changes
amitriptyline (Elavil)	Blue-green
anticoagulants (coumarin and others)	Pink, red, or dark brown (indicative of systemic bleeding)
cascara sagrada	In acid urine, brown; basic urine, yellow to pink; on standing, black
iron salts, dextran, and others	Brown to black
laxatives (danthron, senna)	Pink to red or brown
levodopa (Larodopa, Dopar)	May cause dark urine and sweat
methyldopa (Aldomet, Dopamet 🍁)	Pink, amber to dark urine
metronidazole (Flagyl)	Dark urine
nitrofurantoin (Furadantin, Macrodantin)	Yellow to rusty brown urine
phenazopyridine (Pyridium, Phenazo 🍁)	Orange-red urine; may stain clothing
phenothiazines (chlorpromazine [Thorazine] and others)	Pink, red, or orange urine
phenytoin (Dilantin)	Red-brown or darkening of urine
rifampin (Rifadin, Rofact 🍁)	Red, orange, or brown urine, stool, saliva, sweat, and tears

Medications That May Alter Stool Color

Drug	Possible Color Changes
antacids with aluminum salts (Maalox, Mylanta, and others)	White specks or discoloration of stools
anticoagulants (coumarin and others)	Red, orange, to black because of internal bleeding
bismuth or iron salts	Black
laxative (senna)	Yellow, orange to brown
phenazopyridine (Pyridium and others)	Orange, red

Appendix

D TIME TO DRAW BLOOD FOR SPECIFIC MEDICATIONS

Serum drug levels are used to aid the prescriber in (1) determining dosage adjustments for drugs with a narrow range between therapeutic effect and toxicity and (2) providing information to evaluate a suspected toxicity or noncompliance.

Blood samples are usually drawn according to the pharmacokinetics of the individual drug. For example, to obtain a steady-state serum level, the blood sample should be drawn approximately 5 drug half-lives after instituting therapy.

Gentamicin (Garamycin) has a short half-life; thus peak and trough levels are usually ordered to ensure adequate therapy. The peak serum level (P) is usually obtained 15 to 30 minutes after an IV dose or 1 hour after an IM dose. The trough (Tr) serum level should be drawn just before the next scheduled dose. Trough serum levels are used to predict the risk of adverse reactions; a rising trough level or levels above 2 μg/mL have been associated with increased toxicity.

Therapeutic Ranges of Serum Drug Concentrations

	Serum Concentration		
Drug	**Ther (μg/mL)**	**Tr (μg/mL)**	**Time for Blood Sampling (hours after last dose)***
Antibiotics			
amikacin (Amikin)	15-25	5	See previous discussion on gentamicin.
gentamicin (Garamycin)	4-10	2	See previous discussion on gentamicin.
netilmicin (Netromycin)	6-10	2	See previous discussion on gentamicin.
tobramycin (Nebcin)	4-10	2	See previous discussion on gentamicin.
Anticonvulsants			
carbamazepine (Tegretol)	4-12		SS 1-2 weeks. Before morning dose (Tr).
phenobarbital	10-40		SS 10-30 days. Before morning dose (Tr).
phenytoin (Dilantin)	10-20		SS 1-4 weeks. Oral (Tr), before next dose; IV, 2-4 hours after loading dose.
primidone (Mysoline)	5-12		SS 2-3 days for primidone; phenobarbital as above. Before next dose (Tr).
valproic acid (Depakene, Depakote)	50-100		SS 2-3 days. Before next dose (Tr).
Cardiovascular Drugs			
digoxin (Lanoxin)	0.8-2 ng/mL		SS 1 week. Before next dose (Tr) at least 6 hours after last dose to allow for drug distribution in the body.
lidocaine (Xylocaine)	1.5-5		SS 7-12 hours. Anytime during IV infusion.
procainamide (Pronestyl)	4-10 mg/mL		SS 12-24 hours. Before next dose (Tr).
quinidine (various drugs)	3-6		SS 30 hours. Before next dose (Tr).
Respiratory Drugs			
theophylline (various drugs)	asthma 10-20		SS 1-2 days in adults, up to 1 week in neonates. IV infusion, anytime; oral, before next dose (Tr).

*SS, Time to reach drug steady state (SS time is noted first, then the suggested appropriate time of blood sampling for the specific drug); *Tr,* trough.

Appendix

E ADDITIONAL NEW DRUG PRODUCTS

Generic (Brand Name)	Drug Category	Indication	Usual Dosage	Comments
alemtuzumab (Campath)	Monoclonal antibody	B-cell chronic lymphocytic leukemia	IV infusion; see package insert	Administration is supervised by an experienced physician only. May cause serious infusion reactions, infections, and hematologic toxicity.
arsenic trioxide (Trisenox)	Antineoplastic	Acute promyelocytic leukemia	IV; see package insert	Administration is supervised by an experienced physician only. May cause cardiac abnormalities (complete AV block, QT prolongation); follow ECG and electrolyte monitoring recommendations.
beractant (Survanta) calfactant (Infasurf) colfosceril (Exosurf Neonatal)	Lung surfactant	Infants with RDS	Intratracheal administration based on infant weight	Administration is by trained medical personnel only. Adverse effects of beractant include hypotension or hypertension, pallor, hypercarbia, and apnea; with calfactant, cyanosis, airway obstruction, and bradycardia; with colfosceril, pulmonary damage (e.g., pneumothorax, hemorrhage, pneumonia); nonpulmonary infections, hypotension, seizures, and apnea.

ECG, Electrocardiogram; *GI,* gastrointestinal; *RDS,* respiratory distress syndrome.

Generic (Brand Name)	Drug Category	Indication	Usual Dosage	Comments
epirubicin (Ellence)	Antibiotic Antineoplastic	Breast cancer	IV infusion; see package insert	Avoid extravasation during drug administration; may cause severe tissue necrosis. Dose-related myocardial toxicity may occur during therapy or months/years afterward.
gemtuzumab ozogamicin (Mylotarg)	Antineoplastic	First relapse in older adults with acute myeloid leukemia	IV infusion; see package insert	Approved for clients more than 60 years of age. Common side effect is mucous membrane irritation.
imatinib mesylate (Gleevec)	Protein-tyrosine kinase inhibitor	Chronic myeloid leukemia	PO: 400 mg/day in chronic phase in adults; 600 mg/day for blast crisis in adults	May cause GI upset; take with food and large glass of water. May cause edema and severe fluid retention; monitor closely. May cause hepatotoxicity and hematologic toxicity.
nitric oxide (INOmax)	Vasodilator	Persistent pulmonary hypertension in newborns; acute respiratory distress syndrome in adults	Respiratory inhalant; 20 ppm for up to 2 weeks	Wean client off nitric oxide over several hours or days to avoid rebound effects.
porfimer (Photofrin)	Antineoplastic	Esophageal and endobronchial non–small-cell lung cancer	Photodynamic therapy; requires drug (IV) and laser light; see package insert	Porfimer is a photosensitizing agent; antitumor effects are light and oxygen dependent. May cause chest pain, ocular sensitivity, and respiratory distress.
temozolomide (Temodar)	Antineoplastic	Anaplastic astrocytoma	Oral dosing; see package insert	Most common adverse effects are nausea and vomiting; to reduce this effect, take on an empty stomach; antiemetic may be necessary. Do not open capsules; if accidentally opened, avoid contact with skin or mucous membranes.
triptorelin (Trelstar Depot)	Hormone	Advanced prostate cancer	IM use only; see package insert	Drug is a potent inhibitor of gonadotropin secretion, reducing serum testosterone serum levels to amount seen in castrated man. Monitor with serum levels of testosterone and prostate-specific antigen.

Appendix

F Top 100 Brand-Name Drugs by Prescription

For the complete list of the top 200 brand-name drugs by prescription, as well as the top 200 brand-name drugs by sales, the top 200 generic drugs by sales and prescription, and annual updates, go to www.drugtopics.com..

Top 100 Brand-Name Drugs by Prescription*

Rank	Product	Total Rxs (in thousands)	Rank	Product	Total Rxs (in thousands)
1.	Lipitor	44,714	31.	Toprol XL	11,909
2.	Premarin Tabs	41,876	32.	Ultram	11,708
3.	Synthroid	39,878	33.	Glucotrol XL	11,485
4.	Prilosec	29,603	34.	Flonase	11,484
5.	Norvasc	27,822	35.	Prinivil	11,228
6.	Glucophage	25,858	36.	Celexa	10,680
7.	Claritin	24,497	37.	Neurontin	10,543
8.	Zoloft	23,470	38.	Vasotec	10,283
9.	Zithromax Z-Pak	23,454	39.	K-Dur 20	10,051
10.	Prozac	23,365	40.	Fosamax	10,028
11.	Paxil	22,995	41.	Wellbutrin SR	9,908
12.	Celebrex	22,665	42.	Diflucan	9,720
13.	Prevacid	20,898	43.	Levaquin	9,692
14.	Zestril	21,567	44.	Lotensin	9,265
15.	Augmentin	21,171	45.	Flovent	8,965
16.	Prempro	20,898	46.	Singulair	8,596
17.	Zocor	19,643	47.	Effexor XR	8,493
18.	Vioxx	19,174	48.	Cardura	8,321
19.	Ortho Tri-Cyclen	17,891	49.	Biaxin	8,216
20.	Lanoxin	16,180	50.	Depakote	8,100
21.	Levoxyl	15,747	51.	Zithromax Susp	7,733
22.	Allegra	14,952	52.	Humulin N	7,718
23.	Amoxil	14,858	53.	Nasonex	7,421
24.	Cipro	14,234	54.	Veetids	7,265
25.	Ambien	13,708	55.	Cozaar	7,170
26.	Zyrtec	13,061	56.	Claritin D 12HR	7,130
27.	Coumadin Tabs	12,832	57.	Claritin D 24HR	6,744
28.	Accupril	12,614	58.	Xalatan	6,608
29.	Pravachol	12,412	59.	Adderall	6,405
30.	Viagra	12,266	60.	Serevent	6,403

From Drug Topics Archive, Apr. 16, 2001. Available at: www.medec.drugtopics.com.

Top 100 Brand-Name Drugs by Prescription*—cont'd

Rank	Product	Total Rxs (in thousands)	Rank	Product	Total Rxs (in thousands)
61.	Monopril	6,389	81.	Zyprexa	5,290
62.	Risperdal	6,247	82.	Alesse-28	5,074
63.	Pepcid	6,082	83.	Humulin 70/30	5,049
64.	Plavix	6,075	84.	Lescol	4,967
65.	Allegra-D	6,034	85.	Hyzaar	4,934
66.	Triphasil	6,033	86.	Relafen	4,869
67.	Ortho-Novum 7/7/7	6,000	87.	Combivent	4,804
68.	Cefzil	5,982	88.	Zestoretic	4,723
69.	Ziac	5,969	89.	Levothroid	4,689
70.	Adalat CC	5,956	90.	Serzone	4,613
71.	Dilantin Kapseals	5,881	91.	Ortho-Cyclen	4,556
72.	Diovan	5,622	92.	Necon 1/35	4,443
73.	Oxycontin	5,570	93.	Roxicet	4,422
74.	Evista	5,542	94.	Detrol	4,403
75.	Lotrel	5,487	95.	Macrobid	4,386
76.	Lotrisone	5,400	96.	Klor-Con	4,325
77.	Ceftin	5,350	97.	Imitrex	4,304
78.	Amaryl	5,338	98.	Baycol*	4,292
79.	Avandia	5,312	99.	Bactroban	4,241
80.	Procardia XL	5,302	100.	Cardizem CD	4,173

Modified from Drug Topics Archive, Apr. 16, 2001. Available at: www.drugtopics.com.
*Voluntarily withdrawn from the market August 8, 2001.

Appendix

G Oral Transmucosal Fentanyl

Oral transmucosal fentanyl citrate (Actiq) is a potent opioid analgesic available as a raspberry-flavored lozenge on a stick and is used in managing severe breakthrough cancer pain. This product is indicated only for clients who are already receiving and are tolerant of opioids, that is, clients who are taking at least 60 mg of morphine daily, 50 μg of fentanyl per hour, or an equianalgesic dose of another opioid for a week or more. This product should be prescribed only by oncologists or pain management specialists.

Actiq is available in six strengths (200, 400, 600, 800, 1200 and 1600 μg of fentanyl base), and each drug unit is individually sealed in a child-resistant foil pouch. The unit should be placed in the client's mouth between the cheek and gums; the unit should be moved from one cheek side to the other while twirling the handle. This product needs to be sucked, not chewed, over a 15-minute period (chewed and swallowed fentanyl results in lower fentanyl serum levels). Approximately 25% of the total dose is rapidly absorbed from the buccal mucosa and is available systemically as an analgesic. The other 75% is swallowed and is slowly absorbed from the gastrointestinal tract, with only a third of this dose being available systemically. After 15 minutes of sucking, peak fentanyl serum levels are usually achieved within 20 to 40 minutes.

Inform the client and family that Actiq can be fatal to a child or to adults who cannot tolerate opioids. All Actiq units must be kept out of the reach of children, and open units should be properly disposed of in a secured container. If any drug matrix is present after use, place it under hot running water until the entire matrix is dissolved. The handle should be properly disposed of and kept out of the reach of children.

Actiq is not indicated for the treatment of acute or postoperative pain and should not be used for anyone with an unknown opioid tolerance. It also should not be used in clients who are receiving or who have received an MAO inhibitor within the previous 2 weeks. Extensive information on this drug is available from the drug manufacturer and can also be found on the manufacturer's Internet site (Abbott Laboratories, 1998).

Information from Abbott Laboratories. (1998). Actiq (oral transmucosal fentanyl citrate), Reference 58-0645-R2; www.actiq.com (5/10/00).

Appendix

H System Used to Rate HIV Treatment Recommendations

Rating	Strength of Recommendation
A	Both strong evidence for efficacy and substantial clinical benefit support recommendation for use. **Should always be offered.**
B	Moderate evidence for efficacy—or strong evidence for efficacy but only limited clinical benefit—supports recommendation for use. **Should generally be offered.**
C	Evidence for efficacy is insufficient to support a recommendation for or against use, or evidence for efficacy might not outweigh adverse consequences (e.g., drug toxicity, drug interactions) or the cost of chemoprophylaxis or alternative approaches. **Optional.**
D	Moderate evidence for lack of efficacy or for adverse outcome supports a recommendation against use. **Should generally not be offered.**
E	Good evidence for lack of efficacy or for adverse outcome supports a recommendation against use. **Should never be offered.**
	Quality of Evidence Supporting the Recommendation
I	Evidence from at least one properly randomized, controlled trial.
II	Evidence from at least one well-designed clinical trial without randomization, from cohort or case-controlled analytic studies (preferably from more than one center), or from multiple time-series studies; or dramatic results from uncontrolled experiments.
III	Evidence from opinions of respected authorities based on clinical experience, descriptive studies, or reports of expert committees.

From 1999 USPHS/IDSA Prevention of Opportunistic Infections Working Group, U.S. Public Health Service and Infectious Diseases Society of America. (1999). *USPHS/IDSA guidelines for the prevention of opportunistic infections in persons infected with human immunodeficiency virus.* *48*(RR10), 1-59; www.cdc.gov/epo/mmwr/preview/mmwrhtml/rr4810al.htm (2/17/00).

Appendix

I DRUG THERAPY IN END-OF-LIFE CARE

Many physicians and nurses have been educated in the medical and scientific advances or the technologically sophisticated approach to medicine. When these approaches (often referred to as therapeutic techniques) fail to cure or contain an advanced disease stage, health care professionals often abandon, ignore, or pay less attention to an individual with an unfavorable prognosis and no known cure. Such persons are referred to as terminally ill, and their care is primarily palliative, end-of-life care.

End-of-life care requires an organized approach of palliative and supportive care for dying individuals and their families. The need for a comprehensive, multidisciplinary approach of total care for the dying person evolved in the hospice movement in the United States. Total palliative care has been defined as the provision of medical, nursing, psychosocial, and spiritual services for clients and their families both during illness and during bereavement (Woodruff, 1993).

The following two quotes best describe the key issues involved in caring for these patients:

> In our system, it is easier to get open-heart surgery than Meals on Wheels, easier to get antibiotics than eyeglasses, and certainly easier to get emergency care aimed at rescue than to get sustaining, supportive care (Lynn, 2001).
>
> Good care of the dying person means making the body as comfortable as possible so that the patient can prepare for death mentally and spiritually. It will mean allowing the patient to live as fully as possible up until he dies (Favaro, 2002).

End-of-life care must address and expand on these issues.

PHYSICAL ISSUES

The physical issues present during the end-of-life stage may be extensive. Some of the most common physical problems include pain, dyspnea, constipation, nausea and vomiting, myoclonus, and delirium. The dying person may also experience anorexia and dehydration, which is of greater concern to the family than to the individual. Favaro (2002) states that it is perfectly natural for a patient to stop eating when preparing to die. There is a gradual decrease in eating habits, with meats generally being refused first, then vegetables, then a preference for softer foods, then liquids only. Although this is one of the hardest concepts for the family to accept, it should be accepted that it is acceptable not to eat.

Health care professionals should be knowledgeable about the proper use of pharmacology or drug therapy in end-of-life care; therefore this section will be devoted to the pharmacologic aspects of palliative care.

PAIN

Pain is one of the most common problems that, if left uncontrolled, may cause physical and mental distress that results in disabling of the individual. (See Chapter 14 for a thorough review of analgesics and pain management.) Pain assessment is the most important aspect in developing a treatment plan. The health care provider must be aware that many factors can cause pain and that the key to proper treatment is determination of the cause whenever possible. One should never assume that increased pain always results from advancement of the underlying disease process. Bone fractures, nerve injuries or compression, arthritis or inflammatory pain, or pain secondary to severe constipation may be overlooked and thus improperly treated in this population. Whenever possible, treat the cause of the pain.

The use of analgesics provides many pharmacologic approaches available to treat pain. Treatment should be individualized and, whenever necessary, aggressive. Fear of inducing opioid addiction is of little or no concern in this population.

Be aware that persons unable to report pain may also be in severe pain. When nonverbal pain signs are overlooked, the client will be undertreated. Some of the nonverbal signs and symptoms of pain may include increased irritability, decreased activity, whining or crying easily, tight gripping of an object, restlessness, anxiety, or favoring (protecting) of a body area. The use of an analgesic is appropriate to see if the signs and symptoms decrease.

Pain Management

The World Health Organization recommends a three-step approach to pain management (Agency for Health Care Policy and Research, 1994):

1. ***Step One***, nonopioid analgesic +/− adjuvant* for mild pain
   - acetaminophen (APAP, Tylenol) 500 mg 2 tablets qid (maximum 4 g daily)
   - ibuprofen (Motrin), 400 to 800 g qid
   - nabumetone (Relafen) 500 mg, 1 g hs or in two divided doses
   - naproxen (Naprosyn), 250 to 500 mg bid
2. ***Step Two***, nonopioid +/− opioid combination +/− adjuvant* for moderate pain
   - codeine (15 to 60 mg) with acetaminophen 325 mg, up to 60 mg codeine q4h
   - hydrocodone 5 mg with acetaminophen 500 mg (Lortab, Vicodin), 1 to 2 tablets q4-6h
   - oxycodone 5 mg with acetaminophen 500 mg (Percocet), 1 to 2 tablets q6h
3. ***Step Three***, Strong opioid +/− adjuvant* for severe pain
   - morphine† 10 to 30 mg q2-4h (PO, rectal, SC or IV)
   - morphine controlled release tablet† (Kadian, Oramorph SR, MS Contin) 15 to 100 mg q12h
   - fentanyl transdermal (Duragesic) 25 to 100 μg/hr dosage forms q72h
   - fentanyl transmucosal (Actiq) 50 to 400 μg lozenge on a stick for breakthrough cancer pain
   - hydromorphone (Dilaudid)† 7.5 mg PO q4h; parenteral 1.5 mg (IM, SC, IV) q4-6h
   - oxycodone (OxyContin, Roxicodone)† available in immediate release (5 to 30 mg q4-6h) and controlled release (OxyContin, 10 to 80 mg q12h)

Drug Selection

The selection of an analgesic depends on the level of the client's pain. The proper drug may be selected with the use of a pain scale (0 [no pain] to 10 [severe pain]) and the three-step approach as previously noted. A typical report scale for pain is Step 1, Mild Pain (1-3); Step 2, Moderate Pain (4-6); and Step 3, Severe Pain (7-10). When a sustained-release dosage form is used around-the-clock (ATC), a shorter acting analgesic (whenever possible, the same analgesic) should also be prescribed for breakthrough pain. Frequent use (4 times daily or more) of the rescue drug indicates the need to increase the dose of the long-acting ATC opioid with a continuance of the immediate release analgesic on a PRN basis. The calculated rescue dose is often 5% to 15% of the total daily dose of the sustained-release analgesic administered every 2 to 4 hours as necessary (Breakthrough Pain, 1999; Favaro, 2002).

*Adjuvant analgesics include antidepressants for neuropathic pain, anticonvulsants for neuropathic, lancinating, or tic-like pain; glucocorticoids or steroids for tumor-related pain or tumor infiltration in nerve or bone; and local anesthetics for neuropathic pain not responsive to antidepressants or anticonvulsants.

†No ceiling dose. Analgesic is prescribed according to the client's requirement and response, then titrated to effect.

Opioid Analgesic Equivalency

All analgesics are compared with 10 mg IM of morphine to determine an analgesic dosage equivalent. Equianalgesic information (i.e., the dose of one drug that produces approximately the same analgesic effect as the dose of another drug) is very useful information for the health care provider (see Table 1).

Analgesic Tips

1. Pain is best managed if the analgesic medication is given early or before the pain becomes severe.
2. Meperidine (Demerol) and the mixed agonist-antagonist agents (e.g., pentazocine, butorphanol) have limited (if any) use in this population (Foley, 2001).
3. Nonpharmacologic approaches (e.g., relaxation exercises, imagery, biofeedback, music therapy) and adjuvant drugs are used in conjunction with the opioid analgesics. These techniques and medications can be very helpful in select patients.
4. Myoclonus (muscle spasms, tremors, jerking of extremities) first requires an assessment for underling causes (e.g., renal or hepatic failure, hyponatremia, hypercalcemia, hypoxia). It may also be induced by opioids, which may require the prescriber to switch to a different opioid analgesic. The addition of a benzodiazepine such as clonazepam (Klonopin) may also be helpful (Collins & Cheong, 2001).

TABLE 1 Opioid Analgesic Equivalency

Analgesic	Oral Dose (mg)	IM Dose (mg)
morphine	30-60*	10
codeine	200	—
hydrocodone	30	—
hydromorphone	7.5	1.5
levorphanol	4	2
meperidine	300	75
methadone	20	10
oxycodone	15-30	—
transdermal fentanyl	25 μg patch is equivalent to 45-135 mg of oral morphine/day.	

Data from McCaffery, M., & Pasero, C. (1999). *Pain clinical manual* (2nd ed.). St. Louis: Mosby; and Weissman, D., Dahl J.L., & Dinndorf, P.A. (1996). *Handbook of cancer pain management* (5th ed.). Madison, WI: Wisconsin Cancer Pain Initiative.

*For a single dose or intermittent use. Chronic administration may decrease the oral dose to approximately 30 mg equivalent.

5. The following interventions may be considered for severe dyspnea (Foley, 2001):
   a. Place the client in an upright position and leaning forward, with the arms supported by a bed table *or*
   b. Use oxygen in hypoxemic individuals *or*
   c. Use small doses of oral or intravenous morphine *or*
   d. In some instances, a benzodiazepine of chlorpromazine may also be helpful
6. Children and older adults are often untreated or inadequately treated for pain. Pain assessment and management requires close supervision and monitoring. (See Chapter 14 for specific recommendations.)
7. Inappropriate analgesics for older adults include meperidine (Demerol), propoxyphene (Darvon, Darvocet), pentazocine (Talwin), and indomethacin (Indocin). These agents should be avoided; safer and more effective drugs are available (McCaffery & Pasero, 1999).

ADDITIONAL DRUGS USED IN END-OF-LIFE CARE

In addition to pain management, many other conditions may require end-of-life treatment. The majority of the following agents are discussed elsewhere in this text, and therefore the following is a listing with the typical dosages commonly used. The nurse should be aware that drug dosages may range widely depending on the client's condition, stage of disease, and individual requirements (Collins & Cheong, 2001; *Drug Facts and Comparisons*, 2001; Foley, 2001).

Anxiety

alprazolam (Xanax) 0.25-0.5 mg tid
diazepam (Valium) 2.5-10 mg qid
hydroxyzine (Atarax, Vistaril) 25 mg tid
lorazepam (Ativan) 0.5-1 mg tid

Oral Candida

clotrimazole (Mycelex) troche 5 times daily for 2 weeks
ketoconazole (Nizoral) 200-400 mg daily
nystatin (Mycostatin) suspension 4-6 ml, or troches qid

Constipation

Stool Softeners

docusate (Colace, Surfak) 100 mg 1-3 times daily

Stimulant Laxatives

senna or sennosides (Senokot) 2-4 tablets once or twice daily
bisacodyl (Dulcolax) 5 mg 1-3 tablets daily

See Chapter 11 for additional laxatives. The reader should also be aware that clients receiving large doses of opioid analgesics may require larger dosages of laxatives than listed.

Depression

sertraline (Zoloft) 50-150 mg once daily
nefazodone (Serzone) 200-600 mg daily
venlafaxine (Effexor) 75-225 mg daily

If sleep disturbance is significant with depression, then
amitriptyline (Elavil) 50-150 mg q hs *or*
doxepin (Sinequan) 50 to 150 mg q hs

Diarrhea

diphenoxylate (Lomotil) 5 mg qid
loperamide 2-4 mg dose according to package insert

Gastrointestinal anticholinergic/antispasmodic:
dicyclomine (Bentyl) 20 mg qid
scopolamine 0.4 mg PO as ordered or scopolamine transdermal patch applied behind ear q 3 days

Hypnotics

Many anxiolytic benzodiazepines are effective hypnotic agents. When a client is receiving a benzodiazepine such as alprazolam or lorazepam during the day and a hypnotic drug is necessary, an equivalent dose of the same drug may be considered. For example, 0.5 mg alprazolam or 1 mg of lorazepam is considered to be approximately equivalent to 15 mg flurazepam (Dalmane), 15 mg temazepam (Restoril), or 0.25 mg triazolam (Halcion). In this text, see p. 329 and Chapter 16 for additional information.

Muscle Spasms

baclofen (Lioresal) 5-20 mg tid
diazepam (Valium) 5 mg tid
tizanidine (Zanaflex) 4-8 mg tid

Nausea and/or Vomiting

meclizine (Antivert, Bonine) 25 mg qid
metoclopramide (Reglan) 10 mg qid
prochlorperazine (Compazine) 5-10 mg qid
promethazine (Phenergan) 25 mg tid

Peptic Ulcers/Gastroesophageal Reflux

famotidine (Pepcid) 20 mg q hs
metoclopramide (Reglan) 10 mg qid
ranitidine (Zantac) 150 mg bid

CASE STUDY

For a Case Study that will help ensure mastery of this chapter content, go to www.mosby.com/MERLIN/McKenry/.

BIBLOGRAPHY

Agency for Health Care Policy and Research. Public Health Service. (1994). *Clinical Practice Guideline: Management of cancer pain.* Rockville, MD: Department of Health and Human Services.

Breakthrough pain: Not as simple as it sounds (1999). In *Partners Against Pain News,* 4(1):2.

Collins, P., & Cheong, S. (2001). Improving care at end of life: Essential issues, self-study. Miami: Baptist Health Systems of South Florida.

Drug Facts and Comparisons (2001). St. Louis: Facts and Comparisons.

Favaro, M.K.A. (2002). *Pharmacology: An introductory text* (9th ed.). Philadelphia: W.B. Saunders.

Foley, K. (2001). Pain and symptom control in the dying ICU patient. In J.R. Curtis & G.D. Rubenfeld (Eds.), *Managing death in the ICU,* Oxford University Press.

Lynn, J. (2001). Travels in the valley of the shadow. In P. Collins & S. Cheong (Eds.), *Improving care at end of life: Essential issues, self-study.* Miami: Baptist Health Systems of South Florida.

McCaffery, M., & Pasero, C. (1999). *Pain clinical manual* (2nd ed.). St. Louis: Mosby.

Weissman, D., Dahl, J.L., & Dinndorf, P.A. (1996). *Handbook of cancer pain management* (5th ed.). Madison, WI: Wisconsin Cancer Pain Initiative.

Woodruff, R. (1993). *Palliative medicine.* Melbourne: Asperula Ptys Ltd.

Appendix

J HORSE CHESTNUT AND ARTICHOKE LEAF

HORSE CHESTNUT

Horse chestnut is used in seed extract, leaf, branch bark, and flower forms. It is used for the treatment of varicose veins, hemorrhoids, phlebitis, diarrhea, soft-tissue swelling, fever, and enlarged prostate. Although there is insufficient reliable information available about the effectiveness of horse chestnut for its other uses, clinical studies have shown that horse chestnut seed extract is effective in chronic venous insufficiency. Leg volume and circumference and edema were reduced (Pittler & Ernst, 1998a). The usual daily dose of horse chestnut seed extract is 1 to 3 250-mg capsules daily; there is no typical dosage for the leaf, branch bark, or flower forms of the drug.

ARTICHOKE LEAF

Artichoke leaves and extracts are sometimes used in foods as flavoring agents. Medicinally, artichoke leaf is used as a general tonic and for the treatment of dyspepsia, nausea, irritable bowel syndrome (IBS), and hyperlipidemia. There is preliminary evidence to suggest that artichoke leaf extract may be beneficial in reducing total cholesterol in patients with elevated total cholesterol (Pittler & Ernst, 1998b). It is thought that artichoke inhibits the oxidation of low-density lipoprotein and reduces cholesterol biosynthesis. Further study is required to demonstrate this and other benefits of artichoke leaf. The usual dosage is 12:1 dried leaf extract 500 mg daily.

Pittler, M.H., & Ernst, E. (1998a). Horse-chestnut seed extract for chronic venous insufficiency: A criteria-based systematic review. *Archives of Dermatology* 134:1356-1360.

Pittler, M.H. & Ernst, E. (1998b). Artichoke leaf extract for serum cholesterol reduction. *Perfusion* 11:338-340.

DISORDERS INDEX

Page numbers followed by *t* indicate tables; *italics* indicates illustrations.

I

J

K

L

Q

R

Comprehensive Index

Page numbers in **bold** indicate drug monographs. Page numbers followed by *f* indicate figures; *b* indicates boxes, *t* indicates tables, and ♣ indicates Canada-only drugs.

B

D

E

F

O

Q

S

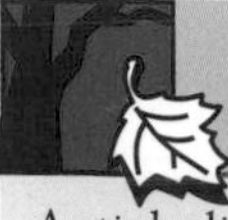

Special Considerations for Older Adults

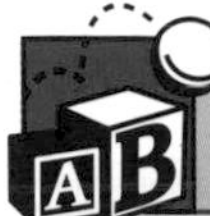

Special Considerations for Children

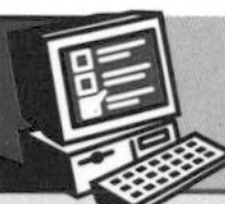

Nursing Research

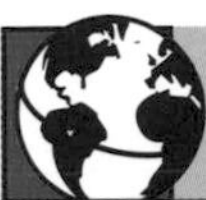

Cultural Considerations

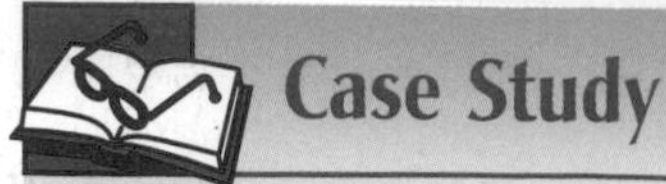

Case Study

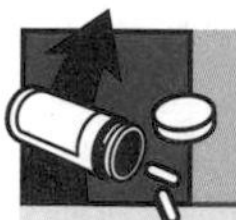

Management of Drug Overdose

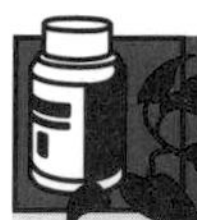

Complementary and Alternative Therapies

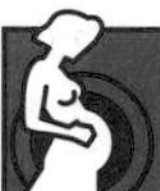

Pregnancy Safety